PATHOLOGY
OF THE
GASTROINTESTINAL TRACT

PATHOLOGY
OF THE
GASTROINTESTINAL
TRACT

edited by

SI-CHUN MING, M.D.
Professor of Pathology
Department of Pathology
School of Medicine
Temple University
Philadelphia, Pennsylvania

HARVEY GOLDMAN, M.D.
Chairman, Department of Pathology
New England Deaconess and New England Baptist Hospitals
and
Professor of Pathology
Harvard Medical School
Boston, Massachusetts

W. B. SAUNDERS COMPANY
Harcourt Brace Jovanovich, Inc.
Philadelphia ■ London ■ Toronto ■ Montreal ■ Sydney ■ Tokyo

W. B. SAUNDERS COMPANY
Harcourt Brace Jovanovich, Inc.

The Curtis Center
Independence Square West
Philadelphia, Pennsylvania 19106

Library of Congress Cataloging-in-Publication Data

Pathology of the gastrointestinal tract / [edited by] Si-Chun Ming, Harvey Goldman.

p.   cm.

ISBN 0-7216-6398-2

1. Gastrointestinal system—Diseases.   2. Gastrointestinal system—Histopathology.   I. Ming, Si-Chun.   II. Goldman, Harvey.
  [DNLM: 1. Gastrointestinal Diseases.   2. Gastrointestinal System—physiology.   WI 100 P29772]

RC802.9.P373   1992

616.3'3—dc20

DNLM/DLC   91-18371

Editor: Jennifer Mitchell
Developmental Editor: Kathleen McCarthy
Designer: Joan Wendt
Production Manager: Linda R. Garber
Manuscript Editors: Jessie Raymond and Judith Redding
Illustration Coordinator: Peg Shaw
Indexer: Roger Wall
Cover Designer: Dorothy Chattin

PATHOLOGY OF THE GASTROINTESTINAL TRACT   ISBN 0-7216-6398-2

Copyright © 1992 by W. B. Saunders Company

All rights reserved.   No part of this publication may be reproduced or transmitted in any form or by any means, electronic or mechanical, including photocopy, recording, or any information storage and retrieval system, without permission in writing from the publisher.

Printed in the United States of America

Last digit is the print number: 9   8   7   6   5   4   3   2   1

*With love
to
Pen-Ming, Carol, Ruby, Stephanie,
Jeffrey, Michael, and Eileen
and to
Eleonora, Palko, Sasha, and Vierka*

Contributors

GERALD D. ABRAMS, M.D.
Professor of Pathology, University of Michigan Medical School, and Pathologist, University Hospitals, University of Michigan, Ann Arbor, Michigan
Infectious Disorders of the Intestines

DONALD A. ANTONIOLI, M.D.
Associate Professor of Pathology, Harvard Medical School, and Director of Anatomic Pathology, Beth Israel Hospital, Consultant in Gastrointestinal Pathology, The Children's Hospital, Consultant in Gastrointestinal Pathology, New England Deaconess Hospital, Boston, Massachusetts
Functional Anatomy of the Gastrointestinal Tract

HENRY D. APPLEMAN, M.D.
Professor of Pathology, University of Michigan, and Staff Pathologist, University of Michigan Hospitals, Ann Arbor, Michigan
Mesenchymal Tumors of the Gastrointestinal Tract

JAMES B. AREY, M.D., Ph.D.
(Deceased)
Emeritus Professor of Pathology (in Pediatrics), Temple University School of Medicine, and Consulting Pathologist, St. Christopher's Hospital for Children, Philadelphia, Pennsylvania
Embryology and Developmental Disorders

CARLO CAPELLA, M.D., Ph.D.
Professor of Pathology, University of Pavia, II Faculty of Medicine, Department of Human Pathology, and Head, Surgical Pathology Service, Multizonal Hospital, Varese, Italy
Disorders of the Endocrine System

HARRY S. COOPER, M.D.
Professor of Pathology, Hahnemann University School of Medicine, and Director of Anatomical Pathology, Hahnemann University Hospital, Philadelphia, Pennsylvania
Benign Polyps of the Intestines

ELEANOR E. DESCHNER, Ph.D.
Associate Member, Laboratory for Digestive Tract Carcinogenesis, Memorial Sloan-Kettering Cancer Center, New York, New York
Cell Renewal in Health and Disease

ROBERTO FIOCCA, M.D.
Senior Assistant, Surgical Pathology Service, IRCCS Policlinico San Matteo, Pavia, Italy
Disorders of the Endocrine System

HARVEY GOLDMAN, M.D.
Professor of Pathology, Harvard Medical School, Chairman, Department of Pathology, New England Deaconess Hospital and New England Baptist Hospital, Boston, Massachusetts
General Concepts and Methods of Examination; Chemical and Physical Disorders; Allergic Disorders; Systemic and Miscellaneous Disorders: Gastritis; Stress Ulcer and Chronic Peptic Ulcer Disease; Mucosal Hypertrophy and Hyperplasia of the Stomach; Ulcerative Colitis and Crohn's Disease; Other Inflammatory Disorders of the Intestines

RODGER C. HAGGITT, M.D.
Professor of Pathology and Adjunct Professor of Medicine, University of Washington, and Director of Hospital Pathology, University of Washington Medical Center, Seattle, Washington
Endoscopy and Endoscopic Biopsy

STANLEY R. HAMILTON, M.D.
Associate Professor of Pathology and Oncology, Department of Pathology,

The Johns Hopkins University School of Medicine and Hospital, Baltimore, Maryland
Esophagitis

TERUYUKI HIROTA, M.D.
Head, First Histopathology Section, Pathology Division, National Cancer Center Research Institute, Tokyo, Japan
Early Gastric Carcinoma

DAVID F. KEREN, M.D.
Adjunct Professor of Biology, Eastern Michigan University, Ypsilanti, Michigan, and Medical Director, Warde Medical Laboratory, Ann Arbor, Michigan
Structure and Function of the Immunologic System of the Gastrointestinal Tract

THOMAS LEHNERT, M.D.
Department of Surgery, University of Heidelberg, Heidelberg, Germany
Cell Renewal in Health and Disease

KLAUS J. LEWIN, M.D., F.R.C. (Path.)
Professor of Pathology and Medicine, University of California, Los Angeles, School of Medicine, Los Angeles, California
Disorders of the Lymphoid System

FU-SHENG LIU, M.D.
Professor, Beijing Union Medical College, and Chairman of Department of Pathology, Cancer Institute and Hospital, Chinese Academy of Medical Sciences, Beijing, People's Republic of China
Squamous Cell Carcinoma of the Esophagus

JAMES L. MADARA, M.D.
Associate Professor of Pathology, Harvard Medical School, and Pathologist and Director, Division of Gastrointestinal Pathology, Brigham and Women's Hospital, Boston, Massachusetts
Functional Anatomy of the Gastrointestinal Tract

PEN-MING L. MING, M.D.
Professor of Pathology and of Obstetrics and Gynecology, Temple University School of Medicine, and Director of Cytogenetics Laboratory, Temple University Hospital, Philadelphia, Pennsylvania
Genetic and Cytogenetic Aspects

SI-CHUN MING, M.D.
Professor of Pathology, Department of Pathology, Temple University School of Medicine, Philadelphia, Pennsylvania
General Concepts and Methods of Examination; Adenocarcinoma and Other Epithelial Tumors of the Esophagus; Epithelial Polyps of the Stomach; Early Gastric Carcinoma; Adenocarcinoma and Other Malignant Epithelial Tumors of the Stomach; Diverticular Disease of the Colon; Adenocarcinoma and Other Malignant Epithelial Tumors of the Intestines

FRANK A. MITROS, M.D.
Professor of Pathology, University of Iowa College of Medicine, and Co-director of Surgical Pathology, University of Iowa Hospitals and Clinics, Iowa City, Iowa
Motor and Mechanical Disorders

H. THOMAS NORRIS, M.D.
Professor and Chairman, Department of Pathology and Laboratory Medicine, East Carolina University School of Medicine, and Chief of Pathology, Pitt County Memorial Hospital, Greenville, North Carolina
Vascular Disorders

ROBERT R. RICKERT, M.D.
Clinical Professor of Pathology, University of Medicine and Dentistry of New Jersey, Newark, New Jersey, and Co-chairman, Department of Pathology, Saint Barnabas Medical Center, Livingston, New Jersey
Disorders of the Anal Region

GUIDO RINDI, M.D.
Research Fellow, Surgical Pathology Unit, Department of Human Pathology, University of Pavia, Pavia, Italy
Disorders of the Endocrine System

CRISTINA RIVA, M.D.
Assistant, Surgical Pathology Service, Multizonal Hospital, Varese, Italy
Disorders of the Endocrine System

CYRUS E. RUBIN, M.D.
Professor of Medicine and Adjunct Professor of Pathology, University of Washington, Attending Physician, University of Washington Medical Center, Seattle, Washington
Endoscopy and Endoscopic Biopsy

FAUSTO SESSA, M.D.
Assistant, Surgical Pathology Service, IRCCS Policlinico San Matteo, Pavia, Italy
Disorders of the Endocrine System

ENRICO SOLCIA, M.D., Ph.D.
Professor of Pathology, University of Pavia, I Medical Faculty, Department of Human Pathology, and Head, Surgical Pathology Service, IRCCS Policlinico San Matteo, Pavia, Italy
Disorders of the Endocrine System

SANDOR SZABO, M.D.
Associate Professor of Pathology, Harvard Medical School, and Pathologist, Brigham and Women's Hospital, Boston, Massachusetts
Chemical and Physical Disorders

CHIK-KWUN TANG, M.D.
Professor of Pathology, Temple University School of Medicine, and Acting Chief of Service and Chief of Surgical Pathology, Temple University Hospital, Philadelphia, Pennsylvania
Disorders of the Vermiform Appendix

PATRIZIA TENTI, M.D.
Assistant, Surgical Pathology Service, IRCCS Policlinico San Matteo, Pavia, Italy
Disorders of the Endocrine System

MARIE VALDES-DAPENA, M.D.
Professor of Pathology and Pediatrics, University of Miami School of Medicine, Miami, Florida
Embryology and Developmental Disorders

QI-LU WANG, M.D.
Professor, Peking Union Medical College, and Vice-Chairwoman, Medical Oncology Department, Cancer Institute and Hospital, Chinese Academy of Medical Sciences, Beijing, People's Republic of China
Squamous Cell Carcinoma of the Esophagus

SIEGFRIED WITTE, M.D.
Professor of Internal Medicine, Medizinische Fakultät, Universität Freiburg, Freiburg, Germany, and Chief, Department of Medicine, Diakonissen-Krankenhaus, Karlsruhe, Germany
Cytologic Techniques and Diagnosis

JOHN H. YARDLEY, M.D.
Baxley Professor and Director, Department of Pathology, The Johns Hopkins University School of Medicine, Baltimore, Maryland
Malabsorptive Disorders

Preface

This book is intended to provide a comprehensive compilation of the many disorders, both primary and secondary, that affect the human alimentary tract from the esophagus through the anal region. Particular emphasis is placed on detailed analysis and presentation of the pathologic features of each disorder, and specific attention is directed to the etiology and evolution of these diseases. Included are critical and practical descriptions of the examination and interpretation of biopsies and surgical specimens, and the differential diagnostic features of the early and late lesions are stressed. Pertinent information regarding the nature of each disorder as well as correlations with diagnostic tests, pathophysiologic alterations, and the clinical course are also provided.

The book is divided into six parts and 34 chapters. The first part offers information of a general nature, with seven chapters on the general concepts and methods of examination, on the functional anatomy of the various parts of the tract, on the uses of endoscopy and endoscopic biopsy, on cytologic techniques and diagnoses, on the characteristics of the gut immune system, on genetic and cytogenetic aspects, and on the cell renewal process. In the second part, the disorders that can occur in multiple parts of the gastrointestinal tract are grouped by their common nature and etiology. Included are nine chapters on embryology and developmental anomalies, on diseases due to chemical and physical agents, on allergic conditions, on disorders of a motor and mechanical nature, on the vascular lesions, on disorders of the endocrine and lymphoid systems, on mesenchymal tumors, and on the various systemic and miscellaneous conditions that can affect the gut. The other four parts of the book consist of chapters detailing the many inflammatory conditions and tumors that primarily affect and are concentrated in one segment of the gut, including three chapters on the esophagus, six on the stomach, seven on the intestines, and two on the appendix and anal region. There are also extensive cross-references and multiple presentations of the disorders affecting the several gut segments throughout the book.

The diseases are presented in a fairly standard fashion throughout the book, with information provided on their nature, etiology and pathogenesis, pathologic features, and functional and clinical correlates. The book should serve to record the essential pathologic characteristics of each disorder and its various stages and also to provide for a systematic approach to the analysis of pathologic specimens. It is intended to aid pathologists in formulating a logical approach to the study of gastrointestinal disorders, to provide insights into the natural history of the various lesions, and to hone diagnostic skills. The book should also assist the clinical gastroenterologist in understanding the various pathologic changes and their relationship to the clinical presentations and courses.

HARVEY GOLDMAN, M.D.
SI-CHUN MING, M.D.

Contents

PART 1

GENERAL PRINCIPLES 1

CHAPTER 1

General Concepts and Methods of Examination 3
Harvey Goldman, M.D., and Si-Chun Ming, M.D.

- GENERAL CONCEPTS OF GASTROINTESTINAL DISORDERS 4
  - Categories of Diseases 4
  - Responses to Injury: Effects on Epithelium 7
  - Responses to Injury: Inflammatory Effects 8
  - Patterns and Stages of Diseases 9
- METHODS OF EXAMINATION 10
  - The Nature of the Specimen 10
  - Gross Preparation and Examination 11
  - Microscopic Examination 11
  - Other Techniques 12
  - Pathology Reports 12

CHAPTER 2

Functional Anatomy of the Gastrointestinal Tract 14
Donald A. Antonioli, M.D., and James L. Madara, M.D.

- GENERAL ORGANIZATION OF THE GASTROINTESTINAL TRACT 14
- ESOPHAGUS 15
  - Gross Anatomy 15
  - Esophageal Functions 16
  - Histologic Features 16
- STOMACH 19
  - Gross Anatomy 19
  - Gastric Functions 19
  - Histology of the Gastric Mucosa 20
- SMALL INTESTINE 24
  - Gross Anatomy 24
  - Organization of the Mucosal Vasculature 24
  - Epithelial Structure: General Aspects 24
  - Epithelial Structure: Individual Cell Types 26

COLON	33
Gross Anatomy	33
Organization of the Colonic Wall	34
Epithelial Structure: General Features	34
Colonic Mucosal Epithelial Cells	34

CHAPTER 3

Endoscopy and Endoscopic Biopsy 37
Rodger C. Haggitt, M.D., and Cyrus E. Rubin, M.D.

HISTORY OF GASTROINTESTINAL ENDOSCOPY	37
MODERN ENDOSCOPY	38
TECHNICAL FACTORS AND METHODS FOR HANDLING ENDOSCOPIC BIOPSY SPECIMENS	39
Orientation	39
Fixation	40
Processing	41
Embedding	41
Sectioning	41
Staining	42
Special Procedures	43
INTERPRETATION OF BIOPSY FINDINGS	44
Artifacts	44
Factors Affecting the Accuracy of Endoscopic Biopsy	45
Value of Good Technique and Optimum Interpretation to the Patient	46
SUMMARY	46

CHAPTER 4

Cytologic Techniques and Diagnosis 48
Siegfried Witte, M.D.

COLLECTION OF MATERIAL	49
Esophagus	49
Stomach	49
Duodenum	50
Colon and Rectum	50
METHODS OF MICROSCOPIC EXAMINATION	50
Fresh Unfixed Preparations	50
Staining Techniques	52
Quantitative Methods	53
CYTOMORPHOLOGY AND CYTODIAGNOSIS	54
Esophagus	54
Stomach	55
Duodenum	60
Colon and Rectum	61
STATISTICAL EVALUATION OF CYTODIAGNOSES	63
Esophagus	63
Stomach	64
Duodenum	66
Colon and Rectum	67

CHAPTER 5

Structure and Function of the Immunologic System of the Gastrointestinal Tract 69
David F. Keren, M.D.

    CONCEPT OF A MUCOSAL IMMUNE SYSTEM 69
    ANATOMY OF THE GUT IMMUNE SYSTEM 70
    MUCOSAL LYMPHOID CELLS 72
    ANTIGEN PROCESSING IN THE GUT 74
    CHARACTERISTICS OF SECRETORY IGA 76

CHAPTER 6

Genetic and Cytogenetic Aspects 81
Pen-Ming L. Ming, M.D.

    PATTERN OF INHERITANCE 82
        Mendelian Inheritance 82
        Multifactorial Inheritance 83
    GENETIC MARKERS 84
        HLA Antigens 84
        Blood Groups 84
    CHROMOSOMAL SYNDROMES AFFECTING THE GASTROINTESTINAL TRACT 84
        Trisomy 21 Syndrome 85
        Trisomy 18 Syndrome 85
        Trisomy 13 Syndrome 85
        Other Chromosomal Syndromes 85
    GENETICS OF NONNEOPLASTIC DISEASES OF THE GASTROINTESTINAL TRACT 85
        Peptic Ulcer 85
        Celiac Disease 86
        Inflammatory Bowel Disease 86
        Hirschsprung's Disease 87
        Congenital Hypertrophic Pyloric Stenosis 87
    GENETICS OF NEOPLASTIC DISEASES OF THE GASTROINTESTINAL TRACT 88
        Esophageal Tumors 88
        Gastric Tumors 88
        Intestinal Tumors 89

CHAPTER 7

Cell Renewal in Health and Disease 98
Eleanor E. Deschner, Ph.D., and Thomas Lehnert, M.D.

    ESOPHAGUS 99
        Normal Proliferation 99
        Proliferation in Disease States 99
    STOMACH 100
        Normal Proliferation 100
        Proliferation in Disease States 101

SMALL INTESTINE...102
    Normal Proliferation 102
    Proliferation in Disease States 103

LARGE INTESTINE..104
    Normal Proliferation 104
    Preneoplasia...105
    Proliferation in Disease States 105

PART 2

DISORDERS COMMON TO THE GASTROINTESTINAL TRACT..111

CHAPTER 8

Embryology and Developmental Disorders 113
James B. Arey, M.D., Ph.D., and Marie Valdes-Dapena, M.D.

    ESOPHAGUS 113
        Embryology..113
        Tracheoesophageal Fistula and Esophageal Atresia.....................114
        Esophageal Stenosis 115
        Double Esophagus..115
        Neurenteric Cysts 115
        Esophageal Cysts...116

    STOMACH 116
        Embryology..116
        Pyloric Atresia...116
        Congenital Pyloric Stenosis 116
        Heterotopic Pancreatic Tissue 117
        Spontaneous Rupture of the Stomach..117

    INTESTINES 118
        Embryology..118
        Aganglionic Megacolon (Hirschsprung's Disease) 119
        Intestinal Atresia and Stenosis...122
        Anomalies of Intestinal Rotation and Volvulus 124
        Hernias 126
        Omphalocele and Gastroschisis..128
        Omphalomesenteric Duct Remnants 129
        Congenital Diverticula of the Intestines 131
        Meconium Ileus and Related Conditions 131
        Spontaneous Perforation of the Intestine......................................133

    DUPLICATIONS OF THE ALIMENTARY TRACT.............................133
        Pathologic Features 135

    RECTUM AND ANUS..135
        Embryology..135
        Imperforate Anus and Related Conditions 136
        Cloacal Exstrophy 137

    CYSTS OF MESENTERY AND OMENTUM 137
        Mesenteric Cysts (Cystic Hygromas) 137
        Omental Cysts...138

CHAPTER 9

Chemical and Physical Disorders...141
Harvey Goldman, M.D., and Sandor Szabo, M.D.

- MECHANISMS OF CELLULAR INJURY..142
- CHEMICAL AND DRUG DISORDERS..142
  - Definitions and Classification 142
  - Pathogenesis..143
  - General Pathologic Features...144
  - Clinical Features and Diagnosis..145
  - Etiologic Agents 146
  - Specific Organ Involvement...152
- RADIATION EFFECTS AND INJURY..156
  - General Aspects...157
  - General Pathologic Features...158
  - Clinical Features 161
  - Diagnosis and Differential Diagnosis 162
  - Specific Organ Involvement...162
- OTHER PHYSICAL INJURY..165
  - Thermal Effects 165
  - Trauma...165

CHAPTER 10

Allergic Disorders 171
Harvey Goldman, M.D.

- GENERAL ASPECTS AND TERMINOLOGY....................................171
- PATHOGENETIC MECHANISMS 172
- ALLERGIC EFFECTS IN OTHER ORGANS....................................173
- EOSINOPHILIC GASTROENTERITIS...173
  - Mucosal Type 173
  - Mural Type 173
  - Serosal Type..174
- ALLERGIC GASTROENTERITIS...175
  - Definitions...175
  - Clinical and Laboratory Features 175
  - General Pathologic Features and Diagnosis 176
  - Specific Organ Features and Differential Diagnosis 177
- ALLERGIC PROCTITIS AND COLITIS..182
  - Definitions...182
  - Childhood Cases 183
  - Adult Cases...184
- MUCOSAL BIOPSY 185

CHAPTER 11

Motor and Mechanical Disorders...188
Frank A. Mitros, M.D.

- NORMAL ANATOMY..188
- MECHANICAL OBSTRUCTION 194
  - Causes and Effects 194
  - Special Forms of Obstruction 195

PSEUDO-OBSTRUCTION 196
   Introduction 196
   Primary Intestinal Pseudo-obstruction 197
   Secondary Intestinal Pseudo-obstruction 204

CONCLUSION 211

CHAPTER 12

Vascular Disorders 214
H. Thomas Norris, M.D.

DIAGNOSIS OF GASTROINTESTINAL BLEEDING 215
METHODS OF EXAMINATION OF SPECIMENS 216
   Injection Studies of Blood Vessels 216
   Lymphatics 216

ANATOMY OF GASTROINTESTINAL VASCULATURE 217
ACQUIRED AND CONGENITAL VASCULAR MALFORMATIONS 217
   Varices 217
   Vascular Abnormalities of the Gastrointestinal Tract 219

TUMORS AND TUMOR-LIKE PROLIFERATIONS OF VESSELS 224
   Hemangiomas 224
   Malignant Vascular Tumors 225
   Lymphangiomas 225

VASCULITIS 225
   General Considerations 225
   Histologic Features and Differential Diagnosis 226
   Utility of Mucosal Biopsy and Other Studies in Establishing the
   Diagnosis of Vasculitis 226
   Vasculitic Lesions in the Gastrointestinal Tract 226

ISCHEMIC DISEASES 229
   General Consideration 229
   Pathophysiologic Effects of Ischemia 229
   Nomenclature and Classification 230
   General Pathology 230
   Etiology of Bowel Infarcts 230
   Ischemic Bowel Disease 230
   Entities of Ischemic Bowel Disease 233

CHAPTER 13

Disorders of the Endocrine System 240
Enrico Solcia, M.D., Ph.D., Carlo Capella, M.D., Ph.D., Roberto Fiocca, M.D., Patrizia Tenti, M.D., Fausto Sessa, M.D., Cristina Riva, M.D., and Guido Rindi, M.D.

NORMAL STRUCTURE AND FUNCTIONS 240
GENERAL ASPECTS OF ENDOCRINE CELL HYPERPLASIA
   AND TUMORS 241
   Diagnosis 241
   Classification 243
   Prognosis 243

GASTRIC ARGYROPHIL (ECL-CELL) TUMORS AND HYPERPLASIAS 244
   In Normal or Hypertrophic Mucosa 245
   In Chronic Atrophic Gastritis 246
   Clinicopathologic Aspects 248

GASTRIN CELL GROWTHS 248
    Gastrin Cell Hyperplasia 248
    Gastrin Cell Tumors 248

SOMATOSTATIN CELL GROWTHS 249
GANGLIONEUROMATOUS PARAGANGLIOMA 251
ARGENTAFFIN (EC-CELL) TUMORS 253
    Small Intestine 253
    Appendix 253

HINDGUT TRABECULAR (L-CELL) TUMORS 255
INAPPROPRIATE ENDOCRINE TUMORS 255
OTHER GUT ENDOCRINE TUMORS 255
POORLY DIFFERENTIATED ENDOCRINE (NEUROENDOCRINE)
    CARCINOMAS 256
ENDOCRINE-EXOCRINE TUMORS 258
    Combined Tumors 258
    Composite Tumors 259

CHAPTER 14

Disorders of the Lymphoid System 264
Klaus J. Lewin, M.D., F.R.C. (Path.)

    FUNCTIONAL ANATOMY 264
        Normal Distribution of Gut-Associated Lymphoid Tissue 264
        Intestinal Host Defense Mechanisms 265

    IMMUNODEFICIENCY DISORDERS OF THE GASTROINTESTINAL TRACT .. 265
        General Features of Immunodeficiency Disorders 265
        Primary Immunodeficiency Disorders 271
        Acquired Immunodeficiency Disorders 274

    LYMPHOPROLIFERATIVE DISORDERS 281
        Lymphoid Hyperplasia 281
        Malignant Lymphoma 290

CHAPTER 15

Mesenchymal Tumors of the Gastrointestinal Tract 310
Henry D. Appelman, M.D.

    GENERAL FEATURES OF MESENCHYMAL TUMORS 310
        Cell Origin and Differentiation 311
        Site Specificity 312
        Clinical Features 312
        Dissection of Gastrointestinal Stromal Tumors 312
        Gross Characteristics 313
        General Microscopic Features 314
        Diagnosis of Malignancy 315
        Role of Frozen Section and Operating Room Consultation 320

    STROMAL TUMORS PECULIAR TO SPECIFIC SITES IN THE
        GASTROINTESTINAL TRACT 320
        Stromal Tumors of Esophagus 320
        Stromal Tumors of Stomach 321

Stromal Tumors of Intestine 326
Tiny Stromal Tumor of Muscularis Propria/Myenteric Plexus............ 335

TUMORS AND TUMOR-LIKE PROLIFERATIONS OF ADIPOSE TISSUE 336
Lipoma and Liposarcoma 336
Lipomatous Hypertrophy of the Ileocecal Valve 336

TUMORS AND TUMOR-LIKE PROLIFERATIONS OF VESSELS 338
Glomus Tumors 338
Other Vascular Tumors 338

TUMORS AND TUMOR-LIKE PROLIFERATIONS OF FIBROUS TISSUE...... 339
Inflammatory Fibroid Polyps 339
Giant Fibrovascular Polyp of Esophagus.................................. 342

TUMOR AND TUMOR-LIKE PROLIFERATIONS OF NERVOUS TISSUE 342
Intramural Neurofibroma.. 344
Ganglioneuroma and Ganglioneuromatosis.............................. 344
Granular Cell Tumors 346

CHAPTER 16

Systemic and Miscellaneous Disorders.................................... 351
Harvey Goldman, M.D.

DISEASES OF OTHER ORGANS AND SYSTEMS............................. 351
Cardiovascular System 352
Respiratory System.. 352
Kidneys and Urinary System 352
Hematologic System 353
Endocrine System 355
Reproductive System.. 356
Skin and Soft Tissues and Other Systemic Conditions 356
Pancreas, Biliary Tract, and Liver.. 358

VITAMIN DISORDERS 359
Fat-Soluble Vitamins 359
Water-Soluble Vitamins 360

DEPOSITIONS 360
Conditions That May Simulate Storage Diseases 361
Lipoprotein Disorders 362
Glycolipid Storage Diseases 362
Lipid Pigment Disorders.. 364
Other Storage Diseases 365
Other Pigment Depositions 365
Amyloidosis... 365

GRANULOMATOUS DISORDERS 368
Infections.. 368
Crohn's Disease 369
Foreign Body Granulomas 369
Isolated Granulomas 369
Sarcoidosis.. 369
Chronic Granulomatous Disease.. 370
Malacoplakia 371
Histiocytosis X.. 372
Miscellaneous Granulomatous Conditions 373

PART 3
ESOPHAGUS ... 381

CHAPTER 17

Esophagitis ... 383
Stanley R. Hamilton, M.D.

- PATHOLOGIC FINDINGS ... 383
- NORMAL HISTOLOGIC VARIANTS ... 385
  - Glycogenic Acanthosis ... 385
  - Ectopic Sebaceous Glands ... 386
  - Melanocytic Proliferation ... 386
- ESOPHAGITIS DUE TO INFECTIOUS AGENTS ... 386
  - Fungal Esophagitis ... 387
  - Viral Esophagitis ... 393
  - Bacterial Esophagitis ... 396
  - Spirochetal (Syphilitic) Esophagitis ... 400
  - Parasitic Esophagitis ... 401
- ESOPHAGEAL INJURY DUE TO EXOGENOUS CHEMICALS ... 401
  - Lye, Acids, Detergents, and Other Household Products ... 401
  - Drug Contact ... 402
  - Sclerotherapy for Esophageal Varices ... 402
  - Chemotherapeutic Agents ... 402
- ESOPHAGEAL TRAUMA ... 404
- ESOPHAGEAL INJURY DUE TO PHYSICAL AGENTS ... 405
  - Radiation Esophagitis ... 405
  - Thermal Injury ... 406
- HIATAL HERNIA (Si-Chun Ming, M.D.) ... 406
  - Sliding Hiatal Hernia ... 406
  - Paraesophageal Hernia ... 406
  - Other Diaphragmatic Hernias ... 407
- GASTROESOPHAGEAL REFLUX ... 407
  - Low-Grade Changes ... 408
  - High-Grade Changes ... 409
  - Barrett's Esophagus ... 411
- MOTOR AND RELATED DISORDERS OF THE ESOPHAGUS ... 423
  - Achalasia ... 423
  - Rings and Webs ... 423
  - Diverticula ... 424
- ESOPHAGEAL INVOLVEMENT BY SYSTEMIC DISEASES ... 424
  - Collagen Vascular–Connective Tissue Diseases ... 424
  - Crohn's Disease ... 425
  - Behçet's Disease ... 426
  - Eosinophilic Gastroenteritis and Esophagitis ... 426
  - Dermatologic Diseases ... 427
  - Sarcoidosis ... 427
  - Immunodeficiency ... 427
  - Graft-versus-Host Disease ... 427
  - Amyloidosis ... 428
- CONCLUDING COMMENTS ... 428

CHAPTER 18

Squamous Cell Carcinoma of the Esophagus 439
Fu-Sheng Liu, M.D., and Qi-Lu Wang, M.D.

- EPIDEMIOLOGY 440
  - Age Distribution 440
  - Sex Distribution 440
  - Geographic Distribtuion 440
  - Mass Surveys in China 441
  - Migrant Studies 442
  - Incidence in the Fowl in China 442
- ETIOLOGY 442
  - Dietary Factors 442
  - Trace Elements 443
  - Dietary Habits in High-Risk Regions in China 443
  - Nitrosamines 443
  - Alcohol Consumption and Smoking 443
  - Genetic Factors 443
- ASSOCIATED CONDITIONS AND PRECANCEROUS LESIONS 443
  - Associated Conditions 443
  - Precancerous Lesions 444
- PATHOLOGY 445
  - Location 445
  - Early Esophageal Carcinoma 446
  - Advanced Esophageal Carcinoma 448
  - Variants of Squamous Cell Carcinoma 450
  - Staging 451
  - Spread and Metastasis 452
  - Pathologic Factors Affecting Prognosis 452
- CLINICOPATHOLOGIC CORRELATION 453
  - Clinical Presentation and Diagnosis 453
  - Complications and Causes of Death 453
  - Treatment 454

CHAPTER 19

Adenocarcinoma and Other Epithelial Tumors of the Esophagus 459
Si-Chun Ming, M.D.

- ADENOCARCINOMA 460
  - Adenocarcinoma in Barrett's Esophagus 460
  - Adenocarcinoma Not Associated with Barrett's Epithelium 469
- ADENOACANTHOMA, ADENOSQUAMOUS CARCINOMA, MUCOEPIDERMOID CARCINOMA, AND ADENOID CYSTIC CARCINOMA 469
- CARCINOSARCOMA 470
- CARCINOID AND SMALL-CELL CARCINOMA 471
- MALIGNANT MELANOMA 472
- CHORIOCARCINOMA 473
- SECONDARY AND METASTATIC TUMORS 473
- BENIGN TUMORS AND TUMOR-LIKE LESIONS 473
  - Squamous Cell Papilloma 473
  - Adenoma 474
  - Polyps 474
  - Cysts 474

PART 4
STOMACH ... 479

CHAPTER 20
Gastritis ... 481
Harvey Goldman, M.D.

- ACUTE GASTRITIS ... 482
- CHRONIC GASTRITIS ... 485
  - Types ... 485
  - General Pathologic Features ... 485
  - Chronic Antral Gastritis ... 489
  - Chronic Fundic Gastritis ... 492
  - Postgastrectomy Gastritis ... 495
  - Chronic Erosive Gastritis ... 496
  - Chronic Hypertrophic Gastritis ... 497
  - Complications ... 497
- CORROSIVE GASTRITIS ... 499
- INFECTIONS OF THE STOMACH ... 500
  - Viral Infections ... 500
  - Bacterial Infections ... 500
  - Fungal Infections ... 503
  - Parasitic Infections ... 503
- MISCELLANEOUS CONDITIONS OF THE STOMACH ... 504
  - Mallory-Weiss Syndrome ... 504
  - Gastritis due to Physical and Chemical Agents ... 505
  - Eosinophilic Gastritis ... 506
  - Gastritis Associated with Motor and Mechanical Disorders ... 506
  - Gastritis Associated with Vascular Diseases ... 506
  - Granulomatous Diseases of the Stomach ... 507
  - Gastritis Cystica Profunda ... 508
  - Other Conditions ... 509
- MUCOSAL BIOPSY ... 509

CHAPTER 21
Stress Ulcer and Chronic Peptic Ulcer Disease ... 517
Harvey Goldman, M.D.

- STRESS ULCER ... 517
  - Definition, Etiology, and Pathogenesis ... 517
  - Clinical Features ... 518
  - Pathology ... 518
  - Differential Diagnosis ... 519
- CHRONIC PEPTIC ULCER DISEASE ... 519
  - Definition ... 520
  - Epidemiology ... 520
  - Etiology and Pathogenesis ... 521
  - Clinical Features ... 522
  - Pathology ... 523
  - Differential Diagnosis ... 526
  - Complications ... 528
  - Other Ulcer Conditions ... 530
- MUCOSAL BIOPSY ... 532

CHAPTER 22

Mucosal Hypertrophy and Hyperplasia of the Stomach 537
Harvey Goldman, M.D.

    FOCAL MUCOSAL HYPERTROPHY OF THE STOMACH 537
        Polyps 537
        Inflammatory Lesions 538
        Heterotopic Pancreatic Tissue 538

    DIFFUSE MUCOSAL HYPERTROPHY OF THE STOMACH 538
        Zollinger-Ellison Syndrome 539
        Ménétrier's Disease 540
        Other Types of Hypertrophic, Hypersecretory Gastropathy 543
        Inflammatory and Neoplastic Conditions 543

CHAPTER 23

Epithelial Polyps of the Stomach 547
Si-Chun Ming, M.D.

    DEFINITION AND INCIDENCE 547
    CLINICAL ASPECTS 547
    HISTOLOGIC DIAGNOSIS AND TISSUE SAMPLING 548
    HISTORICAL REVIEW 548
    HISTOLOGIC CLASSIFICATION OF EPITHELIAL POLYPS 549
    ADENOMAS 550
        Incidence 550
        Histogenesis 550
        Subtypes and Pathology 550
        Malignancy and Adenoma 554

    HYPERPLASTIC (REGENERATIVE) POLYP 557
        Histogenesis and Various Forms 557
        Pathology 557
        Malignant Potential 560

    HAMARTOMATOUS POLYP 561
        Peutz-Jeghers Syndrome 561
        Juvenile Polyposis Syndrome 563
        Fundic Gland Polyp 564
        Foveolar Polyp 564

    INFLAMMATORY POLYP 565
    HETEROTOPIC POLYP 565
        Heterotopic Pancreas 565
        Brunner's Gland Hyperplasia 566
        Adenomyoma 566

CHAPTER 24

Early Gastric Carcinoma 570
Teruyuki Hirota, M.D., and Si-Chun Ming, M.D.

    HISTORY 570
    PROGRESS IN CLINICAL DIAGNOSIS 571
    AGE AND SEX OF PATIENTS 571
    DEFINITIONS 572
    PATHOLOGY 572
        Location and Frequency of Tumor 572
        Macroscopic Features 573

Histologic Features and Classification 575
Ulceration in Early Gastric Cancer 581
Multiple Occurrence of Early Gastric Cancer 581
Metastasis to Lymph Nodes 581

NATURAL HISTORY 581

Histogenesis 581
Growth Pattern 582
Growth Rate 582

PRECANCEROUS LESIONS 582
RECURRENCE OF CANCER AFTER SURGERY AND PROGNOSIS 582

CHAPTER 25

Adenocarcinoma and Other Malignant Epithelial Tumors of the Stomach 584
Si-Chun Ming, M.D.

FREQUENCY AND CELL TYPES OF GASTRIC TUMORS 584
CLINICAL MANIFESTATIONS AND DIFFERENTIAL DIAGNOSIS OF
  GASTRIC TUMORS 585
ADENOCARCINOMA 586

Epidemiology and Etiology 586
Precursors 587
Experimental Gastric Carcinogenesis 595
Natural History 595
Pathology 596
Histologic Classifications 603
TNM Staging 605
Clinical Aspects 605

ADENOCARCINOMA OF THE GASTRIC CARDIA AND THE
  ESOPHAGOGASTRIC JUNCTION 606
SQUAMOUS CELL CARCINOMA, ADENOSQUAMOUS CARCINOMA, AND
  MUCOEPIDERMOID CARCINOMA 607
TERATOMA AND CHORIOCARCINOMA 608
CARCINOSARCOMA 608
SMALL CELL CARCINOMA 609
MULTIPLE PRIMARY AND METASTATIC TUMORS 609

PART 5

SMALL INTESTINE, COLON, AND RECTUM 619

CHAPTER 26

Infectious Disorders of the Intestines 621
Gerald D. Abrams, M.D.

THE GASTROINTESTINAL TRACT AS AN ECOSYSTEM 621

The Normal Microbial Flora 621
Stabilizing Factors in the Gastrointestinal Ecosystem 623
Perturbations of the Gastrointestinal Ecosystem 624

EXOGENOUS INFECTION 626

Virulence Factors 626
Patterns of Host-Microbe Interaction 627

PATHOLOGY OF INTESTINAL INFECTIONS 628
    General Considerations 628
    Viral Infections 629
    Chlamydial Infections 631
    Bacterial Infections 631
    Fungal Infections 636
    Protozoan Infections 638
    Helminthic Infections 640

CHAPTER 27

Ulcerative Colitis and Crohn's Disease 643
Harvey Goldman, M.D.

ULCERATIVE COLITIS 643
    General Aspects 643
    Etiology and Pathogenesis 644
    Clinical Features 644
    Pathology 645
    Differential Diagnosis 652
    Complications 653
    Dysplasia and Carcinoma 655

CROHN'S DISEASE 663
    General Aspects 663
    Etiology and Pathogenesis 664
    Clinical Features 664
    Pathology 665
    Differential Diagnosis of Intestinal Disease 672
    Disease of Other Parts of the Alimentary Tract 673
    Complications 674
    Dysplasia and Carcinoma 676

COMPARATIVE FEATURES 677
    Pathologic and Diagnostic Features 677
    Indeterminate Colitis 678
    Clinical Course 678

MUCOSAL BIOPSY 678
    Rectal and Colonic Biopsy 679
    Ileal Biopsy 681

CHAPTER 28

Other Inflammatory Disorders of the Intestines 689
Harvey Goldman, M.D.

DUODENITIS 689
    Peptic Duodenitis 689
    Other Types of Duodenitis 693

MISCELLANEOUS INFLAMMATORY DISORDERS OF THE SMALL
    INTESTINE 696
    Ulcerative Jejunoileitis 696
    Bypass Enteritis 696
    Enteritis Cystica Profunda 696
    Other Ulcers of the Small Intestine 697

MISCELLANEOUS INFLAMMATORY DISORDERS OF THE COLON 697
    Microscopic (Lymphocytic) Colitis 697
    Collagenous Colitis 698

Diversion-Related Colitis 700
Acute Self-Limited Colitis 702
Colitis Cystica Profunda 702
Solitary Rectal Ulcer Syndrome 703
Effects of Laxatives and Enemias 706
Other Ulcers of the Colon 708
Irritable Bowel Syndrome 709

OTHER TUMOR-LIKE LESIONS OF INTESTINES 709
Pneumatosis Intestinalis 709
Endometriosis 711
Gastric Heterotopia 713
Foreign Body Reactions 715

CHAPTER 29

Malabsorptive Disorders ... 725
John H. Yardley, M.D.

BIOPSY—SPECIAL CONSIDERATIONS 725
CLINICOPATHOLOGIC CONSIDERATIONS 727
PROTEIN-LOSING ENTEROPATHY 727
DISEASES ASSOCIATED WITH NORMAL MUCOSAL HISTOLOGY 727
DISEASES PRIMARILY SHOWING NONSPECIFIC INFLAMMATION AND
  MUCOSAL ALTERATIONS 728
Celiac Disease 728
Celiac-Related Conditions 735
Tropical Sprue (Postinfective Tropical Malabsorption) 739
Stasis (Blind Loop) Syndrome 741
Deficiency States 743
Unclassified Nonspecific Inflammatory Lesions 744

INFECTION-ASSOCIATED MUCOSAL LESIONS 745
Viral Infections 745
Bacterial Infections 745
Fungal Infections 749
Protozoan Parasitosis 749
Metazoan Parasitosis 751

MUCOSAL LESIONS ASSOCIATED WITH ALTERED IMMUNE RESPONSE .. 753
Idiopathic AIDS Enteropathy 754
Autoimmune Enteropathy 754

MISCELLANEOUS DISEASES ASSOCIATED WITH CHARACTERISTIC
  MUCOSAL LESIONS 755
Mastocytosis 756
Microvillus Inclusion Disease 757
Primary Intestinal Lymphangiectasia 758
Waldenström's Macroglobulinemia 759

CHAPTER 30

Diverticular Disease of the Colon ... 768
Si-Chun Ming, M.D.

EPIDEMIOLOGY 769
ETIOLOGY AND PATHOGENESIS 770
Defects in the Colonic Wall 770
Abnormalities of the Muscular Layer 770
Intraluminal Pressure 772

Dietary Fiber 772
Other Factors 772

PATHOLOGY 773

Handling of Gross Specimens 773
Gross Features of Diverticulosis 773
Histologic Features of Diverticulosis 773
Classification 774
Diverticula of the Right Colon 779

CLINICOPATHOLOGIC CORRELATION 779

Clinical Features 779
Complicated Diverticulitis with Perforation 780
Hemorrhage 780
Obstruction 781
Coexisting Colonic Conditions 781
Associated Extracolonic Conditions 782

CHAPTER 31

Benign Polyps of the Intestines 786
Harry S. Cooper, M.D.

DEFINITION AND CLASSIFICATION 786
NONNEOPLASTIC POLYPS 786

Hyperplastic Polyps 786
Peutz-Jeghers Polyp 790
Inflammatory Polyps 792
Juvenile Polyp 793
Lymphoid Polyps 795

NEOPLASTIC POLYPS 796

Adenoma 796
Adenoma with Cancer 804
Adenoma with Pseudoinvasion 806

POLYPOSIS SYNDROMES 807

Familial (Adenomatosis) Polyposis Coli 807
Gardner's Syndrome 808
Turcot Syndrome 809
Juvenile Polyposis 809
Peutz-Jeghers Syndrome 810
Cronkhite-Canada Syndrome 810
Cowden's Disease 811
Intestinal Ganglioneuromatosis 811
Lymphoid Polyposis 811

CHAPTER 32

Adenocarcinoma and Other Malignant Epithelial Tumors of the Intestines 816
Si-Chun Ming, M.D.

INCIDENCE AND TYPES OF INTESTINAL TUMORS 817
ADENOCARCINOMA OF THE INTESTINES 818

General Considerations 818
Experimental Carcinogenesis 827
Pathology 827
Small-Intestinal Adenocarcinoma 836
Colorectal Adenocarcinoma 838

SQUAMOUS CELL CARCINOMA AND ADENOSQUAMOUS CARCINOMA ... 843

ENDOCRINE (NEUROENDOCRINE) CARCINOMA..........................844
    Composite Adenocarcinoma and Carcinoid and Adenocarcinoid..........844
    Small Cell Carcinoma 844
    Pleomorphic (Giant Cell) Carcinoma..845

OTHER RARE CARCINOMAS AND METASTATIC TUMORS 846

PART 6

APPENDIX AND ANAL REGION 859

CHAPTER 33

Disorders of the Vermiform Appendix 861
Chik-Kwun Tang, M.D.

ANATOMY AND EMBRYOLOGY..861
DEVELOPMENTAL ABNORMALITIES 863
    Congenital Absence (Agenesis) 863
    Duplication 863
    Diverticula..863
    Malposition 863
    Miscellaneous Conditions 863

INFLAMMATORY DISORDERS 863
    Acute Appendicitis 863
    Chronic Appendicitis 866
    Ulcerative Colitis and Crohn's Disease 866
    Acquired Diverticulum and Diverticulitis....................867
    Infections...867

EPITHELIAL HYPERPLASIA 870
NEOPLASIA..870
    Adenoma and Cystadenoma 870
    Adenocarcinoma and Cystadenocarcinoma................871
    Mucocele and Pseudomyxoma Peritonei 873
    Carcinoid Tumor 874
    Adenocarcinoid (Goblet Cell Carcinoid Tumor, Mucinous Carcinoid
    Tumor, Crypt Cell Carcinoma) 875
    Other Tumors 877

MISCELLANEOUS LESIONS 878
    Fibrous Obliteration 878
    Sarcoidosis..878
    Periappendicitis...878
    Intussusception 878
    Endometriosis 878
    Arteritis...878
    Cystic Fibrosis 878
    Septa 879
    Other Lesions 879

CHAPTER 34

Disorders of the Anal Region... 882
Robert R. Rickert, M.D.

ANATOMY 882
DEVELOPMENTAL ABNORMALITIES 883

HEMORRHOIDS 884
PROLAPSE 885
INFLAMMATORY AND INFECTIOUS DISORDERS 886
    Fissure 886
    Fistula and Abscess 886
    Hidradenitis Suppurativa 887
    Anal Lesions in Inflammatory Bowel Disease 887
    Sexually Transmitted Diseases 888
    Tuberculosis 889
    Other Conditions 890

BENIGN TUMORS AND TUMOR-LIKE LESIONS 890
    Condyloma Acuminatum 890
    Bowenoid Papulosis 890
    Adnexal Tumors 890
    Keratoacanthoma 892
    Granular Cell Tumor and Neurilemmoma 892
    Leiomyoma 892
    Oleogranuloma 892

MALIGNANT TUMORS 892
    General Considerations 892
    Carcinoma *in Situ* 894
    "Cloacogenic" Carcinoma 895
    Squamous Cell Carcinoma 896
    Adenocarcinoma 898
    Malignant Melanoma 898
    Extramammary Paget's Disease 899
    Basal Cell Carcinoma 900
    Other Malignant Tumors 900

Index 905

PART 1

GENERAL PRINCIPLES

CHAPTER 1

General Concepts and Methods of Examination

HARVEY GOLDMAN, M.D.
SI-CHUN MING, M.D.

GENERAL CONCEPTS OF GASTROINTESTINAL DISORDERS **Categories of Diseases** Developmental Disorders Motor and Mechanical Disorders Vascular Disorders Endocrine and Metabolic Disorders Inflammatory Disorders Tumors	Responses to Injury: Effects on Epithelium Degeneration and Regeneration Metaplasia Dysplasia and Neoplasia **Responses to Injury: Inflammatory Effects** Standard Reaction Special Features **Patterns and Stages of Diseases**	**METHODS OF EXAMINATION** **The Nature of the Specimen** Mucosal Biopsies Surgical and Autopsy Specimens **Gross Preparation and Examination** **Microscopic Examination** **Other Techniques** Cytology Electron Microscopy Immunocytochemistry Special Techniques **Pathology Reports**

The book is divided into six sections dealing with general principles and methods of study; with disorders involving multiple portions of the gastrointestinal tract; and with those diseases primarily affecting individual segments—the esophagus, the stomach, the intestines, the appendix, and the anal region.

This chapter concentrates on a general presentation of the nomenclature, classifications, pathologic processes, and methods of examination used in the study of disorders of the various segments of the gastrointestinal tract. Although it is appreciated that for each of the components of the gut as well as for many of the diseases within that particular portion, an intrinsic terminology has evolved and is often employed, the present chapter attempts to provide the general framework and principles involved in the study and definition of these components and diseases. In the specific organ chapters and disease sections, the relevant or commonly used terms are repeated or introduced as needed to allow for the detailed presentation of the characteristics of a particular disorder. The reader may find it useful on occasion to refer back to this general chapter for an elaboration or presentation of the rationale for any particular concepts or terms.

For each of the diseases presented in the subsequent chapters, information is provided regarding definition, epidemiology, prevalence, etiology, and pathogenesis. The greatest emphasis is placed on a detailed analysis and presentation of the pathologic alterations, which include the citing of the specific nomenclature and classification used for that disorder and a detailed description of the early and late alterations, both gross and microscopic, that can be perceived. Wherever relevant, the use and description of additional, less ordinary studies (such as cytochemistry, ultrastructure) are provided. Particular attention is applied to the examination and interpretation of the pathologic specimen, to include analysis of any biopsy material and immediate or frozen sections. For each disease, a description is given of the features that are essential for diagnosis at any particular stage of the disease; and this is accompanied by a reasonable listing of the differential features that serve to distinguish the disorder. The complications, again including a detailed description of the structural alterations, together with information regarding the clinical course, are provided. In addition, there are brief descriptions of the essential pathophysiologic consequences as well as the immediately relevant clinical aspects of the disorder. Consideration is also given to any age-related differences, particularly in the disorders affecting infants and children.

GENERAL CONCEPTS OF GASTROINTESTINAL DISORDERS

As mentioned above, the authors appreciate and accept that a large array of terms have come to be used in the description of a particular disorder of a single organ. In fact, in describing the same disease affecting a different organ, or closely related ones, one might employ modified or sometimes strikingly different terms. Although this serves as a testimony to the richness of the language, basic concepts and principles may be obscured. We therefore believe it to be a worthwhile exercise to give in this chapter the general tenets and foundations for the description of diseases. This also helps in understanding the order and manner of presentation of the material in the subsequent chapters. As in any attempt at classification, there is an element of arbitrariness, and it should be remembered that the effort is aimed primarily at providing uniformity and constancy in the presentation.

Categories of Diseases

It has proven convenient to separate disorders into broad categories of developmental anomalies (including the relation to embryology and anatomy), motor and mechanical disturbances (including predominant dysfunctions of nerves and muscles), vascular disorders, endocrine and metabolic diseases, the many inflammatory lesions, and tumors (Table 1–1). Although all injuries ultimately evoke a standard and stereotyped inflammatory reaction, the term *inflammatory disorders* has come to be used for those conditions that have a predominant, often primary, element of inflammatory reaction and its effects in their presentation. This may range from appreciation of many inflammatory cells on a slide to the clinical attention to a high fever or an elevated leukocyte count. Although it is appreciated that inflammatory reactions may be present, most disorders of a developmental, mechanical, vascular, or neoplastic nature are excluded from the category of inflammatory disorders. Within each of these broad categories of disease, subgroups can be formed for particular etiologies, common pathogenetic or functional pathways, or anatomic divisions.

Developmental Disorders

When one considers the large volume of the gut and its embryologic complexity, it is not surprising to note a large array of congenital and developmental anomalies affecting all portions. The major effects are in the form of persistent masses due to cysts; interference with luminal flow caused by stenoses and atresias or by extrinsic compression due to hernias; and inflammation or bleeding caused by localized diverticula. The functional anatomy of the gut is detailed in Chapter 2 and the embryology and developmental anomalies are covered in Chapter 8.

Motor and Mechanical Disorders

Food must pass through the gut at a steady and appropriate rate to permit optimal function of the tract. There is a large assortment of congenital and acquired, primary and secondary conditions that can interfere with this flow. These include mechanical disorders, in which there is a discernible physical obstruction such as an inflammatory stricture or tumor, and motor disturbances (pseudo-obstruction) in which no such obstructive element can be identified. The motor disorders may be due to local infiltrations (such as amyloid or tumor) or to specific diseases, either primary or secondary, of the bowel wall musculature or its nerve supply. Many specific and descriptive terms are applied in an attempt to define or at least to qualify a particular disorder. Within the esophagus, for example, we denote a great dilation as a mega-esophagus, discern between a causation by mechanical obstruction for whatever reason as opposed to a motor disturbance (adding the term *achalasia*), and continue the pursuit for the particular cause (e.g., Chagas' disease or of unknown etiology, the latter renamed "primary" or "idiopathic").

The term *mechanical disorder* implies causation by

Table 1–1 CATEGORIES OF GASTROINTESTINAL DISEASES

Developmental disorders

Motor and mechanical disorders
  Muscular and nervous diseases
  Obstructions, diverticula, hernias

Vascular disorders
  Varices and malformations
  Vasculitis
  Ischemic/hypoxic lesions

Endocrine and metabolic disorders

Inflammatory disorders
  Infections
  Physical injury
  Chemical injury
  Immunologic disorders
  Idiopathic disorders

Tumors
  Heterotopias
  Polyps
  Neoplasms

gross physical disturbance. Included as causes are trauma; foreign bodies; obstruction by any mass or other grossly visible lesion; and other alterations of anatomy that may interfere with normal flow or other function, such as diverticula and hernias. Such structural alterations may be congenital or acquired; and this information, together with knowledge of particular location and pathogenetic data, forms the basis for special classifications of disorders within each organ. A diverticulum represents simply a localized outpouching of the gut lumen and has been classified as a true diverticulum (with a wall containing all of the inherent structures, though often attenuated) or a pseudodiverticulum (with a wall missing some of the intrinsic elements). This histologic distinction would appear to be an unnecessary separation functionally, since the term *diverticulum* at a practical level denotes the gross presence of a localized pouch. More useful classifications include designation as congenital versus acquired and division into those resulting from the action of pressure, normal or elevated, applied to a weaker than normal portion of the wall (pulsion type) as opposed to those due to an extrinsic inflammatory process with subsequent retraction or pulling on the gut wall (inflammatory or traction type). Whatever the broad classification, it is important to note the particular etiology and pathogenesis as well as the pathophysiologic consequences for such diverticula within each of the organ systems. Thus, problems emanate from regurgitation of diverticula in the upper esophagus, from potential maldigestion related to multiple diverticula in the small bowel, and from perforation or hemorrhage of colonic diverticula. Similarly, hernias are categorized in a variety of ways on the basis of anatomic location, etiology, content, and morphology.

It should be appreciated that there are many other disorders that start with a gross mechanical event, but this event may be superseded by significant vascular obstruction or effects of inflammation. In such cases, we often discuss the condition under the heading with the greater amount of pathologic effect, i.e., as a vascular or inflammatory disorder. It is not surprising that the listing of causes of intestinal obstruction becomes in turn part of the listing of causes of vascular insufficiency of the gut; and this in turn is superseded by a designation of some of the disorders with a name that implies inflammation. Thus, persistent obstruction of a segment of bowel may lead to local vascular compromise and destruction of tissue; and if this condition should persist and be followed by a wave of inflammation, it may be designated as an example of ischemic enteritis or colitis. The general presentation of motor and mechanical disorders is provided in Chapter 11, and of colonic diverticula in Chapter 30.

Vascular Disorders

Vascular disorders can be separated into simple dilations or varices; other vascular malformations of a congenital or acquired nature; the vasculitides; and ischemic and anoxic disorders. The details of the pathology and the designations of the various clinicopathologic entities of hypoxic damage of the gut are presented in Chapter 12. It would be worthwhile here to consider the general principles underlying this damage, with particular reference to the need for greater clarity in nomenclature and classification. There is probably no other condition of the gut characterized by as much confusion—almost all unnecessary—in the terminology and categorization of ischemic or hypoxic disorders. The confusion appears to emanate from the many attempts to "tell the whole story" in the classification. These become marred by a generous admixture of terms dealing with particular location, causes, proposed pathogenetic mechanisms, standard pathologic effects, differences in morphologic forms usually due to various complicating factors, duration of events, clinical features, and subsequent outcome. It would be more orderly and ultimately wiser to consider and critically analyze each of these factors separately (Table 1–2). As noted, causes of hypoxic injury of the gut result from actual or mechanical obstruction of the blood vessels, including large or small arteries or veins, or other factors resulting in reduced blood flow.[1] In an individual case, there may be a single factor, a dominant one, or any combination. An important cause, of increasing incidence, is reduced perfusion in the absence of any mechanical vascular occlusion. Such decreased splanchnic perfusion may result from any cause of shock (e.g., cardiogenic, hemorrhagic) and any major operative procedure.

Whatever the particular cause of hypoxia, it should be appreciated that the pathogenetic pathway, mechanism of injury, and ultimate effects on the gut are limited in expression. In simplest terms, there evolves a critical reduction in nutrients, particularly in the supply of oxygen; and the cells and tissues undergo hypoxic damage. The bowel injury may differ in speed of occurrence, incidence of complicating events, and therefore different functional and clinical effects, but the initial event of hypoxic damage is the same. Hypoxia of short duration or of a mild degree may cause only a reversible functional derangement without structural damage, characterized by pain and altered absorption

Table 1–2 CAUSES AND EFFECTS OF ISCHEMIC/HYPOXIC DISEASE

Causes
    Arterial occlusion by plaques, thrombi, and emboli
    Venous occlusion by thrombi
    Venous compression associated with adhesions, hernias, volvulus, etc.
    Low perfusion state
    Obstruction and distention of gut lumen

Promoting factors
    Anemia
    Cardiac and pulmonary diseases

Effects
    Functional effects of pain and diarrhea, without necrosis
    Mucosal infarct
    Mural infarct
    Transmural infarct

and/or secretion. With persistent and severe hypoxia, ultimately there is necrosis of the cells and tissues, called an *infarct*. Based on the severity and duration of the hypoxia, the infarction may be limited to the inner lining *(mucosal infarct)* and be largely reversible, without permanent damage; extend into the wall *(mural infarct)*, resulting in inflammatory and fibrous complications; or involve all layers *(transmural infarct)*, leading to the potential for perforation.[2] There are many synonyms employed, of historical interest but of uncertain utility, including *hemorrhagic necrosis, hemorrhagic enteropathy, reversible ischemia,* and *shock* or *low flow lesion* for the mucosal infarct; *chronic ischemia, ischemic enteritis* or *colitis*, and *ischemic stricture* for the mural infarct; and *strangulation, gangrene,* or even the unqualified word *infarct* for the transmural infarct.

To summarize, independent of the specific cause of hypoxia to the gut wall, the effect will be a stereotyped one, consisting of a functional derangement or actual necrosis, which may be called an *infarct*. The infarct, depending primarily on the extent and duration of the ischemia, can be separated into stages of mucosal, mural, and transmural infarction. In any analysis of ischemic disorders, it would be best to list separately the particular location involved, the specific cause or combination of factors, the basic morphologic effects, and the clinical and functional sequelae (both acute and chronic). The bowel infarction may be complicated by secondary events leading to a change in morphologic appearance, including prominent inflammation and inflammatory pseudopolyps, pseudomembrane formation, pneumatosis, and other effects of sepsis or perforation.

Endocrine and Metabolic Disorders

Most hormonal and metabolic disturbances exhibit some effect on the gastrointestinal tract, ranging from an altered motility to the presence of depositions or inflammatory lesions. These are described throughout the book but mainly in Chapter 13, on endocrine disorders, and Chapter 16, on systemic and miscellaneous disorders.

Inflammatory Disorders

This category typically embraces conditions that manifest a prominent degree of tissue necrosis and inflammation, evident both at a structural level and at a clinical level. As indicated previously, it is customary to exclude from this category those disorders that have a primary mechanical, vascular, or tumorous cause. Major causes of inflammatory lesions are infections, radiation, drugs and chemical agents, and allergic and other immunologic processes. Within the gut, there are several conditions lacking a known definitive cause that are referred to as primary or idiopathic inflammatory disorders. These are very common and include reflux esophagitis, chronic peptic ulcer disease, Crohn's disease, and ulcerative colitis. The inflammatory reactions in the idiopathic lesions are often of a nonspecific, stereotyped nature; and precise diagnoses are dependent on history, location of disease, and exclusion of other specific disorders such as infections. There is extensive presentation of inflammatory lesions throughout the book. Concentrating on the etiology, there is information on disorders due to chemical and physical agents in Chapter 9, on allergic diseases in Chapter 10, on other immunologic conditions in Chapters 5 and 14, and on systemic disorders in Chapter 16. In addition, diseases mainly affecting particular parts of the gut are covered in Chapter 17, on the esophagus; Chapters 20 and 21, on the stomach; and Chapters 26 to 29, on the intestines.

Tumors

These are commonly noted in the gastrointestinal tract and present as masses that protrude into the lumen or that infiltrate the gut wall. Included are heterotopic (ectopic) foci of gastric or pancreatic tissues; polyps, representing projections from the mucosal surface, that can be of an inflammatory, hamartomatous, hyperplastic, or neoplastic nature; and a wide variety of benign and malignant neoplasms originating from the many cellular and tissue elements present in the gut. It is essential that the epithelial polyps be properly separated, because only the neoplastic type, the adenoma, is a proven precursor of carcinoma. Most important, because of their high prevalence and clinical significance, are the epithelial neoplasms; but tumors of the mesenchymal elements, of the lymphoid system, and of the endocrine cells are also commonly observed.

Because the mesenchymal tissues of the various parts of the gastrointestinal tract have similar cell types and organization, tumors of these tissues share equivalent pathologic features. The tumors may differ, however, in their behavior and clinical presentation, largely dependent on the particular segment of the gut involved; these are discussed in detail in Chapter 15. The different types and functions of the normal lymphoid cells in the gut are described in Chapter 5. Both lymphoid hyperplasias and malignant lymphomas, principally of the non-Hodgkin's type, can be seen in all parts of the gastrointestinal tract; and these are collectively presented in Chapter 14. A large variety of endocrine cells are present throughout the gut and are defined by their immunocytochemical reactions and ultrastructural features. The distribution of these endocrine cells and their disorders, including hyperplasias and neoplasms, as well as the functional syndromes are detailed in Chapter 13.

There is considerable heterogeneity in the structure and function of the epithelial cells of the different parts of the gastrointestinal tract, and changes in their appearance result from the frequent occurrence of metaplasia, as described below in the section on effects on epithelium. As a result of this mixture of normal and metaplastic elements, the composition of many of the epithelial tumors is complex, particularly in the stomach and lower esophagus. There has been increasing awareness of the existence and importance of precancerous conditions and lesions, particularly of dysplasia, in all parts of the gut, leading to endoscopic surveillance programs that can detect cases of epithelial tumors at an early and potentially curative stage. Although the causative agents of the carcinomas are not yet established, much understanding of possible etiologic factors has been achieved in recent years, largely through epidemiologic studies on esophageal and gastric carcinomas and through experimental studies on colonic carcinoma. Recognition of different pathologic groups of tumors has contributed significantly to the understanding of the biology of carcinoma, especially in the stomach. The vastly expanded knowledge of cytogenetic and oncogenetic influences and interplay in the cell have provided new insights into the mechanism of carcinogenesis in the gastrointestinal tract, particularly in the colon. This new information is beginning to affect the management of these common malignancies. The epithelial tumors of the esophagus are presented in Chapters 18 and 19, tumors of the stomach in Chapters 23 to 25, and tumors of the intestines in Chapters 31 and 32. Genetic and cytogenetic aspects of these tumors are provided in Chapter 6.

Responses to Injury: Effects on Epithelium

The standard pathologic processes affecting epithelia include degeneration as a direct result of the injury, regeneration as part of the reparative response, metaplasia as a sign of chronicity, and dysplasia as a marker of neoplasia and preneoplasia.

Degeneration and Regeneration

Signs of degeneration range from simple swelling of the cell (a reversible situation) to progressive autolysis and necrosis of the cell. The nuclei show disintegration (karyorrhexis and karyolysis), either promptly or after a period of condensation (pyknosis). In some instances, special cytologic features are present that help to indicate a particular etiology. A pronounced degree of nuclear enlargement and hyperchromasia suggests damage by radiation or certain drugs. Many immunologic disorders reveal a marked mononuclear cell infiltrate together with relatively slight light-microscopic evidence of epithelial cell injury. In contrast, more extensive and prompt liquefaction of the cells would be expected in those conditions with a prominent neutrophilic reaction, such as is seen in many infections. It should be stressed that for the most part, these special cellular features are quantitative and not always specific.

Regeneration is recognized by an expansion of the growing immature and less mature cells within a given epithelium. Noted are an increase in the number of mitoses and an enlargement of the regenerative zone, located at the base of squamous epithelium, in the neck region at the bottom of the gastric foveolae (pits), and in the lower portion of the intestinal crypts. The regenerative cells are enlarged and have bigger and rounder than normal nuclei with prominent nucleoli but a relatively faint chromatin pattern. The cytoplasm typically shows a decrease in mature products. It is essential that these cells, because of their larger size and more prominent nuclei, be distinguished from atypical growths (i.e., dysplasia and neoplasia). The latter typically reveal some combination of pleomorphism, hyperchromasia, loss of nuclear polarity, and reduced amount of cytoplasm.

Metaplasia

Metaplasia represents a change in cytoplasmic differentiation from the expected normal to an alternative but mature form. Metaplasia should be distinguished from heterotopia, which is an inborn or developmental misplacement of mature epithelium. This distinction can be made in most instances, because the presence of heterotopic tissue is associated with some developmental anomaly or is not preceded by any inflammatory or degenerative condition, or both. An example of heterotopia is the appearance of mature gastric corpus tissue within Meckel's diverticulum and in other parts of the gut (see Chapters 8 and 16). Acquired metaplasia is much more common and appears to be a consequence of prior inflammatory disease, usually of a chronic nature. After prolonged injury to any portion of the gut, there is a tendency for all epithelial elements of the embryonic tract to appear as part of the regeneration. With time, probably in response to local but unknown stimuli, the native cells for that particular segment of the gut prevail and reconstitute the normal epithelial layer. However, with repeated episodes of injury, the tendency for metaplasia continues in concert with the regenerative signal. The potential importance of metaplasia is that it serves as a marker of a chronic inflammatory condition, which in turn may be prone to the development of carcinoma. This is especially significant in Barrett's esophagus and in chronic gastritis with intestinal metaplasia (see Chapters 17, 19, 20, and 25).

In areas of metaplasia, one encounters and recognizes the elements from other portions of the gut, even within parts of the same organ (Table 1-3). Within the esophagus, after sustained esophagitis, the squamous epithelium may be replaced by glandular tissue, including elements of both the stomach and the intestines, and hybrid forms.[3] Injury within the stomach is

Table 1-3 TYPES OF METAPLASIA IN GUT EPITHELIUM

Location	Metaplasia	Condition
Esophagus	Glandular tissue	Barrett's esophagus
Stomach	Intestinal glands Pyloric glands in corpus	Chronic gastritis Chronic atrophic gastritis Postgastrectomy gastritis
Duodenum	Gastric surface-type mucous cells	Chronic peptic duodenitis
Small intestine	Pyloric glands	Crohn's disease
Colon and rectum	Paneth cells	Ulcerative colitis

commonly associated with a proliferation of pyloric glandular tissue, resulting in replacement of the specialized glandular cells (including parietal and chief cells) within the fundus and corpus; the same process occurs within the antrum but is appreciated as a hyperplasia of pyloric glands because the glands are an element native to that area. Throughout the stomach, there may be metaplasia with an intestinal type of epithelium, including the appearance of columnar absorptive cells, goblet mucous cells, and Paneth cells and, uncommonly, a full development of villi.[4] For the most part, this structurally resembles small-intestinal epithelium, but mucin histochemistry has demonstrated a mixture of small-intestinal and colonic mucous cells.[5,6] Injury to the small intestine is most often associated with pyloric glandular metaplasia, which on occasion is so marked as to produce gross nodules. This has been termed by others as pseudopyloric metaplasia, presumably to emphasize the change in location; however, there are no structural differences between the pyloric glandular cells that are in the native antrum and those in metaplastic sites. Commonly noted in cases of chronic duodenitis is a gastric surface-type mucous-cell metaplasia replacing the intestinal epithelial cells on the villi.[7] Finally, chronic colonic inflammation is invariably associated with Paneth cells,[8] which are indigenous to the small intestine and proximal colon, and less often with pyloric glandular cells. It is rare to find more specialized gastric corpus and small-intestinal absorptive cells within the colon, and it is also very uncommon for squamous metaplasia to occur within any segment of the gut. Further details on metaplastic elements together with information about their precise localization are presented in the organ-specific chapters, with particular reference to diagnosis and clinical significance.

Dysplasia and Neoplasia

The term *neoplasia* should be reserved at all times for the growth of an abnormal cell line. It is cytologically distinct from the other simpler effects of injury (degeneration, regeneration, and metaplasia). Synonyms for the cellular features and process noted in neoplasia include *atypical hyperplasia* and *dysplasia;* and these features can be further quantitated in degree of abnormality to denote a probability for a benign or malignant growth. Unfortunately, the full cellular alterations that may be encountered during simple degeneration or regeneration have not always been appreciated, and there has ensued the fairly common practice of using the term *atypia (atypism, atypical epithelium)* or even *dysplasia* for such cellular changes. At times, to emphasize the probable inflammatory nature of such cellular changes, the terms *inflammatory atypia* and *inflammatory dysplasia* have been used. However, the liberal use of such terms has tended to obscure the real nature of the lesion; furthermore, the information in translation to the clinician may lead to unnecessary concern about a true neoplastic process. Clearly, there will be occasions when one cannot ascertain with certainty whether a cellular alteration is neoplastic or not; in such instances, some narrative statement or a less committed designation (e.g., *cellular atypism*—probably or possibly inflammatory, or of uncertain nature) could be employed. It would be best, however, to avoid using the term *dysplasia* at such times and to reserve that term for the cellular alterations that are clearly a part of neoplasia.[9]

In the assessment of a neoplasm, the designation of *benign* or *malignant* is rendered in part by the degree of cellular alteration (i.e., dysplasia) and tissue organization, and this is made more certain by the demonstration of invasion or metastasis. In some instances, a full range from microscopic dysplasia to grossly evident benign neoplasms and malignancy can be appreciated. Furthermore, the degree of staging of the malignancy can include a true *in situ* state (i.e., malignant tumor that has not transgressed the basement membrane), infiltration of the other mucosal elements (i.e., lamina propria and muscularis mucosae), and invasion into deeper structures. This has been well established for carcinomas of the stomach and probably applies as well to carcinomas of other portions of the gut.

The term *dysplasia* has been used both as a descriptive microscopic term and to indicate a precancerous lesion, such as that in patients with long-standing ulcerative colitis, chronic gastritis, and Barrett's esophagus. This double use of the term, as a cytologic descriptive one and as a particular lesion, has led to some confusion in terminology. As indicated above, this confusion should not be compounded by using the term to designate alterations that are thought to be the sequelae of inflammation alone. In disorders of the gut epithelia, there is an increased tendency to use the word *dysplasia* to signify a neoplastic lesion, to distinguish between microscopic foci and gross lesions, and to limit the rating of dysplasia to low and high grades.[9] This two-tier rating system is particularly helpful in the assessment of microscopic dysplastic lesions noted in patients with chronic inflammatory conditions, with the implication that low-grade lesions require further biopsy and high-grade ones deserve consideration of resection. Further details regarding the dysplastic lesions of the esophagus are in Chapters 17 to 19, of the stomach in Chapter 25, and of the colon in Chapter 27.

Responses to Injury: Inflammatory Effects

Standard Reaction

Inflammation for the most part is a stereotyped response to any injury and is characterized by a combination of the effects of acute inflammation, immunologic response, and repair. Whatever the cause of the disease, if there is destruction of tissue, there is a standard acute inflammatory reaction, consisting of vascular, fluid, and cellular components. Noteworthy are the presence of dilated vessels, edema, and an initial neutrophilic response; in most instances, this is followed in short order by a variable number of macrophages (also termed "histiocytes"). This acute inflammatory reaction is enhanced by causative agents that promote chemotaxis (e.g., microorganisms that act at an extracellular level) or in any disorder with a large amount of necrosis. It should be stressed that this represents differences in degree and not in the quality of the acute inflammatory reaction. In those disorders that proceed to an immunologic response by the body, there are varying quantities of lymphocytes, plasma cells, and eosinophils; also, largely in response to the lymphocytic factors, there are even greater quantities of macrophages present. When the destruction of the tissue exceeds the capacity to provide prompt and orderly regeneration (e.g., when necrosis extends beyond the mucosa into the submucosa), there is also the element of repair tissue, consisting essentially of the small vessels and fibroblasts of granulation tissue and their product collagen. Although each of these processes (acute inflammation, immune response, and repair) may occur in any combination within a particular disorder, each relates independently to a separate stimulus. One should avoid, in this regard, uniting any of these phenomena with the categorization of a disorder as acute or chronic; these latter labels more critically relate to the duration of the disorder. Independent of the duration, whenever there is destruction of tissue, there will be an acute inflammatory reaction (provided the body is capable of mounting it); whenever there is an appropriate immune stimulus, there will be the relevant immune reaction; and whenever there is destruction beyond the ability of the cells to simply regenerate, there will be repair tissue.

Special Features

In some disorders, largely determined by the particular etiologic agent or mechanism, a more restrictive or distinctive pattern of inflammation may be encountered. Examples include prominent cellular alterations without much acute inflammation, as may be seen in microorganisms that operate within the cells; granuloma formation in response to foreign bodies or various hypersensitivity reactions; and differences in the nature and quantity of necrosis. The demonstration of such types of inflammation and their particular subfeatures may assist in the determination of a particular cause or at least in providing a more selective list of causes. It should be emphasized that the only true specific features would include the recognition of a particular microorganism, subject to confirmation by culture if possible, the identification of foreign material, or the unequivocal finding of neoplastic cells. In most instances, the particular features noted of the cellular injury and reactive inflammation are combined with other data (gross, radiologic, clinical) to provide a certain or presumptive diagnosis.

Patterns and Stages of Diseases

The terms *acute* and *chronic* are commonly employed and in the strictest sense relate to the duration of the disorder. It should be stressed that the particular point in time at which a disorder is designated as chronic is largely an empirical one. For example, the duration of an acute bacterial infection is usually measured in a matter of days, whereas the acute timing of some viral infections may be prolonged to weeks or months. Whenever an injury appears to exceed the estimated period for acute disease, it is judged at least tentatively to be a chronic disorder. The pathologist, in this regard, attempts to relate the character of the inflammatory response to this estimate of acute or chronic disease, but there are several limitations to this approach. In dealing with small biopsy specimens, often limited to the mucosa, one may not have an adequate sample to note with precision those features that are more typical of a chronic disorder. Also, there has been a tendency to equate the presence of the cells involved in an immune response with a chronic disorder; this is not strictly accurate, since their presence may signify instead an immune reaction in an acute disorder. Similarly, it is not safe to identify the components of repair tissue with a chronic disorder; again, this may simply indicate, in a given case, healing of an acute disorder. Conversely, the presence of an acute inflammatory reaction typically is in direct response to a particular etiologic agent (e.g., a microorganism, immune complex) or to prominent necrosis; this will be present independent of whether the disorder is an acute one or a chronic disease with ongoing or recurrent stimuli. It should be emphasized again that the standard inflammatory reactions (acute, immune, and repair) occur in response to specific stimuli that are independent of the duration of the disorder. Although there are no absolute qualitative differences, there are clearly differences in degree and, in turn, probability. Thus, a greater degree of immune response and a greater number of elements of repair, or both, usually signify a chronic process. This is supported in many instances by noting combinations of inflammation of apparently different ages that correspond to multiple episodes of injury.

As noted above, an acute injury is defined as one of usually short and certain duration, followed by apparent complete recovery; but it should be stressed that such injuries can recur. The pathologic consequences, depending on both the etiologies and organ responses, would include some combination of cellular degeneration and tissue necrosis, acute inflammatory reaction, immune response, regeneration, and repair. A chronic injury is defined strictly on the notation that the disorder lasts beyond the expected time of recovery. Multiple situations would thus be clearly embraced, including simple prolongation or persistence of the acute disorder, the development of some complication of the acute injury, an uncontrolled tendency for repeated episodes of acute disease, a disorder that cannot be completely eliminated, and any combination of these. The pathologic effects in a given case are highly variable and include any combination of tissue destruction, acute inflammatory and immune reaction, and generation of repair tissue. Because of the extended period of injury, there usually would be a more enhanced immune reaction and products of repair, with ultimately increased distortion of the tissue. For those chronic disorders that wax and wane, corresponding to clinical relapses and remissions, the terms *active* and *inactive* are often employed. In such instances, active disease corresponds to a situation with recurrent or enhanced destruction of tissue; as a consequence, such episodes are associated with increased acute inflammatory reaction. The inactive state usually differs from the completely normal tissue by showing some effects of the repeated injury, in the form of irregular healing of the glands (i.e., some degree of atrophy and metaplasia as well as regeneration) and increased fibrosis. These differences from normal tissue may be used, in some instances, to discern between a complete recovery of an acute injury (e.g., an acute colitis) and an inactive state of a chronic disorder (e.g., chronic ulcerative colitis).[10]

An additional term, *subacute inflammation* or *injury*, has been occasionally used; but it is of doubtful assistance. It appears to have been used in part, largely by clinicians, to signify the duration or degree of a disorder that is greater than expected in ordinary acute disease but does not qualify the disorder as chronic. Some pathologists have employed this term in describing situations of greater destruction or the appearance of some elements of the immune response, including in particular large quantities of eosinophils or plasma cells. The term is at best a tentative one denoting a situation of greater destruction, and it is not clear in a particular case whether it relates to an acute, healing, or chronic disorder. It may be difficult to completely dismiss the term from our jargon, but it must be appreciated that it has different meanings in different situations. Whenever and wherever employed, it must be specifically defined.

METHODS OF EXAMINATION

In all types of pathologic examination, there is a strong need for the relevant clinical information. As described above, the pathologic features are usually not completely specific, and precision in diagnosis demands a combination of these features with the essential functional data. In addition to the quest for a specific diagnosis, a particular biopsy or specimen may be accompanied by additional and varied questions. The information sought may be not only the diagnosis of the underlying condition but rather the severity, activity, or extent of disease. This is especially the case in the examination of small mucosal biopsies. Clearly, in such instances, it is the responsibility of the clinician not only to provide the essential clinical and functional data but also to indicate the special information that is sought in the examination. To this end, special requisition forms, often accompanied by anatomic diagrams, have been recommended; however, this will never supplant the need for the clinician to appreciate how essential this information is to the pathologist, and vice versa. Ideally, whatever the form and manner in which the information is provided on paper, there must be full communication between clinicians and pathologists. This is often best achieved by direct, verbal communication in an individual case, greatly supported by combined conferences between the two groups. We make a constant effort throughout this book to emphasize these points and to indicate the particular clinical or functional data that are required for exact examination.

The Nature of the Specimen

The gastrointestinal specimens examined include a variety of mucosal biopsies obtained by blind aspiration or under direct vision at times of endoscopy, biopsy and resection specimens received at operation, and specimens obtained at autopsy.

Mucosal Biopsies

With the recent advances in technology involving flexible endoscopes, there has been an enormous increase in the number of mucosal biopsy specimens that have been generated for examination.[11,12] These are generally small in size and require special consideration of the best methods for orientation, fixation, modes of examination, and interpretation.[13-17] The pathologist must be prepared to consider this large volume of small and multiple biopsy specimens in the recognition of the earlier stages of many gastrointestinal disorders, in the appreciation of the evolution of the lesions, and in the expansion of the interpretations, to include not only the diagnosis but answers to the other questions posed. We endeavor throughout this book to include information on mucosal biopsies in each organ-specific chapter. At the present time, such endoscopy-derived mucosal biopsy specimens are readily obtained from the esophagus, stomach, first and second portions of duodenum, and all of the colon and rectum and occasionally from the distal ileum. In some of these sites, depending on the clinical circumstances, blind aspiration biopsies may be performed instead; these typically provide a larger specimen, including a larger portion of the submucosa, permitting better orientation and of course a larger sample for study. These aspiration biopsy specimens are the ones that are typically obtained from areas beyond the reach of the conventional endoscopes, such as in the distal duodenum and proximal jejunum.

With all of these small mucosal biopsies, a concern is with the possible need for appropriate orientation of the specimen. This appears to be an essential need in the judging of nonneoplastic conditions of the small bowel, particularly in the determination of the relative and absolute heights of the villi and crypts.[14] Optimal orientation can be readily accomplished by examining the gross specimen with a magnifying lens or dissecting microscope, described in detail in Chapter 29 on malabsorption disorders. Although esthetically desirable, perfect orientation is less important in evaluating mucosal biopsy specimens of the other segments of the gut; by the simple expediency of examining multiple sections of the specimen, areas with reasonable orientation are obtained. The subsequent fixation and processing of the mucosal biopsy specimens are also important considerations. Although standard formalin fixation proves sufficient in most cases, Bouin's and Hollande's solutions have been recommended to improve considerably the cytologic detail. These latter fixatives have been used to a greater degree with small-bowel mucosal biopsies and are probably the preferred fixatives for the detection and typing of highly cellular tumors such as lymphomas. The general subject of endoscopy and endoscopic biopsies is provided in Chapter 3.

Surgical and Autopsy Specimens

Regarding the examination of surgical biopsy and resection specimens, one must remember the tendency for the gut mucosa to undergo fairly rapid autolysis. The overlying epithelial cells are also extremely fragile and subject to excess shedding if there is any manipulation of the mucosa in an unfixed state. For these reasons, it is fairly urgent that the specimen be opened, examined grossly, and immersed in fixative without unnecessary delays. The same rules apply for examination of the gut at the time of autopsy; although one has no control over the interval before the autopsy, the tissue once removed from the body at room temperature should be rapidly examined and fixed.

Gross Preparation and Examination

As indicated above, careful attention to orientation and fixation should be applied to the small biopsy specimens. Sections at multiple levels (usually three) are recommended, serving to provide areas of better orientation, to allow detection of focal findings, and to provide the full range of abnormalities.

The need for prompt examination and fixation of the large specimens, including those obtained from surgery and autopsy, has been discussed. In some instances, it is useful to distend the specimen of gut (prior to its opening) to achieve a clearer anatomic and functional state. This is particularly helpful in obtaining correlations with *in vivo* gross radiographic studies. Examples include specimens with any obstruction, with diverticular disease particularly of the colon, and with sinuses or fistulous tracts. With such studies, one can appreciate better the luminal and muscular alterations and identify with precision any openings in the bowel wall. This specimen preparation is easily accomplished by gently washing out the luminal contents, clamping or tying off one end, and allowing fixative to flow in to completely fill the lumen of the specimen. The other end is then secured, and the entire specimen is immersed in fixative prior to its opening.

Vascular injection, mainly of the arterial segment, can be of use in the full delineation of vascular lesions and in determining the causation of ischemic bowel disease.[18] In vascular lesions, such injection techniques may be of assistance in correlation with *in vivo* angiographic studies, indicate the particular location of the lesion, which is often small and difficult to appreciate by standard gross inspection, and allow appreciation of the full scope and even the pathogenesis of the lesion by providing a three-dimensional model. This is of particular use in defining those vascular lesions that are especially small and do not have extensive communications with the mucosal aspect; these include angiomatous malformations, acquired ectasias, and bleeding points in diverticula. More specialized techniques, involving not only vascular injection but also subsequent clearing by xylol of the gross specimen and examination with the dissecting microscope, have been recommended and are probably essential for the full examination of the very small lesions, such as the vascular ectasias (also termed angiodysplasia) of the right side of the colon in elderly patients.[19] This is discussed further in Chapter 12. Vascular injection may also assist in determining the particular cause of an ischemic bowel disease by providing accurate delineation of the vascular anatomy, including any collaterals, and by noting any areas of narrowing or occlusion. Finally, alterations of the vascular system are being noted in some patients with acquired bowel disease not of an ischemic nature (e.g., some forms of enteritis and chronic colitis)[20]; and it may in the future prove useful to obtain correlative studies with the injected gross specimens.

Special techniques of preparation are also needed to accurately identify the nervous elements within the gut wall. This involves the use of thick sections and silver impregnation, and such studies have provided useful information on many forms of pseudo-obstruction.[21] Details are provided in Chapter 11, on motor and mechanical disorders.

Regarding gross examination in general, the pathologist's attention is usually directed to the *en face* appearance of the mucosa. Noted in particular are any hemorrhages or other discolorations, loss or other alterations of the normal folds, ulcers, and polyps and other tumors. To better appreciate the events occurring in the rest of the bowel wall, these areas should be viewed on profile after appropriate cuts. In such a way, one can better discern the depth of ulcers and of tumor invasion and the presence and extent of any diverticula, sinuses, or fistulas.

Microscopic Examination

As indicated above, there is often an essential need to obtain multiple sections at different levels of the small biopsy specimens. For the larger specimens, the best practice is to obtain sections from any grossly altered area to include representative lesions and any gross variations; these should include the center and edges of tumors and the different areas of inflammatory lesions to denote the character of active and inactive disease. Additional sections from uninvolved areas are often obtained for confirmation of normality or verification of particular anatomic regions.

In addition to the standard hematoxylin and eosin, a large variety of special stains are employed in selected cases. Mucin stains are used for identifying neutral and mildly and strongly acidic types; and these stains may be helpful in determining areas and types of metaplasia, in identifying the differentiation of a tumor, and possibly in the detection of pretumorous states. With such stains, transitional areas between the normal mucosa of the stomach and well-formed areas of intestinal metaplasia can be appreciated; also, the contribution of both gastric and intestinal types of epithelia can be discerned in Barrett's esophagus. As required, additional stains are used in the detection of microorganisms; the identification of various stromal elements, particularly in tumors; the definition of hormone-producing cells; the distinction of pigments; and so on.

Other Techniques

Cytology

Cytologic examination at the time of endoscopy has proved to be an important companion of mucosal biopsy. As currently performed with brushes, it covers a larger area of the mucosa than a single biopsy and provides better access to strictured regions. There is also the potential for more rapid staining, examination, and interpretation. It should be remembered, however, that false-negative cytologic preparations may be obtained from tumors with marked necrosis or those tumors of an infiltrative nature with minimal mucosal abnormality. In the past, when the number of biopsy samples was smaller, cytologic examination was often more critical. This is less the case at present, because multiple mucosal biopsy specimens may be readily obtained with the flexible endoscopes. Nevertheless, it would be wrong to introduce an element of competition between the two examinations. Rather, with the same endoscopic examination, material can be obtained for both cytologic and histologic examination; and this provides the greatest yield with respect to diagnosis of tumors and their particular differentiation. Cytologic examination can also be performed on imprints of tumors from larger specimens, providing finer cellular detail and potentially a more rapid diagnosis. This subject is detailed in Chapter 4, on cytologic techniques and diagnoses.

Electron Microscopy

Ultrastructural examination by standard transmission electron microscopy is helpful in selected instances. To date, electron microscopy has proved of special use in the delineation of some tumors (particularly stromal type, hormonal type, melanocytic, epithelial versus lymphoma), the general definition of hormonal cells, the functional state of a particular cell (e.g., activity of parietal cells), the recognition of early lesions (e.g., surface cell alterations in acute gastritis), the identification of unusual microorganisms (e.g., bacterial rods in Whipple's disease and rare protozoa such as *Cryptosporidia*), and the resolution of storage deposits.

Examination by scanning electron microscopy can be helpful in the demonstration, often exquisite, of topographic markings and detailed microanatomy, but the technique has minimal use in standard diagnoses at present. It has been employed to display the altered villous configurations in small-bowel disorders and to help identify areas of epithelial dysplasia, including squamous cell lesions in the esophagus and glandular dysplasia in cases of long-standing ulcerative colitis.[22]

Immunocytochemistry

There has been an expanding usage of immunologic techniques at a tissue level, including both immunofluorescent and especially immunocytochemical methods. They have been employed to specifically identify particular hormone-producing cells, some microorganisms or their antigens, the various immunoglobulins in the plasma cells, and oncofetal antigens (e.g., carcinoembryonic antigen and oncogene products). The stains can also help to establish monoclonality in lymphomatous cells, to distinguish carcinomas from lymphomas, and to separate the various mesenchymal and nervous tumors.

Special Techniques

As needed, tissues are submitted for appropriate viral, bacterial, or fungal cultures. The recognition of the various parasitic infestations requires the finding of the organisms or their ova in the tissue sections. Histochemical techniques to identify enzymes were previously employed to help in determining the nature of epithelial and stromal populations, but their utility has proved limited, and they have been largely supplanted by ultrastructural and immunocytochemical techniques. Biochemical analyses are used for the more precise identification of the various storage elements and for measurement of enzyme content in selected disorders.

Flow-cytometric analyses are now routinely available for the subtyping of lymphomas and for the identification of the various immunodeficiency disorders. They are also being employed with increasing frequency in the assessment of epithelial and stromal tumors. Aberrations in the chromosomal number and DNA content such as aneuploidy and in the cell cycle fractions can be identified and correlated with the nature of neoplastic tissue and behavior of malignant tumors.[23,24] We are also currently witnessing the rapid application of molecular techniques, such as *in situ* hybridization and gene amplification, to all tissues.[25] These should prove especially helpful in the rapid and specific identification of microorganisms and in the detection of oncogenes in appropriate tissue samples.

Pathology Reports

The manner of reporting the pathologic analysis of a particular specimen cannot be made strictly uniform. We wish, however, to make some suggestions about the type of information that should be routinely included in pathologic reports. First, the diagnosis should be listed clearly; or, in the absence of completely specific features, it may be preceded by some qualifying phrase. The diagnosis can be accompanied, as needed and desired, by a listing of the essential features supporting it. Second, the particular location and extent of the disorder should be indicated, including both the longitudinal amount and the depth of bowel involved. Third, it is worth noting explicitly the areas of the specimen, whether longitudinal or in depth, that are free of disease; this reiteration is of particular assistance to the clinician and surgeon in the evaluation of the disease-free gut. Fourth, any complications of the basic disorder should be recorded. Finally, any other pathologic features of special interest and essential negative statements should be listed. It should be stressed that much of the pathologic description can be readily contracted by the use of precise collective pathologic terms, described in the earlier sections of this chapter. For example, the designation of a chronic active colitis would embrace and make unnecessary the separate listing of "acute and chronic inflammation," "crypt abscesses," "glandular regeneration," and "metaplasia."

It is also necessary to answer any specific questions that are posed by the clinician. This is especially important in analysis of mucosal biopsy specimens, if one considers the multiple potential reasons for the procedure. Sought may be the particular diagnosis, information concerning the extent or activity of the disease, or the presence of complications. It is the obligation of the clinician to provide the particular reason for the procedure and biopsy and the obligation of the pathologist to supply the best available answer.

References

1. Williams LF: Vascular insufficiency of the intestine. Gastroenterology 61:757–777, 1971.
2. Swerdlow SH, Antonioli DA, Goldman H: Intestinal infarctions: A new pathologic classification. Arch Pathol Lab Med 105:218, 1981.
3. Zwas F, Shields HM, Doos WG, et al: Scanning electron microscopy of Barrett's epithelium and its correlation with light microscopy and mucin stains. Gastroenterology 90:1932–1941, 1986.
4. Stemmermann G, Hayashi T: Intestinal metaplasia of the gastric mucosa: A gross and microscopic study of its distribution in various disease states. J Natl Cancer Inst 41:627–634, 1968.
5. Goldman H, Ming SC: Mucins in normal and metaplastic gastrointestinal epithelium: Histochemical distribution. Arch Pathol 85:580–586, 1968.
6. Iida F, Murata F, Nagata T: Histochemical studies of mucosubstances in metaplastic epithelium of the stomach with special reference to the development of intestinal metaplasia. Histochemistry 56:229–237, 1978.
7. James AH: Gastric epithelium in the duodenum. Gut 5:285–294, 1964.
8. Symonds DA: Paneth cell metaplasia in diseases of the colon and rectum. Arch Pathol 97:343–347, 1974.
9. Riddell RH, Goldman H, Ransohoff DF, et al: Dysplasia in inflammatory bowel disease: Standardized classification with provisional clinical applications. Hum Pathol 14:931–968, 1983.
10. Surawicz CM, Belic L: Rectal biopsy helps to distinguish acute self-limited colitis from idiopathic inflammatory bowel disease. Gastroenterology 86:104–113, 1984.
11. Hirschowitz BI: The development and application of fiberoptic endoscopy. Cancer 61:1935–1941, 1988.
12. Goldman H: Era of the mucosal biopsy. In Goldman H, Appelman HD, Kaufman N (eds): Gastrointestinal Pathology. Baltimore, Williams & Wilkins, 1990, pp 1–10.
13. Goldman H, Antonioli DA: Mucosal biopsy of the esophagus, stomach, and proximal duodenum. Hum Pathol 13:423–448, 1982.
14. Perera DR, Weinstein WM, Rubin CE: Small intestinal biopsy. Hum Pathol 6:157–217, 1975.
15. Goldman H, Antonioli DA: Mucosal biopsy of the rectum, colon, and distal ileum. Hum Pathol 13:981–1012, 1982.
16. Whitehead R: Mucosal Biopsy of the Gastrointestinal Tract, 3rd ed. Philadelphia, WB Saunders, 1984.
17. Rotterdam H, Sommers SC: Biopsy Diagnosis of the Digestive Tract. New York, Raven Press, 1981.
18. Ming SC, Bonakdarpour A: The evolution of lesions in intestinal ischemia. Arch Pathol Lab Med 101:40–43, 1977.
19. Mitsudo SM, Boley SJ, Brandt LJ, et al: Vascular ectasias of the right colon in the elderly: A distinct pathologic entity. Hum Pathol 10:585–600, 1979.
20. Wakefield AJ, Sawyerr AM, Dhillan AP, et al: Pathogenesis of Crohn's disease: Multifocal gastrointestinal infarction. Lancet 2:1057–1062, 1989.
21. Krisnamurthy S, Schuffler MD: Pathology of neuromuscular disorders of the small intestine and colon. Gastroenterology 93:610–639, 1987.
22. Shields HM, Best CJ, Goldman H: Distinction of dysplasia from inflammatory changes in ulcerative colitis: A scanning electron microscopy study with quantitative analyses. Surg Pathol 1:183–192, 1988.
23. Haggett RC, Reid BJ, Rabinovitch PS, Rubin CE: Barrett's esophagus. Correlation between mucin histochemistry, flow cytometry, and histologic diagnosis for predicting increased cancer risk. Am J Pathol 131:53–61, 1988.
24. Hood DL, Petras RE, Edinger M, et al: Deoxyribonucleic acid ploidy and cell cycle analysis of colorectal carcinoma by flow cytometry. Am J Clin Pathol 93:615–620, 1990.
25. Grody WW, Gotti RA, Naeim F: Diagnostic molecular pathology. Mod Pathol 2:553–568, 1990.

CHAPTER 2

Functional Anatomy of the Gastrointestinal Tract

DONALD A. ANTONIOLI, M.D.
JAMES L. MADARA, M.D.

GENERAL ORGANIZATION OF THE GASTROINTESTINAL TRACT

ESOPHAGUS
Gross Anatomy
Esophageal Functions
Histologic Features

STOMACH
Gross Anatomy
Gastric Functions
Histology of the Gastric Mucosa
Surface-Foveolar Mucous Cells
Mucous Neck Cells
Epithelial Cells of the Gastric Glands
Oxyntic (Parietal) Cells

Zymogenic (Chief) Cells
Cardiopyloric Mucous Cells
Endocrine Cells

SMALL INTESTINE
Gross Anatomy
Organization of the Mucosal Vasculature
Epithelial Structure: General Aspects
Epithelial Structure: Individual Cell Types
Absorptive Cells
Cytoskeleton
Other Organelles
Undifferentiated Crypt Cells
Goblet Mucous Cells

Endocrine Cells
Paneth Cells
Membranous (M) Cells
Caveolated Cells
Cup Cells

COLON
Gross Anatomy
Organization of the Colonic Wall
Epithelial Structure: General Features
Colonic Mucosal Epithelial Cells
Absorptive Cells
Goblet Mucous Cells
Undifferentiated Columnar Crypt Cells
Other Cells

The objectives of this chapter are to review the general organization of the gastrointestinal tract and to explore the gross and microscopic features of the various segments of that system. Excellent texts on the gross and microscopic anatomy of the gastrointestinal tract are readily available; in this chapter, we will stress histologic features and structural-functional correlations of particular interest to pathologists.

GENERAL ORGANIZATION OF THE GASTROINTESTINAL TRACT

All segments of the gut are organized into four layers. The innermost layer is the *mucosa*, which is structurally and functionally the most complex area. The mucosa rests upon the *submucosa*, beneath which is the *muscularis propria*. The outermost layer is termed the *serosa* or, if it lacks an outer limiting layer of mesothelial cells, the *adventitia* (Figure 2–1).

The mucosa consists of three elements. The portion facing the intestinal lumen is the *epithelium*, which varies in composition in different parts of the gut. The epithelium rests upon and within a mesenchymal compartment termed the *lamina propria*; it contains connective tissue, smooth muscle fibers in some areas, a variety of vascular channels, nerve fibers, and inflammatory cells. The third and deepest layer of the mucosa is the *muscularis mucosae*, a double layer of smooth muscle, consisting of an inner circular and outer lon-

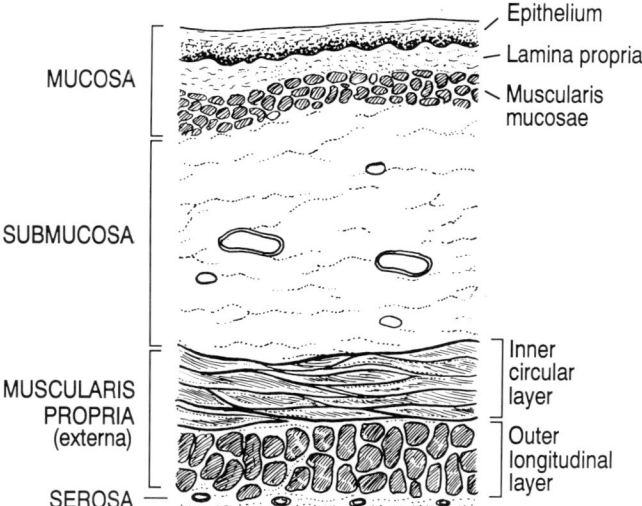

FIGURE 2-1. Schematic representation of the four-layered histologic organization of the digestive tract.

gitudinal band or spiral, that separates the lamina propria from the submucosa.

The submucosa is the branching and distribution zone for muscular arteries that have entered through the muscularis propria; in turn, it is here that small venous channels draining the mucosa converge to form larger veins that exit through the outer muscular layer. The submucosa is rich in lymphatics, a variety of inflammatory cells, autonomic neural fibers, and clusters of ganglion cells that form the submucosal plexus.

In most of the gastrointestinal tract, the muscularis propria consists of smooth muscle organized into a tightly coiled, inner circular layer and a more loosely helical, outer longitudinal layer. The smooth muscle cells are arranged in parallel arrays. Their cytoplasm is normally homogeneous and eosinophilic; however, formalin fixation often introduces an artifactual cytoplasmic vacuolar change that must be distinguished from true muscular degeneration. Specific topographic variations in the organization of the muscularis propria will be discussed in the appropriate subdivisions of this chapter.

Between the two layers of the muscularis propria are prominent autonomic neural fibers and clusters of ganglion cells forming the myenteric plexus. Both layers of the muscularis are additionally innervated by small neural twigs not readily identified by routine hematoxylin and eosin (H&E) preparations but easily demonstrated by immunocytochemical techniques using antibodies to neuron-specific enolase or S-100 protein. Similarly, the capillary network of the muscular layer is inconspicuous, and inflammatory cells are not normally identified in this layer.

The function of the muscularis propria is to propel food through the gut by contractile peristaltic waves initiated and coordinated by neural and hormonal events. Flow is regulated by differing types of peristalsis and by sphincters located in the upper esophagus and in the distal portions of the esophagus, stomach, and ileum and in the anus.

Most of the intestine is lined on its outer surface by a protective layer, the serosa. The serosa is formed of mesenchymal elements (fibroadipose tissue, vessels), lined externally by a single layer of mesothelial cells. In locations where the mesothelial layer is absent, the outermost layer of the gut is termed the adventitia; this occurs in the esophagus, the retroperitoneal portion of the duodenum, the posterior aspect of the ascending colon, and the lower part of the colon and rectum. The serosa forms a natural barrier to the spread of inflammatory and malignant processes. A small number of mononuclear inflammatory cells may normally be identified in this layer.[1]

Please see Chapter 5 for details on the inflammatory cells within the normal gut, Chapter 7 for cell renewal, Chapter 11 for a discussion of the muscular and neural elements, Chapter 12 for further information on the gross vascular supply, and Chapter 13 for a comprehensive review of the endocrine cells.

ESOPHAGUS

Gross Anatomy

The human esophagus is a hollow tube, with a smooth white mucosal surface, that is approximately 25 cm long. It extends from the cricopharyngeal muscle to its junction with the stomach at a point 2 to 3 cm below the diaphragm. On the basis of average endoscopic measurements in adults, the esophagus begins 15 cm distal to the central incisor teeth and ends 40 cm from that dental landmark. It lies behind the tracheobronchial tree, aortic arch, and heart and in front of the vertebral column. At each end, it is demarcated by a sphincter. The upper sphincter is an anatomically definable structure composed of cricopharyngeal skeletal muscle fibers. In contrast, the lower esophageal sphincter, which is formed of smooth muscle, has no clearly defined gross or microscopic identity; rather, it is a zone of increased intraluminal pressure occupying the distal 5 cm of the esophagus.[2,3]

The arterial blood supply to the esophagus is complex, with anastomoses among the various components within the esophageal wall. The upper third of the esophagus is supplied by the inferior thyroid arteries; the mid third by intercostal arteries, the bronchial arteries, and branches directly from the aorta; and the lowest third by the left gastric and inferior phrenic arteries. The accompanying veins form mural complexes that connect the systemic and portal venous systems, thus permitting the possible development of esophageal varices in patients with portal hypertension. The esophagus is well supplied with lymphatics that form a richly anastomosing network in the lamina propria and submucosa. Like the distribution of the arterial supply, lymphatic drainage is related to the three longitudinal segments of the esophagus. Drainage from the upper third of the esophagus is to cervical and paratracheal lymph nodes, from the middle third to bronchial and mediastinal lymph nodes, and from the lowest third to mediastinal nodes and a variety of lymph nodes below the diaphragm. This extensive lymphatic drainage explains the wide dissemination sometimes noted in patients with primary esophageal malignancies.[4]

Esophageal Functions

The primary functions of the normal esophagus are the propulsion of food from the mouth to the stomach and the prevention of significant reflux of gastric contents into the esophagus. The propulsive function is effected by involuntary peristalsis in the muscularis propria, which, unlike the remainder of the digestive tract, is formed of two types of muscle fibers in humans. The upper third consists of skeletal (striated) muscle fibers, the mid third of mixed striated and smooth muscle, and the lowest third of smooth muscle only.[5] Nevertheless, innervation is similar throughout the esophagus, and peristalsis proceeds smoothly and uniformly throughout the organ. This variation in muscular composition accounts for the different types of neuromuscular disorders affecting the upper versus the lower esophagus. Normally closed to prevent reflux of gastric contents into the esophagus, the lower esophageal sphincter relaxes when the peristaltic wave reaches the distal esophagus, thus permitting entry of food into the stomach. Gravity also aids peristalsis in the movement of food to the stomach.

In the resting state, the esophagus is a collapsed tube, its lumen plicated by longitudinal folds. However, it is markedly distensible because of the elastic tissue in its walls. Thus, during swallowing, the lumen dilates and the folds flatten so that the esophagus can normally accommodate the passage of even a large food bolus.

Histologic Features

The esophageal mucosa consists of squamous epithelium, lamina propria, and a thick muscularis mucosae. The inner lining of the esophageal mucosa is a multilayered, nonkeratinizing squamous epithelium that offers protection against injury from hard, jagged, or large food fragments (Figure 2–2). The normal basal (regenerative) zone of the squamous epithelium, composed of cuboidal basophilic cells in an orderly arrangement along the basement lamina, occupies no more than 15% to 20% of the epithelial height, although it may be slightly thicker in the distal esophagus.[6] Mitoses in this zone are usually difficult to identify, perhaps because cell turnover time is relatively long (over 7 days).[7]

Above the basal zone, the postmitotic epithelial cells mature, a process characterized by accumulation of cytoplasmic glycogen, nuclear pyknosis, and a change in cell polarity from vertical to horizontal, the latter accompanied by conversion of the cell shape from round to elliptical. These changes in cell contour and polarity account for the characteristic "basket-weave" appearance of the upper half of the esophageal epithelium. The ratio of the thickness of the basal zone to that of the mature epithelium is an important consideration in evaluating pathologic conditions of the esophagus. A simple method of determining the amount of mature epithelium is to perform the periodic acid–Schiff (PAS) reaction for demonstration of cytoplasmic glycogen.

Ultrastructurally, the basal cells have large nuclei and relatively few cytoplasmic organelles and lack glycogen. In comparison, the maturing, postmitotic squamous cells are characterized by glycogen accumulation in the cytoplasm, increasing amounts of tonofilaments (keratins), especially beneath the cell membrane, and more numerous desmosomes. Cell degeneration occurs in the surface layers.[5] By scanning electron microscopy, the luminal surface of the most superficial squamous cells has a network of microridges. Their function is not precisely known, but they may offer protection by holding a thin layer of mucus for lubrication[8] (Figure 2–3).

Distally, the white esophageal squamous epithelium abruptly converts to the tan to pink gastric cardia glandular epithelium within the high-pressure zone of the lower esophageal sphincter, at a point 2 to 3 cm above the gross anatomic gastroesophageal junction. This sharply defined mucosal junction, called the *Z line*, has a jagged appearance as it extends around the circumference of the esophagus. Recognition of the normal difference in location between the histologic and gross gastroesophageal junctions becomes a point of importance in the diagnosis of Barrett's esophagus (see Chapter 17).

The lowest layers of the squamous epithelium may contain scattered endocrine cells and melanocytes, whereas the lower and middle layers contain T lymphocytes and Langerhans cells[9,10] (Figure 2–4). The latter are antigen-presenting cells that characteristically have elongated, often angulated nuclei and inconspicuous cytoplasm in formalin-fixed and H&E-stained sections. Their presence and their dendritic cytoplasmic processes can be highlighted immunocytochemically by staining the tissue with antibodies to S-100 protein. The presence of T lymphocytes and Langerhans cells in the normal esophageal mucosa suggests an immunoregulatory function for this organ, but mechanisms of its action are as yet undefined.[9,11]

Glandular epithelium on the surface of the esophagus usually represents an acquired metaplastic change, termed *Barrett's epithelium*. However, in the upper 5 to 10 cm of the esophagus, in the area of the cricopharyngeal muscle, islands of the corpus-fundic type of gastric mucosa of congenital origin (gastric heterotopia) have been identified in approximately 4% of patients at endoscopy[12]; see Chapter 17 for further details.

Indigenous mucous glands are also part of the normal esophagus and are of two types. Simple tubular mucous glands (termed *superficial* or *mucosal* mucous

FIGURE 2–2. Normal squamous mucosa of the esophagus. The basal zone occupies less than 20% of the mucosal thickness, whereas the papillae of the lamina propria extend approximately halfway through the height of the mucosa. ($\times$ 150)

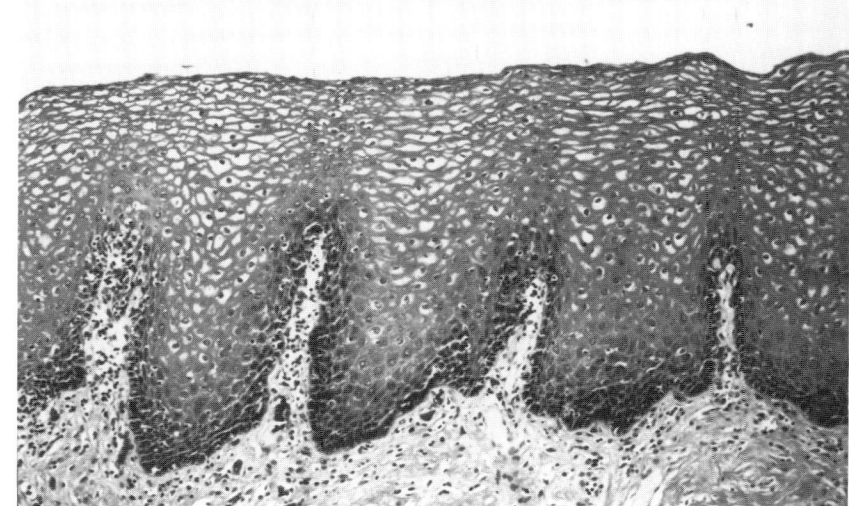

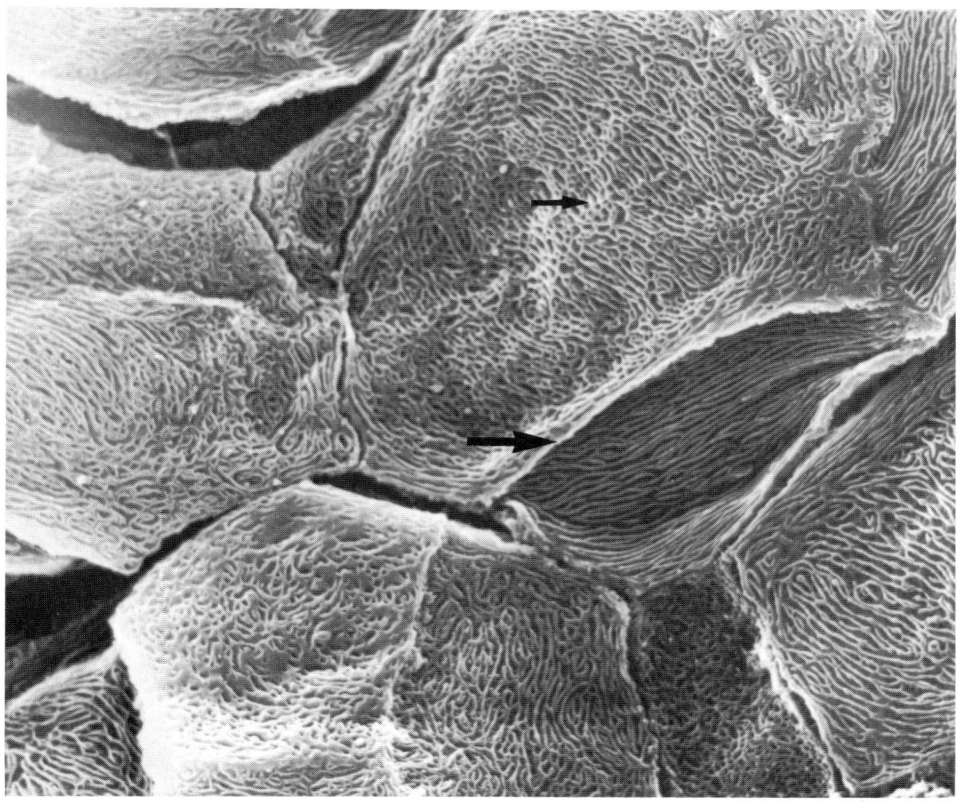

FIGURE 2–3. Scanning electron micrograph of the luminal surface of normal esophageal squamous mucosa, demonstrating the complex pattern of surface microridges (short arrow). Prominent intercellular ridges (long arrow) identify the junction of adjacent squamous cells. (Glutaraldehyde, $\times$ 2800) (Courtesy of Dr. Helen Shields, Beth Israel Hospital, Boston, Mass.)

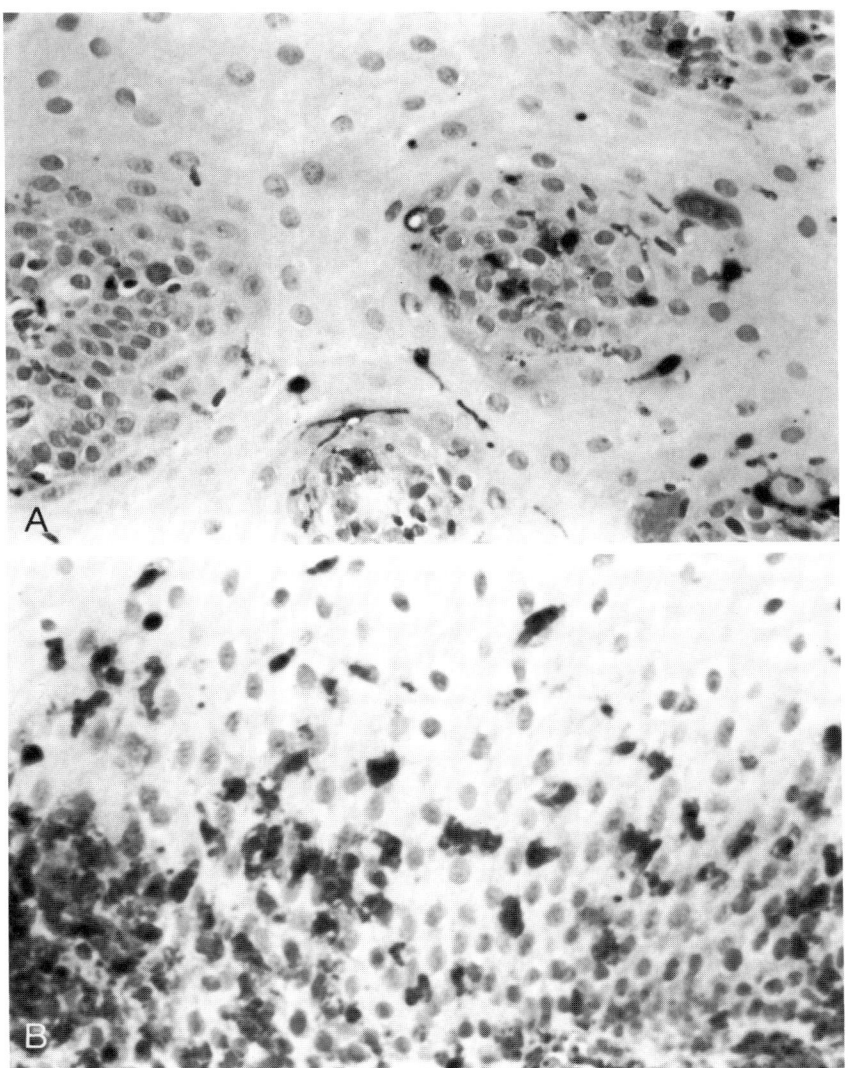

FIGURE 2–4. *A*, Langerhans cells in lower layers of the esophageal epithelium. Note their elongated cytoplasmic processes extending between the squamous cells. (Staining for S-100 protein, PAP technique, × 300) *B*, Lymphocytes are identified within the lower portion of the esophageal epithelium. (Staining for leukocyte common antigen, PAP technique, × 300)

glands) are located in the lamina propria but are confined to narrow zones at the two ends of the esophagus, i.e., adjacent to the cricopharyngeus muscle and next to the gastroesophageal junction. They produce neutral mucins and, because of their similarity to the glands of the gastric cardia, have also been called *cardiac glands*. In contrast, a more complex type of mucous gland (termed *deep* or *submucosal*) is located in variable numbers in the submucosa along the length of the esophagus, with a tendency to a higher concentration in the proximal esophagus (Figure 2–5). These glands, which produce acidic mucins, drain their secretions through the lamina propria and epithelium via ducts lined by columnar epithelium that is surrounded by myoepithelial cells.[5,13,14] The glandular function is presumably to lubricate the luminal surface of the esophagus.

Projections of lamina propria, termed *papillae*, extend into the squamous epithelium at regular intervals along the esophagus (see Figure 2–2). The papillae and lamina propria contain fibrovascular tissue, lymphatics, elastic tissue, and occasional inflammatory cells. The papillae normally do not extend to more than 50% to 60% through the height of the epithelium.[1,6] The lamina propria otherwise lacks specific characteristics; it rests on a two-layered but relatively thick muscularis mucosae that, unlike the muscularis mucosae of the stomach and intestines, consists of longitudinal, rather than spiral, fibers.[14]

Vessels, lymphoid cells, and neural tissue occupy the wide submucosa. Unlike ganglion cells in other parts of the gut, which lie close to the muscularis mucosae, the ganglion cells of the esophageal submucosa are deep and adjacent to the muscularis propria; small nerve twigs extend into the more superficial zones.[5] Thus, it is unusual to identify ganglion cells in the typically small and superficial endoscopically derived grasp biopsy specimens of the esophagus.

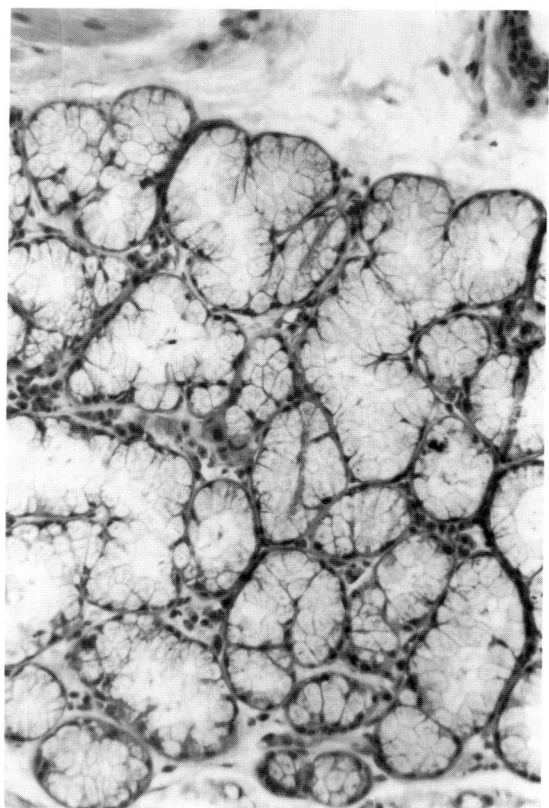

FIGURE 2-5. Complex array of esophageal submucosal mucous glands. (× 150)

STOMACH

Gross Anatomy

The stomach is variable in its gross configuration but is most often J-shaped. Normally located in the left upper quadrant of the abdomen, its upper portion lies beneath the dome of the left hemidiaphragm. Distally, it joins the duodenum at approximately the midline of the peritoneal cavity. As noted in the section on the esophagus, the junction of esophagus with stomach is normally several centimeters below the diaphragm. However, the proximal stomach may extend into the thoracic cavity as a result of defects in the diaphragm, a condition termed *hiatal hernia*.[2,15]

The stomach is divided grossly into four zones, each of which has a specific microscopic mucosal structure. The *cardia* is the narrow (approximately 1.0 cm long) portion of the stomach immediately distal to the gastroesophageal junction. The remainder of the stomach is divided into proximal and distal parts by an imaginary circumferential line drawn through the angle, or notch *(incisura angularis)*, on the lesser curve of the stomach. The proximal portion is called the *body* or *corpus*; the portion of the body that extends above the junction with the esophagus is designated the *fundus*. The distal part of the stomach is termed the *pyloric antrum*, which is demarcated from the duodenum by the pyloric sphincter. The latter is closed in the resting state to prevent the reflux of intestinal contents into the stomach. Particularly in older patients (and perhaps as a consequence of chronic gastritis), the pyloric antral mucosa may extend proximal to the incisura along the lesser curvature, occasionally even reaching the cardia, a process termed *pseudopyloric metaplasia*.[16,17]

In the resting state, the gastric mucosa and submucosa form longitudinal folds, called *rugae*, that lie parallel to, but are absent at, the lesser curvature. These rugae, which tend to be more prominent in the proximal than in the distal stomach, normally flatten during food ingestion to increase the capacity of the stomach. Retention of rugae in the distended stomach may be seen occasionally in normal subjects, but this finding is usually secondary to inflammatory, hyperplastic, and neoplastic processes. In addition to rugae, the mucosa is divided into fixed mosaic-like areas, separated by furrows, called the *areae gastricae*. Unlike normal rugae, they are not changed by alterations in the configuration of the stomach.[16]

The arterial blood supply to the stomach is complex and subject to numerous congenital variations. In brief, the gastric blood supply is derived from three branches of the celiac artery: splenic, common hepatic, and left gastric arteries. These vessels, in turn, give rise to the five major gastric arteries: left and right gastric, left and right gastroepiploic, and short gastric. Because of the rich anastomoses among the intramural gastric arteries, infarction of this organ is extremely rare. Venous drainage from the stomach is through the portal system to the liver. However, as in the esophagus, the potential for systemic-portal anastomoses (left gastric vein–azygos vein) exists in the stomach. Thus, gastric varices may develop in patients with portal hypertension. As discussed later (in the section on histology of the gastric mucosa), lymphatics in the gastric mucosa are located only in the lowermost portion of the lamina propria and in the muscularis mucosae. Deeper in the wall is a rich lymphatic network that drains to regional perigastric lymph nodes and to nodes in the omentum, around the head of the pancreas, and in the splenic hilum.[4]

Gastric Functions

In the stomach, solid food is fragmented and mixed by peristalsis. A semiliquid material (chyme) is formed that is released in small, regulated bursts into the duodenum by rhythmic openings of the pyloric sphincter. In humans, cells in the corpus and fundus of the stomach also produce hydrochloric acid and intrinsic factor, the latter necessary for the absorption of vitamin B_{12} in the terminal ileum. The physiologic roles of hydrochloric acid are not completely defined. It may aid the absorption of iron in the proximal duodenum by providing an acidic environment. Indirect evidence of a bacteriostatic function for hydrochloric acid is the fact that enteric bacterial infections are more prevalent in patients with atrophic gastritis, compared with control subjects. Also, an acid milieu is necessary for the activation of gastric proteolytic enzymes.[18]

Although predominantly a function of the small intestine, some digestion does occur in the stomach. Certain gastric mucosal cells produce pepsinogens, proteolytic enzymes that are secreted in an inactive form but are activated by the acid environment of the gastric lumen during meals. In addition, lipase derived from gastric mucosa is active at a low gastric pH.[19]

Production of the hormone gastrin is another major gastric function. Produced by antropyloric endocrine cells, gastrin causes release of hydrochloric acid as one of its major physiologic effects. Gastric and intestinal endocrine cells are discussed fully in Chapter 13.

Histology of the Gastric Mucosa
(Table 2–1)

The mucosa is structurally and functionally the most complex layer of the gastric wall. The other layers do not contain special anatomic features except for the muscularis propria, which is organized into three (innermost oblique, inner circular, and outer longitudinal), rather than two, layers and which forms a nodular pyloric sphincter at the distal end of the stomach.[16]

The gastric mucosa varies in thickness, being thinnest in the cardia and up to 1.5 mm thick in the corpus.[14] It consists of the usual three components: epithelium, lamina propria, and muscularis mucosae. The epithelial cells vary in different parts of the stomach and functionally are the most important elements in the mucosa. The lamina propria and muscularis mucosae are generally similar histologically to the analogous layers in the esophagus. However, the gastric lamina propria does not contain lymphatics except in its lowermost portion, adjacent to the muscularis mucosae.[20,21] In this regard, it is similar to the lamina propria of the colon but unlike that of the esophagus and small intestine, both of which are rich in lymphatics. The deep location of gastric mucosal lymphatics is an important factor in explaining the low frequency of nodal metastases in gastric carcinomas confined to the mucosa.[20,21]

The lamina propria contains elastic fibers and strands of smooth muscle, the latter derived from the muscularis mucosae and normally identified most prominently in the distal stomach. A small number of inflammatory cells, chiefly mononuclear, are also present in the upper third of the lamina propria in children and adults[16]; however, they are typically absent in newborns and infants. Other common findings noted in endoscopically derived biopsy specimens are edema and variable fresh hemorrhage in the lamina propria. If unaccompanied by epithelial cell necrosis or a polymorphonuclear leukocytic infiltrate, or both, edema and hemorrhage in this location are best considered artifacts secondary to the trauma of the endoscopic procedure.

Surface-Foveolar Mucous Cells

The epithelium of the gastric mucosa forms glands that vary in density and cellular composition in different parts of the stomach. At their upper end, several glands connect with and drain their secretions into conical depressions of the mucosal surface, termed *gastric foveolae* or *pits*. The foveolae and the mucosal surface between them are uniformly lined by surface-foveolar mucous cells, which are columnar cells with a small basal nucleus, pale-staining, apical cytoplasmic mucin, and a straight lateral border (Figure 2–6). These cells produce predominantly neutral glycoproteins,

Table 2–1 GASTRIC EPITHELIAL CELLS: ULTRASTRUCTURAL CHARACTERISTICS AND MAJOR FUNCTIONS

Cell Type	Distinctive Ultrastructural Features	Major Functions
Surface-foveolar mucous cells	Apical stippled granules up to 1 μm in diameter	Production of neutral glycoprotein and bicarbonate to form a gel on the gastric luminal surface; neutralization of HCl*
Mucous neck cell	Heterogeneous granules, 1–2 μm in diameter, dispersed throughout the cytoplasm	Progenitor cell for all other gastric epithelial cells Glycoprotein production Production of pepsinogens I and II
Oxyntic (parietal) cell	Surface membrane invaginations (canaliculi) Tubulovesicle structures Numerous mitochondria	Production of HCl Production of intrinsic factor Production of bicarbonate
Zymogenic (chief) cell	Moderately dense apical granules up to 2 μm in diameter Prominent supranuclear Golgi apparatus Extensive basolateral granular endoplasmic reticulum	Production of pepsinogens I and II
Cardiopyloric mucous cell	Mixture of granules like those in mucous neck and chief cells Extensive basolateral granular endoplasmic reticulum	Production of glycoprotein Production of pepsinogen II
Endocrine cells	See Chapter 13	

*Bicarbonate is produced by other gastric epithelial cells in addition to surface-foveolar mucous cells.

and, thus, the apical cytoplasm stains positively in the PAS reaction.[16] However, the deep foveolar mucous cells also contain acidic mucins. In the corpus-fundic region, these mucins are nonsulfated (N-acylated sialomucins); in the pyloric antrum, sulfated mucins may rarely be identified also[22,23] (Table 2-2). Ultrastructurally, the cells have sparse apical microvilli, beneath which the apical cytoplasm is filled with moderately dense, stippled secretory granules. The cells are adherent to one another by circumferential tight junctions located in the upper third of the lateral cell border[24] (see Figure 2-6).

Surface mucous cells secrete their glycoprotein at a continuous baseline rate by exocytosis; but secretion is increased by vagal stimulation, irritants, prostaglandins, and various hormones. On the cell surface, the mucin forms a tightly adherent gel that contains bicarbonate, the latter also produced by the mucous cells via carbonic anhydrase activity. The gel, with its trapped bicarbonate, is important in neutralizing hydrochloric acid and in maintaining the pH at 7 at the mucosal cell surface. The mucin gel in association with the mucous cell tight junctions forms a mucosal barrier to the back-diffusion of acid.[24–26] In humans, surface mucous cell turnover time is between 2 and 6 days.[7]

Mucous Neck Cells

The mucous neck cell is found throughout the stomach and is located predominantly in the upper portion (neck, or isthmus) of each gland, immediately beneath the glandular junction with the foveolae, but a few neck cells may be scattered along the length of the glands.[27] By light microscopy, these cells are similar in appearance to the surface-foveolar mucous cells but may be distinguished from them by their shorter size, more triangular shape, and slightly basophilic cytoplasm. Also, they stain less strongly than the surface mucous cells with the PAS reaction but may stain with alcian blue at pH 2.5 because they contain some acidic mucins[22,27] (see Table 2-2). They have distinctive features when examined ultrastructurally: compared with surface-foveolar mucous cells, their secretory granules are generally larger and less dense, and they are more evenly dispersed throughout the cytoplasm.[24] Of critical importance, they are the gastric epithelial progenitor cells. In each gland, they form the zone of epithelial cell renewal, giving rise to new surface-foveolar mucous cells as well as to all the cell types within the glands. Despite the cellular renewal function of the neck zone, in adults mitoses are typically not observed in this area in sections of normal stomach. In fact, the presence of mitoses signifies regeneration and is usually accompanied by other evidence of injury and repair.

Table 2–2 MUCIN PROFILES OF GASTRIC EPITHELIAL CELLS

Cell Type	Mucin Type	
	Neutral	Acidic*
Surface-foveolar mucous cells	Predominant	Trace (in cells at base of foveolae)
Mucous neck cells	Predominant	Trace
Cardiopyloric mucous cells	Predominant	Usually negative

*Sialo- and sulfated mucins; see text for details.
Data from Goldman and Ming[22] and Jass and Filipe.[23]

Epithelial Cells of the Gastric Glands

The deeper portions of the gastric epithelial glands vary in their configuration and cellular content. In the

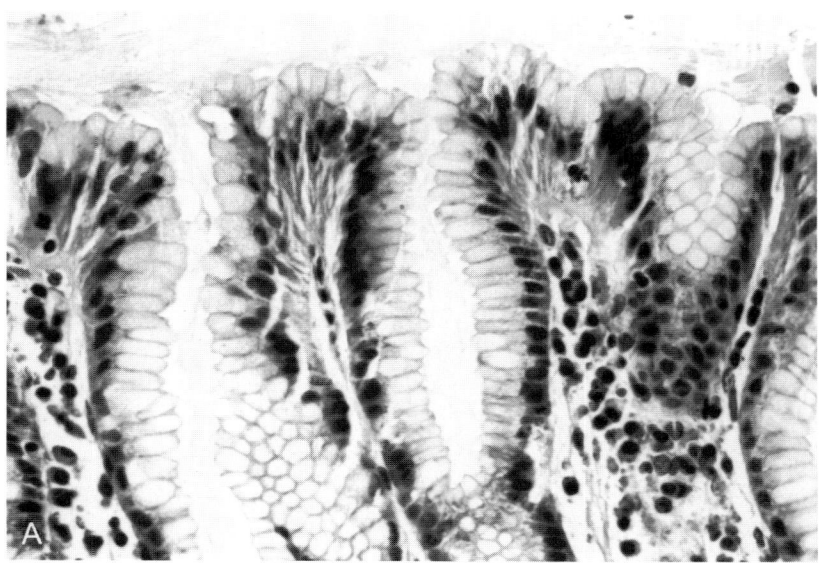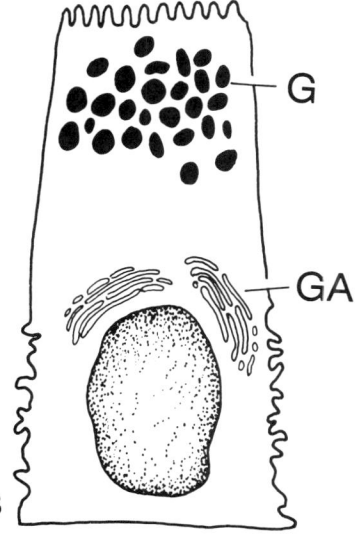

FIGURE 2–6. Gastric surface-foveolar mucous cells. *A*, In routine sections, they are columnar cells with pale granular apical cytoplasm. (× 300) *B*, Schematic representation of their characteristic ultrastructural features: apical granules (G), prominent Golgi apparatus (GA), and complex basolateral cell membrane.

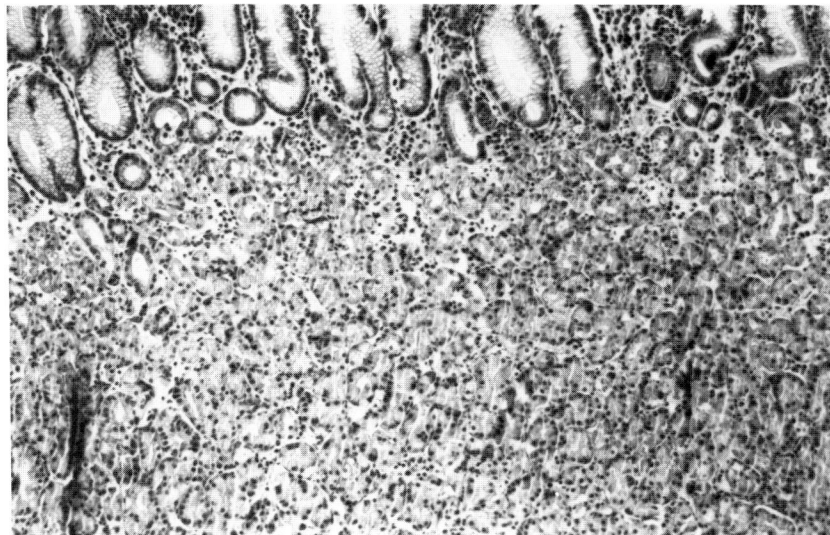

FIGURE 2–7. Architecture of the gastric glands proper. The glands are closely packed, and the foveolae are relatively short. ($\times$ 75)

corpus and fundus, the glands (gastric glands proper, or fundic glands) are long, straight, tightly packed, and associated with relatively short foveolae that form no more than 25% of the mucosal thickness. These are the gastric glands proper; they contain mucous neck, oxyntic (parietal), zymogenic (chief), and endocrine cells (Figure 2–7).

In the cardia and pyloric antrum, the glands (cardiopyloric glands) are shorter, coiled, more loosely arrayed, and associated with longer foveolae that may account for up to 50% of the mucosal height. These cardiopyloric glands are normally lined predominantly by mucous and endocrine cells, but they may contain small numbers of oxyntic cells[28] (Figure 2–8). However, large numbers of oxyntic cells in pyloric mucosa should suggest the possibility of oxyntic cell hyperplasia secondary to hypergastrinemia. Zymogenic cells are not identified outside the corpus and fundus.

The border between the pyloric glands and the gastric glands proper is often not sharp. Rather, it is typically characterized by a transition zone 1 to 2 cm in width that may vary in location in the normal stomach and that contains an admixture of corpus-fundic and cardiopyloric glandular cell types.[16,28] Awareness of the transition zone phenomenon will prevent overinterpretation of corpus mucosa as showing pyloric metaplasia.

Oxyntic (Parietal) Cells

Most oxyntic cells occupy the midportion of the gastric glands, but they may be found in the neck region or at the base. They have a pyramidal shape with a narrowed apex, a centrally placed nucleus, and deeply eosinophilic granular cytoplasm.[16] Their ultrastructural appearance is distinctive. The cells have deep lateral invaginations of the surface membrane, called *canaliculi*, that extend into the cytoplasm. The latter contains numerous cytoplasmic tubulovesicular structures in the

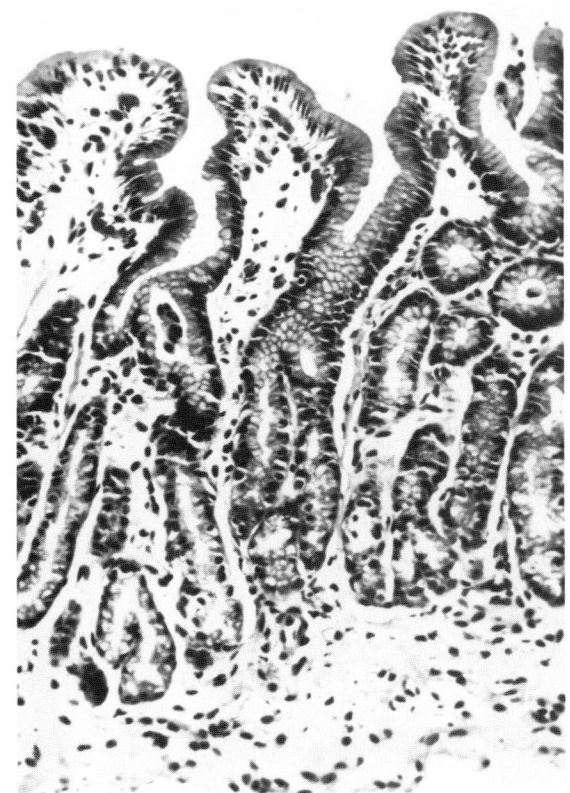

FIGURE 2–8. Architecture of the cardiopyloric glands in a pediatric patient. Compared with the gastric glands proper, the glands are shorter and more irregular and contain a different array of cells (see text for details). The foveoli may occupy up to 50% of the mucosal thickness. ($\times$ 50)

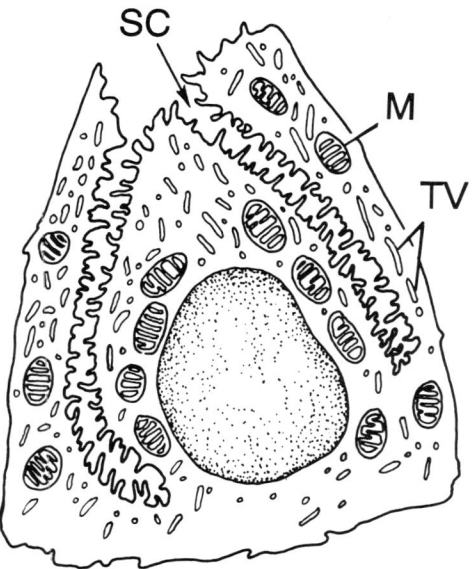

FIGURE 2–9. Schematic drawing to demonstrate the major ultrastructural features of oxyntic cells: surface intracytoplasmic canaliculus (SC), cytoplasmic tubulovesicles (TV), and numerous mitochondria (M).

resting state and many mitochondria, which account for the deep cytoplasmic eosinophilia and granularity noted in H&E-stained sections[24] (Figure 2–9).

Production of hydrochloric acid by the oxyntic cells is effected by several mechanisms, chiefly by vagal stimulation and release of gastrin and histamine. These stimuli eventuate in intracellular energy production (cyclic adenosine monophosphate [cAMP]) and accumulation of calcium. Activation of the oxyntic cells sets into motion a specific hydrogen-potassium-adenosine triphosphatase (ATPase), located on the canalicular and tubulovesicular membranes, that acts as a proton pump for exchange of hydrogen ions for potassium ions across the apical membrane.[18] During acid production, the cytoplasmic tubulovesicles fuse with the canalicular membrane, the latter becoming filled with microvilli, thus increasing the surface area for metabolic exchange. This process of fusion is reversed when acid production ceases.[1,18,20]

Oxyntic cells also contain carbonic anhydrase and produce bicarbonate.[24] In fact, all the major cell types of the gastric glands, except the endocrine cells, contain this enzyme.[29] The release of bicarbonate into the gastric lumen and intercellular spaces presumably contributes to the protection against injury by acid.

In humans, oxyntic cells also produce intrinsic factor, necessary for the ileal absorption of vitamin B_{12}. Intrinsic factor is widely distributed in the oxyntic cell, from the basal rough endoplasmic reticulum to the apical membrane.[30]

Zymogenic (Chief) Cells

Zymogenic cells are concentrated at the base of the gastric glands proper. They are low columnar cells, with basal nuclei and deeply basophilic cytoplasm, that produce two immunologically distinct groups of proteolytic enzymes, termed pepsinogen I and II, in an inactive (proenzyme) form.[31] Ultrastructurally, they are classic protein-synthesizing cells, having extensive subnuclear rough endoplasmic reticulum, a prominent supranuclear Golgi apparatus, and numerous apical, moderately dense secretory granules, the latter accounting for the cytoplasmic basophilia noted in H&E-stained sections (Figure 2–10). When the chief cells are stimulated, the pepsinogens contained in the granules are released from the cells by exocytosis and activated by the low luminal pH during digestion.[24,32] Lipase is also produced in reasonably large amounts in the human gastric corpus, but the precise cell of origin is unclear.[19]

Cardiopyloric Mucous Cells

These cells, which line the cardiopyloric glands, produce predominantly neutral glycoproteins, presumably to aid in neutralizing gastric acid as it enters the duodenum (see Table 2–2). Although these cells superficially resemble surface-foveolar mucous cells at the light-microscopic level, they differ from them ultrastructurally by having mucin granules throughout the cytoplasm rather than confined to the cell apex. Also, the mucin granules are more irregular in size and shape and less dense than those in surface-foveolar mucous cells. Their secretory granules contain pepsinogen II and lysozyme as well as glycoprotein.[24,31,32]

Endocrine Cells

The stomach is rich in endocrine cells, which form part of the diffuse gastrointestinal endocrine system, analyzed in Chapter 13.

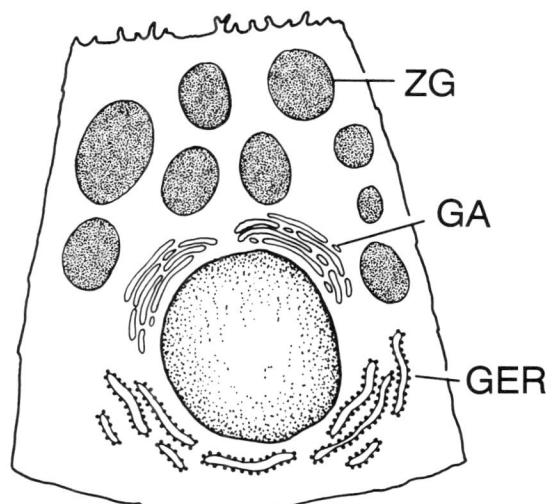

FIGURE 2–10. Schematic drawing to illustrate the chief ultrastructural features of chief cells: basolateral granular endoplasmic reticulum (GER), supranuclear Golgi apparatus (GA), and apical zymogen granules (ZG).

SMALL INTESTINE

Of all the segments of the alimentary tract, the small intestine is perhaps the most crucial, because life may be sustained in the absence of the esophagus, stomach, or colon if direct access to the lumen of the small intestine is maintained. Thus, the fact that endoscopists routinely sample only the two extreme ends of the small intestine should not obviate the need to appreciate the structural detail of this vital organ. Here, we shall present an overview of the vast literature describing small-intestinal structure and function. For more detailed reference, recent reviews may be useful.[33,34]

Gross Anatomy

The first portion of the small intestine, the *duodenum*, extends approximately 25 cm from the pyloric sphincter to a fibrous and muscular band, called the *ligament of Treitz*. From its origin at the distal stomach, the duodenum enters the retroperitoneum, curves, and returns to the peritoneal cavity; thus, it has the contour of a C-shaped loop. Given this appearance, it is not surprising that the duodenum has descriptively (and arbitrarily) been divided into superior, descending, horizontal, and ascending portions. The duodenal loop hugs the head of the pancreas and, focally, is in close apposition to the transverse colon. As a result, processes affecting these latter organs can distort the shape of the duodenal C loop and be recognized by radiologists on upper gastrointestinal (GI) imaging studies.

One feature of duodenal gross anatomy has particular impact on the strategy used by clinicians in obtaining small-intestinal mucosal biopsies. Because the entire duodenum is in a fixed position, the clinician can recognize by endoscopy the site at which an intraluminal biopsy capsule leaves the distal duodenum and enters the mobile proximal jejunum. This site, of course, corresponds to the ligament of Treitz. Recognition of this site permits the endoscopist to reproducibly and serially sample intestinal mucosa in a given patient at the same location.

Between the ligament of Treitz and the ileocecal sphincter lie the *jejunum* and *ileum*. Arbitrarily, the proximal third of this segment of the small intestine is referred to as jejunum and the remainder as the ileum. The structure and function of the jejunum and ileum are substantially different; however, these differences occur gradually, and clear anatomic or functional localization of a precise jejunal-ileal transition site is impossible. One gross alteration occurring along the jejunal-ileal axis that is important to radiologists (and to pathologists attempting to identify an unmarked segment of small intestine) is the presence of circumferential mucosal folds, termed *plicae circulares*. They are densely distributed in the proximal jejunum and, by displacing luminal barium, impart a flocculent appearance to this segment on upper GI series. In contrast, plicae are widely separated in the distal ileum. A second gross feature that permits identification of the ileum is the presence of *Peyer's patches*, which are dense collections of mucosal lymphoid nodules appearing as oval, 1- to 4-cm-long mucosal distortions.

The duodenum is supplied chiefly by the pancreaticoduodenal artery off the celiac axis, with drainage primarily via superior and inferior pancreaticoduodenal veins to the portal system. Lymphatic drainage is to pyloric and lumbar preaortic lymph nodes. The jejunum and ileum are supplied by approximately a dozen branches off the superior mesenteric artery. These branches divide and anastomose several times in the mesentery, forming arcades, the last of which defines a marginal vessel along the small intestine.[4] Because of this series of vascular anastomoses, the risk of small-bowel infarction is greatly diminished if one portion of its proximal blood supply is compromised. The organization of the mucosal vasculature is discussed in the next section.

Venous drainage in the jejunum and ileum parallels the arterial supply, with the superior mesenteric vein joining the splenic vein to form the portal vein. The lymphatic system is highly developed in the small-intestinal mucosa. Each villus contains one or more well-formed vertical lymphatic channels (lacteals) that drain into a complex submucosal lymphatic network. Unlike in the stomach, the lymphatics draining the small intestine are large (up to 1 mm in diameter). Drainage is to periaortic lymph nodes at the mesenteric root. Significant obstruction to the lymphatics may lead to intestinal mural edema and prominent intraluminal loss of protein and fluid.[4]

Organization of the Mucosal Vasculature

The general organization of the wall of the small intestine is the same as described earlier in this chapter. However, because of the potentially major role that the architecture of the mucosal circulation plays in the function of the small intestine, we briefly describe it in more detail here. The mucosal lining is organized into villous projections, each of which is centrally penetrated by an arteriole. This arteriole splays at the villus tip into a network of capillaries that subsequently course down along the sides of the villus. Thus, the villus vasculature is endowed with a hairpin turn that could, in theory, permit countercurrent exchange of gases and solutes similar to that which occurs in the kidney. There is now evidence that exchange between these ascending and descending vascular limbs occurs.[35] Such exchange appears to play a crucial role in determining the distribution of lesions in pathologic disorders, such as ischemia.

Epithelial Structure: General Aspects

The epithelial lining initiates and modulates the basic activities attributed to the small intestine: terminal digestion of nutrients and vectorial transport of nutrients, water, and ions. The epithelial surface is expanded not only by villous processes but also by the

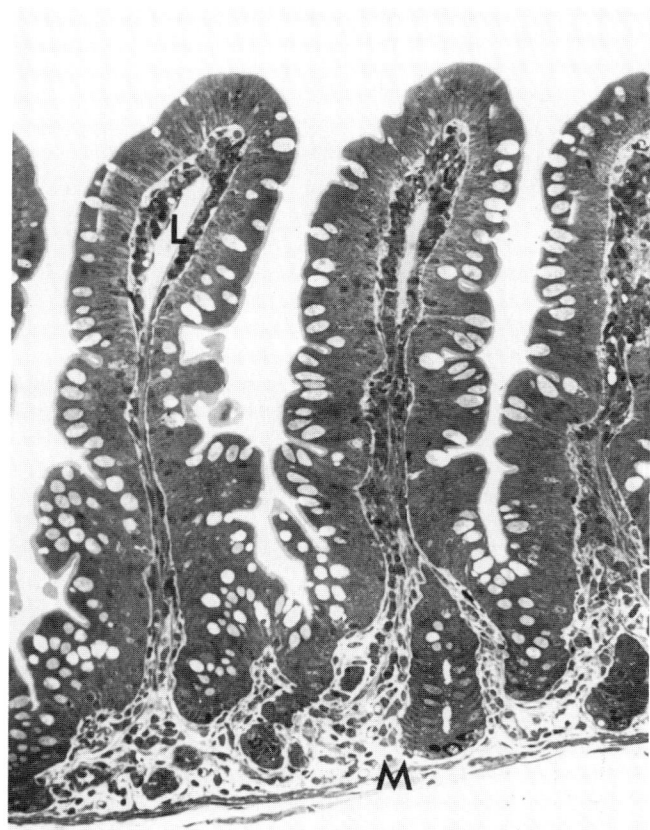

FIGURE 2–11. Light micrograph of small-intestinal mucosa showing tall fingerlike villi and short crypts. Villi are predominantly lined by absorptive cells (cells with a brush border) but also contain several goblet cells (clear goblet-shaped cells). A lymphatic (L) in a villus core can be seen as can a fine wisp of the muscularis mucosae (M). (× 250) (From Madara JL, Trier JS: Functional morphology of the mucosa of the small intestine. In Johnson LR (ed): Physiology of the Gastrointestinal Tract, 2nd ed. New York, Raven Press, 1987, p 1209.)

crypts present between villi (Figure 2–11). The distance from the villus tips to the base of the crypts constitutes the mucosal thickness, since the crypts rest directly on the muscularis mucosae. Normally, the height of the villus, which is approximately 1 mm, exceeds that of the crypt by a factor of 4 to 5. The discrete anatomic nature of crypts and villi is substantiated by the fact that different cell populations reside in these two compartments: Paneth cells, undifferentiated crypt cells, endocrine cells, and goblet cells in the crypt; and absorptive cells, goblet cells, and endocrine cells in the villus. Two additional, minor cell types of unknown function—tuft and cup cells—are present in both compartments.

The anatomic stratification of the epithelium into crypts and villi is paralleled by functional compartmentalization. Crypt cells secrete ions and water, synthesize secretory component, and transport immunoglobulin A (IgA) (synthesized by lamina propria plasma cells) into the lumen. In addition, the crypts are the site at which cell renewal occurs, cell turnover time being approximately 5 to 6 days in the jejunum and 3 days in the ileum (see Chapter 7). In contrast, the villus is the site at which terminal digestion of nutrients and absorption of nutrients, ions, and water occur.[33,34]

Several expectations arise when considering the consequences of the stratification of epithelial function along the crypt-villus axis. Destruction of the crypt, the proliferative unit of this epithelium, should impair or destroy the ability of the small intestine to reconstitute its surface. Expansion of the crypt contribution to total epithelial surface (by enlargement of this compartment or shrinkage of the villus compartment, or both) should result in enhanced secretion of ions and water. Finally, diminution of the villous contribution to epithelial surface should result in abnormal terminal digestion and malabsorption of nutrients, water, and ions. In general, these principles are realized in multiple small-intestinal disease states (see Chapters 26 to 29).

Although crypts and villi constitute the vast majority of the surface area of the small intestine, a third compartment exists that, although small in area, may play an exceedingly important role in intestinal defense mechanisms. Throughout the small intestine, nodules of lymphoid cells distort the mucosal surface contour to produce broad domes rather than discrete villi. In the ileum, aggregates of such structures large enough to be visible macroscopically constitute the previously mentioned Peyer's patches. The so-called follicular dome epithelium overlying these lymphoid nodules (which contain germinal or follicular centers) is comprised predominantly of villous absorptive cells. However, another minor and unique component of this epithelium is the M, or membranous, epithelial cell (described in detail below), which is not found elsewhere (except, perhaps, in progenitor form). Moreover, it is this cell that imparts to the follicular dome epithelium the ability to absorb intact macromolecules and transport such antigenic "samples" to the underlying lymphoid tissue. Thus, the follicular dome epithelium and subjacent lymphoid tissue form the afferent limb of the intestinal immune response.[33,34]

A fourth epithelial compartment deserves brief mention. On the duodenal side of the pyloric sphincter are submucosal mucous glands, termed *Brunner's glands*, lined by cells that are practically indistinguishable from pyloric gland mucous cells. Although present primarily in the duodenum, they may be identified in small numbers in the submucosa up to a foot distal to the ligament of Treitz; thus, their presence does not accurately define whether a biopsy comes from the duodenum or the proximal jejunum. These coiled glands focally penetrate the muscularis mucosae and are in continuity with crypt lumina into which they empty their secretory product. On the basis of ultrastructural, immunochemical, and histochemical evidence, these cells produce and secrete glycoproteins and pepsinogen II by simple exocytosis into their gland lumens. Although it had long been assumed that these cells were also the source of duodenal bicarbonate, which serves to neutralize gastric juice–derived acidity, recent studies indicate that duodenal villous cells are capable of bicarbonate secretion and call into question the Brunner's glands' contribution to duodenal neutralization.[31,36,37]

Epithelial Structure: Individual Cell Types (Table 2–3)

Absorptive Cells

Absorptive cells are the major cell type on the villus. In routine sections, they are characterized by a PAS-positive apical brush border, approximately 1 to 1.5 µm in height (see Figure 2–11). Columnar in shape, these cells display basal, oval nuclei and, in ideal 5-µm sections, a faint supranuclear lucency representing the Golgi apparatus. The remainder of the cytoplasm stains eosinophilic and is granular because of the presence of organelles such as lysosomes and mitochondria. However, the apical cytoplasmic area representing the terminal web is devoid of organelles. The terminal bar, which contains the junctional zone (see below), can be identified as a faint basophilic structure just below the brush border at the interface of adjacent cells by repeatedly focusing through the section. These cellular details are less apparent in formalin-fixed than in Bouin's- or Hollande's-fixed tissue.

The appearance of absorptive cells may change with differing physiologic states. During active absorption, the spaces between absorptive cells (paracellular spaces) may dilate,[38] which causes compression of the cells. In addition, because normal fat metabolism occurs in these cells (i.e., re-esterification of glycerol with absorbed fatty acids in the smooth endoplasmic reticulum and subsequent combination of these lipids with newly synthesized apoproteins, forming chylomicrons), transient intracellular lipid accumulation following a fatty meal may produce vacuoles in absorptive cells.[33] Thus, moderate degrees of absorptive cell vacuolization in an otherwise normal villous epithelium must be interpreted with caution: such a finding may indicate not a disease state such as abetalipoproteinemia (see Chapter 29), but rather the residue of an ill-advised meal eaten shortly before biopsy.

Ultrastructurally, the apical plasma membrane of absorptive cells forms microvilli that regularly measure 0.1 µm in width and approximately 1 µm in height. Conversely, the basolateral membrane is relatively smooth and contains focal fingerlike and sheetlike processes that extend to interdigitate with those of adjacent cells. These two major domains of the plasma membrane also differ strikingly in composition. The protein/lipid ratio of the apical membrane is exceedingly high.[39] Thus, it is not surprising that, when visualized by the freeze-fracture technique, this domain exhibits densely distributed, P-face intramembrane particles[40] that probably represent integral membrane proteins (Figure 2–12). At least 20 different protein bands can be identified in preparations derived from this membrane.[41] This large number is not surprising, considering the array of hydrolases, transporters, and

Table 2–3 SMALL-INTESTINAL AND COLONIC EPITHELIAL CELLS: ULTRASTRUCTURAL CHARACTERISTICS AND MAJOR FUNCTIONS

Cell Type	Distinctive Ultrastructural Features	Major Functions

Absorptive cell (enterocyte)	Dense, tall apical microvilli, with external glycocalyx and internal microfilaments
	Apical terminal web
	Numerous intermediate filaments
	Microtubules
		Small intestine
		  Terminal digestion of nutrients
		  Absorption of nutrients
		  Intracellular lipid metabolism
		Colon
		  Electrolyte uptake; fluid reabsorption

Undifferentiated crypt cell	Short, sparse irregular microvilli Poorly developed terminal web Apical granules, 0.1 to 1.5 µm in diameter	Progenitor cell for all other intestinal cell types Synthesis of secretory component Release of IgA-receptor complex into crypt lumen "Secretion" of chloride and water
Goblet mucous cell	Sparse, irregular microvilli Apical granules that vary in size and density, depending on maturation of the cell (see text)	Production of acidic glycoproteins
Paneth cell	Large, dense apical granules Prominent supranuclear Golgi apparatus Extensive basolateral granular endoplasmic reticulum	Production of lysozyme
M cell	Smooth apical surface Central depression containing lymphoid cells; "inverted glass" appearance Numerous endocytotic vesicles	Uptake of luminal substances; role in intestinal immune response
Caveolated (tuft) cell	Long, wide microvilli containing microfilament bundles Membrane-bound spaces (caveolae) between microfilament bundles	Unknown
Cup cell	Concave brush border with short microvilli Poorly formed terminal web	Unknown
Endocrine cells	See Chapter 13	

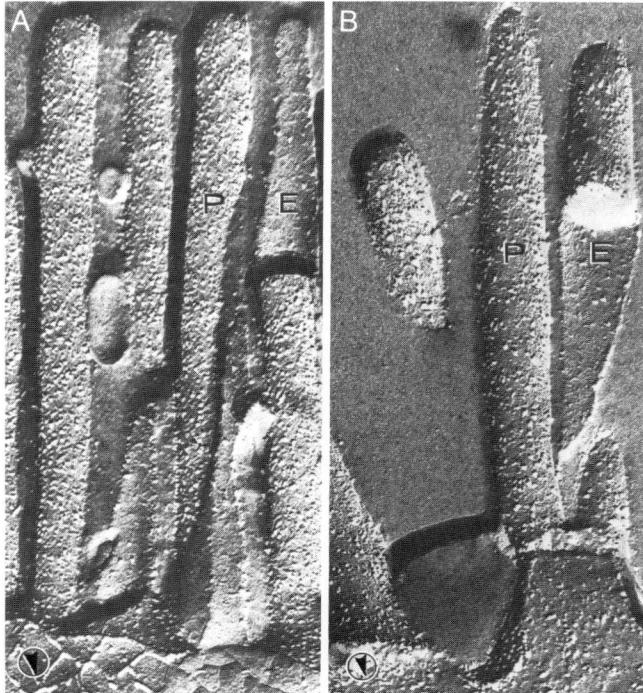

FIGURE 2–12. Freeze-fracture replicas of microvilli of an undifferentiated crypt (A) and a villus absorptive cell (B). The majority of intramembrane particles are associated with the convex membrane half, which covers the microvillus core (protoplasmic, or P, face); fewer particles are associated with the concave membrane half, which abuts the extracellular space (extracellular, or E, face). P-face particles are more numerous in the microvillus membranes of villus cells than in those of crypt cells. E-face particle density is comparable in both sites. (× 135,350) (From Madara JL, Trier JS, Neutra MR: Structural changes in the plasma membrane accompanying differentiation of epithelial cells in human and monkey small intestine. Gastroenterology 78:963, 1980. Copyright 1980, Williams & Wilkins.)

exchangers localized to this site. In contrast, the basolateral membrane exhibits protein and lipid profiles substantially different from those of the apical membrane. These chemical differences no doubt serve as the basis for physical differences between these two membranes, such as discrepant membrane fluidity.[42]

A major basolateral membrane protein is the ATP-driven Na^+/K^+ exchanger (Na^+-K^--ATPase). Na^+-K^+-ATPase–driven sodium extrusion from the cell results in an electrochemical gradient across the plasma membrane that favors sodium entry. This gradient provides the driving force for entry of many ions and nutrients into the cell (and is the reason that nutrient absorption, except that of lipids, is sodium-dependent).[34] Absorption and transport of these substances are vectorial, from the apical membrane through the cell, with extrusion at the basolateral membrane. The highly polarized arrangement of pumps, transporters, and facilitated pathways on the apical and basolateral membranes permits this vectorial transport process to proceed.

Maintenance of the polarity of apical and basolateral membrane domains in absorptive cells is accomplished, in part, by the intercellular tight junction. The tight junction circumferentially belts the apical 0.5-μm portion of the lateral membrane (Figure 2–13). It consists of a series of fusions between the outer membrane leaflets of adjacent cells that seal the lumen from the paracellular space and thus protect the subepithelial compartment from noxious luminal elements. These fusion sites actually are transmitted linearly in the plane of the lateral membrane. Hence, in freeze-fracture replicas, the tight junction appears as an array of anastomosing P-face strands and E-face grooves rep-

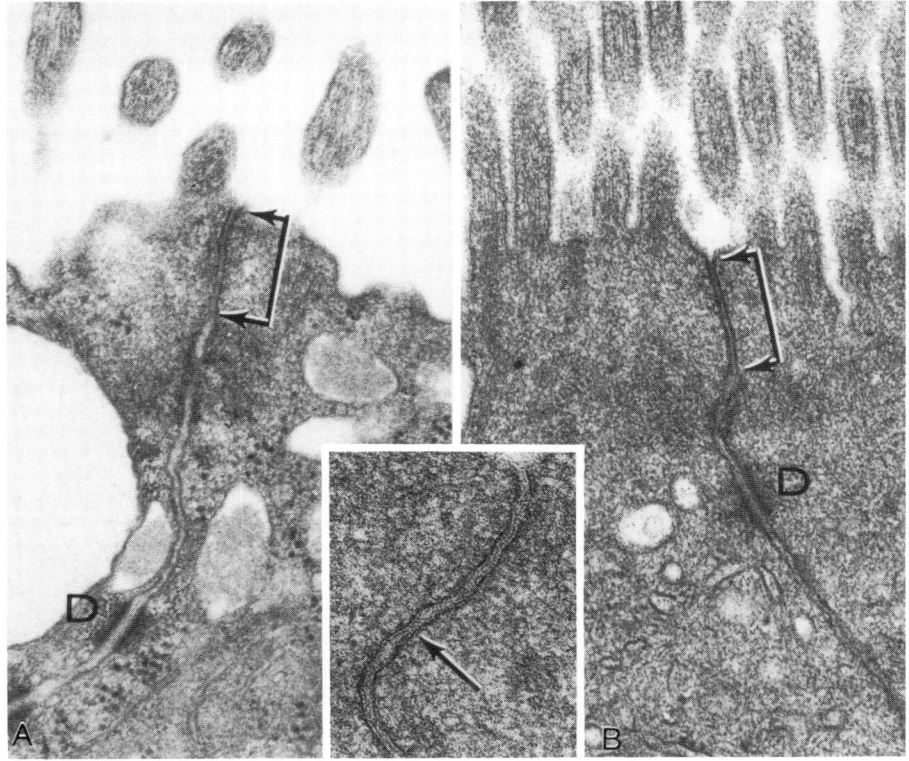

FIGURE 2–13. Thin sections of junctional complexes in the crypt (A) and on the villus (B). The apical junctional complex includes tight junctions (brackets) and desmosomes (D). The organization and structure of tight junctions cannot be fully appreciated in thin sections. (× ~52,700) Inset, Villus tight junction at higher magnification. A point of fusion of the outer membrane leaflets of adjacent cells is indicated (arrow). Fusion points correspond to P-face strands and E-face grooves revealed by freeze-fracture. (× ~78,200) (From Madara JL, Trier JS: Functional morphology of the mucosa of the small intestine. In Johnson LR (ed): Physiology of the Gastrointestinal Tract, 2nd ed. New York, Raven Press, 1987, p 1209.)

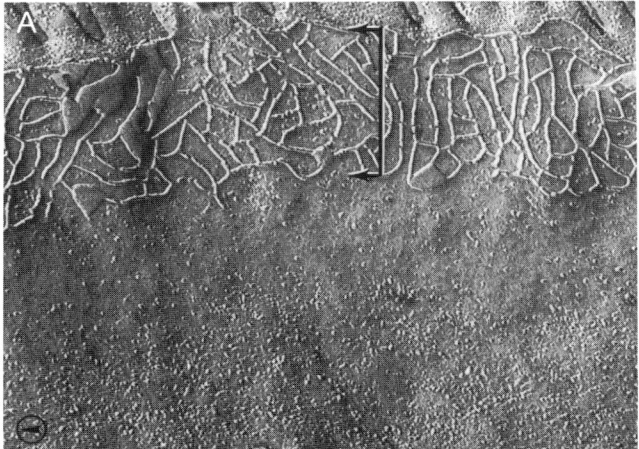

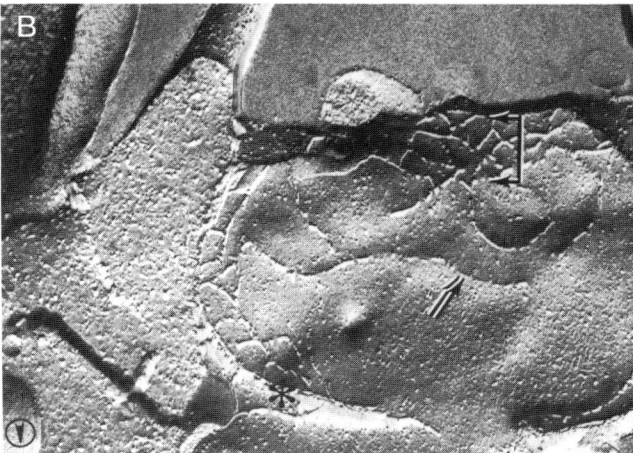

FIGURE 2–14. Freeze-fracture replicas of tight junctions on villus (A) and crypt cells (B). Tight junctions of villus absorptive cells have greater depth (brackets) and are more uniformly organized than those of crypt cells. Unconnected lateral aberrant strands (double arrow) are common in the crypt but rare on the villus. Cells in both crypts and villi show ladderlike specializations at three-cell junctions (*). (× 80,000) (From Madara JL, Trier JS, Neutra MR: Structural changes in the plasma membrane accompanying differentiation of epithelial cells in humans and monkey small intestine. Gastroenterology 78:963, 1980. Copyright 1980, Williams & Wilkins.)

resenting the fusion sites described above (Figure 2–14). The tight junction may also represent a barrier that restricts movement of integral membrane proteins and plasma membrane outer leaflet lipids across it, thus helping to maintain the distinctive chemical profiles of the apical and basolateral membranes.[33]

Although this arrangement in part explains the maintenance of cell polarity, it does not explain the origin of cell polarity. Many constituents of the plasma membrane are replaced several times over the life span of the absorptive cells. For example, the half-life of sucrase-isomaltase may be as short as 4 to 6 hours.[41] However, newly synthesized replacement protein is subsequently found only on the apical domain and is not equally intermixed in the basolateral membrane. This phenomenon, in which newly synthesized membrane components migrate to the appropriate domain, is termed *membrane "addressing."* Currently, it is not a well-understood process, but it obviously lies at the heart of how cells polarize themselves.

As noted earlier, the tight junction not only assists in maintenance of polarity but also acts to impede passive flow of molecules between cells. Although this barrier appears to be absolute for large molecules, it is relative for smaller ones. Indeed, at least 80% of passive ion permeation across ileal epithelium occurs via a transjunctional pathway. However, the distribution of this transjunction "leak" pathway may not be uniform within the mucosa. Rather, in the baseline state, absorptive cells display tight junctions with relatively many strand barriers, whereas undifferentiated crypt cells have fewer strand barriers per junction[43] (see Figure 2–14). The functional significance of less leaky villous epithelium was originally thought to be that the greatest barrier to passive flow of noxious luminal compounds occurs at the site closest to the lumen. However, the results of recent studies indicate that tight junction structure and function may not be static and, thus, the above view may be oversimplified.[44] For example, brief osmotic loads, such as occur in the proximal jejunum during normal digestion, may elicit a reversible increase in the barrier function of the absorptive cell junction and be accompanied by a marked increase in the junction's ability to exclude noxious cations such as hydrogen ion.[45] Conversely, contraction of components of the absorptive cell cytoskeleton may "pull" junctions apart and enhance permeability[46]; such contractile events reversibly occur during physiologic glucose absorption.[38] Thus, paracellular permeation may be transiently enhanced during meal-stimulated cytoskeletal contraction. In disease states, such processes may be magnified or continuously expressed. For example, in active celiac sprue, discontinuities in absorptive cell junctions occur,[47] like those seen with pharmacologically induced cytoskeletal contraction,[46] and are paralleled by abnormalities in mucosal barrier function.

Cytoskeleton

Although all alimentary epithelial cells exhibit a complex cytoskeleton, the absorptive cell has served as a major model for studies of the molecular biology of non–muscle cell cytoskeletal elements.

Each absorptive cell microvillus contains a central bundle of 20 to 30 actin microfilaments[48] (Figure 2–15). These microfilaments insert into a dense apical cap of unknown composition that lies directly under the plasma membrane at the microvillus tip. The ends of the microfilaments associated with this cap material may be viewed as equivalent to the Z bands of skeletal muscle; thus, associations with myosin would be expected at the opposite end. In fact, the distal ends of the parallel microfilaments project as "rootlets" into a "terminal web" of cytoskeletal elements beneath the microvilli (see Figure 2–15). Recent evidence suggests that the actin microfilaments might associate with myosin at this site, but it is not known whether contraction can result.[48]

The actin microfilament bundle is cross-linked by

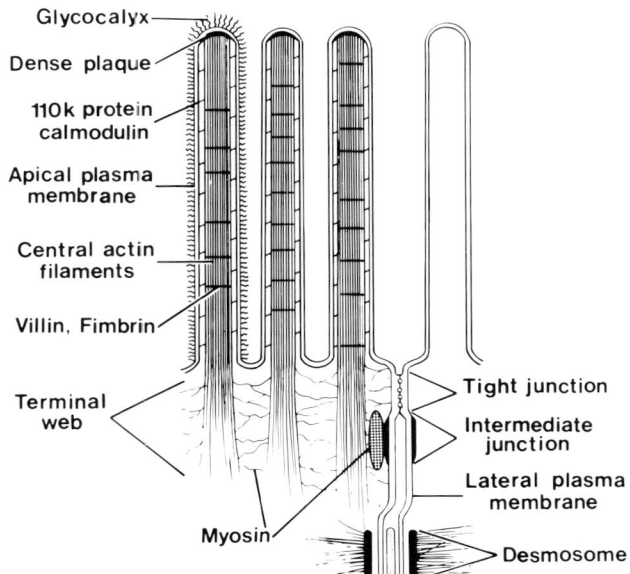

FIGURE 2–15. Schematic diagram of the structural features of the apical plasma membrane, the apical cytoplasm, and the junctional complexes of intestinal absorptive cells. (From Madara JL, Trier JS, Neutra MR: Structural changes in the plasma membrane accompanying differentiation of epithelial cells in human and monkey small intestine. Gastroenterology 78:963, 1980. Copyright 1980, Williams & Wilkins.)

proteins that presumably stabilize its structure (see Figure 2–15). Two proteins—fimbrin and villin—are present at the cross-linking site[48]; the former appears to be the major "bundling" protein, whereas the latter is thought to regulate the physical state of the actin. Lastly, a 110,000-dalton protein, which associates with the calcium regulatory protein calmodulin, appears to link the microvillus core bundle to the lateral microvillus membrane.[48]

The terminal web itself is a distinctive cytoskeletal domain. Proteins identified in the microvillus may be present (villin) or absent (110,000-dalton protein) in the terminal web, whereas other proteins are found here that are not in the microvillus (myosin; spectrin-like TW 260/240 protein). Such proteins assist in tethering other cytoskeletal elements to each other and, probably, also to the plasma membrane. One distinctive structure in the terminal web is the circumferential band of actin-myosin, termed the *contractile ring*. This ring not only can be stimulated to contract in isolated brush borders[49] but experimentally can also be induced to contract in epithelial sheets.[46] Because the ring is tethered to the lateral membrane at the site of the intercellular junction, such contraction pulls tight junctions apart, thus disrupting the barrier function of this crucial structure. Surprisingly, ring contraction is the only clearly described function of brush border contractile proteins.

Cables of 10-nm intermediate filaments composed of keratin-like material course through the cell, loop through the terminal web (presumably stabilizing it), and are anchored to desmosomes on the lateral plasma membrane. Microtubules 25 nm thick also course through the cytoplasm, predominantly in the area between the nucleus and apical membrane. They assist in routing intracellular movement, as evidenced by the fact that lipid movement through the cell is impeded when microtubular function is deranged,[33] and membrane constituents are transported to inappropriate domains under these conditions.[50]

Other Organelles

The remaining organelles in the absorptive cells are similar to those in other cells.[33] However, sequential functional stratification of these organelles exists, as exemplified by intracellular lipid metabolism. After absorption of luminal free fatty acids and monoglycerides, re-esterification of these compounds to triglycerides occurs in the smooth endoplasmic reticulum; the results of this process are visualized as apical lipid droplets. The droplets are then transferred to the Golgi complex, during which time they are combined with apoproteins, cholesterol, and phospholipid to form chylomicrons. Next, chylomicrons are transported in vesicles to the lateral membrane and undergo exocytosis into the lateral intercellular space.

Derangement of one phase of a sequential cellular process during cell injury may result in a cascade of events. For example, in injured absorptive cells, lipid often accumulates in intracellular endoplasmic reticulum–like compartments, producing a vacuolated appearance to the apical cytoplasm by light microscopy. Lipid is passively absorbed, but energy is required for its subsequent intracellular metabolism (re-esterification, chylomicron formation). Thus, the morphologic finding of lipid vacuoles probably represents the "downstream" back-up of internalized lipid in an energy-depleted cell.

Undifferentiated Crypt Cells

This cell is the major component of the crypt. It is called undifferentiated because, in contrast to the absorptive cell, it has sparse, short, often irregular microvilli, a less well developed terminal web (see Figure 2–13), and does not absorb lipid or floridly express functional integral membrane proteins necessary for terminal digestion and absorption of nutrients. However, this is the cell type capable of moving through the cell cycle and thus serves as the progenitor for other cell types in the intestinal epithelium. In addition, these cells perform several unique and sophisticated functions. They synthesize a receptor for IgA, called secretory component, and, with precision, place this receptor on the lateral plasma membrane. After binding the ligand (IgA produced by lamina propria plasma cells), these cells immediately internalize the ligand-receptor complex; shuttle it to the apical membrane; and, by a process in which the receptor is chemically modified, extrude the ligand-receptor complex into the lumen. Thus, these cells are an integral part of the intestinal immune response.[33] Also, in contrast to absorptive cells, these cells are structurally arranged to transport chloride actively into the lumen in response to

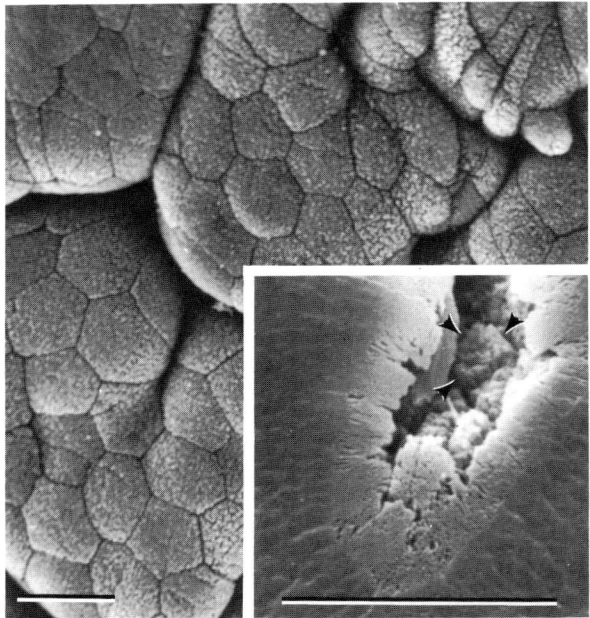

FIGURE 2-16. Scanning electron micrographs of guinea pig ileal villus and crypt *(inset)* epithelium. The villus surface is covered by polygonal absorptive cells that have estimated cell widths of 10 μm and produce the honeycomb appearance of the villus surface. (× 1225) *Inset,* Crypt epithelial cells, such as the one highlighted by the arrowheads, are polygonal in shape but have apical cell widths of only 3.5 μm. Thus the high linear junctional density in the crypt is not due to tortuous cell contours, but to diminished apical cell widths (× 3500). Bars = 10 μm. (From Marcial MA, Carlson SL, Madara JL: Partitioning of paracellular conductance along the crypt-villus axis: A hypothesis based on structural analysis with detailed consideration of tight junction structure-function relationships. J Membr Biol 80:59, 1984.)

secretagogues such as cholera toxin or the heat-labile enterotoxin of *Escherichia coli.*[51]

Undifferentiated crypt cells have other structural modifications that facilitate secretory processes. For example, they have narrow apices (Figure 2-16), causing large amounts of intercellular junction per unit crypt surface (1 cm² of crypt surface has 80 m of junction!).[46] Moreover, in comparison with absorptive cells, they have tight junctions that have fewer strand barriers (see Figure 2-14) and are cation-selective. These anatomic features facilitate the transjunctional movement of paracellular Na$^+$ (driven by the favorable electrical gradient created by the active transcellular chloride secretory process) accompanied by H$_2$O "secretion," thus permitting what, in the extreme, we recognize as secretory diarrhea. Baseline secretion may cleanse the crypt lumen and wash other important crypt products such as IgA into the intestinal lumen proper. Enhanced secretion, as occurs in cholera, may serve to clear the lumen of toxin-producing bacilli and thus shorten the clinical course of the disease. Because modulation of the rate of this normal Cl$^-$ secretory process occurs at the level of the chloride channel, it is not surprising that the intestinal mucosa may be structurally normal by light microscopy in some diarrheal diseases (e.g., cholera).

In general, the other architectural characteristics of undifferentiated crypt cells represent variations on the themes discussed in the absorptive cell section. However, in contrast to absorptive cells, undifferentiated crypt cells prominently display apical secretory vesicles 0.1 to 1.5 nm in diameter. These vesicles contain glycoprotein and exocytose their content when stimulated by cholinergic agonists but have no known function.[33]

Goblet Mucous Cells

Goblet cells are the second major cell population of both crypts and villi.[33] They are more numerous in the ileum than in the jejunum and are relatively sparse on villus tips. They are easily identified in routine sections due to their brandy goblet shape and distended apical cytoplasm filled with pale-stained, 1- to 3-μm mucous granules. A densely staining, thin rim of compressed cytoplasm, termed the *theca,* surrounds this mucous granule mass. There is no brush border.

By electron microscopy, only few, irregular, predominantly perijunctional microvilli, nearly devoid of intramembrane particles, are present on goblet cell apical membranes (Figures 2-17 and 2-18). The mucous granules are membrane-bound and originate from the well-developed supranuclear Golgi apparatus. Although both crypt and villus goblet cells generally share the same structural features, a subclass of less well differentiated goblet cells, called *oligomucous cells,* are found in the crypt. Their distinctive characteristic is that they are capable of cell division.[33]

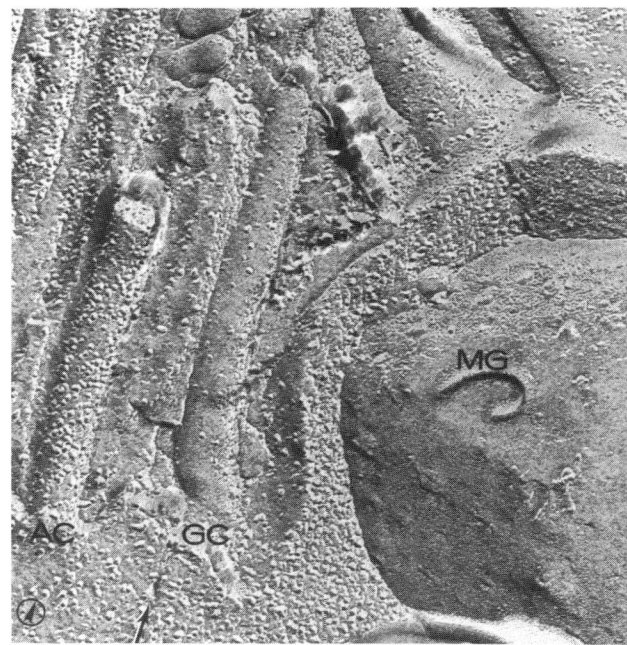

FIGURE 2-17. Freeze-fracture replica of apical cytoplasm of adjacent goblet and villus absorptive cells. The arrow indicates the position of the intercellular space separating the goblet (GC) and the absorptive cell (AC). The P face of a microvillus from each cell is exposed. That of the goblet cell (right) is particle poor, while that of the absorptive cell (left) is particle rich. A mucin granule (MG) can be seen in the goblet cell cytoplasm. (× 146,000) (From Madara JL, Trier JS: Functional morphology of the mucosa of the small intestine. In Johnson LR (ed): Physiology of the Gastrointestinal Tract, 2nd ed. New York, Raven Press, 1987, p 1209.)

FUNCTIONAL ANATOMY OF THE GASTROINTESTINAL TRACT

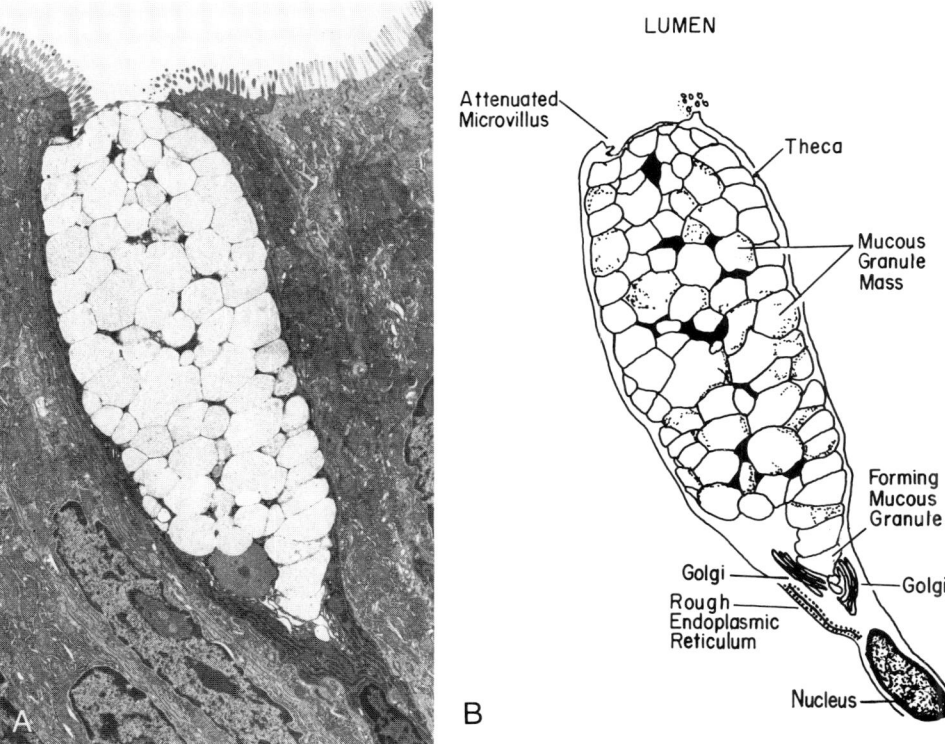

FIGURE 2-18. Electron micrograph (*A*) and trace (*B*) of goblet cell. (From Madara JL: Functional morphology of the epithelium of the small intestine. In Shultz S (ed): Handbook of Physiology. Vol IV, The Gastrointestinal System. Bethesda, American Physiological Association, 1991, p 107.)

Goblet cells release the mucin contained in the secretory vesicles by simple and compound exocytosis.[52] Although the rate of baseline secretion is imprecisely defined, newly synthesized mucin molecules appear to move from the Golgi apparatus, through the vesicle population, and onto the apical surface in approximately 4 hours.[53] If stimulated with a goblet cell secretagogue such as acetylcholine, massive mucin discharge occurs by a process in which multiple vesicles tandemly fuse (compound exocytosis).[52] It is now clear that "apocrine" secretion of goblet cell contents does not occur physiologically but may be artifactually induced by inappropriate tissue handling prior to chemical fixation.

Human small-intestinal mucin contains a high-molecular-weight glycoprotein similar to that produced in the rat[54,55] (2×10^6 daltons, 10% protein plus approximately 85% hexose consisting of at least six hexose species). Lectin labeling patterns are also well described. Lectins bind only the terminal sugars of the long carbohydrate chains and, thus, yield very "superficial" (in a topographical sense, but some would also say in a real sense) information concerning mucin biochemistry. Thus, it should not be surprising if classes of mucins as defined biochemically bear no relationship to classes of mucins defined by lectin staining. Such lectin studies do tell us that goblet cells may be heterogeneous with respect to their secretory product, because goblet cell lectin stain patterns vary from jejunum to ileum. Of interest is the recent observation that goblet cells themselves may secrete lectinlike molecules.[55] By cross-linking terminal sugars, such molecules may stabilize or increase the rigidity of mucus in the intestinal lumen. Goblet cell mucins are acidic and stain positively with alcian blue at pH 2.5. The mucins vary in composition and relative amounts in the small intestine and colon, with more sialomucin found in the small intestine and more sulfomucin in the colon. The sialomucins also vary in the two locations, with N-acetylsialomucins common in the small intestine but O-acetylsialomucins predominant in the colon and most distal ileum[56,57] (Table 2-4).

Table 2-4 MUCIN PROFILES OF INTESTINAL GOBLET CELLS

		Mucin Type*		
Location	Neutral	*Sialomucin* (*N-acetyl*)	*Sialomucin* (*O-acetyl*)	*Sulfomucin*
Small intestine	+	+ (Predominant)	+ (Minor)	−
Colon	+	+	+	+ (Predominant)

*Mucin types also vary along the length of the crypt and/or villus, and in different parts of the small or large intestine (see Filipe and Fenger[57] and Toner et al.[58]).

Mucins may assist intestinal function in a variety of ways. They act as surface lubricants, increase diffusion rates of threatening luminal molecules, and block the epithelial binding sites of bacteria. Of interest in this regard is the observation that exposure to certain bacterial products, particularly enterotoxins, results in massive mucin release.[55]

Endocrine Cells

See Chapter 13 for a discussion of endocrine cells.

Paneth Cells

Located at the base of the crypts, Paneth cells as seen by light microscopy have intensely eosinophilic apical secretory granules. Unlike most other small-intestinal epithelial cells, Paneth cells are renewed only after approximately 20 days[33]; but like other cell types, they appear to originate from undifferentiated crypt cells. Although the ultrastructural appearance of this cell resembles that of the goblet cell, Paneth cells have broader bases and their granules contain a dark, homogeneously staining protein product, with an appearance similar to that in zymogen-producing cells. Paneth cells also exhibit not only baseline secretion but also secretion stimulated by cholinergic agents and inhibited by atropine.[58]

The precise secretory product(s) and function(s) of Paneth cells are unclear. Lysozyme may be one Paneth cell product, and Paneth cells can internalize extracellular matter such as bacteria and immunoglobulin.[33] Such observations have led to the speculation that these cells help to regulate the bacterial microenvironment of the crypt. However, many species (such as cats and dogs) do not have Paneth cells, and these animals do not have any detectable deficiencies in bacteriologic surveillance.

Membranous (M) Cells

Membranous, or M, cells are present only on the epithelium overlying sites where lymphoid follicles protrude from the lamina propria and distort the overlying epithelium into a dome-like contour, hence the name *follicular dome epithelium*.[59,60] Although this epithelium represents only a tiny fraction of the total intestinal surface, and M cells are a numerically minor constituent even in this epithelium, the M cells play a vital role in intestinal immune responses, as outlined earlier.

M cells are difficult to appreciate by light microscopy, but this observation is not surprising in view of their ultrastructural appearance. By electron microscopy (Figure 2–19), M cells have the appearance of an inverted glass: they have thin walls that connect with a confluent surface, and they exhibit a central depression. They also have thin cytoplasmic processes that extend laterally over the basal lamina. Their apical surfaces display small folds or markedly attenuated microvilli (see Figure 2–19); whereas lymphoid cells, which may either be macrophages or mark as B or T cells, reside within the aforementioned hollow.

In addition to the usual allotment of cellular organelles, M cells contain numerous endocytotic vesicles that are crucial to their function. These vesicles internalize luminal matter ranging from macromolecules to virions, bacteria, and parasites and are capable of shuttling such material across the M cell and depositing it

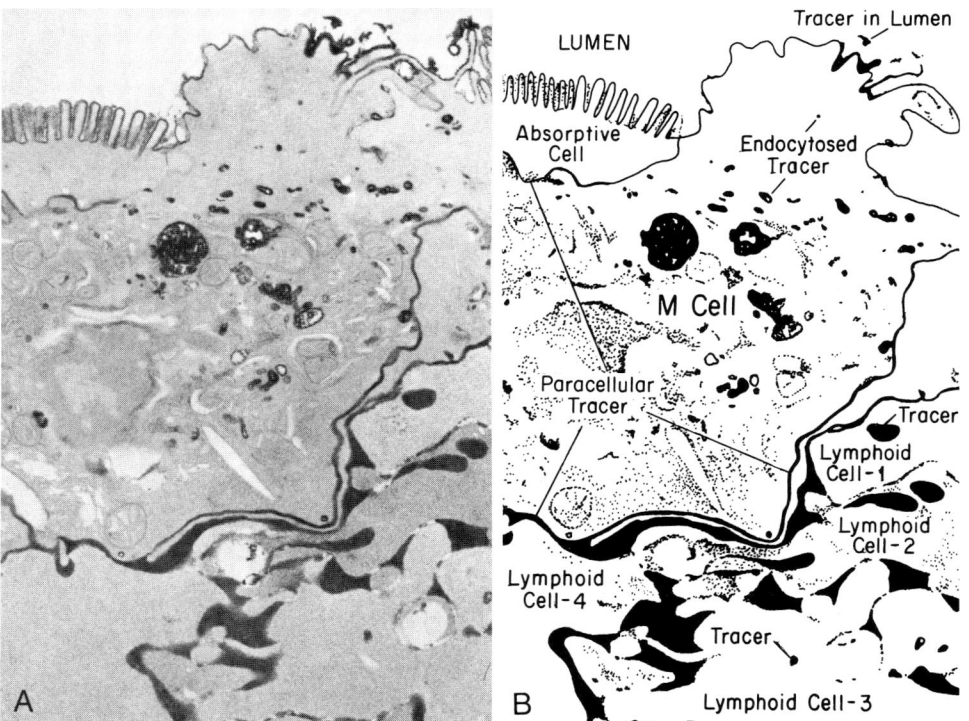

FIGURE 2–19. Unstained electron micrograph (*A*) and a labeled trace illustration (*B*) of follicular dome epithelium exposed on the luminal surface to macromolecule horseradish peroxidase. Dark reaction product indicating presence of this molecule can be seen within the vesicles in the M cell, within spaces surrounding the M cell, and within vesicles of lymphoid cells under the M cell. Comparable transport of this macromolecule across other types of epithelial cells is not known to occur in adult small intestine. ($\times$ 9000) (From Madara JL: Functional morphology of the epithelium of the small intestine. In Shultz S (ed): Handbook of Physiology. Vol IV, The Gastrointestinal System. Bethesda, American Physiological Association, 1991, p 106.)

in the centered hollow, to be engulfed and processed by lymphoid cells.[60] Hence, uptake of luminal substances by M cells appears to be the initial event in the afferent limb of the intestinal immune response.

Although nonselective to some degree, transport of some luminal agents across M cells may be receptor-mediated and, therefore, selective. While this biologic strategy may be of benefit (for example, in initiating a specific IgA response to a luminal organism), this is not always the case. For instance, neurotropic virions may gain entrance to the individual utilizing this same pathway. Of interest, the initial lesions of *Salmonella* infection and of Crohn's disease localize to the region of the follicular dome (see appropriate chapters). Such observations may represent important clues about the initial steps of intestinal injury in these disorders.

Caveolated Cells

Caveolated, or tuft, cells are of necessity defined by their unique structural characteristics, since the function of these cells is completely unknown.[33] They occur in the stomach and throughout the small intestine and colon and are present in crypts and on villi. Although somewhat difficult to identify by light microscopy, they can be recognized in 1-μm sections by the tuftlike brush border that projects above those of adjacent absorptive cells. Ultrastructurally, the microvilli are longer and wider than those of adjacent cells; and as seen by freeze-fracture, relatively few intramembrane particles are present at this site. Each microvillus contains a microfilament bundle that projects deeply into the underlying cytoplasm. Round and tubular membrane-bound spaces, termed *caveolae*, are located between the microfilament bundles. These spaces may be in continuity with the lumen to some degree, but their significance is unknown.[33,34]

Cells with "long rootlets" are often recognized in carcinomas arising from the intestine and have been touted as useful in identifying the origin of a metastatic lesion. Such cells are likely to represent differentiation toward caveolated phenotypes. Further verification of their uniqueness to intestinal carcinomas is needed, because this cell phenotype is also a constituent of other normal epithelia, such as those lining the biliary and respiratory trees.

Cup Cells

A numerically minor class of small-intestinal epithelial cells, cup cells occur in many species, including monkeys, but whether they are present in humans is not specifically known. Often, they are more densely distributed in the ileum than in the jejunum.[33]

In 1-μm sections, they generally display lighter cytoplasmic staining than neighboring absorptive cells. More readily appreciated, however, is the short, concave ("cupped") brush border. By electron microscopy, cup cell microvilli are short but regular; and by freeze-fracture, they have linear P-face particle arrays with complementary E-face grooves. Cup cells also often exhibit thick, poorly defined terminal webs and small mitochondria with dense inner matrices. They do not vigorously absorb lipid, nor do they express significant surface alkaline phosphatase activity. Their function is unknown. However, in guinea pigs, they have been reported to serve as a site for selective attachment of an unidentified species of bacteria.

COLON

The purpose of the colon is to reclaim luminal water and ions. In most instances, this function translates into the absorption of 250 to 270 ml of isotonic fluid per day, a small amount relative to the quantity of fluid and salt absorbed by the small intestine.

The structure of the colon in many respects overlaps that of the small intestine. Thus, some topics will be mentioned briefly here and the reader referred to the immediately preceding section. The appendix is covered in Chapter 33 and the anal canal in Chapter 34.

Gross Anatomy

In adults, the colon is approximately 1.5 meters in length. Anatomic divisions, from proximal to distal, include the cecum (the blind pouch of the large bowel below the ileocecal valve), ascending colon, hepatic flexure, transverse colon, splenic flexure, descending colon, sigmoid colon, rectum, and anus. The posterior-lateral wall of the ascending colon, sigmoid colon, and rectum is not covered with a serosa, and thus has immediate access to the retroperitoneum. It is therefore no surprise that disease processes can penetrate the intestinal wall at these sites and involve retroperitoneal structures or even the joints of the pelvis.

The outer longitudinal layer of the muscularis propria is split into three equidistant visible cables, or *taeniae*, that begin at the cecum, extend along most of the colon, then become one confluent sheet as the colon leaves the peritoneal cavity at the distal sigmoid. Presumably due to tension within the taeniae, the colonic wall displays many prominent pouches, or *haustra*. At the center of such haustra, the colonic lumen will be widest; at the periphery of the haustra, the lumen will be most narrow. These features produce the impression of luminal arclike constrictions or *plicae semilunares*.

The ascending and transverse colon are supplied by three branches of the superior mesenteric artery (ileocolic and right and middle colic arteries), whereas the splenic flexure, descending colon, and sigmoid are nourished by branches of the inferior mesenteric artery (left colic and sigmoid arteries). These vessels form arcades that are less numerous and complex than those in the small-intestinal vasculature. The rectum has a richly anastomosing arterial system derived from the inferior mesenteric and internal iliac arteries.[4]

In general, the venous drainage of the colon parallels its arteries, the right and transverse colonic flow into the superior mesenteric vein and the left colonic drainage into the inferior mesenteric vein. As in the esophagus and stomach, there are systemic-portal anastomoses in the rectum, offering the potential for development of varices in patients with portal hypertension. Also as in the stomach, lymphatic channels in the colonic mucosa are confined to the lowermost portion of the lamina propria and within the muscularis mucosae. For this reason, carcinomas confined to the colonic mucosa have essentially no metastatic potential. Lymph nodes are located adjacent to the colonic wall and along the course of the major arteries. These nodes drain to the superior and inferior mesenteric nodes. The lymphatic drainage from the rectum is complex, with flow to inferior mesenteric and internal iliac nodes.[4]

Organization of the Colonic Wall

As in the small intestine, the mucosa is structurally and functionally the most important layer of the colon. The colonic mucosal surface is flat and peppered with well-like orifices that represent the mouths of the tubular crypts (Figure 2–20). The crypts are exceedingly straight in normal biopsies and are unbranched except during embryologic development, when the colonic surface expands by a process in which crypts bifurcate and subsequently "divide" into two crypts.

Occasionally, light-microscopic sections will show a vaguely nodular pattern to the mucosa produced by the periodic appearance of pairs of crypts that are shorter than their neighbors. At such sites, the colonic surface is gently indented. This is a normal mucosal structural variant, analogous to the areae gastricae in the stomach.

As in the small intestine, lymphoid nodules that distort the normal mucosal architecture are present in the colon. Unlike those in the small intestine, however, such lymphoid nodules are usually not densely clustered enough to become grossly obvious. Like the small intestine, the colonic epithelium renews itself almost weekly, and the undifferentiated crypt cell appears to be the progenitor for all cell types.

Epithelial Structure: General Features

The colonic mucosa may be divided into three compartments that are anatomically and functionally distinct. The surface, which contains columnar absorptive cells and goblet cells, is the site of water and electrolyte resorption and mucin production (see Figure 2–20). The crypt contains undifferentiated columnar cells; goblet cells; endocrine cells; and, in the cecum and ascending colon, scattered, basally located Paneth cells. The crypt is the site of colonic water and electrolyte secretion, mucus secretion, and secretion of poorly characterized non–goblet cell glycoprotein(s). Finally, the epithelium overlying the lymphoid nodules contains M cells and is presumably the site at which luminal antigens can be sampled by the underlying lymphoid stroma.

Colonic Mucosal Epithelial Cells
(see Table 2–3)

Absorptive Cells

In the colon, absorptive cells are tall, columnar structures (see Figure 2–20) with microvilli that are the same diameter as, but shorter and less abundant than, those of small-intestinal absorptive cells. Thus, by light microscopy, it is difficult to identify the colonic microvillous surface as a "brush border." The fine structure of the colonic absorptive cell is otherwise similar to that of its small-intestinal equivalent, but with one subtle variation. The colonic cells have tight junctions with more strands than those of small intestinal absorptive cells, and this difference may, in part, determine the higher resistance to passive transepithelial ion flow exhibited by the colon. In some animals, a subset of colonic absorptive cells exhibit linear P-face microvillous particle arrays reminiscent of those noted in small-intestinal cup cells. Whether these cells represent the colonic cup cell equivalent is unclear.

The colonic absorptive cell exhibits functional differences from its counterpart in the small intestine. The apical membrane proteins involved in terminal diges-

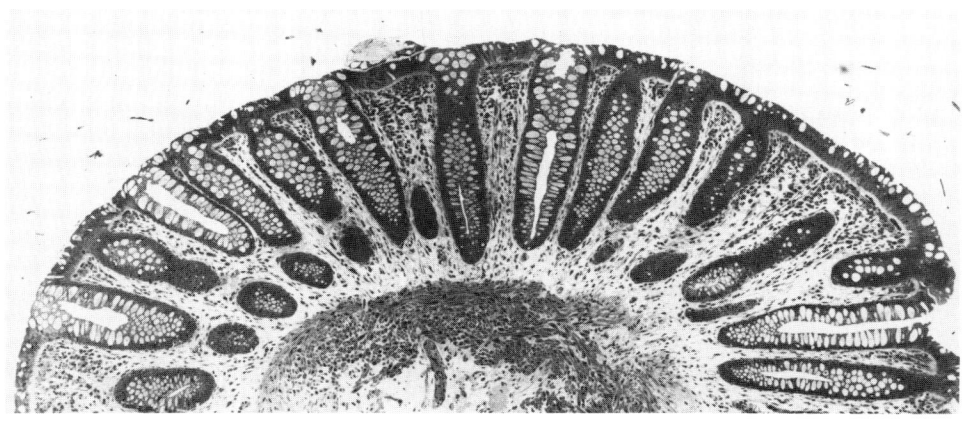

FIGURE 2–20. Section of colonic mucosa obtained by endoscopic biopsy. The specimen is curved because of postbiopsy contraction of the muscularis mucosae. The surface is flat and lined by columnar absorptive and goblet cells. Straight, well-like crypts occupy the depth of the lamina propria. (× 125) (Courtesy of Dr. Marian Neutra, Department of Pediatrics, Harvard Medical School and Children's Hospital, Boston, Mass.)

tion and nutrient uptake are depleted or absent in colonic absorptive cells. Rather, the apical membranes primarily contain transport proteins responsible for electrolyte uptake; specifically, an amiloride-inhibited, aldosterone-stimulated, electrogenic sodium uptake mechanism may dominate the surface of this cell.[61] The importance of this mechanism for pathologists is that upon cellular injury and consequent energy depletion, Na^+-K^+-ATPase is inhibited but a gradient for sodium entry into colonic absorptive cells still transiently exists. This gradient would be diminished as sodium enters the cell through the selective apical membrane pathway. The result might well be sodium accumulation until the gradient favoring sodium entry is dispersed, with a resulting increase in cell volume—i.e., the cells would swell.

Other transport-related molecules present on the apical membrane include a bicarbonate-chloride exchanger that may be of importance in disease states.[61] As previously discussed, secretory diarrheas originating in the small intestine (and in the colon) result from chloride secretion by undifferentiated crypt cells. As this chloride-loaded solution moves into the colon, bicarbonate-chloride exchange at the apical membrane occurs and the luminal content becomes bicarbonate-enriched. This mechanism may well serve as the basis for the bicarbonate loss seen in patients with secretory diarrhea.

Goblet Mucous Cells

Colonic goblet cells are structurally comparable to those of the small intestine. Cholinergic stimulation results in massive exocytosis of mucin secretory granules of crypt, but not of surface, goblet cells.[55] Thus, just as goblet cells vary from region to region and from crypt to surface in the type of mucin they synthesize, so, too, do they vary in expression of basolateral receptors for secretagogues or basolateral innervation, or both. As noted earlier, colonic goblet cell mucin is enriched in sulfomucins, whereas that in the small intestine is mainly sialomucin[62] (see Table 2-4).

Undifferentiated Columnar Crypt Cells

These cells are interposed between crypt goblet cells and are similar in structure to their counterparts in the small intestine, with one major exception. They have numerous membrane-bound vesicles containing flocculent material that presumptively represents a nonmucin glycoprotein. As in the small intestine, these cells are the site of electrogenic chloride secretion.

Other Cells

Caveolated cells, Paneth cells, and M cells are also present in the colonic mucosa and are identical to those described in the small intestine. Endocrine cells are discussed in Chapter 13.

References

1. Fawcett DW: Bloom & Fawcett—A Textbook of Histology, 11th ed. Philadelphia, WB Saunders, 1986, pp 619–640.
2. Pick TP, Howden R (eds): Gray's Anatomy. New York, Bounty Books, 1977.
3. Enterline H, Thompson J: Pathology of the Esophagus. New York, Springer-Verlag, 1984, pp 1–22.
4. Gannon B: The vasculature and lymphatic drainage. In Whitehead R (ed): Gastrointestinal and Oesophageal Pathology. Edinburgh, Churchill Livingstone, 1989, pp 117–160.
5. Geboes K, Mebis J, Desmet V: The esophagus: Normal ultrastructure and pathologic patterns. In Motta PM, Fujita H (eds): Ultrastructure of the Digestive Tract. Boston, Martinus Nijhoff, 1988, pp 17–34.
6. Weinstein WM, Bogoch ER, Bowes KL: The normal human esophageal mucosa: A histological reappraisal. Gastroenterology 68:40–44, 1975.
7. Eastwood GL: Gastrointestinal epithelial renewal. Gastroenterology 72:962–975, 1977.
8. Andrews PM: Microplicae: Characteristic ridgelike folds of the plasmalemma. J Cell Biol 68:420–429, 1976.
9. Geboes K, DeWolf-Peeters C, Rutgeerts P, et al: Lymphocytes and Langerhans' cells in the human oesophageal epithelium. Virchows Arch [A] 401:45–55, 1983.
10. Tateishi R, Taniguchi H, Wada A, et al: Argyrophil cells and melanocytes in esophageal mucosa. Arch Pathol 98:87–89, 1974.
11. Hammar S: Langerhans' cells. Pathol Annu 23(Part 2):293–328, 1988.
12. Jabbari M, Goresky CA, Lough J, et al: The inlet patch: Heterotopic gastric mucosa in the upper esophagus. Gastroenterology 89:352–356, 1985.
13. Hopwood D, Coghill G, Sanders DSA: Human oesophageal submucosal glands: Their detection, mucin, enzyme and secretory protein content. Histochemistry 86:107–112, 1986.
14. Neutra MR, Padykula HA: The gastrointestinal tract. In Weiss L (ed): Modern Concepts of Gastrointestinal Histology. New York, Elsevier, 1984, pp 659–706.
15. Rotterdam H: The normal stomach and duodenum. In Rotterdam H, Enterline HT (eds): Pathology of the Stomach and Duodenum. New York, Springer-Verlag, 1989, pp 1–12.
16. Owen DA: Normal histology of the stomach. Am J Surg Pathol 10:48–61, 1986.
17. Kimura K: Chronological transition of the fundic-pyloric border determined by stepwise biopsy of the lesser and greater curvatures of the stomach. Gastroenterology 63:584–592, 1972.
18. Wolfe MM, Soll AH: The physiology of gastric acid secretion. N Engl J Med 319:1707–1715, 1988.
19. Moreau H, Laugier R, Gargouri Y, et al: Human preduodenal lipase is entirely of gastric fundic origin. Gastroenterology 95:1221–1226, 1988.
20. Lehnert T, Erlandson RA, Decosse JJ: Lymph and blood capillaries of the human gastric mucosa: a morphologic basis for metastasis in early gastric carcinoma. Gastroenterology 89:939–950, 1985.
21. Listrom MB, Fenoglio-Preiser CM: Lymphatic distribution of the stomach in normal, inflammatory, hyperplastic, and neoplastic tissue. Gastroenterology 93:506–514, 1987.
22. Goldman H, Ming S-C: Mucins in normal and neoplastic gastrointestinal epithelium. Arch Pathol 85:580–586, 1968.
23. Jass JR, Filipe MI: The mucin profile of normal gastric mucosa, intestinal metaplasia and its variants and gastric carcinoma. Histochem J 13:931–939, 1981.
24. Helander HF: Fine structure of gastric glands. In Motta PM, Fujita H (eds): Ultrastructure of the Digestive Tract. Boston, Martinus-Nijhoff, 1988, pp 35–51.
25. LaMont JT: Structure and function of gastrointestinal mucus. Viewpoints. Dig Dis 17(2):1–4, 1985.
26. Goldman H, Antonioli DA: Mucosal biopsy of the esophagus, stomach, and proximal duodenum. Hum Pathol 13:423–448, 1982.
27. Toner PG, Watt PCH, Boyd SM: The gastric mucosa. In Whitehead R (ed): Gastrointestinal and Oesophageal Pathology. Edinburgh, Churchill Livingstone, 1989, pp 13–28.

28. Oi M, Oshida K, Sugimura S: The location of gastric ulcer. Gastroenterology 36:45–59, 1959.
29. O'Brien P, Rosen S, Trencis-Buck L, Silen W: Distribution of carbonic anhydrase within the gastric mucosa. Gastroenterology 72:870–874, 1977.
30. Levine JS, Nakane PK, Allen RH: Immunocytochemical localization of human intrinsic factor: The nonstimulated stomach. Gastroenterology 79:493–502, 1980.
31. Samloff IM: Pepsinogens I & II: Purification from gastric mucosa and radioimmunoassay in serum. Gastroenterology 82:26–33, 1982.
32. Basson MD, Modlin IM: Pepsinogen: Prolate ellipsoid or unrecognized pathogen? J Clin Gastroenterol 9:475–479, 1987.
33. Madara JL, Trier JS: Functional morphology of the mucosa of the small intestine. In Johnson LR (ed): Physiology of the Gastrointestinal Tract, 2nd ed. New York, Raven Press, 1987, pp 1209–1249.
34. Madara JL: Functional morphology of the epithelium of the small intestine. In Shultz S (ed): Handbook of Physiology, Volume IV: The Gastrointestinal System. Bethesda, American Physiological Association (In press).
35. Lundgren O, Haglund U: The pathophysiology of the intestinal countercurrent exchanger. Life Sci 23:1411–1422, 1978.
36. Harmon JW, Woods M, Gurll NJ: Different mechanisms of hydrogen ion removal in stomach and duodenum. Am J Physiol 235 (Endocrinol Metab Gastrointest Physiol 4):E692–E698, 1978.
37. Simson JNL, Merhav A, Silen W: Alkaline secretion by amphibian duodenum. I. General characteristics. Am J Physiol 240 (Gastrointest Liver Physiol 3):G401–G408, 1981.
38. Madara JL, Pappenheimer JR: The structural basis for physiological regulation of paracellular pathways in intestinal epithelia. J Membr Biol 100:149–164, 1987.
39. Eichholz A: Structural and functional organization of the brush border of intestinal epithelial cells. III. Enzymic activities and chemical composition of various fractions of Tris-disrupted brush borders. Biochim Biophys Acta 135:475–482, 1967.
40. Madara JL, Trier JS, Neutra MR: Structural changes in the plasma membrane accompanying differentiation of epithelial cells in human and monkey small intestine. Gastroenterology 78:963–975, 1980.
41. Alpers DH: The relation of size to the relative rates of degradation of intestinal brush border proteins. J Clin Invest 51:2621–2630, 1972.
42. Brasitus TA, Schachter D: Lipid dynamics and lipid-protein interactions in rat enterocyte basolateral and microvillus membranes. Biochemistry 19:2763–2769, 1980.
43. Marcial MA, Carlson SL, Madara JL: Partitioning of paracellular conductance along the crypt-villus axis: A hypothesis based on structural analysis with detailed consideration of tight junction structure-function relationships. J Membr Biol 80:59–70, 1984.
44. Madara JL: Loosening tight junctions: Lessons from the intestine. J Clin Invest 83:1089–1094, 1989.
45. Madara JL: Increases in guinea pig small intestinal transepithelial resistance induced by osmotic loads are accompanied by rapid alterations in absorptive-cell tight-junction structure. J Cell Biol 97:125–136, 1983.
46. Madara JL, Moore R, Carlson S: Alteration of intestinal tight junction structure and permeability by cytoskeletal contraction. Am J Physiol 253 (Cell Physiol 22):C854–C861, 1987.
47. Madara JL, Trier JS: Structural abnormalities of jejunal epithelial cell membranes in celiac sprue. Lab Invest 43:254–261, 1980.
48. Mooseker MS: Actin binding proteins of the brush border. Cell 35:11–13, 1983.
49. Rodewald R, Newman SB, Karnovsky MJ: Contraction of isolated brush borders from intestinal epithelia. J Cell Biol 70:541–554, 1976.
50. Pavelka M, Ellinger A, Gangl A: Effect of colchicine on rat small intestinal absorptive cells. I. Formation of basolateral microvillus borders. J Ultrastruct Res 85:249–259, 1981.
51. Field M: Intracellular mediators of secretion in the small intestine. In Binder HJ (ed): Mechanisms of Intestinal Secretion. New York, Alan R. Liss, 1979, pp 83–91.
52. Specian RD, Neutra MR: Acceleration of secretion in colonic goblet cells by acetylcholine. J Cell Biol 85:626–640, 1980.
53. Neutra MR, Leblond CP: Radioautographic comparison of the uptake of galactose-H^3 and glucose-H^3 in the Golgi region of various cells secreting glycoproteins or mucopolysaccharides. J Cell Biol 30:137–150, 1966.
54. Forstner JF, Jabbal I, Forstner GG: Goblet cell mucin of the rat small intestine. Chemical and physical characterization. Can J Biochem 51:1154–1166, 1973.
55. Neutra MR, Forstner JF: Gastrointestinal mucus. In Johnson LR (ed): Physiology of the Gastrointestinal Tract, 2nd ed. New York, Raven Press, 1987, pp 975–1010.
56. Culling CFA, Reid PE, Burton JD, Dunn WL: A histochemical method of differentiating lower gastrointestinal tract mucin from other mucins in primary or metastatic tumors. J Clin Pathol 28:656–658, 1975.
57. Filipe MI, Fenger C: Histochemical characteristics of mucins in the small intestine: A comparative study of normal mucosa, benign epithelial tumours and carcinoma. Histochem J 11:277–287, 1979.
58. Toner PG, Carr KE, Al-Yassin TM: The gastrointestinal tract. In Johanessen JV (ed): Electron Microscopy in Human Medicine. Vol 7, Digestive System. New York, McGraw-Hill, 1980, pp 87–185.
59. Owen RL, Jones AL: Epithelial cell specialization within human Peyer's patches: An ultrastructural study of intestinal lymphoid follicles. Gastroenterology 66:189–203, 1974.
60. Owen RL: Sequential uptake of horseradish peroxidase by lymphoid follicle epithelium of Peyer's patches in the normal unobstructed mouse intestine: An ultrastructural study. Gastroenterology 72:440–451, 1977.
61. Binder HJ, Sandle GI: Electrolyte absorption and secretion in the mammalian colon. In Johnson LK (ed): Physiology of the Gastrointestinal Tract, 2nd ed. New York, Raven Press, 1987, pp 1389–1418.
62. Filipe MI, Branfoot AC: Mucin histochemistry of the colon. Curr Top Pathol 63:143–178, 1976.

CHAPTER 3

Endoscopy and Endoscopic Biopsy

RODGER C. HAGGITT, M.D.
CYRUS E. RUBIN, M.D.

HISTORY OF GASTROINTESTINAL ENDOSCOPY

MODERN ENDOSCOPY

TECHNICAL FACTORS AND METHODS FOR
  HANDLING ENDOSCOPIC BIOPSY SPECIMENS
Orientation
Fixation
Processing
Embedding
Sectioning

Staining
Special Procedures

INTERPRETATION OF BIOPSY FINDINGS
Artifacts
Factors Affecting the Accuracy of Endoscopic Biopsy
Value of Good Techniques and Optimum Interpretation
  to the Patient

SUMMARY

HISTORY OF GASTROINTESTINAL ENDOSCOPY

Attempts to visualize the interior of the esophagus and stomach using a rigid tube passed perorally began more than a century ago in Germany. Whereas visualization of the esophagus was adequate if magnifying lenses were used, and safe if the operator was expert, this was not the case in the stomach. Even in the hands of an expert endoscopist such as the pioneer Rudolph Schindler, a stiff tube occasionally caused perforations while negotiating the esophagogastric junction. Furthermore, the portion of the stomach visualized was extremely limited. Schindler therefore abandoned the rigid gastroscope in 1928 and in collaboration with George Wolf, an instrument maker, designed a new "flexirigid" gastroscope.[1] It was first demonstrated in 1932 and incorporated a flexible optical axis made possible by multiple short focal lenses. This instrument was slightly flexible distally and rigid proximally. Its tip was made of a flexible rubber introducer, and the viewing lens faced laterally just proximal to the flexible rubber tip. The instrument could be passed without causing perforation. The area of stomach visualized was greater than with the rigid tube but still very limited, and the duodenum and several portions of the stomach could not be visualized at all. There was no channel to pass a biopsy forceps for direct sampling of lesions.

The modern era of gastrointestinal endoscopy began in 1957 when Basil Hirschowitz and Lawrence Curtis at the University of Michigan developed the first fiberoptic gastroscope.[2] The technical advances that made the fiberoptic instrument possible actually began in 1927 when Baird proposed the idea of transmitting light along a flexible axis.[3] Hopkins and Kapany constructed a 9-inch-long coherent fiberglass bundle capable of transmitting an image and described their invention in an article that appeared in *Nature* in 1954.[2] Hirschowitz's attention was directed to this invention, and he traveled to London to examine the device at first hand. The image transmitted by the fiber bundle had sufficient definition to make large print readable, but the color was green and the light loss was so great that a long fiber bundle would be impractical. Hirschowitz returned to Ann Arbor and was able to interest his colleagues in the physics department at the University of Michigan in the problem. Lawrence Curtis, a physics student, solved the problem of crosstalk (light loss caused by leakage of light from one fiber into the adjacent one) by inventing a technique for coating the glass fibers with glass of a lower refractive index.[2] This development in 1956 turned out to be the breakthrough that permitted subsequent development of better and better fiberoptic instruments. A usable prototype fiberscope was soon developed, and the first endoscopy was carried out by Hirschowitz on himself: "I took the instrument and my courage in both hands, and swallowed it over the protest of my unanesthetized pharynx and my vomiting center."[2] Some endoscopists to this day retain this penchant for autoendoscopy.[4]

The first fiberoptic endoscopes reached the United States market in 1960. With the stimulus of the American gastroenterologist John Morrissey, the Japanese developed an endoscope that could be passed into the proximal duodenum, and the diagnosis of duodenal ulcer became practical.[5] The control of the tip and the resolution of the image improved substantially with time. A channel for passage of diagnostic biopsy forceps and therapeutic instruments for the control of bleeding assumed increasing importance. Development of fiberoptic colonoscopes followed in 1961, and by 1969 Wolf and Shinya had introduced flexible endoscopic polypectomy for colonic adenomas located beyond the reach of the rigid sigmoidoscope.[6]

Since its introduction nearly 30 years ago, fiberoptic endoscopy has become the most important part of the gastroenterologist's diagnostic armamentarium.

The most recent development in endoscopy has been the introduction of the video endoscope, in which a television chip is substituted for the fiber bundle and the image is revealed on a television screen.

MODERN ENDOSCOPY

Esophagogastroduodenoscopy is the primary method for diagnosing upper gastrointestinal bleeding. In an increasing number of centers in the Western world endoscopy has replaced upper gastrointestinal x-ray as the primary method of diagnosing upper gastrointestinal illness. It plays a large role in the management of peptic ulcer and gastroesophageal regurgitant disease, and it is increasingly being used for surveillance of premalignant conditions of the upper gastrointestinal tract. Flexible sigmoidoscopy is now recommended as a routine screening procedure in patients over 50 to detect colorectal adenomas and unsuspected carcinomas. Colonoscopy has become the prime method of investigation of lower gastrointestinal bleeding of unknown origin.

The ability to pass various instruments via a channel in the endoscope has opened a whole new area of therapeutic endoscopy. Endoscopic techniques have replaced some invasive surgical techniques, e.g., polypectomy via the colonoscope and less frequently via the gastroscope. In the esophagus the channel is used to extract foreign bodies, to dilate strictures, and to sclerose varices. It is also used to palliate esophageal malignancy under direct vision by insertion of an inlying stent after mechanical dilatation or by the opening of a channel through occluding cancer with a laser. A variety of methods have been proposed for the control of bleeding in the stomach and duodenum, such as electrocoagulation devices, heater probes, and various types of lasers. The same methods of bleeding control are now being tested for use in the colon. Gastrostomy can be accomplished percutaneously with the aid of gastroscopy. Tubes can be introduced through the papilla of Vater to visualize the pancreatic and biliary ducts. The papilla of Vater can be incised to release a common duct stone, and balloons can be passed to dilate strictured biliary ducts, which are then kept open with stents inserted via the endoscope.

The importance of being able to biopsy lesions under direct vision cannot be overemphasized. There are, however, limitations because submucosal lesions may not be reached by a biopsy forceps, especially if the lesion is not raised and cannot be excised with a snare. The possibility of follow-up of an unhealed gastric ulcer makes the diagnosis of ulcer-cancer more feasible. The follow-up of inflammatory lesions of the colon can be very useful clinically.

Screening for cancer is most used in the colon in patients with a previous colonic cancer, a family history of colonic cancer, or ulcerative colitis of more than 8 years' duration. Screening of patients with Barrett's esophagus is widely performed, but it is not yet known in which subset of patients screening will prove most cost-effective.

Esophagoscopy, often with biopsy or brush cytology, is essential to the modern diagnosis of esophageal disease. Endoscopy is used in the diagnosis of regurgitant esophagitis, peptic stricture, esophageal ulcer, squamous carcinoma, adenocarcinoma, Mallory-Weiss tear, varices, Barrett's esophagus, hiatal hernia, and a variety of opportunistic infections in the immunosuppressed patient. Gastroscopy within the first 24 hours of bleeding is the best method of finding a bleeding gastric or duodenal source. Gastroscopy is also useful for differentiating a malignant from a benign gastric ulcer and for the diagnosis of the nature of polypoid lesions and various postgastrectomy problems.

Intramural extramucosal lesions may have a characteristic endoscopic appearance with bridging folds from the mass to the surrounding mucosa. Biopsy diagnosis usually fails because the overlying mucosa is uninvolved and the lesion is too deep. Biopsy of the gastric mucosa occasionally determines the diagnosis of specific types of gastritis associated with opportunistic infections with cytomegalovirus and herpes virus or systemic diseases such as Crohn's disease and sarcoidosis. The same is true for the duodenum, but duodenoscopy is primarily useful for the diagnosis of duodenal ulcer. Occasionally periampullary carcinoma can also be diagnosed by biopsy.

All types of fiberoptic endoscopy are contraindicated without informed consent and should never be performed in the uncooperative or combative patient. Patients with acute myocardial infarction can almost always wait for endoscopy at a later period. Acute perforation anywhere in the gastrointestinal tract is also a contraindication.

Complications of endoscopy are rare except in the hands of the inexperienced.[7] Nevertheless, aspiration may occur during upper endoscopy and is catastrophic in the pulmonary cripple. Perforations of the colon occur occasionally during colonoscopy. The more "invasive" therapeutic procedures such as creating a channel through a malignant stenosis of the esophagus with a laser or esophageal sclerosis of varices are associated with a somewhat higher complication rate.

A variety of endoscopes has been designed for specific applications in different organs. The endoscope most commonly used is a forward-looking instrument that can be used for examining the esophagus, the stomach, and duodenum at a single sitting. The side-viewing upper endoscope is used primarily for cannulating the papilla of Vater to visualize the biliary tract and pancreatic tree. The larger endoscopes are used primarily for therapy because they contain a larger size channel. They also are of special use for obtaining biopsy specimens of adequate size that facilitate diagnosis. The colonoscope is longer and has different flexibility characteristics, which enable it to be passed all the way from the anus to the cecum and even into the terminal ileum.

Contemporary endoscopes contain biopsy channels that vary from 2.0 to 3.7 mm in diameter, depending upon the size of the specimen desired and whether the endoscope needs a larger channel for therapy. We believe that an endoscope with the largest channel should be used for obtaining diagnostic biopsy specimens with the largest forceps, if at all possible. All endoscopic biopsy forceps have two cup-shaped jaws that may be either round or elliptical. It is best to use a forceps with a central spike to impale the instrument in the mucosa to assure retrieval of a biopsy specimen of adequate size. In order to take a biopsy specimen, the forceps' jaws are opened and pressed against the mucosa. The forceps' jaws are then closed, and the specimen is pulled off. Typical endoscopic biopsies are about 1 mm in depth and 2 to 5 mm in diameter, depending on the size of the forceps. The specimens usually include only mucosa and a variable amount of the muscularis mucosae; occasionally they include small slivers of submucosa. Thus, the vascular submucosa is avoided, and bleeding is minimal if the patient's coagulation is normal.

The size of the forceps is the most important factor in determining the size of the biopsy specimen. The smallest forceps is 1.8 mm in diameter and obtains biopsy specimens that average 3.3 mg.[8] Such small biopsy specimens are often inadequate for diagnosis. The standard biopsy forceps is 2.4 mm in diameter and obtains specimens averaging 5.9 mg in weight, a size more likely to be diagnostic. The 3.4-mm jumbo forceps obtains specimens averaging 15.5 mg in weight; these large specimens are the best for diagnostic purposes.[8] Elliptical forceps cups consistently obtain larger specimens than round ones. Muscularis mucosae was obtained in only a third of biopsies with the smallest forceps but in two thirds of biopsies with the standard forceps and in almost all biopsies with the largest forceps in the study reported by Danesh and colleagues.[8] Use of the large forceps is not associated with a higher risk of complications.[9]

Some endoscopists obtain biopsy specimens by simply opening the forceps and approximating it to the mucosa, rather than pressing it into the mucosa. The use of pressure on the forceps sufficient to put a slight bend in the cable produces significantly larger specimens with no increase in the risk of complications. Obtaining larger biopsy specimens is critical for making more accurate diagnoses, because larger samples of tissue are less liable to fragment and are easier to orient.

Endoscopic biopsies rarely contain much submucosa and are therefore generally useful only for evaluating conditions that affect the mucosa. Various techniques that overcome this difficulty in sampling the submucosa and in obtaining full-thickness biopsy specimens of the mucosa include fine-needle aspiration biopsy performed under direct vision through the endoscope[10] and the snare biopsy technique, in which an electrosurgical snare is used to obtain a larger specimen.[11] It is only safe to snare a portion of a mass or polyp extending into the lumen. Snare excision of a fold pulled into the snare is more likely to cause bleeding or, on occasion, perforation.[11] Submucosal lesions are difficult to sample.

Another technique applied in the colon is use of an insulated forceps to obtain a biopsy by electrocoagulation, the so-called hot biopsy.[12] In this technique, which is carried out with a standard forceps coated with plastic insulation on its external surface, the mucosa is grasped and tented into the lumen and heated for 1 to 2 seconds by the application of an electrosurgical current before the biopsy is pulled away from the mucosa.[12] This technique is used to obliterate small colonic polyps and yet provide some tissue for histologic examination. The tissue provided is barely adequate, and the technique is not completely safe.

TECHNICAL FACTORS AND METHODS FOR HANDLING ENDOSCOPIC BIOPSY SPECIMENS

Orientation

Correctly oriented biopsy specimens, which permit sections to be taken perpendicular to the mucosal surface, are critical for the diagnosis of reflux esophagitis, for the evaluation of small-intestinal villi, and for the diagnosis of dysplasia in all sites. Although some diagnoses can be confidently made with inadequately oriented biopsy specimens, well-oriented ones are highly desirable because they make all diagnoses easier. Endoscopic biopsy specimens of the small bowel are only adequate if they are properly handled and taken with the largest biopsy forceps.[13,14] In experienced hands, suction biopsy of the small bowel is less expensive and less bothersome for the patient and produces four biopsy specimens that are more likely to be adequate in size and easier to orient. In our experience, specimens taken by suction biopsy are far easier to interpret than those obtained by endoscopy. Unfortunately, far more gastroenterologists are expert in performing endoscopy than are expert in performing suction biopsy.

We prefer to orient endoscopic biopsy specimens before fixation immediately after they are removed from the patient. In our endoscopy unit, this is accomplished by a trained endoscopy assistant. The specimen should be handled gently at all times, preferably with the side, rather than the point, of a dissecting needle. The specimen is gently teased out of the biopsy forceps onto the tip of the index finger. It is placed lumen side down on the finger and then unrolled with the aid of the side of the dissecting needle so that the submucosal, cut side is up. The cut side of the biopsy is then gently pressed onto a plastic monofilament mesh so that the mucosal surface then faces up away from the mesh. The biopsy is then dropped immediately into fixative.[15] Orientation may be facilitated by using magnifying aids such as a hand lens, a ring light with a central magnifying lens, or a jeweler's loupe worn with a headband. Substrates other than plastic mesh can also be used for orientation of the biopsy, including cucumber slices,[16] Gelfoam, Millipore filters, and thin plastic cards. One must perform this operation rapidly and carefully to avoid damaging the mucosa through rough handling. It is far less desirable that the endoscopy assistant simply drop the biopsy into fixative as soon as possible and the orientation be performed during embedding.

An alternative technique for orienting specimens in the laboratory utilizes agar.[17] Liquid agar is dropped onto the fixed specimen while it is held in the correct position on a slide. When the agar solidifies, it is detached from the slide with a blade and placed into a cassette for processing. Although efficacious, this technique is cumbersome when large numbers of biopsy specimens must be processed.

Fixation

The ideal fixative for endoscopic biopsies should be reliable and inexpensive. It should preserve all tissue structures, be compatible with most histochemical and immunohistochemical methods, and not require mixing immediately prior to use. It should have a long shelf life, be relatively safe, and penetrate the tissue deeply and rapidly. Because formalin satisfies many of these requirements, it has been widely adopted as a routine fixative in pathology laboratories. Formalin has a relatively delicate chemical action on proteins, forming methylene bridges between adjacent reactive groups in the protein molecules.[18] Because of the delicate nature of formalin fixation, the tissue is not protected from the disruptive effects of tissue processing, sectioning, deparaffinization, and staining. In contrast, protein precipitant fixatives, such as solutions containing various metallic cations (mercury, copper or zinc) and acids such as picric and acetic, produce a more profound denaturation of cellular proteins and in doing so render the tissue resistant to the harmful effects of processing, sectioning, deparaffinization, and staining.[18] As a result, the sections have much better preservation of tissue detail. In addition, formalin is not a good preservative for nucleoproteins[19] and consequently gives poor nuclear definition, especially in very cellular tissues.[20] Pierre Masson's objection to formalin as a fixative for gastrointestinal tissues is just as valid today as it was when he expressed it in 1928: "Formol itself fixes the granules well but fixes the tissues very badly (I am perhaps alone in this opinion but the greater my experience the more I am convinced of its truth.)"[21] For these reasons, many gastrointestinal pathologists prefer Bouin's fluid, Hollande's modification of Bouin's fluid (Table 3–1), B-5, or others. Alcohol-based fixatives and those containing heavy metals do not preserve Paneth cell and eosinophil granules, and acidic fixatives lake red cells. We prefer the Hollande modification of Bouin's fluid for routine fixation of gastrointestinal biopsy specimens because it produces excellent nuclear detail and minimal tissue shrinkage and preserves red cells and Paneth cell granules.[22,23] The cupric acetate and picric acid in Hollande's probably explain the excellent mordanting (dye fixation of colors) characteristic of Hollande's solution. Picric acid tends to cause tissue shrinkage, and this is counteracted by the swelling action of acetic acid in Bouin's and Hollande's. Formalin-fixed tissues from outlying laboratories can be postfixed in Hollande's, B-5, and so on, for 2 hours with some improvement in histologic appearance.

The shelf life of Hollande's solution is at least 1 year. Specimens should remain in Hollande's solution for a minimum of 2 hours, but not longer than 3 days because they become brittle. Specimens that need to be held for longer periods of time should be transferred to 70% ethanol. Hollande's-fixed tissues should be washed in running tap water until the water becomes clear before they are placed in a tissue processor containing formalin, unless a tissue processor without a formalin step is used. If Hollande's-fixed tissues are placed in phosphate-buffered formalin, a precipitate of small, round, basophilic granules develops, usually in association with mucus, and can be mistaken for fungi or parasites. To obviate this precipitate, unbuffered formalin should be used in the tissue processor. The lack of a buffer in the processor does not cause problems because the solution is changed often.

Table 3–1 FORMULA FOR HOLLANDE'S SOLUTION

Formalin (40% formaldehyde)	100 ml
Glacial acetic acid	15 ml
Picric acid	40 gm
Cupric acetate	25 gm
Water	1000 ml

Dissolve cupric acetate in water without heat; add picric acid slowly with stirring. When dissolved, filter, then add formalin and acetic acid. Hollande's solution has a shelf life of at least 1 year. To avoid storing dry picric acid in the laboratory, you can substitute 1000 ml saturated picric acid solution for the picric acid and water.

The pathologist accustomed to formalin fixation may find that the superior nuclear detail achieved by the various special fixatives requires some initial adjustment of diagnostic criteria.

Processing

Endoscopic biopsy specimens are small enough that most fixatives penetrate them completely within 2 to 3 hours. After fixation, one should leave them on mesh and place them in biopsy cassettes or wrap them in lens paper or place them in embedding bags to ensure that they are not lost during further processing. Polyfoam pads are unsatisfactory because they produce triangular holes in the tissue sections (Figure 3–1).[24]

Most of the standard processing schedules in use on automatic tissue processors should provide satisfactory results with endoscopic biopsy specimens. If the volume of biopsies is large enough that the use of an individual tissue processor for them is possible, the processing cycle can usually be shortened by decreasing the amount of time in each solution.

Embedding

If the specimen was oriented on plastic mesh or some other substrate that cannot be sectioned in the microtome, the biopsy specimen must be carefully removed from the substrate. When the biopsy specimen has been brought to paraffin, it should be turned on edge and embedded in the paraffin block by means of a heated forceps. The long axis of the specimen should be oriented in such a way that in subsequent microtome sectioning the specimen is cut through its longest axis. If two biopsies are to be embedded in the same block, they are easier to cut if they are placed fairly close together with their long axes and cut surfaces oriented in the same direction. We do not recommend placing more than two biopsy specimens in a block because this makes it more difficult to obtain step-serial sections.

If the specimen has been oriented on a cucumber slice or Gelfoam, it may not be necessary to remove it before embedding, because these materials can be sectioned as is tissue: the histotechnologist simply trims the excess substrate, turns the mount on edge, and embeds it intact. Should the Gelfoam or cucumber cause difficulty in ribboning the paraffin sections, the specimen can be removed from the substrate before embedding.

Biopsy specimens that have not been mounted onto a substrate should be oriented during the embedding procedure with the aid of a ring light encompassing a central magnifying lens, a jeweler's loupe, or some other aid. Although orientation in the endoscopy unit is far more desirable, this procedure can deliver acceptable results provided the histotechnologist understands what is required and has the skill, patience, and interest necessary for carrying it out.

In most laboratories, better results can be achieved if only one or two individuals are assigned to handle gastrointestinal mucosal biopsy specimens.

Sectioning

Before sectioning, the blocks are trimmed close to the specimen itself, the upper and lower edges of the block kept as parallel as possible; a rectangle is the desired shape. The reason for trimming the blocks close to the

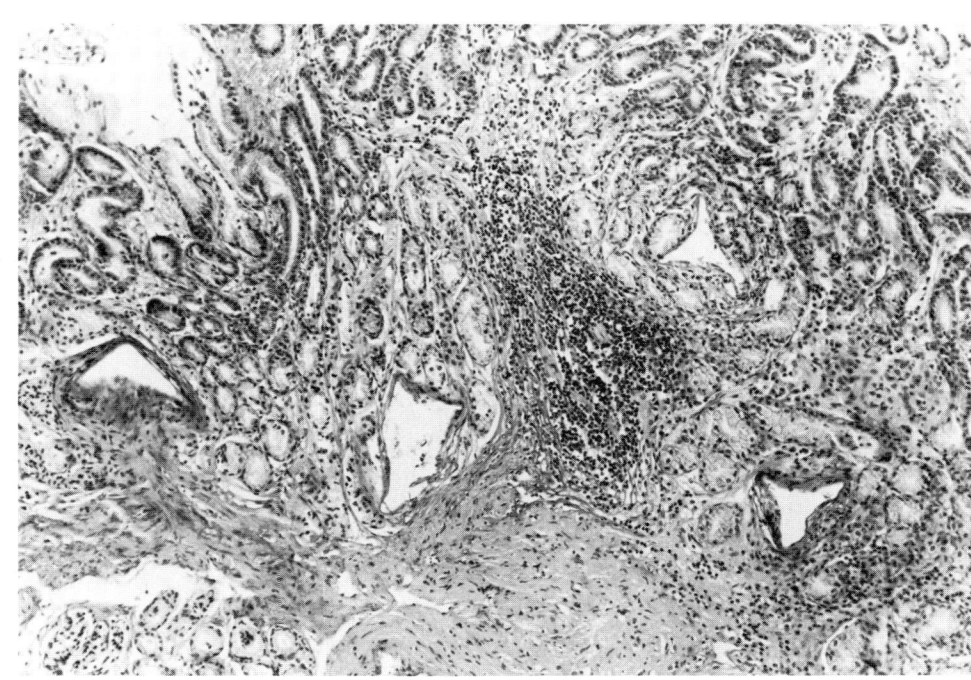

FIGURE 3–1. Gastric biopsies. This specimen was placed in the tissue cassette between two blue polyfoam embedding pads. The triangular holes in the tissue are an artifact caused by irregularities in the surface of the pads. This artifact can create difficulties in interpretation and is easily avoided by using lens paper or embedding bags to secure the specimen from loss during processing. (H&E, × 215)

specimen is that this permits many more sections to be included in a given length of paraffin ribbon and consequently on the glass slide. The cuts made to trim the block should be as shallow as possible, because if the tissue protrudes too far from the underlying paraffin block, it is not stable during sectioning and may fracture.

The biopsy specimens are step-serial-sectioned after the initial portion of the well-oriented area of the biopsy is entered.[25] The specimens can be cut better if the submucosal surface, rather than the luminal surface, meets the knife first during sectioning.

The sections are floated on a 55° to 58° C waterbath in which about 1 teaspoon of gelatin has been dissolved. The water in the bath should be changed daily, and its surface should be cleaned repeatedly during cutting by drawing a tissue across its surface. The slides are allowed to drain dry. After floating the sections onto the slides, the technician must check them to see whether they are in the central oriented core by using a microscope with the condenser diaphragm partially closed. They are then placed in a 62° C oven or into a slide dryer on high temperature for a minimum of one-half hour, or preferably two hours, before staining. We find it better to leave esophageal sections and those containing clot in the oven overnight to keep them from falling off during subsequent staining. We place two ribbons on each slide, leaving an ample margin on each edge of the slide, to avoid the fading from oxidation that occurs near the edge of the coverslip (Figure 3–2). Each ribbon should contain twelve or more sections. We cut five slides, of which three are stained and two are saved for special stains should they be required (see Figure 3–2).[25] For routine work, three stained slides may be enough, provided they were taken from the central, properly oriented core of the biopsy.

We believe that our practice of step-serial sectioning of gastrointestinal biopsies is practical not only for an academic institution but also for the community hospital laboratory. Once the blocks are trimmed, it takes no longer to cut a ribbon or two of serial sections than it does to cut individual step sections. As an absolute minimum, three levels of each block, each containing a ribbon of sections, should be made; additional levels should be obtained liberally in certain situations. Indications for additional levels include incorrect orientation on initial sections, a search for granulomas when clinical or biopsy findings suggest Crohn's disease, biopsy specimens that are negative for malignant tumor thought to be present clinically, findings on initial sections that are equivocal; and any other circumstance where the pathologist's judgment indicates that levels might be helpful.

Staining

We routinely stain all gastrointestinal biopsies with a combination of hematoxylin and eosin (H&E), alcian blue, and saffron (Table 3–2). The rationale for this routine stain is that acid mucins are demonstrated by the alcian blue at pH 2.5, and collagen can be differentiated from smooth muscle by the saffron. When used as a routine stain on gastrointestinal material, this combination results in earlier diagnosis because it eliminates the need for separate special stains for mucin and collagen. Alcian blue has repeatedly proved useful in diagnosing specialized metaplastic columnar epithelium in Barrett's esophagus, in determining the presence of intestinal metaplasia in the stomach, in identifying signet-ring cell carcinoma infiltrating the gastric mucosa, and in determining that giant cells in the lamina propria are foreign-body reactions to mucus. Saffron is useful in diagnosing collagenous sprue in small-bowel biopsies; in identifying the diagnostic fibrosis of

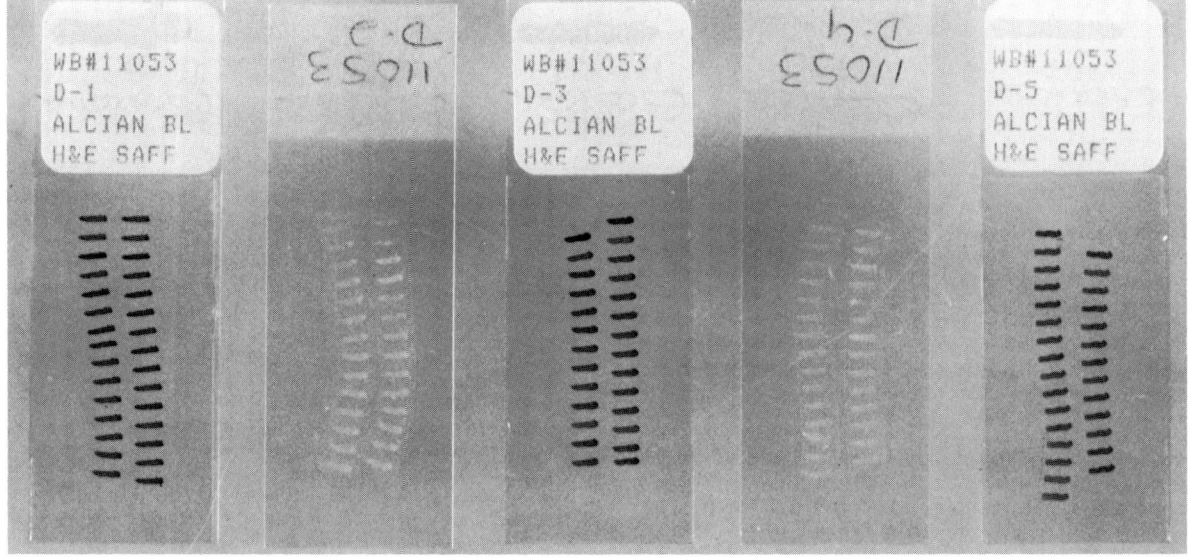

FIGURE 3–2. Step-serial sections of a gastric biopsy. Note that two ribbons of sections have been placed on each slide. Five slides were made, the first, third and fifth of which were stained; the second and fourth were retained unstained.

Table 3–2 METHOD FOR HEMATOXYLIN AND EOSIN, ALCIAN BLUE, SAFFRON STAIN

Rationale
Alcian Blue and saffron used in combination with the routine H&E stain have the added benefits of demonstrating acidic mucins (alcian blue) and staining collagen yellow (saffron). When used as a routine stain on gastrointestinal material, it results in earlier diagnosis as it eliminates the need to use separate special stains for mucin and collagen.

Precautions
Care must be taken not to overstain in saffron. If sections are overstained, decolorize slides in ammonia water, wash well, and restain, starting with eosin.

Results

Nuclei	Blue
Cytoplasm	Pink to red
Mucin	Aqua blue
Collagen	Yellow
Smooth muscle	Salmon pink
Other elements	Shades of pink and blue

Fixation
Any good fixative; excellent results with Hollande's fixed tissues.

Technique
Paraffin sections 4–6 μm.

Solutions

Routine H&E

3% Acetic Acid

Glacial acetic acid	30.0 ml
Distilled water	970.0 ml

1% Alcian Blue

Alcian blue 8 GN	10.0 ml
3% acetic acid	1000.0 ml

Mix until dissolved and add a crystal of thymol as a preservative.

Alcian blue has a normal shelf life of about 3 months, but one must be aware of the more rapid deterioration of solutions when large numbers of slides are stained and change accordingly.

Alcoholic Saffron

Saffron	1.5 gm
Absolute alcohol	100.0 ml
Mix, filter and add: acetic acid	1.0 ml

Keeps well but for consistent staining change once a week.

0.5% Lithium Carbonate

Lithium carbonate	5.0 gm
Distilled water	1000.0 ml

Mix well

The remaining solutions are the routine solutions used in the H&E procedure.

Procedure

1. Deparaffinize and bring to water; remove pigment when necessary	
2. 3% acetic acid	3 minutes
3. Alcian blue	10 minutes
4. Water	wash
5. Check microscopically and dip several times in 3% acetic acid to remove background staining when necessary	
6. Water	Wash
7. Lithium carbonate	1 minute
8. Water	Wash
9. Hematoxylin	6 minutes
10. Water	Wash
11. Acid alcohol	Dip as needed
12. Water	Wash
13. Ammonia water	Dip to blue
14. Water	Wash
15. Check microscopically for nuclear detail	
16. Eosin	2 minutes
17. Water	Wash
18. 95% alcohol	Several dips
19. Absolute alcohol	1 minute
20. Absolute alcohol	1 minute
21. Saffron	30 seconds
22. Absolute alcohol	10 dips
23. Absolute alcohol	10 dips
24. Xylene	10 dips
25. Xylene	2 minutes
26. Xylene	2 minutes
27. Coverslip	

Notes: Metanil yellow (C.I. 13065) can be substituted for saffron for purposes of economy.

Staining time in saffron is variable—5 dips seems to work well with freshly made batches. The solution should be discarded weekly because it gets stronger with age.

---

the lamina propria in solitary rectal ulcer syndrome; and in diagnosing ischemic colitis, collagenous colitis, healed erosions, and ulcers. The use of a routine periodic acid–Schiff (PAS) stain in screening for Whipple's disease is not cost-effective because the foamy macrophages of this rare jejunal lesion are easily recognized by H&E stains; when they are identified, appropriate special studies can then be undertaken to confirm the diagnosis.

Any of the commonly employed special stains can be used on gastrointestinal biopsy specimens as needed. If one has saved unstained slides, these stains can be done much more readily on an *ad hoc* basis, as the need arises.

Special Procedures

The use of Giemsa-stained smears made from mucus teased from the fresh biopsy specimen before fixation can be quite valuable in diagnosing *Giardia lamblia*. Young, Hughes, and Lee advocate touch preparations of biopsy specimens for the diagnosis of gastrointestinal malignancies.[26] They found that such touch preparations had a sensitivity of 100% for carcinoma of the esophagogastric junction. We have not had personal experience with this technique.

Immunohistochemical localization of various antigens is readily performed on gastrointestinal biopsies. Its principal value in a diagnostic setting is for the classification of poorly differentiated malignant tumors, but many other questions can be addressed by the appropriate use of immunohistochemistry. In general, alcohol-based fixatives are better immunopreservatives than formalin-based fixatives. If one knows ahead of time that immunohistochemical techniques will be used, it is a good idea to place one or more biopsies in the modified Carnoy's fixative known as methacarn (60% methanol, 30% chloroform, 10% acetic acid).[27] There are exceptions to the generalization that antibodies work better in alcohol-based fixatives. Lymphocyte cell surface markers require frozen sections of fresh tissue in appropriate tissue culture medium. Hormones and immunoglobulins are generally better preserved by formalin-based fixatives. B-5 is superior for immunoglobulins, and Bouin's is better for hormones, but any formalin-based fixative can be used. The use of antibodies in evaluating gastrointestinal biopsy specimens requires advance knowledge and cooperation between the gastroenterologist and pathologist to ensure that the tissue is appropriately handled.

Electron microscopy likewise requires advance planning so that the specimen can be properly prepared. The indications for electron microscopy have diminished since immunohistochemistry became widely available. The activity of Whipple's disease can be assessed by demonstrating Whipple's bacilli by light microscopy of sections of jejunum fixed in osmic acid and embedded in plastic.

Other techniques that we have employed successfully on endoscopic biopsies include flow cytometry for analysis of nuclear DNA content and cell cycle parameters.[28]

INTERPRETATION OF BIOPSY FINDINGS

Optimal interpretation of endoscopic biopsy findings requires close communication between the endoscopist and pathologist. Endoscopic biopsy specimens challenge the pathologist not only because they are small, but because they pose questions that require more than a diagnosis of "benign" or "malignant"; they require the pathologist to know and recognize diagnostic criteria for a broad spectrum of medical and surgical conditions. The pathologist needs to know the pertinent clinical history and physical findings, the results of roentgenographic and laboratory studies, indications for endoscopy, endoscopic findings, and detailed information concerning the sites of biopsy. Because a complete endoscopy report should contain most of these data, the practice of sending a copy to the laboratory along with each biopsy specimen provides a convenient method of transmitting the necessary information.

The endoscopist should avoid the tendency to group specimens from different locations and place them in the same bottle of fixative. Where this has been done and one biopsy shows equivocal findings that need to be investigated, one does not know which site to target for additional biopsies. In addition, certain diagnoses require information concerning the distribution of pathologic changes in the tissues. A good example of this is idiopathic inflammatory bowel disease. Crohn's disease tends to be segmental and to spare the rectum, whereas ulcerative colitis always involves the rectum and a variable length of contiguous proximal colon in a diffuse and circumferential manner. Well-placed biopsies can detect these distributional phenomena and facilitate the differentiation of ulcerative colitis and Crohn's disease.

Artifacts

Endoscopic biopsy forceps are designed to tear, rather than cut, tissue fragments from the mucosa. Thus, mechanical artifacts are unavoidable. Crush artifacts occur consistently because of the squeezing of the tissue at the point of closure of the biopsy forceps (Figure 3–3). Glandular tissue distorted in this manner

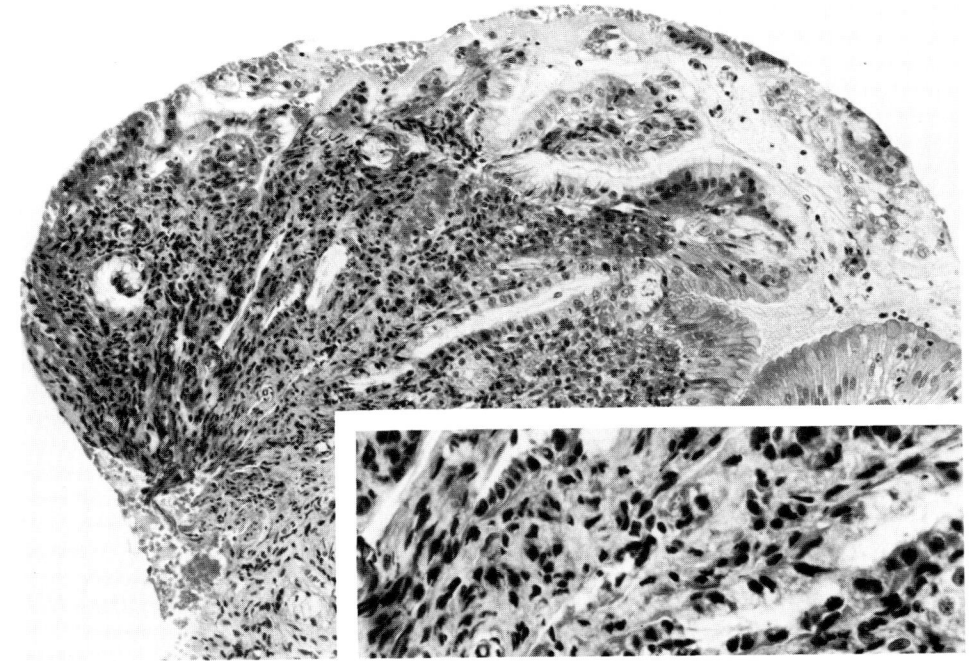

FIGURE 3–3. Gastric biopsy. At the point of closure of the forceps on the tissue, there may be crush artifact, as shown at the edge of this biopsy (left and inset). Benign glandular tissue distorted in this manner can be mistaken for carcinoma. No assessment of the degree of inflammation or fibrosis should be attempted in such distorted tissue. (H&E, alcian blue pH 2.5, saffron, × 215; inset, × 350)

can be mistaken for carcinoma (Figure 3–3). Crush artifact may also compress the component of normal mononuclear cells present at the edges of the biopsy specimens in the small bowel and colon, causing them to appear increased and suggesting inflammation. A similar effect on the normal fibrous tissue may simulate fibrosis. In biopsy specimens that have been oriented onto a substrate, some crush artifact is evident at either end of the specimen (Figure 3–4). In these specimens, the two or three glands at either edge may not be grossly distorted, but the nuclei may be damaged, so that their shape is altered from the normal round to oval configuration to an angulated one. Such nuclei may also become artifactually hyperchromatic, opaque, and distorted, which can mistakenly lead to a diagnosis of dysplasia or carcinoma (see Figure 3–4). Hemorrhages in biopsies are difficult to interpret because the trauma from the biopsy forceps may cause extravasation of blood. Unless there is associated necrosis, fibrin, or hemosiderin deposition, it is difficult to be certain that such extravasates represent true hemorrhage. In the face of uncertainty about the significance of extravasated red cells, one should note their presence and add a comment to the effect that they may represent biopsy artifact.

Enemas and/or laxatives prior to proctosigmoidoscopy and colonoscopy may produce changes in the normal mucosa that can be seen both at endoscopy and on biopsy.[29–32] Endoscopic changes induced by a hypertonic sodium phosphate enema (Fleet Phospho-Soda, Travad) include hyperemia, loss of the normal vascular pattern, production of petechiae, and occasionally production of increased mucosal fragility. Histologically, bisacodyl (Dulcolax) can cause a specific "erased" appearance of the superficial half of the mucosa.[29] All of the above preparations, as well as magnesium citrate and senna derivatives (X-Prep), can produce lamina propria edema, subnuclear vacuoles and nuclear debris in the surface epithelium, separation of the surface epithelium from the basal lamina, and depletion or diminution of goblet cell mucin. Mild hyperplasia of crypt epithelium, with crowding of nuclei and mitoses in the upper region of the crypt, and hemorrhages in the lamina propria may also be seen. Mucosa from patients prepared for colonoscopy with the electrolyte solution known as Golytely does not show these artifacts.[32,33] Thus, the pathologist must factor in the effects of preparation to avoid over-interpretation of the biopsy.

Factors Affecting the Accuracy of Endoscopic Biopsy

Provided that the pathologist knows and is able to identify the diagnostic criteria for each condition being evaluated, the accuracy of endoscopic biopsy depends upon several other factors, foremost among which is the adequacy of tissue sampling. Some disease processes, such as ulcerative colitis and atrophic gastritis, affect the target organ in a diffuse manner, and the site and number of biopsies are less critical than when a discrete lesion is being sampled. In focal or discrete lesions the number of biopsies required to establish or to confidently exclude a diagnosis is important; this depends upon whether a layer of necrotic debris covers the lesion, whether residual benign tissue surrounds the malignant tumor, the size of the lesion (e.g., gastric ulcer), and so forth. Multiple biopsies increase the tissue sample and reduce the incidence of false-negative results. Sancho-Poch and colleagues showed that the positive yield of biopsies for gastric cancers rose from 45% when a single biopsy specimen was taken to 99% for eight or more specimens.[34] Other studies confirm this high positive yield with multiple specimens of gastric cancers[35] and show that the best results are with

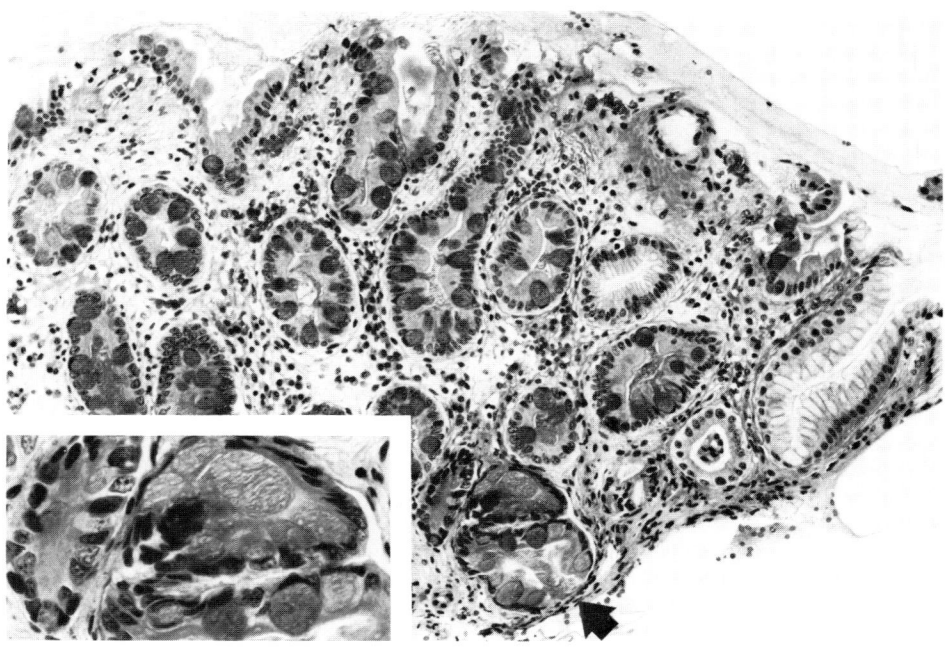

FIGURE 3–4. Barrett's esophagus. This biopsy illustrates "edge" artifact in the absence of gross crushing of the tissue. Note the group of three glands indicated by the arrow. The nuclei in this group of glands *(inset)* appear angulated, irregular, hyperchromatic, or opacified and have lost their polarity. These changes limited to glands at the edge of a biopsy should not be interpreted as dysplasia or carcinoma (H&E, alcian blue pH 2.5, saffron, × 215; *inset,* × 375.

biopsy specimens taken from the rim or edge of an ulcerated carcinoma.[36] Although the rate varies somewhat from organ to organ, increasing the number of biopsy specimens consistently increases the number of positive cancer diagnoses for all sites. Graham and colleagues showed that a minimum of four biopsy specimens, combined with brush cytology, produced a very high diagnostic yield.[37] The endoscopist must be aware that these comments apply equally to lesions that have been interpreted as benign on the basis of their endoscopic and roentgenographic features. Because submucosal lesions such as lipomas and leiomyomas are covered by normal mucosa, the biopsy forceps does not reach them. In these cases needle aspiration via the endoscope may permit a cytologic diagnosis.[10] The same is true of carcinomas that undermine mucosa at their edges or that have benign neoplasm at the edges, as frequently occurs in the colon. In both situations, a snare biopsy may be necessary to confirm the clinical impression of carcinoma[11]; better yet, the whole lesion should be removed with a snare if possible. In certain situations, biopsy cannot confidently exclude a diagnosis; for example, in order to rule out a focus of invasive carcinoma in a colonic adenoma, the entire lesion must be removed and evaluated.[38] The diagnosis of well-differentiated lymphoproliferative disorders may be difficult or impossible with biopsies.

In the hands of a skilled, conservative pathologist, the incidence of false-positive results should be nil. Negative (benign) biopsy results in specimens of clinically suspicious lesions do *not* exclude malignancy. Several studies have shown that a combination of brush cytology and biopsy provides more positive diagnoses of cancer than biopsy alone[39]; however, if *multiple* biopsy specimens are obtained, brush cytology adds little to the diagnostic yield.[35] One study found that brush cytology was poor at establishing the diagnosis of early gastric cancer.[40] Brush cytology generally has a false-positive rate of 4% to 5%.[39] Brush cytology may be useful when biopsies of a clinically malignant lesion are negative or when there is a stricture proximal to the lesion that does not permit passage of the endoscope for biopsy but does allow the cytology brush to be used.[35] Cytology may be more accurate in the diagnosis of lymphoma.[39] Touch smears made from the endoscopic biopsy were shown in one study to have a high sensitivity in diagnosing carcinoma.[26]

Value of Good Technique and Optimum Interpretation to the Patient

The approach to endoscopic biopsy that we have described may seem complicated and not worth the effort to those who are not accustomed to such procedures. In fact, the additional effort required to obtain biopsy specimens of optimum technical quality is relatively small and amply rewarded by the improvement in patient care. The main advantage of this additional effort is more accurate diagnosis. We frequently see biopsy specimens of the esophagus, stomach, or colon for a second opinion, in cases in which the original pathologist was concerned about the possibility of a malignant neoplasm, that, when evaluated with the use of the methods described here, are found to indicate reactive changes caused by inflammation or some other benign condition. Thus, some of the errors in interpretation are attributable to the inadequacy of the material provided to the pathologist or to the inadequacy of its processing in the histology laboratory. Properly processed, expertly interpreted biopsy findings avoid unnecessary operations and foster earlier operative intervention when cancers are potentially curable.

In some clinical situations, it is difficult to differentiate between two related diseases. For example, a patient who has had bloody diarrhea for a month may have chronic idiopathic inflammatory bowel disease or may still have an acute self-limited process, presumably of infectious origin. There are histologic criteria that can be identified in well-processed rectal biopsies that differentiate these two very different conditions with a high degree of accuracy.[41] Similarly, the clinician cannot always differentiate Crohn's colitis from ulcerative colitis. The prognosis and surgical treatment are quite different, and it is therefore helpful to be able to diagnose Crohn's disease with certainty by finding typical epithelioid granulomas in endoscopic colonic biopsy specimens. Granulomas can be quite small and missed when the biopsy is not step-serial sectioned or when only a single biopsy has been taken.[42]

Assessment of villous architecture is the main basis of classifying small bowel biopsy pathology.[15,43] Similarly, crypt architecture is a prime diagnostic feature in differentiating idiopathic inflammatory bowel disease from acute self-limited and infectious colitis. Thus, step-serial sections taken through the central, properly oriented core of the biopsy are essential because it may be impossible to diagnose anything but gross changes in villous or crypt architecture in biopsies not properly oriented or in occasional step sections. Patients, clinicians, and pathologists all benefit from better processing of endoscopic biopsies.

SUMMARY

Over the past decade, practicing pathologists have seen a dramatic increase in the number of endoscopic biopsies of the gastrointestinal tract. Because these biopsies permit earlier diagnosis and aid in the clinical evaluation of many different lesions, one may expect this increase to continue. Accurate interpretation of endoscopic biopsy findings requires close communication with the clinician, technically optimal histologic sections, and the knowledge of and ability to recognize diagnostic criteria for a broad spectrum of medical and surgical conditions. In this chapter, we have discussed some technical pointers and information that we have found helpful in dealing with an ever increasing volume of biopsy specimens.

References

1. Gordon ME, Kirsner JB: Rudolf Schindler, pioneer endoscopist: Glimpses of the man and his work. Gastroenterology 77:354–361, 1979.
2. Hirschowitz BI: A personal history of the fiberscope. Gastroenterology 76:864–869, 1979.
3. Hirschowitz BI: History of fiberoptic endoscopy. (Letter to the editor) Gastroenterology 78:1123, 1980.
4. Jackson FW: Autoendoscopy (letter to the editor). Gastrointest Endosc 77:111, 1981.
5. Morrissey JF: The 1982 A/S/G/E Distinguished Lecture: Gastrointestinal endoscopy—20 years of progress. Gastrointest Endosc 29:53–56, 1983.
6. Wolf WI: Shinya H: Polypectomy via the fiberoptic colonoscope: removal of lesions beyond reach of the sigmoidoscope. N Engl J Med 288:329–332, 1973.
7. Shahmir M, Schuman BM: Complications of fiberoptic endoscopy. Gastrointest Endosc 26:86–91, 1980.
8. Danesh BJZ, Burke M, Newman J, et al: Comparison of weight, depth, and diagnostic adequacy of specimens obtained with 16 different biopsy forceps designed for upper gastrointestinal endoscopy. Gut 26:227–231, 1985.
9. Siegel M, Barkin JS, Rogers AI, et al: Gastric biopsy: A comparison of biopsy forceps. Gastrointest Endosc 29:35–36, 1983.
10. Iishi H, Yamamoto R, Tatsuta M, Okuda S: Evaluation of fine-needle aspiration biopsy under direct vision gastrofiberscopy in diagnosis of diffusely infiltrative carcinoma of the stomach. Cancer 57:1365–1369, 1986.
11. Komorowski RA, Caya JG, Geenen JE: The morphologic spectrum of large gastric folds: utility of the snare biopsy. Gastrointest Endosc 32:190–192, 1986.
12. Williams CB: Diathermy-biopsy—a technique for the endoscopic management of small polyps. Endoscopy 5:215–218, 1973.
13. Achkar E, Carey WD, Petras R, et al: Comparison of suction capsule and endoscopic biopsy of small bowel mucosa. Gastrointest Endosc 32:278–281, 1986.
14. Scott BB, Jenkins D: Endoscopic small intestinal biopsy. Gastrointest Endosc 27:162–167, 1981.
15. Perera DR, Weinstein WM, Rubin CE: Small intestinal biopsy. Human Pathol 6:157–217, 1975.
16. Allen TV, Achord JL: The pickle of proper bowel biopsy orientation. Gastroenterology 72:774–775, 1977.
17. Rosai J: Manual of Surgical Gross Room Procedures. Minneapolis, University of Minnesota Press, 1981, p E1.
18. Banks PM: Technical aspects of specimen preparation and special studies. In Jaffe ES (ed): Surgical Pathology of the Lymph Nodes and Related Organs. Philadelphia, WB Saunders, 1985, p 7.
19. Hopwood D: General principles of fixation. In Filipe MI, Lake BD: Histochemistry in Pathology. Churchill Livingstone, New York, 1983, pp 3–4.
20. Pearse AGE: Histochemistry Theoretical and Applied. Vol 1. New York, Churchill Livingstone, 1980, p 97.
21. Masson P: Carcinoids (argentaffin-cell tumors) and nerve hyperplasia of the appendicular mucosa. Am J Pathol 4:181–211, 1928.
22. Hartz PH: Simultaneous histologic fixation and gross demonstration of calcification. Am J Clin Pathol 17:750, 1947.
23. Haggitt RC: Handling of gastrointestinal biopsies in the surgical pathology laboratory. Laboratory Medicine 13:272–278, 1982.
24. Carson FL: Polyfoam pads—a source of artifact. J Histotechnology 4:33–34, 1981.
25. Surawicz CM: Serial sectioning of a portion of a rectal biopsy detects more focal abnormalities. Dig Dis Sci 27:434–436, 1982.
26. Young JA, Hughes HE, Lee FD: Evaluation of endoscopic brush and biopsy touch smear cytology and biopsy histology in the diagnosis of carcinoma of the lower oesophagus and cardia. J Clin Pathol 33:811–814, 1980.
27. Mitchell D, Ibrahim S, Gusterson BA: Improved immunohistochemical localization of tissue antigens using modified methacarn fixation. J Histochem Cytochem 33:491–495, 1985.
28. Reid BR, Haggitt RC, Rubin CE, Rabinovitch PS: Barrett's esophagus: Flow cytometry complements histology in detection of patients at risk for adenocarcinoma. Gastroenterology 93:1–11, 1987.
29. Saunders DR, Haggitt RC, Kimmey MB, et al: Morphological consequences of bisacodyl on normal human rectal mucosa: Effects of a prostaglandin E_1 analog on mucosal injury. Gastrointest Endosc 36:101–104, 1990.
30. Meisel JL, Bergman D, Graney D, et al: Human rectal mucosa: Proctoscopic and morphological changes caused by laxatives. Gastroenterology 72:1274–1279, 1977.
31. Leriche M, Devroede G, Sanchez G, Rossano J: Changes in the rectal mucosa induced by hypertonic enemas. Dis Colon Rectum 21:227–236, 1978.
32. Pockros PJ, Foroozan P: Golytely lavage versus a standard colonoscopy preparation. Gastroenterology 88:545–548, 1985.
33. David GR, Santa Ana CA, Morawski SG, Fordtran JS: Development of a lavage solution associated with minimal water and electrolyte absorption or secretion. Gastroenterology 78:991–995, 1980.
34. Sancho-Poch FJ, Balanzo J, Ocana J, et al: An evaluation of gastric biopsy in the diagnosis of gastric cancer. Gastrointest Endosc 24:281–282, 1978.
35. Kobayashi S, Yoshii Y, Kasugai T: Biopsy and cytology in the diagnosis of early gastric cancer. Endoscopy 8:53–58, 1976.
36. Hatfield ARW, Slavin G, Segal AW, Levi AJ: Importance of the site of endoscopic gastric biopsy in ulcerating lesions of the stomach. Gut 16:884–886, 1975.
37. Graham DY, Schwartz JT, Cain GD, Gyorkey F: Prospective evaluation of biopsy number in the diagnosis of esophageal and gastric carcinoma. Gastroenterology 82:228–231, 1982.
38. Livstone EM, Troncale FJ, Sheahan DG: Value of a single forceps biopsy of colonic polyps. Gastroenterology 73:1296–1298, 1977.
39. Bemvenuti GA, Hattori K, Levin B, Kirsner JB, Reilly RW: Endoscopic sampling for tissue diagnosis in gastrointestinal malignancy. Gastrointest Endosc 21:159–161, 1975.
40. Ito Y, Blackstone MO, Riddell RH, et al: The endoscopic diagnosis of early gastric cancer. Gastrointest Endosc 25:96–101, 1979.
41. Surawicz CM, Belic L: Rectal biopsy helps to distinguish acute self-limited colitis from idiopathic inflammatory bowel disease. Gastroenterology 86:104–113, 1984.
42. Surawicz CM, Meisel JL, Ylvisaker T, et al: Rectal biopsy in the diagnosis of Crohn's disease: value of multiple biopsies and serial sectioning. Gastroenterology 81:66–71, 1981.
43. Dobbins WO: Small bowel biopsy in malabsorptive states. Contemp Issues Surg Pathol 4:121–165, 1983.

CHAPTER 4

Cytologic Techniques and Diagnosis

SIEGFRIED WITTE, M.D.

COLLECTION OF MATERIAL
Esophagus
Stomach
Duodenum
Colon and Rectum

METHODS OF MICROSCOPIC EXAMINATION
Fresh Unfixed Preparations
Phase Contrast Microscopy
Nomarski Differential Interference Contrast Microscopy
Ultraviolet-Light Microscopy
Fluorescence Microscopy

Staining Techniques
Quantitative Methods
Micromorphometry
Fluorescence Cytophotometry
Flow Cytophotometry
High-Resolution Image Analysis

CYTOMORPHOLOGY AND CYTODIAGNOSIS
Esophagus
Stomach
Duodenum
Colon and Rectum

STATISTICAL EVALUATION OF CYTODIAGNOSES
Esophagus
Stomach
Qualitative Studies
Quantitative Studies
Duodenum
Colon and Rectum

Gastroenterologic cytodiagnosis is based on the desquamation of superficial cells from the mucosa of the gastrointestinal tract. Under pathologic conditions such desquamation can increase markedly. The foremost role of cytology is the identification of malignant tumors. The criteria for recognition of tumor cells by microscopy have been defined in the practice of clinical cytology. These criteria in principle hold for all organs, but there are differences with respect to various tumors. In practice, diagnosis must also take into account organ-specific changes in cells, generally of inflammatory origin, which must be recognized and distinguished from tumor cells.

The yield of cells that can contribute to making a diagnosis is increased when the desquamation of cells is promoted by appropriate technical methods and when cellular material is obtained as specifically as possible. Cytologic samples should be taken only from the suspected regions of the mucosa of only the desired organ, without contamination from other areas. Furthermore, assessment by microscopy requires cells in well-preserved condition and appropriate methods of preparing the cells and of microscopic examination.

Finally, the experience of the cytologist plays an important part. However, even the best cytologist obtains good results only when he or she receives appropriate cellular material from a good endoscopist. At present, the yield of cells almost always depends on endoscopic technique. The cells must be sampled specifically; that is, macroscopically suspected findings must be identified for localization. When indicators of this sort are absent, or when endoscopic investigation cannot be performed, the material must be sampled "blind." In such instances it is necessary to sample as much as possible of the entire mucosal surface of the organ being investigated, as in screening of populations in which certain malignant tumors occur at high rates.

COLLECTION OF MATERIAL

Esophagus

Nonselective esophageal sampling techniques for screening are justified in regions in which esophageal carcinoma is frequent. In China an abrasive balloon is used,[1] a technique whose development is traced back to Panico and Papanicolaou.[2] A gauze sheath is tied in place over an inflatable balloon attached to tubing. After the balloon has been advanced to the chosen level, generally that of the cardia, the balloon is inflated by means of a syringe attached to the oral end of the tubing. This is then pulled back to the level of the proximal esophagus, and the balloon is deflated. The procedure can be repeated. The best yield of cellular material is given by rinsing the balloon in a few milliliters of physiologic saline solution. The sediment obtained by centrifugation can be microscopically examined.

Our own experience has been with the cell-swab method described by Henning.[3] This is a foam-rubber swab fastened to a wire. The wire slides freely within a thin and flexible tube that widens at one end to form a rubber sheath. The swab is introduced while covered by this sheath. At a chosen level the head of the swab is advanced by means of a handle at the oral end of the tube, and the tube is moved backward and forward a few times. The swab is then drawn back into the protective rubber sheath, and the tube is removed. Cellular material is collected from the foam rubber by rinsing in physiologic saline solution and centrifugation, as described above for the abrasive balloon.

The advantage of the abrasive balloon is that it abrades the entire superficial mucosal surface; the disadvantages are that patients find it unpleasant and that it also yields cells from the pharynx and oral cavity. The advantages of the cell-swab method are that the level of sampling is relatively specific, that undesirable contamination is avoided, and that the procedure is rapid.

The high level to which flexible endoscopy has been developed has today made endoscopically guided sampling the optimal and clinically preferred technique for obtaining material. An abrasive brush is used, fastened to a sound that is introduced through the instrument channel of the endoscope. Under direct endoscopic observation, the brush is advanced to the chosen site. By working the guidance lever of the endoscope, one scrapes the brush gently, as tangentially as possible, across the surface of the lesion several times. The brush is then retracted into the protective opening of the instrument channel, and endoscopy is concluded. Any necessary forceps biopsy specimens are taken *before* brush abrasion. After the endoscope is removed from the patient, the brush is again advanced out of the opening of the instrument channel and rinsed in a few milliliters of physiologic saline solution. The cellular sediment is collected by centrifugation.

It is important to perform biopsies before cell-brush abrasion during endoscopy because the tissues are slightly disrupted by the biopsy and the yield of cells on brush abrasion is increased. Additionally, a superficial film of blood affects brush sampling less than it does biopsy.

Stomach

Gastric cell sampling is today performed only under endoscopic observation.[4,5] When attempting cytologically to identify a malignant tumor in the stomach, one must at the same time identify its location. Only in this manner is diagnosis of practical value, leading as it must to surgical treatment to extirpate the tumor. It is generally recognized that even in its early stages gastric carcinoma is manifested as an endoscopically recognizable lesion of the gastric mucosa. It is additionally recognized that in practice the endoscopist generally cannot confirm that a lesion seen at endoscopy is malignant.

The technical conditions under which material is sampled are accordingly of decisive importance for successful diagnosis. They depend on the endoscopist's ability to inspect the entire stomach, to recognize suspicious areas, and to obtain and retrieve material from precisely those areas.

The technique of brush abrasion is in principle the same as that used in the esophagus. Tangential contact with the entire surface of the lesion is necessary, with exertion of light pressure. We avoid pushing the brush away from the instrument; instead, we always draw it toward the endoscope. Strong pressure can cause linear superficial erosions.

If cytologic investigation of more than one gastric lesion during a single session is desired, covered abrasion brushes must be used. They are introduced in plastic tubes that fit within the instrument channel of the gastroscope. The brush is advanced out of the protective tube only in the stomach. After abrasion it is retracted into the tube, and tube and brush are removed together. This permits repeated sampling. However, such covered brushes are smaller than the normal brushes that are used without a cover, and accordingly the yield of cellular material is less. We therefore recommend that the most important lesion be sampled with an uncovered brush at the end of endoscopic investigation.

Needle aspiration can be used for obtaining cells from endoscopically identifiable foci of disease in the submucosa. The injection cannulas used for sclerotherapy of esophageal varices are particularly well suited to this purpose. While one is exerting negative pressure using a 20-ml syringe at the oral end, it is important to move the cannula slightly backward and forward in the tissues several times. However, before the tip of the needle is withdrawn from the mucosa, the vacuum must be released. After the cannula is withdrawn, the syringe is removed, its plunger is drawn back, and the syringe is attached again, for squirting the aspirated cellular material within the tip of the cannula carefully out onto a slide, where it can be smeared as a blood film is smeared.

Duodenum

From a cytologic standpoint, the papilla of Vater is the most important region of the duodenum. We use abrasion brushes in conjunction with duodenoscopy to sample tangentially the papilla or other suspected regions in the proximal horizontal portion, the descending portion, or the distal horizontal portion of the duodenum. The technique is the same as that used in the stomach. With the covered brushes described above, it is possible to enter the lumen of the papilla to obtain cellular material. The particularly important techniques for sampling the excretory ducts of the pancreas and the biliary tree cannot be discussed here, because they lie outside our subject. It should be mentioned, however, that using a probe to aspirate secretions from the immmediate vicinity of the papilla (prepapillary aspiration, with or without stimulation using intravenous secretin) is a routine procedure for cytologic studies of those regions.[6]

Colon and Rectum

In these regions as well we favor endoscopically directed abrasion techniques. We use either the sigmoidoscope or the colonoscope for localization. If polypoid lesions can be removed endoscopically using an electrical snare, that maneuver has diagnostic priority. In such instances the cytologist must content himself or herself with blotting the resected polyp on several microscope slides. In the presence of diffuse inflammatory changes, ulcerative lesions, or polypoid tumors that cannot be endoscopically resected *in toto*, we use brush abrasion. Multiple sampling is possible with the use of covered brushes. We never draw an uncovered brush through the instrument channel of the colonoscope following abrasion. It decreases the cellular yield and soils the instrument channel. For that reason forceps biopsies are always taken *before* brush abrasion.

We obtain cytologic material from the anal canal by means of a firm, dry cotton swab on a wooden stick, introduced through an open proctoscope. The swab is then rolled and blotted on dry microscope slides.

METHODS OF MICROSCOPIC EXAMINATION

Fresh Unfixed Preparations

The cytology laboratory should be in the near neighborhood of the endoscopy suite so that one can make the best use of cytologic diagnosis of unfixed material. In our hospital they open off the same corridor.

The centrifuge tubes containing either the physiologic saline solution, in which the abrasion brushes were rinsed, or the aspirated secretions are sealed and brought to the cytology laboratory, where they are processed within an hour of being obtained by endoscopy.

The tubes are centrifuged for 5 minutes in a normal laboratory centrifuge at a moderate number of revolutions per minute. All of the supernatant is decanted. With a glass rod, the sediment is distributed among three or four dry microscope slides and coverslipped. Careful pressure should produce equal distribution of the material to the rim of the coverslip. One should do this quickly to avoid osmotic changes due to drying. These preparations are then immediately examined under the microscope. They can also be stored for up to approximately 2 hours in a high-humidity container.

Phase Contrast Microscopy

This is the method most frequently used for microscopic examination of unfixed wet smear preparations. We use it routinely in order to scan all preparations.[7] Cell-free preparations can be scanned quickly in this manner. An assessment of cellular content is essential to permit the endoscopist to develop his or her sampling technique as highly as possible. Protozoa, such as *Giardia lamblia*, trichomonads, and amoebae, are immediately recognizable in unfixed preparations because they are motile.

The optical characteristics of phase contrast microscopy (Figures 4–1 and 4–2) permit identification of the following cytologic details: (1) nuclear size (anisokaryosis, alterations in nuclear/cytoplasmic ratio), nuclear shape, nuclear membrane (irregular thickening, double contouring), nucleoli (number, size, shape, definition with regard to the remainder of the optically homogeneous nucleoplasm); (2) cytoplasmic and cellular shape, definition by cellular organelles such as the brush border, fine structure of the cytoplasm (granularity, vacuolation); and (3) *campylobacter (Helicobacter) pylori*,[7a] or protozoa. Thin preparations are optimal for phase contrast illumination. If several cells overlie one another, disturbing halation effects appear in thicker

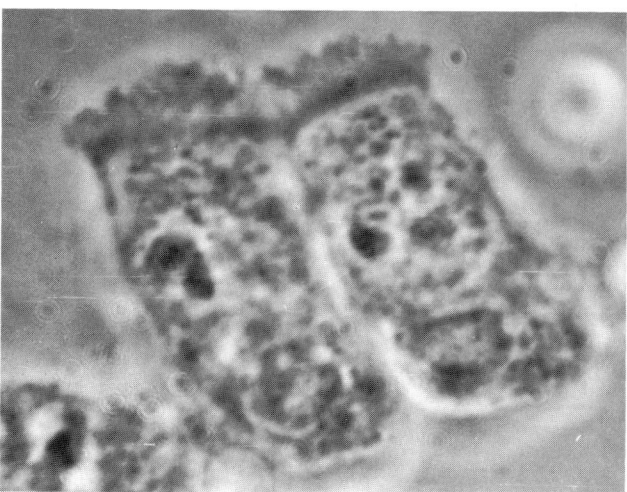

FIGURE 4–1. Jejunal epithelial cells. Gastrectomy. Note the cylindrical cell shape and brush border. (Unfixed wet preparation, phase contrast, ×1250)

CYTOLOGIC TECHNIQUES AND DIAGNOSIS 51

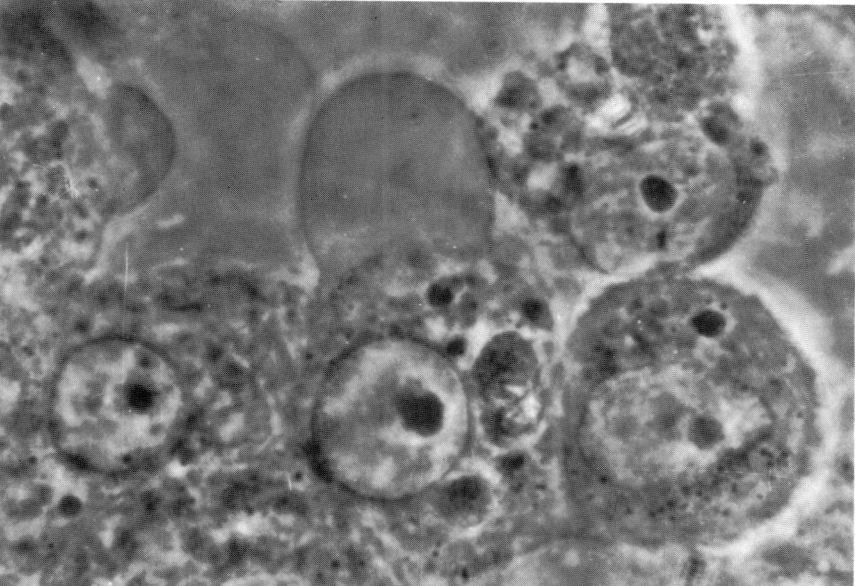

FIGURE 4–2. Tumor cell cluster. Gastric adenocarcinoma. (Unfixed wet preparation, phase contrast, × 1250)

regions. Such instances provide an indication for examination by Nomarski contrast microscopy.

Nomarski Differential Interference Contrast Microscopy[8]

Preparations are made as described above. The technique is somewhat more painstaking than that used for phase contrast microscopy. Its advantage is good resolution even in thick clumps of cells. This is provided by a very narrow depth of focus (Figure 4–3).

Ultraviolet-Light Microscopy[8]

Neither phase contrast nor Nomarski contrast microscopy adequately details nuclear internal structure. This disadvantage is compensated for by ultraviolet-light microscopy, which takes advantage of specific absorbance by nucleic acids and nonhistone proteins on illumination with short-wavelength ultraviolet light. We have been able to demonstrate that the nuclei of unfixed cells display an internal structure that resembles the chromatin structure of fixed and stained cells and that provides information of substantial value in

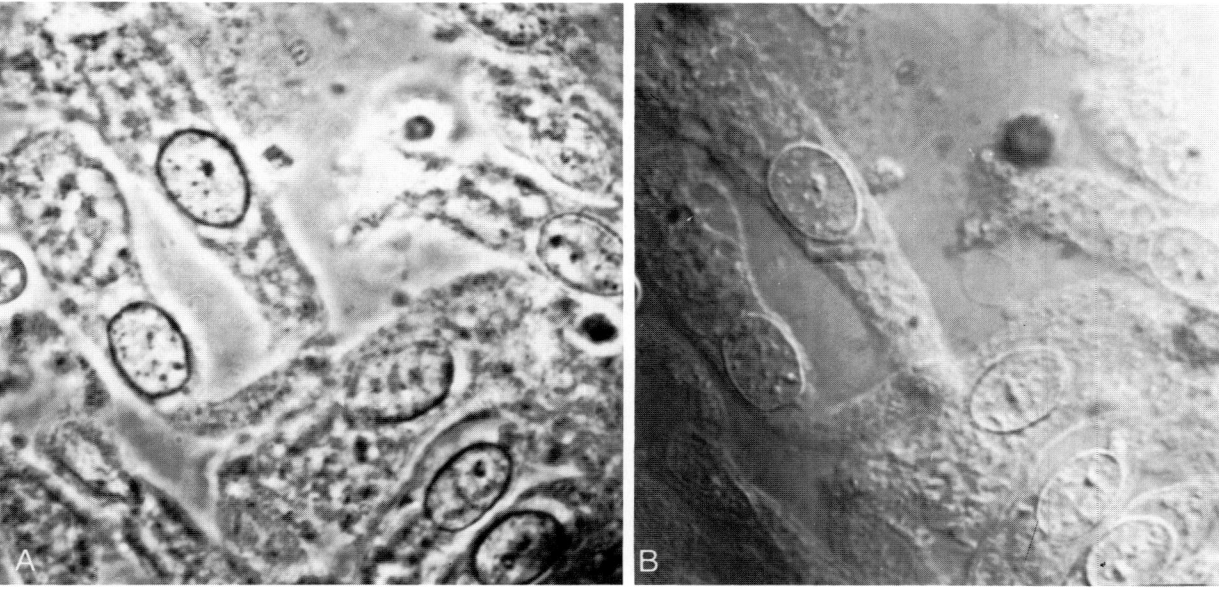

FIGURE 4–3. Normal columnar cells of gastric epithelium. (Unfixed wet preparation, × 800) A, Phase contrast. B, Differential interference contrast.

cytodiagnosis.[8a] Special equipment (quartz optics, monochromatization, image transformers) is required (Figure 4-4).

Fluorescence Microscopy

Staining of unfixed cells with fluorescent dyes like acridine orange also permits chemical differentiation among nucleic acids, in particular distinction of deoxyribonucleic acids within the nucleus from ribonucleic acids within nucleoli and the cytoplasm.[9] This facilitates the recognition of cellular atypia and of tumor cells.

Staining Techniques

After the investigations of unfixed preparations described above have been completed, the same preparations are processed for fixation. To this end the coverslips are pushed sideways across the microscope slides, smearing out the cellular material. The coverslips are removed and the smears are fixed on the microscope slides. We use a fixative spray. Even when microscopic scanning of wet unfixed preparations is not performed, we use the same technique for smearing and fixation. After fixation the preparations are suitable for mailing to a cytologic laboratory.

Routine staining of fixed preparations is performed according to the methods described by Papanicolaou.[10] These methods do not specifically identify tumor cells. They have the advantage, however, of adequately detailing the nuclear features that are particularly important for diagnosis, such as chromatin structure, nucleoli, and the nuclear membrane, even in regions of dense cellularity and in clumps of cells. In addition, distraction due to epithelial mucus staining is only slight.

If the material contains little mucus, hematologic stains such as the May-Grünwald-Giemsa stain also can be used. They provide optimal cytoplasmic differentiation. If the preparations contain abundant mucus or proteinaceous material in the background, they are

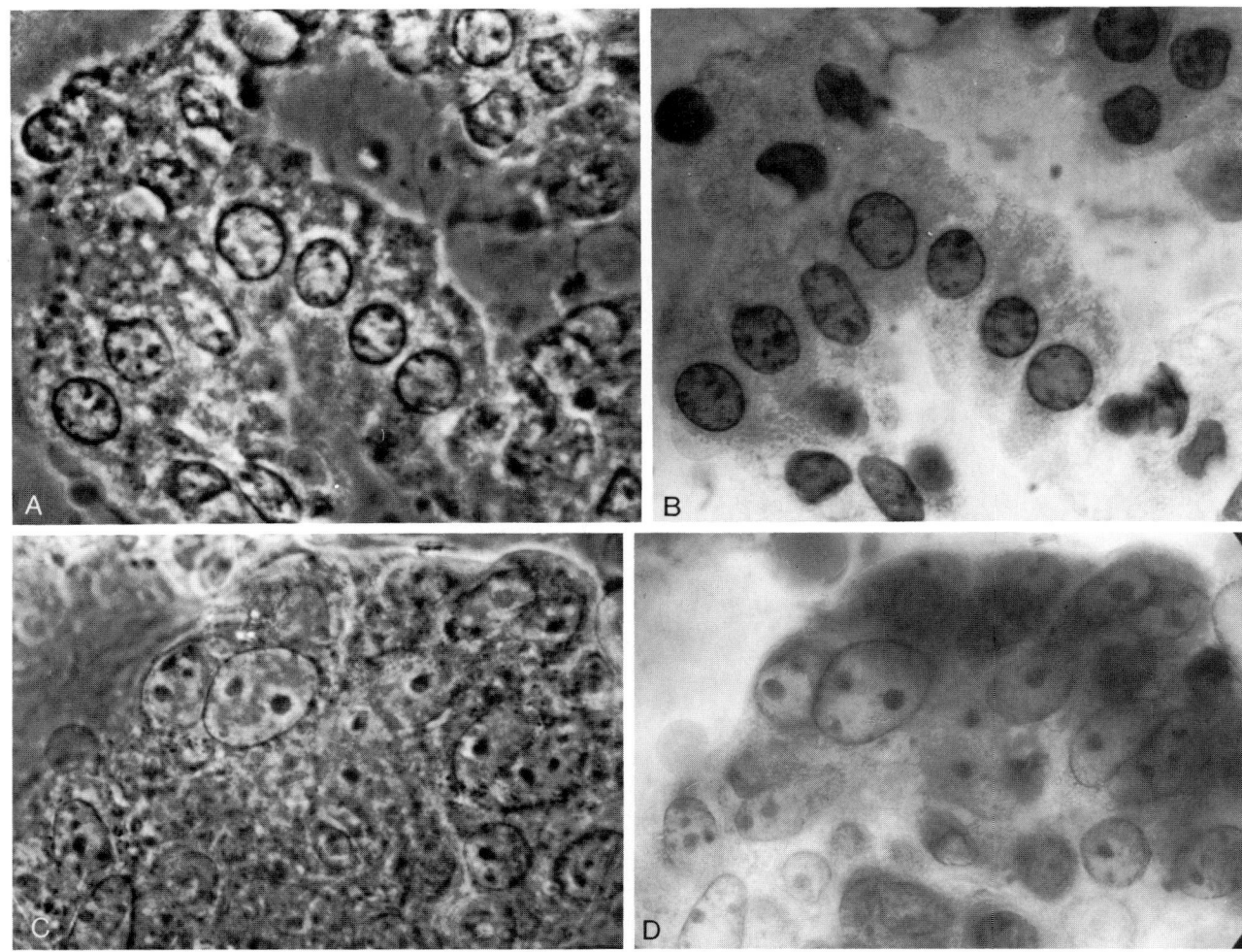

FIGURE 4-4. *A*, Gastric epithelial cells in superficial gastritis. Phase contrast. *B*, Same field, monochromatic ultraviolet microscope. Specific absorbance of nucleic acids, $\lambda = 263$ nm. *C*, Tumor cell cluster. Adenocarcinoma of the rectum. Phase contrast. *D*, Same field. Monochromatic ultraviolet microscopy. Specific absorbance of nucleic acids, $\lambda = 263$ nm. (Unfixed wet preparations, $\times 800$)

generally so overstained by this technique that evaluation is not possible.

Quantitative Methods

Cytologic methods are suited for quantitative studies, a significant advantage over biopsy-histology methods. Even automated techniques for quantitative cytology have recently become available.

Micromorphometry

Individual cells used to be measured subjectively by means of a microscope equipped with an ocular on which a micrometer was engraved. At present micromorphometry is generally performed in combination with projection equipment and a graphics tablet or with a system coupling a video camera and a computer.

Determination of nuclear diameter is the oldest quantitative approach, permitting calculation of nuclear area. This is how significant increases were identified in the dimensions of esophageal and gastric epithelial nuclei in pernicious anemia[11] and tropical sprue.[12] Squamous but not gastric epithelial nuclear measurements returned to normal after therapy with vitamin B_{12}. The area of esophageal squamous epithelial nuclei increases significantly step by step from normal intermediate cells through mild hyperplasia, moderate dysplasia and severe dysplasia, to malignant change.[13]

Among many additional morphometric parameters, one of the most important is standard deviation in nuclear area, which quantitatively describes anisokaryosis. In gastric carcinoma the standard deviation in nuclear area is significantly greater than that in the nuclear area of normal cells. A similar parameter is the nuclear/cytoplasmic ratio, which is smaller for normal gastric epithelium than for malignant cells.[14]

Fluorescence Cytophotometry

Stoichiometric cytochemical demonstration of deoxyribonucleic acid using the Feulgen reaction is the oldest method, and up to now the most important one. It is now generally employed for individual-cell fluorometry, with a fluorescent dye as an indicator. Measurement of intensity of nuclear fluorescence[15] in individual cells, using a fluorescence microscope equipped for photometry, yields a histogram of fluorescence intensities integrated over nuclear areas. With normal diploid cells as standards for comparison, the DNA content of a cytologic smear can be measured, enabling a determination of whether DNA complements are diploid, polyploid, or aneuploid. Statistical evaluation of measured values is necessary for arriving at results of value in diagnosis. The technique is still evolving.

On the basis of our experience,[16] we believe that at present it is not possible to make the diagnosis of cytologic malignancy from DNA histograms alone. Still, quantitative measurement of DNA remains the cornerstone of cytophotometric techniques. Photometry of individual cells is a time-consuming technique. The advantage of being able to assay cells subjectively identified as suspicious is countered by the disadvantage that only a very limited number of cells can be evaluated in a reasonable amount of time.

Flow Cytophotometry

Large numbers of suspensions of individual cells can be assayed in short periods of time by commercially available flow-through systems. A fine stream of liquid transports the cells past one or more ports where fluorescence or light-beam diffraction is measured. Although determination of fluorescence-stained DNA content is important, systems that assay multiple parameters also exist. Flow techniques have definite disadvantages: they have no microscopic optical resolution, microscopic images are not obtained, and permanent preparations for microscopic documentation are not generated. Suspensions of abraded cellular material from clinical sources generally consist of a mixed population of a very great variety of cells, of which only a small proportion can be atypical cells or cells suspected of malignancy. In many instances, therefore, the number of tumor cells is insignificant by comparison with the number of nonmalignant cells. Histogram interpretation is then difficult or inconclusive.[17] The development of cell-sorting methods that deposit enriched populations of atypical cells on permanent substrates would significantly increase the value of flow techniques for our specialty. A new approach is provided by staining with fluorescence-labeled monoclonal antibodies.

High-Resolution Image Analysis

High-power magnification permits quantitative description of cells and, in particular, nuclear structure, using digital video image generation and computer-directed image processing. These methods are suitable for automation and rapid image analysis. Their goal is completely automated evaluation of smear preparations for tumor identification.[18] Preparations can be stained conventionally, with the Papanicolaou stain, or by fluorescence techniques.

We have gained our experience using absorption of monochromatic ultraviolet light by unfixed and unstained cell smears to analyze nucleic acid and nonhistone-protein configurations of nuclei in preparations of gastroenterologic material. Distinction between these nuclear components on high-magnification microscopy is possible with computer-directed image analysis.[19] We have found epithelial cell nuclei that are normal or show inflammatory changes to be readily separable from atypical, neoplastic cell nuclei[20] (Figure 4–5; Table 4–1).

We have learned from our experience that it is necessary to combine quantitative assessments of various characteristics of cells—DNA content, nuclear size, variation in nuclear size—with high-resolution analysis of nuclear texture to identify tumors in cytologic

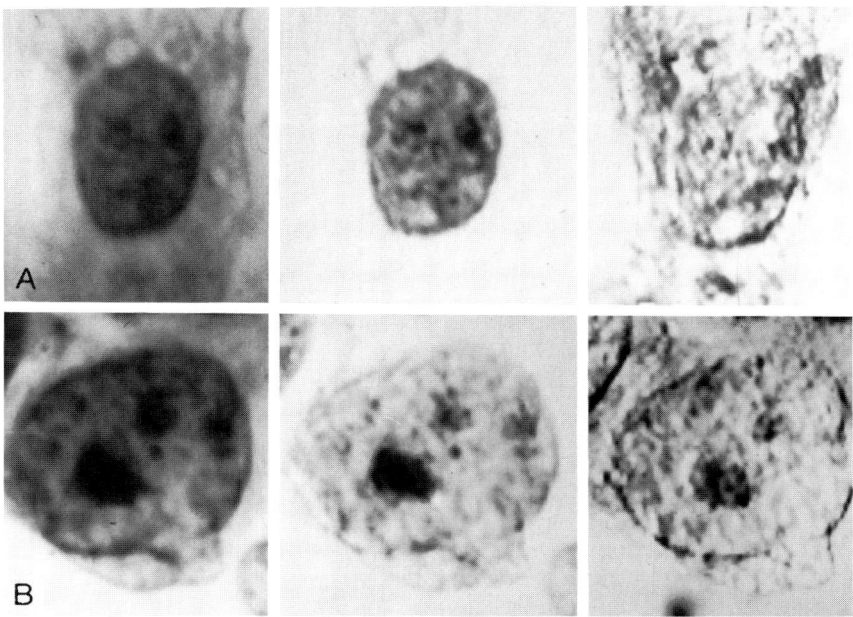

FIGURE 4-5. From left to right, original absorbance, $\lambda = 263$ nm; pure nucleic acid picture; pure nonhistone protein picture. *A*, Atypical colonic epithelial cell in a case of ulcerative colitis. *B*, Tumor cell in a case of adenocarcinoma of the colon. (Monochromatic ultraviolet absorbance of unfixed wet cells, $\times 800$, processed by means of image analysis computer technique)

Table 4-1 COMPARISON OF CYTOLOGIC CLASSIFICATION BY LIGHT MICROSCOPY AND RECLASSIFICATION BY AUTOMATED IMAGE ANALYSIS*

Light Microscopy		Automated Analysis	
Cell Class	Cases	Normal	Pathologic
1	137	129(131)	8(6)
2	51	43(44)	8(7)
3	62	55(57)	7(5)
4	150	67(—)	83(—)
5	174	26(34)	148(140)
6	137	11(5)	126(132)
Total cases	711	331(271)	380(290)

*Misclassified cases by automated analysis: 17% (10%)

Automated, high-resolution image analysis is performed on unfixed, unstained cells, with monochromatic ultraviolet microscopy; wave length, 263 nm.

Six cell classes: 1, normal cylindrical cell; 2, rounded epithelial cell; 3, epithelial cell with nuclear swelling; 4, epithelial cell with slight to moderate nuclear atypia, solitary enlarged nucleolus ("ulcer cells"); 5, cell with severe nuclear atypia; 6, malignant cell.

In automated analysis, normal cells include cells in classes 1 to 3 and pathological cells include cells in classes 4 to 6. Classification after omission of class 4 is given in parentheses.

material objectively, independent of subjective assessments. This is the goal toward which many laboratories are working.

CYTOMORPHOLOGY AND CYTODIAGNOSIS

Esophagus

A cytologic abrasion smear prepared from the normal esophagus shows a uniform pattern of cells, consisting of squamous epithelial cells of the intermediate type. Superficial cells are rare, and no keratinization is present. Hyperplasia is manifested by intermediate cells containing enlarged nuclei with normal finely granular chromatin. In patients with pernicious anemia, we find a tendency toward enlarged, multiple nuclei that regress under vitamin B_{12} therapy. In esophagitis, epithelial cells from deeper layers, the parabasal cells, appear. The nuclei of these cells are larger and their cytoplasm more basophilic and less extensive than that of intermediate cells. In acute esophagitis, intraepithelial leukocytes are found. When severely necrotizing inflammation is present, large numbers of bacteria and/or fungal hyphae and yeasts are seen. A tendency to keratinization is shown by oxyphilic staining of the cytoplasm. This may occur in normal squamous epithelium and also as a sign of atypia in dysplastic cells. Small squamous-type cells with small, round nuclei and bright oxyphilic cytoplasm are termed ductal cells. These cells occur in small groups and are shed from the ducts of mucous glands in the squamous epithelial layer.

Displaced cell types that may be found include gastric columnar cells or even cells from the duodenal mucosa. They demonstrate heterotopy of the corresponding gastric or duodenal mucosa in the esophagus.

Of particular importance are dysplastic squamous cells[21] (Figure 4-6). This term implies a dissociation between the maturation of the nuclei and that of the cytoplasm. Nuclei are enlarged, particularly in relation to the more mature cytoplasm. The nuclei are also hyperchromatic, and the nuclear membrane is emphasized. In moderate dysplasia, the nuclear enlargement is found in the intermediate cells; in more severe dysplasia it also affects the parabasal cells. Hyperchromasia and nuclear enlargement are most marked in such cases. Malignancy is suspected when the smear contains numerous, highly dysplastic, polymorphic parabasal cells. Tumor cells of the squamous epithelium show marked enlargement, anisokaryosis and hyper-

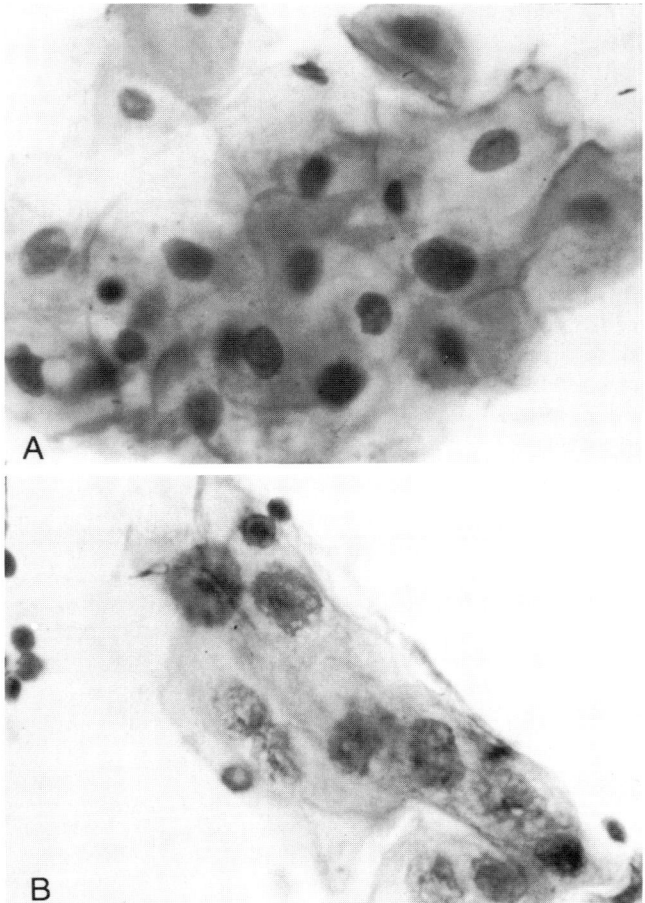

Table 4-2 CYTOLOGIC ASSESSMENT CRITERIA FOR ESOPHAGEAL PREPARATIONS

Cell content
  Squamous cells
    Superficial
    Intermediate
    Parabasal
  Keratinization
    Parakeratosis
    Dyskeratosis
    Hyperkeratosis
  Characteristics of the nucleus
    Size
    Hyperchromasia
    Thickened nuclear membrane
    Chromatin structure
    Number of nucleoli
    Size of nucleoli
  Inflammatory cells
    Count
    Intraepithelial collections
  Bacterial clusters
  Fungi/yeasts

chromia of the nucleus, a thickened nuclear membrane, and a marked shift in the nuclear/cytoplasmic ratio in favor of the nucleus. Enlarged nucleoli are seen in increased numbers. Tumor cells may occur singly or, particularly characteristically, in three-dimensional clumps of cells ("clusters") (Figure 4–7). Rarely, small-cell carcinoma arising from the esophagus can be found.[22] The smears may be assessed in accordance with Table 4–2.

Stomach

The mucosal cells of the stomach are columnar cells. They are rather tall cells, with oval nuclei situated in the basal third of the cells, which often come to a point. The cytoplasm becomes less dense toward the gastric lumen. This secretory area of the gastric mucosa can be seen with particular clarity under phase contrast mi-

FIGURE 4–6. Dysplastic squamous cells of the esophagus. *A*, Slight to moderate dysplasia. *B*, Severe dysplasia. Pernicious anemia. (Papanicolaou, × 500)

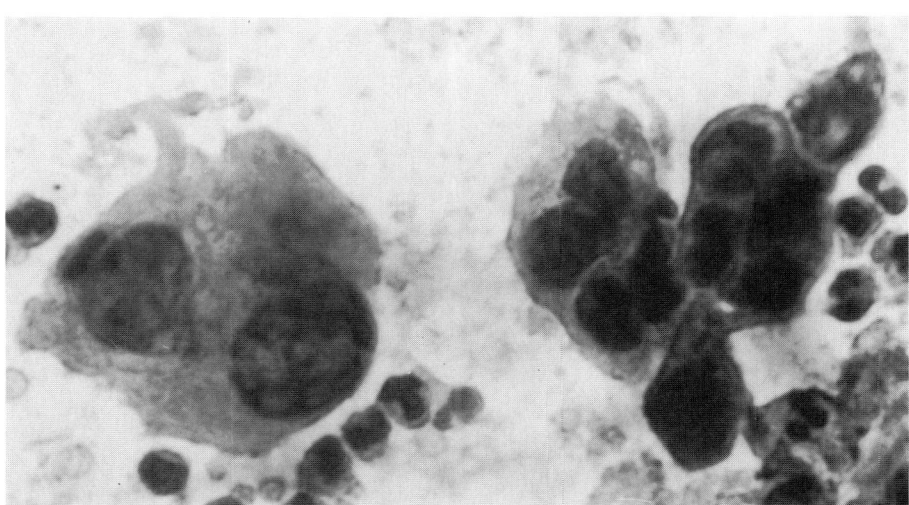

FIGURE 4–7. Tumor cells in squamous carcinoma of the esophagus. Degenerative cell changes after irradiation therapy. (Papanicolaou, × 325)

croscopy. Only a few columnar cells, often lying singly or altered by cytolytic processes, or even free cell nuclei are found in the normal stomach. Columnar cells found in large numbers and in clusters are taken as a sign of shedding of the epithelium from the basement membrane as a result of inflammation. The columnar cells can be recognized in these clusters by elicitation of the so-called honeycomb phenomenon. It is possible to focus the microscope down onto a deep plane, in which the cell nuclei appear sharp and round, and onto a plane lying above these that passes through the foamy cytoplasm and gives a honeycomb-like pattern as the result of the network of interepithelial boundaries (Figure 4–8).

The second variety of epithelial cells is the goblet cells. Their cytoplasm is transformed into a vast homogeneous mucous vacuole with a basal nucleus that is distorted into a semilunar shape. Goblet cells are not found in the normal stomach. They are an accompaniment of chronic gastritis, particularly the atrophic form.

Columnar cells whose short ends do not show the loose density of a vacuole but which have a sharply delineated edge with a thick border of short bristles (cuticular fringe) are usually found only in the small intestine. When they occur in the stomach it is a sign of intestinal metaplasia. Together with other signs of chronic gastritis, they are a sign of metaplastic gastritis. It should be noted that when these intestinal cells are found in the stomach, they are always of a mature type with regular round to oval nuclei and with no signs of cellular atypia (Figure 4–9).

The characteristic representative cells of the glands in the fundus are the parietal cells. They are definitely smaller than the intermediate squamous cells with which they are sometimes confused. They have a relatively extensive cytoplasm and one or more small, round chromatin-rich nuclei. The cell is pyramidal in shape. The main feature is dense, fine-grained, eosinophilic granulation that fills the cytoplasm evenly with the exception of indistinct "roads." The cells mostly occur in groups, sometimes as cell casts, together with small, heavily vacuolated columnar cells with relatively large nuclei, the mucous neck cells. Parietal cells and mucous neck cells in clusters (Figure 4–10), suggestive of the tubular structure of glands, indicate an increased desquamation of glandular cells as the morphologic expression of an increase in the functional activity of the gastric glands, as we have confirmed by bioptic histology.[23] This finding is not present when there is mucosal atrophy of the body of the stomach, but it is found in cases of basal hypersecretion of the stomach and also in cases of duodenal ulcer.

The cells of the mucosal surface are altered in all forms of severe gastritis, and this constitutes therefore the most frequent cytopathologic finding in the stomach. Systematically we must make the following distinction: changes in the cell shape, changes in the cytoplasm, and changes in the nucleus. The cell shape ranges from tall columnar to plump, short columnar and thence to pyramidal, cuboidal, and round. There is thus a marked anisocytosis. The cell content is generally high. The cells lie in clusters. On the other hand, it is characteristic that they are separated from one another, which indicates a loss of cellular adherence. A further characteristic finding in the cytoplasm is the presence of perinuclear vacuoles that indent the pyknotic nucleus from one or both sides. We look upon the cytoplasmic changes as a sign of chronic gastritis and regard the perinuclear vacuoles as a sign of hypoxic cell damage (Figure 4–11).

Nuclear changes are of even greater diagnostic significance than changes in cell shape. The normal oval nuclei may be rounded, often dense, and pyknotic, a

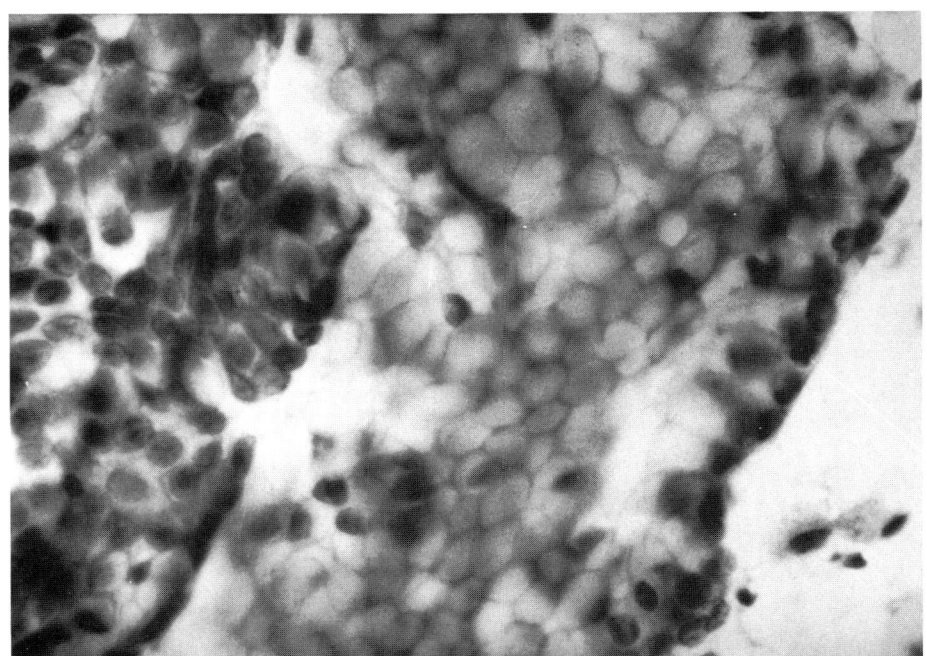

FIGURE 4–8. Columnar epithelial cells from the gastric mucosa. Monolayer sheet with honeycomb pattern. Superficial gastritis. (Papanicolaou, × 108)

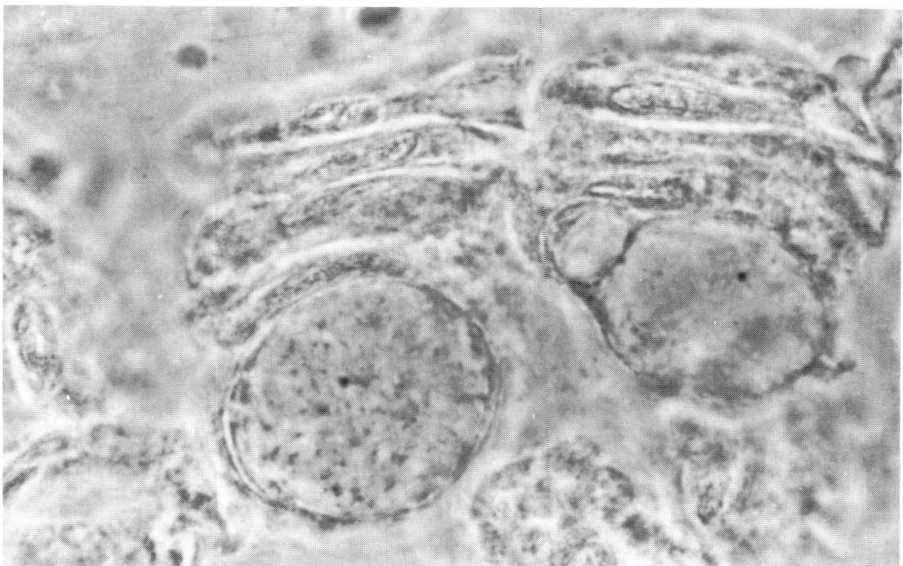

FIGURE 4–9. Goblet cells and elongated cylindrical cells in chronic atrophic gastritis. (Wet unfixed preparation, phase contrast, × 800)

sign of aged, damaged cells. Swollen nuclei with loose chromatin structure may also be found. This leads to anisokaryosis. When the nuclei are enlarged as the result of swelling (edema of the nucleus), the chromatin structure is pale, which indicates a higher level of functional activity associated with increased regeneration. The nucleoli, which are usually not visible or which appear only as dots, are often enlarged in this case and have their own staining characteristics, being copper-colored in Papanicolaou stains. Condensations of chromatin, centromeres, have the violet color of nuclear chromatin (Figure 4–12). These cell changes bring about a shift in the normal nuclear/cytoplasmic ratio in favor of the nucleus. Anisokaryosis and anisocytosis occur simultaneously. In cell clusters the cell boundaries are often no longer visible when the cell changes are advanced (Figure 4–13).

All these variations in the surface epithelium are regarded by us as signs of a maturational disturbance. The normal process of differentiation of the surface epithelium from the less differentiated cells of the regeneration zones in the lacunar region is disturbed or completely abolished. The degree of severity of this maturation disturbance parallels the severity of the gastritis. In superficial gastritis, the cytologic findings are more or less those of normal columnar epithelium. In severe chronic gastritis, generally reported as "atrophic" on histologic examination if the normal glands of the body of the stomach are destroyed, the preponderant cytologic finding is the presence of round cells with marked anisokaryosis. The most severe changes are seen in the surface epithelium of patients with pernicious anemia and include anisomacrokaryosis and

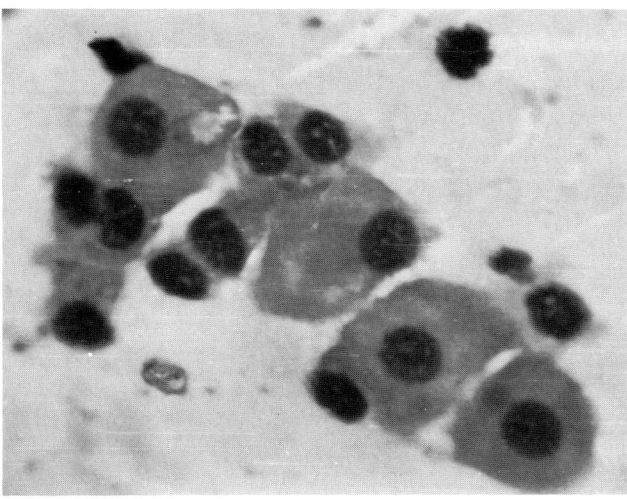

FIGURE 4–10. Parietal cells and mucous neck cells, obtained by gastric brushing, in a case of hyperchlorhydria. (Papanicolaou, × 500)

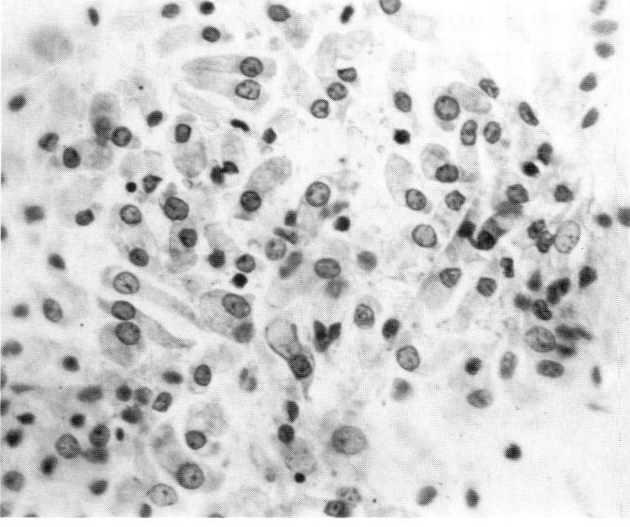

FIGURE 4–11. Anisokaryosis and anisocytosis of gastric epithelial cells. Some perinuclear vacuoles. Chronic superficial gastritis (Papanicolaou, × 108)

58 GENERAL PRINCIPLES

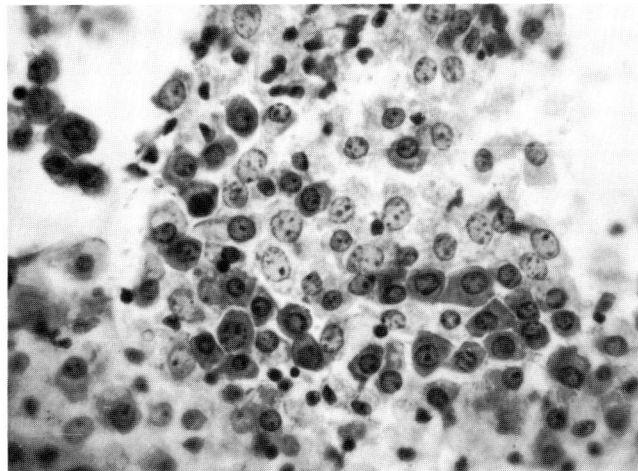

FIGURE 4–12. Gastric epithelial cells with enlarged nuclei, anisokaryosis, enlarged nucleoli, basophilic cytoplasm, cuboid shaped, in a case of chromic gastric erosions. (Papanicolaou, × 325)

enlarged nucleoli. The epithelial changes found in gastritis are irreversible and can be demonstrated constantly over a number of years.

The correlation between the degree of cytologic change in the epithelial cells and the histologic diagnosis of gastritis has been documented impressively by Bigotti and Crespi[24] (Table 4–3).

In peptic ulcer and complete erosions, we have described the so-called ulcer cells at the edge of these lesions as the characteristic cell type of a regenerating surface epithelium. These are large columnar cells with enlarged nuclei and marked anisokaryosis. The chromatin structure is delicate, and the nuclei generally have single, enlarged, sharply demarcated nucleoli. We think it striking that these changes can be demonstrated continuously over a number of months in the case of erosions.

A knowledge of the cell changes just described is a basis for the recognition of tumor cells in cancer of the stomach, because such changes often accompany or

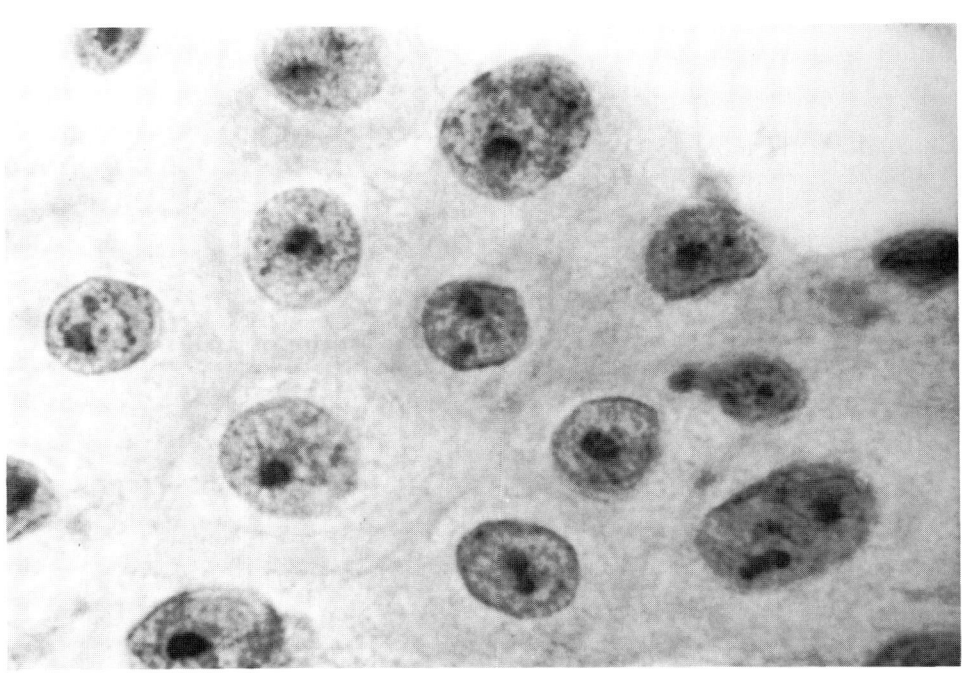

FIGURE 4–13. Gastric epithelial cells with enlarged nuclei, very prominent nucleoli, anisokaryosis, cell borders not visible, in a case of gastric ulcer. (Papanicolaou, × 800)

Table 4–3 COMPARISON OF CYTOLOGIC CHANGES AND HISTOLOGIC DIAGNOSIS OF GASTRITIS

Severity of the Predominant Cell Changes	Number of Cases	Histologic Diagnosis				
		Normal	*Superficial Gastritis*	*Atrophic Gastritis*		*Gastric Atrophy*
				Moderate	Severe	
0 (normal)	29	29	—	—	—	—
I	56	51	5	—	—	—
II	125	4	78	32	11	—
III	129	—	21	45	60	3
IV	45	—	2	2	9	32

even mask malignant cells in cytologic preparations. In order to recognize tumor cells in gastric abrasion smears under the microscope, one needs to take into account a large number of features that can only be assessed in combination (Table 4–4).

Cytologic features of the tumor type exist. Thus, in adenocarcinoma, one almost always finds three-dimensional clusters of cells that are suggestive of tubular structures (Figure 4–14). Large vacuoles in the cytoplasm also belong to the picture. In contrast, greater difficulties are presented by signet-ring cell carcinoma. Here, the tumor cells occur singly as a rule, sometimes being scattered and present only in scanty numbers in the preparation. The characteristic feature is the large mucous vacuole that fills the entire cell, with the result that the cell becomes rounded and the hyperchromic nucleus is distorted and displaced to the edge of the cell (Figure 4–15). Signs of secretory vesicles are seen with particular clarity by phase contrast. Squamous cell carcinomas in the region of the cardia have the following features already noted for the esophagus: relatively extensive cytoplasm and marked anisokaryosis of the hyperchromatic central, round to oval nucleus. Single cell deposits are more frequent than in adenocarcinoma.

The rare mesenchymal tumors of the stomach also furnish typical cytologic findings. Malignant, non-Hodgkin's lymphomas yield single, pathologic lymphatic round cells mostly with a small to moderate amount of homogeneous basophilic cytoplasm. The nuclei have a condensed, coarse-grained chromatin structure and an enlarged, round, solitary nucleolus (Figure 4–16). In highly malignant types of lymphoma, the enlargement and irregularity of the nuclei is very pronounced, as is the cytoplasmic basophilia.[25] The rare Hodgkin's lymphoma can be recognized by the characteristic basophilic cells with giant nuclei and the multinucleated giant cells of the Sternberg type with pale chromatin and marked enlargement of the multiple nucleoli. Leiomyosarcoma is characterized by spindle-shaped or long, drawn-out cells with elliptical nuclei adjacent to basophilic cells with round nuclei.[26]

Tumor-cell–containing smears show secondary cell changes of a regressive type, as the result of necrotic

Table 4–4 CYTOLOGIC CHARACTERISTICS OF GASTRIC CARCINOMA CELLS

Nuclei
  Anisokaryosis
  Tendency to nuclear enlargement
  Hyperchromasia
  Irregular, coarse-grained or lumpy chromatin
  Nuclear membrane thickened irregularly
  Pathologic mitoses
Cytoplasm
  Deviation from the normal shape of epithelial cells ("foreign" cells)
  Anisocytosis
  Increased basophilia
  Shift of nuclear/cytoplasmic ratio in favor of the nucleus

In fixed preparations stained with Papanicolaou stains
  Hyperchromia with coarsened chromatin structure in the nucleus
  Irregular thickening of the nuclear membrane
  Multiplication, enlargement, distortion of the nucleoli
  Shift of the nuclear/cytoplasmic ratio with nuclear enlargement and anisokaryosis
  Three-dimensional arrangement of cells into clusters
  Cell boundaries in the cluster not clearly visible

In unfixed, unstained, phase contrast preparations
  Double contouring of the nuclear membrane with irregular thickening
  Atypical nuclei
  Shift of the nuclear/cytoplasmic ratio with nuclear enlargement and anisokaryosis, granular and vacuolar structures in the cytoplasm
  Honeycomb effect never present in clusters of cells

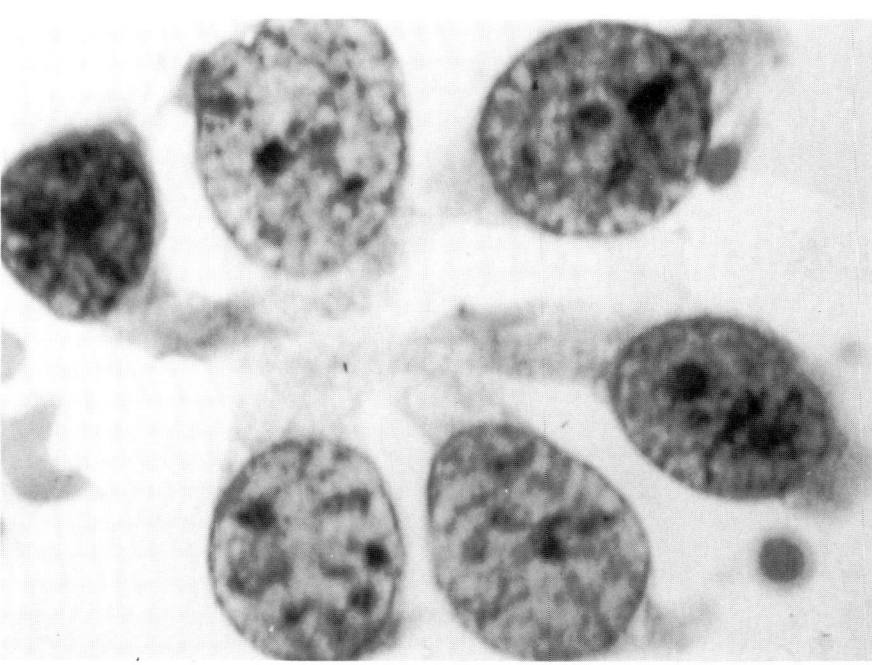

FIGURE 4–14. Tumor cells, cylindrical cell type, in a case of early gastric cancer. (Papanicolaou, × 800)

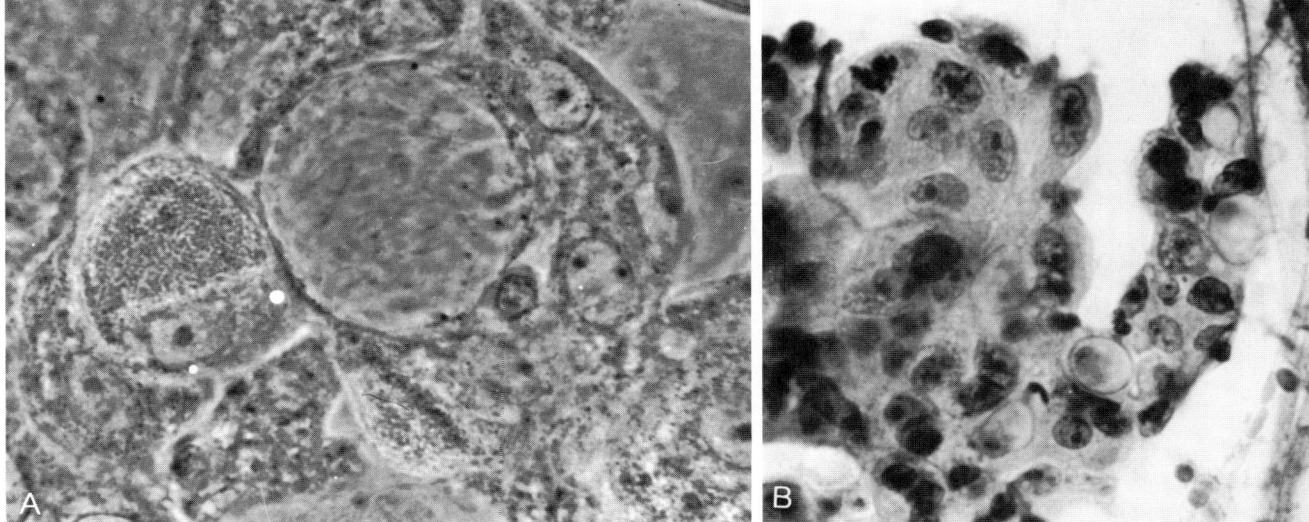

FIGURE 4–15. A and B, Tumor cell clusters, gastric signet-ring cell carcinoma. (A, Unfixed wet preparation, phase contrast, × 800; B, Another case, Papanicolaou, × 400)

phenomena at the tumor surface. The cells take up stain poorly, and the nuclei are reduced to nuclear ghosts. In such cases there are also many leukocytes, mixed bacterial flora, fungal mycelia, and occasional protozoa (usually trichomonads), which are easy to identify in unstained preparations because of their motility but which are more or less impossible to detect in stained preparations. *Campylobacter (Helicobacter) pylori* can be detected with high specificity.[26a] When the tumor growth has produced stenosis, food remnants may be the predominant finding in cytologic preparations.

As a rule, large, necrotic tumors are substantially more difficult to identify cytologically because of the secondary changes just described. Small tumors produce "clean" preparations with well-preserved tumor cells. They are therefore more easy to diagnose on cytologic examination, and this is of relevance to the clinical significance of cytodiagnosis.

Duodenum

The characteristic cell type of the duodenum is the intestinal epithelial cell, a narrow columnar cell with a round or slightly oval chromatin-rich nucleus situated in the basal third of the cell. The cell surface facing the lumen is marked sharply by a borderlike area of condensation on which sits a dense, short cuticular fringe.

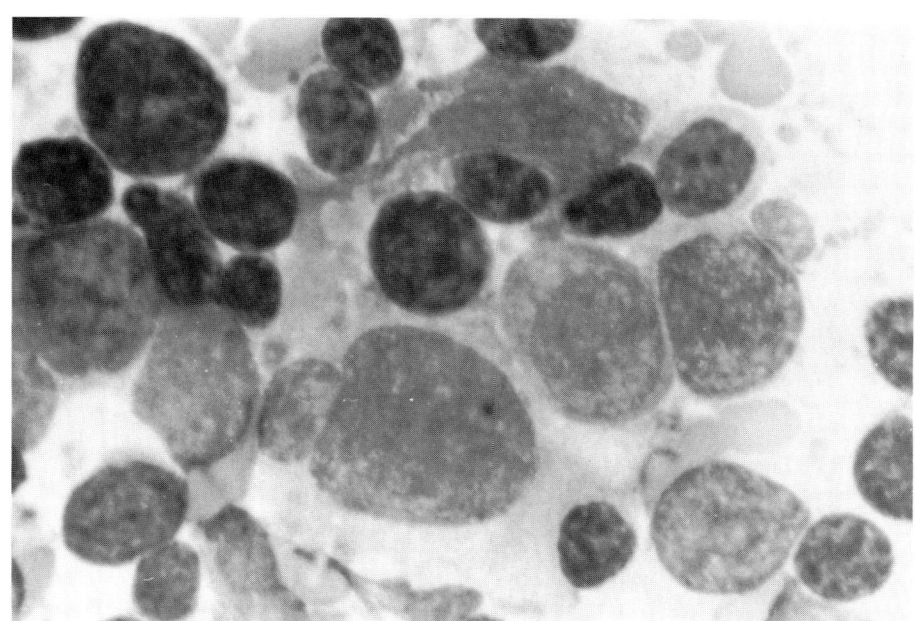

FIGURE 4–16. Malignant non-Hodgkin's lymphoma, high grade, of the gastrointestinal tract. (May-Grünwald-Giemsa, × 800)

In duodenal ulcer, the intestinal cell type disappears. From the edge of the ulcer, regeneration cells are obtained, similar to those described for gastric ulcer, with swollen nuclei and an enlarged, solitary nucleolus. These cells show clear anisokaryosis, in contrast to the intestinal cells with their monomorphic nuclei. Heterotopic gastric mucosa in the duodenum can easily be recognized by the occurrence of parietal cells.

In duodenitis, lymphocytes are mixed with the intestinal cells in greater or lesser numbers.[27] This is particularly the case in the rare Crohn's disease of the duodenum, in which we have also found undifferentiated cells with large nuclei and extensive cytoplasm. Cytologic examination of the unfixed duodenal mucosa by phase contrast microscopy may reveal the presence of *Giardia lamblia*, now present in large numbers, as the cause of long-standing undiagnosed symptoms in the upper abdomen. They manifest a lively motility as a result of the pair of flagella at the hind end and the cilia attached to the pear-shaped, flattened cytoplasm. Motility remains for several hours after sampling if kept in a moist chamber. On Papanicolaou staining, these protozoa can also be recognized, though with greater difficulty, by the pear shape and the two typical eyelike nuclei.

Tumor cells in the duodenum, other than those from the papilla, are a rare finding. These cases are generally the result of a pancreatic adenocarcinoma invading the duodenal wall.

The major papilla has a short, plump columnar epithelium without a cuticular fringe and can thus be distinguished from the duodenal epithelium. Within the pore of the papilla, there is a border zone in which the surface epithelium of the papilla meets the ductal epithelium of the choledochus and pancreatic ducts. Border zones such as this are the most common sites for cell transformation, and they can be investigated satisfactorily by obtaining brush abrasions under endoscopic guidance or by endopapillary aspiration. Most important is the recognition of carcinoma of the papilla, which is susceptible to early cytologic diagnosis and which is more difficult to reach, in our experience, with biopsy forceps. The tumor cells here are of the adenocarcinoma type, or there may also be clusters of papillary tumor cells, which are characterized by a drawn out cytoplasm and an elliptical nucleus with the cytologic criteria of malignancy (Figure 4–17). Atypical columnar cells arranged in a papillary pattern associated with villous papillary adenoma must be differentiated from these cells because they also have elliptical nuclei. Anisokaryosis is, however, rare; and there is no shift in the nuclear/cytoplasmic ratio.[28] We were able to make an early diagnosis of the recurrence of a villous papillary carcinoma, excised at operation, by constantly demonstrating tumor cells in the brush smear of the papilla.

Only brief mention can be made here of the cytologic diagnosis of the biliary tract and pancreatic juice.[29] This is clinically of particular importance because bioptic methods are not available and tumors are becoming more frequent in this area both in our practice and in other countries.

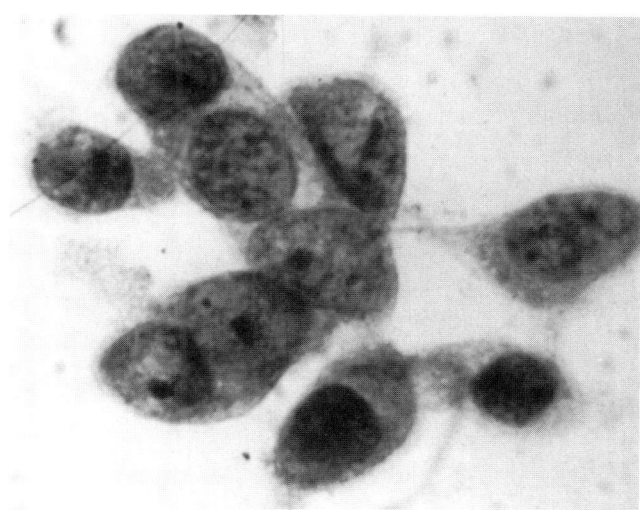

FIGURE 4–17. Tumor cells from an adenocarcinoma of the duodenal papilla. (Papanicolaou, × 800)

Colon and Rectum

The colon is lined with a single layer of tall, blunted columnar cells. The nuclei are large and elliptical and lie within the basal third of the cell. The cytoplasm loses density toward the lumen. There is no cuticular fringe. Only sparse scrapings can be obtained from healthy mucosa. When larger numbers and clusters of single-layered cells are obtained by brush abrasion, we recognize an increased desquamation and friability of the mucosa and regard this finding as cytologic evidence of simple colitis.

The cells that we call colic cells are a singular cytologic finding. These are degenerative forms of intestinal epithelial cells, rounded cells with karyorrhexis, a fragmentation of the pyknotic nucleus into numerous, homogeneous particles of varying size, together with hyaline inclusions in the cytoplasm. These colic cells are the only highly characteristic microscopic feature of the colitic mucosa (Figure 4–18).

In ulcerative colitis, neutrophilic granulocytes predominate in the cytologic picture in the acute stage. In the chronic stages, the surface epithelium shows more or less clear signs of atypia. The nuclei may be enlarged and may show marked anisokaryosis. Confusion with tumor cells is prevented by the absence of hyperchromatic nuclear chromatin and the absence of nucleolar atypia.[30] These nuclear atypias may be present for months. Therefore, careful examination is necessary. It is recognized that such examination may be a difficult undertaking in patients with long-standing active ulcerative colitis.

Crohn's disease is, by way of contrast, more difficult to diagnose cytologically than ulcerative colitis. One feature is the predominance of lymphatic cells. The occurrence of epithelioid cells, pale cells with extensive cytoplasm, large, oval nuclei, and a fine network of chromatin, is characteristic, although rare. The presence of multinucleated giant cells helps to establish the diagnosis (Figure 4–19).

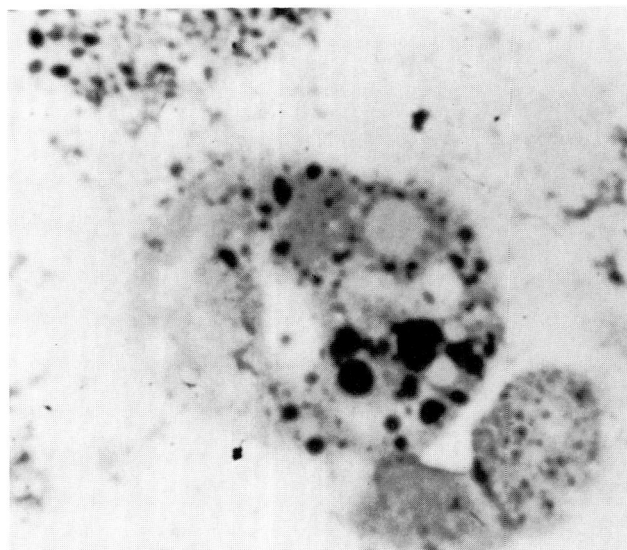

FIGURE 4–18. So-called colic cells, degenerated colonic epithelia, case of colitic mucosa. (May-Grünwald-Giemsa, × 800)

In cancer of the large bowel, tumor cells of the adenocarcinoma type are delivered very regularly, singly and in clusters, generally with accompanying signs of necrosis and collections of leukocytes. Cytodiagnosis is very reliable in these circumstances.[31] This is particularly true of stenosing tumors. Obtaining biopsy specimens from such tumors with forceps under endoscopic control is difficult. In such cases histologic diagnosis of the tumor is secondary to cytologic diagnosis by abrasion. In polypoid tumors, on the other hand, histologic examination of the polyp removed in its entirety by endoscopic snare is favored, for two reasons. Only histologic examination can determine whether the stalk of a polyp has been invaded by tumor, which is an important piece of information in terms of further treatment. Second, the demonstration of a focal malignant transformation in an otherwise nonmalignant polyp is not of particular clinical importance if the polyp has been fully excised. The abrasion form of cytologic examination of smears is therefore of no practical use in colonic polyps that can be removed entirely.

A cytologic swab preparation made from a fully excised polyp provides interesting material for the cytologist nonetheless. It shows clusters of colonic epithelial cells that are characteristic of the various histologic types of polyp. The predominant type in hyperplastic polyp is the normal columnar cell, changed only by a slight nuclear enlargement and anisokaryosis and found in large cell clusters. Adenomatous polyps predominantly produce cuboid cells with large, round nuclei that are arranged in formations suggestive of tubules. Anisokaryosis and enlargement of the solitary nucleolus are variable findings that are regarded as examples of cellular atypia. The more a polyp of the tubular adenomatous variety shows signs of a villous component, the more predominant is cellular atypia. The nuclei show hyperchromasia, irregular condensation of the chromatin. The elliptical nucleus is a general cytologic feature of villous polyps and must be distinguished from the atypical features of the nuclear chromatin that have been mentioned. Polypoid carcinomas, then, show all the nuclear features of malignancy in addition to the lengthening of the cell and the nucleus (Figure 4–20). Thus, it is possible to devise a cytologic spectrum of increasing cellular atypia, embracing hyperplastic polyps; adenomas of the tubular, tubulovillous, and villous types; and polypoid carcinoma.

Mesenchymal malignancies can also be diagnosed cytologically. This is particularly true of lymphosarcomas, whose differentiation requires techniques of mi-

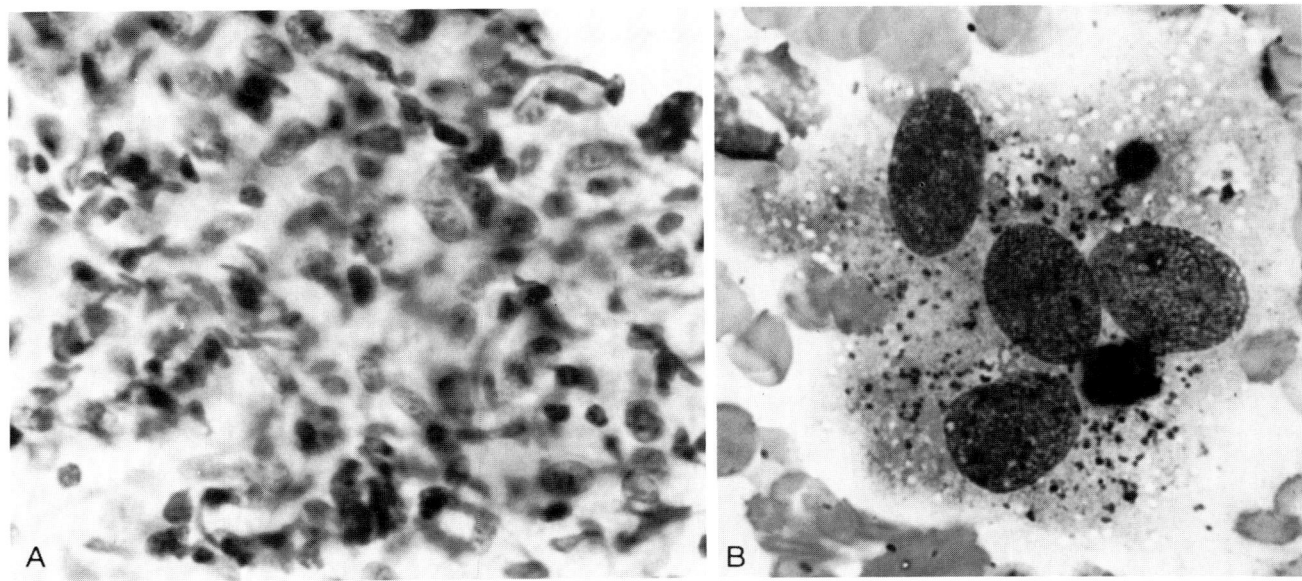

FIGURE 4–19. Crohn's disease of the colon. A, Epitheloid cell granuloma, obtained by endoscopic brushing. (Papanicolaou, ×160) B, Multinucleated giant cell. May-Grünwald-Giemsa, × 800)

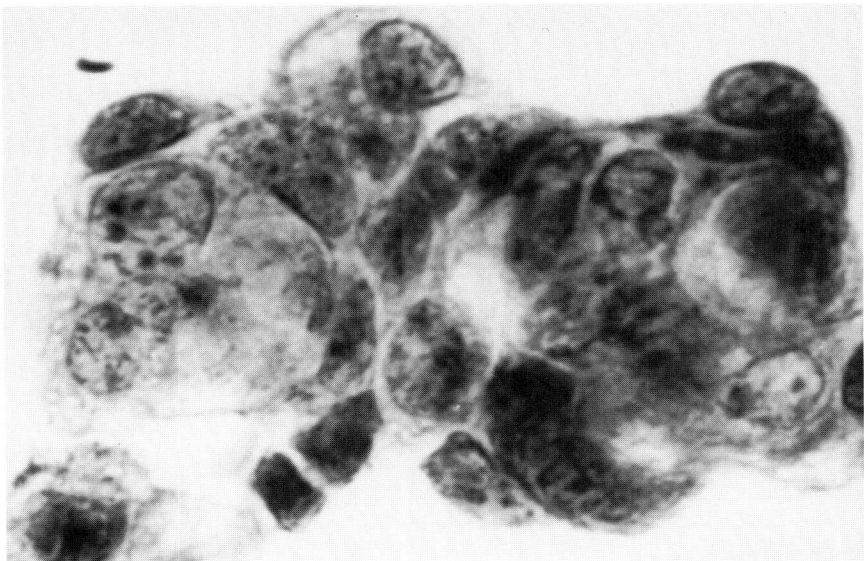

FIGURE 4-20. Tubular adenoma of the colon with severe cellular atypia. (Papanicolaou, × 1000)

croscopy adapted from hematology. The rare, and unfortunately often misdiagnosed, carcinoma of the anus must be mentioned here. This is a squamous cell carcinoma with some signs of keratinization, and it can be diagnosed easily and correctly by the cytologic examination of a smear prepared by means of a cotton wool swab, with or without the aid of a proctoscope.

STATISTICAL EVALUATION OF CYTODIAGNOSES

Esophagus

There is experimental evidence from China concerning the nuclear area in the surface epithelium[13] (Table 4-5). In our own investigations[13] we examined cytologic abrasion smears from the esophagus in a series of patients from two Chinese counties with different incidences of carcinoma of the esophagus (Table 4-6). There is also a high incidence of cancer of the esophagus in South Africa.[32] Among 500 smears from patients without symptoms were 26 showing dysplasia and 15 showing carcinoma.

Among our own patients, in the period from 1981 to 1986 there were 16 cases of cancer of the esophagus. Fifteen of these were correctly diagnosed on endoscopy. Both histologic and abrasion cytologic examinations were positive for tumor in each of 14 cases. In one case, cytology yielded tumor cells when biopsy was falsely negative. In another case the result of histologic examination was positive and that of cytologic examination was negative.

An Italian study involving the combined endoscopic investigation of 173 cases of cancer of the esophagus over a 5-year period used toluidine blue staining of the mucosa for better identification of the lesions.[33] Cytology was positive in 89%; histology, in 84%. Both microscopic examinations had a 3% false-negative rate. In 31 proven cases of esophageal carcinoma, tumor cells were found definitely in 25 cases and probably in 6 over a 5-year period in Australia.[34]

Table 4-5 NUCLEAR AREA OF SQUAMOUS CELLS IN ESOPHAGEAL MUCOSA

	Nuclear Area	
Cell Type	μm^2	RV*
Normal	49.1	1.0
Mild hyperplasia	135.8	2.8
Moderate dysplasia	181.9	3.7
Severe dysplasia	231.9	4.7
"Near carcinoma"	291.2	5.9
Carcinoma	312.8	6.4

*Relative value of nuclear area size as compared with that of the normal cell.

Table 4-6 CYTODIAGNOSIS OF ESOPHAGUS IN PATIENTS FROM TWO CHINESE COUNTIES

			Cytodiagnosis (%)					
					Dysplasia			
County	Rate of Carcinoma	No. of Cases	Normal	Mild Hyperplasia	Moderate	Severe	Near Carcinoma	Carcinoma
Linxian	High	492	52.4	27.3	13.6	2.0	1.2	2.3
Jaoxian	Low	240	74.7	22.5	1.8	0	0	0

In a 6-year period, in a Spanish study, 858 endoscopic examinations of the esophagus and the cardia were performed, including 309 cases with confirmed malignancies.[34a] Cytology was positive for cancer in 93.5%, and no false-positive diagnosis was made in the patients with benign conditions. Biopsies were obtained in only 269 of the tumor cases because of obstructing lesions in 40 patients in whom no satisfactory biopsies could be made, with overall positivity of 77.02%. Cytology increased the yield of biopsy by 20.8%.

A Swiss study[34b] found in 100 cases, including 20 cancers, a sensitivity of 70% for cytology, 80% for histologic biopsy, and 95% for both, with no false-positive results.

A prognostically relevant classification of 37 cases of esophageal carcinoma was undertaken with Feulgen-DNA measurement.[35] In this study, the most favorable prognosis was associated with a predominant hypotriploidy, the least favorable with a hypertetraploidal polyploidy.

Stomach

Qualitative Studies

In the last 5 years we have investigated 145 cases of proven carcinoma of the stomach, comparing material obtained endoscopically for cytology and histology. The endoscopic findings were judged to be neoplastic in 74.5%. Tumor cells were demonstrated cytologically in 70% and histologically confirmed in 89.4% of the tumors. In 17 cases (10.8%), histologic results were positive for tumor, whereas tumor cells were not found cytologically. On the other hand, we had 9 cases (6.2%) with cytologic evidence of tumor in whom no tumor was detectable on histologic biopsy. Tumor cells were described in 3 of 1524 gastroscopic investigations in which no tumor was demonstrable clinically (false-positive rate of cytodiagnosis, 0.2%). From the literature, we had earlier collected 924 cases of proven carcinoma of the stomach in 92.6% in which cytologic examination yielded tumor cells and biopsy showed tumor in 85.1%. In 296 cases of early cancer the corresponding figures for cytologic study and biopsy are 91.6% and 88.9%, respectively.[36,37]

From the recent literature, we collected a further 676 cases of endoscopically demonstrated carcinoma of the stomach (Table 4–7). In this series, cytology yielded tumor cells in 83.6%; and biopsy, with diagnosis of tumor in 85.9%, showed a comparable success rate. We found a false-positive cytologic diagnosis of tumor in 1.8% of 4941 cases in the literature.[37]

In summary, all investigations compared show agreement that the certainty of making a correct diagnosis of tumor is increased if both cytologic and histologic examination is carried out in the same patient. In our experience over a number of years, we have had a false-negative rate for both microscopic methods of between 1% and 2%. In reality, however, there were no true diagnostic failures because these were cases of advanced carcinoma of the stomach that did not permit material suitable for microscopy to be obtained because of advanced necrosis. The diagnoses were, however, readily established visually at endoscopy.

Quantitative Studies

Among the quantitative methods of gastric cytology, a distinction should be made between cytophotometric methods and flow methods. Both are concerned, above all, with measurement of DNA, but micromorphology plays no part in flow methods.

Our own investigations, in association with Sprenger,[16] were performed with the use of single-cell fluorophotometry. For this purpose we first stained the abrasion preparations by Papanicolaou's method and examined them. The same preparations were then decolorized, and DNA was measured with Feulgen-acriflavin staining. Histograms were prepared for each case, together with data on the frequency distribution of DNA values characterized by the following two variables:

(1) The relative mean ploidy (U):

$$U = \frac{\bar{x} \text{ FU in sample population}}{\bar{x} \text{ FU in reference population}}$$

$\bar{x}$ = mean of the measured counts
FU = fluorescent units
Reference population = number of leukocytes, normal intermediate squamous cells, or columnar cells in the preparation
Sample population = number of pathologic cells found in the preparation

(2) The relative frequency of euploid and polyploid DNA values in the sample population (Z):

$$Z = \frac{Nx}{Nx + Ny}$$

N = total number of cells measured
x = all euploid and polyploid cells (mean of the diploid standard population ± 25% or of its multiples ± 25%)
y = all cells not included in x (aneuploid)

We investigated 126 patients with various findings in the gastric mucosa. Histograms of the normal gastric mucosa, of superficial gastritis, and of atrophic gastritis show a peak frequency of diploid cells (stem line). In gastritis, the histogram is expanded as a result of increased cell proliferation to include tetraploid values and, in atrophic gastritis, to include octoploid values (Figure 4–21). Two cases of carcinoma of the stomach (Figure 4–22) show a varying histogram. In the first example, there is an aneuploid stem line at 3c with doubling peaks at 6c and 12c, together with a stem line at 4c. In the second case, a stem line is at 2c with doubling peaks at 4c and 8c. In both histograms there is wide polyploidal scatter up to 32c.

Statistical evaluation of the variables U and Z allows the various groups of cytologic findings and the endo-

Table 4–7 REVIEW OF RECENT REPORTS ON ENDOSCOPICALLY DIAGNOSED GASTRIC CARCINOMA

Reference	Number of Cases	Cytologically Positive	Histologically Positive
Rachail-Arnoux et al.[38]	114	98	104
Simon et al.[39]	72	57	61
Debongnie et al.[40]	96	79	84
Chambers and Clark[41]	163	134	157
Moreno-Otero et al.[42]	194	176	153
Qizilbash et al.[43]	37	33	35
Marbet et al.[34b]	49	30	40
Total	725	607 (83.6%)	634 (85.9%)

scopic diagnostic categories (Figure 4–23) to be separated into significantly different groups. This shows that the relative mean ploidy value (U) is a suitable criterion for differentiating tumor cells from normal cells and from gastric cells that show reactive change. In 20 cases of early gastric cancer, Czernak and associates[44] found two DNA histogram patterns. A diploid type was found in 6 of 7 signet-ring cell carcinomas (diffuse type) and an aneuploid type in 11 of 13 adenocarcinomas of the intestinal type.

Using flow DNA cytometry, we have collected results from 161 examples of gastric abrasion cytology smears.[17] In normal gastric mucosa, most cells are found in the diploid region, only a few in the area between 2c and 4c. Below 2c, there is a fraction representing cell debris. In gastric cancer, the DNA flow histogram is also characterized by a main peak in the diploid region owing to the preponderance of nonmalignant gastric cells in the sample. A second peak at 4c represents a second stem line with scatter to 8c, and this is attributed to tumor cells (Figure 4–24).

We have undertaken a classification of these DNA flow histograms, using discriminance analysis, in benign and malignant and "unsatisfactory" samples and

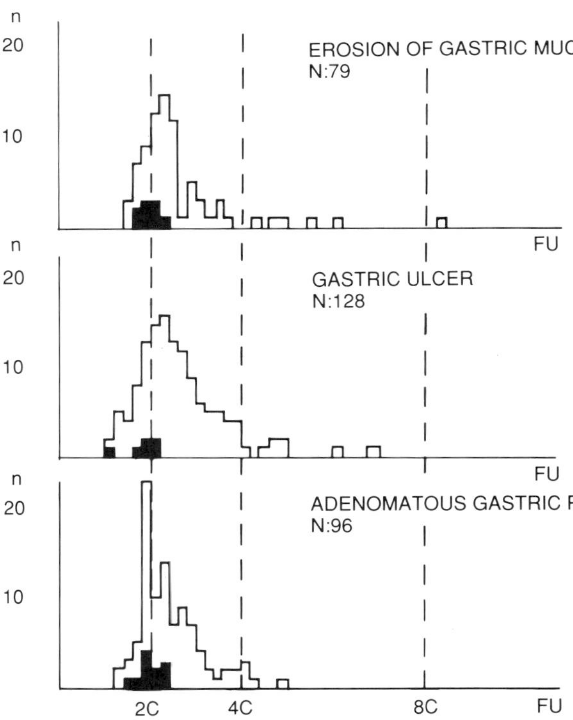

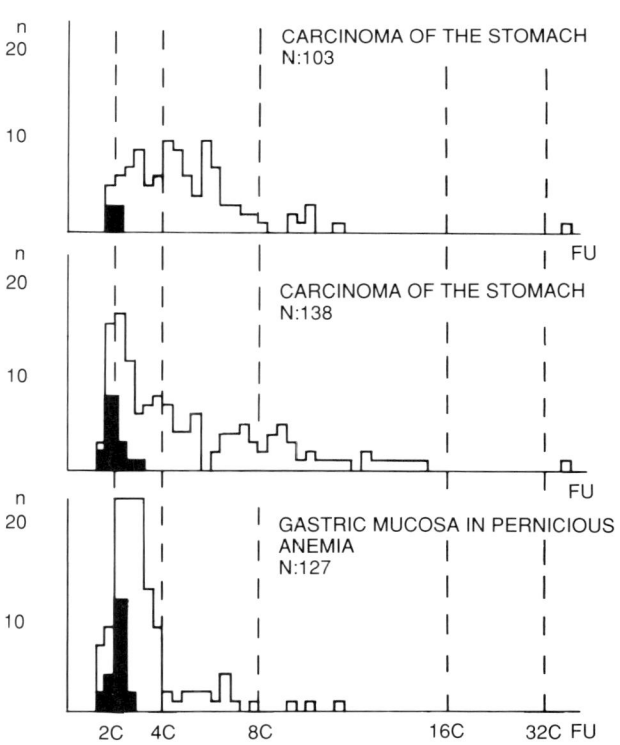

FIGURE 4–21. DNA histograms obtained by single-cell photometry of gastric cell samples from cases of benign gastric lesions. FU, fluorescence units (relative amounts of DNA); n, number of nuclei; 2c, 4c, DNA content, which corresponds to diploid, tetraploid chromosomal set; N, total number of nuclei measured; black columns, white blood cells within the smear as internal standard. (Redrawn from Sprenger E, Witte S: Der diagnostische Wert der Zellkern-DNA-Bestimmung an zytologischen Ausstrichen von gutartigen und bösartigen Veränderungen des Magens. Pathol Res Pract 163:148, 1978.)

FIGURE 4–22. DNA histograms of two cases of gastric carcinoma and a case of pernicious anemia. FU, fluorescence units (relative amounts of DNA); n, number of nuclei; 2c, 4c, DNA content, which corresponds to diploid, tetraploid chromosomal set; N, total number of nuclei measured; black columns, white blood cells within the smear as internal standard. (Redrawn from Sprenger E, Witte S: Der diagnostische Wert der Zellkern-DNS-Bestimmung an zytologischen Ausstrichen von gutartigen und bösartigen Veränderungen des Magens. Pathol Res Pract 163:148, 1978.)

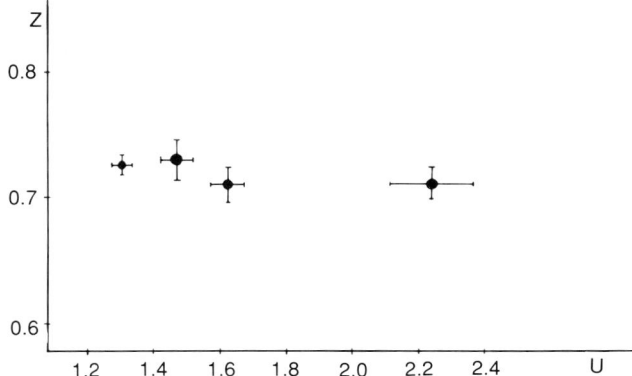

FIGURE 4–23. Mean ploidy DNA values (U) and relative frequency of euploid and polyploid DNA values (Z). Standard deviations of the mean, 126 cases of single-cell DNA measurements in gastric smears. From left to right, cases with normal gastric mucosa, gastric erosions, gastric ulcers, gastric carcinomas. (From Sprenger E, Witte S: Der diagnostische Wert der Zellkern-DNS-Bestimmung an zytologischen Ausstrichen von gutartigen und bösartigen Veränderungen des Magens. Pathol Res Pract 163:148, 1978.)

have compared this with results from conventional cytodiagnosis of the same abrasion smear material (Table 4–8). Of the 37 cases diagnosed as possibly or definitely malignant by conventional techniques, 7 (19%) were not recognized by the DNA flow histogram. Of 122 cases judged to be benign cytologically, 47 (38%) were falsely judged to be positive by the flow method. From these findings it would appear that this method on its own is not capable of achieving a discrimination of practical usefulness between gastric cytograms.

Duodenum

Of 41 cases of papillary carcinoma we were able to diagnose 33 from brush abrasion under endoscopic control by cytologic methods. The histologic biopsy was able to obtain tumor tissue in only 24 cases. In 2 cases, cytologic examination enabled an early diagnosis to be made although they had not been judged to contain malignant tumor on endoscopic examination.

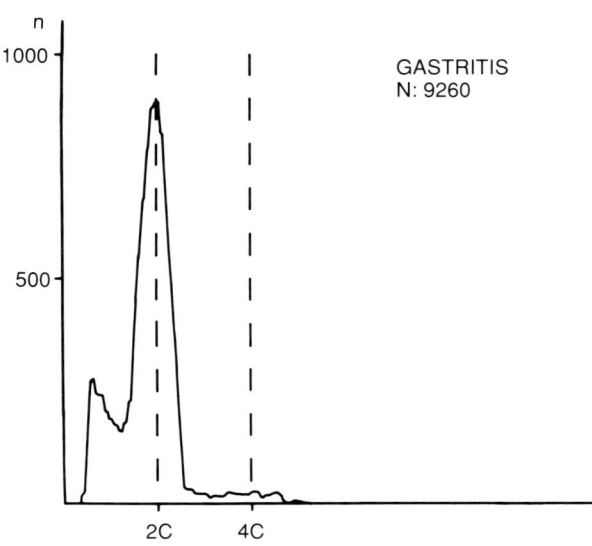

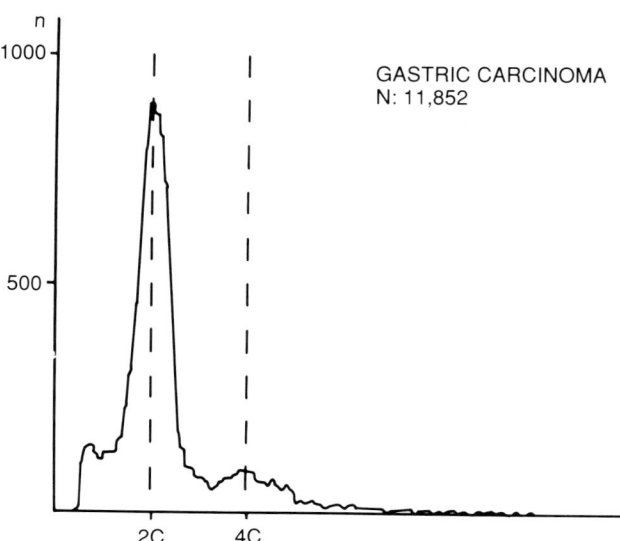

FIGURE 4–24. DNA flow histograms of cell suspensions collected by gastroscopic brushing. Case of superficial gastritis and gastric carcinoma. n, number of nuclei; 2c, 4c, DNA content, which corresponds to diploid, tetraploid chromosomal set; N, total number of nuclei measured. (From Sprenger E, Witte S: The diagnostic significance of flow cytometric nuclear DNA measurement in gastroscopic diagnosis of the stomach. Pathol Res Pract 169:269, 1980.)

Table 4–8 RESULTS OF CONVENTIONAL SMEAR CYTOLOGIC STUDY COMPARED WITH DNA FLOW CYTOMETRY ON CELL SAMPLES OBTAINED BY ROUTINE GASTROSCOPIC BRUSHING

Flow-Cytometric Diagnosis	Cytologic Diagnosis				
	Benign	*Suspicious*	*Malignant*	*Unsatisfactory*	*Total*
Negative	68	6	1	2	77
Positive	47	12	17	0	76
Unsatisfactory	7	1	0	0	8
Total	122	19	18	2	161

Values are calculated by discriminant analysis.[17]
From Sprenger E, Witte S: The diagnostic significance of flow cytometric nuclear DNA measurement in gastroscopic diagnosis of the stomach. Pathol Res Pract 169:269, 1980.

Colon and Rectum

In 182 cases of adenocarcinoma in this region in which biopsy using both brush abrasion and forceps was indicated (in other words, in those cases in which complete polypectomy was not undertaken), we found tumor cells on cytologic examination in 136 cases (75%). The histologic examination resulted in the finding of malignant tumor in 141 (77%). In three of these cases, cytologic results were negative and histologic results positive; and in 8 cases it was the other way around, with cytologic results positive and histologic results negative. In three cases, the preparation for cytology and histology contained only necrotic cells. There were no examples of false-positive cytodiagnosis in our material from 287 endoscopies in nonmalignant disease of the colon.

From the literature we have collected 340 cases of colorectal carcinoma in which cytologic and histologic investigations were undertaken (Table 4–9). The results show that biopsy and cytology have fairly similar diagnostic success, which was improved by cytologic examination in 3% of cases when both methods were used in parallel.

Quantitative investigations of the DNA in cell material from the colon or rectum are only available from the flow analysis of DNA in tissue samples excised or resected for histologic examination, mainly from polyps. Preparations made especially for cytologic study were not evaluated.

In a recent morphometric study[48] of 35 cases with cytologic smears prepared by rectal scraping, including 12 benign adenomas, 14 carcinomas, and 9 irradiated carcinomas free of disease at the time of sampling, a nuclear area of 30 μm^2 was found in 21% of tumor cells but in only 5% of adenoma cells. The nuclear/cytoplasmic ratio, of more than 0.5, showed significant differences between malignant and benign cases and between malignant and treated nonrecurrent cases.

Analysis of chromosomes in abrasion smears taken from the rectum by Xavier and associates[49] showed a normal karyotype in all examples of normal mucosa and in Crohn's disease. In ulcerative colitis, hypotetraploid cells occurred in some cases. In carcinoma, aneuploidy with breakage of chromosomes and marker chromosomes were always present.

References

1. Shu YJ: Cytopathology of the esophagus. Acta Cytol 27:7–16, 1983.
2. Panico FG, Papanicolaou GN, Cooper WA: Abrasive balloon for exfoliation of gastric cancer cells. JAMA 143:1308–1311, 1950.
3. Henning N: Zytodiagnostik von Tumoren. Folia Haematol 70:198–202, 1950.
4. Fukuda T, Shida S, Takita T, Sawada Y: Cytologic diagnosis of early gastric cancer by the endoscopic method with gastrofiberscope. Acta Cytol 11:456–459, 1967.
5. Witte S: Gastroscopic cytology. Endoscopy 2:88–93, 1970.
6. Witte S: Die endoskopische Tumorzelldiagnostik im Bereich des Duodenums. Z Gastroenterol 14:508–514, 1976.
7. Henning N, Witte S: Atlas of Gastrointestinal Cytodiagnosis, 2nd ed. Stuttgart, Georg Thieme, 1970, p 132.
7a. Pinkard KI, Harrison B, Capstick JA, et al: Detection of Campylobacter pyloridis in gastric mucosa by phase contrast microscopy. J Clin Pathol 39:112–113, 1986.
8. Witte S, Ruch F: Moderne Untersuchungsmethoden in der Zytologie. 2. Aufl. Baden-Baden, Gerhard Witzstrock, 1979, p 155.
8a. Witte S, Bloss WH, Schwarzmann P, Strässle G: Quantitative ultraviolet microscopy. In Goeritler K, Feichter GE, Witte S (eds): New Frontiers in Cytology. Berlin, Springer, 1988, pp 140–148.
9. Schümmelfeder N, Ebscher KJ, Krogh E: Acridine orange fluorescence staining. Naturwissensch 44:467, 1957.
10. Papanicolaou GN: Atlas of Exfoliative Cytology. Cambridge, Mass, Harvard University Press, 1954, p 5.
11. Farrant PC: Oral epithelial cells in pernicious anemia. Br Med J 1:1694–1697, 1964.
12. Gardner FH: Cell changes in tropical sprue. J Lab Clin Med 47:529–539, 1956.
13. Witte S: Zytologische Diagnostik des oberen Gastrointestinaltraktes. Leber Magen Darm 14:8–17, 1984.
14. Boon ME, Kurver PHJ, Baak JPA, Thompson HT: The application of morphometry in gastric cytological diagnosis. Virchows Arch [A] 393:159–164, 1981.
15. Böhm N, Sprenger E: Fluorescence cytophotometry, a valuable method for the quantitative determination of nuclear Feulgen-DNA. Histochemie 16:100–118, 1968.
16. Sprenger E, Witte S: Der diagnostische Wert der Zellkern-DNS-Bestimmung an zytologischen Ausstrichen von gutartigen und bösartigen Veränderungen des Magens. Pathol Res Pract 163:148–157, 1978.
17. Sprenger E, Witte S: The diagnostic significance of flow cytometric nuclear DNA measurement in gastroscopic diagnosis of the stomach. Path Res Pract 169:269–275, 1980.
18. Erhardt R, Reinhardt ER, Schlipf W, Bloss WH: FAZYTAN, a system for fast automated cell segmentation, cell image analyses and feature extraction based on TV-image pickup and parallel processing. Anal Quant Cytol Histol 2:25–40, 1980.
19. Witte S, Bloss WH, Reinhardt ER: Differential texture analysis

Table 4–9 COMPARISON OF PARALLEL CYTOLOGIC AND HISTOLOGIC INVESTIGATION AT ENDOSCOPY IN 340 CASES OF PROVEN CARCINOMA OF THE COLON OR RECTUM FROM THE LITERATURE

Reference	Number of Cases	Cytologically Positive	Histologically Positive	Either Positive
Halter[45]	77	70	46	74
Debongnie et al.[46]	60	42	51	56
Watanabe[31]	44	42	38	?
Rachail-Arnoux et al.[38]	86	74	82	83
Miczban and Feher[47]	11	11	11	11
Marbet et al.[34b]	62	51	42	59
Total	340	290 (79.4%)	270 (79.4%)	283* (95.6%)

*These numbers do not include Watanabe's cases.

of short wave length absorbances in unfixed cells. International Conference on High Resolution Cell Image Analysis, North Hollywood, Calif, 1982.
20. Bloss WH, Reinhardt ER, Strässle G, et al: Unpublished data.
21. Shen Q: Diagnostic cytology and early detection. In Huang GJ, Kai WY (eds): Carcinoma of the Esophagus and Gastric Cardia. Berlin-Heidelberg, Springer, 1984, pp 155–190.
22. Horai T, Kobayashi A, Tateishi R, et al: A cytologic study on small cell carcinoma of the esophagus. Cancer 41:1890–1896, 1978.
23. Elster K, Heinkel K, Henning N: Glandular cells in gastric biopsy. Frankf Z Pathol 67:170–176, 1957.
24. Bigotti A, Crespi M: Citopatologia e citodiagnostica apparato digerente. In Cavallero (ed): Trattato di citopatologia e citodiagnostica. Rome, Marrapesa, 1976, pp 387–441.
25. Cabré-Fiol V, Vilardell F: Progress in the cytological diagnosis of gastric lymphoma. Cancer 41:1456–1461, 1978.
26. Sato A, Ishioka K, Kobiyama M, et al: Cytological diagnosis of leiomyogenic tumors of the stomach. Tohoku J Exp Med 132:213–223, 1980.
26a. Gad A: Rapid diagnosis of Campylobacter pylori by brush cytology. Scand J Gastroenterol 24 (Suppl 167):101–103, 1989.
27. Cheli R, Aste H, Nicoló G, Ciancamerla G: Cytological findings in chronic non-specific duodenitis. Endoscopy 6:110–115, 1974.
28. Baczako K, Büchler M, Beger HG, et al: Morphogenesis and possible precursor lesions of invasive carcinoma of the papilla of Vater: Epithelial dysplasia and adenoma. Hum Pathol 16:305–310, 1985.
29. Witte S: Die endoskopische Tumorzelldiagnostik im Bereich des Duodenums. Z Gastroenterol 14:508–514, 1976.
30. Witte S, Göbel D: Zytodiagnostik der Colitis ulcerosa. Leber Magen Darm 3:131–134, 1973.
31. Watanabe H: Cytological diagnosis of cancer of the colon and rectum. Tohoku J Exp Med 154:169–176, 1987.
32. Berry AV, Baskind AF, Hamilton DG: Cytologic screening for esophageal cancer. Acta Cytol 25:135–147, 1981.
33. Norberto L, Cusumano A, Martella B, et al: Evaluation critique des prélèvements cyto-histologiques perendoscopiques après coloration vitale au bleu de Toluidine dans le cancer de l'oesophage. Acta Endosc 15:327–329, 1985.
34. Drake M: Gastro-esophageal Cytology. Basel, S. Karger, 1985, p 267.
34a. Cussó X, Monés-Xiol J, Vilardell F: Endoscopic cytology of cancer of the esophagus and cardia: A long-term evaluation. Gastrointest Endosc 35:321–323, 1989.
34b. Marbet UA, Dalquen P, Stalder GA, Gyr K: Wertigkeit von Biopsie und gezielter Bürstenzytologie bei der gastrointestinalen Karzinomdiagnostik aufgrund der Endoskopien von 1979–1984. Schweiz Med Wochenschr 115:1007–1009, 1985.
35. Hiratsuka R: Clinicopathological studies of DNA content in nuclei of cells isolated from patients with esophageal carcinoma. Fukuoka Acta Med 72:556, 1981.
36. Witte S: Cytologie des Magens. In Demling L (ed): Handbuch der inneren Medizin. 5. Aufl. Berlin, Springer-Verlag, 1974, pp 355–380.
37. Witte S: Magenzytologie. Baden-Baden, Gerhard Witzstrock, 1987, p 80.
38. Rachail-Arnoux M, Aubert H, Zarski J-P, et al: Résultats du cyto-diagnostic dirigé sous contrôle endoscopique dans 248 cas de cancers digestifs. Gastroenterol Clin Biol 7:158–163, 1983.
39. Simon L, Bajtai A, Figus I, Vaskó I: Clinical value of exfoliative and abrasive cytology in the diagnostics of gastric cancer and precanceroses. Arch Geschwulstforsch 47:719–727, 1977.
40. Debongnie I-C, Legros G, Beyaert C: Apport de la cytologie du tractus digestif supérieur dans un hôpital général. Acta Endosc 15:337–342, 1985.
41. Chambers LA, Clark II WE: The endoscopic diagnosis of gastroesophageal malignancy: A cytologic review. Acta Cytol 30:110–114, 1986.
42. Moreno-Otero R, Martinez-Raposo A, Cantero J, Pajares JM: Exfoliative cytodiagnosis of gastric adenocarcinoma. Comparison with biopsy and endoscopy. Acta Cytol 27:485–488, 1983.
43. Qizilbash AH, Castelli M, Kowalski MA, Churly A: Endoscopic brush cytology and biopsy in the diagnosis of cancer of the upper gastrointestinal tract. Acta Cytol 24:313–318, 1980.
44. Czernak B, Herz F, Koss LG: DNA distribution patterns in early gastric carcinomas. Cancer 59:113–117, 1987.
45. Halter F: Brush cytology in colonic malignancies. Hepatogastroenterology 28:178, 1981.
46. Debongnie I-C, Legros G, Beyaert C: Cytologie des lésiens inflammatoires et néoplasiques du colon. Acta Endosc 15:331–336, 1985.
47. Miczban I, Feher M: Die Bedeutung der zytologischen Untersuchungen in der Erkennung der neoplastischen Veränderungen des Rectosigmoideums. Tijdschr Gastroenterol 20(4):237–249, 1977.
48. Gérad F, Guerret S, Gérard J-P, Grimaud I-A: Usefulness of morphometry in the cytologic assessment of rectal tumors. Anal Quant Cytol Histol 12:181, 1990.
49. Xavier RG, Prolla JC, Benvenuti GA, Kirsner JB: Tissue cytogenetic studies in chronic ulcerative colitis and carcinoma of the colon. Cancer 34:684–695, 1974.

CHAPTER 5

Structure and Function of the Immunologic System of the Gastrointestinal Tract

DAVID F. KEREN, M.D.

CONCEPT OF A MUCOSAL IMMUNE SYSTEM

ANATOMY OF THE GUT IMMUNE SYSTEM

MUCOSAL LYMPHOID CELLS

ANTIGEN PROCESSING IN THE GUT

CHARACTERISTICS OF SECRETORY IGA

CONCEPT OF A MUCOSAL IMMUNE SYSTEM

The immune system is known to be important in our bodies' defense against pathogenic microorganisms, their toxic products, and altered states of host cells such as neoplasia. In general, we think of immunity as resulting from a parenteral administration of antigen with a resultant immunoglobulin G (IgG) response in the serum or with development of cell-mediated immunity to this antigen. However, in nature, it is relatively unusual that we are stimulated by foreign antigens in that manner. Our most common exposure to antigens is through the mucosal surface. Daily, we ingest a wide variety of foreign material, most of which is antigenic and does cause the formation of an immunologic response. Because the response does not usually result in the formation of systemic IgG or systemic cell-mediated immunity, it is usually not detected. Antigens given orally elicit the production of secretory IgA in the intestine and along other mucosal surfaces. Further, this route of antigen presentation gives a negative signal that prevents systemic sensitization to antigens that we routinely ingest or inhale.

The concept of a mucosal immune system is not new. Indeed, the first formal experimental study of oral immunization was presented to the Academie des Sciences in Paris in 1880 by Pasteur.[1] In that communication, he noted that chickens became immune to chicken cholera after ingesting food saturated with that agent in an attenuated form. Unfortunately, he obtained inconsistent results when using the oral route to protect sheep from anthrax and decided to discontinue this mode of immunization in his future studies. The idea of protecting humans from infectious agents by oral immunization was proposed by Ferran, who, as early as 1885, found that attenuated cholera vibrios given orally would protect both animals and humans from disease.[2]

That oral immunization might protect against dysentery and other enteric diseases was demonstrated shortly after the turn of the century.[3-5] This work was soon followed up by Besredka's famous work. While studying the immune responses to paratyphoid, Besredka needed more control mice for an experiment, and he was forced to use a mouse that had received paratyphoid orally a month earlier. Much to his surprise, this mouse survived inoculation with a normally lethal dose of paratyphoid.[6] After World War I, Besredka vigorously pursued the study of local immunity and was successful in using oral immunization to protect against dysentery, cholera, and typhoid in both laboratory experiments and clinical trials.[7] The mechanism of this local immunity was found to correlate with agglutinating antibodies in the stool specimens from patients with dysentery and not with serum antibody levels.[8] Fascinating, in part because it antedates by over three quarters of a century the idea of locally stimulated lymphocytes traveling to other mucosal surfaces throughout the body, was the work of Paul Erlich in 1891. He found that antibodies to vegetable poisons could be found in both serum and milk after mice were fed this material.[9,10] Furthermore, these mammary secretions were capable of protecting suckling mice from the poisons for several weeks.

It is now known that systemic (IgG) immunity does not correlate well with protection along mucosal surfaces, however. One of the earliest studies to demonstrate this dichotomy was performed by Elie Metchnikoff in 1894.[11] He noted that although subcutaneous immunization of young rabbits would protect them against an intraperitoneal challenge by *Vibrio cholera* (an artificial experimental method still used today for studying immunity to infectious diseases), these rabbits were not protected from challenge by *V. cholera* via the natural route of oral infection. Further evidence of the divergence of and possibly occasional antagonism between the local and systemic immune responses was provided by Wells and Osborne.[12] They demonstrated that prior daily ingestion of various vegetable proteins would render animals insensitive to subsequent attempts to elicit systemic anaphylactic reactions to the fed antigen.

Clearly, a considerable foundation of the potentials of oral immunization was provided by these early studies. It was, however, the discovery by Tomasi et al. that IgA is the main antibody on mucosal surfaces that provided the key to beginning definitive work to understand the biology of the mucosal immune system.[13] While many surfaces (bronchial mucosa, mammary glands, conjunctiva, genitourinary tract, etc.) other than the gastrointestinal tract are also involved in mucosal immunity, the gastrointestinal tract is the major site of antigenic stimulation and immune response for the secretory IgA system.[14] This chapter will review the gross anatomy, histology, and cellular interactions involved in the local immune response of the gut.

ANATOMY OF THE GUT IMMUNE SYSTEM

The major structures of the gut-associated lymphoid tissue (GALT) consist of Peyer's patches, isolated lymphoid follicles, the appendix, and mesenteric lymph nodes. These structures have in common the presence of lymphocytes that have different functional capabilities from lymphocytes located in peripheral lymph nodes (Table 5–1).

Table 5–1 LYMPHOID POPULATIONS IN GUT-ASSOCIATED LYMPHOID TISSUES

Precursor B cell for the IgA response
Switch T lymphocytes
Helper T cells for the IgA response
Suppressor T cells for the IgA response

Peyer's patches are grossly identifiable aggregates of lymphoid nodules that are most prominent in the ileum, although they are present throughout the small intestine. By defining a Peyer's patch as consisting of at least five lymphoid follicles, Cornes was able to quantify the number and location of these structures in a large series of autopsies (Table 5–2).[15] The average number of Peyer's patches in humans increases from about 50 at 24 to 29 weeks of gestation to almost 250 by adolescence.[15] During adulthood, a gradual decline is seen in the numbers of these structures such that in individuals over 70 years of age less than 100 are usually found. The variation in numbers of Peyer's patches at different ages indicates that this lymphoid tissue is not static, but is continuously involved in a dynamic interaction with the luminal antigens. Development of Peyer's patches has been studied in experimental animals. Primordial structures can first be detected along the intestine about halfway through gestation.[16] Within a few days after their appearance, a striking proliferation of the follicular areas occurs. At birth, Peyer's patches have the greatest density of proliferating lymphoid cells in the body.[16] The increase in numbers of Peyer's patches after birth probably reflects the initial response of the host immune system to the wide variety of environmental antigens that pass through the gastrointestinal tract. As will be discussed later in this chapter, such education is important both to arm the body for a secretory IgA response to the antigen and to disarm the body for a potentially self-destructive systemic IgG, IgE, or cell-mediated immunity to the same antigens.

The size of Peyer's patches can vary greatly. The lower limit of gross visualization is probably at the level of five aggregated follicles,[15] but some patches as large as 30 cm have been described. This also probably reflects the current state of stimulation of these structures. In germ-free animals, for instance, they are quite

Table 5–2 PEYER'S PATCHES IN HUMANS

Age	Average Number of Peyer's Patches*		
	N	Mean	SD
Gestation 24–29 weeks	6	118.50	16.37
Gestation 30 weeks to birth	8	154.75	36.27
Newborn	7	197.43	35.44
6 months	5	266.80	90.86
1–6 years	7	306.86	89.06
12 years	5	478.40	137.97

*N, number of cases; SD, standard deviation.
Data summarized from Cornes.[15]

small but enlarge when the animals are exposed to microorganisms.[17] Histologically, Peyer's patches have been divided into specific areas on the basis of their composition of lymphocytes (Figure 5–1). The large lymphoid follicles are the histologic counterpart of the grossly seen nodules. These areas are rich in B lymphocytes, which are precursors of IgA-secreting plasma cells. The process by which these cells mature to that end will be discussed later. Above the follicles, and just beneath a specialized surface epithelium, is the dome-corona area. The epithelium overlying the dome-corona area contains M cells, which can take up luminal antigens and transport them to adjacent lymphoid tissues.[18] The dome-corona area contains medium-sized lymphocytes and has many macrophages filled with cell debris, lipofuscin-like material, and bacterial remnants. The latter likely reflect the fact that this is the area where luminal antigens are first processed within the GALT. Between the follicles are the T-lymphocyte–dependent areas. This area consists mainly of small lymphocytes with a few macrophages and prominent postcapillary venules (PCVs). These PCVs are sites where lymphocytes travel into the Peyer's patches.[19]

Peyer's patches are enriched in precursor B lymphocytes, which will preferentially mature to become IgA-secreting plasma cells. Although some of the capabilities of these IgA precursor B lymphocytes may be inherent in their genetic programming,[20] it is clear that they are influenced by T lymphocytes present within GALT. Switch T cells, helper T cells, and possibly contrasuppressor cells in GALT encourage B lymphocytes to differentiate and mature as IgA-secreting plasma cells. Suppressor T cells are also present, which inhibit production of systemic immunity to orally administered antigens (see later). Functional macrophages and dendritic cells are prominent within Peyer's patches. The macrophages are phagocytic, and the Ia$^+$ dendritic cells can collaborate with T and B cells in supporting immune responses.[20] Plasma cells are not found within the lymphoid tissues of the Peyer's patch; however, they are abundant in the surrounding lamina propria (Figure 5–2). Because isolated lymphoid follicles are present throughout the gastrointestinal tract, they represent the most abundant discrete lymphoid structure of GALT. Random sections of small intestine or colon will contain one such structure; indeed, colonic biopsies of "small polyps" are frequently nothing more than isolated follicles. In the colon there are an average of three such nodules per square centimeter.[21] Although they look like small Peyer's patches histologically (Figure 5–3), their small size (1 to 3 mm) has precluded their isolation for functional studies *in vitro*. There is some objective evidence, however, that they share functions similar to those of the better characterized Peyer's patches. The epithelium overlying these structures contains the same M cells that can sample luminal antigens as does their counterpart epithelium overlying the dome area of Peyer's patches.[22] Further, other studies of mucosal immunity have implicated these structures in the initiation of a secretory immune response in the gut.[23]

Although in humans the appendix is a relatively small, blind tubular process of the cecum with no digestive function, it may have a role in mucosal immunity. The human appendix does have large lymphoid follicles and a specialized surface epithelium resembling both the Peyer's patches and isolated lymphoid follicles. This overlying epithelium differs considerably from that of the surrounding colon; specialized follicle-associated epithelium with antigen-sampling capabilities has been demonstrated overlying dome-corona areas in the human appendix.[24] Obviously, mesenteric lymph nodes do not share the intimate relationship to the gut lumen that the Peyer's patches, isolated lymphoid follicles, and appendix enjoy. Nonetheless, mesenteric lymph nodes are an important part of GALT. Upon cellular analysis *in vitro*, they can be seen to contain the same types of IgA precursor B lymphocytes

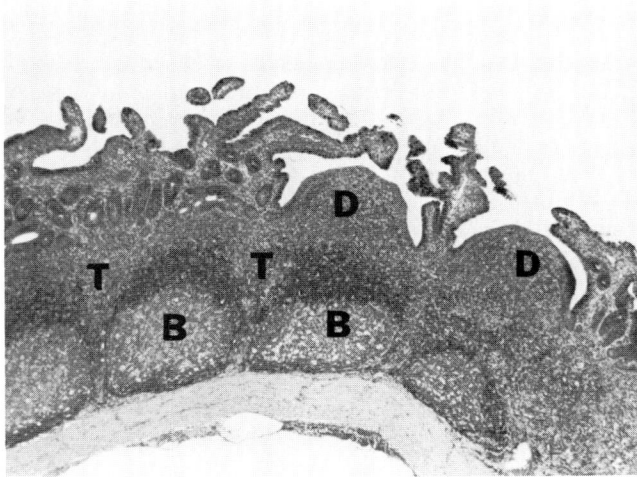

FIGURE 5–1. This Peyer patch shows the characteristic dome-corona area (D) where antigen is first processed, the B-cell follicular areas (B), and the T-cell interfollicular regions (T).

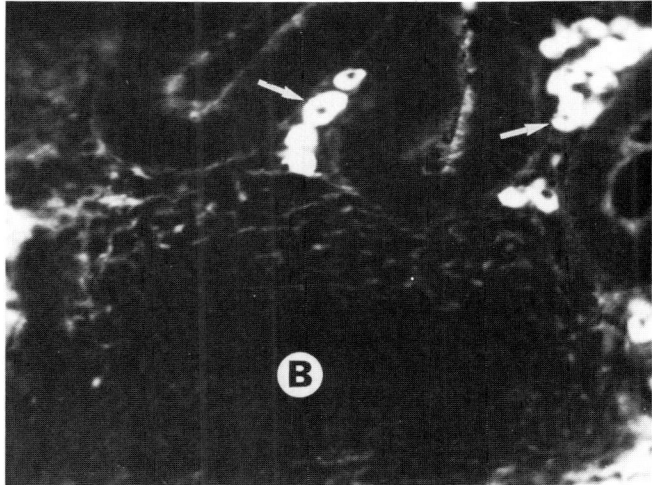

FIGURE 5–2. This Peyer patch was stained with fluorescein-conjugated anti-IgA. Note that the lymphoid nodule that contains precursor B lymphocytes (B) is negative, whereas IgA-containing plasma cells in adjacent villi are clearly evident (arrows).

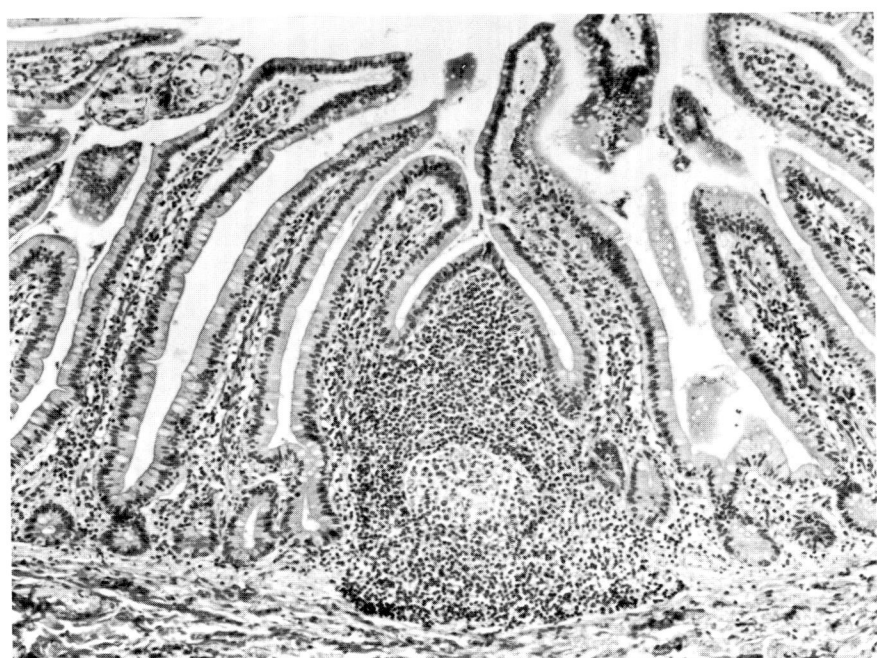

FIGURE 5–3. Isolated lymphoid follicles occur throughout the gastrointestinal tract. They have specialized surface epithelium for antigen uptake, as do Peyer's patches.

that are prominent in Peyer's patches.[25] Further, although they do not receive antigen directly from M cells, they receive lymphatic drainage from the intestine, which contains both GALT lymphocytes and mucosal antigen. In humans, the lymph flow that parallels the course of the superior mesenteric artery drains into lymph nodes within the mesentery itself, whereas the lymph flow that parallels the course of the inferior mesenteric artery supplies the periaortic and superior mesenteric lymph nodes. Despite their unique immunologic composition, histologically, one cannot distinguish these lymph nodes from peripheral lymph nodes throughout the body. It is not clear whether they are merely serving as way stations for lymphocytes that are traveling from the major GALT structures or whether they are unique sources of specialized GALT lymphocytes.

MUCOSAL LYMPHOID CELLS

The intestinal mucosa contains the largest collection of cells actively engaged in immune responses in the body. Included among these cells are plasma cells, lymphocytes, macrophages, granulocytes, and mast cells. Most of these cells are located in the lumina propria; however, some important subpopulations of cells are found between epithelial cells (interepithelial lymphocytes), and other important populations are present within the submucosa. Plasma cells are abundant in the lamina propria throughout the gastrointestinal tract. Human infants usually lack immunoglobulin-containing cells for the first week of life.[26] By the second week, IgM-containing cells predominate, although some IgA-containing plasma cells are present. After 1 month of age, IgA assumes its role as the main immunoglobulin of lamina propria plasma cells (Table 5–3); and after 1 year, adult numbers of plasma cells are attained. Relatively few (about 10%) IgG-containing plasma cells are normally present in the gut. Lamina propria plasma cells are continually replaced in adult life, depending on the local stimulation in the gut. During active inflammatory events, such as active ulcerative colitis, an increase in all three isotypes of plasma cells is commonly seen.[27] In patients with the extremely common IgA deficiency (1 in 700), a compensatory increase in IgM-containing plasma cells is usually seen. In normal adults, there are about 350,000 IgA-, 50,000 IgM-, and 10,000 IgG-containing plasma cells per cubic millimeter along the lumina propria.[28] IgE-containing plasma cells are also normally found in the gut lamina propria,[29] along with IgD-containing cells, representing 1% of the lamina propria plasma cells.[30] Some studies, however, have detected considerably more IgE-containing cells in the upper small intestine.[31] Such variation may represent mild gut allergies, which are known to be associated with increased IgE plasma cells.[32] Further, the number of lamina propria plasma cells is also known to be affected by antibiotic administration in animals.[33]

The lymphocytes within the mucosa can be divided

Table 5–3 DEVELOPMENT OF GUT PLASMA CELLS

Age	IgA Plasma Cells*	IgM Plasma Cells	IgG Plasma Cells
0–1 months	14	26	5
1–3 months	112	53	4
3–6 months	163	59	6
6 months to 2 years	408	137	54

*Cells per high-power field.
Data from Perkkio and Savilahti.[26]

into two major compartments: interepithelial lymphocytes (IELs) and lamina propria lymphocytes (LPLs). Near the turn of the century, pathologists thought that the lymphocytes within the surface epithelium were senescent cells on their way (as it were) out into that great stream of life. Through the use of monoclonal antibody immunohistochemistry and *in vitro* studies, we now know that IELs are a specialized population of lymphocytes that are far from senescent. These cells exist between, not within, epithelial cells (Figure 5–4). They are medium-sized lymphocytes, many of which contain lysosomal granules.[34] Most IELs in humans are T lymphocytes[35] (Table 5–4), which express surface antigens associated with suppressor/cytotoxic T cells (CD8 [formerly T8 or Leu-2a]).[36] From the stomach through the rectum, less than 5% of IELs are B cells, as judged by their expression of the Ia antigen (class II histocompatibility surface antigen).[37] Indeed, this is probably an overestimation of the number of B lymphocytes, because many other cell types (including epithelium itself) can express the Ia antigen. When T cells are activated, they often express Ia. The lack of such expression among the gut IELs suggests that they are not in an activated state. The fact that the same percentage of suppressor/cytotoxic T cells is found in the IELs of experimental animals implies that they serve a specialized (presumably protective) function that is of common importance in evolution.[38]

Several studies have isolated IELs and shown that they are viable cells that can function in a variety of cytotoxic *in vitro* reactions. The exact amount of cytotoxic capability of these cells is still unclear, because the methods used to isolate the cells can have a negative effect on their biologic activity.[39] Nonetheless, IELs have been shown to be capable of several types of cytotoxic activity, including antibody-dependent cell-mediated cytotoxicity (ADCC), spontaneous cell-mediated cytotoxicity (SCMC), and mitogen-induced cellular cytotoxicity (MICC). This activity is always, however, considerably weaker than the activity by peripheral blood lymphocytes. Further, recent studies indicate that known potentiators of cytotoxic activity such as interferon or interleukin-2 do not elicit cytotoxic effects.[40] It is clear that IELs are actively responding to their environment and that they may play a role in some intestinal disorders. For instance, germ-free mice have significantly fewer IELs than conventional mice

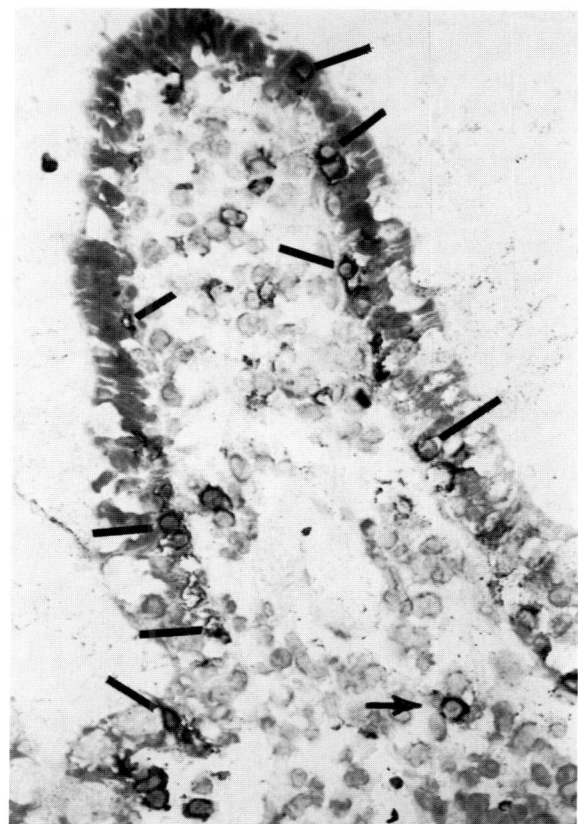

FIGURE 5–4. Interepithelial lymphocytes (indicated) have been identified by anti-CD8 (formerly T8), indicating their suppressor/cytotoxic phenotype. Note the occasional positive cell in the lamina propria (arrow). (Courtesy of Dr. William O. Dobbins, University of Michigan School of Medicine, Ann Arbor, Michigan.)

have,[41] which indicates that these cells respond to the normal flora of the gut. Also, increased numbers of IELs are found in some inflammatory conditions of the gut, including gluten-sensitive enteropathy,[42] but not in inflammatory bowel disease.[43]

The IELs differ considerably from the LPLs, which have the same 2:1 helper/suppressor phenotype as do lymphocytes in the peripheral blood.[40,42–44] Also, although the IELs have only rare lymphocytes in an activated state (with surface Ia and Tac antigen), the LPLs have many T cells with these surface markers.[42,43]

Table 5–4 PHENOTYPES OF MUCOSAL LYMPHOCYTES

Location	T11	T8	T4	T4/T8
Intraepithelial (IEL)*				
Ileum	13.0 + 8.2	13.1 + 6.9	2.0 + 2.1	0.13 + 0.1
Colon	5.1 + 3.6	4.8 + 2.3	0.69 + 1.1	0.20 + 0.1
Lamina Propria (LPL)†				
Ileum	33.6 + 5.5	13.0 + 3.5	24.8 + 3.7	2.0 + 0.6
Colon	27.7 + 6.3	10.8 + 4.1	19.0 + 5.9	1.9 + 0.6

*IEL data expressed as positive lymphoid cells per 100 epithelial cell nuclei.
†LPL data expressed as positive lymphoid cells per 100 mononuclear cells.
From Hirata I, Berrebi G, Austin LL, et al: Immunohistological characterization of intraepithelial and lamina propria lymphocytes in control ileum and colon and in inflammatory bowel disease. Dig Dis Sci 31:593, 1986.

There is good evidence from studies of human colonic mucosa that the LPLs function well in mitogen-induced cell-mediated cytotoxicity with phytohemagglutinin as the mitogen.[45] They do not function as well as peripheral blood lymphocytes in spontaneous cell-mediated cytotoxicity.[45] Overall, LPLs have cell populations and functional capabilities similar to those of peripheral blood lymphocytes, whereas IELs are a selected population of T lymphocytes that play a role in host defense at the mucosal surface.

A third, albeit minor, population of peripheral blood lymphocytes in humans is the natural killer cell. These cells are identified by surface markers and by their ability to destroy certain cell lines *in vitro*. It has been suggested that they may play a role in host defense against neoplasia.[46] Most of these cells react with the Leu-7 (also known as HNK-1) monoclonal antibody. Although many of the IELs are large granulated cells that superficially resemble the large granulated natural killer cells found in the peripheral blood, none of the IELs react with the Leu-7 (HNK-1) antibody.[40] Although this does not rule out the possibility that some of these IELs have a natural killer function, it is clear that there is not a 1:1 correlation of routine histologic structure and surface antigen expression. Some workers have demonstrated a minor natural killer activity of these cells when they are carefully isolated with collagenase and EDTA.[47] While the lamina propria is essentially devoid of these cells when immunohistochemical methods are used,[48] when lymphokines are used to activate the functions of the isolated cells, they can express natural killer activity.[49] The complexities of the techniques to determine the function of these cells plus the fact that they are a minor population even in the peripheral blood limit our present ability to specifically define the role of these cells in the gut.

A complex type of cytotoxic activity involving a collaboration between killer cells (which may be lymphocytes, monocytes, or granulocytes) and antibody has been described in the gastrointestinal tract. This ADCC has been shown to function with secretory IgA directed against specific bacterial pathogens (*Shigella flexneri* and *Salmonella typhi*).[50,51] Although these have all been demonstrated *in vitro*, it is tempting to speculate on the importance of a cytotoxic mechanism that involves the main secretory immunoglobulin of the gut and mucosal cells capable of cytotoxic function. A similar collaboration has been shown in experimental animals for dealing with intestinal parasites. In work by Capron et al., it was found that eosinophils could destroy schistosomes that were coated with a reagenic form of mouse IgG.[52] Such a role for eosinophils in host defense against parasites provides a logical explanation for the eosinophilia commonly observed in patients with parasitic infestations.

Macrophages are present both in the lamina propria and within the organized GALT. Work by Bull and Bookman[53] indicated that the lamina propria macrophages are present in an activated state (Table 5–5). Although some earlier workers doubted the existence of functional macrophages within Peyer's patches, it is quite clear that macrophages are present in these and other GALT structures.[54] Further, they probably play a major role in processing luminal antigens.[55]

Granulocytes are also found in normal human intestine, eosinophils representing as many as 3% of cells isolated from human colonic mucosa.[53] Neutrophils, however, are associated with acute inflammation and are not seen in the uninflamed human bowel. Mucosal mast cells are a heterogeneous group of cells that function at least in response to parasitic infestations.[56] They arise from the bone marrow,[57] are influenced by the microflora of the gut,[58] and are attracted by the production of interleukin-3 by T cells in the mucosa.[59] Experimental work has indicated that these cells are active in expulsion of a variety of intestinal parasites.[60,61] Befus et al. found that these cells could be stained readily when the tissues were fixed in Carnoy's fixative, but not when routine formalin fixation was employed.[62] This implies that in most tissues examined, pathologists considerably underestimate the mast cell content.

Table 5–5 CHARACTERISTICS OF MUCOSAL MACROPHAGES

Characteristic	Macrophage Source	
	Intestinal	*Peripheral Blood*
Granularity	4+	1+
Phagocytosis	4+	1–2+
Pseudopod	Present	Usually absent

Data from Bull and Bookman.[53]

ANTIGEN PROCESSING IN THE GUT

It has been known for many years that orally administered antigen can pass into the systemic circulation. Only recently, however, has evidence been presented that suggests the route by which antigens in the gut lumen stimulate mucosal immune responses under normal physiologic circumstances. Bockman and Cooper demonstrated that the epithelium overlying lymphoid follicles in Peyer's patches, the appendix, or the bursa of Fabricius (in the chick) could imbibe intraluminal antigens.[24] The specific nature of the functional cells was identified by Owen, who observed uptake of macromolecules by these specialized follicle-associated epithelial cells, which he termed M cells.[18] These cells have also been identified overlying isolated lymphoid follicles in the gut, which implies a similar function for these structures.[22] These cells have shorter, more irregular microvilli than adjacent absorptive columnar epithelial cells. They originate from the adjacent crypt epithelium[63] and have more intense esterase but weaker alkaline phosphatase activity than the surrounding cells.[19] In an attempt to explain the unique functions of these cells, Madara et al. found that these cells have a low protein/lipid ratio, compared with absorptive epithelium, and contain abundant morphologically detectable cholesterol, except in areas involved in endocytosis.[64] Adhesion of virus, parasites, and bacteria to these cells is the first step in the processing of luminal antigens by the GALT. The adhesion of these microorganisms may, however, provide an important route for invasion of host cells[65,66] (Figure 5–5).

Paneth cells are poorly characterized cells found in the depth of crypts in the small intestine. Although their location in the bottom of the crypts would not suggest an important role in sampling luminal antigens, it is clear that these cells have phagocytic capabilities *in vivo* and *in vitro*.[67,68] This, together with the Paneth cell hyperplasia that occurs in blind loop syndrome and intestinal bacterial overgrowth, suggests that these cells respond to microorganisms in the gut.[68,69] Finally, these cells contain lysozyme and may function in a specialized way to deal with microorganisms under unusual circumstances.

After antigen has been taken up from the gut lumen, it is transported into the underlying lymphoid tissues in GALT, where it can be processed by dendritic cells and may contact antigen-specific precursors for IgA-secreting plasma cells.[70] There is an elaborate capillary flow in these follicles that may play a role in distributing antigen to the sensitive lymphocytes.[71] The stimulated IgA precursor B lymphocytes leave the GALT shortly after stimulation and travel through the lymphatic drainage to mesenteric lymph nodes.[25] From here, cells enter the lymph that flows into the thoracic duct. By this time, most of the lymphocytes are large, rapidly dividing lymphoblasts. The cells mature further in the spleen, and possibly at other sites.[71,72] It is at these sites that they come under the influence of helper T cells for stimulating the IgA response and suppressor T cells for inhibiting the IgG and IgM responses to the luminal antigen (see later). Thereafter, these cells migrate through the systemic circulation to a variety of mucosal surfaces, including the gut, bronchial mucosa, salivary glands, mammary glands, conjunctiva, and genitourinary secretions. The total time for this journey from the GALT back to the mucosa is about 4 to 6 days. It is clear that a mucosal memory response can be elicited by multiple oral challenges with live microorganisms.[73,74] The reason for this circuitous route is hypothesized to be the arming of all mucosal surfaces to an antigen present in the environment. The paltry defenses of neonates are considerably aided by the secretory IgA in the breast milk. Studies in newborn nurseries have found that babies fed breast milk have a significantly lower rate of enterotoxigenic *Escherichia coli* diarrhea, compared with their counterparts who are fed only formula. Further, the work of Goldblum et al.[75] clearly indicates that the IgA in maternal secretions reflects the specific microorganisms present in their gastrointestinal tract.

It is not completely settled whether antigen in the gut lumen attracts the IgA precursor B lymphocytes. Studies employing isolated ileal (Thiry-Vella) loops in rabbits have shown that mucosal immunity can be detected in loop secretions even when no antigen was directly applied to the loops.[72] Therefore, the oral stimulation serves to arm a wide variety of mucosal surfaces, especially the gut, to antigens readily sampled from the environment. Other work, however, indicates that although all areas of the mucosal immune system may contain secretory IgA, the immune response is stronger in areas containing antigen.[76]

The maturation of the secretory immune response is largely dependent on the collaboration of helper T cells and switch T cells. Although there is good evidence that the B cells within GALT include cells that are genetically programmed to mature into IgA-secreting plasma cells, it is also true that T cells within GALT play a role in this maturation process. By cloning different GALT T-cell populations, Kawanishi et al.[77] demonstrated that some T cells within GALT (switch T

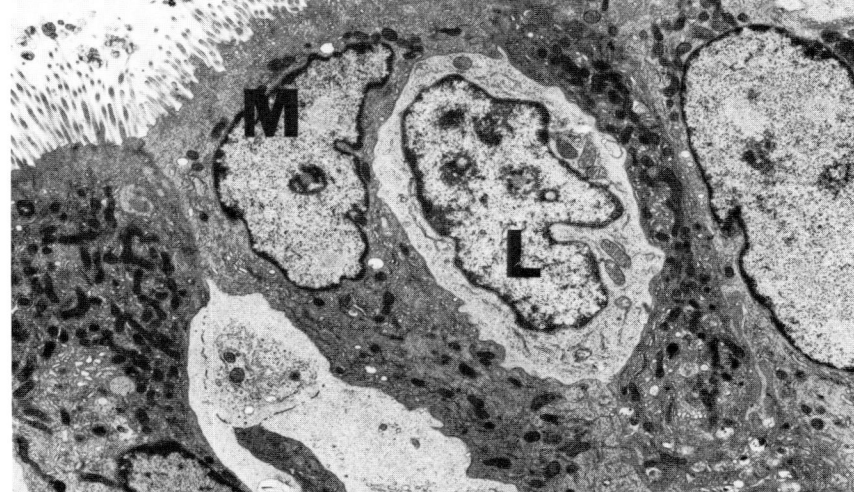

FIGURE 5–5. M cell (M) between two absorptive epithelial cells. Note the irregular microvilli (arrow) and lymphocyte (L) associated with the M cell.

cells) are able to influence directly the isotype expressed by GALT B lymphocytes. Most GALT B cells have surface IgM, indicating their immature stage of development. Under the influence of switch T cells, the surface isotype of these cells is preferentially "switched" to IgA.[77] Similar switch T cells have been detected in some human T-cell neoplasms.[78]

GALT also contains T helper and suppressor cells that have an effect on the isotype of the antigen-specific humoral immune response. After antigen has been taken up by M cells and passed into macrophages or dendritic cells in GALT, it is recognized by T as well as B lymphocytes. Antigen on the surface of macrophages in association with specific major histocompatibility complex class II molecules (Ia) is presented to T lymphocytes. Helper and suppressor T-cell interaction circuits which influence the production of secretory IgA and the systemic immune response, respectively, to these mucosal antigens have been described in GALT.

Since the work of Wells and Osborne,[12] the mechanism by which oral antigen exposure inhibits the subsequent systemic immune response to the same antigen has been sought. Antigen-specific systemic tolerance has been transferred by giving lymphocytes from orally immunized animals to previously unchallenged animals.[79,80] The cells responsible for transferring antigen-induced systemic tolerance in experimental systems are mainly T lymphocytes.[80] These antigen-specific suppressor T cells are found in GALT within 2 days after feeding protein antigen.[81] However, soon thereafter, these cells leave the GALT, so that by 4 days after feeding, the suppressor T cells are absent from Peyer's patches but are present in systemic lymphoid tissues. Elson et al.[82] have shown that T cells responsible for suppressing IgG responses and other T cells that enhance the IgA response are present in GALT, whereas the converse is true in the spleen.

The suppression seen is part of a GALT feedback T-T interaction circuit. Normally during an immune response, at least two T-cell populations are involved, helper and suppressor T cells. The fact that many antigens induce an immune response indicates that the helper reaction usually occurs sooner or is more prevalent than the suppressor reaction. In GALT, after oral antigen administration, precursor T cells are induced to become suppressor T cells to inhibit the production of systemic IgG or IgM to that antigen.[83] It is likely that these suppressor T cells leave the GALT and travel to the spleen in order to act directly on the GALT B cell precursors, which migrate to the spleen soon after antigen stimulation.[81] In humans, suppressor cells for the IgA response have been found to bear surface receptors for IgA.[84,85]

The production of IgA after oral stimulation with antigen involves helper T cells that recognize the antigen presented by the macrophage and augment the production of IgA by specific B lymphocytes.[86,87] However, there is normally a suppressor mechanism that opposes the production of this antibody.[88] For the IgA response to proceed, it requires the existence of a complex contrasuppression circuit. Contrasuppressor cells do exactly what their name implies: they oppose the action of suppressor T cells. As such, they allow helper T cells to proceed with a specific immune response. GALT contains cells that induce contrasuppressor cells to interfere with suppression.[89]

After oral immunization, then, a complex series of cellular interactions occurs. Contrasuppressor cells prevent suppression of the B-cell response to the antigen. Switch T cells influence B lymphocytes to alter their surface isotype from IgM to IgA. These events promote the formation of a secretory IgA response to the administered antigen. Finally, suppressor T cells for the systemic immune response prevent IgG reaction to commonly ingested antigens. The theoretic advantage to the body of the latter is to prevent formation of vigorous systemic immune reactions to myriads of harmless antigens that pass through the gastrointestinal tract and gain entrance, to varying extents, into the systemic circulation.

It is important to note some features of the suppression of systemic immunity following oral immunization. (1) The suppression is largely due to the production of suppressor T cells, although with hypersensitivity responses, suppressor B cells have been described.[90,91] (2) For optimal systemic suppression, the animals must not have been previously immunized systemically with the same antigen. (3) If the animals were previously immunized parenterally, an oral dose of antigen can increase the systemic titer of specific antibody[92]; however, subsequent parenteral administration of antigen has a weaker antibody response than that in unfed animals.[93] (4) Although many antigens follow these rules, exceptions have been described, including cholera toxin and some lipopolysaccharide antigens, that may not elicit systemic tolerance after oral feeding.[94]

CHARACTERISTICS OF SECRETORY IGA

The end result of the cellular interactions described above is the production of an antigen-specific secretory IgA response. Most IgA is produced by plasma cells, which lie in the lamina propria of the gastrointestinal tract, some also deriving from other mucosa. In humans there are two subclasses of IgA, IgA1 and IgA2. Whereas IgA1 predominates in the serum, a disproportionately large amount of IgA2-containing plasma cells are present along the lumina propria of the gastrointestinal tract. IgA is synthesized as a 7S monomeric unit consisting of two α heavy chains and two light chains. IgA monomers preferentially are coupled into a dimeric form (four α chains and four light chains). They are joined together by a small polypeptide (15,000 daltons) called J (joining) chain.

Following secretion by the plasma cells, the dimeric IgA molecules either migrate toward the gut epithelium or pass into the systemic circulation. Those molecules that pass into the bloodstream are taken up by bile duct epithelium and transported into bile.[95] This may provide for mucosal defense in the upper portion of the small intestine. Transportation of IgA into epithelial cells involves the unique collaboration of the immunoglobulin product of lymphoid cells and 60,000-dalton glycoprotein product of epithelial cells termed secretory component (SC) (Figure 5–6). SC is synthesized by epithelial cells in secretory glands and hepatocytes of some species. Ultrastructural studies have shown that SC is present on the cytoplasmic membrane of the epithelial cells.[96,97] It is still unclear why the dimeric secretory IgA-J chain dimers are attracted to these surfaces. However, after attachment to SC, the IgA is endocytosed and packaged into vesicles by the surface epithelium. This is then concentrated at the surface of the epithelial cells and released into the lumen. SC helps to prevent digestion of IgA in the proteolytic environment of the gut lumen. The form released into the lumen, then, is the 11S, 385,000-dalton complex of dimeric IgA-J chain and SC.[98] SC is also able to combine with IgM and provides a similar mechanism of secretion into the gut lumen.

The stimuli responsible for release of IgA-J chain SC into the gut lumen is still unclear, although some studies have suggested that biologically active molecules such as cholera toxin can promote this secretion.[99] Once released into the bowel lumen, secretory IgA has been shown to mediate protection against microorganisms and their toxic products.[100]

The major mechanism by which secretory IgA protects the mucosal surface is by interfering with the uptake of microorganisms and their products. It is known to coat the surface of these antigens, which prevents the adherence of the antigen to the glycocalyx of the surface epithelium. Obviously, microorganisms and toxins that are rendered incapable of binding to the surface epithelium will not be able to damage the tissues. This mechanism has been shown to protect against *Vibrio cholerae* in the gut and in oral mucosa with *Streptococcus sanguis* and *S. mutans*.[101,102]

There is also some evidence that antigen-specific secretory IgA can collaborate with killer cells and damage microorganisms via an antibody-dependent, cell-mediated cytotoxicity (ADCC).[50,51] IgA is a poor activator of complement and does not effectively opsonize antigens for phagocytosis by neutrophils or macrophages.[103–107]

Overall, the mucosal immune response of the gut is a system that deals effectively with the many nonpathogenic microorganisms, food products and occasional pathogens that pass through the gastrointestinal tract. The gut immune system can recognize these many antigens and through a complex network of helper, suppressor, contrasuppressor, and switch regulatory T cells, determine the type and degree of immune response that will be made to the antigen. When functioning properly, it can deal with the occasional pathogens by preventing their attachment or uptake by the surface epithelium or may assist in their destruction via one of the cytotoxicity mechanisms discussed. When not functioning properly, as in immunodeficiency or hyperreactivity states, it permits infection by unusual pathogens (such as *Mycobacterium avium-intracellulare* in acquired immunodeficiency syndrome) or initiates dysfunction as in food allergies, respectively. Much remains to be learned about the role of this host defense system in many disorders of the gastrointestinal tract that have, as a major component of the disease, infiltration of the mucosa by lymphocytes, plasma cells, eosinophils, and mast cells. In poorly understood conditions such as inflammatory bowel disease and gluten-sensitive enteropathy, sorting out whether these infiltrations represent a primary immunopathologic reaction or a secondary phenomenon while the host defense system is trying to fend off an as yet unrecognized pathogen will be the difficult task of future investigations.

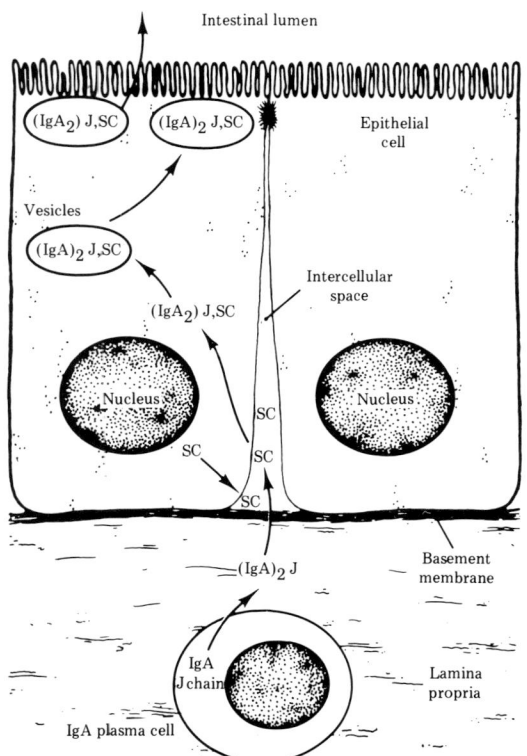

FIGURE 5–6. IgA is synthesized by plasma cells in the lamina propria mainly as a dimer combined with a J chain (also made by the plasma cell). IgA is attracted to the surface epithelial cells, which synthesize secretory component and express it on their basal and lateral borders. The IgA attaches to the secretory component and is taken up by the epithelial cell. This complex is packaged into vesicles, which concentrate near the surface epithelium, and is eventually secreted into the gut lumen. IgM is transported into the lumen by the same mechanism. IgG, IgE, and IgD do not combine with secretory component and do not share this secretory pathway.

References

1. Pasteur L (1880), cited by Calmette A: Les vaccinations microbiennes par voie buccale. Ann Inst Pasteur 37:900–920, 1923.
2. Ferran J: Nota sobre la profilaxis del colera por medio de infecciones hipodermicas de cultivo puro del bacilo virgula. Siglo Med 32:480, 1885.
3. Dopter C: Administration of antidysenteric vaccines by the mouth. Lancet 1:1661, 1908.
4. Courmont J, Rochaix A: L'immunisation par voie intestinale. Vaccination antityphique. Comp Rend Acad Sci 152:797–798, 1911.

5. Wolfe K: Immunesorung per os. Muenchener Mediz Wochenschr 55:270–272, 1908.
6. Besredka A: De la vaccination par voie buccale contre la dysenterie, la fievre typhoide et le cholera. [Oral vaccination against dysentery, typhoid and cholera.] Rev Hyg Med Prevent 49:445–463, 1927.
7. Besredka A: Immunity in Infectious Diseases: A Series of Studies. London, Bailliere, Tindell and Cox, 1930, p 268.
8. Davies A: Serological properties of dysentery stools. Lancet 2:1009–1010, 1922.
9. Erlich P: Experimentelle Untersuchungen über Immunitat. I. Über Ricin. Dtsch Med Wochenschr 17:976–979, 1891.
10. Ehrlich P: Experimentelle Untersuchungen über Immunitat. II. Über Abrin. Dtsch Med Wochenschr 17:1218–1219, 1891.
11. Metchnikoff E (1894), cited by Cantacuzene J: La pathogenie du cholera et la vaccination anticholerigine. Ann Inst Pateur 34:57–87, 1920.
12. Wells HG, Osborne TB: The biological reactions of the vegetable proteins. I. Anaphylaxis. J Infect Dis 9:66–102, 1911.
13. Tomasi TB, Tan EM, Solomon A, Prendergast RA: Characteristics of an immune system common to certain external secretions. J Exp Med 121:101–112, 1965.
14. Brandtzaeg P: Research in gastrointestinal immunology: State of the art. Scand J Gastroenterol [Suppl] 20:S114, 137–156, 1985.
15. Cornes JS: Number, size, and distribution of Peyer's patches in the human small intestine. Gut 6:225–238, 1965.
16. Reynolds JD, Morris B: The evolution and involution of Peyer's patches in fetal and postnatal sheep. Eur J Immunol 13:627–631, 1983.
17. Crabbe PA, Nash DR, Bazin H, et al: Immunohistochemical observations on lymphoid tissues from conventional and germ-free mice. Lab Invest 22:448–460, 1970.
18. Owen RL: Sequential uptake of horseradish peroxidase by lymphoid follicle epithelium of Peyer's patches in normal unobstructed mouse intestine: An ultrastructural study. Gastroenterology 72:440–451, 1977.
19. Bhalla DK, Owen RL: Migration of B and T lymphocytes to M cells in Peyer's patch follicle epithelium: An autoradiographic and immunocytochemical study in mice. Cell Immunol 81:105–112, 1983.
20. Cebra JJ, Cebra ER, Clough ER, et al: IgA commitment: Models for B-cell differentiation and possible roles for T-cells in regulating B-cell development. Ann NY Acad Sci 409:25–38, 1983.
21. Dukes C, Bussey HJR: The number of lymphoid follicles of the human large intestine. J Pathol Bacteriol 29:111–118, 1926.
22. Rosner AJ, Keren DF: Demonstration of M-cells in the specialized follicle-associated epithelium overlying isolated follicles in the gut. J Leukocyte Biol 35:397–404, 1984.
23. Keren DF, Holt PS, Collins HH, et al: The role of Peyer's patches in the local immune response of rabbit ileum to live bacteria. J Immunol 120:1892–1898, 1978.
24. Bockman DE, Cooper MD: Early lymphoepithelial relationships in human appendix: A combined light and electron-microscopic study. Gastroenterology 68:1160–1172, 1975.
25. McWilliams M, Phillips-Quagliata JM, Lamm ME: Mesenteric lymph node B lymphoblasts which home to the small intestine are precommitted to IgA synthesis. J Exp Med 145:866–875, 1977.
26. Perkkio M, Savilahti E: Time of appearance of immunoglobulin-containing cells in the mucosa of the neonatal intestine. Pediatr Res 14:953–995, 1980.
27. Keren DF, Appelman HD, Dobbins WO III, et al: Correlation of histopathologic evidence of disease activity with the immunoglobulin-containing cells in the colon of patients with inflammatory bowel disease. Hum Pathol 15:757–763, 1984.
28. Carbbe PA, Heremans JF: The distribution of immunoglobulin-containing cells along the human gastrointestinal tract. Gastroenterology 51:305–316, 1966.
29. Patterson S, Roebuck P, Platts-Mills TAE, et al: IgE plasma cells in human jejunum demonstration by immune electron microscopy. Clin Exp Immunol 46:301–310, 1981.
30. Slaoui H, Andre C, Dechavanne M, Tolot F: Immunofluorescence study of mucosal B lymphocytes in bile reflux gastritis. Digestion 19:131–133, 1979.
31. Scott BB, Goodall A, Stephenson P, Jenkins D: Duodenal bulb plasma cells in duodenitis and duodenal ulceration. Gut 26:1032–1037, 1985.
32. Rosekrans PCM, Meijer CJLM, Cornelisse CJ, et al: Use of morphometry and immunohistochemistry of small intestinal biopsy specimens in the diagnosis of food allergy. J Clin Pathol 33:125–130, 1980.
33. Cook J, Naqi SA, Sahin N, Wagner G: Distribution of immunoglobulin-bearing cells in the gut-associated lymphoid tissues of the turkey: Effect of antibiotics. Am J Vet Res 45:2189–2194, 1984.
34. Dobbins WO III: Human intestinal intraepithelial lymphocytes progress report. Gut 27:972–985, 1986.
35. Meuwissen SGM, Feltkamp-Vroom TM, de la Reviere AB, et al: Analysis of the lympho-plasmacytic infiltrate in Crohn's disease with special reference to identification of lymphocyte-subpopulations. Gut 17:770–780, 1976.
36. Janossy G, Tidman N, Selby WS, et al: Human T lymphocytes of inducer and suppressor type occupy different microenviroments. Nature 288:81–84, 1980.
37. Selby WS, Janossy G, Jewell DP: Immunohistological characterization of intraepithelial lymphocytes of the human gastrointestinal tract. Gut 22:169–176, 1981.
38. Ernst PB, Petit A, Befus AD, et al: Murine intestinal intraepithelial lymphocytes. II. Comparison of freshly isolated and cultured intraepithelial lymphocytes. Eur J Immunol 15:216–221, 1985.
39. Chiba M, Bartnik W, ReMine SG, et al: Human colonic intraepithelial and lamina proprial lymphocytes: Cytotoxicity in vitro and the potential effects of the isolation method on their functional properties. Gut 22:177–186, 1981.
40. Cerf-Bensussan N, Guy-Grand D, Griscelli C: Intraepithelial lymphocytes of human gut: Isolation, characterization and study of natural killer activity. Gut 26:81–88, 1985.
41. Guy-Grand D, Griscelli C, Vassalli P: The mouse gut T lymphocyte, a novel type of T cell: Nature, origin, and traffic in mice in normal and graft-versus-host conditions. J Exp Med 148:1661–1677, 1978.
42. Selby WS, Janossy G, Bofill M, Jewell DP: Lymphocyte subpopulations in the human small intestine: The findings in normal mucosa and in the mucosa of patients with adult coeliac disease. Clin Exp Immunol 52:219–224, 1983.
43. Hirata I, Berrebi G, Austin LL, et al: Immunohistological characterization of intraepithelial and lamina propria lymphocytes in control ileum and colon and in inflammatory bowel disease. Dig Dis Sci 31:593–603, 1986.
44. Selby WS, Janossy G, Bofill M, Jewell DP: Intestinal lymphocyte subpopulations in inflammatory bowel disease: An analysis by immunohistological and cell isolation techniques. Gut 25:32–40, 1984.
45. Falchuk ZM, Barnhard E, Machado I: Human colonic mononuclear cells: Studies of cytotoxic function. Gut 22:290–294, 1981.
46. Herberman RB (ed): NK Cells and Other Natural Effector Cells. Academic Press, New York, 1982.
47. Targan S, Britvan L, Kendal R, et al: Isolation of spontaneous and interferon-inducible natural killer–like cells from human colonic mucosa: Lysis of lymphoid and autologous epithelial target cells. Clin Exp Immunol 54:14–22, 1983.
48. Csiba A, Whitwell HL, Moore M: Distribution of histocompatibility and leucocyte differentiation antigens in normal human colon and in benign and malignant colonic neoplasms. Br J Cancer 50:699–709, 1984.
49. Hogan PG, Hapel AJ, Doe WF: Lymphokine-activated and natural killer cell activity in human intestinal mucosa. J Immunol 135:1731–1738, 1985.
50. Tagliabue A, Nencioni L, Villa L, Keren DF, Lowell GH, Boraschi D: Antibody-dependent cell-mediated antibacterial activity of intestinal lymphocytes with secretory IgA. Nature 306:184–185, 1983.
51. Tagliabue A, Villa L, Boraschi D, et al: Natural anti-bacterial activity against salmonella typhi by human T4+ lymphocytes armed with IgA antibodies. J Immunol 135:4178–4181, 1985.
52. Capron M, Capron A, Torpier G, et al: Eosinophil-dependent cytotoxicity in rat schistosomiasis: Involvement of IgG2a antibody and role of mast cells. Eur J Immunol 8:127–133, 1978.

53. Bull DM, Bookman MA: Isolation and functional characterization of human intestinal mucosal lymphoid cells. J Clin Invest 59:966, 1977.
54. LeFevre ME, Vanderhoff JW, Laisue JA, Joel DD: Accumulation of 2-μ latex particles in mouse Peyer's patches during chronic latex feeding. Experientia 15:120–123, 1978.
55. Owel RL, Allen CL, Stevens DP: Phagocytosis of Giardia muris by macrophages in Peyer's patch epithelium in mice. Infect Immun 33:591–601, 1981.
56. Guy-Grand D, Dy M, Luffau G, Vassali P: Gut mucosal mast cells: Origin, traffic and differentiation. J Exp Med 160:12–28, 1984.
57. Crowle PK, Reed ND: Bone marrow origin of mucosal mast cells. Int Arch Allergy Appl Immunol 73:242–247, 1984.
58. Wal JM, Meslin JC, Weyer A, David B: Histamine and mast cell distribution in the gastrointestinal wall of the rat: Comparison between germ-free and conventional rats. Int Arch Allergy Appl Immunol 77:308–313, 1985.
59. Kawanishi H: Role of IgE as a mast cell development co-factor in the differentiation of murine gut-associated mast cells in vitro. Eur J Immunol 16:689–692, 1986.
60. Woodbury RG, Miller HRP, Huntley JF, et al: Mucosal mast cells are functionally active during spontaneous expulsion of intestinal nematode infections in rat. Nature 312:450–452, 1984.
61. Handlinger JH, Rothwell TLW: Intestinal mast cell changes in guinea pigs infected with the nematode Trichostrongylus colubriformis. Int Arch Allergy Appl Immunol 74:165–171, 1984.
62. Befus D, Goodacre R, Dyck N, Bienenstock J: The mast cell populations of the human intestine: Selected summaries. Gastroenterology 89:1437–1438, 1985.
63. Smith MW, Jarvis LG, King IS: Cell proliferation in follicle-associated epithelium of mouse Peyer's patch. Am J Anat 159:157–166, 1980.
64. Madara JL, Bye WA, Trier JS: Structural features of and cholesterol distribution in M-cell membranes in guinea pig, rat, and mouse Peyer's patches. Gastroenterology 87:1091–1103, 1984.
65. Wolf JL, Kauffman RS, Finberg R, et al: Determinants of reovirus interaction with the intestinal M cells and absorptive cells of murine intestine. Gastroenterology 85:291–300, 1983.
66. Dhar R, Ogra PL: Local immune responses. Br Med Bull 41:28–33, 1985.
67. Erlandsen SL, Chase DG: Paneth cell function: Phagocytosis and intracellular digestion of intestinal microorganisms. I. Hexamita muris. J Ultrastruct Res 41:296–308, 1972.
68. Kern SE, Keren DF, Dieterle RC: Paneth cell response: Hyperplasia associated with bacterial overgrowth. Lab Invest 52:A34, 1985.
69. Yardley JH, Keren DF: "Precancer" lesions in ulcerative colitis: A retrospective study of rectal biopsy and colectomy specimens. Cancer 34:835–844, 1974.
70. Cebra JJ, Kamat R, Gearhart P, et al: The secretory IgA system of the gut. In Porter R, Knight E (eds): Immunology of the Gut. Ciba Foundation Symposium 46, 1976 (New Series). New York, Elsevier North-Holland, 1977, pp 5–28.
71. Bhalla DK, Murakami T, Owen RL: Microcirculation of intestinal lymphoid follicles in rat Peyer's patches. Gastroenterology 81:481–491, 1981.
72. Tseng J: Expression of immunoglobulin isotypes by lymphoid cells of mouse intestinal lamina propria. Cell Immunol 73:324–326, 1982.
73. Keren DF, Kern SE, Bauer DH, et al: Direct demonstration in intestinal secretions of an IgA memory response to orally administered Shigella flexneri antigens. J Immunol 128:475–479, 1982.
74. Keren DF, McDonald RA, Scott PJ, et al: Effect of antigen form on local immunoglobulin A memory response of intestinal secretions of Shigella flexneri. Infect Immun 47:123–128, 1985.
75. Goldblum RM, Ahlstedt S, Carlson B, et al: Antibody-forming cells in human colostrum after oral immunization. Nature 257:797–798, 1975.
76. Pierce NF: The role of antigen form and function in the primary and secondary immune responses to cholera toxin and toxoid in rats. J Exp Med 148:195–206, 1978.
77. Kawanishi H, Saltzman LE, Strober W: New understanding of regulatory mechanisms of immunoglobulin A secretion by intestinal cells. Selected Summaries. Gastroenterology 85:1219, 1983.
78. Mayer L, Posnett DN, Kunkel HG: Human malignant T cells capable of inducing an immunoglobulin class switch. J Exp Med 161:134–144, 1985.
79. Mowat AM, Lamont AG, Strobel S, Mackenzie S: The role of antigen processing and suppressor T cells in immune responses to dietary proteins in mice. Adv Exp Med Biol 216:709–720, 1987.
80. Richman LK, Chiller JM, Brown WR, et al: Enterically induced immunologic tolerance I. Induction of suppressor T lymphocytes by intragastric administration of soluble protein. J Immunol 121:2429–2434, 1978.
81. Mattingly JA, Waksman BH: Immunologic suppression after oral administration of antigen. I. Specific suppressor cells formed in rat Peyer's patches after oral administration of sheep erythrocytes and their systemic migration. J Immunol 121:1878–1883, 1978.
82. Elson CO, Heck JA, Strober W: T-cell regulation of murine IgA synthesis. J Exp Med 149:632–643, 1979.
83. Elson CO: Inductions and control of gastrointestinal immune system. Scand J Gastroenterol 20:S114:1–15, 1985.
84. Hoover RG, Lynch RG: Isotype-specific suppression of IgA: Suppression of IgA responses in BALB/c mice by T α cells. J Immunol 130:521–523, 1983.
85. Muller S, Hoover RG: T cells with FC receptors in myeloma: Suppression of growth and secretion of MOPC-315 by T α cells. J Immunol 134:644–647, 1985.
86. Kiyono H, McGhee JR, Michalek SM: Lipopolysaccharide regulation of the immune response: Comparison of responses to lips in germ-free, Escherichia coli-monoassociated and conventional mice. J Immunol 124:36–42, 1980.
87. Richman LK, Graff AS, Yarchoan R, Strober W: Simultaneous induction of antigen-specific IgA helper T cells and IgG suppressor T cells in the murine Peyer's patch after protein feeding. J Immunol 126:2079–2083, 1981.
88. Clancy R, Cripps A, Chipchase H: Regulation of human gut B lymphocytes by T lymphocytes. Gut 25:47–51, 1984.
89. Green DR, Gold J, St Martin S, et al: Microenvironmental immunoregulation: Possible role of contrasuppressor cells in maintaining immune responses in gut-associated lymphoid tissues. Proc Natl Acad Sci 79:889–892, 1982.
90. Asherson GL, Zembala M, Perera MACC, et al: Production of immunity and unresponsiveness in the mouse by feeding contact sensitizing agents and the role of suppressor cells in the Peyer's patches, mesenteric lymph nodes and other lymphoid tissues. Cellular Immunol 33:145–154, 1977.
91. Asherson GL, Perera MACC, Thomas WR: Contact sensitivity and the DNA response in mice to high and low doses of oxazolone: Low dose unresponsiveness following painting and feeding and its prevention by pretreatment with cyclophosphamide. Immunology 36:449–459, 1979.
92. Keren DF, Collins HH, Gemski P, et al: Role of antigen form in development of mucosal immunoglobulin A response to Shigella flexneri antigens. Infect Immun 31:1193–1202, 1981.
93. Hanson DG, Vaz NM, Rawlings LA, Lynch JM: Inhibition of specific immune responses by feeding protein antigens. II. Effects of prior passive and active immunization. J Immunol 122:2261–2266, 1979.
94. Elson CO, Ealding W: Cholera toxin feeding did not induce oral tolerance in mice and abrogated oral tolerance to an unrelated protein antigen. J Immunol 133:2892–2897, 1984.
95. Delacroix DL, Malburny GN, Vaerman JP: Hepatobiliary transport of plasma IgA in the mouse: Contribution to clearance of intravascular IgA. Eur J Immunol 15:893–899, 1985.
96. Brown WR, Isobe Y, Nakane PK: Studies on the translocation of immunoglobulins across intestinal epithelium. II. Immunoelectron microscopic localization of immunoglobulins and secretory component in human intestinal mucosa. Gastroenterology 71:985–995, 1976.
97. Brown WR, Isobe Y, Nakane PK, Pacini B: Studies on translocation of immunoglobulins across intestinal epithelium. IV. Evidence for binding of IgA and IgM to secretory component in intestinal epithelium. Gastroenterology 73:1333–1339, 1977.
98. Ahnen DJ, Brown WR, Kloppel TM: Secretory component: The polymeric immunoglobulin receptor. What's in it for the gastro-

enterologist and hepatologist? Gastroenterology 89:667–668, 1985.
99. Hamilton SR, Keren DF, Boitnott JK, et al: IgA content of intestinal epithelium and secreted fluid in experimental cholera: Comparison with net fluid production and goblet cell mucin content. Gut 21:365–369, 1980.
100. Yardley JH, Keren DF, Hamilton SR, Brown GD: Local (IgA) immune response by the intestine to cholera toxin and its partial suppression with combined systemic and intraintestinal immunization. Infect Immun 19:589–598, 1978.
101. Fubara ES, Freter R: Source and protective function of coproantibodies in intestinal disease. Am J Clin Nutr 25:137–142, 1972.
102. Williams RC, Gibbons RJ: Inhibition of bacterial adherence by secretory immunoglobulin A: A mechanism of antigen disposal. Science 177:697–699, 1972.
103. Zipursky A, Brown EJ, Bienenstock J: Lack of opsonization potential of 11S human secretory IgA. Proc Soc Exp Biol Med 142:181–184, 1973.
104. Adinolfi M, Glynn AA, Lindsay M, Milne CM: Serological properties of IgA antibodies to Escherichia coli present in human colostrum. Immunology 10:517–526, 1966.
105. Ishizaka T, Ishizaka K, Borsos T, Rapp H: C'1 fixation by human isoagglutinins: Fixation of C'1 by IgG and IgM but not by IgA antibody. J Immunol 97:716–726, 1966.
106. Iida K, Fujita T, Inai S, et al: Complement fixing abilities of IgA myeloma proteins and their fragments: The activation of complement through the classical pathway. Immunochemistry 13:747–752, 1976.
107. Keren DF: Immunology and Immunopathology of the Gastrointestinal Tract. Chicago, American Society of Clinical Pathologists, 1980.

CHAPTER 6

Genetic and Cytogenetic Aspects

PEN-MING L. MING, M.D.

PATTERN OF INHERITANCE
Mendelian Inheritance
Autosomal Dominant
  Inheritance
Autosomal Recessive
  Inheritance
X-Linked Inheritance
Multifactorial Inheritance

GENETIC MARKERS
HLA Antigens
Blood Groups

CHROMOSOMAL SYNDROMES AFFECTING THE GASTROINTESTINAL TRACT
Trisomy 21 Syndrome
Trisomy 18 Syndrome
Trisomy 13 Syndrome
Other Chromosomal Syndromes

GENETICS OF NONNEOPLASTIC DISEASES OF THE GASTROINTESTINAL TRACT
Peptic Ulcer
Celiac Disease
Inflammatory Bowel Disease
Hirschsprung's Disease
Congenital Hypertrophic Pyloric
  Stenosis

GENETICS OF NEOPLASTIC DISEASES OF THE GASTROINTESTINAL TRACT
Esophageal Tumors
Gastric Tumors

Intestinal Tumors
Clinical Syndromes
Familial Polyposis Syndromes
*Hereditary Nonpolyposis Colorectal
  Cancer*
*Discrete Adenomas and Carcinomas of
  the Colon*
Molecular Genetic and Cytogenetic
  Changes
*Molecular Genetic Changes and Tumor-
  Suppressing Genes*
Cytogenetic Changes
Oncogenes

Genetics plays an important role in many gastrointestinal diseases. Some diseases are hereditary, transmitted in a mendelian dominant or recessive fashion. In either case, family pedigree analysis is essential for determination of the inheritance pattern. In this regard, the hereditary diseases should be distinguished from diseases that occur more frequently within a family than in the general population but are not genetically controlled. Associated with these diseases are strong environmental factors that may be shared by the family members because of their lifestyle or dietary habits. Similarly, the racial or geographic differences in the incidence of many diseases, such as esophageal cancer, can be explained on an environmental, rather than genetic, basis.

The recent advances in molecular biology have made it possible to identify and clone the genes in a number of diseases—such as cystic fibrosis, which affects the mucous cells—including those in the digestive tract. In other diseases, such as colonic tumors, modern recombinant DNA technology has been instrumental in elucidating a sequence of cytogenetic and genetic alterations in the evolution of malignant changes. In addition, changes in gene expression, amplification, and mutation have been found in many types of neoplastic cells. It should be emphasized, however, that such alterations in tumor cells are largely affected by environmental factors, not purely by inherited genetic defects.

Cytogenetic studies of various types of cells demonstrate numeric or structural aberrations, the pattern of which, in many instances, forms the basis for identifying and localizing the specific gene(s) involved in a certain disease. Thus, the combination of cytogenetic and molecular techniques provides a powerful tool for our understanding of cellular as well as genetic changes in many diseases.

PATTERN OF INHERITANCE

The pattern of inheritance can be divided into two major categories: mendelian inheritance and multifactorial inheritance. Mendelian inheritance involves primarily the transmission of a single mutant gene (monogenic). It can be further classified as autosomal dominant, autosomal recessive, or X-linked. Multifactorial inheritance represents the interaction of multiple genes (polygenic) and multiple environmental factors. The risk to relatives is generally lower than that for mendelian disorders except when several family members are affected.

Mendelian Inheritance

Autosomal Dominant Inheritance

Dominant disorders are found in individuals who carry one abnormal gene and one normal gene (heterozygotes). The gene responsible for the disease is located on one of the 22 autosomes in both males and females. Autosomal dominant inheritance is characterized by the following features:

1. Each affected individual has an affected parent (unless the condition is due to a new mutation or the mutant gene has reduced penetrance).
2. Unaffected relatives do not transmit the disease.
3. The children of an affected parent and a normal parent have a 50% chance of being affected.
4. If both parents are affected, their children have a 75% chance of being affected.
5. Males and females are equally affected.

Figure 6–1 shows a typical pedigree of autosomal dominant inheritance. Note the vertical transmission pattern from generation to generation. There are two common clinical features of autosomal dominant inheritance: (1) delayed age of onset—although the mutant gene is present from the time of conception, the disease may not be diagnosed until adulthood; and (2) variability in expression—the severity and extent of disease may vary greatly among affected individuals, resulting in diversified clinical manifestations.

Less commonly, in autosomal dominant inheritance, an individual clearly has inherited a defective gene, there being an affected parent and an affected offspring, but does not have the clinical disease. This phenomenon is known as lack of penetrance. Thus, if a gene is said to have 50% penetrance, only half of the individuals who carry the gene are affected. Some gastrointestinal diseases with autosomal dominant inheritance are summarized in Table 6–1.[1,2]

Autosomal Recessive Inheritance

Unlike autosomal dominant disorders, the autosomal recessive disorders are found in individuals only when both alleles at a particular genetic locus are mutant (homozygotes). As in autosomal dominant inheritance, the gene responsible for an autosomal recessive disorder is located on one of the 22 autosomes; thus, both males and females can be affected. The following are the characteristics of autosomal recessive inheritance:

1. In most instances, both parents are clinically normal but carry the abnormal gene; that is, they are carriers (heterozygotes).
2. If both parents are carriers, one fourth of their children are affected, one half of the children are carriers, and one fourth of the children are normal.
3. If one parent is affected and the other parent is a carrier, one half of their children are affected.
4. Males and females are equally affected.

Figure 6–2 shows a pedigree with autosomal recessive inheritance. Note the horizontal distribution of affected siblings and cousins of the same generation.

Table 6–1 GASTROINTESTINAL DISEASE OF AUTOSOMAL DOMINANT INHERITANCE

Inheritance Proved
Duodenal peptic ulcer with hyperpepsinogenemia I
Familial adenomatous polyposis (FAP)
Familial intestinal neurofibromatosis
Familial juvenile polyposis
Familial tylosis (keratosis plamaris et plantaris) with esophageal cancer
Familial midgut volvulus
Gardner's syndrome
Mucosal neuroma syndromes with endocrine tumors
Olser-Rendu-Weber syndrome
Peutz-Jeghers syndrome

Inheritance Suspected
Anorectal anomalies (anorectal stenosis or imperforate anus)
Duodenal ulcer due to antral G-cell hyperfunction
Familial gastric polyposis
PIV syndrome (polydactyly, imperforate anus, and vertebral anomalies)
Vater associates (vertebral defect, anal atresia, tracheoesophageal fistula, esophageal atresia, and radial dysplasia)

Data from McKusick[1] and Passarge.[2]

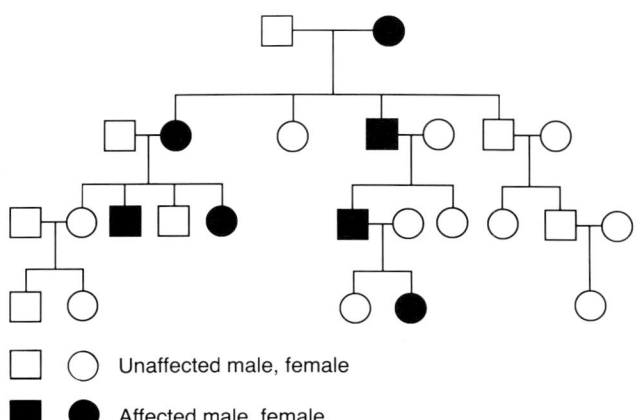

☐ ◯ Unaffected male, female
■ ● Affected male, female

FIGURE 6–1. Pedigree of an autosomal dominant trait.

GENETIC AND CYTOGENETIC ASPECTS 83

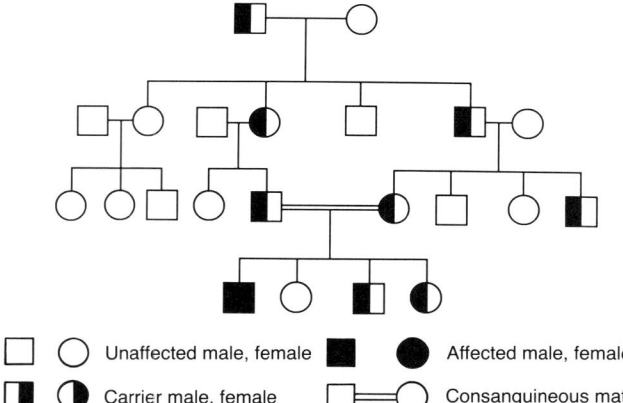

FIGURE 6–2. Pedigree of an autosomal recessive trait.

There are several characteristic clinical features of autosomal recessive inheritance: (1) The disease is usually diagnosed early in life. (2) The clinical manifestations tend to be more uniform than those in dominant disease. (3) Consanguinity increases the frequency of recessive disease, especially when the genes are rare. In general, the rarer the disease, the stronger the likelihood of parental consanguinity. (4) The frequency of homozygotes in a population is much lower than that in heterozygotes (in cystic fibrosis, in Caucasians, the frequency is 1/22 for heterozygotes and 1/2000 for homozygotes). (5) Unless the carrier state is clinically detectable, the parents usually are not alerted to the risk of having affected offspring until a child with the recessive disease is born into the family. Some gastrointestinal diseases with autosomal recessive inheritance are presented in Table 6–2.

X-Linked Inheritance

By definition, the genes responsible for X-linked disorders are located on the X chromosome. Therefore, the risk and clinical expression of the disease are different in the two sexes. The characteristics of X-linked inheritance are as follows:

1. Half of the sons of a female carrier are affected and half of her daughters are carriers.
2. All female offspring of affected males are carriers.
3. Affected males do not transmit the mutant genes to their sons.
4. Unaffected males do not transmit the mutant gene to any offspring.
5. An affected female homozygote can occur only when the father is affected and the mother is a carrier.

Figure 6–3 shows a pedigree with X-linked recessive inheritance. Note the absence of father-to-son transmission. So far, there is no major gastrointestinal disease that clearly follows the pattern of X-linked inheritance. However, it has been reported that some malformations, such as anal atresia, have shown familial aggregation suggestive of an X-linked inheritance.[2]

Genetic heterogeneity is a common phenomenon in genetic diseases. It implies that two or more different mutant genes can produce a similar clinical condition. For instance, congenital deafness can be inherited as autosomal dominant in some families, as autosomal recessive in others, and as X-linked in still others. On the other hand, frequently a hereditary syndrome due to a single mutation may exhibit multiple clinical manifestations. This phenomenon is known as pleiotropism or pleiotropy. For example, in Peutz-Jeghers syndrome, an autosomal dominant disease, the clinical manifestations can be as different as polyposis of the intestine and pigmentation around the mouth.

Multifactorial Inheritance

Several common diseases (such as hypertension) and congenital malformations (such as pyloric stenosis) have been known to "run in families," but they do not follow the pattern of mendelian inheritance. They are usually the result of a number of interacting factors, both genetic and environmental, and, for the most part, still unknown. Many gastrointestinal diseases fit

Table 6–2 GASTROINTESTINAL DISEASE OF AUTOSOMAL RECESSIVE INHERITANCE

Inheritance Proved
Acrodermatitis enteropathica
Congenital chloridorrhea (familial chloride diarrhea)
Disaccharide intolerance, type I (congenital sucrose-isomaltose malabsorption, sucrase-isomaltase deficiency)
Disaccharide intolerance, type II (congenital lactase deficiency)
Disaccharide intolerance, type III (adult lactase deficiency)
Familial esophageal achalasia
Familial intestinal polyatresia syndrome
Familial intestinal pseudo-obstruction, neuronal type

Inheritance Suspected
Crohn's disease and ulcerative colitis
Familial situs inversus viscerum
Groll-Hirschowitz syndrome (familial nerve deafness, mesenteric diverticula of small bowel, and progressive neuropathy)
Hirschsprung's disease (aganglionic megacolon with extensive intestinal involvement)

Data from McKusick[1] and Passarge.[2]

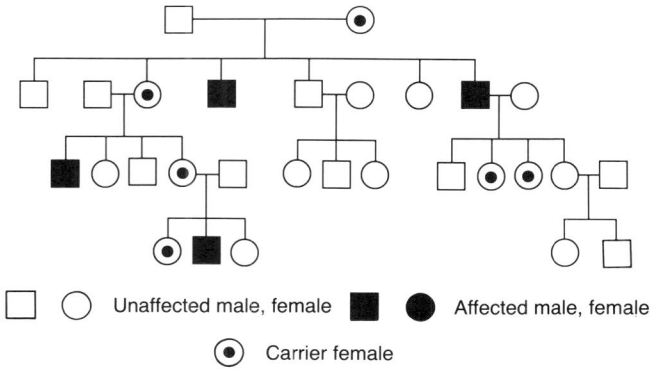

FIGURE 6–3. Pedigree of an X-linked recessive trait.

best into this category. The following features characterize multifactorial inheritance:

1. The interacting genetic and environmental factors must pass beyond the "threshold" to produce clinically overt disease.
2. The recurrent risk varies from family to family and is influenced by the number of affected persons in the family and the severity of the disorder in the affected individuals. In general, the greater the number of affected relatives and the more severe their disease, the greater the risk to other family members.
3. In some multifactorial disorders, the sex of the transmitting parent is a factor in estimating the risk of having an affected offspring. For instance, pyloric stenosis is much more common in males than in females (4:1), and the incidence in male children of affected mothers is notably higher than in male children of affected fathers.[3] These findings indicate that the females are relatively protected from pyloric stenosis. When females are affected, they must carry a heavy "genetic load" and thereby have a higher risk of transmitting the disease to their children.

GENETIC MARKERS

HLA Antigens

The numerous molecules on the cell surface capable of causing rejection of a tissue graft between genetically dissimilar individuals are defined as histocompatibility antigens or transplantation antigens. In the process of rejection, a group of these antigens are particularly important in determining the fate of a graft. This group of antigens is referred to as the major histocompatibility antigens, and the cluster of these genes is known as the major histocompatibility complex (MHC), which has been localized on the short arm of chromosome 6. By international agreement, the MHC in humans is called HLA (human leukocyte antigens), because the MHC-encoded antigens were initially detected on the surface of the white blood cells.

The HLA complex has been known to be associated with a variety of diseases. In some cases, the association is so specific and so significant that the HLA complex can be considered an important genetic marker in the differential diagnosis of the disease.

Among the gastrointestinal diseases, association with HLA has been reported in celiac disease (nontropical sprue, gluten-sensitivity enteropathy), and possibly duodenal ulcer. For example, approximately 80% of patients with celiac disease have HLA-DR3, compared with 24% of controls. Inversely, individuals with DR3 antigens have a risk 11.6 times higher for developing celiac disease than those who do not carry DR3.[4]

In patients with duodenal ulcer, there is an increased frequency of HLA-B5,[5] HLA-B12,[6] and HLA-Bw35.[7] The relative risk of the development of a duodenal ulcer in individuals with HLA-B12 is reported to be 2.16. However, this association has not been consistently found in other reports.

Blood Groups

In 1953, Aird and colleagues[8] first noted that carcinoma of the stomach was more common in individuals of blood group A than in those of other blood groups. This observation was subsequently confirmed among different ethnic groups and in different countries.[9] It has been generally recognized that gastric carcinoma is about 20% more common in persons of blood group A than in those of the remaining blood groups. However, no such association has been found in patients with intestinal metaplasia, which is considered a precursor of gastric cancer. The basis of these observations was recently investigated by Beckman and Angqvist.[10] It was found that the incidence of gastric carcinoma is significantly lower in blood group O women and the survival time longer in group O individuals than in patients of other blood groups. These findings support the hypothesis that gastric cancer cells produce an antigen immunologically related to blood group A, so that group O individuals may have the advantage of preventing tumor growth.

Shortly after the association of blood group A and gastric carcinoma was described, the same group of investigators reported that peptic ulcer was associated with group O.[11] Individuals of blood group O are about 30% to 40% more likely to develop duodenal ulcer than people of the other blood groups.[12,13] In addition, the secretor genes also play a role in determining the relative risk of duodenal ulcer. The nonsecretors are 50% more likely to develop duodenal ulcer than secretors.[14,15] Individuals with both blood group O and nonsecretor status have a 150% increased risk of developing duodenal ulcers. The effect of these two genes, group O and nonsecretor, therefore, seems to be more than additive.[16] The association between blood group antigens and gastric ulcer, however, is not clear.

CHROMOSOMAL SYNDROMES AFFECTING THE GASTROINTESTINAL TRACT

Chromosome imbalance may either be inherited or occur sporadically as a new mutation. It can be recognized by karyotypic analysis as structural or as numeric rearrangement. In general, duplications and deletions of autosomes are more harmful than those of sex chromosomes. With the exception of balanced translocation, these rearrangements usually lead to an abnormal phenotype with a variety of clinical manifestations, including mental and growth retardation, malformation of different organs, and behavioral aberrations. It should be noted that although the balanced translocation can be transmitted from generation to generation without producing deleterious clinical effects, the carrier of such a translocation has a much greater risk than the general population of having offspring with a genetic imbalance.

The gastrointestinal tract is involved in a number of chromosomal syndromes, notably the autosomal trisomies.

Trisomy 21 Syndrome

In trisomy 21, more commonly known as Down's syndrome, 8% of the patients have duodenal atresia.[17] Inversely, about one third of all patients with duodenal atresia have Down's syndrome.[18] The second most common association is with Hirschsprung's disease, which occurs in approximately 2% of patients with Down's syndrome.[19] Of 697 infants studied with anorectal malformation, 10 patients had Down's syndrome.[19] Other less common gastrointestinal malformations include malrotation of the colon, Meckel's diverticulum, tracheoesophageal fistula, and esophageal atresia.

Trisomy 18 Syndrome

The trisomy 18 syndrome is less common but has more severe malformations than Down's syndrome. According to Warkany et al.,[19] in a series of 84 postmortem examinations of infants with trisomy 18, malformations of the gastrointestinal tract were present in 64 (85%). The abnormalities, in decreasing order of frequency, included Meckel's diverticulum, intestinal malrotation, tracheoesophageal fistula, imperforate anus, and pyloric stenosis.

Trisomy 13 Syndrome

Among the autosomal trisomy syndromes, trisomy 13 includes the most severe congenital anomalies, particularly in the central nervous system. Associated gastrointestinal malformations are found in approximately 60% of infants with trisomy 13.[19] These anomalies are listed in decreasing order of frequency as follows: malrotation of the colon, unattached mesentery, Meckel's diverticulum, omphalocele, true diverticula of the appendix, and mesenteric cyst.

Other Chromosomal Syndromes

Gastrointestinal manifestations are a part of many chromosomal syndromes with a variety of malformations involving different sites. These manifestations are summarized in Table 6-3.[19-24]

GENETICS OF NONNEOPLASTIC DISEASES OF THE GASTROINTESTINAL TRACT

As our knowledge and understanding in human genetics have dramatically increased during the last 20 years, more and more clinical disorders have been found to be genetically influenced, if not genetically determined. Gastrointestinal diseases are no exception. In this section, only a few relatively common diseases with a strong genetic basis will be discussed.

Peptic Ulcer

In 1951, Doll and Buch[25] provided the first evidence that genetic factors played a role in the development of peptic ulcer. They demonstrated that both gastric and duodenal ulcers were more commonly found in the siblings of the patients than in the general population. Doll and Kellock[26] further demonstrated that the two types of ulcers had distinct inheritance patterns. The first-degree relatives of gastric ulcer patients tended to have gastric ulcers, whereas the relatives of duodenal ulcer patients tended to have duodenal ulcers. These findings suggested that gastric ulcer and duodenal ulcer were two separate entities with independent segregation. This concept was later supported by the discovery of a strong association of blood group O and nonsecretor status with duodenal ulcer but not with gastric ulcer.[11]

Studies in twins revealed that concordance of peptic ulcer in monozygotic twins is less than 100% but consistently exceeds that in dizygotic twins.[5,13] This differ-

Table 6-3 CHROMOSOMAL SYNDROMES AFFECTING THE GASTROINTESTINAL TRACT

Chromosome Abnormalities	Gastrointestinal Manifestations
Trisomy 1q	Intestinal stenosis and atresia, pyloric stenosis
Deletion of 5p (Cri-du-chat syndrome)	Inguinal hernia
Trisomy 9	Diaphragmatic hernia
Deletion of 9p	Diaphragmatic hernia
Partial trisomy 10q	Malrotation of intestine
Deletion of 11p (Aniridia-Wilms' tumor syndrome)	Inguinal hernia
Trisomy 12q	Malrotation of intestine
Trisomy 13 (Patau's syndrome)	Malrotation of the colon, omphalocele, Meckel's diverticulum, unattached mesentery
Deletion of 13q	Imperforate anus, Hirschsprung's disease
Trisomy 16q	Malrotation of the colon
Trisomy 18 (Edwards' syndrome)	Malrotation of intestine, omphalocele, diaphragmatic or inguinal hernia, pyloric stenosis, Meckel's diverticulum, tracheoesophageal fistula, imperforate anus
Deletion of 18p	Inguinal hernia
Trisomy 19q	Malrotation of intestine
Trisomy 21 (Down's syndrome)	Hirschsprung's disease, duodenal atresia, anal atresia, rectal prolapse, malrotation of colon, Meckel's diverticulum, tracheoesophageal fistula, esophageal atresia
Ring chromosome 21	Pyloric stenosis, inguinal hernia
Partial trisomy 22 (cat eye syndrome)	Malrotation of intestine, anal atresia, Hirschsprung's disease
Monosomy X (Turner's syndrome)	Pyloric stenosis
Triploidy	Malrotation of intestine

Note: p, short arm of chromosome; q, long arm of chromosome.
Data from Warkany et al.,[19] Thompson,[20] DeGrouchy and Turleau,[21] Jones,[22] Beedgen et al.,[23] and Lamont et al.[24]

ence persists even when dizygotic twins are limited to those of like sex. These studies also demonstrated that twins shared either gastric or duodenal ulcer, providing further support for separate genetic transmission of these two types of peptic ulcers.[5] On the other hand, the less than 100% concordance for duodenal ulcer in monozygotic twins points out that there must be other factors involved in the pathogenesis of peptic ulcer.

The association of HLA antigens and duodenal ulcer was alluded to earlier in this chapter. The findings were rather heterogeneous; three separate studies showed an increased frequency of HLA antigens[5-7] in patients with duodenal ulcer, whereas other studies did not find any association.[27] It is therefore possible that each HLA association represents a selected subgroup of patients.[16] In this regard, recent studies with biochemical and physiologic markers have shown that there are indeed discrete genetic subtypes of duodenal ulcer, each with a different genetic basis. According to Rotter[5] and Soll,[16] there are seven major subtypes of familial duodenal ulcer disease: (1) duodenal ulcer with hyperpepsinogenemia I, (2) normopepsinogenemic familial duodenal ulcer, (3) familial duodenal ulcer associated with rapid gastric emptying, (4) familial hypergastrinemic duodenal ulcer related to hyperfunction of antral G cells, (5) childhood duodenal ulcer, (6) combined gastric and duodenal ulcer, and (7) an immunologic form of duodenal ulcer. Among these subtypes, only the first mentioned (duodenal ulcer with hyperpepsinogenemia I) was found to be inherited as an autosomal dominant trait. This was demonstrated by investigations of two large kindreds with segregation for both duodenal ulcer and hyperpepsinogenemia I[28] and later confirmed in a collaborative study between Los Angeles and Liverpool of 123 sibships ascertained for duodenal ulcer[29] and in another study from India.[30] Hyperpepsinogenemia I was present in half of the offspring of hyperpepsinogenemic family members and in none of the offspring of normopepsinogenemic members. Duodenal ulcer occurred in about 40% of the family members with hyperpepsinogenemia I and in none of the normopepsinogenemic family members. Thus, the risk of duodenal ulcer is increased only in the hyperpepsinogenemic siblings.

The other subtypes of duodenal ulcer disease have all shown genetic predisposition, but the definite mode of inheritance has not been established. The predisposing factors include blood group O, nonsecretor, HLA antigens, and even the male sex. It is possible that there is a polygenic background upon which the major predisposing genes act. It has been estimated that about 20% of the first-degree relatives of an ulcer patient will develop peptic ulcer disease during their lifetime.[5]

Celiac Disease

Celiac disease (nontropical sprue) is characterized by generalized malabsorption and abnormal small-intestinal mucosa. The disease is precipitated by ingestion of wheat gluten and similar alcohol-soluble proteins (prolamins) in rye, barley, and oats. In patients with celiac disease, ingestion of these proteins can damage the mucosa of the small intestine and thereby cause atrophy of the villi and elongation of the crypts. This disease is therefore referred to as gluten-sensitive enteropathy.

The tendency for celiac disease to run in families has long been recognized. Several family studies have shown that the incidence of celiac disease in family members is much higher than in the general population, varying from 8.2% to 18.3% in first-degree relatives.[31] The affected relatives appeared in every generation but varied a great deal in disease expression. This led to the suggestion of an autosomal dominant inheritance with variable penetrance.[31] However, celiac disease was found to be concordant in only 70% of monozygotic twins and in about 30% of serologically HLA-identical siblings.[32] About 80% to 90% of celiac disease patients carry the histocompatibility antigens HLA-DR3 and HLA-DQw2, as compared with 20% to 30% of normal adults. Nonetheless, only 1% of the general population with those antigens develop celiac disease.[32] Furthermore, recent studies with molecular probes and analysis of restriction fragment length polymorphism (RFLP) revealed an additional genetic marker in patients with celiac disease.[33,34] Using a DQ beta-chain cDNA probe and the restriction endonuclease RsaI, Howell et al.[33] detected a polymorphic 4.0 kb fragment. Individuals with HLA-DR3, HLA-DQw2, and the 4.0 kb DNA fragment have a risk at least 40 times higher than do those who carry HLA-DR3 and HLA-DQw2 but not the 4.0 kb fragment. These findings indicate that multiple genetic factors are involved in the pathogenesis of celiac disease. In some celiac disease patients, there are increased mucosal antigluten antibody synthesis and increased serum antibody titers to gluten and gliadin, as well as to reticulin and some dietary proteins in milk and eggs.[35-37] In addition, genes linked to the immunoglobulin heavy chain constant region have been proposed as one of the genetic loci associated with celiac disease.[38,39] With all the emerging information, it has now become increasingly clear that the pathogenesis of celiac disease may involve the interplay of multiple genetic factors and an abnormal immunologic response to ingested gluten-related proteins.

Inflammatory Bowel Disease

Inflammatory bowel disease (IBD) refers to a group of chronic inflammatory disorders of unknown etiology involving the gastrointestinal tract. It includes two major diseases: ulcerative colitis and Crohn's disease. Although these two entities can be distinguished by clinical and pathologic characteristics, they share a number of common features. It is possible that each of these two entities encompasses more than a single disease and represents various gradations of a single spectrum.

Family studies of IBD have demonstrated a strong

genetic influence in at least 15% to 20% of patients.[40] It is estimated that 2% to 5% of all patients with IBD will have one or more relatives affected, in most cases a first-degree relative. Monsen et al.[41] investigated 963 patients with IBD in Sweden and found a general prevalence of 7.9% among relatives. The prevalence of ulcerative colitis in first-degree relatives was 15 times higher than that in nonrelatives. The age of onset was significantly lower among patients with a family history of ulcerative colitis. It is interesting to note that ulcerative colitis is more likely than Crohn's disease to occur in the families of probands with ulcerative colitis, and the same relationship holds true for Crohn's disease. However, an intermingling of these two disorders is found in approximately 25% of the familial cases.[40] Case reports have documented concordance in five of eight pairs of monozygotic twins with ulcerative colitis and in seven of eight pairs of monozygotic twins with Crohn's disease.[40]

Serologic assays for HLA antigens failed to show a consistent difference between IBD patients and control groups. However, IBD patients associated with ankylosing spondylitis have a high prevalence of class I HLA-B27.[42] Such association is found in about 3% to 5% of IBD families, either in the same patient or in other members.[40] Other associated conditions include allergic disorders, rheumatoid arthritis, and chronic liver disease.

It has been reported that class II HLA-DR antigens are expressed in intestinal epithelial cells, especially during inflammatory reactions.[43] The pathogenetic mechanism of such antigenic expression is not clearly understood. The accumulated evidence supports a strong genetic influence in the development of IBD, but the exact genetic mechanism has not been identified. It is most likely that both genetic and environmental factors are important in the development of IBD.

Hirschsprung's Disease

Hirschsprung's disease (congenital aganglionic megacolon) is due to absence of intramural ganglion cells in the intestine. It involves the colon and small intestine to varying degrees. Passarge[44] classified the disease into two types. Type I was defined as aganglionosis extending from the rectum to the splenic flexure (short-segment involvement), present in about 90% of patients, and type II was defined as aganglionosis extending beyond the splenic flexure into the transverse colon or even through the entire colon into the small intestine (long-segment involvement).

Approximately 4% of the cases are familial.[45] The risk of recurrence in siblings depends on the length of the aganglionic segment. In general, the longer the involved segment, the higher the risk of recurrence. The sex ratio also varies with the extent of aganglionosis. In cases of long-segment involvement the male-to-female ratio is 1.86:1, whereas in cases of short-segment involvement the male-to-female ratio is 5.2:1.[45] The risk of recurrence, therefore, depends on the length of the aganglionic segment as well as the sex of the affected person. In short-segment disease, the risk of recurrence for siblings of an affected male is about 1% for sisters and 6% for brothers, and that of an affected female is 3% for sisters and 8% for brothers. In long-segment disease, the risk for siblings of an affected male is about 10% for sisters and 7% for brothers, and that of an affected female is 9% for sisters and 18% for brothers.[2] Recently, Badner et al.,[46] on the basis of a study of 487 probands and their families, observed an overall elevated risk for siblings of 4%, as compared with 0.02% for the general population. They further suggested that for cases with aganglionosis beyond the sigmoid colon, the mode of inheritance is compatible with a dominant gene, with incomplete penetrance, whereas for cases with aganglionosis no farther than the sigmoid colon, the pattern of inheritance may be either multifactorial or autosomal recessive, with a very low penetrance gene.

Hirschsprung's disease may be associated with other disorders, notably Down's syndrome. About 2% to 2.5% of Down's syndrome patients have Hirschsprung's disease.[19] Weinberg et al.[47] reported that in a family with deafness in three consecutive generations, Hirschsprung's disease was present in at least two of the affected patients. Other associated conditions include several rare chromosomal syndromes (see Table 6-3), cleft palate, cartilage-hair hypoplasia, pheochromocytoma, rubella embryopathy, colonic atresia,[44] neuroblastoma,[48] Waardenburg's syndrome,[49,50] and Aarskog's syndrome.[51] The association of Hirschsprung's disease with such a wide range of disorders suggests genetic heterogeneity.

Congenital Hypertrophic Pyloric Stenosis

It has long been known that there is a strong genetic influence in congenital hypertrophic pyloric stenosis (CHPS) because it occurs in the siblings of affected children about 12 times more frequently than in the general population.[52] There is a remarkable difference in the distribution of the disease in the two sexes. The incidence in females is 1/750 and in males 1/150. It has been noted that Turner's syndrome patients (monosomy X) have an increased liability to CHPS, indicating that the presence of a second X chromosome has some mitigating effect.[53] When a female does develop CHPS, her offspring has a much higher risk of attracting the disease than the offspring of an affected male. On the average, affected females have affected sons 18.9% of the time and affected daughters 7.0% of the time, whereas affected males have only 5.5% of their sons affected and 2.4% of their daughters affected.[52] It is postulated that females carry a high concentration of the genes determining susceptibility; thus her chance of transmitting these genes to the offspring is greater than that of an affected male. CHPS was the first to illustrate the genetic influence related to the sex of the affected individual.

Twin studies showed higher concordance for monozygotic twins than for dizygotic twins, but the concordance is much lower than 100%.[54] The heterogeneous nature of CHPS is evidenced by its association with a number of other disorders, including chromosomal syndromes (see Table 6–3), phenylketonuria, esophageal atresia, hiatal hernia, peptic ulcer, Smith-Lemli-Opitz syndrome, rubella embryopathy, and Cornelia de Lange's syndrome.

It has been clearly demonstrated that CHPS has a familial distribution, but it does not follow the rules of mendelian inheritance. Multifactorial inheritance is generally considered the best explanation for the distribution pattern of this disease.[55]

GENETICS OF NEOPLASTIC DISEASES OF THE GASTROINTESTINAL TRACT

Esophageal Tumors

Twenty percent of esophageal tumors are benign, mostly leiomyomas. Among the malignant tumors, 90% are squamous cell carcinomas, and 10% are adenocarcinomas. The latter is primarily a complication of Barrett's esophagus secondary to reflux esophagitis. Squamous cell carcinoma of the esophagus has wide geographic variation. The etiology and pathologic features of these tumors are detailed in Chapters 18 and 19. Environmental factors and a history of alcohol intake or tobacco use are the chief causative factors. The only link with genetic predisposition was reported in patients with familial tylosis palmaris et plantaris.[56,57] The patient reported by Shin and Allison[58] had squamous cell carcinoma in what appeared to be Barrett's esophagus. Esophageal carcinoma has also been reported in patients with sporadic tylosis.[59]

The incidence rate of esophageal cancer is very high in the Northern Caspian littoral of Iran. Ghadirian[60] reported a study of family history among Turkoman (high-risk) and non-Turkoman (low-risk) populations in that region. A positive family history was obtained in 47% of the former, of whom 82% were blood relatives and 18% relatives by marriage. In contrast, only 2% of the non-Turkoman group had a positive family history. Thus, there appears to be a genetic factor in the development of esophageal cancer in the high-risk population.

Cytogenetic studies of esophageal cancer cell lines were carried out by Whang-Peng et al.[61] Extensive numeric and structural abnormalities were found involving nearly every chromosome, most frequently chromosomes 1, 9, and 11. The major abnormality is partial deletion. The most frequent break points were 3p14, 11q12, and 9q11. Chromosomal rearrangement at 11p13–15 was found in the adenocarcinomas of the lower esophagus and stomach.[62]

Squamous cell carcinoma of the esophagus has shown amplification of c-myc and epidermal growth factor receptor genes (c-erbB).[63,64] Amplification of hst-1 and int-2 oncogenes were found in 47% of primary esophageal carcinomas and 100% of metastatic lesions.[65] The search for point mutation of ras genes at codon 12 or 13 has been negative.[66]

Gastric Tumors

Over 90% of the neoplasms in the stomach are malignant, mainly adenocarcinomas. Benign neoplasms are nearly equally divided between epithelial and mesenchymal lesions. Adenomas have a high incidence of malignant transformation but are not the main precursor of carcinoma as in the colon. Other precursors include chronic atrophic gastritis (CAG) with or without intestinal metaplasia; chronic gastric ulcer; mucosal hyperplasia, including Ménétrier's disease; postgastrectomy remnants; and, on occasion, nonneoplastic polyps. Detailed information about these conditions is presented in Chapter 25. The most important one is CAG. One of its forms, type A, involving the fundic mucosa, is related to pernicious anemia, which is influenced by a genetic factor with dominant inheritance.[67] The other form of CAG, type B, involving the antral mucosa, is the most important precancerous condition for gastric cancer. A study in Colombia revealed that CAG was transmitted as an autosomal recessive trait with penetrance dependent on the age of the patient and the CAG status of the mother.[68] Homozygous recessives had a penetrance of 72% or 41% at age 30, depending on whether the mother was affected or not.

Gastric carcinoma itself may be affected by genetic factors. Persons with blood groups A have a higher incidence of gastric carcinoma than others do.[69] The increased risk is only 20% over the general population, however. Gastric carcinoma has been reported in patients with ataxia-telangiectasia, an autosomal recessive disease.[70] There have also been reports of clusters of gastric cancers in a family. The best known example is that of Napoleon Bonaparte. Napoleon himself, his grandfather, his father, and five siblings were said to be affected with gastric carcinoma.[71] There appears to be a threefold increased risk among relatives of patients with gastric cancer.[72] Gastric carcinoma also occurs in patients with genetically transmitted intestinal cancers such as familial adenomatous polyposis and cancer family syndrome.

Cytogenetic studies with G-banding on gastric carcinomas revealed many aberrations. Ochi et al.[73] studied five primary stage IV carcinomas and found 67 numeric and 83 structural chromosome anomalies. The most prominent numeric abnormality was a missing Y chromosome in three of four male patients. There were no recurring structural abnormalities. However, break points at 1p22, 3p21, and 19p13 were frequent. It is interesting to note that the modal chromosome number was 43-44 for a signet-ring cell carcinoma, 46/47/48 for a mucin-producing carcinoma, and polyploidy for three other types of carcinomas. The signet-ring cell carcinoma has been found to be mostly diploid by DNA measurement.[74] In another study on two primary gastric carcinomas and three metastatic effusions, karyotypic abnormalities were noted involving mainly chromosomes 1, 7, 8, and 9.[75] Chromosome 9 was the most frequently affected, showing trisomy, i(9q), or 9p+. Chromosome 8 was the next most often affected, showing trisomy and i(8q). In a cytogenetic study on effusions,[76] chromosomes 3, 5, 13, and 17 were involved. Thus, there seem to be no consistent karyotypic changes in gastric carcinoma cells. Allele losses have been found in chromosomes 5,[77] 13,[78] 1,[79] and 12.[79]

By Southern blot hybridization or immunohistochemical staining using antibodies against gene products, several oncogenes were found to be amplified in gastric carcinomas. Ras oncogenes have been investigated by many investigators with varying results. Point mutation has been found in c-Ha-ras in codon 12,[80] c-Ki-ras in codon 12,[81] and c-N-ras in codon 13.[82] Other studies revealed amplified expression of normal allele of the ras gene.[81,83] The frequency of enhanced gene activity varied in different reports and appeared to be related to the depth of invasion of the carcinoma; it was 11.1% in early gastric cancer cases and 43.8% in advanced cases in a report by Tahara et al.[84]

Amplification of c-myc oncogene has been found to be related also to the depth of tumor invasion; none of the early cancers and 36.4% of advanced cancers showed amplification.[85] In a few cases, there was co-amplification of c-myc and c-erbB genes.[86,87] Amplification of c-erbB-2 was found in 40% of tubular adenocarcinomas but not in other histologic types.[88]

The hst-1 (hstf-1) gene, originally identified from cancerous and normal human gastric tissue, was mapped to chromosome band 11q13.[89] It has been found in many different tumors including squamous cell carcinoma of the esophagus.[90] Other genes showing enhanced activity in gastric carcinoma include transforming growth factor,[91] epidermal growth factor and receptors,[91,92] akt-1,[93] c-yes-1,[94] c-fes,[92] c-raf-1,[95] int-2,[89] and pS2.[96]

Intestinal Tumors

In contrast to the esophagus and stomach, benign tumors are common in the intestine, particularly the colorectum. Mesenchymal tumors are common in the small intestine but rare in the large intestine. In the latter, nearly all the primary tumors are epithelial in origin, about two thirds are adenomas, and one third adenocarcinomas. Even though the small intestine is much longer than the colon, carcinomas occur nearly 60 times more often in the colorectum than in the small intestine. Detailed information on tumor types in the intestines is provided in Chapters 31 and 32.

Genetic aberrations play an important role in the development of intestinal adenomas and carcinomas. Several syndromes have been identified in which the major manifestation is the presence of many polyps in the intestine[97-99] (Table 6-4). The polyps are heterogeneous in nature, and their tendency to malignant change varies. The pathologic features of the polyps have been described in Chapter 31. In this section, the genetic aspects of these syndromes are discussed, including the phenotypic characteristics, cytogenetic changes, and molecular genetic alterations.

It has become increasingly obvious that genetics is also a major factor in the development of intestinal cancers in patients without polyposis, including many patients with sporadic tumors.[100,101] In such patients, colorectal carcinoma is the main presentation. Adenomas are also often present, even though they are not numerically or symptomatically significant. Adenomas are nevertheless important components of these cases and may be the seat of malignant transformation.

Polyposis of the intestine is not always hereditary. The Cronkhite-Canada syndrome[102] is such a disease. It affects the elderly, usually over 65 years of age and mostly men. The polyps in this syndrome are inflammatory, not premalignant, in nature and are present throughout the entire gastrointestinal tract. Patients have diarrhea and ectodermal changes, including alopecia, onychotrophia, and pigmentation. In cases of hereditary neoplasm, in contrast, the symptoms are related to the tumor, the patients are young, and there is no sex preference.

Clinical Syndromes

Familial Polyposis Syndromes

Familial Adenomatous Polyposis. Familial adenomatous polyposis[97] (FAP) is also known as familial polyposis coli and adenomatosis coli. The latter terms indicate that the polyps occur primarily in the colon.

Table 6-4 HEREDITARY SYNDROMES OF GASTROINTESTINAL TUMORS

Syndrome	Initial Tumor Type	Other Major Manifestations
Familial Polyposis		
Familial adenomatous polyposis	Adenoma	Upper gastrointestinal lesions
Gardner's syndrome	Adenoma	Osteoma, skin, and soft tissue tumors
Turcot's syndrome	Adenoma	Brain tumor
Peutz-Jeghers syndrome	Hamartoma	Mucocutaneous melanin spots
Familial juvenile polyposis	Hamartoma	None
Nonpolyposis colorectal cancer		
Lynch syndrome I (HSSCC)	Carcinoma	None
Lynch syndrome II (CFS)	Carcinoma	Other cancers in family
Discrete colorectal tumors	Adenoma or carcinoma	None

CFS, cancer family syndrome; HSSCC, hereditary site-specific colorectal cancer.

Recently, there have been many reports of polyps, adenomas, and carcinomas in the stomach[103,104] and small intestine[105,106] (see Chapters 23, 31, and 32). The frequency of this syndrome was estimated to be 1 in 8300 births.[99] It is transmitted as an autosomal dominant trait. The polyps are adenomas and usually diagnosed after the age of 10 years, mostly in the third and early fourth decades. The average age of first diagnosis in symptomatic patients is 35 years,[107] and the average age of cancer diagnosis is 39 years.[108] About 50% of symptomatic and 6% to 12% of asymptomatic patients had carcinoma of the colon at the time of diagnosis.[109,110] It is estimated that by the age of 50, carcinoma is present in all cases. The carcinomas occur mostly in the left colon and are often multiple.

Gardner's Syndrome. In 1951, Gardner reported the genetic study of a family with intestinal polyps and carcinoma.[111] In the next 2 years, osteomas, epidermal cysts, and subcutaneous fibromas of the skin were reported in such cases.[112,113] Additional manifestations include desmoids of the skin and abdomen, cortical thickening and exostosis of the long bone, dental abnormalities, pigmented patches in the retina, and tumors of other organs.[97–99,108,114,115] These extraintestinal manifestations are variable, but the adenomatous polyps of the colon are constant findings. They are morphologically identical to those seen in FAP and have some propensity for malignant change. The disease occurs in 1 of 14,025 births[116] and is transmitted as an autosomal dominant trait, as is FAP. These similarities suggest that Gardner's syndrome and FAP are the result of single gene mutation, but the possibility of additional gene mutation has also been considered.[97]

Turcot's Syndrome. This syndrome is characterized by the presence of brain tumor in patients with colonic adenomatous polyps.[117] The brain tumors are malignant. It is not clear whether this disease is a type of Gardner's syndrome (which may also have brain tumors), or a separate entity, since transmission of Turcot's syndrome has been suggested as an autosomal recessive trait.[107,108]

Hamartomatous Polyposis. The polyps in both Peutz-Jeghers syndrome and familial juvenile polyposis are hamartomatous, but the major tissue components are different. The Peutz-Jeghers polyp is composed of intestinal crypts and villi and smooth muscle bundles in a disorganized fashion. Inflammatory cells are absent or scanty, and the glandular structures are not excessively dilated. The juvenile polyp is composed of dilated intestinal glands and abundant connective tissue of the lamina propria. Smooth muscle elements are usually absent. Lymphoid cells are common. These features closely resemble those of inflammatory retention polyps in children, also known as juvenile polyps, as well as the inflammatory polyps of the Cronkhite-Canada syndrome that occur among the elderly.

Peutz-Jeghers Syndrome. Peutz-Jeghers syndrome[118,119] is characterized by the presence of Peutz-Jeghers polyps throughout the entire gastrointestinal tract and melanin spots on the lip (96%), buccal mucosa (83%), face (36%), and extremities (32%).[118] Small bowel is the favored site of the polyposis. The number of polyps are small. Symptoms of obstruction are produced by the polyp itself or by intussception with a polyp as the leading point. Other associated abnormalities include polyps in the urinary bladder and nasal cavity, bone deformities, congenital heart disease, and retarded development.[120]

The symptoms of Peutz-Jeghers syndrome develop at a younger age than do those in FAP, before the age of 20 in two thirds of cases. The average age at diagnosis is 22.5 years.[108] Peutz-Jeghers polyps are generally not considered to be prone to malignant change. Carcinomas of the gastrointestinal tract have been reported, however, in about 2% to 3% of cases.[121,122] In many reports the relationship between polyp and carcinoma was not clearly stated. When the origin of malignancy was carefully studied, the carcinoma was found to arise in the adenomatous or dysplastic epithelium in the polyp.[123] The carcinomas occurred most commonly in the upper small intestine.

Familial Juvenile Polyposis. Isolated juvenile polyps may occur in the colon and rectum of children.[124] Juvenile polyposis with many such polyps is very rare. In 1966 Veale et al.[125] reported 11 cases in 8 families. Six patients did not have a family history of the disease. The main symptoms were bleeding and prolapse of the polyp from the rectum. The average age at the onset of symptoms was 6 years. Other congenital anomalies were present in four patients without a family history of the disease. The polyps in these patients were mostly in the rectum, and therefore the term *juvenile polyposis coli* was used. Subsequently, polyps have been found in other parts of the gastrointestinal tract.[97,99] Sachatello et al.[126] reported generalized juvenile polyposis involving the entire gastrointestinal tract in infants. As more cases were reported, a wide age range was noted.[127,128] Many patients lack a positive family history,[107,114] but the familial cases were transmitted as an autosomal dominant trait.[108] The incidence of juvenile polyposis coli was estimated to be 1 in 24,000 births.[114]

At first, adenomas and carcinomas of the colon were found in the relatives of the familial cases, but not in the patients themselves.[125] Subsequently, dysplasia and adenomatous changes were found in the polyps,[97] and carcinomas may have developed in them.[127,129] The average age at cancer diagnosis is about 40 years.[97]

Hereditary Nonpolyposis Colorectal Cancer

It is estimated that familial polyposis accounts for only 0.2% of all colorectal carcinomas, whereas hereditary nonpolyposis colorectal cancer accounts for 4% to 6% of cases.[101] The hereditary nonpolyposis colorectal cancer (HNPCC) syndrome includes two major entities: cancer family syndrome (Lynch syndrome II) and hereditary site-specific colorectal cancer (Lynch syndrome I).[72,100,130] In addition, hereditary influence may exist also for discrete colorectal adenomas and cancers.[131]

The Lynch syndromes are characterized by the following: (1) Patients at the time of diagnosis are relatively young, with a mean age of 44.6 years. (2) The first cancer is often found in the right colon (72.3%), whereas only 25% of the first cancers are in the sigmoid or rectum. (3) There is a high incidence of multiple colon cancers: synchronous in 18.1% of cases and metachronous in 24.2%. The risk for developing metachronous cancers within 10 years is 40%. Because of the prevalence of the cancer in the right colon, these cases have been termed *hereditary site-specific colon cancer*.[72] When family members also exhibit cancers of other organs, the term *cancer family syndrome* or *Lynch syndrome II* is applied. When there is no other cancer in the family, it is referred to as *Lynch syndrome I*. The HNPCC syndrome is transmitted as an autosomal dominant trait.[72]

Hereditary site-specific colon cancer was first reported by Woolf and Gardner in 1955.[132] The patients also had discrete polyps. The first family with multiple cancers was reported by Warthin in 1913.[133] Subsequent studies by Lynch and others have greatly expanded the knowledge of these syndromes. Cancers in the Lynch syndrome II can affect the endometrium, ovary, and pancreas and less commonly the brain, bile duct, stomach, small intestine, breast, and urinary system and can include leukemia and lymphoma.[130] The frequency of cancers in the cancer family syndrome was studied in 22 Finnish kindreds by Mecklin et al.[134] Cancers found in 196 family members included colorectal cancer in 61%, undefined intra-abdominal cancer in 15%, endometrial cancer in 10%, gastric cancer in 7%, biliary tract cancer in 3%, and other cancers in 7%. An autosomal dominant pattern of inheritance was shown by the colorectal and uterine cancers. The cumulative risk in the descendants increased to 50% at the age of 69 years.

The Muir-Toore syndrome, which is characterized by multiple intestinal cancers associated with genitourinary and skin tumors, particularly of the sebaceous glands,[135] has been present in some members of a cancer family.[136]

The carcinomas in cancer family patients are more likely to be mucinous and poorly differentiated than are the sporadic colon cancers.[137] Although HNPCC patients do not have polyposis, adenomas do occur in the colon. The incidence of adenoma is not increased, however. On the other hand, some adenomas have a high grade of dysplasia[137] and are precursors of invasive carcinoma.[138] No other lesions have been found to account for the high incidence of colon cancer in these patients.

Discrete Adenomas and Carcinomas of the Colon

Polyposis syndromes are rare. Discrete adenomas in small numbers, on the other hand, are very common, and are estimated to occur in 10% to 50% of the general population. Total colorectal cancer in these patients may affect 3% of the population.[97] The inheritance pattern of these cases is largely unknown. Burt et al.[131] studied a large Utah kindred with clusters of colorectal cancer but no recognizable inheritance pattern. Extensive screening with flexible proctosigmoidoscopy revealed adenomas in 21% of the 191 pedigree members in contrast to 9% of the controls. The excess of adenomas was found to be due to an autosomal dominant inheritance. A subsequent expanded study of 670 persons in 34 kindreds revealed similar results.[139] The estimated prevalence of adenoma at age 60 in related family members was 24%, whereas that in the unrelated spouses was 12%. Such studies emphasize the importance of screening for colorectal tumors in first-degree relatives of patients with these lesions.

Molecular Genetic and Cytogenetic Changes

Molecular Genetic Changes and Tumor-Suppressing Genes

Much progress has been made in the past few years on the understanding of colorectal carcinogenesis. The molecular events in this instance appear to be similar to those found in retinoblastoma (RB). Like colorectal cancer, retinoblastomas occur in either familial or sporadic form. The familial form is transmitted as an autosomal dominant trait with nearly complete penetrance. Based on his study of retinoblastoma, Knudson in 1971[140] proposed the now well-known theory of two mutational events for tumorigenesis. In the familial form, the first mutation is inherited and the second mutation is somatic and occurs in the target tissue. In sporadic cases, both mutations are somatic. The first event in RB is an interstitial deletion of chromosome 13q14, which contains the RB gene.[141] The second event, which may be a mutation, nondisjunction, deletion, or somatic recombination,[142] affects the remaining normal allele of the same gene. The second event is necessary to cause the disease. Thus, retinoblastoma is the result of total loss of the function of the RB gene. The normal allele serves as an antioncogene,[142] or tumor-suppressing gene.[143]

In the colon, a similar sequence of tumorigenesis is found in FAP. First, chromosome 5q was found to be deleted in a patient with Gardner's syndrome by Herrera et al. in 1986.[144] In the following year, the FAP gene was localized on chromosome 5 near 5q21-q22 by Bodmer et al.[145] and others.[146] Chromosome 5 allele loss was found in adenomas from FAP patients[147] and in about 20% of sporadic colorectal carcinomas.[147,148] Law et al.[149] found a low incidence of chromosome 5 allele loss (19%) in 31 colorectal carcinomas but high allele loss on chromosomes 17 (56%) and 18 (52%). Allele losses on chromosomes 17p and 18q were also noted by others.[150–152] Okamoto et al.[153] reported frequent allele loss on chromosome 22 and some losses on chromosomes 5, 6, 12q, and 15. Regional losses have also been found on chromosomes 1q, 4p, 6p, 6q, 8p, 9q, and 22q.[154]

Vogelstein et al.[155] studied these changes and *ras* gene mutations in 172 colorectal tumors at various stages of development. They found that *ras* gene mutation was present in about one-half of large adenomas and carcinomas and 25% of small adenomas. Chromosome 5 allele loss was also found in the late adenomas and carcinomas but not in the early adenomas from FAP cases. Chromosome 18 regional deletion was present in adenomas and carcinomas with an increased frequency in later stages. Chromosome 17p losses were found only in carcinomas. The deleted region was localized to bands 17p12 to p13.3, which contain the gene for p53.[156] P53 is related to normal cell proliferation but may suppress neoplastic growth. In two tumors, the remaining p53 allele was found to be mutated at codons 143 and 175. Loss of the normal tumor-suppressing function of p53 by deletion or mutation may be involved in colonic carcinogenesis.[156] Thus, the development of colorectal tumor involves several tumor-suppressing genes at different stages of development. Mutation of the *ras* oncogene is a significant step in tumorigenesis independent of allele loss. It was postulated by Vogelstein et al. that inactivation of one allele of the FAP gene on chromosome 5, while insufficient to cause adenoma, might stimulate epithelial hyperplasia, and the second event inducing the tumor might be heterogeneous and involve several genetic changes and oncogenes.[154,155]

The diagnostic significance of chromosomal deletions has been evaluated by multivariate analysis in relation to the stage of the carcinoma.[157] Distant metastasis was significantly associated with allele loss and deletions of 17p and 18q but not with the *ras* gene mutation or deletion of 5q.

The clonal origin of colorectal tumors was investigated by means of X-linked restriction fragment length polymorphisms.[158] All tumors examined, including both adenomas and carcinomas, showed a monoclonal pattern of X chromosome inactivation.

Cytogenetic Changes

Cytogenetic changes in the colonic tumors are manifested either numerically or structurally or both. The study of 38 colonic adenomas by Reichmann et al.[159] revealed analyzable karyotypes in 18 tumors. These adenomas showed normal diploid karyotype in five, numeric abnormalities in six, and both numeric and structural abnormalities in seven. The latter included extra chromosome 7, 8, or 13 and marker chromosomes. In one villous adenoma, there were an extra chromosome 8, loss of a Y chromosome, and a marker chromosome 1 with duplication of the long arm.[160] Chromosomal studies in patients with FAP and the HNPCC syndrome and their relatives did not reveal any abnormalities.[161-163]

Levin and Reichmann[164] also studied 49 colonic adenocarcinomas. Only 8% of the tumors had normal karyotypes. Hypodiploidy or hypotriploidy were observed in 50%. Thirty-eight tumors had a total of 257 marker chromosomes, 44% of which had recognizable patterns, most frequently involving chromosomes 1, 5, 8, 9, 13, and 17. Trisomy and double minutes were common. Homogeneous staining regions and abnormal banded regions were also observed. Tumors with marked chromosomal abnormalities were more commonly located in the left colon, whereas tumors with normal karyotypes or few abnormalities were more common in the right colon.

Muleris et al.[165] performed cytogenetic studies on 100 colorectal carcinomas, 14 in the proximal colon, 42 in the distal colon, and 44 in the rectum. Seven tumors had normal karyotypes (NT). Chromosomal abnormalities were classified into three types: (1) monosomic-type near diploid (MD) tumors in 28 cases, characterized by a monosomy of both chromosomes 17 and 18; (2) monosomic-type polyploid (MP) tumors in 42 cases, derived from the MD tumors by endoreduplication; and (3) trisomic-type (TT) tumors in 22 cases, with or without loss of 17p or 18. One tumor could not be classified. The MD and MP tumors were predominantly located in the distal colon and rectum, whereas TT and NT tumors were found mainly in the proximal colon. Structural rearrangements of the chromosomes per tumor in MD and MP tumors were two to three times higher than those in the TT tumors. Sixty percent of the rearrangements were unbalanced and 5% balanced. Deletions occurred in 20% and isochromosomes in 10% to 20%.

Dutrillaux[166] noted that the monosomic-type tumors had losses or deletions involving, in order of frequency, chromosomes 18, 17, 1p, 4, 14, 5, and 21. Trisomy involved chromosomes 7, 12, X, 5, and 8. The study on near diploid tumors showed monosomy 17p, monosomy 18, trisomy 20q, trisomy or tetrasomy 13, monosomy 1p, and trisomy X and 8q.[167]

The feasibility of the application of karyotypic study to clinical diagnosis is exemplified by the report of a rectosigmoid tumor in a 74-year-old man.[168] The biopsy of the tumor was interpreted as histologically benign. The karyotype of the same biopsy specimen showed several chromosomal changes, including trisomy 7, t(3;12), t(1;17), interstitial deletion of 5p, loss of the Y chromosome, and an extra X chromosome. These changes strongly suggested malignancy. A 5-cm well to moderately differentiated adenocarcinoma in Dukes' stage B1 was subsequently excised.

Oncogenes

C-*ras* oncogenes are frequently expressed in colorectal cancers and less frequently in adenomas.[155] Mutations of the *ras* gene were found in 11 of 27 cancers examined by Bos et al.,[169] mainly involving c-Ki-*ras* at codon 12. They were present in both coexisting adenomas and carcinomas within the same lesion in five of six tumors, suggesting a possible role of the mutated genes in the adenoma-carcinoma sequence. However, the presence of the mutant *ras* gene did not correlate with the invasiveness of the tumor.[170] Alexander et al.,[171] on the other hand, did not find rearrangement of the Ki- or N-*ras* genes in the tumors, but one of nine tumors that they examined had a rare allele of the Ha-*ras* gene. They also found no rearrangement of *myc*, N-*myc*, or *fos* oncogenes.

Immunohistochemical studies using antibodies against *ras* oncogene product p21 have been carried out in several laboratories. In an early study, p21 was not detected in the normal colon mucosa and was present in only a few cells in the adenoma.[172] In the carcinoma, the extent of positive reaction paralleled the depth of tumor invasion. Therefore, the *ras* oncogene expression was thought to be a late event. Subsequent studies, however, showed positive reaction in the normal and adenomatous tissue as well as in carcinoma;[155,173,174] and there was no relation between the reaction and tumor stage, histology, or DNA content.[175] In some reports, the reactivity was higher in adenomas than in carcinomas[174] and was further reduced in metastatic lesions.[176] The presence of *ras* oncogene expression in the adenoma suggests that it is an early event before malignant transformation.[154,155] Furthermore, mutation of the *ras* gene in codon 12 was detected in both diploid and aneuploid carcinomas, which suggests that the mutations occurred before ploidy changes.[177]

Monnat et al.[178] investigated the expression of *myc*, *fos*, Ha-*ras*, and Ki-*ras* genes in colonic carcinomas. One-half of the tumors showed increased expression of one or more genes. There was no clear correlation between the degree of expression and pathologic features of the tumors. However, the overexpressed tumors were more aggressive than the nonexpressors. In another report, the expression of *fos* gene was found to be markedly reduced in both adenomas and carcinomas.[179]

The c-*myc* oncogene expression is detectable in both colonic carcinomas and adenomas, with higher expression in the former.[179–181] N-*myc* and L-*myc* are also often overexpressed.[182] Flow-cytometric measurement of c-*myc* protein p62 showed a progressive increase from normal through polyps to carcinoma, and was higher in the better differentiated than in the poorly differentiated carcinomas.[183] The increased c-*myc* expression was correlated with the allele loss on chromosome 5q.[184] In two neuroendocrine cell lines from a colon carcinoma, the amplified c-*myc* expression was located in the homogeneously staining region of the distorted X chromosome.[185] The c-*myc* gene had apparently translocated from its normal site on chromosome 8q24. The carcinomas with elevated c-*myc* expression tended to be located in the left colon (85% of tumors), corresponding with carcinomas in FAP patients, which also had a left-sided predominance.[186] Conversely, the tumors with low expression of c-*myc* gene were located more often in the right colon, which is the case in HNPCC.

Amplified expression of c-*erbB*-2 and allelic deletion of c-Ha-*ras* and c-*myb* oncogenes were found in a small number of colon cancers, but not in adenomas.[187] Amplification of *trk* and *her*-2/*neu* oncogenes in colonic carcinoma have also been reported.[188,189] The c-*src* oncogene and the related c-*yes* and *lck* genes were overexpressed in colon cancer cell lines.[190]

References

1. McKusick VA: Mendelian Inheritance in Man: Catalogs of Autosomal Dominant, Autosomal Recessive and X-linked Phenotypes, 8th ed. Baltimore, Johns Hopkins University Press, 1988.
2. Passarge E: Genetics of the gastrointestinal tract. In Jackson LG, Schimke RN (eds): Clinical Genetics. New York, John Wiley and Sons, 1979, pp 331–347.
3. Dodge JA: Genetics of hypertrophic pyloric stenosis. Clin Gastroenterol 2:523–538, 1973.
4. Carpenter CB: The major histocompatibility gene complex. In Wilson J, Braunwald E, Isselbacher KJ, et al (eds): Harrison's Principles of Internal Medicine. New York, McGraw-Hill, 1991, pp 86–92.
5. Rotter JI: Peptic ulcer. In Emery AEH, Rimoin DL (eds): Principles and Practice of Medical Genetics. New York, Churchill Livingstone, 1983.
6. Ellis A, Woodrow JC: HLA and duodenal ulcer. Gut 20:760, 1979.
7. Goldhard JG, Biemond I, Pena AS, et al: HLA and duodenal ulcer in Netherlands. Tissue Antigens 22:213–218, 1983.
8. Aird I, Bentall HH, Roberts JAF: A relationship between cancer of the stomach and the ABO blood groups. Br Med J 1:799–801, 1953.
9. Langman MJS: Blood group and alimentary disorders. Clin Gastroenterol 2:497–506, 1973.
10. Beckman L, Angqvist KA: On the mechanism behind the association between ABO blood groups and gastric carcinoma. Hum Hered 37:140–143, 1987.
11. Aird I, Bentall HH, Mehigan JA, et al: The blood groups in relation to peptic ulceration and carcinoma of colon, rectum, breast and bronchus. Br Med J 2:315–321, 1954.
12. McConnell RB: The Genetics of Gastrointestinal Disorders. London, Oxford University Press, 1966.
13. McConnell RB: Peptic ulcer, early genetic evidence—Families, twins and markers. In Rotter JI, Samloff IM, Rimoin DL (eds): The Genetics and Heterogeneity of Common Gastrointestinal Disorders. New York, Academic Press, 1980, pp 31–41.
14. Cowan WK: Genetics of duodenal and gastric ulcer. Clin Gastroenterol 2:539–546, 1973.
15. Mourant AE, Kopec AC, Domaniewska-Sobczak K: Blood Groups and Disease: A Study of Associations of Disease with Blood Groups and other Polymorphisms. London, Oxford University Press, 1978.
16. Soll AH: Duodenal ulcer and drug therapy. In Sleisenger MH, Fordtran JS (eds): Gastrointestinal Disease, 4th ed. Philadelphia, WB Saunders, 1989, pp 814–879.
17. Warkany J: Uses and misuses of syndromes. In Shafield ME, Kippel CH Jr (eds): Associated Congenital Anomalies. Baltimore, Williams & Wilkins, 1981, pp 21–23.
18. Shafie ME: Associated anomalies in infants with major congenital surgical malformations. In Shafield ME, Klippel CH Jr (eds): Associated Congenital Anomalies. Baltimore, Williams & Wilkins, 1981, pp 165–174.
19. Warkany J, Passarge E, Smith LB: Congenital malformations in autosomal trisomy syndromes. Am J Dis Child 112:502–517, 1966.
20. Thompson JS: The genetics of multiple congenital anomalies. In Shafie ME, Klippel CH Jr (eds): Associated Congenital Anomalies. Baltimore, Williams & Wilkins, 1981, pp 9–15.
21. DeGrouchy J, Turleau C: Clinical Atlas of Human Chromosomes, 2nd ed. New York, John Wiley and Sons, 1984.
22. Jones KL: Smith's Recognizable Patterns of Human Malformation, 4th ed. Philadelphia, WB Saunders, 1988.
23. Beedgen B, Nutzendel W, Querfeld V, et al: Partial trisomy 22 and 11 due to a paternal 11;22 translocation associated with Hirschsprung's disease. Eur J Pediatr 145:229–232, 1986.
24. Lamont MA, Fitchett M, Dennis NR: Interstitial deletion of distal 13q associated with Hirschsprung's disease. J Med Genet 26:100–104, 1989.
25. Doll R, Buch J: Hereditary factors in peptic ulcer. Ann Eugenics 15:135–146, 1950.
26. Doll R, Kellock TD: The separate inheritance of gastric and duodenal ulcers. Ann Eugenics 16:231–240, 1951.
27. Ellis A: The genetics of peptic ulcer. Scand J Gastroenterol 20, (Suppl 110):25–27, 1985.
28. Rotter JI, Sones JQ, Samloff IM, et al: Duodenal ulcer disease associated with elevated serum pepsinogen I. An inherited autosomal dominant disorder. N Engl J Med 300:63–66, 1979.
29. Rotter JI, Petersen G, Samloff IM, et al: Genetic heterogeneity of hyperpepsinogenemic I and normopepsinogenemic I duodenal ulcer disease. Ann Intern Med 91:372–377, 1979.
30. Habibullah CM, Ali MM, Ishaq M, et al: Study of duodenal

ulcer disease in 100 families using total serum pepsinogen as a genetic marker. Gut 25:1380–1383, 1984.
31. Stokes PL, Asquith P, Cooke WT: Genetics of celiac disease. Clin Gastroenterol 2:547–556, 1973.
32. Cole SG, Kagnoff MF: Celiac disease. Annu Rev Nutr 5:241–266, 1985.
33. Howell MD, Austin RK, Kelleher D, et al: An HLA-D region restriction fragment length polymorphism associated with celiac disease. J Exp Med 164:333–338, 1986.
34. Howell MD, Resner J, Austin RK, et al: Rapid identification of hybridization probes for chromosomal walking. Gene 55:41–45, 1987.
35. Falchuk ZM, Strober W: Gluten-sensitive enteropathy: Synthesis of antigliadin antibody in vitro. Gut 15:947–952, 1974.
36. Kenrick KG, Walker KJ: Immunoglobulins and dietary protein antibodies in childhood celiac disease. Gut 11:635–640, 1970.
37. Maury CP, Teppo AM, Vuoristo M, et al: Autoantibodies to gliadin-binding 90kDa glycoprotein in celiac disease. Gut 37:147–152, 1986.
38. Weiss JB, Austin RK, Schanfield MS, et al: Gluten-sensitive enteropathy: IgG heavy chain (Gm) allotypes and the immune response to wheat gliadin. J Clin Invest 72:96–101, 1983.
39. Kagnoff MF, Weiss JB, Brown RJ, et al: Immunoglobulin allotype markers in gluten-sensitive enteropathy. Lancet 1:952–953, 1983.
40. Kirsner JB: Genetic aspect of inflammatory bowel disease. Clin Gastroenterol 2:556–575, 1973.
41. Monsen U, Brostrom O, Nordenvall B: Prevalence of inflammatory bowel disease among relatives of patients with ulcerative colitis. Scand J Gastroenterol 22:214–218, 1987.
42. Malls EG, Mackintosh P, Asquith P, et al: Histocompatibility antigens in inflammatory bowel disease. Gut 17:906–910, 1976.
43. Paulsen LO, Elling P, Sorensen FB, et al: HLA-DR expression and disease activity in ulcerative colitis. Scand J Gastroenterol 21:364–368, 1986.
44. Passarge E: Genetics of Hirschsprung's disease. Clin Gastroenterol 2:507–513, 1973.
45. Passarge E: Hirschsprung's disease and other developmental defects of the gastrointestinal tract. In Emery AEH, Rimoin DL (eds): Principles and Practice of Medical Genetics. New York, Churchill Livingstone, 1983, pp 886–889.
46. Badner JA, Sieber WK, Garver KL: A genetic study of Hirschsprung's disease. Am J Hum Genet 45:568–580, 1990.
47. Weinberg AG, Currarino G, Besserman AM: Hirschsprung disease and congenital deafness: Familial association. Hum Genet 22:157–161, 1977.
48. Clausen N, Anderson P, Tommerup N: Familial occurrence of neuroblastoma, Von Recklinghausen's neurofibromatosis, Hirschsprung's aganglionosis and Jaw-Winking syndrome. Acta Pediatr Scand 78:736–741, 1989.
49. Omenn GS, McKusick VA: The association of Waardenburg syndrome with Hirschsprung's disease, midgut malrotation and dental anomalies. J Med Genet 17:235–238, 1989.
50. Badner JA, Chakravarti A: Waardenburg syndrome and Hirschsprung disease: Evidence for pleiotropic effects of a single dominant gene. Am J Med Genet 35:100–104, 1990.
51. Hassinger DD, Mulvihill JJ, Chandler JB: Aarskog's syndrome with Hirschsprung's disease, midgut malrotation and dental anomalies. J Med Genet 17:235–238, 1989.
52. Carter CO, Evans KA: Inheritance of congenital pyloric stenosis. J Med Genet 6:233–254, 1969.
53. Benson PF, King MMR: An increased incidence of congenital pyloric stenosis in patients with ovarian dysgenesis. Guy's Hosp Rep 113:354–359, 1964.
54. Carter CO: Congenital pyloric stenosis. In Emery AEH, Rimoin DL (eds): Principles and Practice of Medical Genetics. New York, Churchill Livingstone, 1983, pp 879–885.
55. Chakraborty R: The inheritance of pyloric stenosis explained by a multifactorial threshold model with sex dimorphism for liability. Genet Epidemiol 3:1–15, 1986.
56. Howel-Evans W, McConnell RB, Clarke CA, et al: Carcinoma of oesophagus with keratosis palmaris et plantaris (tylosis). Q J Med (NS) 27:413–458, 1958.
57. Harper PS, Harper RMJ, Howel-Evans AW: Carcinoma of the oesophagus with tylosis. Q J Med (NS) 39:317–333, 1970.
58. Shin I, Allison PR: Carcinoma of the oesophagus with tylosis (kertosis plamaris et plantaris). Lancet 1:951–953, 1966.
59. Parnell DD: Tylosis palmaris et plantaris: Its occurrence with internal malignancy. Am J Dermatol 100:7–9, 1969.
60. Ghadirian P: Familial history of esophageal cancer. Cancer 56:2112–2116, 1985.
61. Whang-Peng J, Banks-Schlegel SP, Lee EC: Cytogenetic studies of esophageal carcinoma cell lines. Cancer Genet Cytogenet 45:101–120, 1990.
62. Rodriguz E, Rao PH, Ladanyi M, et al: 11p13–15 is a specific region of chromosomal rearrangement in gastric and esophageal adenocarcinomas. Cancer Res 50:6410–6416, 1990.
63. Lu SH, Hsieh LL, Luo FC, Weinstein IB: Amplification of the EGF receptor and c-*myc* genes in human esophageal cancers. Int J Cancer 42:502–505, 1988.
64. Hollstein MC, Smits AM, Galiana C, et al: Amplification of epidermal growth factor receptor gene but no evidence of *ras* mutations in primary human esophageal cancers. Cancer Res 48:5119–5123, 1988.
65. Tsuda T, Tahara E, Kajiyama G, et al: High incidence of coamplification of *hst*-1 and *int*-2 genes in human esophageal carcinomas. Cancer Res 49:5505–5508, 1989.
66. Jiang W, Kahn SM, Guillem JG, et al: Rapid detection of *ras* oncogenes in human tumors: Applications to colon, esophageal, and gastric cancer. Oncogene 4:923–928, 1989.
67. Varis K: Family behavior of chronic gastritis. Ann Clin Res 13:123–129, 1981.
68. Bonney GE, Elston EC, Correa P, et al: Genetic etiology of gastric carcinoma. I. Chronic atrophic gastritis. Genet Epidemiol 3:213–224, 1986.
69. McConnel RB: The genetics of carcinoma of the stomach. In Shivas AM (ed): Racial and Geographical Factors in Tumour Incidence. Edinburgh, University Press, 1967, pp 107–113.
70. Haerer AF, Jackson JF, Levers, CG: Ataxia-telangiectasia with gastric adenocarcinoma. JAMA 210:1874–1877, 1969.
71. Sokoloff B: Predisposition to cancer in the Bonaparte family. Am J Surg 40:673–678, 1938.
72. Lynch HT, Lynch PM: Heredity and gastrointestinal tract cancer. In Lipkin M, Good RA (eds): Gastrointestinal Tract Cancer. New York, Plenum, 1978, pp 241–274.
73. Ochi H, Douglass HO Jr, Sandberg AA: Cytogenetic studies in primary gastric cancer. Cancer Genet Cytogenet 22:295–307, 1986.
74. Oda N, Tahara E, Taniyama K: Cytophotometric analysis on nuclear DNA contents of human scirrhous gastric carcinoma. Pathol Res Pract 184:390–401, 1989.
75. Ferti-Passantonopoulou AD, Panani AD, Vlachos JD, Raptis SA: Common cytogenetic findings in gastric cancer. Cancer Genet Cytogenet 24:63–73, 1987.
76. Misawa S, Horiike S, Taniwaki M, et al: Chromosome abnormalities of gastric cancer detected in cancerous effusions. Jpn J Cancer Res 81:148–152, 1990.
77. Michelassi F, Errori F, Angriman I, et al: Chromosome 5 allele loss in human gastric ampullary pancreatic carcinomas. Italian Surg Sci 19:341–344, 1989.
78. Motomura K, Nishisho I, Takai S, et al: Loss of alleles at loci on chromosome 13 in human gastric cancers. Genomics 2:180–184, 1988.
79. Fey MF, Hesketh C, Wainscoat JS, Gendler S, Thein SL: Clonal allele loss in gastrointestinal cancers. Br J Cancer 59:750–754, 1989.
80. Deng GR: A sensitive non-radioactive PCR-RFLP analysis for detecting point mutations at 12th codon on oncogene c-Ha-*ras* in DNAs of gastric cancer. Nucleic Acids Res 16:6231, 1988.
81. Bos JL, Verlaan de Vries M, Marshall CJ, et al: A human gastric carcinoma contains a single mutated and an amplified normal allele of the Ki-*ras* oncogene. Nucleic Acids Res 14:1209–1217, 1986.
82. Nishida J, Kobayashi Y, Hirai H, et al: A point mutation at codon 13 in the N-*ras* oncogene in a human stomach cancer. Biochem Biophys Res Commun 146:247–252, 1987.
83. Fujita K, Ohuchi N, Yao T, Okumura M, et al: Frequent overexpression, but not activation by point mutation, of *ras* genes in primary human gastric cancers. Gastroenterology 93:1339–1345, 1987.

84. Tahara E, Yasui W, Taniyama K, et al: Ha-ras oncogene product in human gastric carcinoma: Correlation with invasiveness, metastasis and prognosis. Jpn J Cancer Res 77:517–522, 1986.
85. Yamamoto T, Yasui W, Ochiai, A, et al: Immunohistochemical detection of c-*myc* oncogene product in human gastric carcinomas: Expression in tumor cells and stromal cells. Jpn J Cancer Res 78:1169–1174, 1987.
86. Nomura N, Yamamoto T, Toyoshima K, et al: DNA amplification of the c-*myc* and c-*erbB*-1 genes in a human stomach cancer. Jpn J Cancer Res 77:1188–1192, 1986.
87. Tsuchiya T, Yeyama Y, Tamaoki N, et al: Co-amplification of c-*myc* and c-*erbB*-2 oncogenes in a poorly differentiated human gastric. Jpn J Cancer Res 80:920–923, 1989.
88. Yokota J, Yamamoto T, Miyajima N, et al: Genetic alterations of the c-*erbB*-2 oncogene occur frequently in tubular adenocarcinoma of the stomach and are often accompanied by amplification of the v-*erbA* homologue. Oncogene 2:283–287, 1988.
89. Yoshida MC, Wada M, Satoh H, et al: Human HST1 (HSTF1) gene maps to chromosome band 11q13 and coamplifies with INT2 gene in human cancer. Proc Natl Acad Sci USA 85:4861–4864, 1988.
90. Tsuda T, Nakatani H, Matsurmura JT, et al: Amplification of the *hst*-1 gene in human esophageal carcinomas. Jpn J Cancer Res 79:584–588, 1988.
91. Yoshida K, Kyo E, Tsujino T, et al: Expression of epidermal growth factor, transforming growth factor-alpha and their receptor genes in human gastric carcinomas: Implication for autocrine growth. Jpn J Cancer Res 81:43–51, 1990.
92. Kitagami S, Itahbashi M, Hirota T, et al: Immunohistochemical study of oncogene-related products in human gastrointestinal malignancies—expression of ras p21, fes p85 and EGF receptor. Gan No Rinsho 32:1950–1958, 1986.
93. Staal SP: Molecular cloning of the *akt* oncogene and its human homologues AKT1 and AKT2: Amplification of AKT1 in a primary human gastric adenocarcinoma. Proc Natl Acad Sci USA 84:5034–5037, 1987.
94. Seki T, Fujii G, Mori S, et al: Amplification of c-*yes*-1 proto-oncogene in a primary human gastric cancer. Jpn J Cancer Res 76:907–910, 1985.
95. Shimuzu K, Nakatsu Y, Sekiguchi M, et al: Molecular cloning of an activated human oncogene, homologous to v-*raf*, from primary stomach cancer. Proc Natl Acad Sci USA 82:5641–5645, 1985.
96. Lugmani Y, Bennett C, Paterson I, et al: Expression of the pS2 gene in normal, benign and neoplastic human stomach. Int J Cancer 44:806–812, 1989.
97. Bussey HJR: Polyposis Syndromes of the Gastrointestinal Tract. New York, Raven Press, 1983, pp 43–51.
98. Murphy EA: Familial polyposis coli. Prog Med Genet 4:59–101, 1980.
99. Weenstrom J, Pierce ER, McKusick VA: Hereditary benign and malignant lesions of the large bowel. Cancer 34:850–857, 1974.
100. Lynch HT, Watson P, Lanspa SJ, et al: Natural history of colorectal cancer in hereditary nonpolyposis colorectal cancer (Lynch Syndrome I and II). Dis Colon Rectum 32:439–444, 1988.
101. Mecklin JP: Frequency of hereditary colorectal carcinoma. Gasteroenterology 93:1021–1025, 1987.
102. Johnson GK, Soergel KH, Hemsley GT, et al: Cronkhite-Canada syndrome: Gastrointestinal pathophysiology and morphology. Gastroenterology 63:140–152, 1972.
103. Utsunomiya J, Maki T, Iwama T, et al: Gastric lesion of familial polyposis coli. Cancer 34:745–754, 1974.
104. Watanabe H, Munetomo E, Yao T, et al: Gastric lesions in familial adenomatosis coli. Hum Path 9:269–283, 1978.
105. Phillips LG: Polyposis and carcinoma of the small bowel and familial colonic polyposis. Dis Colon Rectum 24:478–481, 1981.
106. Ross JE, Mara JE: Small bowel polyps and carcinoma in multiple intestinal polyposis. Arch Surg 208:736–738, 1974.
107. Veale AMO: The polyposes. In Emery AEH, Rimoin DL (eds): Principles and Practice of Medical Genetics. New York, Churchill Livingstone, 1983, pp 890–898.
108. Burt RW, Samowitz WS: The adenomatous polyp and the hereditary polyposis syndromes. Gastroenterol Clin North Am 17:657–678, 1988.
109. Veale AMO: Intestinal Polyposis. Eugenics Laboratory Memoirs, 40. London, Cambridge University Press, 1965.
110. Asman HB, Pierce ER: Familial multiple polyposis—A statistical study of a large Kentucky kindred. Cancer 25:972–981, 1970.
111. Gardner EJ: A genetic and clinical study of intestinal polyposis, a predisposing factor for carcinoma of the colon and rectum. Am J Hum Genet 3:167–176, 1951.
112. Gardner EJ, Plenk HP: Hereditary pattern for multiple osteomas in a family group. Am J Hum Genet 4:31–36, 1952.
113. Gardner EJ, Richards RC: Multiple cutaneous and subcutaneous lesions occurring simultaneously with hereditary polyposis and osteomatosis. Am J Hum Genet 5:139–147, 1953.
114. Bussey HJR: Gastrointestinal polyposis. Gut. 11:970–978, 1970.
115. Boman BM, Levin B: Familial polyposis. Hosp Pract, 21:155–170, 1986.
116. Pierce ER, Weisbord T, McKusick VA: Gardner's syndrome—Formal genetics and statistical analysis of a large Canadian kindred. Clin Genet 1:65–80, 1970.
117. Turcot J, Depres JP, St Pierre F: Malignant tumours of the central nervous system associated with familial polyposis of the colon. Dis Colon Rectum 2:465–468, 1959.
118. Bartholomew LG, Moore CE, Dahlin DC, et al: Intestinal polyposis associated with mucocutaneous pigmentation. Surg Gynecol Obstet 115:1–11, 1962.
119. Staley CJ, Schwarz H: Gastrointestinal polyposis and pigmentation of the oral mucosa (Peutz-Jeghers syndrome). Int Abstr Surg 205:1–15, 1957.
120. Dormandy TL: Gastrointestinal polyposis with mucocutaneous pigmentation (Peutz-Jeghers syndrome). N Engl J Med 256:1093–1103, 1957.
121. Dodds WJ, Schulte WJ, Hensley GT, et al: Peutz-Jeghers syndrome and gastrointestinal malignancy. Am J Roentgenol 115:374–377, 1972.
122. Reid JD: Intestinal carcinoma in the Peutz-Jeghers syndrome. J Am Med Assoc 229:833–834, 1974.
123. Perzin KH, Ridge MF: Adenomatous and carcinomatous changes in hamartomatous polyps of the small intestine (Peutz-Jeghers syndrome): Report of a case and review of the literature. Cancer 49:971–983, 1982.
124. Roth SI, Helwig EB: Juvenile polyps of the colon and rectum. Cancer 16:468–479, 1963.
125. Veale AMO, McCall I, Bussey HJR, et al: Juvenile polyposis coli. J Med Genet 3:5–16, 1966.
126. Sachatello CR, Pickren JW, Grace JT Jr: Generalized juvenile gastrointestinal polyposis: A hereditary syndrome. Gastroenterology 58:699–708, 1979.
127. Stemper TJ, Kent TH, Summers RW: Juvenile polyposis and gastrointestinal carcinoma: A study of a kindred. Ann Intern Med 83:639–646, 1975.
128. Goodman ZD, Yardley JH, Milligan FD: Pathogenesis of colonic polyps in multiple juvenile polyposis: Report of a case associated with gastric polyps and carcinoma of the rectum. Cancer 43:1906–1913, 1979.
129. Grigioni WF, Alampi G, Martinelli G, et al: Atypical juvenile polyposis. Histopathology 5:361–376, 1981.
130. Lynch HT, Lanspa, SJ, Bowman BM: Hereditary nonpolyposis colorectal cancer—Lynch syndromes I and II. Gastroenterol Clin North Am 17:679–713, 1988.
131. Burt RW, Bishop OT, Cannon ML, et al: Dominant inheritance of adenomatous colonic polyps and colorectal cancer. N Engl J Med 312:1540–1544, 1985.
132. Woolf CM, Gardner EJ: Carcinoma of the gastrointestinal tract in a Utah family. J Hered 41:273–276, 1955.
133. Warthin AS: Heredity with reference to carcinoma as shown by the study of the cases examined in the pathological laboratory of the University of Michigan 1895-1913. Arch Int Med 12:545–555, 1913.
134. Mecklin JP, Jarvinen HJ, Peltokallio P: Cancer family syndrome. Gastroenterology 90:328–333, 1986.
135. Anderson DE: An inherited form of large bowel cancer: Muir syndrome. Cancer 45:1103–1107, 1980.
136. Lynch HT, Fusaro RM, Roberts L, et al: Muir-Torre syndrome

in several members of a family with a variant of the cancer family syndrome. Br J Dermatol 113:295–301, 1985.
137. Mecklin JP, Sipponene P, Jarvinen JH: Histopathology of colorectal carcinomas and adenomas in cancer family syndrome. Dis Colon Rectum 29:849, 1986.
138. Love RR: Adenomas are precursor lesions for malignant growth in nonpolyposis hereditary carcinoma of the colon and rectum. Surg Gynecol Obstet 162:8–12, 1986.
139. Cannon-Albright LA, Skolnick MH, Bishop DT, et al: Common inheritance of susceptibility to colonic adenomatous polyps and associated colorectal cancers. N Engl J Med 319:533–537, 1988.
140. Knudson AG Jr: Mutation and cancer: Statistical study of retinoblastoma. Proc Natl Acad Sci 68:820–823, 1971.
141. Yunis JJ, Ramsay N: Retinoblastoma and subband deletion of chromosome 13. Am J Dis Child 132:161–163, 1978.
142. Knudson AG Jr: Etiology of genetically determined cancer, 1989. Genetic analysis of tumor suppression (Ciba Foundation Symposium 142). Chichester, Wiley, 1989, pp 3–19.
143. Friend SH, Dryja TP, Weinberg RA: Oncogenes and tumor-suppressing genes. N Engl J Med 318:618–622, 1988.
144. Herrera L, Kakati S, Gibas L, et al: Brief clinical report: Gardner's syndrome in a man with an interstitial deletion of 5q. Am J Med Genet 25:473–476, 1986.
145. Bodmer WF, Bailey CJ, Bodmer J, et al: Localization of the gene for familial adenomatous polyposis on chromosome 5. Nature 328:614–616, 1987.
146. Leppert M, Dobbs M, Scambler P, et al: The gene for familial polyposis coli maps to the long arm of chromosome 5. Science 238:1411–1413, 1987.
147. Rees M, Leigh SEA, Delhanty JDA, Jass JR; Chromosome 5 allele loss in familial and sporadic colorectal adenomas. Br J Cancer 59:361–365, 1989.
148. Solomon E, Voss R, Hall V, et al: Chromosome 5 allele loss in human colorectal carcinomas. Nature 328:616–619, 1987.
149. Law DJ, Olschwang S, Monpezat J-P, et al: Concerted nonsyntenic allelic loss in human colorectal carcinoma. Science 241:961–965, 1988.
150. Wildrick DM: Molecular genetic studies of colon cancer. Hematol Oncol Clin North Am 3:1–18, 1989.
151. Lothe RA, Nakamura Y, Woodward S, et al: VNTR (variable number of tandem repeats) markers show loss of chromosome 17p sequences in human colorectal carcinomas. Cytogenet Cell Genet 48:167–169, 1988.
152. Fearon ER, Cho KR, Nigro JM, et al: Identification of a chromosome 18q gene that is altered in colorectal cancers. Science 247:49–56, 1990.
153. Okamoto M, Sasaki M, Sugio K, et al: Loss of constitutional heterozygosity in colon carcinoma from patients with familial polyposis coli. Nature 331:273–277, 1988.
154. Fearon ER, Vogelstein B: A genetic model for colorectal tumorigenesis. Cell 61:759–767, 1990.
155. Vogelstein B, Fearon ER, Hamilton SR, et al: Genetic alterations during colorectal-tumor development. N Engl J Med 319:525–532, 1988.
156. Baker SJ, Fearon ER, Nigro JM: Chromosome 17 deletions and p53 mutations in colorectal carcinomas. Science 244:217–221, 1989.
157. Kern SE, Fearon ER, Tersmette KWF: Allelic loss in colorectal carcinoma. JAMA 261:3099–3103, 1989.
158. Fearon ER, Hamilton SR, Vogelstein B: Clonal analysis of human colorectal tumors. Science 238:193–197, 1987.
159. Reichmann A, Martin P, Levin B: Chromosomal banding patterns in human large bowel adenomas. Hum Genet 70:28–31, 1985.
160. Reichmann A, Martin P, Levin B: Karyotypic findings in a colonic villous adenoma. Cancer Genet Cytogenet 7:51–57, 1982.
161. Nielsen KB, Bulow S, Tommerup N: Chromosomal studies in familial polyposis coli. Cancer Genet Cytogenet 17:355–357, 1985.
162. Sandberg AA: Chromosomal abnormalities in patients with familial polyposis and colorectal cancer. Semin Surg Oncol 3:133–136, 1987.
163. Lukeis R, Garson OM, Macrae FA, et al: Chromosome studies in inherited nonpolyposis colon cancer syndrome. Cancer Genet Cytogenet 27:111–124, 1987.
164. Levin B, Reichmann A: Chromosomes and large bowel tumors. Cancer Genet Cytogenet 19:159–162, 1986.
165. Muleris M, Salmon RJ, Dutrillaux B: Cytogenetics of colorectal adenocarcinomas. Cancer Genet Cytogenet 46:143–156, 1990.
166. Dutrillaux B: Recent data on the cytogenetics of colorectal adenocarcinoma. Bull Cancer (Paris) 75:509–516, 1988.
167. Muleris M, Salmon RJ, Dutrillaux AM, et al: Characteristic chromosomal imbalances in 18 near-diploid colorectal tumors. Cancer Genet Cytogenet 29:289–301, 1987.
168. Ferti-Passantonopoulou A, Panani A, Avgerinos A, Raptis S: Cytogenetic findings in a large bowel adenocarcinoma. Cancer Genet Gytogenet 21:361–364, 1986.
169. Bos JL, Fearon ER, Hamilton SR, et al: Prevalence of ras gene mutations in human colorectal cancers. Nature 327:293–297, 1987.
170. Forrester K, Almoguera C, Han K, et al: Detection of high incidence of K-ras oncogenes during human colon tumorigenesis. Nature 327:298–303, 1987.
171. Alexander RJ, Buxbaum JN, Raicht RF: Oncogene alterations in primary human colon tumors. Gastroenterology 91:1503–1510, 1986.
172. Thor A, Hand H, Wunderlich D: Monoclonal antibodies define differential ras gene expression in malignant and benign colonic diseases. Nature 311:562–565, 1984.
173. Kerr IB, Lee FD, Quintanilla M, Balmain A: Immunocytochemical demonstration of p21 ras family oncogene product in normal mucosa and in premalignant and malignant tumours of the colorectum. Br J Cancer 52:695–700, 1985.
174. Williams AR, Piris J, Spandidos DA, Wyllie AH: Immunohistochemical detection of the ras oncogene p21 product in an experimental tumour and in human colorectal neoplasms. Br J Cancer 52:687–693, 1985.
175. Salhab N, Jones DJ, Bos JL: Detection of ras gene alterations and ras proteins in colorectal cancer. Dis Colon Rectum 32:659–664, 1989.
176. Gallick GE, Kuzrock R, Kloetzer WS: Expression of p21 ras in fresh primary and metastatic human colorectal tumors. Proc Natl Acad Sci USA 82:1795–1799, 1985.
177. Burmer GC, Rabinovitch PS, Loeb LA: Analysis of c-Ki-ras mutations in human colon carcinoma by cell sorting, polymerase chain reaction, and DNA sequencing. Cancer Res 49:2141–2146, 1989.
178. Monnat M, Tardy S, Saraga P, et al: Prognostic implications of expression of the cellular genes myc, fos, Ha-ras and Ki-ras in colon carcinoma. Int J Cancer 40:293–299, 1987.
179. Sugio K, Kurata S, Sasaki M, et al: Differential expression of c-myc and c-fos gene in premalignant and malignant tissues from patients with familial polyposis coli. Cancer Res 48:4855–4861, 1988.
180. Calabretta B, Kaczmarek L, Ming P-ML, et al: Expression of c-myc and other cell cycle-dependent genes in human colon neoplasia. Cancer Res 45:6000–6004, 1985.
181. Mariani-Costantini R, Theillet C, Hutzell P, et al: In situ detection of c-myc mRNA in adenocarcinomas, adenomas, and mucosa of human colon. J Histochem Cytochem 37:293–298, 1989.
182. Finley GG, Schulz NT, Hill SA, et al: Expression of the myc gene family in different stages of human colorectal cancer. Oncogene 4:963–971, 1989.
183. Watson JV, Stewart J, Cox H, et al: Flow cytometric quantitation of the c-myc oncoprotein in archival neoplastic biopsies of the colon. Mol Cell Probes 1:151–157, 1987.
184. Erisman MD, Scott JK, Astrin SM: Evidence that the familial adenomatous polyposis gene is involved in a subset of colon cancers with a complementable defect in c-myc regulation. Proc Natl Acad Sci USA 86:4262–4268, 1989.
185. Alitalo K, Schwab M, Lin CC, et al: Homogeneously staining chromosomal regions contain amplified copies of an abundantly expressed cellular oncogene (c-myc) in malignant neuroendocrine cells from a human colon carcinoma. Proc Natl Acad Sci USA 80:1707–1711, 1983.
186. Rothberg PG, Spandorfer JM, Erisman MD, et al: Evidence that

c-*myc* expression defines two genetically distinct forms of colorectal adenocarcinoma. Br J Cancer 52:629–632, 1985.
187. Meltzer SJ, Ahnen DJ, Battifora H, et al: Protooncogene abnormalities in colon cancers and adenomatous polyps. Gastroenterology 92:1174–1180, 1987.
188. Tal M, Wetzler M, Josefberg Z, et al: Sporadic amplification of the *her2/neu* protooncogene in adenocarcinomas of various tissues. Cancer Res 48:1517–1520, 1988.
189. Mitra G, Martin-Zanca D, Barbacid M: Identification and biochemical characterization of p70 *trk*, product of the human *trk* oncogene. Proc Natl Acad Sci USA 84:6707–6711, 1987.
190. Rosen N, Sartor O, Foss FM, et al: Altered expression of c-*src*-related tyrosine kinase in human colon cancer. In Furth M, Greaves M (eds): Molecular Diagnostics of Human Cancer, Cancer Cells. Vol 7. New York, Cold Spring Harbor Laboratory Press, 1989, pp 161–166.

CHAPTER 7

Cell Renewal in Health and Disease

ELEANOR E. DESCHNER, Ph.D
THOMAS LEHNERT, M.D.

ESOPHAGUS
Normal Proliferation
Proliferation in Disease States
Esophagitis
Barrett's Epithelium
Esophageal Carcinoma

STOMACH
Normal Proliferation
Proliferation in Disease States
Atrophic Gastritis

Gastric Ulcer
Gastric Polyps
Ménétrier's Disease
Zollinger-Ellison Syndrome
Gastric Dysplasia
Gastric Carcinoma

SMALL INTESTINE
Normal Proliferation
Proliferation in Disease States

Small-Bowel Resection
Celiac Sprue

LARGE INTESTINE
Normal Proliferation
Preneoplasia
Proliferation in Disease States
Colonic Adenoma
Ulcerative Colitis
Colonic Carcinoma

The inclusion of a chapter on cell proliferation in a book devoted to the pathology of the gastrointestinal tract is entirely appropriate. Our understanding of disease, whether neoplasia or even nonneoplastic conditions, is dependent on the basic behavior of epithelial cells, which includes their proliferation, maturation, and differentiation. The disease state or tumor observed today is the product of a biochemical alteration induced in a stem cell that, in the appropriate environment, perpetuates the defect. If a gastrointestinal abnormality is inherited in the germ line rather than as a somatic mutation, then the likelihood is that the disease state will be expressed earlier. For example, carcinoma of the colon appears earlier in members of families affected by polyposis and colonic cancer than in individuals among the general population.[1]

In broad terms, the health of the digestive system reflects the interaction of the mucosa with substances to which it is continually exposed in the environment. Such substances may be, on the one hand, nutritious and conducive to good health or, on the other hand, hazardous and capable of inducing disease. The latter situation depends on such circumstances as the nature of the substance, the target area of the digestive system, the susceptibility of the epithelial cells, the number of cells at risk, the length of the exposure, and many other factors. Their interaction may result in loss of regulatory control over cell proliferation, and ultimately a pathologic condition arises.

Many disease states of the digestive system have been examined from the point of view of kinetics. Recognition of proliferating cells as mitotic figures was first reported in stomach tissue by Bizzozero.[2] It remained for Howard and Pelc, in 1951,[3] growing the bean root of *Vicia faba* immersed in ^{32}P solution to suggest that only cells synthesizing DNA underwent division and that this synthesis phase (S phase) occupied the middle of interphase. These investigators described the presynthetic phase or G_1 phase as a biochemically active stage for cells preparing to undergo DNA synthesis and the postsynthetic phase as a short preparatory time for 4C cells to undergo mitosis. This fourth phase of the cycle, or mitosis, produces two cells and restores the 2C character to each. Not all cells emerging from mitosis proceed directly from G_1 to S phase; they may alternatively subside into a prolonged resting phase, or

G_0 phase, remaining as a pool of potentially active cells.

These events of the cell cycle occur in a specific region of the gastrointestinal mucosa from which cells migrate out to replace dead and dying cells. S-phase and mitotic cells are part of the proliferative compartment (PC), which in many disease states is altered in size and distribution.

Information concerning the proliferative characteristics of epithelial cells has been gathered with the use of only a limited number of techniques. Radioactive isotopes have played a prominent role in the accumulation of these data. Tritiated thymidine (^{3}HTdR) and ^{14}CTdR are both readily incorporated into the DNA during S phase and allow one to pulse-label proliferative cells.[4] In vitro incubation of biopsies or fragments of surgical specimens can provide data concerning the fraction of cells engaged in S phase, or labeling index (LI), and the distribution of these cells. The LI is the ratio of labeled cells to total cells analyzed. The mitotic index (MI) has been used as a measure of proliferative activity in unlabeled tissue; the MI is the ratio of cells undergoing cell division (mitosis) to the nondividing population analyzed. When two isotopes are employed or double-labeling studies carried out with a high (h) and low (l) dose of ^{3}HTdR, the duration of S phase may be derived. The two different populations of labeled cells (N_h and N_l) are separated by a known interval of time (t) providing a value for S phase (S):

$$\frac{N_h}{N_l} = \frac{S}{t}$$

Knowing the duration of S phase (T_s) and having obtained a value for the LI by a 1-hour incubation, one can estimate the total cell cycle time (T_c):

$$T_c = \frac{T_s}{LI} \times 100$$

In some patients with limited life expectancy and in experimental studies, it has been possible to inject an isotope and follow labeled mitotic cells through the entire cell cycle. This can generate a fraction of labeled mitotic curve, which allows direct measurement of the duration time of the cell cycle and its various phases.

ESOPHAGUS

Normal Proliferation

The PC of this region, which is primarily a squamous epithelium, resides in a basal layer of cells. It is among these cells that random mitotic figures and S-phase cells are observed. One or both of the daughter cells may slowly migrate and differentiate as they proceed toward the lumen, or they may remain basally located.[5] The LI for the proliferative layer of epithelial cells in man as determined in vivo was 8.7% and for the entire mucosa 0.95%, or less than 1% of cells engaged in cell renewal[5] (Table 7–1). This would indicate a slow rate of cell renewal.[6,7] Studies with esophageal biopsies la-

Table 7–1 PROLIFERATIVE INDICES OF EPITHELIAL CELLS IN HUMAN ESOPHAGEAL EPITHELIUM

Specimen	LI (%)	S Phase (hr)	T_c (days)	Reference
Control				
Basal layer	8.7			5
Entire mucosa	0.9			5
Basal layer	10.0	10.6	4.5	7
Basal layer	5.0			6
Severe esophagitis	10.9			6
Barrett's syndrome	23.3	10	<2	7
Carcinoma (not specified)	7.6	22	>10	8

LI, labeling index; T_c, cell cycle time.

beled in vitro showed a range of values for normal esophagus from 6.1% to 11.1% for basal epithelial cells engaged in DNA synthesis. Tissue turnover time estimated by following the migration of the labeled cohort indicated that it took the cells between 4 and 8 days to reach the luminal surface.[5,7]

Proliferation in Disease States

Esophagitis

In vitro studies of various degrees of reflux esophagitis have shown no proliferative differences between patients with mild esophagitis and control patients, but significant alterations were observed between these groups and those with severe esophagitis. Individuals in the latter group had mucosa characterized by severe changes in papillary length and basal-layer thickening, particularly in the distal part of the tissue.[6] In general, biopsies with the highest LI had the thickest basal layer and the longest esophageal papillae. Thus, increased cell renewal correlated with basal-zone hyperplasia.

Barrett's Epithelium

This premalignant condition, believed to arise from reflux esophagitis, is characterized by a mucosa lined by columnar epithelium having an LI two times higher than that of the squamous epithelium.[7] The generation time for this syndrome is estimated to be less than 2 days in duration. Expansion of the PC to the surface has also been observed in a group of patients with this syndrome.

Esophageal Carcinoma

A high risk for esophageal cancer is found in Linxian, China, whereas only a low risk factor exists in Jiaoxian, another county in China. Esophagitis, epithelial atrophy, and dysplasia are more prevalent in biopsies of members of the Linxian population.[8,9] The higher the LI and the closer the S-phase population to the lumen, the more severe were the hyperplasia and dysplasia found to exist.[8,9] Biopsy specimens from patients with dysplasia had a significantly higher LI for the upper five luminal layers of epithelial cells than those from individuals with only hyperplasia had.

Double-labeling studies of two cases of esophageal carcinomas provided an LI of 7.3% to 7.9% and an estimated S-phase duration of 22 hours. The potential tissue doubling time in the absence of cell loss was approximately 10 days or more.[10] Cytophotometric measurements of DNA content in esophageal cancers revealed that when DNA showed a limited dispersion around the normal 2C content, patients had no recurrence of the lesion; but when dispersion extended to the 8C region or greater and/or multiple DNA peaks existed, then patients were prone to recurrence.[11] Such data suggest a predictive potential of cytophotometric studies prior to surgery that may allow channeling of specific cases for more aggressive treatment.

STOMACH

Normal Proliferation

Gastric mucosa consists mainly of two regions with distinct morphologic and functional differences. Fundic mucosa located in the proximal stomach has long, straight glands lined by mucous cells, pepsinogen-producing chief cells, and hydrochloric acid– and intrinsic factor–producing parietal cells. Antral mucosa in the distal parts of the stomach adjacent to the pylorus, in contrast, has shorter coiled glands that consist mainly of mucous cells and gastrin-producing G cells. Both fundic and antral glands empty into gastric pits that are lined by surface mucous cells and border the gastric lumen.

Investigation into the proliferative activity of gastric mucosa has defined distinct differences between fundic and antral epithelium. In fundic mucosa the surface epithelium is derived from immature stem cells located at the isthmus between gastric pits and glands. These stem cells have the ability to divide. Daughter cells then start to differentiate and to migrate toward the luminal surface, where they are eventually shed into the gastric lumen. On their way toward the surface these cells mature and lose their ability to divide. Migration time is approximately 8 days,[12] and autoradiographic studies have shown that 10% to 15% of these cells synthesize DNA. Renewal of antral surface epithelium basically follows the same principles. Labeling studies, however, have indicated that proliferative activity is higher in antral mucosa (Table 7–2).

Replacement of glandular cells also takes place from immature precursor cells located in the progenitor zone at the isthmus. In the fundus, maturing mucous cells migrate downward to the bottom of the glands in a random fashion. This results in a life span that has been estimated at 200 ± 100 days before the cell is lost at the bottom of the gland.[24] Mucous cells in antral glands, however, follow a different pattern of migration. Also derived from immature stem cells at the isthmus, their downward migration follows a pipeline or escalator pattern, resulting in a much shorter life span of only 14 days before they reach the bottom of the glands.[24]

Specialized fundic glandular cells such as parietal cells are also derived from the immature stem cells, a very small percentage possibly self-renewing. Chief cells, on the other hand, are not derived from immature stem cells, but are self-renewing.[25–27] Only in regenerative fundic epithelium may a major portion of

Table 7–2 EPITHELIAL CELL PROLIFERATION IN NORMAL HUMAN GASTRIC MUCOSA

	LI (%)	MI (%)	T_{G_2} (hr)	T_S (hr)	T_{G_1} (hr)	T_C (hr)	Reference
Cardia	13.1	1.3					13
Fundus	11.7		2–4	10.0		48	14
	4.2						5
	9.3	1.0					13
	14.0			9.0		48	15
	10.0	0.8	1.0	7.1	62	72	16
	11.0						17
	7.3–10.7	0.28–0.54					18
	10.9						19
	10.0			6.1		62.7	20
	6.2						21
	7.9						22
Antrum	15.2	1.4					13
	12.8						17
	10.1–13.3	0.36–0.65					18
	12.1						19
	11.7			7.6		65.4	20
	16.0						23
	7.4						22

LI, labeling index; MI, mitotic index; T_{G_2}, T_S, T_{G_1}, time of G_2, S, G_1 phases, respectively; T_c, cell cycle time.

Table 7-3 EFFECT OF HUMORAL FACTORS ON GASTRIC EPITHELIAL CELL PROLIFERATION

	Fundus	Antrum	Reference
Cholecystokinin	Unaltered		32
Cortisone	Depressed	Depressed	35
	Depressed	Depressed	36
	Depressed	Depressed	33
Gastrin	Increased	Depressed	31
	Increased		37
	Increased	Depressed	38
	Depressed	Depressed	33
Histamine	Unaltered		37
Insulin	Depressed	Unaltered	33
Prostaglandin E_2 (PGE_2)	Unaltered		32
	Unaltered	Unaltered	33
Secretin	Unaltered		37
	Unaltered	Unaltered	33
15(R)-15-Methyl-PGE_2	Unaltered	Unaltered	22
PGE_1 analogue	Depressed	Depressed	34

chief cells be renewed by differentiation of immature precursors.[28,29] The same appears to be true for other specialized cells in the fundus. Under normal conditions, gastrin-producing G cells[30] and somatostatin-producing D cells[26] are thought to be self-renewing, whereas in regenerative epithelium these cells may be replaced by differentiation of immature stem cells.[29]

A dynamic process, gastric epithelial renewal is influenced by numerous physiologic stimuli. Gastrin effectively stimulates proliferation of fundic epithelium, whereas antral mucosal proliferation is hardly affected.[31] Cholecystokinin and synthetic prostaglandins had no effect on proliferation in rodents[32,33] and humans[22]; but misoprostol, an analogue of prostaglandin E_1, reduced proliferative activity in both antral and fundic mucosa.[34] A survey of the effects of numerous other humoral factors on gastric epithelial proliferation is given in Table 7-3.

Food intake could not be demonstrated to affect gastric mucosal proliferation in humans,[18] but in dogs a significant increase of fundic proliferation was provoked by oral feeding.[39] Similarly, the antral G-cell mass is reduced by starving but rapidly replenished by refeeding.[40]

Proliferation in Disease States

Atrophic Gastritis

Gastritis has been found to have a prevalence of more than 50% in individuals over the age of 50 years[41,42] and may progress to atrophic gastritis. Such progress is gradual, and the time necessary for superficial gastritis to deteriorate into atrophic gastritis has been calculated to be approximately 17 years.[42]

Support for this concept of gradual progress from superficial gastritis to chronic atrophic gastritis comes from cell kinetics studies. Proliferative activity of gastric mucosa increases with increasing morphologic signs of gastritis. The LI appears to double when normal mucosa is compared with that in atrophic gastritis and again when simple atrophic gastritis is compared with atrophic gastritis with signs of intestinal metaplasia (Deschner, unpublished). In such patients cell cycle times are reduced by 20% to 40%,[20] and the normal replacement time of 8 days is reduced to only 1.25 days.[12] The spatial distribution of labeled cells is changed, and in atrophic gastritis the proliferative zone may expand upward. In the narrowed epithelium of severe atrophic gastritis even superficial epithelium has been found to incorporate ^{3}HTdR, which indicates its proliferative involvement.[23,43]

Gastric Ulcer

This disease state develops when the renewal of surface epithelium cannot keep up with cell loss at the surface. Therefore, either increased cell loss or reduced cell renewal may be responsible for ulcer development. Experimental studies have shown that the proliferative zone in the gastric mucosa narrows when rats are exposed to stress.[44] Ulcerogenic compounds such as cortisone[35,36] and aspirin[45] reduce proliferative activity, whereas others have shown that indomethacin[46] or aspirin[47,48] increase epithelial proliferation. Such different findings may be related to different experimental designs and mirror sequential changes of proliferative activity in the course of ulcer development. When the time sequence of proliferative changes during the development of gastric ulcers was investigated, a 200% increase was noted within 24 hours. Normal activity was present after 48 hours, and after 3 days the ulcer became visible.[49] Therefore, when exposed to an ulcerogenic stimulus, gastric epithelium may respond by increasing cell renewal; but when the damage becomes overwhelming, then regenerative capacity becomes exhausted and the integrity of superficial epithelium cannot be maintained. This concept is supported by the observation of increased proliferation of morphologically normal gastric epithelium in ulcer-bearing individuals as compared with normal subjects.[17,41]

Ulcer healing begins with increased proliferation in the normal epithelium surrounding the ulcer. From here cells migrate over the ulcer crater to form a neo-epithelium that has little proliferative activity itself.[23,50–52]

Gastric Polyps

These entities are of interest in terms of epithelial proliferation, particularly because of their possible association with gastric cancer. The risk of gastric carcinoma developing in an adenomatous polyp may be as high as 70%,[53] whereas no malignant changes have been observed in hyperplastic polyps.

Experimentally, adenomatous hyperplasia was associated with gastric cancer,[54,55] and it has been suggested that the upward expansion of the proliferative zone may be related to the exophytic growth type of some gastric cancers.[56,57]

Ménétrier's Disease

In this rare condition the proliferative activity of gastric epithelium is excessively high. The LIs of antral and fundic mucosa may be raised by 66% and turnover time reduced by 20%.[20] Such increase in cell turnover may be responsible for the protein loss observed in patients with this disease.

Zollinger-Ellison Syndrome

In this syndrome proliferation of gastric mucosa is affected by the excessively high serum gastrin levels produced by gastrinoma. The stimulating effect of gastrin on fundic mucosa and its inhibitory effect on antral epithelial proliferation observed in experimental studies[38] is recognized in these patients.[58] In addition, hyperplasia of fundic parietal and chief cells[58] as well as endocrine cells of the fundus[59] has been observed. Morphologic correlates of such altered proliferative activity are hyperplastic mucosa[60] and reduction of antral area.[58]

Gastric Dysplasia

Severe dysplasia of gastric mucosa must be regarded as a premalignant condition.[61] Recent studies of cell kinetics in this condition have shown that the mitotic activity is shifted toward the base of the glands with increasing degrees of dysplasia. Similarly, the percentage of atypical mitoses increases with severity of dysplasia from 27% in slight dysplasia to 52% in severe dysplasia.[62] In another study on grade III dysplasia of antral mucosa, proliferatively active epithelium was noted in the upper third of the mucosa, forming aberrant proliferative foci of the foveola.[63] Gastric dysplasia, therefore, is defined not only by morphologic characteristics but also by distinct signs of disturbed proliferative activity.

Gastric Carcinoma

Experimental stimulation of gastric mucosa with a carcinogen has indicated that early proliferative changes in the course of cancer development occur in the region between gastric glands and pits, which is precisely the region where gastric mucosal stem cells are located.[56] The concept that gastric cancer originates from such immature stem cells is supported by observations on minute gastric cancer (i.e., gastric cancer less than 5 mm in diameter). In a study of 67 such tumors, all lesions were found in this region between glands and pits.[64]

More information was derived from studies in which morphologically normal gastric mucosa of patients without gastric cancer was compared with normal mucosa from patients with gastric cancer. Labeling indices in the latter were found to be almost three times higher,[65] which indicates a generalized increase in mucosal proliferation in the cancerous stomach. Later in the course of cancer development morphologic changes appear, although the role of intestinal metaplasia, in which the highest proliferative activity is found at the bottom of glands, rather than in an area equivalent to the normal progenitor zone, is not resolved as yet. It may be that the initial increase in proliferative activity is followed by intestinalization of the "incomplete" type. From there, tissue may differentiate into "complete" intestinal metaplasia or undergo malignant change. Well-differentiated cancers frequently are found in areas with intestinalized mucosa, whereas poorly differentiated cancers are less frequently associated with intestinal metaplasia.[66-68] Moreover, gastric carcinoma appears to be more often associated with the less differentiated "incomplete" type of metaplasia.[69]

Early proliferative changes of gastric epithelium exposed to a carcinogen may be related to growth patterns established by advanced gastric carcinomas. The early upward expansion of the proliferative zone may be related to the exophytic, polypoid growth of well-differentiated cancers, whereas expansion in a downward direction may precede the development of primarily infiltrating undifferentiated cancers.[56,57] Such infiltrating cancers have higher nuclear DNA contents as compared with other growth types.[70]

Stathmokinetic studies have indicated that advanced gastric carcinoma in general has lower cell production rates than normal surrounding mucosa,[71,72] thus providing at least one explanation for the failure of radiotherapy or chemotherapy in the treatment of these tumors.

Although some data concerning proliferative activity of gastric cancer are available now, characterization or even classification of cell kinetics is difficult. It appears that the infiltrative peripheral portions of advanced tumors have higher proliferative activity than the center.[72] Some studies indicate a higher mitotic index for poorly differentiated cancers as compared with well-differentiated lesions,[71,72] but more recent studies were unable to confirm this.[73] Similarly, early gastric cancer, i.e., cancer invading the mucosa or submucosa regardless of lymph node metastases, was found to have lower proliferative activity than advanced tumors; but differences were not significant.[73] It is still unclear, therefore, whether early gastric cancer is just a gastric cancer detected at an early stage or is part of a group of particularly slowly growing gastric carcinomas. Further study will therefore be necessary to define the proliferative characteristics of different types of gastric cancer more precisely.

SMALL INTESTINE

Normal Proliferation

Small-intestinal glands are lined by four cell types: columnar cells, mucous cells, Paneth cells, and endocrine cells. All of them are believed to originate from identical stem cells located at the bottom of intestinal crypts.[74]

Under normal conditions the human small intestine sheds approximately 20 to 50 million cells per minute into the lumen of the gut.[75] This loss of epithelial cells is compensated for by continuous renewal of small-intestinal epithelium. Such renewal takes place from the base of intestinal crypts, where immature stem cells are located adjacent to the muscularis mucosae. After division of these stem cells, daughter cells migrate upward to the luminal surface. As they ascend, cells become specialized and lose their proliferative capability as they reach the intestinal villus.

In humans, epithelial cell cycle times range from 42 to 144 hours.[14,76–78] Migration time from the crypt to the villus, where the cells are finally lost into the lumen, is 5 to 6 days in jejunal mucosa[76] and 3 days in the ileum.[14] The labeling index of epithelial cells in the human duodenum was recorded at 15.0%[79] and in the jejunum at 27.4%.[5] Mitotic indices were 2.1% to 3.1%.[5,77,78] Both parameters indicate a faster cell renewal in comparison with gastric or colonic epithelial cell renewal under normal conditions.

Like any dynamic biologic process, small-intestinal epithelial proliferation is subject to a large number of physiologic stimuli. Starvation has long been demonstrated to decrease epithelial proliferation in the intestines of rodents,[80] and a recent case report indicated that refeeding after 30 days of parenteral nutrition caused an immediate increase of epithelial proliferation after only 24 hours of oral feeding.[81] Such an increase of proliferative activity may be mediated by gastrin, which has been found to stimulate ileal DNA synthesis in rats.[37] Epithelial cell proliferation in the small bowel is also increased by serotonin, histamine, and noradrenaline.[37,82–84] Other hormones, in contrast, may suppress intestinal proliferation; and a summary of currently available information on hormonal effects on small-intestinal epithelial cell proliferation is given in Table 7–4. It should be remembered, though, that humoral effects on epithelial cell proliferation may depend on both dosage and route of administration, as well as on the particular target tissue studied.[83,84]

Proliferation in Disease States

Small-Bowel Resection

Humoral factors may also mediate regenerative and adaptive processes after small bowel resection. Morphologically, bowel resection is followed by enlargement of villi, particularly distal to the resection line, which leads to an increase in absorptive capacity of the remaining bowel. Similarly, crypts become deeper and the proliferative zone expands. Autoradiographic studies following a 40% partial resection of small bowel have demonstrated a marked increase of proliferative activity after 2 months.[86] Although in this study no reduction of cell cycle time could be elicited, such shortening of the cell cycle has been described by others fol-

Table 7–4 EFFECT OF HUMORAL FACTORS ON SMALL-INTESTINAL EPITHELIAL CELL PROLIFERATION

Substance	Area	Effect	Reference
Gastrin	Duodenum	Increased	37
	Ileum	Increased	37
Histamine	Duodenum	Unaltered	37
	Ileum	Unaltered	37
	Jejunum	Increased (low dose)	84
		Decreased (high dose)	84
Serotonin	Jejunum	Increased (low dose)	82
		Decreased (high dose)	82
Secretin	Duodenum	Unaltered	37
	Ileum	Unaltered	37
Adrenaline	Jejunum	Decreased	83
Noradrenaline	Jejunum	Increased	83
Hydrocortisone	Duodenum	Decreased	85
Cholecystokinin	Duodenum	Increased	32
16,16 dimethyl-PGE_2	Duodenum	Increased	32

lowing a 70% resection of small bowel.[87] A more recent study also found an increase in the rate of crypt production due primarily to a shorter crypt replication cycle when 30% resection occurred.[88]

Because biliary and, in particular, pancreatic secretions are known to stimulate growth of small intestinal epithelium,[89] the increased concentration of bile and pancreatic juice in the remaining bowel may cause adaptive changes.[90,91] Other studies have shown that oral food intake increases after small bowel resection in rats[92]; therefore, intraluminal food contents may be an important stimulus. In experimental animals that were fed orally, villus height was greater after small bowel resection as compared with that in control animals receiving parenteral nutrition,[93] but no difference was noted between resected rats and rats that underwent sham operation when both groups were fed parenterally.[94] The humoral agent mediating adaption of resected small bowel may be gastrin[95] or, as a more recent study has indicated, enteroglucagon.[96]

Celiac Sprue

The proliferative changes associated with celiac sprue or gluten-induced enteropathy have attracted considerable interest. In this condition intestinal villi are reduced in size or even lost. A threefold increase in intestinal cell loss as compared with that of normal controls has been noted,[97] and proliferative activity is increased. The cell cycle time is reduced to approximately half that of controls, migration time is three times faster, and the proliferative zone expands to comprise the entire length of the crypt. In addition, these crypts contain a large number of cells, so that although the growth fraction is reduced by 25%, the number of renewing cells is increased threefold.[77,78] Treatment of patients with a gluten-free diet leads to reversal of malabsorption; proliferative activity, however, does not return to normal.[98]

Although duodenal ulcer disease is a common condition, few data are available concerning its proliferative characteristics. In one study comprising only a small number of patients, proliferative activity in duodenal biopsies incubated with labeled thymidine was lower than in healthy control subjects.[99] In a more recent report of 15 patients with uncomplicated duodenal ulcer and 10 patients with perforated duodenal ulcer, LIs of nondiseased duodenal mucosa were similar to those of healthy controls. At the ulcer's edge, however, proliferative activity was almost twice as high, probably reflecting regenerative adaption. In the same study higher labeling indices were also reported for patients with duodenitis.[100]

LARGE INTESTINE

Normal Proliferation

During the postnatal development of the colon and even during adult life, the basal region of the crypts is active both as the source of new glands[101] and as the area from which new cells are produced. Basally located cells are responsible for populating the young growing colon with new crypts and for replacing those glands that erode and atrophy during adult life. A fission process involving the formation of a wall effectively bifurcates the existing gland, thus creating two units from the one.

The base of the crypt wherein the stem cells are located also gives rise to the four colonic cell types, columnar, mucous, enteroendocrine, and Paneth cells, in the cecum and ascending colon.[74] The new cells migrate upward to the surface of the mucosa, undergoing maturation and differentiation as they proceed through the middle and upper regions of the crypt. Cells are so regulated that under normal conditions only the lower two thirds of the crypts form the proliferative compartment. Cells in the lower 12 to 14 cell positions are most frequently engaged in cell replication.

The number of epithelial cells per crypt per region is relatively uniform.[101,102] Crypts in the proximal colon are shorter and contain fewer cells than those distally located. The actual number of proliferative cells in the proximal colon is relatively small, compared with the number in the distal colon, i.e., 90 cells in the ascending versus 190 in the descending large bowel.[102] However, the fraction of cells engaged in DNA synthesis, or growth fraction, is approximately the same in both regions (12.3% versus 11.7%, respectively) because of the smaller number of cells in the proximal crypts. Thus, a reasonable explanation for the greater risk for colon cancer in the distal region may be related to the more than twofold greater probability that neoplastic transformation may occur among this larger population of replicating cells.

In the adult Swiss albino mouse approximately 83% of cells are in G_1 phase, 4% in G_2 and mitosis, and 13% in S phase.[103] It is estimated that the time it takes to replace all the cells in the mucosa (turnover time) of this strain is about 62 hours. However, different cell types have different LIs and different turnover times. For example, mucous cells have an LI of 15.8% and an estimated turnover time of 124 hours; whereas Paneth cells have an LI of less than 1% and a turnover time of 3 weeks.[104]

The number of proliferating cells in a particular region of the colon and their distribution is relatively constant for each animal species and strain.[105] There are those mouse strains that exhibit a high LI in the distal colon (greater than 9%), whereas others are significantly lower.[103,105] By and large, those strains with a high LI have a wider proliferative compartment with S-phase cells located futher up the cryptal walls, resulting in more proliferative cells in the middle third of the gland. Nevertheless, under normal conditions, the lower third remains the predominant area of DNA synthesis.

Much of the kinetic data accumulated from human material has shown a remarkable similarity to the general proliferative characteristics described in rodents. The primary source for this data has been colorectal biopsies that were incubated with labeled precursors of DNA. A wide spectrum of LI values was observed among a group of individuals in the general population with no gastrointestinal disease (3.4% to 15.4%).[106] The lower third of the crypts is decidedly the major zone of DNA synthesis, and in this group 54.2% to 76.9% of S-phase cells were located there.

The cell cycle time in colon and rectum as determined *in vivo* is approximately 1 to 2 days, with S-phase duration between 10 and 20 hours, a G_1-phase duration of 14 hours, and a G_2-phase duration less than 6 hours.[14,107] Replacement or turnover time of this tissue is estimated by those using *in vivo* labeling to be as short as 3 to 4 days[14,107] or as long as 6 to 8 days.[108,109] *In vitro* studies with colorectal biopsies show a shorter duration for S-phase (7.2 to 11.2 hours) and a cell cycle time of 2 to 4 days.[110–115]

Several endogenous factors influence epithelial cell proliferation in the large bowel. Variations in LI and mitotic indices (MI) have been observed at different times of the day and night. The phenomenon has been related to fecal production and cell loss at the luminal surface of crypts. The resultant shorter glands induce a cohort of upper crypt cells of the proliferative compartment to enter S phase in a synchronous manner some 8 hours later. The greater the degree of cell loss, the higher the LI and MI induced.[116]

Noradrenergic and cholinergic fibers located near the basal region of colonic crypts may locally stimulate cell proliferation via the production of noradrenaline. When chemical sympathectomy is carried out, MIs decline, which suggests the involvement of this sytem in cell replication.[117]

The biliary system also affects cell replication and

may in fact have a strong trophic effect on the colon. Bile deprivation results in fewer S-phase cells and a slower migration of cells up the crypt walls,[118] whereas it has little or no effect on the small intestine.[89,118] When the reverse condition occurs and bile acids are provided in the diet, there is increased cell proliferation, a widening of the proliferative compartment, and a faster migration of epithelial cells.[119] It is the detergent action of bile acids that is thought to contribute to this faster rate of cell replacement.

Locally produced prostaglandins formed by the metabolism of arachidonic acid via the cyclooxygenase system can suppress proliferation.[120] Administration of indomethacin or aspirin, which suppresses the prostaglandin system, will then stimulate cell renewal. The effect of prostaglandins on tissue level remains to be clarified.

Hormones also may alter replication rates. Exogenous delivery of hormones, e.g., pentagastrin and gastrin, in high doses stimulates cell renewal,[121,122] whereas pancreatic glucagon has no effect.[122] Hydrocortisone, a corticosteroid frequently used in the treatment of ulcerative colitis, significantly reduces the S-phase population in the distal colon but shows little or no effect in the proximal colon.[123]

Dietary factors can also affect colon cell proliferation both directly and indirectly. Obviously high intake of animal fats will increase bile flow and thereby indirectly increase cell replication. Dietary supplementation with wheat bran will also enhance proliferation.[124] But increasing the level of ascorbic acid intake can depress DNA synthesis in the colon.[125] The latter is a site-specific reaction, because proliferation in the small intestine remains unaffected. Other substances shown to lower the proliferation rate are β-sitosterol, a plant sterol, and the food stabilizer butylated hydroxyanisole.[126,127] Both agents reduce the size of the proliferative compartment and the number of S-phase cells per crypt column as well as slow the migration of cells to the luminal surface. Obviously the colonic mucosa receives multiple signals that may modify epithelial cell behavior, and it is the presence of a balanced regulatory system that contributes to the health of the mucosa. We turn now to conditions that imply the existence of an imperfect or unbalanced regulatory system.

Preneoplasia

Unlike untreated rodents, individuals with no colonic disease occasionally show an altered distribution of S-phase cells.[106] There exist cases in which isolated DNA synthesizing cells occur in the upper third and along the luminal surface of the crypts. This is perhaps the first sign of a loss of regulatory control over termination of DNA synthesis. This phenomenon is seen in histologically well-differentiated epithelial cells and appears more frequently in populations having isolated adenomas or a history of familial polyposis, colon cancer, or ulcerative colitis.[128] This deviation from the normal distribution is known as the stage I abnormality.

The second defect seen in normal-appearing colonic mucosa is a shift in the major zone of DNA synthesis from the lower third of glands to the middle and upper third of the crypts. This stage II defect has been recognized in all groups at high risk for adenoma and colon cancer development.[129] A further defect was noted when crypts characterized by the stage I and II abnormality achieved significantly increased LI values. Individuals with no colonic disease rarely have crypts with an LI greater than 15%, but patients in the high risk groups are more likely to have crypts characterized by hyperproliferative activity (stage III defect).[130] These glands have a greater probability of undergoing neoplastic transformation than unaffected or less severely affected crypts. Such glands are thought to be the future site of neoplasia if they do not revert to a less severe stage of abnormality.

Mouse models of colon cancer such as are induced by 1,2-dimethylhydrazine (DMH) and related compounds show similar stages of preneoplasia prior to and simultaneously with the development of adenomas and cancer.[130] Such evidence strengthens the case that these stages do in fact describe the events leading to the formation of microadenomas and adenomas.

Proliferation in Disease States

Colonic Adenoma

The groundwork for the growth and development of the adenoma is laid by the shift of the major zone of DNA synthesis to the middle and upper third of the glands. After neoplastic transformation, that area continues to expand by budding and branching until infolding produces the typical trapezoid shape that is a feature of the adenoma. The new lesion is characterized by more gland openings at the luminal surface while showing little or no increase in cryptal structures in the basal zone near the muscularis mucosa.[131,132] The migration rate during the downward infolding of the adenomatous tissue is estimated at 0.4 of a cell position per hour, compared with 0.3 of a cell position per hour in an upward direction for the normal-appearing mucosa.[133] The histogenesis of adenomas clearly forms an extension of the preneoplastic events described by autoradiographic findings.

The fibroblastic sheath of the adenoma is not well developed at the luminal surface of the lesion; rather, it resembles its immature appearance at the base of the glands.[134] The behavior of this mesenchymal sheath is believed to control the type of adenoma that will develop. That is, if the mesenchymal elements offer little resistance and grow along with the adenomatous tissue, then a villous adenoma is likely to form. On the other hand, if resistance to expansion is present, then a more compact lesion will arise.[131] The greater likelihood of malignancy within a villous adenoma may be related to the greater number of S-phase cells in the continuously expanding lesion.

Basically, the smaller the adenoma, the higher its level of proliferation. The unicryptal microadenomas and microscopic adenomas often seen in the mucosa of animals with chemically induced colonic cancer and in the mucosa of patients with familial polyposis have high replicative activity. In such lesions all the cells participate in DNA synthesis, and their doubling time approximates their cell cycle time. But as the tumor increases in size, the fraction of cells proliferating falls off and the growth rate of the neoplasm decays exponentially. Tumor growth is dependent on three important factors, the percentage of cell loss due to desquamation and necrosis, the growth fraction or percentage of cells proliferating, and the mean cell cycle duration.

A higher and more variable LI is usually observed in adenomas than in normal-appearing colonic mucosa. A range of 5.7% to 35.1% was reported for a group of adenomas observed in a single individual with familial polyposis, whereas a range of 6.2% to 10.5% was seen in the adjacent flat mucosa.[135] S-phase durations estimated from double labeling experiments provide a range of 7.4 to 16.1 hours, with a trend toward longer durations both in the adenoma and adjacent mucosa of individuals with polyps.[136] The estimated cell cycle time is between 1.4 and 6 days,[114,137,138] and the estimated doubling time for adenomatous polyps is about 26 days.[138]

Adenomas in experimental models also have higher LIs and slightly extended cell cycle times than the normal-appearing mucosa.[132,139,140] Heterogeneity among kinetic values is observed even with use of the same carcinogen and the same strain of animal.

Ulcerative Colitis

In general, a more highly proliferating population occurs in the mucosa of those with inflammatory bowel disease, compared with unaffected individuals (Table 7-5). A similar duration of S phase is reported in the two groups, but a shorter turnover time is estimated in patients with colitis (31.2 versus 90.0 hours in control subjects).[113,141] An enlarged proliferative compartment and a faster migration of cells to the luminal surface may explain the immature or undifferentiated appearance of cells seen in the upper third of crypts.[141]

Unlike Biasco et al.,[145] Serafine et al.[142] indicated no difference in LI between patients with colitis in histologic or sigmoidoscopic remission and those with clinically active disease. Extension of the proliferative compartment to the luminal surface (stage I abnormality) as well as a shift of the predominant area of DNA synthesis to the middle and upper third of the glands have been reported (stage II abnormality).[143-145] In the one study, 71% of patients with inflammatory bowel disease for 10 or more years exhibited this defect.[145] Because of the elevated LI expressed in the mucosa of patients with colitis, many of these crypts undoubtedly are characterized by hyperproliferative activity, i.e., an LI greater than 15%, which suggests that the stage III abnormality is also frequently present. It is of interest to note that in another study, 19% of biopsy and colectomy specimens from patients with long-standing disease had foci of adenomatous epithelium.[146]

Another manifestation of a proliferative defect among some individuals with inflammatory bowel disease for 10 years or longer relates to a lack of response on the part of epithelial cells when in the presence of phosphodiesterase inhibitors. Rather than an induced depression in the level of DNA synthesis, no effect is seen which suggests that a related mechanism governing replication is no longer under regulatory control.[147]

The incidence of colonic cancer among patients with inflammatory bowel disease is between 3% and 10%.[148] However, for those with colitis for 20 years or longer, the incidence is four times higher.[149] One possible explanation for this elevated risk for large-bowel cancer may involve the hyperproliferative activity in some isolated crypts. Even in the clinical remission some have LIs over 30%, or more than twice that seen in control tissue (Deschner, unpublished observations). When such replicative activity occurs in a crypt with an abnormal distribution of S-phase cells, there is a strong probability that neoplastic transformation will occur and a tumor arise. Thus the continuous presence of hyperactive crypts in this disease is consistent with the persistent risk in these patients for colonic cancer.

Colonic Carcinoma

Depending on the technique employed, widely divergent kinetic values are obtained. *In vivo* measurements provide values of between 13.0% and 23.1%. *In vitro* studies of 27 specimens have given mean LIs as low as 2.5% (range, 0.1% to 7.0%)[150] and as high as 32.9% for 17 carcinomas.[136] Another recent *in vitro* study covered the entire spectrum from 2.2% to 40.1%, giving a mean LI of 17.8%.[151] Investigators have recognized in some instances that variability from one part of the tumor to another does exist. For example, Lieb and Lisco[152] reported an LI of only 4.8% at the center of one carcinoma and an LI of 31.5% at the periphery. The lack of homogeneity from one area to another may contribute sharply to the poor therapeutic response observed with cycle-specific agents.

Table 7-5 COMPARISON OF LABELING INDEX (LI) IN ULCERATIVE COLITIS (UC) AND CONTROL CASES

Group	Mean LI (%)	Incubation Time (hr)	Reference
UC	25.9	1	113
Control	9.5		
UC	12.9	6	141
Control	4.8		
UC active	19.0	6	142
UC remission	18.9		
Control	13.1		
UC remission	8.1	1	143
Control	7.1		
UC remission	8.9	1	144
Control	7.7		
UC active	24.0	1	145
UC remission	11.0		
Control	9.0		

Cell cycle times for colon carcinomas have been measured successfully on only one occasion.[153] The duration of S phase was 14 hours, G_1 phase 5 hours, and G_2 and mitosis 7 hours, for a total cell cycle time of 26 hours. The estimated growth fraction was about 45%, the cell loss factor 42%, and the doubling time for this specimen 45 days.

Estimates of the cell cycle time of other tumors range from 38 to 125 hours. Extended mitotic times were noted in a study of 19 carcinomas showing almost a twofold increase over the normal tissue values (2.3 versus 1.2 hours).[115] An elongated S phase has also been observed in colonic adenocarcinomas.[136]

Direct volume measurements of 20 cases using radiologic films of the same tumor over long periods have provided doubling times of between 111 and 3430 days (mean, 620 days).[154] The slow growth indicated by these values emphasizes a high cell loss factor, which is obviously a characteristic. Cell loss of over 98% has been estimated in many carcinomas.[115,150] Many exfoliated cells from colorectal tumors are still viable, can synthesize DNA, and can produce metastatic lesions.[155]

Cell proliferation studies have decidedly been of value in our understanding of the evolution of disease in the gastrointestinal system. Overall characteristics leading to abnormal conditions in the entire digestive tract include a widening of the zone of proliferation and an enhancement of the rate of cell replication. Basically, these characteristic abnormalities imply a defect in the mechanisms that control the last stages of differentiation and bring about termination of DNA synthesis. It remains to be determined whether these abnormal conditions can be controlled or reversed so as to slow or eliminate the disease state. This is at least one therapeutic possibility that has emerged from analyses of the kinetic behavior of gastrointestinal epithelial cells.

References

1. Lipkin M, Winawer SJ, Sherlock P: Early identification of individuals at increased risk for cancer of the large intestine. I. Definition of high risk populations. Clin Bull 11:13–21, 1981.
2. Bizzozero G: Über die Regeneration der Elemente der schlauformingen Drusen und des Epithels des Magendarmkanals. Anat Anz 3:781–784, 1888.
3. Howard A, Pelc SR: Nuclear incorporation of P^{32} as demonstrated by autoradiographs. Exp Cell Res 2:178–187, 1951.
4. Messier B, Leblond CP: Cell proliferation and migration as revealed by radioautography after injection of thymidine H^3 into male rats and mice. Am J Anat 106:247–285, 1960.
5. Bell B, Almy TP, Lipkin M: Cell proliferation kinetics in the gastrointestinal tract of man. III. Cell renewal in esophagus, stomach, and jejunum of a patient with treated pernicious anemia. J Natl Cancer Inst 38:615–628, 1967.
6. Livstone EM, Sheahan DG, Behan J: Studies of esophageal epithelial cell proliferation in patients with reflux esophagitis. Gastroenterology 73:1315–1319, 1977.
7. Herbst JJ, Berenson MM, McCloskey DW, Wiser WC: Cell proliferation in esophageal columnar epithelium (Barrett's esophagus). Gastroenterology 75:683–687, 1978.
8. Munoz N. Lipkin M, Crespi M, Wahrendorf J, Grassi A, Shih-Hsien L: Proliferation abnormalities of the oesophageal epithelium of Chinese populations at high and low risk for oesophageal cancer. Int J Cancer 36:187–189, 1985.
9. Yang GC, Wang GC, Wang GQ, et al: Proliferation of esophageal epithelial cells in individuals in Linxian, China. Proc AACR 27:155, 1986.
10. Fabrikant JI: The kinetics of cellular proliferation in human tissues. Determination of duration of DNA synthesis using double labeling autoradiography. Br J Cancer 24:122–127, 1970.
11. Sugimachi K, Ida H, Okamura T, et al: Cytophotometric DNA analysis of mucosal and submucosal carcinoma of the esophagus. Cancer 53:2683–2687, 1984.
12. Oehlert W: Biological significance of dysplasias of the epithelium and of atrophic gastritis. In Herfarth C, Schlag P, (eds): Gastric Cancer. Heidelberg, Springer-Verlag, 1979, p 91.
13. Tanaka J: Autoradiographic studies on the cell proliferation of the human gastric mucosa in supravital condition. Acta Pathol Jpn 18:307–318, 1968.
14. Lipkin M, Sherlock P, Bell B: Cell proliferation kinetics in the gastrointestinal tract of man. II. Renewal in stomach, ileum, colon, and rectum. Gastroenterology 45:721–729, 1963.
15. Bleiberg H, Mainguet P, Vendenhende J: Mesure autoradiographique de la proliferation cellulaire a differente niveaux du tractus digestif normal et pathologique: Utilisation de biopsies incubees in vitro. Rev Europ Etud Clin Biol 16:233–239, 1971.
16. Castrup HJ, Fuchs K, Pieper HJ: Cell renewal of gastric mucosa in Zollinger-Ellison syndrome. Acta Hepatogastroenterologica 22:40–43, 1975.
17. Hansen OH, Pedersen T, Larsen JK: A method to study cell proliferation kinetics in human gastric mucosa. Gut 16:23–27, 1975.
18. Hansen OH, Pedersen T, Larsen JK: Cell proliferation kinetics in normal human gastric mucosa: Studies on diurnal fluctuations and effects of food ingestion. Gastroenterology 70:1051–1054, 1976.
19. Hansen OH, Johansen AA, Larsen JK, et al: Relationship between gastric acid secretion, histopathology and cell proliferation kinetics in human gastric mucosa. Gastroenterology 73:453–456, 1977.
20. Hansen OH, Johansen AA, Larsen JK, Svendsen LB: Cell proliferation in normal and diseased gastric mucosa. Acta Pathol Microbiol Scand [A] 87:217–222, 1979.
21. Assad RT, Eastwood GL: Epithelial proliferation in human fundic mucosa after antrectomy and vagotomy. Gastroenterology 79:807–811, 1980.
22. Tytgat GNJ, Offerhaus GJA, van Minnen AJ, et al: Influences of oral 15(R)-methyl prostaglandin E_2 on human gastric mucosa: A light microscopic, cell kinetic, and ultrastructural study. Gastroenterology 90:1111–1120, 1986.
23. Assad RT, Tedesco FJ, Hardin RD, Brownstein RE: Antral epithelial proliferation in patients with gastric ulcer. Gastroenterology 82:1010, 1982.
24. Fujita S, Hattori T: Cell proliferation, differentiation, and migration in the gastric mucosa: A study on the background of carcinogenesis. In Farber E (ed), Pathophysiology of Carcinogenesis in Digestive Organs, University of Tokyo Press, Tokyo, 1977, p 21.
25. Willems G, Lehy T: Radioautographic and quantitative studies on parietal and peptic cell kinetics in the mouse: A selective effect of gastrin on parietal cell proliferation. Gastroenterology 69:416–426, 1975.
26. Yeomans ND, Trier JS: Epithelial cell proliferation and migration in the developing rat. Dev Biol 53:206–216, 1976.
27. Stoffels GL, Preumont AM, de Reuck M: Cell differentiation in human gastric gland as revealed by nuclear binding of tritiated actinomycin. Gut 20:696–697, 1978.
28. Seelig LL, Winborn WB, Weser E: Changes in gastric glandular cell kinetics after small bowel resection. Gastroenterology 74:1–6, 1978.
29. Hattori T, Helpap B, Gedigk P: Regeneration of endocrine cells in the stomach. Virchows Arch [B] 38:283–290, 1982.
30. Lehy T, Willems G: Population kinetics of antral gastrin cells in mouse. Gastroenterology 71:614–619, 1976.
31. Hansen OH, Pedersen T, Larsen JK, Rehfeld JF: Effect of gastrin on gastric mucosal cell proliferation in man. Gut 17:536–541, 1976.
32. Johnson LR, Guthrie P: Effect of cholecystokinin and 16,16-dimethyl-prostaglandin E_2 on RNA and DNA of gastric and duodenal mucosa. Gastroenterology 70:59–65, 1976.

33. Kawai K, Murakami M, Sasaki S, Misaki F: Cell kinetics of superficial epithelial cells of mouse gastric mucosa. Gastroenterology 84:1204, 1983.
34. Fich A, Arber N, Sestieri M, Zajicek G, Rachmilewitz D: Effect of misoprostol and cimetidine on gastric cell labeling index. Gastroenterology 89:57–61, 1985.
35. Myhre E: Regeneration of the fundic mucosa in rats. V. An autoradiographic study on the effects of cortisone. Arch Pathol 70:476–485, 1960.
36. Avetisyan AA: Effect of hydrocortisone on the mitotic cycle in mucus-forming cells of the gastric fundus epithelium. Biull Eksp Biol Med 76:101–103, 1973.
37. Johnson LR, Guthrie P: Secretin inhibition of gastrin-stimulated deoxyribonucleic acid synthesis. Gastroenterology 67:601–607, 1974.
38. Casteleyn PP, Dubrasquet M, Willems G: Opposite effects of gastrin on cell proliferation in the antrum and other parts of the upper-gastrointestinal tract in the rat. Dig Dis 22:798–804, 1977.
39. Willems G, Vansteenkiste Y, Smets P: Effects of food ingestion on the proliferation kinetics in the canine fundic mucosa. Gastroenterology 61:323–327, 1971.
40. Bertrand P, Willems G: Induction of antral gastrin cell proliferation by refeeding of rats after fasting. Gastroenterology 78:918–924, 1980.
41. Teir H, Räsäen T: A study of mitotic rate in renewal zones of nondiseased portions of gastric mucosa in cases of peptic ulcer and gastric cancer, with observation on differentiation and so-called "intestinalization" of gastric mucosa. J Natl Cancer Inst 27:949–971, 1961.
42. Siurala M, Isokoski M, Varis K, Kekki M: Prevalence of gastritis in a rural population: Bioptic study of subjects selected at random. Scand J Gastroenterol 3:211–233, 1968.
43. Deschner EE, Winawer SJ, Lipkin M: Patterns of nucleic acid and protein synthesis in normal human gastric mucosa and atrophic gastritis. J Natl Cancer Inst 48:1567–1574, 1972.
44. Kuwayama H, Ikeda Y, Tashiro Y, et al: Water immersion restraint stress inhibits epithelial proliferation in rat gastric fundus. Gastroenterology 84:1219, 1983.
45. Takeuchi K, Johnson LR: Effect of cell proliferation and loss on aspirin-induced gastric damage in the rat. Am J Physiol 243:G463–G468, 1982.
46. Kuwayama H, Ikeda Y, Tashiro Y, et al: Effect of chronic indomethacin ingestion on rat fundic, antral and duodenal epithelial proliferation. Gastroenterology 84:1219, 1983.
47. Yeomans ND, St John DJB, de Boer WGRM: Regeneration of gastric mucosa after aspirin-induced injury in the rat. Dig Dis 18:773–780, 1973.
48. Eastwood GL, Quimby GF: Effect of chronic aspirin ingestion on epithelial proliferation in rat fundus, antrum, and duodenum. Gastroenterology 82:852–856, 1982.
49. Andre F, Andre C, Fournier S: Measurement of glycoprotein content and cell kinetics in preulcerous gastric mucosa. Dig Dis Sci 24:667–671, 1979.
50. Stemmermann GN, Hayashi T, Taki M: A study of the morphology and kinetics of epithelial migration in response to gastrointestinal ulceration: A new approach to the cancer-ulcer question. In Farber E (ed): Pathophysiology of Carcinogenesis in Digestive Organs. Tokyo, Tokyo University Press, 1977, p 37.
51. Adair HM: Epithelial mitotic activity in experimental gastric wounds. J Anat 125:401–407, 1978.
52. Helpap B, Hattori T, Gedigk P: Repair of gastric ulcer: A cell kinetic study. Virchows Arch [A] 392:159–170, 1981.
53. Johansen A: Gastric polyps: Pathology and malignant potential. In Sherlock P, Morson BC, Barbara L, Veronei V (eds): Precancerous Lesions of the Gastrointestinal Tract. New York, Raven Press, 1983, p 171.
54. Takahashi M, Shirai T, Fukushima S, et al: Effect of fundic ulcers induced by iodoacetamide on development of gastric tumors in rats treated with N-methyl-N'-nitro-N-nitrosoguanidine. Gann 67:47–54, 1976.
55. Tatematsu M, Furimata C, Katsuyama T, et al: Independent induction of intestinal metaplasia and gastric cancer in rats treated with N-methyl-N'-nitro-N-nitrosoguanidine. Cancer Res 43:1335–1341, 1983.
56. Deschner EE, Tamura K, Bralow SP: Sequential histopathology and cell kinetic changes in rat pyloric mucosa during gastric carcinogenesis induced by N-methyl-N'-nitro-N-nitrosoguanidine. J Natl Cancer Inst 63:171–179, 1979.
57. Schauer A, Kunze E: Relation of adenomatous hyperplasia of the gastric mucosa to carcinogenesis. Pathol Res Pract 164:238–248, 1979.
58. Neuburger P, Lewin M, Bonfils S: Parietal and chief cell populations in four cases of the Zollinger-Ellison syndrome. Gastroenterology 63:937–942, 1972.
59. Bordi C, Cocconi G, Togni R, et al: Gastric endocrine cell proliferation: Association with Zollinger-Ellison syndrome. Arch Pathol 98:274–278, 1974.
60. Ottenjahn R, Gall F, Elster K: Tumorformige hyperplasie der magenschleimhaut bei Zollinger-Ellison syndrom (tumor-like hyperplasia of gastric mucosa in Zollinger-Ellison syndrome). Dtsch Med Wochenschr 92:1538–1546, 1967.
61. Ming SC, Bajtai A, Correa P, et al: Gastric dysplasia: Significance and pathologic criteria. Cancer 54:1794–1801, 1984.
62. Rubio CA, Hirota T, Itabashi T: Atypical mitoses in elevated dysplasias of the stomach. Pathol Res Pract 180:372–376, 1985.
63. Hattori T: Histological and autoradiographic study on development of grade III lesion (dysplasia grade III) in the stomach. Pathol Res Pract 180:36–44, 1985.
64. Nagayo T: Microscopical cancer of the stomach: A study on histogenesis of gastric carcinoma. Inter J Cancer 16:52–60, 1975.
65. Steenbeck L, Wolff G: Histoautoradiographische untersuchungen der menschlichen magenschleimhaut bei chronischer gastritis and magenkarzinom [Histoautoradiographic examinations of human gastric mucosa in chronic gastritis and gastric cancer]. Arch Geschwulstforsch 38:132–138, 1971.
66. Jaervi O, Lauren P: On the role of heterotopias of the intestinal epithelium in the pathogenesis of gastric cancer. Acta Pathol Microbiol Scand 29:26–44, 1951.
67. Nagayo T: Precursors of human gastric cancer: Their frequencies and histological characteristics. In Farber E (ed): Pathophysiology of Carcinogenesis in Digestive Organs. Tokyo, University of Tokyo Press, 1977, p 151.
68. Sowa M, Ohkita H, Nitta M, et al: Evaluation of clinicopathological analysis of early gastric cancer. World J Surg 5:717–720, 1981.
69. Jass JR, Filipe MI: A variant of intestinal metaplasia associated with gastric carcinoma: A histochemical study. Histopathology 3:191–199, 1979.
70. Inokuchi K, Kodama Y, Sasaki O, et al: Differentiation of growth patterns of early gastric carcinoma determined by cytophotometric DNA analysis. Cancer 51:1138–1141, 1983.
71. Wright NA: An in vivo stathmokinetic study of cell proliferation in human gastric carcinoma and gastric mucosa. Cell Tissue Kinet 10:429–436, 1977.
72. Tabuchi Y, Inoue K, Takiguchi Y, et al: Mitotic activity of human gastric cancer cells under stathmokinetic effect of vincristine sulfate. Gann 71:84–93, 1980.
73. Sasaki K, Takahashi M, Ogino T, Okuda S: An autoradiographic study on the labeling index of biopsy specimens from gastric cancers. Cancer 54:1307–1309, 1984.
74. Cheng H, Leblond CP: Origin, differentiation and renewal of the four main epithelial cell types in the mouse small intestine. V. Unitarian theory of the origin of the four epithelial cell types. Am J Anat 141:537–562, 1974.
75. Croft DN, Cotton PB: Gastrointestinal cell loss in man: Its measurement and significance. Digestion 8:144–160, 1973.
76. Shorter RG, Moertel CG, Titus JL, Reitemeier RJ: Cell kinetics in the jejunum and rectum of man. Am J Dig Dis 9:760–763, 1964.
77. Wright N, Watson A, Morley A, et al: Cell kinetics in flat (avillous) mucosa of the human small intestine. Gut 14:701–710, 1973.
78. Wright N, Watson A, Morley A, et al: The cell cycle time in flat (avillous) mucosa of the human small intestine. Gut 14:603–606, 1973.
79. Hendel L, Ammitzboll T, Petri M: Enterocyte-labeling index in the duodenal mucosa of patients with progressive systemic sclerosis. Acta Pathol Microbiol Immun of Scand [A] 94:107–111, 1986.
80. Brown HO, Levine ML, Lipkin M: Inhibition of intestinal epi-

thelial cell renewal and migration induced by starvation. Am J Physiol 205:868–872, 1963.
81. Biasco G, Callegari C, Lami F, et al: Intestinal morphological changes during oral refeeding in a patient previously treated with total parenteral nutrition for small bowel resection. Am J Gastroenterol 79:585–588, 1984.
82. Tutton PJM: The influence of serotonin on crypt cell proliferation in the jejunum of rats. Virchows Arch [B] 16:79–87, 1974.
83. Tutton PJM, Helme RD: The influence of adrenoceptor activity on crypt cell proliferation in rat jejunum. Cell Tissue Kinet 7:125–136, 1974.
84. Tutton PJM: The influence of histamine on epithelial proliferation in the jejunum of the rat. Clin Exp Pharmacol Physiol 3:369–373, 1976.
85. Laguchev SS, Avetisyan AA: Effect of hydrocortisone on time parameters of the mitotic cycle of duodenal epithelial cells. Biull Eksp Biol Med 73:86–88, 1972.
86. McDermott FT, Roudnew B: Ileal crypt cell population kinetics after 40 percent small bowel resection. Gastroenterology 70:707–711, 1976.
87. Hanson WR, Osborne JW: Epithelial cell kinetics in the small intestine of the rat 60 days after resection of 70 percent of the ileum and jejunum. Gastroenterology 60:1087–1097, 1971.
88. Cheng H, McCulloch C, Bjerknes M: Effects of 30% intestinal resection on whole population cell kinetics of mouse intestinal epithelium. Anat Rec 215:35–41, 1986.
89. Williamson RCN, Bauer FLR, Ross JS, Malt RA: Contribution of bile and pancreatic juice to cell proliferation in ileal mucosa. Surgery 83:570–576, 1978.
90. Altmann CG: Influence of bile and pancreatic secretions on the size of the intestinal villi in rats. Am J Anat 1132:167–178, 1971.
91. Weser E, Heller R, Tawil T: Stimulation of mucosal growth in the rat ileum by bile and pancreatic secretions after jejunal resection. Gastroenterology 73:524–529, 1977.
92. Menge H, Gräfe M, Lorenz-Meyer H: Influence of food intake on the development of structural and functional adaption following ileal resection in the rat. Gut 16:468–472, 1975.
93. Feldman FJ, Dowling RH, Naughton J, Peters TJ: Effects of oral versus intravenous nutrition on intestinal adaption after small bowel resection in the dog. Gastroenterology 70:712–719, 1976.
94. Levine GM, Deren JJ, Yezdimir E: Small bowel resection. Oral intake is the stimulus for hyperplasia. Am J Dig Dis 21:542–546, 1976.
95. Junghanns K, Kaess H, Dörner M, Encke A: The influence of resection of the small intestine on gastrin levels. Surg Gynecol Obstet 140:27–29, 1975.
96. Sagor GR, Al-Mukhtar MYT, Ghatei MA, et al: The effect of altered luminal nutrition on cellular proliferation and plasma concentrations of enteroglucagon and gastrin after small bowel resection in the rat. Br J Surg 69:14–18, 1982.
97. Croft DN, Loehry CA, Creamer B: Small bowel cell loss and weight loss in the coeliac syndrome. Lancet 2:68–70, 1968.
98. Trier JS, Browning TH: Epithelial cell renewal in cultured duodenal biopsies in celiac sprue. N Engl J Med 283:1245–1250, 1970.
99. Zagorulko MP, Puzyrev AA: On proliferation of the epithelium of duodenal mucosa in ulcerative disease. Arkh Patol 36:31–35, 1974.
100. Bransom CJ, Boxer ME, Clark JC, et al: Epithelial cell proliferation in duodenal ulcer. Scand J Gastroenterol 19:515–520, 1984.
101. Maskens AP, Dujardin-Loits R: Kinetics of tissue proliferation in colorectal mucosa during post-natal growth. Cell Tissue Kinet 14:467–477, 1981.
102. Appleton DR, Sunter JP, deRodriguez MSB, Watson AJ: Cell proliferation in the mouse large bowel, with details of the analyses of the experimental data. In Appleton DR, Sunter JP, Watson AJ (eds): Cell Proliferation in the Gastrointestinal Tract. Tunbridge Wells, Kent, England, Pitman Medical, 1980, pp 40–53.
103. Cheng H, Bjerkens M: Whole population cell kinetics of mouse duodenal, jejunal, ileal and colonic epithelia as determined by radioautography and flow cytometry. Anat Rev 203:251–264, 1982.
104. Bjerknes M, Cheng H: The stem-cell zone of the small intestinal epithelium. I. Evidence from Paneth cells in the adult mouse. Am J Anat 160:51–63, 1981.
105. Deschner EE, Long FC, Hakissian M, Herrmann SL: Differential susceptibility of AKR, C57BL/6J and CF1 mice to 1,2-dimethylhydrazine induced colonic tumor formation predicted by proliferative characteristics of colonic epithelial cells. J Natl Cancer Inst 70:279–282, 1983.
106. Maskens AP, Deschner EE: Tritiated thymidine incorporation into epithelial cells of normal-appearing colorectal mucosa of cancer patients. J Natl Cancer Inst 58:1221–1224, 1977.
107. Lipkin M, Bell B, Sherlock P: Cell proliferation kinetics in the gastrointestinal tract of man. I. Cell renewal in colon and rectum. J Clin Invest 42:767–776, 1963.
108. Cole JW, McKalen A: Observations of cell renewal in human rectal mucosa in vivo with thymidine-H^3. Gastroenterology 41:122–125, 1961.
109. MacDonald WC, Trier JS, Everrett NB: Cell proliferation and migration in the stomach, duodenum, and rectum of man: Radioautographic studies. Gastroenterology 46:405–417, 1964.
110. Galand P, Mainguet P, Arguello M, et al: In vitro autoradiographic studies of cell proliferation in the gastrointestinal tract of man. J Nucl Med 9:37–39, 1968.
111. Spencer RJ, Huizenga KA, Hammer CS, Shorter RG: Further studies of the kinetics of rectal epithelium in normal subjects and patients with ulcerative or granulomatous colitis. Dis Colon Rectum 12:406–408, 1969.
112. Bleiberg H, Garland P: In vitro autoradiographic determination of cell kinetic parameters in adenocarcinomas and adjacent healthy mucosa of the human colon and rectum. Cancer Res 36:325–328, 1976.
113. Bleiberg H, Mainguet P, Galand P, Chretien J, Dupont-Mairesse N: Cell renewal in the human rectum: In vitro autoradiographic study on active ulcerative colitis. Gastroenterology 58:851–855, 1970.
114. Bleiberg H, Mainguet P, Galand P: Cell renewal in familial polyposis: Comparison between polyps and adjacent healthy mucosa. Gastroenterology 63:240–245, 1972.
115. Camplejohn RS, Bone G, Aherne W: Cell proliferation in rectal carcinoma and rectal mucosa: A stathmokinetic study. Eur J Cancer 9:577–581, 1973.
116. Hamilton E: Diurnal variation in proliferative compartments and their relation to cryptogenic cells in the mouse colon. Cell Tissue Kinet 12:91–100, 1979.
117. Tutton PJM, Barkla DH: The influence of adrenoceptor activity on cell proliferation in colonic crypt epithelium and in colonic adenocarcinomata. Virchows Arch [B] 24:139–146, 1977.
118. Deschner EE, Raicht RF: The influence of bile on kinetic behavior of colonic epithelial cells of the rat. Digestion 19:322–327, 1979.
119. Deschner EE, Cohen BI, Raicht RF: Acute and chronic effect of dietary cholic acid on colonic epithelial cell proliferation. Digestion 21:290–296, 1981.
120. Craven PA, Saito R, DeRubertis FR: Role of local prostaglandin synthesis in the modulation of proliferative activity of rat colonic epithelium. J Clin Invest 72:1365–1375, 1983.
121. Mak KM, Chang WWL: Pentagastrin stimulates epithelial cell proliferation in duodenal and colonic crypts in fasted rats. Gastroenterology 71:1117–1120, 1976.
122. Fatemi SH, Cullan GE, Sharp JG: Evaluation of the effects of pentagastrin, gastrin and pancreatic glucagon on cell proliferation in the rat gastrointestinal tract. Cell Tissue Kinet 17:119–133, 1984.
123. Fath RB, Deschner EE, Winawer SJ, Dworkin BM: Degraded carrageenan-induced colitis in CF_1 mice: A chemical, histopathologic and kinetic analysis. Digestion 29:197–203, 1984.
124. Jacobs LR, Schneeman BO: Effects of dietary wheat bran on rat colonic structure and mucosal cell growth. J Nutr 111:798–803, 1981.
125. Deschner EE, Alcock N, Okamura T, et al: Tissue concentrations and proliferative effects of massive doses of ascorbic acid in the mouse. Nut Cancer 4:241–246, 1983.
126. Deschner EE, Cohen BI, Raicht RF: Kinetics of the protective effect of beta sitosterol against MNU induced colonic neoplasia. J Cancer Res Clin Oncol 103:49–54, 1982.
127. Deschner EE, Wattenberg LW: The proliferative effect of butyl-

128. Deschner EE, Lipkin M: Proliferative patterns in colonic mucosa in familial polyposis. Cancer 35:413–418, 1975.
129. Deschner EE: Cell proliferation as a biological marker in human colorectal neoplasia. In Winawer SJ, Schottenfeld D, Sherlock P, (eds): Colorectal Cancer: Prevention, Epidemiology and Screening. New York, Raven Press, 1980, pp 133–142.
130. Deschner EE, Maskens AP: Significance of the labeling index and labeling distribution as kinetic parameters in colo-rectal mucosa of cancer patients and DMH treated animals. Cancer 50:1136–1141, 1982.
131. Maskens AP: Histogenesis of adenomatous polyps in the human large intestine. Gastroenterology 77:1245–1251, 1979.
132. Wiebecke B, Krey V, Löhrs V, Eder M: Morphological and autoradiographical investigations on experimental carcinogenesis and polyp development in the intestinal tract of rats and mice. Virchows Arch [A] 360:179–193, 1973.
133. Lightdale C, Lipkin M, Deschner E: In vivo measurements in familial polyposis: Kinetics and location of proliferating cells in colonic adenomas. Cancer Res 42:4280–4283, 1982.
134. Kaye GI, Lane N, Pascal RR: Colonic pericryptal fibroblast sheath: Replication, migration, and cytodifferentiation of a mesenchymal cell system in adult tissue. II. Fine structural aspects of normal rabbit and human colon. Gastroenterology 54:852–865, 1968.
135. Deschner EE, Raicht RF: Kinetic and morphologic alterations in the colon of a patient with multiple polyposis. Cancer 47:2440–2445, 1981.
136. Bleiberg H, Byse M, Galand P: Cell kinetic indicators of premalignant stages of colorectal cancer. Cancer 56:124–129, 1985.
137. Bleiberg H, Salhadin A, Galand P: Cell cycle parameters in human colon. Cancer 39:1190–1194, 1977.
138. Lesher S, Schaffer LM, Phanse M: Human colonic tumor cell kinetics. Cancer 40:2706–2709, 1977.
139. Sunter JP: Experimental carcinogenesis and cancer in the rodent gut. In Appleton DR, Sunter JP, Watson AJ, (eds): Cell Proliferation in the Gastrointestinal Tract. Tunbridge Wells, Kent, England, Pitman Medical, 1980, pp 255–277.
140. Chang WWL, Mak KM, MacDonald PMD: Cell population kinetics of 1,2-dimethylhydrazine induced colonic neoplasms and their adjacent colonic mucosa in the mouse. Virchows Arch [B] 30:349–361, 1979.
141. Eastwood GL, Trier JS: Epithelial cell renewal in cultured rectal biopsies. Gastroenterology 64:383–390, 1973.
142. Serafine EP, Kirk AP, Chambers TJ: Rate and pattern of epithelial cell proliferation in ulcerative colitis. Gut 22:648–652, 1981.
143. Lehy T, Mignon M, Abitbol JL: Epithelial cell proliferation in the rectal stump of patients with ileorectal anastomosis for ulcerative colitis. Gut 24:1048–1056, 1983.
144. Deschner EE, Winawer SJ, Katz S, et al: Proliferative defects in ulcerative colitis patients. Cancer Invest 1:41–47, 1983.
145. Biasco G, Miglioli M, Minarini A, et al: Rectal cell renewal as biological markers of cancer risk in ulcerative colitis. In Sherlock P, Morson BC, Barbara L, Veronesi V (eds): Precancerous Lesions of the Gastrointestinal Tract. New York, Raven Press, 1983, pp 261–268.
146. Fenoglio CM, Pascal RR: Adenomatous epithelium, intraepithelial anaplasia, and invasive carcinoma in ulcerative colitis. Dig Dis 18:556–562, 1973.
147. Alpers DH, Philpott G, Grimme NL, Margolis DM: Control of thymidine incorporation in mucosal explants from patients with chronic ulcerative colitis. Gastroenterology 78:470–478, 1980.
148. Greenstein AJ, Sachar DB, Smith H, et al: Patterns of neoplasia in Crohn's disease and ulcerative colitis. Cancer 46:403–407, 1980.
149. Sherlock P, Winawer SJ: Cancer inflammatory bowel disease: Risk factors and prospects for early detection. In Lipkin M, Good RA (eds): Gastrointestinal Tract Cancer. New York, Plenum Medical, 1978, pp 479–488.
150. Ota DM, Drewinko B: Growth kinetics of human colorectal carcinoma. Cancer Res 45:2128–2131, 1985.
151. Meyer JS, Prioleau PG: S-phase fractions of colorectal carcinomas related to pathologic and clinical features. Cancer 48:1221–1228, 1981.
152. Lieb LM, Lisco H: In vitro uptake of tritiated thymidine by carcinoma of the human colon. Cancer Res 36:733–740, 1966.
153. Terz JJ, Curatchet HP, Lawrence W: Analysis of the cell kinetics of human solid tumors. Cancer 28:1100–1110, 1971.
154. Welin S, Youker J, Spratt JS: The rates and patterns of growth of 375 tumors of the large intestine and rectum observed serially by double contrast enema study (Malmo technique). Am J Roentgenol 90:673–687, 1963.
155. Fermor B, Umpleby HC, Lever JV, et al: Proliferative and metastatic potential of exfoliated colorectal cancer cells. J Natl Cancer Inst 76:347–349, 1986.

PART 2

DISORDERS COMMON TO THE GASTROINTESTINAL TRACT

CHAPTER 8

Embryology and Developmental Disorders

JAMES B. AREY, M.D.
MARIE VALDES-DAPENA, M.D.

ESOPHAGUS
Embryology
Tracheoesophageal Fistula and
 Esophageal Atresia
Esophageal Stenosis
Double Esophagus
Neurenteric Cysts
Esophageal Cysts

STOMACH
Embryology
Pyloric Atresia
Congenital Pyloric Stenosis
Heterotopic Pancreatic Tissue
Spontaneous Rupture of the Stomach

INTESTINES
Embryology
Aganglionic Megacolon
 (Hirschsprung's Disease)
Intestinal Atresia and Stenosis
Anomalies of Intestinal Rotation and
 Volvulus
Hernias
Omphalocele and Gastroschisis
Omphalomesenteric Duct Remnants
Congenital Diverticula of the
 Intestines
Meconium Ileus and Related
 Conditions
Spontaneous Perforation of the
 Intestine

DUPLICATIONS OF THE
 ALIMENTARY TRACT
Pathologic Features

RECTUM AND ANUS
Embryology
Imperforate Anus and Related
 Conditions
Cloacal Exstrophy

CYSTS OF MESENTERY AND
 OMENTUM
Mesenteric Cysts (Cystic Hygroma)
Omental Cysts

ESOPHAGUS

Embryology

The esophagus develops from the primitive foregut just caudal to the laryngotracheal groove, a ventromedian fissure in the floor of the foregut caudal to the fourth pharyngeal pouches. This groove deepens and expands to form the laryngotracheal diverticulum, within which paired longitudinal ridges, the tracheoesophageal folds, grow cranially as well as medially toward each other. With fusion of these folds, the tracheoesophageal septum divides the foregut into the ventrally located laryngotracheal tube, the primordium of the larynx, trachea, bronchi, lungs, and the dorsally situated esophagus. This division occurs in a caudocephalad direction, separating first the lung buds and then the trachea from the esophagus. Finally, the only communication between the respiratory and digestive segments of the foregut is the primitive glottis. The epithelium and mucous glands of the esophagus are derived from the endoderm. The striated muscle of the muscularis externa of the upper esophagus develops from mesenchyme in the caudal branchial arches, whereas the smooth muscle and connective tissue are derived from the surrounding splanchnic mesoderm.

Initially the esophagus is only a short, narrow tube passing from the pharynx to the stomach. It rapidly elongates, however, primarily as the result of growth of the embryo, but enhanced by caudal migration of the heart and pericardium and increasing size of the lung buds. Its epithelium proliferates rapidly and almost obliterates the lumen. In contrast to parts of the intestinal tract, however, the esophageal lumen of the human embryo is probably never completely occluded under normal circumstances; and complete canalization normally occurs by the end of embryogenesis, i.e., the eighth week.

The epithelium of the esophagus begins to be ciliated at about the tenth week of gestation, and not until the fifth month does this start to be replaced by stratified squamous epithelium. Even at the time of birth, however, patches of columnar ciliated epithelium may persist in the otherwise continuous stratified squamous epithelium. Islands of gastric mucosa may be present also in the esophagus, usually at the upper end.

Tracheoesophageal Fistula and Esophageal Atresia (Table 8-1)

This condition is the most common anomaly of the esophagus, occurring in about 1 of 3000 livebirths. Its embryogenesis is probably related to posterior deviation of the tracheoesophageal septum or a defective tracheoesophageal septum, or both, as a result of incomplete fusion of the tracheoesophageal folds. Excessive proliferation of esophageal epithelium and failure of vacuolization during the embryonic period might account for some instances of pure esophageal atresia.

Approximately 20% of infants with esophageal atresia and tracheoesophageal fistula are premature by weight, and this frequency is even greater in those with pure esophageal atresia. Other major anomalies are present in 20% to 30% of affected infants, especially those of the cardiovascular system, anorectal malformations, and atresia or stenosis of the small intestine. Down's syndrome occurs with increased frequency in infants with esophageal malformations.

Esophageal atresia with tracheoesophageal fistula accounts for approximately 90% of these malformations (Figure 8–1). In the vast majority the fistula is between the trachea or a bronchus and the distal esophageal segment. The proximal, blind-ending esophageal segment is dilated, hypertrophied, and usually 3 to 4 cm long, terminating at about the level of T2. It resembles a diverticulum lying along the posterior wall of the trachea. The distal segment is usually separated from the proximal one by a distance varying from a few millimeters to 2 or 3 cm. Rarely, the two segments may be in muscular continuity, or the upper one may even overlap the distal one. The distal segment, or tracheoesophageal fistula, usually arises from the trachea at or slightly above the carina. Somewhat less frequently it enters a stem bronchus, usually the right. The fistulous tract passes obliquely inferiorly in the wall of the trachea for a few millimeters before emerging from its posterior aspect to continue as the distal esophagus. It

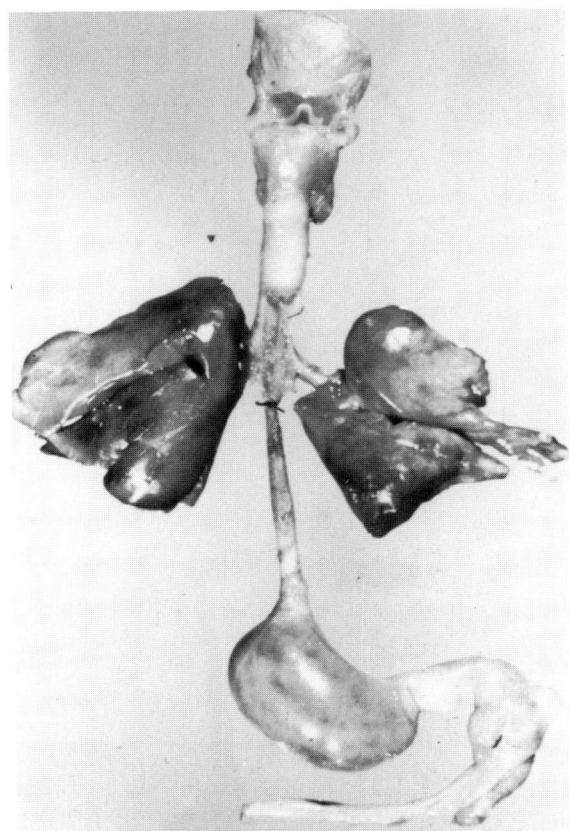

FIGURE 8–1. Esophageal atresia with tracheoesophageal fistula, surgically ligated. From a premature female infant 2 days old who weighed 1580 gm and died of congenital heart disease. Posterior view.

tapers gradually from its relatively normal size at the level of the diaphragm to its point of entrance into the trachea or a bronchus, where it usually does not exceed 0.5 cm in diameter.

A continuous mucous membrane lines the trachea, the esophagus, and the fistulous communication, but in the region of the fistula the nature of the epithelium varies somewhat. The squamous epithelium of the esophagus may end abruptly at its junction with the trachea or may extend upward in the trachea for a short distance. In other instances the esophagus in the region of the fistula may be lined by pseudostratified columnar ciliated epithelium. Ganglion cells are present in the muscularis of the distal esophageal segment, and mixed glands resembling those of the trachea may be present in the region of the fistula.

Pure esophageal atresia without tracheoesophageal fistula accounts for approximately 5% of the cases. Both the upper and lower esophageal segments terminate blindly. There is no fistulous communication of either segment with the tracheobronchial tree. A thin fibromuscular cord devoid of a lumen may be identified connecting the proximal and distal segments of the esophagus. The upper blind segment is dilated and hypertrophied. Early filling of this blind pouch leads to copious drooling, and feedings spill over into the res-

Table 8–1 ESOPHAGEAL ATRESIA AND TRACHEOESOPHAGEAL FISTULA

Combined fistula and atresia	Over 90%
Atresia without fistula	5%
Fistula without atresia	2–3%
Laryngeal cleft	Rare

piratory tract with subsequent gagging, coughing, cyanosis, and aspiration pneumonia. These findings are similar to those with esophageal atresia with a tracheoesophageal fistula, but now the abdomen remains scaphoid because there is no access of air to the gastrointestinal tract.

Tracheoesophageal fistula without esophageal atresia, or the so-called H type of fistula, accounts for only 2% to 3% of this group. The fistulous communication is characteristically a minute one located at a higher level than it is when there is also esophageal atresia; rarely, it is in the neck, just below the cricoid cartilage.[1] Occasionally the proximal "blind" esophageal segment communicates with the trachea by a fistulous tract, the distal esophagus being only a short blind-ending sac arising from the gastric cardia, or both the upper and lower segments communicate with the trachea through separate fistulas but fail to maintain continuity with each other. In the latter anomaly, the proximal fistula is usually located in the neck or at the thoracic inlet, and the distal fistula is also a high one, the upper and lower pouches often overlapping each other.[2]

Laryngeal cleft is a rare anomaly in which a cleft in the midline of the body of the cricoid posteriorly creates a communication between the larynx and the hypopharynx. It may occur as an isolated defect or be associated with esophageal atresia. Even less often a *laryngotracheoesophageal fistula* allows for communication between the trachea and esophagus by a defect including a cleft larynx and extending caudally in the trachea to the carina.

Esophageal Stenosis

Congenital esophageal stenosis may occur at any site along the esophagus. In general, a membranous stenosis or web occurs in the upper esophagus, predominantly in women, just below the level of the cricoid cartilage. At esophagoscopy this condition is seen as simple infolding of the mucosa and submucosa, containing an eccentrically located or, less frequently, central perforation. The web often appears to arise from the anterior wall of the esophagus, the orifice being on its posterior aspect.[3] Because the condition is usually readily treated by dilation, minimal pathologic reports concerning its true nature are available; a few suggest that it simply represents a thin sheet of esophageal mucosa and submucosa, possibly with remnants of muscularis mucosae.[4]

Segmental stenoses of congenital origin, on the contrary, usually involve the distal esophagus of infants and children. They may, however, also occur in adult life and may even be several centimeters above the diaphragm.[5] They are annular in their configuration and involve a segment of the esophagus up to about 2.5 cm in length. Histologically they consist of tracheobronchial elements[6]: pseudostratified columnar ciliated epithelium, mucous glands, smooth muscle, and often lymphoid aggregates[7] and plaques of cartilage.[8,9] They probably represent failure of the normal separation of the respiratory tract from the primitive esophagus.

Esophageal stenosis has also been reported as the result of an annular band of hypertrophic muscle at the esophagogastric junction in an infant with a hiatal hernia. Thin fibrous septa separated the bundles of hypertrophied muscle, and there was evidence of a low-grade inflammatory process, but the predominant finding was that of hypertrophied muscle.[10] Somewhat comparable findings were present in a 5-month-old infant with a segmental esophageal stenosis in the middle third in which the very reduced lumen was surrounded by abundant submucosal smooth muscle and connective tissue,[11] without evidence of inflammation. Extreme hypertrophy of the muscularis mucosae and inner circular muscularis involving virtually all of the esophagus has been noted in a girl 2 years of age.[12]

Double Esophagus

A *double esophagus* is a complete tubular structure passing from the pharynx to the gastric cardia, and the stomach also may be duplicated. The accessory esophagus may communicate with the pharynx, a gastric pouch, or the normal esophagus through a fistulous tract. Although such a lesion has been identified in a newborn infant,[13] more frequently the diagnosis is not established until adult life.[14]

Neurenteric Cysts

These mediastinal cysts have been described as duplications of the esophagus or mediastinal enterogenous cysts. They have commonly been attributed to incomplete or delayed obliteration of the primitive neurenteric (notochordal) canal that passes between the intraembryonic yolk sac and the amniotic cavity. This canal is a short-lived structure passing from the yolk sac through the primitive knot (Hensen's node). Since the tip of the coccyx is the final location of the primitive knot and of the former neurenteric canal, neurenteric remnants or open connections located cranial to this site must represent either accessory neurenteric canals[15] or abnormal connections of the primitive ectodermal and endodermal layers during the presomite period.[16]

The malformations of neurenteric origin are somewhat comparable to the more common remnants of the ventrally located omphalomesenteric duct, e.g., Meckel's diverticulum, umbilical cyst, and persistent omphalomesenteric sinus. In contrast to the omphalomesenteric duct, however, which passes through only the soft tissues of the anterior abdominal wall, the neurenteric canal(s) traverses mesenchymal tissue destined to form the vertebral column. As a result, delayed or incomplete closure of such a canal or abnormal ectoendodermal adhesions at the site of defective or absent mesodermal tissue are responsible for a variety of vertebral anomalies.[17]

Mediastinal cysts of neurenteric origin are observed predominantly in infants. They may be associated with an intra-abdominal duplication of the small intestine.

The triad of vertebral anomalies, posterior mediastinal cyst, and duplication of the small bowel appears to be of neurenteric origin or to result from abnormal ectoendodermal adhesions during the presomite period. The intra-abdominal duplication is usually of the long tubular type and is not continuous with the mediastinal cyst. Infrequently, however, a tubular diverticulum of the small bowel passes through an abnormal hiatus in the diaphragm into the posterior mediastinum.[18]

Clinical manifestations of mediastinal neurenteric cysts are usually related to pressure and displacement of mediastinal structures, e.g., dyspnea and repeated respiratory infections. Hemoptysis has been observed as the result of peptic ulceration of the wall of the cyst and rupture into a bronchus, and melena may occur because of a concomitant intra-abdominal duplication. Infrequently neurologic manifestations may be present because of an intraspinal extension of the mass. The diagnosis should be suspected whenever a posterior mediastinal mass is associated with anomalies of the lower cervical or upper dorsal vertebrae. The mass, however, is usually located caudal to the vertebral lesion, and the latter may not be apparent in routine radiographs of the chest.

The cyst is usually on the right and is a spherical, unilocular structure filled with a mucoid fluid or a reddish brown material. A tubular tract or, more frequently, a fibrous cord may lead from the wall of the cyst to a vertebral body.[15] The wall of the cyst is composed of a thick zone of smooth muscle arranged in two or even three rather distinct layers; myenteric plexuses are often present. A submucosa and muscularis mucosae are present, and the lining epithelium is usually well preserved. It usually consists predominantly of gastric mucosa containing parietal and chief cells; but any combination of gastric, small intestinal, colonic, esophageal, and even pseudostratified columnar ciliated epithelium may be present. Islands of pancreatic tissue are sometimes present. There may be areas of ulceration, and sometimes the lining mucosa is entirely destroyed and replaced by granulation tissue; under such circumstances radiographically demonstrable deposits of calcium may be present in the wall of the cyst. Neural elements have been observed in a few instances, either in the vicinity of the cyst[19] or in its attachment to the vertebral column.[20]

Esophageal Cysts

Esophageal cysts are extremely rare in childhood and are usually asymptomatic until they have enlarged sufficiently to produce dysphagia in early adult life. They are usually small, smooth, hemispherical masses that bulge into the esophageal lumen and move with swallowing. They are embedded in the esophageal wall, and the fibers of muscle within the wall of the cyst are intimately admixed with those of the esophagus. They are lined by a respiratory type of epithelium. Their location within the wall of the esophagus, the presence of a muscularis mucosae, and the absence of cartilage serve to differentiate these from bronchogenic cysts; both probably arise from anomalous buds of the foregut, similar to the true lung buds, which also originate from the foregut.

STOMACH

Embryology

The stomach is discernible during the fourth week of intrauterine life, as a spindle-shaped enlargement of the foregut. Initially located in the region destined to become the neck, it "descends" during the fourth to seventh week to reach its permanent location in the abdomen. During this period the viscus increases in length and its dorsal border grows more rapidly than does the ventral wall, the former forming the convex greater curvature.

The stomach rotates 90 degrees about its long axis until the greater curvature (or the initial dorsal wall) lies on the left, whereas the caudal end is relatively anchored by the short ventral mesentery and bile duct as well as by the vitelline artery. Pits or foveolae appear at 7 weeks, and gastric glands begin to develop at 14 weeks.[21] Pepsin, renin, and probably hydrochloric acid are secreted by the fifth month of fetal life. The pH of the gastric contents at birth is in the vicinity of neutrality, but the reaction becomes remarkably acid between 5 and 24 hours after birth, with an average pH of 1.5. Subsequently the acidity decreases to a temporary low level between the first and second weeks of life.[22]

Pyloric Atresia

Membranous pyloric atresia is a rare malformation with no known association with other diseases. Congenital pyloric atresia resulting from subepithelial separation of the mucosa with subsequent cicatricial obliteration of the lumen is a rare condition that may accompany junctional epidermolysis bullosa.[23]

Congenital Pyloric Stenosis

Clinical Features. Congenital hypertrophic pyloric stenosis is the most important lesion of the stomach in infants. It occurs predominantly in male infants, especially the first-born. Occasionally more than one member of a family is affected. The disease is uncommon in black infants. Vomiting usually begins in the second or third week of life. The vomitus is not bile-stained but may be streaked with blood. With persistent vomiting, severe dehydration, metabolic alkalosis, constipation, and weight loss may occur. Gastric peristaltic waves, originating on the left side, may be observed; and the pyloric mass can be palpated in most instances.

Gross Features. Roentgenographic and fluoroscopic examinations reveal a narrowed, elongated pyloric canal with a threadlike lumen or an enlarged stomach with a blunt antrum and delay in prepyloric opening time as well as in the emptying time of the stomach. Prompt relief of the obstruction follows pyloromyotomy, but the hypertrophy of the pylorus may persist for some time, and in those treated by gastrojejunostomy it may persist into adult life. A hypertrophied pylorus has also been observed in older children and in adults with a history of excessive vomiting since infancy.

At surgery or necropsy the stomach is found to be dilated, often as much as twice normal size. The pylorus is elongated, measuring 1.5 to 3.0 cm in length (the normal length in infants of this age is 1.0 to 1.5 cm).[24] The serosal surface is smooth. The pylorus is thickened; its lumen is narrow, and its wall is pale and almost cartilaginous in consistency. The thickening is the result of an increase in the width of the circular layer of muscle, which varies from 3.0 to 7.0 mm. In infants 1 to 3 months of age without hypertrophic pyloric stenosis, this layer averages only 1.6 mm in width and does not exceed 2.5 mm.[24] Longitudinal section reveals the proximal end of the hypertrophied pyloric musculature to merge with the adjoining musculature of the stomach. Distally, however, it terminates abruptly at the duodenum, the lower end of the mass projecting into the duodenal lumen, resembling the projection of the cervix uteri into the vagina.

Microscopic Features. Histologically, the submucosa may be somewhat edematous, but the characteristic change is in the circular layer of the muscle, which is two to four times as thick as that of a normal adult.[25] The increased mass of muscle results from hypertrophy as well as hyperplasia of individual muscle fibers, the nuclei of which are rather flattened. There is no increase in connective tissue. The enlarged layer of circular muscle presents an irregular pattern, with fibers running in various directions, like those in leiomyoma.

Degenerative changes in the myenteric plexus of the pylorus have been observed by almost all investigators who have studied these structures specifically.[25-29] Although some decrease in the number of myenteric plexuses per unit area of pylorus has been described, this may represent a relative, rather than an absolute decrease; it has not been observed uniformly.[30] In any event, although the presence of degenerative changes in the myenteric plexuses of the pylorus seems to be well established, these changes are not comparable to those observed in congenital aganglionic megacolon. Moreover, it seems highly probable that in the study of isolated sections of the hypertrophied pylorus, the changes in the plexuses might not be apparent without the use of controls.

Pathogenesis. The cause of congenital hypertrophic pyloric stenosis is unknown, and it is not clear whether the changes in the myenteric plexuses represent the primary defect or a secondary phenomenon. Reports of authentic instances of the disease in very young infants are rare, and roentgenographic studies conducted in the immediate newborn period have failed to reveal signs of the disease in infants in whom clinical and roentgenographic evidence of its presence have subsequently developed.[31] Nevertheless, in view of the degree of hypertrophy that is present in infants who are operated upon soon after the onset of symptoms, it seems probable that hypertrophy precedes, rather than follows, the clinical manifestations of obstruction and thus must begin at a very early age. In a very few instances, indeed, there is convincing evidence that it began *in utero*.[32,33] These reports, in addition to an occasional familial occurrence of the disease and the high incidence of involvement of both monovular twins when either is affected, as contrasted with the relative infrequency of involvement of both binovular twins, appear to favor the heritable nature of the disorder.

Heterotopic Pancreatic Tissue

Heterotopic islands of pancreatic tissue are usually only incidental findings at surgery or necropsy. Rarely, however, they may be responsible for clinical symptoms, e.g., pyloric stenosis or intussusception. Symptomatic heterotopias of pancreatic tissue are more common in adults than in infants or children.[34] Aberrant pancreatic tissue may be located at any site along the length of the gastrointestinal tract from the pylorus to the ileocecal valve, along the course of the omphalomesenteric duct, or in the wall of a duplication or neurenteric cyst; pancreatic tissue is present in about 5% of all Meckel's diverticula. Islands of aberrant pancreatic tissue usually do not exceed 1 cm in diameter and appear as sessile, lobulated, yellow, freely movable, subserous or submucous nodules beneath intact surface membranes. When the aberrant tissue is located predominantly in the muscularis, there is often associated hyperplasia of smooth muscle. In the pylorus, such intramural nodules, with their associated hyperplasia of smooth muscle, may be responsible for pyloric stenosis[35,36]; and rarely the clinical and pathologic appearance may be indistinguishable from that of congenital hypertrophic pyloric stenosis.[37] Histologically, the nodules consist of pancreatic acini, sometimes associated with ducts and islets of Langerhans, as well as Brunner's glands and bundles of smooth muscle. In some instances in which only ductal structures and smooth muscle are identified in the initial sections, further sections will reveal distinct acinar elements. Accordingly, no real distinction can be made between such "adenomyomas" and islands of heterotopic pancreatic tissue.[38]

Spontaneous Rupture of the Stomach

Spontaneous rupture of the stomach is rare and occurs almost exclusively in newborn infants. It may be caused by a variety of lesions, and in some instances no cause is apparent. Septicemia with focal areas of necrosis, ulceration, and perforation of the gastric wall, acute gastric ulcers, Rokitansky-Cushing ulcers, and trauma secondary to intubation may all be responsible. Traumatic perforation is probably infrequent, however; and many of the lesions that have been attributed to this are probably secondary to other factors. When traumatic perforations occur, they are usually located on the greater curvature of the stomach opposite the cardioesophageal orifice, where the initial trauma is followed by secondary infection and perforation.[39] Rarely, perforation is associated with a more distally located obstructive lesion; e.g., pyloric or duodenal atresia.[40] In a number of instances, spontaneous perforation of the stomach of a newborn infant has been attributed to congenital absence of the gastric musculature at the site of perforation.[41-45] There is, however, some controversy regarding the validity of this pathogenetic mechanism.[39] These perforations usually occur within the first week of life and are somewhat more frequent in premature infants. Clinically, they are characterized by the sudden appearance of abdominal distention, dyspnea, cyanosis, and often vomiting. Roentgen examination of the abdomen reveals evidence of pneumoperitoneum. The defects vary from 1.5 to 6.0 cm in length and are located principally along the greater curvature of the stomach near the cardia.

Histologic sections reveal absence of muscularis at the edges of the perforation; here the mucosa and muscularis mucosae are intact and the submucosa and serosa appear to be continuous with each other. Little or no inflammatory reaction is present at the edge of the defect.

INTESTINES

Embryology

The proximal duodenum down to the region of the bile duct develops from the foregut and receives blood from the celiac artery. The other parts of the small intestine and the right half of the colon develop from the midgut and receive blood from the superior mesenteric artery. The distal colon is derived from the hindgut and receives blood from the inferior mesenteric artery. The terminal part of the hindgut expands to form the cloaca, from which the rectum and upper portion of the anal canal down to the pectinate line are derived. The lumen of the intestines becomes obliterated during the early embryonic period but recanalizes later by forming vacuoles in the epithelial plug.

The intestine in embryos of 4 weeks is a simple tube beginning at the stomach and ending in the cloaca. In its midportion the tube bends slightly ventrad and is continuous with the attenuated yolk sac. The segments of the intestine above and below the attachment of the yolk sac are referred to as the cranial and caudal limbs of the intestinal loop. The cranial portion will give rise to that part of the duodenum distal to the entrance of the bile duct, to the entire jejunum, and to most of the ileum; whereas the caudal limb will form the distal ileum and all of the colon and rectum. The intestinal tract of the early embryo is suspended in the sagittal plane on a dorsal mesentery.

In the fifth week the intestine elongates more rapidly than the trunk and thus forms a prominent loop, and the yolk sac detaches from the apex of the loop. The subsequent gross changes involve primarily the midgut or that part of the intestine supplied by the superior mesenteric artery; the distal part of the duodenum, the entire small bowel, the cecum, the ascending colon, and the transverse colon near the midline are derived from the midgut.

During the sixth week the elongating intestine, suspended on its dorsal mesentery in the sagittal plane, rotates through an arc of 90 degrees in a counterclockwise direction as one views the embryo from the ventral aspect. The superior mesenteric artery, which passes to the apex of the midgut loop, serves as the axis of this rotation. The cranial limb is then brought to the right and the caudal limb to the left to reach the horizontal plane. At about this same time the elongating intestinal loop, no longer able to be contained within the more slowly growing abdomen, escapes into the extraembryonic coelom in the primitive umbilical cord. The cranial limb continues to elongate and to form multiple coils within the extraembryonic coelom; but the caudal limb, except for development of the cecal diverticulum, changes relatively little during this period.

The return of the bowel to the abdomen is associated with an additional counterclockwise rotation of the midgut through 180 degrees about the axis of the superior mesenteric artery. The entire process of rotation, however, is a continuous one; and at least some of this additional rotation may occur while the bowel is still within the umbilical stalk.[46] At about 10 weeks the abdominal cavity has increased sufficiently in size to accommodate the intestinal loops, which rapidly return to its confines. The proximal coils of the cranial limb are the first to re-enter the abdomen, passing under the root of the mesentery and the superior mesenteric artery to reach the left side of the abdomen. The cecum and adjacent colon are the last to re-enter the abdominal cavity; and as the colon straightens out, it completes its counterclockwise rotation of 180 degrees from the horizontal position it assumed after the initial 90-degree rotation. Thus, with the entire counterclockwise rotation of 270 degrees the duodenum has passed from its initial position in the sagittal plane ventral to the superior mesenteric artery to a position to the right of, then behind, and finally to the left of the origin of this artery. Similarly, the cecum has passed from its initial position in the sagittal plane dorsal to the superior mesenteric artery to a horizontal position to the left of, then anterior to, and finally to the right of this artery.

The final or third stage of "rotation," during midfetal life, includes elongation of the ascending colon with resultant descent of the cecum into the right lower quadrant, as well as fusion of the mesentery of parts of the intestine with the posterior parietal peritoneum, with resultant fixation of these parts. Fusion of the mesentery of the major part of the duodenum with the peritoneum of the dorsal body wall results in the retroperitoneal position of most of this viscus. Finally, the ascending colon and descending colon similarly assume a retroperitoneal position, fixed in their definitive positions. The original mesentery of the midgut, which was attached by only a narrow pedicle at the origin of the superior mesenteric artery, is now attached by a broad base passing obliquely downward from the duodenojejunal junction to the region of the cecum in the right lower quadrant.

Aganglionic Megacolon (Hirschsprung's Disease)

Further details about Hirschsprung's disease and intestinal neuronal dysplasia can be found in Chapter 11.

Definition and Location. Congenital aganglionic megacolon (Hirschsprung's disease) is the result of congenital absence of the ganglion cells of a segment of bowel, usually the rectum or rectosigmoid. The aganglionic segment, in which ganglion cells of both Auerbach's (myenteric) and Meissner's (submucosal) plexuses are absent, varies considerably in length. It may consist of only the distal 4 to 5 cm of rectum or may involve the entire rectum, sigmoid, and descending colon. In less than 10% of cases the aganglionic segment extends proximal to the splenic flexure, sometimes involving all of the colon and a variable length of ileum or even the entire bowel from the duodenojejunal junction through the rectum. Documented instances of "skip areas" are extremely rare; in those few documented instances the aganglionic segments are separated from one another by segments containing normal or diminished ganglion cells.[47] In general, however, in Hirschsprung's disease the bowel is continuously devoid of ganglion cells from its proximal aganglionic level through the distal rectum.

Coordinated peristaltic movements of the bowel are dependent upon intact parasympathetic innervation. Within an aganglionic segment normal peristaltic movements are absent, although mass muscular contractions may occur. The result is functional obstruction within the aganglionic portion. The bowel above the obstructed (aganglionic) segment becomes dilated and hypertrophied, sometimes to a tremendous extent, as it may be above any obstructive lesion.

Clinical Features. Aganglionic megacolon of the usual type is more common in males, whereas females predominate in those with long-segment aganglionosis. The manifestations are often apparent during the first few days of life and consist of failure to pass meconium, vomiting, and abdominal distention. A family history of the disease is sometimes elicited. Roentgenograms of the abdomen reveal fluid levels indicative of intestinal obstruction. Relief of symptoms sometimes occurs after a rectal examination or an enema, after which normal stools may be passed for a short time. In other instances, however, relief of constipation is followed by severe diarrhea, leading to dehydration and even death. Diarrhea is an extremely important complication of aganglionic megacolon in early infancy and may be the initial manifestation. It may occur in infants with relatively long aganglionic segments as well as in those in whom only a short segment is devoid of ganglion cells.

In older children with the disease, now encountered only infrequently because of earlier diagnosis and treatment, there are increasingly severe constipation and abdominal distention. Bowel movements may occur at only weekly or longer intervals, and enemas may be necessary. The abdominal wall becomes tense and thin, and the protuberant abdomen is in striking contrast to the wasted extremities. Rectal examination usually reveals absence of fecal content despite the presence of abundant feces in the more proximal colon. Intermittent attacks of intestinal obstruction often occur as the result of fecal impaction. Intestinal obstruction may lead to death because of volvulus of the sigmoid, water intoxication following the administration of enemas,[48] or inanition and secondary infection. In infants, in whom the disease is now usually encountered, perforation and peritonitis or severe dehydration, following even a brief period of fever, vomiting, and diarrhea may be responsible for death.

Roentgenograms, after the injection of a small amount of barium into the distal rectum, reveal a relatively small, nondilated, distal aganglionic segment, in striking contrast to a more proximal dilated portion of normal colon. This disparity in the size of the aganglionic and ganglionic segments, although sometimes evident even during the neonatal period, is apt to be especially apparent after several months or earlier.

Diagnosis. The diagnosis of aganglionic megacolon usually cannot be established by gross examination in infants who die as neonates. The normal colon of a fetus or infant who has not passed meconium is often 2 to 3 cm in diameter, and the redundant sigmoid may be even larger and lead to the erroneous diagnosis of megacolon. The diagnosis should be suspected, however, in any infant with intestinal obstruction in whom no cause is apparent at laparotomy or upon gross postmortem examination. It should also be suspected whenever periotonitis or intestinal perforation is encountered in the absence of an apparent obstruction, or when the obstruction appears to be the result of multiple hard pellets of meconium in the ileum or colon. Finally, aganglionic megacolon should be suspected in any young infant who dies of an acute enterocolitis associated with multiple areas of ulceration in the colon or the small intestine, or both. Obviously, in not all such cases will the diagnosis be established; but it can be excluded only by histologic examination of selected segments of the bowel, including the distal rectum.

Histologic sections of the distal rectum should always be examined whenever a diagnosis of aganglionic megacolon is considered, because almost without exception the aganglionic segment will include this part of the bowel. If ganglion cells are present in the distal few centimeters of the rectum, the diagnosis of aganglionic megacolon is virtually excluded. If they are not demonstrable here, as they normally are, the diagnosis is established, and an attempt then should be made to determine the extent of the aganglionic segment. This can be done with considerable accuracy if labeled sections from a number of different sites in the bowel are

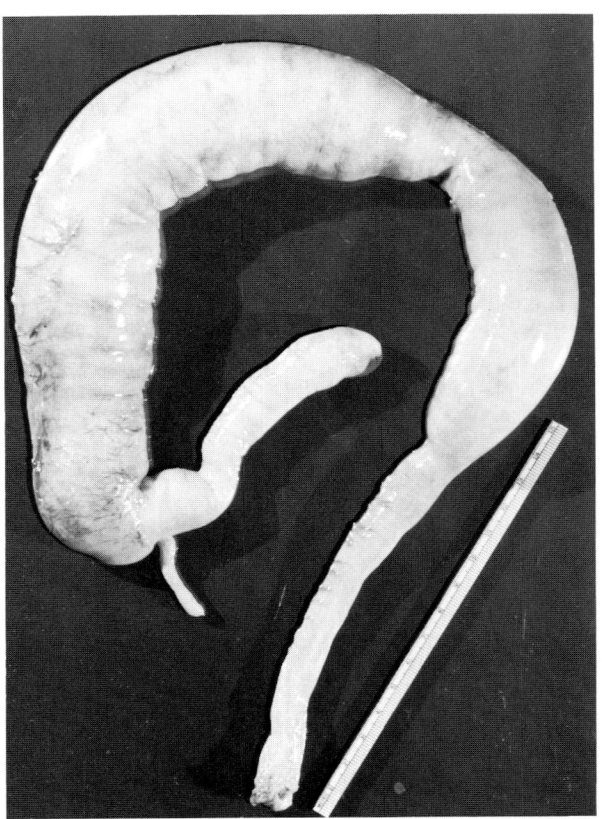

FIGURE 8–2. Aganglionic megacolon from a male infant 1 month old. The narrower aganglionic segment extended almost to the splenic flexure. Multiple mucosal ulcers were present both proximal to and within the aganglionic segment.

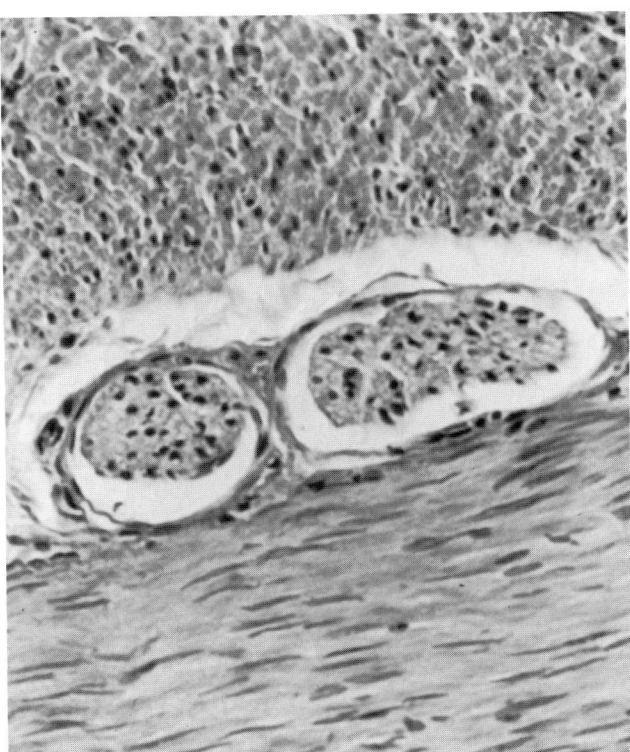

FIGURE 8–3. Nerve fibers but no ganglion cells are present in the muscularis of the aganglionic segment of the same infant as in Figure 8–2. ($\times$ 300)

saved at the time of the postmortem examination, e.g., not only the distal rectum, but also sections 5, 10, and 15 cm above this, the splenic flexure, the hepatic flexure, the ileocecum, and specified levels of the ileum and jejunum.

In the older infant or child, in whom both the clinical and gross morphologic findings are apt to be more obvious, the diagnosis is usually apparent. The aganglionic segment is usually confined to the rectum or rectosigmoid, both of which are of approximately normal size. Above the aganglionic segment, however, the colon enlarges rapidly, here being tremendously dilated, hypertrophied, and filled with fecal material (Figure 8–2). The distention becomes progressively less severe more proximally in the colon and may even be virtually confined to the sigmoid. In others, however, the distention may extend to the splenic flexure or may even involve the entire colon. Multiple stercoral ulcers may be present. The changes in the bowel above the aganglionic segment are thus nonspecific and are those that may be seen with any type of chronic constipation. An unequivocal diagnosis of Hirschsprung's disease can only be made by histologic demonstration of an absence of ganglion cells in the distal, more normal-appearing rectum or rectosigmoid.

Pathology. Auerbach's plexus is normally readily demonstrable from the junction of the middle and upper thirds of the esophagus to a point 2 to 3 cm above the anal mucocutaneous border. It consists of a group of nerve cells and fibers located between the inner and outer layers of the muscularis. Several groups of such plexuses are normally present in any properly oriented section of the intestine more than 1.0 to 1.5 cm in length. In contrast, the submucosal plexuses of Meissner tend to be smaller and more scattered throughout the gastrointestinal tract, and their ganglion cells tend to appear somewhat less mature. Nevertheless, their absence in a series of submucosal biopsies is also diagnostic. In aganglionic megacolon the nerve cells of both Auerbach's and Meissner's plexuses are absent in the aganglionic segment.

In association with the complete absence of ganglion cells, there is an increase in the number and size of the nerve fibers, not only in the muscularis propria but also in the submucosa of the aganglionic segment of bowel (Figure 8–3). Frozen sections stained with acetylcholinesterase enhance their visibility. In many institutions, submucosal biopsies are routinely utilized for definitive diagnosis prior to corrective surgery; both paraffin and frozen sections are then prepared, the former being stained with hematoxylin and eosin and the latter with acetylcholinesterase for confirmation of negative results in the former.

The prominence of nerve fibers in the absence of ganglionic cells is perhaps comparable to an amputation neuroma, the parasympathetic fibers entering the bowel and proliferating aimlessly in the absence of nerve cells with which to make synaptic junctions. Care must be taken, therefore, not to confuse nerve fibers with nerve *cells* in the muscularis and submucosa; it is the latter that are absent in the aganglionic segment.

The affected segment is not strictly confined to the distal nondilated rectum or rectosigmoid, but usually extends a short distance into the dilated and hypertrophied proximal segment of colon. Usually this proximal extension involves only the distal few centimeters of the dilated colon, but infrequently it extends over a longer distance. Proximal to the completely aganglionic segment, a transitional zone 2 to 3 cm in length may reveal an obvious paucity, but not absence of neurons. The zone is not simply the result of separation of plexuses by dilatation of the bowel, but rather an actual decrease in their number. The ganglion cells in this transitional zone are histologically normal. The diagnosis of aganglionic megacolon is dependent upon the demonstration of absence of ganglion cells, not simply a diminution in their number.

The dilated colon is filled with large amounts of inspissated fecal material and its wall is thickened as the result of muscular hypertrophy, especially of the inner circular layer. Scattered ulcers may be present in the mucosa and may also involve the aganglionic segment. Histologically, except for hypertrophy of the muscularis, the dilated colon reveals no distinct changes; its neurenteric plexuses are normal. In some instances, especially in older children, there are scattered macrophages filled with brown pigment in the mucosa of the dilated bowel (melanosis coli).

In infants an associated acute enterocolitis is the most important complication of aganglionic megacolon, sometimes being the initial manifestation; it may even develop after a palliative colostomy. This usually involves only the colon but may be more extensive. Multiple superficial areas of necrosis and ulceration are present; and large patches of mucosa are covered with a yellowish-green membrane composed of necrotic debris, fibrin, and neutrophils. Scattered crypts of Lieberkühn are dilated and filled with neutrophils, and a mild exudate of similar cells may involve the submucosa. The study of any instance of acute colitis or entercolitis at necropsy in a young infant should include not only a description of the alterations in the bowel but also specific note of the presence or absence of ganglion cells in the distal rectum.

Biopsy Interpretation. Today, diagnostic biopsies are often performed by the suction technique. The specimen received is then a tiny disk 2 to 3 mm in diameter and slightly more than 1 mm in thickness. It consists of a rounded cap of mucosa beneath which is a slightly contracted submucosa. This hollowed-out disk is bisected, the cut passing through both ends, and each half is embedded on its largest straight cut edge so that each microscopic section will include mucosa, muscularis mucosae, and submucosa. In any one section, one or two minute, horseshoe-shaped clusters of ganglion cells, each of which is usually closely associated with a prominent capillary, are apparent at the junction of the muscularis mucosae and the submucosa if ganglion cells are present.

These biopsies are often performed on infants, often premature ones, during the neonatal period. At that time the ganglion cells, particularly in Meissner's plexus, are immature and are not easy to identify— without practice. Three features are helpful: (1) most of these cells are located *at* the very junction of the muscularis mucosae and the submucosa; (2) the cells do not appear singly, but in horseshoe-shaped groups; and (3) the individual ganglion cells, although small, do have (*a*) more abundant and slightly bluer staining cytoplasm than other cells in the area and (*b*) prominent nucleoli. Recognition is made a little easier by the use of adjunct acetylcholinesterase stains on frozen sections of these submucosal biopsies; these frozen sections may be prepared at the same time as the paraffin sections. Because the acetylcholinesterase stain can be performed in about 2 hours, a few experienced pathologists will make a rapid diagnosis on the basis of frozen section alone.

In acetylcholinesterase preparations the nerve fibers, which so often become abnormally prominent in aganglionosis, are stained brown; this color is easier to perceive when one lowers the condenser of the microscope. This prominence in size and number of fibers is clearly evident in individual small fibers in the tunica propria. Some pediatric pathologists with abundant experience are comfortable making the diagnosis of aganglionosis on nothing more than the basis of frozen sections so stained. For our part, we feel more secure having both hematoxylin and eosin (H&E) and acetylcholinesterase stains before reaching a decision. We examine between 20 and 40 individual paraffin sections—in ribbons—before establishing a diagnosis of aganglionic megacolon.

Compared with diagnosis in suction biopsies, the diagnosis is usually readily apparent in frozen sections through the muscularis propria at the time of surgery and thus demonstrates the proper level for colostomy or a corrective procedure. Ganglion cells in Auerbach's plexus are larger and have more cytoplasm and larger nucleoli than their counterparts in Meissner's plexus. The specimen is somewhat larger, perhaps as much as 1 to 1.5 cm in length. It must include both the inner and outer layers of the muscularis propria. Sections are cut at right angles to the C-shaped, concave serosa so that the zone between the two muscle layers is clearly visible in frozen and paraffin sections. In properly oriented sections of normally ganglionic colon, several nests of ganglion cells should be visible in any one section through this zone, evidence that this is from above the aganglionic segment and is a site suitable for either colostomy or for the proximal line of resection of the aganglionic segment. Even a few well-defined groups of ganglion cells indicate that the bowel here will have normal peristaltic activity; the determination of a diminished number, rather than complete absence, of ganglion cells is often difficult or impossible. In a few instances, however, even in well-oriented sections only one or two ganglion cells are present; in such instances the biopsy has probably been taken from the transitional zone between the aganglionic and ganglionic segments. Although this transitional zone will probably serve as an adequate site for a colostomy or a proximal line of resection, these are preferably carried out above that level. A second biopsy a few centimeters higher will probably reveal normal numbers of cells. If ganglion cells are absent, the biopsy should be repeated at a higher level until definite nests of ganglion cells are found.

In the interpretation of rectal biopsies of either type, i.e., the submucosal or muscular, it should be recognized that ganglion cells are normally absent for 2 to 3 cm above the mucocutaneous junction at the anus; any biopsy that includes that junction is inadequate and must be repeated at least 3 cm above the mucocutaneous border. If submucosal biopsies are shallow and do not include a generous amount of submucosa deep to the muscularis mucosae, they, too, must be repeated to be of diagnostic value.

Intestinal Atresia and Stenosis

Types and Pathogenesis. The lumen of the duodenum is normally obliterated by proliferation of the lining epithelial cells during the embryonic period. Following this occlusion, vacuoles appear among the epithelial cells and ultimately coalesce to re-establish a lumen. This process passes progressively downward through the entire duodenum between the thirtieth and fiftieth day of gestation.[49] Similar changes have been seen elsewhere in the small bowel and even the colon.[50] Failure of vacuolization along the longitudinal axis of the bowel would result in atresia of this segment. Coalescence of vacuoles in a longitudinal direction, with failure of vacuolization of the more peripherally located epithelium, would result in stenosis rather than atresia. A similar effect might be produced by relatively slight inhibition of epithelial proliferation during the period of rapid elongation of the bowel. Between the fifth week and birth the intestine increases in length 1000 times.[21] During the period of rapid growth, failure of epithelial cells to proliferate in one segment of bowel would result in failure of this segment to keep pace with the growth of the adjoining bowel. Attenuation of the affected segment by continued elongation of the remainder of the bowel might lead to stenosis or atresia of the segment.

Intestinal atresia refers to complete interruption of the continuity of the intestinal lumen, whereas stenosis is narrowing or partial obliteration of the lumen (Figures 8–4 and 8–5). Congenital duodenal obstruction (atresia or stenosis) ranks third after imperforate anus and esophageal atresia as a cause of intrinsic obstruction of the alimentary tract.[49] In the duodenum, stenosis is slightly more common than atresia; more distally, atresia predominates. Approximately 15% to 20% of ileojejunal atresias are multiple.[51] Duodenal atresia, however, accompanied by ileojejunal atresia is rare. Atresia of the colon accounts for only 3% to 4% of intestinal atresias.

There are many differences between duodenal stenosis and atresia and obstructive lesions located more distally. Approximately 25% to 30% of infants with duodenal stenosis or atresia have trisomy 21[52]; and other malformations, e.g., malrotation, esophageal atresia, annular pancreas, and congenital heart disease,[53] occur much more frequently in these infants

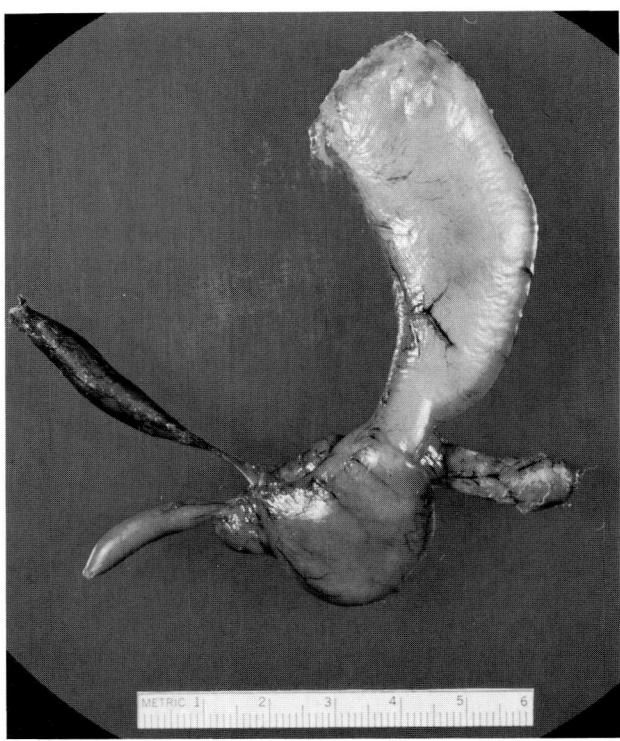

FIGURE 8–4. Annular pancreas and duodenal atresia from a male infant 10 days old with multiple congenital anomalies. An intrinsic atresia of the duodenum was present at the site of the annular pancreas. Note the dilated first portion of the duodenum.

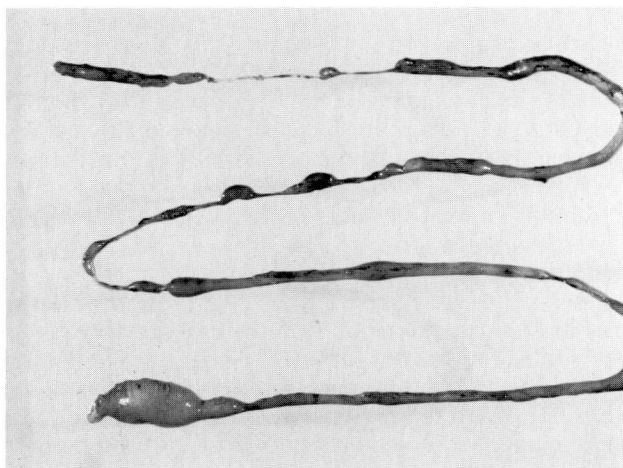

FIGURE 8–5. Multiple jejunal atresias from a female infant 2 days old. Multiple atretic areas are present along a segment of bowel 62 cm long. Note the beadlike appearance resulting from intact, patent bowel intervening among a number of the atretic segments.

than in those with ileojejunal atresia. Duodenal atresia and stenosis have been observed repeatedly in infants damaged by thalidomide.[54] Duodenal stenosis or atresia is usually a membranous or diaphragmatic obstruction; whereas such an obstruction, although it may be produced by a vascular accident,[55] is uncommon in atresias distal to the duodenum.

Thus, no single explanation suffices to explain the pathogenesis of all instances of intestinal atresia or stenosis. Probably most instances of duodenal stenosis or atresia and possibly a few of the diaphragmatic obstructions in the more distal bowel are the result of disturbances in vacuolization of the intestine or impaired epithelial proliferation during embryonic life. Most of the other intestinal atresias and probably also stenoses (excluding anorectal ones) are instead the result of a later fetal accident, with resultant hypoxia of a segment of bowel. The nature of such an accident often is not clear, especially with stenoses; but the presence of deposits of calcium, hemosiderin, meconium, and foreign body giant cells as well as scarring in the affected segment is indicative of previous injury to this area.

Intestinal atresia[56,57] and less often stenosis[58] may be a complication of meconium ileus, resulting from mucosal ulceration with a secondary inflammatory response or, in the case of atresia, from volvulus of a distended loop of bowel. Even in the absence of meconium ileus, severe stenosis has been seen, albeit infrequenty, at the site of a volvulus[59]; and Gross depicts severe stenosis of the distal ileum in a gangrenous segment of bowel that has prolapsed through a mesenteric defect.[60] An intrauterine intussusception similarly may cause atresia.[61] The mesenteric defect that may accompany atresia with blind ends has also been seen with stenosis.[62] An injury to the affected segment of bowel occurring later than the embryonic period (fourth to eighth week) is manifested by the presence of hemosiderin-laden macrophages, meconium, calcium, foreign body giant cells, and scarring in the affected atretic or stenotic segment as well as by the presence of meconium, squamous epithelial cells, and keratin in the bowel distal to an atresia.

The histologic appearance of a number of instances of congenital intestinal atresia or stenosis is comparable to that seen in acquired complete or partial intestinal obstruction in postnatal life following necrotizing enterocolitis, i.e., the presence of granulation tissue, hemosiderin-laden macrophages, and fibrous scars occupying the submucosa and varying portions of the muscularis propria.

Intestinal Atresia. The clinical manifestations of intestinal atresia are obviously dependent upon the site of the obstruction. A history of polyhydramnios is commonly present with duodenal or jejunal atresia, as it is with esophageal atresia. Symptoms of duodenal obstruction may be manifest within a few hours of birth, whereas those of colonic atresia may not be apparent for 24 or 36 hours. Duodenal atresia is responsible for epigastric distention, which may, however, be relieved by persistent vomiting. The vomitus frequently contains bile, because the obstruction is usually below the ampulla of Vater. Atresias of the lower ileum or colon are responsible for more generalized distention; and the vomiting, which appears somewhat later, eventually may become fecal in character. Enormous abdominal distention may occur after rupture of the bowel and escape of air and fluid into the peritoneal cavity. There may be absence of stools, but in some instances what appears to be normal meconium may be passed.

Intestinal atresia may occur in the form of one or more diaphragms or septa that completely occlude the lumen. There may be no visible disturbance of the external contour of the bowel other than severe dilation and hypertrophy proximal to the obstruction and small, collapsed bowel distal to it, the latter unused bowel often being only several millimeters in diameter. Histologically the septum is covered on both surfaces by mucosa with underlying submucosa, Brunner's glands often being absent or misplaced in duodenal septa.[63] Muscularis mucosae may be present beneath the mucosa[64]; and the entire wall, including inner and outer muscularis may be included in the septum[40]. In such instances, in which there is no evidence of an inflammatory reaction, e.g., foreign body giant cells, meconium, or granulation tissue in the septum, this is presumably the result of an early defect in vacuolization or epithelial proliferation. In one unusual case, possibly familial, in which multiple septa were present from the duodenum to the descending colon, the inner and outer muscular layers were intact, and normal neural plexuses were present. The surface of both sides of the septa was lined by epithelium continuous with that of the adjoining bowel. The septa in the colon contained multiple cysts lined by columnar epithelium and goblet cells surrounded by loose mesenchymal tissue and fragmented muscularis mucosae.[65]

In the more frequent type of intestinal atresia secondary to a later intrauterine accident, the muscularis propria at the periphery of the atretic segment may be continuous with that of the adjacent bowel. Within the zone of atresia, however, the muscularis mucosae may be interrupted to a variable extent by sheets of connective tissue. There is no epithelium, and the pre-existing lumen is replaced by a central core of granulation tissue containing deposits of meconium, calcium, and foreign body giant cells (Figure 8–6).

In still other intestinal atresias secondary to an intrauterine accident, the segments of bowel above and below the atretic segment are joined to each other by a thin fibrous or fibromuscular cord of variable length with a histologic appearance similar to that just described, with little or no residual muscularis propria. Finally, the closed end of the upper dilated segment may be completely separated from that of the distal collapsed bowel, no cord of tissue connecting the two. In about 40% of this last type of midgut atresia there is also a defect in the mesentery corresponding to the atretic area.[66]

The length of the atretic bowel varies widely; rarely, the entire colon is absent and represented only by a cord of tissue consisting predominantly of connective tissue following the course usually occupied by the large bowel.[67] The bowel above the atresia is severely

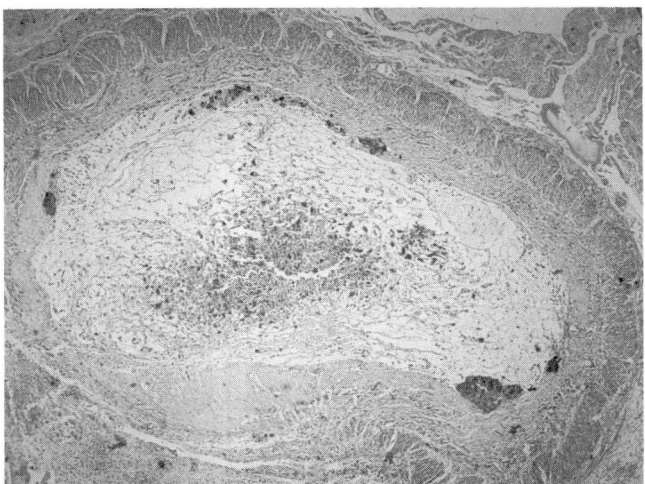

FIGURE 8-6. Atresia of ileum from a male 2 days old. The lumen is replaced by loose connective tissue containing deposits of calcium. There is no residual muscularis mucosae, and much of the inner muscular layer is replaced by fibrous tissue. (× 20)

dilated, whereas distally it is small and collapsed. With multiple atresias the distended bowel may be followed by several small beadlike cysts joined to one another by minute threads of tissue (see Figure 8-5). Perforation of the distended bowel may occur, with resultant generalized peritonitis.

Intestinal Stenosis. This is less common than atresia. The duodenum is the most common site, followed by the ileum and jejunum. Multiple intestinal stenoses are rare, as is colonic stenosis. Clinical manifestations of intestinal stenosis are again dependent upon the site as well as the extent of the obstruction. In about half, the signs of intestinal obstruction are apparent during the first week or two of life and may be indistinguishable from those of atresia. In a small number, however, symptoms may be so mild that the diagnosis is not suspected for months or even years, there being only occasional attacks of vomiting or intermittent abdominal pain.

The bowel proximal to the stenosis is dilated, sometimes to a striking degree if only a minute orifice is present; and its wall reveals varying degrees of hypertrophy. The diaphragmatic type, most frequently seen in the duodenum, is similar to that encountered with diaphragmatic atresias but with a residual orifice of varying size. Segmental stenoses of later intrauterine origin vary from approximately 0.5 cm to relatively long segments that may be mistaken for atresia. Histologically the stenotic segment is similar to that seen with intestinal atresia but, again, with a residual lumen of variable size. The extent of damage to the bowel in stenosis tends to be somewhat less severe than it is in atresia; and parts of the residual lumen may be covered by a low cuboidal or flattened epithelium, beneath which a few glands may be present. Varying amounts of granulation tissue or loose connective tissue expand the submucosa and may extend into the muscularis mucosae and even the muscularis propria, especially the inner circular layer.[68] Again, scattered hemosiderin-laden macrophages, deposits of calcium, meconium, chronic inflammatory cells, and foreign body giant cells may be present in the wall.

Annular Pancreas. In this condition the pancreas either partially or completely encircles the duodenum. This may be entirely asymptomatic, but occasionally it is associated with an underlying intrinsic duodenal stenosis or atresia (see Figure 8-4). With complete interruption of the continuity of the duodenum, the space intervening between the blind ends may be filled with pancreatic tissue. Associated conditions, in addition to duodenal stenosis or atresia, include malrotation, esophageal atresia, and trisomy 21. This malformation probably occurs at about the sixth week of fetal life as the result of a bilobed ventral pancreatic bud, the left bud of which persists and grows around the left side of the duodenum to join the other ventral and the dorsal pancreatic anlage.[69,70]

The annular pancreas usually encircles the second part of the duodenum but occasionally is at about the first or third portion. The ring of pancreatic tissue is usually complete; but if incomplete, the gap is usually anterior. Usually a large pancreatic duct begins anteriorly, passes to the right, and then passes laterally and posteriorly to join either the common bile duct or the main pancreatic duct. Infrequently an annular pancreas may so extensively infiltrate the muscularis of the duodenum as to cause duodenal stenosis. Far more frequently, however, any duodenal stenosis or atresia accompanying an annular pancreas is the result of an intrinsic duodenal obstruction, not of constriction by the encircling pancreatic tissue.

Anomalies of Intestinal Rotation and Volvulus (Table 8-2)

Anomalies of rotation and fixation of the midgut, often collectively referred to as *malrotation*, may be associated with no clinical manifestations or with serious or lethal intestinal obstruction.

Nonrotation. In this condition the midgut, although returning to the abdominal cavity, fails to rotate beyond the horizontal position it occupied after the initial 90-degree counterclockwise rotation (see the section on the embryology of the intestines). The duodenum does not cross the midline, but lies entirely to the right of the superior mesenteric artery. The small intestine is on the right side of the abdomen, and the entire colon on

Table 8-2 ANOMALIES OF INTESTINAL ROTATION

Nonrotation
Mixed rotation (most common)
Reversed rotation (rare)
Incomplete formation of mesocolon or mesentery

the left, the terminal ileum entering the cecum from the right side. Failure of attachment of the mesentery of the midgut to the posterior parietes along a broad base is its most important sequel. The root of the mesentery is a narrow structure confined to the region of the superior mesenteric vessels, and the midgut hangs as a pendulum from this narrow isthmus. Such a position predisposes to the development of volvulus of the midgut. Although this anomaly, with accompanying volvulus, has been recognized in the neonatal period, affected persons may be asymptomatic throughout life; and if clinical manifestations do appear, they usually do so in adult life.

Mixed Rotation. Mixed rotation of the midgut is the most common type of malrotation seen clinically. It resuts from failure of the cranial limb of the midgut to rotate in a counterclockwise direction beyond the initial 90 degrees. The caudal limb, however, continues its rotation an additional 90 degrees, which makes its total rotation 180 degrees. As a result, the distal duodenum and all of the small bowel lie on the right side of the abdomen; the colon lies anterior to the superior mesenteric vessels, as it normally does; and the cecum assumes a subpyloric position, with the ileum entering it from below. The mesentery of the small bowel is continuous with that of the cecum and ascending colon. During the process of fixation, fibrous bands, probably an abortive mesocolon, extend from the cecum and proximal colon to the right posterior parietes, crossing the duodenum anteriorly. These bands may lead to duodenal obstruction; or the cecum, held fast over the duodenum by such bands, may cause intestinal obstruction. In addition, the narrow base of the mesentery, confined to the region of the superior mesenteric vessels, creates a situation conducive to volvulus of the midgut.

Clinical manifestations of duodenal obstruction are usually seen in very early life. Vomiting, often bile-stained, usually starts in the first days of life and is soon followed by abdominal distention. If loops of intestine wrap themselves around the narrow base of the mesentery, the bowel becomes mechanically obstructed at the duodenojejunal junction and at the midtransverse colon. Moreover, if this persists, the torsion of the mesentery partially occludes the superior mesenteric vessels, with resultant infarction of the bowel. The volvulus can be recognized by the fact that the cecum and right half of the colon are hidden from view by the loops of small intestine, which may be discolored from impairment of their blood supply. If all of the midgut is now brought onto the abdominal wall, care being taken not to rotate it, the volvulus can be reduced by rotating the midgut and its mesentery through 180 degrees or even through three or four complete turns. Because the volvulus usually occurs in a clockwise direction, its relief will usually be accomplished by rotation in the counterclockwise direction. After its reduction, the narrow root of the mesentery, confined to the region of the superior mesenteric vessels, can be appreciated. If fibrous bands from the cecum to the right posterior parietes cross the duodenum or hold the cecum against this structure, they can now be severed. The duodenum can now be recognized passing from the pylorus to the jejunum along the right side of the superior mesenteric vessels. The viability of those loops of bowel, perhaps including the entire midgut, can be ascertained.

Duodenal obstruction with mixed rotation may result not only from volvulus but also from the aforementioned fibrous bands or from compression of the duodenum by the cecum, fixed in this position by such bands. Either of these may occur independently; but almost half of the infants presenting with duodenal obstruction and malrotation have a volvulus of the midgut.[71] Associated malformations are present in a significant number of infants with volvulus and include such lesions as intrinsic stenosis or atresia of the bowel, especially the duodenum; diaphragmatic hernia; esophageal atresia; and omphalocele. Approximately one third of the infants with omphalocele have mixed rotation of the midgut.[72]

Volvulus of the midgut is usually a complication of malrotation. It may, however, occur after complete, normal rotation has taken place but fusion of the mesentery with the posterior parietes is incomplete.[73] The ascending colon lies in its normal position, and the duodenum passes posterior to the superior mesenteric vessels normally. The mesenteric root, however, remains a narrow pedicle, predisposing to volvulus. Volvulus of one or more loops of small bowel, unassociated with malrotation, may occur as a loop of bowel lies in a hernial sac, with loops of bowel filled with thick meconium in meconium ileus, or with a loop of bowel caught by a peritoneal adhesion or by a persistent omphalomesenteric duct remnant.

Reversed Rotation. This is a rare disorder that results from a clockwise, rather than the usual counterclockwise, rotation of the midgut during the second stage of rotation. With 180-degree rotation from the horizontal plane in which the respective loops were situated after the initial 90-degree counterclockwise rotation, the result is a total of 90-degree clockwise rotation for each of the loops. The distal duodenum now lies anterior to the superior mesenteric vessels, and the cecum and ascending colon lie on the right. The mesentery of the midgut crosses obliquely in front of the transverse colon and is attached to the posterior peritoneum on the right, leaving a retroarterial tunnel through which passes the transverse colon.[74] The interposition of the dorsally located colon may so impair the dorsal attachment of the mesentery as to lead to volvulus of the ileocecum. In other instances, however, the obstruction may be at the retroarterial (retromesenteric) tunnel, with intermittent signs of compression of the transverse colon by the overlying mesentery and superior mesenteric vessels. Although intestinal obstruction from reverse rotation may occur in the newborn period, it usually does not appear until adult life.

Mobile Cecum. This is a minor anomaly found in approximately 10% of the population. The cecum is normally located but freely moveable, and the ascending mesocolon is not fused with the parietal peritoneum posteriorly. Volvulus of the cecum is a rare sequel of a mobile cecum. Accompanying such abnormal fixation, there may also be failure of fixation of the mesentery of the ileum, with subsequent volvulus of the ileum.

Volvulus of the Sigmoid. This condition may be the result of a sigmoid mesocolon incompletely adherent to the posterior parietes. More frequently, however, it is secondary to some other condition responsible for a large, redundant loop of sigmoid, e.g., unrecognized aganglionic megacolon or chronic constipation in the elderly.

Hernias (Table 8-3)

Mesenteric Hernias. Inclusion of one or more loops of bowel in a defect of the dorsal mesentery, which is to form the descending mesocolon, is responsible for a *left paraduodenal* or *mesentericoparietal hernia*. This is about three times more common than a similar hernia on the right. The orifice of the sac is located posteriorly, just below the ligament of Treitz, and faces toward the right. The inferior mesenteric artery and vein are in the free border of the sac at its orifice. The sac is formed by a leaf of the descending mesocolon and posterior parietal peritoneum. A *right paraduodenal* or *mesentericoparietal hernia* has its orifice in a comparable location, but this now faces toward the left and slightly downward. The superior mesenteric vessels course near the mouth of the sac, which consists of a leaf of the ascending mesocolon and the posterior parietal peritoneum.

Still other hernias through a defect in the transverse mesocolon, *transmesocolic* or *omentomesenteric parietal hernias*[74] are again located in close proximity to the duodenum. The sac, however, is now located above the transverse colon, behind, below, and to the right of the stomach. The middle colic artery lies on the right of the ostium of the sac and posteroinferior to the sac itself.

These mesentericoparietal hernias are congenital defects that occur during the return of the midgut from the umbilical stalk. At that time loops of intestine may rotate into a defect in the mesenteric attachment of the caudal limb of the midgut loop, producing the sac of a left or right mesentericoparietal, or omentomesenteric parietal hernia. Although the defect through which these hernias occur is congenital in nature, symptomatic herniatious usually do not appear until adult life.

Mesenteric defects unrelated to intestinal atresia or stenosis or to anomalies of rotation of the bowel are rare. They may occur at any site in the mesentery but are especially apt to involve the region of the terminal ileum. Such *transmesenteric hernias* are the internal hernias most commonly seen in the pediatric age group.[62]

Diaphragmatic Hernias. The ventral portion of the diaphragm is the first part to appear. It is derived from the septum transversum, a broad partition extending dorsally from the ventral body wall and interposed between the thoracic and abdominal cavities. The cranial part of this septum forms the floor of the pericardial cavity, whereas the caudal part is penetrated by the hepatic bud. The septum is an incomplete one, however, since paired pleural canals pass posterior to it and form communications between the abdominal and thoracic cavities. The pleural cavities become separated from the pericardial cavity about the sixth week of intrauterine life by fusion of the pleuropericardial membranes on each side with the primitive mediastinum. The pleuroperitoneal canals, however, persist until the end of the seventh week, being obliterated gradually by growth of the pleuroperitoneal folds, continuous with the dorsolateral portion of the septum transversum. These folds give rise to the paired dorsolateral parts of the diaphragm. A small dorsomedian part of the diaphragm is derived from the primitive mesentery. Finally, a late ingrowth of muscle from the body wall contributes to the dorsolateral margins of the diaphragm.

Congenital diaphragmatic hernias may be located posterolaterally in the foramina of Bochdalek (the primitive pleuroperitoneal canal), in the region of the esophageal hiatus, or in the retrosternal region. Less frequently, an anterior defect may be present in the midline with a communication between the peritoneal and pericardial sacs (peritoneopericardial hernia).

The majority of congenital diaphragmatic hernias are *pleuroperitoneal hernias* that occur through a persistent pleuroperitoneal canal (foramen of Bochdalek) and are therefore posterolateral in position. They are usually unilateral and involve the left leaf of the diaphragm three or four times as frequently as the right. No hernial sac is present, the defect involving not only the musculature of the diaphragm but also the associated parietal pleura and peritoneum. When a sac is present, composed of the fused pleura and peritoneum, the lesion is referred to as an *eventration of the diaphragm*; in only about 10% of posterolateral diaphragmatic defects is such a sac present.

Clinical manifestations of a congenital posterolateral diaphragmatic hernia are dependent upon the extent of herniation of abdominal contents into the pleural cavity and the associated pulmonary hypoplasia; in a few

Table 8-3 CONGENITAL HERNIAS AFFECTING THE ALIMENTARY TRACT

Mesenteric and mesocolic hernias
   Paraduodenal (mesentericoparietal) hernia
   Transmesocolic hernia
   Transmesenteric hernia

Diaphragmatic hernias
   Pleuroperitoneal hernia
     Eventration of diaphragm
   Hiatal hernias
     Paraesophageal hernia
     Sliding hiatal hernia
   Retrosternal hernia
   Pericardiodiaphragmatic hernia
Epigastric hernia
Inguinal hernia
   Indirect
   Direct
Femoral hernia
Umbilical hernia

instances, signs of intestinal obstruction may also be apparent. Cyanosis and dyspnea are usually present at or shortly after birth and may be associated with vomiting. The respiratory distress is accentuated by the accumulation of air within the bowel. Death may occur suddenly and unexpectedly, or the newborn infant may make only a few gasping respiratory efforts and die before establishing a respiratory pattern. If untreated, the majority of infants with congenital posterolateral diaphragmatic hernias are dead by the end of the first month of life. A few, however, have no symptoms until several months or even years of age, when digestive disturbances or signs of intestinal obstruction may be the first manifestations. Physical examination reveals decreased respiratory movements and diminished or absent breath sounds on the affected side. The heart is displaced to the opposite side, and peristaltic sounds may be audible in the affected hemithorax. The abdomen is characteristically scaphoid.

The extent of herniation of abdominal contents varies with the size of the defect. Defects on the right are apt to be associated with somewhat less extensive displacement of the viscera than those on the left, the liver forming a partial barrier to the ascent of bowel into the right pleural cavity. A narrow, rudimentary mesenteric attachment, sometimes with malrotation of the bowel, is a rather commonly associated malformation and facilitates displacement of the bowel into the pleural space. The stomach, spleen, pancreas, left lobe of the liver, cecum, and ascending and transverse colon may all be herniated into the left pleural cavity (Figure 8-7). The heart is displaced anteriorly and to the unaffected side, and the posterior mediastinum, between the aorta and the esophagus, may form a saclike projection into the unaffected pleural cavity. The lung on the affected side is commonly small, collapsed, and hypoplastic. If the hypoplasia is severe, the bronchi and bronchioles in the affected lung are well developed, whereas alveolar ducts and alveoli are reduced in number. As a result, the bronchi and bronchioles are disproportionally numerous and close to the visceral pleura. The lung on the uninvolved side is often also reduced in size, but less so than that on the side of the defect. Vigorous attempts to expand the hypoplastic lung may induce interstitial emphysema, pneumomediastinum, and pneumothorax. After replacement of the viscera into the abdomen and repair of the defect, if the residual pulmonary tissue is adequate to maintain life, the lung apparently develops normally, eventually attaining normal size and histologic pattern.

The extent of the displacement of the abdominal viscera is usually less severe in infants with eventration of the diaphragm than in those with a true posterolateral diaphragmatic hernia. In some infants only a rounded mass of hepatic tissue herniates into the thorax, and there are no clinical manifestations. Extensive unilateral or even bilateral eventrations are sometimes encountered, however, and may be responsible for symptoms similar to those of a true diaphragmatic hernia; the thin sac composed of fused pleura and peritoneum may be compressed against the inner surface of the thoracic wall and easily overlooked. Unilateral eventration is more common on the left side and may be associated with paradoxical movements of the leaves of the diaphragm similar to those seen with unilateral paralysis following injury of the phrenic nerve. In some instances, however, there is no movement on the affected side.

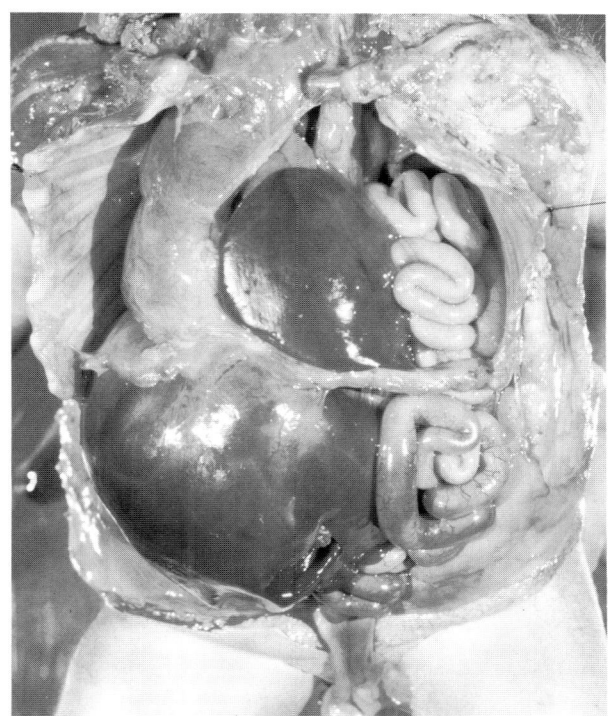

FIGURE 8-7. Left diaphragmatic hernia from a female infant with anencephaly who died 10 minutes after birth. The heart is displaced to the right by the left lobe of the liver, much of the bowel, the spleen, and the stomach, all of which occupied the left pleural cavity. The combined weight of the lungs was 4.2 gm as compared with an expected weight of 33.7 gm.

Hiatal hernias are those in which abdominal viscera, usually only the stomach, extend into the thorax through an abnormally wide esophageal hiatus. They are classified as *paraesophageal* and *sliding hiatal hernias*, the latter being the common hiatal hernia of adults, particularly women; whether those in adults are congenital or acquired lesions is not clear. Although a difference of opinion exists as to whether the contents of each of these hiatal hernias are enclosed within a peritoneal sac,[16,73,75] for practical purposes such a sac, complete or incomplete, always exists and prevents extension of the viscera into either pleural space. In the paraesophageal hernia, the cardioesophageal junction is located normally below the diaphragm, and usually only the fundus of the stomach is present within the hernia. In the sliding hernia the cardioesophageal junction is above the diaphragm, and both the cardia and part of the fundus may be within the thorax. With the exception of those with neurologic defects, hiatal hernias do not usually necessitate a fundal plication. (See Chapter 17 for further details.)

A *retrosternal hernia* is one passing through the foramen of Morgagni, usually that on the right. Occasionally bilateral hernias are present, the orifices of the two defects being separated by fibers of the sternal attachment of the diaphragm. These latter fibers, however, may be absent, and a midline retrosternal defect results. Even with such a defect the hernial sac usually projects to the right. A peritoneal sac is present in about half of the retrosternal hernias, which are limited by the pleural and pericardial surfaces. They usually contain only parts of the transverse colon, liver, and stomach and, rarely, a few loops of bowel. Symptoms, usually vague digestive disturbances, are often absent or do not appear until adult life.

A *pericardiodiaphragmatic hernia* is even less frequent than the usual retrosternal one. The diaphragmatic defect is not simply through one or both foramina of Morgagni, but is the result of defective formation of the septum transversum, which is destined to form the ventral aspect of the diaphragm laterally to the region of the pleuroperitoneal membranes and dorsally to the point of attachment of the liver and diaphragm. The pericardial defect involves that part that normally arises from the somatic mesoderm immediately adjacent to the same mesoderm from which arises the septum transversum. Such defects are more extensive than those through the foramina of Morgagni, to which they are not embryologically related,[76] and are apt to be combined with a supraumbilical midline defect of the abdominal wall, usually an omphalocele, a cleft of the distal sternum, and an intracardiac defect. This combination of five defects (pericardial, diaphragmatic, abdominal wall, sternal cleft, and cardiac), or *pentalogy of Cantrell*, has often been reported as thoracoabdominal ectopia cordis. The intracardiac defect, almost always including a ventricular and often an atrial septal defect,[77] may be associated with tetralogy of Fallot, atrioventricularis communis, bilocular heart,[78] or a diverticulum of the left ventricle. This combination of anomalies may be associated with trisomy 18.[79]

Epigastric Hernias. These hernias are rare. They occur at any point in the linea alba and immediately to either side of the midline between the umbilicus and the xiphoid process. They are small defects, usually devoid of a peritoneal sac, and contain only a protrusion of extraperitoneal fat accompanied by a small artery through the transverse fascia.

Inguinal Hernias. The inguinal canals, through which pass *indirect inguinal hernias,* form pathways for the descent of the testes into the scrotum; smaller canals, the canals of Nuck, occur in females; but the ovaries do not enter these. An evagination of the peritoneum, the processus vaginalis, occurs in the anterior abdominal wall on each side. The opening produced in the transverse fascia by this process forms the deep inguinal ring, and that in the external oblique becomes the superficial inguinal ring. By about 28 weeks of intrauterine life the testes have descended from the posterior abdominal wall to the deep inguinal rings, normally entering the scrotum at about 32 weeks of gestation. During their descent they pass posterior to the processus vaginalis, which, following their complete descent, is narrowed to a slitlike space and normally is obliterated during the perinatal period, leaving only a minute space about the testes. In the female the relatively small inguinal canals are usually completely obliterated long before birth.

Indirect inguinal hernias are much more common in males, and almost all of the inguinal hernias in infants and children are of the indirect type. They may be present at or shortly after birth (congenital inguinal hernia), but many do not appear until later in infancy or even childhood. True cryptorchidism is commonly present in association with a congenital inguinal hernia, both testicular descent and the closure of the entire processus vaginalis apparently having been arrested. A hydrocele resulting from patency of the distal but obliteration of the proximal processus vaginalis is present in about 15% of the infants and children with an inguinal hernia.

Subjective manifestations of an inguinal hernia may be entirely absent. A history of recurrent swelling in the groin is common. The appendix sometimes extends into a right inguinal hernia, and in a female a fallopian tube or ovary rarely can herniate into the sac on either side. As a rule, however, only small intestine is present in the sac. Incarceration is the most important complication, occurring most frequently during the first 6 months of life. It is manifested by a tender, painful, irreducible swelling in the groin accompanied by fretfulness and vomiting; in a number of instances these may be the first indications of the presence of an inguinal hernia. If unrelieved, signs of intestinal obstruction with abdominal distention, persistent vomiting, fever, and leukocytosis develop; but gangrene of the bowel is relatively infrequent. Occasionally pressure against the spermatic vessels alongside an incarcerated hernia is responsible for infarction of the testis, and in girls an incarcerated tube and ovary may be infarcted.

Direct inguinal hernias are hernias that pass only through the superficial inguinal ring without traversing the entire inguinal canal; these are acquired, not developmental, defects.

Femoral hernias. These hernias pass through the femoral canal below the inguinal ligament and are usually acquired defects, occurring more frequently in women.

Umbilical Hernia. These are the result of imperfect closure or weakness of the umbilical ring. They are especially common in black infants and those of low birth weight. They contain only the omentum or a part of the small intestine. Most of those which appear before the age of six months will disappear spontaneously by the age of one year. Corrective surgery may be indicated for those which become strangulated (which is very rare) or which become progressively larger after one or two years of age.

Omphalocele and Gastroschisis

An *omphalocele* is a sac covered by a thin delicate membrane, the amnion, and containing varying amounts of the abdominal viscera (Figure 8–8). It occurs in approximately 1 of every 6000 live births; if stillbirths are included, the frequency is almost twice as great. Its formation is usually attributed to failure of the intestine to return to the abdominal cavity after its

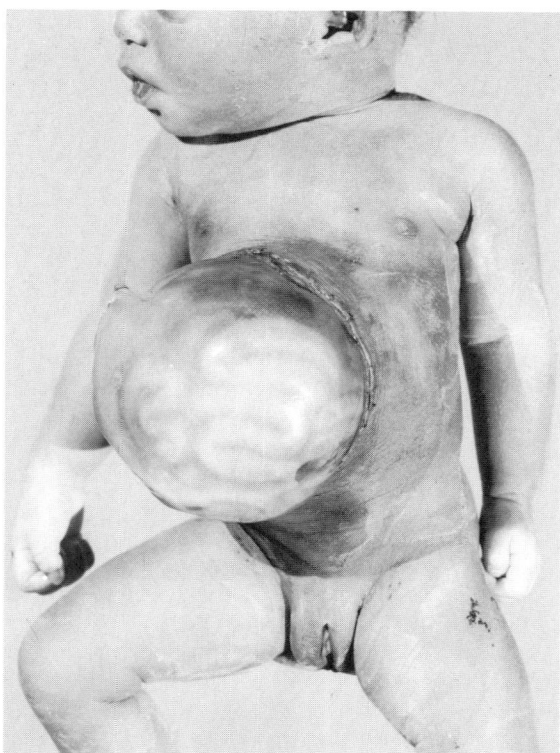

FIGURE 8–8. Omphalocele with pericardiodiaphragmatic hernia from a female infant 1 day old. The loops of bowel as well as part of the liver are apparent within the large omphalocele, and the apex of the heart could be seen extending into the sac through the defect in the pericardium. A small ostium secundum was present at the site of the foramen ovale.

sojourn in the extraembryonic coelom at about the tenth week. However, the basic disturbance may occur much earlier, at the beginning of the third week, at which time failure of formation of the lateral folds of the ventral embryonic wall results in a wide-open umbilical orifice. The prolapse of the intestine into the omphalocele according to this embryologic origin is the result of this earlier defect, rather than its cause.[80]

A small omphalocele is a hernia into the umbilical cord. This may not be apparent until intestinal obstruction and a fecal fistula follow ligation of the cord. The base of the cord is typically somewhat expanded but in normal position, and the cord arises from the apex of the sac.

The usual omphalocele varies considerably in size, large ones sometimes having a capacity greater than that of the infant's abdomen. With large omphaloceles the anterior abdominal wall above the umbilicus may be defective, so that the lesion extends upward, toward the sternum. The sac is a thin, transparent membrane composed of fused peritoneum internally and amnion externally, where patches of mucoid material (Wharton's jelly) may be visible. The abdominal skin may extend a short distance onto the base of the sac, but it is otherwise devoid of skin, in contrast to the much more common umbilical hernia. The umbilical cord is usually attached to the apex of the sac but may be inserted somewhat eccentrically. From here the umbilical arteries and vein course through its wall, which is otherwise remarkably avascular. A single umbilical artery is present in about one third of the infants with a large omphalocele.[81] Although the wall of the sac is initially moist and transparent, within the first 12 to 24 hours it becomes opaque, dry, and somewhat friable and is apt to rupture, which causes evisceration. In some instances the sac is already ruptured at the time of delivery, and the viscera may then be matted together by fibrinous or fibrous adhesions. Bacterial invasion with resultant peritonitis may occur even with an intact sac. Loops of small bowel are almost always present in the sac; and the proximal half of the colon and some parts of the liver, stomach, spleen, and pancreas may also be included.

Associated anomalies are present in over half of the infants. Many of these are not lethal ones; but a few are major ones that may be of immediate significance with respect to survival, e.g., intestinal atresia, diaphragmatic hernia, and congenital heart disease. Malrotation of the intestine, especially mixed rotation and failure of fixation, occurs in a significant number; and the occurrence of vomiting in an infant with an omphalocele suggests the possibility of intestinal obstruction secondary to volvulus or obstructing bands.

Omphalocele may represent one manifestation of the Beckwith-Wiedemann syndrome, which includes large size of the infant; macroglossia; visceromegaly, especially of the liver and kidneys; and omphalocele or umbilical hernia. There is an increased frequency of certain malignant tumors in these children. Some of the infants with an omphalocele and other congenital malformations have chromosomal anomalies, e.g., trisomy 13.[82]

Gastroschisis is much less common than an omphalocele, for which it is sometimes mistaken. It is the result of absence of the ventral abdominal wall at some area other than the umbilicus.[69] There is no sac, and the margins of the defect are smooth. Although it may occur anywhere on the abdominal wall lateral to the linea alba, it is usually located to the right of the umbilicus. The extent of herniation of the viscera varies with the size of the defect. The exposed viscera, having been bathed in amniotic fluid, are boggy and matted together by fibrinous or fibrous adhesions. Although sometimes accompanied by intestinal atresia, as a rule other severe malformations are uncommon.

Omphalomesenteric Duct Remnants
(Table 8–4)

The omphalomesenteric duct (yolk stalk) connects the yolk sac with the apex of the intestinal loop in early embryonic life. It usually detaches itself from the in-

Table 8–4 OMPHALOMESENTERIC DUCT REMNANTS

Type	Persistent Element
Meckel's diverticulum	Enteric end
Umbilical sinus	Umbilical end
Umbilical polyp	Umbilical end
Umbilical cyst	Isolated segment
Umbilical fistula	Entire duct

testine by the end of the fifth week of intrauterine life and normally degenerates and disappears before the intestine returns to the abdomen during the tenth week. The entire duct or any portion of it may, however, remain patent or may persist as a fibrous cord passing between the ileum and the umbilicus or attached to the tip of a Meckel's diverticulum.

Meckel's Diverticulum. This is the most common anomaly of the intestinal tract, being present in 2% to 3% of all persons. It is even more common in those with certain chromosomal anomalies, e.g., in more than 20% of those with trisomy 18 and in approximately 10% of those with trisomy 13.[82] It represents the proximal (enteric) end of the omphalomesenteric duct and may be located anywhere from 10 to 90 cm above the ileocecal valve,[83] arising from the antimesenteric border. In rare instances it may appear to arise from the side of the bowel or to course between the folds of the mesentery, probably as the result of fixation secondary to adhesions. It usually has a broad base and a diameter smaller than that of the adjoining bowel. It varies from 1 to 8 cm in length. The tip may be bifurcated or appear nodular as the result of heterotopic gastric or pancreatic tissue. It is occasionally fixed to the ileum by its own mesentery, which infrequently may be complete as far as the umbilicus. Damage to the omphalomesenteric artery (a direct continuation of the superior mesenteric artery) results in infarction of the diverticulum, the line of demarcation being at the junction of the diverticulum and the ileum.

A fibrous cord that may contain remnants of the omphalomesenteric artery infrequently passes from the tip of the diverticulum to the undersurface of the umbilicus; or this cord, still attached to the diverticular tip, may hang free in the peritoneal cavity and subsequently become attached to another intra-abdominal structure, e.g., the mesentery. Remnants of the omphalomesenteric vein are occasionally observed as a fibrous cord passing from the umbilicus to the base of the mesentery or to the porta hepatis.

The wall of the diverticulum consists of all of the layers of the bowel, and its mucous membrane is usually similar to that of the adjoining ileum. Heterotopic tissues are frequently present, however, especially in those diverticula that are responsible for clinical manifestations. Gastric mucosa is present in about 50% of symptomatic diverticula. It often occurs as one or more patches amid the intestinal mucosa but may line the entire diverticulum or only its fundus. Pancreatic tissue (Figure 8–9) with both acini and islets of Langerhans may be present in the submucosa, muscularis, or subserosa. Colonic or duodenal mucosa, including Brunner's glands, may also be present.

The majority of persons with a Meckel's diverticulum are asymptomatic. Clinical manifestations, however, may appear at any age, especially in infancy and childhood. The predominant signs and symptoms are those of intestinal obstruction, a peptic ulcer with bleeding, or diverticulitis. Intestinal obstruction may be the result of an intussusception, the diverticulum serving as the leading point; or a vestigial band leading from the tip of the diverticulum to the umbilicus or

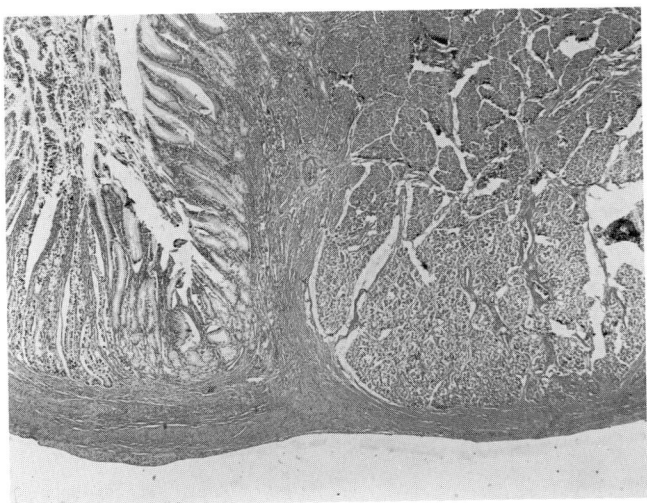

FIGURE 8–9. Aberrant pancreas in Meckel's diverticulum. The diverticulum is lined by small intestinal mucosa. (H&E, × 19)

elsewhere may entrap loops of bowel beneath it, causing an internal hernia. In other instances such a band may provide the axis about which a volvulus of one or more loops of bowel occurs. Hemorrhage from an ulcer secondary to heterotopic gastric mucosa in the diverticulum is especially apt to occur in the young, often presenting before 2 years of age. It is usually not accompanied by pain. The ulcer is in the ileal mucosa and may be in the diverticulum or the immediately adjoining bowel. Hemorrhage may be intermittent or may be so severe as to necessitate transfusions and immediate surgical intervention. Acute diverticulitis is usually preoperatively considered to be acute appendicitis; rupture of the inflamed diverticulum is apt to occur early, with subsequent peritonitis. Meconium peritonitis caused by rupture of a Meckel's diverticulum has been observed in a newborn[84]; and generalized peritonitis from a perforated diverticulum, possibly due to infarction, has been seen in the early neonatal period.[85]

Umbilical Sinus. An umbilical sinus is a mucosa-lined tract leading from the umbilicus for a variable distance into the abdominal wall, from which there is a mucoid discharge. It results from persistence of a portion of the umbilical end of the omphalomesenteric duct, a fibrous remnant of which may be attached to a Meckel's diverticulum.

Umbilical Polyp. This results from persistence of only the umbilical end of the omphalomesenteric duct. There may be no other remnant of the duct, or there may be an umbilical sinus or a fibrous cord passing to the ileum or to a Meckel's diverticulum. The polyp consists of a bright red, firm nodular mass of mucosa in the umbilical fossa, sometimes with a central orifice ending blindly at the base of the polyp or extending a variable distance as an umbilical sinus. Histologically,

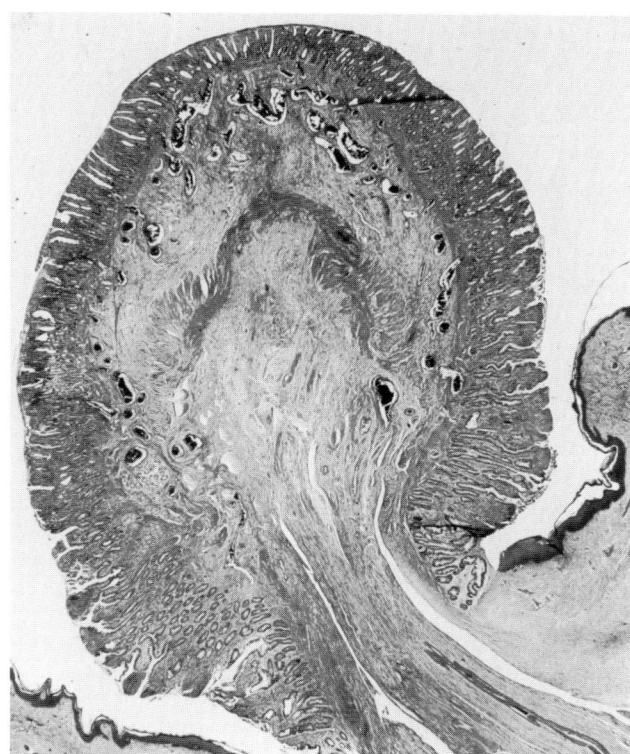

FIGURE 8–10. Umbilical polyp from a male infant 9 weeks old. The polyp is covered by gastric mucosa. Meckel's diverticulum was also present. (H&E, × 9.5)

it frequently consists of gastric mucosa (Figure 8–10), but intestinal mucosa and even pancreatic tissue may be present. It should be differentiated from the more common umbilical granuloma, which consists only of granulation tissue with acute and chronic inflammation.

Umbilical Cyst. This cyst is the result of persistence of an isolated segment of the omphalomesenteric duct. It may be located in the abdominal cavity, attached to the umbilicus or to the convex surface of the ileum by a fibrous cord, or it may be situated within the abdominal wall beneath the umbilicus. Gastric mucosa is frequently present, and perforation of the cyst onto the surface of the skin converts it into an umbilical sinus. It is a very rare lesion, in contrast to epidermal inclusion cysts in the umbilicus.

Umbilical Fistula. This fistula represents persistent patency of the entire length of the omphalomesenteric duct, from the ileum to the umbilicus. The fistulous tract is lined by mucosa similar to that of a Meckel's diverticulum, and intestinal contents may drain from its umbilical orifice. After separation of the umbilical cord, the base of which is usually larger than normal, a bright red, flat or more frequently elevated nodule is apparent in the umbilical fossa. A small orifice is present at the apex of this nodule, from which mucus or intestinal contents may escape. Prolapse of the intestine through the umbilical fistula is an important complication. If only the duct is prolapsed, it will appear as an I-shaped mucosal structure with a single orifice at its apex. With progression of the process loops of bowel proximal and distal to the duct will project through the umbilical orifice, creating a T-shaped mucosal mass with two orifices.[86] The resultant intestinal obstruction, actually an intussusception, is apt to occur in the first month or so of life and requires immediate surgical correction.

Congenital Diverticula of the Intestines

Congenital intestinal diverticula, other than Meckel's, are extremely rare. They are usually solitary and are most common in the ileum and duodenum. Minute hollow buds of the epithelial lining of the primitive intestine extend into the subepithelial tissue or submucosa during embryonic life; these are found chiefly on the antimesenteric surface, especially of the ileum. Normally they disappear; but rarely one may persist, extend through the circular layer of the muscularis, stretch or penetrate the outer longitudinal layer, and expand on the surface of the intestine as a diverticulum or cyst. The wall consists only of mucosa and serosa, sometimes with a few bundles of muscle. Similarly, if the primitive epithelial bud fails to penetrate either of the muscular coats it may expand within the submucosa to form a submucosal cyst.[69] Such cysts may be differentiated from duplications by their lack of distinct muscular walls containing both layers with myenteric plexuses. The diverticula should be differentiated from acquired diverticula, which are usually multiple, involve predominantly the colon, and occur principally in adults, their incidence increasing with age (see Chapter 30).

Congenital diverticulum of the cecum is usually single and possibly has a somewhat different embryologic origin from those of the small intestine. The lesion may be manifested by pain that localizes in the right lower quadrant, occasionally accompanied by a palpable mass. The preoperative diagnosis is usually that of appendicitis.

Meconium Ileus and Related Conditions

Meconium Ileus. This condition is responsible for approximately 15% of intestinal obstructions in the newborn period and is the initial manifestation of cystic fibrosis of the pancreas in about 10% of those with this disease. It is probably always a manifestation of cystic fibrosis of the pancreas, surviving infants usually developing evidence of pulmonary disease within the first few months of life.[87] Severe abdominal distention may be present at birth, especially in those in whom severe meconium peritonitis is present. Manifestations of intestinal obstruction within the first day or two of life should suggest the possibility of meconium ileus in any newborn infant with a history of cystic fibrosis of the pancreas in a sibling.

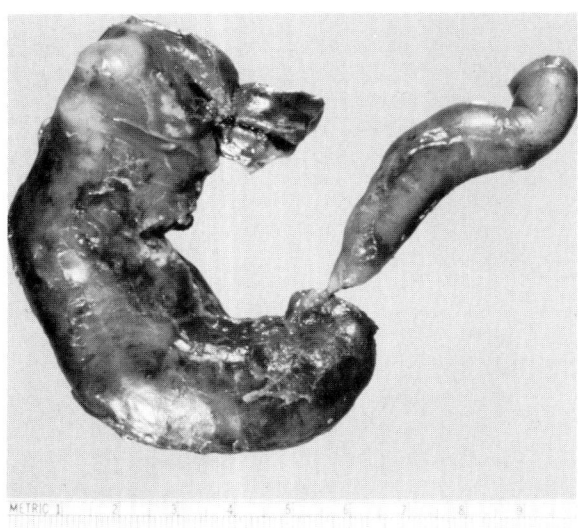

FIGURE 8–11. Meconium ileus with volvulus and intestinal atresia. Meconium peritonitis is also apparent on the serosal surface. From a female infant 7 hours old.

At laparotomy or autopsy the colon is empty and so narrow that it may be erroneously interpreted as a hypoplastic colon. Typically the terminal ileum is relatively small and contains concretions of gray, inspissated meconium with the consistency of dried putty. These may be responsible for a beadlike appearance of this segment of bowel. More proximally, the loops of ileum gradually enlarge until they become enormously dilated and the muscularis hypertrophied. Here the content is a dark, plum-colored, extremely tenacious meconium. Still more proximally the dilation and hypertrophy diminish and the content becomes semiliquid. The meconium, which is both quantitatively and qualitatively abnormal, usually distends a segment of bowel about 30 cm in length, although in some instances only a short segment of bowel is so distended.

Perforation of the bowel may occur prior to or shortly after birth, with a resultant sterile meconium peritonitis; but when it occurs from several hours to a day or more after birth, a bacterial peritonitis results. Perforation of the distended loop of bowel may occur in the absence of any macroscopically demonstrable lesion of the bowel. Moreover, the bulk of the dilated loop of bowel predisposes to an intrauterine volvulus with perforation and meconium peritonitis. The volvulus, moreover, may so impair the blood supply of a segment of bowel as to lead to atresia (Figure 8–11), sometimes with a defect in the adjoining mesentery.[73] Intestinal atresia or, less often, stenosis in the absence of a volvulus may occur as the result of mucosal ulceration, extravasation of meconium into the intestinal wall, meconium granulomas, and intense scarring with partial or complete obliteration of the lumen.[56] In the presence of meconium peritonitis a similar reaction involving the peripheral aspects of the bowel may lead to intestinal obstruction.[56] In some instances perforation of the transverse or even the sigmoid colon may occur.

Other evidences of cystic fibrosis of the pancreas are present at autopsy but are often inadequate to establish this diagnosis macroscopically. The pancreas is usually macroscopically normal. A very hypoplastic gallbladder containing only colorless mucus devoid of bile is present in about 25% of patients of all ages with cystic fibrosis[88] and strongly suggests this diagnosis. The lungs are usually macroscopically normal in those dying of meconium ileus *per se*. In contrast to older children, the vas deferens and seminal vesicles are apparently grossly normal.[89] Histologically, the changes in the pancreas are usually only mild to moderate and in a few instances are so minimal that an unequivocal diagnosis of cystic fibrosis is impossible. Changes in the mucous glands of the larynx, trachea, and major bronchi are usually present; but there is usually no significant emphysema, bronchitis, or bronchiolitis in those dying of meconium ileus. In contrast, the intestinal glands, especially in the small intestine, are usually dilated and contain a stringy, homogeneous, acidophilic material, often continuous with abundant similar acidophilic material in the lumen. This is strongly positive when stained by the periodic acid–Schiff (PAS) technique (Figure 8–12).

Meconium Ileus Equivalent. This condition occurs in older children with cystic fibrosis of the pancreas. It is characterized by intermittent or complete intestinal obstruction as the result of accumulations of inspissated or impacted fecal material in the terminal ileum and cecum. Intermittent, incomplete intestinal obstruction may result; and the presence of these masses in the cecum may suggest the possibility of a neoplasm. Intussusception, usually ileocolic, with incomplete obstruction and crampy abdominal pain, results from the adherent intestinal contents. Morphologically, the involved segment of bowel reveals severe changes in the mucosa similar to those in meconium ileus.

Meconium Peritonitis. This condition is usually a complication of meconium ileus but may follow perforation of the bowel *in utero* or in the first few hours after birth from any cause. In a number of instances there is no evidence of intestinal obstruction, and it may be impossible to demonstrate the site of the perforation. It is a sterile, chemical peritonitis characterized by the presence of dense fibrous adhesions, keratinized epithelial debris derived from ingested amniotic fluid, and a foreign body reaction about particles of meconium. Large amounts of serous or dark green, brown, or turbid fluid may be present in the peritoneal cavity in addition to deposits of fibrin, masses of meconium, and deposits of calcium. With the escape of abundant meconium, the deposits of calcium may be so extensive as to obscure the presence of accumulations of squamous debris. Occasionally the inflammatory reaction is so localized as to produce a pseudocyst within the peritoneal cavity, presenting as a localized abdominal mass.

If the perforation is rapidly sealed after the escape of only a small amount of meconium, the presence of meconium peritonitis may never be known without the fortuitous discovery of calcific particles in roentgenograms of the abdomen. Radiographically demonstrable

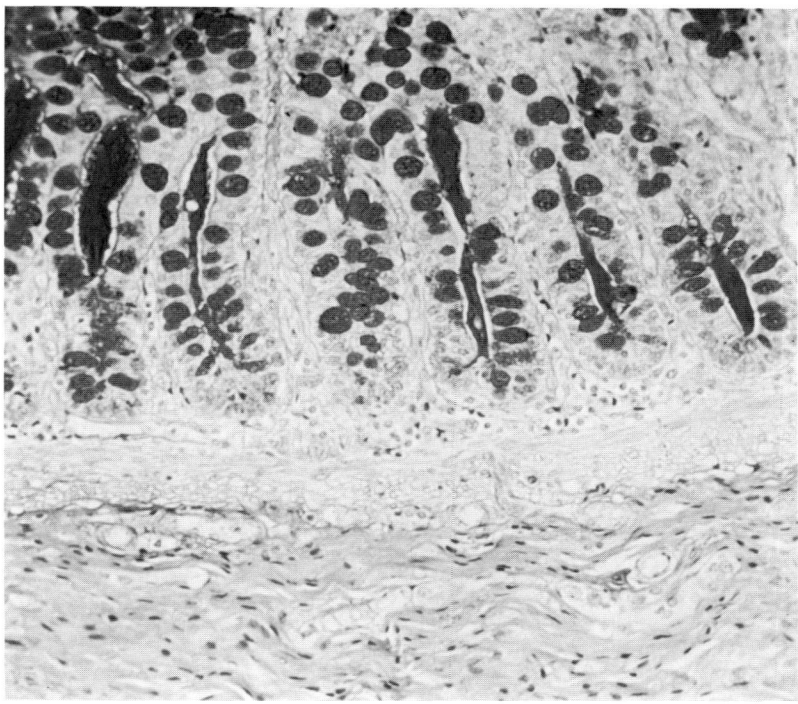

FIGURE 8-12. Histologic section of the bowel from the same infant, stained by the periodic acid–Schiff technique. A number of the glands are somewhat dilated and contain a bright red secretion. Similar material was present in the lumen. (PAS, × 100)

calcification may be present in a remarkably short time, sometimes as early as 24 hours after the perforation.

Meconium Plug Syndrome. A rare cause of intestinal obstruction in the newborn, not related to cystic fibrosis of the pancreas, is a plug of meconium with a lower water content than normal, usually located in the anorectal region. Digital examination under such circumstances is usually followed by expulsion of the plug, relief of the intestinal obstruction, and passage of meconium; infrequently it may be expelled only after an enema. The plug is a long, ribbonlike or tapering structure, the distal narrow end of which is firm, gray, and dry and the proximal portion of which is more normal meconium. Rarely anorectal plugs may cause ulceration and perforation. Even less frequently a plug in the more proximal bowel may cause perforation and meconium peritonitis. The cause of such plugs is unknown, but infants so affected should be carefully followed for the possible presence of aganglionic megacolon.

Spontaneous Perforation of the Intestine

Spontaneous perforation of the intestine is a rare cause of peritonitis in newborn infants. The perforations may be single or multiple, and the cause is usually unknown. Some are the result of a necrotizing enterocolitis secondary to ischemia of the affected segment of bowel.[68] Disruptions of the muscularis and peritoneum with an intact mucosa and submucosa have been described in a few, in addition to the actual perforation. Perforations may involve the small or large bowel, including the cecum. Perforation of the bowel may also occur *in utero* or in the neonatal period as a result of meconium ileus, intussusception, volvulus, or rupture of a Meckel's diverticulum; even acute appendicitis has been described in the neonatal period.[90-94]

DUPLICATIONS OF THE ALIMENTARY TRACT

General Features. Duplications of the alimentary tract (enteric or enterogenous cysts) may occur at any site from the posterior half of the tongue to the anus but are most frequent in the region of the ileum. They are usually spherical or oval masses lying within the mesentery and adherent to the adjoining bowel, with which a portion of their wall usually shares a common muscularis (Figures 8–13 and 8–14). Less frequently, the duplication is a tubular structure that may resemble a giant diverticulum or may lie alongside the bowel, giving the latter a "double-barreled" appearance (Figure 8–15). In some of the latter, only a slight furrow is present between the intestine and the duplication; and even that may be absent, so that the anomaly is not recognized until the bowel has been opened. They are usually solitary, but occasionally multiple duplications are present along a segment of the bowel. They may communicate with the adjoining bowel through one or more openings; but cystic duplications, which are the most common type, usually lack such a communication.

Pathogenesis. The embryologic origin of duplications is not clearly established, but they are usually attributed to defects in recanalization of the bowel after the normal obliteration of its lumen by epithelial pro-

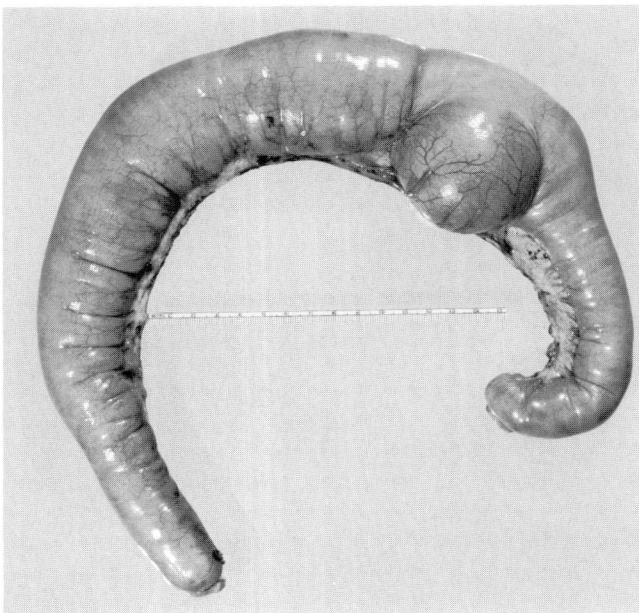

FIGURE 8–13. A spherical mass of duplication of the bowel is present between the leaves of the mesentery. This was lined in part by gastric mucosa and communicated with the adjoining bowel near the proximal end of the duplication. The muscularis of the bowel and that of the duplication were fused over a considerable distance. From a boy 18 months old.

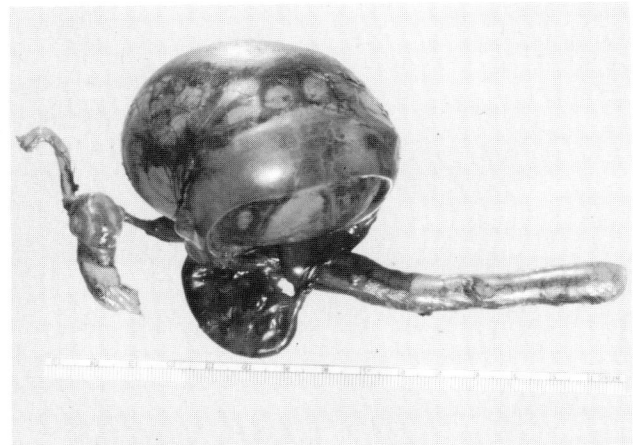

FIGURE 8–14. Duplication of terminal ileum with volvulus and infarction of bowel. From an infant 1 day old.

liferation during the embryonic period (see the section on intestinal atresia and stenosis). Failure of a group of vacuoles to coalesce with the definitive intestinal lumen would result in the formation of a second epithelium-lined space invested with a muscular wall similar to that of the normal alimentary tract. With less complete separation of the two epithelium-lined spaces, however, the duplication may be predominantly in the submucosa, and the muscularis between it and the adjoining bowel may be incomplete. Conversely, with complete separation, each of the two epithelium-lined spaces may develop an independent submucosa, muscularis, serosa, and even mesentery. Such a mechanism may explain the origin of certain duplications but fails to explain their almost constant location on the mesenteric aspect of the bowel. "Duplications" of the foregut that penetrate the diaphragm to reach the posterior mediastinum or those intra-abdominal ones associated with an independent mediastinal cyst are probably of neurenteric origin (see the section on neuroenteric cyst). This may also be true of infrequent colonic duplications associated with vertebral defects and duplications of the lower genitourinary tract, sometimes attributed to partial twinning. Perhaps many duplications are of neurenteric origin, but this can be established only by further study of the frequency of vertebral anomalies in all such patients. Histologic differentiation of neurenteric cysts from other duplications is impossible except in those rare instances in which neural tissue is present in the wall.

Clinical Features. Clinical manifestations are, of course, dependent upon the location of the duplication. They are usually apparent in infancy or early childhood but may be delayed until adult life.[95–97] The manifestations are commonly those of intestinal obstruction, pain, or gastrointestinal hemorrhage, sometimes associated with a palpable abdominal mass. Obstruction results from compression of the adjacent

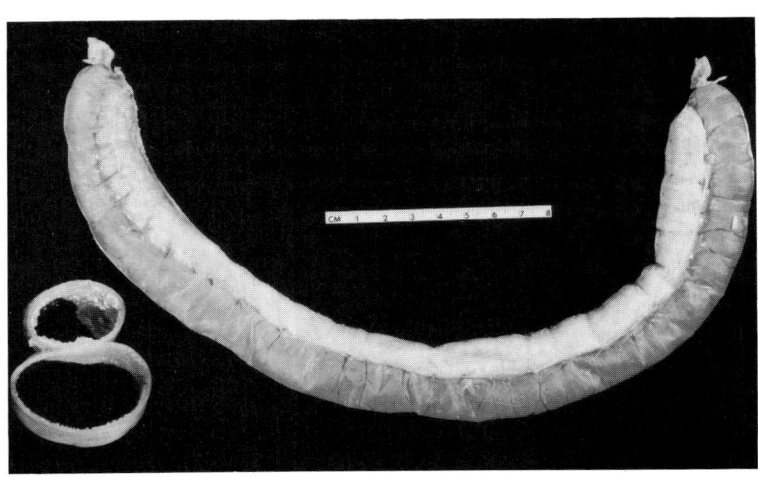

FIGURE 8–15. Tubular duplication of terminal ileum from a male infant 7 months old. The duplication, lying on the mesenteric border of the bowel, is 29 cm long and communicated with the adjoining bowel near its distal end. The duplication, which is the smaller of the two cross sections, was lined largely by gastric mucosa; an ulcer was present within it, near its point of communication with the bowel. An island of aberrant pancreas was also present in its wall.

intestinal lumen by the expanding mass, from intussusception secondary to the presence of the mass, or from an inflammatory stricture of the bowel resulting from escape of gastric juice from the gastric tissue in the duplication into the lumen of the bowel. Pain is caused by distention of the mass, by peptic ulceration, or by intestinal obstruction. Bleeding may be caused by peptic ulceration, by impairment of the blood supply of the bowel as the result of an expanding lesion within the leaves of the mesentery, or by intussusception.

Specific Locations. *Duplications of the esophagus* only infrequently communicate with the lumen of the esophagus and may be entirely asymptomatic. More frequently, however, they manifest themselves as expanding intrathoracic lesions, usually extending into the right hemithorax, associated with cough, atelectasis, pneumonia, and dysphagia. Hemoptysis may occur as a result of erosion into the lung by a duplication containing gastric mucosa. Many so-called duplications of the esophagus probably are neurenteric in origin; such an origin can be established by the presence of vertebral anomalies or by demonstration of a cord of tissue, perhaps containing neural elements, leading from the cyst to a vertebral body.

Duplications of the duodenum are rare lesions that may be responsible for duodenal obstruction. There is usually no communication with the adjoining bowel. They are apt to be submucosal and bulge into the lumen of the adjoining bowel, from which they are separated by only a scanty muscularis.

Duplications of the stomach are usually located along the greater curvature and are manifested by signs of partial obstruction, which may simulate congenital hypertrophic pyloric stenosis.[98] A palpable mass is sometimes present. There is usually no communication with the gastric lumen, and bleeding is infrequent.[99]

Duplications of the small intestine are sometimes palpable and are manifested by intermittent signs of partial intestinal obstruction. They may, however, be responsible for intermittent pain, melena, or intussusception. Infrequently the wall of the duplication is partially calcified and is visible as a curvilinear density on roentgen films of the abdomen.

Duplications of the colon may be asymptomatic but usually compress the adjacent bowel, causing constipation and abdominal distention. Those in the rectum are usually apparent in early infancy and are palpable by rectal examination. Rarely, a cystic mass lined by transitional epithelium may be present as a small lump adjacent to the anus; masses such as these have been referred to as *cloacal cysts* and may represent remnants of the primitive tail gut. Long tubular duplications of the colon and sometimes also the terminal ileum may be associated with other anomalies such as imperforate anus and duplication of the genitalia and the bladder,[100] exstrophy of the bladder, omphalocele, and vertebral defects. Many of these are probably neurenteric in origin. They usually communicate proximally with the colon or terminal ileum, but the external opening of one or both colons is apt to be an abnormal one, e.g., a rectoperineal or rectourethral fistula or an imperforate anus. Associated anomalies in infants and children with duplications are usually confined to the gastrointestinal tract except in instances of complete duplication of the colon.

Pathologic Features

Macroscopically, duplications vary considerably in their appearance but are most frequently unilocular cystic structures lying in the mesentery and intimately adherent to the bowel. Occasionally they are submucosal in location and bulge into the lumen of the bowel. Rarely, almost the entire small intestine or all of the colon and a part of the terminal ileum are duplicated, and triplication of the entire colon has been reported.[101] The contents may be those of the adjoining bowel when there is a communication between the two, but this is true in only about 20% of duplications.[102] More often the lumen contains clear mucus or bloody fluid. The wall of a duplication is thick and muscular, containing one, two, or even three layers of smooth muscle. Auerbach's plexuses are commonly present in the wall, the muscularis of which is usually intimately admixed with that of the adjoining alimentary tract. The mucosa lining the duplication is that of some part of the alimentary tract but need not correspond to that part of the tract from which it arises. Gastric mucosa is commonly present, especially at the blind end of a duplication, and occasionally heterotopic pancreatic tissue is present.[103] Pseudostratified columnar ciliated epithelium similar to that of the early fetal esophagus is occasionally encountered, and several types of mucosa may be present in a single duplication. The mucosa is usually well preserved but may be atrophic or partially destroyed. Peptic ulcers, which may develop when gastric mucosa is present, may be responsible for hemorrhage or perforation of the duplication itself or of the adjacent bowel. These ulcers may occur within the duplication, usually in intestinal mucosa adjoining that of gastric type, but often they are in the contiguous intestine near its communication with the duplication.

RECTUM AND ANUS

Embryology

The rectum is derived from the cloaca, the common endodermal channel that receives the allantois and the dorsally located hindgut. The cloacal membrane, composed of endoderm of the cloaca and surface ectoderm, constitutes the caudal and ventral wall of the cloaca. Linear thickenings of mesenchyme of the lateral body wall form ridges within the cloaca and fuse with each other in a craniocaudal direction. The cloaca is thus divided by the urorectal septum, or fused ridges, into a dorsally located rectum and upper anal canal and a ventral urogenital sinus. In the male, the urogenital sinus gives rise to the epithelium of the urinary bladder, the urethra (except for the fossa navicularis), the glands of the prostate, and the bulbourethral glands; the connective tissue and smooth muscle develop from the adjacent splanchnic mesenchyme. In the female, it gives rise to the urinary bladder, vagina (perhaps cranially formed by the fused paramesonephric or müllerian ducts), the urethra, and the urethral, paraurethral, and greater vestibular glands. During the seventh week the urorectal septum fuses with the cloacal membrane, dividing it into an anal membrane and a larger urogenital membrane; then these membranes rupture, the anal somewhat later than the urogenital. The caudal part of the digestive system is thus brought into communication with the amniotic cavity.[70]

Imperforate Anus and Related Conditions (Table 8–5)

Imperforate anus occurs in approximately one in every 5000 births. The term is used to denote a variety of anorectal malformations, regardless of the presence or absence of an anal opening. With recognition of the imperfections of any classification of such anomalies, they will here be considered as low malformations of the anorectal region, i.e., anal agenesis, anal stenosis, and membranous anal atresia, and high malformations, i.e., anorectal agenesis and rectal atresia.[70]

Imperforate anus may be part of the VATER complex of anomalies.[104] *VATER* is an acronym applied to certain nonrandom association of defects consisting of *v*ertebral anomalies, *a*nal atresia, *t*racheo*e*sophageal fistula with esophageal atresia, *r*enal defects, and *r*adial hypoplasia. Any of these defects may occur together in any combination of two or more and the association is occasionally part of a chromosomal anomaly, e.g., trisomy 18 or the 13q deletion syndrome. A variety of other anomalies may be present as well, including cardiac and genital anomalies, polydactyly, defects of the thumb, duodenal atresia with annular pancreas, and single umbilical artery. Its occurrence is usually sporadic.

Anal agenesis is that anomaly in which the anal canal, the upper portion of which is derived from the hindgut, terminates blindly below the levator ani. There is usually an associated fistula, to the peritoneum in either sex or less frequently to the vaginal fourchette in the female or the scrotum in the male (ectopic anus). The anomaly presumably results from dorsal deviation of the cloaca by the urorectal septum and, if a fistula exists, from incomplete division of the cloaca by this septum.

Alternately, the anomaly may be the result of an arrest in the normal dorsal migration of the anal canal. According to this concept, the upper portion of the anal canal is normally moved posteriorly across the perineum from its initial site in the urogenital sinus by the growth of mesodermal tissue in the caudal portion of the urorectal septum and in the area of fusion of this septum with the cloacal membrane, i.e., the future perineal body. Thus, the rectal opening initially leads into the urogenital sinus until this opening is closed by the urorectal septum. The tip, i.e., the distal portion of the hindgut or upper part of the anal canal then "migrates" posteriorly to its normal position within the external sphincter muscle, which develops independently at the normal position of the anus.[105] Finally, the anal canal communicates with the exterior by rupture of the anal membrane. This dorsal migration of the distal hindgut may be arrested at any point along its course, whereas the rest of the perineum, including the external anal sphincter, develops normally. Thus the fistula may terminate in the perineum at any point anterior to its usual site in either sex, in the scrotum, bladder, or urethra in the male or the vagina in the female.

Anal stenosis rsults from a slight dorsal deviation of the urorectal septum as it grows caudally to fuse with the cloacal membrane. As a result, the anal canal is narrow, sometimes only admitting a small probe.

Membranous anal atresia, a very rare condition, clearly results from failure of the anal membrane to perforate. A thin membrane in the vicinity of the pectinate line bulges upon straining and may appear dark because of the meconium immediately behind it.

Anorectal agenesis is the most common anorectal malformation, constituting about 80% of these anomalies. The rectum terminates blindly some distance above the anal dimple. Usually a fistulous tract in the male passes from the distal rectum to the bladder in the region of the trigone or to the urethra. In the female the fistula usually terminates in the vagina. This anomaly is usually attributed to dorsal deviation of the urorectal septum and, if a fistula exists, incomplete fusion of this septum. Some, however, consider failure of normal dorsal migration of the distal hindgut or upper anal canal as the embryologic event responsible for most instances of imperforate anus with a fistula *(supra vide).*[105] Such an origin is suggested by the fact that the fistulas are lined by a transitional type of epithelium and are enclosed in muscle; i.e., they have the appearance of a hypoplastic anus.

Associated anomalies are present in a significant number of those with anorectal agenesis, and in some instances are directly responsible for death. Among the more frequent are congenital heart disease; malformations of the urinary tract, especially megaloureter and hydronephrosis; anomalies of the skeleton, especially of the sacrococcygeal region; and esophageal or duodenal atresia. Anorectal malformations occur with increased frequency in those with trisomy 18 or 21.[82] Associated malformations are present in almost all of those who come to necropsy.

Rectal atresia is a blind-ending rectal pouch that is separated from the intact distal rectum and anal canal by a variable distance. Its embryologic origin may be similar to that of intestinal atresia involving the small bowel, usually resulting from impaired blood supply, or, infrequently, from failure of vacuolization of the bowel.

Table 8–5 TYPES OF IMPERFORATE ANUS

Low malformations
    Anal agenesis
    Anal stenosis
    Membranous anal atresia
High malformations
    Anorectal agenesis (most common)
    Rectal atresia

Cloacal Exstrophy

Cloacal exstrophy is an uncommon, complicated malformation, the embryologic origin of which is not entirely clear. Just as the cloaca is normally divided into rectum and urogenital sinus by fused linear thickenings of mesenchyme (the urorectal septum), so also paired mounds of mesoderm (the genital swellings), located lateral to the cephalic border of the cloacal membrane, migrate toward the midline along the cephalolateral edge of this membrane. By the fifth week these fuse in the midline, forming the genital tubercle at the cephalic edge of the cloacal membrane. When the anal and urogenital membranes rupture, the urogenital orifice is caudal to the genital tubercle. Proliferation of mesoderm also occurs in the anterior abdominal wall below the umbilicus, leading to a notable increase in the distance between this and the cloacal membrane. In cloacal exstrophy there is probably failure of normal development of many of these mesodermal growths, so that the cloacal membrane remains as a thin ectoentodermal membrane. Following its rupture, the urogenital portion of the entodermal cloaca is exposed. There is also failure of development of the infraumbilical mesoderm so that the ventral abdominal wall between the cloaca and the umbilicus is defective, the distance between the exposed dorsal wall of the bladder (a derivative of the urogenital portion of the cloaca) and the umbilicus being almost nonexistent. Failure of development of the urorectal septum also occurs, as a result of which the dorsal wall of the hindgut is exposed.

The lower ileum, colon, and rectum, derived from the hindgut or caudal limb of the intestinal loop, do not grow normally; and the small intestine opens in a field of intestinal mucosa below the umbilicus and between the two halves of the exposed bladder. The lesion is further complicated by prolapse of the ileum. Below the prolapsed segment, but still in the field of intestinal mucosa,[106] lies a second orifice leading to a short, blind-ending colon. The anus is imperforate. There may be one or two appendices, the appendix may be absent, or a small rudimentary appendix may open in the intestinal field between the small intestinal and colonic orifices.[107] The penis or clitoris often consists of two widely separated halves. There are often multiple other congenital anomalies, including myelocystocele, omphalocele, and malrotation of the midgut.

CYSTS OF MESENTERY AND OMENTUM

Mesenteric Cysts (Cystic Hygromas)

A mesenteric cyst (or cystic hygroma) is not a neoplasm; rather, it is a hamartoma consisting of a local overgrowth of lymphatics, comparable to the cystic lymphangiomas of the cervical, axillary, and inguinal regions. Mesenteric cysts are uncommon lesions, occurring less frequently than duplications of the bowel, from which they must be differentiated.

Clinical Features. They may first become manifest in infancy, childhood, or adult life. The predominant clinical feature is usually progressive, painless abdominal enlargement, sometimes of several years' duration, which may be so extensive as to simulate ascites. Less frequently, recurrent attacks of abdominal pain, sometimes associated with vomiting, may occur; or the manifestations may be those of acute intestinal obstruction.[108] Pain may be caused by partial intestinal obstruction or possibly by traction upon the root of the involved mesentery.[109] Intestinal obstruction results from encroachment on the intestinal lumen by the cystic mass in the adjoining mesentery or from volvulus of that segment of bowel adjoining the cyst. Occasionally, in the presence of malrotation of the bowel or inadequate mesenteric fixation, a mesenteric cyst is associated with volvulus of the entire midgut.[110] A mass that is more freely movable in the lateral than in the vertical direction may be palpable, and sometimes a fluid wave or shifting dullness may be detected. In many instances, however, owing to the flabbiness of the cyst, no mass can be palpated. Roentgenographic examination reveals displacement of the intestines and stomach by a mass with the density of fluid. Differentiation from ascites may be difficult or impossible; but as a rule, the separation of loops of bowel by thin layers of fluid that may be encountered with ascites is not apparent.

Pathologic Features. Mesenteric cysts usually arise in the mesentery of the jejunum or ileum and less frequently in the mesocolon. They vary considerably in size, some containing as much as 3000 ml of fluid.[111] They often assume a saddlelike configuration, projecting on either side of the mesentery and incompletely encircling the adjoining intestine (Figure 8–16). They are usually multilocular and may contain clear, serous fluid resembling plasma or opaque, chylous fluid con-

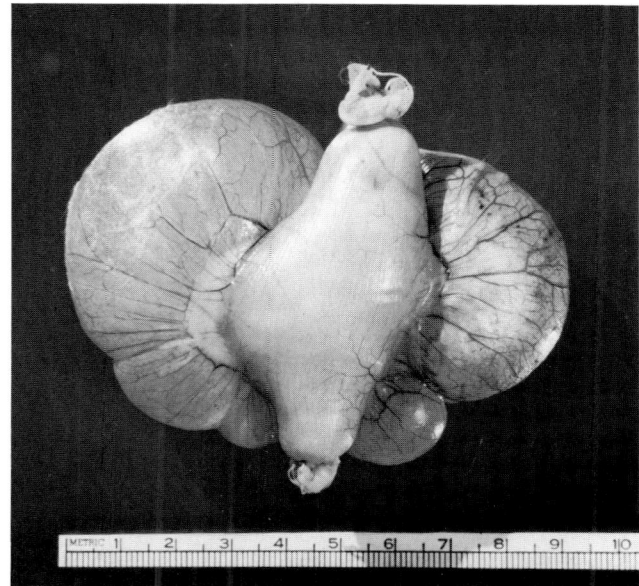

FIGURE 8–16. Mesenteric cyst (cystic hygroma) from a 4-year-old girl. Note the saddlelike configuration of the two larger cysts on the mesenteric aspect of the bowel.

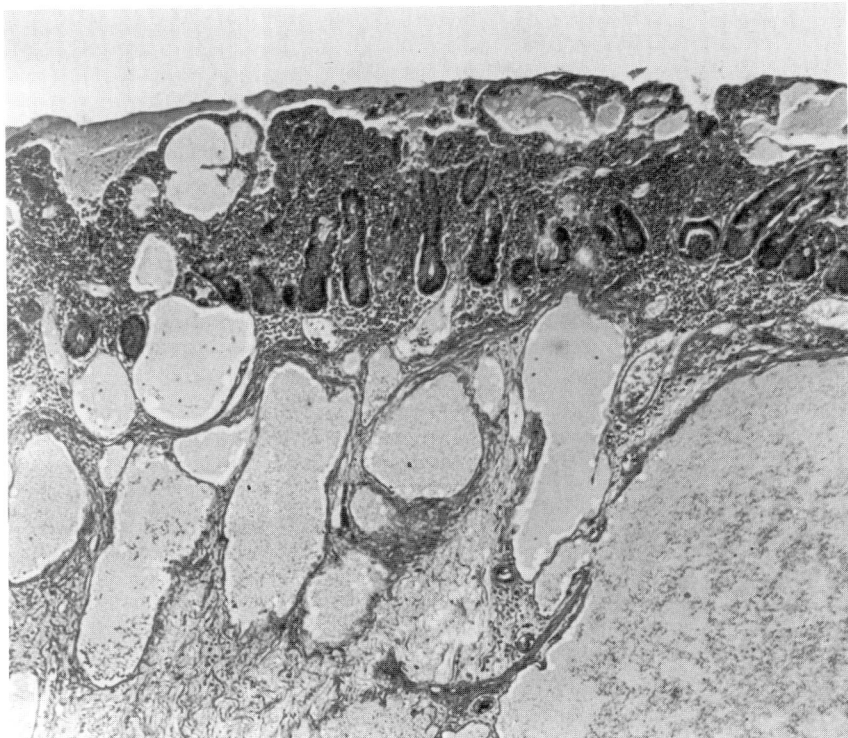

FIGURE 8-17. Mesenteric cyst (cystic hygroma) from a 3-year-old girl. The multilocular cystic mass weighed 3960 gm, and a segment of bowel 25 cm long coursed about the bases of the cysts. Several yellow plaques were present in the mucosa of the bowel adjoining some of these cysts. This is a section of one such area, in which numerous dilated lymphatics are present in the submucosa and lamina propria. ($\times$ 50)

taining less protein and a considerable amount of fat. Hemorrhage into the cyst may transform the contents into a dirty brown fluid.

Histologically, they are composed of multiple, irregular, endothelium-lined spaces with thin walls, some of which contain small bundles of smooth muscle. Focal aggregates of lymphocytes as well as accumulations of vacuolated macrophages, foreign body giant cells, and cholesterol clefts are commonly present. Occasionally multiple dilated lymphatic spaces are present in the submucosa and lamina propria of the adjoining bowel (Figure 8-17), necessitating resection of the involved bowel for complete removal of the mass.

Most mesenteric cysts are isolated lesions involving only a given segment of the mesentery. Rarely, however, the entire mesentery or the major portion of it is irregularly thickened, edematous, and occupied by myriad small nodules and cysts, the latter varying from minute lesions to cystic spaces several centimeters in diameter. Histologically the nodules are composed of aggregates of endothelial cells with only a few developing endothelium-lined spaces. The appearance of the nodular aggregates of cells closely simulates that of many of the rapidly growing cellular hemangiomas of infants, and indeed hamartomatous proliferation of blood vessels as well as of lymphatic vessels may contribute to the overall picture. Nevertheless, the presence of clearly recognizable lymphatic channels and the location of some of the cellular aggregates in regions normally occupied by perineural lymphatics indicate that the lesion is principally lymphatic in origin.

Omental Cysts

Omental cysts are even less common than mesenteric cysts, with which they probably share a common origin. A few, however, may result from inclusions of mesothelium-lined spaces within the omentum rather than from hamartomatous proliferation of lymphatics; rarely, a teratoma or cystic degeneration of a sarcoma may give rise to a cystic lesion in the omentum.[112] Clinically an omental cyst is manifested by progressive abdominal enlargement, which may simulate ascites. Torsion of the cyst may occur with resultant acute abdominal pain; hemorrhage into it is, on occasion, so severe as to be responsible for anemia. The cysts are rounded or lobulated, unilocular or multilocular, and are filled with serous or bloody fluid. Histologically they resemble mesenteric cysts, but the cells lining a unilocular cyst may be so extensively destroyed as to preclude exact determination of the nature of the cyst.

References

1. Kraus M, White H: Congenital tracheoesophageal fistula in the neck without atresia: Report of a case. J Pediatr 51:580–583, 1957.
2. Rehbein F: Oesophageal atresia with double tracheoesophageal fistula. Arch Dis Child 39:138–142, 1964.
3. Shamma'm MH, Benedict EB: Esophageal webs: A report of 58 cases and an attempt at classification. N Engl J Med 259:378–384, 1958.
4. Adler RH: Congenital esophageal webs. J Thorac Cardiovasc Surg 45:175–185, 1963.
5. Bergmann M, Charnas RM: Tracheobronchial rests in the

esophagus: Their relation to some benign strictures and certain types of cancer of the esophagus. J Thorac Surg 35:97–104, 1958.
6. Fonkalsrud EW: Esophageal stenosis due to tracheobronchial remnants. Am J Surg 124:101–103, 1972.
7. Ishida M, Tsuchida Y, Saito S, Tsunoda A.: Congenital esophageal stenosis due to tracheobronchial remnants. J Pediatr Surg 4:339–345, 1969.
8. Kumar R: A case of congenital oesophageal stricture due to a cartilaginous ring. Br J Surg 49:533–534, 1962.
9. Rose JS, Kassner EG, Jurgens KH, Farman J: Congenital oesophageal stricture due to cartilaginous rings. Br J Radiol 48:16–18, 1975.
10. Vargas LL, Britton RC, Goodman EN: Congenital esophageal stenosis: Report of a case of annular muscle hypertrophy at the esophagogastric junction. N Engl J Med 255:1224–1227, 1956.
11. Bonilla KB, Bowers WF: Congenital esophageal stenosis: Pathologic studies following resection. Am J Surg 97:772–776, 1959.
12. Blank E, Michael TD: Muscular hypertrophy of the esophagus: Report of a case with involvement of the entire esophagus. Pediatrics 32:595–598, 1963.
13. Moir JD: Combined duplication of the esophagus and stomach. J Can Assoc Radiol 21:257–262, 1970.
14. Ansell G, Edwards FR: Double oesophagus. J Facul Radiol 9:154–155, 1958.
15. Bremer JL: Dorsal intestinal fistula, accessory neurenteric canal: Diastematomyelia. Arch Pathol 54:132–138, 1952.
16. Warkany J: Congenital Malformations: Notes and comments. Chicago, Year Book Medical Publishers, 1971, pp 700–701.
17. Bentley JFR, Smith JR: Developmental posterior enteric remnants and spinal malformations: The split notochord syndrome. Arch Dis Child 35:76–86, 1960.
18. Gross RE, Neuhauser EBD, Longino LA: Thoracic diverticula which originate from the intestine. Ann Surg 131:363–375, 1950.
19. Beardmore HE, Wiglesworth FW: Vertebral anomalies and alimentary duplications: Clinical and embryological aspects. Pediatr Clin North Am 5:457–474, 1958.
20. Neuhauser EBD, Harris GBC, Berrett A: Roentgenographic features of neurenteric cysts. AJR 79:235–240, 1958.
21. Arey LB: Developmental Anatomy: A Textbook and Laboratory Manual of Embryology, 6th ed. Philadelphia, WB Saunders, 1954, p 244.
22. Smith CA, McKay RJ Jr: Physiology of the newborn infant. In Nelson, WE: Textbook of Pediatrics, 7th ed. Philadelphia, WB Saunders, 1959, pp 286–293.
23. Chang CH, Perrin EV, Bove KE: Pyloric atresia associated with epidermolysis bullosa: Special reference to pathogenesis. Pediatr Pathol 1:449–457, 1983.
24. Wollstein M: Healing of hypertrophic pyloric stenosis after the Fredet-Rammstedt operation. Am J Dis Child 23:511–517, 1922.
25. Belding HH, III, Kernohan JW: A morphologic study of the myenteric plexus and musculature of the pylorus with special reference to the changes in hypertrophic pyloric stenosis. Surg Gynecol Obstet 97:322–334, 1953.
26. Nielsen OS: Histological changes of the pyloric myenteric plexus in infantile pyloric stenosis: Studies on surgical biopsy specimens. Acta Paediatr 45:636–647, 1956.
27. Alarotu H: The histopathologic changes in the myenteric plexus of the pylorus in hypertrophic pyloric stenosis of infants (pylorospasm). Acta Paediatr 45(Suppl 107):1–131, 1956.
28. Ling LL, Ma AC: The pathology and pathogenesis of congenital hypertrophic pyloric stenosis. Chin Med J 78:228–232, 1959.
29. Lane-Roberts PA: Pathology of infantile hypertrophic pyloric stenosis. Proc Roy Soc Med 52:1022–1023, 1959.
30. Friesen SR, Boley JO, Miller DR: The myenteric plexus of the pylorus: Its early normal development and its changes in hypertrophic pyloric stenosis. Surgery 39:21–29, 1956.
31. Wallgren A: Preclinical stage of infantile hypertrophic pyloric stenosis. Am J Dis Child 72:371–376, 1946.
32. Baar HS: Congenital hypertrophic pyloric stenosis. Lancet 2:224, 1951.
33. MacHaffie LP: An early case of congenital pyloric stenosis. Can Med Assoc J 17:946–947, 1927.
34. Martinez NS, Morlock CG, Dockerty MB, et al: Heterotopic pancreatic tissue involving the stomach. Ann Surg 147:1–12, 1958.
35. Krieg EG: Heterotopic pancreatic tissue producing pyloric obstruction. A review and case report. Ann Surg 113:364–370, 1941.
36. MacKinnon D, Nash FW: Pyloric obstruction due to pancreatic heterotopia in a child. Br Med J 1:87–88, 1957.
37. Kernohan RJ, Morison JE: Symptomatic pancreatic heterotopia of the pylorus associated with bilateral renal cortical necrosis in an infant. Arch Dis Child 31:276–278, 1956.
38. Clarke BE: Myoepithelial hamartoma of the gastrointestinal tract: A report of eight cases with comment concerning genesis and nomenclature. Arch Pathol 30:143–152, 1940.
39. Potter EL, Craig JM: Pathology of the Fetus and the Infant, 3rd ed., Chicago, Year Book Medical Publishers, 1975, p 363.
40. Brody H: Ruptured diverticulum in the stomach in a newborn infant associated with congenital membrane occluding the duodenum. Arch Pathol 29:125–128, 1940.
41. Antila LE, Ahvenainen EK: Rupture of the stomach in the newborn infant. Ann Paediatr Fenn 4:49–53, 1958.
42. Vargas LL, Levin SM, Santulli TV: Rupture of the stomach in the newborn infant. Surg Gynecol Obstet 101:417–424, 1955.
43. Moore JB, Chan L: Spontaneous rupture of the stomach in the newborn: A report of two cases. Surgery 42:484–487, 1957.
44. Meyer JL, II: Congenital defect in the musculature of the stomach resulting in spontaneous gastric perforation in the neonatal period: A report of two cases. J Pediatr 51:416–421, 1957.
45. McCormick WF: Rupture of the stomach in children: Review of the literature and a report of seven cases. Arch Pathol 67:416–426, 1959.
46. Snyder WH, Chaffin L: Malrotation of the intestine. Surg Clin North Am 36:1479–1494, 1956.
47. Yunis E, Sieber W, Akers DR: Does zonal aganglionosis really exist? Report of a rare variety of Hirschsprung's disease and review of the literature. Pediatr Pathol 1:33–49, 1983.
48. Richards MR, Hiatt RB: Untoward effects of enemata in congenital megacolon. Pediatrics 12:253–258, 1953.
49. Boyden EA, Cope JG, Bill AH Jr: Anatomy and embryology of congenital intrinsic obstruction of the duodenum. Am J Surg 114:190–201, 1967.
50. Lynn HB, Espinas EE: Intestinal atresia: An attempt to relate location to embryologic processes. Arch Surg 79:357–361, 1959.
51. Shafie ME, Rickham PP: Multiple intestinal atresias. J Pediatr Surg 5:655–659, 1970.
52. Bodian M, White LLR, Carter CO, Louw JH: Congenital duodenal obstruction and mongolism. Br Med J 1:77–78, 1952.
53. Young DG, Wilkinson AW: Abnormalities associated with neonatal duodenal obstruction. Surgery 63:832–836, 1968.
54. Kreipe U: Missbildungen innerer Organe bei Thalidomidembryopathie. Arch Kinderheilk 176:33–61, 1967.
55. Santulli TV, Blanc WA: Congenital atresia of the intestine. Pathogenesis and treatment. Ann Surg 154:939–948, 1961.
56. Bernstein J, Vawter G, Harris GBC, Hillman LS: The occurrence of intestinal atresia in newborns with meconium ileus: The pathogenesis of an acquired anomaly. Am J Dis Child 99:804–818, 1960.
57. Zuelzer WW, Newton WA, Jr.: The pathogenesis of fibrocystic disease of the pancreas: A study of 36 cases with special reference to the pulmonary lesions. Pediatrics 4:53–69, 1949.
58. Donnell GN, Cleland RS: Intestinal atresia or stenosis in the newborn associated with fibrocystic disease of the pancreas. California Med 94:165–170, 1961.
59. Nixon HH: Intestinal obstruction in the newborn. Arch Dis Child 30:13–22, 1955.
60. Gross RE: The Surgery of Infancy and Childhood: Its Principles and Techniques. Philadelphia, WB Saunders, 1953, p 170.
61. Parkkulainen KV: Intrauterine intussusception as a cause of intestinal atresia: A contribution to the etiology of intestinal atresias. Surgery 44:1106–1111, 1958.
62. Murphy DA: Internal hernias in infancy and childhood. Surgery 55:311–316, 1964.
63. Spriggs NI: Congenital intestinal occlusion: An account of twenty-four unpublished cases, with remarks based thereon and upon the literature of the subject. Guy's Hosp Rep 66:143–218, 1912.

64. Feggetter S: Congenital intestinal atresia. Br J Surg 42:378–388, 1955.
65. Kao KJ, Fleischer R, Bradford WD, Woodard BH: Multiple congenital septal atresias of the intestine: Histomorphologic and pathogenetic implications. Pediatr Pathol 1:443–448, 1983.
66. Louw JH, Barnard CN: Congenital intestinal atresia. Observations on its origin. Lancet 2:1065–1067, 1955.
67. Klinefelter EW: Congenital absence of the colon. Am J Dis Child 50:454, 1935.
68. DeSa D: The spectrum of ischemic bowel disease. Perspect Pediatr Pathol 3:273–309, 1976.
69. Bremer JL: Congenital Anomalies of the Viscera: Their Embryological Basis. Cambridge, Harvard University Press, 1957, p 202.
70. Moore KL: The Developing Human: Clinically Oriented Embryology, 4th ed. Philadelphia, WB Saunders, 1988.
71. Kiesewetter WB, Smith JW: Malrotation of the midgut in infancy and childhood. Arch Surg 77:483–490, 1958.
72. Kissane JM: Pathology of Infancy and Childhood, 2nd ed. St. Louis, CV Mosby, 1975, p 198.
73. Grob M: Lehrbuch der Kinderchirurgie. Stuttgart, Georg Thieme Verlag, 1957, pp 336–343.
74. Estrada RL: Anomalies of Intestinal Rotation and Fixation (Including Mesentericoparietal Hernias). Springfield, Ill, Charles C Thomas, 1958, pp 76–97.
75. Waterston D: Hiatus hernia. In Benson C, Mustard WT, Ravitch MM, Snyder WH, Jr, Welch KJ, (eds): Pediatric Surgery, Vol. 1. Chicago, Year Book Medical Publishers, 1962, pp 301–309.
76. Cantrell JR, Haller JA, Ravitch MM: A syndrome of congenital defects involving the abdominal wall, sternum, diaphragm, pericardium and heart. Surg Gynecol Obstet 107:602–614, 1958.
77. Spitz L, Bloom KR, Milner S, Levin SE: Combined anterior abdominal wall, sternal, diaphragmatic, pericardial, and intracardiac defects: A report of five cases and their management. J Pediatr Surg 10:491–496, 1975.
78. Toyama WM: Combined congenital defects of the anterior abdominal wall, sternum, diaphragm, pericardium, and heart: A case report and review of the syndrome. Pediatrics 50:778–792, 1972.
79. Soper SP, Roe LR, Hoyme HE, Clemmons JJ: Trisomy 18 with ectopia cordis, omphalocele, and ventricular septal defect. Pediatr Pathol 5:481–483, 1986.
80. Duhamel B: Embryology of exomphalos and allied malformations. Arch Dis Child 38:142–147, 1963.
81. Kermauner F: Die Missbildungen des Rumpfes. In Schwalbe E (ed.): Die Morphologie der Missbildungen des Menschen und der Tiere. Jena, Gustav Fischer, 1909, vol. 3, pt. 1, pp 41–85.
82. Warkany J, Passarge E, Smith LB: Congenital malformations in autosomal trisomy syndromes. Am J Dis Child 112:502–517, 1966.
83. Söderlund S: Meckel's diverticulum in children. A report of 115 cases. Acta Chir Scandinav 110:261–274, 1956.
84. Gilbert EF, Rainey JR Jr.: Meconium peritonitis caused by a rupture of a Meckel's diverticulum in a newborn infant. J Pediatr 53:597–601, 1958.
85. Hunter WC: Perforated gangrenous Meckel's diverticulum in a new-born infant. Report of a case. Am J Dis Child 35:438–442, 1928.
86. Moore TC: Omphalomesenteric duct anomalies. Surg Gynecol Obstet 103:569–580, 1956.
87. Schwachman H, Pyles CV, Gross RE: Meconium ileus. A clinical study of twenty surviving patients. Am J Dis Child 91:223–244, 1956.
88. Bodian M: Fibrocystic Disease of the Pancreas. A Congenital Disorder of Mucus Production—Mucosis. New York, Grune and Stratton, 1953, p 152.
89. Oppenheimer EH, Esterly JR: Pathology of cystic fibrosis. Review of the literature and comparison with 146 autopsied cases. Perspect Pediatr Pathol 2:241–278, 1975.
90. Hill WB, Mason CC: Prenatal appendicitis with rupture and death. Am J Dis Child 29:86–87, 1925.
91. Shinaberger JH, Tomsovic EJ, Butz WC: Fatal acute appendicitis in a fifteen-day-old infant. J Pediatr 51:422–428, 1957.
92. Potter EL, Craig JM: Pathology of the Fetus and the Infant, 3rd ed. Chicago, Year Book Medical Publishers, 1975, p 367.
93. Waldhausen JA, Herendeen T, King H: Necrotizing colitis of the newborn: Common cause of perforation of the colon. Surgery 54:365–372, 1963.
94. Fonkalsrud EW, Ellis DG, Clatworthy HW Jr: Neonatal peritonitis. J Pediatr Surg 1:227–239, 1966.
95. Roberts DI: Intestinal duplication. Aust NZ J Surg 27:215–218, 1958.
96. Saleeby RG, Zollinger RM, Ellison EH: Acute appendicitis in an adult with two separate vermiform appendices. Surgery 36:306–311, 1954.
97. Nolan JJ, Lee JG: Duplications of the alimentary tract in adults with a report of three cases. Ann Surg 137:342–348, 1953.
98. Stoneman MER: Duplication of the stomach simulating pyloric stenosis. Br Med J 2:781, 1958.
99. Kiesewetter WB: Duplication of the stomach: A case report. Ann Surg 146:990–993, 1957.
100. Ravitch MM. Duplications of the alimentary canal. In Benson CD, Mustard WT, Ravitch MM, et al (eds.): Pediatric Surgery. Vol 2. Chicago, Year Book Medical Publishers, 1962, pp 692–703.
101. Gray AW: Triplication of the large intestine. Arch Pathol 30:1215–1222, 1940.
102. Gross RE, Holcomb GW Jr, Farber S: Duplications of the alimentary tract. Pediatrics 9:449–468, 1952.
103. Burne JC: Pancreatic and gastric heterotopia in a diverticulum of the transverse colon,. J Pathol Bacteriol 75:470–471, 1958.
104. Quan L, Smith DW: The Vater association: Vertebral defects, anal atresia, T-E fistula with esophageal atresia, radial and renal dysplasia: A spectrum of associated defects. J Pediatr 82:104–107, 1973.
105. Bill AH Jr, Johnson RJ: Failure of migration of the rectal opening as the cause for most cases of imperforate anus. Surg Gynecol Obstet 106:643–651, 1958.
106. Johnson TB: Extroversion of the bladder, complicated by the presence of intestinal openings on the surface of the extroverted area. J Anat Physiol 48:89–106, 1913.
107. Zarabi CM, Rupani M: Cloacal exstrophy: A hypothesis on the allantoic origin of the distal midgut. Pediatr Pathol 4:117–124, 1985.
108. Wood K: Lymphatic cysts of the mesentery: A review of the literature and a report of two cases. Br J Surg 43:304–308, 1955.
109. Handelsman JC, Ravitch MM: Chylous cysts of the mesentery in children. Ann Surg 140:185–193, 1954.
110. Bentley JFR, O'Donnell MB: Mesenteric cysts with malrotated intestine. Br Med J 2:223–225, 1959.
111. Moore TC: Congenital cysts of the mesentery: Report of four cases. Ann Surg 145:428–436, 1957.
112. Hastings N, Norris WJ: Unusual abdominal cysts in infants and children. California Med 81:84–86, 1954.

CHAPTER 9

Chemical and Physical Disorders

HARVEY GOLDMAN, M.D.
SANDOR SZABO, M.D.

MECHANISMS OF CELLULAR INJURY

CHEMICAL AND DRUG DISORDERS
Definitions and Classification
Pathogenesis
Physical Events
Toxic Injury
Vascular Lesions
Promotion of Infections
Altered Motility
Foreign Body Deposits
Synergistic Effects
General Pathologic Features
Hemorrhage and Thrombosis
Ulceration
Inflammatory Conditions
Complications
Clinical Features and Diagnosis
Etiologic Agents
Caustic Agents
Ethyl Alcohol
Steroid Hormones
Nonsteroid Anti-inflammatory Drugs (NSAIDs)
Chemotherapeutic and Immunosuppressive Drugs
Antibiotics and Other Antimicrobial Drugs
Antidepressant and Anticholinergic Drugs
Anticoagulant Drugs
Cardiovascular Drugs
Heavy Metals
Enemas and Laxatives
Miscellaneous Drugs
Specific Organ Involvement
Esophagus
Stomach and Duodenum
Jejunum and Ileum
Colon and Rectum

RADIATION EFFECTS AND INJURY
General Aspects
Types of Radiation
Mechanisms of Radiation Injury
Measurements of Radiation
Radiation Sensitivity of the Gastrointestinal Tract
General Pathologic Features
Whole-Body Irradiation
Localized Radiation
Secondary Features
Development of Tumors
Clinical Features
Diagnosis and Differential Diagnosis
Specific Organ Involvement
Esophagus
Stomach
Small Intestine
Colon and Rectum

OTHER PHYSICAL INJURY
Thermal Effects
Trauma

This chapter provides the detailed information on the pathogenesis and morphologic alterations of the gastrointestinal disorders caused by various chemical and physical agents. Included are general concepts, patterns of injury resulting from the many agents, and specific effects on the several components of the gastrointestinal tract. The chapter has been divided into sections dealing with common mechanisms of cellular injury, the chemical and drug disorders, effects of radiation, and other physical conditions. Some of this material is also covered in other parts of the book, including disorders of the esophagus, in Chapter 17; disorders of the stomach, in Chapters 20 and 21; disorders of the intestines, in Chapters 28 and 29; and systemic conditions, in Chapter 16.

There have been extensive investigations of the mechanisms and factors involved in injury due to chemicals, drugs, and radiation. Noteworthy are the concept of gastric cytoprotection,[1-4] the elucidation of the potent actions of free radicals,[5-7] the role of effects on the microcirculation and extracellular matrix components, and the interactions of exogenous agents and gut secretions and microbial flora in the production of disease.[8] A proper understanding of the etiology and pathogenesis of various disorders should help in the construction of appropriate pharmacologic agents that can be used in the prevention and treatment of these diseases. This approach has been successful with other organ systems and will probably improve our knowledge and control of gastrointestinal disorders as well.

MECHANISMS OF CELLULAR INJURY

Most of the deleterious effects of chemicals, drugs, and ionizing radiation are initiated by damage to the mucosal epithelial cells, either direct or mediated by vascular insufficiency. The common factors and mechanisms involved in this injury are summarized in this section. It should be stressed that the steps leading to the lesions do not involve new biochemical reactions, but, rather, are derangements of existing processes. The features are generally nonspecific and occur independent of the particular etiology.[6,7,9]

Oxygen is of central importance in the mechanisms of cell injury. Lack of oxygen causes cell injury (e.g., ischemia); and excess or unused cellular oxygen can be rendered toxic by the generation of free radicals, which are the highly reactive species of oxygen.

Free radicals are chemicals with unpaired electrons and are usually the result of incomplete reduction of oxygen to water. This reaction is normally performed by the mitochondrial electron transport system and catalyzed by cytochrome oxidase. The free radicals can be induced by many chemicals and drugs and by ionizing radiation. The altered reduction of oxygen results in the generation of superoxide and hydrogen peroxide. Interaction of hydrogen peroxide with superoxide or ferrous ions produces hydroxyl radicals, which are probably the most toxic species among free radicals. Hydroxyl radicals alone, but especially in the presence of ferric ions, promote lipid peroxidation or disulfide formation of membrane proteins, leading to the membrane injury and increased permeability and representing the first steps in the cellular damage.

Until recently, lipid peroxidation was regarded as the major mechanism responsible for irreversible cell injury, but it is now accepted that the process is often just a secondary event. In the pathogenesis of gastric mucosal injury caused by ethanol, HCl, NaOH, or aspirin, four biochemical methods revealed virtually no detectable elevation of malondialdehyde, conjugated dienes and trienes, or fluorescent products despite the fact that pretreatment with superoxide dismutase, catalase, and antioxidants decreased the extent of mucosal injury.[6,10] These results were interpreted as indicating that free radicals are involved in the pathogenesis of chemically induced gastric mucosal lesions but that their targets are primarily the structural or enzyme proteins rather than the membrane lipids.

Some of the oxygen radicals contribute to tissue damage indirectly, by causing vascular smooth muscle contraction or through interaction with nitric oxide.[11,12] The resulting ischemia may then be one of the major causes of the ensuing tissue injury and necrosis. Free radicals can also stimulate the synthesis of other potent toxic agents such as hypochlorous acid.[9] It appears that free radicals have a dominant role in the pathogenesis of cell and tissue injury, irrespective of whether it is caused by ischemia, chemicals, or physical agents.

Calcium also exerts a major regulatory role in cell damage. When isolated hepatic or gastric mucosal cells are incubated in the presence or absence of calcium and of toxic concentrations of phalloidin, ethanol, or indomethacin, the viability of cells is much higher in the medium with little or no calcium.[13] After membrane injury by different mechanisms, the influx of calcium from the extracellular medium is a major rate-limiting step. Calcium, however, not only comes from outside the cell but very often is mobilized within the cell; e.g., the endoplasmic reticulum sequestrates calcium in a concentration gradient two or three orders of magnitude larger than the cytoplasm. Calcium may activate enzymes such as phospholipases and calcium-dependent cysteine (thiol) proteases, which then attack the protein component of plasma membrane and other structural or enzyme proteins and initiate or accelerate the membrane damage.

Adenosine triphosphate (ATP) production is related to the functional status of the mitochondria. Selective depletion of ATP or prevention of its synthesis is usually not sufficient to cause severe cell injury. The decrease in ATP production associated with other mitochondrial dysfunction in electron transport and membrane damage, however, will lead to a loss of ion gradients, release of calcium from intracellular stores and influx from extracellular sources, and acceleration of loss of membrane integrity. This is aggravated by glycolysis and intracellular acidification, which are also the consequences of diminished ATP synthesis, followed by alterations in adenosine pool.[14]

Proteases, derived from lysosomes and activated in the cytosol, also have a major role in both cell and tissue injury.[15] These enzymes, released by parenchymal cells or neutrophils that are attracted after initial cell damage, may attack the intracellular and extracellular structural proteins and cell adhesion molecules and activate procollagenase. The proteases are normally controlled by endogenous inhibitors, but the latter can be inactivated by free radicals, which lead to the potentiation of the proteases.

CHEMICAL AND DRUG DISORDERS

Only the toxic effects of chemicals and drugs leading to inflammatory lesions are addressed in this chapter. The roles of chemicals in the initiation and promotion of tumors of the esophagus are discussed in Chapters 18 and 19; of the stomach, in Chapter 25; and of the intestines, in Chapter 32.

Definitions and Classification

There are over 6 million chemicals registered, inorganic and organic as well as naturally occurring and synthetic substances. The number has risen exponentially since the 1940s; this increase was triggered by the discovery of a synthetic process for producing artificial rubber from acrylonitrile and butadiene, which was needed during World War II. As a result, the frequency of lesions due to chemicals and drugs has also dramatically increased and now rivals the occurrences of other injuries such as ischemia and infectious diseases.

It is estimated that about 50,000 chemicals are employed in industry, agriculture, the household, and medicine, including dentistry and veterinary medicine. The Index Medicus lists over 10,000 organic and inorganic chemicals that have been tested in toxicologic and/or pharmacologic evaluations, including 3000 to 4000 drugs.[16] Drugs represent a subgroup of chemicals that are used in medicine for treatment, prevention, and diagnostic tests; and their effects are emphasized in this chapter. About 5% of patients receiving drugs experience some form of adverse reaction,[17] and these account for 5% of hospital admissions.[18] Of all drug injuries noted, 18% to 33% affect one or more portions of the gastrointestinal tract.[19,20]

The actions of chemicals that are not established drugs are observed in persons with a particular addiction (e.g., ethyl alcohol) or after exposure of an accidental, occupational, or suicidal nature. The lesions tend to occur regularly and to have a standard appearance. In contrast, the effects of drugs are more variable, with respect to frequency, mechanism of injury, and type of lesion.

Pathogenesis

The principal ways that a chemical or drug can induce injury of the gut are summarized in Table 9–1. In many situations the specific pathogenic event is not clearly established. This is particularly a problem with drugs that may act either as toxic agents or as mediators of an immunologic reaction. Furthermore, the lesions observed may be due to a combination of the drugs with an underlying condition or with other modes of therapy such as radiation. The intracellular factors and events involved are detailed in the section above on Mechanisms of Cellular Injury. After irreversible cell injury, there ensue necrosis and reactive acute inflammation. Most lesions due to chemicals and drugs undergo complete resolution, after elimination of the offending agent. Repeated exposure, however, can cause the lesions to persist in the form of erosions, ulcers, or chronic inflammatory conditions. Complications are generally uncommon and include fibrous stricture formation, deep mural necrosis leading to perforation, pseudo-obstruction from altered motility, and malabsorption.

Physical Events

Some drugs cause injury by the simple entrapment of a pill or capsule in the mucosa, before it has been dissolved, resulting in a localized ulceration. This is most often noted in the esophagus but can be seen rarely in the stomach and small intestine. It has been observed with emepronium biomide, potassium chloride, barbiturates, tetracycline, and many other antibiotics and drugs (see Esophagus section for details). Obstruction due to a mass of undissolved pills, representing a type of bezoar, can occasionally occur; this is facilitated by the taking of an excessive number of pills and by the presence of narrowed regions of the gut.

Toxic Injury

This is the common mechanism for most chemicals and drugs, with effects ranging from inhibition of cell growth to necrosis. Water-soluble agents typically act directly on the cells, whereas lipid-soluble substances generally operate by the induction of free radicals. The majority of the chemicals and drugs are lipid-soluble and become toxic through metabolic activation. Acetaminophen does not directly damage the liver, but during the metabolic process toxic intermediates are formed that interact with glutathione, the endogenous protective peptide. As the concentration of hepatic glutathione decreases, the toxicity of the drug increases, leading to massive necrosis.[21] The decrease of gastric mucosal glutathione by fasting also seems to contribute to the gastrotoxicity of ethanol, acrylonitrile, nonsteroidal anti-inflammatory drugs (NSAIDs), and stress.[22]

The indirect toxicity of a chemical to the stomach is further illustrated by the example of aspirin. Depending on the acid concentration in the stomach (the pK of aspirin is 3.5), the drug may cause mucosal injury either directly or indirectly. If the gastric pH is 3.5 or higher, most of the aspirin is not dissociated and damages the superficial epithelium directly as a physical agent in crystallized form.[8,23] Injury is caused indirectly if the gastric acidity is below pH 3.5; most of the aspirin is in lipid-soluble form and so is absorbed by the stomach, causing the formation of salicylate, which is a potent mitochondrial poison. In this case, the depletion of mucosal prostaglandins, due to the inhibition of cyclooxygenase, might contribute to the gastrotoxicity, but studies have not revealed a definite correlation between the mucosal levels of prostaglandins and the damaging actions of NSAIDs in the stomach.[8,24] The

Table 9–1 CHEMICAL AND DRUG DISORDERS—PATHOGENETIC MECHANISMS

Physical events
  Pill entrapment in mucosa
  Bezoar
Chemical injury
  Cellular toxicity
  Allergic reaction
Vascular lesions
  Hemorrhage and thrombi
  Vasoconstriction and low perfusion
  Vasculitis
Promotion of infections
Altered motility
Foreign body reactions

pathogenesis of toxic injury in the gastrointestinal tract is complex and involves either direct cytotoxicity by chemicals (e.g., ethanol, HCl, ammonia, bile acids, and aspirin) or indirect actions through the metabolism and release of endogenous tissue and vascular mediators of damage (e.g., free radicals and proteins).

Efforts have been made to distinguish between a direct toxic effect on the tissues and damage that is mediated by an immunologic event. Toxic injuries are characterized by the ability to achieve reproducible lesions in animals, by a dose-related effect with fairly specific timing of the events, and by the development of a standard lesion. In contrast, immunologic injury is typically not a regular and reproducible one: it cannot routinely be induced in animals, it is not dose-related, it has more variable timing, and the lesion produced may differ even within the same host. There is mounting evidence, however, that the majority of chemical and drug lesions are due to direct cytotoxicity or mediated by the release of free radicals or by changes in the local microvasculature. All parts of the gut may be involved; examples include corrosive substances, ethanol, aspirin and other anti-inflammatory agents, and chemotherapeutic drugs.

Vascular Lesions

Vascular lesions include hemorrhages due to treatment with anticoagulants or thrombolytic agents and due to drug-induced thrombocytopenia (see Chapter 16); vasculitis, which can be caused by many drugs and is usually of a generalized nature, with sporadic involvement of the gastrointestinal tract[25]; embolic events in the course of injection treatment of tumors or bleeding disorders[26,27]; vascular thrombosis due to estrogens and progesterones, leading to ischemic lesions[28]; and reduced splanchnic blood flow resulting from the action of vasoconstrictor, hypotensive, and hypovolemic drugs.[29]

Promotion of Infections

Many antibiotics and chemotherapeutic agents can be associated with the development of pseudomembranous colitis, due to the preferential growth of *Clostridium difficile* and elaboration of its toxins. Drugs can also lead rarely to agranulocytosis, favoring the appearance of neutropenic colitis, an infection resulting usually from *Clostridium septicum*, and to a more general immunosuppression, leading to the promotion of numerous opportunistic infections by such agents as herpes virus, cytomegalovirus, *Mycobacterium avium*, fungi, *Giardia*, and *Cryptosporidia* (see Chapters 14 and 26).

Altered Motility

A variety of drugs acting on the nerves, ganglia, and muscles of the gut can interfere with the motility, causing a pseudo-obstruction that is usually dominant in the colon.[30] Examples include anticholinergic, antidepressant, and chemotherapeutic drugs, ganglionic blockers, and narcotics (see Chapter 11).

Foreign Body Deposits

Foreign body deposits are usually due to barium and to oils and are concentrated in the lower colon and rectum[31,32] (see Chapter 28, Figures 28–25 and 28–26).

Synergistic Effects

Many of the patients with advanced tumors receive multiple chemotherapeutic agents and radiation, and the lesions encountered are probably a consequence of the multiple agents and enhanced by the debilitated nature of the patients. Certain drugs such as Adriamycin and actinomycin D are radiomimetic, serving to exaggerate the radiation effects.[33-35] Local, potentially toxic secretions may also act in conjunction with the chemicals and drugs to evoke the lesions; the presence of gastric acid appears to be essential for the full development of lesions due to ethanol and to aspirin.

General Pathologic Features

All of the features noted in chemical and drug disorders are nonspecific, and the diagnosis is dependent on the history and on the exclusion of other conditions. The large variety of lesions involving the several segments of the gut have been compiled and reviewed by Riddell[29] and others.[20,36,37] The types of inflammatory lesions are briefly described here (Table 9–2), and further details are provided in the sections dealing with specific agents and with the parts of the gut involved.

Hemorrhage and Thrombosis

Solitary hemorrhages are typically fresh and concentrated in the mucosa and submucosa. They vary in size from simple streaks to relatively large hematomas, and the bigger lesions can be discerned as projecting lumps on radiographic examination. Hemorrhages are more often seen in conjunction with the inflammatory conditions, particularly in cases of gastritis and duodenitis.

Table 9–2 CHEMICAL AND DRUG DISORDERS—GENERAL PATHOLOGIC FEATURES

Hemorrhages and thromboses

Ulcerations

Inflammatory conditions

Complications
  Perforation
  Stricture

Other features (uncommon)
  Infarction
  Pseudo-obstruction
  Foreign body deposits
  Pneumatosis

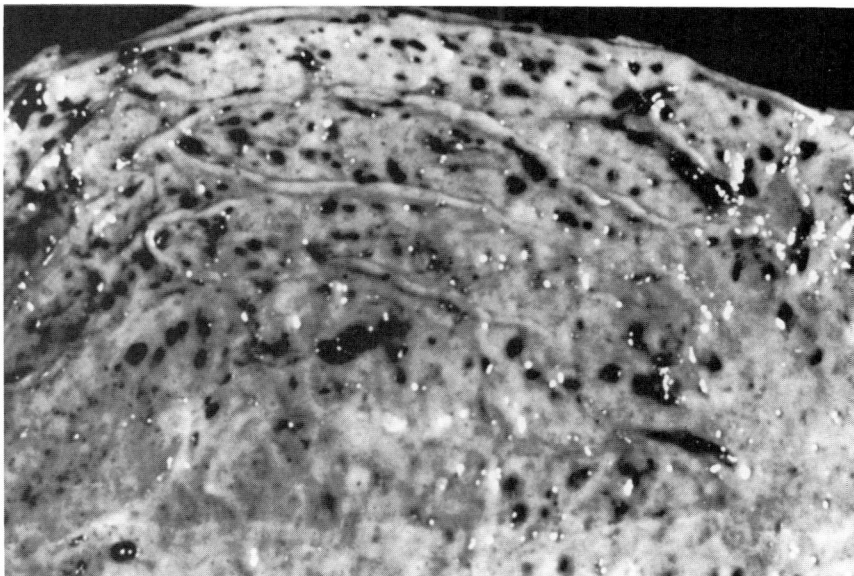

FIGURE 9–1. Mucosal surface of stomach, revealing numerous small and hemorrhagic erosions. This appearance is typical of gastric injury due to ethyl alcohol, aspirin, other NSAIDs, and acute stress ulcers. (Courtesy of Dr. Karoly Balogh, New England Deaconess Hospital, Boston, Mass.)

Venous thrombosis is uncommonly noted in patients receiving estrogens or progesterone; they usually cause local hemorrhages but on occasion can lead to more extensive vascular insufficiency and infarction.

Ulceration

This is a common manifestation of chemical and drug injury and may represent a solitary lesion or be part of a more diffuse inflammatory condition. It can be caused by any of the pathogenetic mechanisms, including physical pressure, cytoxic damage, vasculitis, or infection. The ulcers are usually superficial, and noted are necrosis and a variable amount of acute inflammation. Deeper ulcers and greater inflammation can be seen, especially in cases due to corrosive substances or to chemotherapeutic agents. Drugs can also promote recurrences of chronic peptic ulcers of the stomach and duodenum.

Inflammatory Conditions

This is the typical effect seen with most chemicals and drugs in the gastroduodenal region and in the colon. There is usually a diffuse involvement of the mucosa, with prominent acute inflammation and hemorrhage; erosions and ulcerations are noted in the more severe cases (Figure 9–1). A chronic inflammatory condition is rarely observed with most agents, presumably because the exposure to the drugs is discontinued. It is possible that some of the cases of chronic antral gastritis and chronic duodenitis are due to repeated episodes of injury from ethanol, aspirin, and other anti-inflammatory drugs. The cases affecting the upper tract are typically limited to the mucosa, whereas those in the distal small intestine and colon can be associated with more extensive involvement and simulate cases of ischemic disease and idiopathic inflammatory bowel disease. Rare cases of enteritis and colitis with granulomas have been noted due to naproxen (an anti-inflammatory agent) and to clofazimine (a drug used in the treatment of leprosy).[38,39]

Complications

More extensive necrosis, inflammation, and fibrosis of any part of the gut can be seen in patients who have received combined chemotherapy, alone or in conjunction with radiation, for malignant tumors. Fibrous strictures due to drug reactions are relatively rare but can develop in cases with deeper ulceration. They are seen most often in the esophagus as a result of lye injury and in the distal small intestine related to potassium chloride and exceptionally to anti-inflammatory drugs. Perforation is also uncommon and limited to the cases with extensive caustic damage, to the tumor cases, and to the severe forms of colitis. In patients with tumors, it is usually difficult or impossible to determine which effects are due to the drugs, the radiation, secondary infections, or the underlying condition. Other uncommon features include vascular insufficiency and infarction of the intestines due usually to vasculitis or venous thrombi, pseudo-obstruction from drug damage to the nerves or muscles of the gut, localized deposits of barium and oils, and pneumatosis cystoides intestinalis.

Clinical Features and Diagnosis

The particular clinical features depend on the location of the injury within the gut, on the nature and extent of the lesion, and on the appearance of any complications.[20,29,36] Symptoms in the early stages typically relate to the degree of hemorrhage, ulceration, and inflammation and are identical to those seen in conditions with other causes. Less commonly noted are signs of obstruction due to a fibrous stricture or a motility disorder; malabsorption of fats, vitamin B_{12} or folate; and a more severe form of enteritis or colitis that can mimic ischemic disease, Crohn's disease, and ulcerative colitis. There are no specific features noted on radiographic, gross endoscopic, or histologic examinations; the diagnosis of a chemical or drug injury is reliant on the history. These studies with biopsy are occasionally obtained to exclude other conditions such as recurrent tumor, infections, radiation injury, and the more common inflammatory conditions affecting the gut. Further details are provided in the sections dealing with specific organ involvement.

Etiologic Agents

Considering the huge number of existing chemicals and drugs, it is not feasible to cite all of the reported injuries affecting the gut. Major examples are stressed, and the reader is referred to the extensive reviews on this subject for further details.[20,29,36,37] The material is presented in two parts, with the emphasis on the causative agents and on the general effects in the gastrointestinal tract in this section, and concentration on the diseases involving particular segments of the gut in the next section. Most chemicals and drugs do not uniformly affect the entire gastrointestinal tract. Caustic agents and alcohol, for example, primarily damage the esophagus and stomach. Among the steroid hormones, glucocorticoids in large doses can induce gastric and duodenal ulcers, whereas estrogens and progesterones in oral contraceptives may damage the intestinal tract. All of the NSAIDs cause injury to the stomach and duodenum, but some of the agents can also cause ulcers and strictures of the more distal small intestine. The antibiotics, antineoplastic agents, and vasoactive drugs can injure any part of the tract, although the mechanism of action and nature of the lesions varies in the different regions.

Many drugs of all types can cause a vasculitis.[25] This is typically the result of an immunologic injury, and the vasculitis tends to be generalized or have major effects in the skin, lungs, or kidneys. Involvement of the gastrointestinal tract by drug-induced vasculitis is relatively uncommon. It can lead to areas of ischemic necrosis, usually in the form of focal ulcers and rarely resulting in larger areas of infarction; and the lesions tend to be concentrated in the intestinal tract (see Chapter 12).

Studies of chemical and drug effects have the advantage of quantification. The dose and time of exposure can usually be determined with precision, which permits an elucidation of the pathogenesis and evolution of the lesions. It is also possible to promptly effect treatment by removal of the offending agent, change of the dose, or administration of appropriate antidotes or pharmacologic antagonists in most cases. The categories of the various chemicals and drugs, together with examples of the major alterations in the gut, are summarized in Table 9–3.

Caustic Agents

Caustic agents include strong alkali (lye), acids, and bleaches that are present in common household cleaning products (Table 9–4).[29,40] Injury results from the accidental ingestion of the substances by children or from suicidal efforts, and the lesions are generally confined to the oropharynx, esophagus, or stomach.[41-43] The location and degree of damage depend on the amount, concentration, and nature (whether crystalline or liquid) of the substance as well as the time of exposure. In general, the crystalline products tend to affect the more proximal regions and are promptly expelled, whereas the liquids reach and act throughout the esophagus and stomach. The lesions are in the form of burns, which may be limited to the mucosa and resolve rapidly or, more often, extend into the wall, causing persistent ulceration.[44,45] They reveal necrosis, reactive inflammation, and the formation of granulation tissue and fibrosis in cases with deeper involvement. Early perforation due to transmural involvement is uncommon, whereas the later development of fibrous strictures is a frequent event. Also noted in the esophagus is the rare occurrence of Barrett's esophagus, localized to the strictured area, and an increased incidence of squamous cell carcinoma.[46]

Most of the esophageal cases are due to the liquid alkaline solutions, with effects seen throughout the middle and distal portions. Contraction of the lower sphincter serves to protect the stomach in some instances. The esophageal squamous epithelium appears to be relatively resistant to acids but can be damaged by high concentrations. In contrast, both acids and alkali commonly damage the stomach, with greatest effects in the antral region. The diagnosis of caustic injury is typically afforded by the history, and treatment may include glucocorticoid hormones in an attempt to limit the edema and stricture formation and antibiotics for secondary infections. Additional tests, including endoscopy, are employed to determine the extent of the disease, and the strictures are controlled by luminal dilation or by surgery. Further details are provided in Chapter 17, on esophagitis, and Chapter 20, on gastritis.

Ethyl Alcohol

There is extensive evidence in humans and animal experiments that alcohol can regularly damage the gastric mucosa, causing an acute erosive or nonerosive gastritis[47-49] (see Chapter 20). As a lipid-soluble agent, the alcohol dissolves in and damages the surface epithelial cell membranes, rendering the tissue more permeable to the back diffusion of hydrogen ions.[50,51] The ions, in turn, can cause vasoconstriction of the mucosal microcirculation, promoting larger areas of injury.[52] The lesions are dominant in the antrum but can also involve the corpus of the stomach. Noted are a superficial necrosis, prominent acute inflammation and hemorrhages in the lamina propria, and erosions in most cases (see Figure 9–1). After elimination of the exposure, there is typically a prompt renewal of the mucosa

Table 9–3 EFFECTS OF CHEMICALS AND DRUGS

Category	Examples of Lesions
Caustic agents	Ulcers and strictures of esophagus and stomach Proctitis from enema (hydrogen peroxide)
Ethyl alcohol	Gastritis and duodenitis Mild effects on small intestine Proctitis from accidental enemas
Steroid hormones	
Glucocorticoids	Gastric and duodenal ulcers Promotion of infections
Estrogen and progesterone	Hemorrhage, thrombosis, and ischemia of intestines
Nonsteroid anti-inflammatory drugs	Focal esophageal ulcers from pills Gastritis and duodenitis Focal ulcers and strictures of small intestine Rare colitis and proctitis (suppository)
Chemotherapeutic and immunosuppressive drugs	Ulcers and inflammation of all parts Synergism with radiation (Adriamycin, actinomycin D) Malabsorption (methotrexate, colchicine) Pseudo-obstruction (vincristine)
Antibiotic and antimicrobial drugs	Focal esophageal ulcers from pills Pseudomembranous colitis Malabsorption (neomycin, p-aminosalicylate) Other enteritis and colitis (flucytosine, clofazimine)
Anticholinergic and antidepressant drugs	Pseudo-obstruction
Anticoagulant drugs	Hemorrhages and hematomas
Cardiovascular drugs	Focal esophageal ulcers from pills (quinidine, vasopressin) Gastric and duodenal ulcers (reserpine, ethacrynic acid) Ischemic lesions of intestines (vasoconstrictor, hypovolemic and hypotensive drugs) Malabsorption (methyldopa) Pseudo-obstruction (ganglion blockers)
Heavy metals	Focal esophageal ulcers from pills (iron salts) Gastric ulcers (iron and zinc salts) Enteritis and colitis (gold salts)
Enemas and laxatives	Proctitis from enemas (Fleet, bisacodyl, soaps) Cathartic colon
Miscellaneous drugs	Focal esophageal ulcers from pills Malabsorption and pseudo-obstruction Rare cases of allergic colitis Gastric and ileal ulcers and strictures (KCl) Possible ulcers of stomach and duodenum (bromocriptine, spironolactone) and pneumatosis intestinalis (lactulose and practolol)

and complete recovery within a few days. It is probable that repeated episodes of alcoholic injury can result in chronic antral gastritis, although the evidence is conflicting, with estimates of incidence ranging from 3% to 10% of cases. Alcoholic patients also have an increased prevalence of chronic peptic ulcers of the antrum and duodenum of about 15% to 20%, most cases related to the presence of hepatic cirrhosis and enhanced by shunt procedures[53]; this is believed to be due to reduced inactivation of gastric acid stimulants such as histamine and gastrin by the damaged or shunted liver.

Alcohol can also affect the small intestinal mucosa,[54,55] although the changes are usually mild as a result of lesser exposure in this region, and clinical problems are uncommon. An increase in goblet mucous cells and gastric mucous cell metaplasia, indicative of chronic injury, have been noted in the duodenum. Cases with greater enteritis, in the form of reduced villi, are usually due to associated nutritional problems such as folate deficiency. The lower part of the intestinal tract is ordinarily not involved. Cases of superficial proctitis have been observed following the accidental inclusion of alcohol in enema preparations.[56] The diagnosis of alcoholic injury is typically established by the history, and endoscopic study may be performed to exclude other causes of hemorrhage from the upper gastrointestinal tract.

Table 9–4 CAUSTIC AGENTS

Alkali	Acids
Sodium hydroxide	Hydrochloric acid
Potassium hydroxide	Sulfuric acid
Ammonium hydroxide	Nitric acid
Sodium metasilicate	Phosphoric acid
Sodium perborate	Acetic acid
Potassium monopersulfate	Oxalic acid
Bleaches	Fixatives
Hydrogen peroxide	Formalin
Sodium hypochlorite	Zenker's solution

Steroid Hormones

There has been considerable controversy about the potential toxicity of glucocorticoid hormones in the gastrointestinal tract.[57-59] They probably enhance the recurrence rate of chronic peptic ulcers and worsen the extent of the lesions by retarding the healing process. The hormones can reduce the mucous secretion in the stomach, either directly or by inhibition of the regenerative cells; and the evidence suggests a slight increase of acute gastric and small-intestinal ulcer formation, particularly in the treatment of patients with rheumatoid arthritis.[20,60] It is often difficult, however, to discriminate between the actions of the steroids and those of other medications taken by these patients; and the possibility of additive effects from the drugs exists. The ulcers are usually superficial and promptly reversible, but deeper lesions leading to perforation have been noted, especially in the small intestine.[61] Prolonged use of corticosteroids can also promote the development of secondary opportunistic infections in all parts of the gut. Most often noted are infections due to herpes virus, cytomegalovirus, and fungi; and these infections can worsen an underlying disorder such as peptic ulcers and ulcerative colitis, leading to an increased chance of perforation.

Estrogens and progesterone compounds, including oral contraceptive drugs, can cause ischemic lesions of the small intestine and colon,[28,62-66] although the incidence is probably low. They are more common in older patients, and other risk factors include cigarette smoking and systemic arterial hypertension. The lesions usually develop in persons who have taken at least 0.5 gm of the drug per day for more than 1 year. The drugs cause injury by promoting the formation of thrombi in the mesenteric arteries or veins, leading to segmental areas of hemorrhage or hemorrhagic infarction of the intestines, simulating other causes of ischemic enteritis and colitis or Crohn's disease.[28,67,68] Rarely, the cases show more extensive colonic disease and resemble ulcerative colitis.[69] There is otherwise no definite evidence that these drugs promote recurrences of existing cases of idiopathic inflammatory bowel disease. The lesions are usually reversible after elimination of the drugs; but complications, including fibrous strictures and, rarely, bowel perforations, can occur. The pathologic features are essentially identical to other cases of infarction due to vascular thromboses, and the diagnosis is based on the history. The propensity for thrombosis is more widespread, and the patients may develop lesions in other sites, especially venous thrombi in the legs and pulmonary emboli.

Nonsteroid Anti-inflammatory Drugs (NSAIDs)

These include aspirin (acetylsalicylic acid) and other salicylates, indomethacin, phenylbutazone, and derivatives; and an ever-expanding group of other anti-inflammatory agents that are primarily used in the treatment of patients with rheumatoid arthritis and degenerative joint disease (Table 9-5).[70-73] The major

Table 9-5 EXAMPLES OF NONSTEROID ANTI-INFLAMMATORY DRUGS (NSAIDs)

Alclofenac	Mefanamic acid
Aspirin	Naproxen
Diclofenac	Niflumic acid
Diflunisal	Oxyphenbutazone
Fenoprofen	Phenylbutazone
Floctafenine	Piroxicam
Glafenine	Salsalate
Ibuprofen	Sulindac
Indomethacin	Tolfenamic acid
Ketoprofen	Tolmetin
Meclofenamate	

effects are in the gastric antrum and proximal duodenum in the form of a diffuse hemorrhagic inflammation, erosions and ulcers (Figures 9-2 and 9-3). Furthermore, these drugs can activate the recurrence of a chronic peptic ulcer in this area. Aspirin has been available for the longest time and has been most extensively investigated.[20,29,74-77] Over half of patients presenting with hemorrhage from the upper gastrointestinal tract offer a history of aspirin ingestion; and with chronic use of the drug, there is increasing blood loss, which may exceed ten times the normal amount in the stool. Endoscopic evidence of gastric ulcers has been noted in 20% of cases, erosions in 40%, and mucosal erythema in 75%.[77] Of interest, most of the patients with documented blood loss or abnormal endoscopic findings do not have symptoms. Some patients exhibit a gastric adaptation, characterized by the healing of lesions despite the continued use of aspirin[78]; and it is thought that this might be due to the regeneration of prostaglandins in the tissues.

The anti-inflammatory effect of aspirin, and probably of most of the NSAIDs, is due to the inhibition of cyclooxygenase, leading to reduced prostaglandin synthesis from arachidonic acid. High concentrations of prostaglandins, especially PGE_2 and PGI_2, are present in the normal gastric and duodenal mucosa, where they act to inhibit gastric acid secretion and to increase mucus production. The toxic action of aspirin probably involves multiple factors, including the depletion of mucosal prostaglandins, damage to the membranes of the surface epithelial cells leading to enhanced back-diffusion of hydrogen ions and overall increased membrane permeability, and inhibition of platelet aggregation favoring an increase in bleeding. The back-diffusion is probably a vital component, because the presence of gastric acid is needed to produce the more florid lesions. The presence of other toxic agents such as ethanol and bile salts increase the injury caused by aspirin, whereas the administration of prostaglandins can act to prevent or ameliorate the lesions.

Because of the regularly observed toxicity of aspirin, a large number of alternative analgesic and anti-inflammatory drugs have been introduced and promoted. Buffered forms of aspirin and other salicylate compounds appear to cause less gastric lesions but equivalent damage to the duodenum,[79] whereas the effects of acetaminophen are minimal. The phenylbutazone compounds have been largely discarded because

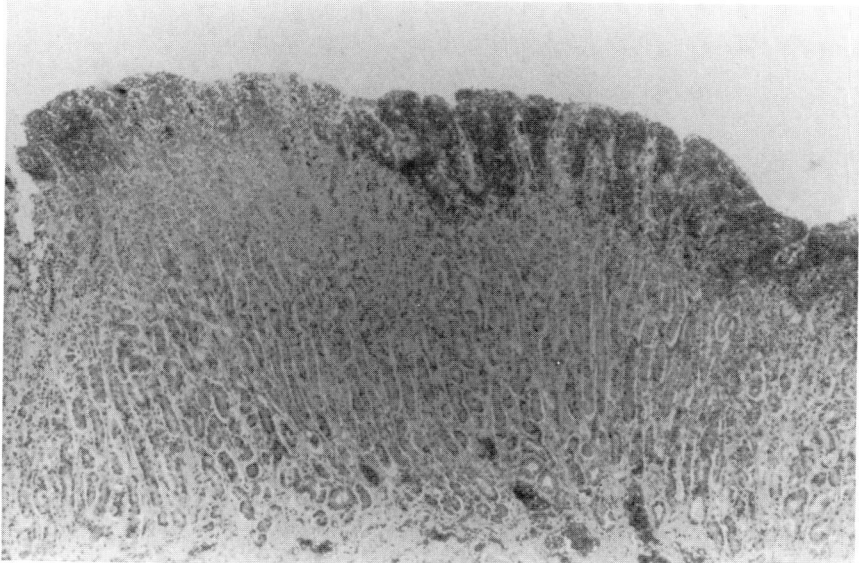

FIGURE 9–2. Gastric corpus mucosa in an early case of aspirin injury, with a fragment of the muscularis mucosae at the bottom. There is fresh hemorrhage limited to the superficial foveolar region, and the corpus glands are normal. (H&E, × 80) (Courtesy of Dr. Karoly Balogh, New England Deaconess Hospital, Boston, Mass.)

of their hematologic as well as gastrointestinal toxicity. Indomethacin and the other NSAIDs have all been shown to cause equivalent lesions in the stomach and duodenum, although the amount of bleeding might be less. It has, therefore, been recommended that none of the NSAIDs should be used as analgesic agents and that the drugs be employed at the minimum dosage to achieve the anti-inflammatory effect.[73] The lesions due to aspirin and the other NSAIDs are similar, revealing superficial necrosis and hemorrhage of the gastric and duodenal mucosa with focal erosions or ulcers and relatively slight inflammation. Indeed, the finding of minimal or no inflammation in the mucosa next to an ulcer helps to identify that the lesion is one primarily caused by a drug, rather than an established chronic peptic ulcer, in which a marked degree of inflammation is invariably present.[80,81] After elimination of the drug, there is typically a prompt recovery with renewal of the mucosa; there is no definite evidence to support that these drugs can cause a chronic gastritis. Further details on the pathology and course of gastritis are provided in Chapter 20, and peptic ulcers are discussed in Chapter 21.

There is mounting evidence that these drugs can cause necrosis and ulceration of the mucosa of the jejunum and ileum, although the exact frequency is not known.[82-85] The pathologic features are generally nonspecific, and most cases are promptly reversible. Perforation from areas of transmural necrosis and strictures from the development of marked submucosal fibrosis are infrequent events. Rare cases have been recorded of enteritis with granulomas due to naproxen[38]; of colitis due to meclofemanate, mefenamic acid, and sulfasalazine[86-88]; and of proctitis secondary to the use

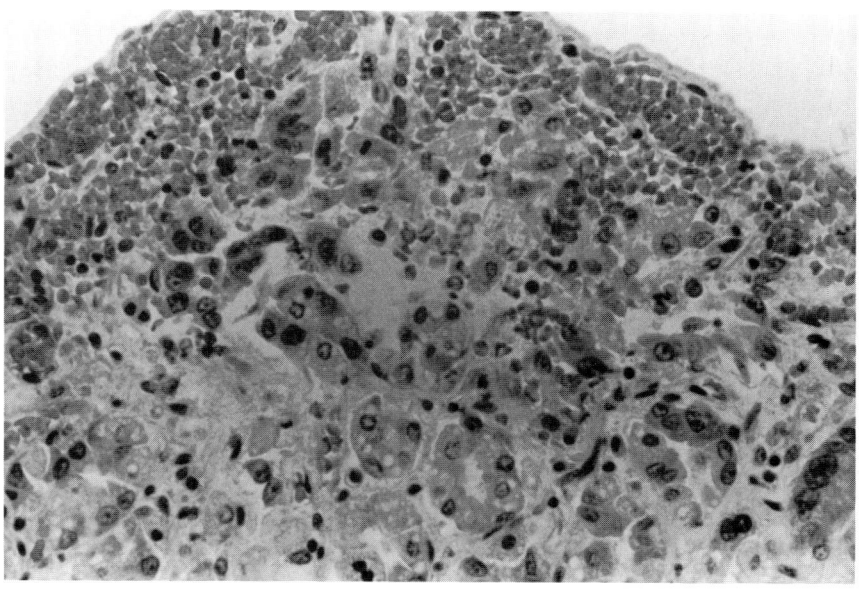

FIGURE 9–3. Same case as in Figure 9–2, with the luminal surface at top, showing the hemorrhage, together with necrosis of the surface and foveolar (pit) epithelial cells. There is minimal inflammation at this early stage. (H&E, × 200) (Courtesy of Dr. Karoly Balogh, New England Deaconess Hospital, Boston, Mass.)

of suppositories containing NSAIDs.[89] Focal ulcers of the esophagus due to the localized entrapment of pills in the mucosa have been noted due to aspirin, indomethacin, phenylbutazone, tolectin, and various compounds containing a mixture of NSAIDs.[90] Overall, the diagnosis of a gut injury due to NSAIDs is primarily determined by the history, and treatment ordinarily consists of stopping the drug or decreasing its amount. Prostaglandins, H_2-blocking agents, and other gastric protective drugs such as sucralfate are occasionally provided to facilitate healing or to lessen the effects of the NSAIDs. Endoscopy with biopsy is often employed to localize the lesion, to determine the extent of the injury, and to monitor the clinical course following the cessation of the drug or a reduction in its dosage.

Chemotherapeutic and Immunosuppressive Drugs

The gastrointestinal tract is regularly affected by the many drugs that are used in the treatment of malignant tumors of the gut and of the other organs and tissues of the body (Table 9–6).[20,29,37,91–94] Some of these drugs are also being used with increasing frequency for immunosuppressive therapy in transplant patients and in patients with advanced inflammatory conditions. Because all of these agents operate primarily by the inhibition of mitotically active cells, the dominant effects are noted in the mucosal epithelial cells throughout every portion of the tract. The toxicity in the individual patient is highly variable and dependent on the number of drugs used and their dosage, the time of exposure, the added effects of radiation therapy and surgery, and the extent of tumor involvement. The major lesions are ulceration and inflammation, with the greatest effects from 5-fluorouracil and its analogues as well as from combinations of drugs. Lesser amounts of injury are observed with some of the agents, such as cyclophosphamide, cisplatin, and daunorubicin.

The small intestinal mucosa is probably the most sensitive region, and a reduction in mitoses and the early ultrastructural signs of cellular injury are seen about 3 hours after exposure to the drugs.[95,96] Noted are clumping of the nuclear chromatin, fragmentation of mitochondria, and dilatation of the endoplasmic reticulum and Golgi region in the villous epithelial cells. The injury becomes maximal after 1 day and persists for the duration of the drug usage. There is usually only patchy damage of the villi in cases treated with single drugs, whereas more extensive injury with ulceration results from the use of combination therapy. There is concomitant regeneration of the epithelial cells, which may appear atypical; and this process persists until the drugs are discontinued. The mucosal epithelial cells are replenished within a few days to 2 weeks, but there can be continued inflammation and vascular dilation with the potential for further bleeding for 3 to 4 weeks.[97,98]

Some of the cases, particularly in the later stages of their diseases, are compounded by the coincident development of ischemia and shock, the additive effects of radiation therapy, the promotion of complicating infections, and the progression of tumor growth.[99] In such instances, it becomes very difficult or impossible to sort out the particular effects of the drugs. An autopsy study revealed ulcerations of the esophagus in 55%, of the stomach in 20%, of the small intestine in 33%, and of the colon in 70%.[97] Multiple lesions were noted in one third of the cases, and commonly present were complicating infections, pneumatosis intestinalis, and ischemic lesions. The infecting organisms are often of the opportunistic type and include *Candida* and other fungi, cytomegalovirus and herpesvirus, *Mycobacterium avium-intracellulare*, *Cryptosporidia*, and *Strongyloides*. Bleeding is frequently observed and is usually due to tumor, to drug or radiation ulcers, or to thrombocytopenia. Bowel perforation can occur and is typically seen in patients with extensive tumor necrosis and in patients receiving glucocorticoid hormones; the latter may be associated with ruptured diverticula, probably related to their thin walls. Fibrous strictures are relatively uncommon and are usually located in the esophagus.

The degree of esophageal injury is relatively large, related to the aggressive treatment of tumors in the thorax, to the limited size of the lumen, and to the frequent combination of drugs and radiation therapy. Adriamycin and actinomycin D inhibit DNA repair and, therefore, greatly enhance the effects of radiation.[33–35,100] These agents exhibit a recall phenomenon, in which the drugs evoke further radiation-type damage after the prior administration of relatively low doses of radiation. Other drugs used that seem to increase the effects of radiotherapy in the esophagus include 5-fluorouracil, bleomycin, hydroxyurea, procarbazine, and vinblastine. After the hepatic arterial infusion of potent drugs such as 5-fluoro-2'-deoxyuridine or of 5-fluorouracil combined with mitomycin C for the treatment of malignant tumors in the liver, in 10% to 50% of the cases prominent necrosis of the stomach and duodenum develops.[101–106] Often present in these cases is a marked atypia of the mucosal epithelial cells, characterized by the presence of enlarged and irregularly hyperchromatic nuclei; and this is distinguished from tumor by the prominent inflammation and the lack of signs of invasion.

A variety of complicating conditions are noted in the colon, including the development of ischemic lesions secondary to shock and thrombosis, of pseudomembranous colitis that is typically the result of antibiotic use, and of neutropenic colitis.[20,99] The last of these occurs in patients that have agranulocytosis and is due to

Table 9–6 EXAMPLES OF CHEMOTHERAPEUTIC DRUGS

Actinomycin D	5-Fluoro-2'-deoxyuridine
Adriamycin	Hydroxyurea
Bleomycin	Methomazine
Cisplatin	Methotrexate
Colchicine	Mitomycin C
Cyclophosphamide	Procarbazine
Cytosine arabinoside	Vinblastine
Daunorubicin	Vincristine
5-Fluorouracil	

a secondary infection with virulent bacteria such as *Clostridium septicum*; the lesions are concentrated in the cecum (typhlitis) and right colon and reveal extensive, often transmural necrosis with the potential for perforation.[107-109] Examples of other effects that have been observed in the intestines are a protein-losing enteropathy from cytosine arabinoside and from combination therapy,[97] a malabsorption syndrome from methotrexate and from colchicine,[110,111] a pseudo-obstruction from vincristine,[112] and a toxic megacolon from methotrexate.[113] There is also an increased prevalence of second tumor development, particularly of malignant lymphomas.[114]

Antibiotics and Other Antimicrobial Drugs

Some patients exhibit prompt intolerance to a variety of antibiotics, particularly erythromycin, in the form of abdominal pain, nausea and vomiting, and occasional diarrhea. This is probably mediated by the nervous or hormonal systems, and signs of mucosal damage are rare. The major injurious effects of antibiotics are pill-induced esophagitis and pseudomembranous colitis, and these are described in the later sections on specific organ involvement. Several drugs can induce vasculitis, including penicillin, ampicillin, tetracycline, isoniazid, and chloramphenicol.[25] Examples of other uncommon events are a malabsorption syndrome due to neomycin, p-aminosalicylate, and some antimalarial agents[20]; a direct toxicity leading to an ulcerative enteritis or colitis from flucytosine,[115] an antifungal drug, and from clofazimine used in the treatment of leprosy[39]; and the lesions of the Stevens-Johnson syndrome in the esophagus due to co-trimoxazole.[116]

Antidepressant and Anticholinergic Drugs

The chronic use of these drugs can retard intestinal motility and prompt the development of a pseudo-obstructive disorder, discussed in the section below on colonic involvement.

Anticoagulant Drugs

Drug-associated gastrointestinal hemorrhage can occur in patients with reduced platelets, a condition usually due to chemotherapeutic agents, and in those receiving thrombolytic therapy; most cases, however, are due to anticoagulants. Although hemorrhages and intramural hematomas have been noted in 30% to 40% of patients taking anticoagulants, the lesions are usually small and asymptomatic. More significant bleeding has been detected in 1.2% of patients taking heparin and 0.2% of those receiving coumadin.[117] They are three to four times more commonly noted in males, and hematomas can occur in any part of the gut.[118] One series of intestinal lesions revealed 9% in the duodenum, 59% in the jejunum, 25% in the ileum, and 7% in the colon.[119] The patients can present with pain; a mass; or signs of obstruction, including blockage of the pancreatic or bile ducts. Massive bleeding is rare. Treatment consists mainly of cessation of the drug or a change in its dose, and surgery is occasionally required for a persistent obstruction.

Cardiovascular Drugs

A large number of drugs used in the treatment of patients with cardiac diseases and that act primarily on vessels can cause damage in the gastrointestinal tract (Table 9-7).[20,29,37,120] The principle mechanisms involved are a sustained vascular spasm, a volume depletion, or hypotension leading to reduced splanchnic blood flow. This can result in the development of ischemic lesions that mainly involve the small intestine and colon, and it is probable that the drug effects are facilitated by the underlying cardiac and vascular disorders. In these instances, it is often difficult to sort out the damage caused by the drugs (e.g., digoxin, diuretics, and antihypertensive medications) from the direct effects of heart failure.[121,122] The lesions are usually observed in elderly patients, the population taking these drugs, and are relatively infrequent. Most often noted are patchy areas of hemorrhage or hemorrhagic infarction that are confined to the mucosa or submucosa; deeper involvement leading to strictures or perforation is rare. Nevertheless, their appearance with hemorrhage can seriously affect the patients who already have significant cardiac disease.

The vasoconstrictive action of vasopressin is greatest in patients that receive the drug in a selective artery for the control of some other cause of bleeding but can also develop after systemic administration.[20,123] The ergot compounds, including ergotamine tartrate and ergonovine, are largely employed in the treatment of migraine. Although they are generally safe, examples of ischemic enteritis and colitis with rare perforations and strictures have been recorded.[124-126] The use of ergot drugs as suppositories can cause localized ulcers of the rectum and anal region, resembling those seen in the solitary rectal ulcer syndrome, but the lesions heal promptly.[127] A variety of other effects from the cardiovascular drugs have been noted. Gastric bleeding has been observed in about 5% of patients receiving ethacrynic acid alone and in 10% of patients when glucocorticosteroids are added.[117] Reserpine is linked to an increased recurrence of chronic peptic ulcers, probably related to enhanced gastric acid production.[29,128] Methyldopa can cause a reversible colitis that is associated with a rash and peripheral eosinophilia and is thought to be an immunologic reaction.[129] Examples of other lesions include pill-induced esophagitis from quinidine and vasopressin,[90] rare cases of vasculitis from several of the drugs,[25] malabsorption from meth-

Table 9-7 EXAMPLES OF CARDIOVASCULAR DRUGS

α-adrenergic blockers	Ganglion blockers
Antihypertensive drugs	Methyldopa
Catecholamines	Methylsergide
Digoxin	Quinidine
Diuretics	Reserpine
Ergot compounds	Vasopressin
Ethacrynic acid	

yldopa,[130] and pseudo-obstruction from ganglionic blocking agents such as pentolinium and hexamethonium.[29,131]

Heavy Metals

The native forms of the metals are inert, but damage to the gastrointestinal tract can infrequently occur due to some of the salts, principally those of iron and gold. The iron compounds, such as ferrous sulfate, appear to cause injury by a physical attachment of the pills to the mucosa, leading to a localized ulceration. These are seen most often in the esophagus[90] and in rare cases involve the stomach[132,133] and the small intestine.[134] Most of the lesions are superficial and promptly reversible, but deeper ulcers resulting in fibrous strictures have been recorded, mainly in the small intestine.

Gold salts are used in the treatment of patients with rheumatoid arthritis, and injuries to the gastrointestinal tract have been noted after both parenteral and oral administration of several medications, including the thiomalate, thiosulfate, thioglucose, thiopropanol sulfate, and triethylphosphine compounds.[135-141] The lesions are rare, only about 30 cases having been reported by 1986; are usually seen in women; and are localized to the small intestine and colon. They typically begin within 3 months after the start of the drug, and the total dosage received by the patients is less than 500 mg. Because of the short exposure, the occasional association with a rash and peripheral eosinophilia, and the response to cromolyn sodium in some cases, the gold injuries are thought to have an allergic basis; but the exact mechanism of the injury is not known.[142] The patient typically presents with abdominal pain, fever, and diarrhea, which can range from watery to hemorrhagic, which probably reflects the severity of the lesions.[138] The pathologic features vary from scattered mucosal petechiae to widespread inflammatory involvement of the small intestine and/or colon, the latter simulating cases of ulcerative colitis.[136] Earlier reports noted a mortality in one quarter of the cases, but this has sharply declined in recent years with the prompt recognition and treatment of the disorder.

Reactions to other metals are rare. Noted have been a gastritis with focal ulcers due to zinc sulfate pills, a foreign body reaction to mercury derived from a broken thermometer in the intestine, and an inflammatory mass of the cecum following intraperitoneal installation of radioactive zirconium phosphate.[29] Bismuth does not cause damage to the gut, but the inclusion of salicylates in some of the proprietary compound products can be injurious.[143]

Enemas and Laxatives

The effects of the various enema solutions and laxatives and the cathartic bowel condition are detailed in Chapter 28. Briefly summarized, laxatives are associated with the increased deposition of macrophages containing a lipofuscin type of pigment in the lamina propria of the colonic mucosa (see Chapter 28, Figures 28-14 and 28-15). When marked, this results in a uniformly dark brown surface and is termed melanosis or pseudomelanosis coli.[144,145] There are no symptoms or other deleterious effects. More extensive use of laxatives, however, can in rare cases cause damage to the muscle and intrinsic nervous tissue of the colon, leading to mucosal atrophy and a marked shortening of the segment, called cathartic colon.[146,147] Most preparatory enemas in current use lead to increased edema fluid in the lamina propria but do not otherwise damage the mucosa.[148] A mild and reversible proctitis has been noted that is due to enemas containing Fleet solution and especially bisacodyl salts[149,150] (see Chapter 28, Figure 28-16), and more marked lesions with the potential for fistulas and perforations have been noted due to cleansing enemas[151,152] and to the accidental inclusion of hydrogen peroxide[153] or ethyl alcohol.[56]

Miscellaneous Drugs

Many other drugs of all types can injure the gastrointestinal tract. These are briefly cited here and further detailed in the sections on specific organ involvement. Enteric-coated potassium chloride pills can cause ulcerations of the esophagus, stomach, and small intestine; and the action is probably due to the localized entrapment of the pills in the mucosa and to the sustained release of the toxic substances from the special capsules.[154-156] Compared with other pills, potassium chloride is more often associated with deeper ulcers leading to fibrous strictures of both the esophagus and the small intestine.[157] As a result of this complication, this particular form of medication is no longer regularly employed. Emepronium bromide, an anticholinergic drug that is commonly employed in England, is one of the more frequent causes of pill-induced esophagitis.[90,157,158] Noted are focal ulcers, and the lesions are generally reversible and rarely lead to complications. Many other drugs can produce similar ulcers of the esophagus because of localized attachment of the pill and injury to the mucosa; and there are isolated reports of the lesions due to barbiturates, chloral hydrate, pantogar, estramustine phosphate, alprenolol chloride, ascorbic acid, and Clinitest tablets.[29] Further details are provided in the section on specific organ involvement in the esophagus.

Other examples of drug damage to the gut are described in the next section, including gastric ulcers from bromocriptine and spironolactone; rare reports of colitis from isoretinonin, cocaine, and penicillamine; malabsorption from phenytoin, clofibrate, and cholestyramine; and a pseudo-obstructive disorder from morphine, clonidine, omeprazole, cimetidine, *Amanita* toxin, and loperamide. Rare cases of pneumatosis intestinalis related to practolol and in a patient with ulcerative colitis receiving lactulose have been recorded, but a definite association has not been established.[29,159]

Specific Organ Involvement

As noted above, most chemicals and drugs can affect multiple portions of the gastrointestinal tract, although the dominant actions may be more restrictive. For each of the gut segments described in this section, the major injuries caused by every subgroup of agents are briefly reviewed, more complete information is provided on the lesions that are concentrated in or peculiar to the region, and the clinical and diagnostic applications are considered. Additional details are available on the esophagus in Chapter 17, the stomach in Chapters 20 and 21, and the intestines in Chapters 28 and 29.

Esophagus

The most common type of drug damage in the esophagus is that resulting from the focal entrapment of a pill in the mucosa, leading to a localized burn and ulceration (Table 9–8).[90,157,158,160-163] This can be caused by a wide variety of drugs, and the only common feature is the relatively large size of many of the pills. Most cases in the United States are caused by antibiotics, whereas emepronium bromide is more often noted in the United Kingdom. Development of the lesions is facilitated by the ingestion of multiple tablets, by the inadequate consumption of liquids, by the taking of the medication in the supine position, and by the presence of cardiomegaly or any intrinsic narrowing of the esophagus. The lesions can involve any part but tend to be concentrated in the lower half, and they usually appear as a single, well-circumscribed ulcer with adjacent edema of the mucosa and without evidence of a more diffuse esophagitis. The patients typically present with burning pain, and dysphagia due to the prominent edema is observed in about 20% of cases. The ulcers can be readily identified by endoscopic study, and the diagnosis is ordinarily established by the finding of residual fragments of the pill, which is uncommon, or simply by the history. The histologic features of the ulcers are entirely nonspecific, revealing necrosis and acute inflammation in the active phase and granulation tissue and regenerative epithelium in the healing stage. Those conditions considered in the differential diagnosis include the common form of peptic esophagitis, which reveals a diffuse inflammation and always involves the distal portion, and other causes of localized ulceration such as infections. Mucosal biopsies of the ulcer edge and intact mucosa can help in identifying the extent of the inflammation and the presence of herpes viral inclusions.[164] Most pill-induced ulcers are superficial and promptly heal, and the occurrence of deeper lesions leading to perforation or to stricture formation is uncommon in the esophagus and usually due to potassium chloride.

The local injection of sclerosing agents has been used recently in the treatment of esophageal varices, particularly in patients with advanced cirrhosis.[20,165-167] Examples of sclerosants used include ethanolamine oleate, polidocanol, and sodium tetra-decyl sulfate. These substances regularly produce vascular thrombi and necrosis, leading to ulceration and fibrosis. A wide variation in the degree of damage has been noted, probably reflecting the strengths of the agents and the experience with the procedure. Persistent ulcers are seen in only 2% to 6% of some series and in 15% to 20% of other cases. Most lesions heal spontaneously, but transmural necrosis and perforation occurs in 1% to 5% of patients and fibrous strictures in 1% to 7%. Other alterations include the presence of mucosal bridges and hematomas as well as the appearance of minor motor abnormalities.

The other causes of chemical and drug injury in the esophagus are much less common and are detailed in the section above on etiologic agents. Included are caustic damage that is mainly from strong alkaline (lye) solutions[29,40]; ulceration from chemotherapeutic drugs such as actinomycin D, Adriamycin, and 5-fluorouracil, often in conjunction with radiation effect and secondary opportunistic infections[33-35,100]; and rare allergic reactions as part of the Stevens-Johnson syndrome, which represents erythema multiforme involving the mucous membranes (e.g., from the antibiotic co-trimoxazole).[116] Injury from most antibiotics, NSAIDs, vasoactive drugs, and inorganic salts, as noted above, is attributed to the direct effects of the pills on the mucosa.

Stomach and Duodenum

The major causes of chemical and drug injury in the stomach and duodenum are ethyl alcohol,[47-49] aspirin,[74-77] indomethacin, and the other NSAIDs.[70-73] These regularly damage the mucosa, leading to hemorrhage and acute inflammation, erosions, and ulcers (Figures 9–1 to 9–3; also, see Chapter 20, Figures 20–2 to 20–4). They also enhance recurrences of chronic peptic ulcers in these regions. The lesions of acute gastritis and duodenitis are confined to the mucosa and promptly heal after cessation of the offending agent. It is possible, however, that some cases of chronic antral gastritis are due to repeated episodes of alcohol- or drug-induced injury. The patients typically present with burning epigastric pain and bleeding, and the diagnosis is ordinarily provided by the history. The differential diagnosis includes other causes of acute or chronic gastritis and duodenitis, principally peptic disease, stress lesions, and *Helicobacter pylori* infection.

Table 9–8 EXAMPLES OF CAUSES OF PILL-INDUCED ESOPHAGITIS

Antibiotics	Miscellaneous drugs
Clindamycin	Alprenolol hydrochloride
Doxycycline	Ascorbic acid
Erythromycin	Barbiturates
Lincomycin	Chloral hydrate
Minocycline	Clinitest tablets
Oxytetracycline	Cromolyn
Penicillin	Emepronium bromide
Tetracycline	Estramustine phosphate
Tinidazole	Ferrous salts
Anti-inflammatory drugs	Pantogar
Aspirin	Potassium chloride
Indomethacin	Quinidine
Phenylbutazone	Vasopressin
Tolmetin	
Combinations	

Modified from Lewis JH: Gastrointestinal injury due to medicinal agents. Am J Gastroenterol 81:819–834, 1986, © by The American College of Gastroenterology.

Endoscopic examination can help to determine the extent of the disease, to identify infectious agents, and to monitor the clinical course.[164] Treatment consists mainly of eliminating the toxic agent and can be facilitated by the use of H_2-blocking drugs, prostaglandins, and other gastric protective medications. Complete details are provided on gastritis in Chapter 20, on stress lesions and peptic ulcers in Chapter 21, and on duodenitis in Chapter 28.

Both corticosteroid hormones and reserpine are associated with an increased frequency and recurrence rate of chronic peptic ulcers.[58,128] Ulcer formation has also been noted in patients with acromegaly who received high doses of bromocriptine and in patients with hepatic cirrhosis treated with spironolactine.[168,169] However, the ulcers may be related instead to the underlying clinical conditions; and the causative effect of these drugs has not been clearly established.[29] The H_2-blocking agents, such as cimetidine and ranitidine, lead to a sustained reduction in gastric acid. Concerns have been expressed about the potential promotion of infections and tumors, but this has not as yet proved to be a problem. During the infusion of chemotherapeutic agents (5-fluorouracil and derivatives) into the hepatic artery for the treatment of malignant tumors in the liver, some of the substances can enter the branches supplying the stomach and duodenum. Lesions occur in 10% to 50% of the cases and consist usually of ulcerations with marked atypia of the epithelial cells and uncommon perforations.[102-107]

Other examples of effects in this region are described in the previous section Etiologic Agents and include caustic injury in the stomach from either strong alkaline solutions or acids[29,40] (also see Chapter 20); hematomas from reduced platelets or anticoagulant drugs[117-119]; bleeding from ethacrynic acid, abetted by corticosteroids[20,117]; and gastric ulcers from ferrous salts, zinc sulfate, and potassium chloride.[29,132,133,154-156] Rarely observed in the stomach are the extension of the sclerosing agents used in the treatment of esophageal varices and the formation of bezoars from sticky substances such as sucralfate and cholestyramine.[20,170]

Jejunum and Ileum

Most of the chemical and drug injuries affecting the small intestine are described in the section Etiologic Agents and are briefly reviewed here. The caustic agents do not ordinarily reach this region, and the effects of ethyl alcohol and most antibiotics are minimal. The prolonged use of corticosteroid hormones favors the development of secondary infections and other ulcers, and one study noted that 10% of small-bowel perforations were related to these drugs.[61] Aspirin and all of the other NSAIDs can damage the mucosa, causing focal ulcers and occasional strictures.[82-85] The small-intestinal mucosa is readily damaged by chemotherapeutic agents, with focal lesions noted from single agents and more extensive damage resulting from combined therapy.[95-98] Furthermore, these cases are often complicated by secondary infections, shock, and tumor growth; and it may be difficult to discern the particular effect of the drug.[99]

Table 9-9 EXAMPLES OF DRUG CAUSES OF MALABSORPTION

Antimalarial drugs	Methotrexate
Cholestyramine	Methyldopa
Clofibrate	Neomycin
Colchicine	p-Aminosalicylate
Diphenylhydantoin	Phenformin
Metformin	

Modified from Lewis JH: Gastrointestinal injury due to medicinal agents. Am J Gastroenterol 81:819-834, 1986, © by The American College of Gastroenterology.

Ischemic lesions can result from vascular thrombi due to estrogens and progesterone compounds,[28,62-66] from vasculitis due to many drugs,[25] and from a variety of agents used in the treatment of vascular and cardiac disorders.[20,29,37,120] The latter consist of vasoconstrictors such as vasopressin and ergots; of digoxin and antiarrhythmia drugs; and of the potential hypovolemic and hypotensive agents, including diuretics and blocking drugs.[121-127] The lesions range from reversible hemorrhages of the mucosa to more extensive infarction of the bowel wall, and it is often difficult to distinguish the drug actions from the effects of the underlying cardiac condition. Most of the ischemic lesions subside without sequelae, and perforations and strictures are relatively infrequent.

A malabsorptive disorder involving fats and vitamin B_{12} or folates has been observed with a variety of drugs (Table 9-9).[20,171] The possible mechanisms involved are a direct injury to the mucosal epithelial cells and a motility derangement favoring the promotion of excess bacteria and bile salt deconjugation, but the actual events are usually not known. The disorder is typically mild and promptly reversible, and chronic effects are not seen. Cyclosporin can cause a transient ileus that is eliminated by reduction of the dosage.[172] Rare cases of granulomatous inflammation have been recorded due to naproxen and to clofazimine.[38,39] Other examples of small-intestinal injury, described above, include hematomas from anticoagulant drugs,[117-119] ulcers and strictures from enteric-coated potassium chloride pills,[154-157] and rare cases of enteritis and colitis due to flucytosine[116] and to gold salts.[135-141]

Colon and Rectum

The most common type of drug damage in the large intestine is pseudomembranous colitis due to antibiotic and other antimicrobial drugs (Table 9-10).[20,29,173,174] Practically all of the antibiotics can be associated with this condition, with the exception of vancomycin and bacitracin. In the early 1950s, severe cases of colitis due to *Staphylococcus aureus* were noted from the use of penicillin, tetracycline, chloramphenicol, and neomycin, particularly in postoperative patients, but this organism has been controlled and is no longer a major problem.[175] The present cases are due to the selective overgrowth of *Clostridium difficile* in the colonic lumen and the effects of its toxins. The precise mechanism is not known and probably involves both the cytotoxic and vasoconstrictive effects of the different toxins. The timing is highly variable, some cases appearing after

Table 9-10 EXAMPLES OF DRUGS THAT CAUSE PSEUDOMEMBRANOUS COLITIS

Ampicillin	Minocycline
Amoxicillin	Nafcillin
Carbenicillin	Neomycin
Cephalosporins	Oxacillin
Chloramphenicol	Oxytetracycline
Chlorpropamide*	Penicillin
Clindamycin	Rifampin
Doxycycline	Streptomycin
Dicloxacillin	Sulfamethoxazale/trimethoprim
Erythromycin	Sulfasalazine*
Gentamicin	Tetracycline
Lincomycin	Ticarcillin
Metronidazole	Tinidazole
Miconazole	

*Nonantibiotic drug.
Modified from Lewis JH: Gastrointestinal injury due to medicinal agents. Am J Gastroenterol 81:819–834, 1986, © by The American College of Gastroenterology.

only a single dose of the drug and about one third occurring after the medicine is stopped. Diarrhea is present in all cases and is associated with colitis and hemorrhage in 20%, and about 30% of the lesions are limited to the right side of the colon.

The characteristic lesions in the colitis cases can be identified at endoscopy, revealing small slightly raised yellow membranes.[176] Biopsies taken from the edges of the early lesions are distinctive, revealing a sharply defined area of extreme acute inflammation (Figure 9–4), whereas examination of older cases show a more diffuse inflammation that is similar to other forms of colitis particularly of ischemic colitis (Figure 9–5).[177–180] The diagnosis is established by a positive assay for the toxin, and treatment consists of removal of the offending drug and the administration in severe cases of vancomycin or metronidazole.[181] Most cases rapidly subside, although recurrences are noted in 20%. More severe examples leading to toxic megacolon have been observed, particularly in older cases before the etiology and therapy were known but also in current cases that are unrecognized or compounded by other conditions (Figures 9–6 and 9–7). These show greater necrosis and extreme edema of the colonic wall and usually require colectomy.[182] The general subject of antibiotic-associated colitis is also discussed in Chapter 26, and the role of secondary C. difficile infection in ulcerative colitis and Crohn's disease is discussed in Chapter 27.[183]

A pseudo-obstructive disorder with major effects in the colon has been noted due to a variety of anticholinergic, antidepressant and other drugs (Table 9–11).[29,30,97,112,131,184–190] These typically occur after prolonged use of the drugs and are thought to be caused by damage to the myenteric plexus or muscles in the colonic wall.[191] This topic is covered in Chapter 11. The other types of colonic damage due to drugs are described in previous sections on etiologic agents and on the jejunum and ileum and are briefly reviewed in this section. Long-term use of corticosteroids can promote secondary infections, such as those caused by herpesvirus and cytomegalovirus in cases of ulcerative colitis; whereas estrogens and progesterone drugs infrequently cause vascular thrombi and ischemic lesions of the small and large intestines that can simulate cases of Crohn's disease and ulcerative colitis.[28,62–69] The NSAIDs do not ordinarily affect the colon, but rare cases of colitis thought to have an allergic basis have been noted due to meclofenamate and mefanamic acid,[86] and proctitis can occur after the use of suppositories containing salicylates.[89] There have been many other isolated reports of colitis that are usually associated with rashes and eosinophilia and considered to be due to an allergic etiology; included are cases due to isoretinonin,[192] penicillamine,[37] methyldopa,[129] clofazimine,[39] and sulfasalazine.[87,88] These allergic cases are generally reversible and do not cause strictures, although severe cases with toxic megacolon have been observed.

Patients receiving chemotherapeutic and immunosuppressive drugs often exhibit colonic lesions that can be due to the primary agents but more frequently are related to other factors, including the development of secondary opportunistic infections, pseudomembra-

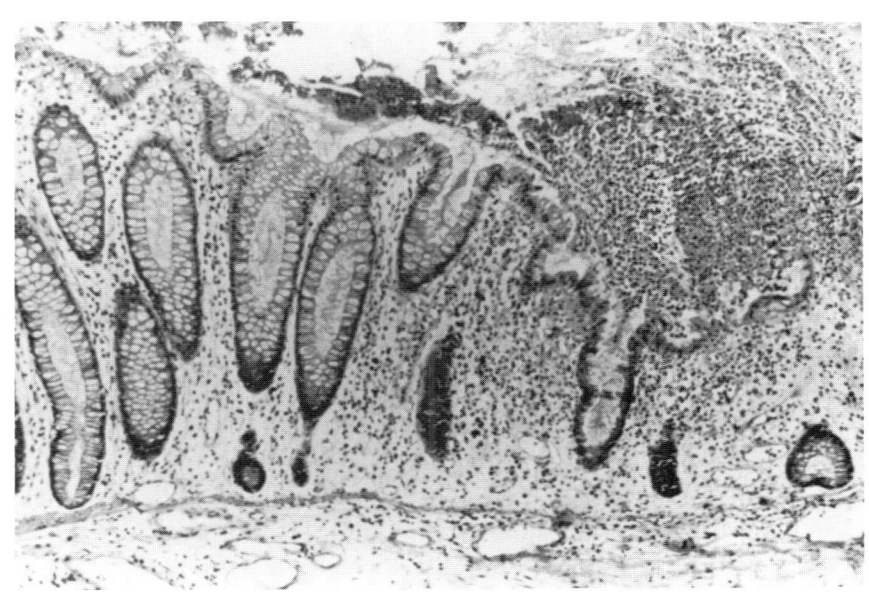

FIGURE 9–4. Colonic mucosal biopsy in a case of antibiotic-associated pseudomembranous colitis, revealing the characteristic early lesion. The biopsy was taken from the edge of a gross membrane and shows the junction of the normal mucosa (on the left) with the exuberant acute inflammation reaction. The latter is concentrated in the superficial part of the mucosa and consists of a massive infiltrate of neutrophils and fibrin in the dilated crypts and on the surface (upper right). The rest of the mucosa and submucosa (at the bottom) is edematous. (H&E. × 80) (From Goldman H, Antonioli DA: Mucosal biopsy of the rectum, colon and distal ileum. Hum Pathol 13:981–1012, 1982.)

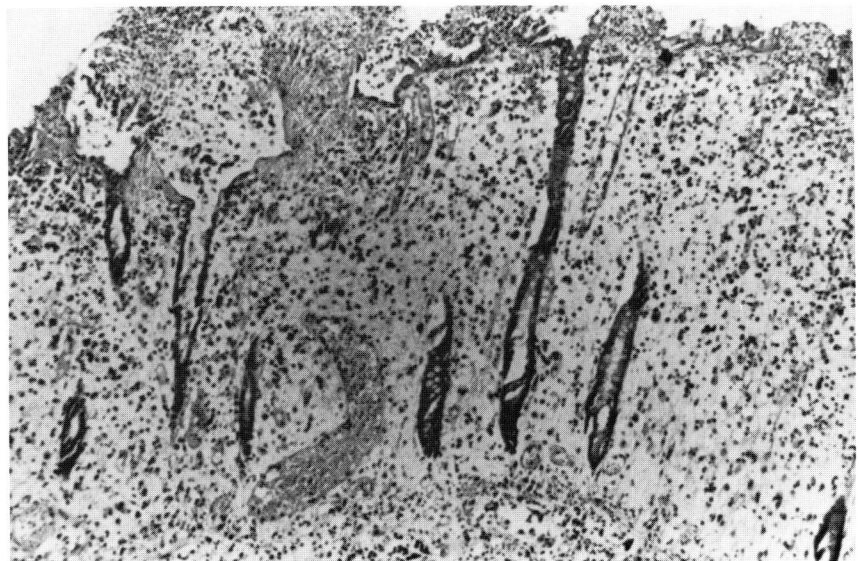

FIGURE 9-5. Colonic mucosa from a later stage of antibiotic-associated pseudomembranous colitis, with the luminal surface at the top. Compared with Figure 9-4, there is more extensive necrosis and inflammation involving the entire mucosa. The surface is diffusely eroded and inflamed. (H&E, × 80) (From Goldman H, Antonioli DA: Mucosal biopsy of the rectum, colon and distal ileum. Hum Pathol 13:981–1012, 1982.)

nous colitis from the concomitant administration of antibiotics, ischemic lesions from thrombi or low perfusion, neutropenic colitis in cases with agranulocytosis, and tumor necrosis.[20,97,99] Indeed, multiple factors are probably involved in many of the lesions.

A marked proctitis resulting from the use of enema solutions containing cleansing agents or the accidental presence of ethyl alcohol and hydrogen peroxide have been described.[56,151–153] The other effects of enemas and laxatives are summarized in the section above on etiologic agents and detailed in Chapter 28.[148–150] Localized reactions to barium and to oils can result in nodule formation usually in the rectum.[31,32] and these are also described in Chapter 28. Other examples of drug damage in the large intestine, described above, include hematomas due to anticoagulants[117–119]; focal ulcers of the rectum and anal region due to suppositories containing ergot compounds[127]; ischemic lesions of the small and large intestines due to other vasoconstrictor, hypovolemic and hypotensive agents[37,120–125]; allergic reactions to gold salts[135–141]; and possibly pneumatosis intestinalis due to lactulose and practolol.[29,159] There are also reports of colitis due to cocaine and to other narcotics that were hidden in the tract but accidentally released, and these may be mediated by a localized vasoconstriction.[193]

RADIATION EFFECTS AND INJURY

Biologic substances tend to decay, which results in the production of less stable atomic nuclei and in the release of radiation energy, either in the form of electromagnetic waves or of particulate matter (Table 9-

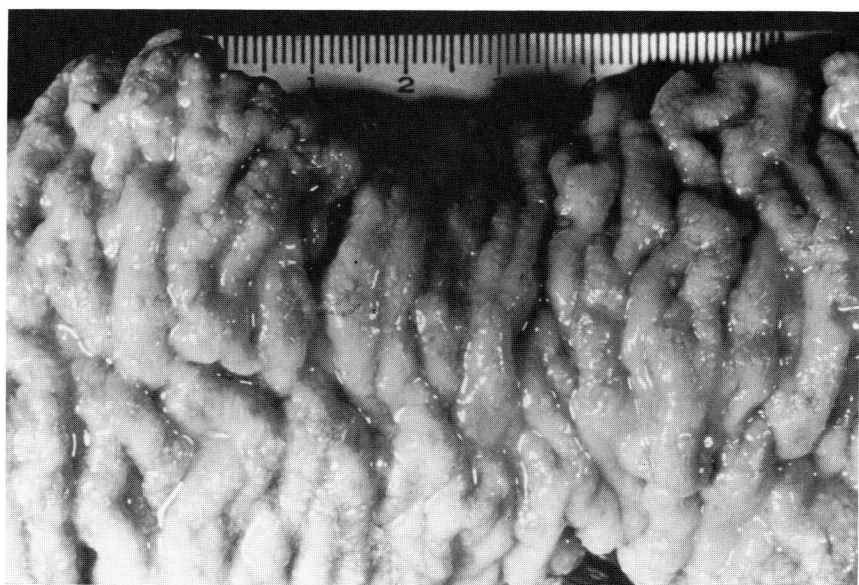

FIGURE 9-6. Mucosal surface of the colon in a case of severe pseudomembranous colitis. There is marked edema, resulting in the appearance of prominent folds, rather than the normal haustra. Scattered throughout are tiny patches of inflammatory membrane.

CHEMICAL AND PHYSICAL DISORDERS 157

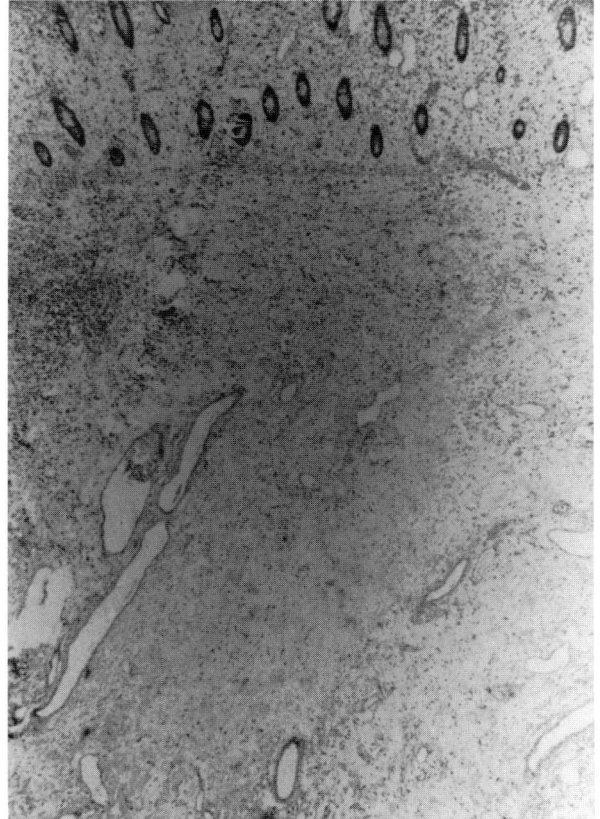

FIGURE 9–7. Same case as in Figure 9–6, with the mucosa at the top. There is marked edema, which greatly expands the submucosa. (H&E, × 31)

Table 9–11 EXAMPLES OF DRUG CAUSES OF PSEUDO-OBSTRUCTION

Anticholinergic drugs	Miscellaneous drugs
Benztropine	Cimetidine
Trihexyphenidyl	Clonidine
Antidepressant drugs	Hexamethonium
Amitriptyline	Loperamide
Chlorpromazine	Methadone
Imipramine	Morphine
Nortriptyline	Omeprazole
Thioridazine	Oxprenolol
Trifluoperazine	Pentolinium
	Vincristine

of the gastrointestinal tract, principally tumors, and also for neoplasms of adjacent structures, including especially the lungs, lymph nodes, genital structures, and urinary bladder.

General Aspects

Types of Radiation

There are two forms of radiation, electromagnetic waves and particles (see Table 9–12). The electromagnetic waves have no mass or electrical charge, and each type has its own wave length and frequency; examples consist of electrical, radio, and light waves; cosmic rays; and gamma rays, including x-rays. They tend to penetrate tissue deeply but generally have low to moderate energy. Radiation particles have mass and variable charges and include beta particles (electrons), protons, alpha particles (helium nuclei), and neutrons. The particles generally exhibit higher energy and less penetration of tissues. The most commonly involved type of radiation is in the form of x-rays, which are low- or moderate-energy photons (i.e., a type of gamma rays) and are characterized by relatively high penetration of tissue, measured as several centimeters to a meter or more. Less frequently involved types of radiation include alpha particles, which are high-energy, slow-moving helium nuclei with low penetration in tissue, typically less than a few millimeters but of high local intensity; and beta particles, which are rapidly moving, moderate- or low-energy electrons with an intermedi-

12). Sources of radiation include cosmic rays, the earth's crust, building materials, and substances within our bodies such as phosphorus in the bones; accidental exposure as a result of occupational hazards and nuclear explosions; and the cummulative effects of diagnostic tests employing radiographic techniques and of radiotherapy.[194,195] The amount of radiation due to background sources has been estimated to be about 0.1 rad per year. By far, the most significant source of radiation leading to potential damage is radiation therapy. Such therapy may be used for various disorders

Table 9–12 TYPES OF RADIATION

Type	Major Source	Atomic			Relative Feature	
		Substance	*Mass*	*Charge*	*Energy*	*Tissue Penetration*
Electromagnetic waves						
Cosmic rays	Background	Photon	0	0	Low to Moderate	Deep
Gamma rays	Isotope	Photon	0	0	Low to Moderate	Deep
X-rays	Machine	Photon	0	0	Low to Moderate	Deep
Particulate matter						
Beta	Isotope	Electron	0.00055	−1	Moderate	Intermediate
Proton	Isotope	Proton	1	+1	Moderate	Intermediate
Alpha	Isotope	Helium nucleus	4	+2	High	Superficial
Neutron	Isotope	Neutron	1	0	High	Superficial

Mechanisms of Radiation Injury

Unlike chemical and biologic agents, there are no structural barriers at the tissue and cellular levels to the penetration of most forms of radiation.[194] There is an initial atomic collision ("direct hit") between the radiation wave or particle and the macromolecules, concentrated in the cellular nuclei, resulting either in the excitation or the ionization (from the release of an electron) of the molecules; and ultimately the energy is dissipated as heat. The released electrons can collide with other molecules ("indirect hit"), causing further damage; some radiation forms such as neutrons act solely by this mechanism. Because most of the body substance is composed of water, there is also extensive ionization and dissociation of its molecules, causing the further production of free radicals, including uncharged hydrogen atoms and hydroxyl groups as well as charged molecules of water and hydrogen peroxide. Most of the effects and injury from radiation are due to the ionization of the various molecules and production of free radicals, leading to a localized chain reaction before the energy is lost. The mechanisms of action of the unstable free radicals are described above in the section Mechanisms of Cellular Injury.

Although all macromolecules within the cells and in the tissues are theoretically targeted by the radiation, the effects on the nuclear DNA are more lasting and produce the greatest damage.[194-196] With the exception of germ cells and lymphocytes, very high doses of radiation (over 10,000 rads) are needed to kill cells that are in interphase. In contrast, the largest effect of radiation occurs during the G_2 (postsynthesis gap) and M (mitotic) phases of the cell cycle and, therefore, is noted in cells that are continually dividing, such as most hematopoietic and epithelial cells. Large tumors that develop hypoxic regions can be rendered more sensitive to radiation by increasing the oxygen supply to such areas; this increased oxygen does not appear to affect the sensitivity of the normal tissues.

Measurements of Radiation

The quantity of radiation to which a patient is exposed can be measured in terms of roentgens (R), with 1 R producing 2.08×10^9 electrons and an equal number of positive charges when passing through and ionizing 1 cm^3 of air. A much more useful and the standard measure of the effect of radiation is in the form of the doses or units of absorption known as rads, where one rad equals 100 ergs of energy absorbed per 1 gm of tissue. Other standards employed include the linear energy transfer (LET), which represents the amount of energy lost or transferred per unit distance that the radiation wave or particle travels, and the relative biologic effectiveness (RBE), which is determined by the particular type and dose of radiation as well as the duration of exposure. The term *rem* is used for comparing the biologic effects of the various radiation types, with the number of rems equal to the number of rads times the RBE. At a practical level, the RBE for x-rays is 1, resulting in an equivalence of rads and rems, whereas the RBE and number of rems is greater for the particulate types of radiation.

Radiation Sensitivity of the Gastrointestinal Tract

During the radiotherapy of tumors, the deleterious effects of radiation on the normal tissues can be restricted by using divided or fractionated doses of no more than 800 to 1000 rads per week. To estimate the potential severity of the radiation, tolerance doses for the various human tissues have been empirically obtained.[197] These are usually expressed as the incidence of toxic damage occurring after 5 years; the dose that would be expected to effect 1% to 5% of persons is termed the "minimum tolerance dose," and that which would effect 25% to 50% of patients by that time is the "maximum tolerance dose." The minimum and maximum tolerance doses that have been calculated for the human gut are 6000 to 7500 in the esophagus, 4500 to 5000 in the stomach, 4500 to 6500 in the small intestines and colon, and 5500 to 8000 in the rectum. These tolerance doses relate mainly to the effects on the more sensitive elements of each of these organs, namely, the epithelia and the vascular endothelial cells. Less appears to be known about the doses for some of the later effects, principally the proliferative vascular changes and tumor induction.[198,199]

The potential for significant tissue injury depends not only on the innate sensitivity but also on the particular dose applied. Consequently, although the esophagus and rectum may seem more resistant, these areas often receive high tumoricidal doses and therefore represent sites of major radiation damage. Furthermore, it has been suggested that the radiation damage may be promoted by a variety of conditions, including prior surgery to the area, poor nutrition, concomitant use of various chemotherapeutic agents, and the presence of pre-existing chronic inflammatory or vascular disorders.[200] Overall, the incidence of significant radiation damage to the gut is not known; with recognition of the tolerance doses for each area and the use of fractionation, it can be kept to the minimum levels.[201] Clearly, the theoretic potential for damage is lessened by the reduced survival of many of the patients with tumors.

General Pathologic Features

As noted above, the principal effects of radiation are due largely to the interactions with the nuclear DNA, especially in dividing cells, resulting either in the stoppage of mitosis and death of the cell or in the production of a mutation.[194,195] These changes can be potentiated by the concomitant administration of radiomimetic drugs such as Adriamycin, actinomycin D, and bleomycin.[33-35] The cellular alterations noted are a simplification of the surface membrane structures, vacuolization of the mitochondria and other cytoplasmic organelles, and aberrations in the chromosomal number and components.[202] Of interest, there may be a delay or latency period between the radiation exposure and the death of the cell, typically seen after doses of under 1000 rads. Also, cells with enlarged nuclei can persist for several weeks; this is presumably due to continued nuclear synthesis but lack of mitoses. There is much less understanding of the mutational events that include the initiation of tumors. It is probable that most of the radiation effects are ameliorated or totally reversed by the actions of reparative enzymes such as nucleases within the cells and by the regeneration of the surviving, unaffected cells; but these built-in protective mechanisms can be overcome by repeated radiation exposure.

The amount of injury relates to the type and potency of the radiation energy as well as to the dose. For a given volume of tissue, the potential for injury is greatest for the alpha particles, intermediate for the beta particles, and least for the gamma rays, including x-rays; however, because the x-rays are capable of greater penetration and represent the principle source of application to human tissues, these are the key cause of radiation damage. There is always some interaction between the radiation and the tissues, and it is useful to separate and classify those changes at a cellular level that are not accompanied by any important tissue or functional derangement as "radiation effect." When there is more significant destruction of tissue with permanent structural and clinical sequelae, it is termed "radiation injury."

Whole-Body Irradiation

For whole-body irradiation in excess of 500 rads, a particular sequence of events involving the gastrointestinal tract has been established.[203,204] There is an initial and transient phase with marked nausea and vomiting, which appears to be attributed to an effect on the central nervous system. This is followed after a few days by significant destruction of the gastrointestinal mucosa as well as the bone marrow elements, leading in most cases to death. The gastrointestinal tract shows extensive destruction and ulceration of the mucosa, and this is a consequence of damage to the generative epithelial cells in all components. With lower doses of total body radiation, the effects are milder and reversible after a few weeks. These are usually seen in patients being prepared for a bone marrow transplant, and the changes are maximal in the small intestinal mucosa which is the most sensitive region of the gut to radiation.

Localized Radiation

The changes noted after localized radiation are separated into early or acute and late or chronic stages, and these are summarized in Table 9-13.[205-209] There is a prompt elimination of the lymphocytes, which are concentrated in the lamina propria of both the small and large intestines; whereas the other inflammatory

Table 9-13 HISTOLOGIC FEATURES OF RADIATION INJURY

Acute (early) features
   Epithelial cell degeneration
   Mucosal and submucosal edema
   Small and reversible ulcerations

Chronic (late) features
   Common
     Telangiectasia
     Atypical fibroblasts
     Submucosal fibrosis
     Large and persistent ulcerations
   Uncommon
     Vascular inflammation and intimal thickening
     Deep mural necrosis and fistulas
     Development of secondary tumors

cells persist. The other early effects are on the mucosal epithelial cells, principally the mitotic cells, and on the vascular endothelial cells.[202,210,211] Initially, these cells show irregular enlargement of their nuclei, with increased chromatin. This leads in the epithelia to reduced maturation and a simplification of the surface epithelial structures, such as blunting of the small intestinal villi. Coincident with the cellular alterations of the endothelial cells, there is a marked increase in permeability resulting in the transfer of edema fluid, mainly into the submucosa. This edematous fluid is often accompanied by large quantities of fibrin. It is interesting that in the stomach, the chief and parietal cells appear to be more sensitive than the mitotic cells in the neck region. Indeed, external irradiation has been used in the past to reduce their content in patients with peptic ulcer disease; unfortunately, this appears to be a transient effect, because the cell population is replenished from the surviving neck mitotic cells. The only gross alterations noted at this early stage are a swelling of the mucosa and submucosa, attributed to the increased vascular permeability, and small areas of ulceration. With relatively low doses of irradiation, all of these early effects appear to be reversible and unassociated with any significant sequelae.[201]

With increasing doses of radiation, there is persistence and extension of the ulcerations, and additional features are noted, including the irregular dilation of the small vessels (telangiectasia) (Figure 9-8); a progressive increase in granulation tissue and collagen formation that is in excess of the amount expected in relation to the inflammatory response (Figure 9-9); and the appearance of fibroblasts with enlarged, irregular, hyperchromatic nuclei, termed atypical fibroblasts (see Chapter 20, Figure 20-25). In some cases, there is also an endothelial inflammation and an increase in muscle and fibroblastic proliferation in the small arteries and veins, leading to narrowing of their lumina (Figure 9-10).[212,213] The other mesenchymal elements and nervous tissue in the gut wall are relatively radioresistant but can be secondarily damaged.[198] The later effects of irradiation consist of progressive changes in the epithelia resulting in atrophy, of increasing fibrosis leading to stricture formation, and of vascular narrowing occasionally associated with thrombosis causing secondary

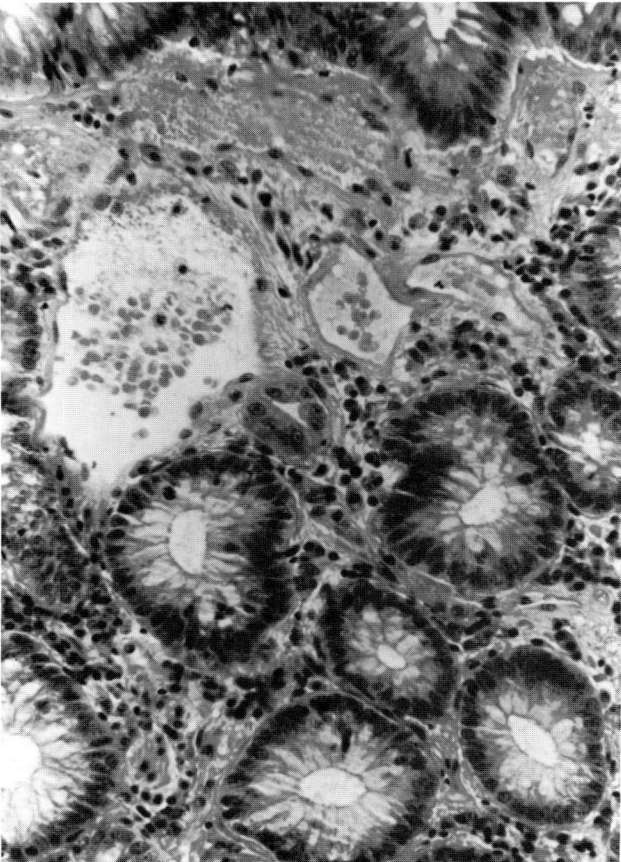

FIGURE 9–8. Colonic mucosal biopsy, with the luminal surface at the top, showing the effects of radiation. Noted are prominent dilation of venules (telangiectasia) and increased fibrous tissue in the superficial part of the lamina propria. There is no increase in inflammatory cells. (H&E, × 200)

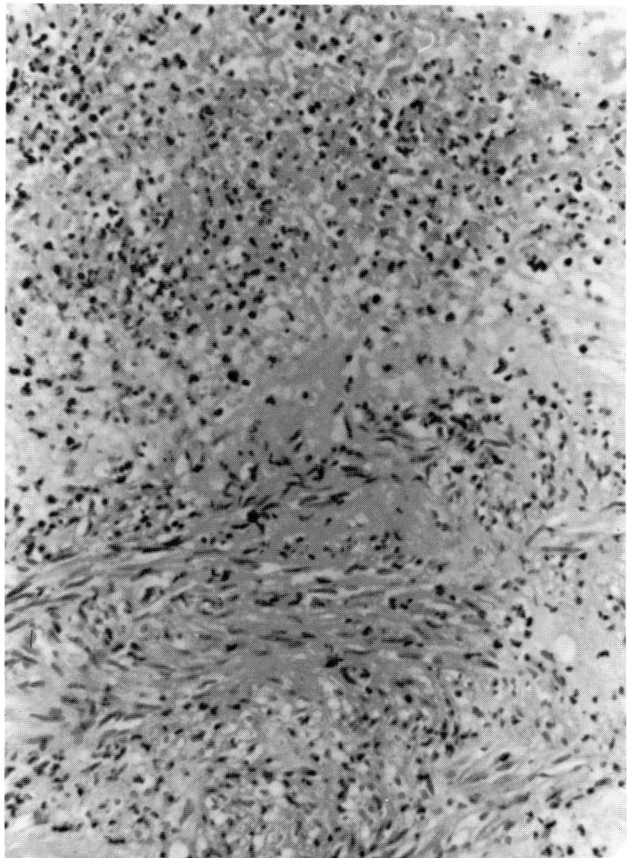

FIGURE 9–9. Section of an ulcer in a case of radiation damage, showing necrosis and acute inflammation in top portion and prominent fibrous tissue at the base of the lesion. (H&E, × 80)

ischemic damage. Grossly, the tissues involved may show narrowings from the strictures, foci of mucosal destruction and ulceration, and secondary areas of ischemic necrosis in the form of localized fistulas or more extensive infarction. These can lead to intestinal obstruction and on rare occasions to focal areas of perforation.

Secondary Features

Many patients with radiation injury are debilitated or immunosuppressed as a result of their underlying tumors and/or the effects of drug and radiation therapy. Therefore, a variety of opportunistic infections may appear in the gastrointestinal tract, due mainly to herpesvirus and cytomegalovirus and to numerous types of fungi and protozoa. Indeed, the overall damage to the gut and the patient may consist of a complex mixture of the effects of chemicals, radiation, and infectious agents; of nutritional deficiencies and metabolic disturbances; and of residual or recurrent tumor.

Development of Tumors

A potential late effect of radiation is the development of a secondary tumor of the epithelial or stromal elements in the gastrointestinal tract.[214–216] This effect is limited by the relatively poor survival of many of the patients due to their primary tumors, especially those of the lungs. Nevertheless, it has been estimated that about 3% of carcinomas appearing in the gut may be a consequence of prior radiation, 2.5% due to natural and accidental radiation exposure and 0.5% related to cumulative diagnostic and therapeutic radiation.[217,218] Indeed, caution has been expressed about the use of repeated radiographic tests in patients with chronic inflammatory disorders of the intestines. The carcinomas tend to occur in sites in which those tumors naturally develop, particularly the colon and rectum; they usually have the same histologic features and appear at the same age as in patients without prior radiation. The tumors can also develop in regions that have not shown significant radiation damage. It was suggested that radiation could induce dysplastic lesions of the epithelium, similar to those seen in ulcerative colitis; but this has not been substantiated.[219,220] Rather, the epithelial changes noted, consisting of irregular glands with mildly hyperchromatic nuclei (Figure 9–11), typically appear early in the course after radiation exposure and are reversible. Overall, the increased risk of neoplasms developing in the gut following radiation appears to be slight and is mainly related to the large intestine, but additional long-term surveillance programs are needed.

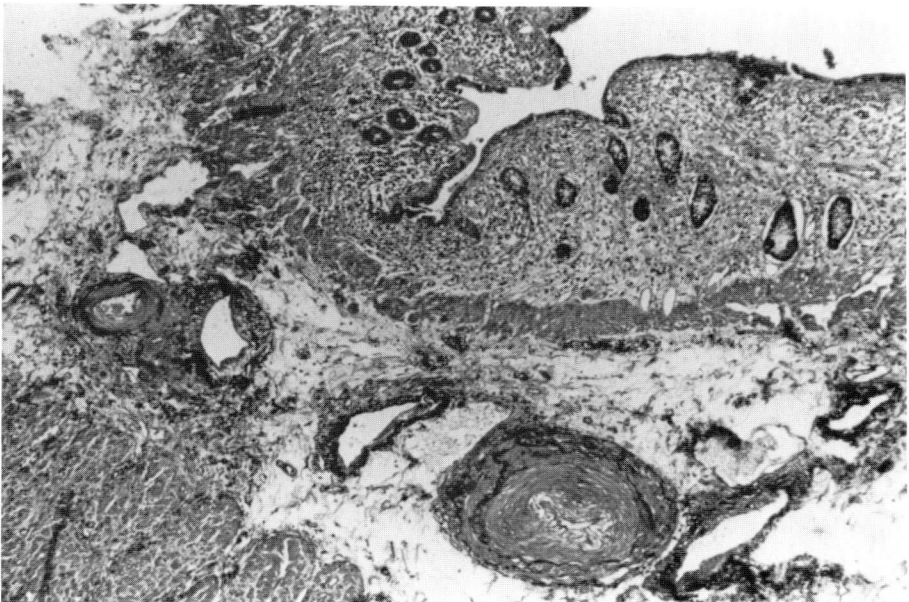

FIGURE 9–10. Section of the colonic wall in a case of radiation colitis. The mucosa at the top is atrophic, and there is an artery with marked narrowing due to fibromuscular proliferation of its intima in the submucosa (lower right). A portion of the muscularis propria is at the lower left. (van Gieson elastic stain, × 31) (Courtesy of Dr. Karoly Balogh, New England Deaconess Hospital, Boston, Mass.)

The exact mechanism by which radiation causes neoplasms is not established. There is considerable support, in humans and experimental animals, for there being direct DNA mutations that are oncogenic.[194] Alternatively, the mutations may favor the activation of viral proto-oncogenes, or the radiation might lead to immunosuppression, thereby fostering the promotion of tumors.

Clinical Features

The presenting symptoms and signs of radiation injury are determined by the particular segment of gut involved and the pathologic stage.[201,221–223] They relate mainly to the presence of luminal obstruction and focal ulcerations and exceptionally to the development of fistulas and perforation. Aside from pain, most often noted are dysphagia with lesions of the esophagus and gastric cardia, abdominal distention and diarrhea with involvement of the intestines, and masses or peritoneal signs in cases of deep mural necrosis. The clinical diagnosis is typically determined by the history, and radiographic tests and endoscopy with biopsy may be employed for purposes of excluding complications of any associated surgery and detecting other disorders, particularly infections and recurrent tumor.[164,180] In addition, in patients with a remote history of radiation, the late complications, including secondary cancers, must be distinguished from the other common inflam-

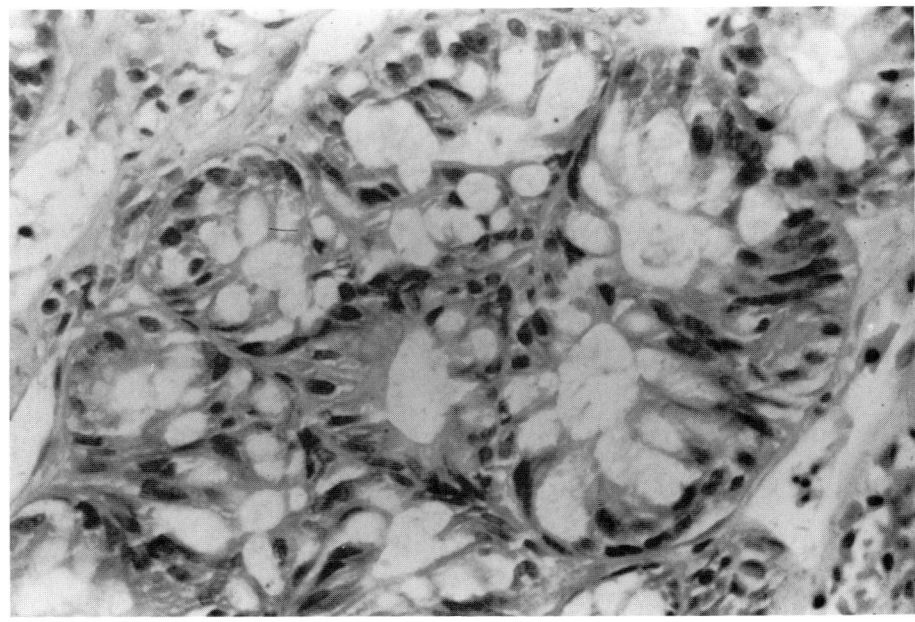

FIGURE 9–11. Colonic mucosal biopsy specimen in a case of radiation colitis, showing a focus of closely packed glands that vary in size and mucin production. The nuclei of the epithelial cells are generally small and lack prominent pleomorphism or hyperchromatism. (H&E, × 200)

matory and neoplastic disorders of the gastrointestinal tract that can occur in any patient.

The treatment is largely supportive and various anti-inflammatory and radioprotective drugs are used.[222,224-228] Endoscopic manipulations and surgery are reserved for cases with permanent fibrotic strictures, fistulas, and deep ulcerations that do not otherwise resolve.[229-231]

Diagnosis and Differential Diagnosis

It should be stressed that all of the features noted in cases of radiation injury are nonspecific. The prominent granulation tissue and fibrosis, atypical fibroblasts, and vascular changes have all been observed in more ordinary wounds.[209] This lack of specificity is compounded, in many instances, by the patient's having an underlying disorder or receiving adjuvant therapy that may lead to some of these alterations, such as mucosal atrophy and ulceration and increasing fibrosis. The diagnosis is secured by noting the combination of the history with compatible morphologic features. In many instances, because radiation therapy was given for a prior tumor, tissue examination is performed to distinguish between the presence of tumor elements and the nonspecific features of radiation damage. In such cases, it is extremely important to appreciate the cellular, particularly the nuclear, alterations that may be seen in the epithelial cells, fibroblasts, and endothelial cells as a consequence of the radiation.[196] This can be especially difficult in small endoscopic biopsies, and great caution must be applied in their assessment. The differential diagnosis of radiation injury includes determination of the presence of residual or recurrent tumor; other causes of mucosal destruction such as concomitant drugs, nutritional problems, or infection; and the coincidental development of ischemic damage, particularly in older patients.

Specific Organ Involvement

Esophagus

Radiation damage to the esophagus typically occurs in patients who have received radiotherapy for tumors of the esophagus and contiguous structures such as the lungs, mediastinal lymph nodes, and thymus.[232-235] Injury and functional effects are common because of the frequent use of radiation therapy for these tumors and the relatively narrow lumen of the esophagus. The early changes consist mainly of submucosal edema and focal, superficial ulcerations, which are largely reversible after several weeks. Radiographic evidence of a chronic narrowing, due to a fibrous stricture and often associated with persistent ulceration, has been noted in up to 30% of the cases.[201,236] Any part of the esophagus can be involved, related to the site of maximal radiation exposure, but the lesions tend to be more common in the proximal and middle thirds because of the greater dependence on radiotherapy for lesions in these areas. Rare complications include the presence of more extensive mural necrosis, the development of fistulas that can extend into the bronchi or aorta, the development of diverticula, and perforation leading to a mediastinitis. The appearance of mucosal bridges, similar to the inflammatory pseudopolyps in patients with chronic colitis, has also been noted; these consist of a core of inflamed lamina propria covered by hyperplastic squamous epithelium.[237]

The diagnosis of radiation-induced esophagitis is primarily dependent on the history and on the exclusion of other disorders. The latter include reflux esophagitis, if the lesion is concentrated in the distal portion; esophagitis due to infections or retained pills, which tend to be more circumscribed; and residual or recurrent tumor. The development of secondary tumors related to the radiation is rare; these are mainly squamous cell carcinomas and appear more than 10 years after the original therapy.[235,238-240] When one considers the small number of cases and the lack of distinguishing features, however, it is difficult to be certain that they are related to the radiation. Alternatively, they may represent *de novo* tumors occurring in a tissue that is prone to carcinoma formation. Support for a radiation causation is provided by noting that the original tumor was not in the esophagus and that there are no other risk factors present, such as a history of excess smoking and ethanol consumption.[235] See Chapters 17 to 19, on the esophagus, for further details.

Stomach

Low-dose irradiation to reduce the parietal and chief cells was formerly used in patients with peptic ulcer disease who were considered poor candidates for surgery.[241,242] The effect is transient and usually reversed by regeneration after a few weeks to months, however. This technique is no longer in vogue; see Chapter 20, on gastritis, for further details. Cases with more extensive radiation damage to the stomach are relatively uncommon, compared with other parts of the gut.[201,243] This relates mainly to the fact that high-dose radiation therapy is infrequently employed for most tumors of the stomach and its contiguous structures. Also, the functional consequences may be less because of the relative spaceousness of the gastric lumen. The types of lesions are standard and include focal ulcerations, which are usually superficial, and fibrous strictures, particularly in naturally narrow regions such as the cardia and pylorus.[244,245] Rarely observed are cases with more extensive mural necrosis, fistulas, and perforation. The diagnosis is based primarily on the history and on the exclusion of other common gastric conditions such as ordinary gastritis, peptic ulcer disease, infections, and recurrent tumor.

Of interest, there is very little information in the literature on secondary, radiation-associated tumors. Primary gastric carcinomas and lymphomas are relatively common lesions, and their occurrence could easily mask the appearance of a radiation-induced lesion. Overall, most of the cases with significant radiation injury to the stomach were recorded many years ago when the therapeutic instruments and techniques were in the developmental stage. With modern procedures, including greater attention to dose and tissue shielding, the occurrence of radiation effects on the stomach has been greatly reduced.[201] This subject is also covered in part in Chapter 20.

Small Intestine

This region is the most sensitive to radiation and the most extensively investigated.[198,222,223,246-252] Because primary malignant neoplasms of the small intestine are rare, excepting lymphomas, most cases of radiation enteritis occur in patients who have undergone radiotherapy for tumors involving the mesentery and retroperitoneum, including lymphomas, germ cell tumors, Wilms' tumor, neuroblastoma, and other mesenchymal lesions. In addition, parts of the mobile small bowel, especially the fixed terminal ileum, can be exposed to radiation given for the pelvic tumors of the genital organs and urinary bladder. A decreasing order of sensitivity from the proximal duodenum to the distal ileum has been claimed,[223] but all regions are subject to damage.[253,254] Predisposing and potentiating factors include the fixation of a segment of intestine, typically a consequence of prior surgery; the concomitant administration of chemotherapy; and the presence of cardiovascular disease, limiting the vascular supply to the gut.[200]

Acute injury to the small intestine following radiation is probably a regular event; but the lesions are usually mild, reversible, and not productive of major clinical problems.[201] The occurrence is dose-dependent, 90% in patients receiving over 3000 rads, 40% in those receiving 1000 to 3000 rads, and 20% in those receiving less than 1000 rads.[210] The very early changes in the small intestinal mucosa were described by Trier et al.[202] Observed within 12 hours after a dose of 2500 to 3000 rads were an inhibition of the epithelial cell mitoses, clumping and enlargement of their nuclei, and shortening of the columnar absorptive cells. Marked villous shortening followed by 7 days, but restitution began by day 14. There was also depletion of the mucosal lymphocytes, whereas the other inflammatory cells persisted. Ultrastructural studies showed shortening of the microvilli, vacuolization of the mitochondria, and nuclear aggregation in the affected epithelial cells. These changes offer an explanation for the transient gastrointestinal symptoms noted in most patients after radiation. Beyond this period, there are usually no further problems; seen in a minority of the cases are small ulcers associated with prominent edema, which can be appreciated on radiographic examination[255]; and more severe involvement during the acute stage is rarely observed.

The development of chronic radiation enteritis is highly variable. It was noted in 5 of 14 (36%) children who had received high doses of radiation, and all of these 5 patients had evident acute disease.[256] Most other series, mainly of adults, have failed to demonstrate any direct relation to prior acute damage, however; and the incidence of chronic disease has varied from 0.5% to 17%, with a general projected average of 5.2%.[200,201] It has also been observed that there can be a considerable and variable delay between the radiation exposure and the appearance of chronic enteritis, ranging from 1 to 6 years[222,246,247]; and it is thought that these changes are principally due to the vascular thickening leading to a localized area of vascular insufficiency. Once the chronic lesion is established, about 40% of cases progress and further complications develop.[257] Most often seen is a localized area of intestinal obstruction, due to a fibrous stricture with overlying ulceration or to peritoneal adhesions, the latter related to prior surgery or radiation damage of the mesentery, or both. Less frequent, occurring in about 15% to 20% of the chronic cases, are fistulas, which usually communicate with another segment of small intestine but can also connect with the colon and other hollow viscera such as the urinary bladder. More extensive infarction and perforation are rarely observed.[258]

A very uncommon finding is persistence of villous loss in the small intestinal mucosa, leading to a prolonged malabsorption disorder.[259-261] Possible causes include persistent damage to the dividing epithelial cells in the crypts, abetted by vascular insufficiency, and a stagnant bowel, favoring the appearance of a bacterial proliferation syndrome. In such cases, the mucosa typically shows a marked shortening, but not a complete loss, of the villi[262]; and the crypts are normal or slightly reduced in height (Figure 9-12). This appearance is in marked contrast to the mucosa in enteritis and malabsorption with other causes, such as ce-

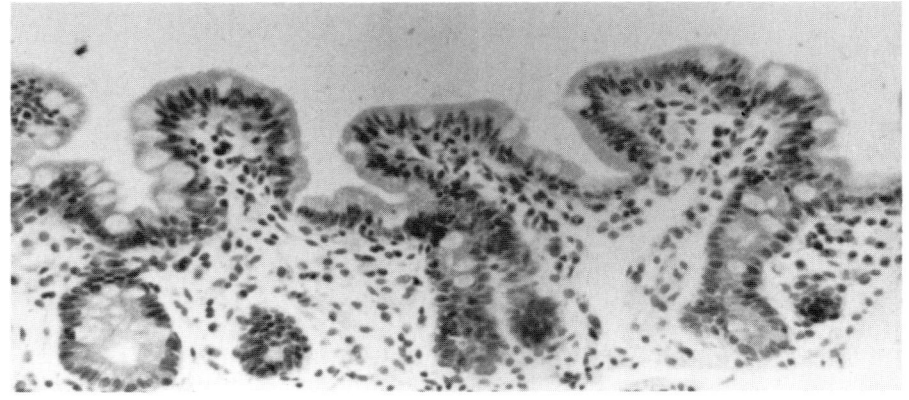

FIGURE 9-12. Jejunal mucosal biopsy specimen showing features of chronic radiation injury, with the luminal surface at the top. There is marked shortening of the villi, and most of the epithelial cells are goblet mucous cells, rather than absorptive cells. The crypts are probably of normal height but reduced in number. Compared with most cases of enteritis due to other causes (e.g., celiac disease), there is a striking absence of crypt hyperplasia. (H&E, × 80)

liac disease, in which there is a prominent, reactive hyperplasia of the crypts. The difference reflects the primary site of the injury, which is the crypts in radiation disease and the villous epithelial cells in celiac disease. The pattern of primary crypt damage is relatively uncommon but has also been observed in vascular insufficiency, some drug injuries, severe nutritional deficiency in infants, and a rare hereditary form of enteritis.[263]

The diagnosis of radiation enteritis is typically established by the history.[200,222,246] Radiography, endoscopy, and biopsy may be required for identification or exclusion of other disorders that can occur in these patients, particularly the effects of drugs, infections, and tumor. As in other parts of the gut, treatment is largely supportive, with surgery reserved for cases with persistent areas of obstruction and fistulas. There does not appear to be any significant increase of small-intestinal tumors following radiation exposure. Further information on radiation enteritis is provided in Chapter 29, on malabsorptive disorders.

Colon and Rectum

Although this region of the gut is relatively radioresistant, the incidence of radiation damage here is the greatest because of the very high doses of radiation employed in the treatment of tumors in this area and the fixed position of the sigmoid colon and rectum.[201,252,264–267] Radiation at moderate doses is used as adjuvant therapy for many rectal carcinomas, but most cases of damage occur instead in patients receiving therapy for tumors of adjacent structures, including the uterus and cervix, prostate, testes, and urinary bladder. After treatment of testicular tumors, damage to the transverse colon was noted in 16% of patients receiving 4500 rads and 37% of those exposed to 6000 rads.[268] Radiotherapy of cervical carcinoma is associated with about a 10% incidence of chronic damage to the large intestine, with rectal lesions seen in half and other colonic involvement in three fourths of the cases.[269]

As in other parts of the gastrointestinal tract, the acute changes at a clinical level, occurring after treatment with 4000 rads or more, tend to be mild and disappear after the therapy is stopped.[201,270] Nevertheless, persistent histologic features were demonstrated in a sequential study of rectal mucosal biopsies taken from patients who received 5000 to 8800 rads for pelvic malignancies.[211] The biopsy specimens obtained during treatment revealed loss of epithelial cell mitoses, enlarged nuclei, and focal fibroblastic proliferation in the lamina propria; the vessels appeared to be normal at this stage. In contrast, biopsy specimens taken after 4 months showed intact epithelial cells, subintimal fibrosis of the arterioles, telangectasia of the capillaries and venules, endothelial cell degeneration, and greater fibrosis of the lamina propria with distortion of the crypts. Further studies are needed to determine whether these persistent alterations at a mucosal level presage the future development of chronic radiation damage. In some cases, the collagen deposition is con-

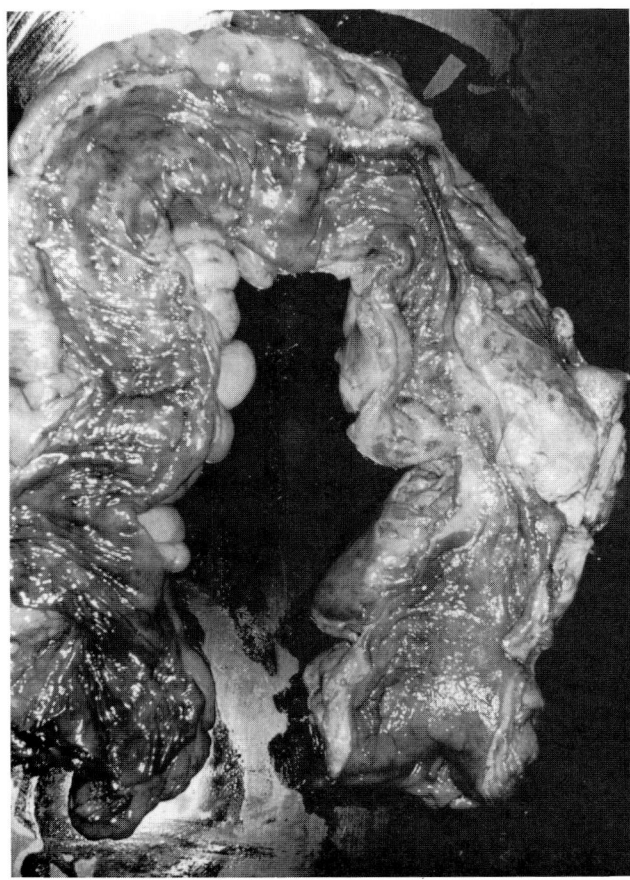

FIGURE 9–13. Colon segment, with a small portion of the attached terminal ileum at the lower left, in a case of radiation colitis. There is a localized fibrotic stricture in the descending colon portion (at the right). (Courtesy of Dr. Karoly Balogh, New England Deaconess Hospital, Boston, Mass.)

centrated in the region beneath the surface epithelium, simulating the lesion noted in collagenous colitis (see Figure 9–8). The crypts may also reveal a marked proliferation mimicking dysplasia, but there is a lack of prominent pleomorphism and hyperchromasia of the epithelial cell nuclei (see Figure 9–11), and the glandular alteration eventually disappears.

Evidence of chronic damage to the colon and rectum is seen in up to 10% of patients who were exposed to high doses of radiation and typically appears after 6 to 12 months. Usually noted is a chronic active colitis limited to the lower colon and rectum or a localized ulcer on the anterior wall of the rectum.[222,270–272] The latter is most often seen after treatment of cervical carcinoma and may be associated with a rectovaginal fistula. Compared with other regions of the gut, obstruction due to an inflammatory or fibrous stricture seems to be less common, occurring in only 1% to 4% of cases (Figure 9–13).[265] Rarely observed are examples of more extensive colitis.[201] The diagnosis is typically provided by the history, and the early edematous features can be well visualized by radiographic examination.[255] Because of the ease of access, endoscopy and biopsies are often obtained and permit exclusion of other disorders, especially infections and recurrent tumor. It may be difficult to distinguish the chronic active colitis seen in the cases of radiation from that noted in chronic ulcerative colitis.[180] In such instances, the findings of patchy involvement, the vacular features, and the increased collagen help to support the diagnosis of radiation colitis or proctitis.[211]

There appears to be an increased risk of carcinoma,[215,218,273-279] and possibly of lymphoma,[280] of the colon and rectum after radiation exposure. This subject has been studied mostly in patients treated for gynecologic malignancies, and the risk factor for carcinoma was estimated to be 2.0 to 3.6.[215] Most cases occur more than 10 years after the radiation, and the tumors are usually in the rectosigmoid region.[215,274] In one study, 58% of the tumors were of the mucinous or colloid type, in contrast to 10% of the tumors unrelated to radiation.[276] This preponderance of mucinous carcinomas has also been seen in patients with chronic ulcerative colitis. Further support for a link between radiation and colon cancer is provided by noting an increase of tumors in persons exposed to atomic explosions and to radium at work.[199,204,218,281,282] Overall, the number of cases due to medical uses of radiation is probably less than 1%, but this becomes significant when one considers that there are almost 150,000 new cases of large-bowel carcinoma each year in the United States. For comparison, the cases of carcinoma complicating ulcerative colitis also constitute about 1% of the total. Accordingly, high-risk groups such as patients who were treated for gynecologic tumors, and possibly for other neoplasms, might be considered candidates for a surveillance program, especially after 10 years. However, the prior development of a dysplastic lesion that can serve to identify patients with early or preinvasive tumors has not been definitely identified in the radiation cases.

OTHER PHYSICAL INJURY

Thermal Effects

Systemic alterations in temperature, in the form of hyperthermia or hypothermia, can be associated with effects on gastrointestinal function, principally on acid secretion and motility. These appear to be mediated by the autonomic nervous system. With prolonged duration, there may ensue those lesions that are usually associated with a stressful situation, including acute stress ulcers of the stomach and duodenum (see Chapter 21) and mucosal areas of hemorrhagic necrosis of the intestines (see Chapter 12); these are probably related to sustained reductions in splanchnic circulation. Most of these effects of systemic temperature alterations are of a transient nature, and there are no long-term or permanent complications.

Local areas of thermal damage to the tissue are noted as a result of freezing or application of lasers. The introduction of freezing solutions into the gastric lumen was formerly tried to reduce acid secretion[283-285] (see Chapter 20), and more recently lasers have been used in an attempt to obliterate sites of mucosal bleeding. In either case, local areas of coagulative necrosis typically confined to the mucosa are seen. When carefully conducted, this is not associated with any deeper areas of necrosis or complications. Because of the highly localized nature of the lesion, there is no potential for any chronic effects.

Trauma

The several segments of the gastrointestinal tract can be injured by blunt trauma or penetrating wounds. Depending on the location and severity of the wounds, possible effects include hematomas, with the potential for obstruction, and perforations, leading to inflammation of adjacent serous cavities or other structures.

Iatrogenic lesions can result from the use of balloons to compress varices, the use of rigid dilators to expand strictured areas, and the use of endoscopy and radiography. Complications due to flexible endoscopy are uncommon, probably because of the superficial nature of the biopsy. Hemorrhage most often occurs in removing polyps with long stalks, and the rare perforations tend to be seen in cases of deep ulcerations (see Chapter 3).

References

1. Robert A: Cytoprotection by prostaglandins. Gastroenterology 77:761–767, 1979.
2. Miller TA, Jacobson ED: Gastrointestinal cytoprotection by prostaglandins: Progress report. Gut 20:75–88, 1979.
3. Wallace JL: Cytoprotection: Define or dispose of it. Dig Dis Sci 31:667–668, 1986.
4. Szabo S: Critical and timely review of the concept of gastric cytoprotection. Acta Physiol Hung 73:115–127, 1989.
5. Szabo S: Biology of disease: Pathogenesis of duodenal ulcer disease. Lab Invest 51:121–147, 1984.
6. Pihan G, Regillo C, Szabo S: Free radicals and lipid peroxidation in ethanol- or aspirin-induced gastric mucosal injury. Dig Dis Sci 32:1395–1401, 1987.
7. Cotran RS, Kumar V, Robbins SL: Robbins' Pathologic Basis of Disease, 4th ed. Philadelphia, WB Saunders, 1989, pp 1–38.
8. Szabo S, Spill WF, Rainaford KD: Non-steroidal anti-inflammatory drug-induced gastropathy: Mechanisms and management. Med Toxicol Adv Drug 4:77–94, 1989.
9. Werns S, Lucchesi BR: Free radicals and ischemic tissue injury. Trans Pharmacol Sci 11:161–166, 1990.
10. Kusterer K, Pihan G, Szabo S: Role of lipid peroxidation in gastric mucosal lesions induced by HCl, NaOH or ischemia. Am J Physiol 252:G811–G816, 1987.
11. Katusic ZS, Vanhoutte PM: Superoxide anion is an endothelium-derived contracting factor. Am J Physiol 257:H33–H37, 1989.
12. McCall TB, Boughton-Smith NK, Palmer RMJ, et al: Synthesis of nitric oxide from L-arginine by neutrophils. Biochem J 261:293–296, 1989.
13. Xu YL, Spill W, Szabo S: Time and temperature-dependent toxicity of indomethacin to isolated gastric mucosal cells. Proc Intl Conf Gastroenterol Biol, Los Angeles, 1988.
14. Mozsik G, Javor T: A biochemical and pharmacological approach to the genesis of ulcer disease: A model study of ethanol-induced injury to gastric mucosa in rats. Dig Dis Sci 33:92–105, 1988.
15. Weiss SJ: Tissue destruction by neutrophils. N Engl J Med 320:365–376, 1989.
16. The Merck Index, 10th ed. Rahway, NJ, Merck and Co, 1983.

17. Jick H, Miettinen OS, Shapiro S, et al: Comprehensive drug surveillance. JAMA 213:1455–1460, 1970.
18. Barr DP: Hazards of modern diagnosis and therapy—the price we pay. JAMA 159:1452–1456, 1967.
19. Benson JA Jr. Gastroenterology reactions to drugs. Am J Dig Dis 16:357–362, 1971.
20. Lewis JH: Gastrointestinal injury due to medicinal agents. Am J Gastroenterol 81:819–834, 1986.
21. Smilkstein MJ, Knapp GL, Kulig KW, et al: Efficacy of oral N-acetylcysteine in the treatment of acetaminophen overdose: Analysis of the national multicenter study (1976 to 1985). N Engl J Med 319:1557–1562, 1988.
22. Dupuy D, Roza A, Szabo S: The role of endogenous nonprotein and protein sulfhydryls in gastric mucosal injury and protection. In Szabo S, Pfeiffer C (eds): Ulcer Disease: New Aspects of Pathogenesis and Pharmacology. Boca Raton, Fla, CRC Press, 1989, pp 421–432.
23. Domschke S, Domschke W: Gastroduodenal damage due to drugs, alcohol and smoking. Clin Gastroenterol 13:405–437, 1984.
24. Taha AS, McLaughlin S, Holland PJ, et al: Effect on gastric and duodenal mucosal prostaglandins of repeated intake of therapeutic doses of naproxen and etodolac in rheumatoid arthritis. Ann Rheum Dis 49:354–358, 1990.
25. McAllister HA Jr, Mullick FG: The cardiovascular system. In Riddell RH (ed): Pathology of Drug-Induced and Toxic Diseases. London, Churchill Livingstone, 1982, pp 207–210.
26. Bradley EL III, Goldman ML: Gastric infarction after therapeutic embolization. Surgery 79:421–424, 1976.
27. Shapiro N, Brandt L, Sprayregan S, et al: Duodenal infarction after therapeutic gelfoam embolization of a bleeding duodenal ulcer. Gastroenterology 80:176–180, 1981.
28. Tedesco FJ, Volpicelli NA, Moore FS: Estrogen- and progesterone-associated colitis: A disorder with clinical and endoscopic features mimicking Crohn's colitis. Gastrointest Endosc 28:247–249, 1982.
29. Riddell RH: The gastrointestinal tract. In Riddell RH (ed): Pathology of Drug-Induced and Toxic Diseases. London, Churchill Livingstone, 1982, pp 515–606.
30. Anuras S, Shirazi SS: Colonic pseudoobstruction. Am J Gastroenterol 79:525–532, 1984.
31. Lewis JW, Kerstein MD, Koss N: Barium granuloma of the rectum: An uncommon complication of barium enema. Ann Surg 181:418–423, 1975.
32. Mazier WP, Sun MK, Robertson WG: Oil-induced granuloma (oleoma) of the rectum: Report of four cases. Dis Colon Rectum 21:292–294, 1978.
33. Hagemann RF, Concannon JP: Mechanism of intestinal radiosensitization by actinomycin D. Br J Radiol 46:302–308, 1973.
34. Phillips TL, Fu KK: Quantification of combined radiation therapy and chemotherapy effects on critical normal tissues. Cancer 37:1186–1200, 1976.
35. Rubin P: Late effects of chemotherapy and radiation therapy. Radiat Oncol Biol Phys 10:5–34, 1984.
36. Cooke AR: Drug damage to the gastroduodenum. In Sleisenger MH, Fordtran JS (eds): Gastrointestinal Disease, 2nd ed. Philadelphia, WB Saunders, 1978, pp 807–826.
37. Fortson WC, Tedesco FJ: Drug-induced colitis: A review. Am J Gastroenterol 79:878–883, 1984.
38. Baas EU, Ewe K, Hohn P: Granulomatose kolitis nach naproxen. Dtsch Med Wochenschr 101:1434, 1976.
39. Karat ABA: Long-term follow-up of clofazimine (Lamprene) in the management of reactive phases of leprosy. Lepr Rev 46(Suppl):105–109, 1975.
40. Loeb PM, Eisenstein AM: Caustic injury to the upper gastrointestinal tract. In Sleisenger MH, Fordtran JS (eds): Gastrointestinal Disease: Pathophysiology, Diagnosis, Management, 4th ed. Philadelphia, WB Saunders, 1989, pp 203–210.
41. Tewfik TL, Schloss MD: Ingestion of lye and other corrosive agents: A study of 86 infants and child cases. J Otolaryngol 9:72–77, 1980.
42. Allen R, Thoshinsky M, Stallone R, et al: Corrosive injuries of the stomach. Arch Surg 100:409–413, 1970.
43. Davis LL, Raffensperger J, Novak GM: Necrosis of the stomach secondary to ingestion of corrosive agents: Report of three cases requiring total gastrectomy. Chest 62:48–51, 1972.
44. Dafoe CS, Ross CA: Acute corrosive oesophagitis. Thorax 24:291–294, 1969.
45. Cello JP, Fogel RP, Boland CR: Liquid caustic ingestion: Spectrum of injury. Arch Intern Med 140:501–504, 1980.
46. Appelqvist P, Salmo M: Lye corrosion carcinoma of the esophagus: A review of 63 cases. Cancer 45:2655–2658, 1980.
47. Wynn-Williams A: Effects of alcohol on gastric mucosa. Br Med J 1:256–259, 1956.
48. Valencia-Parparcen J: Alcoholic gastritis. Clin Gastroenterol 10:389–399, 1981.
49. Laine L, Weinstein WM: Histology of alcoholic hemorrhagic "gastritis": A prospective evaluation. Gastroenterology 94:1254–1262, 1988.
50. Davenport HW: Back diffusion of acid through the gastric mucosa and its physiological consequences. In Glass GBJ (ed): Progress in Gastroenterology. Vol 2. New York, Grune & Stratton, 1970.
51. Smith BM: Permeability of the human gastric mucosa: Alteration by acetylsalicylic acid and ethanol. N Engl J Med 285:716–721, 1971.
52. Szabo S, Pihan G, Trier JS: Alterations in blood vessels during gastric injury and protection. Scand J Gastroenterol 22(Suppl 125):92–96, 1986.
53. Bode JC: Alcohol and the gastrointestinal tract. Adv Intern Med Pediatr 45:1–75, 1980.
54. Gottfried EB, Korsten MA, Lieber CS: Alcohol-induced gastric and duodenal lesions in man. Am J Gastroenterol 70:587–592, 1978.
55. Millan MS, Morris GP, Beck IT, et al: Villous damage induced by suction biopsy and by acute ethanol intake in normal human small intestine. Dig Dis Sci 25:513–525, 1980.
56. Herreiros JM, Munioin MA, Sanchez S, Garrido M: Alcohol-induced colitis. Endoscopy 15:121–122, 1983.
57. Conn HO, Blitzer BL: Nonassociation of adrenocorticosteroid therapy and peptic ulcer. N Engl J Med 294:473–479, 1976.
58. Messer J, Reitman D, Sacks HS, et al: Association of adrenocorticosteroid therapy and peptic ulcer disease. N Engl J Med 309:21–24, 1983.
59. Spiro HM: Is the steroid ulcer a myth? N Engl J Med 309:45–47, 1983.
60. Prillaman WW, Hurst DC, Ball GV, et al: Intestinal complications in rheumatoid arteritis and their relationship to corticosteroid therapy. J Chron Dis 27:475–481, 1974.
61. Remine SG, McIlrath DC: Bowel perforation in steroid-treated patients. Ann Surg 192:581–586, 1980.
62. Kilpatrick ZM, Silverman JF, Betancourt E, et al: Vascular occlusion of the colon and oral contraceptives. N Engl J Med 278:438–440, 1968.
63. Brennan MF, Clarke AM, MacBeth WAAG: Infarction of the midgut associated with oral contraceptives: Report of two cases. N Engl J Med 279:1213–1214, 1969.
64. Cotton PB, Thomas ML: Ischemic colitis and the contraceptive pill. Br Med J 3:27–28, 1971.
65. Bernardino ME, Lawson TL: Discrete colonic ulcers associated with oral contraceptives. Dig Dis Sci 21:503–506, 1976.
66. Hoyle M, Kennedy A, Prior AL, et al: Small bowel ischaemia and infarction in young women taking oral contraceptives and progestational agents. Br J Surg 64:533–537, 1977.
67. Gelfand MD: Ischemic colitis associated with a depot synthetic progesterone. Dig Dis Sci 17:275–277, 1972.
68. Rhodes JM, Cockel R, Allan RN, et al: Colonic Crohn's disease and use of oral contraception. Br Med J 288:595–596, 1984.
69. Bontils S, Hervoir V, Girodet J, et al: Acute spontaneously recovering ulcerating colitis (ARUC): Report of 6 cases. Dig Dis Sci 22:429–436, 1977.
70. Pemberton RE, Strand LJ: A review of upper gastrointestinal effects of the newer non-steroidal anti-inflammatory agents. Dig Dis Sci 24:53–64, 1979.
71. McIntyre RL, Irani MS, Piris J: Histological study of the effects of three anti-inflammatory preparations on the gastric mucosa. J Clin Pathol 34:836–841, 1981.
72. Larkai EN, Smith JL, Lidsky MD, Graham DY: Gastroduodenal mucosa and dyspeptic symptoms in arthritic patients during chronic nonsteroidal anti-inflammatory drug use. Am J Gastroenterol 82:1153–1158, 1987.
73. Graham DY, Smith JL: Gastroduodenal complications of

chronic NSAID therapy. Am J Gastroenterol 83:1081–1084, 1988.
74. Kuiper DH, Overholt BF, Fall DJ, et al: Gastroscopic findings and fecal blood loss following aspirin administration. Am J Dig Dis 14:761–769, 1969.
75. Langman MJS: Epidemiological evidence for the association of aspirin and acute gastrointestinal bleeding. Gut 11:627–634, 1970.
76. Metzger WH, McAdam L, Bluestone R, Guth PH: Acute gastric mucosal injury during continuous or interrupted aspirin ingestion in humans. Am J Dig Dis 21:963–968, 1976.
77. Silvoso GR, Ivey KJ, Butt JH, et al: Incidence of gastric lesions in patients with rheumatic disease on chronic aspirin therapy. Ann Intern Med 91:517–520, 1979.
78. Graham DY, Smith JL, Dobbs SM: Gastric adaptation occurs with aspirin administration in man. Dig Dis Sci, 28:1–6, 1983.
79. Lima MAS: Duodenal ulcers associated with salsalate therapy. Gastrointest Endosc 32:356–357, 1986.
80. McDonald WC: Correlation of mucosal histology and aspirin intake in chronic gastric ulcer. Gastroenterology 65:381–389, 1973.
81. Hamilton SR, Yardley JH: Endoscopic biopsy diagnosis of aspirin-associated chronic gastric ulcers. (Abstract) Gastroenterology 78:1178, 1980.
82. Davies DR, Brightmore T: Idiopathic and drug-induced ulceration of the small intestine. Br J Surg 57:134–139, 1970.
83. Freeman HJ: Sulindac-associated small bowel lesion. J Clin Gastroenterol 8:569–571, 1986.
84. Eliakim R, Ophir M, Rachmilevitz D: Duodenal mucosal injury with nonsteroidal anti-inflammatory drugs. J Clin Gastroenterol 9:395–399, 1987.
85. Bjarnson I, Price AB, Zanelli G, et al: Clinicopathological features of nonsteroidal anti-inflammatory drug-induced small intestinal strictures. Gastroenterology 94:1070–1074, 1988.
86. Doman DB, Goldberg HJ: A case of meclofenamate sodium-induced colitis. Am J Gastroenterol 81:1220–1221, 1986.
87. Schwartz AG, Targan SR, Saxon A, et al: Sulfasalazine-induced exacerbation of ulcerative colitis. N Engl J Med 306:409–412, 1982.
88. Ruppin H, Domschki S: Acute ulcerative colitis—a rare complication of sulfasalazine therapy. Hepatogastroenterology 31:192–193, 1984.
89. Lantheir P, Detry R, Debongnic JL, et al: Solitary rectal lesions due to suppositories containing acetylsalicylic acid and paracetamol. Gastroenterol Clin Biol 11:250–253, 1987.
90. Mason SJ, O'Meara TF: Drug-induced esophagitis. J Clin Gastroenterol 3:115–120, 1981.
91. Floch MH, Hellman L: The effect of 5-fluorouracil in rectal mucosa. Gastroenterology 48:430–437, 1965.
92. Miller SS, Muggia AL, Spiro HM: Colonic histologic changes induced by 5-fluorouracil. Gastroenterology 43:391–399, 1962.
93. Gwavava NJT, Pinkerton CR, Glasgow JFT, et al: Small bowel enterocyte abnormalities caused by methotrexate treatment in acute lymphoblastic leukaemia of childhood. J Clin Pathol 34:790–795, 1981.
94. Cunningham D, Morgan RJ, Mills PR, et al: Functional and structural changes of the human proximal small intestine after cytotoxic therapy. J Clin Pathol 38:265–270, 1985.
95. Trier JS; Morphologic alterations induced by methotrexate in the mucosa of the human proximal intestine. I. Serial observations by light microscopy. Gastroenterology 42:295–305, 1962.
96. Trier JS: Morphologic alterations induced by methotrexate in the mucosa of human proximal intestine. II. Electron microscopic observation. Gastroenterology 43:407–424, 1962.
97. Slavin RE, Dias MA, Sarai R: Cytosine arabinoside induced gastrointestinal toxic alterations in sequential chemotherapeutic protocols: A clinico-pathologic study of 33 patients. Cancer 42:1747–1759, 1978.
98. Mitchell EP, Schein PS: Gastrointestinal toxicity of chemotherapeutic agents. Semin Oncol 9:52–64, 1982.
99. Dosik GM, Luna M, Valdivieso M, et al: Necrotizing colitis in patients with cancer. Am J Med 67:646–656, 1979.
100. Boal DK, Newburger PE, Teele RL: Esophagitis induced by combined radiation and adriamycin. AJR 132:567–570, 1979.
101. Petras RE, Hart WR, Bukowski RM: Gastric epithelial atypia associated with hepatic arterial infusion chemotherapy: Its distinction from early gastric carcinoma. Cancer 56:745–750, 1985.
102. Jewell LD, Fields AL, Murray CJW, Thomson ABR: Erosive gastroduodenitis with marked epithelial atypia after hepatic infusion chemotherapy. Am J Gastroenterol 80:421–424, 1985.
103. Wells JJ, Nostrant TT, Wilson JAP, Gyver JW: Gastroduodenal ulcerations in patients receiving selective hepatic artery infusion chemotherapy. Am J Gastroenterol 80:425–429, 1985.
104. Shike M, Gillin JS, Kemeny N, et al: Severe gastroduodenal ulcerations complicating hepatic artery infusion chemotherapy for metastatic colon cancer. Am J Gastroenterol 81:176–179, 1986.
105. Hirakawa M, Iida M, Aoyagi K, et al: Gastroduodenal lesions after transhepatic arterial chemo-embolization in patients with hepatocellular carcinoma. Am J Gastroenterol 83:837–840, 1988.
106. Schuger L, Peretz T, Goldin E, et al: Duodenal epithelial atypia. A specific complication of hepatic arterial infusion chemotherapy. Cancer 61:663–666, 1988.
107. Wagner ML, Rosenberg HS, Fernbach DJ, et al. Typhlitis: a complication of leukemia in childhood. AJR 109:341–350, 1970.
108. Koep LJ, Peters TG, Starzl TE: Major colonic complications of hepatic transplantation. Dis Colon Rectum 22:218–220, 1979.
109. Ryan ME, Morrissey JF; Typhlitis complicating methimazole-induced agranulocytosis. Gastrointest Endosc 29:299–302, 1983.
110. Craft AW, Kay HEM, Lawson DM, et al: Methotrexate-induced malabsorption in children with acute lymphoblastic leukemia. Br Med J 4:1511–1512, 1977.
111. Race TF, Paes IC, Faloon WW: Intestinal malabsorption induced by oral colchicine: Comparison with neomycin and cathartic agents. Am J Med Sci 259:32–41, 1970.
112. Sandler SG, Tobin W, Henderson ES: Vincristine-induced neuropathy: A clinical study of fifty leukemic patients. Neurology 19:367–374, 1969.
113. Atherton LD, Leib ES, Kaye MD: Toxic megacolon associated with methotrexate therapy. Gastroenterology 86:1583–1588, 1984.
114. Hoover R, Fraumeni JF: Drug-induced cancer. Cancer 47:1071–1080, 1981.
115. White CA, Traube J: Ulcerating enteritis associated with flucytosine therapy. Gastroenterology 83:1127–1129, 1982.
116. Heer M, Altorfer J, Burger H-R, Walti M: Bullous esophageal lesions due to cotrimoxazole: An immune-mediated process? Gastroenterology 88:1954–1957, 1985.
117. Jick H, Porter J: Drug-induced gastrointestinal bleeding: Report from The Boston Collaborative Drug Surveillance Program, Boston University Medical Center. Lancet 2:87–89, 1978.
118. Birns MT, Katon RM, Keller F: Intramural hematoma of the small intestine presenting with major upper gastrointestinal hemorrhage: Case report and review of the literature. Gastroenterology 77:1094–1100, 1979.
119. Herbert DC: Anticoagulant therapy and the acute abdomen. Br J Surg 55:353–357, 1968.
120. Granger DN, Richardson PDI, Kvietys PR, Mortillaro NA: Intestinal blood flow. Gastroenterology 78:837–863, 1980.
121. Ferrer MI, Bradley SE, Wheeler HO, et al: The effect of digoxin in the splanchnic circulation in ventricular failure. Circulation 32:524, 1965.
122. Lely AH, van Enter CHJ: Non-cardiac symptoms of digitalis intoxication. Am Heart J 83:149–152, 1972.
123. Renert WA, Button KF, Fuld SL, et al: Mesenteric venous thrombosis and small bowel infarction following infusion of vasopressin into the superior mesenteric artery. Radiology 102:299–302, 1972.
124. Greene FL, Ariyan S, Stansel HC: Mesenteric and peripheral vascular ischemia secondary to ergotism. Surgery 81:176–179, 1977.
125. Stillman AE, Weinberg M, Mast WC, Palpant S: Ischemic bowel disease attributable to ergot. Gastroenterology 72:1336–1337, 1977.
126. Wormann B, Hochter W, Seib HJ, Ottenjann R: Ergotamine-induced colitis. Endoscopy 17:165–166, 1985.
127. Eckardt VF, Kanzler G, Remmele W: Anorectal ergotism: Another cause of solitary rectal ulcers. Gastroenterology 91:1123–1127, 1986.

128. Hollister LE: Hematemesis and malena complicating treatment with raulwolfia alkaloids. Arch Intern Med 99:218–221, 1957.
129. Graham CF, Gallagher K, Jones JK: Acute colitis with methyldopa. N Engl J Med 304:1044–1046, 1981.
130. Shneerson JM, Gazzard BG: Reversible malabsorption caused by methyldopa. Br Med J 2:1456–1457, 1977.
131. Gibson DS: A case of intestinal obstruction following the administration of pentapyrrolidinium bitartrate ("Ansolysen"). Med J Aust 2:860–861, 1957.
132. Filpi RG, Majd M, LoPresto JM: Reversible gastric stricture following iron ingestion. South Med J 66:845–846, 1973.
133. Carne-Ross IP: Pyloric stenosis and sustained-release iron tablets. Br Med J 2:642–643, 1976.
134. Knott LH, Miller RC: Acute iron intoxication with intestinal infarction. J Pediatr Surg 13:720–721, 1978.
135. Stein HB, Urowitz MB: Gold-induced enterocolitis: Case report and literature review. J Rheumatol 3:21–26, 1976.
136. Sckolnick BR, Katz LA, Kozower M: Life-threatening enterocolitis after gold salt therapy. J Clin Gastroenterol 1:145–148, 1979.
137. Reinhart WH, Kapeller M, Halter F: Severe pseudomembranous and ulcerative colitis during gold therapy. Endoscopy 15:70–72, 1983.
138. Nagler J, Paget SA: Nonexudative diarrhea after gold salt therapy: Case report and review of the literature. Am J Gastroenterol 78:12–14, 1983.
139. McCormick PA, O'Donoghue D, Lemass B: Gold-induced colitis: Case report and literature review. Irish Med J 78:17–18, 1985.
140. Jackson CW, Haboubi NY, Whorwell RJ, Schofield PF: Gold-induced enterocolitis. Gut 27:452–456, 1986.
141. Geltner D, Sternfeld M, Becker SA, Kori M: Gold-induced ileitis. J Clin Gastroenterol 8:184–186, 1986.
142. Martin DM, Goldman JA, Gilliam J, Nasrallah SM: Gold-induced eosinophilic enterocolitis: Response to oral cromolyn sodium. Gastroenterology 80:1567–1570, 1981.
143. Gorbach SL: Bismuth therapy in gastrointestinal diseases. Gastroenterology 99:863–875, 1990.
144. Wittoesch JH, Jackman RJ, MacDonald JR: Melanosis coli: General review and study of 887 cases. Dis Colon Rectum 1:172–180, 1958.
145. Steer HW, Colin-Jones DG: Melanosis coli: Studies of the toxic effects of irritant purgatives. J Pathol 115:199–205, 1975.
146. Smith B: Pathology of cathartic colon. Proc R Soc Med 65:288, 1972.
147. Urso FP, Urso MJ, Lee CH: The cathartic colon: Pathological findings and radiological/pathological correlation. Radiology 116:557–559, 1975.
148. Pockros PJ, Foroozan P: Golytely lavage versus standard colonoscopy preparation: Effect on normal colonic mucosal histology. Gastroenterology 88:845–848, 1985.
149. Meisel JL, Bergman D, Graney D, et al: Human rectal mucosa: Proctoscopic and morphological changes caused by laxatives. Gastroenterology 72:1274–1279, 1977.
150. Leriche M, Devroede G, Sanchez G, et al: Changes in the rectal mucosa induced by hypertonic enemas. Dis Colon Rectum 21:227–236, 1978.
151. Hardin RD, Tedesco FJ: Colitis after Hibiclens enema. J Clin Gastroenterol 8:572–575, 1986.
152. Jonas G, Mahoney A, Murray J, Gertler S: Chemical colitis due to endoscopic cleansing solutions: A mimic of pseudomembranous colitis. Gastroenterology 95:1403–1408, 1988.
153. Meyer CT, Brand M, DeLuca VA, Spriro HM: Hydrogen peroxide colitis: a report of three patients. J Clin Gastroenterol 3:31–35, 1981.
154. Weiss SM, Rutenberg HL, Paskin DL, Zeren HA: Gut lesions due to slow-release KCl tablets. N Engl J Med 296:111–112, 1977.
155. Lambert JR, Newman A: Ulceration and stricture of the esophagus due to oral potassium chloride (slow release tablet) therapy. Am J Gastroenterol 73:508–511, 1980.
156. Barloon T, Moore SA, Mitros FA: A case of stenotic obstruction of the jejunum secondary to slow-release potassium. Am J Gastroenterol 81:192–194, 1986.
157. Collins FJ, Matthews HR, Baker SE, et al: Drug-induced esophageal injury. Br Med J 1:1673–1676, 1979.
158. Barrison JG, Trewby PN, Kane SP: Esophageal ulceration due to emepronium bromide. Endoscopy 12:197–199, 1980.
159. Thein SL, Asquith P: Pneumatosis coli: Complication of practolol. Br Med J 1:268, 1977.
160. Doman DB, Ginsberg AL: The hazard of drug-induced esophagitis. Hospital Practice 16:17–25, 1981.
161. Winckler K: Tetracycline ulcers of the oesophagus: Endoscopy, histology and roentgenology in two cases, and review of the literature. Endoscopy 13:225–228, 1981.
162. Kikendall JW, Friedman AC, Oyewole MA, et al: Pill-induced esophageal injury. Case reports and review of the medical literature. Dig Dis Sci 28:174–182, 1983.
163. Bott S, Prakach C, McCallum RW: Medication-induced esophageal injury: Survey of the literature. Am J Gastroenterol 82:758–763, 1987.
164. Goldman H, Antonioli DA: Mucosal biopsy of the esophagus, stomach, and proximal duodenum. Hum Pathol 13:423–448, 1982.
165. Evans DMD, Jones DB, Cleary BK, Smith PM: Oesophageal varices treated by sclerotherapy: a histopathological study. Gut 23:615–620, 1982.
166. Galambos JT: Endoscopic sclerotherapy. Ann Intern Med 98:1009–1011, 1983.
167. Marzuk PM, Schwartz JS: Endoscopic sclerotherapy for esophageal varices. Ann Intern Med 100:608–610, 1984.
168. Wass JAH, Thorner MO, Besser GM, et al: Gastrointestinal bleeding in patients on bromocriptine. Lancet 2:851, 1976.
169. Goodman MJ: Gastric ulceration induced by spironolactone. Lancet 1:752–753, 1977.
170. Goldstein SS, Lewis JH, Rothstein R: Intestinal obstruction due to bezoars. Am J Gastroenterol 79:313–318, 1984.
171. Faloon WW: Drug production of intestinal malabsorption. NY State J Med 70:2189–2192, 1970.
172. Cohen DJ, Loertscher R, Rubin MF, et al: Cyclosporin: a new immunosuppressive agent for organ transplantation. Ann Intern Med 101:667–682, 1984.
173. Tedesco FJ, Barton RW, Alpers HD: Clindamycin-associated colitis. Ann Intern Med 81:429–433, 1974.
174. Bartlett JG, Chang TW, Gurwith M, et al: Antibiotic-associated pseudomembranous colitis due to toxin-producing clostridia. N Engl J Med 198:531–534, 1978.
175. Goulston SJM, McGovern VJ: Pseudomembranous colitis. Gut 6:207–212, 1965.
176. Gebhard RL, Gerding DN, Olson MM, et al: Clinical and endoscopic findings in patients early in the course of Clostridium difficile-associated pseudomembranous colitis. Am J Med 78:45–48, 1985.
177. Medline A, Shin DH, Medline NM: Pseudomembranous colitis associated with antibiotics. Hum Pathol 7:693–703, 1976.
178. Price AB, Davies DR: Pseudomembranous colitis. J Clin Pathol 30:1–12, 1977.
179. Totten MA, Gregg JA, Fremont-Smith, P, Legg M: Clinical and pathological spectrum of antibiotic-associated colitis. Am J Gastroenterol 69:311–319, 1978.
180. Goldman H, Antonioli DA: Mucosal biopsy of the rectum, colon, and distal ileum. Hum Pathol 13:981–1012, 1982.
181. Bartlett JG: Treatment of Clostridium difficile colitis. Gastroenterology 89:1192–1195, 1985.
182. Schnitt SJ, Antonioli DA, Goldman H: Massive mural edema in severe pseudomembranous colitis. Arch Pathol Lab Med 107:211–213, 1983.
183. Trynka YM, LaMont JT: Association of Clostridium difficile toxin with symptomatic relapse of chronic inflammatory bowel disease. Gastroenterology 80:693–696, 1980.
184. Faulk, DL, Anuras S, Christensen J: Chronic intestinal pseudoobstruction. Gastroenterology 74:922–931, 1978.
185. Warnes H, Lehmann HE, Ban TA: Adynamic ileus during psychiatric medication. Can Med Assoc J 96:1112–1113, 1967.
186. Milner G: Gastro-intestinal side-effects of psychotropic drugs. Med J Aust 2:153–155, 1969.
187. Evans DL, Rogers JF, Peiper SC: Intestinal dilatation associated with phenothiazine therapy: A case report and literature review. Am J Psychiatry 136:970–972, 1979.
188. Bauer GE, Hellestrand KJ: Pseudoobstruction due to clonidine. Br Med J 1:769, 1976.

189. Butterfield WC: Surgical complications of narcotic addiction. Surg Gynecol Obstet 134:237–240, 1972.
190. Spira IA, Rubenstein R, Wolff D, Wolff WI: Fecal impaction following methadone ingestion simulating acute intestinal obstruction. Ann Surg 181:15–19, 1975.
191. Smith B: The Neuropathology of the Alimentary Tract. London, Edward Arnold, 1972.
192. Martin P, Manley PN, Depew WT, Blakeman JM: Isotretinonin-associated proctosigmoiditis. Gastroenterology 93:606–609, 1987.
193. Nalbundian H, Sketh N, Dietrich R, et al: Intestinal ischemia caused by cocaine ingestion: Report of two cases. Surgery 97:374–376, 1985.
194. Little JB: Cellular effects of ionizing radiation. I and II. N Engl J Med 278:308–315, 1968.
195. Rubin P, Casarett GW (eds): Clinical Radiation Pathology. Philadelphia, WB Saunders, 1968.
196. Fajardo LF, Berthrong M: Radiation injury in surgical pathology. Part I. Am J Surg Pathol 2:159–199, 1978.
197. Rubin P, Cassarette GW: A direction for clinical radiation pathology. In Vaeth JN (ed): Frontiers of Radiation Therapy and Oncology. Vol 6. Baltimore, University Park Press, 1972:1–16.
198. Bloomer WD, Hellman S: Normal tissue responses to radiation therapy. N Engl J Med 293:80–83, 1975.
199. Committee on the Biological Effects of Ionizing Radiation: The effects on populations of exposures to low levels of ionizing radiation. Washington DC, National Academy Press, 1980, pp 367–372.
200. Sher ME, Bauer J: Radiation-induced enteropathy. Am J Gastroenterol 85:121–128, 1990.
201. Novak JM, Collins JT, Donowitz M, et al: Effects of radiation on the human gastrointestinal tract. J Clin Gastroenterol 1:9–39, 1979.
202. Trier JS, Browning TH: Morpholigic response of the mucosa of human small intestine to x-ray exposure. J Clin Invest 45:194–204, 1966.
203. Key CR: Studies of the acute effects of the atomic bombs. Hum Pathol 2:475–484, 1971.
204. Prasad KN: Radiation Syndrome in Human Radiation Biology. Hagerstown, Harper & Row, 1972, pp 176–183.
205. Warren S, Friedman NB: Pathology and pathologic diagnosis of radiation lesions in the gastrointestinal tract. Am J Pathol 18:499–507, 1942.
206. Friedman NB: Effects of radiation on the gastrointestinal tract, including the salivary glands, the liver and the pancreas. Arch Pathol 34:749–787, 1942.
207. Mulligan RM: The lesions produced in the gastrointestinal tract by irradiation. Am J Pathol 18:515–525, 1942.
208. Ackerman LV: The pathology of radiation effect of normal and neoplastic tissue. Am J Roentgenol Rad Ther Nucl Med 14:447–459, 1972.
209. Berthrong M, Fajardo LF: Radiation injury in surgical pathology. II. Alimentary tract. Am J Surg Pathol 5:153–178, 1981.
210. Tarpila S: Morphological and functional response of human small intestine to ionizing radiation. Scand J Gastroenterol 6(Suppl 12):1–52, 1971.
211. Haboubi NY, Schofield PF, Rowland PL: The light and electron microscopic features of early and late phase radiation-induced proctitis. Am J Gatroenterol 83:1140–1144, 1988.
212. Kirkpatrick JB: Pathogenesis of foam cell lesions in irradiated arteries. Am J Pathol 50:291–309, 1967.
213. Hasleton PS, Carr N, Schofield, PF: Vascular changes in radiation bowel disease. Histopathology 9:517–534, 1985.
214. Sadove M, Block M, Rossof HH, et al: Radiation carcinogenesis in man: Primary neoplasms in fields of prior radiation. Cancer 48:1139–1143, 1981.
215. Sandler RS, Sandler DP: Radiation-induced cancers of the colon and rectum: Assessing the risk. Gastroenterology 84:51–57, 1983.
216. Lieber MR, Winans CS, Griem ML, et al: Sarcomas arising after radiotherapy for peptic ulcer disease. Dig Dis Sci 30:593–599, 1985.
217. Jablon S, Bailas JC III: The contribution of ionizing radiation to cancer mortality in the United States. Prev Med 9:219–226, 1980.
218. Schottenfeld D: Radiation as a risk factor in the natural history of colorectal cancer. (Editorial) Gastroenterology 84:186–190, 1983.
219. Shamsuddin AKM, Elias EG: Rectal mucosa: Malignant and premalignant changes after radiation therapy. Arch Pathol Lab Med 105:150–151, 1981.
220. Haggitt RC, Appelman HD, Correa P, et al: Dysplasia in Crohn's disease. (Letter) Arch Pathol Lab Med 106:308–309, 1982.
221. Wood IJ, Ralston M, Kurrle GR: Irradiation injury to gastrointestinal tract: Clinical features, management and pathogenesis. Australas Ann Med 12:143–152, 1963.
222. DeCosse JJ, Rhodes RS, Wentz WB, et al: The natural history and management of radiation injury of the gastrointestinal tract. Ann Surg 170:369–384, 1969.
223. Roswit B: Complications of radiation therapy: The alimentary tract. Semin Roentgenol 9:51–63, 1974.
224. Stewart JR, Gibbs FA: Prevention of radiation injury. Annu Rev Med 33:385–395, 1982.
225. Mennie AT, Dalley VM, Dinneen LC, et al: Treatment of radiation-induced gastrointestinal distress with acetylsalicylate. Lancet 1:942–943, 1975.
226. Ambrus JL, Ambrus CM, Lillie DB, et al: Effect of sodium meclofenamate on radiation induced esophagitis and cystitis. J Med 15:81–91, 1984.
227. Nicolopoulos N, Mantidis A, Stathopoulos E, et al: Prophylactic administration of indomethacin for irradiation esophagitis. Radiother Oncol 3:23–28, 1985.
228. Shofield PF, Carr ND, Holden D: Pathogenesis and treatment of radiation bowel disease. J R Soc Med 79:30–32, 1986.
229. Cram AE, Pearlman NR, Jochlmsen PR: Surgical management of radiation injured gut. Am J Surg 133:551–553, 1977.
230. Russel JC, Welch JP: Operative management of radiation injuries of the intestinal tract. Am J Surg 137:433–442, 1979.
231. Lillemoe KD, Brigham RA, Harmon JW, et al: Surgical management of small bowel radiation enteritis. Arch Surg 118:905–907, 1983.
232. Seamen WB, Ackerman LV: The effect of radiation on the esophagus. Radiology 68:534–540, 1957.
233. Jennings FL, Arden A: Acute radiation effects on the esophagus. Arch Pathol 69:407–412, 1960.
234. Chowhan NM: Injurious effects of radiation on the esophagus. Am J Gastroenterol 85:115–120, 1990.
235. Vanagunas A, Jacob P, Olinger E: Radiation-induced esophageal injury: A spectrum from esophagitis to cancer. Am J Gastroenterol 85:808–812, 1990.
236. Goldstein HM, Rogers LF, Fletcher GH, et al: Radiological manifestations of radiation-induced injury to the normal upper gastrointestinal tract. Radiology 117:135–140, 1975.
237. Papazian A, Capron J-P, Ducroix J-P, et al: Mucosal bridges of the upper esophagus after radiotherapy for Hodgkin's disease. Gastroenterology 84:1028–1031, 1983.
238. Goffman TE, McKeen EA, Curtis RE, et al: Esophageal carcinoma following irradiation for breast cancer. Cancer 52:1808–1809, 1983.
239. Sheril DJ: Radiation-associated malignancies of the esophagus. Cancer 54:726–728, 1984.
240. Marchese MJ, Liskow A, Chang CH: Radiation therapy-associated cancer of the esophagus. NY St J Med:152–153, 1986.
241. Levin E, Clayman CB, Palmer WL, Kirsner JB; Observations on the value of gastric radiation in the treatment of duodenal ulcer. Gastroenterology 32:42–51, 1957.
242. Clayman CB, Palmer WL, Kirsner JB: Gastric irradiation in the treatment of peptic ulcer. Gastroenterology 55:403–407, 1968.
243. Kellum JM, Jaffe BM, Calhoun T, Ballinger WF: Gastric complications after radiotherapy for Hodgkin's disease and other lymphomas. Am J Surg 134:314–317, 1977.
244. Hamilton FE: Gastric ulcer following radiation. Arch Surg 55:394–399, 1947.
245. Goldgraber MB, Rubin CE, Palmer WL, et al: The early gastric response to irradiation: A serial biopsy study. Gastroenterology 27:1–20, 1954.
246. Schier J, Symmonds RE, Dahlin DC: Clinicopathologic aspects of actinic enteritis. Surg Gynecol Obstet 119:1019–1025, 1964.
247. Wellwood JM, Jackson BT: The intestinal complications of radiotherapy. Br J Surg 60:814–818, 1973.

248. Poddar PK, Bauer JJ, Gelerent I, et al: Radiation injury to the small intestine. Mt Sinai J Med 49:144–149, 1982.
249. Haddad GK, Grodsinsky C, Allen H: The spectrum of radiation enteritis. Dis Colon Rectum 26:590–594, 1983.
250. O'Brien PH, Jenette JM, Garvin AJ: Radiation enteritis. Am Surg 53:501–504, 1987.
251. Yeoh EK, Horowitz M: Radiation enteritis. Surg Gynecol Obstet 165:373–376, 1987.
252. Schofield PF: Radiation damage of the bowel. In Taylor I (ed): Progress in Surgery. Edinburgh, Churchill Livingstone, 1987, pp 142–156.
253. Abrahamson R: Radiation ileitis. Arch Surg 81:55–59, 1960.
254. Burn JI: Radiation duodenitis. Proc R Soc Med 64:395–396, 1971.
255. Mason GR, Dietrich P, Friedland, et al: The radiological findings in radiation-induced enteritis and colitis. Clin Radiol 21:232–247, 1970.
256. Donaldson SS, Jundt S, Ricour C, et al: Radiation enteritis in children: A retrospective review, clinicopathologic correlation, and dietary management. Cancer 35:1167–1178, 1975.
257. Galland RB, Spencer J: The natural history of clinically established radiation enteritis. Lancet 1:1257–1258, 1985.
258. Dencker H, Holmdahl KH, Lunderquist A, et al: Mesenteric angiography in patients with radiation injury of the bowel after pelvis irradiation. Am J Roentgenol Rad Ther Nucl Med 114:476–481, 1972.
259. Greenberger NJ, Isselbacher KJ: Malabsorption following radiation injury to the gastrointestinal tract. Am J Med 36:450–456, 1964.
260. Tankel HI, Clark DH, Lee FD: Radiation enteritis with malabsorption. Gut 6:560–569, 1965.
261. Duncan W, Leonard JC: The malabsorption syndrome following radiotherapy. Q J Med 34:319–329, 1965.
262. Wiernik G: Changes in the villous pattern of the human jejunum associated with heavy irradiation damage. Gut 7:149–153, 1966.
263. Whitehead R: Mucosal Biopsy of the Gastrointestinal Tract, 3rd ed. Philadelphia, WB Saunders, 1985.
264. May J, Lowenthal J: Irradiation injury to the colon. Gut 6:444–447, 1965.
265. Villasanta U: Complications of radiotherapy for carcinoma of the uterine cervix. Am J Obstet Gynecol 119:727–732, 1974.
266. Weisbrodt IM, Liber AF, Gordon BS: The effects of therapeutic radiation on colonic mucosa. Cancer 36:931–940, 1975.
267. Schmitz RM, Chao JH, Bartolome JS: Intestinal injuries to irradiation of carcinoma of the cervix of the uterus. Surg Gynecol Obstet 138:29–32, 1984.
268. Friedman M: Calculated risks of radiation injury of normal tissue in the treatment of cancer of the testis. In American Cancer Society: Proceedings of the Second National Cancer Conference, New York. National Cancer Institute, USPHS Federal Science Agency, 1952, pp 390–400.
269. Stockbrine, MF, Hancock JE, Fletcher GH: Complications in 831 patients with squamous cell carcinoma of the intact uterine cervix treatment with 3000 rads or more whole pelvis irradiation. AJR 108:293–304, 1970.
270. Gelfand MD, Tepper M, Katz LA, et al: Acute radiation proctitis in man. Gastroenterology 54:401–411, 1968.
271. Colcock BP, Hume A: Radiation injury to the sigmoid and rectum. Surg Gynecol Obstet 108:306–312, 1959.
272. Gilensky NH, Burns DG, Barbezat GO, et al: The natural history of radiation-induced proctosigmoiditis: An analysis of 88 patients. Q J Med 202:40–53, 1983.
273. Smith JC: Carcinoma of the rectum following irradiation of cancer of the cervix. Proc R Soc Med 55:701–702, 1962.
274. Black WC, Ackerman LV: Carcinoma of the large intestine as a late complication of pelvic radiotherapy. Clin Radiol 16:278–281, 1965.
275. MacMahon CE, Rowe JW: Rectal reaction following radiation therapy of cervical carcinoma: Particular reference to the subsequent occurrence of rectal carcinoma. Ann Surg 173:264–269, 1971.
276. Castro EB, Rowen PP, Quan SHQ: Carcinoma of large intestine in patients irradiated for carcinoma of cervix and uterus. Cancer 31:45–52, 1973.
277. Cunningham MD, Wilhoite R: Radiation-induced carcinoma of the transverse colon: Report of a case. Dis Colon Rectum 16:145–148, 1973.
278. Qizilbash AH: Radiation-induced carcinoma of the rectum: A late complication of pelvic irradiation. Arch Pathol 98:118–121, 1974.
279. O'Connor TW, Rombeau JL, Levine HS, Turnbull RB: Late development of colorectal cancer subsequent to pelvic irradiation. Dis Colon Rectum 22:123–128, 1979.
280. Sibly TG, Keane RM, Lever JV, et al: Rectal lymphoma in radiation injured bowel. Br J Surg 72:879–880, 1985.
281. Gilbert ES, Marks S: An analysis of the mortality of workers in a nuclear facility. Radiat Res 79:122–148, 1979.
282. Kato H, Schull WJ: Studies of the mortality of A-bomb survivors. VII. Mortality, 1950–1978. Part I. Cancer Mortality. Radiat Res 90:395–432, 1982.
283. McIlrath DC, Hallenbeck GA: Review of gastric freezing. JAMA 190:715–718, 1964.
284. Barnes HB, Collins CH, Jones TI, Garlick TB: Morphology of human stomach after therapeutic freezing. Arch Surg 90:358–362, 1965.
285. Perry GT, Dunphy JV, Fruin RC, Littman A: Gastric freezing for duodenal ulcer. A double blind study. Gastroenterology 47:6–9, 1964.

CHAPTER 10

Allergic Disorders

HARVEY GOLDMAN, M.D.

GENERAL ASPECTS AND TERMINOLOGY

PATHOGENETIC MECHANISMS

ALLERGIC EFFECTS IN OTHER ORGANS

EOSINOPHILIC GASTROENTERITIS
Mucosal Type
Mural Type
Pathologic Features and Diagnosis
Differential Diagnosis
Serosal Type

ALLERGIC GASTROENTERITIS
Definitions
Clinical and Laboratory Features
General Pathologic Features and Diagnosis
Specific Organ Features and Differential Diagnosis
Esophagus
Stomach
Small Intestine
Colon and Rectum

ALLERGIC PROCTITIS AND COLITIS
Definitions
Childhood Cases
Clinical and Laboratory Features
Pathologic Features
Diagnosis and Differential Diagnosis
Adult Cases
Ulcerative Proctitis and Colitis
Isolated Cases

MUCOSAL BIOPSY

This chapter deals with the major manifestations of the allergic disorders due to food sensitivity that can affect the various parts of the gastrointestinal tract. The category of eosinophilic gastroenteritis, including both the allergic and nonallergic forms, is also included. Details of the normal structure and function of the immunologic system are contained in Chapter 5; and some of the allergic conditions are presented in part in the specific chapters dealing with diseases of the esophagus (Chapter 17), the stomach (Chapter 20), and the intestines (Chapter 28 and 29). Reactions to nonfood substances, including chemicals and drugs, are covered in Chapter 9.

GENERAL ASPECTS AND TERMINOLOGY

Persons may react to ingested foods for a variety of reasons (Table 10–1), including the presence of heavy metals and other toxic chemicals, food poisoning due to pathogenic bacteria and their exotoxins, selective enzyme deficiencies such as primary lactose intolerance, celiac disease (gluten enteropathy), and other more generalized malabsorptive disorders. An abnormal response may also occur in patients with anorexia nervosa and psychologic disorders and may result simply from a dislike of a particular food. All of these conditions and circumstances must be excluded before one can consider that the patient has a specific allergic reaction or sensitivity to an ingested food substance.

Allergic disorders due to foods are much more commonly seen in infants and children,[1,2] but they may occur in persons of all ages and especially in young adults.[3,4] Indeed, a delay in the making of a diagnosis of an allergic condition, sometimes up to several months or years, is not unusual in an adult patient, principally because of the failure to consider the diagnostic possibility.

The specific diagnosis of a food allergy or sensitivity affecting the gastrointestinal tract is dependent on a combination of compatible clinical and pathologic features, the exclusion of other potential causes such as infections and various malabsorptive diseases, and the

Table 10–1 CAUSES OF FOOD REACTIONS IN THE GUT

Allergic diseases
Contamination by toxic chemicals
Infectious food poisoning
Malabsorptive disorders
Anorexia nervosa
Psychologic reactions

beneficial response to an elimination diet or to treatment with corticosteroid hormones. The patient often exhibits an elevation of the peripheral blood eosinophil count and a rise in the serum level of immunoglobulin E (IgE), but other more specific tests to support an allergic basis are ordinarily not available. Ideally, the diagnosis should be substantiated by an oral rechallenge with the suspected food allergen; and one should note the return of symptoms or the reappearance of alterations in a mucosal biopsy specimen. Such documentation has been achieved in selected cases, especially in those due to cow's milk protein[5]; but it has proved difficult in many of the more generalized cases of allergic gastroenteritis to establish the particular allergens involved. Furthermore, in most cases of allergic proctitis, the association with a single allergen such as milk or soy protein seems so certain that it has not been a standard clinical practice recently to perform a rechallenge study.[6]

There are a variety of terms used to connote different aspects of allergic diseases of the gut due to foods, based on the particular antigens and pathogenetic mechanisms involved, on the distribution of the lesions in the different segments of the alimentary tract, and on the overall severity and behavior of the lesions. Thus, if the disorder appears to be related to a single food allergen such as cow's milk, soy protein, or wheat protein, the disease is often referred to by the particular etiologic agent as well as the distribution of the lesions if known.[7–11] For example, terms used include *cow's milk protein allergy, sensitivity, hypersensitivity, intolerance, enteritis,* or *colitis.* When the disorder involves multiple antigens and is associated with more widespread effects in the gut segments, it has usually been referred to as *eosinophilic gastroenteritis* or *allergic gastroenteropathy.*[12–15] As noted below, it is important to sort out the mucosal form of eosinophilic gastroenteritis, which has a definite or presumed allergic cause, from the mural type, which lacks an allergic basis. Because there is considerable overlap in the antigens and pathogenetic mechanisms and ambiguity in the use of the term *eosinophilic gastroenteritis,* the author has divided the allergic cases affecting the gut into two major groups[2] based primarily on the dominant localization of the lesions: (1) allergic gastroenteritis, in which the lesions may affect any part of the gut but tend to be concentrated in the esophagus, stomach, and proximal small intestine; and (2) allergic proctitis or colitis, in which the lesions are predominantly or solely present in the large bowel. This separation helps to explain the functional effects and overall clinical behavior of the allergic disorders.

PATHOGENETIC MECHANISMS

The potential immunologic mechanisms involved in gastrointestinal allergy[16] are summarized in Table 10–2, and further details are provided in Chapter 5. Serum antibodies of the IgG class to food proteins are normally present in young infants but are often further elevated and associated with IgE antibodies, both in the serum and in the gut lumen, in patients with food allergy. There is, however, no constant correlation between the presence of food antibodies and the activity of the allergic condition. Most cases of food allergy appear to involve the type I, or immediate hypersensitivity, form of immunologic reaction. This is supported in such cases by an elevation of the serum IgE level and positive radioallergosorbent test (RAST) response to numerous food substances, including cow's milk protein, eggs, fish, soy, nuts, and wheat. These patients also frequently exhibit other signs of type I reaction such as asthma, rhinitis, and urticaria. Furthermore, an increase in IgE-producing plasma cells has been identified in the gut mucosa by immunohistochemical staining in selected patients, including those with milk protein allergy affecting the small intestines[17,18] and a subset of patients with ulcerative proctitis and colitis that have responded to anti-allergic medication.[19–21] Injury probably results from the triggering of the IgE-coated mast cells in the gastrointestinal mucosa leading to their release of histamine, prostaglandins, and other inflammatory mediators.

The type III, or humoral, form of immunologic mechanisms appears to be involved in a minority of allergy cases and is characterized by the presence of circulating and mucosal immune complexes, consisting of foreign protein, complement, and immunoglobulins of the IgG and IgM classes. A delayed type of hypersensitivity with activated lymphocytes has also been demonstrated in a few cases but is not thought to be a dominant factor, at least as a primary cause, of gastrointestinal allergy. The exact immunologic mechanism is

Table 10–2 IMMUNOLOGIC MECHANISMS IN GASTROINTESTINAL FOOD ALLERGY

Type of Reaction	Occurrence in GI Allergy	Mechanism of Injury
I. Immediate hypersensitivity Anaphylactic reaction	Yes	Degranulation of IgE-coated mast cell
II. Cytotoxic reaction	No	—
III. Humoral immunity Immune complex disease	Probable	Deposition of immune complexes, causing activation of complement
IV. Cell mediated immunity Delayed hypersensitivity	Probable	Release of lymphokines from activated lymphocytes

usually not documented in an individual clinical case but may be inferred by the speed of onset of symptoms following exposure to the food protein, with a short duration supportive of a type I reaction and a more prolonged start indicative of a humoral or other delayed reaction. Also, the immediate reactions are often associated with similar signs of hypersensitivity in the respiratory tract and skin.

One of the major histologic features of allergic reactions is the presence of abundant eosinophils, and both mast cell mediators[22,23] and lymphokines released from activated lymphocytes[24,25] have been shown to attract and to affect the migration of eosinophils in tissues. Although it has been customary to consider the eosinophil as a scavenger of immune complexes and as a general modulator of an inflammatory reaction, recent evidence indicates that some of the products of eosinophils, such as eosinophil granule protein, may be directly toxic to the tissues.[26-29]

ALLERGIC EFFECTS IN OTHER ORGANS

There have been numerous attempts to relate food allergy to the development of diseases of various organ systems, alone or in conjunction with gastrointestinal disease.[16] It would appear, however, that a strong association exists only for the appearance of pulmonary symptoms and cutaneous disorders, which are seen in about half of the patients with allergic gastroenteritis. The symptoms in most cases are those that would be expected in a type I or immediate hypersensitivity reaction and include wheezing, rhinorrhea, and urticaria. Although still debated, it is thought that some cases of eczema or atopic dermatitis have an allergic basis, and a beneficial response to milk-free and egg-free diets has been noted. There are also rare reports that link allergic disease in the gut with bronchitis and eosinophilic pneumonia.[30]

EOSINOPHILIC GASTROENTERITIS

Eosinophilic gastroenteritis and *gastroenteropathy* are generic terms that have been used in the past to indicate a disorder characterized by tissue damage and a prominent reaction with eosinophils. It is now apparent that the term has been employed to embrace a large number of etiologically and morphologically varied conditions. Indeed, abundant eosinophils can be seen in many conditions, and it is imperative that one exclude more specific disorders such as reflux esophagitis, parasitic infections, toxic reactions to drugs, idiopathic inflammatory bowel disease, and the various collagen-vascular disorders from consideration. The remaining cases of eosinophilic gastroenteritis have been divided[12,31] into three distinct forms (mucosal, mural, and serosal) on the basis of their dominant location in the gut wall (Table 10–3).

Table 10–3 TYPES OF EOSINOPHILIC GASTROENTERITIS

Type	Location of Disease	Etiology	Functional Effect
Mucosal	Mucosa	Allergic	Bleeding, protein loss and malabsorption
Mural	Submucosa and muscularis propria	Unknown	Mass lesion resulting in obstruction and rare perforation
Serosal	Serosa	Unknown	Ascites

Mucosal Type

In this form, the injury is concentrated in the mucosal layer, although the inflammation may extend into the upper submucosa. The lesions are often multiple and can be seen in any part of the gut, including the esophagus, stomach (particularly the antrum), and both the small and large intestines. The patients typically present with some combination of malabsorption, iron-deficiency anemia, and protein-losing gastroenteropathy, and it is believed that these cases have an allergic cause.[12,13,15,32,33] This mucosal form of eosinophilic gastroenteritis is described in detail in the following section on allergic gastroenteritis.

Mural Type

This form of eosinophilic gastroenteritis is characterized by the localization of tissue injury and inflammatory reaction with abundant eosinophils in the submucosa and muscularis propria.[34] It appears to be more common in children but can occur in any age group.[35] The lesions may affect any part of the gut but are more often noted in the gastric antrum, usually in the prepyloric region, and in the distal small intestine. They are most often single and produce an obstructive mass[36,37]; exceptionally, there may be extensive ulceration and necrosis leading to perforation, especially in the intestines.[38-40] There is no relation between this mural type and the mucosal form of eosinophilic gastroenteritis, there is no evidence of an allergic etiology, and the pathogenesis of the mural lesions is not known.

Considering the inflammatory nature of the lesion, an infectious cause has been often considered but not proved; and there is no constant evidence of a vasculitis. Despite the uniform histologic features, it is probable that the lesions are a heterogenous lot and will prove to have varied causes. In the past, the term *eosinophilic granuloma* has been applied to some of these lesions, particularly those involving the stomach. This is a poor term because there are no granulomas and there is no relation between this mural form of eosinophilic gastroenteritis and histiocytosis X, which can include isolated lesions called eosinophilic granuloma.

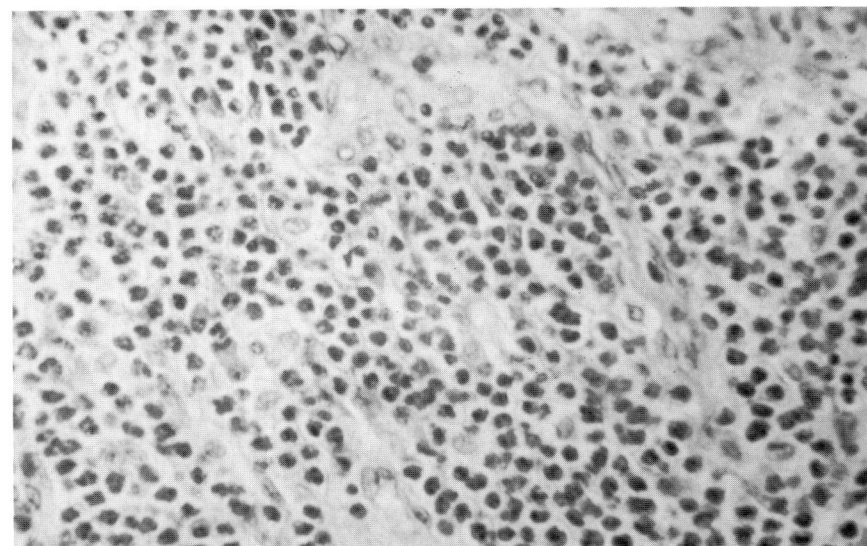

FIGURE 10–1. Mural type of eosinophilic gastroenteritis. Section of lesion showing large sheet of mature eosinophils admixed with small blood vessels. (H&E, × 400)

Pathologic Features and Diagnosis

Surgery is usually required because of the obstructive symptoms and the uncertainty of the nature of the mass lesion,[31,41] and the diagnosis is based on the histologic finding of a nonspecific inflammatory reaction with many eosinophils and on the exclusion of other specific disorders. The lesions are usually single and composed of an ill-defined mass, from a few to several centimeters in diameter, that is located in the wall of the affected portion of the gut[34–36]; the overlying mucosa may show focal ulceration. Histologic examination reveals extensive inflammation with a dominance of mature eosinophils (Figure 10–1) and either patchy or confluent areas of liquefaction or coagulation necrosis. The eosinophilic reaction may encircle areas of necrosis but there are no prominence of macrophages or well formed granulomas. Uncommonly, the necrosis may be more severe and extend through the gut wall, causing a perforation, especially in lesions of the intestines.[39,40]

Differential Diagnosis

At a clinical level, the major considerations are a tumor of the gut wall, such as a leiomyoma or leiomyosarcoma, and a chronic inflammatory condition with stricture formation. Before rendering a diagnosis of the mural form of eosinophilic gastroenteritis, it is imperative that one considers the other disorders that can be associated with mural necrosis and a prominent eosinophilic inflammatory reaction. These include toxic reactions to some chemicals and drugs and especially chronic parasitic infections such as anisakiasis and that due to *Strongyloides*. Accordingly, stool examination and multiple tissue sections must be surveyed for worm fragments and eggs. Crohn's disease may present with obstruction due to an inflammatory stricture in any part of the gut and can be associated with a marked eosinophilic infiltrate. Features supportive of Crohn's disease would include the presence of inflammatory sinus tracts and fistulas, the appearance of multiple lesions in the distal ileum and colon, signs of chronic enteritis in the form of prominent pyloric metaplasia and neuronal hyperplasia, and the identification of well-formed granulomas. Other less common conditions that can be associated with a prominent tissue eosinophilia include occasional tumors, amyloidosis, and chronic granulomatous disease, all of which would show other characteristic features on histologic examination.

Finally, just about any condition affecting the gut can be exceptionally complicated by the unexplained appearance of numerous eosinophils in the inflammatory reaction. For example, some cases of ordinary peptic ulcer disease of the gastric antrum or duodenum may reveal an extraordinary eosinophilic response (Figure 10–2), and there is no correlation between this finding and the overall behavior of the lesion. It must be stressed that the appearance of tissue eosinophils even when abundant is still a nonspecific finding. Certain conditions, as outlined above, should be considered; but one may simply be left with a common diagnosis such as peptic ulcer disease or a particular infection without a ready explanation for the enhanced eosinophilic reaction. Accordingly, the diagnosis of the mural form of eosinophilic gastroenteritis should be made only after there has been an extensive effort to rule out other disorders. Even then, it should be appreciated that the mural form of eosinophilic gastroenteritis is probably not a single entity; it simply describes a particular type of inflammatory mass without an apparent cause. In making the diagnosis, it is exceedingly important that one stress the mural nature of the lesion so that it is not confused with the allergy-associated mucosal form of eosinophilic gastroenteritis.

Serosal Type

The serosal type of eosinophilic gastroenteritis is the rarest. It is characterized by diffuse eosinophilic infil-

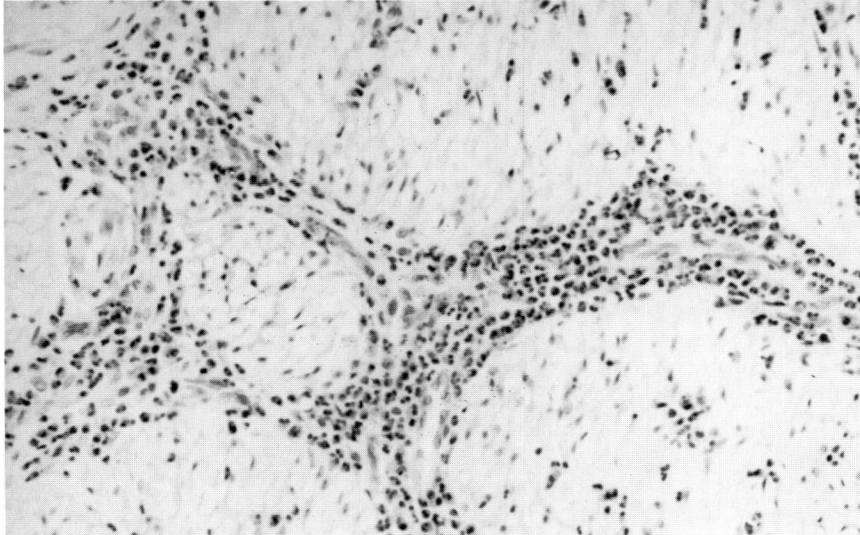

FIGURE 10–2. Case of chronic peptic ulcer of stomach. Section of muscularis propria beneath the ulcer revealing clumps of eosinophils insinuated between the muscle bundles. (H&E, × 100)

trates of the gut serosa and a prominent ascites.[12,31,42] Its etiology is unknown, and it is unlikely that this form represents a single entity. Indeed, considering its rarity and uncertain nature, one could question whether the condition is deserving of a special name. It should be separated from the mucosal and mural forms of eosinophilic gastroenteritis, because there is no relation between any of these types.

ALLERGIC GASTROENTERITIS

Definitions

The term *allergic gastroenteritis* is used to describe those cases of food allergy in which the lesions are often multiple and can affect any part of the gut from the esophagus to the colon. The severity of the disease is highly variable and appears to depend on the magnitude of the food allergens involved. Thus, cases due to a single food substance, such as cow's milk or soy protein, typically present with less severe disease, which possibly reflects early diagnosis; and the disorder is readily reversed by an elimination diet. Conversely, in cases involving multiple food allergens, the clinical course is more protracted, and the patients often require corticosteroid therapy. Indeed, the particular constellation of offending food substances may not be completely identified in half of these more severe cases.[2] Because of these differences in behavior, many investigators have preferred to designate the milder and more restrictive cases by the particular offending food with such terms as *cow's milk protein allergy* or *soy protein allergy* (or *sensitivity*) and to use the term *eosinophilic gastroenteritis* (or *gastroenteropathy*) for the more complex cases. As noted above, the latter would correspond to the mucosal form of eosinophilic gastroenteritis, in contrast to the mural and serosal forms.[12]

The author prefers to use the collective term *allergic gastroenteritis* for both the milder cases and the severe cases for the following reasons: (1) The pathologic pattern of injury in the mucosa is identical, consisting of epithelial and glandular degeneration with a prominence of eosinophils. (2) The distribution of lesions in the gut is the same. (3) The pathogenetic mechanisms involved appear to be similar or, at least, to overlap. (4) There are no differences in the frequency of other allergic symptoms in the patients and their families. (5) The other differences in clinical features and laboratory results simply reflect the degree of injury to the mucosa and the duration of the disorder. (6) Finally, one can avoid the use of the generic term *eosinophilic gastroenteritis* and the potential confusion between the mucosal and mural forms. Admittedly, there will be some cases in which an allergic etiology is not firmly established; these are included because of the lack of any other known cause, the similarity in their clinical and pathologic features to those of the definite allergic cases, and their beneficial response to corticosteroid therapy.

Clinical and Laboratory Features

The disorder can affect either sex and persons of all ages but is more commonly seen in children and young adults. The patients typically present with some combination of bleeding or iron-deficiency anemia, a protein-losing state, and malabsorptive symptoms.[12,15,32] In a study of 38 cases in children,[2] the major presenting symptoms were growth failure with diarrhea and vomiting in 26, anemia in six, asthma in three, the hyper-IgE syndrome in two, and overt rectal bleeding in only one case. Overall, diarrhea was noted in 67%, vomiting in 51%, weight loss in 40%, abdominal pain in 33%, and rectal bleeding in 25% of the patients; most symptoms were more commonly noted in the older children, probably reflecting the longer duration of the illness. A history of other allergic findings in the patients and their families is noted in about half of the cases and includes mainly asthma, rhinitis, and eczema. Occasionally, the patients have dominant symptoms referable to involvement of a particular part of the upper tract, and they may present with features simulating ordinary peptic esophagitis[43] or hypertrophic pyloric stenosis.[44]

The peripheral blood eosinophil count is elevated at some time in the great majority of cases and is often marked, with counts ranging from 5% to 15%. An increase in the serum IgE levels is noted in about three quarters of the cases and is often associated with abnormal results in the RAST. Anemia of the iron deficiency type is present in a quarter to half of the patients and is usually of a mild degree. As with the clinical features, the abnormal laboratory test results are more commonly noted in older children and adults. Other signs of malabsorption and mucosal injury are present in about one third of cases and include excess protein excretion, reduced serum albumin and IgG, abnormal lactose and xylose tolerance test results, and prominence of gastric and intestinal folds in radiographic and endoscopic examinations.

Patients with disease due to one or two food allergens such as cow's milk and soy protein typically respond promptly to an elimination diet, and there are no recurrences.[45,46] Most patients, especially children, appear to lose the capacity to react to the food substances after several years. This is possibly due to maturity in the development of the mucosal immune system, resulting in more effective production of IgG and IgA, which may neutralize ingested antigens, and a reduction in the synthesis of IgE. In contrast, the cases due to multiple antigens and those in which the offending foods cannot be completely identified require corticosteriod or other immunosuppressive therapy and are prone to multiple relapses.[47] Exceptionally, there are adult cases wherein the condition is refractory to medical therapy and sustained malabsorption develops, which can lead in rare cases to death.

General Pathologic Features and Diagnosis

The lesions of allergic gastroenteritis are usually multiple and can affect any part of the gut but are least common in the colon and rectum. Although most investigators and clinical studies have concentrated on disease of the small bowel,[13,17] it has become evident that lesions are often present and frequently more prominent in the esophagus and the stomach, especially the antral portion.[48] The reason for the localization in an individual case is not known, and the finding of disease in a particular tissue site does not indicate any special pathogenesis, but, rather, determines the clinical features observed and the area that should be selectively biopsied.

The pathologic features of the lesions in allergic gastroenteritis are generally the same, regardless of their location in the gut, and differ only in severity. Focal disease is observed in cases due to a single food allergen such as cow's milk protein; more extensive involvement is seen in patients with disease due to multiple antigens (the so-called mucosal form of eosinophilic gastroenteritis). The lesions always affect the mucosa and are characterized by variable degrees of epithelial damage and an inflammatory infiltrate that is usually rich in mature eosinophils. The eosinophils not only are present in the lamina propria but also extend into the epithelial layers on the surface and in the glands. The lesions may be patchy, especially in the small intestine, and multiple sections may be needed for identification.[13] Occasionally, the lesions are more extensive and confluent, resulting in prominent edema of the mucosal folds; these can be visualized by endoscopic and radiographic examination of the stomach and intestines.[49] Ulceration of the surface of the mucosa is exceptionally present[50]; when seen, however, it is important to consider and exclude disorders that more frequently have ulceration, such as infections, idiopathic inflammatory bowel disease, and tumors. The inflammation may extend into the submucosa, but there is no involvement of the deeper parts of the gut wall. Neutrophils are rarely prominent and usually restricted to the cases with ulceration. An increase in plasma cells, especially those producing IgE, and occasional prominence of mast cells have been noted in the lamina propria of the intestines in some cases.[17,18] There does not appear to be a regular increase in the numbers of other mononuclear inflammatory cells in the lamina propria.

Although the presence of abundant eosinophils is a characteristic finding, there are cases in which the number of eosinophils is not especially striking. This can be a special problem in the analysis of the intestinal mucosa, which normally contains some eosinophils in the lamina propria[51,52]; only a marked increase with aggregates should be considered abnormal. Ideally, quantitative methods should be applied; but these are not readily available in ordinary clinical practice. It is probably best to require that there be evidence of epithelial damage and extension of the eosinophils into the epithelial layer for the more precise diagnosis of an allergic lesion. With healing of the lesions, following an elimination diet or the use of corticosteroid therapy, there is prompt regeneration of the epithelium, which may exhibit numerous mitoses; but the eosinophilic infiltrate in the lamina propria may linger for several days (Figure 10-3).

The diagnosis of allergic gastroenteritis depends on the exclusion of other disorders—as described below in the section on differential diagnosis (Table 10-4)—that have a prominent eosinophilic reaction; on the finding of compatible clinical, laboratory, and pathologic features; and on the beneficial response to an elimination diet or to corticosteroid therapy. Food rechallenges have been often recommended but are rarely employed in standard clinical practice, probably because of the ready availability of alternative formulas and diets.[6,45,46] The cases caused by one or two food allergens are effectively eliminated by a dietary change. Relapses may be seen in cases caused by multiple antigens, and the lesions observed are identical in appearance to the original disease and usually involve the same portions of the gut. Despite repeated recur-

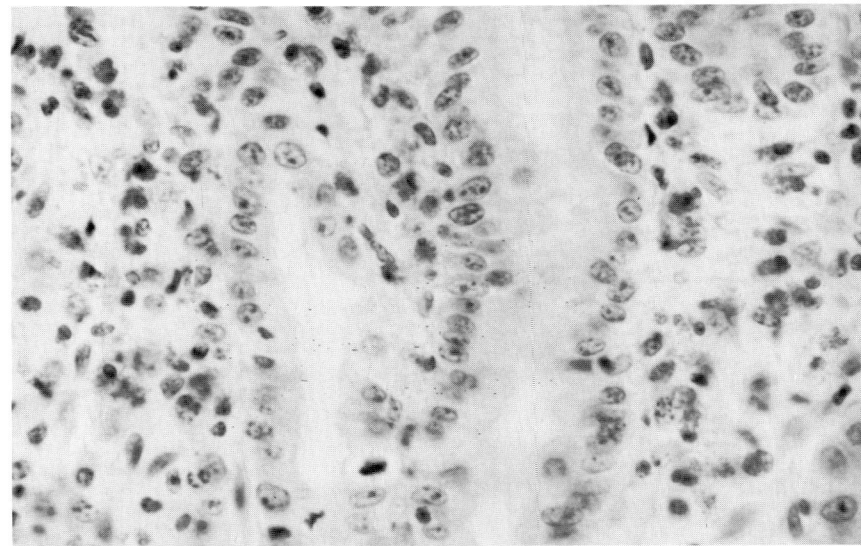

FIGURE 10–3. Gastric antral mucosa in case of healing allergic gastroenteritis. There are regenerating gastric pits with several mitoses (center) and persistence of eosinophils in the lamina propria. (H&E, × 400)

rences, the development of fibrosis, glandular atrophy, or other signs of chronic disease has not been described in cases of allergic gastroenteritis.

Specific Organ Features and Differential Diagnosis

It should be re-emphasized that the finding of a prominent eosinophilic infiltrate in the gut mucosa is not a specific feature and does not by itself indicate an allergic disorder. Mucosal injury with an exaggerated eosinophilic response can be seen in many other conditions of the gastrointestinal tract (see Table 10–4), including reflux esophagitis,[53–55] toxic reactions to some chemicals and drugs such as gold salts,[56] parasitic infections,[57] the idiopathic inflammatory bowel diseases ulcerative colitis and Crohn's disease,[58] chronic granulomatous disease,[59] connective tissue disorders,[60] amyloidosis, and some tumors.[4]

Esophagus

Although the esophagus was formerly thought to be rarely involved in food allergy,[61–63] it appears that this notion was due to a lack of examination of the esophagus. At least in children, frequent and sometimes extensive lesions have been noted in the esophageal mucosa[2,43,55]; these lesions usually coexist with disease affecting other parts of the gut, such as the stomach and small intestine, but may occasionally be the dominant feature in a case of allergic gastroenteritis. It is established that there is esophageal involvement in the severe form of allergic gastroenteritis, but its frequency in the milder cases due to a single antigen is not known.

The lesions are concentrated in the distal esophagus—which may reflect the tendency for this area to be selectively sampled by endoscopic biopsy—and are characterized by a basal zone hyperplasia of the squamous epithelial layer and a pronounced infiltrate of mature eosinophils within the epithelium (Figure 10–4). There is usually a large number of eosinophils also in the lamina propria, but it is more difficult to evaluate this criterion because such cells may be present in this compartment in the normal esophagus.[52]

The major differential diagnosis is that of reflux esophagitis, which is a much more common disorder and which reveals the identical histologic feature of basal zone hyperplasia[64] and infiltration of eosinophils within the squamous epithelium.[53–55] In limited studies to date, it appears that the number of intraepithelial eosinophils observed is much greater and associated with large aggregates on the surface in cases of allergic disease[2]; but confirmatory quantitative studies have not been performed (Figure 10–5). The diagnosis of esophageal involvement in allergic gastroenteritis is supported by an elevated blood eosinophil count and the finding of mucosal lesions in other parts of the gut such as the gastric antrum and small intestine. In contrast, cases of reflux esophagitis would reveal a normal blood eosinophil count, would lack lesions in other parts of the tract, and would show abnormalities in a pH probe and manometric examination of the esophagus. Other causes of esophagitis, including various infections and injury from entrapped pills, typically re-

Table 10–4 CAUSES OF INCREASED EOSINOPHILS IN THE GUT MUCOSA

Allergic disease
Reflux esophagitis
Toxic reactions to chemicals and drugs
Parasitic infections
Idiopathic inflammatory bowel diseases
    Ulcerative colitis
    Crohn's disease
Vasculitis
Amyloidosis
Chronic granulomatous disease
Tumors

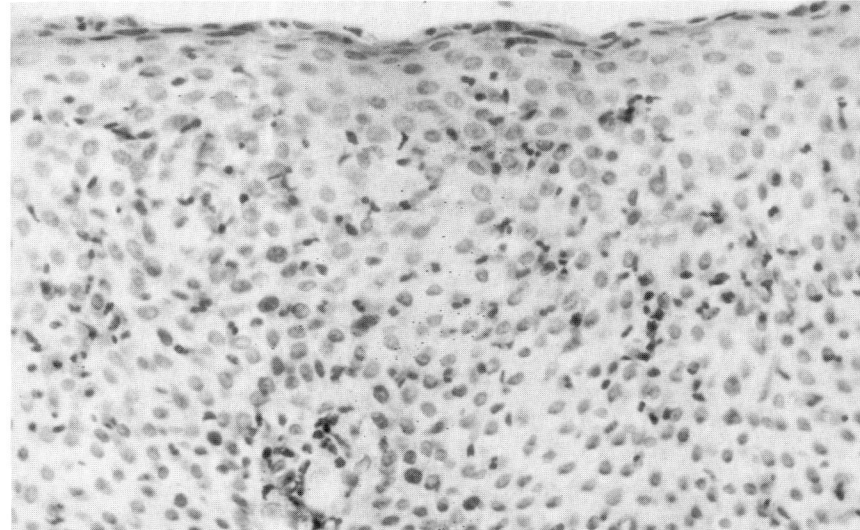

FIGURE 10–4. Esophageal mucosa in allergic gastroenteritis. There is marked basal zone hyperplasia of the squamous epithelium. There are also many eosinophils within the epithelial layer. (H&E, × 400)

veal more focal lesions and are not usually associated with a prominent eosinophilic reaction.

Stomach

It has become evident that the stomach, particularly the antral portion, is a very common site for the appearance of allergic lesions and that they are often pronounced in this region.[2,48,65] This observation was first noted in children but also appears to occur in adults. The cause of this preferential localization is not known, but it is clear that the gastric antral lesions can contribute to the blood loss and excess protein excretion observed in patients with allergic disease. Furthermore, since the gastric lesions seem to be more constantly found than disease in other parts of the gut, mucosal biopsy of the gastric antrum has proven to be an effective tool in the identification of patients with food allergy. Gastric involvement has been noted both in the milder cases due to a single food allergen and in the severe form of allergic gastroenteritis.

The mucosal lesions are generally more pronounced in the antrum than in the corpus or fundus of the stomach. Milder lesions are more typically seen in patients with disease due to a single allergy such as cow's milk protein and consist of the presence of numerous eosinophils in the lamina propria and focal extension of the eosinophils into the surface and glandular epithelium (Figure 10–6). Occasionally, the lesions are patchy, perhaps reflecting a very mild insult or partial treatment; multiple samples of the antrum may need to be examined. More often, and especially in the severe cases of allergic gastroenteritis, the gastric lesions are florid and reveal a diffuse and very marked infiltrate of eosinophils, which may form aggregates and extend into the regions of the muscularis mucosae and upper

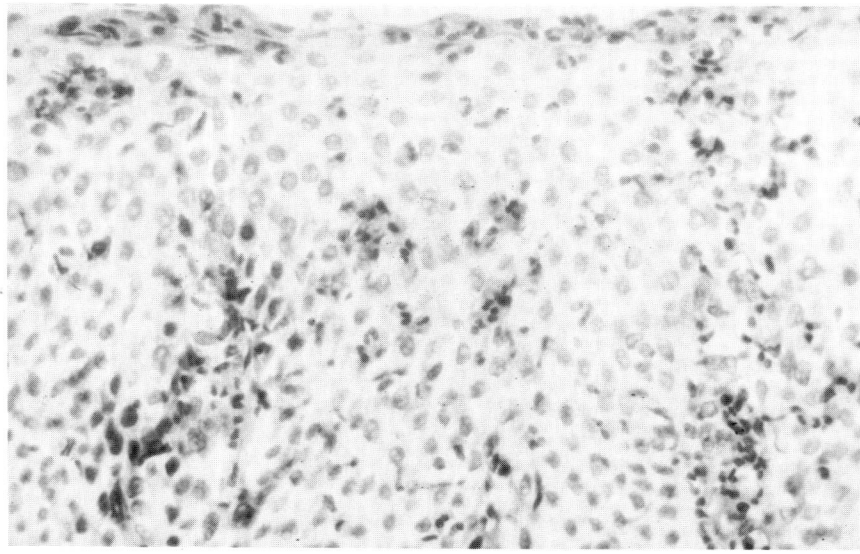

FIGURE 10–5. Esophageal mucosa in allergic gastroenteritis. There are large clumps of eosinophils within the epithelium and on its surface. (H&E, × 400)

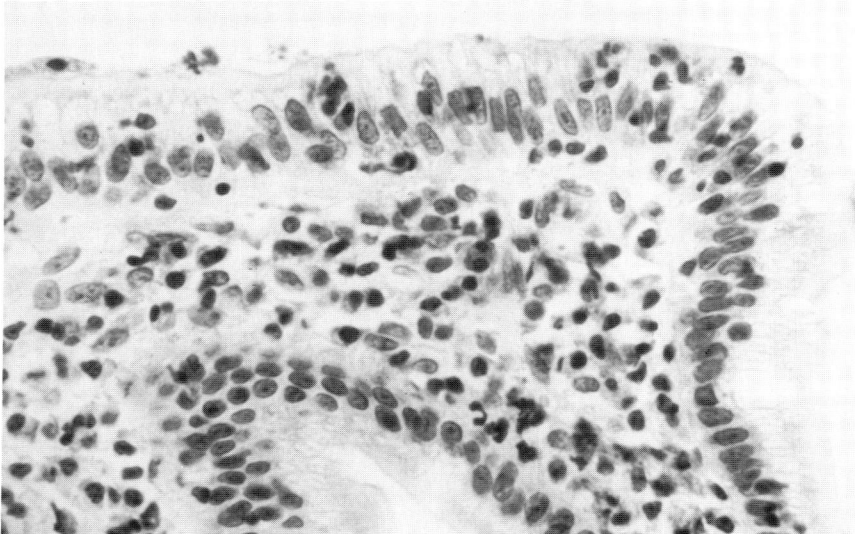

FIGURE 10–6. Gastric antral mucosa in allergic gastroenteritis. Numerous eosphinophils are present in the lamina propria, and there is focal extension into the surface epithelial layer (top right). (H&E, × 400)

submucosa (Figures 10–7 and 10–8). There is destruction of the surface and glandular epithelium with the presence of clusters of eosinophils within the lumina of the gastric foveolae (pits). Exceptionally, there is the appearance of marked mucosal edema and surface erosions (Figure 10–9), and this can be visualized by endoscopic and radiographic examinations.[49] Small foci of intestinal metaplasia have been observed in the chronic cases, but there is no development of atrophic gastritis. Lesions of the corpus and fundic mucosa tend to be more focal and much milder in appearance, consisting of only a small number of eosinophils in the lamina propria and rare extension of the eosinophils into the epithelial layer; the corpus mucosa is typically normal in the milder cases due to a single food allergen.

Only a rare eosinophil is noted in the lamina propria of the normal gastric mucosa, and the cells do not ordinarily penetrate the epithelial layer. An additional advantage of looking for evidence of allergic disease in the gastric antrum is that there are very few disorders due to other causes with a similar histologic appearance. Thus, although a prominent eosinophilic infiltrate can be seen in the gastric mucosa in some cases of parasitic infections, vasculitis, Crohn's disease, amyloidosis, and occasional tumors, these disorders can be readily distinguished by the finding of other more specific features. The more common causes of gastritis, including those due to alcohol, medications, and bile reflux are associated with glandular destruction, but the inflammatory infiltrate is typically composed of neutrophils and mononuclear types without a prominence of eosinophils. Occasional cases of any gastritis and the mucosa adjacent to a chronic peptic ulcer may reveal scattered clusters of eosinophils in the lamina propria, causing particular concern in a mucosal biopsy

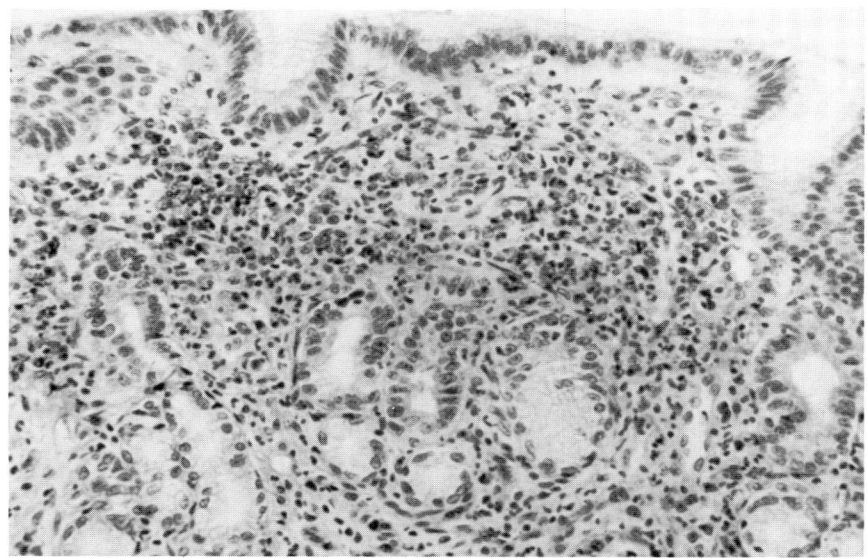

FIGURE 10–7. Gastric antral mucosa in allergic gastroenteritis. There is an extensive infiltrate of eosinophils associated with damage to the gastric glands. (H&E, × 100)

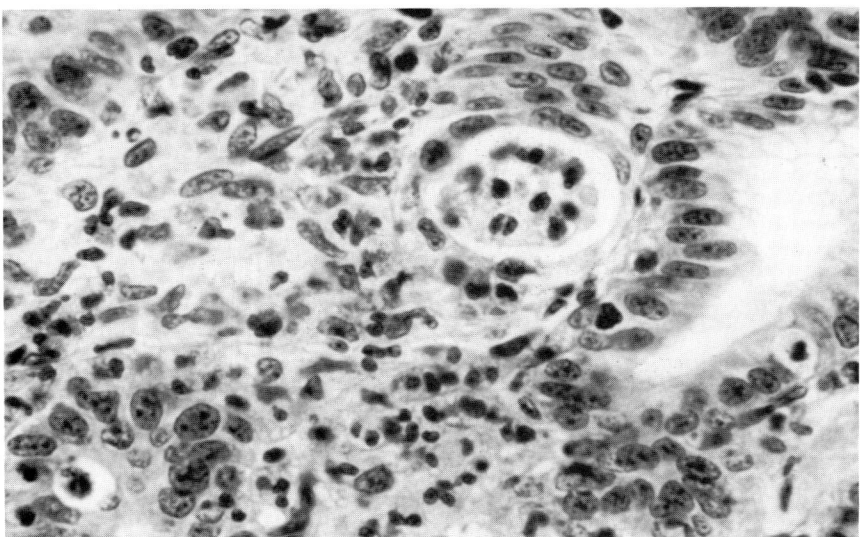

FIGURE 10-8. Gastric antral mucosa in allergic gastroenteritis, showing damaged gastric pit with numerous eosinophils within its lumen. (H&E, × 400) (From Goldman H, Antonioli DA: Mucosal biopsy of the esophagus, stomach, and proximal duodenum. Hum Pathol 13:423, 1982.)

sample; in such cases, however, there is rarely any extension of the eosinophils into the epithelium and glandular lumina. Enlarged gastric folds can be observed in Ménétrier's disease,[66] both in children and in adults; but these are invariably confined to the proximal stomach, in contrast to the antrum, where they are found in allergic disease. As described above in the section on eosinophilic gastroenteritis, the mural form commonly affects the gastric antrum. This disorder, however, is characterized by an inflammatory mass that is concentrated in the wall of the stomach, with at most a focal ulceration of the overlying mucosa. In this disorder, in contrast to allergic disease, there is no diffuse injury of the gastric mucosa or signs of damage to other parts of the gut mucosa, and there is no elevation of the serum IgE level or other signs of allergy in these patients.

Many of the patients with allergic gastroenteritis have signs of malabsorption, leading to a consideration of other more common disorders such as celiac disease (gluten enteropathy) and prolonged viral enteritis. In these cases, examination of the gastric antrum can be especially useful in establishing an allergic condition, because the stomach is not directly affected in the other intestinal disorders.

Small Intestine

Lesions are commonly noted in the small-intestinal mucosa in patients with allergic gastroenteritis, both the mild type due to a single food allergen and the severe form.[12-15,32,33] The lesions have been most commonly noted in the duodenum and jejunum and least often in the ileum, but this may reflect in part the access by endoscopy and selective biopsy of the more proximal portion of the small bowel. The allergic lesions in the small intestine are most often focal, even in the severe cases due to multiple antigens; and numerous biopsy samples are usually required for their detection.[13]

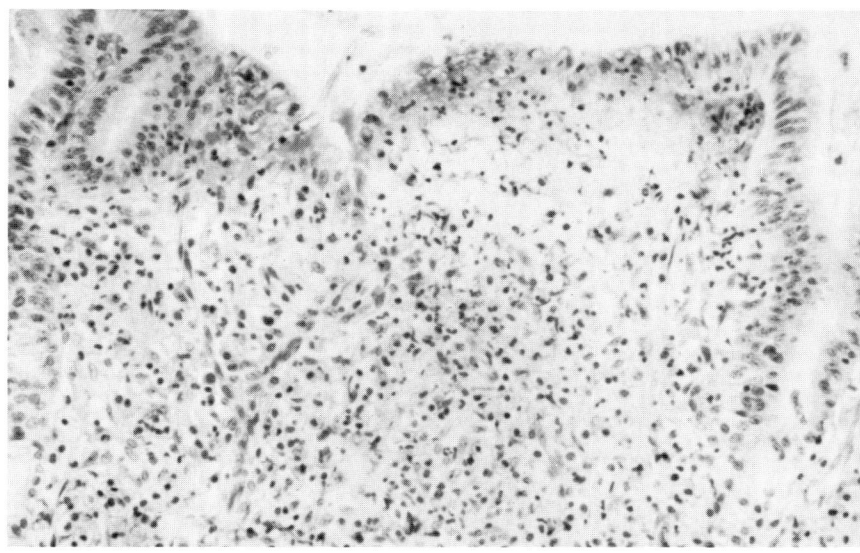

FIGURE 10-9. Gastric antral mucosa in allergic gastroenteritis. There are extensive destruction of the glands, edema, and superficial erosion. This can result in grossly enlarged folds. (H&E, × 60)

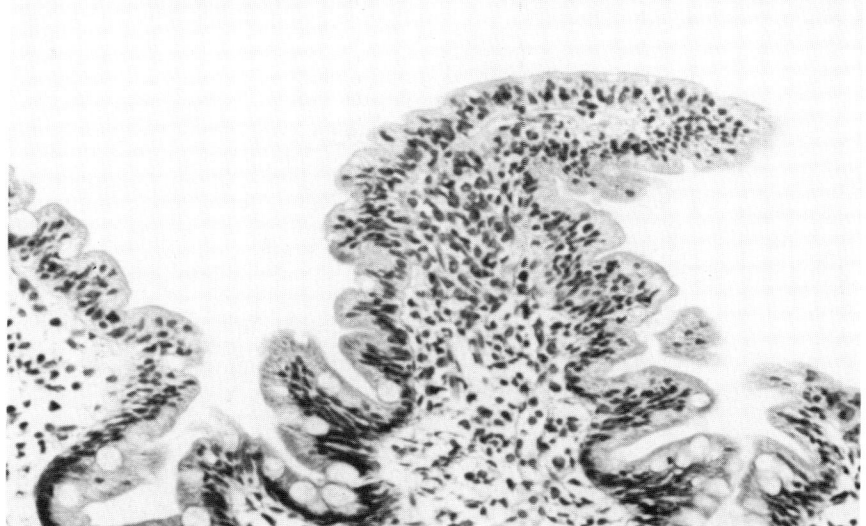

FIGURE 10–10. Small-intestinal mucosa in allergic gastroenteritis. There is a mild lesion, characterized by focal and partial shortening of the villi. A large cluster of eosinophils is noted in the lamina propria, with focal extension into the epithelial layer (the left side of the villus). (H&E, × 400)

In most instances, there is only a partial blunting of the villi, a focal infiltrate of eosinophils in the lamina propria of the villous cores, and extension of a few eosinophils into the surface epithelial layer (Figure 10–10). There also may be increased lymphocytes in the surface layer; and the epithelium often shows evidence of damage in the form of a less well-formed brush border, corresponding to a shortening and diminution of the microvilli, and the presence of numerous small lipid vacuoles in the cytoplasm.[51] The lipid nature of these vacuoles is ordinarily inferred because of the lack of reaction with various mucin stains but has been substantiated in electron-microscopic studies. In these milder lesions, there is usually only a slight crypt hyperplasia and no great increase of other inflammatory cells in the lamina propria. More marked or advanced lesions are observed in only about 10% of the cases and reveal greater shortening or complete loss of the villi, together with more pronounced damage of the surface epithelium, crypt hyperplasia, and mononuclear inflammatory cells in the lamina propria and surface epithelial layer (Figures 10–11 and 10–12). The quantity of eosinophils in these marked lesions is variable; there may be only a few small clusters or a diffuse infiltrate.

There are problems in trying to establish allergic disease in the small intestine. A small number of eosinophils is normally present in the lamina propria, both between the crypts and in the villous cores.[51,52] In the absence of quantitative measurements that are ordinarily not available,[67] only the presence of a considerable increase of eosinophils with the formation of large clusters or aggregates and their extension into the epithelial layer, together with signs of epithelial damage, can be considered evidence of an active enteritis that may be due to allergic disease. Furthermore, the num-

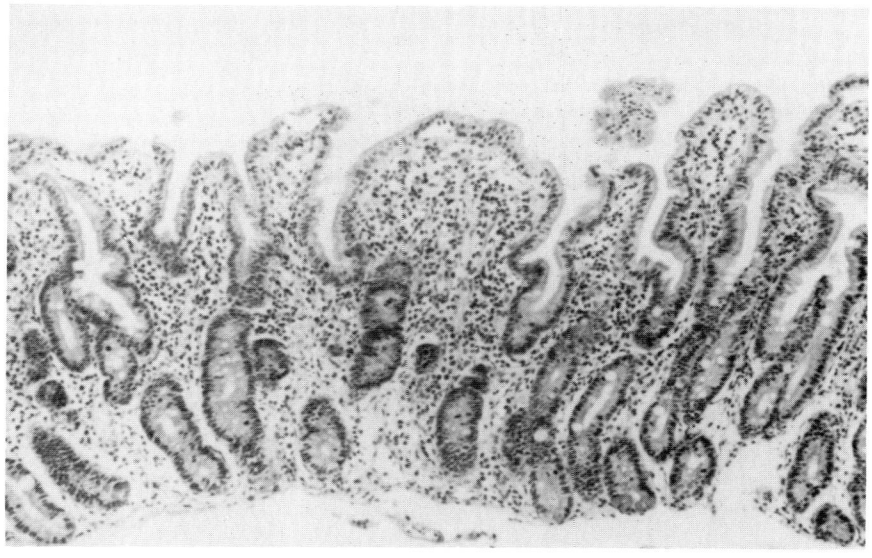

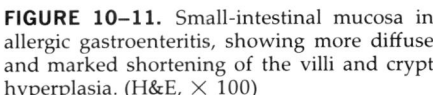

FIGURE 10–11. Small-intestinal mucosa in allergic gastroenteritis, showing more diffuse and marked shortening of the villi and crypt hyperplasia. (H&E, × 100)

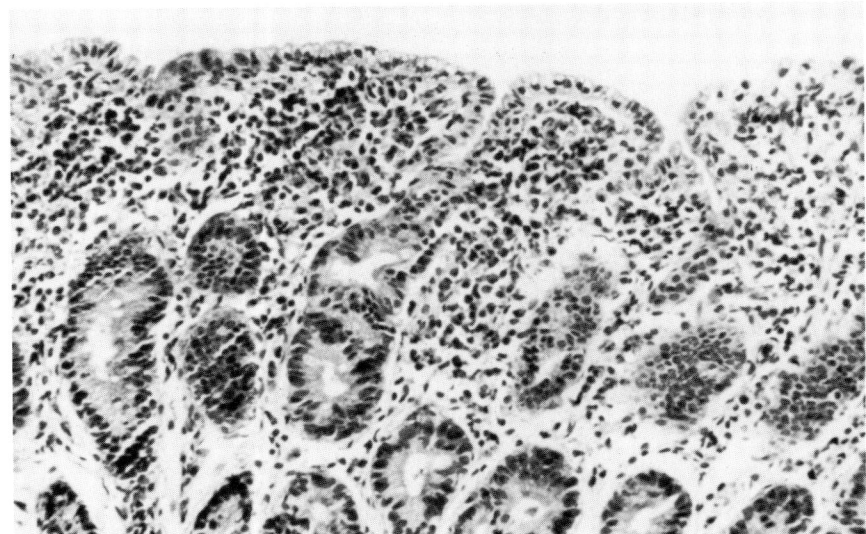

FIGURE 10–12. Small-intestinal mucosa in allergic gastroenteritis. There is complete loss of villi and marked flattening and degeneration of the surface epithelium, simulating the appearance of active celiac disease (gluten enteropathy). (H&E, × 250)

ber of eosinophils that can be present in an allergic lesion is highly variable, and there are some cases, including those with marked villous shortening, that may not reveal a conspicuous eosinophilic infiltrate; this is a special problem in the evaluation of the relatively small mucosal biopsy specimens. Finally, even if there is marked tissue eosinophilia, the histologic findings are not specific, because an equivalent increase in eosinophils can be seen in many other conditions affecting the small-bowel mucosa. Accordingly, the diagnosis of allergic disease affecting the small intestine must always be made in accord with compatible clinical and laboratory features. As described above, it may prove useful to add examination of the gastric antrum and, perhaps, the esophageal mucosa in such cases, because the differential diagnosis is more limited in those areas.

In patients with allergic disease of the small intestine resulting in malabsorption or a protein-losing enteropathy, the principal differential diagnoses are celiac disease (gluten enteropathy), prolonged infections, and a variety of immunologic disorders; these are covered in Chapter 29. Mucosal biopsy may reveal a specific disorder such as Whipple's disease, lymphangiectasia, or amyloidosis; but this is a rare event. The stool and biopsy samples should be examined for evidence of a protozoan or helminthic infection, and toxic reactions to ingested chemicals and drugs should be excluded. In celiac disease and in tropical sprue, the lesions are always diffuse; and a focal lesion observed in a mucosal biopsy can serve to exclude them. Conversely, occasional cases of allergic disease reveal diffuse lesions with variable quantities of eosinophils, and the distinction from celiac disease may require a trial of a gluten-free diet. Crohn's disease may also show an increase of mucosal eosinophils; but there are usually signs of more extensive damage, with ulcerations, sinuses, and strictures as well as occasional granulomas; furthermore, the disease is most often concentrated in the distal ileum and colon. Patients with vascular-connective tissue disorders such as lupus erythematosus and polyarteritis nodosa may disclose an increase in eosinophils, typically located in an inflammatory band just above the muscularis mucosae.[60] Rarely, cases of allergic disease of the small bowel can develop superficial ulcerations[50] simulating refractory sprue or an occult lymphoma, and an operative biopsy may be required for the distinction.

Colon and Rectum

The large bowel is least involved in cases of generalized allergic gastroenteritis, whether due to a single antigen or to multiple antigens. The lesions are typically minor, consisting of patchy infiltrates of eosinophils in the lamina propria and only rare damage of the surface and crypt epithelium. There are usually no functional disturbances that can be directly related to the involvement of the colonic mucosa, and both endoscopic and radiographic examinations of the large intestine are typically normal in patients with the diffuse form of allergic gastroenteritis.[2]

It should be stressed, however, that both the rectum and the colon can be involved with food sensitivity but that the cases are usually limited to this region and unassociated with disease affecting the upper part of the gastrointestinal tract. These cases are described in the following sections.

ALLERGIC PROCTITIS AND COLITIS

Definitions

The terms *allergic proctitis* and *allergic colitis* are used to indicate cases in which the lesions are predominantly confined or limited to the large intestine. The great majority of cases affect infants and young chil-

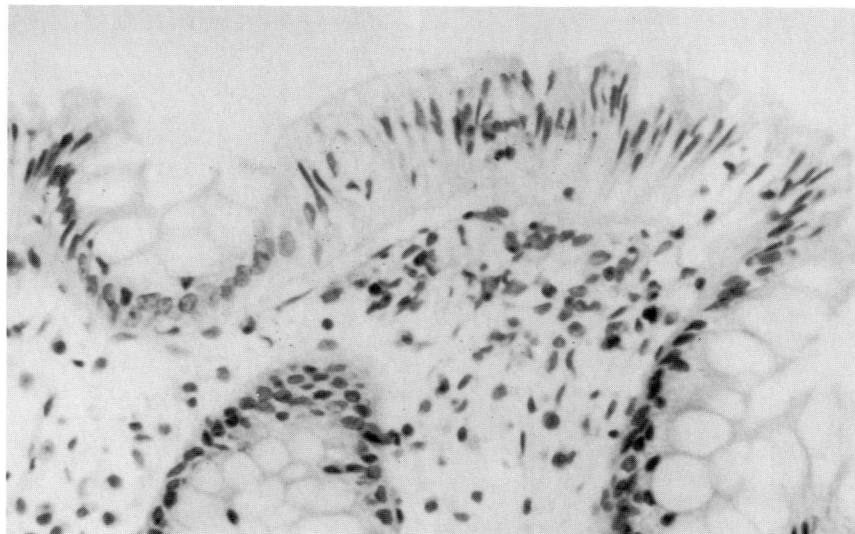

FIGURE 10-13. Rectal mucosa in allergic proctitis, showing a cluster of eosinophils in the upper lamina propria with extension into the surface epithelium. (H&E, × 400)

dren; whereas there are only isolated reports of disease involving the colon, alone or in conjunction with ileitis, in adults.

Childhood Cases

Clinical and Laboratory Features

Isolated food allergy affecting the rectum and colon is probably the leading cause of colitis in infants.[1] Most cases are due to cow's milk protein,[7,8,10,68,69] alone or together with soy protein[9,10,70]; and the patients promptly respond to an elimination of these foods from the diet. Although rechallenge studies have been recommended,[5] they are ordinarily not performed because of the clear association with the offending foods and the ready availability of alternative formulas.[6,45,46] As noted above, most patients lose the particular food sensitivity after several years and appear to be able to ingest the substance without problems as adults.

The disorder appears to be more common in males, and most cases present in the first 6 months of age and practically all before 2 years of age.[1] In a personal series of 15 childhood cases,[2] the average age at onset was 5 months and the median age 2 months. Almost all cases have overt rectal bleeding, alone or together with diarrhea. Other symptoms, including vomiting, abdominal pain, and weight loss, are uncommon; and only a rare patient or family member reveals allergic symptoms referable to other organ systems. The blood eosinophil count is usually elevated to levels of 10% to 20%, but the serum IgE is only mildly increased, and RAST responses are typically negative. Anemia is also uncommon, and it is probable that the low frequency of general symptoms and abnormal laboratory test results is related to the very young age of the patients. Compared with cases of allergic gastroenteritis, patients with allergic proctitis and colitis are generally much younger, present with more rectal bleeding and diarrhea, and have a lower incidence of other symptoms and altered laboratory results. The colitis cases are also more often due to a single antigen, and therefore the patients fare better.

Pathologic Features

Most of the information has been obtained by examination of rectal mucosal biopsies, but limited studies suggest that there is equivalent involvement in the colonic mucosa.[1,2,10,70] The exact distribution of the disease, whether it is patchy or diffuse and whether it is concentrated in the left portion or more universal, however, is not known. The abnormal findings are generally similar in the rectal and colonic mucosa and consist mainly of a diffuse increase of eosinophils in the lamina propria and very focal damage of the surface epithelium and crypts (Figure 10–13). The area of epithelial injury is usually very small and may be limited to one or two crypts in a biopsy sample, which emphasizes the need to examine multiple levels of such specimens. The injured epithelium is associated with an almost pure eosinophilic reaction, with eosinophils noted in the epithelial layer and rarely in the crypt lumina (Figure 10–14). More marked cases are less often noted and show an even greater increase of eosinophils, which may extend into the region of the muscularis mucosae and upper submucosa, and more necrosis with a neutrophilic reaction. The overall mucosal architecture remains normal, and signs of a chronic colitis[71] are not seen. The underlying bowel wall is not involved. Because the mucosal lesions in the colon and rectum are generally mild, there are usually no gross abnormalities, and radiographic studies are typically normal. Endoscopic examination is also usually normal or may reveal scattered petechiae or a rare erosion.

Occasionally mucosal biopsy specimens of the small intestine show a minor abnormality, but this is not clinically significant. There are usually no alterations in the

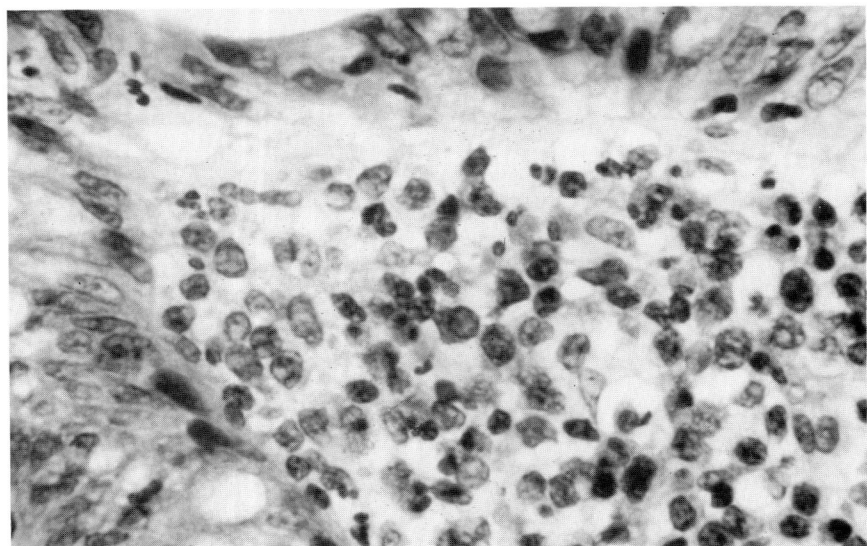

FIGURE 10–14. Rectal mucosa in allergic proctitis. There is a marked infiltrate of eosinophils in the lamina propria, with extension into the crypt (left) and surface (top) epithelium. (H&E, × 400)

mucosa of the proximal gut in cases of allergic proctitis or colitis.

Diagnosis and Differential Diagnosis

As is the case in the small intestine (see Allergic Gastroenteritis), it may be difficult to evaluate the finding of eosinophils in the colonic mucosa, because a small number are present in the normal lamina propria.[72,73] Indeed, one may encounter a rare eosinophil in the surface epithelium of the colonic mucosa in an otherwise normal person. Quantitative measurements have varied, but an average of up to six eosinophils per high-power field of the colonic mucosa is generally considered to be within the normal range.[74] In a comparative evaluation of rectal biopsies in children with allergic proctitis, those with infections and those who were normal, the finding of greater than 60 eosinophils per 10 high-power fields and infiltration of the muscularis mucosae by eosinophils were the two features that best correlated with the allergic cases.[75] The penetration of eosinophils into the surface and crypt epithelium can be seen in infections and in other colitides, but this feature is usually more prominent and other inflammatory cells such as neutrophils are lacking in most cases of allergic proctitis or colitis. As with allergic disease in other parts of the gut, the diagnosis of allergic proctitis requires the finding of compatible clinical and biopsy features and the exclusion of other causes of colitis, notably infections. It is not sufficient to relate the onset of disease to the introduction of a new food to the patient, because this may be merely coincidental. The diagnosis is ordinarily confirmed by noting the clinical resolution after withdrawal of the offending food.

The principal differential diagnoses in these young patients with allergic proctitis are infections and the obstructive type of colitis that can occur in cases of aganglionic megacolon. Colonic infections are often associated with more diffuse lesions and a greater neutrophilic reaction, which may be evident in the dysenteric stool; eosinophils are rarely a dominant feature. Nevertheless, one should always exclude an infectious cause of a proctitis or colitis by appropriate stool examination before making a diagnosis of allergic disease. The colitis that may complicate aganglionosis usually reveals a relatively bland hemorrhagic necrosis without a prominent tissue eosinophilia, and the primary diagnosis is secured by noting the absence of submucosal ganglia in the constricted portion. An increase in mucosal eosinophils is commonly noted in cases of chronic ulcerative colitis and Crohn's disease of the colon,[58] but there are also other features of a chronic colitis, in the form of an irregular crypt architecture, with budding and atrophy, and Paneth cell metaplasia[71,72]; furthermore, the idiopathic inflammatory bowel diseases are rare in patients under the age of 5 years. Other conditions that can affect the colonic mucosa and can be associated with tissue eosinophils include some of the vasculitides and chronic granulomatous disease[59]; these are distinguished by the finding of more specific features. Patients with necrotizing exterocolitis are typically much sicker and often reveal obstruction and signs of peritonitis.

Adult Cases

Allergic disease due to food in adults that is limited to the colon or to the colon and ileum appears to be a rare event.

Ulcerative Proctitis and Colitis

A subset of patients that were originally thought to have idiopathic ulcerative colitis was shown to contain an increased number of IgE-producing plasma cells and mast cells in the mucosa.[19] The lesions were concentrated in the rectum, and the patients responded selectively to antiallergy medications with a reduction in the symptoms and the number of mucosal inflammatory cells. Similar proliferations of IgE-bearing cells have been noted in other cases of proctitis and colitis,[20,21] but the provocative antigens are not known, and there have been no studies of long-term follow-up in these cases. It is not evident whether the allergic lesions are primary or not and whether the antigens are foods or other substances.

Isolated Cases

There have been isolated reports in adolescents and adults of presumed allergic disease confined to the colon[74,76] or to the ileum and colon.[77-79] Some of the cases appear to be the mural form of eosinophilic gastroenteritis (see the previous section), which can affect and be limited to the intestines; these must be sorted out because they do not have an allergic cause. The allergic cases present with abdominal pain and diarrhea, which may be bloody; and the peripheral eosinophil count is elevated. Enlarged folds and an inflamed mucosal surface are demonstrated by radiographic and endoscopic examination, and mucosal biopsies typically show mucosal damage with an intense eosinophilic reaction; over 60 eosinophils in a single high-power field have been noted.[74,79] The gross lesions usually appear to be segmental, but there have been no extensive biopsy studies showing whether more diffuse disease is possible. Although the particular food allergen is usually not known, patients typically respond to antiallergy therapy with complete recovery.

As described above, there are many other causes of enteritis and colitis that can have a prominent eosinophilic infiltrate in the mucosa, and these must be excluded before a diagnosis of allergic disease can be entertained. When one considers the age of the patients and the apparent segmental distribution of the lesions, the principal differential diagnoses are Crohn's disease, parasitic infections, and an occult lymphoma in the underlying wall of the intestine. Other common disorders that may present with segmental lesions of the colon include ischemic colitis and diverticular disease, but these are not associated with a prominent eosinophilic reaction.

MUCOSAL BIOPSY

The general techniques and uses of endoscopy and endoscopic biopsy are covered in Chapter 3. These procedures are invariably performed in cases of gastrointestinal food allergy in assisting in the diagnosis and in monitoring the course after therapy.[51,52,72] The allergic lesions are essentially confined to the mucosa; but they are often focal, necessitating the need for multiple samples and the examination of several levels of a biopsy specimen.

The biopsy results in a series of 38 cases of allergic gastroenteritis in children are summarized in Table 10-5.[2] Although biopsy of the small intestine, including the duodenum and proximal jejunum, has been most frequently performed, the lesions are usually focal and of a mild degree. In contrast, disease of the gastric antrum can be documented in a higher percentage of cases, even with only a single biopsy, and the lesions tend to be more florid. Also, because the differential diagnosis of an eosinophilic infiltrate appears to be more limited in the stomach, an antral biopsy would be the preferred choice in trying to establish whether a patient has an allergic disorder. It is important that the antral mucosa be selectively sampled, because lesions in the gastric corpus or fundus are usually sparse. It has also become evident that allergic disease of the esophagus is more common than formerly thought. The features observed in esophageal mucosal biopsies are similar to those seen in the much more prevalent disorder reflux esophagitis, resulting in the need to use other tests such as a pH probe or manometric studies to distinguish the two conditions in uncertain cases. The fact that the blood eosinophil count is normal in cases of reflux esophagitis and elevated in most patients with allergic gastroenteritis is helpful.

In cases of allergic gastroenteritis, rectal and colonic involvement in the absence of lesions in the proximal part of the gut is exceedingly uncommon, and it is unlikely that biopsy samples of the large bowel need be obtained in such cases. Conversely, the colon and rectum are preferentially involved in the cases of allergic proctitis, and biopsy of this area should be performed in patients that present with rectal bleeding or greater diarrhea, especially in infants.

Table 10-5 BIOPSY OF ALLERGIC GASTROENTERITIS IN CHILDREN

Tissue	Biopsy Cases (%)	Positive Biopsies (%)	Marked Alteration (%)
Esophagus	39	60	53
Gastric corpus	55	52	10
Gastric antrum	58	100	73
Small intestine	89	79	12
Rectum	21	13	0

Modified from Goldman H, Proujansky R: Allergic proctitis and allergic gastroenteritis in children: Clinical and mucosal biopsy features in 53 cases. Am J Surg Pathol 10:75, 1986.

References

1. Jenkins HR, Pincott JR, Soothill JF, et al: Food allergy: the major cause of infantile colitis. Arch Dis Child 59:326-329, 1984.
2. Goldman H, Proujansky R: Allergic proctitis and allergic gastroenteritis in children: clinical and mucosal biopsy features in 53 cases. Am J Surg Pathol 10:75-86, 1986.
3. Kaplan SM, Goldstein F, Kowlessar OD: Eosinophilic gastroenteritis: Report of a case with malabsorption and protein-losing enteropathy. Gastroenterology 58:540-545, 1970.
4. Cello JP: Eosinophilic gastroenteritis—A complex disease entity. Am J Med 87:1097-1104, 1979.
5. Goldman AS, Anderson DW Jr, Sellers WA, et al: Milk allergy. I. Oral challenge with milk and isolated milk proteins in allergic children. Pediatrics 32:425-443, 1963.
6. Sumithran E, Iyngkaran N: Is jejunal biopsy really necessary in cow's milk protein intolerance? Lancet 2:1122-1123, 1977.
7. Grybowski JD: Gastrointestinal milk allergy in infants. Pediatrics 40:354-360, 1967.

8. Shiner M, Ballard J, Brook CGD, et al: Intestinal biopsy in the diagnosis of cow's milk protein intolerance without acute symptoms. Lancet 2:1060–1063, 1975.
9. Ament M, Rubin CE: Soy protein—Another cause of the flat intestinal lesion. Gastroenterology 62:227–234, 1972.
10. Halpin RC, Byrne WJ, Ament ME: Colitis, persistent diarrhea and soy protein intolerance. J Pediatr 91:404–410, 1977.
11. Eastham EJ, Walker WA: Adverse effects of milk formula ingestion on the gastrointestinal tract: An update. Gastroenterology 70:364–374, 1979.
12. Klein NC, Hargrove RL, Sleisenger MH, Jeffries GH: Eosinophilic gastroenteritis. Medicine 49:299–319, 1970.
13. Leinbach GE, Rubin CE: Eosinophilic gastroenteritis: A simple reaction to food allergens? Gastroenterology 59:874–889, 1970.
14. Jacobson LB: Diffuse eosinophilic gastroenteritis: An adult form of allergic gastroenteropathy: Report of a case with probable protein-losing enteropathy. Am J Gastroenterol 54:580–588, 1970.
15. Waldmann TA, Wochner RD, Laster L, Gordon RS: Allergic gastroenteropathy. N Engl J Med 276:761–769, 1967.
16. Stern M, Walker WA: Food allergy and intolerance. Ped Clin North Am 32:471–492, 1985.
17. Shiner M, Ballard J, Smith ME: The small intestinal mucosa in cow's milk allergy. Lancet 1:136–140, 1975.
18. Rosekrans PC, Meijer CG, van der Wal AM, Lindeman J: Use of morphometry and immunohistochemistry of small intestinal biopsy specimens in the diagnosis of food allergy. J Clin Pathol 33:125–130, 1980.
19. Rosekrans PC, Meijer CG, van der Wal AM, Lindeman J: Allergic proctitis: A clinical and immunopathological entity. Gut 21:1017–1023, 1980.
20. Heatley RV, Calcroft BJ, Fifield R, et al: Immunoglobin E in rectal mucosa of patients with proctitis. Lancet 2:1010–1012, 1975.
21. Murdock DL, Piris J: Immunoglobulin E in non-specific proctitis and ulcerative colitis: Studies with a monoclanal antibody. Digestion 25:201–204, 1983.
22. Ogawa H, Kunkel SL, Fantone JC, Ward PA: Comparative study of eosinophil and neutrophil chemotaxis and enzyme release. Am J Pathol 105:149–155, 1981.
23. Uden AM, Palmblad J, Lindgren JA, Malmsten C: Effects of novel lipoxygenase products on migration of eosinophils and neutrophils in vitro. Int Arch Allergy Appl Immunol 72:91–93, 1983.
24. Weller PF, Dvorak JA, Whitehouse WC: Human eosinophil stimulation promoter lymphokine: Production by antigen stimulated lymphocytes and assay with a new electro-optical technique. Cell Immunol 40:91–102, 1978.
25. Hirashima M, Tashiro K, Skata K, Hirashima M: Isolation of an eosinophil chemotactic lymphokine as a natural mediator for eosinophil chemotaxis from concanavalin A-induced skin reaction sites in guinea-pigs. Clin Exp Immunol 57:211–219, 1984.
26. Gleich GH, Frigas E, Leogering DA, Wassom DL, Steinmuller D: Cytologic properties of the eosinophil major basic protein. J Immunol 123:2925–2927, 1979.
27. Dvorak AM: Ultrastructural evidence for release of major basic protein-containing crystalline cores of eosinophil granules in vivo: Cytotoxic potential in Crohn's disease. J Immunol 125:460–462, 1980.
28. Weller PF, Lee CW, Foster DW, et al: Generation and metabolism of 5-lipoxygenase pathway leukotrienes by human eosinophils: Predominant production of leukotriene C_4. Proc Natl Acad Sci 80:7626–7630, 1983.
29. Keshavarzian A, Saverymuttu SH, Tai P-C, et al: Activated eosinophils in familial eosinophilic gastroenteritis. Gastroenterology 88:1041–1049, 1985.
30. Marnocha KE, Maglinte DDT, Kelvin FM, et al: Eosinophilic enteritis associated with chronic eosinophilic pneumonia. Am J Gastroenterol 81:1205–1208, 1986.
31. Talley NJ, Shorter RG, Zinsmeister AR: Eosinophilic gastroenteritis: A clinicopathological study of patients with disease of the mucosa, muscle layer, and subserosal tissues. Gut 31:54–58, 1990.
32. Greenberger NJ, Tennenbaum L, Ruppert RD: Protein-losing enteropathy associated with gastrointestinal allergy. Am J Med 43:777–784, 1967.
33. Kuitunen P, Visakorpi JK, Savilahti E, Pelkonen P: Malabsorption syndrome with cow's milk intolerance. Arch Dis Child 50:351–356, 1975.
34. Ureles AL, Alschibaja T, Lodico D, Stabins SJ: Idiopathic eosinophilic infiltration of the gastrointestinal tract, diffuse and circumscribed: A proposed classification and review of the literature, with two additional cases. Am J Med 30:899–908, 1961.
35. Jona JZ, Belin RP, Burke JA: Eosinophilic infiltration of the gastrointestinal tract in children. Am J Dis Child 130:1136–1139, 1976.
36. Johnstone JM, Morson BC: Eosinophilic gastroenteritis. Histopathology 2:335–348, 1978.
37. Caldwell JH, Mekhjian HS, Hurtubise PE, Berman FM: Eosinophilic gastroenteritis with obstruction: Immunological studies of seven patients. Gastroenterology 74:825–829, 1978.
38. Russell JY, Evangelow G: Eosinophilic infiltration of the stomach and duodenum complicated by perforation. Postgrad Med J 41:30–33, 1965.
39. Felt-Bersma RJ, Neuwissen SG, van Velzen D: Perforation of the small intestine due to eosinophilic gastroenteritis. Am J Gastroenterol 79:442–445, 1984.
40. Lysey J, Eid A: Eosinophilic gastroenteritis with small bowel perforation. J Clin Gastroenterol 8:694–695, 1986.
41. Higgins GA, Lamm ER, Yutzy LV: Eosinophilic gastroenteritis. Arch Surg 92:476–483, 1966.
42. Levinson JD, Romanathan VR, Nozick JH: Eosinophilic gastroenteritis with ascites and colon involvement. Am J Gastroenterol 68:603–607, 1977.
43. Katz AJ, Goldman H, Flores AF, Twaroq FJ: Esophageal involvement in allergic (eosinophilic) gastroenteritis. Gastroenterology 88:1438, 1985.
44. Snyder JD, Rosenblum N, Wershil B, et al: Pyloric stenosis and eosinophilic gastroenteritis in infants. J Ped Gastroenterol Nutr 6:543–547, 1987.
45. Zeiger RS, Heller S, Mellon M, et al: Effectiveness of dietary manipulation in the prevention of food allergy in infants. J Allergy Clin Immunol 78:224–238, 1986.
46. Sogn D: Medications and their use in the treatment of adverse reactions to foods. J Allergy Clin Immunol 78:238–243, 1986.
47. Katz AJ, Twaroq FJ, Zeiger RS, Falchuk ZM: Milk-sensitive and eosinophilic gastroenteropathy: Similar clinical features with contrasting mechanisms and clinical course. J Allergy Clin Immunol 74:72–78, 1984.
48. Katz, AJ, Goldman H, Grand RJ: Gastric mucosal biopsy in eosinophilic (allergic) gastroenteritis. Gastroenterology 73:705–709, 1977.
49. Teele RL, Katz AJ, Goldman H, Kettell RM: The radiographic features of eosinophilic gastroenteritis (allergic gastroenteropathy) of childhood. Am J Radiol 132:575–580, 1979.
50. Lucak BK, Sansaricq C, Snyderman SE, et al: Disseminated ulcerations in allergic eosinophilic gastroenterocolitis. Am J Gastroenterol 77:248–252, 1978.
51. Perera DR, Weinstein WM, Rubin CE: Small intestinal biopsy. Hum Pathol 6:157–217, 1975.
52. Goldman H, Antonioli DA: Mucosal biopsy of the esophagus, stomach, and proximal duodenum. Hum Pathol 13:423–448, 1982.
53. Winter HS, Madara JL, Stafford RJ, et al: Intraepithelial eosinophils: A new diagnostic criterion for reflux esophagitis. Gastroenterology 83:818–823, 1982.
54. Brown LF, Goldman H, Antonioli DA: Intraepithelial eosinophils in endoscopic biopsies of adults with reflux esophagitis. Am J Surg Pathol 8:889–905, 1984.
55. Lee RG: Marked eosinophila in esophageal mucosal biopsies. Am J Surg Pathol 9:475–479, 1986.
56. Martin DM, Goldman JA, Gilliam J, Nasrallash SM: Gold-induced eosinophilic enterocolitis: Response to oral cromolyn sodium. Gastroenterology 80:1567–1570, 1981.
57. Haggitt RC: Granulomatous diseases of the gastrointestinal tract: In Iochim HL (ed): Pathology of Granulomas. New York, Raven Press, 1983, pp 257–305.
58. Heatley RV, James PD: Eosinophils in rectal mucosa. Gut 20:787–791, 1978.
59. Ament ME, Ochs HD: Gastrointestinal manifestations of chronic granulomatous disease. N Engl J Med 288:382–387, 1973.

60. DeSchryver-Kecskemeti K, Clouse RE: A previously unrecognized subgroup of "eosinophic gastroenteritis": Association with connective tissue diseases. Am J Surg Pathol 8:171–180, 1984.
61. Dobbins JW, Sheahan DG, Behar J: Eosinophilic gastroenteritis with esophageal involvement. Gastroenterology 72:1312–1316, 1977.
62. Picus D, Frank PH: Eosinophilic esophagitis. AJR 136:1001–1003, 1981.
63. Matzenger MA, Daneman A: Esophageal involvement in eosinophilic gastroenteritis. Pediatr Radiol 13:35–38, 1983.
64. Weinstein WM, Bogoch ER, Bowes KL: The normal esophageal mucosa: A histologic reappraisal. Gastroenterology 68:40–44, 1975.
65. Reimann H-J, Lewin J: Gastric mucosal reactions in patients with food allergy. Am J Gastroenterol 83:1212–1219, 1988.
66. Baker A, Volberg F, Summer T, Moron R: Childhood Menetrier's disease: Four new cases and discussion of the literature. Gastrointest Radiol 11:131–134, 1986.
67. Peckkio M, Savilahti E, Kuitunen P: Morphometric and immunohistochemical study of jejunal biopsies from children with intestinal soy allergy. Fin Eur J Pediatr 137:63–69, 1981.
68. Wilson JF, Lahey ME, Heiner DC: Studies on iron metabolism. V. Further observations on cow's milk-induced gastrointestinal bleeding in infants with iron-deficiency anemia. J Pediatr 84:335–344, 1974.
69. Walker-Smith JA, Harrison M, Kilby A, et al: Cow's milk-sensitive enteropathy. Arch Dis Child 53:375–380, 1978.
70. Powell GK: Milk and soy-induced enterocolitis of infancy. J Pediatr 93:553–561, 1978.
71. Surawicz CM, Belic L: Rectal biopsy helps to distinguish acute self-limited colitis from idiopathic inflammatory bowel disease. Gastroenterology 86:104–113, 1984.
72. Goldman H, Antonioli DA: Mucosal biopsy of the rectum, colon and distal ileum. Hum Pathol 13:981–1012, 1982.
73. Levine DS, Haggitt RC: Normal histology of the colon. Am J Surg Pathol 13:966–984, 1989.
74. Moore D, Lichtman S, Lentz J, et al: Eosinophilic gastroenteritis presenting in an adolescent with isolated colonic involvement. Gut 27:1219–1222, 1986.
75. Winter HS, Antonioli DA, Fukagawa N, et al: Allergy-related proctocolitis in infants: Diagnostic usefulness of rectal biopsy. Modern Pathol 3:5–10, 1990.
76. Naylor AR, Pollett JE: Eosinophilic colitis. Dis Colon Rectum 28:615–618, 1985.
77. Haberkern CM, Christie DL, Haas EE: Eosinophilic gastroenteritis presenting as ileocolitis. Gastroenterology 74:896–899, 1978.
78. Schulze K, Mitros FA: Eosinophilic gastroenteritis involving the ileocecal area. Dis Colon Rectum 72:47–50, 1979.
79. Tedesco FJ, Huckaby CB, Hamby-Allen M, Ewing GC: Eosinophilic ileocolitis. Dig Dis Sci 26:943–948, 1981.

CHAPTER 11

Motor and Mechanical Disorders

FRANK A. MITROS, M.D.

NORMAL ANATOMY

MECHANICAL OBSTRUCTION
Causes and Effects
Special Forms of Obstruction

PSEUDO-OBSTRUCTION
Introduction
Chronic Disorders
Acute Disorders
Clinical Features
Primary Intestinal Pseudo-obstruction
Myopathy
Familial Cases

Sporadic Cases
Pathologic Features
Prognosis and Therapy
Neuropathy
Familial Cases
Sporadic Cases
Secondary Intestinal Pseudo-obstruction
Muscle Diseases
Scleroderma
Myotonic Dystrophy and Progressive Muscular Dystrophy
Ceroidosis
Small-Intestinal Diverticulosis
Amyloidosis

Neural Diseases
Hirschsprung's Disease
Neuronal Intestinal Dysplasia
Chagas' Disease
Parkinson's Disease
Others
Endocrine Disorders
Diabetes Mellitus
Hypothyroidism
Others
Pharmacologic Agents
Miscellaneous Lesions

CONCLUSION

Although the study of the gastrointestinal tract has been an area of intense interest to pathologists for many years, that interest has been until recently rather superficial, that is, limited largely to the mucosa. Although the smooth muscle and controlling neural apparatus constitute the bulk of the alimentary tube, these areas are relatively poorly studied, at least with regard to changes in human disease processes. Many of the diseases studied so carefully in mucosal biopsies are caused by underlying neuromuscular dysfunction. Gastroesophageal reflux and its consequences and the small-intestinal mucosal alterations in the stasis syndromes are two examples. As always, the morphologically oriented pathologist must struggle to gain an appreciation of the normal anatomy to better understand some of the changes seen in the disease process. For this reason, we will begin with a brief overview of the normal anatomy, concentrating on some of the peculiarities of the various segments of the gastrointestinal tract.

NORMAL ANATOMY[1]

With the exception of the proximal esophagus, the muscle of the gastrointestinal tract is smooth muscle. The myocytes of the gastrointestinal tract average about 500 to 700 μm in length and 6 μm in thickness; they are capable of up to a fourfold change in length. The general organization is into two layers, an inner circular and an outer longitudinal layer. There are regional variations, but the circular layer tends to be the thicker of the two. This is not surprising, because the circular layer controls the luminal diameter, and its rhythmic contractions provide the main propulsive force to move along the luminal contents. More is understood about the physiology of gastrointestinal motility than about its morphology[1]; these aspects are beyond the province of this chapter. Suffice it to say that there needs to be an integration of myogenic, neural, and hormonal influences; the muscle provides the major impetus for coordinated movement, and the

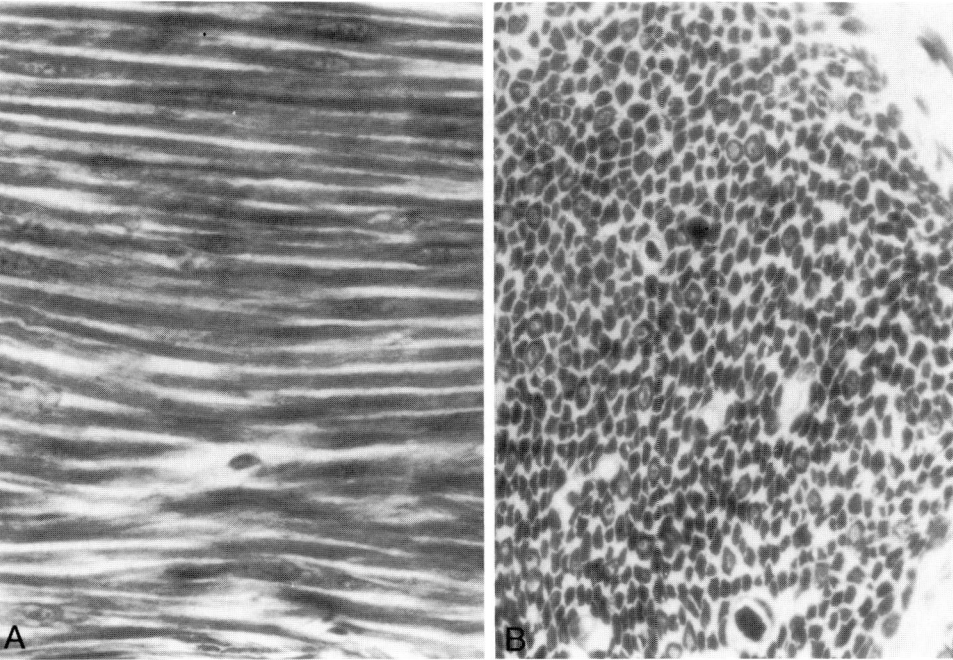

FIGURE 11–1. Well-oriented longitudinal (A) and cross (B) sections of the circular muscular layer of jejunum reveal a striking uniformity of the myocytes. Pericellular connective tissue is scant. (Trichrome, × 132)

neural and hormonal influences provide the fine tuning. There is a striking degree of uniformity in cell size in the normal muscularis propria. There is also only scant collagen around the individual smooth muscle cells. These features are best appreciated in a carefully oriented cross section through the muscle fibers (Figure 11–1).

The neural control of the gastrointestinal tract is exercised at three levels: the central nervous system, the prevertebral ganglia, and the intrinsic intramural neural structures. The last of these is the most amenable to study by morphologic methods; nevertheless, our knowledge is scanty. The intramural plexuses have two well-known components, the submucosal plexus (Meissner's) and the myenteric plexus (Auerbach's). The standard histologic section provides only a slitlike window for viewing the wonders of these plexuses (Figure 11–2). The techniques pioneered by Barbara Smith[2] and applied to human motility disorders by Schuffler[3] provide a new insight into these structures.

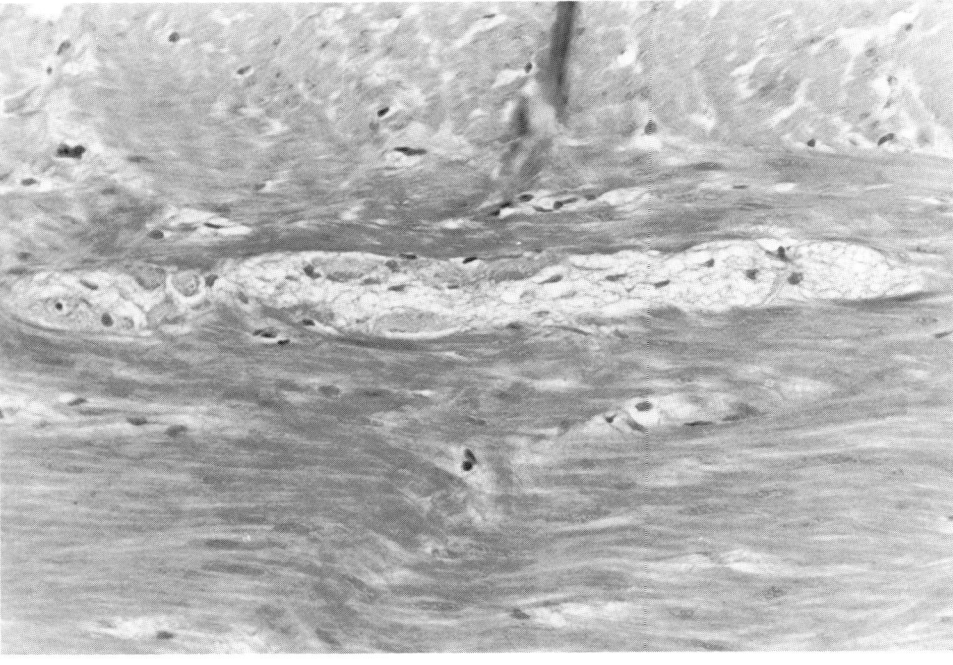

FIGURE 11–2. The standard view in a longitudinal section of colon provides only a glimpse at the myenteric plexus. Several mature ganglion cells and nerve fibers are visible. (H&E, × 66)

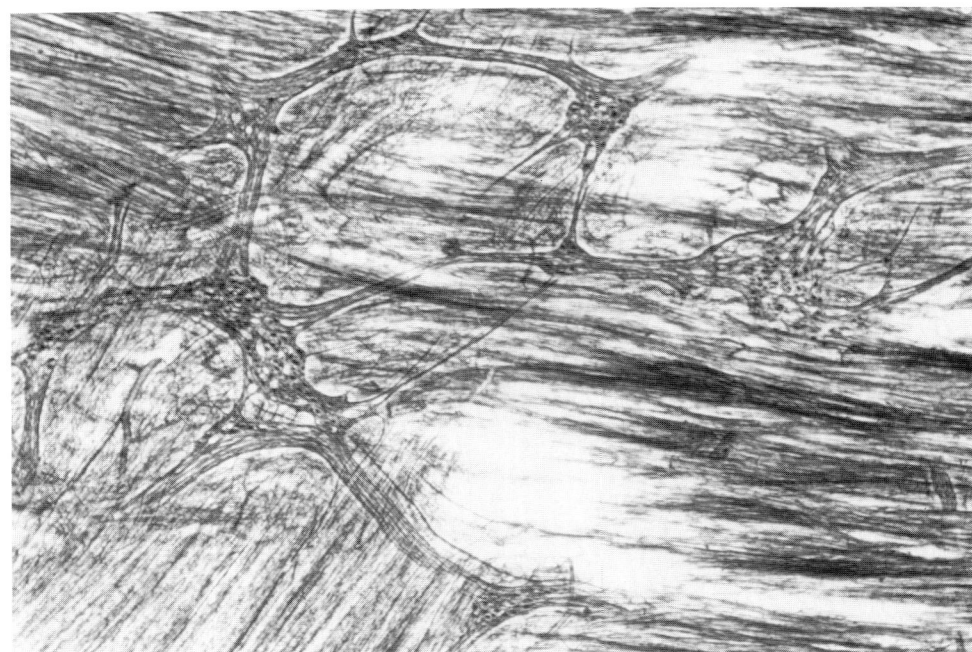

FIGURE 11–3. Myenteric plexus of normal colon viewed in a 50-μm section in the tangential plane. This provides some insight into the variability of the ganglia and the complexity of their interconnections. Note criss-crossing muscle fibers in the background. (Silver, × 7) (From a section prepared in the laboratory of Dr. M. D. Schuffler.)

Briefly, frozen sections of formalin-fixed bowel are cut on a sledge microtome in a plane tangential to the serosal surface at 50 μm until the plane of the myenteric plexus is reached. This plane is recognized by the trained eye by the crisscrossing of the muscle fibers of the two layers of the muscularis propria. These sections are then stained by a careful and experienced technologist with a silver stain, which unfortunately is quite difficult. When successful, the results of this procedure are extraordinary (Figures 11–3 and 11–4). The appearance of the ganglia is radically different from that in standard sections, and the interconnections between the ganglia can begin to be appreciated. Neurons are crudely broken down into two categories, argyrophil and argyrophobe, although it is immediately obvious that there is a good deal more heterogeneity than that. The argyrophilic neurons stain darkly because of the large number of neurofilaments that they contain; the argyrophobic cells stain a light brown and tend to be indistinct.[4] Glial cells are not well visualized. The functional correlates of this variable argyrophilia are not understood. Because of its more diffuse nature, the submucosal plexus is not amenable to such study.

It is becoming clear that there is a great deal of variability in the segments of the gastrointestinal tract with regard to the structure and presumably the function of the plexuses. Specialized structures, such as thickened bundles of nerve fibers ("shunt fascicles"), are beginning to be recognized in human tissues.[5] Obviously, a great deal of experience is needed to understand and interpret these various neural structures in the human disease process. Because the silver techniques are difficult and are not readily available in most centers, it is uncertain that they will ever play a major role in diagnostic pathology.

Standard immunoperoxidase techniques, particularly those employing antibodies against S-100 protein and neuron-specific enolase (NSE), are widely available, and are beginning to be employed for examination of a number of practical problems.[6] The neurons can be identified with certainty even in difficult situations, and the nerve bundles can be seen quite readily (Figure 11–5). Surprises remain in store for those beginning to apply these stains to the neuromuscular structures of the gut. Witness the numerous cells of apparent neural origin occupying a substantial position in the muscular layers (Figure 11–6). These mysterious structures, which have largely eluded the notice of even the most observant surgical pathologist, are the interstitial cells of Cajal.[6,7] The function of these cells is unknown, although it is clear that they are likely to play a major role in a number of human diseases.

Now we examine some of the features of the muscular and neural apparatus that are peculiar to the individual segments of the gastrointestinal tract, because the differences can interfere with interpretation of surgical specimens.

The *esophagus* contains abundant skeletal muscle, which forms the typical circular and longitudinal layers proximally. The circular layer extends intact somewhat beyond the longitudinal layer into the middle third, where an admixture with smooth muscle occurs. It is not certain that these fibers are strictly under voluntary control; the myenteric plexus is present even in areas composed largely of skeletal muscle. The physiologically distinctive and important lower esophageal sphincter is not readily recognizable morphologically, showing only subtle ultrastructural differences from the surrounding smooth muscle. The muscularis mucosae of the esophagus is extraordinarily thick (200 to

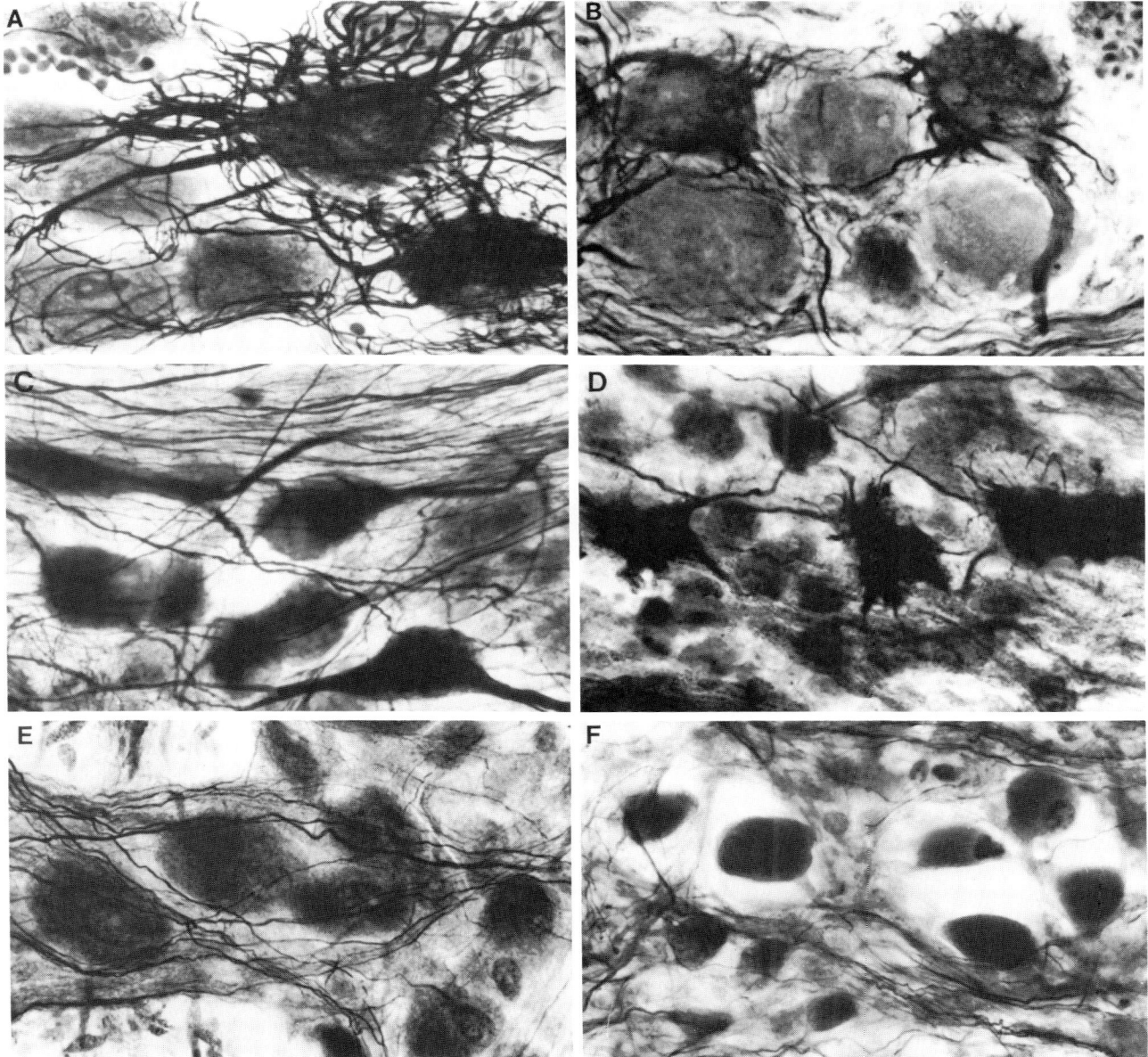

FIGURE 11-4. The normal esophagus, with complex argyrophilic (*A*) and rounded argyrophobic (*B*) neurons. The argyrophilic neurons of normal jejunum are smaller and less complex (*C*); the argyrophilic neurons of normal colon are small and quite irregular in shape (*D*). The normal argyrophobic neurons of jejunum (*E*) and of colon (*F*) have few visible processes (Silver stain, × 1360) (From Krishnamurthy S, Schuffler MD: Pathology of neuromuscular disorders of the small intestine and colon. Gastroenterology 93:610, 1987. Copyright 1987 by The American Gastroenterological Association. Reprinted by permission.)

400 μm), which often leads to a startling appearance and some concern in peroral biopsies. As is true of its counterpart in the rest of the gastrointestinal tract, nothing is known of its function. Ganglia tend to be small and are often located outside the plane of the large nerve bundles (parafascicular ganglia). The final peculiarity of the esophagus is the virtual absence of a submucosal neural plexus.

The muscularis propria of the *stomach* is distinctive, in that it contains a third layer, the inner oblique layer, which appears to be in continuity with the lower esophageal sphincter; it diminishes in the distal portion of the stomach. The circular layer exists only up to the pylorus, whereas the longitudinal layer is continuous with that of the duodenum. The muscle of the antrum is quite thick. The pyloric sphincter serves to prevent duodenal reflux and acts as a barrier to the distal passage of the large food particles.

Despite its great physiologic complexity with regard to motility, the structure of the neuromuscular portion of the *small intestine* is simple and uniform throughout. There are no obvious specializations of the muscularis propria or neural plexuses on standard hematoxylin and eosin (H&E) sections. The muscularis mucosae

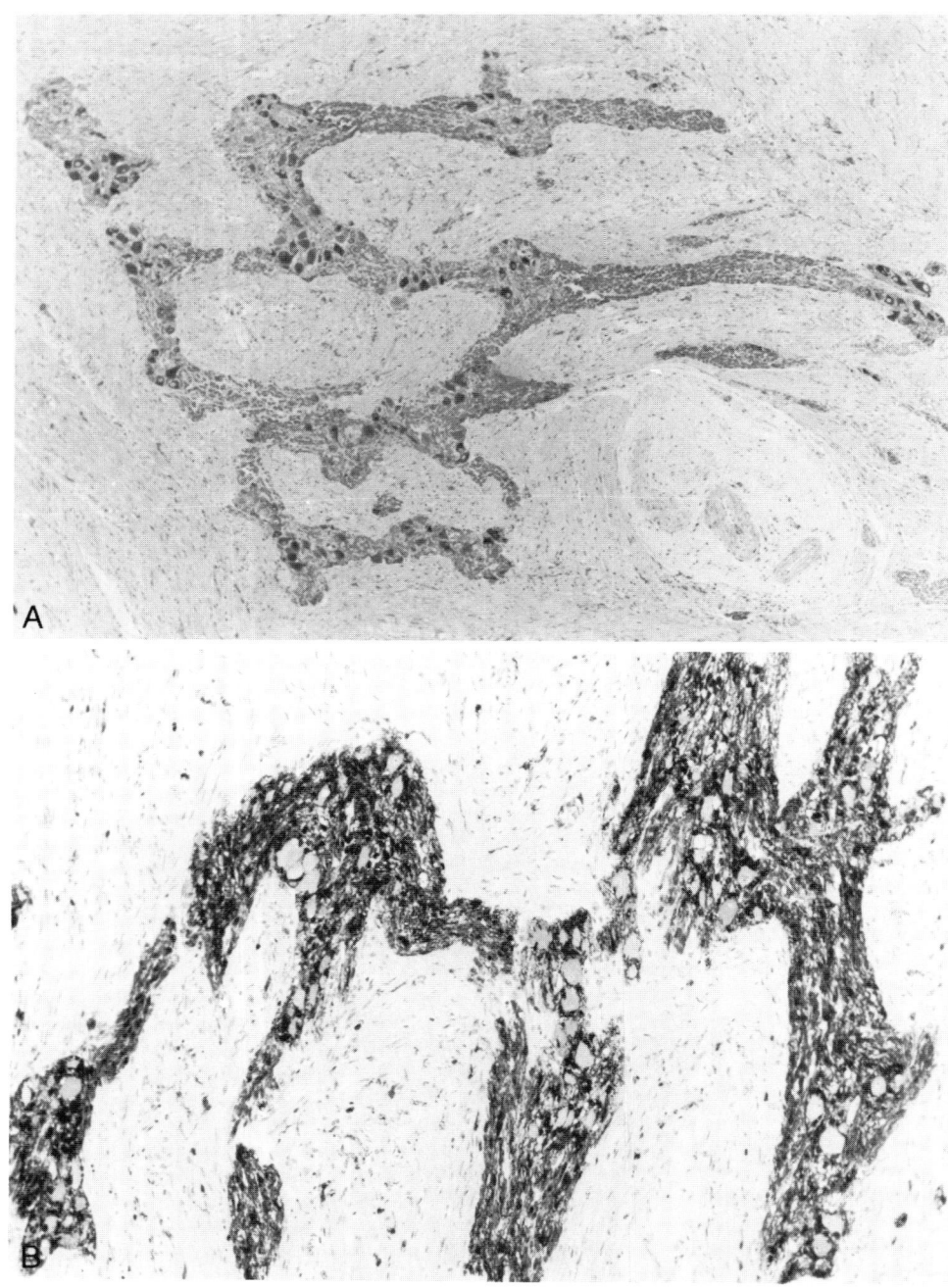

FIGURE 11–5. *A,* Neurons and nerve fibers are well appreciated in this 6-μm tangential section of normal colon. (Immunoperoxidase, NSE, × 16) *B,* Nerve fibers interconnecting ganglia in tangential section of normal colon. Immunologic methods are more widely available and less technically demanding than silver stain methods, but experience in their interpretation needs to be gained. (Immunoperoxidase, S-100, × 25)

does send numerous smooth muscle cells up into the lamina propria of the villi, which act to alter the villous configuration and surface area. The muscle of the ileocecal valve has a distinctive configuration, and routinely shows some excess collagen encircling individual muscle cells at its free edge (Figure 11–7).

The most obvious specialization in the *colon* is the formation of three taeniae coli by the longitudinal layer; these taeniae are present from cecum to proximal rectum. They can lead to a deceptive idea about the thickness of the external layer on longitudinal sections. There is normally a definite increase in collagen around myocytes in the taeniae, which can lead to a mistaken impression of fibrosis (Figure 11–8). Muscle fibers of the longitudinal layer, particularly the taeniae, may pass into the circular layer and fuse with it. It does not appear that study of the neuromuscular structures of the *appendix* provides useful information about the nerve or muscle in the rest of the gastrointestinal tract.

Because the smooth muscle cells can change their length and thickness greatly and rapidly under physiologic and nonphysiologic conditions (surgical excision, death, formalin fixation), absolute values of length and thickness of the muscularis propria are of little use. If the neuromuscular apparatus is to be examined, the segment of gut should be opened fresh

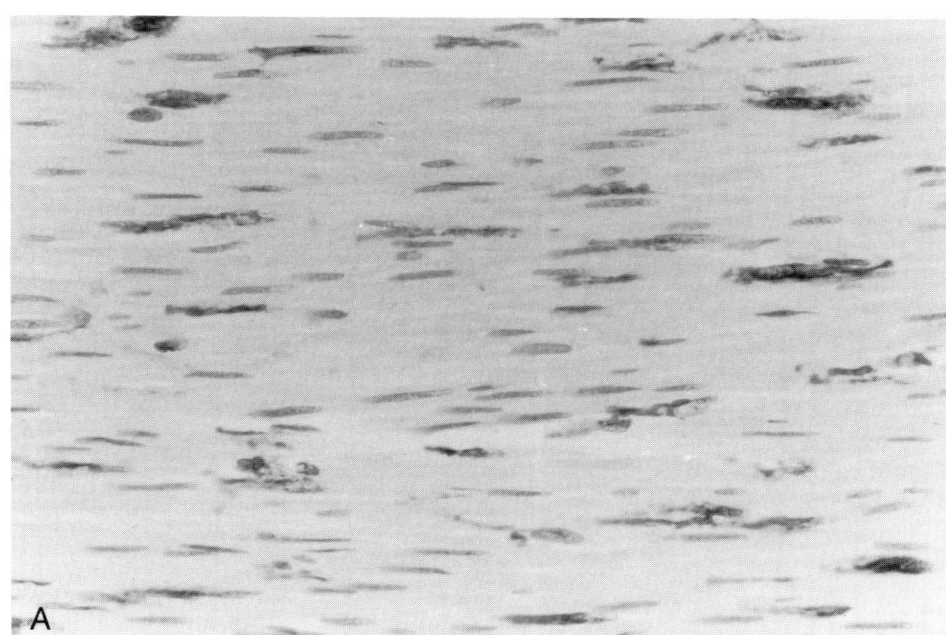

FIGURE 11–6. *A,* The interstitial cells of Cajal, which stain with both NSE and S-100, occupy a substantial portion of the muscularis propria throughout the gastrointestinal tract. (Immunoperoxidase, S-100, × 100) *B,* The nuclei of these cells are shorter and more rounded than those of the myocytes. The cytoplasm may be branched, and appears pale and slightly vacuolated on H&E sections. (Immunoperoxidase, S-100, × 330)

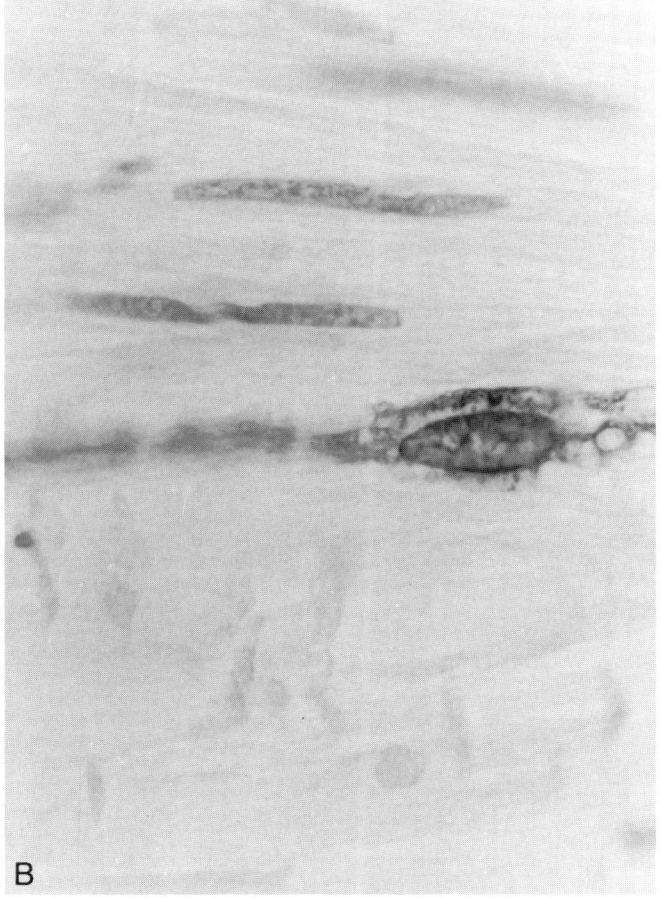

and pinned out flat on paraffin or corkboard. Both longitudinal and cross sections should be taken. In addition, tangential sections (mucosa, submucosa, and mesentery trimmed away) may provide an opportunity for an interesting perspective on the myenteric plexus.

Formalin-fixed tissue should be saved for potential examination in referral centers with experience in performing and interpreting silver-stained sections of plexus. Standard trichrome techniques are useful in evaluating the integrity of the smooth muscle.

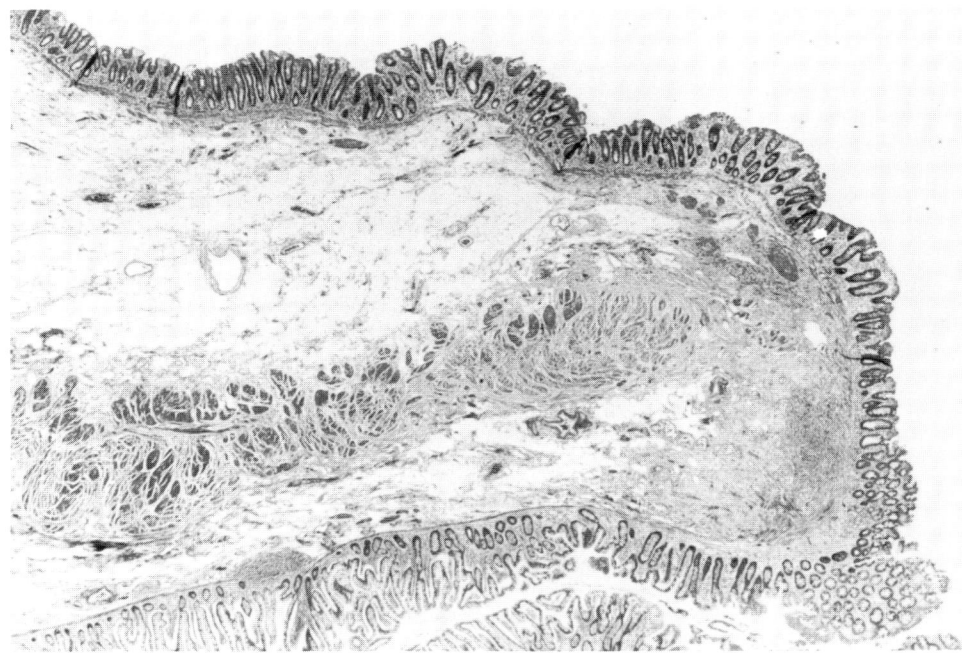

FIGURE 11-7. Section of normal ileocecal valve, with ileal mucosa at the bottom and colonic mucosa at the top. The attenuated muscle fibers at the tip of the ileocecal valve are richly invested by collagen fibers, giving an appearance that can be confused with damage seen in visceral myopathies. (Trichrome, × 4)

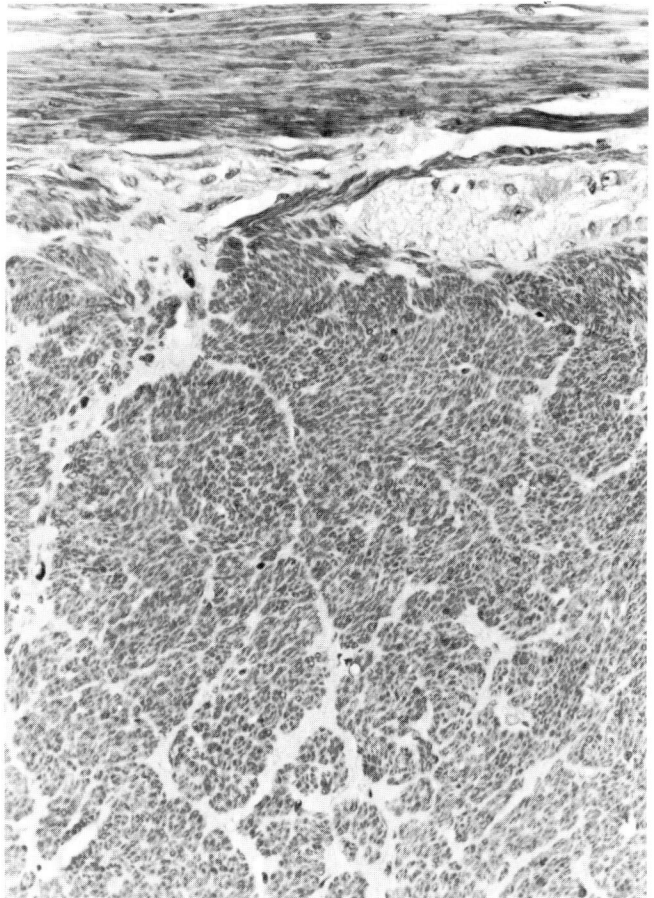

FIGURE 11-8. Muscularis propria of normal colon. Along with the ileocecal valve, the taeniae coli (bottom) physiologically contain abundant collagen, both around individual myocytes and around groups of myocytes. (Trichrome, × 66)

MECHANICAL OBSTRUCTION

The major mechanical problem affecting the gastrointestinal tract is obstruction. Mechanical obstruction implies that there is a readily definable structural alteration comprising luminal diameter and hindering passage of intestinal contents. The small intestine and the colon are the two major segments involved. For the pathologist confronted with a specimen from a patient with intestinal obstruction, the chief tasks are identifying and defining this structural alteration and determining the degree of secondary damage to the involved segment.

Causes and Effects

The causes of obstruction are legion, but over the years the two most common have been hernia and adhesions.[9-12] Because of the earlier recognition and repair of hernias in the last few decades, they have now become a less common cause of obstruction; whereas the concomitant increase in abdominal surgery has led to an increased frequency of adhesions as a cause of obstruction.[10,11] Cancer is the next most common cause, and must be carefully excluded in each case, particularly in adults.[9,11] Volvulus, intussusception, inflammatory conditions, including diverticulitis, foreign bodies, and congenital malformations are other reasonably common causes of obstruction.[11,12]

Once obstruction occurs, the accumulation of secretions, swallowed food and air, and interference with absorption lead to distention. As noted previously, the structure of the intestine allows for remarkable distensibility. When the pressure within the obstructed loops reaches that in the arterial circulation, strangulation occurs, causing ischemic damage to the bowel and possible bacterial penetration and infection due to loss of structural integrity.[9,12] This pathophysiologic sequence accounts for the clinical manifestations of obstruction. The key symptoms are pain, vomiting, and obstipation. The pain tends to be episodic and colicky; when constant, it suggests strangulation and its consequences. The temporal relationship of the onset of vomiting to that of the pain can provide a clue as to the level of the obstruction, as can the character of the vomitus. Feculent vomiting implies a lesion in the mid or low small intestine; the term *feculent* is a misnomer, however, because the character of the dark, foul-smelling material reflects stasis with rapid bacterial overgrowth and decomposition of intestinal contents. Obstipation can be partial or complete, reflecting the character of the obstruction. Distention is the main physical sign. Hyperactive high-pitched peristaltic rushes and metallic tinkling sounds are commonly heard. Absence of peristaltic sounds implies peritoneal irritation.

Special Forms of Obstruction

Several specific forms of mechanical obstruction deserve further note. Intussusception is a particularly common cause of intestinal obstruction in children. As the invagination of one portion of the gastrointestinal tract (the intussusceptum) into that more distal (the intussuscipiens) occurs, the ischemic compromise that results may necessitate operative intervention (Figure 11–9). About 80% of childhood intussusceptions are ileoileal.[13] The lymphoid tissue in Peyer's patches is often prominent (Figure 11–10). A response to a viral infection has been postulated, but the lymphoid prominence may be merely physiologic. The situation is more ominous in adults, with an obvious cause present in the majority. This is typically a tumor mass, which may be malignant (Figure 11–11). This is particularly true with colocolic intussusception, a rare occurrence.

Volvulus results from a twisting of the bowel upon

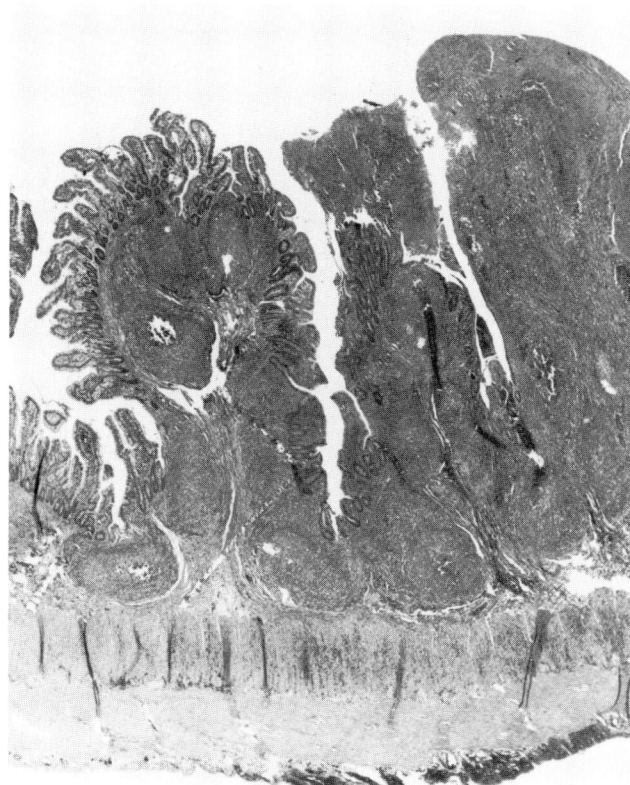

FIGURE 11–10. The prominent lymphoid tissue in this intussuscepted ileum shows ischemic damage, characterized by mucosal erosion (right) and hemorrhage in the wall and serosa. (H&E, × 5)

itself. This produces a simultaneous closed-loop obstruction and proximal open-loop obstruction.[9] Characteristically, the degree of distention is enormous. Because this phenomenon requires a long mesenteric attachment, its sites of occurrence are predictable. Areas of predilection, roughly in order of descending frequency, include sigmoid, cecum, small bowel (all or

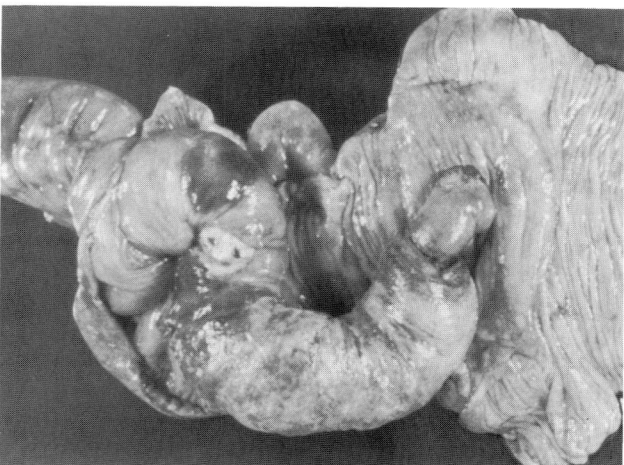

FIGURE 11–9. Ileoileal intussusception in a child. The intussuscepted bowel (center), seen just proximal to the ileocecal valve, shows evidence of ischemic damage.

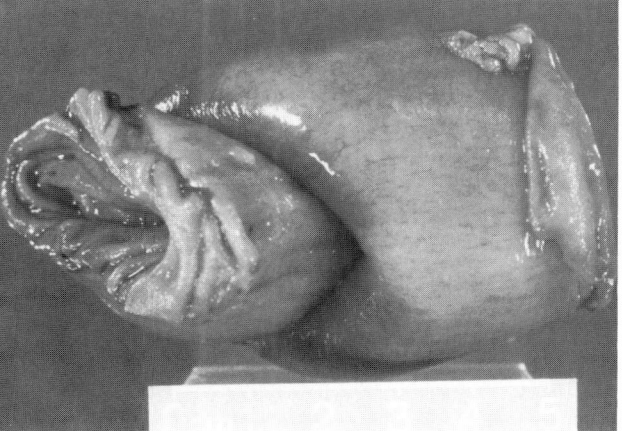

FIGURE 11–11. This intussusception of small bowel in an adult was the result of a submucosal mass (not shown) formed by a metastasis from a large-cell undifferentiated carcinoma of the lung. The proximal entering segment is on the left.

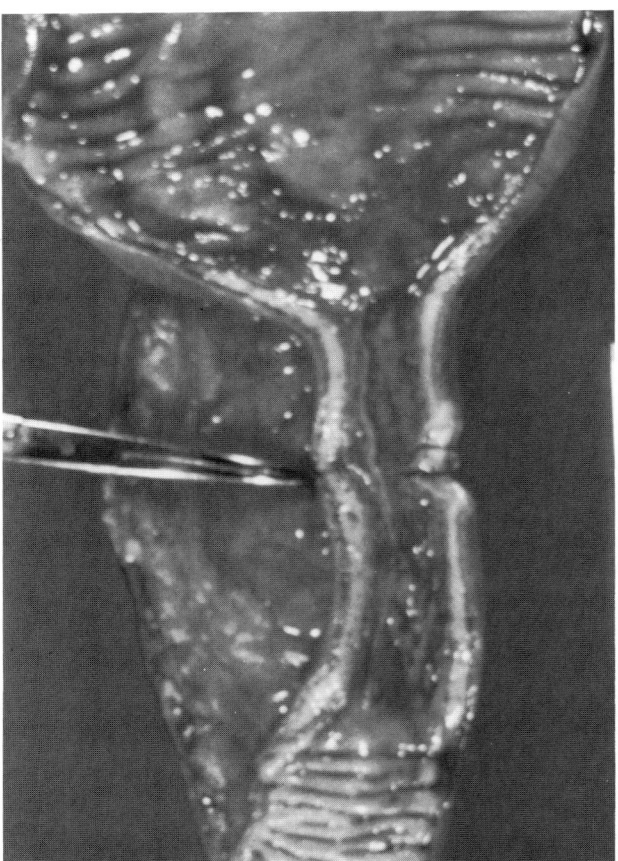

FIGURE 11–12. This slowly forming small-bowel stricture secondary to Crohn's disease resulted in both dilatation and hypertrophy of the muscularis propria in the proximal segment of small intestine (top).

a portion thereof), stomach, and (rarely) transverse colon. Sudden onset of pain and rapid distention are characteristic.[9]

Intraluminal mechanical obstruction may result from gallstone impaction. So-called gallstone ileus is thought to result from bouts of cholecystitis with formation of a cholecystoenteric fistula (usually cholecystoduodenal). The stone must be of a size (about 3 cm) that will cause obstruction; such stones typically occur in the ileum. Enteroliths formed spontaneously in the gastrointestinal tract may act in a similar manner; they are recognized by their occurrence in the absence of gallbladder disease.[9] Other intraluminal causes of obstruction include bezoars (usually mixtures of hair and vegetable material), parasites *(Ascaris, Taenia, Trichuris),* and ingested foreign bodies.[11]

Apart from the offending lesion (adhesive band, tumor) and the ischemic damages, the neuromuscular apparatus of the gastrointestinal tract is usually unremarkable. In long-standing cases of incomplete mechanical obstruction, dilatation and muscular hypertrophy do occur (Figure 11–12). Experimental evidence supports the hypertrophic response of intestinal smooth muscle in the presence of obstruction.[14,15]

PSEUDO-OBSTRUCTION

Introduction

The term *intestinal pseudo-obstruction* denotes a syndrome in which typical signs and symptoms of intestinal obstruction as described above occur but in which a typical mechanical lesion cannot be demonstrated.

Chronic Disorders

Much of the recent interest has focused on chronic cases. Most of these cases are secondary to disease processes that are systemic and can affect the neuromuscular apparatus of the gastrointestinal tract. The prime example of such disease processes is scleroderma, but there are many diseases that behave in a similar way (see below). An ever increasing number of cases appear to be due to primary disorders of the neuromuscular apparatus. Previously undescribed lesions affecting the smooth muscle of the myenteric plexus have recently been recognized and are discussed in several excellent reviews.[4,16–22] Of the primary diseases affecting muscle or nerve, both familial and sporadic forms have been described (Table 11–1).[17,21] It is not clear whether the majority of such cases are of muscle or nerve; because lesions within the enteric nervous system are more difficult to identify morphologically than those affecting smooth muscle, it is likely that many neuropathies go unrecognized. Likewise, many early reports clearly document cases of chronic intestinal pseudo-obstruction clinically but say that no pathologic lesions were identified.[23–26] This may merely reflect the lack of availability of the refined morphologic techniques necessary for their detection.

Acute Disorders

Acute forms of intestinal pseudo-obstruction also exist. These are more commonly known as adynamic ileus or Ogilvie's syndrome. These processes are by definition self-limited and do not usually come to the attention of the morphologic pathologist. Briefly, *adynamic ileus* is a form of functional obstruction that is quite common. To one degree or another, it follows vir-

Table 11–1 PRIMARY INTESTINAL PSEUDO-OBSTRUCTION

Myopathies
    Familial forms
        Autosomal dominant (type I)
        Autosomal recessive (types II and III)
    Sporadic cases

Neuropathies
    Familial forms
        Autosomal recessive
        Autosomal dominant
    Sporadic cases
        Degenerative, noninflammatory
        Degenerative, inflammatory
        Isolated axonopathy
        Idiopathic constipation

MOTOR AND MECHANICAL DISORDERS

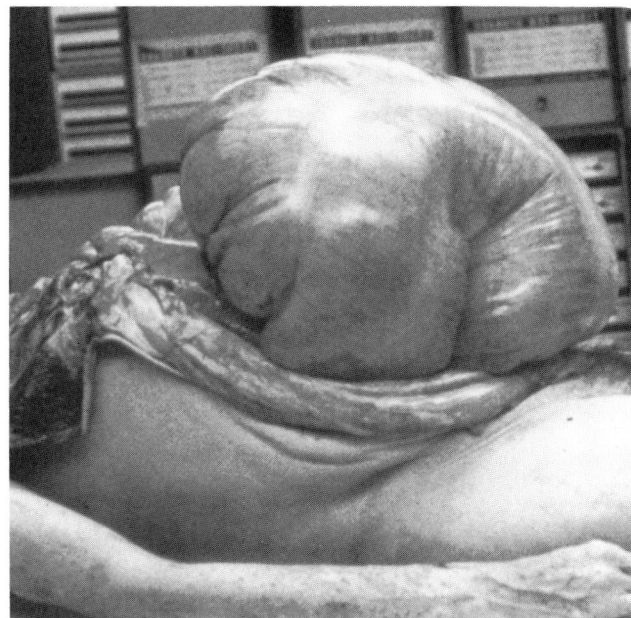

FIGURE 11–13. Unusually prominent colonic dilatation in an autopsy of a patient with pseudo-obstruction, a testimony to the remarkable distensibility of the gastrointestinal tract and to the potentially lethal nature of these disease processes. (Courtesy of Dr. C. E. Foucar, Presbyterian Hospital, Albuquerque, New Mexico.)

tually every abdominal operation. In addition, trauma, peritonitis, ischemia, spinal cord injury, and systemic infection can all produce the distention and absence of peristaltic sounds characteristic of ileus. The nature and severity of the underlying disease determine the outcome. A particular form of acute pseudo-obstruction limited to the colon has been referred to as *Ogilvie's syndrome*.[27,28] Affected patients are often in the sixth decade; men predominate. Again, there are various underlying disease processes. Some of the more common include trauma (operative and nonoperative), infection, myocardial infarction, and respiratory or renal failure. Other than dilatation and its consequences, there are no morphologic lesions in adynamic ileus or in Ogilvie's syndrome.

Clinical Features

In the chronic forms of pseudo-obstruction, the symptoms are, by definition, those that are associated with mechanical obstruction. In most cases, these symptoms begin in childhood and are recurrent over a prolonged period, but a few patients do not begin to have symptoms until middle age, and some patients are asymptomatic. Abdominal distention, pain, and vomiting predominate. The degree of distention varies but is usually quite significant and can be enormous when substantial portions of the small intestine and colon are involved (Figure 11–13). Loud borborygmi and succussion splashes are common. Vomiting is of high volume. The pain is usually epigastric or periumbilical and correlates with the degree of distention. Alternating diarrhea and constipation, rather than obstipation, is the rule. This may reflect small-bowel bacterial overgrowth, an important factor in many patients (see below).[22] These patients often have lost from 15 to 30 kg of body weight prior to diagnosis.

Primary Intestinal Pseudo-Obstruction

Myopathy

Visceral myopathy is characterized by degeneration, thinning, and fibrous replacement of the smooth muscle of the gastrointestinal tract; in some cases involvement of the muscle of the urinary tract has also been documented (Figure 11–14).[29]

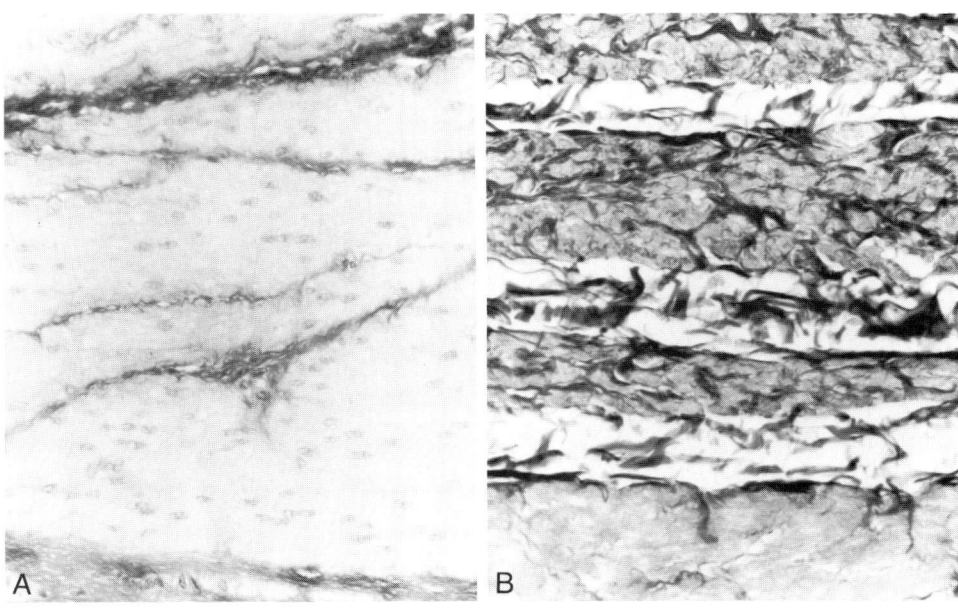

FIGURE 11–14. *A,* Normal intrafascicular collagen in a control urinary bladder. *B,* Increased intrafascicular and pericellular collagen in a urinary bladder from a patient with familial visceral myopathy; elastic fibers may also be increased. (Trichrome, × 325) (Courtesy of Dr. S. M. Bonsib, Department of Pathology, University of Iowa Hospitals and Clinics, Iowa City, Iowa.)

Familial Cases

The majority of the cases of visceral myopathy tend to be familial. At least 12 families have been described.[23–25,30–41] The histologic appearance of the affected gastrointestinal segments tends to be very similar in all these families. However, the pattern of distribution of the involved segments, the presence or absence of gastrointestinal manifestations, and the mode of inheritance have led to the recognition of several subtypes.[4,12]

Type I appears to be the most common.[23–25,32,37,39–41] It is characterized by autosomal dominant inheritance.[39–41] Esophageal dilatation, megaduodenum, redundant colon, and megalocystis are all common. Megaduodenum is particularly common. The onset of symptoms is usually after the first decade of life, but over half of the involved family members are asymptomatic. Uterine inertia has been observed on occasion. In one family, members of three generations have had dysplastic nevus syndrome and multiple basal cell carcinomas in addition to the myopathy.[42]

Type II familial visceral myopathy is autosomal recessive.[31,33–35] There is distinct gastric dilatation, as well as slight dilatation of the entire small intestine, which often has diverticula. Over 75% of the patients are symptomatic, and symptoms tend to start during the teenage years; abdominal pain tends to be severe. Ptosis and external ophthalmoplegia are common.

Type III familial visceral myopathy is also autosomal recessive.[30] The entire gastrointestinal tract, from esophagus to rectum, is markedly dilated. However, the symptoms of intestinal pseudo-obstruction tend not to appear until middle age. No areas of involvement of muscle outside the gastrointestinal tract have been noted.

Sporadic Cases

There have been a number of clear-cut cases of visceral myopathy reported that are apparently nonfamilial.[21,43,44] Because some affected family members may be asymptomatic, and because an accurate family history can be difficult to obtain, care must be exercised before considering a case to be sporadic. In general, these cases tend to resemble the autosomal recessive familial type III visceral myopathy,[12] in that they tend to have severe involvement of the entire gastrointestinal tract. Megalocystis may be present.

Pathologic Features

The morphologic appearance of the visceral myopathies is quite distinctive. The gross appearance, other than the dilatation, is unremarkable (Figure 11–15); this dilatation tends to be segmental, particularly in the more common type I. The histologic appearance is characteristic.[4,38] The process of smooth muscle degeneration and fibrosis involves the muscularis propria but tends to spare the muscularis mucosae, although recently some cases with muscularis mucosae involvement have been reported.[45] The longitudinal layer is usually more severely involved, and the damage may be limited to this layer (Figure 11–16). The circular layer alone may be involved in the sporadic cases (Fig-

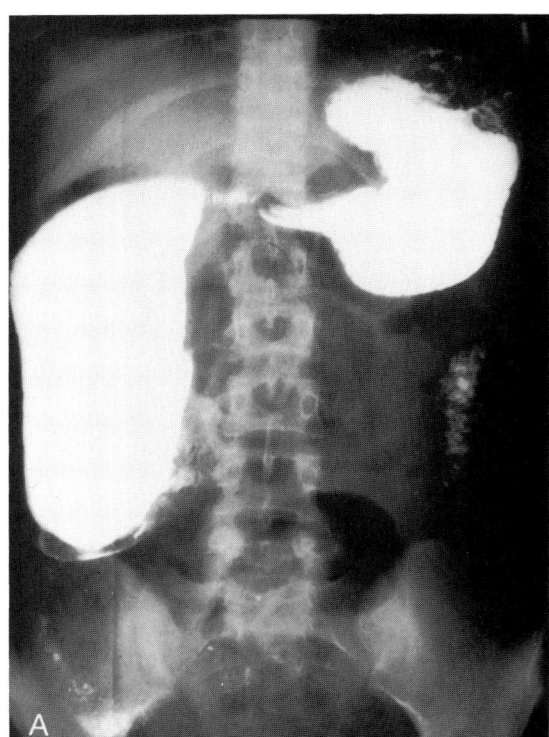
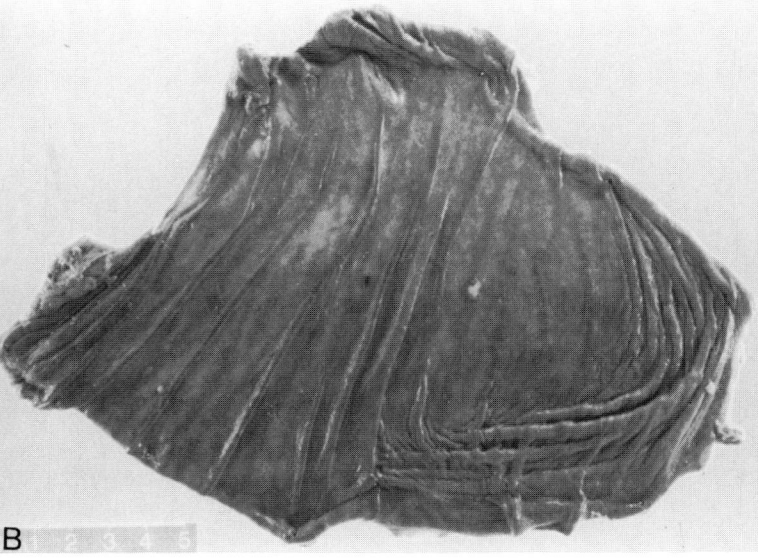

FIGURE 11–15. *A*, Megaduodenum in a patient with type I familial visceral myopathy; the massive dilatation of duodenum terminated just proximal to the ligament of Treitz. *B*, Massively dilated duodenum from a patient with visceral myopathy.

FIGURE 11-16. *A*, Cross section of duodenum from type I familial visceral myopathy. (Trichrome, × 16) *B*, Longitudinal section of jejunum from a patient with type II familial visceral myopathy. (Trichrome, × 8) Both show involvement limited to the longitudinal layer of the muscularis propria (bottom), which is the typical early pattern.

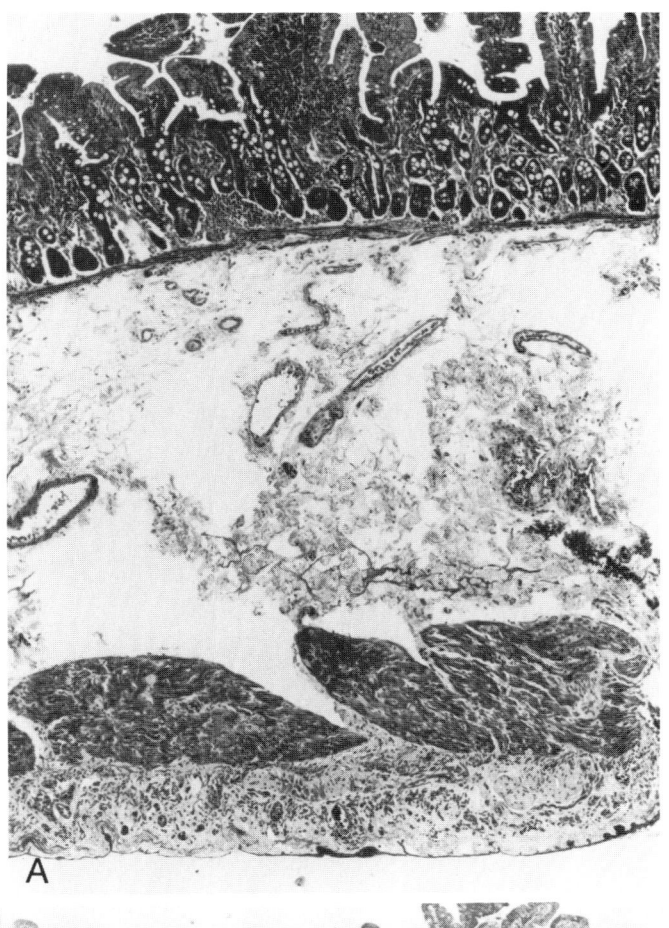

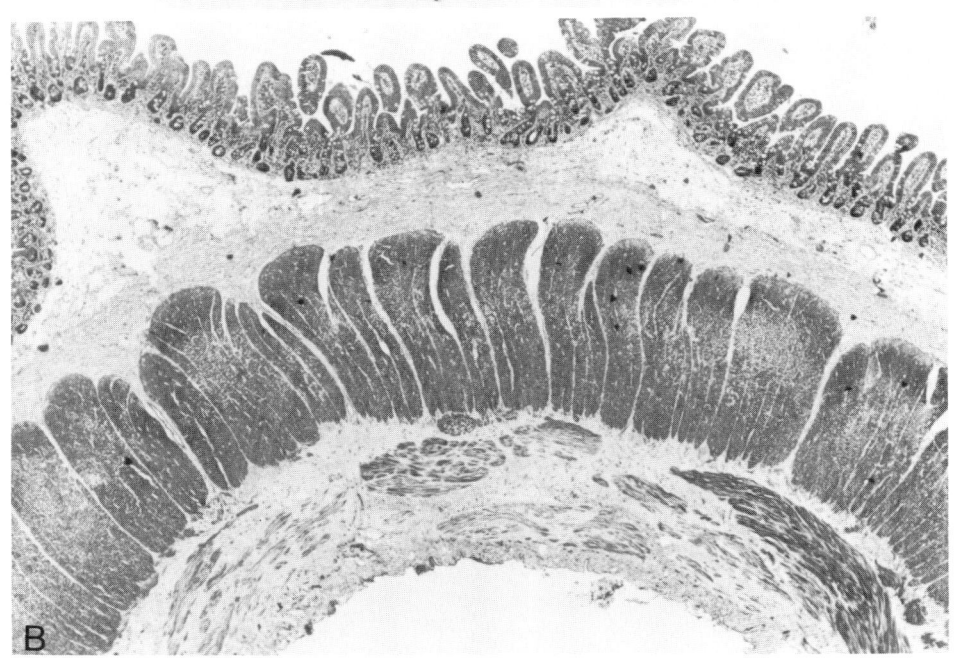

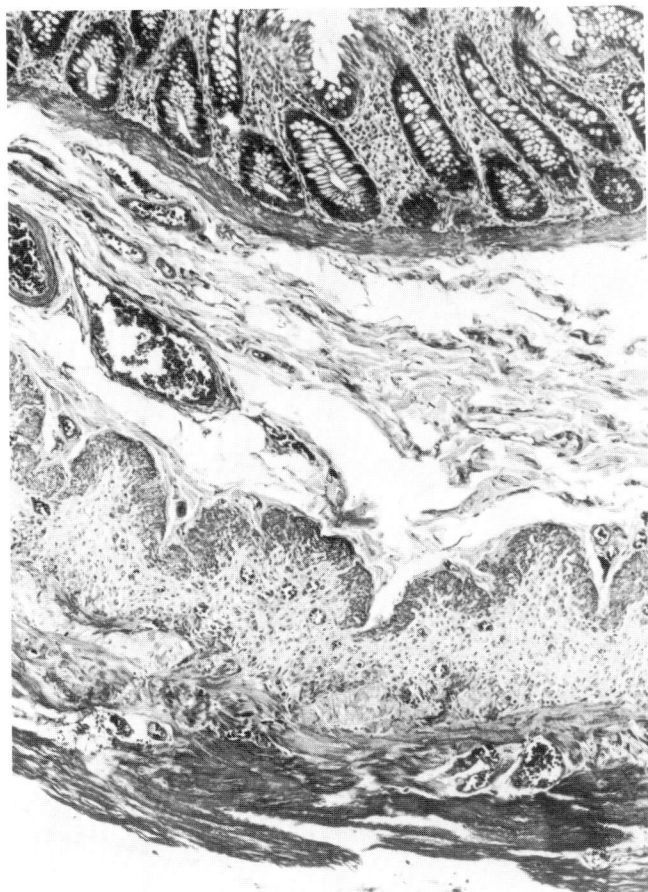

FIGURE 11–17. Colon from a child with sporadic visceral myopathy, who mistakenly carried a diagnosis of Hirschsprung's disease for many years. Ganglion cells were intact, but the circular layer of the muscularis propria (bottom) was clearly damaged. This is an atypical pattern of distribution for visceral myopathy. (Trichrome, × 25)

ure 11–17). There may be a striking variability in the diameter of the muscle fibers; this is best appreciated on carefully oriented cross sections (Figure 11–18). As the degeneration of muscle fibers continues and dense collagen is laid down around the damaged fibers, a honeycomb appearance results. This characteristic feature, referred to as vacuolar change (Figure 11–19), serves to distinguish the myopathies from other forms of muscle fibrosis. The scarring of the muscularis propria in conditions such as scleroderma (see below), ischemia (Figure 11–20), and Crohn's disease (Figure 11–21), tends to obliterate completely the muscle fibers in the affected areas and shows no preferential involvement of the longitudinal layer. For recognition of mild lesions, careful attention to proper orientation and utilization of trichrome stains are necessary.

Electron microscopy confirms the smooth muscle degeneration and collagen deposition but provides no further insight into the nature of the damage. The myenteric plexus structures are normal as seen with light microscopy, electron microscopy, silver stains, and acetylcholinesterase stains in the visceral myopathies.[4,38]

Prognosis and Therapy

The treatment of these disorders is symptomatic. Of paramount importance is the consideration of small-intestinal bacterial overgrowth. It has been noted that this process can result in striking alteration in small-intestinal mucosal architecture (Figure 11–22), leading to significant malabsorbtion with steatorrhea.[46] In fact, one member of the type II families succumbed to inanition after years of being considered to have "refractory sprue"; at autopsy, the characteristic fibrosis of visceral myopathy was evident. Patients with type I

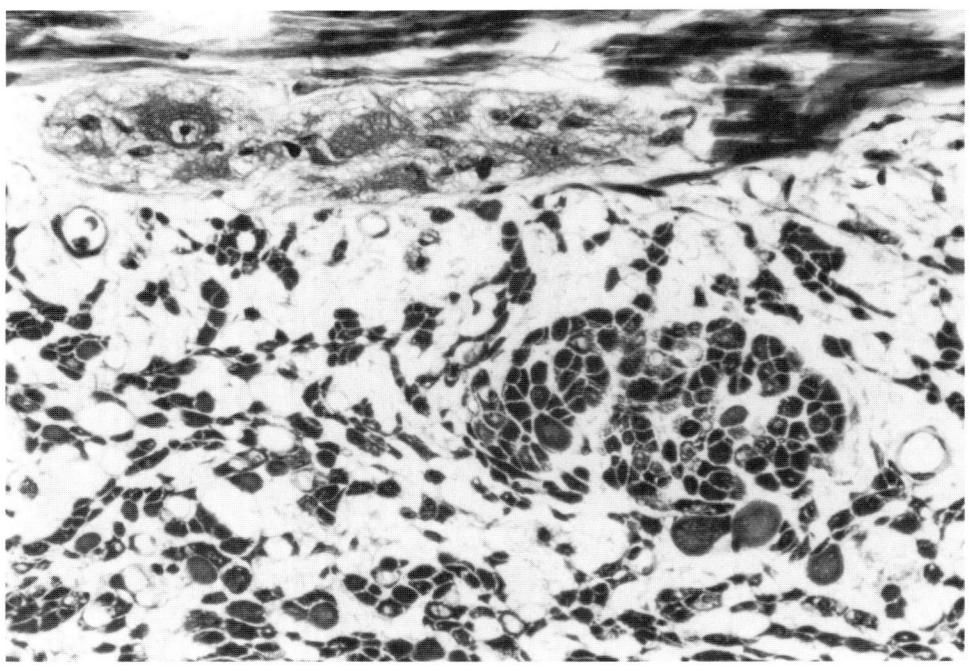

FIGURE 11–18. The longitudinal layer of a slightly dilated ileal segment from a patient with type I familial visceral myopathy. Ganglion cells (top) are intact, but many myocytes are enlarged, and there is excess pericellular collagen. (Trichrome, × 100)

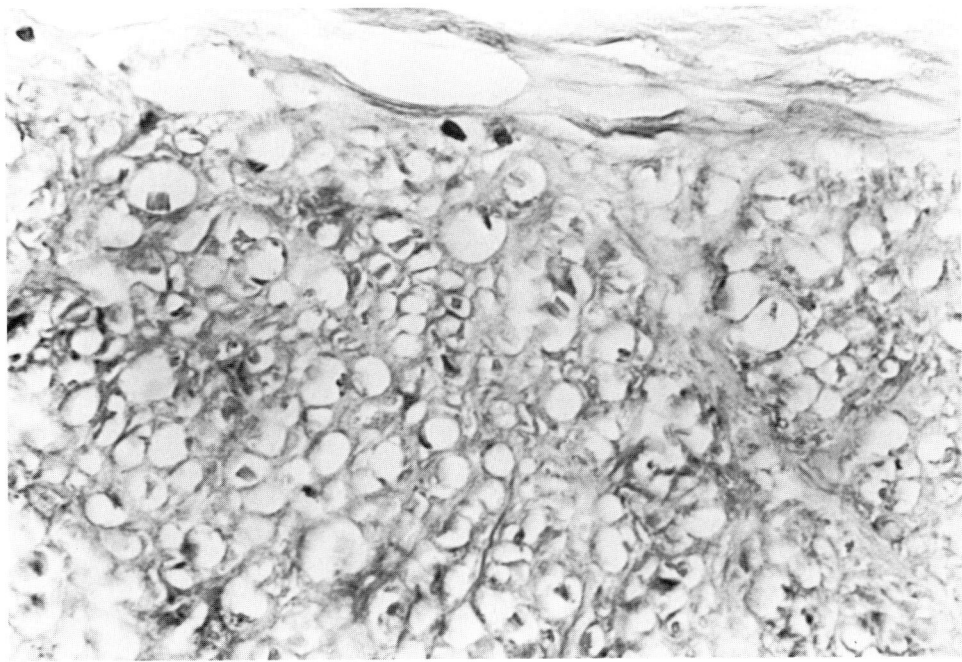

FIGURE 11-19. Vacuolar change in longitudinal muscle layer in type II familial visceral myopathy. In this advanced lesion, myocyte enlargement and vacuolization are prominent; individual cells are surrounded by collagen. (Trichrome, × 400)

myopathy have a relatively good prognosis, perhaps related to the relatively limited area of involvement; their disease process is amenable to surgery, such as side-to-side duodenojejunostomy or partial resection of the duodenum. It is imperative that antibiotic therapy be given in consideration of the large volume of bacteria in these static bowels and the consequent high incidence of postoperative peritonitis.[47] Patients with type II and III and sporadic visceral myopathy have a poorer prognosis. Often their demise is an indirect result of their severe nutritional difficulties, but in some the cause of death is more mysterious.[43]

Neuropathy

Visceral neuropathy is characterized by damage directed against the neural apparatus, with sparing of the smooth muscle structures. It may be recognized in some of the cases by noting decreased numbers of neurons on standard H&E sections; this requires the em-

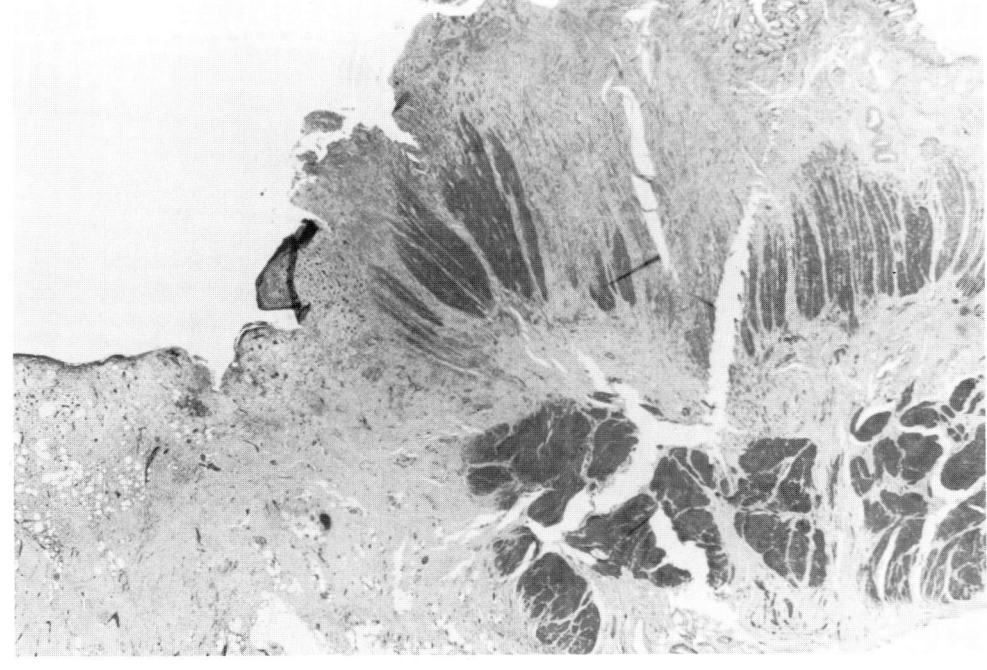

FIGURE 11-20. Section of colon, with the mucosal surface at the top. Ischemic colonic stricture, with focally transmural fibrosis. Individual degenerating fibers and vacuolar change are not present. (Trichrome, × 2.5)

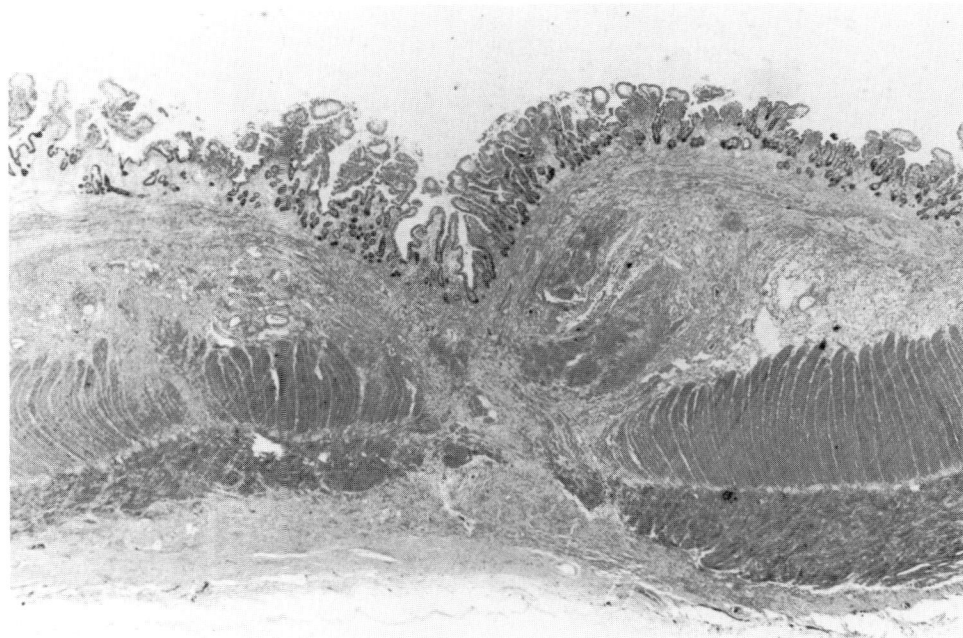

FIGURE 11–21. Section of small intestine with the mucosal surface at the top. Abrupt focus of transmural fibrosis (center) in a stricture of small intestine secondary to Crohn's disease. (Trichrome, × 3.3)

ployment of fastidious neuron-counting techniques.[48] In some cases, neurons may contain intranuclear inclusions visible on standard sections.[48] In most cases, damage to the neurons or interconnecting nerve bundles cannot be appreciated unless the difficult silver stain techniques described above are utilized.[3] The portions of the neural apparatus outside the gut important to controlling the movement of the gut are not amenable to ready morphologic analyses. These factors have probably led to a significant underrecognition of neural causes of motility disorders. There may be clues to the neural nature of the problem if there is involvement of the central, autonomic, or peripheral nervous system elsewhere, but this is not always the case. The suggestion has been made that there might be different motility patterns appreciable manometrically in the neuropathic versus myopathic processes,[48–50] a hypoactive pattern being suggestive of myopathy and a hyperactive pattern being suggestive of neuropathy.

Familial Cases

A family documented to have a neuropathy significantly affecting the movement of the gastrointestinal

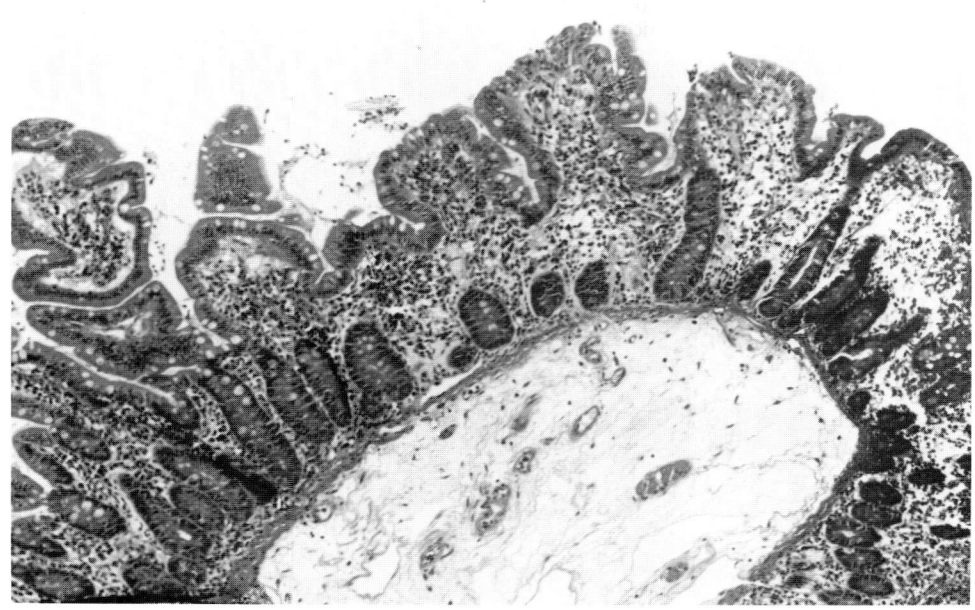

FIGURE 11–22. Partial and patchy villous atrophy, from the jejunum of a patient with scleroderma. Small-bowel bacterial overgrowth can be a major problem regardless of the cause of the motility disturbance. (H&E, × 25)

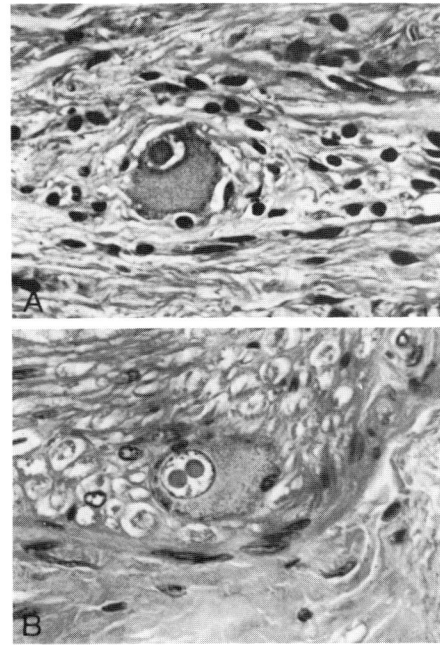

FIGURE 11-23. *A* and *B*, The round eosinophilic intranuclear inclusions within ganglionic nerve cells seen in some forms of familial visceral neuropathy. (H&E, × 460) (From Krishnamurthy S, Schuffler, MD: Pathology of neuromuscular disorders of the small intestine and colon. Gastroenterology 93:610, 1987. Copyright 1987 by The American Gastroenterological Association. Reprinted with permission.)

tract was elegantly described by Schuffler,[48] who noted two siblings with intestinal pseudo-obstruction who also had neurologic abnormalities, including mild autonomic deficiency and denervation hypersensitivity of pupillary and esophageal smooth muscle. Inheritance is apparently recessive.[12] The number of neurons in Auerbach's plexus was strikingly decreased compared with that of control subjects, and about one third of these remaining neurons contained characteristic eosinophilic intranuclear inclusions (Figure 11-23). These did not resemble viral inclusions and were shown to be a proteinaceous and filamentous material by histochemistry and electron microscopy. They were also found in Meissner's plexus neurons, as well as in neurons of the brain, spinal cord, dorsal root, and celiac plexus ganglion. Subsequently similar inclusions have been noted by several observers in the neurons of patients with a variety of neurologic diseases, but without significant gastrointestinal dysfunction.[4,51-53] This phenomenon has been referred to as neuronal intranuclear inclusion disease. The plexus was free of inflammatory cells; silver stains revealed a decrease in both argyrophilic and argyrophobic neurons and markedly decreased numbers of fibers in the nerve tracts.

Another family with an apparently autosomal recessive mode of inheritance for what appears to be a visceral neuropathy has been reported.[54] Four siblings with pseudo-obstruction and malabsorbtion were also noted to have mental retardation and basal calcification. Silver stains showed a diminution in the number of argyrophilic neurons in the colon and some apparent damage to the argyrophobe neurons.

Two families with an autosomal dominant mode of transmission have also been reported.[55,56] The area of involvement seems to center on the myenteric plexus of the small intestine. Neurons appeared degenerated and decreased in number; no inclusions were noted. Some nerve fibers showed swelling and scattered beading, appreciable only on the silver stains. There was no evidence of extraintestinal involvement.

Sporadic Cases

Given the difficulties in identifying lesions within the enteric and extraenteric nervous system previously described, it is likely that a large number of patients with gastrointestinal motility disorders will eventually prove to have neural lesions. Krishnamurthy and Schuffler have done much in recent years to begin to clarify this situation; we shall use the provisional classification from their studies in considering this group of diseases.[4]

Degenerative noninflammatory neuropathies show two basic patterns of damage. In one, the disease process centers on the colon, where even H&E-stained sections reveal a decreased number of neurons in Auerbach's plexus.[3] This abnormability is also apparent on silver staining; in addition, there are fragmentation and loss of axons as well as glial proliferation. Many neurons are swollen and have a decreased number of processes. Many of the remaining processes are thickened and have areas of swelling along their length (Figure 11-24). In the second type, there is a central pallor to argyrophil and argyrophobe neurons on silver staining; there is some disorganization, but there are no dendritic swellings or glial proliferation.[4]

Degenerative inflammatory neuropathies appear to represent a more varied array of conditions. The morphologic hallmark of the condition is a lymphocytic and plasma cell infiltrate within the myenteric plexus (Figure 11-25). Some of these cases appear to be idiopathic[57,58]; however, care must be taken to exclude the paraneoplastic syndrome[59] or infection, e.g., Chagas' disease[60,61] or cytomegalovirus,[62,63] in which the myenteric plexus may have a similar appearance. This problem demonstrates the difficulties in separating idiopathic pseudo-obstruction from pseudo-obstruction secondary to systemic diseases. Indeed, this separation is to a good degree artificial but must remain so until the pathophysiologic mechanisms of the "idiopathic" cases are more completely understood. In addition to these types of cases, a curious case of rapidly progressive and lethal pseudo-obstruction showed normal neurons on silver sections but had peculiar beading and fragmentation of axons.[64] This has been referred to as an isolated axonopathy.[4]

The problem of *severe idiopathic constipation*,[65] also known as Arbuthnot Lane's disease,[66] can be considered to be a distinct subset of sporadic visceral neuropathy. It is one of the more common motility disorders encountered in the average pathology laboratory. This condition is almost exclusively limited to young

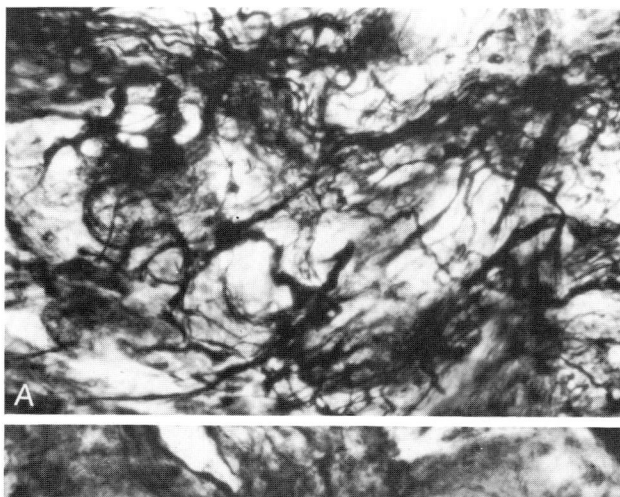

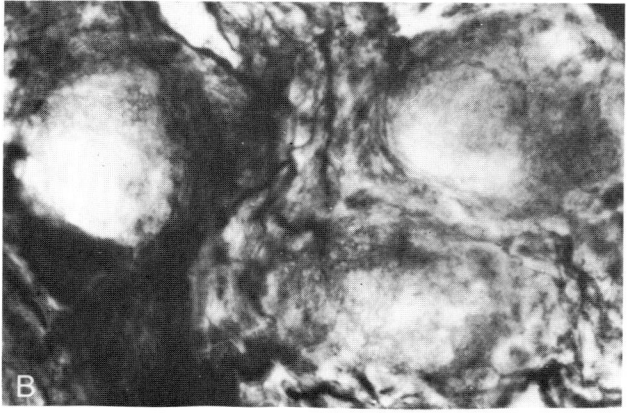

FIGURE 11–24. Indistinct argyrophilic neurons with axonal disorganization (*A*) and swollen degenerating argyrophilic neurons (*B*) from the ileum of a patient with degenerative noninflammatory neuropathy. (Silver stain, × 1360) (From Krishnamurthy S, Schuffler MD: Pathology of neuromuscular disorders of the small intestine and colon. Gastroenterology 93:610, 1987. Copyright 1987 by The American Gastroenterological Association. Reprinted with permission.)

women who have a prolonged history of severe constipation but do not seem to have significant alimentary tract involvement beyond the colon. The severity of the constipation often results in colectomy. The colectomy specimens show little change in standard sections except for the occasional occurrence of melanosis coli. Silver stains reveal a distinctive abnormality consisting of reduced numbers of argyrophilic neurons in colonic myenteric plexuses that are otherwise populated by large numbers of cells with prominent nuclei of variable size and faint cytoplasm (Figure 11–26); these are thought to represent either glial cells or abnormal (? immature) neurons. Because these patients with severe constipation all had at least some laxative usage, the question of whether or not the myenteric plexus changes represent the effect of the laxatives, i.e., "cathartic colon,"[67,68] must be raised. First, it must be said that the very existence of "cathartic colon" must be questioned,[65] because heavy users of laxatives probably all have some pre-existing disorder of the neuromuscular apparatus awaiting definition. Also, the changes described in this characteristic clinical situation are not those seen in patients with the other motility disorders described in this chapter who may have equally impressive histories of laxative use.

Secondary Intestinal Pseudo-Obstruction (Table 11–2)

Patients with secondary intestinal pseudo-obstruction are defined as those having certain reasonably well-defined conditions or systemic diseases that cause the motility problem observed in the gastrointestinal tract.[16,17] It is admitted that the categorization as to pri-

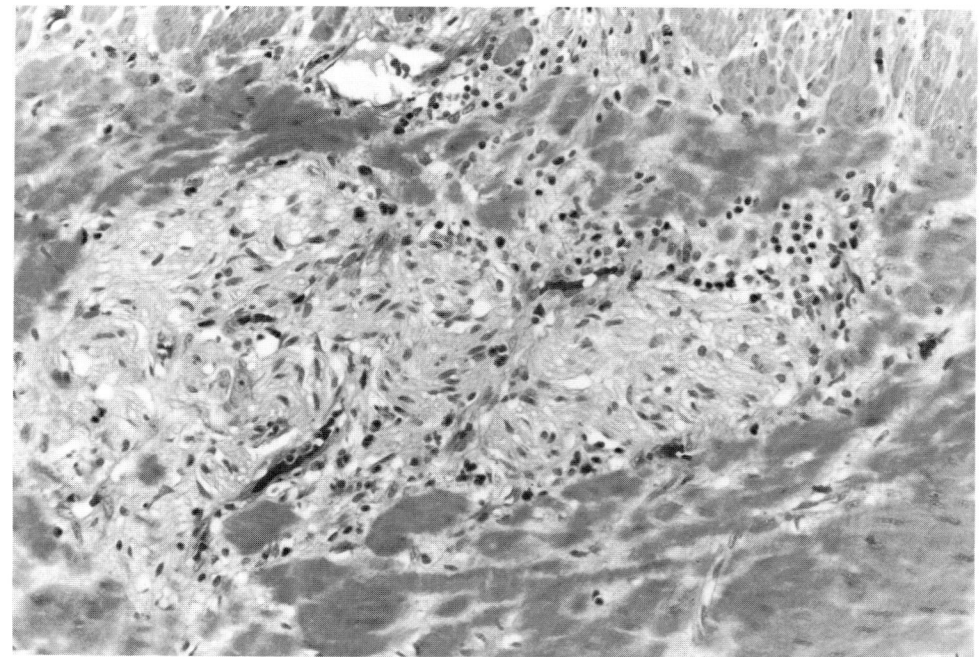

FIGURE 11–25. Myenteric plexus from a patient with degenerative inflammatory neuropathy. There is a lymphocytic and plasma cell infiltrate, along with decreased numbers of neurons. (H&E, × 50)

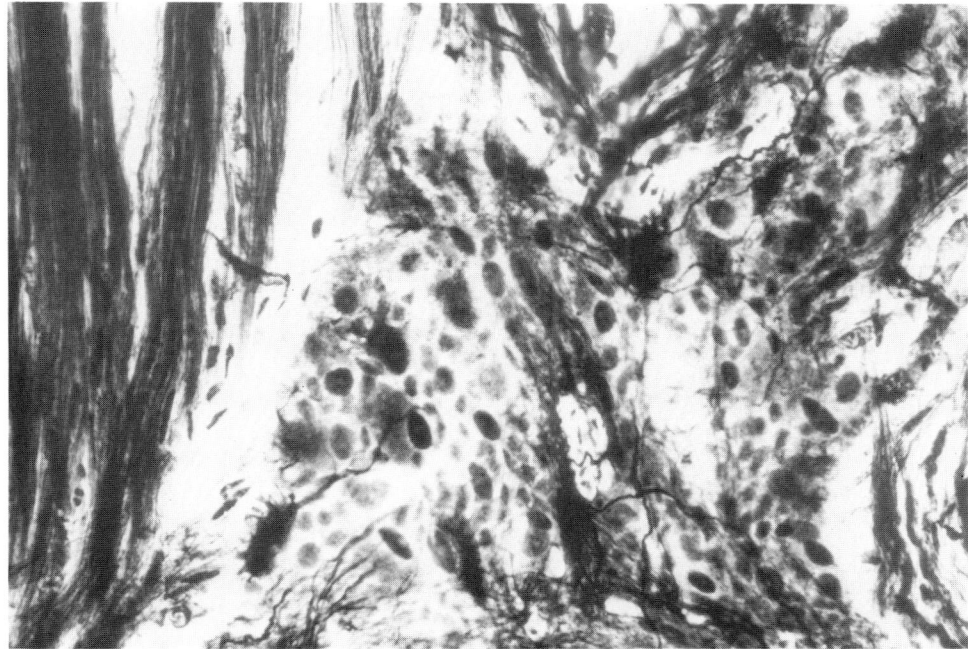

FIGURE 11–26. Colonic myenteric plexus in severe idiopathic constipation with increased numbers of poorly staining cells and decreased numbers of normal argyrophilic neurons. (Silver stain, × 100) (From a section prepared in the laboratory of Dr. M. D. Schuffler.)

mary and secondary is somewhat arbitrary. Some diseases considered primary or idiopathic will certainly be found to be secondary to some other process as our understanding expands. Likewise, the motility problems present in such well-known clinical entities such as Hirschsprung's disease or Parkinson's disease have traditionally been considered among the secondary

Table 11–2 SECONDARY INTESTINAL PSEUDO-OBSTRUCTION

Diseases affecting smooth muscle
   Collagen vascular disease (chiefly scleroderma)
   Muscular dystrophies
   Ceroidosis
   Jejunal diverticulosis
   Amyloidosis

Diseases affecting neural structures
   Developmental abnormalities
      Hirschsprung's disease
      Neuronal dysplasia
   Chagas' disease
   Parkinson's disease
   Familial autonomic dysfunction
   Jejunal diverticulosis
   Amyloidosis

Endocrine disorders
   Diabetes mellitus
   Hypothyroidism
   Hypoparathyroidism
   Pheochromocytoma

Pharmacologic agents

Miscellaneous
   Jejunoileal bypass
   Radiation
   Eosinophilic gastroenteritis
   Diffuse lymphoid infiltration

causes of pseudo-obstruction,[16,17] although a cogent argument can be made for considering them under the classification of primary visceral neuropathies. Of the large number of conditions associated with damage to the neuromuscular apparatus of the gastrointestinal tract, those a morphologic pathologist is most likely to encounter are scleroderma, diabetes mellitus, and Hirschsprung's disease.

Muscle Diseases

Scleroderma

Scleroderma, or progressive systemic sclerosis, is the most common of the diseases affecting the musculature of the gastrointestinal tract to such a degree as to cause a clinically significant motility disorder.[21,69] The frequent occurrence of gastrointestinal involvement in scleroderma is well known,[70–72] about half of all patients having some significant gastrointestinal problem. All portions of the gastrointestinal tract can be involved, but esophageal problems predominate. The clinical features usually allow ready distinction from the primary visceral myopathies, but there are significant morphologic differences as well.[38,69] Although both scleroderma and the primary myopathies can involve the entire muscularis propria, the longitudinal layer often is preferentially involved in the latter. In scleroderma, if there is preferential involvement of one layer, it is the circular muscle that is affected (Figure 11–27). In scleroderma, the collagenous replacement of the muscle tends to be nearly complete, often with an abrupt line of demarcation with adjacent normal muscle. In fact, this phenomenon accounts for the peculiar square-mouthed diverticula that are characteristic for sclerodermatous involvement of the colon (Figure 11–

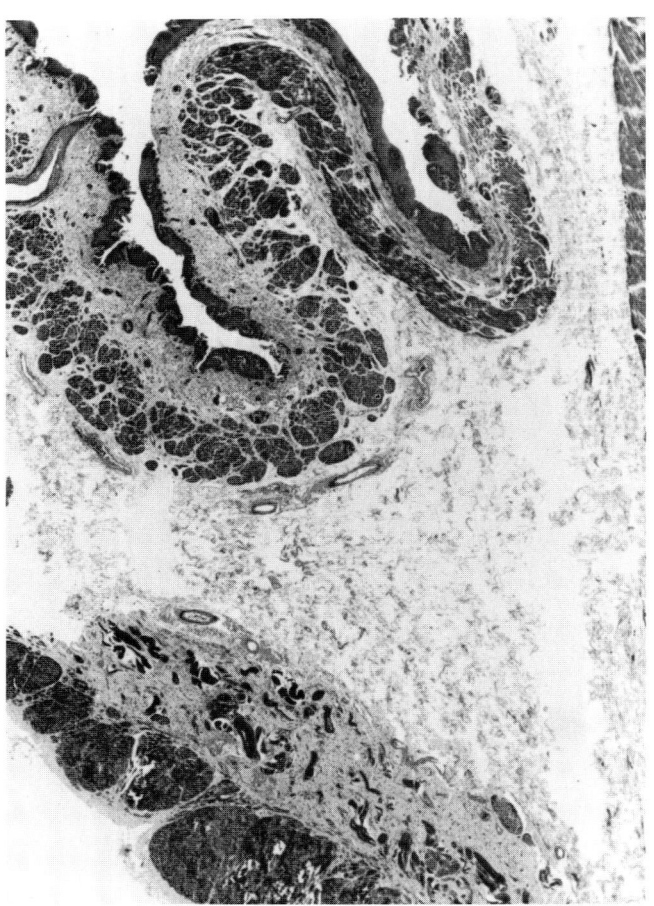

FIGURE 11-27. Mid esophagus in a case of scleroderma, with the mucosal surface at the top. There is almost complete fibrous replacement of the smooth muscle in the circular layer of the muscularis propria. (Trichrome, × 7)

28).[73] These differ from the banal diverticula so commonly seen which are herniations of mucosa through muscularis propria. The vacuolar change described above is not present. Indeed, the presence of the broad swaths of scarring and the frequent observation of vascular abnormalities have led some to postulate on ischemic component of the sclerodermatous gut.[74,75] Much of the clinically obtained biopsy material in patients with scleroderma reveals only those disease processes secondary to the impaired musculature, namely, the consequences of gastroesophageal reflux (esophagitis and Barrett's esophagus) or the small-intestinal villous architectural abnormalities secondary to bacterial overgrowth. Pseudo-obstruction with muscle damage has also been seen in dermatomyositis/polymyositis and systemic lupus erythematosus; in the latter particularly, an underlying vasculitis is evident as the pathogenetic mechanism.[16]

Myotonic Dystrophy and Progressive Muscular Dystrophy

In both *myotonic dystrophy* and in *progressive muscular dystrophy*, signs and symptoms suggestive of pseudo-obstruction may be present.[4,16,76,77] A number of reports have described some swelling, atrophy, and degeneration of smooth muscle fibers; but a clear picture of the morphologic alterations of the muscularis propria has not yet emerged.

Ceroidosis

Ceroidosis of the gastrointestinal tract, or the "brown bowel syndrome," results from the deposition of a granular light brown, lipofuscin-like pigment within the myocytes of the musculature of the gastrointestinal

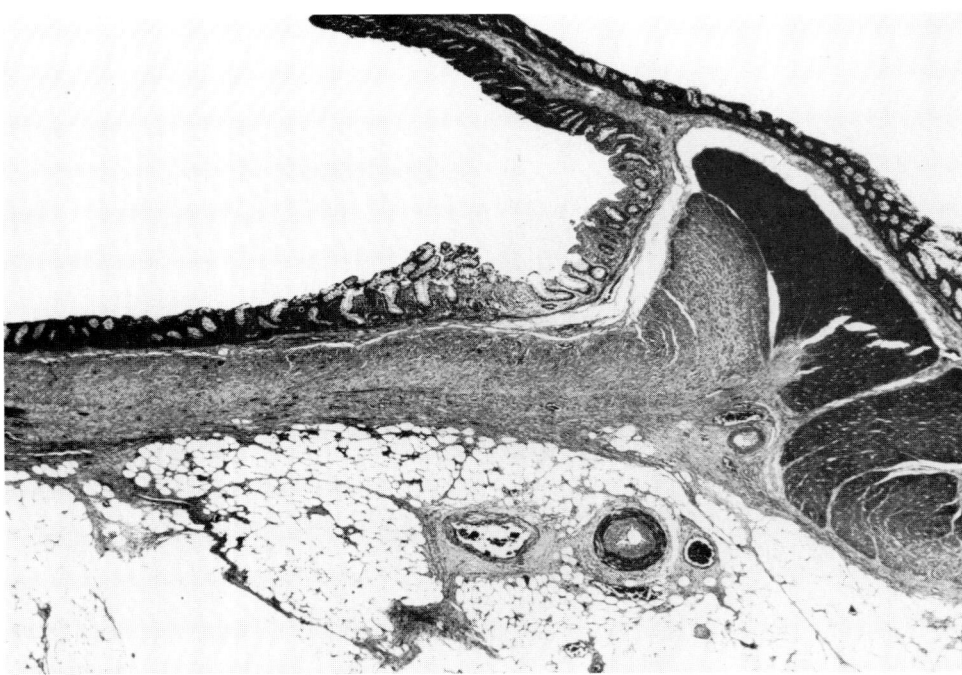

FIGURE 11-28. Mucosal surface at the top. Transmural obliteration and fibrosis of muscle in the colon in scleroderma. One mesenteric artery (bottom right) has abnormal intimal proliferation. (Trichrome, × 7)

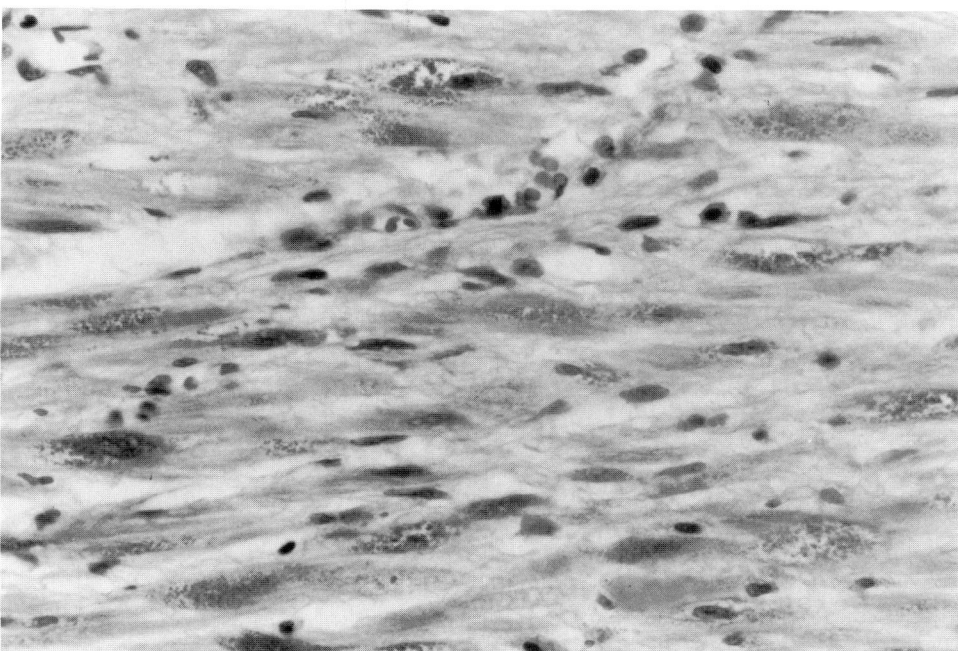

FIGURE 11–29. Ceroidosis of the bowel. Most of myocytes in the muscularis propria contain fine-granular brown pigment. (H&E, × 100)

tract (Figure 11–29). Both muscularis mucosae and muscularis propria of any segment of the gastrointestinal tract may be involved. Ultrastructural examination has shown osmiophilic granular aggregates of electron-dense material containing myelin figures associated with abnormal distorted mitochondria.[78] It is clear that the deposition of ceroid pigment is associated with lack of vitamin E; and pigment is seen in many processes associated with malabsorption, including celiac disease, Whipple's disease, and chronic pancreatitis.[79,80] What is not clear is whether or not the deposition of this pigment is ever a marker for a disease process primarily damaging smooth muscle[81] (see Chapter 16).

Small-Intestinal Diverticulosis

Small-intestinal diverticulosis—the most prominent area of involvement being the jejunum—may be the marker for a variety of disease processes affecting the neuromuscular apparatus (Figure 11–30). In those cases with damaged muscle, the abnormal areas may resemble those seen in either the familial visceral myopathies or in scleroderma.[82] The diverticula tend to result from the outpouching of a segment of jejunal wall with transmural fibrosis.[4] In those patients with scleroderma-like changes in the muscle, scleroderma is not usually clinically overt, but there is a high frequency of Raynaud's phenomenon. Jejunal diverticulosis can also

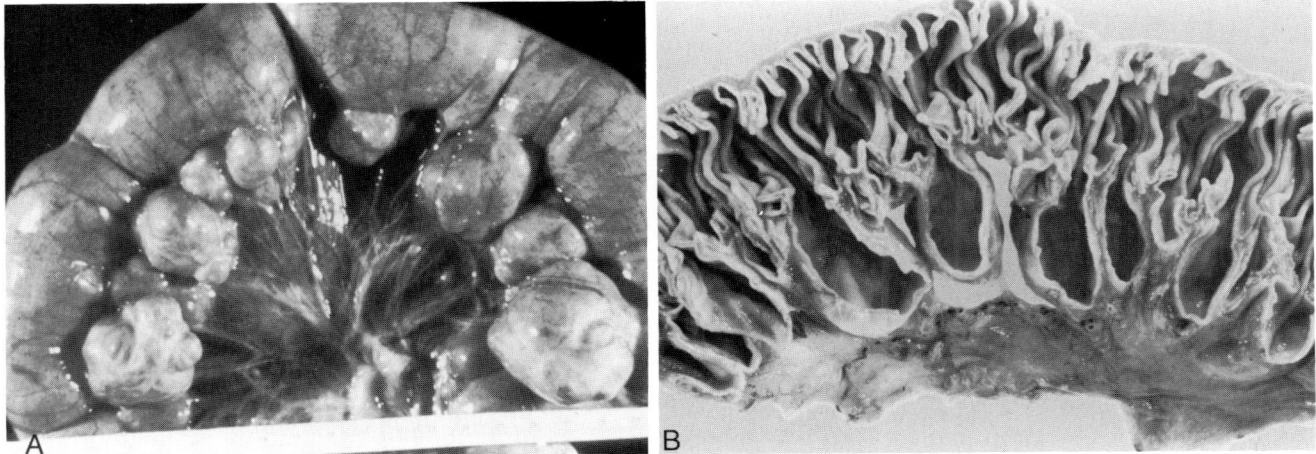

FIGURE 11–30. *A*, Jejunal diverticulosis. In this case, the diverticula occur on the mesenteric side. *B*, Opening the bowel revealed large diverticula with relatively large mouths.

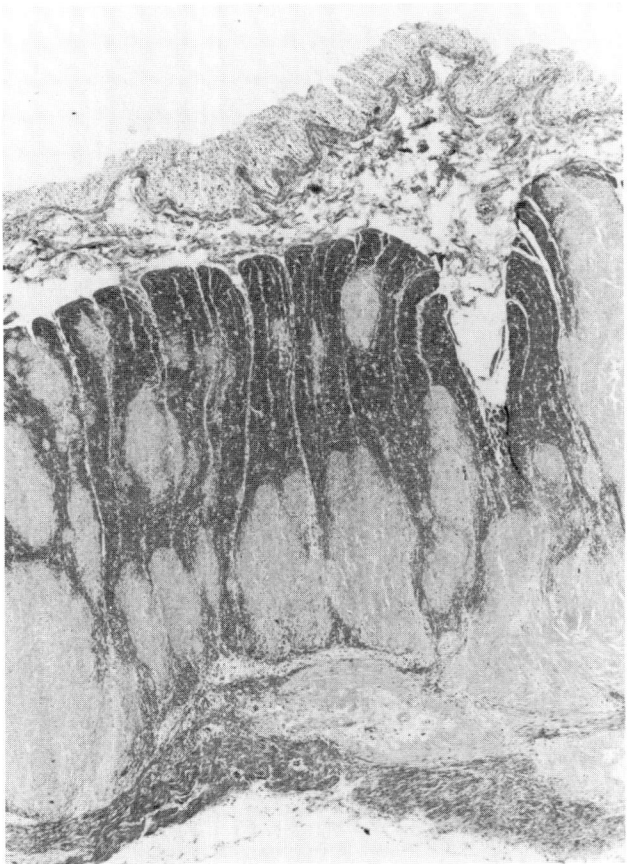

FIGURE 11–31. Mucosal surface at the top. Amyloidosis with multiple large, pale-staining deposits of amyloid in the muscularis propria and myenteric plexus in a patient with pseudo-obstruction syndrome. (Trichrome, × 8)

be caused by lesions affecting the myenteric plexus. In such instances, herniations of mucosa and submucosa similar to the false diverticula commonly seen in the colon are produced. Some cases appear to be secondary to known neurologic disease processes, such as *Fabry's disease*[83]; in others, the myenteric plexus shows changes on silver staining similar to some of those seen in the familial visceral neuropathies.[4] Interestingly, it should be noted that small-intestinal diverticula have occurred in patients with type II visceral myopathy. The commonly encountered duodenal diverticula, which are usually single or few in number, are not usually associated with motility problems.

Amyloidosis

In a manner analogous to that of jejunal diverticulosis, *amyloidosis* can involve both the muscular and neural structures of the gut, leading to severe motility problems.[4,16,84,85] The effect on muscle usually predominates. The clinical picture is dominated by features typical of amyloidosis. Within the wall of the gastrointestinal tract, large deposits of amyloid can be found in the muscularis propria and can even lead to gross mural thickening (Figure 11–31). While the gastrointestinal tract is frequently involved in amyloidosis, clinically significant pseudo-obstruction appears to occur in the minority of cases (see Chapter 16).

Neural Diseases

Hirschsprung's Disease

The main disease process in this group is *Hirschsprung's disease*, a developmental abnormality (see Chapter 8). Much has been written concerning this process as a clinicopathologic entity,[86] and the discussion here will only serve to fit it into the framework of the other neuromuscular disorders of the gastrointestinal tract. Unlike the other processes described in this chapter, there is a stereotypical localization of the involved segment, namely, the most distal portion. Even the uncommon long-segment cases involve the distal portion in continuity. The defect is primarily neural, with an absence of ganglion cells in the distal portions of Auerbach's and Meissner's plexuses. The muscle is normal except for the expected hypertrophy[14,15] in the segment proximal to the distal aganglionic segment, which causes a functional obstruction. The standard of diagnosis for many years has been the demonstration of the absence of ganglion cells in the myenteric plexus in full-thickness or seromuscular biopsy specimens. Parasympathetic nerve fibers, representing ramifications of lumbosacral preganglionic fibers, are increased in numbers in the muscularis mucosae and lamina propria of the aganglionic areas of the colon in children with Hirschsprung's disease.[87] Acetylcholinesterase is present in high concentration in such fibers and can be readily demonstrated histologically in frozen sections of mucosal biopsies. With the advent of the widespread application of acetylcholinesterase techniques,[88] suction biopsies of rectal mucosa and submucosa have become increasingly useful.[89] The increased caliber and number of fibers in involved areas are in striking contrast to the staining pattern in the ganglionic areas (Figure 11–32). When these findings are combined with manometric and other clinical data, the need for biopsy specimens including myenteric plexus can often be obviated. We have applied this technique to the biopsies from a number of our patients with primary myopathies and to some with primary neuropathies (primarily idiopathic constipation) and have seen only normal staining patterns thus far. Immunoperoxidase staining for neuron-specific enolase, S-100 protein, and neurofilament protein has proved useful in identifying neural structures, even immature ganglion cells,[6] but to date has not clearly demonstrated the proliferation of acetylcholinesterase-rich parasympathetic fibers. It is to be expected that continued widespread application of such techniques will enhance our understanding of this disorder and others affecting the enteric neuromuscular apparatus.

Neuronal Intestinal Dysplasia

Neuronal intestinal dysplasia is another developmental disorder affecting the colonic neural structures and

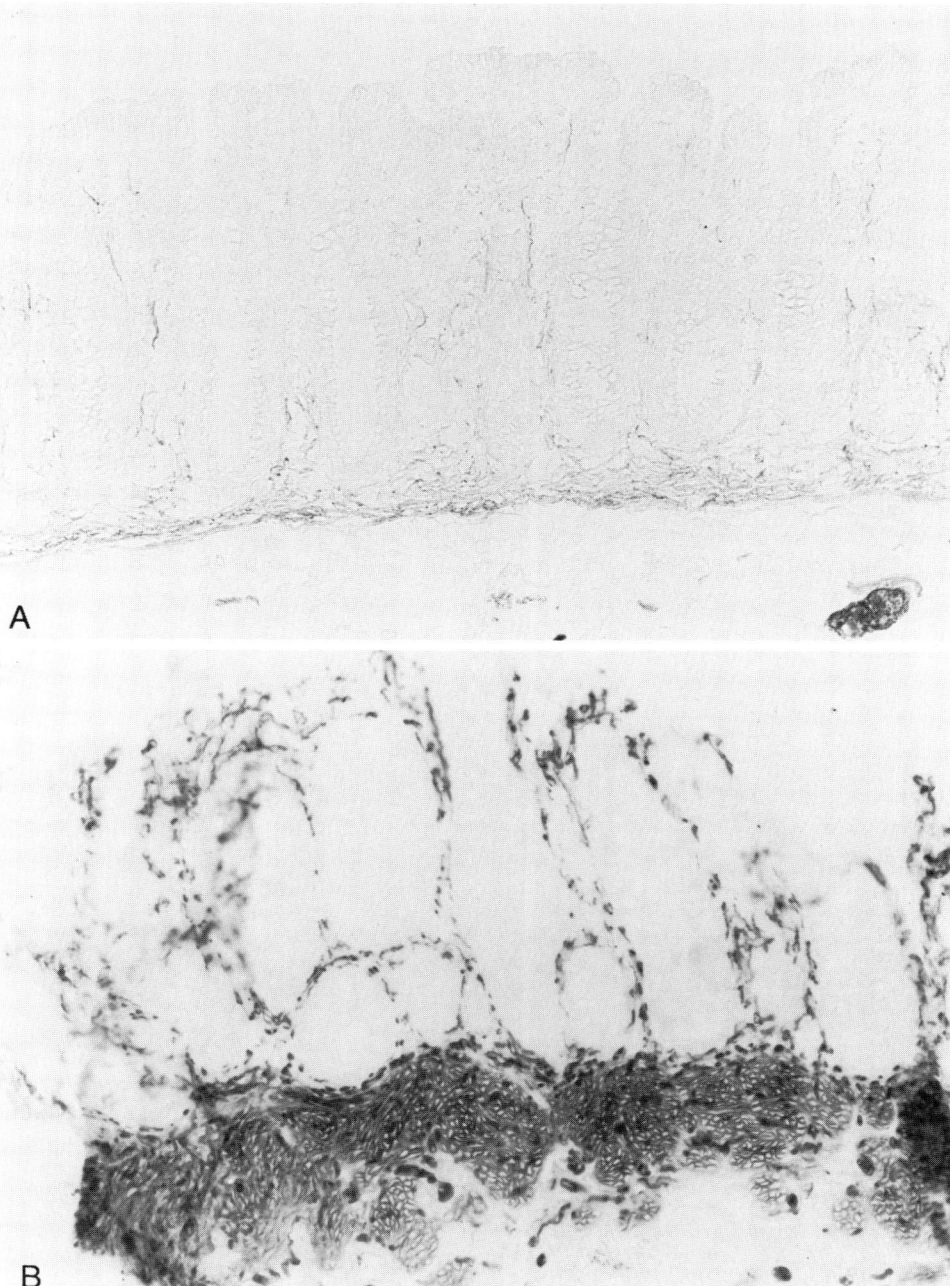

FIGURE 11–32. *A*, The normal colonic mucosa (surface at the top) contains only delicate twigs of parasympathetic fibers in the lamina propria between the crypts; staining of the muscularis mucosae is light. (Acetylcholinesterase, × 40) *B*, In the aganglionic colonic segment in Hirschsprung's disease, the parasympathetic fibers form thick, ramifying branches in the lamina propria, and staining in the muscularis mucosae is intense. (Acetylcholinesterase, × 40)

can mimic Hirschsprung's disease in many ways.[86] Although the appearance on acetylcholinesterase staining is quite similar to that of Hirschsprung's disease, mature ganglion cells can be found in the submucosa.[90,91] In fact, the characteristic feature of the disease process is hyperplasia of the submucosal and myenteric plexuses. Giant ganglia may be formed, and ganglion cells may even be found in the lamina propria (Figure 11–33). Multiple segments throughout the gastrointestinal tract may be involved. The process is most commonly associated with von Recklinghausen's disease[92] or multiple endocrine neoplasia syndrome type IIB[93] but apparently occurs occasionally in isolation.

Chagas' Disease

The syndrome of intestinal pseudo-obstruction has long been known to be associated with *Chagas' disease*. This disease, caused by infection with the parasitic agent *Trypanosoma cruzi*, is limited to South America. The damage to the myenteric plexus has been shown to be related to an immunologic reaction to this agent.[61] Esophageal involvement is common, resulting in acha-

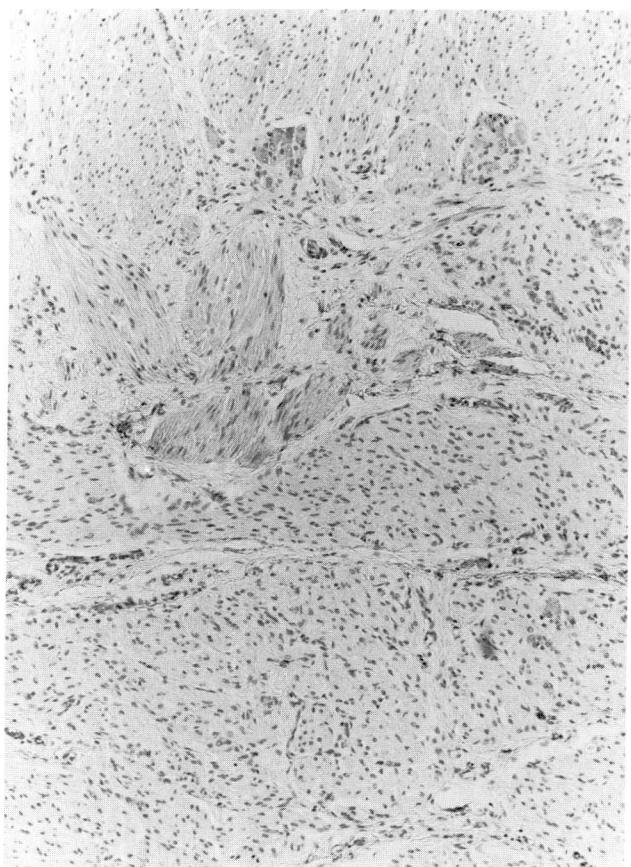

FIGURE 11-33. Neuronal intestinal dysplasia with a giant ganglion, occupying a substantial portion of the colonic muscularis propria in this case (bottom two thirds of the photograph). Fragments of muscle are at the top. (H&E, × 25)

lasia; megacolon is also quite common.[93,94] The organisms are not visualized in the plexus. Rather, there is plasma cell and lymphocytic infiltrate of the myenteric plexus with a loss of neurons, and there is secondary hypertrophy of the muscular layers.[4]

Parkinson's Disease

Pseudo-obstruction has been reported to occur in patients with *Parkinson's disease*,[94,95] although it is probably not possible to exclude the effect of therapeutic anticholinergic agents in these patients.[16] A distinct morphologic lesion has not been described.

Others

Familial autonomic dysfunction[96] and *Shy-Drager syndrome*[97] are two disease processes with widespread neurologic consequences that have been implicated in motility disorders.[4,16] There may be some damage to enteric neurons,[98] but diagnosis rests primarily on the associated clinical findings.

As described above, in some instances jejunal diverticulosis and amyloidosis may interfere with gastrointestinal motility because of damage to the myenteric plexus.

Endocrine Disorders

There are many gastrointestinal hormones that have profound effects on the secretions and motility of the gastrointestinal tract. These include gastrin, cholecystokinin, secretin, glucagon, vasoactive intestinal polypeptide, gastric inhibitory peptide, motilin, enterogastrone, somatostatin, and substance P.[99] Although it seems certain that many of these substances play pivotal roles in the motility disorders of the gastrointestinal system, progress similar to that which has been made recently (see above) in understanding clinicopathologic correlates of the enteric neural and muscular system has not been made with regard to the enteric endocrine system. This section will deal only with the effects on the gastrointestinal tract of known systemic disorders (see Chapter 16).

Diabetes Mellitus

Diabetes mellitus, because of its frequency, is one of the most common disorders thought to be related to gastrointestinal motility disorders. There are a number of mechanisms by which the gastrointestinal tract is affected. Foremost among these is visceral autonomic neuropathy, although some role may be played by microangiopathy, an altered electrolyte state, increased susceptibility to secondary infections, and abnormal production of insulin and glucagon.[100] Subclinical involvement of the esophagus is common; when esophageal disease is clinically apparent, it usually presents as typical reflux esophagitis. Esophageal candidiasis is common. Gastroparesis can be a more disabling problem. Huge atonic stomachs may necessitate surgical intervention; no characteristic lesion is seen in the neuromuscular apparatus. Some reports have described changes in the autonomic nerves and in the prevertebral and paravertebral ganglia.[101] The impaired motility resulting from such damage can lead to small-bowel bacterial overgrowth and diarrhea. Care must be taken to exclude celiac disease, which appears with an increased frequency in diabetics.[102] Constipation can also be a problem in diabetics, but no specific lesion has been found in the colon.

Hypothyroidism

Intestinal pseudo-obstruction can be significant in patients with *hypothyroidism* and may precede the other symptoms.[103] Colonic distention may be striking, and the muscularis propria may show an infiltration by mucopolysaccharide.[104]

Others

Hypoparathyroidism[105] and *pheochromocytoma*[106] have been reported to be associated with pseudo-obstruction, although this appears to be uncommon. In the latter instance, the effect on motility was probably the result of catecholamine production by the tumor.

Pharmacologic Agents

A variety of pharmacologic agents can have a profound effect on gastrointestinal motility, and may produce the clinical picture of pseudo-obstruction. Foremost among these are the phenothiazines, tricyclic antidepressants, ganglionic blockers, clonidine, and antiparkinsonian medications.[16]

Naturally occurring toxins, such as that of *Amanita phalloides*, can also dramatically alter motility.[16]

Miscellaneous Lesions

Megacolon may develop following jejunoileal bypass[107]; it appears in some way to be related to an effect of the altered bacterial flora in the blind loop draining into the colon.[108]

A variety of disease processes with obvious alterations in the muscle wall may present as pseudo-obstruction. Eosinophilic gastroenteritis[109] is a well-known process in which the motility problem may predominate. Likewise, the fibrosis and alteration of the intestinal musculature seen in radiation may have a similar effect.[110] A peculiar lymphoid infiltrate of the muscularis propria resulting in pseudo-obstruction has recently been described.[111]

CONCLUSION

It is obvious that much needs to be learned about the structure and function of the enteric neuromuscular apparatus. Although standard techniques are sufficient for examination of the smooth muscle, those necessary for examination of the enteric nervous system are difficult at best. The silver stain techniques used in examining the myenteric plexus are capricious and require experience and expertise for proper interpretation. As recognition and knowledge of these diseases grow, the widespread application of readily available immunoperoxidase techniques should add several pieces to the puzzle. Although many of the devastating primary forms of pseudo-obstruction are rare, more subtle alterations of the neuromuscular apparatus are common. A greater understanding of such processes could conceivably change substantially our perceptions of such common diseases as reflux esophagitis and diabetes. The long-neglected muscle and nerve of the gastrointestinal tract certainly deserve greater attention.

References

1. Christensen, J, Wingate DL: A guide to gastrointestinal motility. Bristol, UK, Wright and Sons, 1983, pp 1–214.
2. Smith BF: The neuropathology of the alimentary tract. London, Edward Arnold, 1972, pp 3–16.
3. Schuffler MD, Jonak Z: Chronic intestinal pseudo-obstruction caused by a degenerative disorder of the myenteric plexus: The use of Smith's method to define the neuropathology. Gastroenterology 82:476–486, 1982.
4. Krishnamurthy S, Schuffler MD: Pathology of neuromuscular disorders of the small intestine and colon. Gastroenterology 93:610–639, 1987.
5. Kumar D, Phillips SF: Human myenteric plexus: Confirmation of unfamiliar structures in adults and neonates. Gastroenterology 96:1021–1028, 1989.
6. Mackenzie JM, Dixon MF: An immunohistochemical study of the enteric neural plexi in Hirschsprung's disease. Histopathology 11:1055–1066, 1987.
7. Faussone-Pellegrini M: Comparative study of interstitial cells of Cajal. Acta Anat 130:109–126, 1987.
8. Kobayashi S, Suzuki M, Endo T, et al: Framework of the enteric nerve plexuses: An immunocytochemical study in the guinea pig jejunum using antiserum to S-100 protein. Arch Histol Jpn 49:159–188, 1986.
9. Berk JE: Bockus Gastroenterology. Philadelphia, WB Saunders, 1985, pp 2056–2092.
10. Ellis H: The causes and prevention of intestinal adhesions. Br J Surg 69:241–243, 1982.
11. Mucha P: Small intestinal obstruction. Surg Clin North Am 67:597–620, 1987.
12. Fielding LP, Welch JP: Intestinal obstruction. New York, Churchill Livingstone, 1987, pp 32–41, 153–162.
13. Orloff MV: Intussusception in children and adults. Surg Gynecol Obstet 102:313–329, 1956.
14. Gabella G: Hypertrophy of intestinal smooth muscle. Cell Tissue Res 163:199–214, 1975.
15. Brent L: The response of smooth muscle cells in the rabbit colon to anal stenosis. Pathology 5:209–218, 1973.
16. Faulk DL, Anuras S, Christensen J: Chronic or intestinal pseudo-obstruction. Gastroenterology 74:922–931, 1978.
17. Anuras S, Christensen J: Recurrent or chronic intestinal pseudo-obstruction. Clin Gastroenterol 10:177–190, 1981.
18. Golladay ES, Byrne WJ: Intestinal pseudo-obstruction. Surg Gynecol Obstet 153:257–273, 1981.
19. Hirsh EH, Brandenburg D, Hersh T, Brooks WS: Chronic intestinal pseudo-obstruction. J Clin Gastroenterol 3:247–254, 1981.
20. Hanks JB, Meyers WC, Andersen DK: Chronic primary intestinal pseudo-obstruction. Surgery 89:175–182, 1981.
21. Schuffler MD, Rohrmann CA, Chaffee RG: Chronic intestinal pseudo-obstruction. Medicine 60:173–196, 1981.
22. Schuffler MD: Chronic intestinal pseudo-obstruction syndromes. Med Clin North Am 65:1331–1358, 1981.
23. Weis W: Zur Atiologic des Megaduodenums. Deutsch Z Chir 251:317–330, 1938.
24. Law DH, Ten Eyck EA: Familial megaduodenum and megacystis. Am J Med 33:911–922, 1962.
25. Newton WT: Radical enterectomy for hereditary megaduodenum. Arch Surg 96:549–553, 1968.
26. Byrne WJ, Cipel L, Euler AR: Chronic idiopathic intestinal pseudo-obstruction syndrome in children. J Pediatr 90:585–589, 1970.
27. Vanek VW, Al-Salti M: Acute pseudo-obstruction of the colon (Ogilvie's syndrome). Dis Colon Rectum 29:203–210, 1986.
28. Anuras S, Shirazi SS: Colonic pseudo-obstruction. Am J Gastroenterol 79:525–532, 1984.
29. Bonsib SM, Fallon B, Mitros FA, Anuras S: Urological manifestations of patients with visceral myopathy. J Urol 132:1112–1116, 1984.
30. Anuras S, Mitros FA, Milano A, et al: A familial visceral myopathy with dilatation of the entire gastrointestinal tract. Gastroenterology 90:385–390, 1986.
31. Anuras S, Mitros FA, Nowak TV: A familial visceral myopathy with external ophthalmoplegia and autosomal recessive transmission. Gastroenterology 84:346–353, 1983.
32. Faulk DL, Anuras S, Gardner GD, et al: A familial visceral myopathy. Ann Intern Med 89:600–606, 1978.
33. Ionasescu V: Oculogastrointestinal muscular dystrophy. Am J Med Genet 15:103–112, 1983.
34. Ionasescu V, Thompson SH, Ionasescu R: Inherited opthalmoplegia with intestinal pseudo-obstruction. J Neurol Sci 59:215–228, 1983.
35. Ionasescu V, Thompson SH, Aschenbrenner C, Anuras S: Late

onset oculogastrointestinal muscular dystrophy. Am J Med Genet 18:781–788, 1984.
36. Jacobs E, Andichvili D, Perissino A, et al: A case of familial visceral myopathy with atrophy and fibrosis of the longitudinal muscle layer of the entire small bowel. Gastroenterology 77:745–750, 1979.
37. Lewis TD, Daniel EE, Sarna SK, et al. Idiopathic intestinal pseudo-obstruction: Report of a case, with intraluminal studies of mechanical and electrical activity, and response to drugs. Gastroenterology 74:107–111, 1978.
38. Mitros FA, Schuffler MD, Teja K, Anuras S: Pathology of familial visceral myopathy. Hum Pathol 13:825–833, 1983.
39. Schuffler MD, Lowe MC, Bill AH: Studies of idiopathic intestinal pseudo-obstruction clinical and pathological studies. Gastroenterology 73:327–338, 1977.
40. Schuffler MD, Pope CE: Studies of idiopathic intestinal pseudo-obstruction. II. A hereditary hollow visceral myopathy: Family studies. Gastroenterology 73:339–344, 1977.
41. Shaw A, Shaffer H, Teja K, et al: A perspective for pediatric surgeons: Chronic idiopathic intestinal pseudo-obstruction. J Pediatr Surg 14:719–727, 1979.
42. Foucar CE, Lindholm J, Anuras S, et al: A kindred with dysplastic nevus syndrome associated with visceral myopathy and multiple basal cell carcinomas. Lab Invest 52:23A, 1985.
43. Anuras S, Mitros FA, Shirazi SS, et al: Cardiac arrest in two children with nonfamilial chronic intestinal pseudo-obstruction on total parenteral nutrition. J Pediatr Gastroenterol 1:137–144, 1982.
44. Puri P, Lake BD, Gorman F, et al: Megacystic microcolon intestinal hypoperistalsis syndrome: A visceral myopathy. J Pediatr Surg 18:64–68, 1983.
45. Alstead EM, Murphy MN, Flanagan AM, et al: Familial autonomic visceral myopathy with degeneration of muscularis mucosae. J Clin Pathol 41:424–429, 1988.
46. Schuffler MD, Kaplan LR, Johnson L: Small intestinal mucosa in pseudo-obstruction syndromes. Am J Dig Dis 23:821–830, 1978.
47. Anuras S, Shirazi S, Faulk DL, et al: Surgical treatment in familial visceral myopathy. Ann Surg 189:306–310, 1979.
48. Schuffler MD, Bird TD, Sumi SM, Cook A: A familial neuronal disease presenting as intestinal pseudoobstruction. Gastroenterology 75:889–898, 1978.
49. Schuffler MD, Rohrmann CA, Templeton FE: The radiological manifestations of idiopathic intestinal pseudoobstruction. AJR 127:729–736, 1976.
50. Summers RW, Anuras S, Green J: Jejunal manometry patterns in health, partial intestinal obstruction, and pseudoobstruction. Gastroenterology 85:1290–1300, 1983.
51. Palo J, Haltia M, Carpenter S, et al: Neurofilament subunit-related proteins in neuronal intranuclear inclusions. Ann Neurol 15:322–328, 1984.
52. Patel H, Norman MG, Perry TL, Berry KE: Multiple system atrophy with neuronal intranuclear hyaline inclusions. J Neurol Sci 67:57–65, 1985.
53. Monoz-Garcia D, Ludwin SK: Adult onset neuronal intranuclear hyaline inclusion disease. Neurology 36:785–790, 1986.
54. Cockel R, Hill EE, Rushton DI, et al: Familial steatorrhea with calcification of the basal ganglia and mental retardation. Q J Med 168:771–783, 1973.
55. Roy AD, Bharucha H, Nevin NC, Odling-Smee GW: Idiopathic intestinal pseudo-obstruction: A familial visceral neuropathy. Clin Genet 18:291–297, 1980.
56. Mayer EA, Schuffler MD, Rotter JI, et al: Familial visceral neuropathy with autosomal dominant transmission. Gastroenterology 91:1528–1535, 1986.
57. Erskine JM: Acquired megacolon, megaesophagus and megaduodenum with aperistalsis: A case report. Am J Gastroenterol 40:588–600, 1963.
58. Horoupian DS, Kim Y: Encephalomyeloneuropathy with ganglionitis of the myenteric plexuses in the absence of cancer. Ann Neurol 11:628–631, 1982.
59. Schuffler MD, Baird HW, Fleming CR, et al: Intestinal pseudo-obstruction as the presenting manifestation of small cell carcinoma of the lung: A paraneoplastic neuropathy of the gastrointestinal tract. Ann Intern Med 98:129–134, 1983.
60. Earlam RJ: Gastrointestinal aspects of Chagas' disease. Dig Dis Sci 17:559–571, 1972.
61. Wood JN, Hudson L, Jessell TM, Yamamoto M: A monoclonal antibody defining antigenic determinants on subpopulations of mammalian neurones and Trypanosoma cruzi parasites. Nature 296:34–38, 1982.
62. Press MF, Riddell RH, Ringus J: Cytomegalovirus inclusion disease: Its occurrence in the myenteric plexus of a renal transplant patient. Arch Pathol Lab Med 104:580–583, 1980.
63. Sonsino E, Mouy R, Foucaud P, et al: Intestinal pseudo-obstruction related to cytomegalovirus infection of the myenteric plexus. N Engl J Med 311:196–197, 1984.
64. Krishnamurthy S, Schuffler MD, Belic L, Schweid AI: An inflammatory axonopathy of the myenteric plexus causing rapidly progressive intestinal pseudoobstruction. Gastroenterology 90:754–758, 1986.
65. Krishnamurthy S, Schuffler MD, Rohrmann CA, Pope CE: Severe idiopathic constipation is associated with a distinctive abnormality of the colonic myenteric plexus. Gastroenterology 88:26–34, 1985.
66. Preston DM, Hawley RR, Lennard-Jones JE, Todd IP: Results of colectomy for severe idiopathic constipation in women (Arbuthnot Lane's disease). Br J Surg 71:547–552, 1984.
67. Smith B: Effect of irritant purgatives on the myenteric plexus in man and the mouse. Gut 9:139–143, 1968.
68. Smith B: Pathologic changes in the colon produced by anthraquinone purgatives. Dis Colon Rectum 16:455–458, 1973.
69. Schuffler MD, Beegle RG: Progressive systemic sclerosis of the gastrointestinal tract and hollow visceral myopathy: Two distinguishable disorders of intestinal smooth muscle. Gastroenterology 77:664–671, 1979.
70. Poirier TJ, Rankin GB: Gastrointestinal manifestations of progressive systemic sclerosis based on a review of 364 cases. Am J Gastroenterol 58:30–44, 1972.
71. Goldgraber MB, Kirsner JB: Scleroderma of the gastrointestinal tract. Arch Pathol 64:255–265, 1957.
72. D'Angelo WA, Fries JF, Masi AT, Shulman LE: Pathologic observations in systemic sclerosis (scleroderma). Am J Med 46:428–440, 1969.
73. Heinz ER, Steinberg AJ, Sackner MA: Roentgenographic and pathologic aspects of intestinal scleroderma. Ann Intern Med 59:822–826, 1983.
74. Norton WL, Nardo JM: Vascular disease in progressive systemic sclerosis (scleroderma). Ann Intern Med 73:317–324, 1970.
75. Morson BC: Gastrointestinal pathology. London, Blackwell Scientific Publications, 1979, pp 694–695.
76. Nowak TV, Ionasescu V, Anuras S: Gastrointestinal manifestations of the muscular dystrophies. Gastroenterology 82:800–810, 1982.
77. Leon SH, Schuffler MD, Kettler M, Rohrmann CA: Intestinal pseudo-obstruction as a complication of Duchenne's muscular dystrophy. Gastroenterology 90:455–459, 1986.
78. Horn T, Svendsen LB, Johansen A, Backer O: Brown bowel syndrome. Ultrastruct Pathol 8:357–361, 1985.
79. Braustein H: Tocopherol deficiency in adults with chronic pancreatitis. Gastroenterology 40:224–231, 1961.
80. Fox B: Lipofuscinosis of the gastrointestinal tract in man. J Clin Pathol 20:806–813, 1967.
81. Foster CS: The brown bowel syndrome: A possible smooth muscle mitochondrial myopathy? Histopathology 3:1–17, 1979.
82. Krishnamurthy S, Kelly MM, Rohrmann CA, Schuffler MD: Jejunal diverticulosis: A heterogenous disorder caused by a variety of abnormalities of smooth muscle or myenteric plexus. Gastroenterology 85:538–547, 1983.
83. Friedman LS, Kirkham SE, Thistlethwaite JR, et al: Jejunal diverticulosis with perforation as a complication of Fabry's disease. Gastroenterology 86:558–563, 1984.
84. Legge DA, Wollaeger EE, Carlson HC: Intestinal pseudoobstruction in systemic amyloidosis. Gut 11:764–767, 1970.
85. Wald A, Kichler J, Mendelow H: Amyloidosis and chronic intestinal pseudoobstruction. Dig Dis Sci 26:462–465, 1981.
86. Holschneider AM: Hirschsprung's disease. New York, Thieme-Stratton, 1982, pp 62–71.
87. Weinberg AG: Acetylcholinesterase and Hirschsprung's disease. J Pediatr Gastroenterol 5:837–843, 1986.

88. Lake BD, Puri P, Nixon HH, Claireaux AE: Hirschsprung's disease: An appraisal of histochemically demonstrated acetylcholinesterase activity in suction rectal biopsy specimens as an aid to diagnosis. Arch Pathol Lab Med 102:244–248, 1978.
89. Huntley CC, Shaffner L, Challa VR, Lyerly AD: Histochemical diagnosis of Hirschsprung's disease. Pediatrics 69:755–761, 1982.
90. Scharli AF, Meier-Ruge W: Localized and disseminated forms of neuronal intestinal dysplasia mimicking Hirschsprung's disease. J Pediatr Surg 16:164–170, 1981.
91. MacMahon RA, Moore CCM, Cussen LJ: Hirschsprung-like syndromes in patients with normal ganglion cells on suction rectal biopsy. J Pediatr Surg 16:835–839, 1981.
92. Feinstat T, Testnk H, Schuffler MD, et al: Megacolon and neurofibromatosis: A neuronal intestinal dysplasia. Gastroenterology 86:1573–1579, 1984.
93. Demos TC, Blonder J, Schey WL, et al: Multiple endocrine neoplasia (MEN) syndrome type IIB: gastrointestinal manifestations. Am J Roentgenol 140:73–78, 1983.
94. Lewitan A, Nathanson L, Slade WR: Megacolon and dilatation of the small bowel in Parkinsonism. Gastroenterology 17:367–374, 1951.
95. Caplan LH, Jacobson JG, Rubinstein BM, Rotman MZ: Megacolon and volvulus in Parkinson's disease. Radiology 85:73–78, 1965.
96. Grossman HJ, Limosani MA, Shore M: Megacolon as a manifestation of familial autonomic dysfunction. J Pediatr 49:289–296, 1956.
97. Shy GM, Drager GA: A neurological syndrome associated with orthostatic hypotension. Arch Neurol 2:511–516, 1960.
98. Smith B: The neuropathology of pseudo-obstruction of the intestine. Scand J Gastroenterol 17(Suppl 71):103–109, 1982.
99. Ouyang A, Cohen S: Effects of hormones on gastrointestinal motility. Med Clin North Am 65:111–127, 1981.
100. Yang R, Arem R, Chan L: Gastrointestinal tract complications of diabetes mellitus. Arch Intern Med 144:1251–1256, 1984.
101. Hensley GT, Soergel KH: Neuropathologic findings in diabetic diarrhea. Arch Pathol 85:587–597, 1968.
102. Green PA, Wollaegen EE, Sprague RG: Diabetes mellitus associated with non-tropical sprue: Report of 4 cases. Diabetes 11:388–392, 1962.
103. Chadha JS, Ashby SW, Cowan WK: Fatal intestinal atony in myxoedema. Br Med J 3:398–401, 1969.
104. Abbassi AA, Douglas RC, Bissell GW, Chen Y: Myxedema ileus: A form of intestinal pseudo-obstruction. JAMA 234:181–183, 1975.
105. Taybi H, Keele D: Hypoparathyroidism: A review of the literature and report of two cases in sisters, one with steatorrhea and intestinal pseudo-obstruction. AJR 88:432–442, 1962.
106. Mullen JP, Cartwright RC, Tisherman SE, et al: Case report: Pathogenesis and pharmacologic management of pseudo-obstruction of the bowel in pheochromocytoma. Am J Med Sci 290:155–158, 1985.
107. Barry RE, Benfield JR, Nicell P, Bray GA: Colonic pseudo-obstruction: A new complication of jejunoileal bypass. Gut 16:903–908, 1975.
108. Barry RE, Chow AW, Billesdon J: Role of intestinal microflora in colonic pseudo-obstruction complicating jejunoileal bypass. Gut 18:356–359, 1977.
109. Johnstone JM, Morson BC: Eosinophilic gastroenteritis. Histopathology 2:335–348, 1978.
110. Berthrong M, Fajardo LF: Radiation injury in surgical pathology. Part II. Alimentary tract. Am J Surg Pathol 5:153–178, 1981.
111. McDonald GB, Schuffler MD, Kadin ME, Tytgat GNJ: Intestinal pseudoobstruction caused by diffuse lymphoid infiltration of the small intestine. Gastroenterology 89:882–889, 1985.

CHAPTER 12

Vascular Disorders

H. THOMAS NORRIS, M.D.

DIAGNOSIS OF GASTROINTESTINAL BLEEDING

METHODS OF EXAMINATION OF SPECIMENS
Injection Studies of Blood Vessels
Gelatin-Barium Mixture
Silicone Rubber
Other Techniques
Lymphatics

ANATOMY OF GASTROINTESTINAL VASCULATURE

ACQUIRED AND CONGENITAL VASCULAR MALFORMATIONS
Varices
Associated with Portal Hypertension of Hepatic Origin
Pathophysiology
Location
Associated with Portal Hypertension of Extrahepatic Origin
Hemorrhoids
Vascular Abnormalities of the Gastrointestinal Tract
Classification
Arteriovenous Malformation
Angiodysplasia
Submucosal Arteriovenous Malformation
Telangiectasia
Congenital: Osler-Weber-Rendu Disease and Turner's Syndrome
Acquired: CRST Syndrome

Disorders of Connective Tissue Affecting Blood Vessels
Pseudoxanthoma Elasticum
Ehlers-Danlos Syndrome
Uncommon Vascular Lesions
Congenital Arteriovenous Malformations
Aneurysms
Gastric Antral Vascular Ectasia

TUMORS AND TUMORLIKE PROLIFERATIONS OF VESSELS
Hemangiomas
Classification, Pathology, and Location
Syndromes Involving Gastrointestinal Hemangiomas
Diffuse Intestinal Hemangiomatosis
Universal (Miliary) Hemangiomatosis
Blue Rubber Bleb Nevus Syndrome
Peutz-Jeghers Syndrome
Klippel-Trenaunay-Weber Syndrome
Malignant Vascular Tumors
Kaposi's Sarcoma
Primary Angiosarcoma
Lymphangiomas

VASCULITIS
General Considerations
Histologic Features and Differential Diagnosis
Utility of Mucosal Biopsy and Other Studies in Establishing the Diagnosis of Vasculitis
Vasculitic Lesions in the Gastrointestinal Tract
Polyarteritis Nodosa
Systemic Lupus Erythematosus
Rheumatoid Arthritis

Hypersensitivity Angiitis
Churg-Strauss Syndrome
Allergic Granulomatous Angiitis
Henoch-Schönlein Purpura
Wegener's Granulomatosis
Hemolytic-Uremic Syndrome
Ulceration of the Stomach
Differentiation from Other Diseases of Unknown Etiology That May Have Vasculitis as a Component

ISCHEMIC DISEASES
General Considerations
Pathophysiologic Effects of Ischemia
Nomenclature and Classification
General Pathology
Etiology of Bowel Infarcts
Ischemic Bowel Disease
Spectrum and Clinical Features
Experimental Studies
Proposed Mechanisms of Pathogenesis
Superoxide Radicals
Intracellular Calcium Homeostasis
Intra-arterial Platelet Activating Factor and Bacterial Endotoxin
Therapeutic Considerations
Entities of Ischemic Bowel Disease
Ischemic Colitis
Necrotizing Enterocolitis of the Premature Infant
Pseudomembranous Colitis
Hemorrhagic Necrosis
Stress Ulceration
Radiation Injury
Other Disorders
Effect of Chronic Narrowing of Splanchnic Vessels

This chapter on vascular disorders of the gastrointestinal tract is an attempt to cover the vast number of diseases involving the vessels that can be found throughout the gastrointestinal tract. Pathologic factors as diverse as emboli into the orifices of major arteries to vasculitis occurring in the smallest vessels all have a profound effect on the functioning of an organ. The gastrointestinal tract is not exempt from these changes. This chapter will utilize as resource material predominantly those references that have provided new knowledge during the last 5 to 10 years.

Symptoms referable to abnormalities of the gastrointestinal vasculature provide three main types of clinical findings—pain, obstruction to flow of gastrointestinal contents, and hemorrhage. One of the major advances of the last 10 years is greater definition of the site of bleeding.

DIAGNOSIS OF GASTROINTESTINAL BLEEDING

Dramatic changes have occurred in the diagnosis and management of gastrointestinal tract bleeding during the past decade. In the past, the cause and source of gastrointestinal bleeding often remained obscure even after extensive study. Currently, with the widespread application of fiberoptic endoscopy and advances in radiologic techniques, fewer cases now occur in which the cause of the gastrointestinal bleeding remains obscure or occult.[1]

A three-step approach is often used for investigation of suspected gastrointestinal bleeding. The first step in determining the source of bleeding is taking an adequate history and performing a thorough physical examination. Included in the examination is confirmation that the patient has actually experienced a gastrointestinal hemorrhage. This is usually accomplished by the use of a guaiac test for occult blood. Once it has been established that the patient has had a gastrointestinal hemorrhage, the next step is to determine whether the source of bleeding is from the upper or lower gastrointestinal tract. For purposes of this discussion, the dividing point of these two areas will be the ligament of Treitz. An upper gastrointestinal source of bleeding, that is, proximal to the ligament of Treitz, is suggested clinically by hematemesis. If the clinical situation is unclear, gastric aspiration may be of help in confirming the source of the hemorrhage. A gastric aspirate positive for blood suggests an upper tract source, whereas a negative study suggests a lower tract source. The third step is to as closely as possible identify the specific site of bleeding. The approach usually includes endoscopy, followed by contrast radiography, radionuclide scans, or arteriography, or a combination. With contemporary endoscopic techniques, in 70% to 90% of patients currently the source of the upper gastrointestinal bleeding can be identified by endoscopy.[2]

As noted above, the presence of occult blood in the stools or a negative gastric aspirate suggests lower gastrointestinal bleeding. In patients with lower gastrointestinal bleeding (colonic hemorrhage), flexible fiberoptic sigmoidoscopy should be the first procedure undertaken. However, appropriate preparation of the patient is essential for this study to have a successful outcome. The development of newer and smaller endoscopes have made examination of infants and children a practical diagnostic procedure.

Radiologic evaluation usually begins with plain films to exclude bowel obstruction and/or free intra-abdominal gas. This is followed by upper gastrointestinal tract studies, small-bowel series, or barium enemas, depending upon the suspected source of hemorrhage. Radiologic evaluation may be of limited usefulness in the diagnosis of certain vascular disorders. However, a double-contrast barium study may still detect bleeding lesions that are predominantly submucosal in location and thus difficult to see on colonoscopy.

Radionuclide studies have the advantage of documenting the presence of active bleeding in the gastrointestinal tract, although they may give only general information about the location of the site of active bleeding. These studies are of great benefit, especially when the bleeding is intermittent or of a subacute nature. Radionuclide studies certainly help in the appropriate timing of angiographic studies.

With the increased use of the flexible endoscope to ascertain the source of bleeding, angiography has undergone a concomitant decline as a diagnostic tool. Endoscopy during massive bleeding may be impossible. However, angiography in these instances continues to serve as a very useful diagnostic procedure. Angiography can detect active bleeding with flow rates as low as 0.5 ml/min, although the accuracy increases with the rate of bleeding. Angiography has a special role in demonstrating lesions that may not be currently bleeding but are caused by abnormal vessels, e.g., vascular malformations, telangiectasias, and hemangiomas. However, the role of angiography in treatment is becoming more evident. The infusion of either vasoconstrictive agents such as vasopressin or embolization therapy has either significantly decreased or stopped bleeding in certain cases.

During upper gastrointestinal tract endoscopy, the cause of bleeding usually can be placed in one of two categories. The first category includes mucosal lesions such as erosions, ulcerations, esophagitis, gastritis, and tears (Mallory-Weiss tears). The second major category is bleeding from upper gastrointestinal tract varices.

The major vascular causes of lower gastrointestinal bleeding include hemorrhoids, fissures, acute diverticulitis, and ischemic colitis. In patients over 60 years of age, angiodysplasia is the most frequent cause.

Therapy can also be accomplished during the endoscopic examination. Therapeutic interventions include the neodymium:yttrium-aluminum-garnet (Nd:YAG) laser, the heater probe, and electrocoagulation.

All of these advances have resulted in a general benefit to the patient. The site of bleeding can now be ascertained with much greater accuracy. In the past, it was assumed that gastrointestinal bleeding usually came from one specific single site. One of the advances in understanding that we have obtained using the flexible endoscope is that in upwards of a third of the cases, multiple potential sites or sources of bleeding can be found. With advances in technique and instruments, therapeutic endoscopy is being used with greater frequency during active bleeding. If these therapeutic attempts fail, definitive surgery may result in a cure.

METHODS OF EXAMINATION OF SPECIMENS

The type of vascular lesions affecting the gastrointestinal tract may be obvious. However, in many cases, the type of vascular lesion may not be readily apparent. In these latter cases, specific types of studies are often very helpful. The input of the clinician, surgeon, and radiologist with regard to the suspected type of lesion is essential before the studies are undertaken.

Injection Studies of Blood Vessels

The documentation and demonstration of the various vascular abnormalities of the gastrointestinal tract may require a variety of approaches. It is not difficult to make the diagnosis on a histopathologic basis once the lesion has been found. Finding the lesion is often the most challenging aspect of the examination for the pathologist. Special techniques may not be necessary. The most important part of the examination is close visual inspection of the mucosal surface. Most vascular abnormalities are usually less than 1 cm in size.

There are a variety of injection techniques that have been useful in the study of vascular lesions. The best special studies leave the specimen in a state that can be studied by subsequent radiologic and histologic techniques. These techniques demand that the vasculature be flushed with a solution to remove as much of the blood and small clots as possible. The artery to the specimen is cannulated, and this vessel is flushed until no clots are seen coming from the adjacent vein. Approximately 200 to 300 ml of warm saline or heparinized saline is usually effective. Occasionally, over 500 ml of solution is necessary.

Gelatin-Barium Mixture

A method that yields a specimen very amenable to both radiologic and pathologic techniques is the infusion of a mixture of gelatin and barium.[3,4] This mixture usually allows filling of the capillaries. The mixture is prepared by adding 3 ml of liquefied phenol and 2 ml of liquefied 2-octanol to 600 ml of hot tap water. This solution is placed in a blender and 100 gm of Knox Type 2136 gelatin is added slowly and blended for 1 minute. Then, 400 gm of Micropaque powder is added and blended for 2 minutes. This mixture is allowed to gel overnight and then is stored in the refrigerator. The solution is rewarmed and infused into the appropriate artery at the patient's systolic pressure. (This solution will not re-liquefy if it has come in contact with formalin.) If the vein does not fill, the vein is then subsequently infused with the same solution at similar pressures. Color can be added to the mixture if the distribution of individual vessels is to be studied. The addition of monastral red or monastral blue imparts a red or blue color, respectively, to the injection mixture. The specimen is then fixed in 10% formalin for 24 hours before appropriate radiologic and histopathologic studies are undertaken.

Whether the specimen has been injected or not, close examination of the mucosa is essential. Inspection may demonstrate small erosions or ulcerations. Pinpoint hemorrhages and small petechial lesions may be the only changes present on the surface. Occasionally, the lesions are linear. The presence of tiny clots on the surface of the mucosa is an extraordinarily helpful marker. The judicious application of India ink to suspected lesions on the mucosa will allow the examiner to return to the areas of interest and concern without causing significant morphologic alteration, which can occur with the use of pins and other sharp objects. India ink also helps localize the suspected area of abnormality in histologic section.

Silicone Rubber

Another technique is the injection of silicone rubber or silicone rubber with a radiopaque material added to it.[5] The injected specimen is refrigerated at 4.5°C for 24 hours, dehydrated in ethyl alcohol, and cleared in methyl salicylate. This results in a transparent specimen with an accentuated vascular bed. Although these specimens are very good for radiologic studies, they yield less than optimal results when studied histologically.

Other Techniques

Still another technique is the injection of the specimen with 5 ml of "biologic" *colloidal carbon* suspension filtered through Whatman paper No. 1.[6]*

A variety of other techniques have been used, especially during surgery, when there is concern about the location of the malformation. One such technique is the injection of indigo carmine solution during operation into the appropriate artery, which has been cannulated.[6] Methylene blue has also been used intraoperatively.[7]

Lymphatics

Demonstration of the lymphatics of the gastrointestinal tract is a much more challenging project. The author, personally, has only had success on an experimental basis when substances rich in lipid, such as melted butter, were placed in the lumen of the small

---

*Peliken Company, Hanover, Germany (Batch No. C11/1431a, sold in the United States as Biologic Ink by John Herschel and Co. Inc., 425 Fourth Avenue, New York, New York, 10016).

bowel during *in vivo* studies. The appearance of the lipid substance in the serosal lacteals was observed. One study suggests that the use of cedar oil mixed with a dye (color in oil) such as Prussian blue can be helpful in attempting to delineate lymphatic vessels.[8]

ANATOMY OF GASTROINTESTINAL VASCULATURE

Although the anatomy of the vasculature—arterial, venous and lymphatic—was studied extensively in the past, new diagnostic techniques and new therapeutic procedures have stimulated renewed interest in this subject. The vascular anatomy of the gastrointestinal tract is covered in further detail in Chapter 2. Several recent articles have reviewed the subject in detail.[9-12] These studies reiterate that a substantial anastomotic network is present involving both the arteries and the veins of the gastrointestinal tract. The extensive arterial anastomotic network and collateral circulation provide significant protection against ischemic episodes. The *marginal artery of Drummond* in the colon is one such anastomotic connection. This artery is derived from the middle colic branch of the superior mesenteric artery and the ascending division of the left colic branch of the inferior mesenteric artery.

The extensive anastomotic and collateral circulation present in the gastrointestinal venous network is usually not evident until there are altered pathophysiologic conditions within the portal venous system. With increased portal venous pressure, changes in venous blood flow patterns occur. Significant variation in the position of veins has an impact on the segment of bowel that develops acquired venous abnormalities. While the larger veins are usually located in the submucosa, occasionally they are located in the lamina propria. This is especially true at the junction of the esophagus and stomach. It is these areas that are thought to manifest varices earliest after an increase in portal venous pressure occurs.

ACQUIRED AND CONGENITAL VASCULAR MALFORMATIONS

Varices

Associated with Portal Hypertension of Hepatic Origin

Pathophysiology

Varices are dilated veins—the result of increased pressure in vessels that are collateral connections between portal and systemic venous circulation. Hayes et al. point out that portal hypertension develops when the pressure in the portal venous system is raised above the normal range of 10 to 15 mm Hg and becomes clinically important when portal venous pressure is above 15 mm Hg.[13] The liver has a dual blood supply, receiving about 1 L/min through the hepatic portal vein and the hepatic artery. The hepatic portal vein supplies 75% of the hepatic blood flow. Functional interactions occur between these two vascular systems as well as anatomic connections. An increase in blood flow through one circuit produces an increase in vascular resistance in the other. The consequence of portal hypertension is the development of an abnormal collateral venous circulation between the portal and systemic venous systems.

Location

Esophagus. The anastomosis that is clinically most important is at the lower end of the esophagus (Figure 12–1). Larger varices are associated with an increased risk of hemorrhage. Despite many years of speculation, we remain almost completely ignorant about the factors responsible for rupture of a varix and subsequent variceal hemorrhage. Increased portal venous pressure may have a direct bearing on the potential for bleeding.[14]

Spence speculates that the reason that the lower esophagus is the site of varix formation is that there is a unique anatomic variation in the 2 to 5 cm above the esophagogastric junction.[15] Here, the veins lie mainly

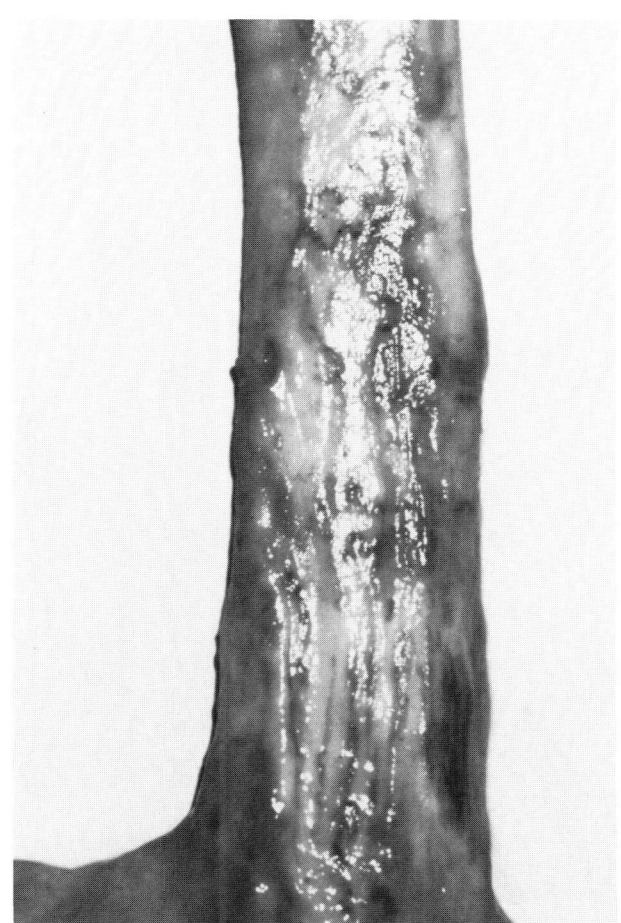

FIGURE 12–1. Gross photograph of esophageal varices. The dilated and tortuous veins are best demonstrated by turning the specimen inside out.

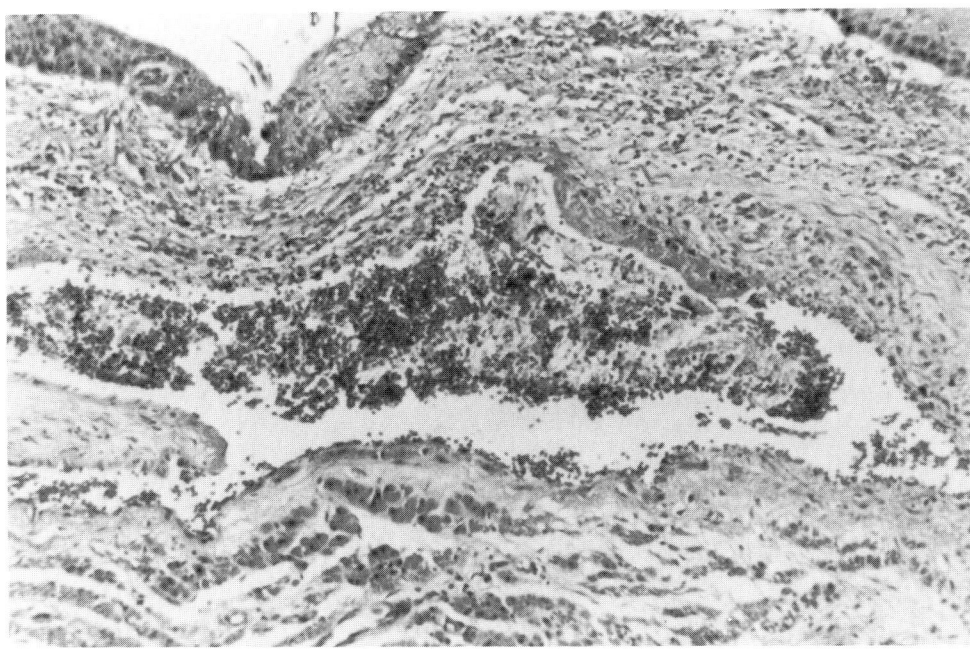

FIGURE 12-2. Low-power photomicrograph of esophageal varix. An unusually large dilated and congested vein is located immediately beneath the epithelium. ($\times$ 40)

in the lamina propria. In the stomach and proximal esophagus, the veins lie mainly within the submucosa. The close proximity of the veins in the esophagogastric junction to the lumen of the gastrointestinal tract with loss of structural support results in varix formation with increase in portal venous pressure (Figure 12-2).

Esophageal varices are caused most frequently by portal hypertension associated with alcoholic cirrhosis. There are other causes, but these are discussed separately. Bleeding esophageal varices due to alcoholic liver disease is a very grave sign. Over one third of these patients die soon after hospital admission for massive upper gastrointestinal hemorrhage.[16]

Other Sites. In addition to esophageal varices, rectal varices, anal varices (hemorrhoids), mesenteric serosal varices, dilated periumbilical veins (caput medusae), and spontaneous retroperitoneal splenorenal venous shunts may develop in patients with substantial portal hypertension. These latter types of varices are only rarely associated with significant hemorrhage.

The portal hypertension may be so high that varices occur in the *colon* (Figure 12-3). They are frequently

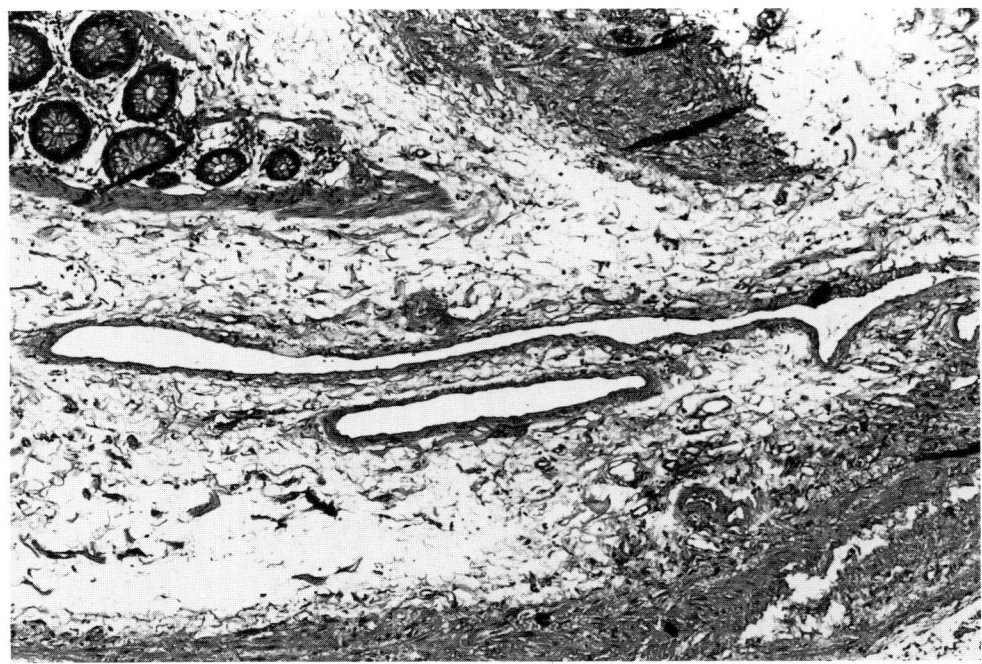

FIGURE 12-3. Colon varix. The vein in the submucosa collapsed during dissection. ($\times$ 20)

found on the right side of the colon. Rarely, the colonoscopist may be confronted with vascular malformations that appear to be varices but are actually capillary hemangiomas.[17] A unique anastomosis between portal veins on the right colon and the right ovarian veins has been documented.[18] Although most colonic varices occur in relation to portal hypertension, there are isolated reports of colonic varices occurring in families having no evidence of portal hypertension.[19] These may represent inherited venous dysplastic disorders.

An infrequent complication of patients with a *gastrointestinal stoma* is the development of stomal varices. These patients have associated alcoholic or other forms of cirrhosis.[20] Conservative treatment of the stomal varices appears to be most appropriate in these cases. Because the bleeding from the stomal varices is frequently mild, it may require only observation or adjustment of the stomal appliance.

Associated with Portal Hypertension of Extrahepatic Origin

There are other diseases besides cirrhosis that cause varix formation. Included in this group are certain extrahepatic etiologies of portal hypertension; specifically, thrombosis or cavernous transformation of the portal vein and schistosomiasis.[21] These conditions may lead to the development of varices via increased portal hypertension. The pattern and consequences of bleeding associated with varices secondary to extrahepatic portal hypertension are distinctly different from those in patients in whom the varices are the result of hepatic disease. Recurrent bleeding episodes are common. Although there is a high incidence of recurrent bleeding, there is a low incidence of exsanguination as a consequence of initial or recurrent bleeding varices. There is a reasonable success rate with treatment by classic shunting procedures, both in children over 5 years and adults, and a negligible increase in true encephalopathy. In addition to portal vein thrombosis, splenic vein thrombosis can also lead to generalized portal hypertension.[22] Hepatic vein thrombosis and pylephlebitis are additional causes of varices.

It must also be pointed out that in diseases other than alcoholic cirrhosis the development of portal hypertension may occur in a segmental fashion with only isolated portions of the portal venous system being involved. This is particularly documented by patients that have ileal varices after surgery for ulcerative colitis.[23] Additional examples of segmental varices are those in other unusual locations such as the small intestine. These all occurred in sites of postoperative intestinal adhesions.[24] In these cases, all of the patients had portal hypertension. The bleeding points were traced to mucosal erosions over large submucosal varices within the bowel. Rare cases in which tumors have invaded specific areas of the colonic vasculature have also resulted in varix formation.[25]

Hemorrhoids

The development of hemorrhoids may signal the presence of portal hypertension with both cirrhotic and noncirrhotic causes. A complete evaluation of the case is therefore necessary before hemorrhoid surgery is undertaken.

Vascular Abnormalities of the Gastrointestinal Tract

Classification

Vascular anomalies affecting the gastrointestinal tract are extraordinarily rare.[26] The older literature cites an incidence of 1 in 14,000 individuals. A great deal of confusion has been generated over this subject because there is no consistent and uniform classification for these lesions. Developments in radiology over the last two decades have further confused the picture by the introduction of radiologic terms to lesions that may represent one or more pathologic entities. Camilleri et al. have recently proposed a new classification of vascular anomalies of the intestine.[26]

For the sake of clinical utility, an even simpler classification could be used clinically. Such a classification is proposed (Table 12–1). The latter classification is very similar to that proposed by Moore et al. in 1976.[27]

The vast majority of vascular malformations of the gastrointestinal tract fall into two main groups—angiodysplasias and telangectasias. Hemangiomas are briefly discussed later in this chapter and also in Chapter 15.

Arteriovenous Malformation

Angiodysplasia

Vascular ectasias occur most frequently on the right side of the colon. They are also referred to, regrettably, as angiomas.[28] They are all arteriovenous malforma-

Table 12–1 PROPOSED CLASSIFICATION OF VASCULAR ABNORMALITIES OF THE GASTROINTESTINAL TRACT

Malformations
  Arteriovenous malformations
  Telangectasia
    Acquired
      Calcinosis-Raynaud's-sclerodactyly-telangiectasia (CRST) syndrome
    Hereditary
      Hereditary hemorrhagic telangiectasia (Osler-Weber-Rendu)
      Turner's syndrome

Disorders of connective tissue affecting blood vessels
  Pseudoxanthoma elasticum
  Ehlers-Danlos syndrome

Hemangioma
  Capillary hemangioma
  Cavernous hemangioma—single or diffuse
  Mixed capillary-cavernous hemangioma
  Diffuse intestinal hemangiomatosis
  Universal (miliary) hemangiomatosis
  Blue rubber bleb nevus syndrome
  Peutz-Jeghers syndrome
  Klippel-Trenaunay-Weber syndrome

Angiosarcoma and Kaposi's sarcoma

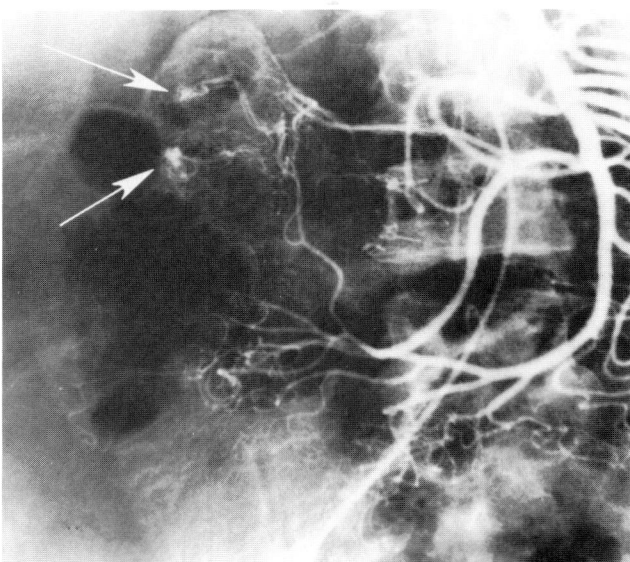

FIGURE 12–4. Angiogram of angiodysplasia of the colon. Two tuft-like collections of contrast media (arrows) are present. In addition, there were prominent early draining veins in the hepatic flexure. (From Johnsrude IS, Jackson DC: A Practical Approach to Angiography, 2nd ed. Boston, Little, Brown, 1987.)

tions (Figure 12–4). These lesions are usually irregularly shaped clusters of ectatic *small arteries, small veins,* and their capillary connections. Angiodysplasias are usually located in the mucosa and submucosa of the intestine. They are multiple, rather than single, and usually less than 5 mm in diameter (Figure 12–5). Microscopically, angiodysplastic lesions are dilated, distorted, thin-walled vessels (small arteries, capillaries, and veins) (Figure 12–6). The amount of smooth muscle in the vessel wall can be quite variable. The vessel wall can become so thinned that it appears to be composed only of endothelium. Elastic tissue stains may demonstrate the loss of elastic tissue in small arteries as they become incorporated into the ectatic mass (Figure 12–7). Angiodysplastic lesions are found most frequently on the right side of the colon, i.e., the cecum and ascending colon in elderly patients. Lesions occur with less frequency in the jejunum and stomach and may be the cause of bleeding at these sites in younger patients, including adolescents.[29] They are not associated with angiomatous lesions of the skin or other viscera. In the past, hemorrhage in association with diverticulosis was thought to be the major cause of gastrointestinal hemorrhage in the older age group.[5] With the advent of selective gastrointestinal angiography, colonic angiodysplasia has gained a predominant role as the cause of lower gastrointestinal bleeding in the elderly.[28] Angiodysplasias are probably the most frequent cause of recurrent lower gastrointestinal tract bleeding after age 60. Angiodysplastic lesions may present either as acute colonic hemorrhage or more often as chronic blood loss leading to iron deficiency anemia. Gastric lesions tend not to cause persistent hemorrhage after an initial bleeding episode. Colonic angiodysplasia may be associated with aortic valve stenosis, but no other somatic features have been recognized. Renal insufficiency appears more prevalent in patients with gastric angiodysplasia.[29]

The etiology of angiodysplasia is unknown, but the lesions are considered degenerative lesions.[30] One common speculation is that chronic intermittent increases in intraluminal pressure cause obstruction to the submucosal veins as they pierce the muscular layer of the bowel, which results in increased pressure within the vessels and consequent dilatation.[28] Angiography is the mainstay of diagnosis, although colonoscopic diagnosis[31,32] with coagulation of the lesion is feasible. There continues to be controversy about the frequency of angiodysplastic lesions in the colon. Some studies indicate that these lesions are very common. Some reports document that as many as 25% of patients over 60 have these lesions and are without any evidence of bleeding.[28,30] Other studies deny finding these lesions in control patients.[3]

Submucosal Arteriovenous Malformation

Arteriovenous malformations also occur in the submucosa (Figures 12–8 to 12–11). These lesions rarely involve the muscular layer. They may be a cause of significant gastrointestinal bleeding.[6]

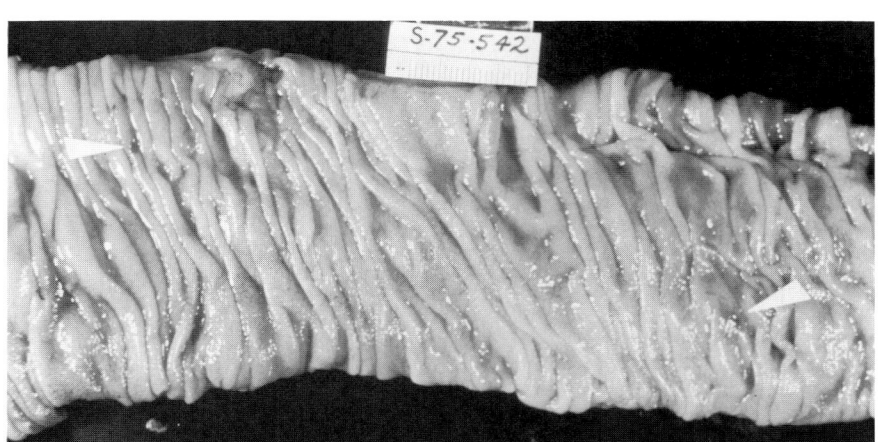

FIGURE 12–5. Segment of colon with two angiodysplastic lesions. The surface representation may be merely localized areas of discoloration (arrows).

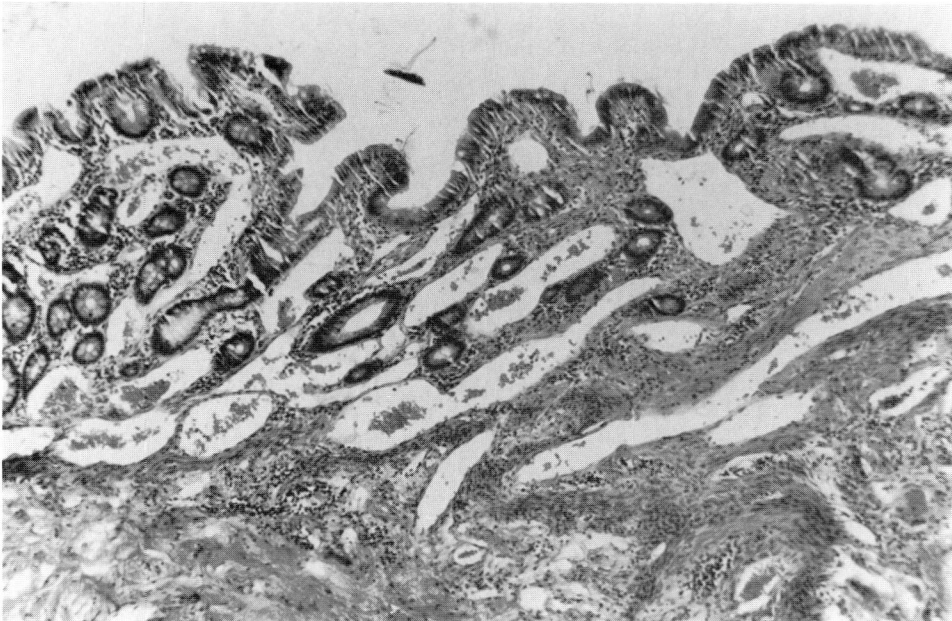

FIGURE 12–6. Histologic section of angiodysplasia of the colon. The abnormal vessels involve both the mucosa and the submucosa. (× 100)

Telangiectasia

Telangiectasia is a localized dilatation of *arterioles, capillaries,* and *venules*. Multiple lesions may occur in the gastrointestinal tract in the Osler-Weber-Rendu syndrome and Turner's syndrome. Acquired lesions occur in the calcinosis-Raynaud's-sclerodactyly-telangiectasia (CRST) syndrome.

Congenital: Osler-Weber-Rendu Disease and Turner's Syndrome

Hereditary hemorrhagic telangiectasia (Osler-Weber-Rendu disease) is inherited as an autosomal dominant disorder. These telangiectasias occur in many locations, including the skin, mucous membranes, and internal organs, resulting in recurrent hemorrhage (Figure 12–12). Telangiectasias arise from simple dilatation of normal vascular structures because of congenital thinning of the muscular coat and/or elastic fibers in the arteriolar walls. The vascular lesions may be stellate or nodular. They are punctate, red to purple in color, and noncompressible and vary in size from 1 to 4 mm. The mucocutaneous lesions usually become clinically apparent in the second and third decades. The earliest symptom is epistaxis, which can occur in childhood. Gastrointestinal bleeding occurs in

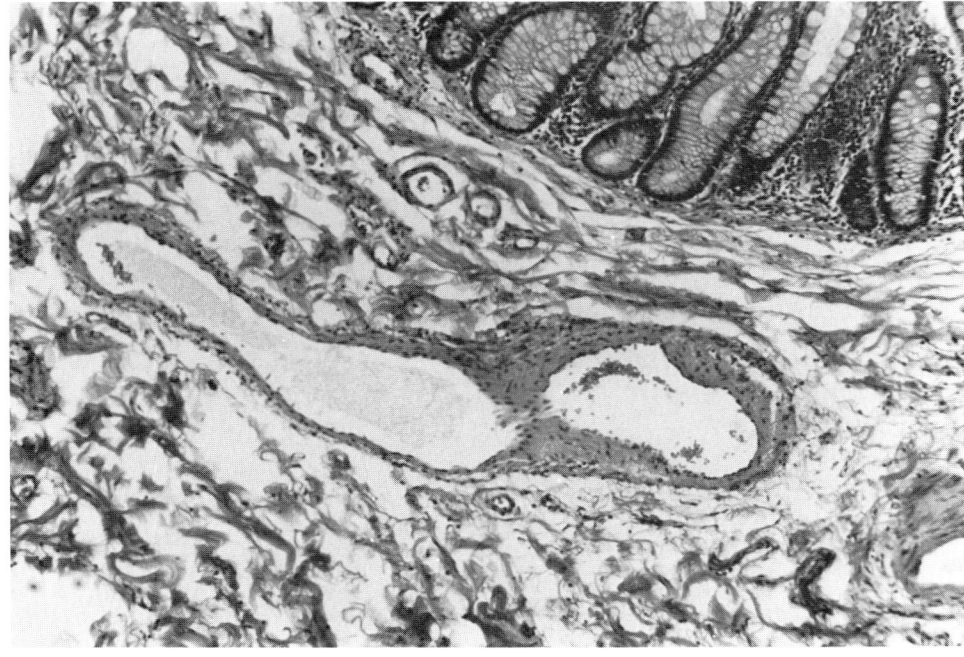

FIGURE 12–7. Arteriovenous malformation in the submucosa of colon of a patient with angiodysplasia. Elastic tissue stains can confirm the transition from artery to vein in many of these cases. (× 150)

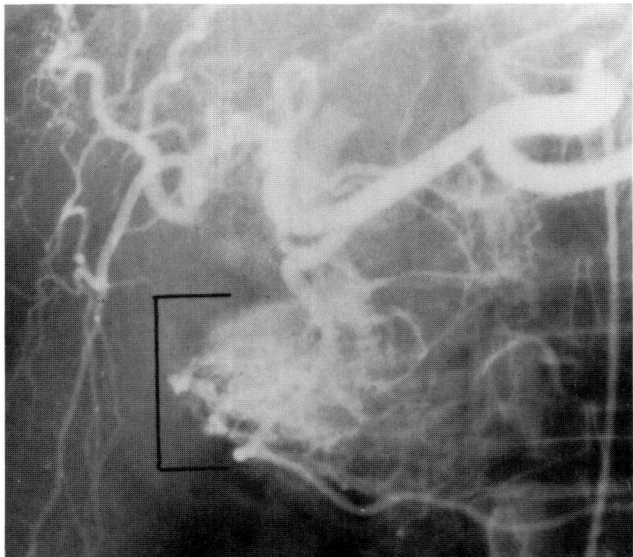

FIGURE 12–8. Angiogram of a large arteriovenous malformation of the duodenum. (From Johnsrude IS, Jackson DC: A Practical Approach to Angiography, 2nd ed. Boston, Little, Brown, 1987.)

about 15% of patients. It is usually chronic and becomes manifest later in life, usually in the fourth decade. It should be noted that vascular anomalies also occur in other organs—the meninges, spinal cord, eye, liver, and genitourinary tract. Arteriovenous malformations also occur in this disease. Fibrosis and atypical cirrhosis of the liver have been reported in these pa-

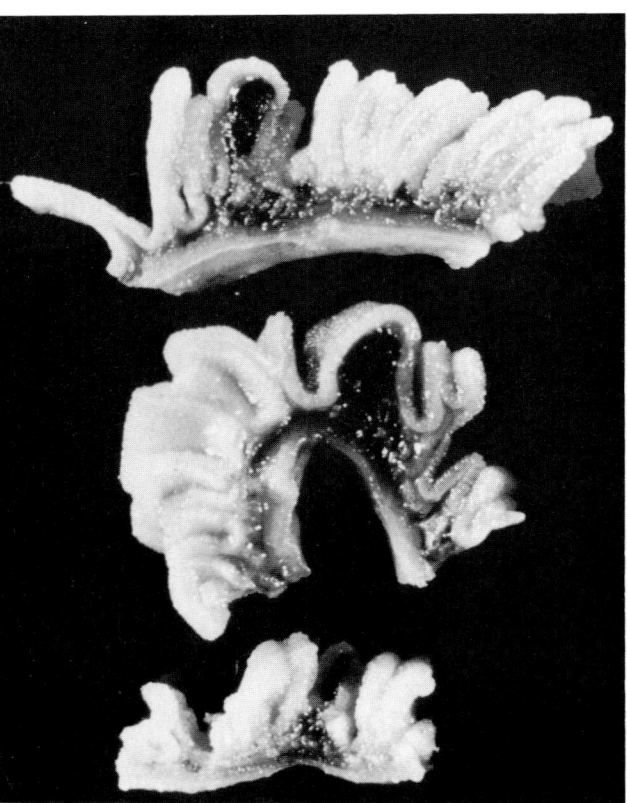

FIGURE 12–10. Gross photograph of an arteriovenous malformation of the small bowel. This vascular lesion was predominantly in the submucosa.

tients.[33] Hemorrhagic defects are also associated with the Osler-Weber-Rendu syndrome.[34]

Turner's syndrome (ovarian dysgenesis) is associated with gastrointestinal hemorrhage from telangiectasia that may be found throughout the small and large bowel and mesentery but occurs most frequently in the small intestine. These vascular lesions tend to regress spontaneously; therefore, a conservative approach is generally warranted.[26]

Acquired: CRST Syndrome

Telangiectasias are also present in systemic sclerosis, especially the calcinosis-Raynaud's-sclerodactyly-telangiectasia (CRST) variant. Lesions are most frequently found on the hands, lips, face, and tongue. Gastrointestinal hemorrhage may result from telangiectasias located in the stomach, rectum, and colon.[26] Frequently, endoscopy with electrocoagulation, heater probe, or Nd:YAG laser can adequately treat these lesions.

Disorders of Connective Tissue Affecting Blood Vessels

Pseudoxanthoma Elasticum

Pseudoxanthoma elasticum is associated with marked clinical variability, due to genetic heterogeneity. This disorder is thought to be due to deranged elas-

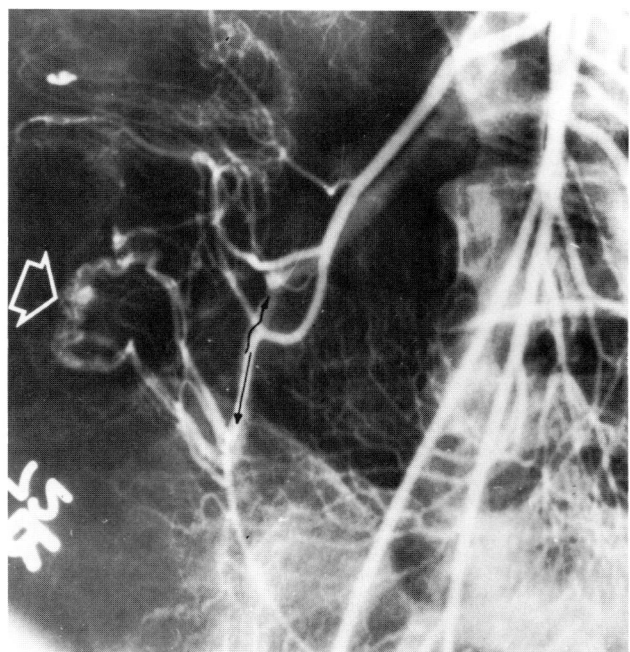

FIGURE 12–9. Angiogram of arteriovenous malformation of the cecum (open arrow). The arterial branch is quite prominent (straight arrow), and premature venous return is present (curved arrow). (From Johnsrude IS, Jackson DC: A Practical Approach to Angiography, 2nd ed. Boston, Little, Brown, 1987.)

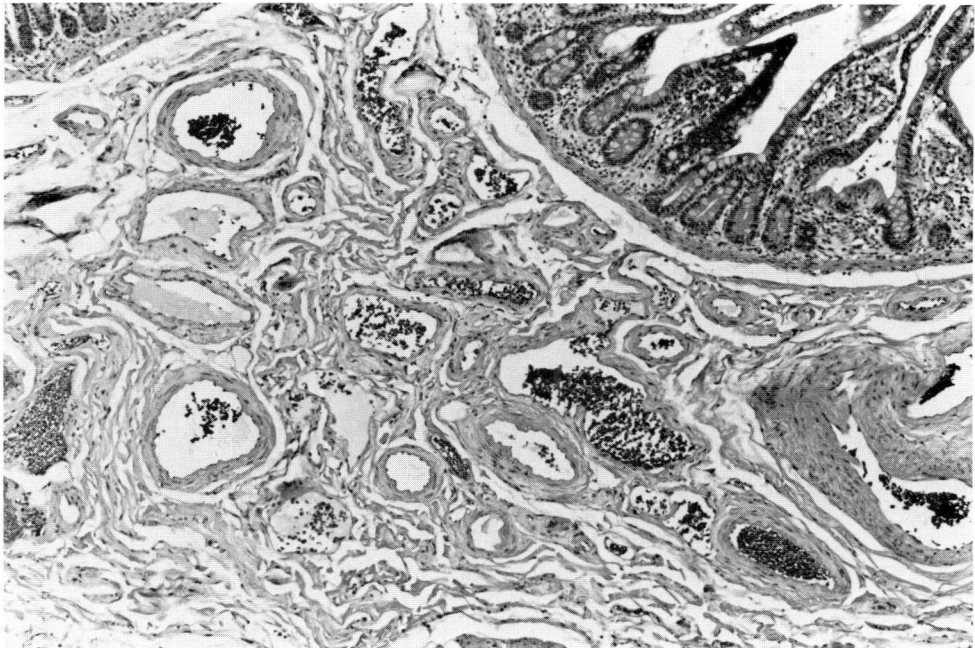

FIGURE 12–11. Photomicrograph of the arteriovenous malformation of the small bowel shown in Figure 12–10. Distinctly abnormal vascular complex composed of moderate size arteries and veins is present in the submucosa. Many of the vessels are ectatic and filled with blood. Elastic tissue stains demonstrate the transition from arteries to veins. (× 40)

tin metabolism, affecting many tissues, including the heart, kidneys, skin, mucosa, eyes, and blood vessels in the gastrointestinal tract. Hemorrhage, the most frequent finding with gut involvement, may occur in childhood. Bleeding from the stomach is frequent. It is the result of spontaneous vascular rupture. Failure of calcified vessels to contract after injury may prolong the hemorrhagic episode. The gastric and rectal mucosa has a characteristic appearance on endoscopy. Angiography demonstrates abnormal tortuous, narrowed mesenteric vessels and vascular malformations within the gastrointestinal tract.[26]

Ehlers-Danlos Syndrome

The Ehlers-Danlos syndrome is another group of disorders that is characterized by marked variation in severity because of genetic heterogeneity. They have a common defect in collagen synthesis. The gastrointestinal involvement includes spontaneous rupture of arteries in the gastrointestinal tract and dilatation of the bowel wall at all levels of the gastrointestinal tract. Hemorrhage from the gastrointestinal tract can also be the result of hiatal hernia or peptic ulceration.[26]

Uncommon Vascular Lesions

Congenital Arteriovenous Malformations

Congenital arteriovenous malformations occur anywhere in the body and have been reported in the colon.[28] Gastric malformation (Dieulafoy's disease) is another rare condition, in which massive gastric hemorrhage can occur.[35] This condition typically affects middle-aged and elderly men, although younger men and women can be affected. See Chapter 20 for further details.

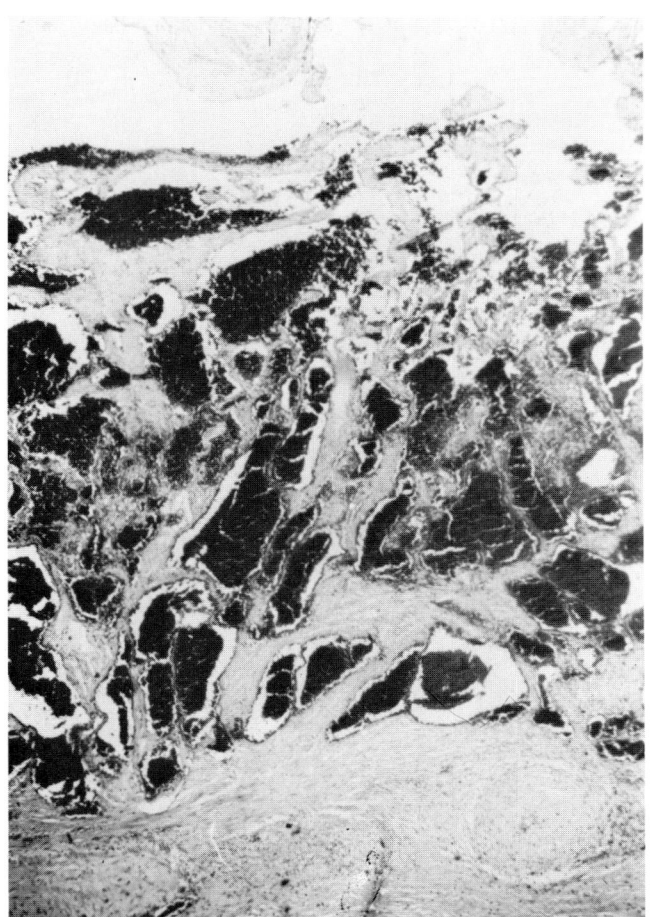

FIGURE 12–12. Telangiectasia in a patient with Osler-Weber-Rendu disease. The vessels are lined by endothelium. The vessels are quite dilated. Hyalinized material is present between the vascular spaces. (× 40)

Aneurysms

Aneurysms can occur in the human gastrointestinal tract. They are rare and usually involve the small bowel (Figure 12-13).

Gastric Antral Vascular Ectasia

Gastric antral vascular ectasia presents a unique picture to the endoscopist or pathologist at gross examination because of nearly parallel red stripes traversing the top of the mucosal folds of the gastric antrum. Because of their unique pattern, the lesion was referred to as "watermelon stomach" by Jabbari et al.[36] The red stripes are caused by ectatic and congested capillaries and small vessels in the lamina propria of the antral mucosa. See Chapter 20 for further details.

TUMORS AND TUMORLIKE PROLIFERATIONS OF VESSELS

Hemangiomas

Classification, Pathology, and Location

There continues to be controversy over whether hemangiomas found in the gastrointestinal tract are true neoplasms or whether they represent hamartomas. This issue is not addressed in this discussion. Hemangiomas are usually classified into three types—cavernous, capillary, or mixed. Most hemangiomas are small, varying in size from a few millimeters to 1 to 2 cm. Larger lesions do occur. Bleeding from these lesions is usually slow, producing anemia or melena from occult blood loss. Rarely, large hemangiomas cause massive hemorrhage. Grossly, the large hemangiomas are usually polypoid or moundlike reddish purple lesions seen through the mucosa. Histologically, numerous dilated irregular blood-filled spaces within the mucosa and submucosa are encountered. Occasionally these lesions will extend through the muscular layer into the serosal surface. As would be expected, the channels are lined by flat endothelial cells.

Intestinal hemangiomas are rare and not hereditary. They account for about 10% of all benign small-intestinal tumors. The majority of hemangiomas are solitary localized lesions. Approximately 40% are multiple. Most hemangiomas of the small bowel occur in the jejunum and ileum.[26] Capillary hemangiomas are usually single lesions. Cavernous hemangiomas can often give the appearance of varices, especially in the colon.[17] Cavernous hemangiomas occasionally occur in the anus.[37] Histologic confirmation of hemangiomas is often difficult in tissue obtained by mucosal biopsy because of the amount of hemorrhage that may occur with this procedure. Therefore, the appearance during endoscopy takes on an even greater importance.[38] Hemangiomas of the stomach[39] and of the esophagus[40-42] have also been reported, but they are infrequent.

A unique form of colonic hemangioma is the cavernous hemangioma of the rectum. These are usually not associated with other gastrointestinal hemangiomas, but they may extensively involve the entire rectum or a portion of the rectosigmoid.[28]

Syndromes Involving Gastrointestinal Hemangiomas

Diffuse Intestinal Hemangiomatosis

Diffuse intestinal hemangiomatosis is an entity in which as many as 100 lesions involving the stomach,

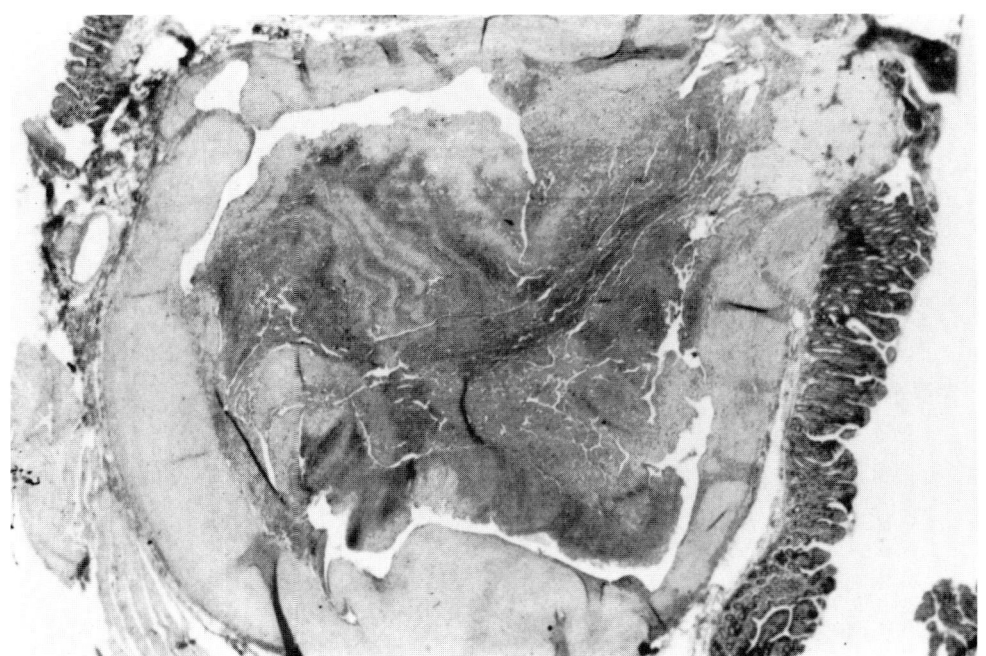

FIGURE 12-13. Aneurysm of the small bowel. Aneurysm formation of the gastrointestinal tract is extraordinarily rare but appears to have a predilection for the small bowel. ($\times$ 10)

small bowel, and colon are encountered. Bleeding or anemia in childhood usually leads to this diagnosis. Hemangiomas of the skin and soft tissue of the head and neck are often present. The gastrointestinal hemangiomas may be large enough to cause intussusception.[28] In diffuse neonatal hemangiomatosis, early angiography is probably the most reliable means of detecting the lesion.[43]

Universal (Miliary) Hemangiomatosis

Universal (miliary) hemangiomatosis is an extraordinarily rare syndrome usually fatal in infancy with hundreds of hemangiomas involving all organs.[28]

Blue Rubber Bleb Nevus Syndrome

The blue rubber bleb nevus syndrome (cutaneous and intestinal cavernous hemangioma) was recognized in the last century because of the association of cutaneous vascular nevi, intestinal lesions, and gastrointestinal bleeding. The lesions in this syndrome are unique. The hemangiomas vary in size from 0.1 to 5.0 cm, are blue and raised, and have a wrinkled surface. Direct pressure on the lesion causes emptying of the blood, leaving a wrinkled sac. These lesions are most frequent in the small bowel but may be present in any part of the gastrointestinal tract. In the colon, they are most common on the left side and in the rectum. Microscopically, they are cavernous hemangiomas.[26,28]

Peutz-Jeghers Syndrome

In the Peutz-Jeghers syndrome, intestinal hemangiomas without the presence of intestinal polyps have been reported. These cases are thought to represent incomplete penetrance of the gene responsible for the syndrome.[26]

Klippel-Trenaunay-Weber Syndrome

A sporadic disorder of children and young adults, the Klippel-Trenaunay-Weber syndrome is characterized by soft tissue and bony hypertrophy, varicose veins, and port wine hemangiomas, which may be unilateral. It is not an inherited disorder. There is accompanying atresia, hypoplasia, or obstruction of the deep venous system. Involvement of the gastrointestinal tract is by vascular malformations of the mixed or cavernous hemangioma type.[26,44]

Malignant Vascular Tumors

Kaposi's sarcoma and angiosarcoma are the two malignant lesions usually associated with the vasculature. The occurrence of these malignancies within the gastrointestinal tract is very rare, although an increased incidence of Kaposi's sarcoma has been reported in patients with acquired immunodeficiency syndrome.[45] For additional information, see Chapter 14.

Kaposi's Sarcoma

The gastrointestinal tract is the most common area of visceral involvement by Kaposi's sarcoma. The small bowel is affected more frequently than the colon, rectum, or stomach.[45,46] Such manifestations can occasionally precede the cutaneous manifestations of this disease.[46] On colonoscopy, the lesions have been described as macular, angiodysplastic with a uniform appearance, polypoid, volcano-like, and maculopapular.[47] Histologically, Kaposi's sarcoma is composed of neoplastic spindle cells in which erythrocytes are incorporated with "vascular" clefts between the cells. The process extends into the mucosa; therefore, confirmation of the disease by mucosal biopsy is feasible.

Primary Angiosarcoma

Primary angiosarcomas of the gastrointestinal tract are very rare. Angiosarcoma following irradiation in the gastrointestinal tract has been reported. The terminal ileum is the area most frequently involved by this disease.[48,49]

Lymphangiomas

Lymphangiomas of the gastrointestinal tract are also extremely rare. They usually present as polypoid lesions which are submucosal in location with cystically dilated lymph vessels seen on microscopic examination.[50] By colonoscopy, they appear as smooth, soft polypoid lesions on a broad base.[51] Lymphangiomas have also been reported in the esophagus,[52] stomach, and jejunum.[53] They seem to appear more frequently in the small intestine than in the large intestine, although occasionally are encountered in the colon as a result of barium enema examination.

VASCULITIS

General Considerations

No subject is more confusing and challenging than vasculitis and its classification. Some classifications are based upon the size of the predominant vessel involved; whereas other classifications are based on the most serious clinical expression, that is, the predominant site or location when a variety of vessels are involved. The mechanism and etiology of vasculitis are poorly understood. The majority of vasculitides are associated with immunopathogenic mechanisms, i.e., the interaction of antigens and antibodies forming immune complexes, which in association with complement can cause injury to the vascular wall.[54,55] Hypersensitivity states, including those produced in reaction to drugs and certain environmental exposures, also induce vasculitis. In patients with systemic vasculitis, the gastrointestinal tract is infrequently involved.[56] The four major organs predominantly involved in systemic vasculitis are skin, muscle, peripheral nervous tissue, and kidneys.

The fundamental pathologic consequence of vasculitis is ischemia in the area supplied by the involved vasculature. If the vessels of the mucosa and submucosa are affected, then there is mucosal ischemia with erosions, ulceration, transmural infarction, and ultimately perforation.

Pneumatosis intestinalis has been associated with almost all diseases caused by vasculitis that affect the gastrointestinal tract. With the loss of mucosal integrity, enteric organisms gain access to the bowel wall.[57] The etiology of the vasculitic process is based on clinical as well as histologic data. The histologic response, however, can be a guide in establishing the diagnosis.

Histologic Features and Differential Diagnosis

Diseases that involve the gastrointestinal tract and have as a common denominator involvement of the vessels by a vasculitic process are listed in Table 12–2.

Polyarteritis nodosa is characterized by acute inflammation and fibrinoid necrosis of the medium-sized and small arteries. In polyarteritis nodosa, lesions are found in all stages of development.

In the Churg-Strauss syndrome, there is necrotizing vasculitis of small arteries and veins with extravascular granulomas and infiltration of the vessels and perivascular tissue with eosinophils.

The distinction, microscopically, between classic polyarteritis nodosa and the Churg-Strauss syndrome depends on the size of the vessel involved. In polyarteritis nodosa, the vessels involved are usually medium-sized and small arteries, whereas in the Churg-Strauss syndrome, the vessels involved are small arteries and veins. In polyarteritis nodosa, the cellular infiltrate is predominantly neutrophilic leukocytes; eosinophils predominate in the Churg-Strauss syndrome.

Henoch-Schönlein purpura is an example of hypersensitivity vasculitis involving predominantly the small arterioles and capillaries in children. Deposition of immunoglobulins, predominantly IgA, complement components, and fibrin have been noted in involved vessels in the gastrointestinal tract.

Severe necrotizing vasculitis affecting the small and medium-sized arteries of the submucosa are frequently encountered in systemic lupus erythematosus. Fibrinoid necrosis occurs; and the inflammatory infiltrate, while perivascular in location, is composed of both neutrophils and eosinophils.

Vasculitis is a common manifestation in rheumatoid disease. Small arteries and arterioles are involved in Wegener's granulomatosis. Histologically, the coagulative or liquefactive necrotizing epithelioid granulomas in Wegener's granulomatosis differ morphologically from the more fibrinoid necrotizing (allergic) epithelioid and eosinophilic granulomas seen in the Churg-Strauss syndrome. The diagnosis is made by finding characteristic histologic lesions in the small arteries and veins. The involved vessel, often located adjacent to the granuloma, undergoes fibrinoid necrosis with mononuclear cell infiltration.

Utility of Mucosal Biopsy and Other Studies in Establishing the Diagnosis of Vasculitis

It is often difficult to make the diagnosis of vasculitis by mucosal biopsy[58] (Figure 12–14). However, it is possible to document necrotizing arteritis when the biopsy is deep enough to include portions of the submucosa (Figure 12–15). Necrotizing vasculitis affects the bowel in polyarteritis, lupus erythematosus, rheumatoid arthritis, and Henoch-Schönlein purpura. There is usually involvement of the small arteries or veins in the wall with patchy necrosis and inflammation of the overlying mucosa. The smaller biopsies may be too superficial to demonstrate the vasculitis. Patients with hemolytic uremic syndrome may have focal areas of marked mucosal edema and hemorrhage that can even be evident on gross endoscopic examination. In hypersensitivity angiitis, bowel biopsies, both of large and small intestines, demonstrate extravascular tubercular granulomas without necrosis.

The use of ^{111}In-granulocyte scanning may give significant additional information when studying the involvement of the gastrointestinal tract by collagen vascular disease.[59] This procedure, although not commonly used, helps establish the diagnosis of gastrointestinal vasculitis.

Vasculitic Lesions in the Gastrointestinal Tract

Polyarteritis Nodosa

Polyarteritis nodosa causes a variety of changes in the gastrointestinal tract. Involvement of the mesenteric artery can lead to aneurysm formation and occasionally rupture with exsanguination.[60] In polyarteritis nodosa, approximately two thirds of the patients have symptomatology referable to the gastrointestinal tract.[61] The manifestations of gastrointestinal involvement all relate to the ischemia caused by occlusion of the affected vessels.

Mesenteric infarction with gut ischemia and perforation has been reported frequently in polyarteritis no-

Table 12–2 DISEASES WITH VASCULITIC PROCESSES THAT AFFECT THE GASTROINTESTINAL TRACT

Polyarteritis nodosa
Churg-Strauss syndrome
Henoch-Schönlein purpura
Systemic lupus erythematosus
Rheumatoid disease
Wegener's granulomatosis
Hemolytic-uremic syndrome

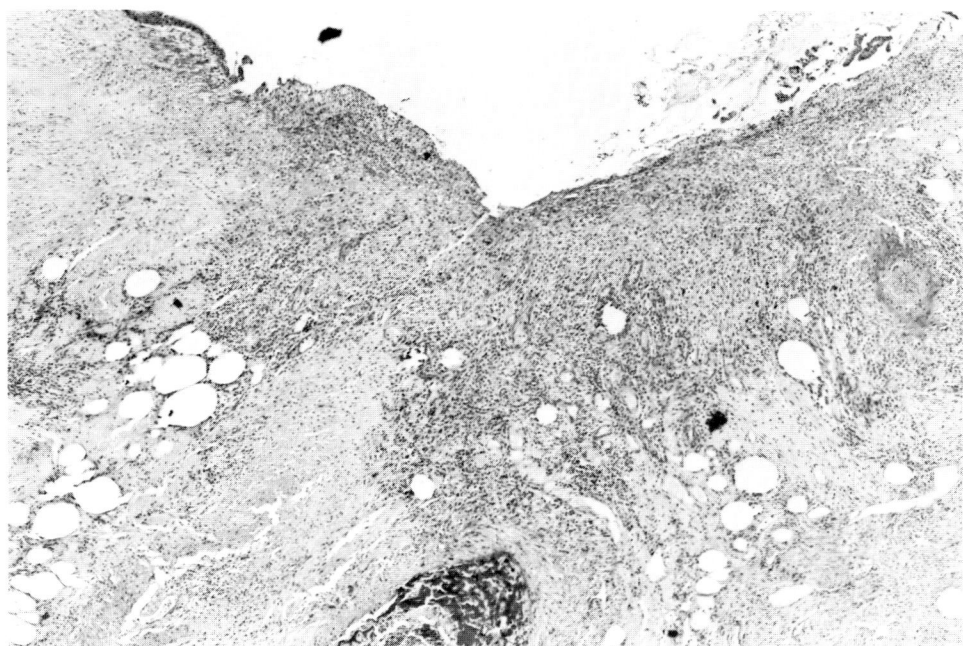

FIGURE 12–14. Base of colonic ulcer in a patient with periarteritis nodosa. The vessels with definitive vasculitis are present in the deeper portions of the ulcer. (× 20)

dosa.[62] Patients with polyarteritis nodosa have also demonstrated necrotizing vasculitis of the gallbladder and appendix.[63]

Gastrointestinal ulceration, intraluminal hemorrhage, perforation, and pyloric obstruction are well recognized, with localized or diffuse gangrene.[61] Ischemic colitis is fairly frequently reported in polyarteritis nodosa.[64,65] The degree of involvement can be very diffuse to quite isolated and specific.[66]

Systemic Lupus Erythematosus

The gastrointestinal manifestations of systemic lupus erythematosus can be quite varied; however, mesenteric arteritis and serositis occur frequently.[67] Serositis occurs in 60% to 70% of cases of systemic lupus erythematosus. Serositis takes a variety of forms, including peritoneal inflammation, adhesions between bowel loops, perihepatitis, and perisplenitis. Small-vessel ar-

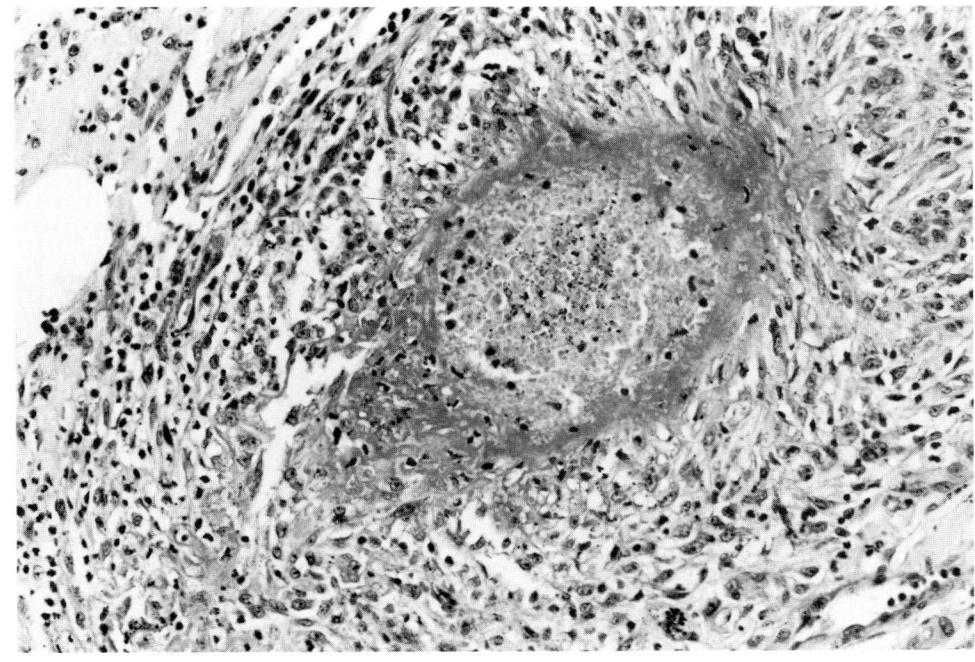

FIGURE 12–15. High-power illustration of the colon shown in Figure 12–14. There is severe vasculitis and the development of fibrinoid necrosis in the wall as well as infiltration by a variety of inflammatory cells. (× 100)

teritis leads to involvement of the small bowel by lupus enteritis. Because of the difficulty in making this diagnosis, some cases have been mistakenly diagnosed as Crohn's disease.[68] In addition to lupus enteritis, lupus gastritis, ischemic colitis, and esophagitis have been reported.[69] To further complicate the picture, in lupus, arteritis of the mesenteric arteries has also been reported. Intestinal venulitis is thought to be a possible explanation for the protein-losing enteropathy seen in some of these patients.[70] Considerable overlap occurs in the complications of systemic lupus erythematosus and polyarteritis as they affect the gastrointestinal tract.[71]

Rheumatoid Arthritis

The vasculitis associated with rheumatoid arthritis can lead to involvement of the colon,[72] with gastrointestinal bleeding, interperitoneal bleeding, ischemic mucosal ulceration, small- and large-bowel infarction, and bowel perforation.[73,74] Occasionally, in rheumatoid arthritis instead of vasculitis, there is a proliferative endarteritis characterized by intimal proliferation without vessel wall necrosis or inflammation.[74]

Hypersensitivity Angiitis

Churg-Strauss Syndrome

The classic features of this syndrome are systemic vasculitis in the setting of bronchial asthma and eosinophilia. Although the lungs, peripheral nerves, and skin are frequently involved, involvement of the gastrointestinal tract does occasionally occur.[75] The gastrointestinal complications have varied from gastric ulceration to pseudopolyp formation in the colon.

Although some authors consider the Churg-Strauss syndrome a distinct entity, others consider it a subdivision of polyarteritis nodosa. Necrotizing extravascular granulomas are usually not seen in polyarteritis nodosa. A history of asthma is the rule in the Churg-Strauss syndrome, but it is only infrequently encountered in polyarteritis nodosa. Differentiating the Churg-Strauss syndrome from Wegener's granulomatosis may also be difficult. In this case, clinical history also plays a large role, because allergy is typical in the Churg-Strauss syndrome and infrequently in Wegener's granulomatosis.

Allergic Granulomatous Angiitis

Involvement of the bowel by allergic granulomatous angiitis has been reported.[76] Part of this spectrum is the finding of eosinophilic infiltration in the gastrointestinal tract.[77] This process can be either diffuse or localized and perhaps, therefore, a part of the disease spectrum of the Churg-Strauss syndrome. In the infiltrative form, the affected segment of bowel shows an ill-defined transmural thickening simulating intestinal lymphoma or Crohn's disease. The lesions may be multiple. This has been referred to as diffuse eosinophilic infiltration, eosinophilic gastroenteritis, and eosinophilic granuloma. In the circumscribed form, a well-delineated and polypoid mass can be encountered, commonly confined to the submucosa. This form is not associated with blood eosinophilia or an allergic history and is currently referred to as inflammatory fibroid polyp or eosinophilic granuloma. Controversy exists over whether these two different presentations are reflecting two different separate and unrelated conditions or whether they are part of the same spectrum. The infiltrative form can be found in either the small or the large bowel. Microscopically, the hallmark of both presentations is an eosinophilic infiltrate admixed with a variety of chronic inflammatory cells, including plasma cells, lymphocytes, and histiocytes, within a loose network of vascularized fibroblastic connective tissue. Granulomatous nodules are occasionally encountered. Omental nodules show the same histologic picture. See also Chapter 10 for further details.

Henoch-Schönlein Purpura

Henoch-Schönlein purpura is characterized by a nontraumatic, nonthrombocytopenic hemorrhagic diathesis resulting in bleeding at the joints, skin, and viscera singly or in combination. Purpuric lesions can occur in the gastrointestinal tract, and occasionally intussusception of the ileum or ileocecal region has occurred in Henoch-Schönlein purpura.[78] Superficial ulceration can occur with the development of a pseudomembrane. While Henoch-Schönlein purpura may involve any portion of the gastrointestinal tract, the jejunum and ileum are the most frequently affected. Complications include massive bleeding,[79] intussusception, infarction with perforation,[80] and chronic small-bowel obstruction. The primary lesion is found in the small arteries, arterioles, and capillaries. The colon is also involved in this disease.[81]

On endoscopy, if the stomach is involved, coalescing erythematous lesions are encountered with large areas of purpura.[82] Further studies have documented the presence of IgA and C3 by immunofluorescence examination in the small-bowel (duodenum and proximal jejunum) blood vessels in Henoch-Schönlein purpura.[83]

Wegener's Granulomatosis

Wegener's granulomatosis is a disease of unknown etiology characterized by necrotizing granulomatous lesions of the upper or lower respiratory tract, vasculitis, and glomerulonephritis. Involvement of the gastrointestinal tract has been extremely rare in this disease, although involvement in virtually all areas of the gastrointestinal tract now is being reported. Clinically, with gastrointestinal involvement, patients complain of a blood-stained mucous diarrhea. The disease in the gastrointestinal tract responds to appropriate therapy.[84] Wegener reported an ulcerating necrotizing process in the ileum, colon, and rectum with marked edema and leukocyte infiltration in the submucosa. Multiple gastric ulcers have also been reported in Wegener's.[86] The process can progress to small-bowel perforation[86] when intense necrotizing vasculitis is present.[87] Occasionally, the process can be confused with ulcerative colitis.[88,89]

Hemolytic-Uremic Syndrome

The hemolytic-uremic syndrome consists of microangiopathic hemolytic anemia, acute renal failure, and thrombocytopenia following a prodromal illness of gastroenteritis or upper respiratory infection. Signs and symptoms referable to the gastrointestinal tract frequently herald the beginning of this syndrome. They include abdominal pain, abdominal tenderness, or peritoneal signs. The symptoms can be so severe that patients undergo laparotomy. When the colon is resected, hemorrhagic infarction is usually encountered with full-thickness hemorrhage and necrosis of the colon wall. Extensive fibrin thrombi and fibrinoid necrosis can be seen in the capillaries of the peritoneum and submucosa of the colon.[91] In some cases, only the mucosa and submucosa are involved. Clinical presentations include bloody diarrhea or a pseudomembranous colitis-like picture.[92] Currently, it is believed that the degree of gastrointestinal involvement in this syndrome is underestimated. Basically, two histologic forms occur in the colon—ischemic or pseudomembranous colitis. Some researchers feel that ischemic colitis may precede the full development of the hemolytic-uremic syndrome.[93] Late manifestations of the hemolytic-uremic syndrome include persistent colitis as well as bowel stenosis.[94]

Hemolytic-uremic syndrome needs to be differentiated from appendicitis, ulcerative colitis, cecal polyp, pseudomembranous colitis, and intussusception.[95–97] This disease entity may be due to a localized Shwartzman type of reaction with deposition of fibrin strands on the capillary endothelium.[95]

Ulceration of the Stomach

Virtually all diseases thought to be caused by vasculitis have caused changes in the stomach. These include erosions, stress ulcers, and peptic ulcer disease.

Differentiation from Other Diseases of Unknown Etiology That May Have Vasculitis as a Component

There is significant overlap in patients with rheumatoid disease and gastrointestinal symptoms and patients with gastrointestinal diseases such as ulcerative colitis and Crohn's disease that have arthritic symptoms.[90] In rheumatoid disease, lesions in the gut are frequent and are caused by arteritis. The arteritis can affect the alimentary tract at any point. The arteritis results in erosion, ulceration, bleeding, perforation, infarction, and gangrene. Peptic ulcers are extremely frequent; next in frequency are ischemic ulcers of the intestine, which can either bleed or perforate. If the lesions are of the larger arteries, segmental or extensive bowel gangrene can occur. Malabsorption also occurs in patients with rheumatoid arthritis.

Involvement of the gut in systemic lupus erythematosus occurs frequently, but less so than in polyarteritis nodosa. The lesions are again similar because of the arteritis that occurs. Ileus may occur along with an acute abdomen from bowel ischemia, infarction, or perforation. In lupus, an appendicitis-like picture or terminal ileitis that can mimic Crohn's disease has been reported. Also, in systemic lupus erythematosus, an ulcerative colitis–like presentation can occur.

The picture is further complicated in that these patients may be partially immunosuppressed. In this clinical setting, the cytomegalovirus can cause mechanical occlusion of small vessels with ulceration of the overlying mucosa.

ISCHEMIC DISEASES

General Considerations

The focus of the chapter now changes to one of the more frequent causes of bowel disease, ischemia, and its most severe consequence, infarction. Bowel ischemia has three main causes: (1) occlusion of the arteries supplying an area, (2) occlusion of the veins supplying an area, and (3) low-flow states in which a specific mechanical factor cannot be implicated or can only minimally be implicated.

Pathophysiologic Effects of Ischemia

Significant decrease in blood flow can cause three main types of responses in the human gastrointestinal tract. If the episode is transient, focal mucosal necrosis occurs, followed by restitution of tissue architecture. There is no significant loss of tissue when this response occurs. If the episode is of greater magnitude, the patient develops ulceration of the gastrointestinal tract but recovers from the acute episode, with healing by fibrosis and resultant stricture formation, which usually develops 6 to 8 weeks after the initial episode. If the episode is severe, transmural infarction with perforation and peritonitis can occur.

The pathophysiologic effects of ischemia depend upon the severity of the episode, the length of time the effect lasts, and the amount of tissue involved. The episodes generally fall into two main categories—acute and chronic presentations. In the acute form, there is a dramatic loss of function of the segment of the gastrointestinal tract affected. Clinical signs and symptoms also mirror the acute nature of the insult. In the acute presentations, a single specific etiologic agent can usually be identified. In the chronic form, the changes in pathophysiology are much more diffuse. In the more chronic forms, a variety of factors are all at work at the same time. In the older adult, atherosclerosis of vessels is frequently one of several factors that are at work concomitantly.

Nomenclature and Classification

Because transmural infarcts of the duodenum, stomach, and esophagus are very rare, classifications usually relate only to infarcts of the rest of the small bowel and of the large intestine. Transmural infarcts of the small and large intestines are usually classified in the following manner:

1. Those due to superior mesenteric artery occlusion
2. Those due to inferior mesenteric artery occlusion, mesenteric vein thrombosis, or arteritis
3. Those due to nonocclusive causes[98]

A new classification has been proposed:

1. Acute intestinal ischemia either with arterial occlusion or nonocclusion
2. Chronic arterial obstruction
3. Focal ischemia of the small bowel or of the colon[99]

As with all ischemic processes, the metabolic needs of the organ are not being met by the blood supply with concomitant loss of function. With either classification, the literature relating to this subject is often listed under acute mesenteric ischemia.[98]

General Pathology

Histologic consequences of ischemia are quite uniform, whatever the cause. The mucosa is the most sensitive to the ischemia because of its high oxygen demands. The mucosa responds with the usual response to any deprivation of oxygen supply—increases in vascular permeability, edema formation, and concomitant coagulative necrosis with sloughing of the devitalized tissue. The earliest morphologic changes are seen just beneath the surface epithelium, where coagulation necrosis of the lamina propria occurs (Figure 12–16). The vessels of the lamina propria become congested. In the small bowel, the earliest changes are seen in the lamina propria beneath the tip of the villus.[100] The ischemic process is initially limited to the mucosa, where there is edema formation in the lamina propria and loss of integrity of the microvasculature of the lamina propria with extravasation of erythrocytes. Necrosis of the epithelium is now readily apparent. This can be followed by similar changes in the submucosa, the muscular layer, and the serosa as the process extends into the wall of the bowel. If the process is severe enough, transmural infarction will occur. In the least severe forms, bloody diarrhea may be the only presenting symptomatology. In the more severe forms, abdominal pain and the presence of occult blood may herald the presence of the condition. In the most severe form, full-fledged signs and symptoms of tissue necrosis with perforation are usually present. Recent developments in angiography have significantly altered the natural history of the disease, because earlier diagnosis is the most important factor in lowering mortality. Angiography is also playing a therapeutic role, because it is the method by which vasodilating drugs are often infused in an attempt to modify the degree of occlusion.

Etiology of Bowel Infarcts

Acute occlusion of the superior mesenteric artery causes 50% of the cases of transmural gastrointestinal infarct.[98] It is due equally to thrombosis or embolism (Figure 12–17). The degree of revascularization following either embolectomy, endarterectomy or bypass graft is hard to estimate even when sophisticated studies such as fluorescein injection and Doppler monitoring are used. Second-look operations are often planned for 12 to 24 hours after definitive surgery.

Twenty-five percent of all bowel infarcts are due to occlusion of the inferior mesenteric artery, mesenteric vein thrombosis, or arteritis. Occlusion of the inferior mesenteric artery rarely leads to colonic infarction when it has an atherosclerotic basis. Most cases have been reported after ligation for aortic aneurysm surgery.

Thrombosis or compression of the superior mesenteric vein may have a variety of causes. One of the most frequent is a portion of the bowel becoming incorporated into an irreducible hernia (Figure 12–18). Extension of a thrombus from the portal vein, especially with rapidly enlarging hepatic tumors, can also cause venous infarcts. There are, however, a large number of cases in which no specific predisposing cause is found.

Nonocclusive infarction accounts for 25% of the infarcts of the small and large bowel. The pathogenesis of infarction without occlusion is much more complicated. Although this process affects small and large bowel, it can also cause similar changes in the upper gastrointestinal tract. These pathologic lesions are often grouped under the heading of ischemic bowel disease.

Ischemic Bowel Disease

Spectrum and Clinical Features

Recent studies have continued to define the concept and clarified the spectrum of ischemic bowel disease. Ischemic bowel disease results from a sequential series of changes following anoxia. The etiology is multifactorial, involving the state of the vessels, the duration of the anoxic or hypoxic episode, and the virulence of bacteria located in the lumen of the affected gastrointestinal tract.[100]

Profound changes occur in the hemodynamics of the bowel wall. Complete occlusion is usually absent, and thromboembolic phenomena are only rarely seen. Ischemic bowel disease affects all age groups and can be found in any area of the gastrointestinal tract. The pathogenesis of this lesion is dependent upon enough blood being supplied to prevent complete death of the involved segment but insufficient blood flow to meet the metabolic needs of the injured bowel. After necrosis, there is bacterial invasion as the mucosal barrier becomes ineffective.

The basic pathologic response is coagulative necrosis. The mucosal layer, the layer of the gastrointestinal tract most susceptible to anoxia, is affected first. The

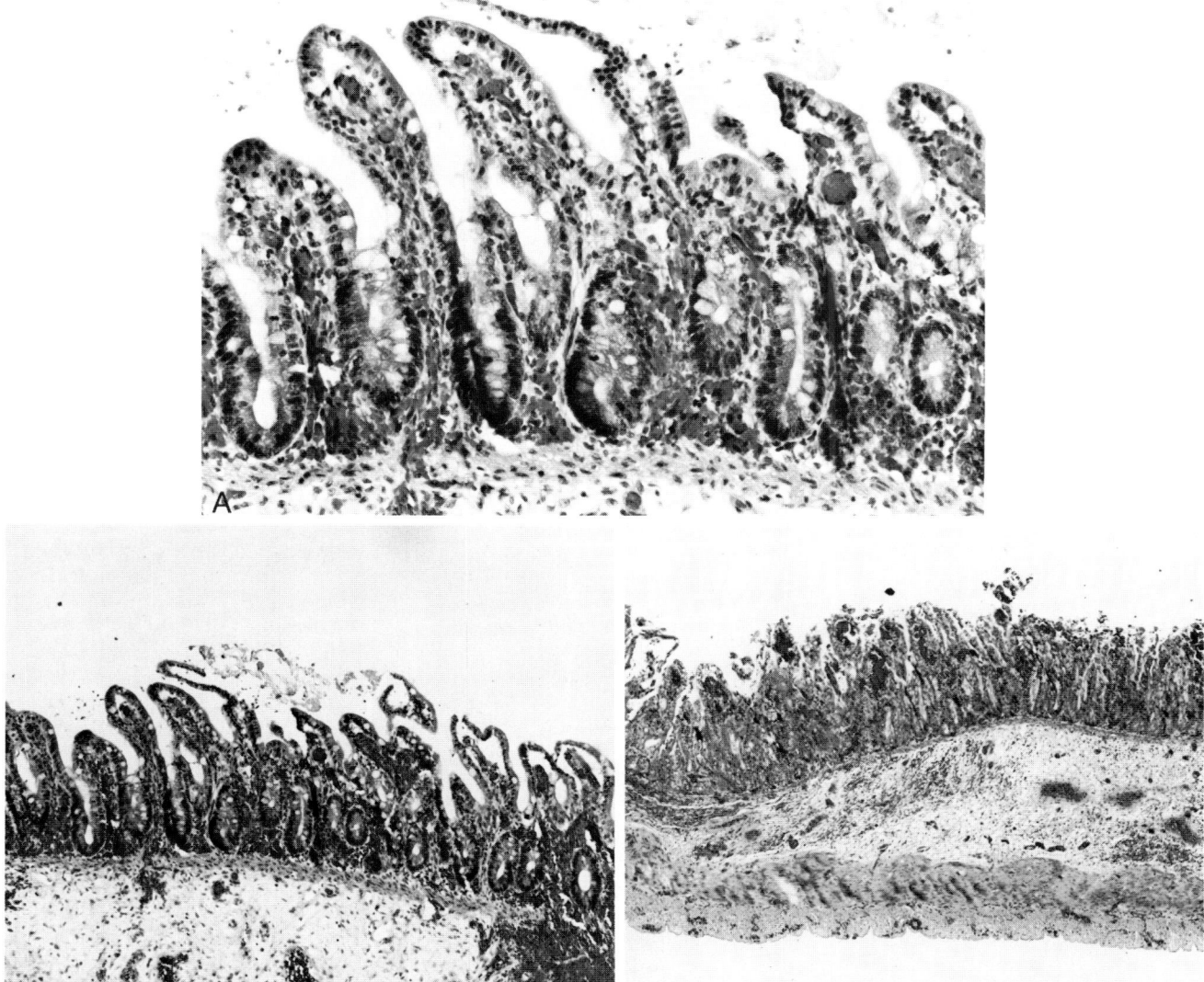

FIGURE 12-16. Stages in the progression of ischemic bowel disease. A, The earliest changes in ischemic bowel disease occur at the tip of the villus, just beneath the epithelium. The vessels become congested, the adjacent lamina propria develops edema, and there is extravasation of erythrocytes into the lamina propria. ($\times$ 100) B, With early necrosis of the mucosal layer, the submucosa becomes edematous and the vasculature becomes congested. ($\times$ 40) C, Later stage in ischemic bowel disease. The mucosa and superficial submucosa are now necrotic and beginning to slough. The remainder of the wall of the gastrointestinal tract is edematous, congested, and undergoing the earliest stages of necrosis. ($\times$ 20)

spectrum of ischemic bowel disease includes the entities listed in Table 12-3.

The clinical picture in chronic arterial obstruction is extraordinarily complex. The disease itself is very rare.[101,102] Postprandial pain, weight loss, and disturbances of bowel habits do not occur in all cases. What is well accepted, however, is that when there is significant atherosclerosis in the vessels supplying the gastrointestinal tract, there is also severe atherosclerosis affecting many other organs.

It is thought that the small bowel has a much better collateral circulation than the large bowel. Hence, focal ischemia in the large intestine is more frequently encountered. Initial studies of patients with intestinal arterial occlusion have shown that there is no relationship between intestinal performance when studied by measuring insorptive and exsorptive functions and the degree of potential chronic ischemia suggested by angiography.[103] Recent studies have shown that a decrease in the intramural pH below the usual pH of 6.86 was a good indicator of early colonic ischemia.[104] The symptoms, diagnosis, and therapy of ischemic intestinal syndromes have been extensively reviewed.[101,102]

Experimental Studies

Most of our knowledge of intestinal blood flow has been obtained from invasive techniques used in a variety of experimental models and rarely in man. What is really needed is a noninvasive clinical method of

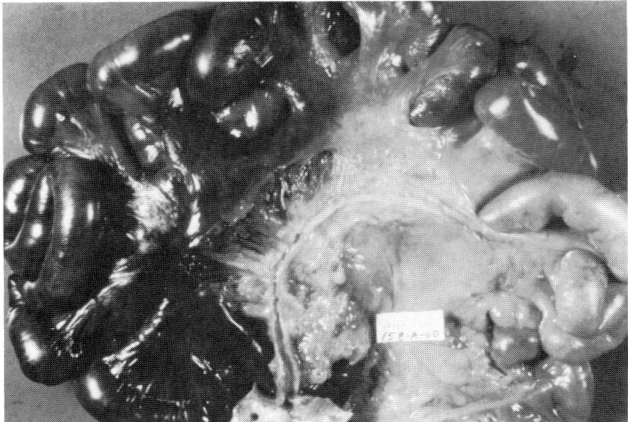

FIGURE 12–17. Infarct of the small bowel. Severe atherosclerosis is present around the orifice of the superior mesenteric artery (bottom center).

Table 12–3 ENTITIES OF ISCHEMIC BOWEL DISEASE

Ischemic colitis
Necrotizing enterocolitis of the premature infant
Hemorrhagic necrosis of the gastrointestinal tract
Pseudomembranous enterocolitis
Staphylococcal enterocolitis
Radiation enterocolitis—delayed form
Uremic colitis
Potassium-induced stenotic ulcer
Stress ulceration

measuring intestinal blood flow.[105] With invasive techniques, total blood flow to the small intestine is estimated to be 500 to 600 ml/min. Transcutaneous Doppler ultrasound allows the identification of intestinal arteries and the measurement of blood flow within them with minimal distress for the patient.[105] With this noninvasive method, similar rates of flow are obtained. Physiologic challenge indicates that blood flow can increase by more than 100% after a meal. Studies using noninvasive techniques in pathologic states are under way. Current studies of ischemia show that the spectrum of clinical situations encountered on the basis of this lesion are much more complex than previously thought.[99]

Review of the changes that occur in blood flow in the gastrointestinal tract during shock reveals that these changes are many. With shock, the amount of tissue perfused and the volume and distribution of blood flow through the gastrointestinal tract change dramatically. There are, however, two main significant changes.[106] First, less than 50% of the bowel perfused during normal conditions is perfused during shock. Second, and of greater importance, is that the decrease in perfusion is not equitably distributed to all layers. The mucosa and submucosa, the layers of the bowel with the highest metabolic demands, suffer a disproportionate decrease in both area perfused and volume of blood flowing through the area. Only 20% of the mucosa and submucosa perfused during normal conditions is perfused during shock, and the volume of blood flow through the mucosa and submucosa in shock is decreased to 16% of normotensive levels. These changes in hemodynamics are similar to those encountered in aquatic animals that are able to dive to great depths—the diving reflex.

Proposed Mechanisms of Pathogenesis

Over the last 3 years, three different perspectives have been brought to the question of pathogenesis. The first implicates the superoxide radical as the initiator.[107] The second perspective focuses on changes in intracellular calcium homeostasis,[108] and the third brings the perspective of the action of platelet activating factor and endotoxin when it is administered intraarterially.[109]

Superoxide Radicals

The superoxide radical concept is championed by Granger and Park. This concept gives us further insight into the biochemical basis of ischemia and is the concept that has received the most recent study.[107]

Granger and Park and their co-workers have implicated the superoxide radical generated during reperfusion of the ischemic bowel as the culprit.[110] Prior to their studies, it was thought that hypoxia *per se* was the cause. The superoxide radical, an unstable and cytotoxic form of molecular oxygen, is thought to alter vascular permeability of the endothelial cell and cause necrosis of the epithelial cells by peroxidation of the cell membranes. The source and action of the superoxide radical is thought to be quite different from the superoxide radical's well-known role in the neutrophil-mediated acute inflammatory response.[111] The basic change these investigators found following ischemia was an increase in vascular permeability.

The major source of the superoxide radical in the ischemic bowel appears to be the enzyme xanthine ox-

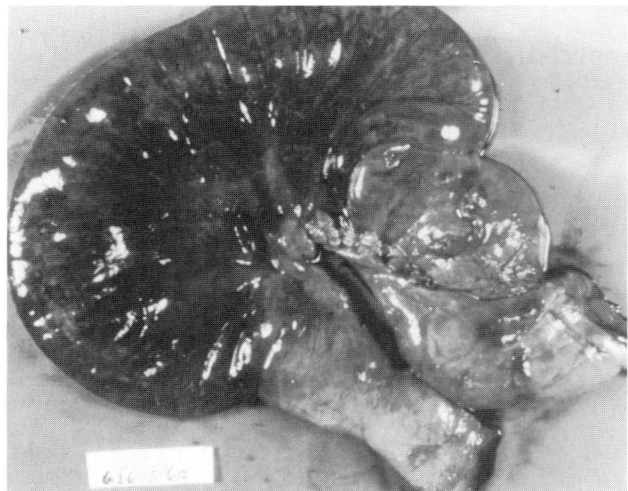

FIGURE 12–18. Venous infarct of the small bowel due to an adhesive band. The venous portion of the vasculature is affected first. Significant congestion occurs before the arterial blood supply is compromised.

idase.[112] The liver and small intestine are the two richest sources of this enzyme in the human. Interestingly, in the small bowel, most of the enzyme is concentrated in the villus tip. Obviously, a substrate is necessary, and the substrate in this model is hypoxanthine. The amount of xanthine oxidase present in the large intestine is much smaller than in the small bowel.[113]

Intracellular Calcium Homeostasis

The second concept implicates changes in intracellular calcium homeostasis as the culprit. This latter work is the result of looking at the pathogenesis of experimental stress ulceration in the stomach and its amelioration with drugs.[114,115]

Recently, the effects of changes in intracellular calcium homeostasis and ischemic injury have received significant attention. With ischemia, it has been shown that there is a significant increase in intracellular calcium and that perhaps the increased amount of intracellular calcium has a primary role in mediating irreversible ischemic injury.[108]

Intra-arterial Platelet Activating Factor and Bacterial Endotoxin

The third concept resulted from an attempt to develop another experimental model that mimicked necrotizing enterocolitis of the premature infant. This is the first model where vascular hypoperfusion, exsanguination, or other mechanisms of decreased blood flow are not utilized.[109] This third experimental model is beginning to give us additional insight into the pathogenesis of ischemic bowel disease. This model was developed by Gonzalez-Crussi and his co-workers.[109] This experimental model is produced by the intra-aortic injection of synthetic platelet activating factor or a combination of platelet activating factor and bacterial endotoxin in the rat.[116]

Therapeutic Considerations

A variety of pharmacologic agents have been recently tested in ischemic bowel disease for determination of whether they enhance the pathology or reduce the pathology. It appears that indomethacin may potentiate bowel ischemia, whereas prostaglandin E_1 (PGE_1) and ibuprofen may have a significant effect on decreasing the degree of bowel necrosis.[117] The manner in which prostaglandins are protective of mucosa appears to involve several different and complex mechanisms, including production of a shielding, gelatinous layer formed by mucus and exfoliated surface epithelial cells; flow of mucosal fluid in the lumen, which dilutes noxious agents; and a rapidly healing superficial mucosal layer, which quickly reconstitutes the physical barrier between the lumen and the lamina propria.[118]

Slow calcium channel blockers such as verapamil prevent or significantly attenuate experimentally produced stress ulcers in the stomach.[114,115]

In experimental models of necrotizing enterocolitis, it has been shown that both polycythemia and increased blood viscosity may add to the risk of the development of necrotizing enterocolitis.[119]

Entities of Ischemic Bowel Disease

Ischemic Colitis

In the 1960s, Marston et al. described three syndromes that resulted from ischemic processes in the colon.[120] The clinical course depended upon the degree of pathologic change in the visceral arteries supplying the colon, the duration of hypotension and the virulence of bacteria present in the bowel lumen. In the most severe form, transmural infarction developed. In the intermediate form, healing by fibrosis resulted in colonic stricture; and in the least severe form, bloody diarrhea developed, with subsequent healing and restitution of normal structure.

The gross pathology of the ischemic portion demonstrates mucosal ulceration and severe congestion beneath the surface. In addition, expansion of the distance between the mucosa and the muscular layers is present, due to edema formation. Microscopically, the

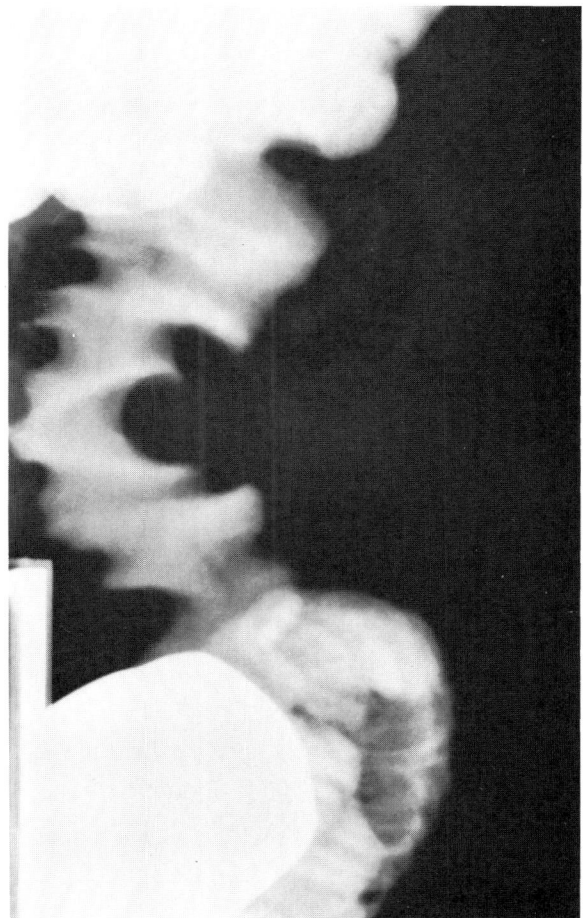

FIGURE 12–19. Barium enema in a patient with ischemic bowel disease. The barium column is irregular because of numerous indentations caused by focal edema of the mucosa and submucosa—the thumbprint sign.

picture is that of coagulative necrosis with severe congestion beneath the necrotic epithelium. The process frequently extends into the submucosa with extensive edema formation. Pseudopolyp formation is the hallmark of the disease. Pseudopolyps are the result of focal severe edema of the mucosa and submucosa. On barium enema, they can be seen as indentations of the barium column (Figure 12–19). The most frequent area of involvement in ischemic colitis is the splenic flexure—the watershed or anastomotic area between the superior and inferior mesenteric arteries. In addition to presenting as transient, strictured, and gangrenous forms, ischemic colitis can also present as megacolon in the elderly.[121]

It is being appreciated that ischemic colitis in the elderly can mimic ulcerative colitis and granulomatous colitis clinically.[122] Studies indicate that as many as 75% of the patients over the age of 50 who are initially thought to have ulcerative colitis, Crohn's colitis, or nonspecific colitis have ischemic bowel disease.[123] For further information, see Chapter 27.

Necrotizing Enterocolitis of the Premature Infant

Necrotizing enterocolitis, in the past, was thought to be due to perinatal gastrointestinal ischemia, which facilitated the invasion of enteric bacteria in an underdeveloped gastrointestinal tract, which had, as yet, little immune protective mechanism. Recent studies have challenged these traditional thoughts about the pathogenesis and have introduced data supporting the predominant role of an infectious agent.[124] Controlled studies, unfortunately, have demonstrated no consistent risk factor among infants with necrotizing enterocolitis when compared with unaffected infants. Current thought indicates that neonatal necrotizing enterocolitis is a single pathologic response whereby the immature intestine reacts to injury. The immature bowel may only have a limited manner in which it can respond to injury. The unique mucosal pathologic response may be initiated by multiple factors or microbiologic agents acting either alone or in concert.[124] The incidence of this disease is markedly increased in premature infants. It usually starts between the third and the tenth day of life. In patients, the diagnosis can only be confirmed by demonstration on an abdominal roentgenogram of abnormal intestinal bacterial gas formation or pneumatosis intestinalis. Currently, there is considerable debate about the importance of composition and the rate of administration of milk in the subsequent development of necrotizing enterocolitis. Likewise, ischemia as a risk factor is still undergoing intensive reinvestigation. Many organisms have been associated with necrotizing enterocolitis, including *Escherichia coli*, *Klebsiella*, *Enterobacter*, *Pseudomonas*, *Salmonella*, *Clostridium perfringens*, *Clostridium difficile*, and a variety of viruses (and their toxins).

Necrotizing enterocolitis develops only if a threshold of injury sufficient to initiate intestinal necrosis is exceeded.[125] The three leading events still continue to be (1) intestinal ischemia, (2) colonization by pathogenic bacteria, and (3) excess protein substrate in the intestinal lumen. Whether a single event or multiple events are necessary still is undergoing debate. Certainly, the premature infant appears at higher risk than the full-term infant of normal birth weight. In a similar manner, the presence of umbilical catheters in the pathogenesis of this disease via formation of thrombi that embolize, while raised in the past, appears at the moment to be receiving relatively little interest. Infants of less than 28 weeks' gestation and those with low birth weights, less than 1500 gm, had increased mortality rates due to this disease.[126]

Necrotizing enterocolitis has also occurred immediately after cardiac surgery, which gives more emphasis to the theory that local perfusion inadequacy plays a predominant role in the pathogenesis of this disease.[127]

Necrotizing enterocolitis has also been observed in older infants, children, and adolescents. Unfortunately, this diagnosis is usually made only at autopsy. The majority of these patients had either an altered immune state or evidence of low-flow situations or hypoxemia.[128]

Very recent studies show that there is no increased incidence of necrotizing enterocolitis in those receiving early enteral feeding.[129] When the mesenteric veins are examined, bubbles of gas are frequently found. Attempts are being made at the present time to find methods of measuring the amount of hydrogen in exhaled breath in hopes that an earlier diagnosis of necrotizing enterocolitis will be possible.[124] Microscopically, coagulative necrosis is the hallmark of the disease process. The initial stages are characterized by congestion in the lamina propria. This is followed by extravasation of erythrocytes into the lamina propria and submucosal congestion. The ischemic process then continues with necrosis of the submucosa. By this time, the mucosa is severely infarcted and ulcerated. The process then continues with coagulative necrosis of the subjacent layers. The degree of involvement of the bowel by pneumatosis can be quite extensive. These findings can often be lost if the tissue is not handled properly and promptly after removal at surgery.

Stricture formation also occurs in this disease. Stricture usually occurs within 5 to 8 weeks after the acute episode. Externally, the stricture is easy to demonstrate; and on opening this bowel, significant dilatation of the proximal intestine is readily apparent (Figure 12–20). Necrotizing enterocolitis most frequently affects the ileum and ascending colon. The ascending colon is the location of most frequent stricture formation. Histologically, the degree of fibrosis is often difficult to appreciate with hematoxylin and eosin stains; however, with trichrome stains, the degree of fibrosis becomes readily apparent. The end stage of necrotizing enterocolitis may be the development of colonic atresia.[130]

Pseudomembranous Colitis

That pseudomembranous colitis can follow the administration of a variety of antibiotics and be associated with the toxin of *C. difficile* has been appreciated

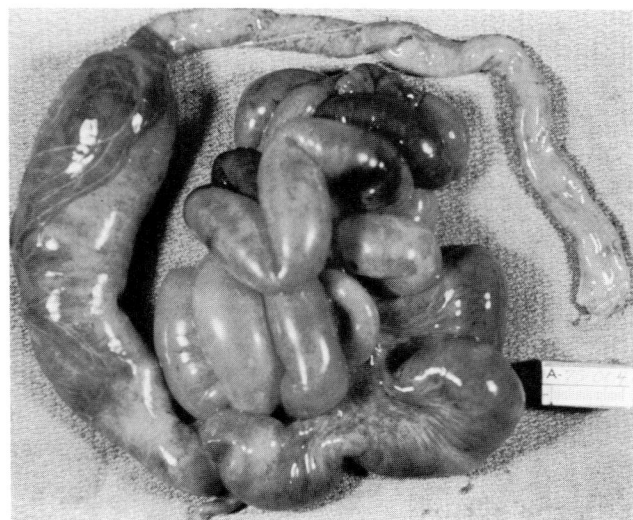

FIGURE 12-20. Necrotizing enterocolitis of the premature infant. Gross photograph at autopsy showing an area of stenosis with dilated bowel proximal to this area. The patient 5 weeks before death experienced an episode of necrotizing enterocolitis.

Hemorrhagic Necrosis

Not all ischemic processes occurring in the gastrointestinal tract result in a primary symptom complex. Some years ago, Ming summarized cases of hemorrhagic necrosis of the gastrointestinal tract studied at autopsy occurring as secondary phenomena in patients with severely compromised cardiovascular status, shock, or severe infection.[135] The histologic picture is identical to that previously described. Frequently, at autopsy, small areas of hemorrhagic necrosis are encountered (Figure 12-21). Microscopically, once again, severe coagulative necrosis of the mucosa is present (Figure 12-22).

Stress Ulceration

While the pathogenesis of stress ulceration in the stomach is still controversial, the leading cause of this phenomenon appears to be mucosal ischemia associated with cellular hypoxia but perhaps can be multifactorial in cause[136] (Figure 12-23). For additional details, see Chapter 20.

Radiation Injury

Radiation has a wide variety of effects on the gastrointestinal tract from the esophagus through the small intestine.[137] Although mucosal injury is very frequent, the ability of the mucosa to regenerate often leaves this area of the gastrointestinal tract without sequelae. Clinically, however, ischemic necrosis with concomitant massive fibrosis are sequelae of radiation injury, the picture mimicking ischemic injury to the gastrointestinal tract.[137] Profound effects occur on the microvasculature.[138] For more information, see Chapter 9.

since the mid 1970s.[131] Evidence indicates that pseudomembranous colitis continues to be due to the administration of antibiotics[132]; however, other organisms seem also to be able to cause pseudomembranous colitis (*Yersinia*).[133] There continues, however, to be a spectrum of patients in whom pseudomembranous colitis develops whose condition is not associated with antibiotic therapy.[134] Whether these cases are due to an initial episode of low perfusion or to bacterial toxins remains speculative. The pseudomembrane is a reflow phenomenon in which injured vessels respond with acute inflammation when circulation is re-established. For additional information, see Chapter 26.

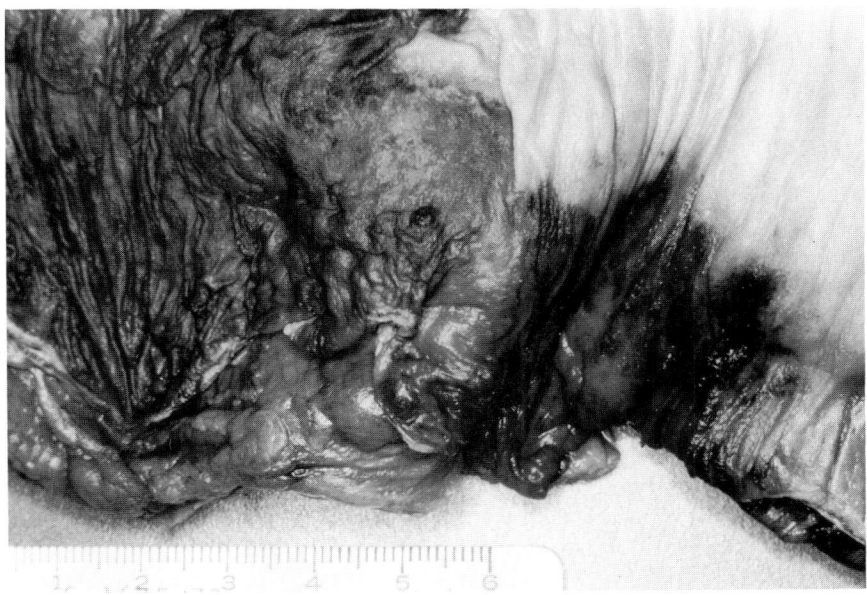

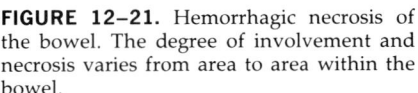

FIGURE 12-21. Hemorrhagic necrosis of the bowel. The degree of involvement and necrosis varies from area to area within the bowel.

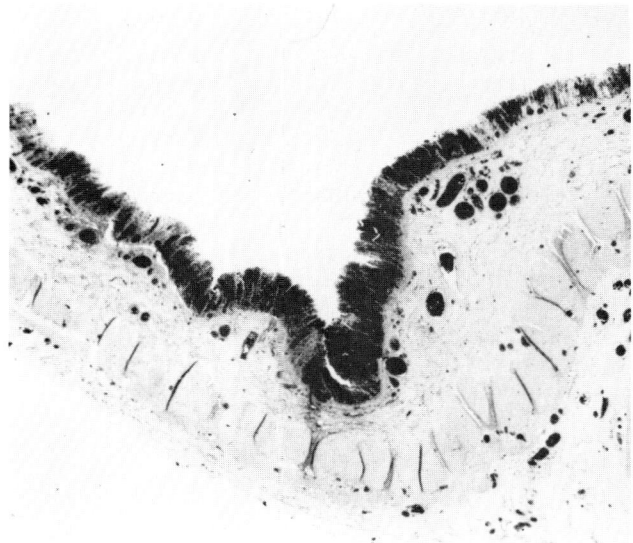

FIGURE 12-22. Histologic section of hemorrhagic necrosis of the bowel. The mucosa is severely congested and necrotic. The submucosa is congested and edematous. The deeper layers, however, are viable. (× 20)

Other Disorders

Other causes of gastrointestinal ischemia have been associated with the release of *potassium chloride* into the small bowel in the form of nonenteric coated tablets.[139,140] Recent studies have reiterated their injurious effect.[141] See Chapter 9 for additional information. Chronic *uremia* has also been associated with ischemic colitis.[142] This disease is quite frequent in patients after bilateral nephrectomy or renal transplantation.[142,143] For further information, see Chapter 16. Finally, it must be reiterated that various species and toxins of *staphylococci* have also been associated with enterocolitis.[144,145] Ischemia is thought to play a significant role in the mechanism of pathogenesis.

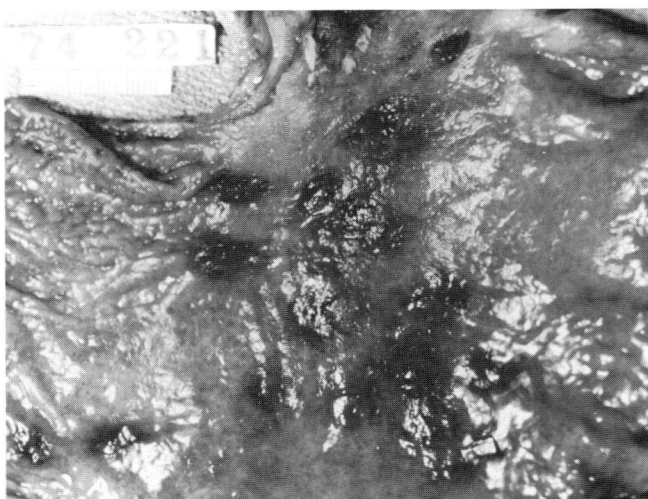

FIGURE 12-23. Multiple stress ulcers present in the stomach, another form of ischemic bowel disease.

Effect of Chronic Narrowing of the Splanchnic Vessels

Partial obstruction of the celiac artery and superior mesenteric artery has been associated with the clinical syndrome of chronic intestinal ischemia. Occasionally, histopathologic consequences of these findings have been documented. Patients with these findings have associated erosions of the stomach and duodenum.[146,147]

Acknowledgments. Special thanks to Mr. James Ebert, who researched the references, and to Ms. Roberta Herring, who typed the manuscript.

References

1. Hyams JS, Leichtner AM, Schwartz AN: Recent advances in diagnosis and treatment of gastrointestinal hemorrhage in infants and children. J Pediatr 106:1–9, 1985.
2. Raskin JB: Upper gastrointestinal hemorrhage: Early diagnostic approaches. Comp Ther 9:31–34, 1983.
3. Baer JW, Ryan S: Analysis of cecal vasculature in the search for vascular malformations. AJR 126:394–404, 1976.
4. Pounder DJ, Rowland R, Pieterse AS, et al: Angiodysplasias of the colon. J Clin Pathol 35:824–829, 1982.
5. Talman EA, Dixon DS, Gutierrez FE: Role of arteriography in rectal hemorrhage due to arteriovenous malformations and diverticulosis. Ann Surg 190:203–213, 1979.
6. Crawford ES, Roehm JOF, McGavran MH: Jejunoileal arteriovenous malformation: Localization for resection by segmental bowel staining techniques. Ann Surg 191:404–409, 1980.
7. Fogler R, Golembe E: Methylene blue injection: An intraoperative guide in small bowel resection for arteriovenous malformation. Arch Surg 113:194–195, 1978.
8. Papamiltiades MN: Injection of lymphatics: With colored cedar oil; With plastic. Stain Technol 36:241–246, 1961.
9. Hamilton SR: Structure of the colon. Scand J Gastroenterol Suppl 93:13–23, 1984.
10. Williams DB, Payne WS: Observations on esophageal blood supply. Mayo Clin Proc 57:448–453, 1982.
11. Bulkley GB, Womack WA, Downey JM, et al: Characterization of segmental collateral blood flow in the small intestine. Am J Physiol 249 (Gastrointestinal Liver Physiology 12): G228–G235, 1985.
12. Granger DN, Barrowman JA: Microcirculation of the alimentary tract. I. Physiology of transcapillary fluid and solute exchange. Gastroenterology 84:846–868, 1983.
13. Hayes PC, Shepherd AN, Bouchier IAD: Medical treatment of portal hypertension and oesophageal varices. Br Med J [Clin Res] 287:733–736, 1983.
14. Fleig WE, Stange EF, Hunecke R, et al: Prevention of recurrent bleeding in cirrhotics with recent variceal hemorrhage: Prospective, randomized comparison of propranolol and sclerotherapy. Hepatology 7:355–361, 1987.
15. Spence RAJ: The venous anatomy of the lower oesophagus in normal subjects and in patients with varices: An image analysis study. Br J Surg 71:739–744, 1984.
16. Navab F, Schiller TD, Slaton D: Management of variceal hemorrhage. South Med J 77:1302–1307, 1984.
17. Lieberman DA, Krippaehne WW, Melnyk CS: Colonic varices due to intestinal cavernous hemangiomas. Dig Dis Sci 28:852–858, 1983.
18. Cello JP, Crass RA, Federle MP: Colonic varices: An unusual source of lower gastrointestinal hemorrhage. West J Med 136:252–255, 1982.
19. Hawkey CJ, Amar SS, Daintith HAM, Toghill PJ: Familial varices of the colon occurring without evidence of portal hypertension. Br J Radiol 58:677–679, 1985.
20. Grundfest-Broniatowski S, Fazio V: Conservative treatment of bleeding stomal varices. Arch Surg 118:981–985, 1983.
21. Grauer SE, Schwartz SI: Extrahepatic portal hypertension: A retrospective analysis. Ann Surg 189:566–571, 1979.

22. Roder OC: Splenic vein thrombosis with bleeding gastroesophageal varices: Reports of two splenectomized cases and review of the literature. Acta Chir Scand 150:265–268, 1984.
23. Ricci RL, Lee KR, Greenberger NJ: Chronic gastrointestinal bleeding from ileal varices after total proctocolectomy for ulcerative colitis: correction by mesocaval shunt. Gastroenterology 78:1053–1058, 1980.
24. Moncure AC, Waltman AC, Vandersalm TJ et al: Gastrointestinal hemorrhage from adhesion-related mesenteric varices. Ann Surg 183:24–29, 1976.
25. Granqvist S: Colonic varices caused by carcinoid tumor. Gastrointest Radiol 9:269–271, 1984.
26. Camilleri M, Chadwick VS, Hodgson HJF: Vascular anomalies of the gastrointestinal tract. Hepatogastroenterology 31:149–153, 1984.
27. Moore JD, Thompson NW, Appelman HD, Foley D: Arteriovenous malformations of the gastrointestinal tract. Arch Surg 111:381–389, 1976.
28. Boley SJ, Brandt LJ, Mitsudo SM: Vascular lesions of the colon. Adv Intern Med 29:301–326, 1984.
29. Clouse RE, Costigan DJ, Mills BA, Zuckerman GR: Angiodysplasia as a cause of upper gastrointestinal bleeding. Arch Intern Med 145:458–461, 1985.
30. Boley SJ, Sammartano R, Adams A, et al: On the nature and etiology of vascular ectasias of the colon: Degenerative lesions of aging. Gastroenterology 72:650–660, 1977.
31. Stamm B, Heer M, Buhler H, Ammann R: Mucosal biopsy of vascular ectasia (angiodysplasia) of the large bowel detected during routine colonoscopic examination. Histopathology 9:639–646, 1985.
32. Max MH, Richardson JD, Flint LM, et al: Colonoscopic diagnosis of angiodysplasias of the gastrointestinal tract. Surg Gynecol Obstet 152:195–199, 1981.
33. Martini GA: The liver in hereditary haemorrhagic telangiectasia: An inborn error of vascular structure with multiple manifestations: A reappraisal. Gut 19:531–537, 1978.
34. Ahr DJ, Rickles FR, Hoyer LW, et al: Von Willebrand's disease and hemorrhagic telangiectasia: Association of two complex disorders of hemostasis resulting in life-threatening hemorrhage. Am J Med 62:452–457, 1977.
35. Mower GA, Whitehead R: Gastric hemorrhage due to ruptured arteriovenous malformation (Dieulafoy's Disease). Pathology 18:54–57, 1986.
36. Jabbari M, Cherry R, Lough JO, et al: Gastric antral vascular ectasia: The watermelon stomach. Gastroenterology 87:1165–1170, 1984.
37. Sweeney K, Petrelli N, Herrera L, et al: Cavernous hemangioma of the anus. J Surg Oncol 27:286–288, 1984.
38. Pontecorvo C, Lombardi S, Mottola L, et al: Hemangiomas of the large bowel: Report of a case. Dis Colon Rectum 26:818–820, 1983.
39. Oswalt CE, Kasal NG: Gastric hemangioma in a 15-year-old girl. Texas Med 79:37–39, 1983.
40. Govoni AF: Hemangiomas of the esophagus. Gastrointest Radiol 7:113–117, 1982.
41. White IL, Dunkelman D: Obstructive cervical esophageal hemangioma. Ear Nose Throat J 60:324–327, 1981.
42. Hanel K, Talley NA, Hunt DR: Hemangioma of the esophagus: An unusual cause of upper gastrointestinal bleeding. Dig Dis Sci 26:257–263, 1981.
43. Stillman AE, Hansen RC, Hallinan V, Strobel C: Diffuse neonatal hemangiomatosis with severe gastrointestinal involvement: Favorable response to steroid therapy. Clin Pediatr 22:589–591, 1983.
44. Ghahremani GG, Kangarloo H, Volberg F, Meyers MA: Diffuse cavernous hemangioma of the colon in the Klippel-Trenaunay syndrome. Radiology 118:673–678, 1976.
45. Weber JN, Carmichael DJ, Boylston A, et al: Case report: Kaposi's sarcoma of the bowel, presenting as apparent ulcerative colitis. Gut 26:295–300, 1985.
46. Bianco J, Pratt-Bianco L: Kaposi's sarcoma of the rectum: A case report. Mt Sinai J Med 50:278–280, 1983.
47. Weprin L, Zollinger R, Clausen K, Thomas FB: Kaposi's sarcoma: Endoscopic observations of gastric and colon involvement. J Clin Gastroenterol 4:357–360, 1982.
48. Chen KTK, Hoffman KD, Hendricks EJ: Angiosarcoma following therapeutic irradiation. Cancer 44:2044–2048, 1979.
49. Nanus DM, Kelsen D, Clark DGC: Radiation-induced angiosarcoma. Cancer 60:777–779, 1987.
50. Nakagawara G, Kojima Y, Mai M, et al: Lymphangioma of the transverse colon treated by transendoscopic polypectomy: Report of a case and review of the literature. Dis Colon Rectum 24:291–295, 1981.
51. Camilleri M, Satti MB, Wood CB: Cystic lymphangioma of the colon: Endoscopic and histologic features. Dis Colon Rectum 25:813–816, 1982.
52. Liebert CW Jr: Symptomatic lymphangioma of the esophagus with endoscopic resection. Gastrointest Endosc 29:225–226, 1983.
53. Colizza S, Tiso B, Bracci F, et al: Cystic lymphangioma of stomach and jejunum: Report of one case. J Surg Oncol 17:169–176, 1981.
54. Fauci AS (moderator), Haynes BF, Katz P (discussants): The spectrum of vasculitis: Clinical, pathologic, immunologic and therapeutic considerations. Ann Intern Med 89 (Part 1):660–676, 1978.
55. Holman HR, Calin A: Rheumatology. In Rubenstein E, Fedderman D (eds): Scientific American Medicine. Section VIII, The Vasculitides: Fibrositis. New York, Scientific American, 1987, pp 1–10.
56. Camilleri M, Pusey CD, Chadwick VS, Rees AJ: Gastrointestinal manifestations of systemic vasculitis. Q J Med 52:141–149, 1983.
57. Kleinman P, Meyers MA, Abbott G, Kazam E: Necrotizing enterocolitis with pneumatosis intestinalis in systemic lupus erythematosus and polyarteritis. Radiology 121:595–598, 1976.
58. Goldman H, Antonioli DA: Mucosal biopsy of the rectum, colon, and distal ileum. Hum Pathol 13:981–1012, 1982.
59. Keshavarzian A, Saverymuttu SH, Chadwick VS, et al: Noninvasive investigation of the gastrointestinal tract in collagen-vascular disease. Am J Gastroenterol 79:873–877, 1984.
60. Han SY, Jander HP, Laws HL: Polyarteritis nodosa causing severe intestinal bleeding. Gastrointest Radiol 1:285–287, 1976.
61. Harvey MH, Neoptolemos, JP, Fossard DP: Abdominal polyarteritis nodosa—a possible surgical pitfall? Br J Clin Pract 38:282–283, 1984.
62. Gorton M, John JF Jr: Polyarteritis overlap syndrome with extensive bowel infarction. Am J Gastroenterol 74:153–156, 1980.
63. Fayemi AO, Ali M, Braun EV: Necrotizing vasculitis of the gallbladder and the appendix: Similarity in the morphology of rheumatoid arteritis and polyarteritis nodosa. Am J Gastroenterol 67:608–612, 1977.
64. Lee EL, Smith HJ, Miller GL, et al: Ischemic pseudomembranous colitis with perforation due to polyarteritis nodosa. Am J Gastroenterol 79:35–38, 1984.
65. Wood MK, Read DR, Kraft AR, Barreta TM: A rare cause of ischemic colitis: Polyarteritis nodosa. Dis Colon Rectum 22:428–433, 1979.
66. Meyer GW, Lichtenstein J: Isolated polyarteritis nodosa affecting the cecum. Dig Dis Sci 27:467–469, 1982.
67. Hoffman BI, Katz WA: The gastrointestinal manifestations of systemic lupus erythematosus: A review of the literature. Sem Arthritis Rheum 9:237–247, 1980.
68. Gladman DD, Ross T, Richardson B, Kulkarni S: Bowel involvement in systemic lupus erythematosus: Crohn's disease or lupus vasculitis? Arthritis Rheum 28:466–470, 1985.
69. Zizic TM, Shulman LE, Stevens MB: Colonic perforations in systemic lupus erythematosus. Medicine 54:411–425, 1975.
70. Weiser MM, Andres GA, Brentjens JR, et al: Systemic lupus erythematosus and intestinal venulitis. Gastroenterology 81:570–579, 1981.
71. Zizic TM, Classen JN, Stevens MB: Acute abdominal complications of systemic lupus erythematosus and polyarteritis nodosa. Am J Med 73:525–531, 1982.
72. Burt RW, Berenson MM, Samuelson CO, Cathey WJ: Rheumatoid vasculitis of the colon presenting as pancolitis. Dig Dis Sci 28:183–188, 1983.
73. Tsai JT: Perforation of the small bowel with rheumatoid arthritis. South Med J 73:939–940, 1980.
74. McCurley TL, Collins RD: Intestinal infarction in rheumatoid arthritis. Arch Pathol Lab Med 108:125–128, 1984.

75. Chumbley LC, Harrison EG, DeRemee RA: Allergic granulomatosis and angiitis (Churg-Strauss syndrome): Report and analysis of 30 cases. Mayo Clin Proc 52:477–484, 1977.
76. Modigliani R, Muschart JM, Galian A, et al: Allergic granulomatous vasculitis (Churg-Strauss Syndrome): Report of a case with widespread digestive involvement. Dig Dis Sci 26:264–270, 1981.
77. Suen KC, Burton JD: The spectrum of eosinophilic infiltration of the gastrointestinal tract and its relationship to other disorders of angiitis and granulomatosis. Hum Pathol 10:31–43, 1979.
78. Case records of the Massachusetts General Hospital: Weekly clinicopathological exercises. Case 14-1980. N Engl J Med 302:853–858, 1980.
79. Weber TR, Grosfeld JL, Bergstein J, Fitzgerald J: Massive gastric hemorrhage: An unusual complication of Henoch-Schönlein purpura. J Pediatr Surg 18:576–578, 1983.
80. Smith HJ, Krupski WC: Spontaneous intestinal perforation in Schönlein-Henoch purpura. South Med J 73:603–606, 1980.
81. Novy SB, Weaver RM, Jensen KM, O'Donnell WW: Henoch-Schönlein purpura of the colon: An unusual gastrointestinal manifestation. South Med J 70:884–886, 1977.
82. Goldman LP, Lindenberg RL: Henoch-Schoenlein purpura: Gastrointestinal manifestations with endoscopic correlation. Am J Gastroenterol 75:357–360, 1981.
83. Morichau-Beauchant M, Touchard G, Maire P, et al: Jejunal IgA and C3 deposition in adult Henoch-Schönlein purpura with severe intestinal manifestations. Gastroenterology 82:1438–1442, 1982.
84. Haworth SJ, Pusey CD: Severe intestinal involvement in Wegener's granulomatosis. Gut 25:1296–1300, 1984.
85. Hashikata Y, Nishioka K: Multiple gastric ulcers in Wegener's granulomatosis: A follow-up report. (Letter) Dermatologica 166:325–327, 1983.
86. McNabb WR, Lennox MS, Wedzicha JA: Small intestinal perforation in Wegener's granulomatosis. Postgrad Med J 58:123–125, 1982.
87. Oddis CV, Schoolwerth AC, Abt AB: Wegener's granulomatosis with delayed pulmonary and colonic involvement. South Med J 77:1589–1591, 1984.
88. Kedziora JA, Wolff M, Chang J: Limited form of Wegener's granulomatosis in ulcerative colitis. AJR 125:127–133, 1975.
89. Sokol RJ, Farrell MK, McAdams AJ: An unusual presentation of Wegener's granulomatosis mimicking inflammatory bowel disease. Gastroenterology 87:426–432, 1984.
90. Hawkins C: Rheumatic diseases and the alimentary tract. Practitioner 220:59–65, 1978.
91. Smith CD, Schuster SR, Gruppe WE, Vawter GF: Hemolytic-uremic syndrome: A diagnostic and therapeutic dilemma for the surgeon. J Pediatr Surg 13:597–604, 1978.
92. Case records of the Massachusetts General Hospital: Weekly clinicopathological exercises. Case 12-1981. N Engl J Med 304:715–721, 1981.
93. Kawanami T, Bowen A, Girdany BR: Enterocolitis: Prodrome of the hemolytic-uremic syndrome. Radiology 151:91–92, 1984.
94. Sawaf H, Sharp MJ, Youn KJ, et al: Ischemic colitis and stricture after hemolytic-uremic syndrome. Pediatrics 61:315–316, 1978.
95. Whitington PF, Friedman AL, Chesney RW: Gastrointestinal disease in the hemolytic-uremic syndrome. Gastroenterology 76:728–733, 1979.
96. Dillard RP: Hemolytic-uremic syndrome mimicking ulcerative colitis: Lack of early diagnostic laboratory finding. Clin Pediatr 22:66–67, 1983.
97. Tochen ML, Campbell JR: Colitis in children with the hemolytic-uremic syndrome. J Pediatr Surg 12:213–219, 1977.
98. Ottinger LW: Mesenteric ischemia. N Engl J Med 307:535–537, 1982.
99. Marston A: Ischaemia. Clin Gastroenterol 14:847–862, 1985.
100. Norris HT: Reexamination of the spectrum of ischemic bowel disease. In Norris HT (ed): Pathology of the Colon, Small Intestine and Anus. New York, Churchill-Livingstone, 1983, pp 109–120.
101. Brandt LJ, Boley SJ: Ischemic intestinal syndromes. Adv Surg 15:1–45, 1981.
102. Boley SJ, Brandt LJ, Veith FJ: Ischemic disorders of the intestines. Curr Prob Surg 15:1–85, 1978.
103. Marston A, Clarke JMF, Garcia-Garcia J, Miller AL: Alimentary and pancreas: Intestinal function and intestinal blood supply: A 20 year surgical study. Gut 26:656–666, 1985.
104. Fiddian-Green RG, Amelin PM, Herrmann JB, et al: Prediction of the development of sigmoid ischemia on the day of aortic operations: Indirect measurements of intramural pH in the colon. Arch Surg 121:654–660, 1986.
105. Qamar MI, Read AE: Intestinal blood flow. (Editorial) Q J Med 56:417–419, 1985.
106. Norris HT, Sumner DS: Distribution of blood flow to the layers of the small bowel in experimental cholera. Gastroenterology 66:973–981, 1974.
107. Granger DN, Parks DA: Role of oxygen radicals in the pathogenesis of intestinal ischemia. Physiologist 26:159–164, 1983.
108. Cheung JY, Bonventre JV, Malis CD, Leaf A: Calcium and ischemic injury. N Engl J Med 314:1670–1676, 1986.
109. Gonzalez-Crussi F, Hsueh W: Experimental model of ischemic bowel necrosis: The role of platelet-activating factor and endotoxin. Am J Pathol 112:127–135, 1983.
110. Parks DA, Granger DN, Bulkley GB, Shah AK: Soybean trypsin inhibitor attenuates ischemic injury to the feline small intestine. Gastroenterology 89:6–12, 1985.
111. McCord JM, Roy RS: The pathophysiology of superoxide: Roles in inflammation and ischemia. Can J Physiol Pharmacol 60:1346–1352, 1982.
112. Bulkley GB, Kvietys PR, Parks DA, et al: Relationship of blood flow and oxygen consumption to ischemic injury in the canine small intestine. Gastroenterology 89:852–857, 1985.
113. Parks DA, Bulkley GB, Granger DN: Role of oxygen-derived free radicals in digestive tract diseases. Surgery 94:415–422, 1983.
114. Wait RB, Leahy AL, Nee JM, Pollock TW: Verapamil attenuates stress-induced gastric ulceration. J Surg Res 38:424–428, 1985.
115. Ogle CW, Cho CH, Tong MC, Koo MWL: The influence of verapamil on the gastric effects of stress in rats. Eur J Pharmacol 112:399–404, 1985.
116. Hsueh W, Gonzalez-Crussi F, Arroyave JL: Platelet-activating factor–induced ischemic bowel necrosis: An investigation of secondary mediators in its pathogenesis. Am J Pathol 122:231–239, 1986.
117. Grosfeld JL, Kamman K, Gross K, et al: Comparative effects of indomethacin, prostaglandin E_1, and ibuprofen on bowel ischemia. J Pediatr Surg 18:738–742, 1983.
118. Lacy ER: Prostaglandins and histological changes in the gastric mucosa. Dig Dis Sci 30:83S–94S, 1985.
119. Dunn SP, Gross KR, Scherer LR, et al: The effect of polycythemia and hyperviscosity on bowel ischemia. J Pediatr Surg 20:324–327, 1985.
120. Marston A, Pheils MT, Thomas ML, Morson BC: Ischaemic colitis. Gut 7:1–15, 1966.
121. Margolis IB, Faro RS, Howells EM, Organ CH: Megacolon in the elderly: Ischemic or inflammatory? Ann Surg 190:40–44, 1979.
122. Eisenberg RL, Montgomery CK, Margulis AR: Colitis in the elderly: Ischemic colitis mimicking ulcerative and granulomatous colitis. AJR 133:1113–1118, 1979.
123. Brandt L, Boley S, Goldberg L, et al: Colitis in the elderly: A reappraisal. Am J Gastroenterol 76:239–245, 1981.
124. Kliegman RM, Fanaroff AA: Necrotizing enterocolitis. N Engl J Med 310:1093–1103, 1984.
125. Kosloske AM: Pathogenesis and prevention of necrotizing enterocolitis: A hypothesis based on personal observation and a review of the literature. Pediatrics 74:1086–1092, 1984.
126. Cikrit D, Mastandrea J, West KW, et al: Necrotizing enterocolitis: Factors affecting mortality in 101 surgical cases. Surgery 96:648–655, 1984.
127. Silane MF, Symchych PS: Necrotizing enterocolitis after cardiac surgery: A local ischemic lesion? Am J Surg 133:373–376, 1977.
128. Moss TJ, Adler R: Necrotizing enterocolitis in older infants, children, and adolescents. J Pediatr 100:764–766, 1982.
129. Ostertag SG, LaGamma EF, Reisen CE, Ferrentino FL: Early enteral feeding does not affect the incidence of necrotizing enterocolitis. Pediatrics 77:275–280, 1986.
130. Beardmore HE, Rodgers BM, Outerbridge E: Necrotizing enterocolitis (ischemic enteropathy) with the sequel of colonic atresia. Gastroenterology 74:914–917, 1978.

131. Tedesco FJ, Barton RW, Alper DH: Clindamycin-associated colitis: A perspective study. Ann Intern Med 81:429–433, 1974.
132. Parry MF, Rha C-K: Pseudomembranous colitis caused by topical clindamycin phosphate. Arch Dermatol 122:583–584, 1986.
133. Brown R, Tedesco FJ, Assad RT, Rao R: *Yersinia* colitis masquerading as pseudomembranous colitis. Dig Dis Sci 31:548–551, 1986.
134. Moskovitz M, Bartlett JG: Recurrent pseudomembranous colitis unassociated with prior antibiotic therapy. Arch Intern Med 141:663–665, 1981.
135. Ming S-C: Hemorrhagic necrosis of the gastrointestinal tract and its relation to cardiovascular status. Circulation 32:332–341, 1965.
136. Pruitt BA Jr, Goodwin CW Jr: Stress ulcer disease in the burned patient. World J Surg 5:209–222, 1981.
137. Berthrong M, Fajardo LF: Radiation injury in surgical pathology. Part II. Alimentary tract. Am J Surg Pathol 5:153–178, 1981.
138. Carr ND, Pullen BR, Hasleton PS, Schofield PF: Microvascular studies in human radiation bowel disease. Gut 25:448–454, 1984.
139. Allen AC, Boley SJ, Schultz L, Schwartz S: Potassium-induced lesions of the small bowel. II. Pathology and pathogenesis. JAMA 193:1001–1006, 1965.
140. Leijonmarck C-E, Raf L: Ulceration of the small intestine due to slow-release potassium chloride tablets. Acta Chir Scand 151:273–278, 1985.
141. McMahon FG, Akdamar K, Ryan JR, Ertan A: Upper gastrointestinal lesions after potassium chloride supplements: A controlled clinical trial. Lancet 2:1059–1061, 1982.
142. Aubia J, Lloveras J, Munne A, et al: Ischemic colitis in chronic uremia. Nephron 29:146–150, 1981.
143. Margolis DM, Etheredge EE, Garza-Garza R, et al: Ischemic bowel disease following bilateral nephrectomy or renal transplant. Surgery 82:667–673, 1977.
144. Bass JW: The spectrum of staphylococcal disease: From Job's boils to toxic shock. Postgrad Med 72:58–64, 69–73, 75, 1982.
145. Gruskay JA, Abbasi S, Anday E, et al: Staphylococcus epidermidis-associated enterocolitis. J Pediatr 109:520–524, 1986.
146. Force T, MacDonald D, Eade OE, et al: Ischemic gastritis and duodenitis. Dig Dis Sci 25:307–310, 1980.
147. Allende HD, Ona FV: Celiac artery and superior mesenteric artery insufficiency: Unusual cause of erosive gastroduodenitis. Gastroenterology 82:763–766, 1982.

CHAPTER 13

Disorders of the Endocrine System

ENRICO SOLCIA, M.D., Ph.D.
CARLO CAPELLA, M.D., Ph.D.
ROBERTO FIOCCA, M.D.
PATRIZIA TENTI, M.D.
FAUSTO SESSA, M.D.
CRISTINA RIVA, M.D.
GUIDO RINDI, M.D.

NORMAL STRUCTURE AND FUNCTION

GENERAL ASPECTS OF ENDOCRINE CELL HYPERPLASIA AND TUMORS
Diagnosis
Classification
Prognosis

GASTRIC ARGYROPHIL (ECL-CELL) TUMORS AND HYPERPLASIAS
In Normal or Hypertrophic Mucosa
In Chronic Atrophic Gastritis
Clinicopathologic Aspects

GASTRIN CELL GROWTHS
Gastrin Cell Hyperplasia
Gastrin Cell Tumors

SOMATOSTATIN CELL GROWTHS

GANGLIONEUROMATOUS PARAGANGLIOMA (NEUROCARCINOID)

ARGENTAFFIN (EC-CELL) TUMORS
Small Intestine
Appendix

HINDGUT TRABECULAR (L-CELL) TUMORS

INAPPROPRIATE ENDOCRINE TUMORS

OTHER GUT ENDOCRINE TUMORS

POORLY DIFFERENTIATED ENDOCRINE (NEUROENDOCRINE) CARCINOMAS

ENDOCRINE-EXOCRINE TUMORS
Combined Tumors
Composite Tumors

NORMAL STRUCTURE AND FUNCTION

A manifold population of endocrine cells is scattered in the epithelium lining the gastric glands and the intestinal crypts and villi. Together with endocrine cells scattered in other endodermal derivatives such as the pancreas, biliary tree, lung, thyroid, and urethra, gut endocrine cells form the so-called diffuse endocrine system (DES).

Studies on these cells are largely dependent on their selective detection by refined morphologic techniques staining endocrine granules, histochemical techniques for secretory peptides or amines, and electron microscopy. When the whole endocrine cell population of a tissue is to be studied, Grimelius' silver, lead-hematoxylin, and neuron-specific enolase (NSE) or chromogranin immunohistochemistry are the techniques of choice.[1-5] However, the same techniques are of little help when the exact type of endocrine cell is to be identified. This goal is better achieved by means of

Acknowledgments. Supported by grants from the Italian National Research Council (National Gastroenterology Group and Special Oncology and Biomedical Technology Projects) and Ministry of Health (to IRCCS Policlinico S. Matteo).

Table 13–1 HUMAN GASTROENTEROPANCREATIC ENDOCRINE CELLS

			Stomach		Intestine					
					Small				Large	
Cell	Main Product	Pancreas	Oxyntic	Antral	Duodenum	Jejunum	Ileum	Appendix	Colon	Rectum
P	Unknown	f	+	+	+	f	f		f	f
EC	5-HT + peptides	f	+	+	+	+	+	+	+	+
EC$_1$ subtype	5-HT + substance P				+	+	+	+	+	+
D	Somatostatin	+	+	+	+	+	f	+	f	+
L	GLI + PYY				f	+	+	+	+	+
A	Glucagon	+	a							
PP (F/D$_1$)	Pancreatic peptide	+								
B	Insulin	+								
X	Unknown		+							
ECL	Histamine		+							
G	Gastrin			+	+					
CCK	CCK				+	+	f			
VL/TG	C-t G/CCK				+	+	f			
S	Secretin				+	+				
GIP	GIP				+	+	f			
M	Motilin				+	+	f			
N	Neurotensin				f	+	+			

f, few; a, fetus and newborn; CCK, cholecystokinin; EC, enterochromaffin; GIP, gastric inhibitory polypeptide; GLI, glucagon-like immunoreactants: glicentin, glucagon-37, glucagon-29; PP, pancreatic peptide; PYY, PP-like peptide with N-terminal tyrosine and C-terminal tyrosine amide; C-t G/CCK, C-terminal gastrin/CCK immunoreactivity lacking N-terminal and mid-part gastrin and CCK reactivities; EC, enterochromaffin; ECL, enterochromaffin-like; 5-HT, 5-hydroxytryptamine; VL/TG, very large granule/tetragastrin.

hormone immunohistochemistry and electron microscopy.

As a rule, secretory granules of endocrine cells are concentrated in the basal part of the cytoplasm, whereas the Golgi complex is supranuclear. In the pyloric and intestinal mucosa, most cells reach the lumen in a narrow, specialized area showing tufts of microvilli, coated vesicles, and a centriole; it is likely that this area acts as a receptor surface facing luminal contents. Such a pattern suggests some functional polarity of the cell. In the fundic mucosa, endocrine cells lack luminal contacts and show less evident polarity.[6]

Secretory granules are released at the basal surface of the cell or along the lower part of its lateral surface, where intervening cells may form interstitial spaces and canaliculi. In the upper (juxtaluminal) part of the epithelium, these spaces are closed by junctional complexes with neighboring cells. Granule release at the luminal surface has never been observed.

Both endodermal and neuroectodermal origins of gut endocrine cells have been considered. Their origin from nervous elements, first put forward by Danisch, has been supported by Pearse and co-workers, who suggested the involvement of neural crests or neurally programmed cells of epiblastic origin.[7] However, graft experiments accurately performed in embryos show that gut endocrine cells are not derived from neural crests or the epiblast.[8] At present, their endodermal origin seems likely.

Because of sequence homologies among gut hormonal peptides, reliable immunohistochemical localization of secretory products in gut endocrine cells can be obtained only by using a battery of antisera or monoclonal antibodies of different specificity and comparing their results with those of hormone characterization in extracts of gastrointestinal mucosa. The identification of different cell types among gut endocrine cells depends, in addition, on (1) the detection of hormone or prohormone and related fragments in the cell; (2) the ultrastructural characterization of the cell itself, with special reference to its secretory granules, and (3) the co-localization of different hormonal (such as glicentin and PYY [see Table 13–1] in intestinal L cells) and nonhormonal products (chromogranins, membrane glycoproteins, and various enzymes) stored in the same granules. As many as 15 gastro-enteropancreatic (GEP) endocrine cells were considered in the Lausanne 1977 classification, approved by 18 specialists working in the field and further revised during subsequent meetings.[9,10] This classification, rearranged and improved according to recent immunohistochemical and electron-immunocytochemical investigations,[11-19] is presented in Table 13–1. The main structural and histochemical features of the various cell types are summarized in Table 13–2.

GENERAL ASPECTS OF ENDOCRINE CELL HYPERPLASIA AND TUMORS

Diagnosis

Endocrine cells of the gut may increase in number and become hyperplastic while remaining intraglandular, as scattered elements or forming rows, tubules, microacini, and micronodules.[20] Sometimes, budding of small clusters of hyperplastic endocrine cells from the base of glandular epithelium is found. Minute extraglandular micronodules made up of small clusters of endocrine cells, usually surrounded by a thin basement

Table 13-2 MAIN HISTOCHEMICAL AND ULTRASTRUCTURAL FEATURES OF HUMAN GASTROENTEROPANCREATIC ENDOCRINE CELLS

Cell	Hormone Histochemistry	Other Stains	Secretory Granule Ultrastructure		
			Size	*Shape*	*Inner Structure*
P		Grimelius, chrom A	100–150	Round	Thin-haloed
EC	Serotonin	Grimelius, chrom A, PbH	150–500	Pleomorphic	Heavily osmiophilic
EC_1	Serotonin, substance P	Grimelius, chrom A, PbH	150–300	Pleomorphic	Heavily osmiophilic
D	Somatostatin	Davenport's silver, PbH	200–400	Round	Poorly osmiophilic, homogeneous
L	Glicentin/glucagon-37, PYY	PbH, Grimelius, chrom C > A	150–300	Round	Solid, fairly dense
A	Glucagon (C-t IR)	Grimelius, chrom A > C	200–350	Round	Target-like
PP	Pancreatic polypeptide	Grimelius, chrom C, A	D_1: 40–200	Round	Homogeneous, moderately dense
			F: 200–400	Variable	Variable
B	Insulin	Aldehyde fuchsin	200–400	Round	Vesicular with crystalloids
X		PbH, Grimelius	160–280	Round	Solid, fairly dense
ECL	Histamine, serotonin	Grimelius, chrom A	160–300	Round	Vesicular, coarsely granular core
G	Gastrin (Non C-t IR)	Grimelius, chrom A	150–350	Round	Vesicular, flocculent core
CCK	Cholecystokinin (Non-C-t IR)		150–250	Round	Thin haloed, fairly dense
VL/TG	Gastrin/CCK C-t IR		200–500	Variable	Moderately dense
S	Secretin	Grimelius, chrom A	200–350	Round to angular	Solid to target-like
GIP	Gastrin inhibitory peptide		200–300	Round	Solid, fairly dense
M	Motilin		150–220	Round	Solid, fairly dense
N	Neurotensin	Grimelius, chrom A	250–350	Round	Solid, fairly dense

PbH, lead-hematoxylin; chrom, chromogranin; C-t IR, C-terminal immunoreactivity; >, heavier staining than.

membrane and barely exceeding the size of the glands, may be found in the lamina propria of the mucosa, especially in areas of chronic inflammation.[21] Reactive proliferation of endocrine cells surviving gland damage and entrapped in the connective tissue might be involved in the genesis of such micronodules. Only in occasional cases have all intermediate patterns between hyperplastic micronodules and frank endocrine tumors, including enlargement and fusion of the micronodules with loss of basement membrane, been observed, especially in a pathologic condition of the stomach called microcarcinoidosis showing very numerous intramucosal foci of hyperplasia, dysplasia, and tumor growth.[20]

In most cases the histologic features of endocrine tumors in the gut are distinctive enough to permit their identification. However, pseudoglandular (tubuloacinar) structures with true lumina may be rather prominent in some tumors, such as gastrin and somatostatin cell tumors, which on purely histologic grounds may be difficult to distinguish from usual adenomas and adenocarcinomas.[22,23] Distinguishing some endocrine tumors with solid sheets or broad trabeculae and atypical changes from solid carcinomas with moderate atypia may also be difficult. Selective staining techniques for endocrine granules, such as Grimelius' silver and lead-hematoxylin, are helpful in proving the endocrine nature of such tumors. The immunohistochemical detection of neuron-specific enolase, chromogranins, and specific glycoproteins of secretory granule membrane may also provide useful and more specific markers of neuroendocrine tumors.[24-28] In particular, chromogranins A, B, and C, a family of anionic intragranular proteins, possibly involved in hormone posttranslational biosynthesis, storage, and release, seem closely related to the argyrophil and basophilic component of secretory granules, which accounts at least in part for their reactivity with selective stains such as Grimelius' silver, and lead-hematoxylin and masked metachromasia.[5]

Endocrine peptides and monoamines are the most specific markers of gut endocrine tumors and represent useful tools for their characterization and classification. The immunohistochemical detection of hormones and related prohormones allows for precise correlation of tumor cell differentiation and function with tumor-associated hyperfunctional syndromes.[14,20,27,29-31] Because of the frequent occurrence in the same tumor of multiple cell types producing different hormones, problems may arise in classifying endocrine tumors purely on functional grounds. Thus, it seems opportune to restrict the use of functional labelings as *gastrinoma, vipoma,* or *somatostatinoma* to those tumors that, besides showing the appropriate peptide in tumor cells, also develop a related hyperfunctional syndrome (Table 13-3). Tumors lacking any hyperfunctional syndrome may be classified on the basis of the prevalent tumor cell type (as, for instance, *gastrin [G] cell tumor, somatostatin [D] cell tumor, G/D-cell tumor,* or *enterochromaffin-like [ECL] cell tumor*) or even on the basis of more conventional morphologic criteria, such as histologic pattern, reactivity to silver techniques, site of origin,

Table 13-3 MAIN GUT-RELATED ENDOCRINE SYNDROMES

Syndrome	Increased Blood Hormone(s)	Symptoms	Cause
Carcinoid			
Classical	5-HT, substance P, kallikrein-bradykinin	Red-blue flushing, diarrhea	EC-cell argentaffin carcinoid
Atypical	Histamine, 5-HT/5-HTP; ↑ by gastrin	Red flushing	ECL-cell argyrophil carcinoid
Zollinger-Ellison or gastrinoma	Gastrin; ↑ by secretin	Peptic ulcer, hyperchlorhydria	G-cell tumor
G-cell hyperfunction	Gastrin; ↓ by secretin, ↑ by meal	Peptic ulcer, hyperchlorhydria	G-cell hyperplasia
Somatostatinoma	Somatostatin	Diabetes, steatorrhea, cholelithiasis	D-cell tumor
Glucagonoma	Glucagon	Skin rash, diabetes	A-cell tumor
Verner-Morrison or vipoma	VIP, PHM, PP	Watery diarrhea, hypokalemia, ana/hypochlorhydria (WDHA)	Epithelial endocrine or neurogenic vipoma

VIP, vasoactive intestinal peptide; PHM, peptide with N-terminal histidine and C-terminal methionine; ↑, enhanced; ↓, decreased; 5-HT, 5 hydroxytryptamine; 5-HTP, 5-hydroxytryptophan.

and so forth (as, for instance, *gastric argyrophil carcinoid, rectal trabecular carcinoid*, or *intestinal argentaffin carcinoid*).

Classification

A classification of gut endocrine tumors into *foregut* (stomach, pancreas, duodenum, and upper jejunum), *midgut* (lower jejunum, ileum, appendix, cecum), and *hindgut* (colon, rectum), with considerable clinicopathologic differences among the three groups, was introduced decades ago by Williams and Sandler[32] and supported recently by hormone histochemical studies.[30] In the case of foregut tumors, the usefulness of such a classification in practical diagnostic work remains limited by its failure to characterize individual tumor entities with well-defined histologic, cytologic, hormonal, and/or clinicopathologic profiles. However, because gut endocrine tumors express cell types and hormones that are largely coherent with those expressed by their tissues of origin, knowledge of the exact site of origin is often of help in suggesting the nature of the tumor, to be ascertained by subsequent histochemical and ultrastructural investigations. Thus, midgut tumors are mostly 5-hydroxytryptamine (5-HT) and substance P–producing argentaffin EC-cell carcinoids, whereas hindgut tumors show mainly glicentin/glucagon-37-, PP-, and/or PYY-producing L cells. Pyloric and duodenal tumors are mainly gastrin and somatostatin cell tumors. Finally, argyrophil ECL cells largely predominate in gastric argyrophil carcinoids arising in the body-fundus mucosa.[14,33]

A general classification of carcinoids based on structural patterns has been developed by Soga and Tazawa.[34] It comprises four pure patterns (A, solid nest or insular; B, trabecular; C, glandular; and D, undifferentiated) and several mixed patterns (A + C, A + B, B + C, B + D, A + B + C). The various structural patterns have been found to be significantly related with the primary site of the tumor. For instance, A or A + C patterns largely prevail in the ileum and appendix, and B and B + C patterns prevail in the rectum. At least in part, structural patterns are linked with the endocrine cell type(s) composing the tumor growth, for instance, A-type carcinoids are, as a rule, EC-cell carcinoids[34,35] whereas rectal trabecular carcinoids are mainly L-cell tumors.[36] In patients with metastatic disease, these structural patterns have been found to have significantly different survival rates.[37]

Thus, combination of the site and structural patterns of a gut endocrine tumor may provide useful information, although it can hardly fulfill all the requirements for fruitful clinicopathologic correlation. For practical purposes, the classification of gut endocrine tumors in Table 13-4, covering most available histopathologic, histochemical, ultrastructural, and clinicopathologic data, is recommended.

Prognosis

In the case of gut endocrine tumors, factors known to be of prognostic relevance include site, size, multicentricity, level of invasion, regional lymph node or distant metastases, histologic pattern, clinical symptoms (with special reference to functional syndromes), and association with other neoplasms.

The better outcome of appendiceal tumors and, to some extent, rectal tumors in comparison with colonic, midgut, or foregut tumors is well known.[38-40] This results in part from their smaller size, and lower invasive level and spread at the time of discovery. The good prognosis of tumors less than 1 cm in size has been well documented; most tumors above 2 or 2.5 cm have shown malignant behavior.[40-42]

At all levels in the gut, patients with tumors with invasion limited to the mucosa-submucosa or muscularis propria ("superficially invasive" or "intramural" tumors) show much better survival than those with tumors invading the gastrointestinal wall deeply (serosa or beyond). In the extensive study of Hajdu and co-

Table 13-4 CLASSIFICATION OF GUT ENDOCRINE TUMORS

Tumor	Preferred Site	Prevalent Structural Pattern	Prevalent Cell Type	Main Hormonal Products	Associated Syndrome or Pathologic Condition
Well-differentiated					
Gastric argyrophil carcinoid	Body/fundus	Microlobular-trabecular	ECL	Histamine, 5-HT/5-HTP	CAG, ZES ± MEN I, G cell hyperplasia, atypical carcinoid syndrome
Gastrin cell tumor	Duodenum, antrum, jej.	Trabecular-glandular	G	Gastrin	ZES, ECL-cell growth
Somatostatin cell tumor			D	Somatostatin	Cholelithiasis
Gangliocytic paraganglioma	Duodenum	Trabecular + neuroid	PP, D	Somatostatin, PP	Neurofibromatosis
Argentaffin carcinoid	Appendix, ileum, jejunum, cecum	Solid nest	EC	5-HT, substance P	Carcinoid syndrome
Hindgut trabecular carcinoid	Rectum, colon	Trabecular-glandular	L	Glicentin/glucagon-37, PP, PYY	
Inappropriate tumors	Stomach, intestine			ACTH/MSH, VIP, calcitonin	Cushing's syndrome, vipoma syndrome
Poorly differentiated					
Neuroendocrine carcinoma	Esophagus, stomach, intestine	Undifferentiated, poorly trabecular or diffuse sheets	Protoendocrine	Variable	Variable

MSH, melanocyte stimulating hormone; CAG, chronic atrophic gastritis; ZES, Zollinger-Ellison syndrome; MEN I, multiple endocrine neoplasia syndrome, type I.
Other abbreviations, see Tables 13-1 and 13-3.

workers,[40] less than 1% of "superficially invasive" tumors metastasized and caused death; whereas of the deeply invasive tumors, 85% metastasized and 65% were fatal. None of 32 carcinoids (mostly intestinal) confined to the mucosa-submucosa showed associated metastatic disease, whereas 7% of 29 tumors invading the muscularis propria and 69% of 13 cases showing serosal involvement demonstrated metastatic spread.[43] None of 45 patients who had intramural carcinoids died in the 5-year period after excision of the tumor; whereas of the 39 patients whose tumor extended into the serosa or beyond, only two (5%) lived longer than 5 years.[44]

Half of patients presenting with metastases restricted to regional lymph nodes, but only 8% of patients with distant metastases, were among survivors at the end of the study.[40] In patients with metastatic disease, both the anatomic site of the primary tumor and the histologic pattern of the tumor were significantly and independently correlated with survival. In particular, mixed A + C, pure A, pure B, mixed A + B, other mixed types, pure C, and pure D patterns ranked in a progressively decreasing order of median survival time.[37]

In general, endocrine tumors diagnosed because of clinical symptoms have a poorer prognosis than those discovered by chance during clinical examination, most of which are intramural.[44] In particular, tumors associated with hyperfunctional syndromes have a poorer prognosis than those lacking the syndrome. Coexistence of other malignant neoplasms was found in as many as 29% of patients with carcinoids of the small intestine, a fact that may greatly influence survival rates.[38,41,43]

In the large series of cases analyzed by Godwin,[39] 5% of carcinoids in the appendix were nonlocalized (1.4% in the series of Moertel et al.[38]), 14% in the rectum and rectosigmoid, 55% in the stomach (17% to 39% in Brodman and Pai's review of the literature[45]), 64% in the ileum and jejunum, and 71% in the colon; 5-year relative survival rates were 99%, 83%, 52%, 54%, and 52%, respectively.

GASTRIC ARGYROPHIL (ECL-CELL) TUMORS AND HYPERPLASIAS

Gastric carcinoids account for about 0.3% of all gastric tumors and 3% of all gastrointestinal carcinoids in the old literature.[39] Their possible multifocality, up to patterns of diffuse gastric *carcinoidosis*,[46,47] and their association with chronic atrophic gastritis (CAG) with or without anemia, hypergastrinemia, and peptic ulcer disease have been outlined.[6,46,48] After the identification of different endocrine cell types in the human gastric mucosa[6,49] (Table 13-1), several attempts were made to characterize cytologically gastric endocrine growths and to clarify their natural history.[6,20,29,50-54] Tumors and hyperplasias associated with chronic atrophic gastritis have been separated from those arising in normal or hypertrophic mucosa (Table 13-5).

Table 13-5 PERSONALLY INVESTIGATED GASTRIC ENDOCRINE TUMORS (38 CASES)

Diagnosis	Cell Type	Site			Number of Cases	Cases with CAG
		Body-Fundus	Whole Stomach	Antrum-Pylorus		
Well-differentiated		28	2	3	33	24
Argyrophil carcinoids		27	2	1	30	22
	ECL	24			24	16
	EC	1		1	2	2
	P	1			1	1
	Unknown	1	2		3	3
G cell tumors	G ± D	1		2	3	2
Poorly differentiated	Protoendocrine	1		4	5	4

CAG, chronic atrophic gastritis.

In Normal or Hypertrophic Mucosa

Diffuse *hyperplasia* and *hypertrophy* of argyrophil endocrine cells has been found regularly in the hypertrophic fundic glands of hypergastrinemic patients with gastric hypersecretion and peptic ulcer disease, due to pancreatic and/or duodenal gastrinoma (Zollinger-Ellison syndrome [ZES]) or even to pyloric gastrin cell hyperplasia.[6,22,55,56] The argyrophil cells were identified mostly as ECL cells, with secretory granules ranging from vesicular to haloed or solid, round to irregularly shaped, with a more or less apparent, coarsely granular texture in the core. Enlarged Golgi complexes as well as increased and dilated endoplasmic reticulum were often observed.

In the hypertrophic gastropathy of hypergastrinemic patients with ZES or gastrin cell hyperplasia, the argyrophil cells show a tendency to increase in number progressively from the renewal zone to the bottom of the glands (simple hyperplasia), where they may accumulate and form hyperplastic chains (linear hyperplasia) at the base of the epithelium, a distinctive pattern in some ZES patients with long-standing, severe hypergastrinemia that the authors have investigated (Figure 13-1).

Among argyrophil *carcinoids* arising in nonatrophic fundic mucosa reported so far in the literature only a few cases have been characterized cytologically at the ultrastructural level,[30,51,57] all of which proved to be ECL cell tumors. Ultrastructurally proven ECL-cell tumors were characterized histologically by their microlobular-trabecular structure, intense argyrophilia with both Grimelius' and Sevier-Munger's silver (the latter technique, somewhat more selective for ECL cells, is, however, less reproducible), consistent chromogranin A immunoreactivity in the absence of chromogranin B and C reactivity, no or poor staining with lead-hematoxylin, no reactivity with argentaffin and diazonium techniques, and no reactivity or weak reactivity with serotonin and known peptides (Figure 13-2).

Of the authors' eight ECL-cell tumors arising in nonatrophic mucosa (Table 13-5), one was associated with pyloric G-cell hyperplasia and two with gastrinomas, ZES, and hyperparathyroidism (multiple endocrine neoplasia syndrome [MEN], type I, or Wermer's syndrome). It seems interesting to note that, including the authors' two cases, 14 cases of gastric carcinoids (mostly carcinoidoses) coupled with ZES have been observed, 12 with MEN I also involving the parathyroids. In five other cases, three with MEN I, gastric carcinoids were associated with hyperparathyroidism in the absence of ZES.

In addition to simple and linear hyperplasia, the body-fundus mucosa of ZES + MEN patients also showed micronodular hyperplasia as well as dysplasia of argyrophil cells. Hyperplastic micronodules develop mainly in the deep part of the glands, inside their basement membrane, apparently from proliferation of endocrine cells, coupled with simultaneous loss of exocrine cells. Such micronodules may remain intraglandular or accumulate in the lamina propria just above the muscularis mucosae, where they may form adenomatoid patterns of growth. Dysplastic micronodules were characterized by their increasing size (more than 150 μm in diameter) and tendency to fuse with

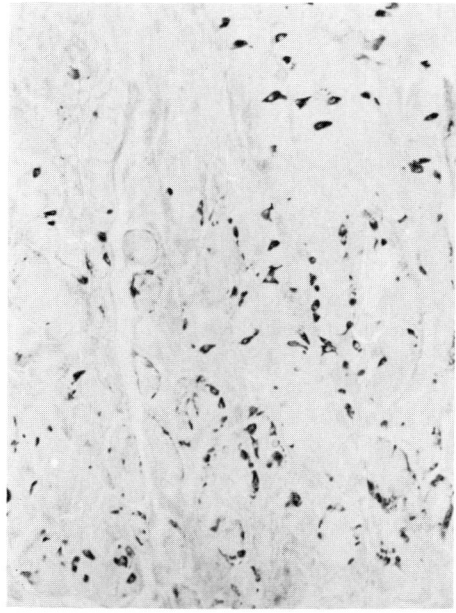

FIGURE 13-1. Diffuse, chain-forming hyperplasia of argyrophil cells in the oxyntic glands of a patient with antropyloric G-cell hyperplasia and hyperfunction (see Figure 13-5). (Grimelius' silver, × 110)

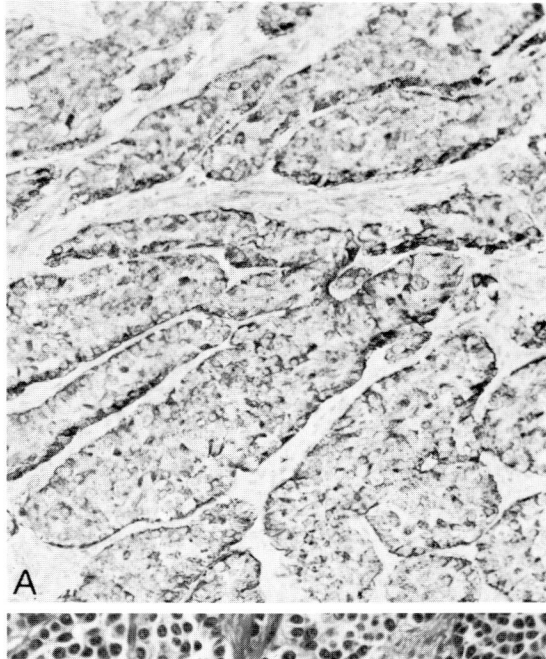
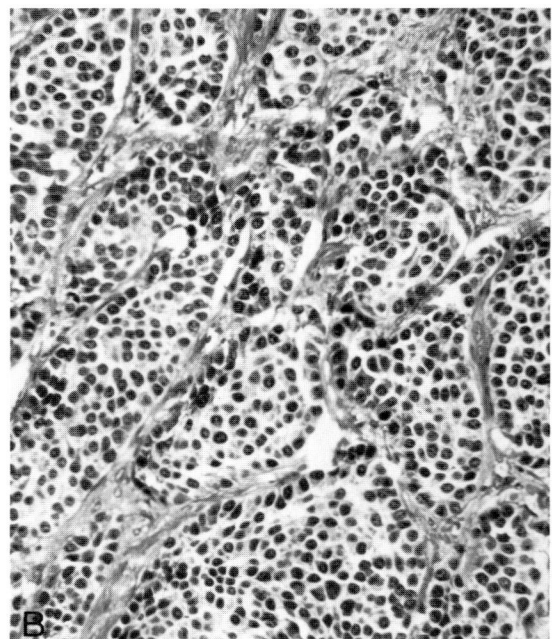
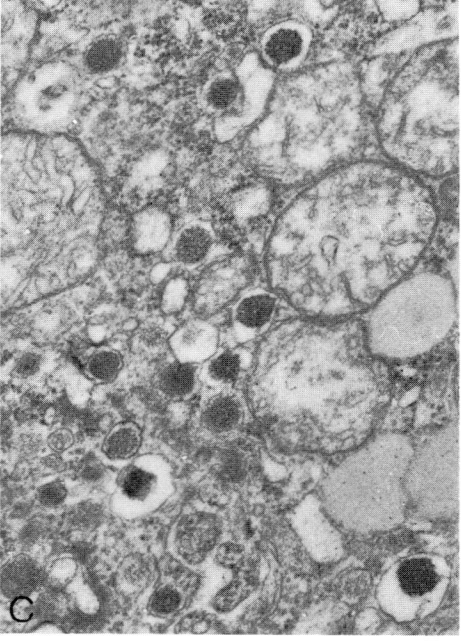

FIGURE 13-2. Invasive, submucosal part of a gastric argyrophil carcinoid metastatic to the liver, coupled with atypical carcinoid syndrome. Note the argyrophilia (A) (Grimelius' silver, × 140) of monomorphic tumor cells forming trabeculae and microlobules (B) (H&E, × 220). (C) Electron microscopy (× 28,000) shows vesicular granules containing a fairly dense core, often with coarsely granular substructure.

each other. Other dysplastic lesions were formed by irregular clusters or stripes of argyrophil cells arising at any level in the glands, from the neck to the bottom, and growing outside the basement membrane to infiltrate the lamina propria or even the muscularis mucosae. Dysplastic micronodules and microinfiltrative growths probably represent the starting points of the multiple intramucosal tumor growths typical of microcarcinoidosis (Figure 13–3).

In Chronic Atrophic Gastritis

Scattered and micronodule *hyperplasia* of endocrine cells has been noted several times during histologic, histochemical, and ultrastructural studies of CAG with or without pernicious anemia (PA) and/or hypergastrinemia.[20,21,54,55,58,59] Intestinal endocrine cells, including enterochromaffin (EC), cholecystokinin, enteroglucagon, secretin, and somatostatin cells, have been identified in intestinal metaplasia associated with CAG.[20,50,54,60] Occasionally these cells, with special reference to EC cells, accumulated at the bottom of the crypts, forming hyperplastic palisades. Irregularly scattered, linear, and micronodular hyperplasias of argyrophil ECL cells, together with EC and P cells, have been observed in surviving acidopeptic glands and regenerating neck region of mucous tubules of CAG, especially in hypergastrinemic patients.[20,57,59,61]

In areas of gland atrophy and sclerosis, small endo-

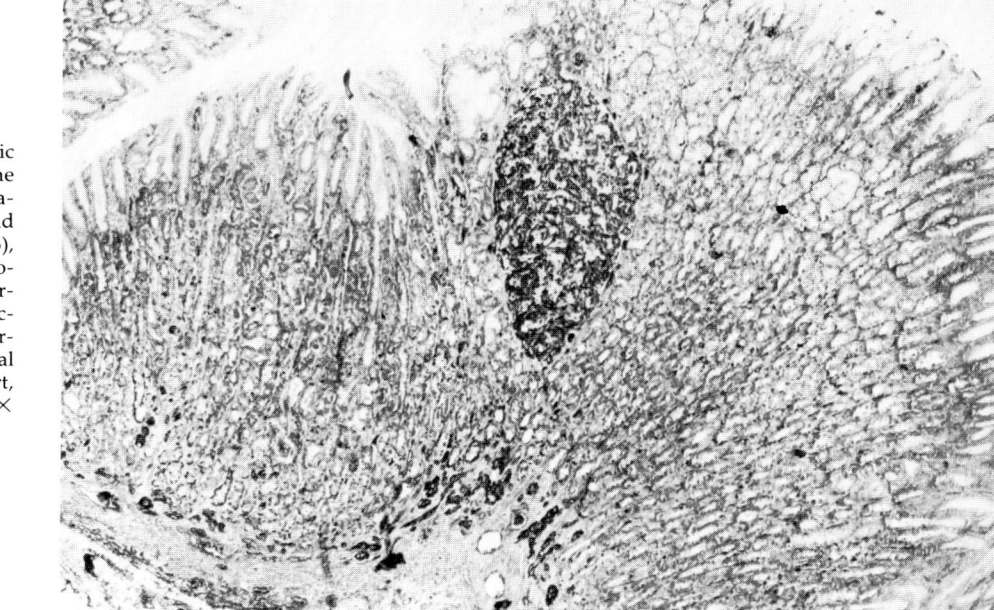

FIGURE 13–3. Hypertrophic gastropathy in multiple endocrine neoplasia (MEN) type I with parathyroid adenoma, pancreatic and duodenal gastrinomas (with ZES), and gastric carcinoidosis. A microcarcinoid and numerous hyperplastic micronodules are selectively stained with Sevier-Munger's silver in the superficial to middle part and the basal part, respectively, of the mucosa. (× 65)

crine cell clusters forming minute micronodules, with a diameter barely exceeding that of tubular glands, were frequently observed in the lamina propria (Figure 13–4A). They showed a prevalence of ECL, EC, or P cells, sometimes admixed with poorly granular or immature mucous cells, and they seemed to represent the product of a self-limiting, reactive growth of endocrine cells which had survived gland atrophy and been entrapped in the inflamed lamina propria.[20,57]

In the body-fundus mucosa, diffuse hyperplasia of argyrophil cells has been found in 65% of PA patients with CAG; minute micronodular hyperplasia, either intraglandular or stromal, has been detected in 30% of the same patients.[54] In the antral mucosa affected by CAG the authors have frequently observed diffuse and micronodular hyperplasia of gastric EC cells, with poor 5-HT content, and irregularities in gastrin cell distribution.

As many as 79 *carcinoids* associated with CAG have been reported in the literature.[53,54,57] Most of these were argyrophil tumors arising in the body-fundus region, in the majority of cases due to type A (corpus-fundus)

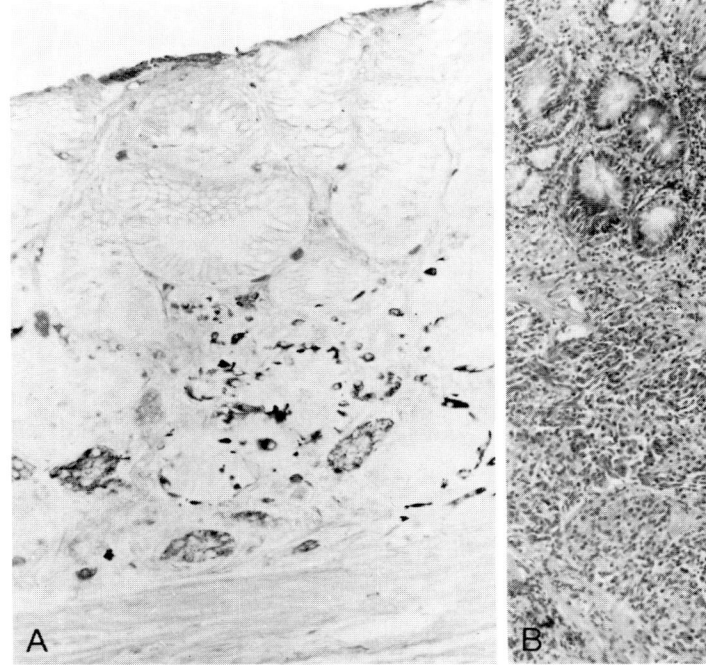

FIGURE 13–4. Type A chronic atrophic gastritis with hypergastrinemia. *A*, Irregular hyperplasia of endocrine cells forming intraglandular chains and extraglandular micronodules in the deep scleroatrophic mucosa. Note lack of endocrine cells in the hyperplastic foveolae forming the upper half of the mucosa. (Grimelius' silver, × 150) *B*, Microcarcinoid in the deep, atrophic mucosa covered by polypoid foveolar hyperplasia. (H&E, × 110)

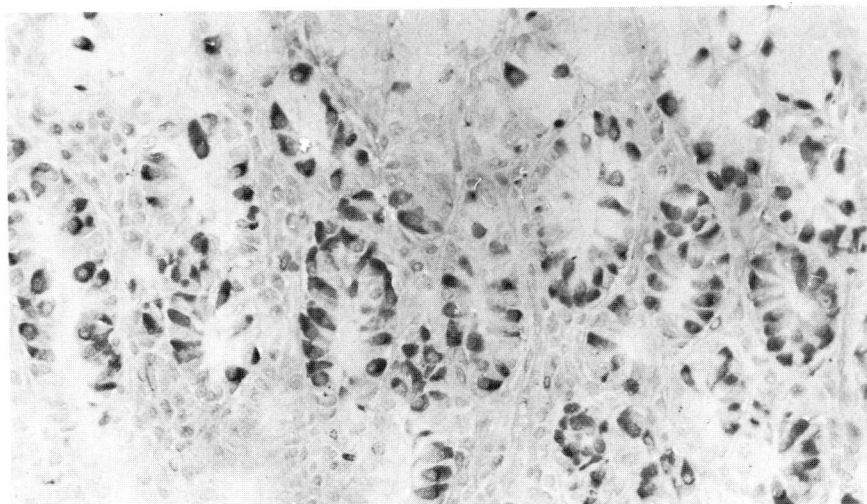

FIGURE 13-5. Gastrin-cell hyperplasia in the pyloric mucosa of a patient with food-enhanced hypergastrinemia, hyperchlorhydria, and peptic ulcer disease. Same patient as in Figure 13-1. (N-terminal gastrin-34 antiserum A30, CRB, Cambridge, U.K..) (Immunoperoxidase-hematoxylin, × 200)

CAG associated with PA and hypergastrinemia (Figure 13-4). Most cases investigated, including 16 cases of the authors (Table 13-5), have been characterized histochemically and ultrastructurally as ECL-cell tumors.[30,50,51,53,57,62]

Clinicopathologic Aspects

Only 18% of 61 cases arising in type A CAG[53] and 23% of 35 cases associated with both CAG and PA[54] have been reported to show metastases, mostly in regional lymph nodes. Only 3 of 74 (4%) cases with nonantral CAG showed distant metastases.[57] It seems possible that gastric carcinoids arising in a background of CAG, mostly diagnosed endoscopically at present, have a more favorable prognosis than those arising in nonatrophic mucosa. Whether earlier tumor diagnosis due to CAG-related symptoms or an intrinsically more benign nature of CAG-associated tumor growths contributes to this difference remains to be ascertained. Metastases to regional lymph nodes and liver were demonstrated in 17% to 39% of cases, mostly surgical or autopsy, in the old literature.[45]

An "atypical carcinoid syndrome" with red cutaneous flushing and without diarrhea has been reported rarely in association with gastric carcinoids, as a rule without mention of CAG, PA, ZES, or hypergastrinemia, usually coupled with liver metastases and production of histamine and 5-hydroxytryptophan,[63-65] a secretory pattern closely reminiscent of ECL cells.[6,66] In both of the authors' patients with ECL cell tumors, unassociated with CAG, that metastasized to the liver, the atypical carcinoid syndrome developed, with long-lasting flushing, without diarrhea; whereas in none of the remaining 22 patients with ECL-cell tumors (or the 28 patients with gastric argyrophil carcinoids) with or without gastritis did the syndrome or metastases develop.

A dermatosis with the pattern of acanthosis nigricans has been found in association with a malignant ECL-cell tumor.[67] Whether ECL-cell products had any role in the genesis of the dermatosis, which subsided after tumor excision, remains uncertain.

GASTRIN CELL GROWTHS

Gastrin Cell Hyperplasia

G-cell hyperplasia is known to occur in the pyloric mucosa of patients with peptic ulcer disease (often recurrent and resistant to medical therapy), hyperchlorhydria, and severe food-stimulated hypergastrinemia.[6,22,55,68-70] In five cases the authors have investigated (Figure 13-5) the average number of G-cells per millimeter of pyloric mucosa (counted in 5-μm-thick histologic sections) from muscularis mucosae to luminal surface ranged from 140 to 250, in comparison with 40 to 90 in control subjects who lacked G-cell hyperfunction and peptic ulcer disease. Borderline cases between severely hyperfunctioning, massive G-cell hyperplasia and common duodenal ulcer disease lacking G-cell hyperplasia and hypergastrinemia were also observed.

Bombesin, which is present in intrinsic nerves running in the lamina propria adjacent to pyloric G cells,[71] might have a role in the genesis of this primary G-cell hyperplasia. In fact, bombesin treatment has been found to stimulate gastrin cell proliferation.[72] Secondary G-cell hypertrophy, hyperplasia, and hyperfunction have been reported in the pyloric mucosa of achlorhydric patients with type A CAG, with or without pernicious anemia.[73-76]

Gastrin Cell Tumors

G-cell tumors associated with hypergastrinemia and peptic ulcer disease have been found only rarely in the stomach,[29,77-81] generally as multifocal lesions coupled with diffuse or micronodular G-cell hyperplasia. The single case we have observed also showed somatostatin cells in the tumor (Table 13-5). Moreover, we observed two mixed ECL-cell G-cell tumors in association with CAG, one arising in a nongastritic pyloric mucosa also showing G-cell hyperplasia[82] and the other in gastritic mucosa of the corpus showing focal pyloric-type metaplasia (see Table 13–5). Two G-cell tumors without peptic ulcer or CAG, one pyloric and one of the corpus, have also been reported.[30]

G-cell tumors are found much more frequently in the duodenal mucosa, coupled with hypergastrinemia and peptic ulcer disease (13% of all cases of ZES)[83] or with nonfunctional tumor signs, or even as unexpected findings during surgery, endoscopy, X-ray analysis, and autopsy.[84,85] We have collected 22 cases of gastrin cell tumors, of which 14 were in patients with peptic ulcer disease and 8 were unexpected findings (4 in the duodenal cuff of gastrectomy specimens resected for gastric cancer and 4 found at endoscopic or radiologic examination).

Duodenal G-cell tumors are nodular or polypoid lesions arising in the Brunner glands or deep crypts, where G cells normally occur, and expanding into the submucosa. Associated G-cell hyperplasia, sometimes chain-forming or micronodular, may be found in nontumor Brunner glands or crypts, especially in cases with multiple tumor foci.[22,86] Deep infiltration of the muscularis propria seems relatively uncommon (3 of 12 cases according to Solcia et al.[22] and 1 of 19 cases in the series of Lasson et al.[85]) and is usually absent in clinically silent tumors. Metastases in periduodenal lymph nodes have been found more frequently (4 of Lasson's 19 cases), especially in functioning tumors: in 26 of 74 (35%) ZES cases free of pancreatic growth in the surgical series of Hofmann et al.[83]

An overall malignancy rate of 38% has been reported in 103 ZES patients with duodenal tumor, 24 of which (23%) had associated pancreatic tumor; whereas 62% of 697 pancreatic gastrinomas without duodenal tumor have been found to be malignant.[83] Frequent multiplicity and association with pancreatic tumors, MEN syndrome, and G-cell hyperplasia limits the value of local tumor excision for duodenal gastrinomas with overt ZES.[83] This therapeutic procedure is recommended for duodenal endocrine tumors that are less than 2 cm in size, lack invasion of the muscularis propria, and are free of metastases.[85]

A fairly distinctive gyriform ribbon structure with scattered pseudorosettes (Soga's B pattern) has been observed in most G-cell tumors from the duodenum, jejunum, and stomach.[22] Poorly formed solid nests and sheets have also been observed. Tumor cells are usually medium-sized and polygonal, with faintly granular, eosinophilic cytoplasm stained blue-black with lead-hematoxylin and yellow-brown with Grimelius' silver.

Gastrin immunohistochemistry is essential for appropriate diagnosis of these tumors and for distinguishing them from somatostatin-producing D-cell tumors, serotonin-producing argentaffin carcinoids, and other endocrine growths occurring in the same area (Figure 13–6). For this purpose, N-terminal–directed gastrin antibodies should be preferred to C-terminal antibodies, which may cross-react with cholecystokinin (CCK) because of structural homology with gastrin at its C-terminal end. In fact, both gastrin and CCK cells have been found to react with most C-terminal gastrin, CCK, and cerulein antibodies, either polyclonal or monoclonal; whereas gastrin and CCK cells were specifically detected with the use of N-terminal gastrin-34 antibodies devoid of any CCK cross-reactivity and with N-terminal CCK-33 antibodies lacking gastrin cross-reactivity.[87] However, so far, only a few cells in a single tumor, among the 12 cases the authors have investigated, showed specific CCK immunoreactivity free of gastrin cross-reactivity (see Figure 13–6B).

Ultrastructural studies of these tumors[88–90] showed a variety of cellular patterns, ranging from classic G cells with vesicular granules of floccular content, storing mainly gastrin-17, to cells with small, round, solid granules (see Figure13–6D) storing mainly gastrin-34 (so-called intestinal gastrin or IG cells)[91] and cells with large, solid, often irregularly shaped granules (so-called VL cells).[20,22] The latter may correspond to the C-terminal gastrin or "tetragastrin" (TG) immunoreactive cells lacking gastrin N-terminal reactivity detected in the small intestine.[12,87,92,93]

Mixed gastrin cell/somatostatin cell (G/D-cell) tumors have been reported in the stomach,[30,57] duodenum,[22,85,89] and jejunum,[94] some of which are associated with peptic ulcer disease but none with the "somatostatinoma" syndrome. Association of G and EC cells has been observed in a jejunal tumor with ZES[95] and of G cells with substance P–immunoreactive argentaffin cells in a tumor of the proximal duodenum.[29]

SOMATOSTATIN CELL GROWTHS

Increased density of somatostatin D cells, coupled with a decreased G/D-cell ratio, has been observed in the pyloric mucosa of patients with gastrinoma, probably due to long-standing hyperchlorhydria.[76] An increased number of somatostatin cells has also been observed in the crypts of the small intestine affected by celiac disease.[96] A case of extreme, possibly congenital, somatostatin cell hyperplasia of the gastroduodenal mucosa, coupled with dwarfism, obesity, and goiter apparently due to severe long-standing somatostatin cell hyperfunction, has been recently described.[97]

A small number (at least 30 cases, mostly from the ampullary region) of duodenal tumors mainly or exclusively composed of well-differentiated, immunohistochemically and/or ultrastructurally proven, somatostatin D cells have been reported in the literature.[23,85,98–102] The majority of them were deeply infiltrating tumors metastatic to paraduodenal lymph nodes. None of the patients developed the full features of the somatostatinoma syndrome (diabetes mellitus, diarrhea, steatorrhea, hypo- or achlorhydria, anemia, and gallstones), which has been reported in association with some pancreatic D-cell tumors,[103–105] although association with diabetes and/or gallstones has been noted in some cases. Admixed gastrin, substance P, VIP, and insulin-immunoreactive cells have been found in a few cases.

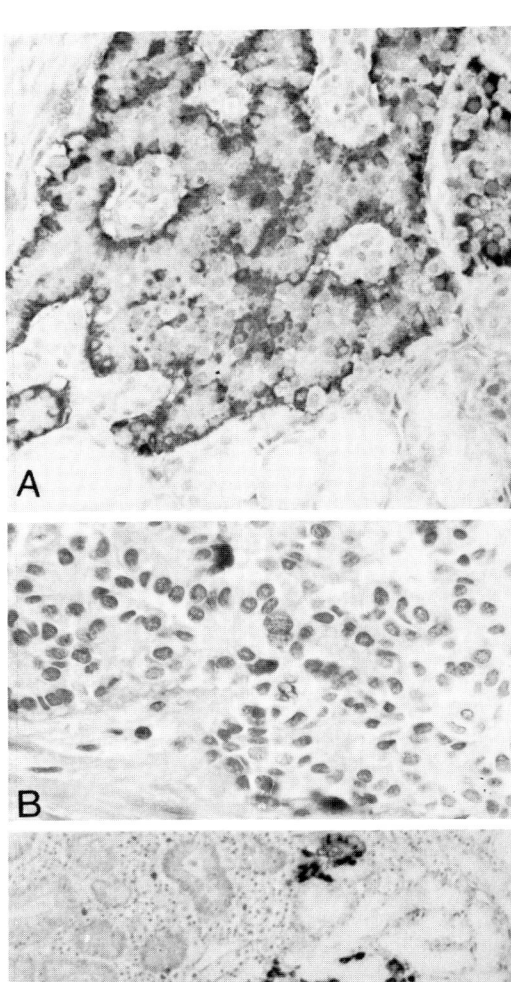

FIGURE 13-6. Multiple duodenal gastrinomas and gastrin cell hyperplasia in a ZES patient. Gastrin immunoreactivity of most tumor cells (A) (immunoperoxidase-hematoxylin, × 150) and rare CCK-immunoreactive cells (B) (serum AB01 from CRB) (immunoperoxidase-hematoxylin, × 280) in a small gastrinoma growing in the Brunner gland area. C, Multifocal, chain-forming hyperplasia of gastrin cells in nontumor Brunner glands. (Immunoperoxidase-hematoxylin, × 110) Note a few gastrin cells in the deep crypts (top left). D, Ultrastructural immunolocalization of gastrin in small (~180 nm), round, solid granules of a tumor cell. (Immunogold technique, × 45,000)

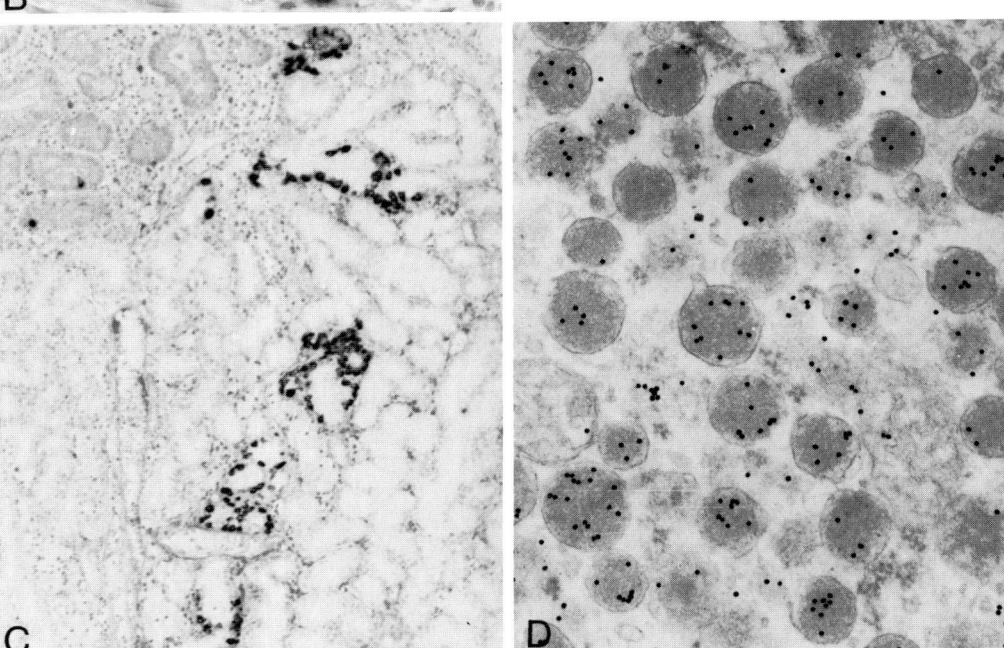

We have personally investigated two duodenal D-cell tumors, both from the ampullary region, one of which was associated with a prominent neuromatous component, and two mixed D/G-cell tumors. Histologically, the D-cell tumors show a prominent glandular or type C structure, with well-formed acini lined by a single row of cuboidal cells, intimately admixed with trabecular and solid-nest foci.[23] Besides somatostatin immunoreactivity, tumor cells show intense lead-hematoxylin staining, consistent argyrophilia with the Davenport (or Hellman-Hellerstrom) technique, and no or scarce argyrophilia with the Grimelius technique. Ultrastructurally, tumor cells are filled with moderately dense, large granules closely resembling those of the D cells observed in normal human duodenum (Figure 13-7).

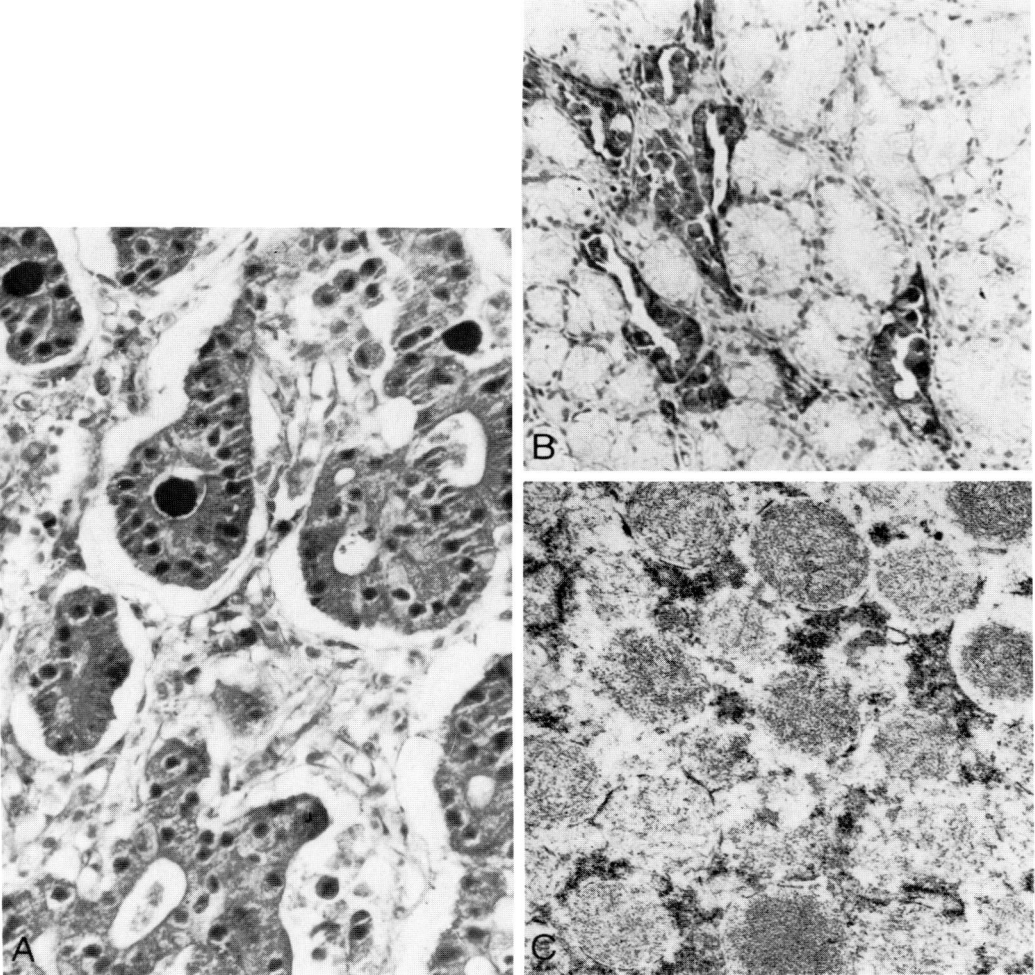

FIGURE 13–7. Duodenal D-cell tumor with cholelithiasis and diabetes (somatostatinoma). *A*, Type C, microglandular arrangement of tumor cells with cytoplasmic granules and intraluminal psammoma bodies. (Lead-hematoxylin, × 230). *B*, Somatostatin-immunoreactivity of tumor cells apparently arising from Brunner glands. (Immunoperoxidase-hematoxylin, × 150) *C*, Large, poorly dense, D-type granules filling the cytoplasm of a tumor cell. Electron microscopy specimen fixed in routine, non-buffered formalin. (× 28,000)

A striking feature of several of these duodenal tumors is the presence of endoluminal (sometimes interstitial or intracellular) psammoma bodies. These concentrically lamellated, heavily periodic acid–Schiff (PAS)-positive, and partly calcific bodies fail to react with both hormone and amyloid tests, contrary to the extracellular deposits found in other endocrine tumors, such as pituitary prolactin cell tumor, thyroid medullary carcinoma, and pancreatic insulinoma, while showing a distinctive substructure characterized by small, radiating, needle-shaped crystals embedded in a granular matrix.[23]

Interestingly, an association between *Von Recklinghausen's multiple neurofibromatosis* and intestinal nonargentaffin carcinoids has been reported in nine cases, eight of which with duodenal tumor (five in the ampullary region) and one in the ileum.[123] Of three cases investigated for hormonal peptides, two showed somatostatin and the other calcitonin immunoreactivity.[31] A tenth case of ampullary tumor associated with neurofibromatosis we have studied showed a gland-forming epithelial endocrine component, made up mostly of somatostatin cells, together with a minority of gastrin cells, as well as a neuromatous component intimately surrounding the endocrine nests (Figure 13–8B). The epithelial nature and endodermal origin of the endocrine component was confirmed by the finding of tumor foci inside the epithelium of ampullary glands.

GANGLIONEUROMATOUS PARAGANGLIOMA (NEUROCARCINOID)

This is a rare tumor resulting from an admixture of (1) polygonal, cuboidal, or columnar epithelial endocrine cells arranged in solid nests and ribbons or forming small tubuloacini, resembling more nonargentaffin carcinoids than nonchromaffin paragangliomas; (2) mature ganglion cells; and (3) Schwann-like spindle cells enveloping nerve cells, axons, and epithelial cells or forming small fascicles.[106–109] Most tumors develop in the submucosa (with or without a mucosal compo-

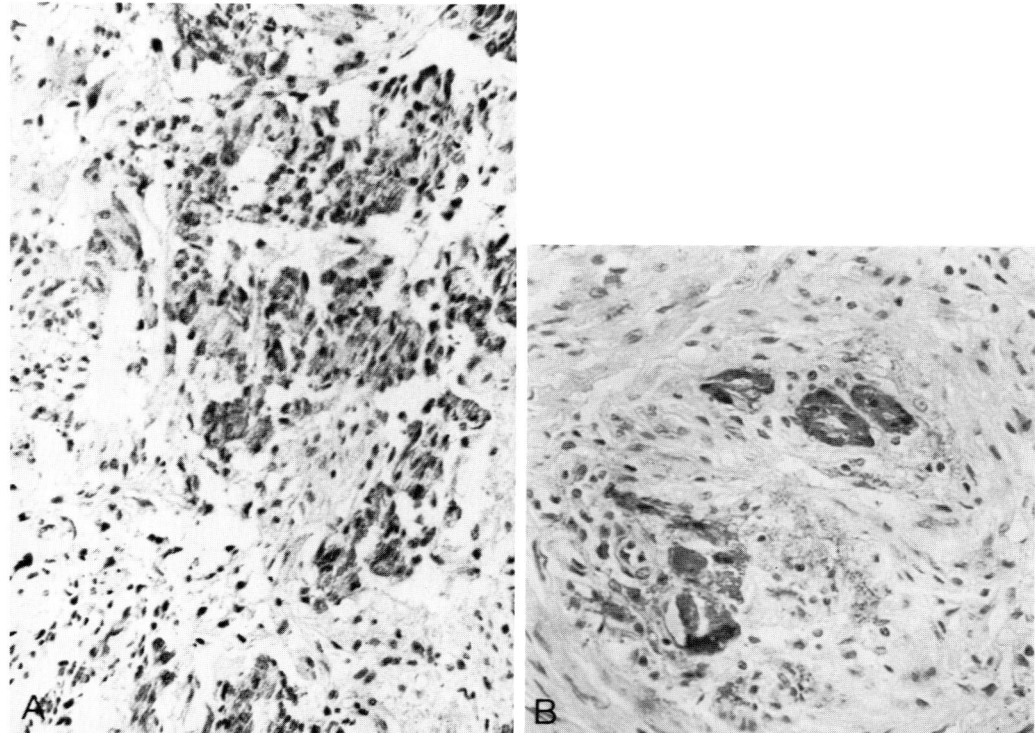

FIGURE 13–8. Two duodenal neuroendocrine tumors whose neuromatous component in one case (A) surrounds solid nests and cords of PP-immunoreactive epithelial cells (ganglioneuromatous "paraganglioma"), whereas in the second case (B) it envelops microglands formed of somatostatin-immunoreactive epithelial cells ("neurosomatostatinoma"). (Immunoperoxidase-hematoxylin, A, × 150; B, × 175)

nent and infiltration of the muscularis propria) of the duodenum, especially in the periampullary region. Occasional cases have been observed in the upper jejunum[110] and stomach.[111]

Because of its usually benign behavior,[109] the tumor seems to be distinguished from purely endocrine tumors (such as gastrin and somatostatin cell tumors and argentaffin or nonargentaffin carcinoids) arising in the same area and known to have some malignant potential. However, a single case with local lymph node metastasis due to its carcinoid-like component has been reported.[112]

The presence, among a manifold population of peptide- and serotonin-immunoreactive cells, of PP-, somatostatin-, and occasionally, glucagon-, insulin-, and gastrin-immunoreactive cells, suggests some relationship with pancreatic endocrine tumors[113,114] or with the ventral pancreatic anlage.[109] An intestinal, rather than a pancreatic, origin of these tumors, on the other hand, is supported by (1) the abundance in the lamina propria of the human intestine during early fetal development of epithelial endocrine cells intimately related with nerves,[115] (2) the occurrence of a few such cells, enveloped by Schwann-like cells together with nerve axons, even in the human adult duodenum and stomach,[15] and (3) the presence of cells immunoreactive to somatostatin, PP/PYY, serotonin, gastrin, and cholecystokinin in both the duodenal (fetal) mucosa and the "paraganglionic" component of reported tumors. In particular, a relationship with the "endodermal-neuroectodermal" complexes described by van Campenhout in fetal duodenum[116] and reputed to be homologous with the "neuroinsular" complexes reported in the pancreas seems attractive.

One of the four cases the authors observed developed around an ectopic growth of pancreatic ducts in the submucosa of the proximal duodenum. This case, together with that occurring around an anomalous common bile duct located in the upper jejunum[110] and with the periampullary origin of many other cases,[106,109,117] suggests that endocrine cells migrate during early fetal development from the intraduodenal part of pancreatic-biliary ducts, from the ampulla, and from periampullary duodenal epithelium into the surrounding mesenchyme, where they interact with the abundant nerves and ganglion cells of the Meissner plexus to form endodermal-neuroectodermal complexes.

The origin of ganglioneuromatous "paragangliomas" from these complexes and from scattered subepithelial endocrine cells would be in keeping with the alleged origin of some appendiceal "neurocarcinoids" from subepithelial endocrine cells forming neuroendocrine complexes scattered in the lamina propria.[118–121] In any case, the epithelial endodermal nature of the endocrine component of the duodenal tumors[109,113,122] is confirmed by its PP and PP-icosapeptide immunoreactivity, with lack of neuropeptide Y (NPY) immunoreactivity, in one of our personally investigated cases (Figure 13–8A). To designate such tumors, the term *neurocarcinoid*, coined by Masson (1924) for their appendiceal counterpart, seems more appropriate than the currently used term *paraganglioma*.

ARGENTAFFIN (EC-CELL) TUMORS

The argentaffin nature of classic midgut carcinoids and their origin from EC cells were first recognized by Gosset and Masson,[124] and their production of 5-HT was discovered by Lembeck.[125] They account for nearly all endocrine tumors arising in the ileum, appendix, and Merkel's diverticulum; the majority of those arising in the jejunum and cecum; and a minority of those occurring in the duodenum, stomach, colon and rectum. In the ileum, they account for 46% of all tumors found at autopsy and 19% of tumors found at surgery.[41]

Small Intestine

Carcinoid tumors of the small intestine have been found in 0.65% of all autopsies at the Mayo Clinic, most of these (133 out of 137 cases) as incidental findings; only 9% showed metastases. On the other hand, 52 of the 72 surgical cases were clinically symptomatic; nearly all metastasized. Intermittent intestinal obstruction was present in 57% of symptomatic patients. The well-known *carcinoid syndrome*, with flushing, diarrhea, valvular involvement, and so forth, was found in only 14 patients (7% of the whole series of 209 cases); all had metastases, 12 of which involved the liver.[41]

The primary tumor, multiple in about one fourth of the cases, usually appears as a deep mucosal-submucosal nodule with apparently intact or slightly eroded overlying mucosa. An origin of ileal multiple EC-cell carcinoids from proliferation of EC cells scattered in the lamina propria, rather than from intraepithelial EC cells of the crypts, has been suggested.[126] Deep infiltration of the muscular wall and peritoneum is a frequent finding. Extensive involvement of the mesentery stimulates considerable fibroblastic reaction with resulting contraction, kinking of the bowel, and obstruction of the lumen. Thus, obstruction, the most frequent and significant among presenting symptoms, is shown only by invasive and relatively advanced disease.[41]

A close relationship was found between the size of the primary lesion and the incidence of metastases. Only 2% of lesions less than 1 cm in diameter, about 50% of those from 1 to 2 cm, and about 80% of those 2 cm or larger showed metastases.[41] The invasive level of the tumor is also significant in this respect. There were no metastases found in 17 superficially invasive tumors, but there were metastases in 23 of 26 deeply invasive cases.[40]

Solid nests or islets of tumor cells, often with peripheral palisading, represent the typical, highly diagnostic (type A) histologic pattern in most argentaffin EC-cell tumors of the midgut (Figure 13–9A). In some cases, glandlike structures of the rosette type appear within the solid nests; this variant of the fundamental structure has been designated as mixed insular and glandular (A + C) structure and seems prognostically more favorable than the pure type A structure.[37] In areas of deep invasion with abundant sclerosis, the cell nests are sometimes compressed into cords and trabeculae.[35] Practically all tumor cells are intensely argyrophilic, lead-hematoxylin–positive, and reactive with chromogranin A antibodies.

The characterization of tumor cells as EC cells can be obtained with a variety of histochemical methods for serotonin, including argentaffin, diazonium, formaldehyde-induced fluorescence, and immunohistochemical tests (Figure 13–9A). Because of the occurrence of serotonin in some non-EC cells and related tumors, as, for instance, in lung bombesin cells and related carcinoid tumors[14,127] or in a fraction of gastric ECL cells and related tumors,[57] electron-microscopic examination of serotonin-immunoreactive tumors (especially those failing to react with the argentaffin test) is necessary to confirm their EC-cell nature, by detecting characteristic pleomorphic, intensely osmiophilic granules (Figure 13–9B).[6,20]

Substance P and other tachykinins, such as eledoisin, physalemin, kassinin, and substance K, have been found to be reliable markers of a fraction (EC_1 cells) of intestinal EC cells as well as of midgut EC-cell carcinoids,[128–133] whereas foregut EC cells and related tumors remain mostly unreactive. Minority populations of enkephalin, somatostatin, gastrin, ACTH, calcitonin, motilin, neurotensin, glucagon/glicentin, and PP-like immunoreactive cells, unassociated with pertinent hyperfunctional signs, have been reported in some ileal and jejunal tumors mostly composed of argentaffin cells.[31,130,132,134] Dopamine and norepinephrine have also been detected, in addition to serotonin, in a type A argentaffin carcinoma of the ileum.[135]

Our experience in nine cases of ileal argentaffin carcinoids agrees with that of Märtensson et al.[132] in that no other hormone apart from serotonin and substance P or related tachykinins is detected in most such tumors. However, we have observed an ileal trabecular nonargentaffin carcinoid with large prevalence of glicentin/PP-immunoreactive L cells over argentaffin EC cells.

Appendix

Most carcinoids of the appendix have been shown to be EC-cell argentaffin tumors of type A or A + C structure,[34,35,124] arising, at least in part, from subepithelial endocrine cells scattered in the deep lamina propria, in close connection with nerves and ganglion cells of the

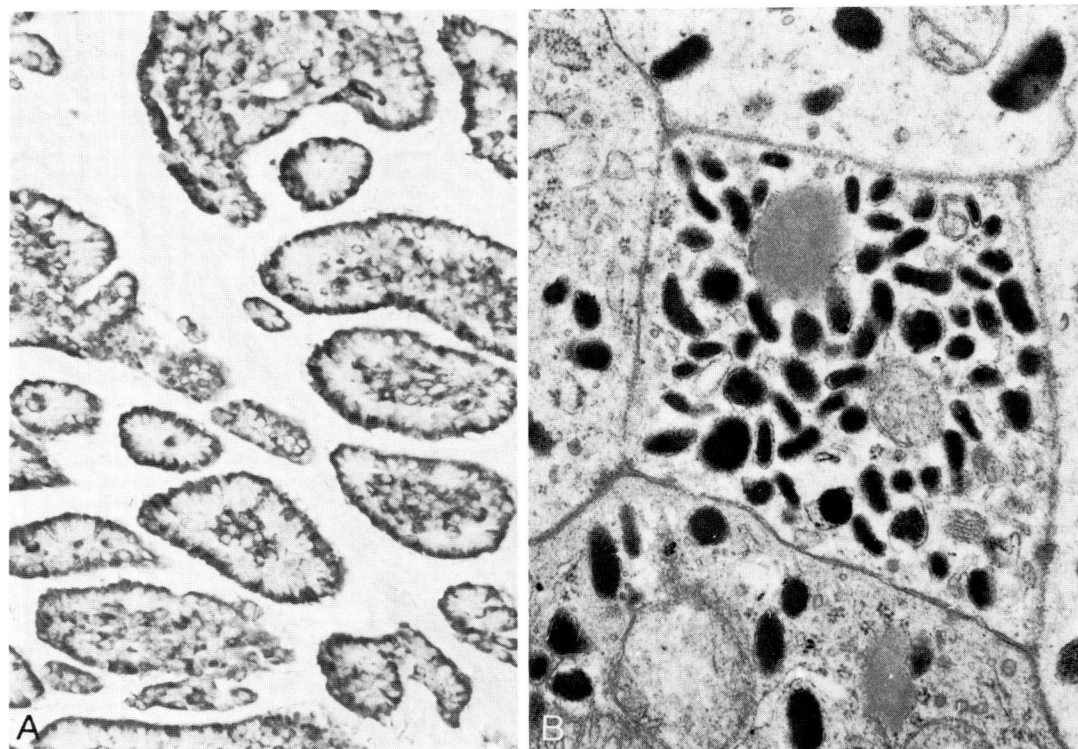

FIGURE 13–9. Argentaffin EC-cell carcinoid of the ileum. A, Argentaffinity of serotonin-storing tumor cells arranged in solid nests with peripheral palisading. (Masson-Fontana method, × 150) B, Ultrastructure of tumor cells to show medium-sized, rod to pyriform, heavily osmiophilic granules characteristic of EC_1 cells. Substance-P immunoreactivity of tumor cells was obtained in paraffin sections. (× 28,000)

Meissner plexus.[118–121,136] Nearly all are small (usually less than 1 cm) tumors, either discovered by chance at operation, incidentally with pelvic or gallbladder surgery,[38] or found in patients undergoing surgery because of symptoms of acute appendicitis.[137] They account for about half the entire group of benign and malignant tumors of the appendix, with sharp predilection (71%) for the tip of the organ[38] (see also Chapter 33).

Most tumors show muscular and lymphatic invasion or perineural involvement; two thirds of cases in Moertel's series also showed invasion of peritoneum, probably through endolymphatic growth. Despite these signs of apparent aggressivity and histologic malignancy, and as is not the case with ileal carcinoids, lymph node or distant metastases were exceptional (1.4% of Moertel's series; 35 cases until 1968 in the world literature), as were associated carcinoid syndromes (5 cases in the literature reviewed by Moertel et al.)[38]; and most cases were cured by appendectomy, without recurrence.[137] Metastatic cases were usually of primary tumors larger than 2 cm.

Argentaffin EC cells of the EC_1 subtype, producing both serotonin and substance P, usually arranged in solid nests with some peripheral palisading (type A structure), occasionally with microlumina (type A + C), have been observed in most cases investigated histochemically and ultrastructurally, including 11 cases from the authors' files. Thus, no relevant histologic, cytologic, or cytochemical difference has been detected between most ileum and appendix carcinoids, despite their very different clinical behavior.

Very small (usually 2 to 3 mm) nonargentaffin tumors with prevalence of type B or B + C structure have been also observed in the appendix.[138] A few such cases the authors have investigated showed glicentin- and PP-immunoreactive cells ultrastructurally resembling L cells,[139] thus reproducing some patterns of rectal L-cell carcinoids. L cells, together with EC and somatostatin cells, are a regular component of the crypt epithelium of the appendix.[121] However, most of the nonargentaffin "carcinoids" described by Dische,[138] with special reference to those showing frank glandular structure, seem to be interpreted as "muco-carcinoids" (see Endocrine-Exocrine Tumors).

Of special interest are the three cases of appendiceal argentaffin microcarcinoid admixed with neuromatous growth observed by Masson,[118] the so-called neurocarcinoid. According to Masson, these growths take origin from "neuro-argentaffin hyperplasia," frequently observed in chronic appendicitis. The intimate relationship of such subepithelial endocrine cells and related carcinoids with nerves of Meissner's plexus has been confirmed by ultrastructural investigations.[120,121,136] A homology of Masson's appendiceal neurocarcinoids with duodenal "paragangliomas" seems obvious (see Ganglioneuromatous Paraganglioma). Intimate relationships of endocrine cells with Schwann cells and nerve axons have been also reported in some rectal carcinoids.[120]

HINDGUT TRABECULAR (L-CELL) TUMORS

Most of these carcinoids arise in the rectum, a few have been reported in the colon, and occasionally even in the pelvic soft tissue posterior to the rectum. They are characterized by predominance of a type B "looped ribbon"[35] pattern, often admixed with type C (tubuloacini or broad, irregular trabeculae with rosettes) and occasionally with type A (solid nest) areas.

Rectal carcinoids account for 12% to 27% of all gastrointestinal carcinoids,[39,43,44] and usually present as submucosal nodules with apparently intact overlying epithelium, sometimes with a polypoid appearance.[140,141] The large majority of these tumors are diagnosed when asymptomatic and measuring less than 1 cm in diameter, usually during investigation of another gastrointestinal lesion. In a 1962 review of the literature, Bates found 234 cases measuring less than 1 cm, 77 between 1 and 2 cm, and 45 more than 2 cm in diameter, whose malignancy rates were 1.7%, 10%, and 82%, respectively.[142] An overall malignancy rate of 15% has been calculated in another study.[39]

As malignancy criteria, invasion of the muscularis propria, regional lymph node metastases, and distant metastases have been considered. Of practical interest is the high correlation found between invasion of the muscularis propria and lymph node metastases, a finding suggesting the use of histologically proven muscular invasion to discriminate invasive tumors, to be treated with radical surgery, from noninvasive tumors, requiring only local excision.[141]

In a series of 62 rectal tumors from routine surgical pathology files that have been investigated immunohistochemically, 48 (77%) have been found to display glucagon/glicentin- and/or PP/PYY-related immunoreactivities typical of intestinal L cells, whereas only 21 (32%) showed 5-HT immunoreactivity and 12 (18%) somatostatin immunoreactivity, usually of few tumor cells.[36,134,143–146] Glucagon-29, glucagon-37, glicentin, proglucagon cryptic fragments, PYY, PP, and pro-PP-icosapeptide, all proved useful immunochemical markers of rectal carcinoids.[36] Minority populations of substance P-, insulin-, enkephalin-, β-endorphin-, neurotensin-, and motilin-immunoreactive cells have been observed in occasional tumors.[134,145] Recently, 16 of 24 rectal carcinoids tested (67%) showed immunoreactivity for prostatic acid phosphatase, a finding relatively unusual in other gut endocrine tumors and possibly related with the common origin of rectum and prostate from cloacal hindgut.[147]

Thus, L cells seem to represent the dominant tumor cell component in rectal carcinoids and to be positively related with their type B or B + C structure (Figure 13–10). A relationship between type A solid-nest areas of both rectal and colonic tumors and serotonin-producing EC cells has also been noted.[35,36] A similar correlation of histologic patterns, tumor cell types, and hormones produced has been observed in the appendix, small bowel, and ovary, where L-cell trabecular carcinoids with glicentin/PP-related immunoreactivities occur rarely,[14] in addition to the prevalent type A serotonin-producing EC-cell tumors.[148]

Colonic carcinoids are relatively rare, with preference for the cecum. In comparison with rectal tumors, they are larger in size (mean, 4.9 cm) and with a higher relative frequency of 5-HT-producing tumors, sometimes with the classic syndrome.[149]

No definite hyperfunctional syndrome has been identified in association with L-cell tumors producing enteroglucagon (glucagon-37, glicentin) and PP/PYY-related hormonal peptides, with the exception of an "enteroglucagon-producing" tumor found in the kidney[150] and proven to consist of L cells,[20] which was associated with reduced intestinal motility and absorption as well as hypertrophy of the intestinal mucosa.[151] Constipation was also one of the main complaints of patients bearing trabecular rectal tumors.[141] The classic carcinoid syndrome has been reported only exceptionally in association with rectal carcinoids, which proved to be of 5-HT–producing argentaffin type.[152]

INAPPROPRIATE ENDOCRINE TUMORS

Differentiated endocrine tumors producing inappropriate hormones, such as calcitonin,[153,154] adrenocorticotropic hormone/melanocyte-stimulating hormone (ACTH/MSH),[155–157] growth hormone (GH), gonadotropin-releasing factor (GRF),[158] vasoactive intestinal peptide (VIP),[159] and related hyperfunctional syndromes have rarely been observed in the gut.[135] Minority populations of inappropriate cells, including insulin, ACTH, calcitonin, VIP, human chorionic gonadotropin (hCG), and related α-chain, in the absence of pertinent functional or pathologic signs, have been found more frequently.[31,134,145] It should be recalled that β-endorphin–, β-lipotropin–, and pro-α-MSH–immunoreactive endocrine cells have been observed in normal human intestine,[12] so that β-endorphin–producing tumors occasionally found in the rectum[145] are not necessarily to be interpreted as "inappropriate." Moreover, although in man VIP is exclusively found in nerves, VIP-producing epithelial endocrine cells have been reported in the gut of other species.[160]

OTHER GUT ENDOCRINE TUMORS

Tumors lacking functional or cytologic characterization are frequently diagnosed as "carcinoids," especially "nonargentaffin carcinoids," by pathologists. Most of such tumors, when appropriately investigated, will fit in one of the tumor entities of Table 13–4. However, a few such tumors may escape final identification because of inappropriate fixation or processing of tumor tissue. For these tumors the generic diagnosis of "carcinoid," a time-honored and noncommittal labeling, should be retained. Clinically nonfunctioning argyrophil tumors showing ultrastructural resemblance

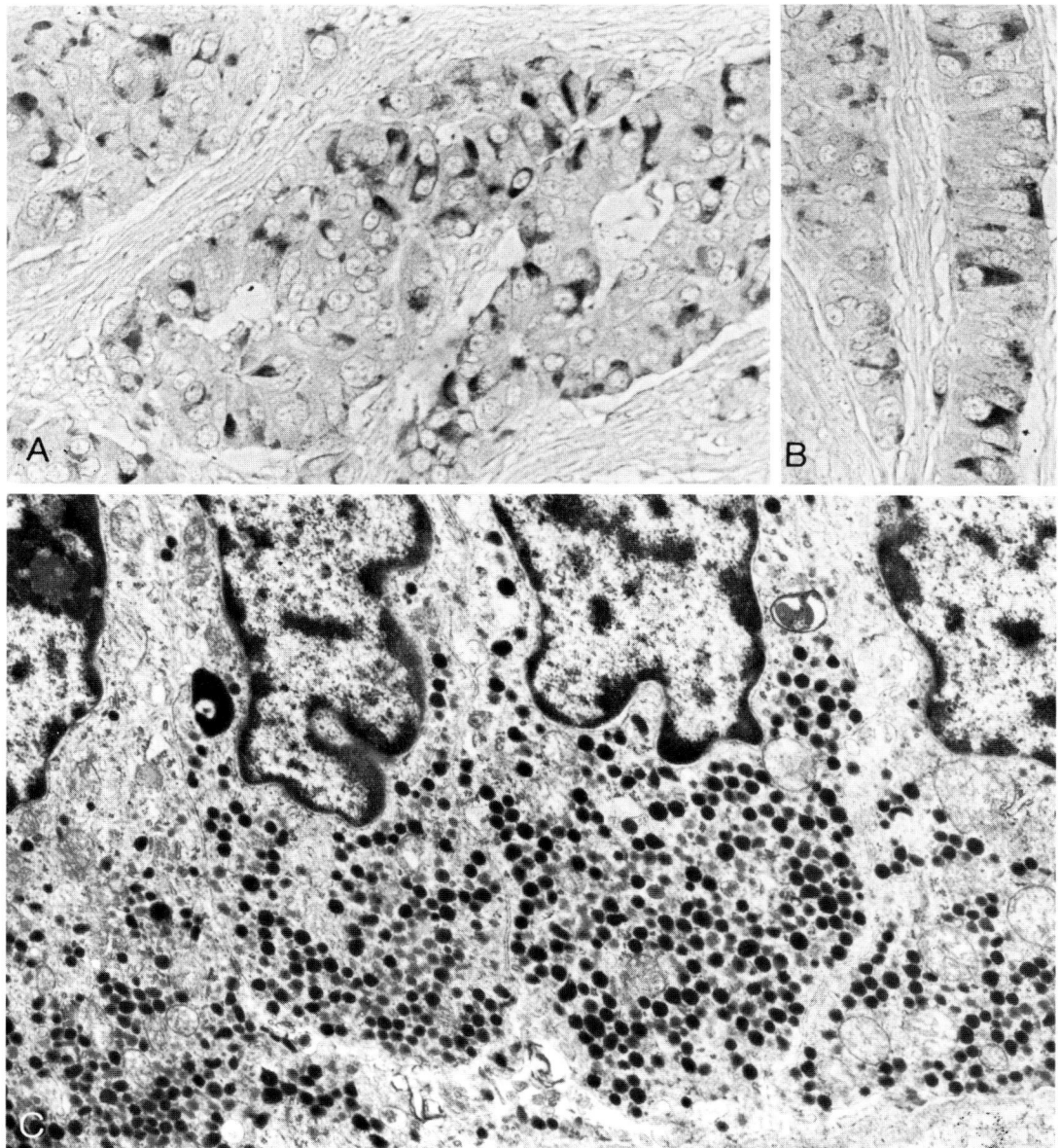

FIGURE 13-10. Rectal carcinoid. *A*, Glicentin C-terminus immunoreactivity of many tumor cells (serum R4804 from Prof. N. Yanaihara, Shizuoka, Japan). (Immunoperoxidase, × 360) *B*, PP-immunoreactive cells in a tumor trabecula. (Immunoperoxidase, × 360) *C*, Round to slightly angular secretory granules filling the "basal" cytoplasm of tumor cells aligned perpendicularly in a trabecula. (× 13,700)

to gut P cells, with small thin-haloed granules and no known hormone reactivity, have seldom been observed in the stomach and duodenum.

A small mucosal-submucosal tumor composed of small, heavily argyrophilic (with both Grimelius' and Sevier-Munger's techniques) cells arising from the crypts of the duodenal bulb has been observed in a patient with long-standing, severe hyperchlorhydria and peptic ulcer disease due to pancreatic gastrinoma (Figure 13-11). PP and neurotensin immunoreactivity has been detected in some tumor cells. Nonargentaffin cells of the duodenal mucosa reacting heavily with both Grimelius' and Sevier-Munger's techniques have been recently identified as secretin cells.[17] Severe hypersecretinemia has been reported in hyperchlorhydric ZES patients,[161] probably due to HCl-stimulated secretin cell hyperfunction and, possibly, hyperplasia.

A glucagon-immunoreactive tumor associated with the "glucagonoma" syndrome has been reported in the duodenum.[162]

POORLY DIFFERENTIATED ENDOCRINE (NEUROENDOCRINE) CARCINOMAS

The occurrence in the esophagus of small- to intermediate-cell carcinomas resembling oat cell carcinoma of the lung has been known for a long time.[163] That at

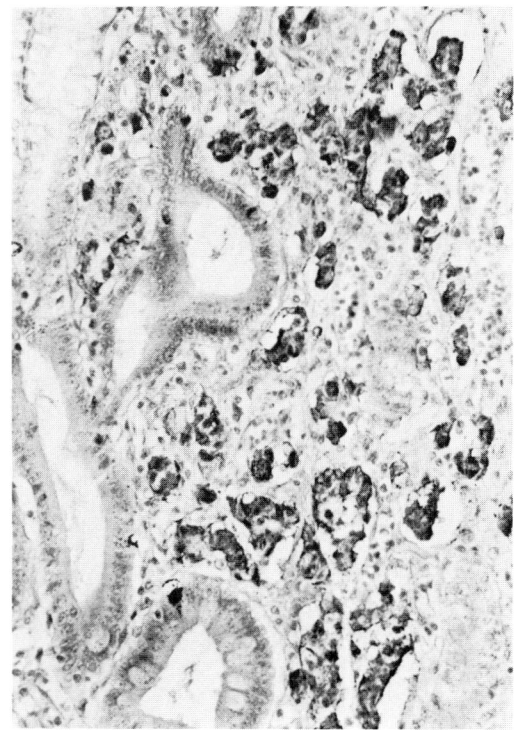

FIGURE 13–11. Strongly argyrophil nonargentaffin tumor cords and small nests arising from duodenal crypts in a patient with ZE syndrome due to a pancreatic gastrinoma. PP and neurotensin immunoreactivity was obtained in some cells. Diagnosis: argyrophil non-argentaffin carcinoid with PP and neurotensin cells. (Grimelius' silver, × 150)

least part of these tumors show histologic, histochemical, and ultrastructural signs of endocrine or neuroendocrine (i.e., storage of amines and peptides normally produced by both endocrine and neural structures) differentiation has been recognized more recently.[164,165] Similar tumors have been reported in the stomach[57,166,167] and colon.[168]

Under conventional light microscopy (Figure 13–12A) poorly differentiated endocrine carcinomas are characterized by small to intermediate-sized, round to spindle-shaped cells with indistinct nucleoli and scanty cytoplasm arranged in poorly defined solid nests and sheets, often with necrotic centers (Soga's type D structure). Scattered argyrophilic cells or cell processes were observed in many cases when stained with Grimelius' silver; serotonin and appropriate or inappropriate hormonal peptides (calcitonin, ACTH, etc.) have been detected more rarely. Ultrastructurally, a few, small (100 to 200 nm in diameter) secretory granules resembling those of immature "protoendocrine" cells of early fetal development[169] have been observed (Figure 13–12B), often concentrated in thin cell processes not seen with conventional light-microscopic study.[57,170]

None of the tumors so far reported was associated with an overt endocrine syndrome, even when hormonelike immunoreactivities were detected in tumor tissue, possibly because of the scarce amount of hormone produced or because inactive prohormones, rather than active molecular species, were produced. All the tumors studied by Gould and co-workers had histologic signs suggestive of high malignancy (high

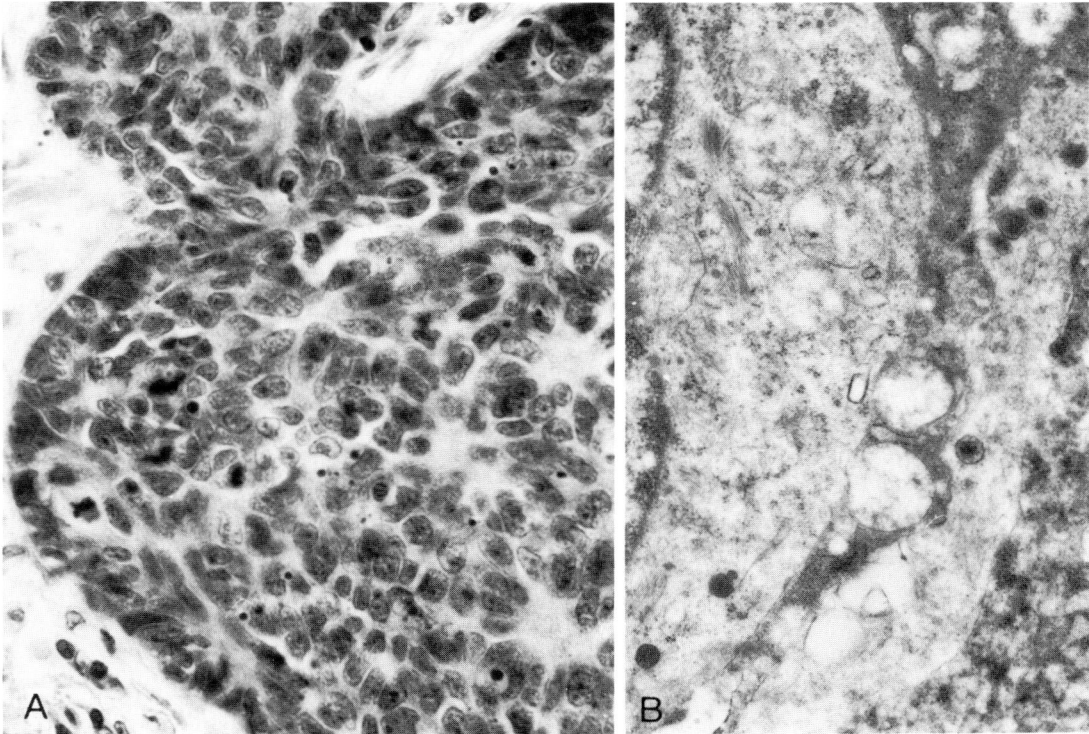

FIGURE 13–12. A, Small- to intermediate-cell endocrine carcinoma of the stomach. Note the arrangement of tumor cells to form some rosettelike structures and attempts at peripheral palisading. No hormone reactivity was obtained apart from scattered hCG immunoreactivity. (H&E, × 400) B, Ultrastructure of the same tumor to show a few, small "protoendocrine" granules. (× 14,000)

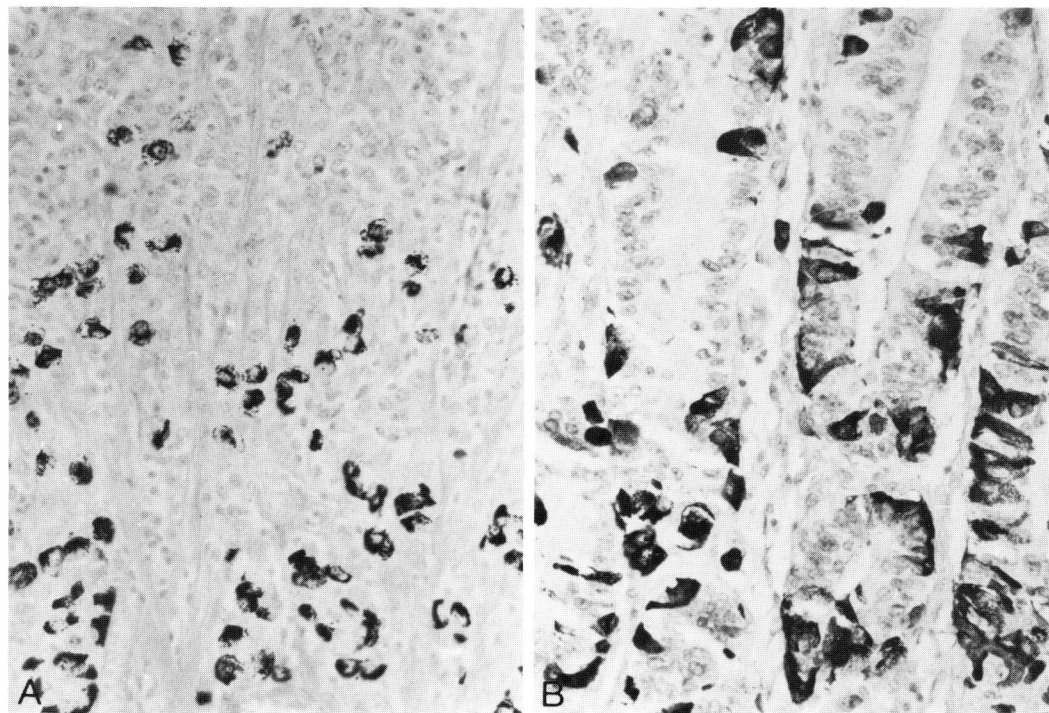

FIGURE 13–13. Argyrophil endocrine cells in gastric combined carcinoma of diffuse (A) and glandular (B) type. (Grimelius' silver, × 220)

mitotic rate, extensive tissue infiltration, angioinvasion); nearly all metastasized; and all of the patients died within 1 to 16 months from diagnosis.[170]

In fact, these poorly differentiated carcinomas with focal signs of abortive endocrine differentiation appear to display the same aggressive behavior as poorly differentiated carcinomas lacking endocrine differentiation. Abortive foci of squamous (esophagus) or glandular (stomach, colon) differentiation may also be found in such tumors, suggesting that we are dealing essentially with undifferentiated tumor cells undergoing focal and abortive multidirectional differentiation, of which endocrine differentiation seems to occur more frequently, in keeping with the early development of endocrine cells from the immature gut epithelium.[169]

ENDOCRINE-EXOCRINE TUMORS

Sporadic differentiation of one or more lines of endocrine cells inside nonendocrine neoplasms of the gut has been observed frequently—for instance, in 13% of gastric carcinomas[171] and 9% of intestinal adenomas.[172] Endocrine cells occur more frequently in association with mucopeptic, rather than foveolar, growths of the stomach[173] and more with diffuse than with glandular carcinomas.[174,175] As a rule, the lines of endocrine cell differentiation are coherent with the exocrine cell lines, both occurring in the normal tissue mimicked by the tumor growth.

No apparent change of tumor prognosis or clinical behavior has been reported for most of these tumors, compared with histologically similar tumors of the same site lacking endocrine cells. However, their endocrine component may well explain clinically relevant hyperfunction occasionally reported in association with ordinary carcinoma, such as the skin melanosis associated with a MSH-producing gastric papillary adenocarcinoma[176] or the ZES due to a gastrin-producing mucinous cystadenocarcinoma of the ovary.[177]

Mixed endocrine-exocrine tumors in which the endocrine component forms a major cell population, either intimately and diffusely admixed with the nonendocrine component (combined tumors) or occurring in separate areas of the same tumor (composite tumors), are also known.

Combined Tumors

In gastric combined tumors (Figure 13–13) the endocrine cells (including gastrin, somatostatin, argentaffin, and ECL cells) seem more frequently associated with "poorly differentiated" scirrhous and mucin-producing growths,[178,179] although a mucin-producing tubular carcinoma resembling pyloric glands has also been reported.[180] In cases of scirrhous argyrophil carcinoma the authors have also investigated the nonendocrine component and found either group II (mostly in the absence of group I) pepsinogen, a known marker of pyloric type mucopeptic differentiation, or intestinal crypt markers.[173] The lysozyme, M_2 glycoprotein antigen, and gastrin immunoreactivities observed in these combined tumors[178,179] also suggest pyloric gland or intestinal crypt differentiation. Interestingly, in early gastric cancers argyrophil cells have been found mainly in deeply situated mucopeptic or intestinal crypt growths, rather than in juxtaluminal foveolar growths of either glandular or signet-ring type.[173,181]

Abundant endocrine cells occur more rarely in well-differentiated intestinal adenocarcinomas.[182] Diffusely infiltrating goblet cell carcinomas, with or without signet-ring change, containing numerous endocrine cells have been observed.[174,183] These may represent the more malignant counterpart of the so-called goblet cell carcinoid,[184,185] goblet cell carcinoma,[186] goblet cell adenocarcinoid,[187] or crypt cell carcinoma[188] frequently observed in the appendix (see also Chapter 33). This is a low-grade microglandular and cord-forming tumor showing goblet cells, columnar cells, lysozyme-producing and secretory component–producing cells as well as endocrine cells of EC, L, or D type, often representing a consistent minority (up to 30%) of tumor cells. Because of its distinctive morphology and behavior, this well-differentiated "organoid" growth mimicking intestinal crypts is to be separated from both true, endocrine carcinoids and ordinary adenocarcinomas.[187,188]

Composite Tumors

Composite adenocarcinoma-carcinoid tumors have been observed in the large intestine,[189,190] small intestine,[191] and stomach.[192,193] These tumors, even in the presence of lymph node metastases, might have a more favorable prognosis than ordinary adenocarcinoma, thus approaching the prognosis of differentiated malignant carcinoids.[193] Care must be taken, by means of appropriate histochemical and ultrastructural investigations, to distinguish the endocrine component of composite tumors from trabecular and solid carcinomas showing areas of peripheral palisading or basaloid patterns, mimicking histologically an endocrine growth but lacking histochemical and ultrastructural signs of true endocrine differentiation.

Occasionally, *amphicrine cells* showing both exocrine and endocrine granules in their cytoplasm, often at opposite poles of the cell, as a result of simultaneous differentiation toward endocrine and exocrine lines, have been reported in adenocarcinomas from the stomach, intestine, appendix, and esophagus.[194–196]

References

1. Grimelius L: A silver nitrate stain for α_2 cells in human pancreatic islets. Acta Soc Med Upsal 73:243–270, 1968.
2. Solcia E, Capella C, Vassallo G: Lead-haematoxylin as a stain for endocrine cells: Significance of staining and comparison with other selective methods. Histochemie 20:116–126, 1969.
3. Bishop AE, Polak JM, Facer P, et al: Neuron specific enolase: A common marker for the endocrine cells and innervation of the gut and pancreas. Gastroenterology 83:902–915, 1982.
4. Lloyd RV, Wilson BS: Specific endocrine tissue marker defined by a monoclonal antibody. Science 222:628–630, 1983.
5. Rindi G, Buffa R, Sessa F, et al: Chromogranin A, B and C immunoreactivities of mammalian endocrine cells: Distribution, distinction from costored hormones/prohormones and relationship with the argyrophil component of secretory granules. Histochemistry 85:19–28, 1986.
6. Solcia E, Capella C, Vassallo G, Buffa R: Endocrine cells of the gastric mucosa. Int Rev Cytol 42:223–286, 1975.
7. Pearse AGE, Polak JM: The diffuse neuroendocrine system and the APUD concept. In Bloom SR (ed): Gut Hormones. Edinburgh, Churchill Livingstone, 1978, pp 33–39.
8. Le Douarin NM: The embryological origin of the endocrine cells associated with the digestive tract: Experimental analysis based on the use of a stable cell marking technique. In Bloom SR (ed): Gut Hormones. Edinburgh, Churchill Livingstone, 1978, pp 49–56.
9. Solcia E, Polak JM, Pearse AGE, et al: Lausanne 1977 classification of gastroenteropancreatic endocrine cells. In Bloom SR (ed): Gut Hormones. Edinburgh, Churchill Livingstone, 1978, pp 40–48.
10. Solcia E, Creutzfeldt W, Falkmer S, et al: Human gastroenteropancreatic endocrine-paracrine cells: Santa Monica 1980 classification. In Lechago J, Grossman MI, Walsh JH (eds): Cellular Basis of Chemical Messengers in the Digestive System. New York, Academic Press, 1981, pp 159–165.
11. Fiocca R, Sessa F, Tenti P, et al: Pancreatic polypeptide (PP) cells in the PP-rich lobe of the human pancreas are identified ultrastructurally and immunocytochemically as F cells. Histochemistry 77:511–523, 1983.
12. Sjölund K, Sandén G, Håkanson R, Sundler F: Endocrine cells in human intestine: An immunocytochemical study. Gastroenterology 85:1120–1130, 1983.
13. Böttcher G, Sjölund K, Ekblad E, et al: Coexistence of peptide YY and glicentin immunoreactivity in endocrine cells of the gut. Reg Pept 8:261–266, 1984.
14. Solcia E, Capella C, Buffa R, et al: Cytology of tumours in the gastroenteropancreatic and diffuse (neuro)endocrine system. In Falkmer S, Håkanson R, Sundler F (eds): Evolution and Tumour Pathology of the Neuroendocrine System. Amsterdam, Elsevier, 1984, pp 453–480.
15. Solcia E, Capella C, Buffa R, et al: Endocrine cells of the digestive system. In Johnson LR (ed): Physiology of the Gastrointestinal Tract. 2nd ed. New York, Raven Press, 1986, pp 111–130.
16. Usellini L, Buchan AMJ, Polak JM, et al: Ultrastructural localization of motilin in endocrine cells of human and dog intestine by the immunogold technique. Histochemistry 81:363–368, 1984.
17. Usellini L, Capella C, Frigerio B, et al: Ultrastructural localization of secretin in endocrine cells of the dog duodenum by the immunogold technique. Comparison with ultrastructurally characterized S cells of various mammals. Histochemistry 80:435–441, 1984.
18. Usellini L, Capella C, Solcia E, et al: Ultrastructural localization of gastric inhibitory polypeptide (GIP) in a well characterized endocrine cell of canine duodenal mucosa. Histochemistry 80:85–89, 1984.
19. Usellini L, Capella C, Malesci A, et al: Ultrastructural localization of cholecystokinin in endocrine cells of the dog duodenum by the immunogold technique. Histochemistry 83:331–336, 1985.
20. Solcia E, Capella C, Buffa R, et al: Endocrine cells of the gastrointestinal tract and related tumors. Pathobiol Annu 9:163–203, 1979.
21. Feyrter F: Uber die peripheren endocrinen (parakrinen) Drüsen des Menschen. Wien-Düsseldorf, W Maudrich, 1953.
22. Solcia E, Capella C, Buffa R, et al: Pathology of the Zollinger-Ellison syndrome. In Fenoglio CM (ed): Progress in Surgical Pathology. Vol. 1. New York, Masson Publishing USA, 1980, pp 119–133.
23. Dayal Y, Nunnemacher G, Doos WG, et al: Psammomatous somatostatinomas of the duodenum. Am J Surg Pathol 7:656–665, 1983.
24. Carlei F, Polak JM: Antibodies to neuron-specific enolase for the delineation of the entire diffuse neuroendocrine system in health and disease. Semin Diagn Pathol 1:59–70, 1984.

25. O'Connor DT, Burton D, Deftos LH: Immunoreactive human chromogranin A in diverse polypeptide producing human tumors and normal endocrine tissues. J Clin Endocrinol Metab 57:1084–1086, 1983.
26. Lloyd RV, Warner TFC, Mervak T, et al: Immunohistochemical detection of chromogranin and neuron-specific enolase in pancreatic endocrine neoplasms. Am J Surg Pathol 8:607–614, 1984.
27. Solcia E, Capella C, Buffa R, et al: Antigenic markers of neuroendocrine tumors: Their diagnostic and prognostic value. In Fenoglio CM, Weinstein RS, Kaufman N (eds): New Concepts in Neoplasia as Applied to Diagnostic Pathology. Baltimore, Williams and Wilkins, 1986, pp 242–261.
28. Widenmann B, Franke WW, Kuhn C, et al: Synaptophysin: A novel marker protein for neuroendocrine cells and neoplasms. Proc Natl Acad Sci USA 83:3500–3504, 1986.
29. Wilander E, Grimelius L, Lundquist G, Skoog V: Polypeptide hormones in argentaffin and argyrophil gastroduodenal endocrine tumors. Am J Pathol 96:519–530, 1979.
30. Alumets J, Sundler F, Falkmer S, et al: Neurohormonal peptides in endocrine tumors of the pancreas, stomach, and upper small intestine. I: An immunohistochemical study of 27 cases. Ultrastruct Pathol 5:55–72, 1983.
31. Dayal Y, Wolfe H: Regulatory substances in clinically nonfunctioning gastrointestinal carcinoids. In Falkmer S, Håkanson R, Sundler F (eds): Evolution and Tumour Pathology of the Neuroendocrine System. Amsterdam, Elsevier, 1984, pp 497–517.
32. Williams ED, Sandler M: The classification of carcinoid tumours. Lancet 1:238–239, 1963.
33. Solcia E, Capella C, Buffa R, et al: The contribution of immunohistochemistry to the diagnosis of neuroendocrine tumors. Semin Diagn Pathol 1:285–296, 1984.
34. Soga J, Tazawa K: Pathologic analysis of carcinoids. Histologic reevaluation os 62 cases. Cancer 28:990–998, 1971.
35. Dawson IMP: The endocrine cells of the gastrointestinal tract and the neoplasms which arise from them. Curr Top Pathol 63:222–258, 1976.
36. Fiocca R, Rindi G, Capella C, et al: Glucagon, glicentin, proglucagon, PYY, PP and proPP-icosapeptide immunoreactivities of rectal carcinoid tumors and related non-tumor cells. Regul Pept 17:9–29, 1987.
37. Johnson LA, Lavin P, Moertel CG, et al: Carcinoids: The association of histologic growth pattern and survival. Cancer 51:882–889, 1983.
38. Moertel CG, Dockerty MB, Judd ES: Carcinoid tumors of the vermiform appendix. Cancer 21:270–278, 1968.
39. Godwin JD: Carcinoid tumors: An analysis of 2837 cases. Cancer 36:560–569, 1975.
40. Hajdu S, Winawer SJ, Myers WPL: Carcinoid tumors. A study of 204 cases. Am J Clin Pathol 61:521–528, 1974.
41. Moertel CG, Sauer G, Dockerty MB, Baggenstoss AH: Life history of the carcinoid tumor of the small intestine. Cancer 14:901–912, 1961.
42. Greenwood SM, Huvos AG, Erlandson RA, Malt SH: Rectal carcinoid and rectal adenocarcinoma: A case report and review of the literature. Dis Colon Rectum 17:644–655, 1974.
43. Zeitels J, Naunheim K, Kaplan EL, Straus F: Carcinoid tumors: A 37-year experience. Arch Surg 117:732–737, 1982.
44. Zakariai YM, Quan SH, Hajdu SI: Carcinoid tumors of the gastrointestinal tract. Cancer 35:588–591, 1975.
45. Brodman HR, Pai BN: Malignant carcinoid of the stomach and distal esophagus: Review of literature and case report. Am J Dig Dis 13:677–681, 1968.
46. Pestana C, Beahrs OH, Woolner LB: Multiple (seven) carcinoids of the stomach: Report of a case. Proc Mayo Clin 38:453–456, 1963.
47. Black WC, Haffner HE: Diffuse hyperplasia of gastric argyrophil cells and multiple carcinoid tumors: An historical and ultrastructural study. Cancer 21:1080–1099, 1968.
48. Lattes R, Grossi C: Carcinoid tumors of the stomach. Cancer 9:698–711, 1956.
49. Vassallo G, Capella C, Solcia E: Endocrine cells of the human gastric mucosa. Z Zellforsch 118:49–67, 1971.
50. Larsson LI, Rehfeld JF, Stockbrügger R, et al: Mixed endocrine gastric tumors associated with hypergastrinemia of antral origin. Am J Pathol 93:53–68, 1978.
51. Capella C, Polak JM, Frigerio B, Solcia E: Gastric carcinoids of argyrophil ECL cells. Ultrastruct Pathol 1:411–418, 1980.
52. Hodges JR, Isaacson P, Wright R: Diffuse enterochromaffin-like (ECL) cell hyperplasia and multiple gastric carcinoids: A complication of pernicious anaemia. Gut 22:237–241, 1981.
53. Carney JA, Go VLW, Fairbanks VF, et al: The syndrome of gastric argyrophil carcinoid tumors and nonantral gastric atrophy. Ann Intern Med 99:761–766, 1983.
54. Borch K, Renvall H, Liedberg G: Gastric endocrine cell hyperplasia and carcinoid tumors in pernicious anemia. Gastroenterology 88:638–648, 1985.
55. Solcia E, Capella C, Vassallo G: Endocrine cells of the stomach and pancreas in states of gastric hypersecretion. Rendic Gastroenterol 2:147–158, 1970.
56. Bordi C, Cocconi G, Togni R, et al: Gastric endocrine cell proliferation: Association with Zollinger-Ellison syndrome. Arch Pathol 98:274–278, 1974.
57. Solcia E, Capella C, Sessa F, et al: Gastric carcinoids and related endocrine growths. Digestion 35(Suppl 1):3–22, 1986.
58. Rubin W: Proliferation of endocrine-like (enterochromaffin) cells in atrophic gastric mucosa. Gastroenterology 57:641–648, 1969.
59. Bordi C, Gabrielli M, Missale G: Pathological changes of endocrine cells in atrophic gastritis. Arch Pathol Lab Med 102:129–135, 1978.
60. Bordi C, Ravazzola M: Endocrine cells in the intestinal metaplasia of gastric mucosa. Am J Pathol 96:391–398, 1979.
61. Bordi C, Ravazzola M, De Vita O: Pathology of endocrine cells in gastric mucosa. Ann Pathol (Paris) 3:19–28, 1983.
62. Bordi C, Senatore S, Missale G: Gastric carcinoid following gastrojejunostomy. Am J Dig Dis 21:667–671, 1976.
63. Sandler M, Snow PJD: An atypical carcinoid tumour secreting 5-hydroxytryptophan. Lancet 1:137–139, 1958.
64. Oates JA, Sjoerdsma A: A unique syndrome associated with secretion of 5-hydroxytryptophan by metastatic gastric carcinoids. Am J Med 32:333–342, 1962.
65. Roberts LJ, Bloomgarden ZT, Marney SR, et al: Histamine from a gastric carcinoid: Provocation by pentagastrin and inhibition by somatostatin. Gastroenterology 84:272–275, 1983.
66. Håkanson R, Owman CH, Sjöberg NO, Sporrong B: Amine mechanisms in enterochromaffin and enterochromaffin-like cells of gastric mucosa in various mammals. Histochemie 21:189–220, 1970.
67. Hage E, Hage J: A gastric carcinoma identified as an ECL-oma associated with acanthosis nigricans. In Fujita T (ed): Endocrine Gut and Pancreas. Amsterdam, Elsevier, 1976, pp 359–363.
68. Polak JM, Stagg B, Pearse AGE: Two types of Zollinger-Ellison syndrome: Immunofluorescent, cytochemical and ultrastructural studies of the antral and pancreatic gastrin cells in different clinical states. Gut 13:501–512, 1972.
69. Keuppens F, Willems G, Degraef J, Woussen-Colle MC: Antral gastrin cell hyperplasia in patients with peptic ulcer. Ann Surg 191:276–281, 1980.
70. Friesen SR, Tomita T: Pseudo-Zollinger-Ellison syndrome: Hypergastrinemia, hyperchlorhydria without tumor. Ann Surg 194:481–491, 1981.
71. Buffa R, Solovieva I, Fiocca R, et al: Localization of bombesin and GRP (gastrin releasing peptide) sequences in gut nerves or endocrine cells. Histochemistry 76:457–467, 1982.
72. Lehy T, Accardy JP, Labeille D, Dubrasquet M: Chronic administration of bombesin stimulates antral gastrin cell proliferation in the rat. Gastroenterology 84:914–919, 1983.
73. Creutzfeldt W, Arnold R, Creutzfeldt C, et al: Gastrin and G-cells in the antral mucosa of patients with pernicious anaemia, acromegaly, and hyperparathyroidism and in a Zollinger-Ellison tumour of the pancreas. Eur J Clin Invest 1:461–479, 1971.
74. Stockbrugger R, Larsson LI, Lundqvist G, Angervall L: Antral gastrin cells and serum gastrin in achlorhydria. Scand J Gastroenterol 12:209–213, 1977.
75. Solcia E, Frigerio B, Capella C: Gastrin and related endocrine cells modulating gastric secretion. In Rehfeld JF, Amdrup E (eds): Gastrin and the Vagus. London, Academic Press, 1979, pp 31–39.

76. Arnold R, Hülst MV, Neuhof CH, et al: Antral gastrin-producing G-cells and somatostatin-producing D-cells in different states of gastric acid secretion. Gut 23:285–291, 1982.
77. Royston CMS, Brew DSJ, Garnham JR, et al: The Zollinger-Ellison syndrome due to an infiltrating tumour of the stomach. Gut 13:638–642, 1972.
78. Larsson LI, Ljungberg O, Sundler F, et al: Antropyloric gastrinoma associated with pancreatic nesidioblastosis and proliferation of islets. Virchows Arch [A] 360:305–314, 1973.
79. Bhagavan BS, Hofkin GA, Woel GM, Koss LG: Zollinger-Ellison syndrome: Ultrastructural and histochemical observations in a child with endocrine tumorlets of gastric antrum. Arch Pathol 98:217–222, 1974.
80. Soulé JC, Potet F, Mignon FC, et al: Syndrome de Zollinger-Ellison dû à un gastrinome gastrique. Arch Fr Mal Appar Dig 65:215–225, 1976.
81. Berger B, Chayvialle JA, Berger F: Ulcère duodénal associé à un microgastrinome pylorique et à une gastrinose focale antropylorique. Nouv Presse Méd 7:1937–1940, 1978.
82. Russo A, Buffa R, Grasso G, Giannone G, Sanfilippo G, Sessa F, Solcia E: Gastric gastrinoma and diffuse G cell hyperplasia associated with chronic atrophic gastritis. Digestion 20:416–419, 1980.
83. Hofmann JW, Fox PS, Milwaukee SDW: Duodenal wall tumors and the Zollinger-Ellison syndrome. Arch Surg 107:334–338, 1973.
84. Berger G, Patricot LM, Guillaud MT, et al: Les gastrinomes silencieux pyloro-duodénaux: A propos de trois observations. Ann Anat Pathol (Paris) 22:5–20, 1977.
85. Lasson Å, Alwmark A, Nobin A, Sundler F: Endocrine tumors of the duodenum: Clinical characteristics and hormone content. Ann Surg 197:393–398, 1983.
86. De Lellis RA, Gagel RF, Kaplan MM, Curtis LE: Gastrinoma of duodenal G-cell origin. Cancer 38:201–208, 1976.
87. Capella C, Usellini L, Riva C, et al: Light and electron immunocytochemical characterization of cholecystokinin (CCK), gastrin, mixed gastrin/CCK and C-terminal gastrin/CCK cells in the human small intestine. In preparation.
88. Creutzfeldt W, Arnold R, Creutzfeldt C, Track NS: Pathomorphologic, biochemical and diagnostic aspects of gastrinomas (Zollinger-Ellison syndrome). Hum Pathol 6:47–76, 1975.
89. Berger G, Berger F, Boman F, et al: Localisation of C-terminal gastrin immunoreactivity in gastrinoma cells. Virchows Arch [A] 406:223–236, 1985.
90. Berger G, Berger F, Boman F, Feroldi J: Light and electron microscope localization of G-17- and G-34-like immunoreactivities of human gastrinomas. Ultrastruct Pathol 8:305–318, 1985.
91. Buchan AMJ, Polak JM, Solcia E, Pearse AGE: Localization of intestinal gastrin in a distinct endocrine cell type. Nature 277:138–140, 1979.
92. Larsson LI, Jørgensen LM: Ultrastructural and cytochemical studies on the cytodifferentiation of duodenal endocrine cells. Cell Tissue Res 194:79–102, 1978.
93. Larsson LI, Rehfeld JF: A peptide resembling COOH-terminal tetrapeptide amide of gastrin from a new gastrointestinal endocrine cell type. Nature 277:575–578, 1979.
94. Alumets J, Ekelund G, Håkanson R, et al: Jejunal endocrine tumour composed of somatostatin and gastrin cells and associated with duodenal ulcer disease. Virchows Arch [A] 378:17–22, 1978.
95. Solcia E, Capella C, Buffa R, et al: The diffuse endocrine paracrine system of the gut in health and disease: Ultrastructural features. Scand J Gastroenterol 16(Suppl 70):25–36, 1981.
96. Sjölund K, Alumets J, Berg NO, et al: Duodenal endocrine cells in adult coeliac disease. Gut 20:547–552, 1979.
97. Holle GE, Spann W, Eisenmenger W, et al: Diffuse somatostatin-immunoreactive D-cell hyperplasia in the stomach and duodenum. Gastroenterology 91:733–739, 1986.
98. Weichert RF, Roth LM, Harkin JC: Carcinoid-islet cell tumor of the duodenum and associated multiple carcinoid tumors of the ileum: An electron microscopy study. Cancer 27:910–918, 1971.
99. Murayama H, Imai T, Kikuchi M, Kamio A: Duodenal carcinoid (APUDOMA) with psammoma bodies: A light and electron microscopic study. Cancer 43:1411–1417, 1979.
100. Kaneko H, Yanaihara N, Ito S, et al: Somatostatinoma of the duodenum. Cancer 44:2273–2279, 1979.
101. Greider MH, De Schryver-Kecskemeti K, Kraus FT: Psammoma bodies in endocrine tumors of the gastroenteropancreatic axis: A rather common occurrence. Semin Diagn Pathol 1:19–29, 1984.
102. Taccagni GL, Carlucci M, Sironi M, et al: Duodenal somatostatinoma with psammoma bodies: An immunohistochemical and ultrastructural study. Am J Gastroenterol 81:33–37, 1986.
103. Ganda OP, Weir GC, Soeldner JS, et al: "Somatostatinoma": A somatostatin-containing tumor of the endocrine pancreas. N Engl J Med 296:963–967, 1977.
104. Larsson LI, Hirsch MA, Holst JJ, et al: Pancreatic somatostatinoma: Clinical features and physiologic implications. Lancet 1:666–668, 1977.
105. Krejs GJ, Orci L, Conlon JM, et al: Somatostatinoma syndrome: Biochemical, morphologic and clinical features. N Engl J Med 301:285–292, 1979.
106. Taylor HB, Helwig EB: Benign non-chromaffin paragangliomas of the duodenum. Virchows Arch [A] 335:356–366, 1962.
107. Kepes JJ, Zacharias DI: Gangliocytic paragangliomas of the duodenum: A report of two cases with light and electron microscopic examination. Cancer 27:61–70, 1971.
108. Beltrami CA, Montironi R, Cinti S: Gangliocytic paraganglioma of the duodenum: Case report. Tumori 66:637–641, 1980.
109. Perrone T, Sibley RK, Rosai J: Duodenal gangliocytic paraglioma: An immunohistochemical and ultrastructural study and a hypothesis concerning its origin. Am J Surg Pathol 9:31–41, 1985.
110. Savio OS, Gonzalez BN, Cortes FG, et al: Paraganglioma no cromafinico del yeyuno. Rev Cubana Cir 13:497–505, 1974.
111. Delamarre J, Potet F, Capron JP, et al: Chémodectoma gastrique: Étude d'un cas et revue de la literature. Arch Fr Mal App Dig 64:339–346, 1975.
112. Buchler M, Malfertheiner P, Baczako K, et al: A metastatic endocrine-neurogenic tumor of the ampulla of Vater with multiple endocrine immunoreaction: Malignant paraganglioma? Digestion 31:54–59, 1985.
113. Kermarec J, Duplay H, Lesbros F: Paraganglioma gangliocytique du duodenum: Une observation, avec étude ultra-structurale. Arch Anat Cytol Pathol 24:261–268, 1976.
114. Guarda LA, Ordonez NG, del Junco GW, Luna MA: Gangliocytic paraganglioma of the duodenum: An immunocytochemical study. Am J Gastroenterol 78:794–798, 1983.
115. Osaka M, Kobayashi S: Duodenal basal-granulated cells in the human fetus with special reference to their relationship to nervous elements. In Fujita T (ed): Endocrine Gut and Pancreas. Amsterdam, Elsevier, 1976, pp 145–158.
116. Van Campenhout E: Contribution au problème des connexions neuro-entoblastiques. Acad R Med Belg 5:189–201, 1940.
117. Ljungber O, Jarnerot G, Rolny P, Wickbom G: Human pancreatic polypeptide (HPP) immunoreactivity in an infiltrating endocrine tumour of the papilla of Vater with unusual morphology. Virchows Arch [A] 392:119–126, 1981.
118. Masson P: Appendicite neurogene et carcinoides. Ann Anat Pathol 1:3–59, 1924.
119. Rode J, Dhillon AP, Papadaki L, Griffiths D: Neurosecretory cells of the lamina propria of the appendix and their possible relationship to carcinoids. Histopathology 6:69–79, 1982.
120. Auböck L, Höfler H: Extraepithelial intraneural endocrine cells as starting-points for gastrointestinal carcinoids. Virchows Arch [A] 401:17–33, 1983.
121. Höfler H, Kasper M, Heitz U: The neuroendocrine system of normal human appendix, ileum and colon, and in neurogenic appendicopathy. Virchows Arch [A] 399:127–140, 1983.
122. Reed RJ, Daroca PJ, Harkin JC: Gangliocytic paraganglioma. Am J Surg Pathol 1:207–216, 1977.
123. Hough DRH, Chan MA, Davidson MH: Von Recklinghausen's disease associated with gastrointestinal carcinoid tumors. Cancer 51:2206–2208, 1983.
124. Gosset A, Masson P: Tumeurs endocrines de l'appendice. Presse Med 25:237–240, 1914.
125. Lembeck F: 5-hydroxytryptamine in a carcinoid tumour. Nature 172:910–911, 1953.
126. Sherman SP, Li CY, Carney JA: Microproliferation of entero-

chromaffin cells and the origin of carcinoid tumors of the ileum. Arch Pathol Lab Med 105:639–641, 1979.
127. Wharton J, Polak JM, Cole GA, et al: Neuron-specific enolase as an immunocytochemical marker for the diffuse neuroendocrine system in human fetal lung. J Histochem Cytochem 29:1359–1364, 1981.
128. Pearse AGE, Polak JM: Immunocytochemical localization of substance P in mammalian intestine. Histochemistry 41:373–379, 1975.
129. Alumets J, Håkanson R, Ingemansson S, Sundler F: Substance P and 5-HT in granules isolated from an intestinal argentaffin carcinoid. Histochemistry 52:217–222, 1977.
130. Wilander E, Grimelius L, Portela-Gomes G, et al: Substance P and enteroglucagon-like immunoreactivity in argentaffin and argyrophil midgut carcinoid tumors. Scand J Gastroenterol 14(Suppl 53):19–25, 1979.
131. Norheim I, Theodorsson-Norheim E, et al: Antisera raised against eledoisin and kassinin detect elevated levels of immunoreactive material in plasma and tumor tissues from patients with carcinoid tumors. Regul Pept 9:245–257, 1984.
132. Mårtensson H, Nobin A, Sundler F, Falmer S: Endocrine tumors of the ileum: Cytochemical and clinical aspects. Pathol Res Pract 180:356–363, 1985.
133. Conlon JM, Schäfer G, Schmidt WE, Lazarus HD, Becker HD, Creutzfeldt W: Chemical and immunochemical characterization of substance P-like immunoreactivity and physalaemin-like immunoreactivity in a carcinoid tumour. Regul Pept 11:117–132, 1985.
134. Yang K, Ulrich T, Chen GL, Lewin KJ: The neuroendocrine products of intestinal carcinoids. Cancer 51:1918–1926, 1983.
135. Goedert M, Otten U, Suda K, Heitz PU, Stalder GA, Obrecht JP, Holzach P, Allgöwer M: Dopamine, norepinephrine and serotonin production by an intestinal carcinoid tumor. Cancer 45:104–107, 1980.
136. Auböck L, Ratzenhofer M: "Extraepithelial enterochromaffin cell-nerve-fibre complexes" in the normal human appendix, and in neurogenic appendicopathy. J Pathol 136:217–226, 1982.
137. Ryden SE, Drake RM, Ralph A, Franciosi A: Carcinoid tumors of the appendix in children. Cancer 36:1538–1542, 1975.
138. Dische FE: Argentaffin and non-argentaffin carcinoid tumours of the appendix. J Clin Pathol 21:60–66, 1968.
139. Cristina ML, Mendonga ME, Tenti P, et al: L cell microcarcinoids of the appendix with glicentin and PP immunoreactivity. In preparation.
140. Caldarola VT, Jackman RJ, Moertel GC, Dockerty MB: Carcinoid tumors of the rectum. Am J Surg 107:844–849, 1964.
141. Orloff MJ: Carcinoid tumors of the rectum. Cancer 28:175–180, 1971.
142. Bates HR Jr: Carcinoid tumors of the rectum. Dis Colon Rectum 5:270, 1962.
143. Wilander E, Portela-Gomes G, Grimelius L, et al: Enteroglucagon and substance P-like immunoreactivity in argentaffin and argyrophil rectal carcinoids. Virchows Arch [B] 25:117–124, 1977.
144. Fiocca R, Capella C, Buffa R, et al: Glucagon-, glicentin- and pancreatic polypeptide-like immunoreactivities in rectal carcinoids and related colorectal cells. Am J Pathol 100:81–92, 1980.
145. Alumets J, Alm P, Falkmer S, et al: Immunohistochemical evidence of peptide hormones in endocrine tumours of the rectum. Cancer 48:2409–2415, 1981.
146. O'Briain DS, Dayal Y, De Lellis RA, et al: Rectal carcinoids as tumors of the hindgut endocrine cells: A morphological and immunohistochemical analysis. Am J Surg Pathol 6:131, 1982.
147. Sobin LH, Hjermstad BM, Sesterhenn IA, Helwig EB: Prostatic acid phosphatase activity in carcinoid tumors. Cancer 58:136–138, 1986.
148. Robboy SJ, Scully RE, Norris HJ: Insular carcinoid primary in the ovary: A clinico-pathologic analysis of 48 cases. Cancer 36:404–418, 1975.
149. Berardi RS: Carcinoid tumors of the colon (exclusive of the rectum): Review of the literature. Dis Colon Rectum 15:383–391, 1972.
150. Bloom SR: An enteroglucagon tumour. Gut 13:520–523, 1972.
151. Gleeson MH, Bloom SR, Polak JM, et al: Endocrine tumour in kidney affecting small bowel structure, mobility, and absorptive function. Gut 12:773–782, 1971.
152. Gross M: Tumeurs carcinoides du rectum. Helv Chir Acta 35:239–248, 1968.
153. Cattan D, Pappo E, Dervichian M, et al: Tumeur carcinoide de l'intestin grêle avec métastases hépatiques riches en thyrocalcitonine associée a un adénome benim à cellule C de la glande thyroide. Arch Fr Mal Appar Dig 62:141, 1973.
154. Weder W, Saremaslani P, Maurer R: Calcitoninbildendes duodenalkarzinoid bei neurofibromatose von Recklinghausen. Schweiz Med Wschr 113:885–892, 1983.
155. Johnson W, Waisman J: Carcinoid tumor of the vermiform appendix with Cushing's syndrome. Cancer 27:681–686, 1971.
156. Hirata Y, Sakamoto N, Yamamoto H, et al: Gastric carcinoid with ectopic production of ACTH and β-MSH. Cancer 37:377–385, 1976.
157. Marcus FS, Friedman MA, Callen PW, Churg R, Harbour J: Successful therapy of an ACTH-producing gastric carcinoid APUD tumor. Cancer 46:1263–1270, 1980.
158. Leveston SA, McKeel W, Buckley PJ, et al: Acromegaly and Cushing's syndrome associated with a foregut carcinoid tumor. J Clin Endocrinol Metab 53:682–689, 1981.
159. Capella C, Polak JM, Buffa R, et al: Morphological patterns and diagnostic criteria of VIP-producing endocrine tumours: A histological, histochemical, ultrastructural and biochemical study of 32 cases. Cancer 52:1860–1874, 1983.
160. Larsson LI, Polak JM, Buffa R, et al: On the immunocytochemical localization of the vasoactive intestinal polypeptide. J Histochem Cytochem 27:936–938, 1979.
161. Straus E, Yalow RS: Hypersecretinemia associated with marked basal hyperchlorhydria in man and dog. Gastroenterology 72:992–994, 1977.
162. Roggli VL, Judge DM, McGavran MH: Duodenal glucagonoma: A case report. Hum Pathol 10:350–353, 1979.
163. McKeown F: Oat cell carcinoma of the esophagus. J Pathol Bacteriol 64:889–891, 1952.
164. Tateishi R, Taniguchi K, Horai T, et al: Argyrophil cell carcinoma (apudoma) of the esophagus: A histopathologic entity. Virchows Arch [A] 371:283–294, 1976.
165. Reyes CV, Chejfec G, Jao W, Gould VE: Neuroendocrine carcinomas of the esophagus. Ultrastruct Pathol 1:367–376, 1980.
166. Chejfec C, Gould V: Malignant gastric neuroendocrinomas. Hum Pathol 8:433, 1977.
167. Sweeney EC, McDonnell L: Atypical gastric carcinoids. Histopathology 4:215–224, 1980.
168. Gould VE, Chejfec G: Neuroendocrine carcinomas of the colon: Ultrastructural and biochemical evidence of their secretory function. Am J Surg Pathol 2:31–38, 1978.
169. Capella C, Hage E, Solcia E, Usellini L: Ultrastructural similarity of endocrine-like cells of the human lung and some related cells of the gut. Cell Tissue Res 186:25–37, 1978.
170. Gould VE, Jao W, Chejfec G, et al: Neuroendocrine carcinomas of the gastrointestinal tract. Semin Diagn Pathol 1:13–18, 1984.
171. Azzopardi JG, Pollock DJ: Argentaffin and argyrophil cells in gastric carcinoma. J Pathol Bacteriol 86:443–451, 1963.
172. Bosman FT: Neuroendocrine cells in non-neuroendocrine tumours. In Falkmer S, Håkanson R, Sunder F (eds): Evolution and Tumour Pathology of the Neuroendocrine System. Amsterdam, Elsevier, 1984, pp 519–543.
173. Fiocca R, Villani L, Tenti P, et al: Characterization of four main cell types in gastric cancer: Foveolar, mucopeptic, intestinal columnar and goblet cells: An histopathologic, histochemical and ultrastructural study of "early" and "advanced" tumours. Pathol Res Pract 182:308–325, 1987.
174. Kubo I, Watanabe H: Neoplastic argentaffin cells in gastric and intestinal carcinomas. Cancer 27:447–454, 1971.
175. Proks C, Feit V: Gastric carcinoma with argyrophil and argentaffin cells. Virchows Arch [A] 395:201–206, 1982.
176. Waldum HL, Burhol PG, Johnson JA, Smith AG: MSH-producing gastric tumour. Acta Hepatol Gastroenterol 24:386–388, 1977.
177. Cocco AE, Conway SJ: Zollinger-Ellison syndrome associated with ovarian mucinous cystadenocarcinoma. N Engl J Med 298:144–146, 1978.
178. Pradé M, Bara J, Gadenne C, et al: Gastric carcinoma with ar-

gyrophilic cells: Light microscopic, electron microscopic, and immunochemical study. Hum Pathol 13:588–592, 1982.
179. Tahara E, Hisao I, Nakagami K, et al: Scirrhous argyrophil cell carcinoma of the stomach with multiple production of polypeptide hormones, amine, CEA, lysozyme, and HCG. Cancer 49:1904–1915, 1982.
180. Soga J, Tazawa K, Aizawa O, Wada K, Tuto T: Argentaffin cell adenocarcinoma of the stomach: An atypical carcinoid? Cancer 28:999–1003, 1971.
181. Tahara E, Ito H, Shimamoto F, et al: Argyrophil cells in early gastric carcinoma: An immunohistochemical and ultrastructural study. J Cancer Res Clin Oncol 103:187–202, 1982.
182. Ulich RT, Cheng L, Glover H, et al: A colonic adenocarcinoma with argentaffin cells. A immunoperoxidase study demonstrating the presence of numerous neuroendocrine products. Cancer 51:1483–1489, 1983.
183. Shousha S: Signet ring cell adenocarcinoma of rectum: A histological, histochemical and electron microscopic study. Histopathology 6:341–350, 1982.
184. Klein HZ: Mucinous carcinoid of the vermiform appendix. Cancer 33:770–777, 1974.
185. Warner TFCS, Seo IS: Goblet cell carcinoid of appendix. Cancer 44:1700–1706, 1979.
186. Abt AB, Carter SL: Goblet cell carcinoma of the appendix. Arch Pathol Lab Med 100:301–306, 1976.
187. Cooper PH, Warkel RC: Ultrastructure of the goblet cell type of adenocarcinoid of the appendix. Cancer 42:2687–2695, 1978.
188. Isaacson P: Crypt cell carcinoma of the appendix (so-called adenocarcinoid tumour). Am J Surg Pathol 5:213–224, 1981.
189. Bates HR Jr, Belter LF: Composite carcinoid tumour (argentaffin adenocarcinoma) of the colon: Report of two cases. Dis Colon Rectum 10:467–470, 1967.
190. Hernandez FL, Reid JD: Mixed carcinoid and mucus-secreting intestinal tumors. Arch Path 88:489–496, 1969.
191. Goldberg SL, Toker C: Composite tumor of small intestine. Mt Sinai J Med NY 43:153–156, 1976.
192. Parks TG: Malignant carcinoid and adenocarcinoma of the stomach. Br J Surg 57:377–379, 1970.
193. Rogers LW, Murphy RC: Gastric carcinoid and gastric carcinoma. Morphologic correlates of survival. Am J Surg Pathol 3:195–202, 1979.
194. Ratzenhofer M, Auböck L: The amphicrine (endoexocrine) cells in the human gut with a short reference to amphicrine neoplasia. Acta Morphol Acad Sci Hung 28:37–58, 1980.
195. Höfler H, Köppel G, Heitz U: Combined production of mucus, amines and peptides by goblet-cell carcinoids of the appendix and ileum. Pathol Res Pract 178:555–561, 1984.
196. Chejfec G, Capella C, Solcia E, et al: Amphicrine cells, dysplasias and neoplasias. Cancer 56:2683–2690, 1985.

CHAPTER 14

Disorders of the Lymphoid System

KLAUS J. LEWIN, M.D., F.R.C. PATH.

FUNCTIONAL ANATOMY
Normal Distribution of Gut-Associated Lymphoid Tissue
Intestinal Host Defense Mechanisms

IMMUNODEFICIENCY DISORDERS OF THE GASTROINTESTINAL TRACT
General Features of Immunodeficiency Disorders
Types of Immunodeficiency Disorders
Clinical Aspects
Pathology
Primary Immunodeficiency Disorders
Predominant Antibody Defects
Common Variable Hypogammaglobulinemia
Selective IgA Deficiency
Secretory Component Deficiency
Infantile X-Linked Agammaglobulinemia
Miscellaneous B-Cell Disorders
Predominant Cell-Mediated Immunodeficiency
Severe Combined Immunodeficiency
Chronic Mucocutaneous Candidiasis
Immunodeficiency Associated with Other Defects
DiGeorge's Syndrome

Wiskott-Aldrich Syndrome and Ataxia Telangiectasia
Phagocytic Dysfunction
Chronic Granulomatous Disease
Acquired Immunodeficiency Disorders
Bone Marrow Transplantation
Transplantation Regimen
Infection
Graft-Versus-Host Disease
Gastrointestinal Manifestations of the Acquired Immunodeficiency Syndrome
Opportunistic Infections
Kaposi's Sarcoma
Workup of the Immunodeficient Patient

LYMPHOPROLIFERATIVE DISORDERS
Lymphoid Hyperplasia
Focal Lymphoid Hyperplasia of the Stomach
Value of Endoscopic Biopsy in the Diagnosis of Gastric Lymphoid Hyperplasia
Focal Lymphoid Hyperplasia of the Small Intestine

Focal Lymphoid Hyperplasia of the Rectum
Nodular Lymphoid Hyperplasia
Focal Nodular Lymphoid Hyperplasia of the Terminal Ileum and Appendix
Diffuse Nodular Lymphoid Hyperplasia of the Intestine
Malignant Lymphoma
Conditions Associated with Increased Risk of Lymphoma
Celiac Sprue
Immunoproliferative Small-Intestinal Disease
Lymphoid Hyperplasia and Primary Immunodeficiency Disorders
Inflammatory Bowel Disease
Primary Lymphoma of the Gastrointestinal Tract and Mesentery in Adults
Childhood Lymphomas
Secondary Malignant Lymphomas and Leukemias
IPSID and IPSID-Associated Lymphoma (Mediterranean Lymphoma and Alpha-Chain Disease)
Solitary Plasmacytomas
Workup of Gastrointestinal Lymphomas

FUNCTIONAL ANATOMY

Normal Distribution of Gut-Associated Lymphoid Tissue

Lymphoid tissue is normally abundant throughout the mucosa of the gastrointestinal tract, with the exception of the gastric fundus and body. It first appears in the lamina propria of the bowel at the 80-mm stage (10 weeks).[1] At 14 weeks lymphoid follicles develop, and plasma cells appear at birth but are very scanty.[1] The lymphoid tissue is arranged in three forms[2]: (1) diffuse lymphoplasmacytic infiltrate, which is distributed evenly throughout the intestinal mucosa of the small and large intestine; (2) solitary lymphoid nodules, which are present throughout the gastrointestinal tract but are most frequent in the distal colon[3]; and (3) aggregate lymphoid nodules, which occur in the appen-

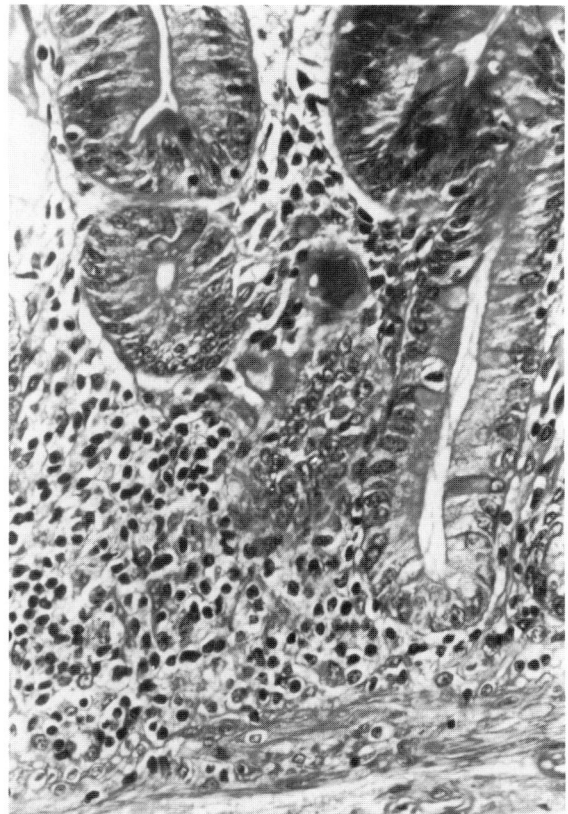

FIGURE 14–1. Photomicrograph illustrating the distribution of the diffuse lymphoid tissue within the lamina propria. Note the lymphoplasmacytic cell infiltrate in the intercrypt area.

Intestinal Host Defense Mechanisms

The gastrointestinal tract has a unique role in that its major function is the selective absorption of nutrients, while at the same time it excludes large amounts of potentially harmful ingested substances, such as microorganisms, toxins, and toxic breakdown products of ingested material.[13] Both immune and nonimmune defense mechanisms are important in the exclusion of harmful substances from the body.

The main function of the gut immune system is to provide (1) a barrier to the absorption of undesirable antigens from the gut while at the same time allowing for the absorption of nutrients and (2) to prevent bacterial, viral, and parasitic infections. This protection is provided within the lumen by secretory IgA[13] (originating from the intestine or bile) and within the mucosa by the lymphocytes and macrophages. Secretory IgA has been likened to an antiseptic paint lining the bowel mucosa and acting as a protective layer against the intestinal contents. It has four antigen combining sites and is very efficient at agglutinating bacteria and viruses and preventing their adherence to mucosal surfaces.[14,15] Also, by combining with toxins or food, it interferes with the absorption of macromolecules, which could initiate harmful systemic immune responses. Those antigens (particulate and soluble products) that escape the action of secretory IgA and penetrate the surface epithelium may form immune complexes, which are then cleared by the liver and excreted in the bile; alternatively, they may be dealt with by locally sensitized lymphocytes, by combination with preformed antibodies, or by ingestion by macrophages.[16]

The important nonimmunologic mechanisms in gut host defense include (1) intestinal mucus, which may impair antigen binding and allow antigen degradation by intestinal enzymes; (2) competition with resident microbial flora; (3) the physical integrity of the mucosa; (4) the action of acid and pepsin, which causes bacterial and dietary antigen degradation; (5) the action of bile acids, which suppress microbial proliferation; and (6) bowel motility, which produces regular cleansing of the intestinal tract.[17]

From the above-mentioned list it is evident that many major intestinal disorders, for example, atrophic gastritis, inflammatory bowel disease, and motility disorders, as well as extraintestinal diseases such as pancreatic and liver disorders, and iatrogenic causes such as antibiotic medication can cause a breakdown of intestinal host defense mechanisms with resultant secondary intestinal manifestations.

IMMUNODEFICIENCY DISORDERS OF THE GASTROINTESTINAL TRACT

General Features of Immunodeficiency Disorders

The gastrointestinal tract is frequently an important target organ in both the primary and the secondary immunodeficiency disorders, since the gastrointestinal

dix and small intestine. In the small intestine, these aggregates are referred to as Peyer's patches and are most frequent in the distal ileum.[4] The lymphoid tissue in the ileocecal valve is unique in that it is arranged circumferentially.[5] The mesenteric lymph nodes are also usually considered part of the gut-associated lymphoid tissue. In common with gut, mesenteric lymph nodes are exposed to considerable antigenic material via the lymphatic flow from the small and large bowel and are populated by predominantly IgA precursor B lymphocytes.

The diffuse lymphoid tissue is contained in two separate compartments.[6,7] One is located within the epithelial layer of the mucosa, the so-called intraepithelial lymphocytes or theliolymphocytes (Figures 14–1 and 14–2). Although these cells appear to be sparse in number in any one section, when the entire intestine is considered, they are in fact very numerous and are said to equal in the aggregate the number of lymphocytes in the spleen. They consist primarily of T lymphocytes.[1,8–10] In inflammatory states, neutrophils and eosinophils may also enter this area.[11] The second compartment of the diffuse lymphoid system is contained within the lamina propria and contains numerous plasma cells, the majority of which are IgA-producing, and a heterogeneous group of B and T lymphocytes, macrophages, and a small number of eosinophils and mast cells (Figure 14–2).[12]

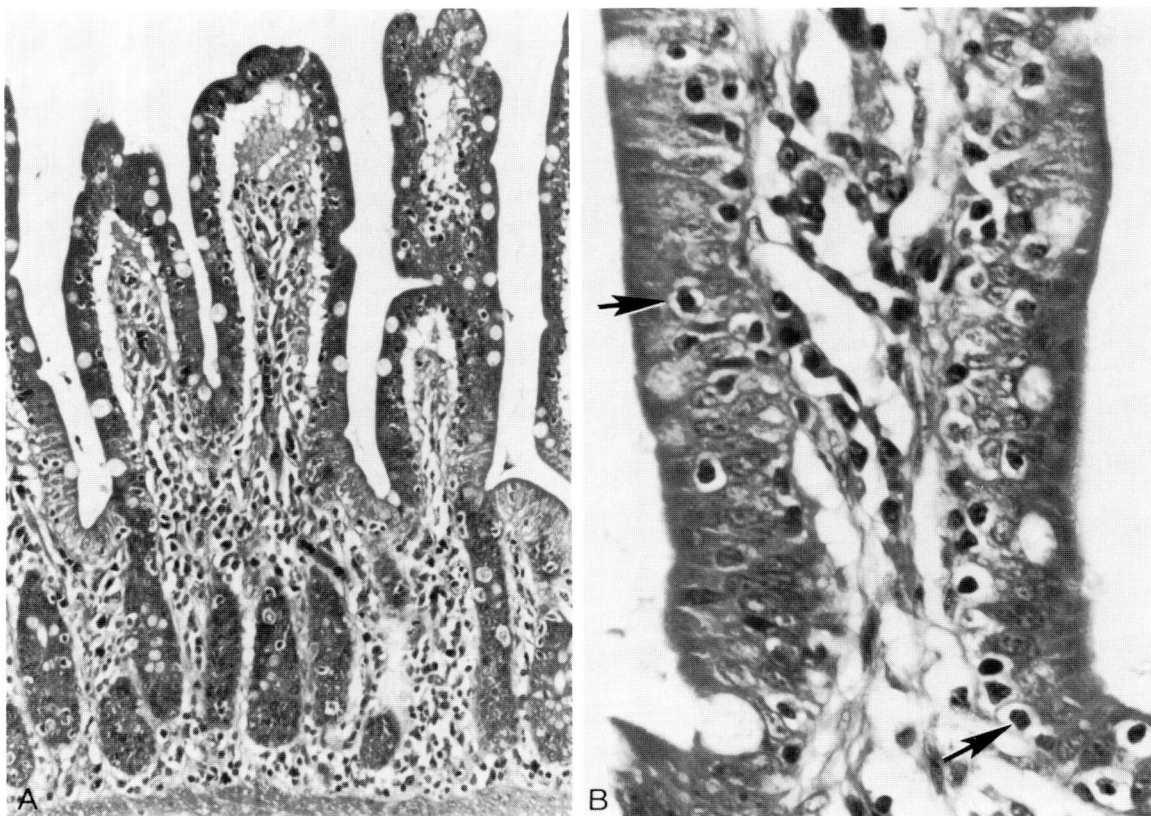

FIGURE 14-2. Photomicrograph demonstrating the intraepithelial lymphocytes (theliolymphocytes). *A,* Low-power view of the mucosa. *B,* Higher magnification of an intestinal villus illustrating the characteristic dark hyperchromatic nucleus surrounded by a clear halo. The lymphocytes lie between the basement membrane and the columnar absorptive cells and also between the absorptive cells (arrows).

tract is constantly exposed to a heavy antigen load. The diagnosis of immunodeficiency disease is often suspected by the clinician because these patients commonly have a history of prolonged infections by unusual organisms in unusual sites. The pathologist's role consists mainly in confirming and identifying the frequent complications of immunodeficiency, of which infection and neoplasia are the most important. Sometimes, however, unexpected histologic changes may be found in the gut, such as giardiasis or coccidiosis, which should lead one to suspect an immunodeficiency disorder in a clinically unsuspected case.

Types of Immunodeficiency Disorders

There are two major categories of immunodeficiency disorders, primary and secondary.

The primary immunodeficiency disorders are a large and varied group of diseases resulting from impairment of the B- and T-cell systems and abnormalities of phagocytic function. The functional interaction of B and T cells and monocytes in the expression of the immune system makes the division of immunodeficiency diseases into B- and T-cell disorders somewhat artificial.[18,19] Nevertheless, usually either the antibody defects or cell-mediated abnormalities predominate, which allows a practical subdivision of the immunodeficiency disorders. In addition, genetic defects have recently been described in which there are specific abnormalities in responsiveness to certain antigens. In these disorders, there appears to be poor antigen clearance leading to immune complex disease or hypersensitivity reaction.[20,21]

In adults, common variable or late-onset immunodeficiency and selective IgA deficiency are by far the most common immunodeficiency disorders. In children, severe combined immunodeficiency disease is the most common. It usually presents soon after birth; and it is important that it be diagnosed so that the sequelae of acute and chronic infection can be prevented.

Secondary immunodeficiency disorders are becoming an increasingly more common and important group. Some develop naturally with increasing age or after certain infections; others are iatrogenic complications of immunosuppressive therapy, radiation therapy, or bone marrow transplantation. However, the most important disorder to emerge in the last few years is the *acquired immunodeficiency syndrome (AIDS),* which is causally related to human immunodeficiency virus (HIV) infection.

Clinical Aspects

Clinically, impairment of the immune system is characterized by a decreased resistance to infection, the nature of which depends on the specific defect. Thus, patients with impaired B-cell function are most susceptible to bacterial infections; whereas those with impaired T-cell function have defective cell-mediated immunity and a susceptibility to prolonged viral, fungal, and mycobacterial infections. The major clinical manifestations of these infections depend on the primary site of involvement of the gastrointestinal tract. They consist of dysphagia, diarrhea, and malabsorption, and in children, failure to thrive.[22]

The diagnosis of the primary immunodeficiency disorders is usually no problem. Patients commonly have a history of recurrent and prolonged opportunistic infections, and there is frequently a family history of immunodeficiency disease. The finding of associated lesions, such as autoimmune disorders, helps greatly in determining the precise immunologic abnormality.

The diagnosis and categorization of the immunodeficiency disorders are based primarily on the following immunologic tests for humoral (B-cell) and cellular (T-cell) immunity.[18,19]

1. Serum immunoglobulins
2. Serum antibody levels and antibody response to immunization
3. The nature and number of circulating B cells
4. The nature and number of circulating T cells, including helper/suppressor ratios
5. T-cell function as expressed in cell-mediated immune responses

In addition, the family history, clinical features, and associated lesions help greatly in determining the precise immunologic abnormality.

Pathology

The pathologic changes accompanying the immunodeficiency disorders are variable and depend in part on the specific immunologic defect (Table 14–1). It should be stressed that in some cases there may be no

Table 14–1 PATHOLOGY OF THE GASTROINTESTINAL TRACT IN PRIMARY IMMUNODEFICIENCY DISORDERS

No change
Specific morphologic changes
  Altered lymphoplasmacytic content of lamina propria:
    Absence of inflammatory cells
    Altered B- or T-cell subsets
  Diffuse nodular lymphoid hyperplasia
Nonspecific morphologic changes due to bacterial overgrowth, infections, or other injury.
  Esophagitis
  Mucosal erosions
  Atrophic gastritis
  Mucosal lesions (villous atrophy)
  Enterocolitis
  Demonstration of organisms, particularly:
    Candida, cytomegalovirus, herpesvirus, *Giardia, Trichomonas*, Coccidia, and *Cryptosporidium*
Neoplasia
  Carcinoma
  Lymphoma

significant histologic alteration. The most frequently seen histologic lesions are the result of complications, namely, infections; and intrinsic lesions of immunodeficiency are uncommon. The histologic changes fall into four major categories.

No Change. In a number of cases there may be no significant morphologic mucosal alterations other than an altered inflammatory cell content of the lamina propria (Figure 14–3). Normally, the lamina propria of the intestinal tract is infiltrated by large numbers of IgA-containing cells and lesser numbers of IgM- and IgG-containing plasma cells.[17] In the B-cell deficiency states, there is an absence or paucity of IgA-containing cells, sometimes compensated for by an increase in number of the other plasma cells, especially IgM-containing ones. Immunoperoxidase staining of sections is helpful because it shows the specific cell type that is altered—for example, a diminution in number of IgA-containing

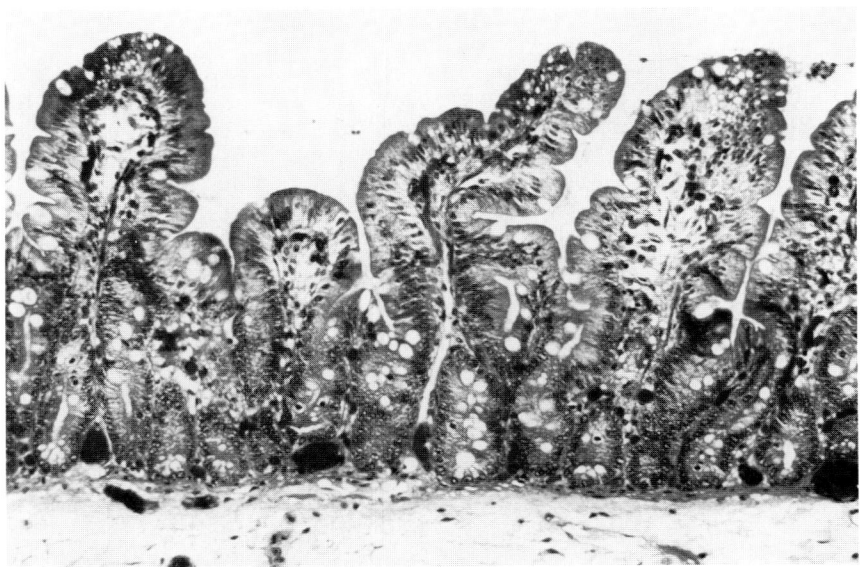

FIGURE 14–3. Small-intestinal mucosa in a patient with severe combined immunodeficiency disease (SCID). There is a virtual absence of inflammatory cells in the lamina propria and mild villous shortening but otherwise no abnormality.

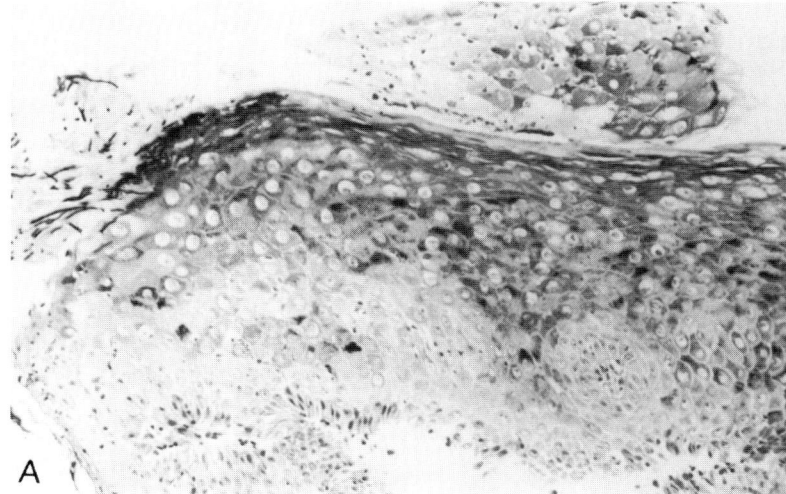
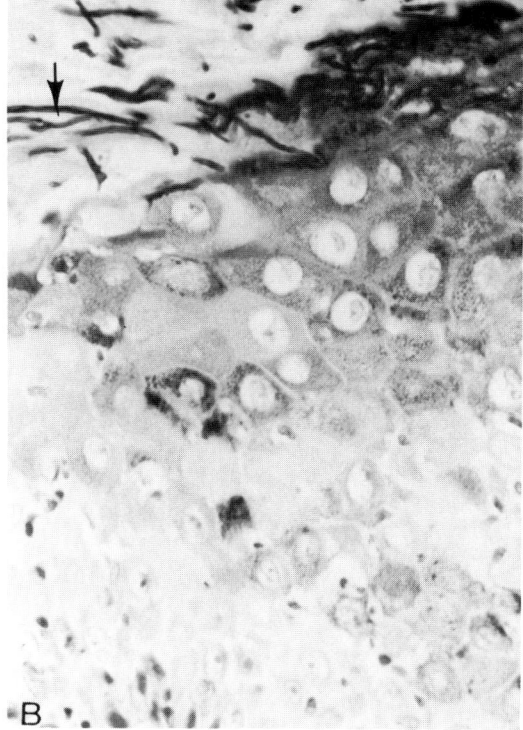

FIGURE 14–4. Esophageal biopsy from a patient with mucocutaneous candidiasis. *A*, Hyperkeratosis, focal epithelial degeneration, and pseudohyphae growing in the degenerating squamous epithelium. Note the absence of significant inflammation of the mucosa. *B*, Higher magnification showing the pseudohyphae within the degenerating epithelium (arrow).

plasma cells in selective IgA deficiency or an absence of plasma cells in severe combined immunodeficiency disease.

Mucosal Lesions Resulting from Infections or Bacterial Overgrowth. Patients with immunodeficiency disorders are especially prone to infections by one or more organisms of low virulence that are not normally pathogenic to man.[2] These include the normal commensals of the gastrointestinal tract,[23] fungi such as *Candida*[24] (Figure 14–4) and viruses such as cytomegalovirus (Figures 14–5 and 14–6) and herpes virus.[20,25] These patients are also susceptible to unusual organisms not normally found in the gastrointestinal microflora, such as *Giardia lamblia* (Figure 14–7), *Trichomonas hominis, Coccidia,* and *Strongyloides*.[26–29] An awareness of these uncommon infections in immunodeficient patients has led to the discovery of other unusual infecting organisms in the gastrointestinal tract in recent years, for example, *Cryptosporidium,* which is a coccidian protozoon commonly found in the intestines of animals (Figure 14–8).[30,31]

The histologic changes in the immunocompromised patient differ from those found in the normal patient, mainly in that the inflammatory response is often muted. The specific histologic changes resulting from infections vary somewhat with the site of involvement. In the esophagus, stomach, and large intestine, the lesions consist primarily of mucosal erosions and inflammation.[22–24] In candidal infections, the organism is present in the superficial necrotic debris and may invade the mucosa and occasionally extend through the bowel wall. For example, invasive candidiasis present in homosexual males is virtually diagnostic of AIDS.[32] In virus infections, the viral inclusions tend to be scant and are frequently missed, unless serial sections are carefully screened. The viral inclusions are commonly associated with mucosal erosions and ulcerations, often with minimal inflammation in the early stages.[25] Herpes can be especially difficult to diagnose. The edges of herpetic ulcers frequently contain desquamated cells with a tombstone-like appearance, a useful low-power clue. The presence of the more traditional features of herpetic infections, such as a nuclear ground-glass appearance and the presence of intranuclear inclusions and multinucleate giant cells, may then be sought. In AIDS the herpetic infections may be particularly intractable.[31] Sometimes viral inclusions, especially cytomegalovirus, are found in an otherwise unremarkable mucosa. It is these findings that have given rise to the debate as to whether the virus is a cause of mucosal injury or merely a passenger in a mucosa injured by some other organism or process. Finally, it should be noted that multiple organisms may be found in the lesions of these patients.

In the small intestine, bacterial overgrowth or parasitic infestations characteristically produce a sprue-like picture. However, unlike gluten enteropathy, the mucosal lesion is often patchy, of mild or moderate severity, and lacking an inflammatory infiltrate.[23] Occasionally, crypt abscesses and a neutrophilic infiltrate of the lamina propria are seen.[22] Giardiasis is the most common parasitic infection and characteristically is found predominantly in the intestinal mucus (see Figure 14–7) or is adherent to the epithelial cell microvillous sur-

FIGURE 14–5. Gastric biopsy from a patient with AIDS illustrating gastric erosions associated with cytomegalovirus infection. *A*, Gastric erosion and cystically dilated gastric glands in the adjacent mucosa. *B*, Higher magnification of the gastric erosion showing degeneration of glandular epithelium, the characteristic intranuclear viral inclusions surrounded by a clear halo (arrow) and a moderately severe inflammatory infiltrate.

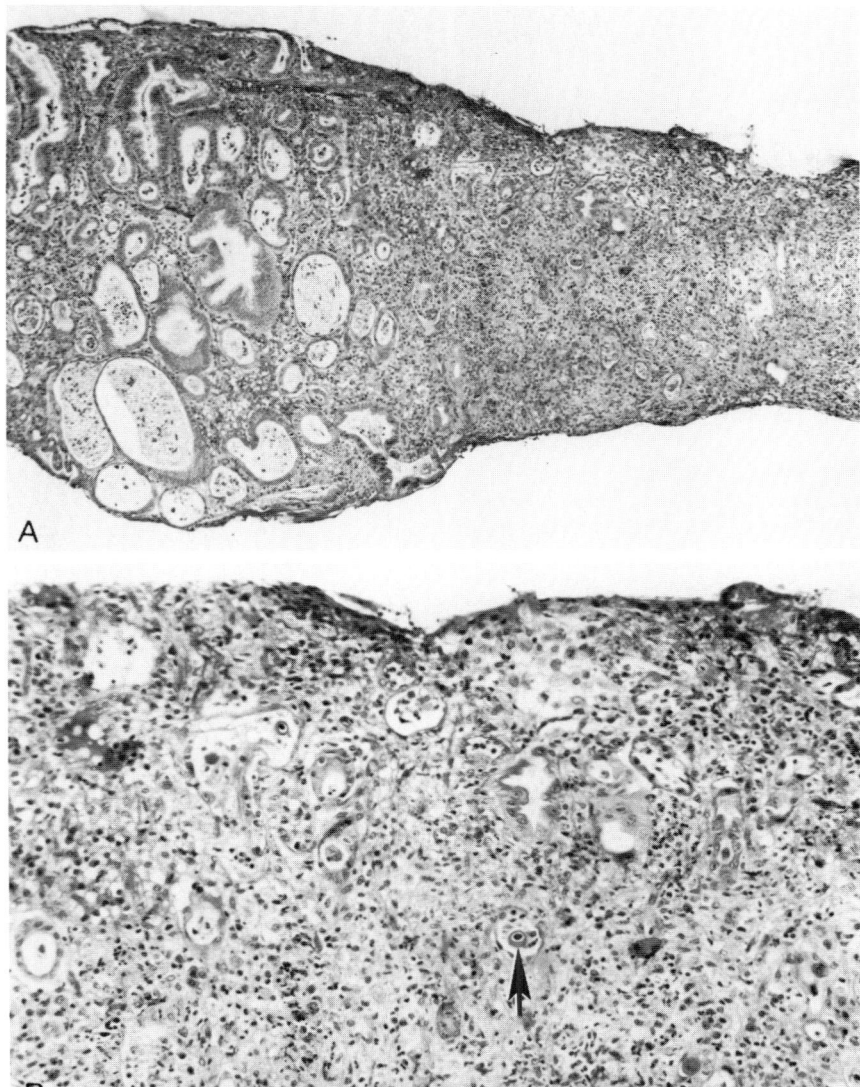

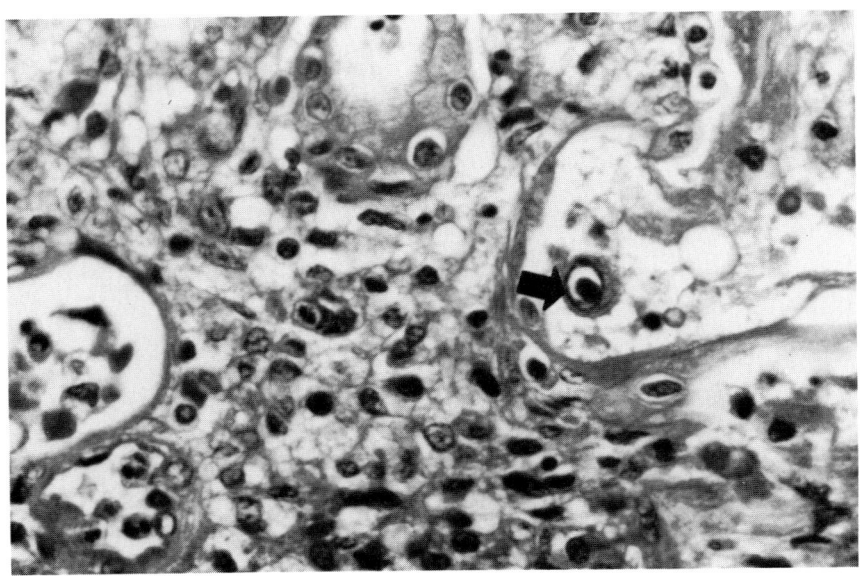

FIGURE 14–6. Higher magnification of Figure 14–5B, illustrating a degenerating gastric gland with a nuclear viral inclusion (arrow) and the surrounding inflammatory infiltrate.

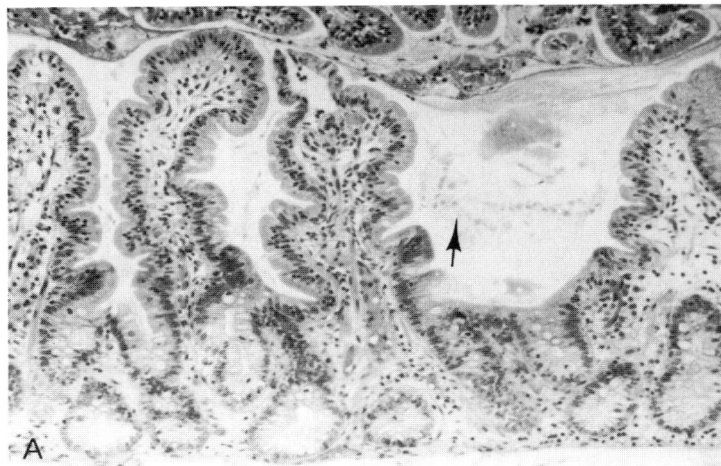
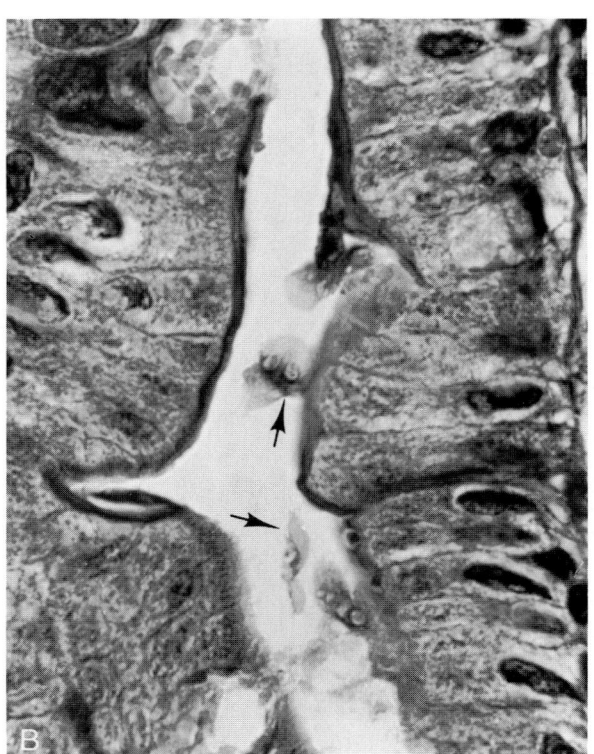

FIGURE 14–7. *Giardia lamblia* in a small-intestinal biopsy from a patient with common variable hypogammaglobulinemia and malabsorption. *A,* Low-power view showing relatively normal mucosa but numerous giardial parasites in the mucus between the intestinal villi (arrow). *B,* Higher-power magnification showing the characteristic owl-eyed nuclei of giardia (arrows).

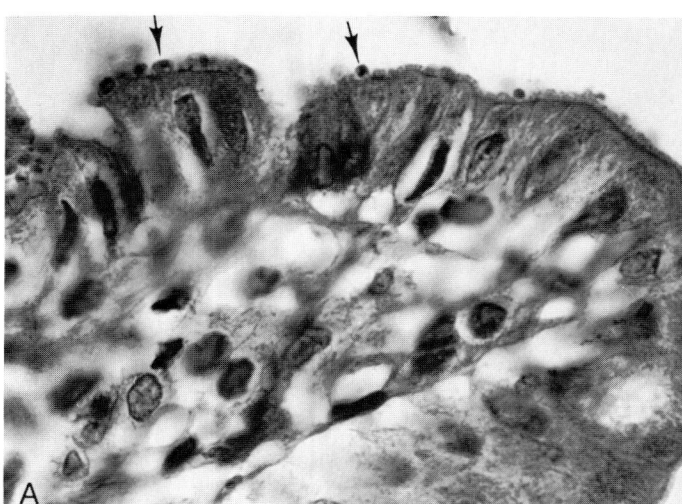
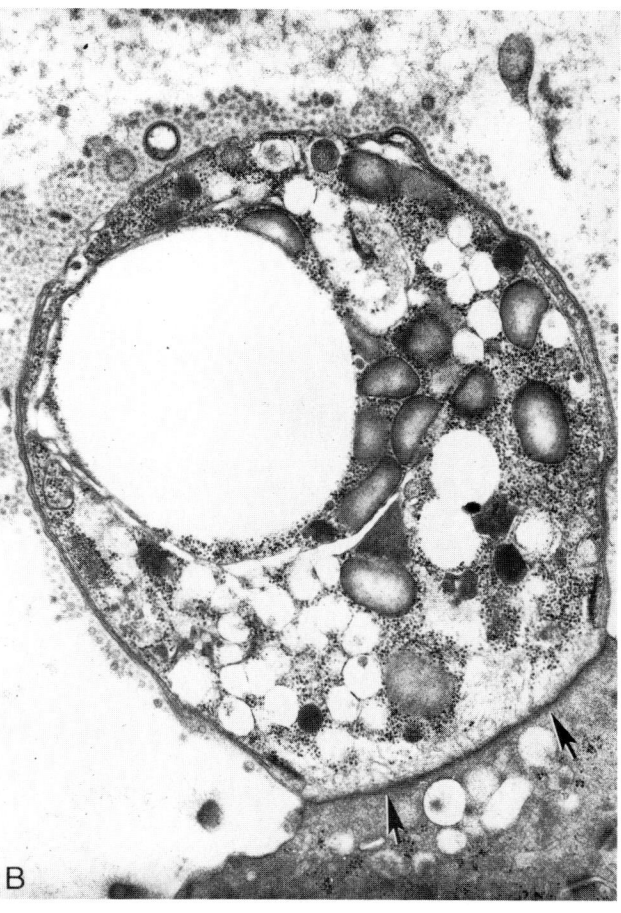

FIGURE 14–8. *Cryptosporidium* in a patient with AIDS. *A,* The organisms are attached to the columnar absorptive cell brush border (arrows). *B,* Electron micrograph of the organism showing the dense attachment site on the columnar epithelium (arrows), osmiophilic granules typical of a macrogamete, and the surrounding pellicle, which is thought to be of host origin.

face.[33,34] Although giardiasis can be diagnosed histologically in sections of small bowel, the diagnosis is best made by identification of cysts in the stools and vegetative forms in smears of mucus taken from the mucus adherent to the peroral biopsy specimens. The only other significant protozoal infections described are the coccidial infections. Coccidia are common parasites in the intestinal tract of animals and are generally transmitted by ingestion of contaminated food or water.[30,35,36] Such infections in man were thought to be very uncommon and usually associated with immunodeficiency states. However, recent reports have shown that they may be a common cause of gastroenteritis in children and veterinarians.[37] In *Isospora* infections (*hominis* and *belli*) the parasites are found within the epithelial cell cytoplasm of the mucosa, and all stages of its life cycle are observed. *Cryptosporidium* is a coccidial protozoan related to *Isospora* but differs from it in that it exclusively inhabits the striated or microvillous border of the small intestinal epithelium[29,30,38] (see Figure 14–8) and may be found in the gastric and rectal mucosa. The organism is rapidly cleared in the normal population but in the immunodeficient patient is very resistant to eradication.

Intrinsic and Associated Morphologic Changes. Although the mucosal injury in the immunodeficient patient is frequently the result of superimposed infection, in a number of cases it appears to result from an accompanying immune injury. For example, some cases of IgA deficiency have been described, which have an associated gluten-sensitive enteropathy unresponsive to a gluten-free diet. Some of these patients were found to have an IgG anti–epithelial cell antibody.[39] In the stomach, pernicious anemia with gastric atrophy is found in some late-onset immunodeficiency syndromes. It occurs in younger patients (20 to 30 years versus 40 to 60), lacks plasma cells in the atrophic mucosa, and also lacks antibodies to intrinsic factor and parietal cells.[23,40] Occasionally, however, typical lesions are seen that are characteristic of immune disorders, such as those in nodular lymphoid hyperplasia and graft-versus-host disease. These will be described in greater detail in the sections dealing with these disorders.

Gastrointestinal Neoplasms. The immunodeficiency disorders show an increased incidence of gastrointestinal neoplasia. The majority of these neoplasms are lymphomas, but in about 20% of cases, carcinomas occur. Some immunodeficiency disorders appear to be associated with a particular tumor, for example, Kaposi's sarcoma with AIDS.[38]

Primary Immunodeficiency Disorders

These result from defects along the discrete steps of maturation of the immune system. As previously mentioned, the functional interaction of B and T cells and the monocytes makes the division of immunodeficiency disorders somewhat artificial. Nevertheless, usually either antibody defects or cell-mediated abnormalities predominate, allowing for a practical subdivision.[17,18] This is the basis of the World Health Organization (WHO) classification of immunodeficiency disorders.[19] In addition, the WHO has included a third category, which is characterized by the association of nonimmunologic defects. Finally, there is a fourth category, characterized by a primary disorder of phagocytic function. Common variable hypogammaglobulinemia and selective IgA deficiency are the two major adult immunodeficiency disorders[17,18,41,42] and severe combined immunodeficiency disease the most common childhood disorder.[19,23] The other abnormalities are relatively uncommon. The gastrointestinal manifestations of these diseases are listed in Table 14–2.

Predominant Antibody Defects

Common Variable Hypogammaglobulinemia

Pathogenesis and Clinical Features. This is a heterogeneous group of immunologic disorders.[23,43] Three major immunologic abnormalities have been described to date, namely, an intrinsic B-cell defect, an immunoregulatory T-cell abnormality, and rarely the production of autoantibodies to T and B cells, all of which lead to impairment of immunoglobulin secretion.[18,19] The disorder occurs at any age and is often familial, but no mode of inheritance has been discerned. There is a high incidence of lupus, hemolytic anemia, and idiopathic thrombocytopenia in first-degree relatives.[19] Patients have panhypogammaglobulinemia and tend to present in one of two ways, either with recurrent respiratory tract infections or with chronic diarrhea and malabsorption,[44] most commonly due to giardiasis, although bacterial overgrowth and other infections may occur.[19,23,28,29] A third of patients develop pernicious anemia, and there is a high incidence of gastrointestinal tumors.[19]

Pathology. Histologically, there is a decrease in number of plasma cells and lymphoid follicles (see Figure 14–3); otherwise, the gastrointestinal tract is often normal. However, sometimes the small intestine may show a mild to severe mucosal lesion with villus blunting, usually in association with giardiasis or bacterial overgrowth. The large intestine may show an acute colitis with crypt abscesses and neutrophilic infiltration of the lamina propria. In addition, a variety of other gastrointestinal abnormalities have been reported, such as pernicious anemia, hypogammaglobulinemic sprue, nongranulomatous ulcerative jejunoileitis, nodular lymphoid hyperplasia, and malignancy.[23,26,28]

Pernicious anemia in cases of common variable hypogammaglobulinemia differs from classic pernicious anemia in that there is an absence of plasma cells from the atrophic gastric mucosa, autoantibodies are not found, and serum gastrin levels are not elevated.[40,45–47]

In *hypogammaglobulinemic sprue*, the small intestinal mucosa resembles celiac sprue: the mucosa is flat (total villous atrophy). However, in contrast to the usual gluten enteropathy, there is an absence or paucity of plasma cells in the lamina propria. The cause of the

Table 14-2 GASTROINTESTINAL MANIFESTATIONS OF PRIMARY IMMUNODEFICIENCY DISORDERS

Type	Postulated Defect	Main Gastrointestinal Features
Predominant Antibody Defects		
Common variable immunodeficiency	Predominant B-cell defect Immunoregulatory T-cell disorder Autoantibodies to B and T cells	Diarrhea and malabsorption most commonly due to *Giardia* or bacterial overgrowth, pernicious anemia, nodular lymphoid hyperplasia, nongranulomatous ulcerative jejunoileitis, and gastrointestinal lymphoma and carcinoma
Selective IgA deficiency	Defective IgA B-cell maturation	Malabsorption due to bacterial overgrowth or parasite infestation, esp. *Giardia*, nodular lymphoid hyperplasia. Increased incidence of pernicious anemia, celiac disease, Crohn's disease, and ulcerative colitis
Selective deficiency of other immunoglobulin isotypes, IgM, IgE, IgD	Differentiation defect of IgM B-cell to isotype-specific plasma cells	Association with celiac disease, ulcerative colitis, and Crohn's disease
Infantile Y-linked agammaglobulinemia (Bruton's agammaglobulinemia)	Intrinsic defect of pre-B to B-cell differentiation	Malabsorption and chronic diarrhea due to persistent gastrointestinal infections with rotavirus and *Giardia*
X-linked immunodeficiency with increased IgM	Defect in isotype switch prevents normal maturation of IgM B-cells to IgG, IgA and IgE cells	Diarrhea, *Candida* infections, and malignancies
Transient hypogammaglobulinemia of infancy	Delayed B-cell maturation ?due to defect in T-cell–dependent stimulation	Malabsorption and diarrhea due to bacterial overgrowth and *Giardia* infestation
Kappa light chain deficiency	Unknown	Malabsorption and diarrhea; cystic fibrosis
Immunodeficiency with thymoma	Deficiency of pre-B cells ?Defective development of stem cells	Infections
Secretory component deficiency		Diarrhea, *Candida* infections
Predominant Defects of Cell-Mediated Immunity		
Severe combined immunodeficiency disease (includes Nezelof's syndrome)	Lymphoid maturation defect T-cell defect due to adenosine deaminase deficiency Purine nucleoside phosphorylase deficiency	Malabsorption and intractable diarrhea, repeated gastrointestinal viral and fungal infections (herpes, varicella and *Candida*); mucosal lesion with Whipple's-like features
Chronic mucocutaneous candidiasis	Uncertain—may be secondary to drugs	*Candida* infection of mouth, esophagus, and small bowel
Immunodeficiency Associated with Other Defects		
Wiskott-Aldrich syndrome	Cell membrane defect affecting all hemopoietic stem cell derivatives	Recurrent bloody diarrhea and malabsorption
DiGeorge syndrome (congenital thymic aplasia)	Abnormal thymic development with resultant T-cell defects	Malabsorption, intractable diarrhea, severe malnutrition
Ataxia telangiectasia	Defective T-cell maturation	Nodular lymphoid hyperplasia and vitamin B_{12} malabsorption
Phagocyte Dysfunction		
Chronic granulomatous disease	Macrophages unable to kill phagocytosed organisms	Gastrointestinal obstruction, malabsorption, and diarrhea

mucosal lesion in hypogammaglobulinemic sprue is uncertain and may be multifactorial; patients may respond to antibiotics, gammaglobulin injections, and steroids, either singly or in combination.[48-57]

Nodular lymphoid hyperplasia is said to occur in up to 60% of patients with common variable hypogammaglobulinemia.[23] Recurrent sinopulmonary infection is the most common mode of presentation, followed by steatorrhea.[56] The lesion usually involves the small intestine, although the colon and stomach may be affected. On the basis of immunologic findings, it has been postulated that the lymphoid hyperplasia that occurs in these patients is a compensatory proliferation of lymphocytes, which are unable to undergo full maturation to immunoglobulin-secreting B cells or T cells.[44,58,59] Giardiasis commonly accompanies this lesion and appears to be responsible for the diarrhea in many patients.

Selective IgA Deficiency

Pathogenesis and Clinical Features. This is the most common congenital immunodeficiency syndrome. It occurs in about 1 of every 700 people,[19,41,42,60] usually sporadically, although rare hereditary cases have been reported.[61] The cause of selective IgA deficiency is not understood, nor is its relationship to celiac disease, although the finding of IgG anti-epithelial cell antibodies in some cases suggests an immunologic mechanism.[39,62] Whether IgA deficiency results purely from a failure of maturation of the B-cell precursor or the action of suppressor T cells or some other mechanism remains to be elucidated.[23]

Most patients are asymptomatic,[63] the IgA abnormality compensated for in part by enhanced production of secretory IgM. Those that are symptomatic suffer from a variety of gastrointestinal disorders, food allergies, and recurrent pulmonary infections. These patients also have a higher incidence of collagen vascular disease, autoimmune disease,[23,39,64] pernicious anemia, celiac disease, ulcerative colitis, and Crohn's disease.[65-67]

The gastrointestinal manifestations are primarily malabsorption and steatorrhea and resemble those of celiac sprue (and may even respond to a gluten-free diet)[26,67-72] and less commonly nodular lymphoid hyperplasia, chronic bacterial infection, and giardiasis.

Pathology. The gastrointestinal tract in most cases is unremarkable other than for a paucity of IgA-containing plasma cells within the lamina propria (sometimes compensated for by increased numbers of IgM- and IgG-containing plasma cells). There is a concomitant absence of secretory IgA, and serum IgA levels are also greatly reduced (<0.5 gm/L).[41]

Secretory Component Deficiency

So far this abnormality is limited to one case report.[73] The patient suffered from chronic intestinal candidiasis. Serum IgA levels were normal, but secretory IgA could not be detected in the saliva or jejunal fluid.

Infantile X-Linked Agammaglobulinemia[17-19]

This is a sex-linked disorder due to a maturation block in the pre-B-cell to B-cell differentiation resulting in failure to make antibody and clear antigen. It usually presents at about the sixth week of life, with recurrent pyogenic infections such as bronchitis, otitis media, and meningitis. This period of life coincides with the disappearance of the maternally derived IgG antibodies. The gastrointestinal manifestations are rare; consist of vomiting, steatorrhea, and diarrhea; and are probably due to bacterial overgrowth or giardial infestation.[74] The patients have a virtual absence of serum immunoglobulins of all classes. The small intestine is usually normal but may show a nonspecific mucosal lesion of variable severity with villus blunting and virtual absence of plasma cells and lymphoid follicles. Crypt abscesses have been described in the colonic mucosa. Patients with this disorder have an increased risk of malignancy, usually lymphoma and leukemia.[75]

Miscellaneous B-Cell Disorders[17-19]

A number of other B-cell disorders, namely, transient hypogammaglobulinemia of infancy, deficiency of kappa light chain, X-linked immunodeficiency with hyper-IgM, and selective IgM, E, or D deficiency, occasionally have gastrointestinal manifestations[23] due to infections and bacterial overgrowth. Patients with these disorders are also more susceptible to celiac disease, ulcerative colitis and Crohn's disease, cystic fibrosis, and malignancies. The specific intestinal manifestations are listed in Table 14-2.

Predominant Cell-Mediated Immunodeficiency

Severe Combined Immunodeficiency

This is the second most common primary immune deficiency disease. It is usually a hereditary disorder transmitted as either an autosomal recessive or a Y-linked disease.[23] Occasionally sporadic cases are seen. Severe combined immunodeficiency results from a stem-cell disorder and in fact consists of a heterogeneous group of disorders. Recent work suggests that there are at least three abnormalities[17-19,76]:

1. A failure of T- and B-cell maturation due to failure of thymic epithelium to mature (consisting of endodermal cells devoid of Hassall's corpuscles and lymphocytes)
2. A T-cell defect associated with adenosine deaminase deficiency
3. A T-cell defect associated with purine nucleoside phosphorylase deficiency

Combined immunodeficiency associated with an embryonic thymus and normal B cells and immunoglobulins has been called *Nezelof syndrome*. It does not appear to be a distinct entity and has been classified as a variant of severe combined immunodeficiency disease in the latest World Health Organization classification.[17-19]

Clinical Manifestations of Combined Immunodeficiency. The disease afflicts predominantly male neonates between 3 and 6 months of age, and they rarely survive beyond 5 years.[23] The children usually develop a morbilliform rash at birth, which is thought to be due to a graft-versus-host reaction to maternal lymphocytes. Subsequently, they suffer from repeated viral and fungal infections, especially those caused by cytomegalovirus, herpesvirus, *Pneumocystis*, and *Can-*

dida, resulting in pneumonia and an encephalitis that may lead to severe dementia. Ninety percent of these patients develop an irreversible enterocolitis with intractable diarrhea.[23] The cause of the diarrhea is not always clear, because symptoms may persist after eradication of the infection.

Pathology. Histologically, the intestinal tract shows the usual features of immunodeficiency. Plasma cells and lymphocytes are absent from the lamina propria, and there may be flattening of the small-intestinal mucosa (see Figure 14–3). The colon may be friable, edematous, and focally ulcerated. In addition, large vacuolated macrophages similar to those seen in Whipple's disease but much fewer in number, have been described.[77] Although this condition was invariably fatal in the past, recent bone marrow, thymic, and fetal liver transplants offer hope for some degree of restoration of the immune system.[17–19,78]

Chronic Mucocutaneous Candidiasis

Chronic mucocutaneous candidiasis is characterized by chronic candidal infection of the skin, nails and mucous membranes and is frequently associated with endocrinopathies, such as Addison's disease, and hypothyroidism. It is thought to result from a defect of the cellular immune system either as a primary disorder, or secondary to immune suppression by drugs or disease.[23,79]

Clinically, gastrointestinal lesions consist of white plaques in the mouth which produce pain and discomfort on mastication and esophageal lesions resulting in dysphagia and occasionally strictures. Gastric lesions produce epigastric pain and vomiting.

Histologically, the esophageal lesions are typically superficial and consist of mild epithelial degeneration or necrosis, with pseudohyphae growing in the necrotic epithelium (see Figure 14–4). In rare cases more extensive tissue destruction and stricture formation are found. There is only a mild inflammatory infiltrate. It should be stressed that on biopsy alone it may be difficult to separate commensal colonization by *Candida* from infection, and the diagnosis rests on the combined clinical and pathologic findings.

Immunodeficiency Associated with Other Defects[19]

This group of disorders is characterized by the accompanying nonimmunologic defects.

DiGeorge's Syndrome[80]

DiGeorge's syndrome is a very rare condition characterized by thymic aplasia or hypoplasia and the absence of the parathyroid glands. Other congenital abnormalities have also been described, such as nasal clefts, hypertelorism, and anomalies of the great vessels. Patients present with neonatal hypocalcemia and are susceptible to fungal, viral, and occasionally bacterial infections. They may develop intractable diarrhea, which is sometimes associated with severe malnutrition and death.[22] Histologically, the intestinal changes are characterized by a nonspecific mucosal lesion with crypt abscesses. The T-cell defect is seldom absolute and at autopsy remnants of thymus may be demonstrated. Humoral immune response is normal. Thymic transplant with restoration of cell-mediated immunity has been successful in some patients.[81]

Wiskott-Aldrich Syndrome and Ataxia Telangiectasia

The other disorders in this group consist of the *Wiskott-Aldrich syndrome* (eczema and thrombocytopenia), and *ataxia telangiectasia* (cerebellar ataxia and telangiectasia of the conjunctivae and flexor surfaces of the arms). The gastrointestinal manifestations consist mainly of candidiasis and malabsorption.[23] In ataxia telangiectasia there is IgA deficiency, and there may be a nodular lymphoid hyperplasia.[23,26,74]

Phagocytic Dysfunction

Chronic Granulomatous Disease

Chronic granulomatous disease is an X-linked inherited disorder in which there is an inability to kill certain organisms that have been phagocytosed by polymorphonuclear leukocytes and macrophages. The disease involves mainly young male children and is characterized by recurrent infections involving the skin, lymph nodes, and gastrointestinal tract.[82–84]

Clinically, gastrointestinal manifestations are primarily diarrhea and vomiting and less commonly steatorrhea and vitamin B_{12} malabsorption. In one instance gastric obstruction due to chronic granulomatous inflammation of the antrum was reported. Most patients also have lymphadenopathy and hepatosplenomegaly.

Pathologically, lipid-laden pigmented histiocytes similar to those seen in Whipple's disease have been described in the small intestinal and rectal mucosa. Other changes that have been reported are ulcerative stomatitis, rectal granulomas, and perianal fistulas and abscesses.[83,84] See Chapter 16 for further details.

Acquired Immunodeficiency Disorders

Acquired immunodeficiency disorders are a heterogeneous group of disorders that may be acquired in a number of different ways. For example, T-cell dysfunction may develop naturally with increasing age; is sometimes associated with certain malignancies such as Hodgkin's disease[85]; or may complicate severe infections, such as tuberculosis, lepromatous leprosy, and some viral infections, notably *HIV III* infection.[86,87] B-cell dysfunctions with dysgammaglobulinemia may occur in malignancies, such as multiple myeloma and certain lymphomas, for example, alpha-chain disease. Hypogammaglobulinemia can also result from secondary loss of antibody in disease of the kidney, the protein-losing enteropathies, and intestinal lymphangiectasia.[88] Still other causes of acquired immunodeficiency are the iatrogenic complications of immunosuppressive and steroid therapy, given for the treatment of autoimmune disease, neoplasia, and organ transplantation.

The pathologic manifestations in the gastrointestinal tract consist primarily of *infection* and an increased risk of *neoplasia*. These morphologic changes are similar to those previously described in the primary immunodeficiency diseases. The state of the patient after bone marrow transplantation and AIDS are two unique forms of acquired immunodeficiency that have emerged in the last few years. These will be described in greater detail.

Bone Marrow Transplantation

Bone marrow transplantation is now an established form of treatment for certain disorders, notably severe aplastic anemia, hematologic malignancies, congenital immunodeficiency syndromes, and enzyme deficiency disorders. Long-term survival is excellent in some of these conditions, especially acute nonlymphoblastic leukemia and severe combined immunodeficiency and approaches 50% in aplastic anemia.[89] However, injury to the gastrointestinal tract is common after bone marrow transplantation and results from three major causes: (1) the transplantation regimen, (2) infections complicating immunosuppression, and (3) the graft-versus-host reaction. Differentiating among these three major causes of injury in bone marrow transplantation is obviously important, because specific therapies can improve one condition but worsen another.

Transplantation Regimen

The transplantation regimen usually consists of chemotherapy and total body irradiation, which are given to immunosuppress the patient for prevention of graft rejection; to create space in the marrow for the allograft; and in the case of acute leukemia, to eradicate tumor cells. By itself, the dose of chemotherapy does not usually cause any mucosal injury; but in conjunction with the radiation, it does.[89] The changes in the small and large bowel are similar and indistinguishable from radiation enteritis. In the bowel the injury is characterized by atypia of crypt cell nuclei, decreased mitoses, degeneration and later flattening of crypt epithelium, abnormal surface cells, and stunted villi in the small bowel. Extensive necrosis of intestinal crypts may follow. The mucosal injury is usually transient, lasting about 3 weeks, with complete resolution.[89]

Infection

After conditioning therapy bone marrow transplant patients are susceptible to bacterial, viral, and fungal infections and parasitic infestations (Table 14–3), a reflection of the severe, though transient immunodeficiency and granulocytopenia.[90] The greatest risk for infection is at the time of acute graft-versus-host disease

Table 14-3 COMMON GI INFECTIONS AND PARASITIC INFESTATIONS IN BONE MARROW TRANSPLANTATION AND AIDS

Esophagitis
  Candida species
  Herpes simplex virus
Gastroduodenal erosions and ulcers
  Candida species
  Aspergillus
  Herpes simplex virus
Enterocolitis
  Intestinal overgrowth by aerobic gram-negative bacteria
  Candida and *Aspergillus*
  Cytomegalovirus
Pseudomembranous colitis
  Clostridium difficile
Neutropenic colitis
  Probably due to multiple causes
Parasitic infestations
  Giardia
  Cryptosporidium
  Disseminated strongyloidiasis

(GVHD), and consequently the mucosal changes due to infection may be compounded by the changes resulting from the GVHD reaction.

Graft-Versus-Host Disease

The pathogenesis of GVHD is not clearly understood, but there are three possible mechanisms that may be acting in concert with one another. These are (1) a cell-mediated cytotoxic reaction of the donor's T lymphocytes against the host's mucosa,[91,92] (2) infectious injury associated with a deficiency of intestinal immunity induced by acute GVHD,[93,94] and (3) "innocent bystander" injury to the mucosa following immune response to the infiltrating lymphocytes.[95]

Clinicopathologically, GVHD has two forms of presentation, acute and chronic.

Acute GVHD. Acute GVHD usually starts 3 to 4 weeks after bone marrow transplantation (range, 2 to 10 weeks) and is characterized by the abrupt onset of an erythematous rash, severe watery diarrhea, crampy abdominal pain, and intestinal hemorrhage. The severity of the intestinal lesion parallels the skin involvement.[88]

Pathology. The brunt of the injury is found in the ileum and right colon, the stomach and rectum usually being spared. Endoscopic changes range from normal to patchy erythema to extensive mucosal sloughing.[89] The early histologic changes are unique[89,96,97] and consist of focal crypt cell necrosis. The necrotic foci are characterized by lacunae containing cellular debris lying between the basement membrane[89,96] and the crypt epithelium, so-called popcorn lesions (Figures 14–9 and 14–10). These lacunae have been called apoptotic bodies and although also rarely found in inflammatory bowel disease (IBD), lack the inflammatory response characteristic of IBD. In more severe GVHD the epithelial necrosis extends to involve the whole crypt, which results in the dropping out of entire

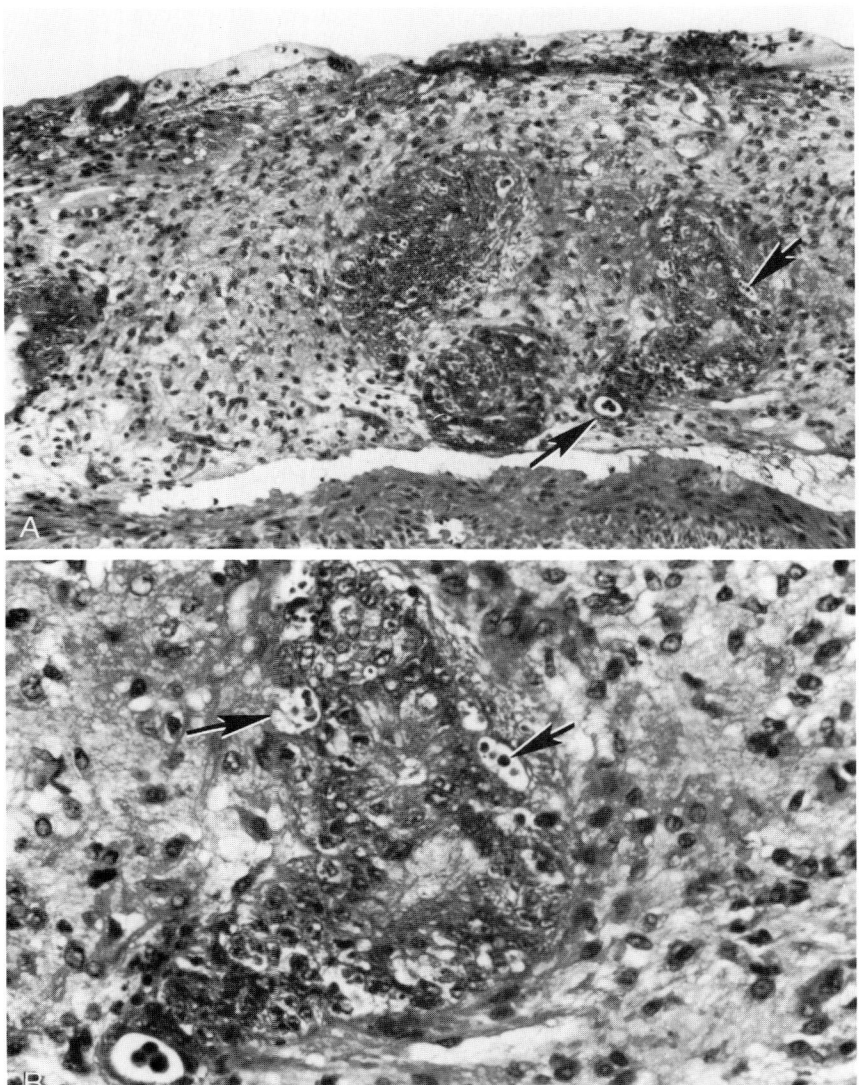

FIGURE 14–9. Colonic mucosa in acute graft-versus-host disease (GVHD). *A*, Low-power view showing degenerating crypts with so-called popcorn lesions (arrows). *B*, High-power magnification of popcorn lesions characterized by lacunae containing cellular debris.

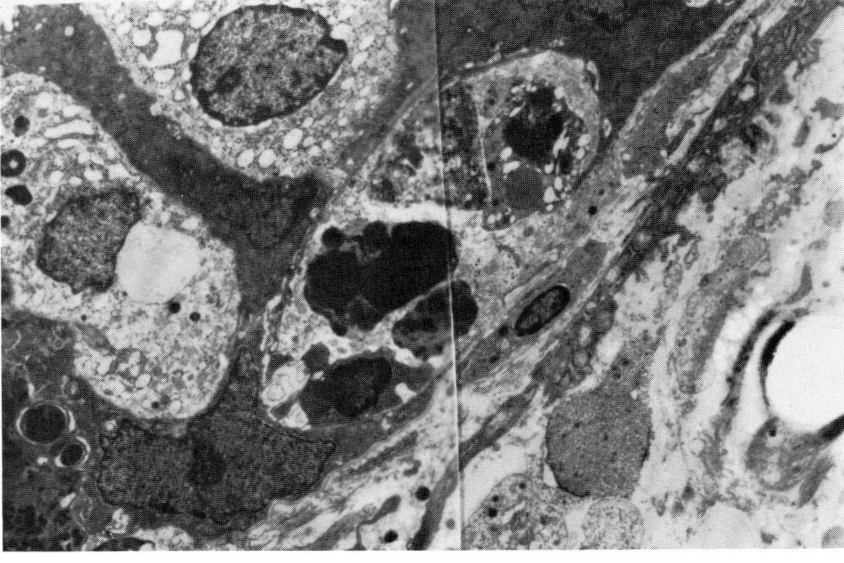

FIGURE 14–10. Low-power electron micrograph of a popcorn lesion of acute GVHD showing a lacuna lying between the basement membrane and the glandular epithelium. The lacuna contains lymphocytes and macrophages.

crypts. At this stage apoptotic bodies are difficult to find. In advanced cases there is extensive ulceration, edema, and fibrosis.

Chronic GVHD. This is a multisystem syndrome that resembles autoimmune disease and develops 80 to 400 days after marrow transplantation in about 30% of long-term survivors.[89] Most patients with chronic GVHD have had preceding acute GVHD. Clinically, patients have many features in common with scleroderma, such as skin pigmentation and contractures, oral mucositis, oral and ocular sicca, polyserositis, and esophagitis.

Pathology. The esophagus is primarily involved; only rarely are the small and large bowel involved.[89,98] In the esophagus there are desquamation and ulceration of the mucosa and submucosal fibrosis, which may produce stricture. The intestinal mucosa is usually spared; on rare occasions, however, it may develop submucosal and subserosal fibrosis.

Gastrointestinal Manifestations of AIDS

The gastrointestinal tract is a major target organ in AIDS, second only to the lung. The major features are opportunistic infections[99] and less commonly certain neoplasms such as Kaposi's sarcoma,[100] lymphoma,[101,102] condylomas, and carcinomas of the anus[103] and carcinoma of the tongue.[104] It should be stressed that a lesion unique to the HIV virus has not been observed and that all pathologic changes represent the secondary manifestations of infection and neoplasm in an immunocompromised host.

Opportunistic Infections

The most common opportunistic infections seen in the gut in AIDS patients are *Candida* esophagitis, disseminated cytomegalovirus (CMV) infection (see Figures 14-5 and 14-6), *Mycobacterium avium-intracellulare* (MAI) infection (Figures 14-11 and 14-12) and

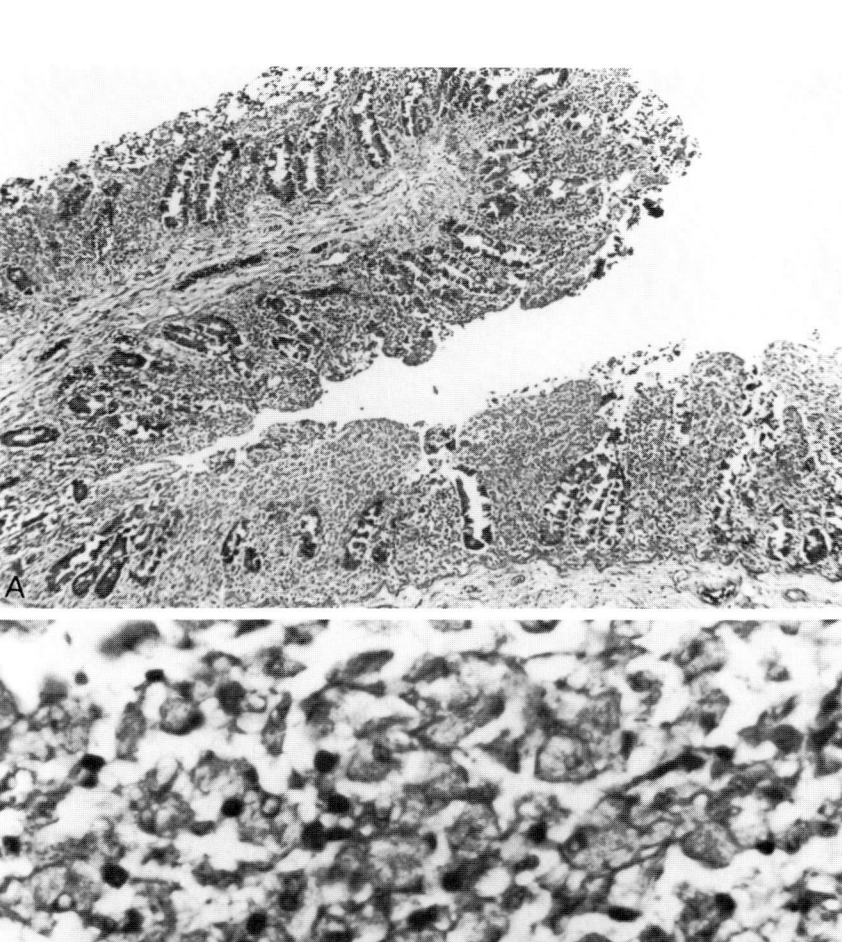

FIGURE 14-11. Mycobacterium avium-intracellulare in a patient with AIDS. *A*, Low-power magnification showing lamina propria packed with pale-staining macrophages. The surface epithelium is absent because of autolysis. This lesion resembles Whipple's disease but lacks the lymphangiectasia, a common feature in the latter. *B*, High-power magnification illustrating the densely packed foamy macrophages.

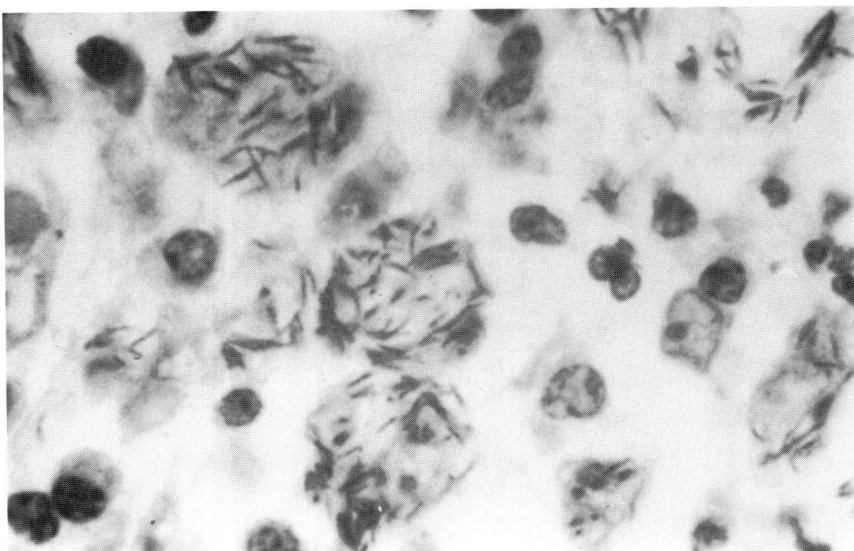

FIGURE 14-12. High-power magnification under oil immersion demonstrating numerous mycobacteria within macrophages (acid-fast stain).

cryptosporidiosis (see Figure 14-8). Although all of these infections were observed prior to the AIDS epidemic, their clinical and pathologic manifestations often differ in AIDS.[105] For example, *Candida* infection is common in lymphoma and leukemia. In these patients there is usually widespread intestinal infection, in contrast to AIDS patients, in whom it is usually limited to the oral mucosa and esophagus. *M. avium* was previously seen primarily as a low-grade pulmonary infection associated with obstructive lung disease, whereas in AIDS it usually shows widespread dissemination.

***Candida* Infection.**[31,106-108] This infection is common in AIDS, involving almost exclusively the oral and esophageal mucosa. It is commonly present at the outset of the disease or during the course of therapy for other opportunistic infections. The endoscopic findings are striking, with diffuse erythema and mucosal plaques. Histologically there is superficial ulceration with necrotic squamous epithelium infiltrated by numerous fungal hyphae. Sometimes deep esophageal ulceration is found. These cases are usually associated with a second offending organism, commonly cytomegalovirus. To date, *Candida*-associated esophagitis is the most treatable finding in the gastrointestinal tract of patients with AIDS. It may occur even in the absence of oral lesions and may be asymptomatic. Earlier recognition of this complication has led to more prompt therapy.

Cryptosporidiosis. This is a common infection in animals, especially calves, and may occur in healthy individuals as a self-limited infection.[37,109,110] In AIDS it is a serious problem, produces a severe watery diarrhea, and contributes directly to morbidity and mortality.[111] Because the parasite does not produce any significant mucosal lesion, it is thought that the secretory diarrhea results from toxin. Histologically, this tiny (4 to 5 µm) protozoan parasite inhabits the microvillous regions of epithelial cells[30] and can be seen in routinely stained sections as small round structures attached to the microvillous border (see Figure 14-8). It is patchily distributed in the small bowel and colon and occasionally in the stomach. In the small bowel the parasite is clustered at the tip of the villus. In the rectum it is located primarily in the rectal crypts. There is usually no significant underlying inflammation. Diagnosis of cryptosporidiosis can be made by screening tissue sections for cryptosporidia, but this method is laborious. The most sensitive method is searching for the organisms in fresh stool specimens.[112,113]

Cytomegalovirus Infection. CMV infection in AIDS is always widespread throughout the gastrointestinal tract and other organs, and patients usually have high serum antibody titers. Histologically there is a wide spectrum of mucosal abnormalities, often without an associated inflammatory reaction. The most frequent lesions occur in the colon, usually in the cecum,[114,115] and consist of multiple shallow ulcers set in a hyperemic mucosa (Figure 14-13). Sometimes the colonic infection is severe and may perforate. Histologically, CMV inclusions are prominent mainly within histiocytes, endothelial cells, and fibroblasts. Capillary thrombosis with secondary ischemic change may occur. Other lesions that have been described with CMV are localized ulceration of the small intestine, low-grade gastritis, and esophagitis[106]; we have seen several examples of hypertrophic gastritis in which numerous viral inclusions were found within gastric epithelial cells (see Figure 14-6).

Mycobacterium Avium-Intracellulare Infection. MAI infection is an obligate intracellular acid-fast bacillus previously found in the Southern United States as a low-grade pulmonary disease associated with obstructive lung disease or tuberculosis. AIDS patients may have an immunologic defect that particularly favors this mycobacterium over other atypical mycobacteria,[116-117] and it is commonly found as a disseminated

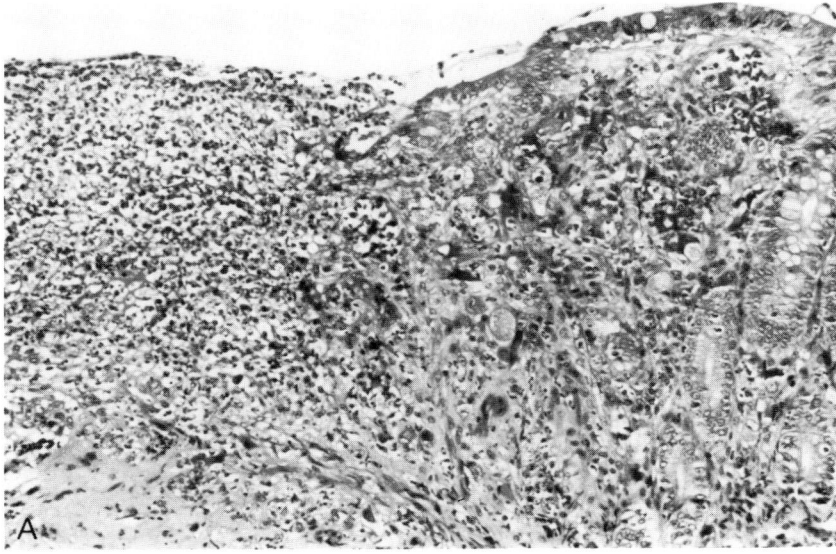
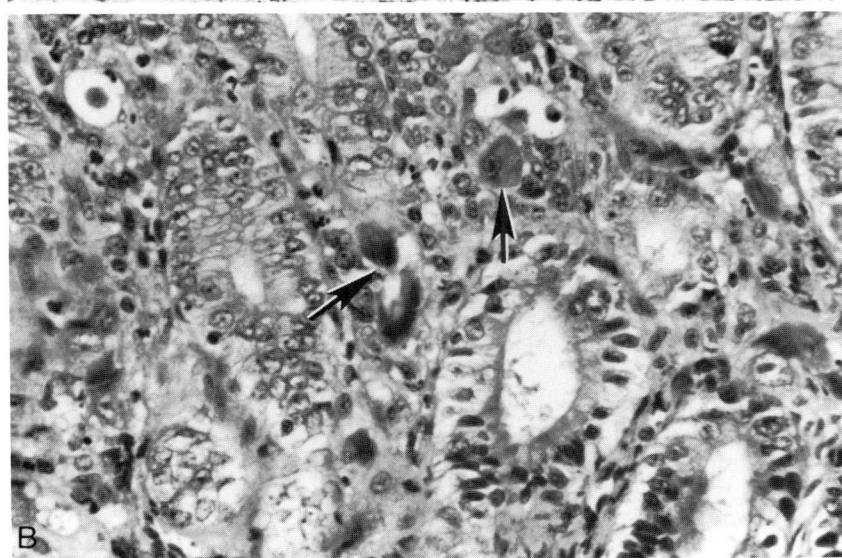

FIGURE 14–13. Cytomegalovirus-associated colitis. *A,* Low-power view showing severe inflammation and focal ulceration. *B,* Higher-power magnification of the mucosa adjacent to the mucosal ulcer showing the viral inclusions (arrows).

infection just before death.[116,118] MAI infection involves mainly the small intestine and grossly appears as small yellow-white plaques. The characteristic histology consists of an infiltrate within the mucosa of foamy macrophages (reminiscent of Whipple's disease, although lymphangiectasia is absent), which are weakly periodic acid–Schiff (PAS)-positive and packed with acid-fast bacteria (see Figures 14–11 and 14–12). There is a poor tissue response, and granuloma formation is generally absent.[119]

Other Infections. Gastrointestinal investigation in patients with AIDS may also uncover other pathogens, such as herpes virus, *Giardia, Amoeba, Salmonella,* intestinal spirochetes (Figure 14–14), *Isospora belli,* and microsporidial organisms, known to occur with increased frequency in homosexuals (Table 14–3).[120,121] Perianal herpesvirus infection and herpes proctitis may be more intractable in AIDS patients than in the homosexual population at large. The diagnosis is best established with culture of mucosal swabs. The typical herpeslike cells may be seen in smears or biopsy sections.

Other Lesions. In the opportunistic infection group, other unexplained findings have been reported.[31] These include mild to moderate villous abnormalities in the small bowel of uncertain etiology and diffuse multifocal nodular lymphoid hyperplasia of the colon associated with incidentally discovered granulomas in both antral and fundic gland mucosa.

Kaposi's Sarcoma

There is extensive visceral involvement in Kaposi's sarcoma (KS)[122–125] in AIDS. This is in distinct contrast to the more indolent dermal tumors that occur in elderly Caucasian males with KS. The gastrointestinal tract appears to be affected in approximately 50% of patients who present with skin involvement, although the majority of cases are clinically silent, and occasionally the gut lesions antedate the skin lesions. In the

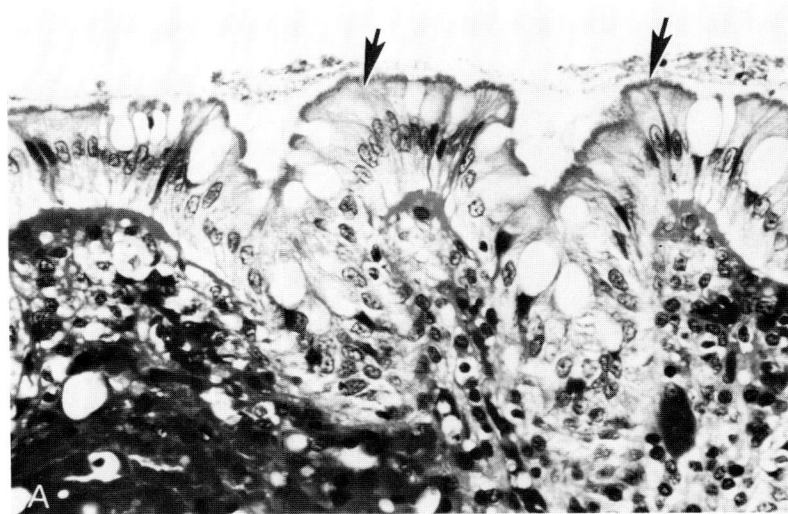
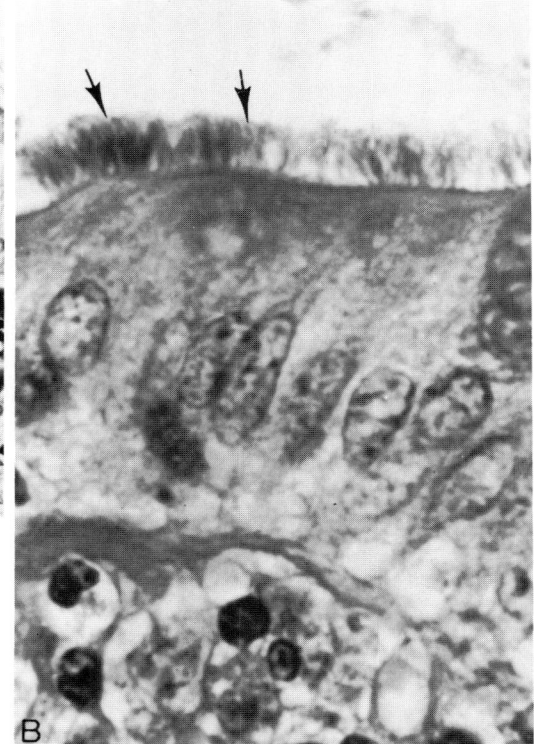

FIGURE 14-14. Intestinal spirochetosis in a rectal biopsy from a patient with AIDS. Low-power view illustrating organisms adherent to surface epithelium producing a brush border–like appearance (arrows). *B*, Higher magnification illustrating cilia-like organisms adherent to surface epithelium (arrows). (Courtesy of M. Janssen, M.D., California.)

upper gastrointestinal tract, the gastric antrum, body, and proximal duodenum appear to be equally susceptible. In the large bowel, lesions are more common in the left colon, approximately 75% being located within the distal 60 cm. Grossly, the lesions are rounded, bright red, smooth sessile nodules, averaging 0.5 to 1.0 cm in diameter (Figure 14–15). Larger lesions have a reticulated white surface, and the largest lesions have central umbilication. Histologically, the lesions show the characteristic features of KS, namely, spindle cell proliferation, extravasated red blood cells, and interlacing thin-walled vascular structures (see Figure 14–15). However, histologic confirmation of KS is possible in only a minority of endoscopic biopsies, because the le-

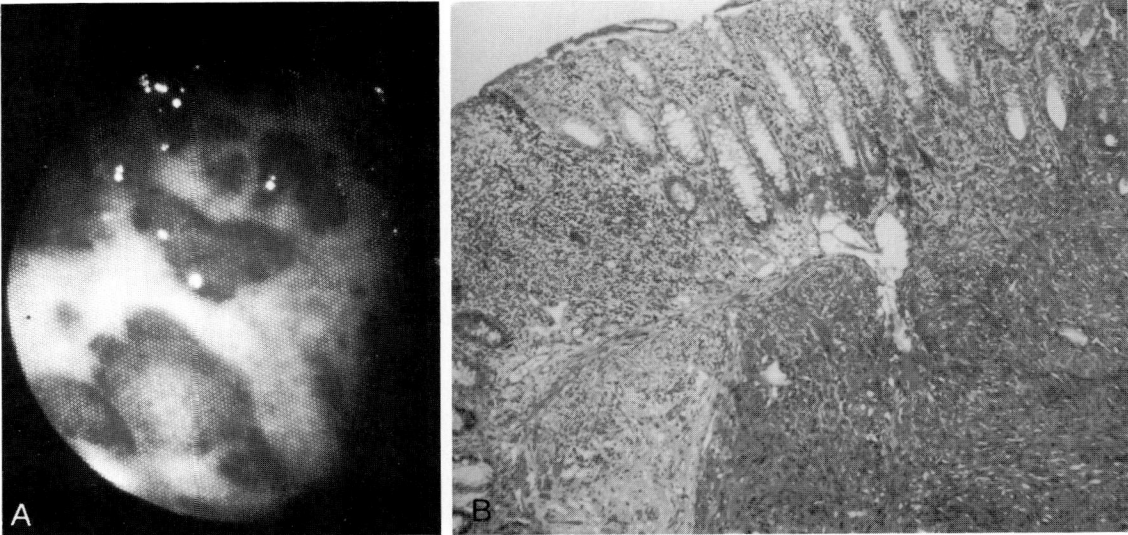

FIGURE 14-15. Kaposi's sarcoma in the rectum from a patient with AIDS. *A*, Endoscopic appearance characterized by smooth, raised, reddish, mucosal nodules. *B*, Low-power photomicrograph showing the characteristic spindle-cell proliferation within the submucosa extending up into the mucosa.

DISORDERS OF THE LYMPHOID SYSTEM

Table 14-4 LABORATORY WORKUP OF THE IMMUNODEFICIENCY PATIENT

Tests for immunologic function	Serum immunoglobulin
	Nature and number of circulating B and T cells
	T-cell function as expressed in cell-mediated immune response
Stools	1. Stool concentrates for ova and parasites, especially
	Giardia
	Cryptosporidium
	Strongyloides
Aspirate or suction trap	2. Selective culture media
	Mycologic—*Candida*
	Viral—herpes and cytomegalovirus (CMV)
	Mycobacteria
	Bacteria—commensal and pathogenic
Endoscopy	3. Direct smear—special stains and immunofluorescence
	Candida
	Giardia
	Herpes
	CMV
	4. Biopsy
	a. No change—immunoperoxidase for plasma cell isotype
	b. Infections—identify pathogens
	H&E and PAS for most organisms and viral inclusions (*Candida, Giardia, Cryptosporidium,* herpesvirus, and CMV)
	c. Immunoperoxidase and DNA hybridization for viruses, e.g., herpesvirus and CMV
	d. Tumors
	Lymphoma and lymphoid hyperplasia
	Immunoperoxidase for lymphoma workup and determination of isotypes of lymphoid cell
	Carcinoma and Kaposi's sarcoma

sions are primarily submucosal and also because it can be difficult to differentiate mucosal ulceration and granulation tissue from early KS.

Workup of the Immunodeficient Patient
(Table 14-4)

As previously mentioned, the major complication of the immunodeficiency diseases, as they involve the gut, is infection. The infections will vary, depending on the type of immunodeficiency.

In recent years, new techniques have been developed to optimize the detection and isolation of pathogens in the gastrointestinal tract. These include (1) special concentration techniques for stool specimens for the isolation of specific pathogens, e.g., *Cryptosporidium*[110,112,113]; (2) direct swabbing of lesions seen at endoscopy; (3) the use of suction traps attached to endoscopes for the aspiration of selected lesions; (4) the use of carrier media; and (5) the use of selective media. The pathologist should be aware of these techniques and should work closely with the endoscopist and the microbiologist to maximize the diagnostic yield from the specimen.

LYMPHOPROLIFERATIVE DISORDERS

The gastrointestinal tract is a common site for lymphoproliferative disorders. This is not surprising, in view of the extensive lymphoid tissue normally present in the mucosa of the gastrointestinal tract. The lymphoproliferative disorders may occur in the confines of existing lymphoid structures (as solitary or diffuse lesions) but frequently extend beyond the areas normally populated by the lymphoid cells, namely, transmurally by direct extension and beyond to mesenteric lymph nodes.

Lymphoid Hyperplasia

Lymphoid hyperplasia occurs in virtually all parts of the gastrointestinal tract. Most cases are either focal or diffuse and can be assigned to one of five distinct clinicopathologic groups:

1. Focal lymphoid hyperplasia of the stomach (gastric pseudolymphoma)
2. Focal lymphoid hyperplasia of the small intestine
3. Focal lymphoid hyperplasia of the rectum (benign lymphoid polyp, rectal tonsil)
4. Focal nodular lymphoid hyperplasia of the terminal ileum and appendix
5. Diffuse nodular lymphoid hyperplasia of the intestine

On rare occasions lymphoid hyperplasia has been described in unusual locations such as the esophagus and colon.[126,127] Familiarity with the various forms of gastrointestinal lymphoid hyperplasia is important for the proper evaluation of the lesion and, in particular, its distinction from malignant lymphoma of the gastrointestinal tract.

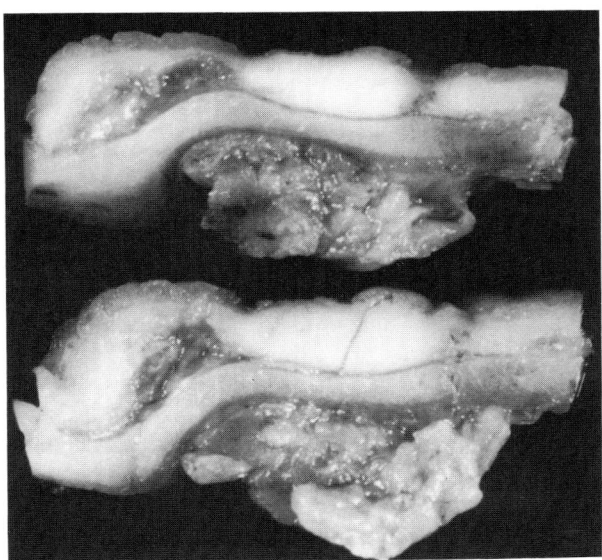

FIGURE 14–16. Gastrectomy specimen of gastric lymphoid hyperplasia. Note the thickening of the antral submucosa with a smooth lower border abutting on the muscle coat (cross-sectional cut).

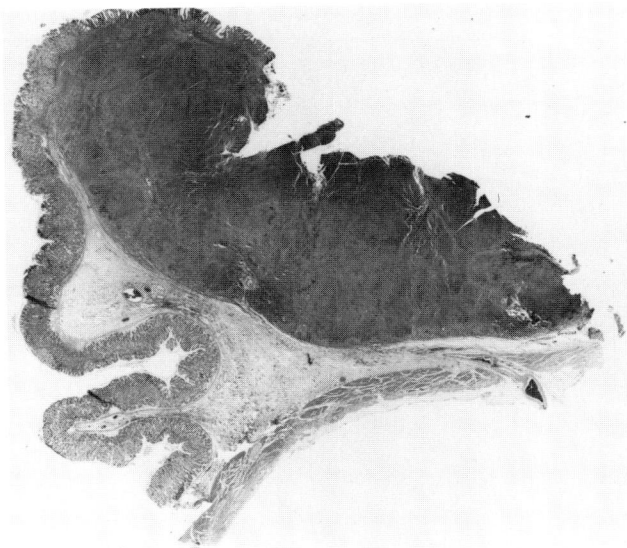

FIGURE 14–17. Gastric lymphoid hyperplasia. Low-power view demonstrating an exophytic tumor-like mass. The lymphoid infiltrate has a smooth "pushing" border, and the nodularity of the admixed lymphoid follicles can just be made out.

Lymphoid hyperplasia may also occur as a secondary component in a number of disorders, including nonerosive gastritis, Crohn's disease, and ulcerative colitis, and may sometimes cause difficulty in diagnosis. However, in primary lymphoid hyperplasia, the proliferation of lymphoid tissue is the predominant or only pathologic feature responsible for producing topographical and structural change.

Focal Lymphoid Hyperplasia of the Stomach

The term *gastric pseudolymphoma* has been widely used for focal lymphoid hyperplasia of the stomach, and understandably so, because it may closely simulate lymphoma.[128–134] This lesion occurs in adults, most frequently during the fourth to sixth decades, and affects men more commonly than women. Patients usually present with symptoms suggestive of gastric ulcer disease. Clinically, patients with gastric lymphoid hyperplasia may have the radiologic and endoscopic features of a peptic ulcer[130,132,134,135]; and it is only on histologic examination that the excessive lymphoid infiltrate causes concern. More frequently, however, gastric lymphoid hyperplasia simulates a malignant neoplasm both radiologically and endoscopically.[129–132,135–139]

Pathology. On gross examination the stomach is usually ulcerated; these ulcers may mimic tumors because of their raised margins and thickened rugal folds (Figures 14–16). Histologically, gastric lymphoid hyperplasia may have two architectural forms.[128,132,134] The most common type is a chronic gastric ulcer with a lymphoid infiltrate at the margins and the floor of the ulcer (Figure 14–17). In the second variety (which is less common) there is gastric thickening and cobblestoning of the gastric mucosa, due to lymphocytic infiltration predominantly in the mucosa and submucosa. Mucosal ulceration, when present, is superficial (Figure 14–18). However, other combinations are occasionally seen, such as exophytic masses and deep ulceration (Figure 14–19).

Histologically, the typical lesions show mucosal ulceration, a dense polymorphous inflammatory infiltrate, admixed lymphoid follicles, and fibrosis (Figures 14–20 and 21).[132] The inflammatory infiltrate is composed predominantly of small mature lymphocytes with round or mildly indented nuclei, admixed with lesser numbers of immunoblasts, plasma cells, and eosinophils, especially near the ulcerated surface (Figure 14–22). Lymphoid follicles with or without obvious germinal centers are scattered throughout the lymphoid infiltrate and are best formed and most abundant superficially in the mucosa and upper submucosa.[132] Since reactive lymphoid follicles may be found at the margins of gastric lymphomas, it is important that they be clearly identified within the lymphoid infiltrate. Fibrosis is a common accompaniment of lymphoid hyperplasia, especially beneath the ulcerated areas. It is often characterized by dense acellular collagen bundles separating columns of intact lymphocytes in a single-file pattern (see Figures 14–20 and 21).[126] On rare occasions, two variants of lymphoid hyperplasia, namely, nodular lymphoid hyperplasia and angiofollicular hyperplasia, are found in the stomach.[130]

Differential Diagnosis. Malignant lymphoma is the most important lesion to exclude, and the most important distinguishing features relate to the nature of the lymphoid infiltrate (Table 14–5). Whereas in lymphoid hyperplasia it is polymorphous with admixed lymphoid follicles, it is monomorphous in lymphoma, commonly causing destruction of mucosal glands (Figure 14–23); and when lymphoid follicles are seen, they

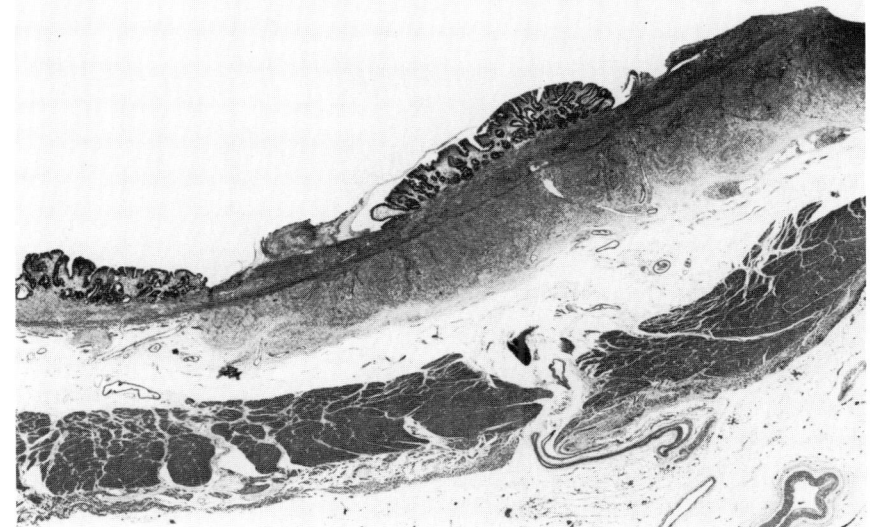

FIGURE 14–18. Gastric lymphoid hyperplasia. Low-power view demonstrating dense lymphoid infiltrate of mucosa and superficial submucosa. Although there are mucosal erosions, the typical features of chronic gastric ulcer, namely, fibrosis and destruction of muscle coats, are absent.

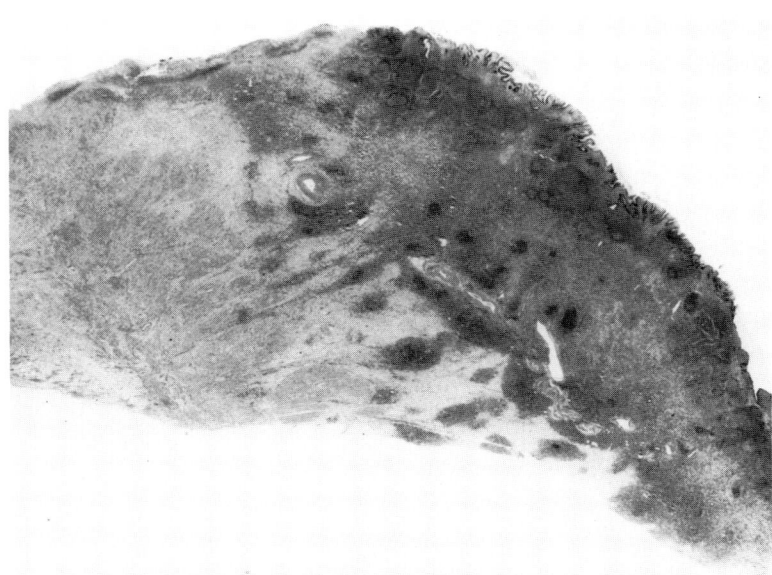

FIGURE 14–19. Gastric lymphoid hyperplasia. Low-power view demonstrating the heavy lymphoid infiltrate at the margin of a gastric ulcer. The lymphoid infiltrate is localized primarily in the mucosa and submucosa and has an "infiltrative" lower margin. (Courtesy of Dr. M. Ranchod, Good Samaritan Hospital, San Jose, Calif.)

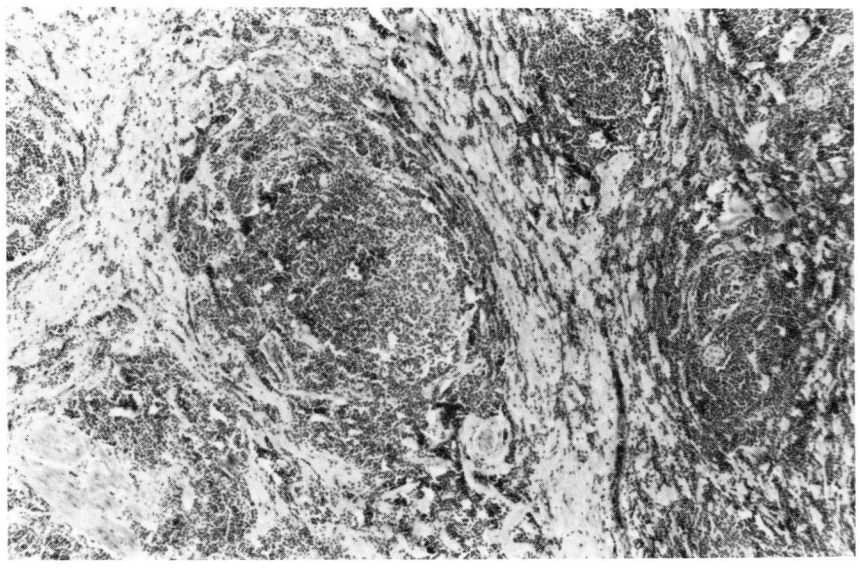

FIGURE 14–20. Gastric lymphoid hyperplasia. Low-power view showing dense lymphoid infiltration, admixed lymphoid follicles, and fibrosis.

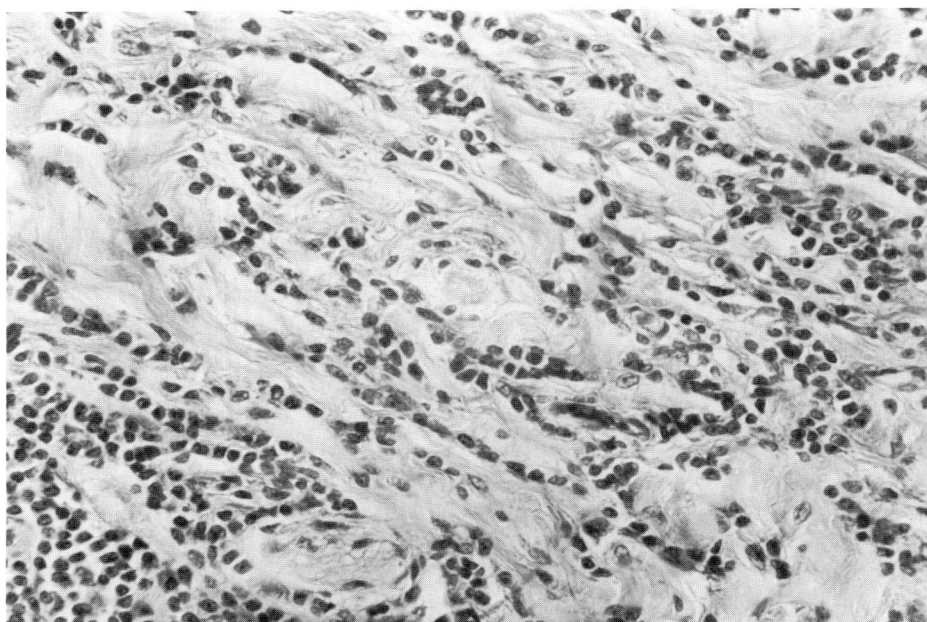

FIGURE 14–21. Gastric lymphoid hyperplasia demonstrating dense collagenous fibrosis and intervening single-file columns of mature lymphocytes.

are found at the periphery of the lesion. The cytology of the infiltrate also differs. Because the majority of gastric lymphomas are of the large-cell "histiocytic" variety or the small-cell cleaved variety, the distinction between lymphoma and lymphoid hyperplasia is usually readily made. However, in the rare well-differentiated lymphocytic lymphomas and in suboptimally fixed specimens, distinction from lymphoid hyperplasia can be difficult. In these cases immunohistochemical studies with the demonstration of a polyclonal immunoglobulin pattern in the lymphoid infiltrate, is very helpful.[140,141] However, it is of interest that several cases of gastric lymphoid hyperplasia have been described with monotypic cytoplasmic immunoglobulin. Whether these cases represent a prelymphomatous state remains to be determined.[142]

The form of gastric lymphoid hyperplasia most familiar to pathologists is that which is present at the margins of a typical chronic peptic ulcer. However, it is important to stress that on rare occasions gastric lymphoma may also have this architectural arrangement; thus, careful examination of the lymphoid infiltrate is essential for distinguishing between lymphoid hyperplasia and lymphoma.[128,132] Furthermore, lymphoid hyperplasia may be unassociated with a chronic peptic ulcer and may produce diffuse thickening of the mucosa, often accompanied by narrowing and distortion of the affected segment of the stomach, thus simulating

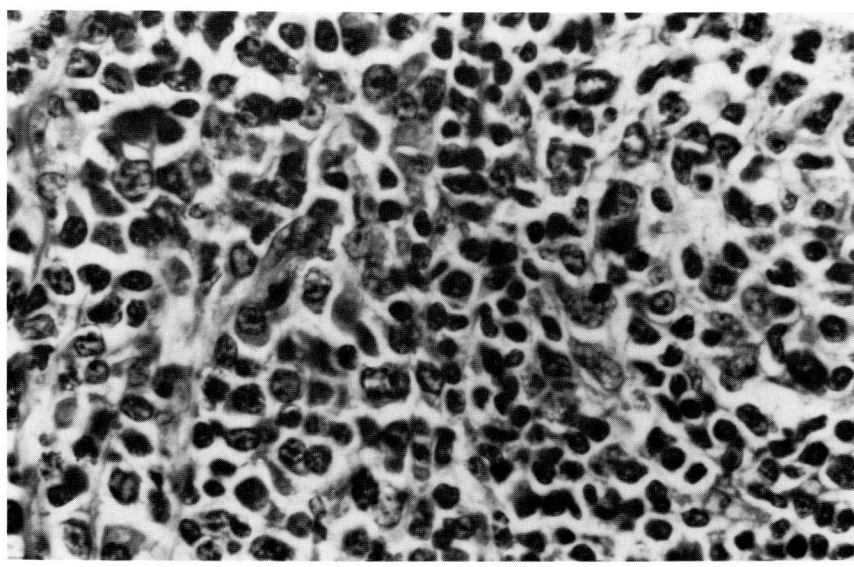

FIGURE 14–22. Gastric lymphoid hyperplasia demonstrating the characteristic polymorphous infiltrate composed of mature lymphocytes, plasma cells, immunoblasts, and histiocytes.

Table 14–5 HISTOLOGIC FEATURES DIFFERENTIATING GASTRIC LYMPHOID HYPERPLASIA FROM LYMPHOMA

	Lymphoid Hyperplasia	Lymphoma
Cellular Infiltrate	Polymorphous nature with admixed neutrophils, eosinophils and histiocytes	Monomorphous with cytologic atypia*
	Admixed reactive lymphoid follicles	Lymphoid follicles, if present, at periphery of lesion
Peptic Ulceration	In 90%	Superficial ulceration but typical peptic ulceration rare
	Collagenous fibrosis separating columns of mature lymphocytes	Fibrosis unusual; if present, at base of lesion
Mucosal Glands	Intact, other than if involved in peptic ulceration	Infiltration and destruction by atypical lymphoid infiltrate

*Rare cases of well-differentiated lymphocytic lymphoma show minimal cytologic atypia.

a malignant neoplasm both radiologically and on gross pathologic examination.[131] It is probable that some of these lesions represent the aftermath of a healed gastric ulcer.

The lymphoid infiltrate in gastric lymphoid hyperplasia may be confined to the mucosa and submucosa; but in a substantial number of cases, the lymphoid infiltrate has an infiltrating pattern involving the full thickness of the gastric wall (see Figures 14–17 to 14–19). Conversely, a significant number of gastric lymphomas may show involvement of the mucosa and submucosa only with a uniform "pushing" margin. The degree of involvement of the gastric wall, therefore, is of no aid in distinguishing between lymphoid hyperplasia and malignant lymphoma.

Malignant Predisposition of Gastric Lymphoid Hyperplasia. Does gastric lymphoid hyperplasia predispose to gastric lymphoma? There have been a few documented cases of gastric lymphoid hyperplasia showing this association.[128,143–145] Whether these cases represent sporadic aberrations, rather than consistent precursor lesions of lymphoma, remains to be determined.

Value of Endoscopic Biopsy in the Diagnosis of Gastric Lymphoid Hyperplasia

With the recent development of the large-particle biopsy forceps, sufficient material may be obtained in some cases to make a presumptive diagnosis of lymphoid hyperplasia (Figure 14–24). However, we would caution that interpretation needs to be carefully correlated with the endoscopic findings and follow-up. The reason for advising caution in the endoscopic diagnosis

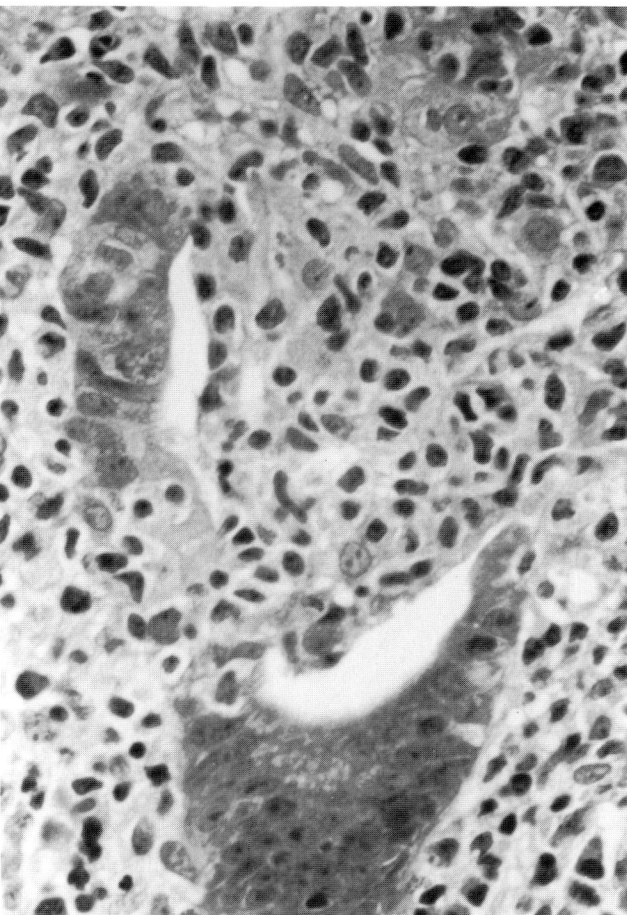

FIGURE 14–23. Gastric lymphoma illustrating the monomorphous nature of the infiltrate and the infiltration and destruction of the gastric glands.

of lymphoid hyperplasia is that many cases of gastric lymphoid hyperplasia and gastric lymphoma are superficially ulcerated, and only this part may undergo biopsy. Thus, laparotomy may be necessary for diagnosis of these cases.

Focal Lymphoid Hyperplasia of the Small Intestine

This is an exceedingly uncommon condition with few acceptable cases in the literature that could clearly be distinguished from lymphoma.[132,146] We have seen three cases, one located in the duodenum and two in the mid small intestine.[132] Patients usually present with recurrent abdominal pain. Upper gastrointestinal examination shows a focal constricting lesion radiologically. Grossly, there is nodular thickening of the mucosa, which may be circumferential. In contrast to gastric lymphoid hyperplasia, here the mucosa is not ulcerated. The lymphoid infiltrate may be superficial, involving only the mucosa and submucosa, or involve the full thickness of the intestinal wall. This lesion can be distinguished from lymphoma by the mature and

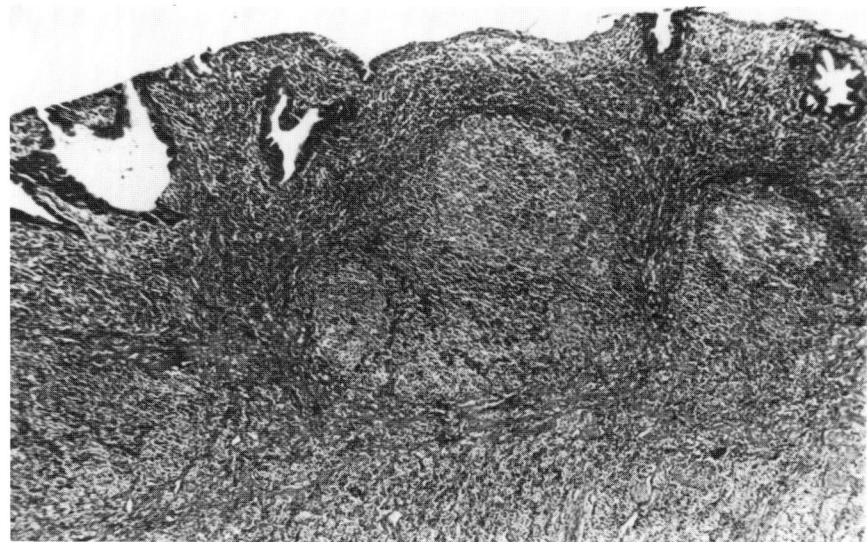

FIGURE 14-24. Endoscopic biopsy of gastric lymphoid hyperplasia obtained with the large-particle biopsy forceps. Note the dense lymphoid infiltrate with admixed lymphoid follicles and intact mucosa.

bland nature of the lymphoid infiltrate and the presence of follicles with germinal centers throughout the lesion.[7]

Focal Lymphoid Hyperplasia of the Rectum[147,148,149]

Focal lymphoid hyperplasia of the large intestine (lymphoid polyp, rectal tonsil) appears to be located almost exclusively in the rectum.[150-152] It occurs in all age groups but is most common in the second to fifth decades. Patients with lymphoid polyps have a variety of symptoms, including rectal bleeding, constipation, anal discomfort, prolapse of a rectal mass, and diarrhea, and frequently have associated anorectal lesions, such as hemorrhoids, anal fissures, and colonic carcinoma. When barium enemas have been performed, most patients have had no evidence of lymphoid polyps or nodular lymphoid hyperplasia in the proximal colon.

Pathology. Focal lymphoid hyperplasia of the rectum usually affects the lowermost portion of the rectum.[132] About 60% to 80% of the lesions present as single polyps, and multiple polyps usually number less than six. However, the polyps may be numerous on occasion and impart a cobblestone appearance to the rectal mucosa.[153] The polyps are most commonly sessile and have a smooth surface and, endoscopically, a pale yellow or white color. They range from a few millimeters to 5 cm in diameter.[132,149,150]

Microscopically, a heavy lymphoid infiltrate is present in the lamina propria and submucosa (Figure 14-25). Large follicles with prominent germinal centers are always present, although they may be difficult to identify in poorly prepared tissue. The majority of polyps are covered by intact, although at times attenuated, colonic epithelium (see Figure 14-25). Low-lying polyps may be covered by anal squamous epithelium.[132,147,149,150] The lymphoid nodules straddle the mucosa and submucosa and are therefore in a location similar to that of the solitary lymphoid nodules found in the normal colon. The muscularis mucosae shows irregular proliferation. Focal lymphoid hyperplasia of the rectum must be differentiated from malignant lym-

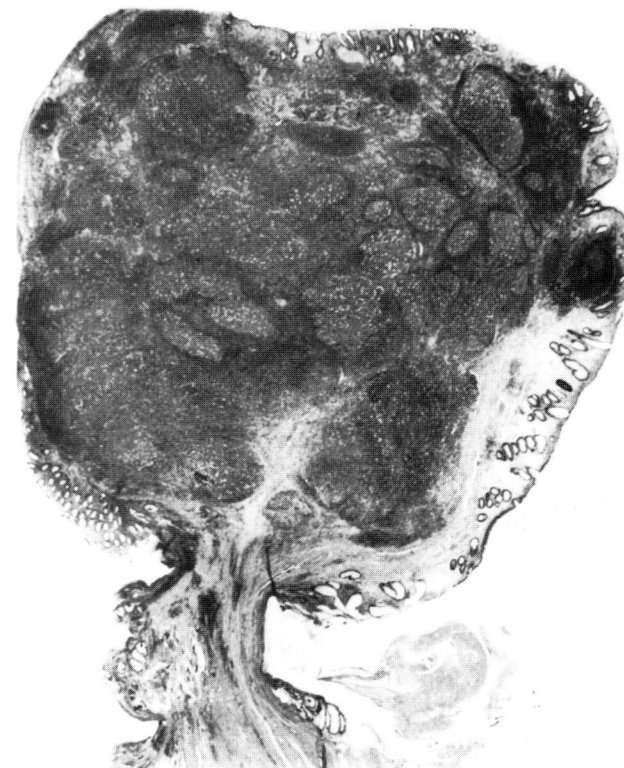

FIGURE 14-25. Focal lymphoid hyperplasia of the rectum (lymphoid polyp) demonstrating the polypoid appearance of the lesion. The polyp is covered by intact, focally attenuated colonic epithelium and contains large lymphoid follicles with prominent germinal centers.

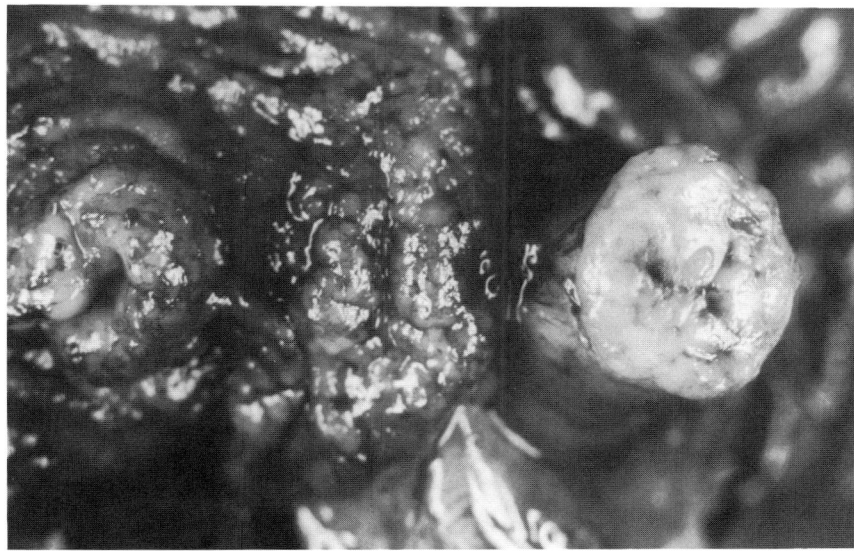

FIGURE 14-26. Focal lymphoid hyperplasia of the terminal ileum and appendix from a patient with symptoms of acute appendicitis. Gross appearance showing cobblestoning of ileal mucosa and marked thickening of the transected appendix with luminal obliteration.

phoma, although it should be noted that the latter is exceedingly rare at this site.[154]

Lymphoid polyps of the rectum should be treated by excisional biopsy for diagnostic purposes. If the lesions are multiple and the patient is asymptomatic, complete excision is probably not necessary, because there is evidence that these lesions regress spontaneously. The incidence of local recurrence is low, even after incomplete excision.[132,149]

Nodular Lymphoid Hyperplasia

Nodular lymphoid hyperplasia may be focal or diffuse and is associated with a number of distinct clinicopathologic entities. However, focal nodular lymphoid hyperplasia may represent a localized form of the diffuse disease.

Focal Nodular Lymphoid Hyperplasia of the Terminal Ileum and Appendix

Lymphoid tissue is abundant in the terminal ileum and appendix, and it is not surprising that lymphoid hyperplasia should be reported. On the other hand, involvement of the appendix is rarely mentioned and is confined to case reports.[155,156] The reason for the rarity of diagnosis of appendiceal lymphoid hyperplasia is probably that pediatric appendices normally have abundant active lymphoid tissue, and the question arises as to what constitutes abnormal lymphoid proliferation. It is our belief that pathologic features that have the potential for producing symptoms, such as thickening and swelling of the appendix with luminal narrowing, should be seen before a diagnosis of focal lymphoid hyperplasia is made (Figure 14-26).

Lymphoid hyperplasia of the terminal ileum and appendix may occur either together (see Figure 14-26) or separately and is usually found in children or young adults,[155-160] although the lesion may occur in older patients.[155] These patients usually present with ileocecal intussusception or a clinical syndrome that simulates acute appendicitis.[161-165] Roentgenograms show variable luminal narrowing of the terminal ileum; and in patients with intussusception, a filling defect may be present in the cecal area. The recent isolation of various adenovirus strains from patients with ileocecal intussusception[166,167] and the occasional demonstration of adenovirus in intussuscepted tissue[167] suggests that at least some cases of ileocecal lymphoid hyperplasia may have an infective cause. Nodular lymphoid hyperplasia of the terminal ileum has been described in patients with familial polyposis and Gardner's syndrome.[168,169]

On gross examination, the mucosa of the terminal ileum is thickened and may have a cobblestone or papillary appearance (see Figure 14-26). Lymphoid hyperplasia of the appendix is characterized by marked swelling and thickening of the mucosa and submucosa and luminal obliteration (see Figure 14-26).

Histologically, both the terminal ileum and the appendix show marked hyperplasia of the lymphoid tissue in the mucosa and submucosa (Figures 14-27 to 14-29). There are many lymphoid follicles with conspicuous germinal centers (see Figure 14-27) and many with only a thin mantle of mature lymphocytes, which may be confused with nodular lymphoma.

Diffuse Nodular Lymphoid Hyperplasia of the Intestine

Diffuse nodular lymphoid hyperplasia is characterized by the presence of numerous small, discrete lymphoid nodules involving a variable segment of the small intestine or large intestine, or both (Figure 14-30). The term *gastrointestinal pseudoleukemia* has been used for this lesion,[170] but it is confusing and should be abandoned. Diffuse nodular lymphoid hyperplasia of the gastrointestinal tract can be divided into two major

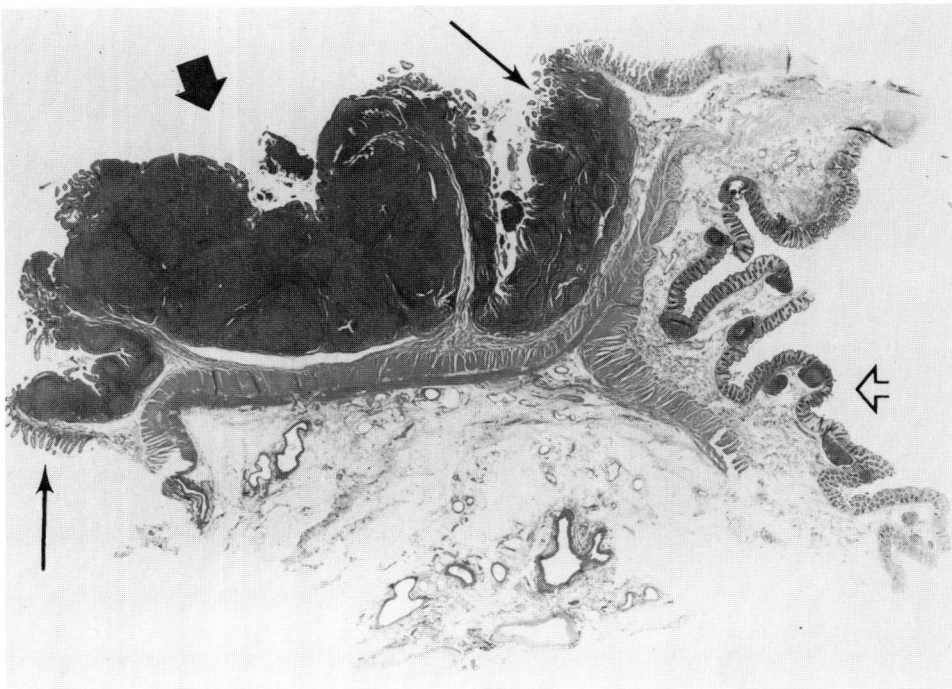

FIGURE 14–27. Focal lymphoid hyperplasia of the terminal ileum and appendix. Note the follicular hyperplasia of a Peyer's patch in the terminal ileum (between thin arrows) extending into the appendix (thick arrow).

clinicopathologic groups: those cases with acquired hypogammaglobulinemia and those without.

Diffuse Nodular Lymphoid Hyperplasia with Hypogammaglobulinemia. Nodular lymphoid hyperplasia occurs most commonly with late-onset hypogammaglobulinemia, and occasionally in isolated IgA deficiency.[171–173] However, it should be stressed that only a small portion of patients with late-onset hypogammaglobulinemia have nodular lymphoid hyperplasia. Patients present most commonly in the second to fifth decades,[172] and have decreased serum IgG and normal, decreased or absent serum IgA and IgM in various combinations. Recurrent sinopulmonary infections are the most common mode of presentation, followed by diarrhea, sometimes accompanied by steatorrhea. In patients with late-onset hypogammaglobulinemia a variety of other maladies may also develop, including pernicious anemia, cholelithiasis, thyrotoxicosis, myxedema, a variety of skin lesions, arthritis, keratoconjunctivitis, splenomegaly, and sarcoidosis.[174] Most important, however, is the increased risk of the development of gastrointestinal neoplasms.[172,175,176] In 24% of patients in the series of Hermans et al.[172] neoplasms developed, carcinoma of the gastrointestinal tract being the most frequent.

Pathology. Nodular lymphoid hyperplasia with hypogammaglobulinemia usually affects the small intestine only, but occasionally colonic and rarely gastric involvement occur.[132,172,177,178] On gross examination, the mucosa is studded with sessile or polypoid nodules, which measure up to 5 mm in diameter[132,172,179] and are readily detectable on barium studies as multiple translucencies.[172] The nodules are composed of one or a cluster of hyperplastic lymphoid nodules. When large, these nodules may produce blunting of the overlying villi, but mucosal ulceration is absent (Figure 14–31). The lymphoid nodules are confined to the lamina propria and superficial submucosa (see Figure 14–31). A decrease or absence of plasma cells is often noted in the lamina propria. Some patients appear to have normal numbers of plasma cells in hematoxylin and eosin–stained sections of the jejunal mucosa. However, immunoperoxidase staining for specific lymphocyte isotypes reveals an absence or paucity of IgA marking cells and compensatory hyperplasia of IgM or IgG isotypes. Based on immunologic findings, it has been postulated that the lymphoid hyperplasia that occurs in these patients is a compensatory proliferation

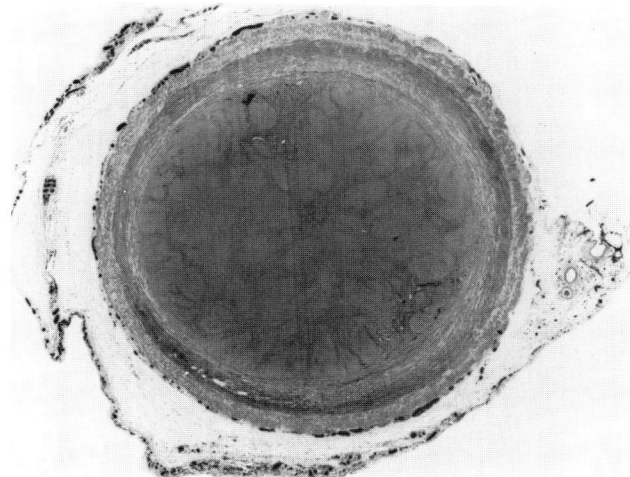

FIGURE 14–28. Focal lymphoid hyperplasia of the appendix. Low-power photomicrograph of cross-sectional cut demonstrating marked mucosal thickening, follicular hyperplasia, and luminal obliteration.

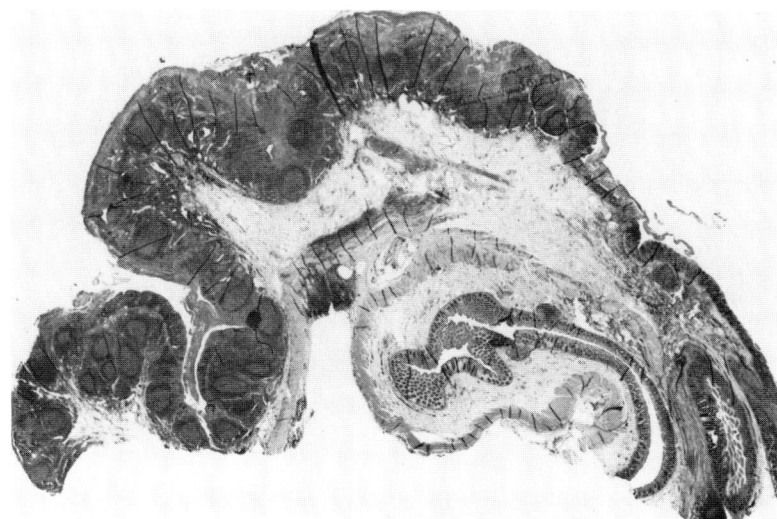

FIGURE 14–29. Low-power photomicrograph of focal lymphoid hyperplasia of the terminal ileum, which produced intussusception. Note the thickened, superficially ulcerated mucosa of the terminal ileum with marked lymphoid hyperplasia. The intussuscepted ileum is seen at the lower right margin.

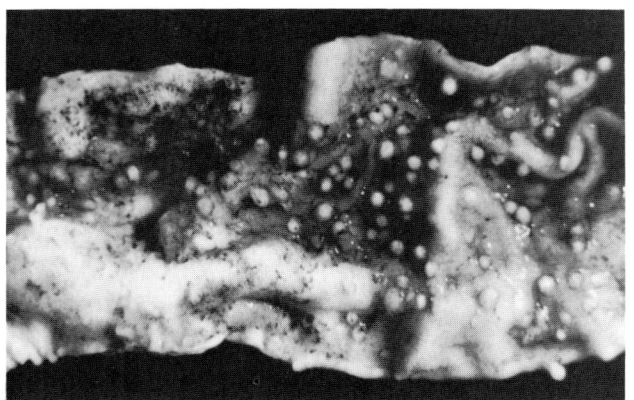

FIGURE 14–30. Nodular lymphoid hyperplasia of the large intestine showing mucosa studded with small sessile polyps measuring approximately 2 mm.

of lymphocytes, which are unable to undergo full maturation to immunoglobulin-secreting cells.[58,180,181] Lymphoid hyperplasia similar to that found in the mucosa is commonly found in mesenteric lymph nodes.

Giardiasis is commonly present and appears to be responsible for the diarrhea in many but not all patients.[58,172,177,180,182,183] Hermans et al.[172] have postulated the existence of some other factor (epithelial defect?) to explain the diarrhea in the latter. In those patients whose diarrhea responds to metronidazole and antibiotic therapy, there is no corresponding disappearance of the lymphoid nodules in the gastrointestinal tract.[172]

Diffuse Nodular Lymphoid Hyperplasia Without Hypogammaglobulinemia. Diffuse nodular lymphoid hyperplasia of the intestine often occurs in the absence of hypogammaglobulinemia and is much more frequent than nodular lymphoid hyperplasia associated

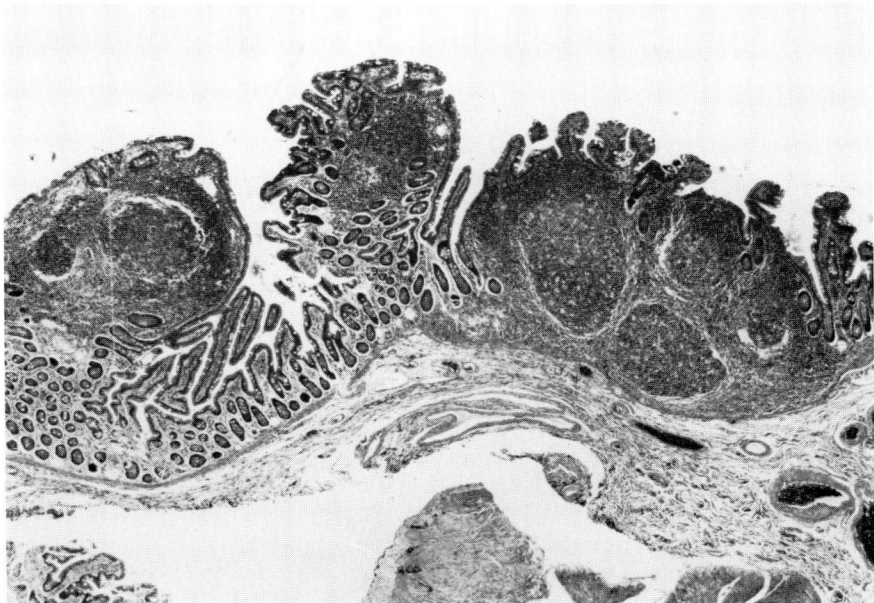

FIGURE 14–31. Nodular lymphoid hyperplasia with hypogammaglobulinemia showing clustered hyperplastic lymphoid follicles within the mucosa. Note blunting of intestinal villi over lymphoid follicles.

with late-onset hypogammaglobulinemia. Robinson et al.[184] in a study of 1000 consecutive autopsies, found 30 cases of nodular lymphoid hyperplasia. The small intestine alone was involved in 13% of cases, the large intestine alone in 40%, and the small and large intestine together in 47% of cases. These patients died of a variety of causes, and none had gastrointestinal symptoms, or giardiasis, or hypogammaglobulinemia. Robinson et al.[184] have used the term *enterocolitis lymphofollicularis* for this lesion, but we prefer the term *diffuse nodular lymphoid hyperplasia* because of the morphologic similarity of this lesion to that seen in late-onset hypogammaglobulinemia. Furthermore, the term *enterocolitis* is misleading for a process that is characterized by an absence of classical inflammation and mucosal destruction.

Nodular lymphoid hyperplasia of the colon has been observed in children who have had barium enemas for a variety of gastrointestinal complaints, and it is clear that it is a common incidental finding on barium enema and unrelated to the patient's symptoms.[185,187] Serum immunoglobulin levels were measured in three of Capitanio and Kirkpatrick's patients and were found to be normal.[185]

Pathology. The lesions are grossly visible as mucosal nodules and normally measure up to 0.4 cm in diameter, although occasionally they may be as large as 2 cm.[188] Histologically, the mucosal nodules are similar to those seen in nodular lymphoid hyperplasia with hypogammaglobulinemia except that the lamina propria contains normal numbers of plasma cells. It is probable that the lymphoid nodules represent hyperplasia of the solitary lymphoid follicles normally present in the gastrointestinal tract.

Clinical Implications. It is clear that diffuse nodular lymphoid hyperplasia may occur in the small intestine and the large intestine without associated hypogammaglobulinemia and giardiasis. Furthermore, it may be found incidentally during radiologic examination of the gastrointestinal tract or at autopsy and should not be immediately incriminated for any gastrointestinal symptoms the patient may have. An awareness that diffuse nodular lymphoid hyperplasia may give rise to multiple filling defects in the colon will allow inclusion of this lesion in the differential diagnosis of multiple polypoidal lesions in the colon. This is especially important in patients who are being evaluated for familial polyposis, where unnecessary colonic resection may be performed.[175,180,189] Because patients with nodular lymphoid hyperplasia without hypogammaglobulinemia are asymptomatic, and there are well-documented cases of spontaneous regression,[185-187] treatment of these lesions is unnecessary.

Nodular lymphoid hyperplasia has to be distinguished from multiple lymphomatous polyposis of the intestine,[190] especially if the lymphoma is follicular and lymphocytic in type. This distinction is easily made in most cases, because the nodules in nodular lymphoid hyperplasia are small, are largely confined to the lamina propria, and contain prominent germinal centers. In the rare instances when the lymphoid nodules are poorly formed, immunoperoxidase staining to determine clonality may be necessary.

Rarely, patients with nodular lymphoid hyperplasia without hypogammaglobulinemia develop lymphoma.[175,191] Matuchansky et al.[175] reported a patient with nodular lymphoid hyperplasia who developed a jejunal lymphoma. Their case is of interest because they demonstrated immunohistochemically a transition from a hyperplastic lymphoid follicle to a neoplastic one.

Malignant Lymphoma

Conditions Associated with Increased Risk of Lymphoma

A number of gastrointestinal lesions are found in association with or appear to predispose to malignant gastrointestinal lymphomas. These include the following:

1. Celiac sprue including dermatitis herpetiformis
2. Immunoproliferative small-intestinal disease (IPSID) (Mediterranean lymphoma and alpha-chain disease)
3. Lymphoid hyperplasia of the gastrointestinal tract, especially gastric lymphoid hyperplasia and diffuse nodular lymphoid hyperplasia (with and without hypogammaglobulinemia)
4. Immunodeficiency disorders of the gastrointestinal tract
   a. Primary, especially common variable immunodeficiency and selective IgA deficiency
   b. Acquired, especially AIDS, and transplantation
5. Ulcerative colitis and Crohn's disease

Celiac Sprue

Patients with celiac sprue have an increased risk of developing gastrointestinal lymphoma and carcinoma, and this complication is a major cause of death in these patients.[192-197] The characteristic clinical setting is that of a patient with known celiac sprue, usually in his fifties, who deteriorates for no apparent reason.[195] There is usually a recurrence of his malabsorption in addition to fever, abdominal pain, and weight loss. Fewer patients present with intestinal perforation. However, it should be stressed that in some patients with intestinal lymphoma, the associated celiac sprue is clinically occult.[196]

Pathology. Grossly, lesions may be single or diffuse and involve primarily the small intestine. Occasionally, the stomach or mesenteric nodes alone are involved, with sparing of the small intestine. The diseased bowel is usually thickened and may ulcerate and resemble benign ulcers. A number of these lesions in the past were mistakenly diagnosed as ulcerative jejunoileitis when they were in fact lymphoma. The ulcerated lesions may hemorrhage, perforate, or cause obstruction.[193,194,197]

Histology. Lymphomas complicating celiac disease have a variable appearance. Some are monomorphous, of the diffuse large-cell type, Rappaport's so-called histiocytic lymphoma. Others are pleomorphic and sometimes overshadowed by accompanying inflammatory cells composed of mature lymphocytes, plasma cells, histiocytes, and eosinophils.[197-199] It is these lesions that are sometimes misdiagnosed as ulcerative jejunoileitis. The atypical lymphoid cells have large, multilobulated, indented or folded nuclei, prominent nucleoli and frequently exhibit phagocytosis (erythrocytes, platelets and cell debris). Some of the tumor cells occasionally resemble Reed-Sternberg cells. On the basis of immunohistochemical studies, performed on the atypical pleomorphic tumor, it was postulated that these tumors were of true histiocytic origin.[197-199] However, recent studies indicate that they may be T-cell lymphomas.[200]

The early lymphomatous lesions may be difficult to diagnose, especially in endoscopic biopsy material, because of the polymorphous infiltrate.[193,201] Histologic features, which should alert one to the possibility of lymphomatous change in celiac disease, are the finding of a dense inflammatory infiltrate, which separates the base of the gland crypts from the muscularis mucosae and which extends beyond the muscularis mucosae into the submucosa. The presence of scattered "atypical lymphocytes" within the inflammatory infiltrate is more definite evidence of early malignant change.

Treatment. Because lymphoma complicating celiac disease and ulcerative nongranulomatous jejunoileitis may be indistinguishable clinically and because there is some evidence that in ulcerative jejunoileitis lymphoma may develop,[195] the treatment of both conditions is the same, namely, segmental resection and staging. To date, there is no evidence that a gluten-free diet protects against the development of lymphoma in celiac disease.[195] Finally, it should be mentioned that in the past it was believed that intestinal lymphoma could give rise to a flat mucosa, but there is no good evidence for this view.

Immunoproliferative Small-Intestinal Disease

IPSID is a proliferative lymphoplasmacytic disorder localized to the mucosa and may last for years.[202] Eventually in many, if not most, cases an associated lymphoma develops. These diseases are discussed further in the next section.

Lymphoid Hyperplasia and Primary Immunodeficiency Disorders

The association of lymphoid hyperplasia and the primary immunodeficiency disorders with lymphomas has already been discussed.

Inflammatory Bowel Disease

Lymphoma has also been described in association with ulcerative colitis and Crohn's disease,[203-205] although the exact incidence and significance remain unclear.

Primary Lymphoma of the Gastrointestinal Tract and Mesentery in Adults

Definition. Primary intestinal lymphomas are defined as those lymphomas presenting in the gastrointestinal tract of patients in whom there is no evidence of liver, spleen, and peripheral or mediastinal lymph node involvement at the time of presentation. Also included with the primary gastrointestinal lymphomas are those lymphomas originating in the mesenteric lymph nodes.[206] They are included because of their similarity in clinical presentation and also because some of them may be causally related to the prelymphomatous intestinal diseases such as celiac sprue and IPSID.[203,207] Problems in definition arise in those cases of lymphoma that present with gastrointestinal manifestations but on workup are found to have microscopic dissemination. Are these cases of primary gastrointestinal lymphoma with secondary dissemination (which we know can occur in roughly 50% of cases), or do they represent nodal lymphoma with intestinal involvement? We prefer to regard them as gastrointestinal lymphomas with dissemination, although from a practical point of view the question is somewhat moot, because they need to be managed as disseminated lymphomas.

Etiology and Pathogenesis. The etiology and pathogenesis of gastrointestinal tumors remain uncertain, although a number of interesting associations are emerging. As has already been noted, a number of gastrointestinal diseases, such as immunoproliferative small-intestinal disease, celiac disease, diffuse and focal gastrointestinal lymphoid hyperplasia, and immunodeficiency disorders, are associated with an increased risk of lymphoma. Also, Isaacson notes that these lymphomas share the specific homing patterns characteristic to gut-associated lymphoid tissue, which, he postulates, confer on these tumors specific characteristics, such as invasion of gastrointestinal glands and their tendency to remain localized to the gut for long periods.[208]

The cell of origin of primary gastrointestinal lymphomas has been the subject of some controversy. Particularly contentious has been the notion of true histiocytic lymphomas, which some investigators have claimed to be relatively frequent in the gastrointestinal tract.[209] However, recent immunohistochemical studies have shown that these tumors stain positively for B- or, less often, T-cell markers, which indicates that their derivation is in fact from lymphoid cells.[210-213] In light of these findings, we believe that true histiocytic lymphomas are extremely rare.

Clinical Presentation. Lymphomas of the gastrointestinal tract involve predominantly the middle-aged of either sex and, with the exception of the Mediterranean lymphomas, show no significant racial distribution.[203,214-218] Clinically, the patients present with ulcer symptoms or intestinal obstruction accompanied by pain and hemorrhage and rarely with perforation and intussusception.[203,206,213,216,217] Malabsorption is uncommon except in those cases complicating celiac sprue and IPSID.[203]

Location and Gross Pathology. The gastrointestinal tract is the most common site for primary extranodal lymphomas[203,215,219] and is secondarily involved in about 10% of cases of disseminated nodal lymphoma.[220,221] The most frequent site of involvement is the stomach (50%), followed by the small intestine

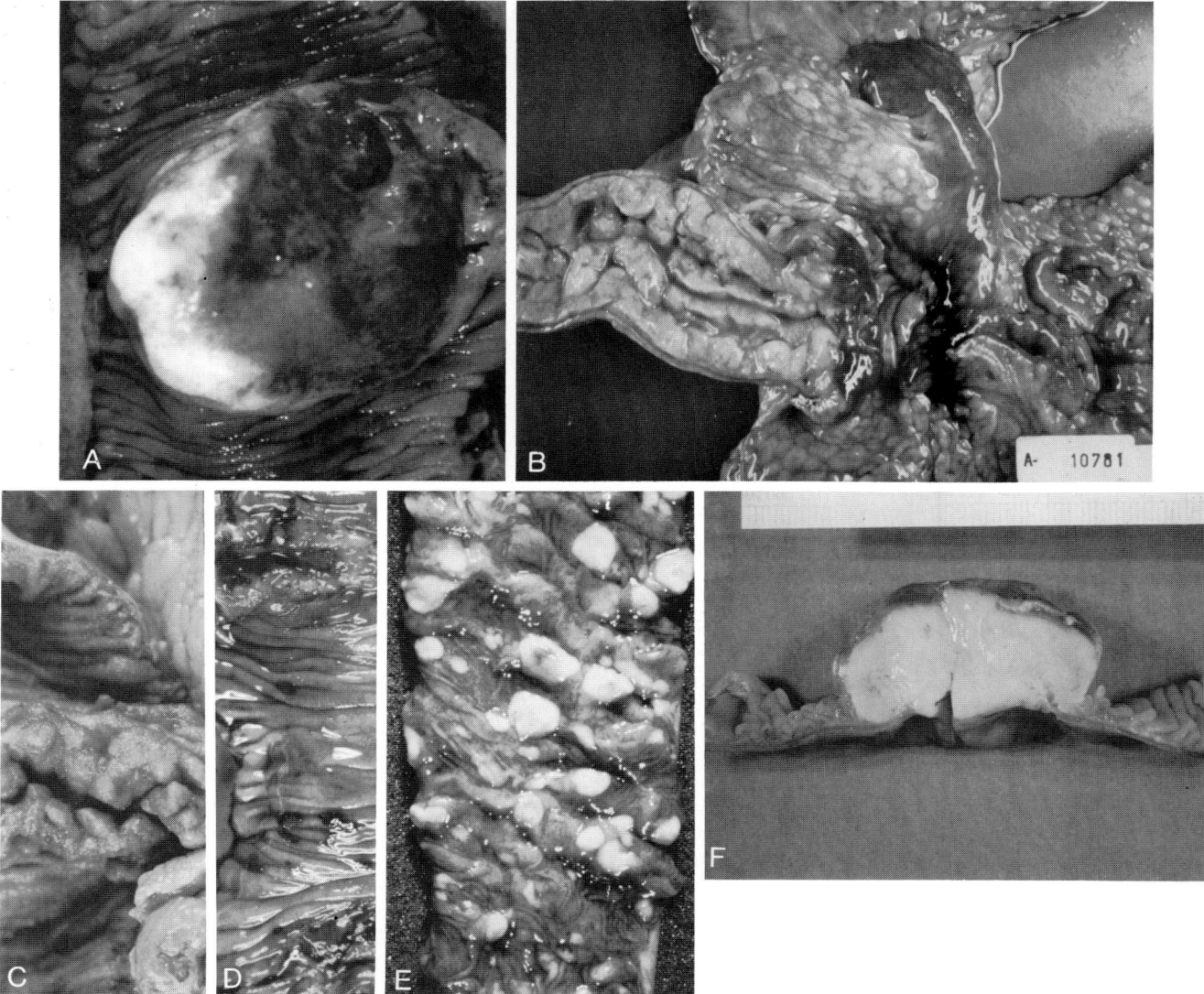

FIGURE 14–32. Malignant lymphoma of the gastrointestinal tract demonstrating the varied gross appearances, namely, (A) a solitary intraluminal mass with a hemorrhagic surface, (B) diffusely infiltrative, producing encephaloid folds, (C) focally nodular, (D) ulcerated, (E) diffusely polypoid, and (F) diffuse pinkish white appearance on cross section.

(37%) and the ileocecal region (13%).[203,216–219,222,223] Involvement of the remainder of the intestinal tract and mesentery is uncommon.[215,218] Lymphomas of the small intestine characteristically involve the ileum and only rarely the jejunum.[203]

In about half of all cases, the lymphoma is confined to the affected viscus at the time of presentation.[78,94,96] Involvement of regional nodes is quite common, occurring in about one third of all cases.[203,213,216,218] About 20% of patients have more widespread dissemination of disease, although this is not always apparent from initial clinical examination unless adequate workup and staging have been undertaken.[203]

Primary gastrointestinal lymphomas are most commonly single. Multiple lesions are unusual in the stomach but may occur in up to 20% of intestinal lymphomas.[203,206,217] They number from two to six lesions and are usually found in the same general areas.[203] Diffuse lymphomatous polyposis is an uncommon form of primary intestinal lymphoma.[206,224,225] Primary mesenteric lymphoma often involves the gastrointestinal tract secondarily in multiple sites by direct extension.[203]

Gastrointestinal lymphomas are usually quite large at the time of diagnosis, averaging about 7.9 cm in greatest diameter.[203] On cut section they have a characteristic white or yellow appearance. Grossly, they form exophytic polypoid masses or infiltrative lesions with localized mucosal ulceration and raised margins. The infiltrative growths cause either uniform thickening of the bowel or, less commonly, an annular napkin-ring lesion mimicking carcinoma. However, occasionally we have seen atypical ulcerative lesions without apparent thickening of the bowel wall (Figure 14–32). Because lymphomas of the gastrointestinal tract are at times associated with destruction of the full thickness of the bowel wall without an associated des-

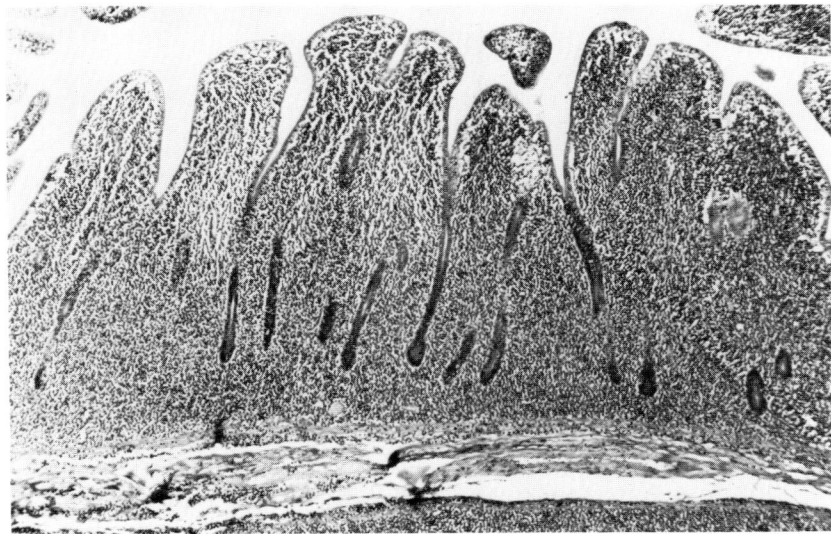

FIGURE 14-33. IPSID. Low-power photomicrograph showing separation of gland crypts and lifting of base of crypts from the muscularis mucosae by the lymphoid infiltrate.

moplastic reaction, it is not surprising that a number of these neoplasms perforate.[213,226] The frequency of this complication varies from 1% to 28% in the literature.[203,213,217,227] In rare instances intussusception is seen.

Microscopic Features. In general, gastrointestinal lymphomas are characterized by a monomorphous lymphoid infiltrate showing marked cytologic atypia. Occasionally, however, the infiltrate may be polymorphous and may be confused with the lymphoid hyperplasias.[203,228]

The early cases of lymphoma tend to be limited to the mucosa and superficial submucosa. The lymphoid infiltrate causes expansion and thickening of the mucosa. The glands are pushed apart from one another and from the underlying muscularis mucosae (Figure 14-33), and there is transmigration of the atypical lymphocytes through the glands and surface epithelium. The infiltrate also separates the muscle fibers of the muscularis mucosae. A helpful feature in the biopsy diagnosis of these cases is the infiltration and destruction of mucosal glands by the lymphomatous process (Figure 14-34).

The more advanced gastrointestinal lymphomas are commonly associated with mucosal ulceration and more extensive infiltration of the viscus. The latter may take one of two forms:

1. Invasion in a band-like manner, with a pushing border and often associated with underlying fibrosis (Figure 14-35).
2. Invasion with an irregularly infiltrating margin unassociated with a desmoplastic reaction (Figure 14-36). The lymphoma commonly invades the muscle coats separating individual muscle fibers (Figure 14-37). A similar invasion of muscle fibers may be seen involving the vasculature. Eventually the muscle undergoes atrophy, resulting in marked weakening of the viscus and propensity to perforation.

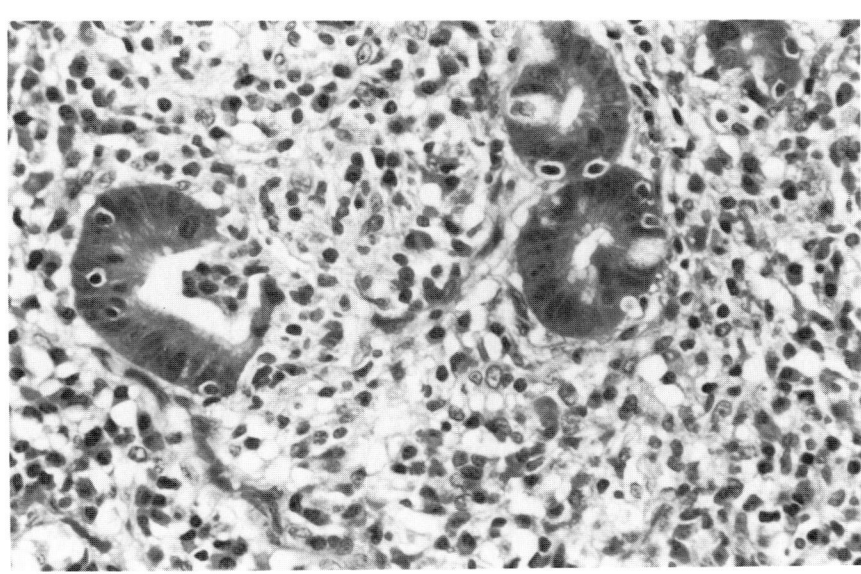

FIGURE 14-34. Malignant lymphoma, small-cell cleaved type. High magnification showing lymphoepithelial lesion with infiltration and destruction of glands by the atypical lymphocytes.

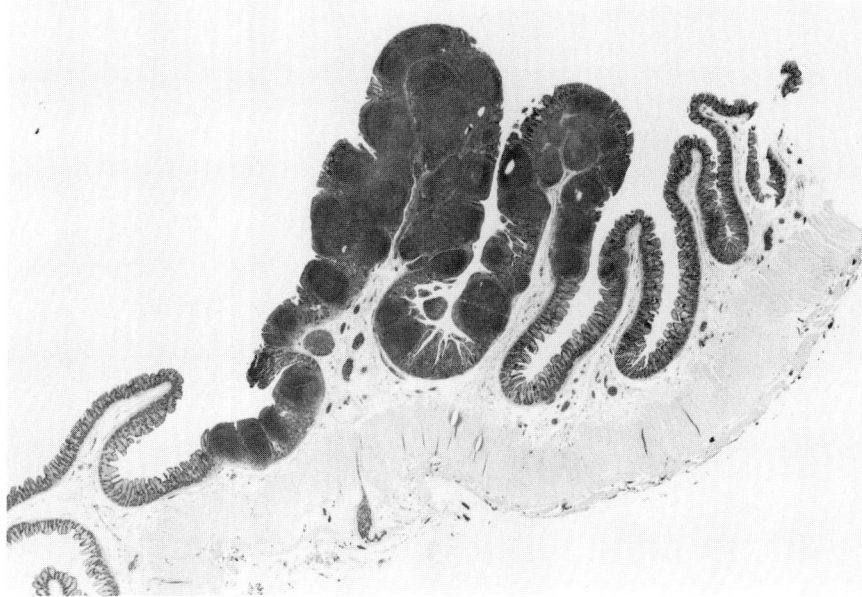

FIGURE 14–35. Nodular lymphoma of the ileum. The lymphoma is confined largely to the mucosa and has a smooth "pushing" border.

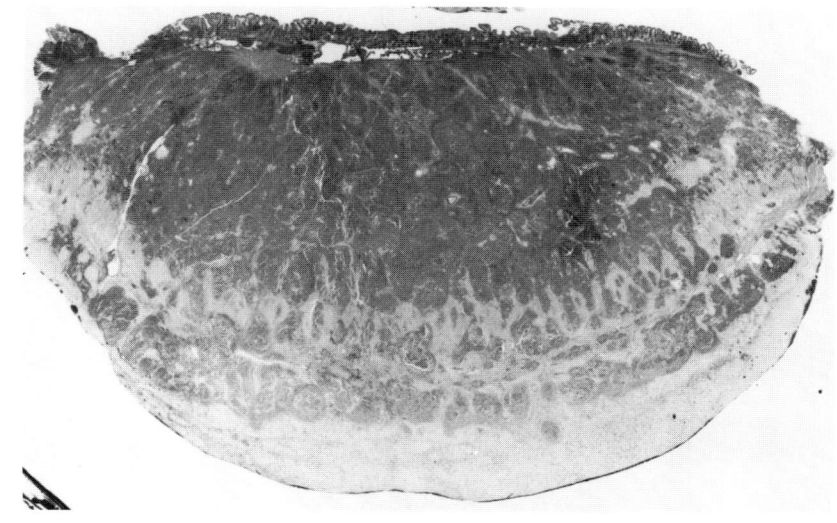

FIGURE 14–36. Malignant lymphoma of the ileum. Scanning power photomicrograph to show marked submucosal thickening caused by the lymphomatous infiltrate. Note the irregular infiltrative lower margin infiltrating the muscularis propria.

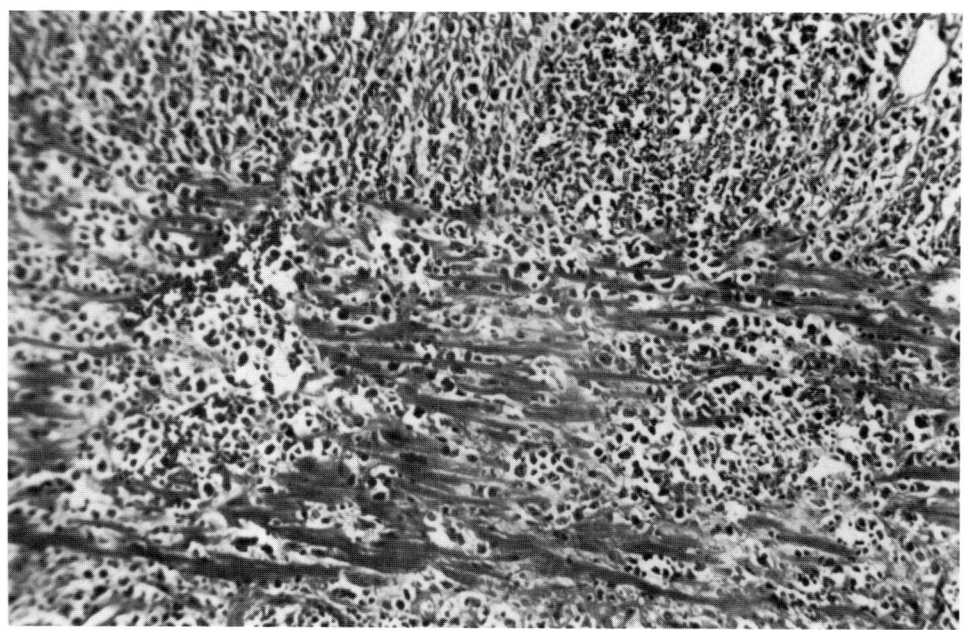

FIGURE 14–37. Malignant lymphoma of the small intestine showing separation of the muscle fibers of the muscularis propria by the lymphomatous infiltrate.

Table 14–6 GASTROINTESTINAL LYMPHOMAS: HISTOLOGIC CLASSIFICATION

Working Formulation	Rappaport	Incidence (%)
Large-cell	Histiocytic	
Diffuse	Diffuse	55
Immunoblastic	Pleomorphic	4
Small cleaved	Poorly differentiated lymphocytic	
Follicular	Nodular	9
Diffuse	Diffuse	8
Diffuse mixed small- and large-cell	Diffuse mixed histiocytic and lymphocytic	3
Small lymphocytic	Well-differentiated lymphocytic	4
Small noncleaved (Burkitt's)	Burkitt's	8
Miscellaneous		
IPSID* and IPSID-associated lymphoma (Mediterranean lymphoma and alpha-chain disease†)		4
Composite lymphoma		1
Hodgkin's disease		2
Solitary plasmacytoma		?
Unclassified		2

Modified from Lewin KJ, Ranchod M, and Dorfman RF: Lymphomas of the gastrointestinal tract; a study of 117 cases presenting with gastrointestinal disease. Cancer 42:693, 1978.
*Immunoproliferative small-intestinal disease.
†Incidence varies with geographic location.

The histologic types of gastrointestinal lymphomas, classified according to the working formulation of the National Cancer Institute,[229] are shown in Table 14–6. With the exception of Burkitt's lymphoma and IPSID-associated lymphoma (Mediterranean lymphoma), they are similar to those encountered in lymph nodes.[203] Also, none of the intestinal lymphomas, except for the IPSID-associated lymphomas, to be described later, show a particular site of predilection for the gastrointestinal tract.

Most gastrointestinal lymphomas are diffuse, only 10% being nodular (Figure 14–36). As with other sites of extranodal lymphoma, the majority of gastrointestinal lymphomas are of the large-cell type (Figure 14–38)[215] (Rappaport's so-called histiocytic lymphoma or Luke's large noncleaved follicular center cell lymphoma). A few of these tumors are characterized by a polymorphous and pleomorphic infiltrate, sometimes with sclerosis (Figure 14–39), composed of plasmacytoid cells and atypical immunoblasts, some of which resemble Reed-Sternberg cells, and an accompanying inflammatory cell infiltrate composed of mature lymphocytes, plasma cells, histiocytes, and sometimes eosinophils[203] (Rappaport's pleomorphic histiocytic lymphoma or Luke's immunoblastic sarcoma).

Lymphomas of the small-cell type constitute the sec-

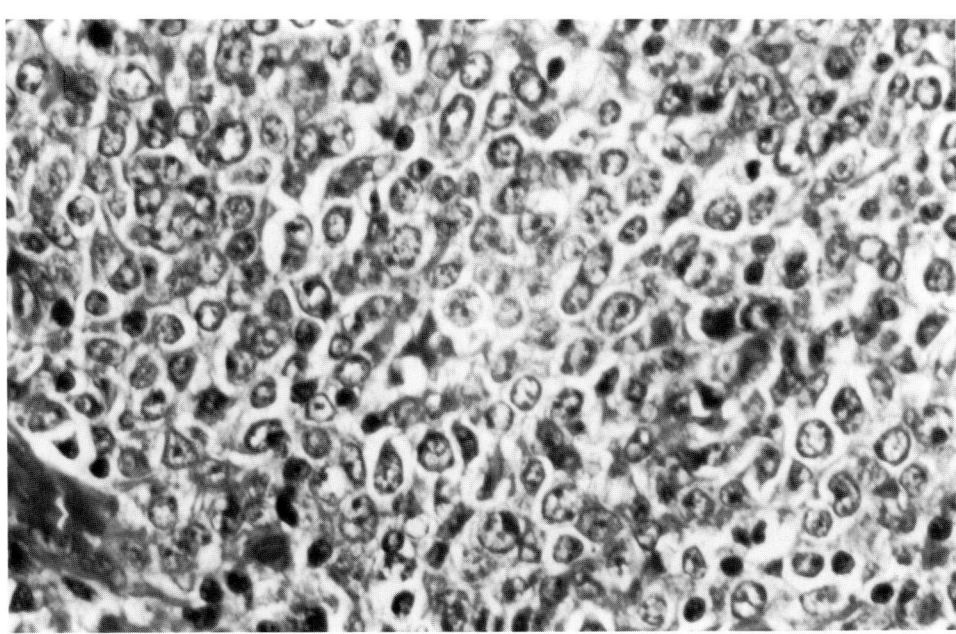

FIGURE 14–38. Malignant lymphoma, diffuse large-cell type, illustrating monomorphous infiltrate of atypical large lymphoid cells with large, round, vesicular nuclei and prominent nucleoli.

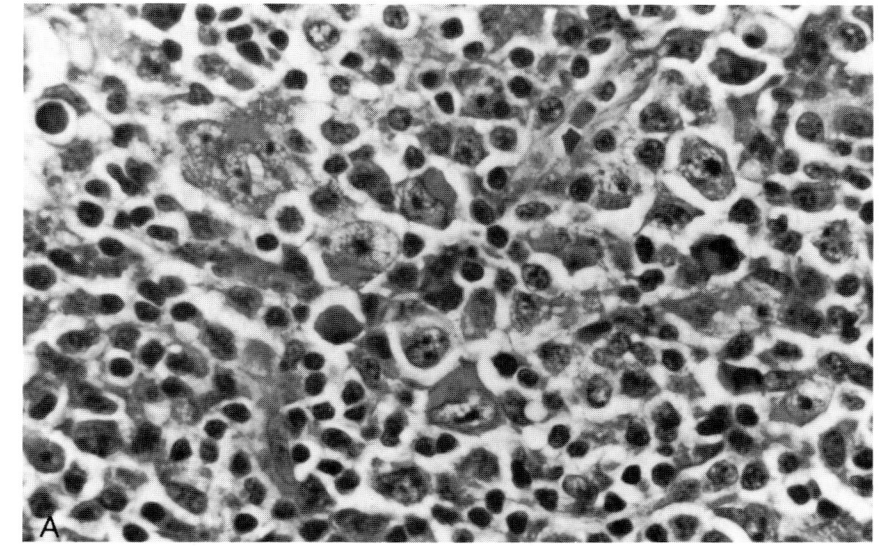
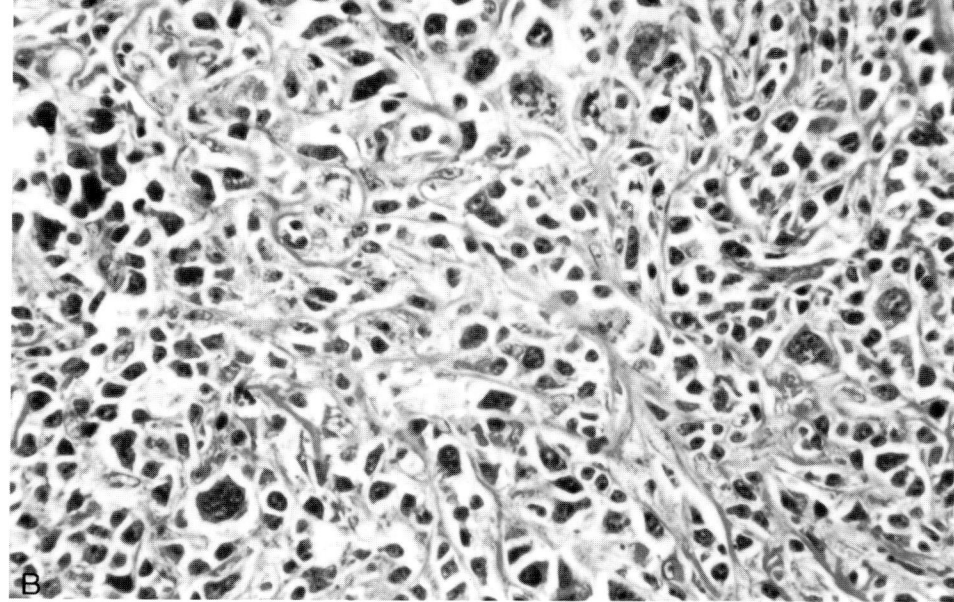

FIGURE 14–39. Malignant lymphoma, pleomorphic large-cell type. *A*, Pleomorphic infiltrate composed of immunoblasts and admixed mature lymphocytes. *B*, Similar features, together with diffuse sclerosis.

ond most common type of gastrointestinal lymphomas and are usually of the cleaved type (Rappaport's poorly differentiated lymphocytic lymphoma). A number of these show both nodular and diffuse patterns.[230] Because nodular lymphomas are known to evolve into diffuse lymphomas with the passage of time,[231] the occurrence of this evolutionary process in one lesion is not surprising. However, it is important to recognize residual nodular areas because they may be of prognostic value. Malignant lymphomas of the small lymphocytic type (well-differentiated lymphocytic lymphomas) are uncommon. They are usually diffuse and may show plasmacytoid change and, rarely, a signet-ring cell pattern; and as is true for these lymphomas elsewhere, it is important first to exclude a lymphocytic leukemia (Figure 14–40).

The gastrointestinal tract is one of the sites of predilection for the rare cases of American Burkitt's lymphoma.[203,226,232] These tumors occur primarily in children and although they may occur anywhere in the bowel, are found most commonly around the ileocecal region and in the mesenteric nodes. They characteristically have a "starry sky" pattern and consist of undifferentiated lymphoid cells with scant cytoplasm, regular round nuclei, finely dispersed chromatin, and numerous small nucleoli (Figure 14–41). Less typical forms characterized by more prominent mitotic activity, variation in nuclear size, and irregular parachromatin clearing also are seen and do not appear to behave any differently. Occasionally Burkitt's lymphoma has a nodular pattern.[203] This is in keeping with recent evidence that nonendemic Burkitt's lymphoma is of B-cell origin and may selectively involve B-cell areas such as Peyer's patches and solitary lymphoid follicles.[233]

Primary Hodgkin's disease of the gastrointestinal tract is vanishingly rare.[203] Care should be taken not to

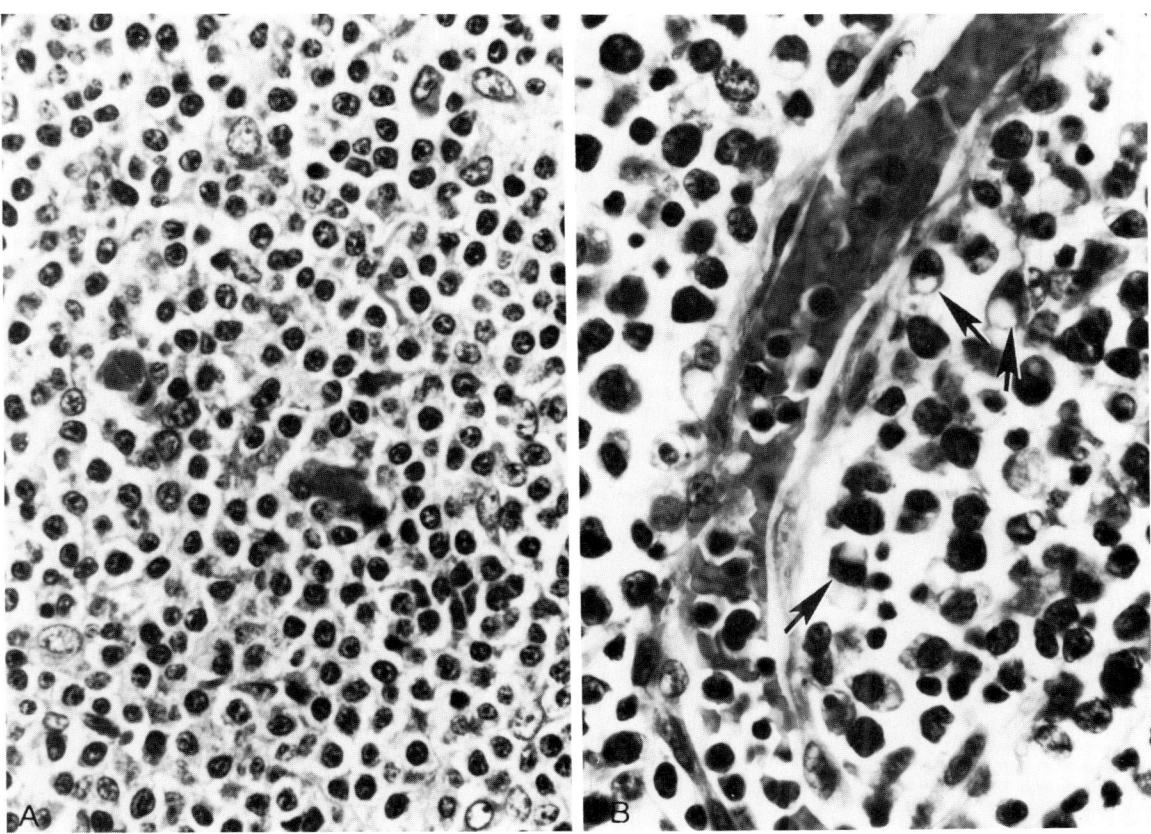

FIGURE 14–40. Malignant lymphoma, diffuse small-cell type (well-differentiated lymphocytic). A, Diffuse monomorphous infiltrate composed of mature-looking lymphocytes. B, Cytoplasmic vacuolation producing a signet-ring cell pattern (arrows).

erroneously misdiagnose pleomorphic large-cell lymphoma, Mediterranean lymphoma, and malignant histiocytosis of the intestine, which may resemble Hodgkin's, because of the admixed inflammatory cells and Reed-Sternberg–like cells.

Other histologic patterns, which are occasionally encountered, are mixed small- and large-cell lymphomas and composite lymphomas.[203] It should be noted that at times gastrointestinal lymphomas are difficult to classify because of poor fixation.

Differential Diagnosis. The major problems in diagnosis are encountered in differentiating some lymphomas from lymphoid hyperplasia and poorly differentiated adenocarcinoma, especially in the stomach. Most lymphomas are readily differentiated from focal lymphoid hyperplasia because of their monomorphous infiltrate and clear-cut cytologic atypia. However, difficulty may arise in the rare cases of malignant lymphoma of small lymphocytic type (well-differentiated) because of the mature nature of the lymphoid infiltrate. However, the monomorphous nature of the infiltrate should lead to a correct diagnosis, aided, if necessary, by immunohistochemistry. Further problems in diagnosis may occur with some lymphomas, such as pleomorphic large-cell lymphoma, and IPSID-associated lymphoma because these are characterized by a polymorphous infiltrate in which the inflammatory cells may predominate (thus mimicking the lymphoid hyperplasia) and obscure the atypical lymphoid cells. The clinical setting should alert one to the possibility of lymphoma and lead to a careful search for large bizarre lymphoid cells. In those cases where difficulty in diagnosis remains, immunohistochemistry may be very helpful. Because most lymphomas are of B-cell origin, many show a monotypic immunoglobulin staining pattern, whereas the lymphoid hyperplasias are characterized by a polyclonal pattern.[141]

Poorly differentiated carcinoma can on occasion be almost indistinguishable from lymphoma. However, it is important to differentiate between them because treatment protocols and prognosis are different for these two conditions. Multiple sections (taken especially from the margins of the tumor) should be examined for evidence of glandular differentiation and a transition zone of tumor arising from atypical glands. With the development of immunohistochemical techniques for the detection of keratins, carcinoembryonic antigen (CEA), and common leukocyte antigen, the differential diagnosis between carcinoma and lymphoma is rarely a problem.

The rare cases of multiple lymphomatous polyposis need to be distinguished from cases of nodular lymphoid hyperplasia.[203,206,225,234] This distinction is easily made, because the nodules in nodular lymphoid hyperplasia are small, are largely confined to the lamina propria, and often contain prominent germinal centers.

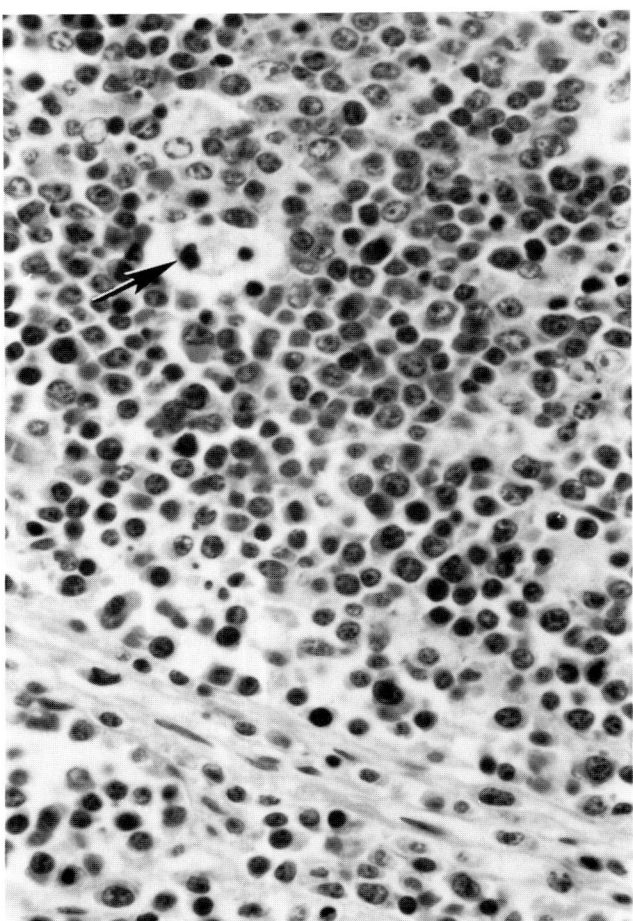

FIGURE 14–41. Burkitt's lymphoma of the terminal ileum showing small lymphocytes with scant cytoplasm, regular round nuclei, and small nucleoli. A vacuolated macrophage, responsible for the starry-sky pattern, is present to the left of center (arrow).

Course of Disease and Prognosis. Progression of lymphoma is not uncommon, occurring in about 60% of cases.[203,214,218,235] There is usually local extension of tumor to adjacent soft tissues and involvement of draining lymph nodes, such as the mesenteric and periaortic nodes. Involvement of other abdominal viscera may also occur.[203,213,218,236] Extra-abdominal spread occurs in up to 50% of cases, involving most commonly the peripheral lymph nodes, lung, brain, and meninges.[203] However, few organs are spared.[203,237] There appears to be no correlation between the propensity for extra-abdominal dissemination and the initial site or stage of the tumor.[203] The majority of relapses occur within 1 year of diagnosis; this is an ominous sign, because most patients die within 1 year of relapse.

The overall survival of gastrointestinal lymphomas is relatively good; these tumors tend to remain localized for prolonged periods,[237] the five-year survival being about 45%.[203,236–239] Prognosis appears to correlate best with the stage of the disease at the time of presentation. Two-year actuarial survival is about 75% for tumors localized to the viscus and regional nodes and 0% for the more widespread dissemination.[203] There is also some evidence that stage 1 lesions (that is, lymphoma localized to the viscus) have a better prognosis than those with accompanying involvement of regional lymph nodes (stage 2), but the reports in the literature are conflicting.[203,228,237,239–242] This discrepancy may be related to the inadequacy of staging procedures employed.[203] The prognostic relevance of local extension of tumor to adjacent soft tissues and of involvement of para-aortic lymph nodes is still unclear. The site of the primary lesion may also be of prognostic significance. Gastric and cecal lymphomas appear to have a better 5-year survival than tumors of the small intestine and rectum.[203,213,216,226,227]

The histologic type of lymphoma may also affect prognosis, recent reports indicating that nodular lymphomas and diffuse small (well-differentiated) lymphocytic lymphomas carry a better prognosis than diffuse large-cell histiocytic lymphomas.[234,238,239,243]

Treatment. Patients treated with surgery and postoperative radiotherapy and/or chemotherapy appear to have a significantly better prognosis than those treated with surgery alone.[237–239,244] It has been suggested that resection before definitive radiation therapy is unnecessary.[245] However, we believe that resection of the primary lesion is important for achieving local control and preventing the high risk of bleeding and perforation that may complicate radiotherapy. Finally, it is important to reiterate that because prognosis is related to the extent of the disease at the time of diagnosis, one should undertake a proper staging procedure to determine the full extent of the disease.[203,214,236,245] This should include sampling of mesenteric and para-aortic lymph nodes, biopsy of the liver, and careful inspection of the spleen. Careful evaluation should also be done for nodal lymphoma to exclude the possibility of the intestinal lesion being a manifestation of disseminated lymphoma.

Childhood Lymphomas

In comparison with lymphomas in adults, those in children show a number of notable differences with respect to sex distribution, site of involvement, and histopathologic characteristics.[203] Whereas the adult lymphomas of the ileum and ileocecal region show a 3:1 male predominance, in children the tumor occurs almost exclusively in males. The clinical features of the tumors are similar in the two groups, with the exception of a palpable abdominal mass, which is found most commonly in children. This may in part be due to the fact that abdominal masses are easier to palpate in children. The childhood lymphomas occur almost exclusively in the ileum and ileocecal region, in contrast to adult lymphomas, where other sites, notably the stomach, are commonly involved. The histopathologic types are also different from those of adults. In common with adults, large-cell lymphoma is the most frequent histologic type; however, small-cell lymphomas are rare. These findings are in accordance with the types of childhood lymphomas encountered in other sites.[78] The overall survival figures for children are comparable to those for adults.[203]

Secondary Malignant Lymphomas and Leukemias

The clinical features of patients who have disseminated lymphoma with secondary gastrointestinal involvement do not differ significantly from those with primary intestinal lymphoma.[213,245,246] However, the secondary lymphomas tend to produce marked ulcers in the stomach and involve multiple gastrointestinal sites more frequently. There is also a marked difference in overall survival between the two groups, namely, 3% for secondary as opposed to 45% for primary lymphomas.

Gastrointestinal complications of leukemia are common, occurring in up to 25% of cases.[247-253] The changes in the gastrointestinal tract mirror the complications of leukemia generally, namely

1. Tumorous infiltration of the bowel with ulceration and obstruction
2. Opportunistic infection, which is usually localized to the esophagus and large bowel but may become disseminated[248]
3. Neutropenic enterocolitis, a form of enterocolitis occurring in neutropenic patients, which may result in perforation and gram-negative septicemia.[248,249,252,253]
4. Massive hemorrhage secondary to septicemia

IPSID and IPSID-Associated Lymphoma (Mediterranean Lymphoma and Alpha-Chain Disease)

IPSID was first described in a group of Oriental Jews and Arabs with primary small-bowel lymphoma.[254,255] However, subsequently it became apparent that this disease had a more widespread distribution; and it has since been encountered in many parts of the world.[203,207,254-261] Since 1968 cases of IPSID have been found in which an abnormal paraprotein, consisting of α chains devoid of light chains, was secreted into the serum and jejunal juices. These cases were designated as α-chain disease.[207,262-268] The amount of the abnormal secretion varied greatly from case to case and sometimes could be demonstrated only immunocytochemically within the plasma cell cytoplasm. IPSID can occur *ab initio* with or without lymphoma,[202,207] lymphoma does not invariably develop in these cases,[202,269] and IPSID with or without lymphoma need not necessarily produce an abnormal paraprotein. About 30% to 50% of cases will produce α heavy chain[269-271] or rarely other abnormal gammaglobulins such as γ heavy chain.[272,273]

Clinically, cases of IPSID with and without α-chain protein are indistinguishable. It is a disease of young patients, with no sex differences. It is characterized by malabsorption, with chronic diarrhea, weight loss, and abdominal pain. Sometimes patients present with an acute abdomen due to obstruction or intestinal perforation.[207,254]

Etiology. The causes of IPSID are unclear. Most cases have been reported in patients of low socioeconomic status, with poor hygiene, malnutrition, and a high degree of intestinal infections.[207,274] Also, a number of these patients are of HLA-AW19 and HLA-12 types.[207,260] These findings indicate that genetic and environmental factors may be operative in these conditions. Because some patients with plasma cell infiltration apparently remit spontaneously or reportedly respond to antibiotic therapy and because α heavy chain is not usually demonstrated in the malignant infiltrate,[198] it has been postulated that plasma cell infiltration is a benign proliferative response to antigenic stimulation, possibly in genetically predisposed individuals. This later undergoes malignant dedifferentiation, perhaps due to some oncogenic agent. However, it is of note that clonal immunoglobulin gene rearrangements have been detected even in the initial plasma cell infiltration stage (prior to histologically overt lymphoma),[275] and so it may be incorrect to consider this strictly a benign process. Others have suggested that the antigenic response initiates an immunodeficient state that predisposes the patient to lymphoma.

Pathology. IPSID can be morphologically divided into two stages:

1. A benign-appearing diffuse plasmacytic cell infiltration of the lamina propria (PCI) (Figure 14-42).
2. Malignant lymphoma superimposed on the diffuse

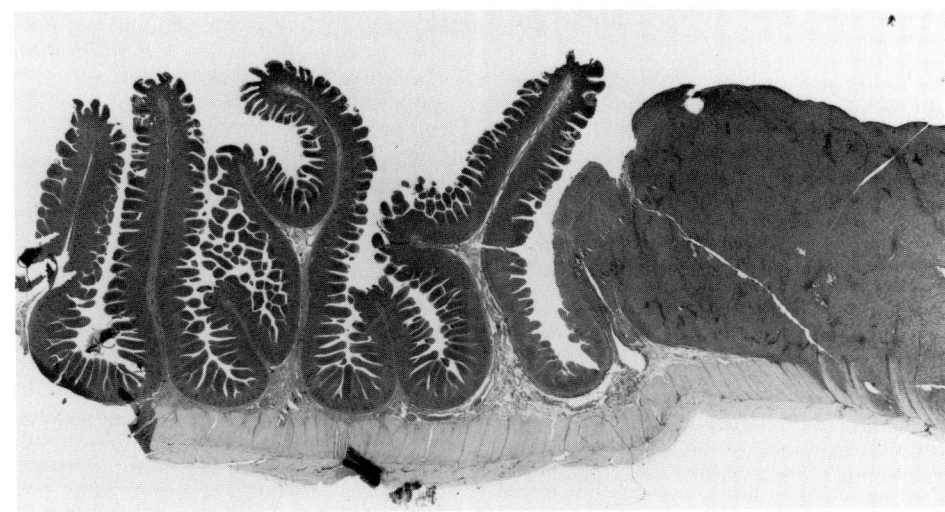

FIGURE 14-42. IPSID and associated lymphoma. Low-power magnification showing dense lymphoid infiltrate confined to the mucosa on the left and a transmural lymphomatous infiltrate on the right.

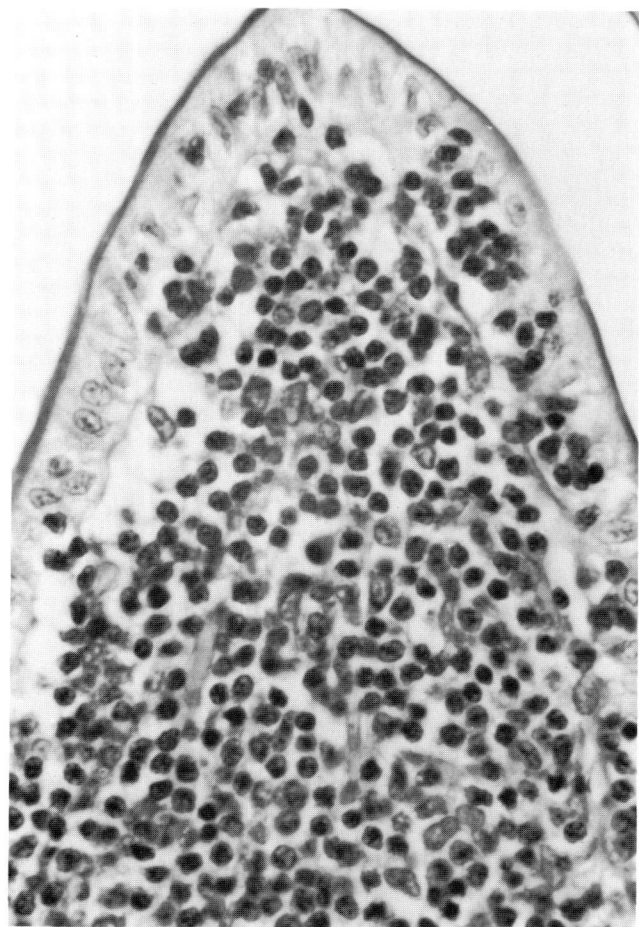

FIGURE 14–43. IPSID. High-power magnification showing monomorphous infiltrate of mature-appearing lymphocytes at the tip of an intestinal villus. Note also lymphocytes transmigrating through absorptive columnar cells.

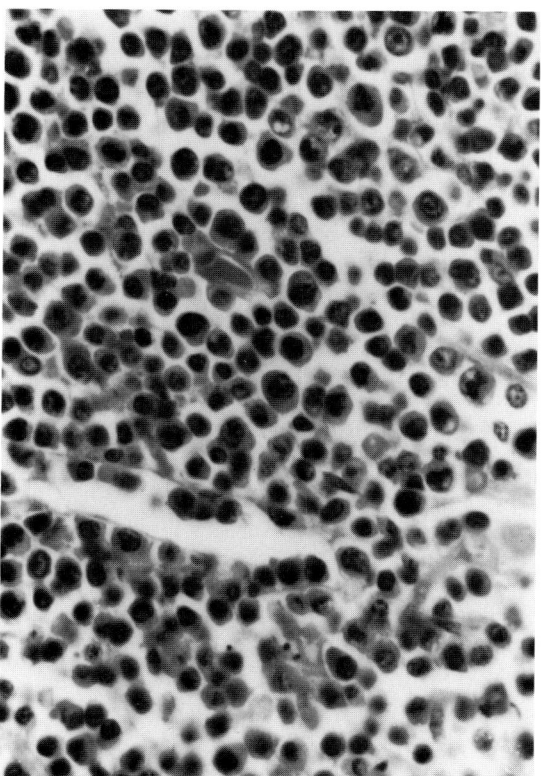

FIGURE 14–44. IPSID. High-power magnification showing monomorphous infiltrate of mature-appearing plasma cells.

plasmacytic infiltrate. This has been designated as IPSID-associated lymphoma (IAL)[269] and also Mediterranean lymphoma (see Figures 14–33 and 14–42).

Cases of IPSID are histologically indistinguishable from α-chain disease, although the abnormal paraprotein may be demonstrated within the plasma cells immunohistochemically in the latter.[269,276]

Stage 1 (plasma cell infiltrate) is characterized by diffuse involvement of the jejunum with frequent extension to the ileum. Gastric and large-bowel involvement are rare. On gross examination there is dilatation of the small bowel and thickening of the mucosal folds, a reflection of the plasmacytic infiltrate. Microscopically, the lymphoid infiltrate is confined to the lamina propria and is usually composed of mature-appearing plasma cells and less commonly of mature lymphocytes (Figures 14–43 and 14–44; see also Figure 14–33).[202,207] Whether the latter represent variants of IPSID or not is currently unknown. The crypts are widely separated and frequently displaced upward away from the muscularis mucosae by the infiltrate (see Figure 14–33). There is variable villous blunting, ranging from a mild shortening to a flat mucosa. With time (probably the majority of cases, although it may take many years) atypical large lymphoid cells are seen scattered among the plasmacytic infiltrate (Figure 14–45). Eventually the infiltrate becomes atypical and extends beyond the muscularis mucosae, and a florid lymphoma develops.

Malignant lymphoma complicating plasma cell infiltration may be multifocal and is grossly characterized by diffuse thickening of the viscus.[222,254,259] Ulcerated lesions, some with raised margins, may also be seen.[207] Microscopically, most cases of lymphoma have a fairly characteristic appearance, namely, a polymorphous infiltrate composed of a spectrum of cells consisting of atypical small lymphoid cells, plasmacytoid cells, and Reed-Sternberg–like cells, admixed with mature plasma cells, lymphocytes, and eosinophils (Figure 14–46).[207] However, we and others[269] have seen cases that do not conform to this typical pattern, being monomorphous and resembling the diffuse large-cell noncleaved lymphoma (Figure 14–47). Once lymphoma supervenes, the abnormal cytoplasmic immunoglobulins are rarely demonstrable in cases with α-chain protein.

Although the lymphoma usually involves the jejunum, it may spare the small intestine and involve only the mesenteric lymph nodes. In these cases the pattern of nodal infiltration is unusual, in that preservation of the medullary sinuses is a common finding.[207]

Diagnosis and Differential Diagnosis. Immunoproliferative small-intestinal disease has a distinctive

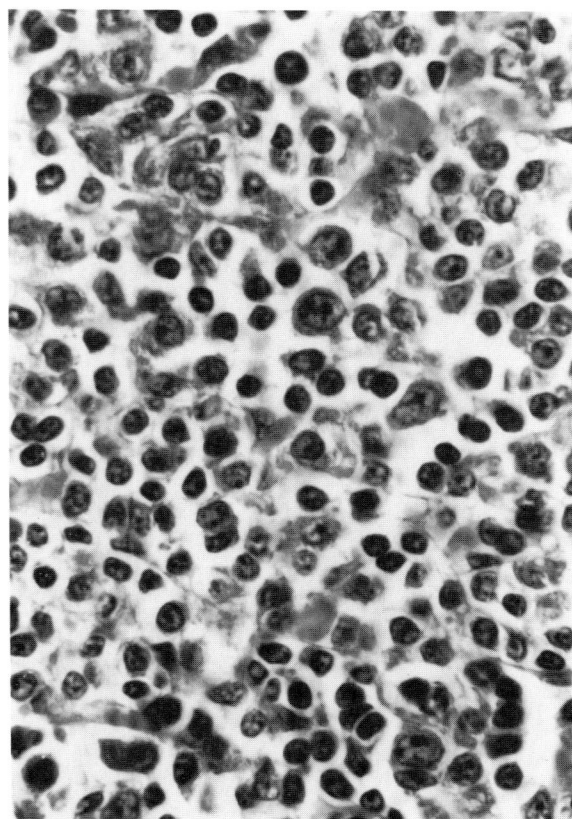

FIGURE 14–45. IPSID with atypia. High-power magnification showing many atypical lymphocytes admixed with more mature lymphocytes and plasma cells.

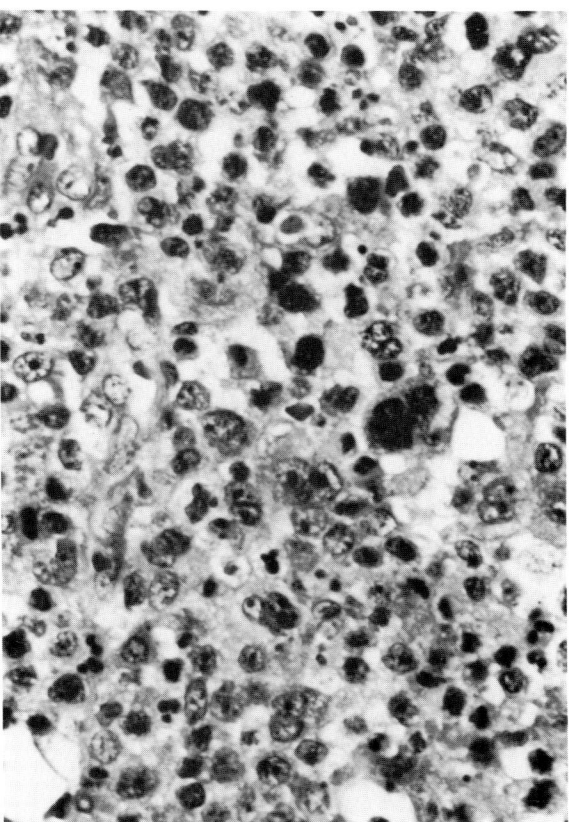

FIGURE 14–46. IPSID-associated lymphoma. High-power magnification illustrating the pleomorphic lymphoid infiltrate with scattered bizarre multinucleated giant cells.

morphologic pattern, and diagnosis rests on finding the characteristic diffuse plasmacytic infiltrate of the lamina propria. Once lymphoma supervenes, it is important to demonstrate the massive plasmacytic infiltration in the adjacent mucosa in order to sustain the diagnosis. Occasionally we have found massive plasmacytic infiltration to occur predominantly in the stomach. Should these cases be designated as IPSID? In our opinion, they should, because they have the typical histologic features of this disorder, albeit in an unusual site. Whether these lesions behave in a manner similar to that of the more typical lesions remains to be determined. Once IPSID is suspected, it should be determined whether the patient has α-chain disease. The paraprotein should be sought in the serum, urine, and jejunal juices and also by the use of immunoperoxidase in tissue sections. It should be noted that in many cases the abnormality is not detected by routine immunoelectrophoresis with polyvalent antiserum to normal serum, and thus monospecific antiserum to IgA is essential.[254]

Histologically, the nonspecific mucosal lesions, exemplified by celiac disease, infectious gastroenteritis, kwashiorkor, and tropical sprue, must be differentiated from massive plasmacytic infiltration, because all of these disorders are characterized by villous blunting and increased plasmacytic infiltration of the lamina propria.[207] Normally, the differentiation poses no problem, because in IPSID the dominant feature is the dense plasma cell infiltration, in contrast to the other conditions, where this is a secondary feature. The clinical setting is also of importance and frequently helps to differentiate the various diseases.[207]

The usual gastrointestinal lymphomas seen in the United States, the so-called "Western type" of lymphomas, differ in many respects from the IPSID-associated lymphomas. They are located mainly in the stomach and ileum, in contrast to the jejunum, and also lack the massive plasma cell infiltrate in the lamina propria adjacent to the tumor.[82] Occasionally "Western type" lymphomas have been reported to produce α heavy chain[277] but they lack the other clinicopathologic features of IPSID.

IPSID-associated lymphoma may also be confused with Hodgkin's disease because of the finding of Reed-Sternberg–like cells. However, Hodgkin's disease of the bowel is very uncommon, and does not involve atypical lymphocytes.

Prognosis and Management. The long-term outcome of IPSID remains unclear. However, it is becoming apparent that this disorder may persist for years[261] (up to 7 years in one report[202]); and patients may go into remission on antihelminthic and antibiotic therapy.[269] However, when the lymphomatous phase supervenes, the prognosis is generally poor. In one study, the mortality rate of IPSID with lymphoma was 11 of

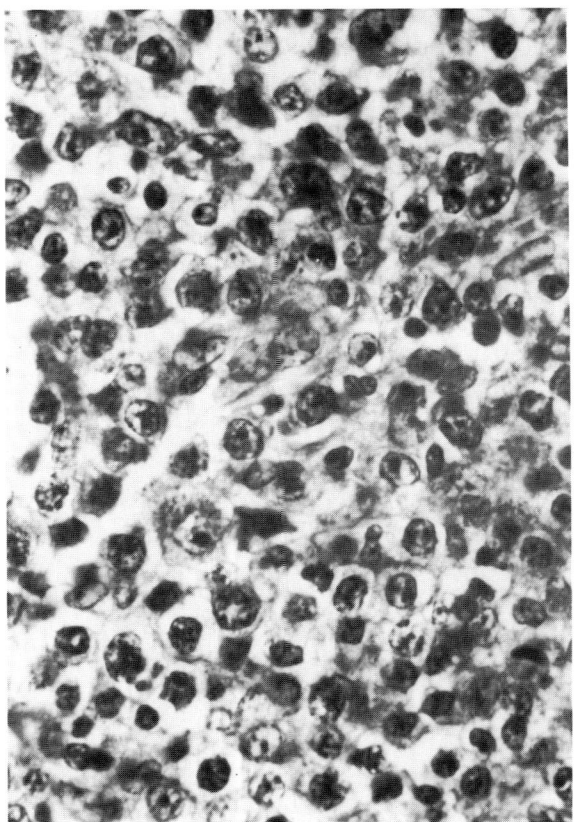

FIGURE 14-47. IPSID-associated lymphoma. In this patient the infiltrate was of a more monomorphous nature, being composed of atypical large cells.

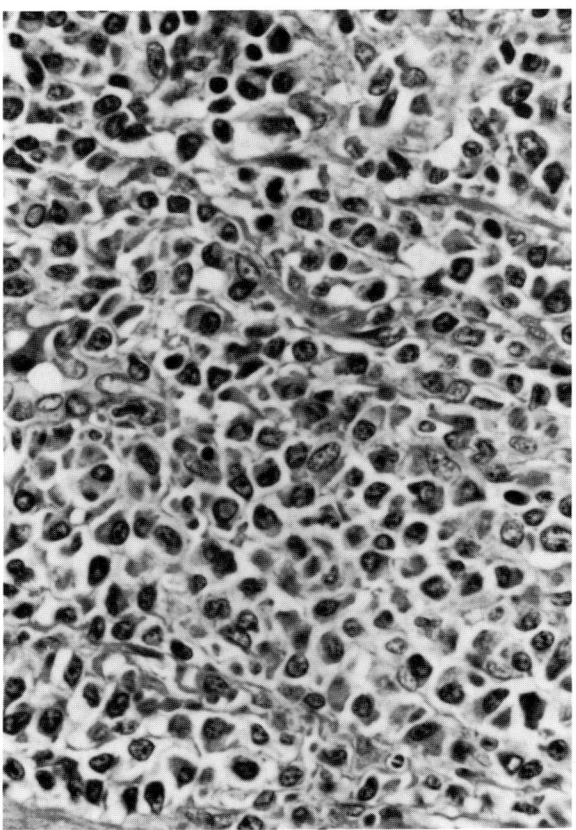

FIGURE 14-48. Gastric plasmacytoma showing monomorphous infiltrate of predominantly mature-looking plasma cells.

14 patients with an average survival of 32 months. Because patients seldom have evidence of disease above the diaphragm, the treatment of choice is widefield abdominal radiation.[269] However, because bowel that is macroscopically infiltrated by lymphoma is in danger of perforation after radiation and chemotherapy, resection of tumor may first be necessary.[207]

Solitary Plasmacytomas

Solitary plasmacytomas of the gastrointestinal tract are uncommon, accounting for approximately 4% to 12% of extramedullary plasmacytomas.[278-281] Clinically, they have many of the features of myelomas, being more common in middle-aged and elderly men,[279] and are sometimes associated with a monoclonal protein spike in the serum or urine.[280,282]

Pathology. The majority are located in the stomach and small bowel,[280,281,283,284] but cases have also been described in the colon.[285] Histologically, they are typically composed of a monomorphous infiltrate of mostly plasma cells. However, sometimes they may be pleomorphic; we have seen an unusual case with numerous bizarre Russell bodies (Figures 14-48 to 14-50).[285,286] The lesions may contain extracellular amyloid deposition. The gastrointestinal plasmacytomas must be differentiated from localized extramedullary manifestations of multiple myeloma, inflammatory pseudotumors (plasma cell granulomas),[279,283,287-289] and the massive plasmacytic cell infiltration associated with Mediterranean lymphoma and α-chain disease.[207] Histologically, plasmacytomas are differentiated from pseudotumors by demonstration of a monomorphic population of plasma cells with little admixture of inflammatory cells or granulomatous change (in contrast to the polymorphous infiltrate of the pseudotumors).[279,285,287] The plasma cells may contain crystalline inclusions,[281,290] and those cases are invariably associated with dysproteinemia. In addition, the neoplastic nature of the lesion can be shown immunohistochemically by the demonstration of a single immunoglobulin in the plasma cells.[284,285,290,291] The lack of bone marrow plasmacytosis indicates that the tumor is not a localized manifestation of multiple myeloma. Also, bone marrow aspirations from several sites and a reasonable period of follow-up should differentiate these two diseases.[279] The distinction from lymphoma can be made on morphologic grounds. Although these tumors may be related histogenetically, they have sufficiently characteristic clinicopathologic features to warrant distinction from lymphomas with plasmacytoid features.[207]

Surgery with or without local radiotherapy appears to be the treatment of choice for solitary plasmacytomas of the gastrointestinal tract, although some authorities have advocated chemotherapy.[279]

DISORDERS OF THE LYMPHOID SYSTEM

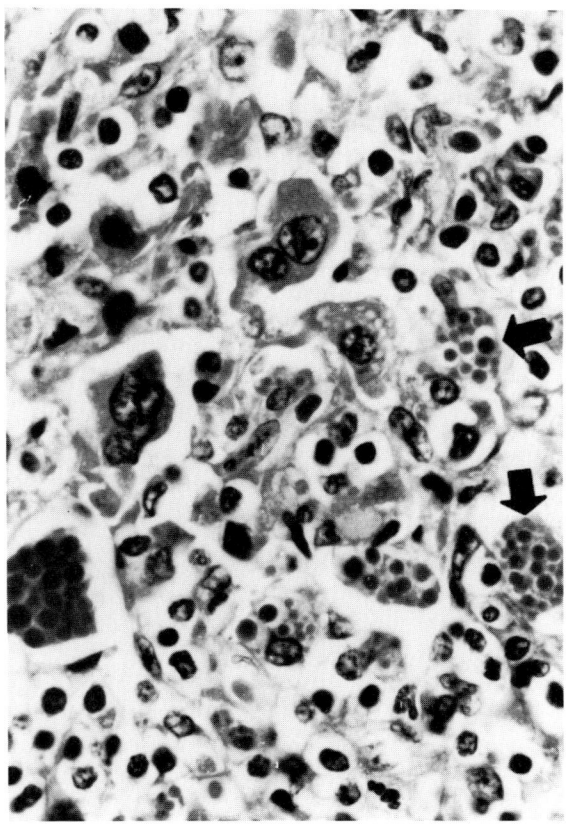

FIGURE 14-49. Pleomorphic gastric plasmacytoma. High-power magnification showing infiltrate composed of mature and immature plasma cells. Some of the atypical plasma cells contain numerous bizarre Russell bodies (arrows).

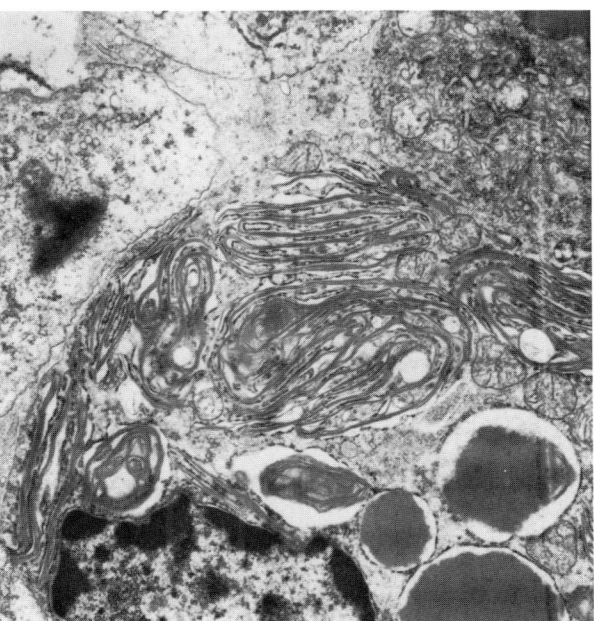

FIGURE 14-50. Electron micrographs of the Russell bodies illustrated in Figure 14-49. These consist of numerous cytoplasmic granules composed of an aggregate of membranes. (Courtesy of M. Janssen, M.D., San Bernardino, Calif.)

Workup of Gastrointestinal Lymphomas

Endoscopic Biopsy (Table 14-7). If the biopsy specimen is adequate in size, not crushed, and not from a deeply ulcerated area, a diagnosis of malignant lymphoma can frequently be confirmed by endoscopy. The problem arises in small, frequently crushed biopsy specimens and in suboptimally fixed tissues. Difficulty of interpretation may also occur in those biopsy specimens showing necrosis and a mixed inflammatory infiltrate, because these findings may be seen in superficial biopsy specimens of ulcerated lymphomas and in gastric lymphoid hyperplasias that are commonly associated with peptic ulceration. In these cases it is important to perform repeat biopsies from multiple sites and the endoscopist should be careful to avoid unnecessary crush artifact when removing the tissue from the biopsy forceps. In addition, he should be encouraged to use one of the large particle forceps now available, because they yield superior specimens subject to much less distortion (see Figure 14-37). Finally, separate biopsy material should be taken and frozen specifically for immunohistochemistry (see Figure 14-36.) If repeat biopsies do not resolve the issue of lymphoma versus lymphoid hyperplasia, laparotomy is necessary.

Laparotomy Workup (Table 14-8). It should be stressed that once laparotomy is undertaken, lym-

Table 14-7 WORKUP OF LYMPHOPROLIFERATIVE DISORDERS OF THE GASTROINTESTINAL TRACT BY ENDOSCOPIC BIOPSY

1. *Polymorphous infiltrate without cytologic atypia*
   Consistent with lymphoid hyperplasia if compatible with clinical history. Repeat biopsy after therapy.
2. *Polymorphous infiltrate with cytologic atypia*
   Lymphoma. Confirm with immunochemistry (on frozen tissue).
3. *Necrosis and poorly defined polymorphous infiltrate*
   Dangerous to interpret.
   Repeat biopsy.
   If in repeat biopsies not clearly lymphoid hyperplasia or lymphoma, proceed to laparotomy and frozen section. If lymphoma, proceed with lymphoma workup.
4. *Monomorphous infiltrate*
   Confirm with immunohistochemistry.
   Exclude undifferentiated carcinoma and carcinoid tumor from lymphoma.

Table 14-8 WORKUP PROCEDURE OF GASTROINTESTINAL LYMPHOMA ON TISSUES TAKEN AT LAPAROTOMY

1. Snap-freeze for routine immunohistochemistry lymphoma workup
2. Glutaraldehyde fixation; hold for electron microscopy if necessary.
3. Staging:
   Mesenteric lymph nodes
   Para-aortic lymph nodes
   Liver
   Bone marrow
   Spleen

phoma staging is essential for determination of the extent of the disease. This should include sampling of mesenteric and para-aortic lymph nodes, biopsy of the liver and careful inspection of the spleen. Also, frozen tissue should be taken specifically for determination of the type of lymphoma, or, in the case of undifferentiated tumors, to aid in the differential diagnosis.

References

1. Kraft SC: Intraepithelial lymphocytes revisited. In Selected Summaries. Gastroenterology 78:180–181, 1980.
2. Weiss L, Greep RO: Histology. 4th ed. New York, McGraw-Hill, 1977, p 663.
3. Dukes C, Bussey HJR: The number of lymphoid follicles of the human large intestine. J Pathol Bacteriol 29:111–116, 1926.
4. Cornes JS: Number, size and distribution of Peyer's patches in the human small intestine. Gut 6:225–233, 1965.
5. Perrin WS, Lindsay EC: Intussusception: A monograph based on 400 cases. Br J Surg 9:46–71, 1921–1922.
6. Mowat A McI: The cellular basis of gastrointestinal immunity. In Marsh MN (ed): Immunopathology of the Small Intestine. New York, John Wiley and Sons, 1978, pp 41–42.
7. Rudzik O, Bienenstock J: Isolation and characteristics of gut mucosal lymphocytes. Lab Invest 30:260–266, 1974.
8. Dobbins WO: Human intestinal intraepithelial lymphocytes: Progress report. Gut 27:972–985, 1986.
9. Bockman DE, Cooper MD: Early lymphoepithelial relationships in human appendix: A combined light and electron-microscopic study. Gastroenterology 68:1160–1168, 1975.
10. Fichtelius KE, Sundstrom C, Kullgren B, Linna J: The lympho-epithelial organs of Homo sapiens revisited. Acta Path Microbiol Scand 77:103–116, 1969.
11. Eade OE, Andre-Ukena S, St Moulton C, et al: Lymphocyte sub-populations of intestinal mucosa in inflammatory bowel disease. Gut 21:675–682, 1980.
12. Bull DM, Bookman MA: Isolation and functional characterization of human intestinal mucosa lymphoid cells. J Clin Invest 59:966–974, 1977.
13. Walker WA, Isselbacher KJ, Bloch KJ: The role of immunization in controlling antigen uptake from the small intestine. Adv Exp Med Biol 45:295–303, 1974.
14. Williams RC, Gibbons RJ: Inhibition of bacterial adherence by secretory immunoglobulin A: A mechanism of antigen disposal. Science 177:697–699, 1972.
15. Tomasi TB: Structure and function of mucosal antibodies. Ann Rev Med 21:281–295, 1970.
16. Warshaw AL, Walker WA, Cornell R, et al: Small intestinal permeability to macromolecules: Transmission of horseradish peroxidase into mesenteric lymph and portal blood. Lab Invest 25:675–684, 1971.
17. Walker WA: Host defense mechanisms in the gastrointestinal tract. Pediatrics 57:901–916, 1976.
18. Rosen FS: The primary immunodeficiencies. New Engl J Med 311:235–242, 300–310, 1984.
19. Rosen FS, Wedgwood RJ, Aiuti F, et al: Primary immunodeficiency diseases: Report prepared for the WHO by a scientific group on immuno-deficiency. Clin Immun Immunopathol 28:450–475, 1983.
20. McDevitt HO, Benacerraf B: Genetic control of specific immune responses. Adv Immunol 11:31–74, 1969.
21. Thompson RA: Immunological mechanisms. In Asquith P (ed): Immunology of the Gastrointestinal Tract. New York, Churchill Livingstone, 1979, pp 14–22.
22. Ament ME: Immunodeficiency syndromes and gastrointestinal disease. Pediatr Clin North Am 22:807–825, 1975.
23. Ross IN, Asquith O: Primary immune deficiency. In Asquith P (ed): Immunology of the Gastrointestinal Tract. New York, Churchill Livingstone, 1979, p 152.
24. Eras P, Goldstein MJ, Sherlock P: Candida infection of the gastrointestinal tract. Medicine 51:367–379, 1972.
25. Foucar E, Mukai K, Foucar K, et al: Colon ulceration in lethal cytomegalovirus infection. Am J Clin Pathol 76:788–801, 1981.
26. Ament ME, Ochs HD, David SD: Structure and function of the gastrointestinal tract in primary immunodeficiency syndromes: A study of 39 patients. Medicine 52:227–248, 1973.
27. Boram LH, Keller KF, Justus DE, et al: Strongyloidiasis in immunosuppressed patients. Am J Clin Pathol 76:778–781, 1981.
28. Hermans PE, Diaz-Buxo JA, Stobo JD: Idiopathic late-onset immunoglobulin deficiency: Clinical observations in 50 patients. Am J Med 61:221–237, 1976.
29. Meisel JL, Perera DR, Meligro C, et al: Overwhelming watery diarrhea associated with Cryptosporidium in an immunosuppressed patient. Gastroenterology 70:1156–1160, 1976.
30. Lasser KH, Lewin KJ, Ryning FW: Cryptosporidial enteritis in a patient with congenital hypogammaglobulinemia. Hum Pathol 10:234–240, 1979.
31. Matthew JS, Gottlieb MS, Lewin KJ, Weinstein WM: Gastrointestinal (GI) lesions in homosexual men with acquired cellular immunodeficiency. (Abstract) Gastroenterology 82:1126, 1982.
32. Klein RS, Harris CA, Butkus-Small C, et al: Oral candidiasis in high-risk patients as the initial manifestation of the acquired immunodeficiency syndrome. N Engl J Med 311:354–358, 1984.
33. Owen RL, Nemanic PC, Stevens DP: Ultrastructural observation on giardiasis in a murine model: 1. Intestinal distribution, attachment, and relationship to the immune system of Giardia muris. Gastroenterology 76:757–769, 1979.
34. Brandborg LL, Tankersley CB, Gottlieb S, et al: Histological demonstration of mucosal invasion by Giardia lamblia in man. Gastroenterology 52:143–150, 1967.
35. Brandborg LL, Goldberg SB, Bridenbach WC: Human coccidiosis—a possible cause of malabsorption. N Engl J Med 283:1306–1312, 1970.
36. Trier JS, Moxey PC, Schimmel EM, et al: Chronic intestinal coccidiosis in man: Intestinal morphology and response to treatment. Gastroenterology 66:923–935, 1974.
37. Current WL, Heyman MB, Weinstein WM: Human cryptosporidiosis in immunocompetent and immunodeficient persons: Studies of an outbreak and experimental transmission. N Engl J Med 308:1252–1257, 1983.
38. Gottlieb MS, Groopman JE, Weinstein WM, et al: The acquired immunodeficiency syndrome. Ann Intern Med 99:208–220, 1983.
39. Petty RE, Haddow M, Oen K, et al: Antibodies to nucleic acid antigens in selective IgA deficiency. Clin Immunol Immunopathol 13:182–186, 1979.
40. Twomey JJ, Jordan PH, Laughter AH, et al: The gastric disorder in immunoglobulin deficient patients. Ann Intern Med 72:499–504, 1970.
41. Bull DM, Tomasi TB: Deficiency of immunoglobulin A in intestinal disease. Gastroenterology 54:313–320, 1968.
42. Johansson SGO, Hogman CF, Killander J: Quantitative immunoglobulin determination. Acta Pathol Microbiol Scand 74:519–530, 1968.
43. Geha RS, Schneeberger E, Merler E, et al: Heterogeneity of "acquired" or common variable agammaglobulinemia. N Engl J Med 291:1–10, 1974.
44. Dobbins WO: Gut immunophysiology: A gastroenterologist's view with emphasis on pathophysiology. Am J Physiol 242:G1-G8, 1982.
45. Hughes WS, Brooks FP, Conn HO: Serum gastrin levels in primary hypogammaglobulinemia and pernicious anemia. Studies in adults. Ann Intern Med 77:746–750, 1972.
46. James D, Asherson, Chanarin I, et al: Cell-mediated immunity to intrinsic factor in autoimmune disorders. Br Med J 4:494–496, 1974.
47. Conn HO, Binder H, Burns B: Pernicious anaemia and immunologic deficiency. Ann Intern Med 68:603–612, 1968.
48. Binder HJ, Reynolds RD: Control of diarrhea in secondary hypogammaglobulinemia by fresh plasma infusions. N Engl J Med 277:802–803, 1967.
49. Diaz-Buxo JA, Hermans PE, Huizenga KA: Gastrointestinal dysfunction in immunoglobulin deficiency: Effect of corticosteroids and tetracycline. JAMA 233:1189–1191, 1975.
50. Ament ME, Rubin CE: Relation of giardiasis to abnormal intes-

tinal structure and function in gastrointestinal immunodeficiency syndromes. Gastroenterology 62:216–226, 1972.
51. Eidelman S: Intestinal lesions in immune deficiency. Hum Pathol 7:427–434, 1976.
52. Mann JG, Brown WR, Kern F: The subtle and variable clinical expressions of gluten-induced enteropathy (adult celiac disease, nontropical sprue). Am J Med 48:357–366, 1970.
53. Swift PN: Hypogammaglobulinemia, steatorrhoea and megaloblastic anaemia: Response to gluten-free diet and folic acid. Postgrad Med J 38:633–639, 1962.
54. Hughes WS, Cerda JJ, Holtzapple P, et al: Primary hypogammaglobulinemia and malabsorption. Ann Intern Med 74:903–910, 1971.
55. Editorial: Temporary gluten intolerance. Lancet 2:555, 1976.
56. Visakorpi JK, Immonen P: Intolerance to cow's milk and wheat gluten in the primary malabsorption syndrome in infancy. Acta Paediatr Scand 56:49–56, 1967.
57. Walker-Smith J: Transient gluten intolerance. Arch Dis Child 45:523–526, 1970.
58. Johnson BL, Goldberg LS, Pops MA, et al: Clinical and immunological studies in a case of nodular lymphoid hyperplasia of the small bowel. Gastroenterology 61:369–374, 1971.
59. Waldmann TA, Strober W, Blaese RM: Immunodeficiency disease and malignancy: Various immunologic deficiencies of man and the role of immune processes in the control of malignant disease. Ann Intern Med 77:605–628, 1972.
60. Bachmann R: Studies on the serum gamma-A-globulin level. III. The frequency of A-gamma-A-globulinemia. Scand J Clin Lab Invest 17:316–320, 1965.
61. Koistinen J: Familial clustering of selective IgA deficiency. Vox Sang 30:181–190, 1976.
62. McCarthy DM, Katz SI, Gazze RL, et al: Selective IgA deficiency associated with total villous atrophy of the small intestine and an organ-specific anti-epithelial cell antibody. J Immunol 120:932–938, 1978.
63. Ammann AJ, Hong R: Selective IgA deficiency: Presentation of 30 cases and a review of the literature. Medicine 50:223–236, 1971.
64. Niwa Y, Kanoh T: Immune deficiency states and immune imbalance in systemic lupus erythematosus and other autoimmune diseases. Clin Immunol Immunopathol 12:289–300, 1979.
65. Bergman L, Johansson SGO, Krause U: The immunoglobulin concentrations in serum and bowel secretion in patients with Crohn's disease. Scand J Gastroenterol 8:401–406, 1973.
66. Falchuk KR, Falchuk ZM: Selective immunoglobulin A deficiency, ulcerative colitis, and gluten-sensitive enteropathy—a unique association. Gastroenterology 69:503–506, 1975.
67. Soltoft J, Peterson L, Kruse P: Immunoglobulin A deficiency and regional enteritis. Scand J Gastroenterol 7:233–236, 1972.
68. Anderson KE, Finlayson NDC, Deschner EE: Intractable malabsorption with a flat jejunal mucosa and selective IgA deficiency. Gastroenterology 67:709–716, 1974.
69. Crabbe PA, Heremans JF: Selective IgA deficiency with steatorrhoea: A new syndrome. Am J Med 42:319–326, 1967.
70. Crabbe PA, Heremans JF: Lack of gamma A-immunoglobulin in serum of patients with steatorrhoea. Gut 7:119–127, 1966.
71. Hoskins LC, Winawer SJ, Broitman SA, et al: Clinical giardiasis and intestinal malabsorption. Gastroenterology 53:265–279, 1967.
72. Hobbs JR, Hepner GW: Deficiency of gamma M-globulin in coeliac disease. Lancet 1:217–220, 1968.
73. Strober W, Krakauer R, Klaeverman HL, et al: Secretory component deficiency: A disorder of the IgA immune system. N Engl J Med 294:351–356, 1976.
74. Ochs HD, Ament ME, Davis SD: Giardiasis with malabsorption in X-linked agammaglobulinemia. N Engl J Med 287:341–342, 1972.
75. Kirkpatrick CH: Cancer and immunodeficiency diseases. Birth Defects: Original Article Series 12:61–78, 1976.
76. Dosch HM, Lee JWW, Gelfand EW, et al: Severe combined immunodeficiency disease: A model of T-cell dysfunction. Clin Exp Immunol 34:260–267, 1978.
77. Horowitz S, Lorenzsonn VW, Olsen WA, et al: Small intestinal disease in T-cell deficiency. J Pediatr 85:457–462, 1974.
78. Buckley RH, Whismant JK, Schiff RI, et al: Correction of severe combined immunodeficiency by fetal liver cells. N Engl J Med 294:1076–1081, 1976.
79. Kirkpatrick CH, Smith TK: Chronic mucocutaneous candidiasis: Immunologic and antibiotic therapy. Ann Intern Med 80:310–325, 1974.
80. DiGeorge AM: Congenital absence of the thymus and its immunologic consequences: Concurrence with congenital hypoparathyroidism. In Good RA, Bergsma D (eds): Immunologic Deficiency Diseases in Man. Birth Defects: Original Article Series 4:116–121, 1968.
81. Pahwa R, Pahwa S, O'Reilly R, et al: Treatment of the immunodeficiency diseases: Progress towards replacement therapy emphasizing cellular and macromolecular engineering. Springer Semin Immunopathol 1:355–404, 1978.
82. Baehner RL: The growth and development of our understanding of chronic granulomatous disease. In Bellanti JA, Dayton DM (eds): The Phagocytic Cell in Host Resistance. New York, Raven Press, 1975, pp 173–200.
83. Johnston RB, McMurray JS: Chronic familial granulomatosis: report of five cases and review of the literature. Am J Dis Child 114:370–378, 1967.
84. Johnston RB, Baehner RL: Chronic granulomatous disease: Correlation between pathogenesis and clinical findings. Pediatrics 48:730–739, 1971.
85. Twomey JJ, Laughter AH, Farrow S, et al: Hodgkin's disease: An immunodepleting and immunosuppressive disorder. J Clin Invest 56:467–475, 1975.
86. Fauci AS: The human immunodeficiency virus: infectivity and mechanisms of pathogenesis. Science 239:617–622, 1988.
87. Rodgers VD, Fassett R, Kagnoff MF: Abnormalities in intestinal mucosal T-cells in homosexual populations including those with lymphadenopathy syndrome and acquired immunodeficiency syndrome. Gastroenterology 90:552–558, 1986.
88. Strober W, Wochner RD, Carbone PP, et al: Intestinal lymphangiectasia: A protein-losing enteropathy with hypogammaglobulinemia, lymphocytopenia and impaired homograft rejection. J Clin Invest 46:1643–1656, 1967.
89. McDonald GB, Shulman HM, Sullivan KM, Spencer GD: Intestinal and hepatic complications of human bone marrow transplantation. Part I. Gastroenterology 90:460–477, 1986. Part II. Gastroenterology 90:770–784, 1986.
90. Elfenbein GJ, Saral R: Infectious disease during immune recovery after bone marrow transplantation. In Allen JC (ed): Infection and the Compromised Host, Clinical Correlations and Therapeutic Approaches. Baltimore, Williams & Wilkins, 1981, pp 157–196.
91. Mowat AM, Ferguson A: Hypersensitivity reactions in the small intestine. 6. Pathogenesis of the graft-versus-host reaction in the small intestinal mucosa of the mouse. Transplantation 32:238–243, 1981.
92. Selby WS, Janossy G, Goldstein G, et al: T lymphocyte subsets in human intestinal mucosa: The distribution and relationship to MHC derived antigens. Clin Exp Immunol 44:453–458, 1981.
93. Beschorner WE, Yardley JH, Tutschka PJ, et al: Deficiency of intestinal immunity with graft-vs.-host disease in humans. J Infect Dis 144:38–46, 1981.
94. Beschorner WE, Tutschka PJ, Santos GW: Sequential morphology of graft-versus-host disease in the rat radiation chimera. Clin Immunol Immunopathol 22:203–224, 1982.
95. Elson CO, Reilly RW, Rosenberg IH: Small intestinal injury in the graft-versus-host reaction: An innocent bystander phenomenon. Gastroenterol 72:886–889, 1977.
96. Epstein RJ, McDonald GB, Sale GE, et al: The diagnostic accuracy of the rectal biopsy in acute graft-versus-host disease: A prospective study of thirteen patients. Gastroenterol 78:764–771, 1980.
97. Sale GE, Shulman HM, McDonald GB, et al: Gastrointestinal graft-versus-host disease in man: A clinicopathologic study of the rectal biopsy. Am J Surg Pathol 3:291–299, 1979.
98. Shulman HM, Sullivan KM, Weiden PL, et al: Chronic graft-versus-host syndrome in man: A long term clinicopathologic study of 20 Seattle patients. Am J Med 69:204–217, 1980.
99. Smith PD, Lane HC, Gill VJ, et al: Intestinal infections in pa-

tients with Acquired Immunodeficiency Syndrome (AIDS): Etiology and response to therapy. Ann Intern Med 108:328–333, 1988.
100. De Jarlais DC, Marmor M, Thomas P, et al: Kaposi's sarcoma among four different AIDS risk groups. (Letter) N Engl J Med 310:1119, 1984.
101. Burkes RL, Meyer PR, Gill PS, et al: Rectal lymphoma in homosexual men. Arch Intern Med 146:913–915, 1986.
102. Ziegler JL, Beckstend JA, Volberding A, et al: Non-Hodgkin's lymphoma in 90 homosexual men. N Engl J Med 311:565–570, 1986.
103. Daling JR, Weiss NS, Hislop TG, et al: Sexual practices, sexually transmitted diseases, and the incidence of anal cancer. N Engl J Med 317:973–977, 1987.
104. Haeney MR: Acquired immune deficiency syndrome (AIDS) and the gastrointestinal tract. In Marsh MN (ed): Immunopathology of the Small Intestine. John Wiley and Sons, 1987, pp 333–368.
105. Mobley C, Rotterdam HZ, Lerner CW, Tapper ML: Autopsy findings in the acquired immune deficiency syndrome. Pathol Annu 20:45–65, 1985.
106. Waisman J, Niedt GN, Rotterdam H, et al: AIDS: An overview of the pathology. Pathol Res Pract 182:729–754, 1987.
107. Mildvan D, Mathur U, Enlow RW, et al: Opportunistic infections and immune deficiency in homosexual men. Ann Intern Med 96:700–704, 1982.
108. Gottlieb MS, Schroff R, Schanker HM, et al: Pneumocystis carinii pneumonia and mucosal candidiasis in previously healthy homosexual men: Evidence of a new acquired cellular immunodeficiency. N Engl J Med 305:1425–1431, 1981.
109. Centers for Disease Control: Unexplained immunodeficiency and opportunistic infections in infants—New York, New Jersey, California. MMWR 31:665–668, 1982.
110. Reese NC, Current WL, Ernst JV, et al: Cryptosporidiosis of man and calf: A case report and results of experimental infections in mice and rats. Am J Trop Med Hyg 31:226–229, 1982.
111. Connolly GM, Dryden MS, Shanson DC, et al: Cryptosporidial diarrhoea in AIDS and its treatment. Gut 29:593–597, 1988.
112. Garcia LS, Bruckner DA, Brewer RC, Shimizur Y: Techniques for the recovery and identification of cryptosporidium oocysts from stool specimens. J Clin Microbiol 18:185–190, 1983.
113. Ma P, Soave R: Three-step stool examination for cryptosporidiosis in ten homosexual men with protracted watery diarrhea. J Infect Dis 147:824–828, 1983.
114. Hinnant HL, Rotterdam H, Bell E, Tapper M: Cytomegalovirus infection of the alimentary tract: Clinico-pathologic correlations. Am J Gastroenterol 81:944–950, 1986.
115. Jacobson MA, Mills J: Serious cytomegalovirus disease in the acquired immunodeficiency syndrome (AIDS): Clinical findings, diagnosis, and treatment. Ann Intern Med 108:585–594, 1988.
116. Greene JB, Sidhu GS, Lewin S, et al: Mycobacterium avium-intracellulare: A cause of disseminated life-threatening infection in homosexuals and drug abusers. Ann Intern Med 97:539–546, 1982.
117. Mufarrij AA, Greco A, Antopol SC, et al: The histopathology of cervical lymphadenitis caused by Mycobacterium avium-Mycobacterium intracellulare complex in an immunocompromised host. Hum Pathol 13:78–81, 1982.
118. Zakowski P, Fligiel S, Berlin GW, Johnson BL: Disseminated Mycobacterium avium-intracellulare infection in homosexual men dying of acquired immunodeficiency. JAMA 248:2980–2982, 1982.
119. Roth RI, Owen RL, Keren DF, et al: Intestinal infection with Mycobacterium avium in acquired immune deficiency syndrome (AIDS): Histological and clinical comparison with Whipple's disease. Dig Dis Sci 30:497–504, 1985.
120. Quinn TC, Corey L, Chaffee RG, et al: The etiology of anorectal infections in homosexual men. Am J Med 71:395–406, 1981.
121. Goodell SE, Quinn TC, Mkrtrician E, et al: Herpes simplex virus proctitis in homosexual men: Clinical, sigmoidoscopic and histopathological features. N Engl J Med 308:868–871, 1983.
122. Friedman-Kien AE, Laubenstein LJ, Rubinstein P, et al: Disseminated Kaposi's sarcoma in homosexual men. Ann Intern Med 96:693–700, 1982.
123. Bernal A, Del Junco GW, Gibson SR: Endoscopic and pathologic features of gastrointestinal sarcoma: A report of four cases in patients with acquired immunodeficiency disease. Gastrointest Endosc 31:74–77, 1985.
124. Saltz RK, Kurtz RC, Lightdale CJ, et al: Gastrointestinal involvement in Kaposi's sarcoma. (Abstract) Gastroenterology 82:1168, 1982.
125. Friedman SL, Wright TL, Altman DF: Kaposi's sarcoma in patients with acquired immunodeficiency syndrome: Endoscopic and autopsy findings. Gastroenterology 89:102–108, 1985.
126. Sheahan DG, West AB: Focal lymphoid hyperplasia (pseudolymphoma) of the esophagus. Am J Surg Pathol 9:141–147, 1985.
127. Strodel WE, Cooper R, Eckhauser F, et al: Pseudolymphoma masquerading as colonic malignancy. Dis Colon Rectum 26:68–72, 1983.
128. Brooks JJ, Enterline HT: Gastric pseudolymphoma: Its three subtypes and relation to lymphoma. Cancer 51:476–486, 1983.
129. Buchholz RR, Reid RA: Pseudolymphoma of the stomach. Surg Clin North Am 52:485–491, 1972.
130. Jacobs DS: Primary gastric malignant lymphoma and pseudolymphoma. Am J Clin Pathol 40:379–394, 1963.
131. Perrillo RP, Tedesco FJ: Gastric pseudolymphoma: A spectrum of presenting features and diagnostic considerations. Am J Gastroenterol 65:226–230, 1976.
132. Ranchod M, Lewin KJ, Dorfman RF: Lymphoid hyperplasia of the gastrointestinal tract: A study of 26 cases and review of the literature. Am J Surg Pathol 2:383–400, 1978.
133. Watson RJ, O'Brien MT: Gastric pseudolymphoma (lymphofollicular gastritis). Ann Surg 171:98–106, 1970.
134. Wright CJE: Pseudolymphoma of the stomach. Hum Pathol 4:305–318, 1973.
135. Chiles JT, Platz CE: The radiographic manifestation of pseudolymphoma of the stomach. Radiology 116:551–556, 1975.
136. Eras P, Winawer SJ: Benign lymphoid hyperplasia of the stomach simulating gastric malignancy. Am J Dig Dis 14:510–515, 1969.
137. Faris TD, Saltzstein SL: Gastric lymphoid hyperplasia: A lesion confused with lymphosarcoma. Cancer 17:207–212, 1964.
138. Perez CA, Dorfman RF: Benign lymphoid hyperplasia of the stomach and the duodenum. Radiology 57:505–510, 1966.
139. Tandon RK, Tandon HD, Singh DS, Berry M: Benign lymphoid hyperplasia of the stomach mimicking gastric malignancy. Am J Gastroenterol 66:36–41, 1976.
140. Saraga P, Hurlimann J, Ozzello L: Lymphomas and pseudolymphomas of the alimentary tract: An immunohistochemical study with clinicopathologic correlations. Hum Pathol 12:713–723, 1981.
141. Barge J, Molas G, Potet I: Lymphoid stromal reaction in gastrointestinal lymphomas: Immunohistochemical study of 14 cases. J Clin Pathol 40:760–765, 1987.
142. Eimoto T, Futami K, Naito H, et al: Gastric pseudolymphoma with monotypic cytoplasmic immunoglobulin. Cancer 55:788–793, 1985.
143. Wolf JA, Spjut HJ: Focal lymphoid hyperplasia of the stomach preceding gastric lymphoma: A case report and review of the literature. Cancer 48: 2518–2523, 1981.
144. Scoazed JY, Brousse N, Potet F, Jeulain JF: Focal malignant lymphoma in gastric pseudolymphoma: Histologic and immunohistochemical study of a case. Cancer 57:1330–1336, 1986.
145. Murayama H, Kikuchi M, Eimoto T, et al: Early lymphoma co-existing with reactive lymphoid hyperplasia of the stomach. Acta Pathol Jpn 34:679–686, 1984.
146. Gudjonsson H, Jonas M, Krawilt EL, Kaye MD: Pseudolymphoma of the jejunum. Dig Dis Sciences 32:1314–1318, 1987.
147. Sniderman BF: Benign lymphoma of the rectum. Am J Surg 82:611–615, 1951.
148. Harwood RA, Abreu FB: Benign lymphoma and diffuse lymphoid hyperplasia: A case report. Am J Proctol 26:63–66, 1975.
149. Cornes JS, Wallace H, Morson BC: Benign lymphomas of the rectum and anal canal: A study of 100 cases. J Pathol Bacteriol 82:371–382, 1961.
150. Helwig EB, Hansen J: Lymphoid polyps (benign lymphoma) and malignant lymphoma of the rectum and anus. Surg Gynecol Obstet 92:233–243, 1951.

151. Holtz F, Schmidt LA: Lymphoid polyps (benign lymphoma) of the rectum and anus. Surg Gynecol Obstet 106:639–642, 1958.
152. Keeling WM, Beatty GL: Lymphoid polyps of the rectum: Report of three cases in siblings. Arch Surg 73:753–756, 1956.
153. Meissner WW: Benign lymphoma of the rectum: Review of the literature and report of fifteen additional cases. J Int Coll Surg 26:739–749, 1956.
154. Heule BV, Taylor CR, Terry R, Lukes RJ: Presentation of malignant lymphoma in the rectum. Cancer 49:2602–2607, 1982.
155. Molas G, Potet F, Nogig P: Hyperplasie lymphoide focale (pseudo-lymphome) de l'ileon terminal chez l'adulte. Gastroenterol Clin Biol 9:630–633, 1985.
156. Nathans AA, Merenstein H, Brown SS: Lymphoid hyperplasia of the appendix. Clinical Study. Pediatrics 12:516–524, 1953.
157. Charlesworth D, Fox H, Mainwaring AR: Benign lymphoid hyperplasia of the terminal ileum. Am J Gastroenterol 53:579–584, 1970.
158. Cornes JS, Dawson IMP: Papillary lymphoid hyperplasia at the ileocecal valve as a cause of acute intussusception in infancy. Arch Dis Child 38:89–91, 1963.
159. Selke AC, Jona JZ, Belin RP: Massive enlargement of the ileocecal valve due to lymphoid hyperplasia. Am J Roentgenol 127:518–520, 1976.
160. Stout AP: Isolated lymphoid hyperplasia in the cecum and appendix of children. Am J Dis Child 34:797–806, 1927.
161. Fieber SS, Schaefer HJ: Lymphoid hyperplasia of the terminal ileum—a clinical entity? Gastroenterology 50:83–98, 1966.
162. O'Sullivan WD, Child CG: Ileocecal intussusception caused by lymphoid hyperplasia. J Pediatr 38:320–324, 1951.
163. Sarason EL, Prior JT, Prowda RL: Recurrent intussusception associated with hypertrophy of Peyer's patches. N Engl J Med 253:905–908, 1955.
164. Swartley RN, Stayman JW: Lymphoid hyperplasia of the intestinal tract requiring surgical intervention. Ann Surg 155:238–240, 1962.
165. Perrin WS, Lindsay EC: Intussusception: A monograph based on 400 cases. Br J Surg 9:46–71, 1921–1922.
166. Clark EJ, Phillips IA, Alexander ER: Adenovirus infection in intussusception in children in Taiwan. JAMA 208:1671–1674, 1969.
167. Yunis EJ, Hashida Y: Electron microscopic demonstration of adenovirus in appendix vermiformis in a case of ileocecal intussusception. Pediatrics 51:566–570, 1973.
168. Dorazio RA, Whelan TJ: Lymphoid hyperplasia of the terminal ileum associated with familial polyposis coli. Ann Surg 171:300–302, 1970.
169. Gruenberg J, Mackman S: Multiple lymphoid polyps in familial polyposis. Ann Surg 175:552–554, 1972.
170. Cosens CG: Gastrointestinal pseudoleukemia: A case report. Ann Surg 148:129–133, 1958.
171. Hermans PE, Huizenga KA, Hoffman HN, et al: Dysgammaglobulinemia associated with nodular lymphoid hyperplasia of the small intestine. Am J Med 40:78–89, 1966.
172. Hermans PE, Diaz-Buxo JA, Stobo JD: Idiopathic late-onset immunoglobulin deficiency: Clinical observations in 50 patients. Am J Med 61:221–237, 1976.
173. Gryboski JD, Self TW, Clemett A, Herskovic T: Selective immunoglobulin A deficiency and intestinal nodular lymphoid hyperplasia: Correction of diarrhea with antibiotics and plasma. Pediatrics 42:833–836, 1968.
174. Davis SD, Eidelman S, Loop JW: Nodular lymphoid hyperplasia of the small intestine and sarcoidosis. Arch Intern Med 126:668–672, 1970.
175. Matuchansky C, Morichau-Beauchant M, Touchard G: Nodular lymphoid hyperplasia of the small bowel associated with primary jejunal malignant lymphoma. Gastroenterology 78:1587–1592, 1982.
176. Aquilar FP, Alfonso V, Rivas S: Jejunal malignant lymphoma in a patient with adult-onset hypogammaglobulinemia and nodular lymphoid hyperplasia of the small bowel. Am J Gastroenterol 82:472–475, 1987.
177. Bird DC, Jacobs JB, Silbiger M, Wolff SM: Hypogammaglobulinemia with nodular lymphoid hyperplasia of the intestine: Report of a case with rectosigmoid involvement. Radiology 92:1535–1536, 1969.
178. De Smet AA, Tubergen DG, Martel W: Nodular lymphoid hyperplasia of the colon associated with dysgammaglobulinemia. Am J Roentgenol 127:515–517, 1976.
179. Penny R: Nodular lymphoid hyperplasia of the small intestine and hypogammaglobulinemia. Gastroenterology 56:982–985, 1969.
180. Hodgson JR, Hoffman HN, Huizenga KA: Roentgenologic features of lymphoid hyperplasia of the small intestine associated with dysgammaglobulinemia. Radiology 88:883–888, 1967.
181. Waldmann TA, Broder S, Blease RM, et al: Role of suppressive T cells in pathogenesis of common variable hypogammaglobulinemia. Lancet 2:609–613, 1974.
182. Ajdukiewicz AB, Youngs GR, Bouchier IAD: Nodular lymphoid hyperplasia with hypogammaglobulinemia. Gut 13:589–595, 1972.
183. Milano AM, Lawrence LR, Horowitz L: Nodular lymphoid hyperplasia of the small intestine and colon with giardiasis: A case with borderline serum IgA levels. Am J Dig Dis 16:735–737, 1971.
184. Robinson MJ, Padron S, Rywlin AM: Enterocolitis lymphofollicularis: Morphologic, pathologic, and serum immunoglobulin patterns. Arch Pathol 96:311–315, 1973.
185. Capitanio MA, Kirkpatrick JA: Lymphoid hyperplasia of the colon in children: Roentgen observations. Radiology 94:323–327, 1970.
186. Franken WA: Lymphoid hyperplasia of the colon. Radiology 94:329–334, 1970.
187. Theander G, Tragardh B: Lymphoid hyperplasia of the colon in childhood. Acta Radiol Diagn 17:631–640, 1976.
188. Louw JH: Polypoid lesions of the large bowel in children with particular reference to benign lymphoid polyposis. J Pediatr Surg 3:195–209, 1968.
189. Collins JO, Falk M, Guibone R: Benign lymphoid polyposis of the colon: A case report. Pediatrics 38:897–899, 1966.
190. Cornes JS: Multiple lymphomatous polyposis of the gastrointestinal tract. Cancer 14:249–257, 1961.
191. Kahn LB, Novis BH: Nodular lymphoid hyperplasia of the small bowel associated with primary small bowel reticulum cell lymphoma. Cancer 33:837–844, 1974.
192. Asquith P, Haeney MR: Celiac disease. In Asquith P (ed): Immunology of the Gastrointestinal Tract. Edinburgh, Churchill Livingstone, 1979, p 69.
193. Swinson CM, Slavin G, Coles EC, Booth CC: Coeliac disease and malignancy. Lancet 1:111–115, 1983.
194. Roehrkasse RL, Roberts IM, Wald A, et al: Celiac sprue complicated by lymphoma presenting with multiple gastric ulcers. Gastroenterology 91:740–745, 1986.
195. Cooper BT, Holmes GKT, Ferguson R, Cooke WT: Celiac disease and malignancy. Medicine 59:249–261, 1980.
196. Freeman HJ, Weinstein WM, Shnitka TK, et al: Primary abdominal lymphoma: Presenting manifestation of celiac sprue or complicating dermatitis herpetiformis. Am J Med 63:585–594, 1977.
197. Isaacson P, Jones DB, Sworn MJ, Wright DH: Malignant histiocytosis of the intestine: Report of three cases with immunological and cytochemical analysis. J Clin Pathol 35:510–516, 1982.
198. Isaacson P, Wright DH, Judd MA, Mepham BL: Primary gastrointestinal lymphomas: The classification of 66 cases. Cancer 43:1805–1819, 1979.
199. Isaacson P: Primary gastrointestinal lymphoma. Editorial. Virchows Arch [A] 391:1–8, 1981.
200. Salter DM, Krajewski AS, Dewar AE: Immunophenotype analysis of malignant histiocytosis of the intestine. J Clin Pathol 39:8–15, 1986.
201. Klaeveman HL, Gebhard RL, Sessoms C, et al: In vitro studies of ulcerative ileojejunitis. Gastroenterology 68:572–582, 1975.
202. Gilinsky NH, Novis BH, Mee AS, et al: Immunoproliferative small-intestinal disease: follow-up of an alpha-chain negative, lymphoma-free group. J Clin Gastroenterol 5:421–428, 1983.
203. Lewin KJ, Ranchod M, Dorfman RF: Lymphomas of the gastrointestinal tract: A study of 117 cases presenting with gastrointestinal disease. Cancer 42:693–707, 1978.
204. Loehr WJ, Mujahed Z, Zahn FD, et al: Primary lymphoma of the gastrointestinal tract: Review of 100 cases. Ann Surg 170:232–238, 1969.

205. Baker D, Chirprut RO, Rimer D, et al: Colonic lymphoma in ulcerative colitis. J Clin Gastroenterol 7:379–386, 1985.
206. Dawson IMP, Cornes JS, Morson BC: Primary malignant lymphoid tumors of the intestinal tract: Report of 37 cases with a study of factors influencing prognosis. Br J Surg 49:80–89, 1961.
207. Lewin KJ, Kahn LB, Novis BH: Primary intestinal lymphoma of "Western" and "Mediterranean" type, alpha-chain disease and massive plasma cell infiltration. Cancer 38:2511–2528, 1976.
208. Isaacson P, Wright DH: Malignant lymphoma of mucosa-associated lymphoid tissue: A distinctive type of B-cell lymphoma. Cancer 52:1410–1416, 1983.
209. Isaacson P, Wright DH, Jones DB: Malignant lymphoma of true histiocytic (monocyte/macrophage) origin. Cancer 51:80–91, 1983.
210. Otto HF, Bettman I, Weltzien JV, Gabbers JO: Primary intestinal lymphomas. Virchows Arch [A] 391:9–31, 1981.
211. Yamanaka N, Ishii Y, Hoshiba H, et al: A study of surface markers in gastrointestinal lymphoma. Gastroenterology 79:673–677, 1980.
212. Grody WW, Magidson JG, Weiss LM, et al: Gastrointestinal lymphomas: Immunohistochemical studies on the cell of origin. Am J Surg Pathol 9:328–337, 1985.
213. Berger F, Coiffier B, Bonneville C, et al: Gastrointestinal lymphomas: Immunohistochemical study of 23 cases. Am J Clin Pathol 88:707–712, 1987.
214. Gray GM, Rosenberg SA, Cooper AD, et al: Lymphomas involving the gastrointestinal tract. Gastroenterology 82:143–152, 1982.
215. Freeman C, Berg JW, Cutler SJ: Occurrence and prognosis of extranodal lymphomas. Cancer 29:252–260, 1972.
216. Allen AW, Donaldson G, Sniffen RC, Goodale F Jr: Primary malignant lymphoma of the gastrointestinal tract. Ann Surg 140:428–438, 1954.
217. Faulkner JW, Docherty MB: Lymphosarcoma of the small intestine. Surg Gynecol Obstet 95:76–84, 1952.
218. Frazer JW: Malignant lymphomas of the gastrointestinal tract. Surg Gynecol Obstet 108:182–190, 1959.
219. Bush RS: Primary lymphoma of the gastrointestinal tract. JAMA 228:1291–1294, 1974.
220. Goffinet DR, Warnke R, Dunnick NR, et al: Clinical and surgical (laparotomy) evaluation of patients with non-Hodgkin's lymphomas. Cancer Treat Rep 61(6):981–992, 1977.
221. Hande KR, Fisher RI, DeVita VT, et al: Diffuse histiocytic lymphoma involving the gastrointestinal tract. Cancer 41:1984–1989, 1978.
222. Vanden Heule B, Taylor CR, Terry R, Lukes RJ: Presentation of malignant lymphoma in the rectum. Cancer 49:2602–2607, 1982.
223. Joseph JI, Lattes R: Gastric lymphosarcoma: Clinicopathologic analysis of 71 cases and its relation to disseminated lymphosarcoma. Am J Clin Pathol 45:653–669, 1966.
224. Cornes JS: Multiple lymphomatous polyposis of the gastrointestinal tract. Cancer 14:249–257, 1961.
225. Ruppert GB, Smith VM: Multiple lymphomatous polyposis of the gastrointestinal tract. Gastrointest Endosc 25:67–79, 1979.
226. Usher FC, Dixon CF: Lymphosarcoma of the intestines. Gastroenterology 1:160–178, 1943.
227. Burman SO, van Wyke FAK: Lymphomas of the small intestine and cecum. Ann Surg 143:349–359, 1956.
228. Shepherd NA, Blackshaw AJ, Hall PA, et al: Malignant lymphoma with eosinophilia of the gastrointestinal tract. Histopathology 11:115–130, 1987.
229. Rosenberg SA, Berard CW, Brown BW, et al. National Cancer Institute sponsored study of classifications of non-Hodgkin's lymphomas: Summary and description of a working formulation for clinical usage: The non-Hodgkin's lymphoma pathologic classification project. Cancer 49:2112–2135, 1982.
230. Warnke RA, Kim H, Fuks Z, Dorfman RF: The coexistence of nodular and diffuse patterns in nodular non-Hodgkin's lymphomas: Significance and clinicopathologic correlation. Cancer 40:1229–1233, 1977.
231. Rappaport H, Winter WJ, Hicks EB: Follicular lymphoma: A re-evaluation of its position in the scheme of malignant lymphoma based on a survey of 253 cases. Cancer 9:792–821, 1956.
232. Levine PH, Kamaraja LS, Connelly RR, et al: The American Burkitt's Lymphoma Registry: Eight years' experience. Cancer 49:1016–1022, 1982.
233. Mann RB, Jaffe ES, Braylan RC, et al: Nonendemic Burkitt's lymphoma: A B-cell tumor related to germinal centers. N Engl J Med 295:685–691, 1976.
234. Sheehan DG, Martin F, Bagkinsky S, et al: Multiple lymphomatous polyposis of the gastrointestinal tract. Cancer 28:408–425, 1971.
235. Isaacson P, Wright D: Extranodal malignant lymphoma arising from mucosa associated lymphoid tissue. Cancer 53:2515–2524, 1984.
236. Weingrad DN, Decosse JJ, Sherlock P, et al: Primary gastrointestinal lymphoma: A thirty year review. Cancer 49:1258–1265, 1982.
237. Cox JD: Prognostic factors in malignant lymphoreticular tumors of the small bowel and ileocecal region: A review of 50 case histories. Int J Radiat Oncol Biol Phys 5:185–190, 1979.
238. Shimm DS, Dosoretz DE, Anderson T, et al: Primary gastric lymphoma: An analysis with emphasis on prognostic factors and radiation therapy. Cancer 52:2044–2048, 1983.
239. Filippa DA, Lieberman PH, Weingrad DN, et al: Primary lymphomas of the gastrointestinal tract: Analysis of prognostic factors with emphasis on histological type. Am J Surg Pathol 7:363–372, 1983.
240. Jones RE, Willis S, Inne DJ, Wanebo HJ: Primary gastric lymphoma: Problems in staging and management. Am J Surg 55:118–123, 1988.
241. Dragosics B, Bauer P, Radaszkiewicz T: Primary gastrointestinal non-Hodgkin's lymphomas: A retrospective clinicopathologic study of 150 cases. Cancer 55(5):1060–1073, 1985.
242. Maor MH, Maddux B, Osborne BM, et al: Stages IE and IIE non-Hodgkin's lymphomas of the stomach: Comparison of treatment modalities. Cancer 54:2330–2337, 1984.
243. Aozasa K, Ueda T, Jurata A, et al: Prognostic value of histologic and clinical factors in 56 patients with gastrointestinal lymphomas. Cancer 61:304–315, 1988.
244. Nelson DF, Cassady JR, Traggis D, et al: The role of radiation therapy in localized resectable intestinal non-Hodgkin's lymphoma in children. Cancer 39:89–97, 1977.
245. Hermann R, Panahon AM, Barcos MP, et al: Gastrointestinal involvement in non-Hodgkin's lymphoma. Cancer 46:215–222, 1980.
246. Rosenfelt F, Rosenberg SA: Diffuse histiocytic lymphoma presenting with gastrointestinal tract lesions: The Stanford experience. Cancer 45:2188–2193, 1980.
247. Cornes JS, Gwynfor T, Fisher GB: Leukaemic lesions of the gastrointestinal tract. J Clin Pathol 15:305–313, 1962.
248. Prolla JC, Kirsner JB: The gastrointestinal lesions and complications of the leukemias. Ann Intern Med 61:1084–1103, 1964.
249. Moir DH, Bale PM: Necropsy findings in childhoood leukaemia emphasizing neutropenic enterocolitis and cerebral calcification. Pathology 8:247–258, 1976.
250. Dewar GJ, Lim CNH, Michalynshyn B, et al: Gastrointestinal complications in patients with acute and chronic leukemia. Can J Surg 24:67–71, 1981.
251. Sherman NJ, Williams K, Woolley MM: Surgical complications in the patient with leukemia. J Pediatr Surg 8:235–244, 1973.
252. Kies MS, Luedke DW, Boyd JF, McCue MJ: Neutropenic enterocolitis. Cancer 43:730–734, 1979.
253. McCarthy D, Holland I, Lavender JP, Catousky D: Pneumatosis coli in adult acute myeloid leukaemia. Clin Radiol 30:175–178, 1979.
254. Alpha-chain disease and related small intestinal lymphoma: Report of a WHO meeting of investigators. Arch Fr Mal App Dig 65:591–607, 1976.
255. Seijffers MJ, Levy M, Hermann G: Intractable watery diarrhea, hypokalemia and malabsorption in a patient with Mediterranean type of abdominal lymphoma. Gastroenterology 55:118–124, 1968.
256. Eidelman S, Parkins RA, Rubin CE: Abdominal lymphoma presenting as malabsorption: A clinicopathologic study of nine

257. Ramot B, Shahin N, Bubis JJ: Malabsorption syndrome in lymphoma of the small bowel. Isr J Med Sci 1:221–226, 1965.
258. Al-Saleem T, Al-Bahrani Z: Malignant lymphoma of the small intestine in Iraq (Middle East lymphoma). Cancer 31:291–294, 1973.
259. Nasr K, Haghighi P, Bakhashandeh K, Haghshenas M: Primary lymphoma of the upper small intestine. Gut 11:673–678, 1970.
260. Novis BH, Banks S, Marks IN, et al: Abdominal lymphoma presenting with malabsorption. Quart J Med 40:521–540, 1971.
261. Asselah F, Slavin G, Sowter G, Asselah H: Immunoproliferative small intestinal disease in Algerians: Light microscopic and immunochemical studies. Cancer 52:227–237, 1983.
262. Rambaud JC, Bognel C, Prost A, et al: Clinicopathological study of a patient with "Mediterranean" type of abdominal lymphoma and a new type of IgA abnormality ("alpha chain disease"). Digestion 1:321–336, 1968.
263. Rambaud JC, Matuchansky C: Alpha-chain disease pathogenesis and relation to Mediterranean lymphoma. Lancet 1:1430–1432, 1973.
264. Isaacson P: Middle East lymphoma and alpha-chain disease: An immunohistochemical study. Am J Surg Pathol 3:431–441, 1979.
265. Seligmann M, Mihaesco E, Hurez D, et al: Immunochemical studies in 4 cases of alpha chain disease. J Clin Invest 48:2374–2389, 1968.
266. Seligmann M: Immunochemical, clinical and pathological features of alpha-chain disease. Arch Intern Med 135:78–82, 1975.
267. Seligmann M, Mihaesco E: Studies on alpha-chain disease. Ann NY Acad Sci 190:487–500, 1971.
268. Shahid MJ, Alami SY, Nassar VH, et al: Primary intestinal lymphoma with paraproteinemia. Cancer 35:848–858, 1975.
269. Gilinsky NH, Chaimowitz G, Van Standen ML: Immunoproliferative small-intestinal disease with lymphoma. Diagnostic difficulties and pitfalls. S Afr Med J 69:260–262, 1986.
270. Monges H, Aubert L, Chamlian A, et al: Maladie des chaines alpha a forme intestinale. Presentation d'un cas traite par antibiotherapie avec remission clinique, histologique et immunologique. Arch Fr Mal App Dig 64:223–231, 1975.
271. Ramot B, Shahin N, Bubis JJ: Malabsorption syndrome in lymphoma of the small intestine: A study of 13 cases. Isr J Med Sci 1:221–226, 1965.
272. Bender SW, Danon F, Preud'homme JL, et al: Gamma heavy chain disease simulating alpha chain disease. Gut 19:1148–1152, 1978.
273. Papac RJ, Rosenstein RW, Richards F, Yesner R: Gamma heavy chain disease seen initially as gastric neoplasm. Arch Int Med 138:1151–1153, 1978.
274. Roge J, Druet P, March C: Lymphome Mediterranéen avec maladie des chaines alpha: Triple remission clinique, anatomique et immunologique. Pathol Biol 18:851–858, 1970.
275. Smith WJ, Price SK, Isaacson PG: Immunoglobulin gene rearrangement in immunoproliferative small intestinal disease (IPSID). J Clin Pathol 40:1291–1297, 1987.
276. Coulbois J, Galian P, Galian A, et al: Gastric form of alpha-chain disease. Gut 27:719–725, 1986.
277. Cho C, Linscheer WG, Bell R, Smith R: Colonic lymphoma producing alpha-chain disease protein. Gastroenterology 83:121–126, 1982.
278. Isaacson P, Buchanan R, Mepham BL: Plasma cell granuloma of the stomach. Hum Pathol 9:355–358, 1978.
279. Wiltshaw E: The natural history of extramedullary plasmacytoma and its relation to solitary myeloma of bone and myelomatosis. Medicine 55:217–238, 1976.
280. Nahanishi I, Kajikawa K, Migita S, et al: Gastric plasmacytoma. An immunologic and immuno-histochemical study. Cancer 49:2025–2028, 1982.
281. Ferrer-Roca O: Primary gastric plasmacytoma with massive intracytoplasmic crystalline inclusions: A case report. Cancer 50:755–759, 1982.
282. Douglas HO, Sika JV, LeVeen HH: Plasmacytoma: A not so rare tumor of the small intestine. Cancer 28:456–460, 1971.
283. Asselah F, Crow J, Slavin G, et al: Solitary plasmacytoma of the intestine. Histopathology 6:631–645, 1982.
284. Rygaard-Olsen C, Boedker A, Emus HC, Olsen HAR: Extramedullary plasmacytoma of the small intestine: A case report studied with electron microscopy and immunoperoxidase technique. Cancer 50:573–576, 1982.
285. Gleason TH, Hammar SP: Plasmacytoma of the colon. Cancer 50:130–133, 1982.
286. Remigio PA, Klaum A: Extramedullary plasmacytoma of stomach. Cancer 27:562–568, 1971.
287. McCaffrey J, Kingston CW, Hasker WE: Extramedullary plasmacytoma of the gastrointestinal tract. Aust NZ J Surg 41:351–353, 1972.
288. Sharma KD, Shrivastav JD: Extramedullary plasmacytoma of gastrointestinal tract: With a case report of plasmacytoma of the rectum and a review of the literature. Arch Pathol 71:229–233, 1961.
289. Soga J, Saito K, Suzuki N, Sakai T: Plasma cell granuloma of the stomach: A report of a case and review of the literature. Cancer 25:618–625, 1970.
290. Funakoshi N, Kanoh T, Kobayashi Y, et al: IgM-producing gastric plasmacytoma. Cancer 54:638–643, 1984.
291. Scott FET, Dupont PA, Webb J: Plasmacytoma of the stomach: Diagnosis with the aid of immunoperoxidase technique. Cancer 41:675–681, 1978.

CHAPTER 15

Mesenchymal Tumors of the Gastrointestinal Tract

HENRY D. APPELMAN, M.D.

GENERAL FEATURES OF
    MESENCHYMAL TUMORS
Cell Origin and Differentiation
Site Specificity
Clinical Features
Dissection of Gastrointestinal
    Stromal Tumors
Gross Characteristics
General Microscopic Features
Diagnosis of Malignancy
Role of Frozen Section and
    Operating Room Consultation

STROMAL TUMORS PECULIAR
    TO SPECIFIC SITES IN THE
    GASTROINTESTINAL TRACT
Stromal Tumors of Esophagus
Leiomyoma
Leiomyosarcoma
Stromal Tumors of Stomach
Cellular Spindle Cell Tumor (Cellular
    Leiomyoma)

Epithelioid Leiomyoma and Epithelioid
    Leiomyosarcoma
Gastric Sarcomas of Miscellaneous
    Patterns
Stromal Tumors of Intestine
Leiomyoma and Leiomyosarcoma of
    Small Intestine
Leiomyoma and Leiomyosarcoma of
    Colon
Leiomyoma of Muscularis Mucosae
    (Leiomyomatous Polyp) of Rectum
    and Sigmoid Colon
Deep Intramural Leiomyoma and
    Leiomyosarcoma of Rectum
Tiny Stromal Tumor of Muscularis
    Propria/Myenteric Plexus

TUMORS AND TUMOR-LIKE
    PROLIFERATIONS OF ADIPOSE
    TISSUE
Lipoma and Liposarcoma

Lipomatous Hypertrophy of the
    Ileocecal Valve

TUMORS AND TUMOR-LIKE
    PROLIFERATIONS OF VESSELS
Glomus Tumors
Other Vascular Tumors

TUMORS AND TUMOR-LIKE
    PROLIFERATIONS OF FIBROUS
    TISSUE
Inflammatory Fibroid Polyps
Giant Fibrovascular Polyp of
    Esophagus

TUMORS AND TUMOR-LIKE
    PROLIFERATIONS OF
    NERVOUS TISSUE
Intramural Neurofibroma
Ganglioneuroma and
    Ganglioneuromatosis
Granular Cell Tumors

GENERAL FEATURES OF MESENCHYMAL TUMORS

The gastrointestinal tract is a long tube endowed with a variety of motile activities that are the responsibility of a huge mass of smooth muscle, mainly situated in a deep double layer, the muscularis propria. In addition, there are other smooth muscles, such as the thin double layer that separates the mucosa from the submucosa, the muscularis mucosae. From here, occasional muscle slips extend perpendicularly into the mucosa, especially in the small intestine. Furthermore, there are blood vessels in all layers, the larger of which have considerable smooth muscle in their walls.

Other than this impressive smooth muscle mass, there is relatively little stroma of other types. Nerves with their Schwann cell support traverse all layers and are concentrated mostly in two plexuses, one in the muscularis propria, and the other in the submucosa, except for the esophagus, which has only a muscular plexus. Scattered adipose cells are found in the submucosa, especially in the right colon. Fibroblasts are ubiquitous, because collagen is ubiquitous. Obviously, if there are blood vessels and lymphatic vessels, then there are endothelial cells to line them. Finally, the serosal surfaces throughout the gut are covered by mesothelium.

Cell Origin and Differentiation

Two classes of stromal tumors arise in the gastrointestinal tract. The first group, the smaller of the two, consists of some stromal tumors identical to those arising in other sites. These neoplasms clearly develop within or from either easily definable layers, such as muscularis and submucosa, or structures such as nerves. Some of these are typical leiomyomas, identical in every morphologic aspect to those arising elsewhere; they occur in the esophagus and less frequently in the rectum. Amazingly, only on rare occasions will typical totally differentiated leiomyomas or leimyosarcomas be discovered in the stomach, small bowel, or colon. Submucosal lipomas composed of mature adipocytes arise throughout the gut. Patients with von Recklinghausen's disease are likely to form neurofibromas in any location within the gut. By this time, probably at least one of every imaginable stromal tumor, benign and malignant, has been found somewhere in the gut and reported, one of the latest being a jejunal osteosarcoma.[1]

The second and larger group of gut stromal tumors arises in the stomach and intestines and consists predominantly of spindle cell tumors that do not really resemble typical tumors outside the bowel. These neoplasms do not obviously arise from definable normal structures. Certainly, with all the smooth muscle in the gastrointestinal tract, it would be foolish to avoid designating all of these spindle cell stromal tumors as either of smooth muscle origin, smooth muscle differentiation, or both, unless there were compelling reasons to do so. The early students of gut stromal tumors were no fools, because they usually referred to these tumors as leiomyomas or leiomyosarcomas.[2,3] These designations were based upon the light-microscopic suggestion of fibrillar cytoplasm in the cells of many of these gut stromal tumors and the pericellular reticulin fibers that seemed to indicate smooth muscle differentiation, as did the blunt-ended nuclei, which were considered at one time to be a hallmark of the smooth muscle cell.

The fact that some gastrointestinal stromal tumors contained rounded or polygonal cells, called epithelioid cells, as well as spindle cells, added confusion to the smooth muscle issue. Clearly, these round cells did not look like any normal stromal component. In some tumors, especially in the stomach, epithelioid cells dominated.

Then, as if to confuse us even more, every so often, some gastric neoplasm contained spindle cells arranged in the most spectacular palisades imaginable. Who could blame any sane pathologist for deciding such a tumor was a schwannoma or a neurilemmoma? Thus, there is a body of literature that refers to such a subset of spindled, palisaded gastric tumors as nerve sheath lesions of one type or another.

More accurate analysis of differentiation awaited the next two technical developments, namely, electron microscopy and immunohistochemical demonstration of cytoplasmic filaments or cellular proteins. These highly sophisticated techniques would seem to be ready-made to tell us exactly what kind of differentiated cells were making up these peculiar tumors. Much to the dismay of the students in this field, neither technique gave completely satisfactory performances. On electron-microscopic evaluation, it appeared that most of the cells of most of the stromal tumor cells had amazing deficient cytoplasmic sophistication.[4-11] There were mitochondria, occasional profiles of endoplasmic reticulum of both smooth and granular types, scattered ribosomes, an occasional filament or two, but nothing dramatic. A rare cell might have some features that suggested smooth muscle differentiation, such as a few pinocytotic vesicles or an increase in the number of cytoplasmic microfilaments, with occasional aggregation into dense bodies. A rare cell might even contain a subplasmalemmal linear density. However, none of these cells were even close to normal smooth muscle cells in terms of cytoplasmic differentiation.

In the cells of some tumors there were even suggestions of Schwann cell differentiation, including elongated processes, which seemed to be tightly applied to one another, and occasionally even bits of basement membrane.[5] Nevertheless, the overwhelming cellular constituent was neither differentiated Schwann cells nor differentiated smooth muscle cells. In fact, it was not even a well-differentiated fibroblast.

Recently immunohistochemical studies have yielded equally conflicting results, probably as a result of the use of different fixatives, different antibodies, different sets of technologists, and different interpretations.[12-16] Common to most studies is a fairly impressive demonstration of vimentin as an intermediate filament protein in most stromal tumor cells. The problem with vimentin is that it does not help to determine cell type; it seems to be a nonspecific marker of stromal cells in general. In some studies, there was a prominent staining for desmin in some of the tumors, suggesting muscle differentiation.[16] In other studies, there were variable reaction patterns with antibody to the S-100 protein, depending upon the site of origin of the tumor.[14,15] Thus, gastric tumors were likely to have scattered S-100–positive cells, perhaps trapped Schwann cells from the myenteric plexus. The stromal tumors of the small intestine were more likely to have large geographic patterns of S-100 staining mixed or alternating with similar patches of S-100 negativity. Of course, the cells that were staining positively and the cells that were staining negatively looked exactly alike by light microscopy and apparently by electron microscopy as well. To further complicate matters, in a recent study of two large solitary small-intestinal stromal tumors, both occurring in patients with von Recklinghausen's disease, ultrastructurally and immunohistochemically these tumors were exactly the same as the common variety of small-intestinal stromal tumors that occurred in patients without the syndrome, although in these two patients Schwann cell tumors were the type to be expected.[17]

These highly sophisticated approaches to the demonstration of differentiation of gastrointestinal stromal tumors indicate that these tumors are composed predominantly of undifferentiated cells and that the benign tumors and the malignant ones have exactly the same cellular constituents. Although the concept of a benign undifferentiated tumor is a chilling thought for traditionally oriented pathologists, nevertheless, it is a concept that must be accepted in gastrointestinal stromal tumor pathology.

Since these tumors are composed of such primitive cells, what should we call them? They have been designated mainly as smooth muscle tumors and occasionally as neural tumors, but is this really fair to the non-differentiated stromal cell? Since the *leiomyo-* prefix is the one most commonly and widely accepted by surgeons, radiologists, and gastroenterologists, as well as by pathologists, why introduce a new set of names? In this chapter, these tumors will be referred to as *leiomyoma* and *leiomyosarcoma*, but it is recognized that these names are only nicknames or pseudonyms as far as the gut is concerned.

Site Specificity

Certain tumors prefer to arise in certain sites.[4,18] Even the stromal neoplasms, both benign and malignant, composed mainly of the undifferentiated cells, are not the same in all areas of the gastrointestinal tract. Furthermore, a particular type of stromal tumor in one site may be predictably benign; whereas a similar, although not necessarily identical, tumor arising in a second site may be predictably malignant. This type of local variability has been well known and totally accepted for stromal tumors arising in extragastrointestinal sites. For instance, we appreciate the fact that certain bone tumors arise commonly in certain bones and rarely or never in other bones. We know that rhabdomyosarcomas of the head and neck are likely to be of the embryonal subtype, whereas those of the peripheral soft tissues more commonly have the alveolar pattern. Similarly, the esophageal mesenchyme seems capable of producing a cast of stromal tumors different from that produced by the mesenchyme in the immediately distal neighbor, the stomach.

The following is a summary of this site specificity for gut stromal tumors:

1. In the esophagus, generally small typical leiomyomas arise in the two muscle layers. Muscle sarcomas are rare. Granular cell tumors occur here more than anywhere else.
2. The stomach is the primary site for over half of all the gut stromal tumors. It houses the glomus tumor almost exclusively. Epithelioid cell stromal tumors and all their variants, both benign and malignant, are the most common tumors in the stomach. The next most common, the cellular spindle cell tumor with perinuclear vacuoles, almost never arises elsewhere. Furthermore, although all gastric stromal tumors are found mostly in the body of the stomach, some are likely to arise in the cardia and fundus, while others are rarely found there. Thus, there is site specificity even within this single viscus.
3. The small intestine, including the duodenum, contains about one third of the tumors; and it is the site of origin for a group of spindle cell tumors with organoid vascular patterns and large lumps of collagen. Such tumors are not found elsewhere, except, on rare occasions, in the proximal colon. Small-bowel sarcomas tend to be highly cellular and composed of uniform small spindle cells.
4. The colon, excluding the rectosigmoid, is an unusual site for stromal tumors, so unusual, in fact, that there are very few published data. This may be the only gut site for truly pleomorphic sarcomas.
5. The rectum and, to a lesser extent, the sigmoid colon contain two quite characteristic neoplasms. One is a small nodular expansion of the muscularis mucosae, the leiomyomatous polyp. The second is the deep intramural cellular spindle cell tumor, which superficially resembles the benign spindle cell lesion in the stomach but is highly likely to be a sarcoma.

Clinical Features

These tumors usually are discovered in patients of both sexes during the fourth through the seventh decades with slight variation in peak incidence from one site to another. Signs and symptoms depend upon size, site of origin, location within the wall, and whether the tumor is benign or malignant. Thus, a relatively small intramural tumor, perhaps 1.5 to 2 cm across, arising in a part of the gut with a narrow lumen, such as the pylorus or the small bowel, may cause obstruction with pain and vomiting. A large tumor attached to the greater curvature of the body of the stomach not involving the mucosa may cause no symptoms or may be detected as an abdominal mass during a physical examination or by the patient. A tumor of any size anywhere that presses on the mucosa as it pushes or protrudes into the lumen is likely to become secondarily ulcerated and bleed or cause pain, or both. Such lumps may even form the leading end of an intussusception. Weight loss is frequently associated with sarcomas. Small sarcomas of the small intestine may present with their metastases, such as with hepatomegaly. In general, tumors in the small bowel, with its smaller diameter, are likely to cause symptoms when they are smaller than those in the stomach, which has a much larger diameter.

Dissection of Gastrointestinal Stromal Tumors

The proper gross handling of these neoplasms is predicated upon determining whether they are benign

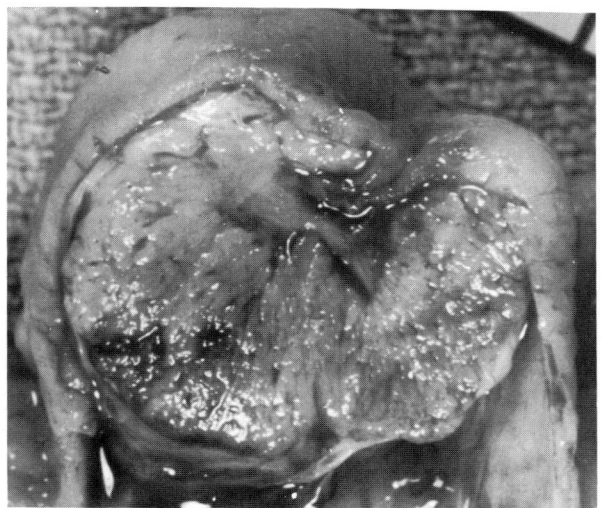

FIGURE 15–1. This gastric leiomyoma is intramural, and the overlying mucosa (top) is compressed and ulcerated. (Courtesy of Dr. Aina Silenieks, Lincoln, Neb.)

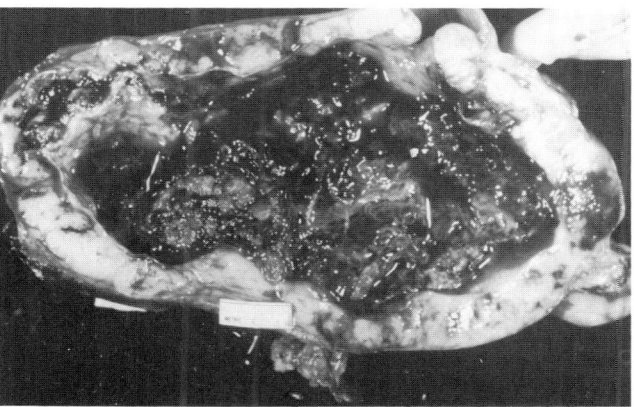

FIGURE 15–3. A huge small intestinal sarcoma forms a circumscribed mass mainly outside the wall of the bowel. There is a small ulcer (top right center) that communicates with a giant central hemorrhagic and necrotic cavity.

or malignant. First, size is critical because of its association with the ability to metastasize. Second, adequate sampling of large tumors is important in picking up small malignant areas in otherwise histologically benign neoplasms. Such sampling includes mucosa over the tumor or at the edge of any ulcer for the purpose of looking for mucosal infiltration, a good marker of malignancy. Then, it is important to concentrate on the solid, nonnecrotic and nonhemorrhagic foci. In large tumors, most samples should be taken from the deeper aspects, because those are the areas where sarcomatous components are most likely to be found. There are no rules for the number of sections to be examined per centimeter of tumor diameter. Possibly a reasonable rule would be to examine one section per centimeter of diameter up to 10 cm. It seems unlikely that ten sections will not pick up any significant sarcomatous component.

Gross Characteristics

Gut stromal tumors usually produce single masses situated anywhere within the wall of the viscus. Most will expand the wall and push toward the lumen, elevating the mucosa, which, in turn, may become secondarily ulcerated (Figures 15–1 and 15–2). Some tumors expand outwardly into the subserosa (Figure 15–3). In fact, on occasion, especially with large gastric tumors, the mass may be almost totally outside the wall, with only a tiny attachment to the muscularis propria. Some tumors have both intramural and extramural components constricted at the muscularis propria, producing the classic "dumbbell" shape (Figure 15–4).

Most tumors are circumscribed; even the malignant tumors are likely to have easily identifiable perimeters (Figures 15–5 and 15–6). Only rarely will a tumor, usually a sarcoma, appear to invade the wall or adjacent structures (Figure 15–7). Most tumors are solitary

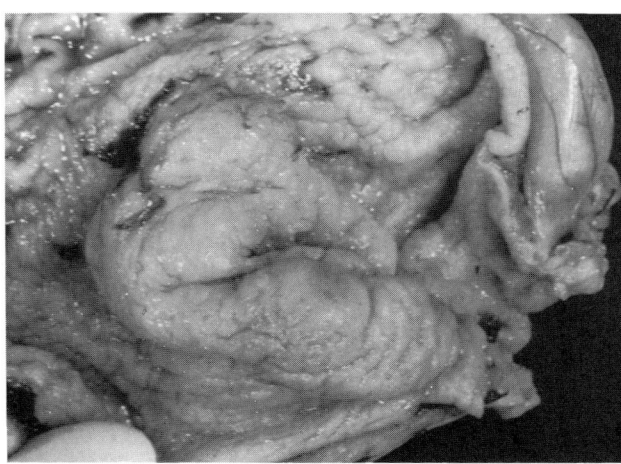

FIGURE 15–2. This lobulated gastric sarcoma has elevated the mucosa and has produced several huge knobby folds.

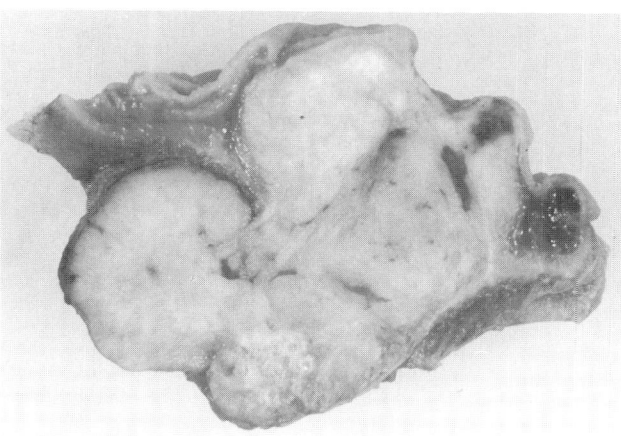

FIGURE 15–4. This is a duodenal leiomyoma 3 cm in diameter that has submucosal and subserosal components, separated by a constriction at the muscularis propria.

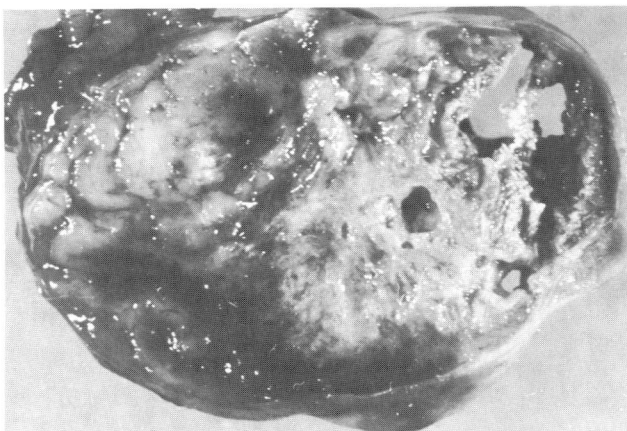

FIGURE 15-5. A gastric leiomyoma forms a circumscribed intramural nodule that has several dark areas of hemorrhage and a central cyst, the result of liquefactive necrosis. (Courtesy of Dr. James K. Billman, Jr., Moline, Ill.)

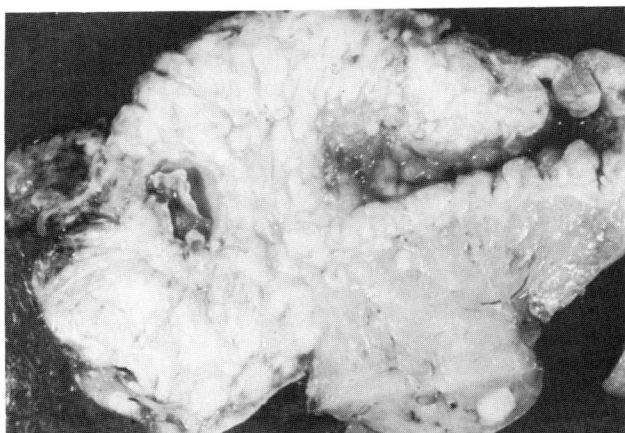

FIGURE 15-7. The unusual infiltrative pattern of a gut sarcoma that forms a large mass on the left and nodules that thicken the wall toward the center. (Courtesy of Dr. Aina Silenieks, Lincoln, Neb.)

round or oval, occasionally lobulated, masses (Figures 15-8 and 15-9).

The one tumor without the appearance of a solitary mass is the multinodular or multifocal epithelioid cell tumor of the stomach (Figure 15-10) associated with pulmonary chondromas and extra-adrenal pheochromocytomas usually occurring in young women—a triad described by Carney.[19,20]

On cross section, the esophageal leiomyomas are identical to uterine leiomyomas; however, stromal tumors in other gastrointestinal sites are quite different. For instance, they do not bulge when cut across, and they do not appear whorled. Instead, the cut surface lies flat and appears granular and pockmarked by vessels and patches of collagenization, lysis, and hemorrhage (see Figures 15-1 and 15-4; Figure 15-11). At times, these degenerative changes dominate the cross-sectional appearance, with the formation of cysts and broad zones of hemorrhagic necrosis (Figure 15-12), which may communicate with the overlying ulcers (see Figure 15-3). There is a tendency for the sarcomas to be more hemorrhagic and necrotic than their benign counterparts; however, this may be more a manifestation of size than of malignancy, since the bigger benign tumors are also extensively degenerated. In general, the benign tumors and the sarcomas are so similar in appearance that they cannot be distinguished. Large size may be the only hint that a tumor is malignant.

General Microscopic Features

Whereas the gross characteristics of the solitary gut stromal tumors of stomach and intestines tend to be much the same no matter the type and the site, the microscopic features are quite site specific. Therefore, these specific microscopic patterns are described separately and related to the individual locations in which

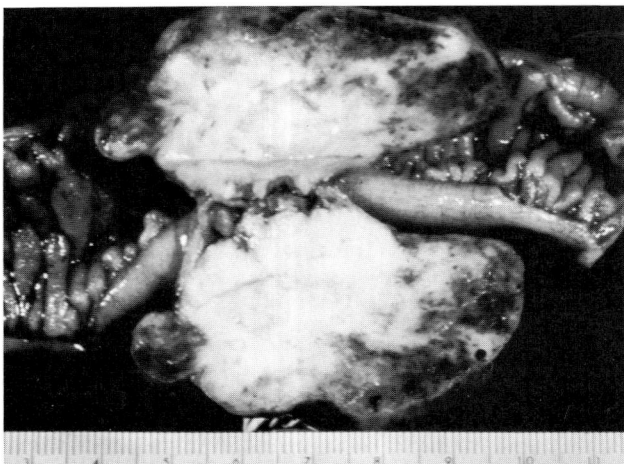

FIGURE 15-6. A small bowel stromal tumor 6.5 cm in diameter is slightly lobulated and well circumscribed and forms a mass that protrudes outward into the peritoneal cavity. The tumor has been cut across, and both halves can be seen.

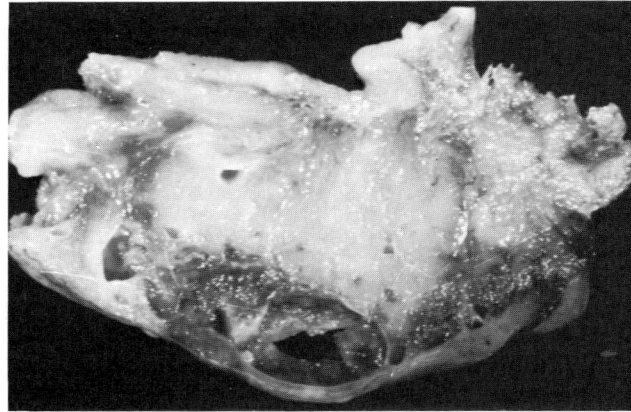

FIGURE 15-8. A slightly lobulated discrete 3-cm intramural jejunal leiomyoma fills the submucosa. Note the liquefactive cysts at the bottom in the center.

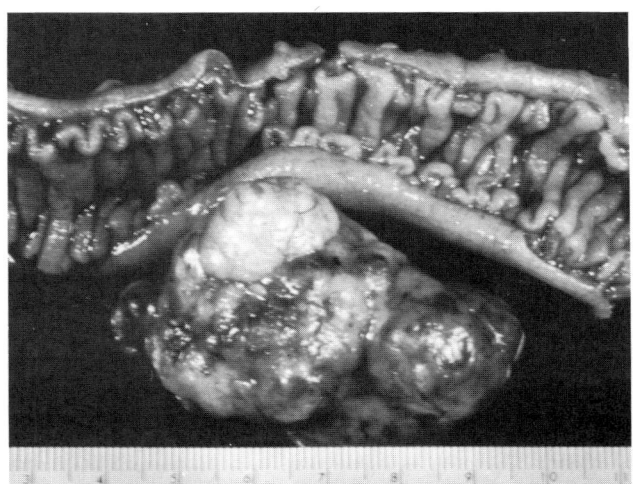

FIGURE 15-9. A lobulated outwardly protruding small-intestinal borderline stromal tumor.

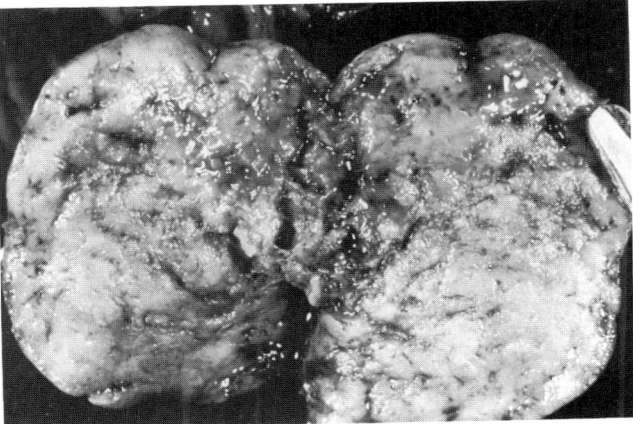

FIGURE 15-11. The cut surface of a typical gastric or intestinal stromal tumor is pale and pockmarked by vessels and degenerative changes. There is no whorling or gristle-like appearance so typical of uterine leiomyomas.

they occur. However, there are some common histologic characteristics that are outlined first.

Tumors in all sites are likely to be situated within either the submucosa or the muscularis propria, or most likely both (Figure 15-13). The muscle of the muscularis tends to be hypertrophic and often hyalinized at the edges of a tumor, and muscle bundles may penetrate the tumor, forming muscular septa that subdivide the mass into smaller units or lobules (Figures 15-14 and 15-15). This lobulation is more accentuated in gastric than in intestinal tumors (Figure 15-16). On the other hand, in an occasional small-bowel leiomyoma, the muscularis propria will pass across the tumor like a sling, with the fibers separated by fascicles of neoplastic spindle cells (Figure 15-17). Sometimes the hypertrophied muscle completely or partly surrounds the tumor like a capsule, even blending with fibers of the muscularis mucosae. There is never a transition between normal smooth muscle cells and tumor cells, although quite often there is an interdigitation of tumor cells and muscle cells creating the appearance of tumor infiltrating muscularis.

Diagnosis of Malignancy

Based upon analysis of tumors with proven metastases, the following generalizations may be made: (1) Malignant gut stromal tumors tend to be larger, more densely cellular, and more mitotically active than their benign counterparts in all locations.[4,21,22] (2) What is larger, more cellular, and more mitotically active differs from one site to another. (3) The risk of metastasis increases with increasing size and increasing mitotic rate at all locations.[23] (4) Using anaplasia as a criterion of malignancy is pointless, because these tumors are composed predominantly of undifferentiated cells, whether they are benign or malignant. Highly pleo-

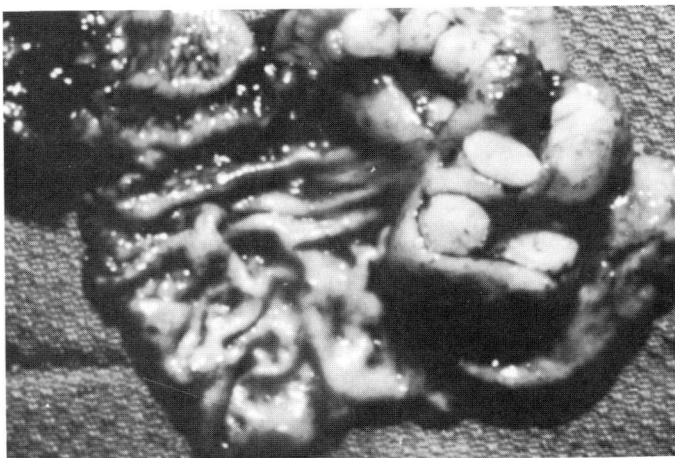

FIGURE 15-10. A multinodular epithelioid gastric tumor characteristic of Carney's triad. (Courtesy of Dr. Donald Antonioli, Boston, Mass.)

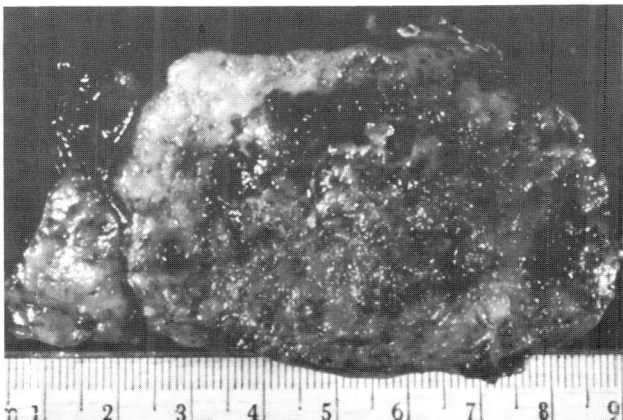

FIGURE 15-12. The cut surface of this leiomyoma of the stomach is dominated by irregular zones of hemorrhage and necrosis.

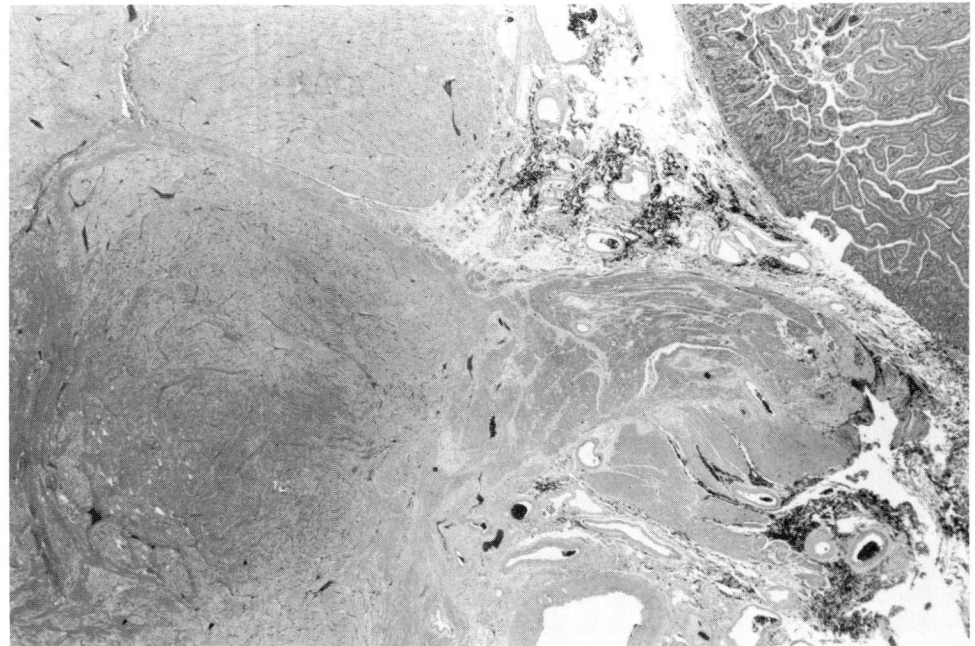

FIGURE 15–13. At the edge of this small intestinal leiomyoma, which fills the left side of the field, the muscularis propria becomes thick with the dark muscle bundles separated by pale collagen (right center). (×13)

morphic sarcomas are uncommon.[21,22] (5) Gross invasion of adjacent organs is clear evidence of malignancy. (6) Somewhat similar tumors occurring in different sites do different things. For example, a highly cellular tumor of the gastric wall composed of uniform tightly packed spindle cells arranged in fascicles, palisades, and whorls is predictably benign. A comparable tumor deep in the rectal wall usually recurs multiple times and eventually metastasizes. Another example is an epithelioid cell tumor of the stomach composed of fairly large cells with plentiful cytoplasm, which is predictably benign; whereas a comparable tumor of the small bowel with nearly identical cells has a much higher mitotic rate and will probably metastasize. A tumor 6 cm in diameter in the stomach rarely metastasizes, no matter what its microscopic appearance. This reflects the fact that almost all 6-cm gastric stromal tumors are histologically benign.

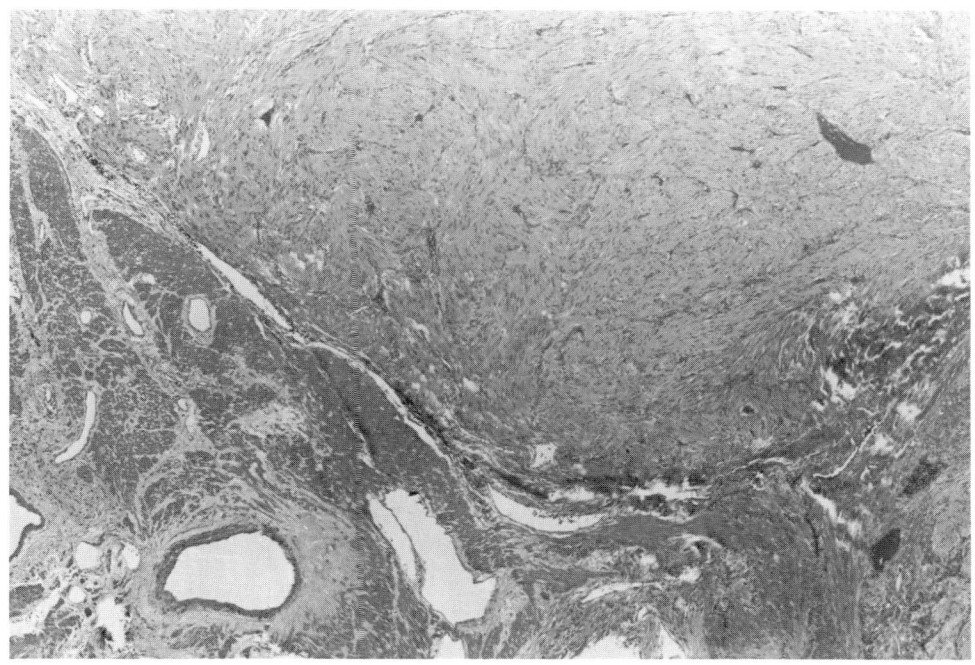

FIGURE 15–14. At the edge of this small bowel leiomyoma, which fills the upper part of this field, the muscularis propria becomes thick and partly encapsulates the tumor. (×33)

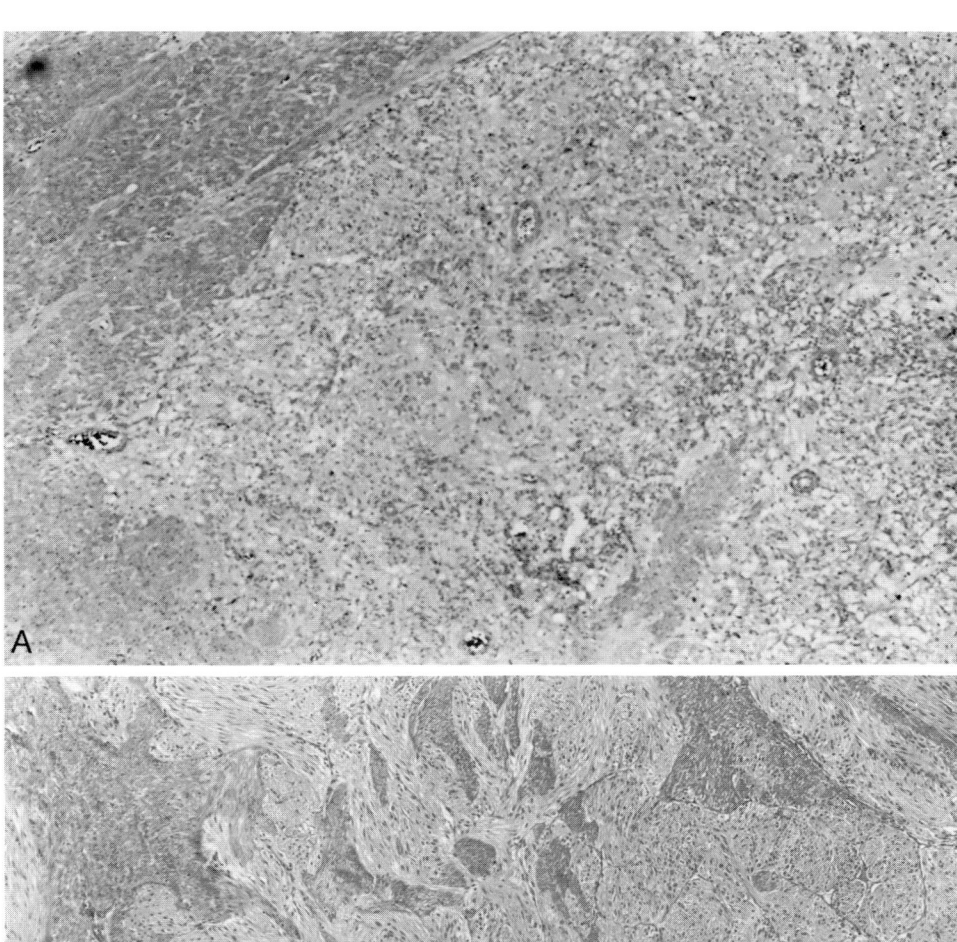

FIGURE 15–15. *A*, At the edge of this gastric leiomyoma, the muscularis propria (left side of field) forms a partial muscular capsule from which a muscular trabeculum penetrates the tumor as a septum (lower right center). (×53) *B*, Muscular trabeculae extend from the muscular capsule into the center of this small bowel leiomyoma. The normal smooth muscle (dark) and the tumor cells (light) stain completely differently. (×53)

A 6-cm tumor in the small intestine can be predicted to metastasize 50% of the time on the basis of size alone, a reflection of the fact that half or more small-bowel stromal tumors of that size are sarcomas when studied by light microscopy. (7) Microscopic invasion of the mucosa with separation of epithelial elements by stromal cells indicates malignancy (Figure 15–18). However, the likelihood of finding this is small because of the broad ulcers that obliterate mucosal involvement. (8) Tumor necrosis may be a useful marker of malignancy, but too many benign tumors have necrotic foci.

Therefore, there are no specific criteria for malignancy which are applicable across the board to all tumors arising in all sites.[4,21] In general, there are a few rules that may be useful. These are based upon analysis of multiple features within an individual tumor, including site, size, cellularity, mitotic rate, and invasive characteristics. In the stomach, an epithelioid cell tumor with small, solidly packed cells and easily found mitoses that is over 6 cm in diameter is a potentially metastasizing tumor. The same tumor, but smaller than 6 cm across, has a minimal metastatic risk. Also in the stomach, a densely packed spindle cell tumor with uniform cells, especially with perinuclear vacuoles, will probably not metastasize no matter what the size. A spindle cell tumor without the vacuoles and with a

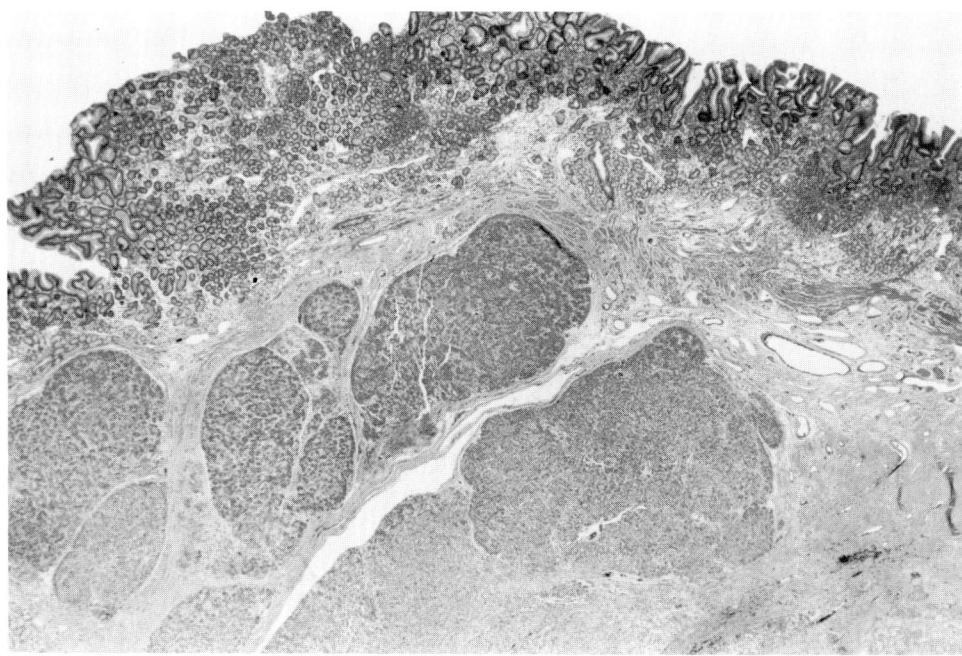

FIGURE 15–16. Discrete tumor lobules in the submucosal aspect of this gastric leiomyoma are separated by bands of collagen. (×53)

high mitotic rate measuring over 6 cm across has a definite metastatic risk that increases with increasing size. In the small intestine or colon, any cellular spindle cell tumor over 2 cm across which has mitoses carries a metastatic risk. Any relatively pure epithelioid tumor in the small intestine is probably malignant. A deeply situated, highly cellular spindle cell tumor of the rectum is likely to be malignant and should be treated aggressively from the beginning.

Mitotic rates in many metastasizing gastrointestinal sarcomas are much lower than would be required for the diagnosis of a sarcoma in another primary site, such as the uterus. Leiomyosarcomas of the uterus generally have at least five to ten mitoses per ten high-power fields. Such numbers would be extremely high for the gut, where any tumor with no more than one mitosis per ten high-power fields is likely to be malignant. Thus, it must be remembered that the criteria for malignancy in gut stromal tumors are not necessarily the same as those for stromal tumors in other sites.[21]

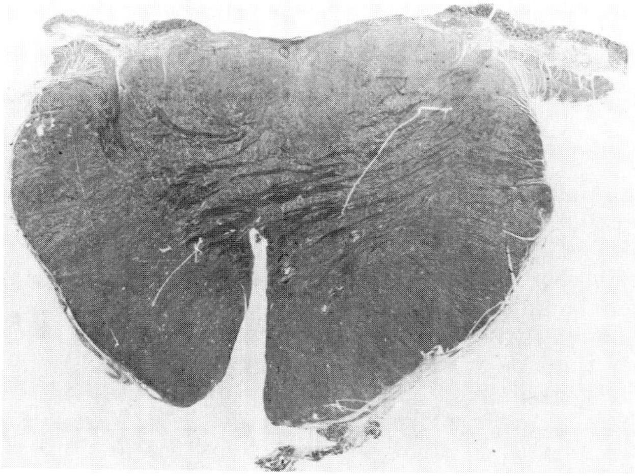

Histologic grading systems for gastrointestinal sarcomas have been developed at different institutions, based upon tumor cellularity, mitoses, nuclear cytoplasmic ratio, and pleomorphism.[22,24,25] These seem to have some validity in their correlation with frequency of metastases or rapidity of metastases and death from tumor, at least in the institutions in which they are used.

Quite often, in tumors that have histologically malignant areas, there will also be areas that are equally obviously benign. Usually these benign foci are situated in the submucosa, whereas the malignant foci are deeper. This occurrence is frequent enough to suggest that sarcomas evolve from pre-existing benign stromal tumors, essentially a stromal dysplasia-sarcoma sequence. We do not know what determines metastasizing ability in such cases, whether it is the size of the tumor as a whole or simply the size of the sarcomatous component.

Finally, the need to use multiple factors to determine malignancy has led to the recognition of a group of tumors that have conflicting or overlapping features and are thus not easily definable as either benign or malignant. Such tumors may be referred to as possessing "borderline" features or features of "undetermined malignant potential." An example is a tumor that has unfamiliar features, with which no one has had experience. A benign tumor with a small malignant component also falls within this category, as do a tumor

FIGURE 15–17. In this small intestinal leiomyoma, the fibers of the muscularis propria (dark staining) traverse the tumor like a sling. (×8)

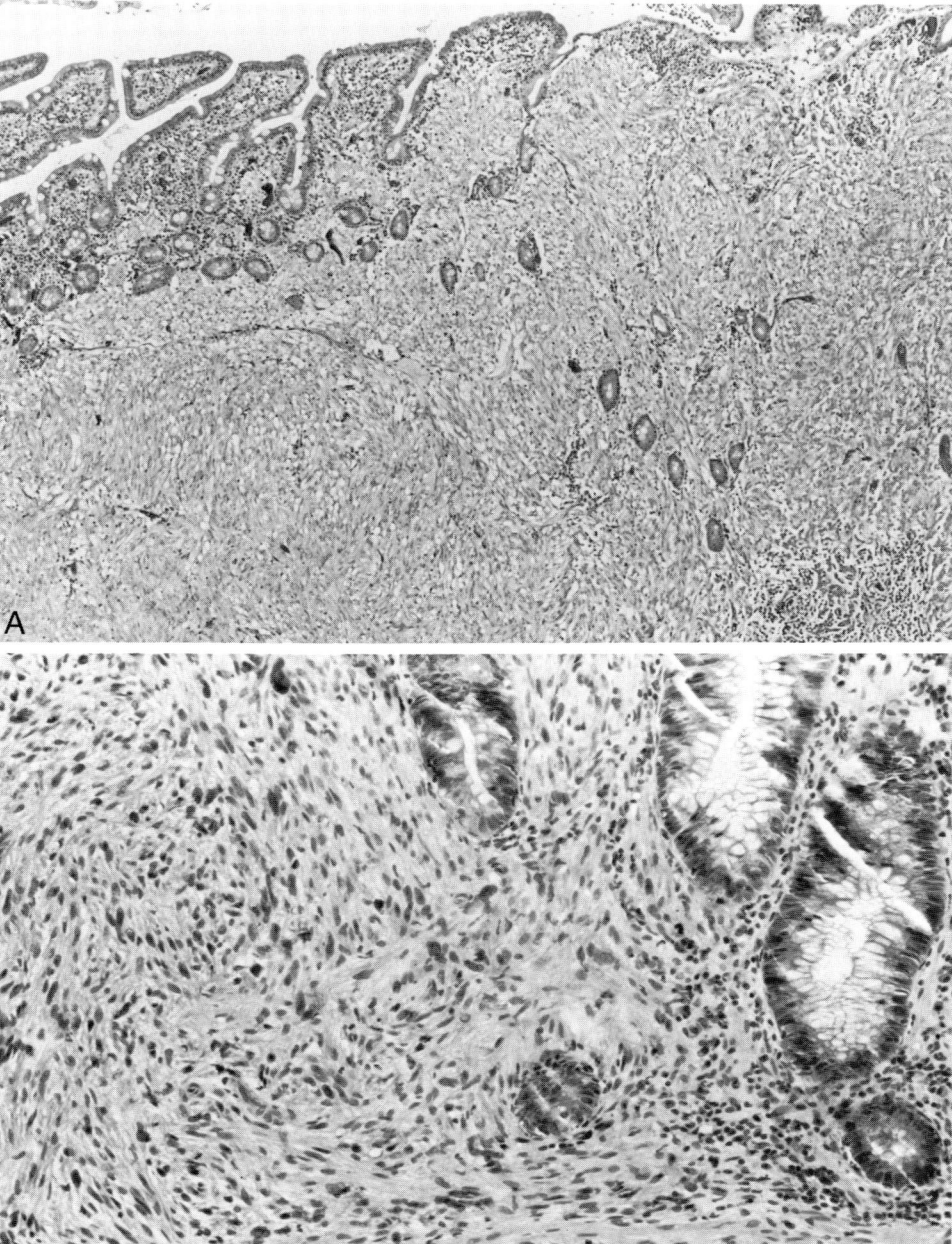

FIGURE 15–18. Mucosal invasion with separation of the epithelial elements by tumor cells is an excellent criterion for malignancy. A, Small-bowel sarcoma. (×53) B, Rectal sarcoma. (×132)

with benign cellularity but a high mitotic rate and a tumor with a degree of cellularity that is not easily definable as either benign or malignant. Presumably, tumors belonging to this borderline or undetermined group will gradually become categorized more specifically as experience with them accumulates.

The patterns of metastases for almost all of the sarcomas throughout the gastrointestinal tract are pretty much the same. There are two primary sites of metastasis, the liver and the peritoneal surfaces. Sometimes the metastases are larger than the primary tumor, especially for small-intestinal sarcomas, some of which are quite small. Peritoneal studding is extremely common; and in advanced cases, the entire peritoneal surface can be covered by large tumor nodules. As a result of this peritoneal distortion, it is unusual to find metastases that are obviously within lymph nodes. Lymph node metastases do occur but can be demonstrated in only about 10% of the sarcomas that metastasize. Another intra-abdominal site of metastasis is the retroperitoneal soft tissues, again possibly but not always clearly within lymph nodes. Rarely do gastrointestinal sarcomas leave the abdomen. When they do, they are likely to involve the lung in perhaps 10% of the cases, the subcutaneous tissues in another 10%, and elsewhere throughout the rest of the body in gradually diminishing degrees of frequency.

Role of Frozen Section and Operating Room Consultation

When a surgeon encounters a mass in the gastrointestinal tract, that surgeon is likely to want to know what it is, usually because subsequent surgical treatment will be dictated by the diagnosis. At the moment, the available data suggest that the proper treatment for a gastrointestinal tract stromal tumor is gross total removal, whether the tumor is benign or malignant.[23,24,26] It is not known how wide a margin of resection is necessary, but it does not appear that major resections such as total gastrectomies offer a greater chance of cure than does local resection. Therefore, is there a place for frozen-section diagnosis of gastrointestinal stromal tumors, and can a frozen section give enough information for determining whether a tumor is benign or malignant? The answer to these questions is not well established, but certain use can be made of frozen sections or of operating room consultation. When a tumor is submitted from the operating room for analysis, the pathologist should first measure it, because the size alone of a gastrointestinal stromal tumor can be a reasonably good predictor of its behavior. A frozen section can then be performed for two reasons, probably neither of which is critical for immediate management. The first reason is verification that the tumor is of stromal type. However, the gross characteristics of gut stromal tumors are so different from those of any other neoplasm that this may be unnecessary in terms of information. The one exception is the tiny nodule of the muscularis propria/myenteric plexus, which can look, to the surgeon, like a metastasis from a carcinoma. The second reason for frozen section is to see whether the tumor is obviously malignant; that is, whether it is highly cellular and mitoses are easily identified on the frozen section. This may help the surgeon when he or she discusses the situation with the patient and the family shortly after the operation, but is not likely to dictate definitive treatment. The information given to the surgeon, therefore, is that the tumor is stromal; whether it is obviously malignant or the pathologist cannot tell if it is malignant; and finally, the size of the tumor as a potential prognosticator. It must be remembered that it is impossible to determine whether many gastrointestinal stromal tumors are benign or malignant on the basis of frozen section alone. Too many sarcomas have very low mitotic rates, and many benign tumors are characteristically highly cellular, depending upon the site of origin.

Finally, a word of caution is in order. Occasionally the cells of an epithelioid leiomyoma of the stomach form clusters or cords, which, on frozen section, look very much like a diffuse spreading carcinoma. The gross features clarify the issue, because the carcinoma produces a diffuse mural thickening, whereas the leiomyoma forms a discrete mass. However, the sample submitted for frozen section may not be the whole tumor, but only a biopsy of it, and a potential error becomes more likely. The surgeon should be asked to describe the gross characteristics in such cases.

It is obvious from the foregoing discussion that the diagnosis of a gut stromal tumor and the malignant aspects of that tumor are really permanent-section issues.

STROMAL TUMORS PECULIAR TO SPECIFIC SITES IN THE GASTROINTESTINAL TRACT

Stromal Tumors of Esophagus

Leiomyoma

The esophagus is the only site within the gut where, with few exceptions, the common stromal tumors are typical, classic, ordinary leiomyomas.[18] Most of these arise within the muscularis propria, although occasional leiomyomas develop within the muscularis mucosae. An exhaustive survey of the world's literature on smooth muscle tumors of the esophagus through 1971 was compiled by Seremetis et al., and the data they accumulated are still valid.[27] In their study, over half of the leiomyomas arose in the lower third, about 30% arose in the middle third, and the rest arose in the upper. However, this distribution probably reflects the location of the large, often symptomatic tumors; and it corresponds to the relative amounts of smooth muscle within the muscularis propria, which consists totally of smooth muscle in the lower third, mixed smooth and skeletal muscle in the middle, and mainly skeletal muscle proximally. Actually, most esophageal leiomyomas are tiny, subclinical lesions that lie within one of the muscle layers, and almost two thirds of these arise in the region of the esophagogastric junction. Such tiny tumors have been designated as "seedling leiomyomas."[28] They occur in close to 10% of adult esophagi, and they may be multiple (Figure 15–19). The large leiomyomas are likely to produce symptoms of dysphagia or pain, depending upon their size and whether they obstruct the lumen. Most reported cases are between 2 and 5 cm in diameter, but occasional giant tumors occur, some weighing over 1000 gm. Some become calcified. Grossly, on cut section, esophageal leiomyomas are pale or white, firm, rubbery, whorled, and well circumscribed.

Histologically, the esophageal leiomyoma contains normal-appearing or hypertrophic smooth muscle cells arranged in fascicles or whorls. The tiny seedling lesions look like localized expansions of the muscularis. In fact, at times it is impossible to tell a tiny seedling leiomyoma from a bundle of hypertrophic smooth muscle, especially in the middle third of the esophagus, where skeletal and smooth muscle fibers are mixed in the muscularis propria.

Circumferential leiomyomas have been reported. These are probably examples of an entity known as "diffuse leiomyomatosis of the esophagus," a rare dis-

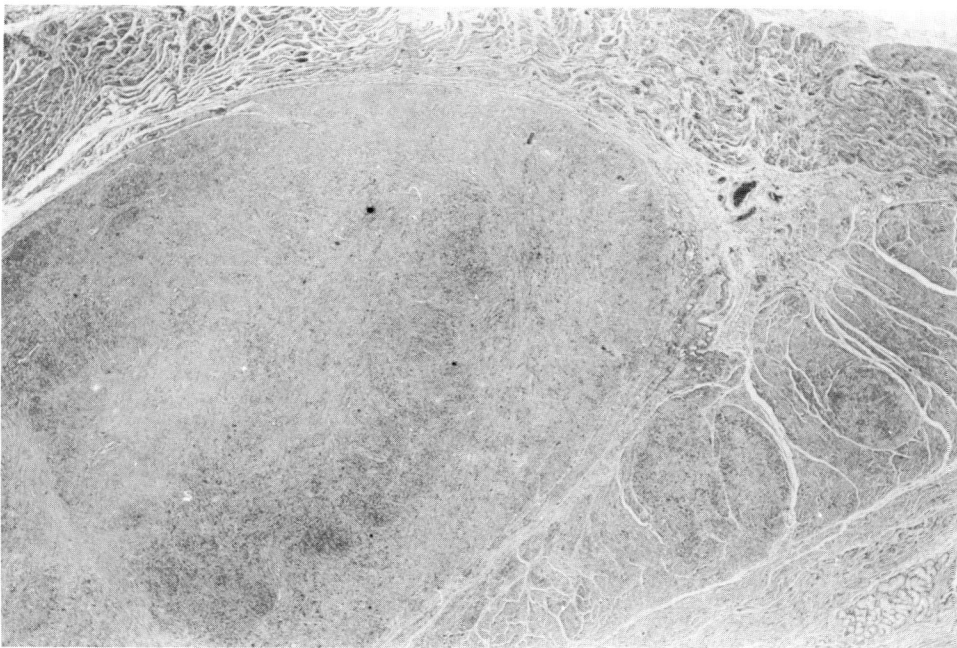

FIGURE 15–19. Three seedling leiomyomas of the esophageal muscularis propria, a large one on the left and two smaller ones on the right.

order, mainly of young women who have long-standing dysphagia.[29,32] The lower esophagus and usually proximal stomach have an eccentric nodular thickened muscularis propria, which looks like a confluence of leiomyomas. Occasionally such cases have been associated with vulvar leiomyomas as well.

Leiomyosarcoma

In the massive literature series of Seremetis et al., only 40 published cases of leiomyosarcoma were uncovered, compared with 838 cases of leiomyoma.[27] Not many have been reported more recently.[33–35] Furthermore, clear-cut ultrastructural and immunohistochemical demonstration of smooth muscle differentiation in these reported sarcomas is lacking. Finally, these cases resemble the pseudosarcomatous carcinomas in terms of clinical presentation, patient sex and age, location in the esophagus, gross characteristics, and prognosis (see Chapter 19). For instance, cases of so-called esophageal leiomyosarcoma with adjacent or overlying squamous cell carcinoma have been reported.[34] Quite likely, many or even most cases are really pseudosarcomatous squamous cell carcinomas. Therefore, although there is no reason to expect that leiomyosarcomas of the esophagus do not occur, they are probably even rarer than the number of published cases would indicate. Presumably, a leiomyosarcoma of the esophagus will be a malignant spindle cell neoplasm with mitoses and variable pleomorphism that has definite ultrastructural and/or immunohistochemical smooth muscle characteristics, that invades and/or metastasizes, and that has no marginal or overlying squamous cell carcinoma. It appears from the literature that these requirements are met by very few tumors.

A few cases of rhabdomyosarcoma of the esophagus have been reported, perhaps as many as five.[36]

Stromal Tumors of Stomach

Cellular Spindle Cell Tumor (Cellular Leiomyoma)

This tumor is composed of uniform spindle cells arranged in whorls, cartwheels, or fascicles, often with prominent nuclear palisades[37] (Figures 15–20 and 15–21). Broad areas of liquefaction and hyalinization are likely to be present, so that very cellular areas alternate with sparsely cellular foci. In most tumors, many of the cells have a vacuole that compresses or indents the nucleus at one pole (Figure 15–22). These vacuoles may be artifactual, because they do not stand out ultrastructurally. Peculiarly, these perinuclear vacuoles do not occur in sarcomas, and so they seem to be a very specific benign marker. Mitotic figures are found scattered about but usually are no more frequent than one per ten high-power fields. The only tumor of this histologic appearance that has been reported as metastasizing measured 17 cm across and had five mitoses per 50 high-power fields.

Epithelioid Leiomyoma and Epithelioid Leiomyosarcoma

In the early 1960s, Martin et al., in France, and Stout, in the United States, identified a group of gastric stromal tumors that were composed mainly of rounded or polygonal cells, many of which had clear cytoplasm.[38,39] Stout even coined a new name for this type of tumor, the *leiomyoblastoma*, a noncommittal term that had neither benign or malignant connotations, because Stout was not certain how these tumors behaved.[39] It now appears that in the stomach, epithelioid cell tumors are the most common stromal tumors. The clear cytoplasm is actually an artifact of fixation.[6]

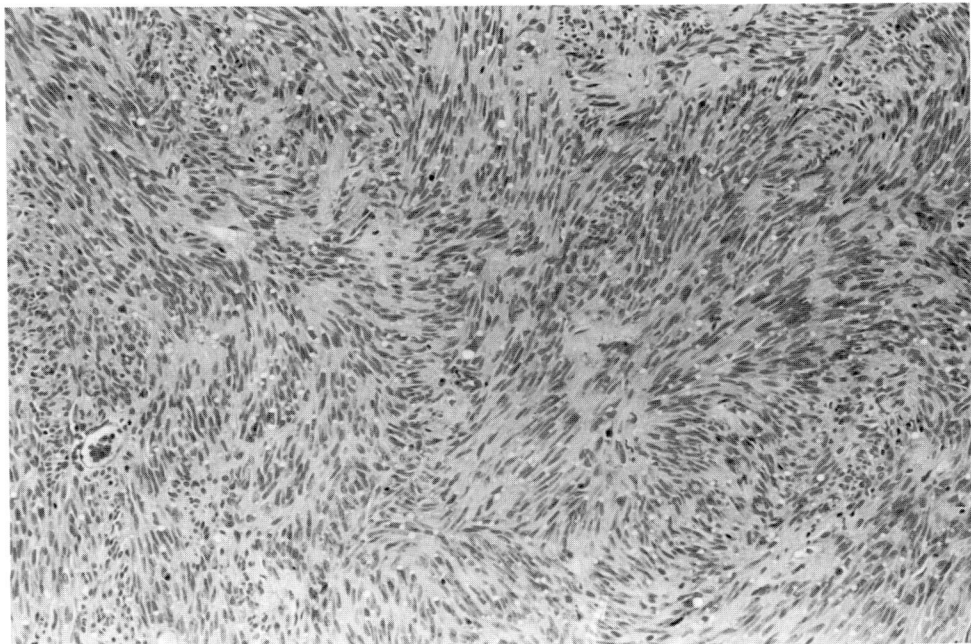

FIGURE 15-20. A cellular leiomyoma of the stomach. Spindle cells are in fascicles and in palisades. (×132)

The cells do contain a cytoplasmic rim condensed about the nucleus after formalin fixation, but on frozen section the cells have eosinophilic cytoplasm and are not clear (Figure 15-23). Very few tumors are composed totally of epithelioid cells.[26] Most have a mixture of epithelioid and plump spindle cells (Figure 15-24). Multinucleated cells and cells with giant nuclei are frequent and are found in the benign tumors, rather than in the malignant ones (Figure 15-25). These tumors are often multinodular, and commonly there are different types of cells and different patterns of growth in different nodules (Figure 15-26).

The epithelioid cells are arranged in sheets, but occasionally prominent perivascular orientation is found, suggesting a recapitulation of vascular smooth muscle[26] (Figure 15-27). As a result, areas within these tumors may resemble glomus tumors or hemangiopericytomas. Liquefaction and hyalinization are common features (Figure 15-28).

The malignant variants, or epithelioid leiomyosarcomas, contain smaller cells with less cytoplasm than do the benign lesions (Figure 15-29). The sarcoma cells are also more uniform, so that multinucleated and pleomorphic cells are unusual. Furthermore, in the sar-

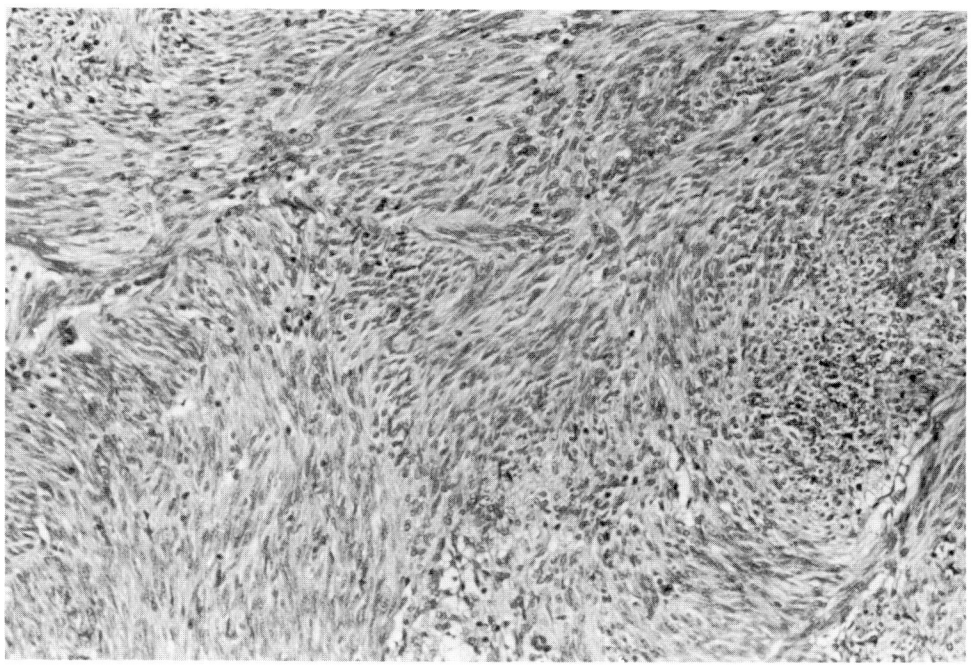

FIGURE 15-21. Cellular leiomyoma of the stomach. The spindle-cell fascicles have a storiform pattern. (×132)

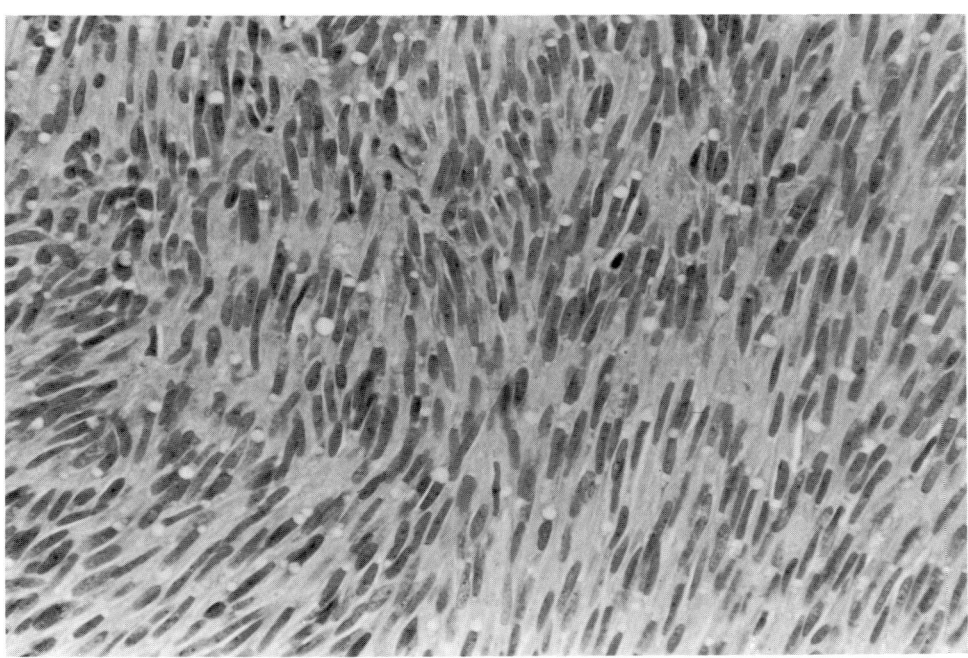

FIGURE 15–22. Cellular leiomyoma of the stomach. Many spindle cells have round, clear vacuoles indenting the nucleus at one pole. (×330)

comas, the epithelioid cells frequently form small clusters or groupings resembling alveoli, often embedded in an acid mucopolysaccharide-rich stroma. Sometimes foci of small, tightly packed palisaded spindle cells in a comparable stroma will also be found. Frequently, both benign- and malignant-appearing areas are present in the same tumor.

Both epithelioid leiomyomas and leiomyosarcomas most commonly arise in the body of the stomach. However, peculiarly, almost half of the sarcomas arise in the cardia and fundus and rarely in the antrum, whereas almost half of the leiomyomas arise in the antrum but rarely occur in the proximal stomach. A subset of the epithelioid sarcomas constitutes one of the components of a peculiar multiorgan abnormality occurring mainly in young women described originally by Carney.[19,20] In this syndrome, the gastric epithelioid sarcoma tends to occur as multiple discrete tumor lumps that have a microscopic organoid appearance and a low metastatic rate. The other components of the syndrome are pulmonary chondromas and extra-adrenal functioning paragangliomas.

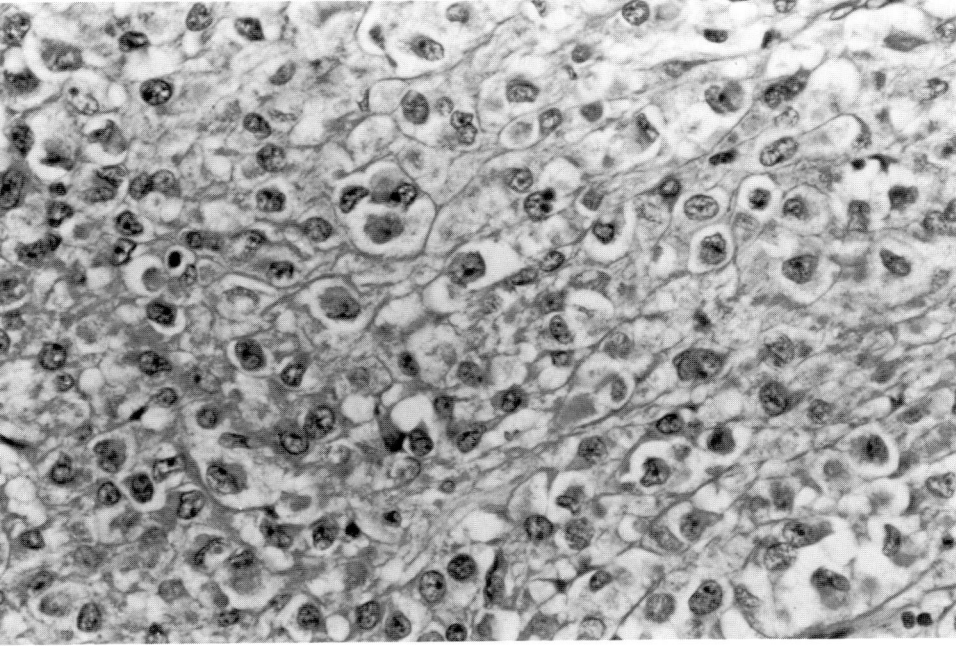

FIGURE 15–23. Epithelioid leiomyoma. Many of the rounded cells have clear peripheral cytoplasm and condensed darker cytoplasm adherent to the nuclei. (×330)

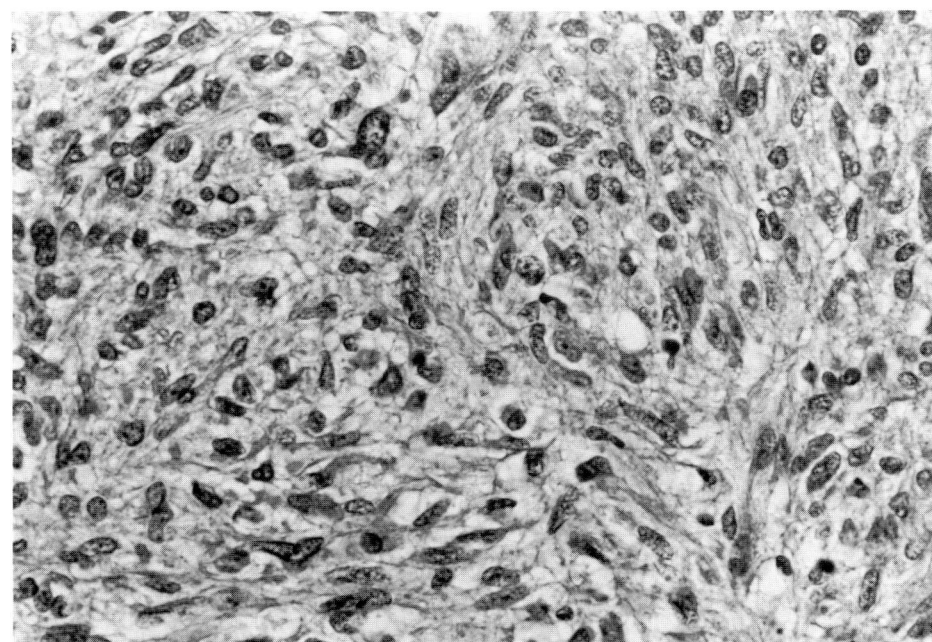

FIGURE 15–24. Epithelioid gastric leiomyoma. In this field there is a mixture of epithelioid cells and plump spindle cells. (×330)

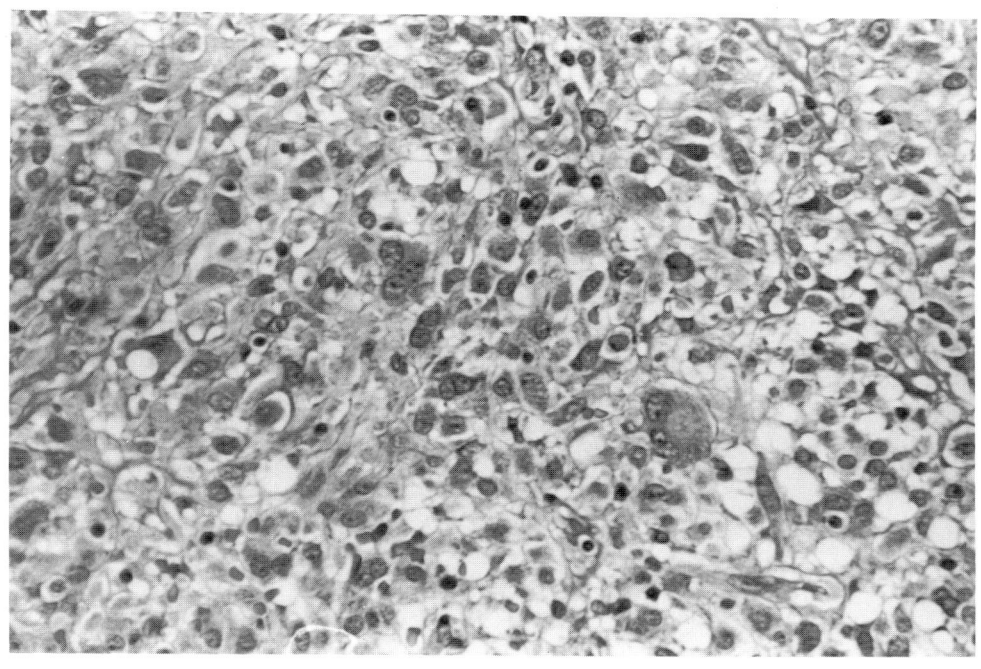

FIGURE 15–25. Cellular pleomorphism with variable nuclear sizes and multinucleated giant cells are common in the benign, but not the malignant, epithelioid gastric tumors. (×330)

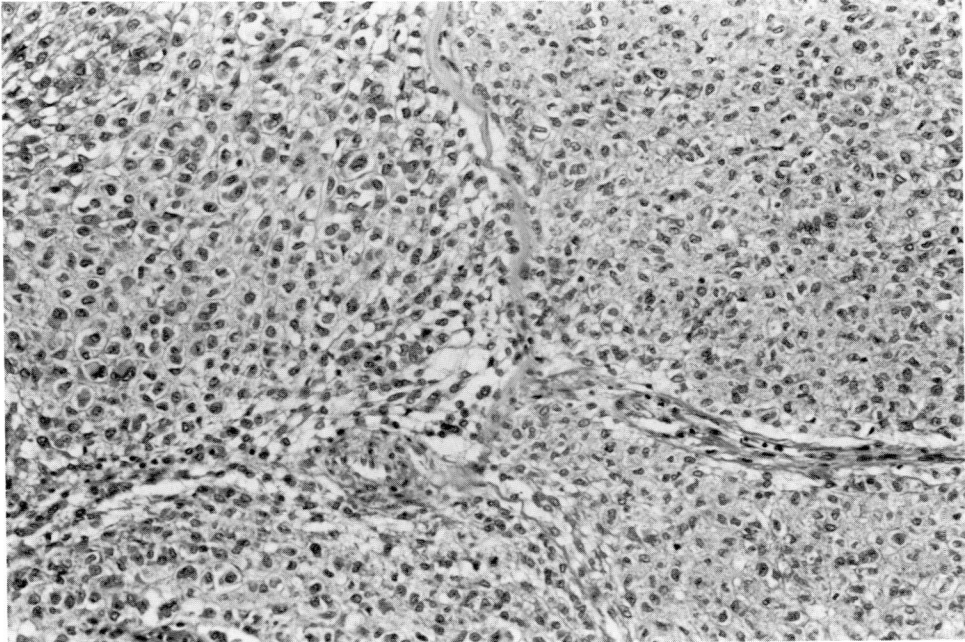

FIGURE 15-26. An example of variation in growth pattern and cellular composition in adjacent nodules of an epithelioid gastric leiomyoma. The nodule at the left has only epithelioid cells, whereas the nodule on the right has a mixture of epithelioid and plump spindle cells. (×132)

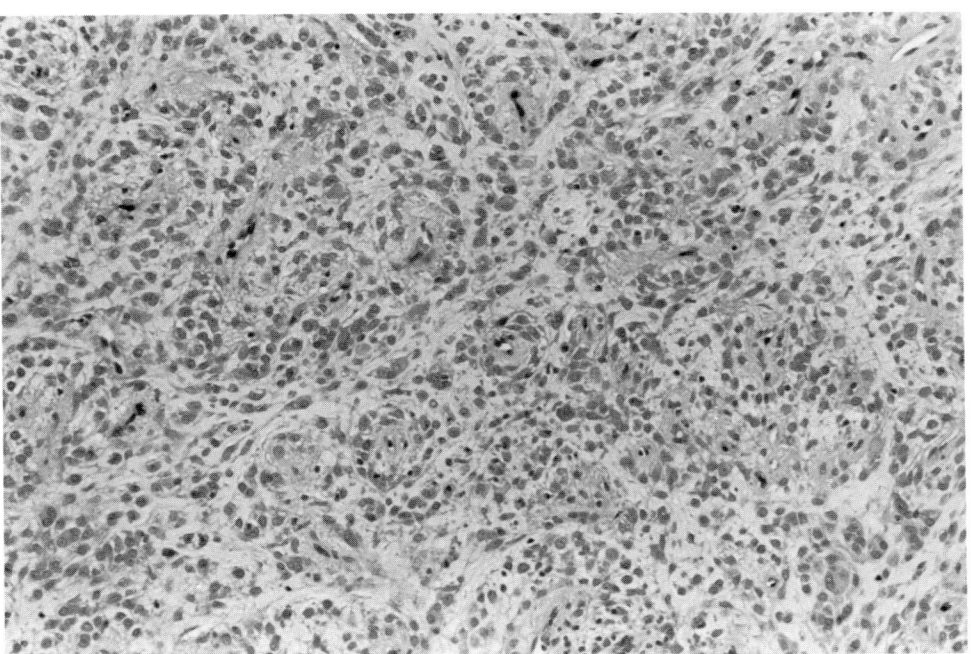

FIGURE 15-27. The perivascular or perithelial pattern of growth in a gastric epithelioid leiomyoma. (×132)

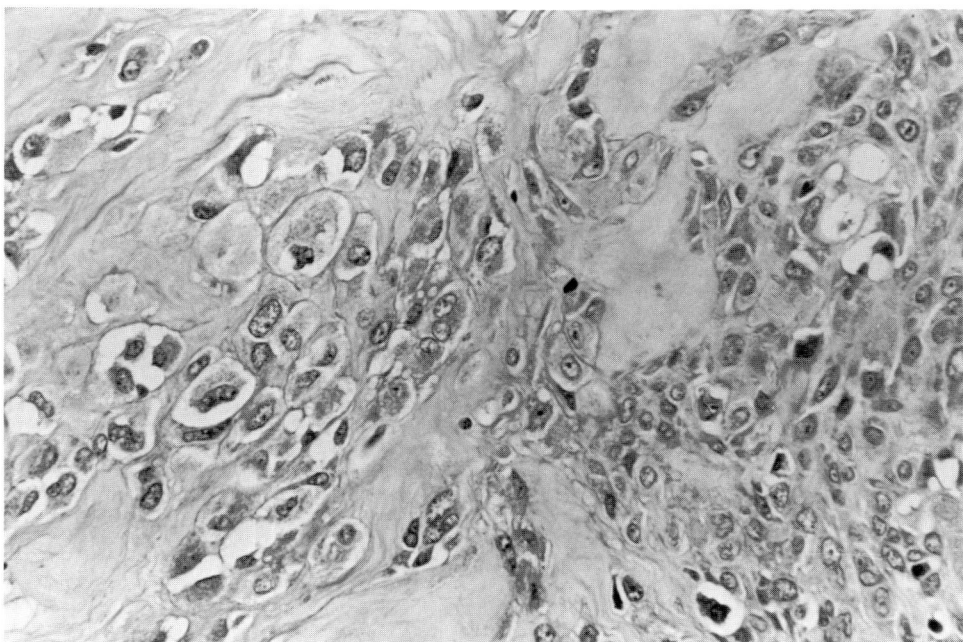

FIGURE 15-28. Broad zones of hyalinization separate cell strands, clusters, and sheets in a gastric epithelioid leiomyoma. (×330)

The epithelioid cell composition of a benign gastric tumor really does not impart to that tumor any unusual qualities that make it different from other benign gastric stromal tumors. It looks the same grossly. However, as will be mentioned below, the epithelioid sarcomas are somewhat different from other gastric sarcomas from a prognostic standpoint.

Gastric Sarcomas of Miscellaneous Patterns

Although the most common gastric sarcomas are the epithelioid cell variants, there is a group of sarcomas of large size and various microscopic patterns, usually composed of spindle cells, sometimes with considerable pleomorphism and invariably with a high mitotic rate[25,40] (Figure 15-30). These tumors are so diverse that it has not been possible to subdivide them on the basis of specific histologic patterns and accumulate enough tumors of any one pattern for statistically significant data. As a result, they are grouped together in a miscellaneous category. What they share is the fact that they are highly aggressive tumors that metastasize rapidly and widely throughout the abdomen. Patients with this group have a median survival of only about 9 to 10 months after diagnosis, whereas patients with sarcomas of epithelioid cell type have a median survival of slightly over 5 years.

There have been a number of attempts at grading sarcomas of the stomach on the basis of cellularity, mitoses, and pleomorphism. These grading systems may vary from one study to another. It appears that some cellular leiomyomas and some benign epithelioid leiomyomas are likely to have been included among the sarcomas in some studies.

Stromal Tumors of Intestine

Leiomyoma and Leiomyosarcoma of Small Intestine

In the small bowel, including the duodenum, the stromal tumors are quite different from those that occur in the stomach. Almost all are composed of spindle cells; predominantly epithelioid cell tumors are rare (Figure 15-31). In the leiomyomas, the spindle cells tend to be organized into short fascicles, and quite often the fascicles are separated into small nodules by fine fibrovascular septa, which creates a distinctly organoid appearance[4,18] (Figure 15-32). This is more likely to be present in the submucosal aspect of a tumor than deeper; but some tumors, especially small ones, may be completely organoid. Small-bowel leiomyomas frequently contain dense hyaline balls or blobs that lie among the cells in no particular orientation, but they tend to be more obvious and more numerous deeper in the tumor and are less likely to be found closer to the mucosa (Figure 15-33). Ultrastructurally, these blobs are clumps of normal collagen fibers.[17] Whether they are produced by tumor cells or by other cells is not known.

The spindle cells of the leiomyomas are long and have plentiful cytoplasm, which may appear longitudinally fibrillar (Figure 15-31). Sarcomas have smaller, shorter, plumper, spindle cells with much less cytoplasm, which resemble the cells of the mesenchymal condensations about the central epithelial core in the embryonic gut (Figure 15-34). In the benign tumors, mitoses are so infrequent that a search of 100 high-power fields may not yield a single one. In the sarcomas, mitoses also may be rare; yet a tumor with no

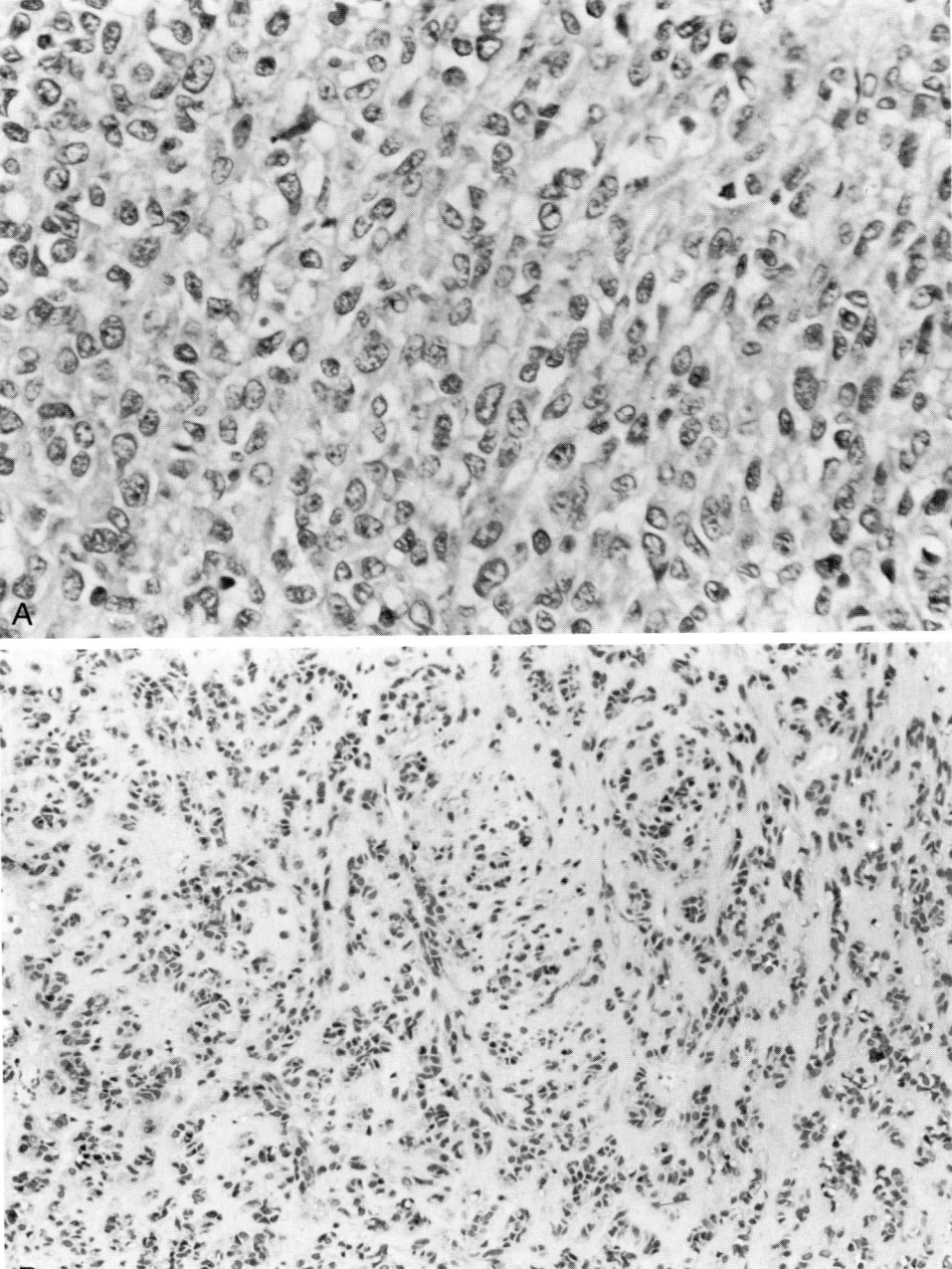

FIGURE 15-29. *A*, The gastric epithelioid leiomyosarcoma contains cells that are smaller, have less cytoplasm, and are thus more tightly packed than does the comparable leiomyoma. Compare with Figure 15-23. (×330) *B*, In this field from an epithelioid leiomyosarcoma, the cells are clustered in a pale stroma full of acid mucopolysaccharide. (×132)

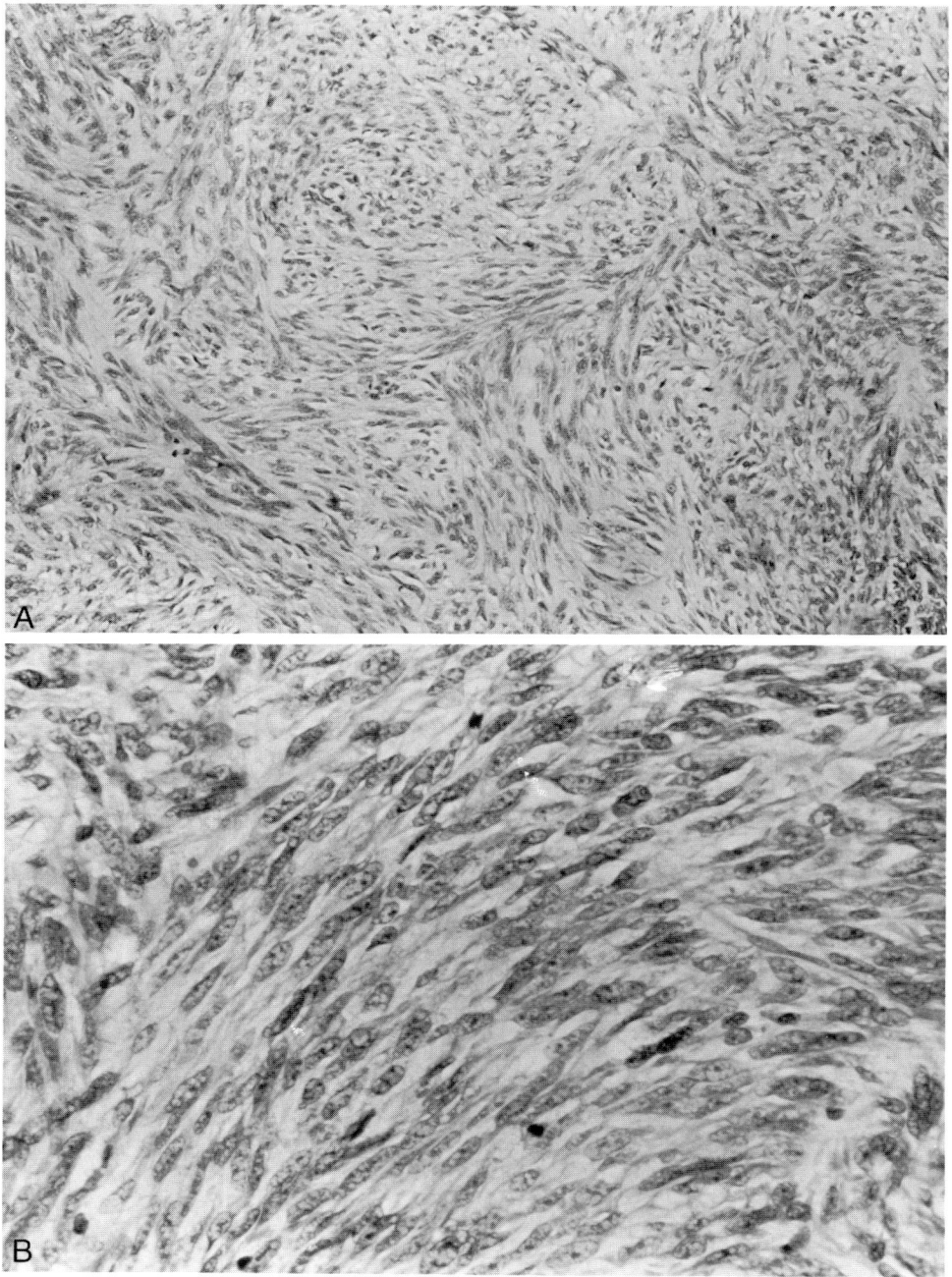

FIGURE 15–30. Gastric sarcoma of miscellaneous pattern, in this case spindle-cell, with storiform arrangement. *A*, Low-power magnification. (×132) *B*, High-power magnification of the large spindle cells. There are two mitoses in this field (top and bottom center). (×332)

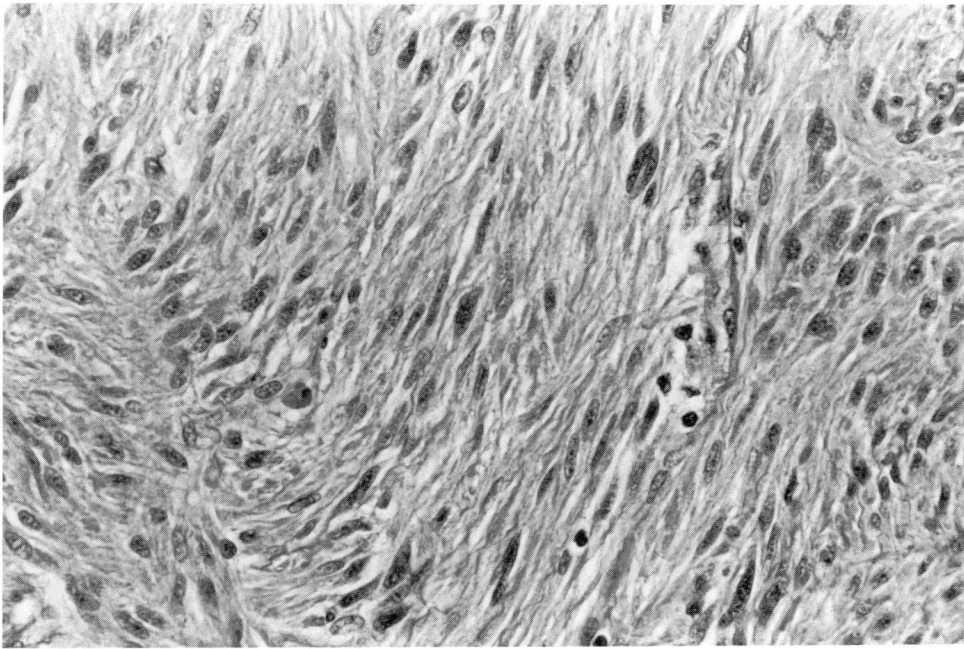

FIGURE 15–31. The typical leiomyoma of small intestine has spindle cells with plentiful fibrillar cytoplasm. (×330)

more than one mitosis per 20 high-power fields is capable of metastasis if the cellularity and cell type are characteristic for sarcoma.[21,22] Pleomorphism in small-intestinal sarcomas is not common.[21] Small-intestinal, dumbbell-shaped tumors may have benign areas located submucosally, whereas the component outside the intestinal wall may have a completely sarcomatous appearance. Purely epithelioid tumors in the small intestine are quite likely to be malignant regardless of their cellularity.

Stromal tumors occur throughout the small bowel, perhaps somewhat more frequently in the ileum than in the jejunum. A disproportionately large number occur in the duodenum, considering its short length. There are a number of cases reported as arising in a Meckel's diverticulum. Some of these may be sarcomas of the ileum with central cavitation. Others actually may be tumors of the diverticulum itself.

Leiomyoma and Leiomyosarcoma of Colon

The colon, exclusive of the rectum, is quite an unusual site for stromal tumors. For instance, in the largest series of sarcomas of the intestines reported to date covering the period from 1911 to 1974, there were 106 small-bowel tumors and 26 rectal tumors, but only 15 tumors that arose in the abdominal colon.[22] There are so few published data on colonic stromal tumors that we really have very little concept of how they behave and what they look like.[41] Most seem to arise in the ascending and transverse colon. Most reported tumors are considered by the author to be malignant, rather than benign; but this does not really tell us the relative frequencies of leiomyomas and sarcomas in the colon.

In general, the colonic sarcomas appear to be highly aggressive tumors that either metastasize soon after diagnosis or are discovered after they have metastasized.

Grossly, some colonic sarcomas grow as multiple confluent nodules in a longitudinal fashion, a pattern virtually never encountered elsewhere in the gut (Figure 15–35). However, most seem to produce the solid or lobulated localized mass appearance characteristic of gastrointestinal sarcomas in other sites. Leiomyomas are generally smaller than sarcomas and are circumscribed single nodules, comparable to those in the stomach and small intestine.

Compared with rectal sarcomas, which tend to be fairly uniform in cell composition, colonic sarcomas are likely to be pleomorphic, with cells and nuclei of variable size and shape, bizarre mitotic figures, and a more haphazard, rather than fascicular, growth pattern (Figure 15–36). The leiomyomas are less cellular and contain uniform long spindle cells with much cytoplasm.

Appendiceal leiomyomas and leiomyosarcomas are very rare (see Chapter 33).

Leiomyoma of Muscularis Mucosae (Leiomyomatous Polyp) of Rectum and Sigmoid Colon

The muscularis mucosae of the gastrointestinal tract is a continuous smooth muscle with inner circular and outer longitudinal layers comparable to those in the much thicker muscularis propria. This muscle has considerable bulk; yet it is surprising that only one tumor arises predictably from this layer with any frequency; and that tumor is confined to the rectum and sigmoid colon, where it produces a rounded elevation or bump, seen by the endoscopist as a small sessile polyp.[42] These leiomyomatous polyps are generally too small to produce symptoms, since their median size is only about 5 to 6 mm. Every so often, one of them will grow to a centimeter or even a centimeter and a half in diameter. The age and sex distribution is really meaning-

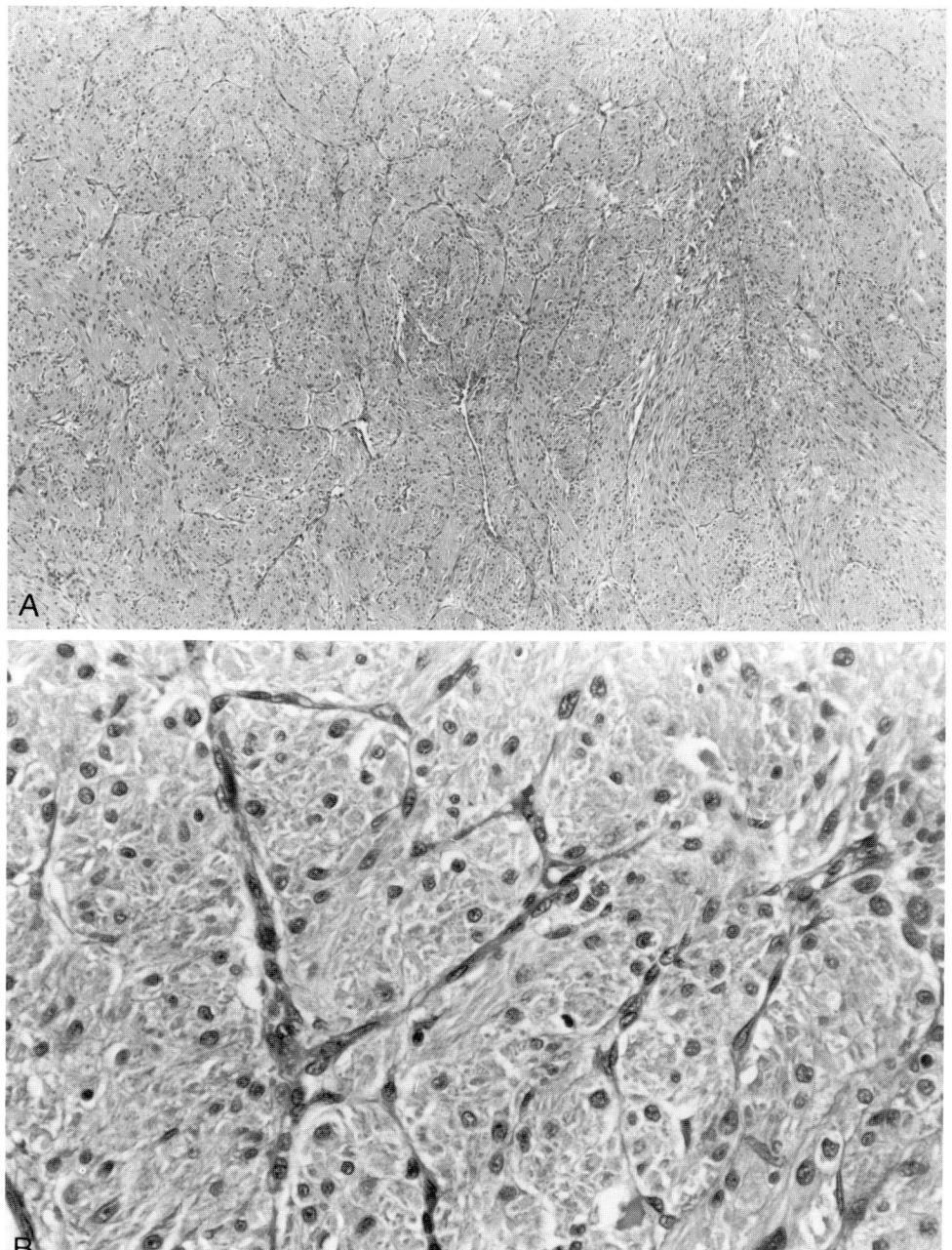

FIGURE 15-32. Many small-intestinal leiomyomas have this organoid pattern with small fascicles of cells surrounded by thin vascular septa. *A,* Low-power magnification. (×53) *B,* High-power magnification. (×330)

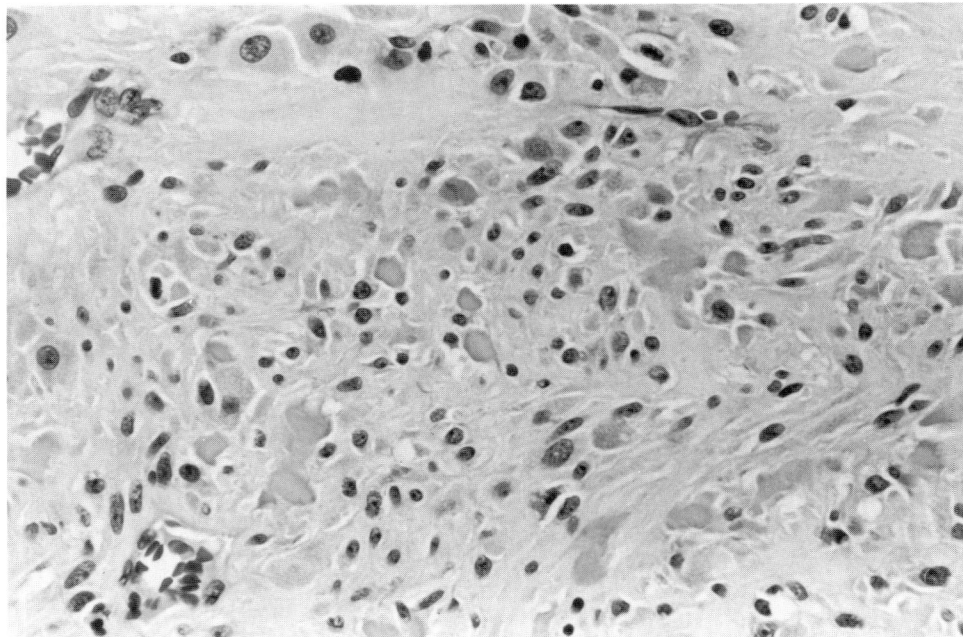

FIGURE 15–33. Collagen balls are frequently interspersed randomly among the cells in small-bowel leiomyomas. (×330)

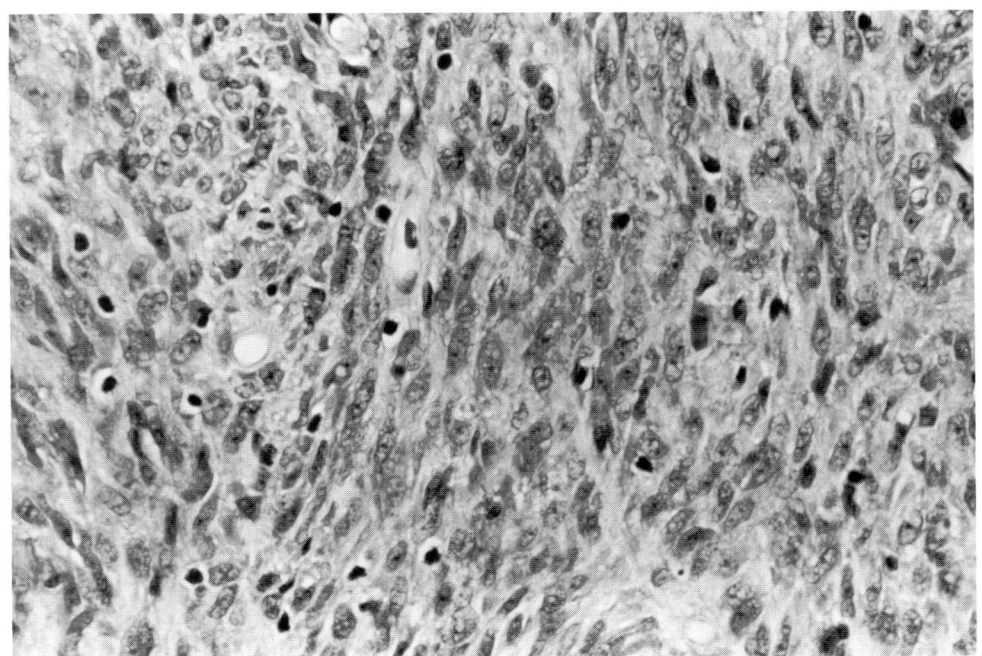

FIGURE 15–34. The small-intestinal leiomyosarcomas are composed of small, uniform, more crowded cells than are the leiomyomas. Compare with Figure 15–31. (×330)

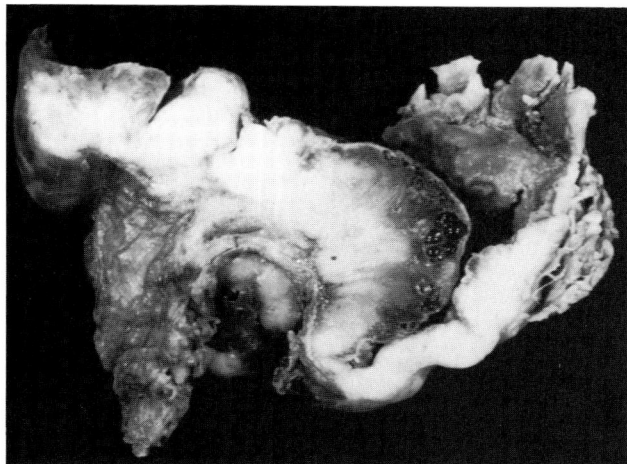

FIGURE 15–35. This colonic sarcoma forms both a dominant mass and extensive diffuse mural thickening, a picture rarely seen outside the colon.

FIGURE 15–36. Comparison of a colonic leiomyoma (*A*) with uniform spindle cells and a leiomyosarcoma (*B*) with pleomorphism, a mitosis, and a mixture of spindle and epithelioid cells. (×330)

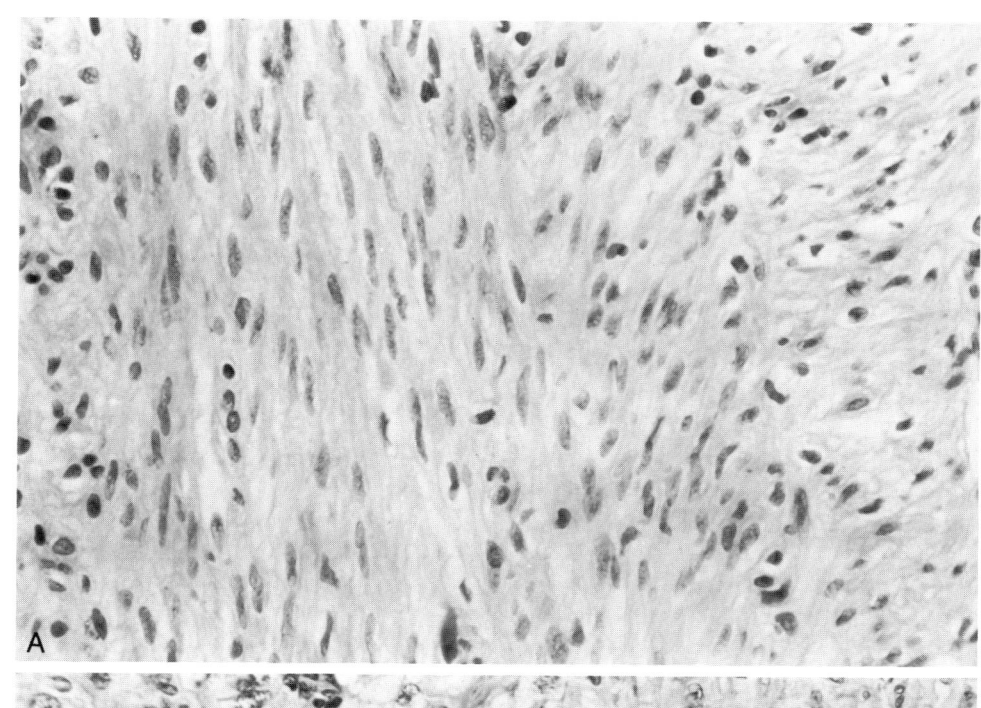

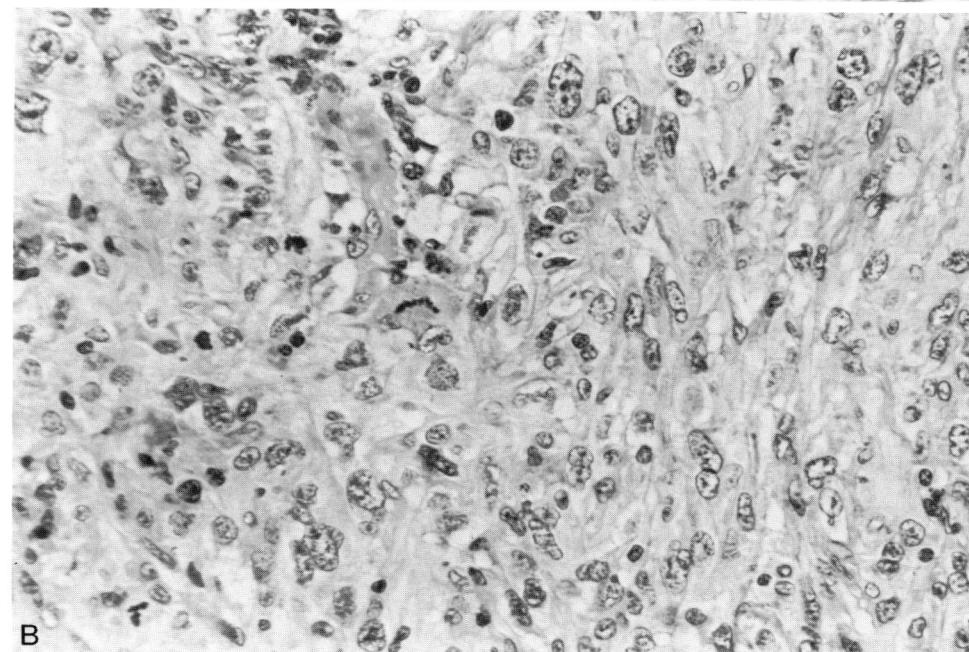

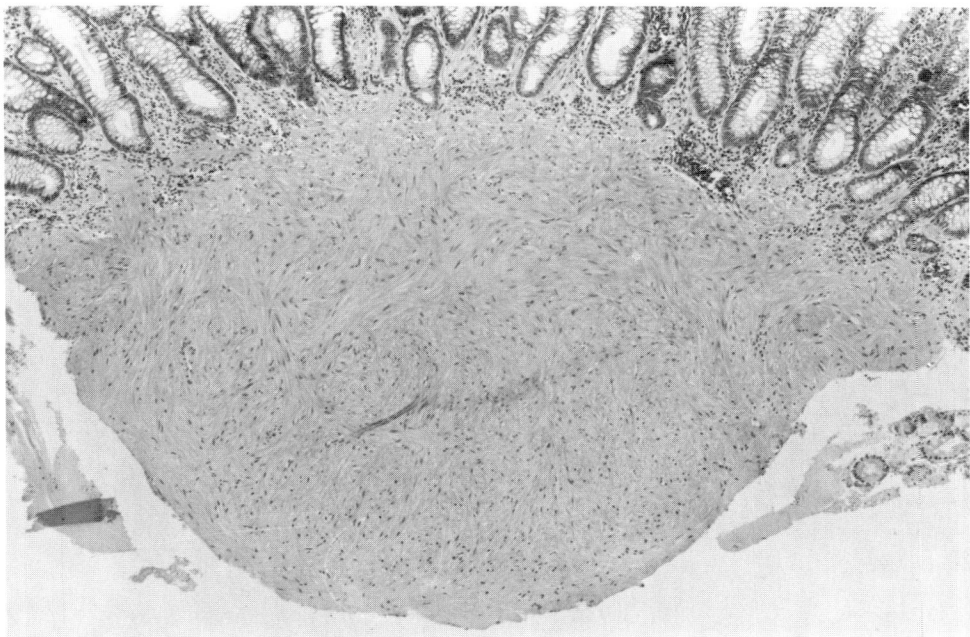

FIGURE 15-37. The leiomyoma of the rectosigmoid muscularis mucosae typically forms a ball of muscle beneath the mucosa. (×53)

less, since it is much the same as the age and sex distribution for patients who have routine lower endoscopic examinations, simply because these lumps do not produce symptoms and are detected as incidental findings.

Besides the esophageal leiomyomas, the rectal nodule is the only other tumor of the gastrointestinal tract composed of typical mature smooth muscle. The muscularis mucosae seems to undergo a nodular expansion in which the smooth muscle cells lose their normal bilayer orientation and form small bundles that seemingly proliferate randomly within the nodule (Figures 15-37 and 15-38). These nodules are covered by normal or slightly attenuated colonic mucosa.

Deep Intramural Leiomyoma and Leiomyosarcoma of Rectum

In the rectum, generally in the muscularis propria, often extending into the submucosa, are a small group of spindle cell tumors some of which have a unique set of behavioral characteristics. They have a tendency to recur after initial and subsequent excisions; and, after several recurrences over a number of years, metastases

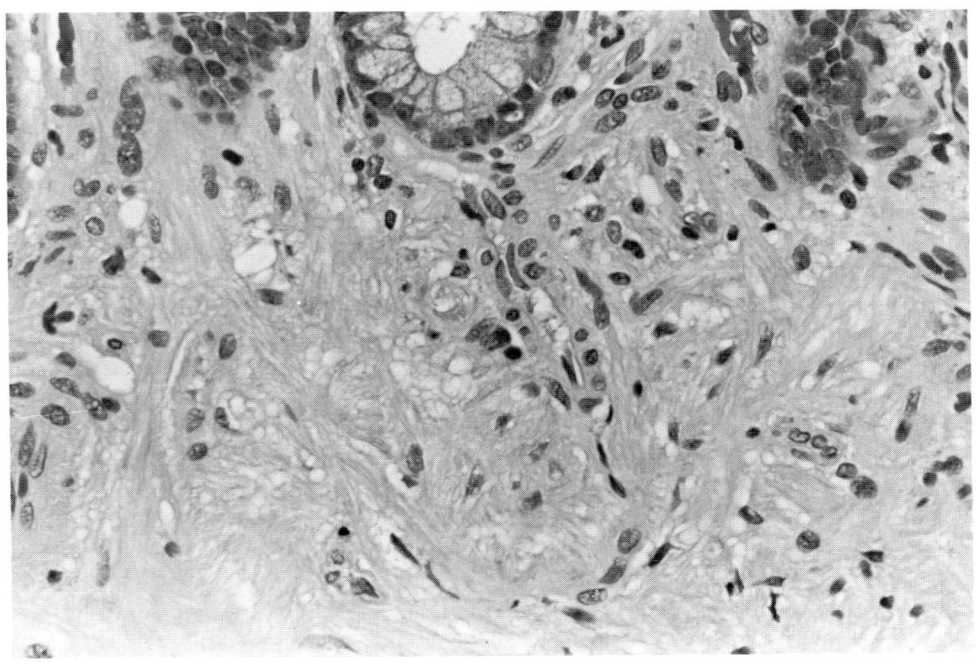

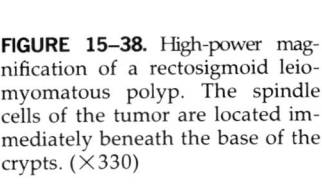

FIGURE 15-38. High-power magnification of a rectosigmoid leiomyomatous polyp. The spindle cells of the tumor are located immediately beneath the base of the crypts. (×330)

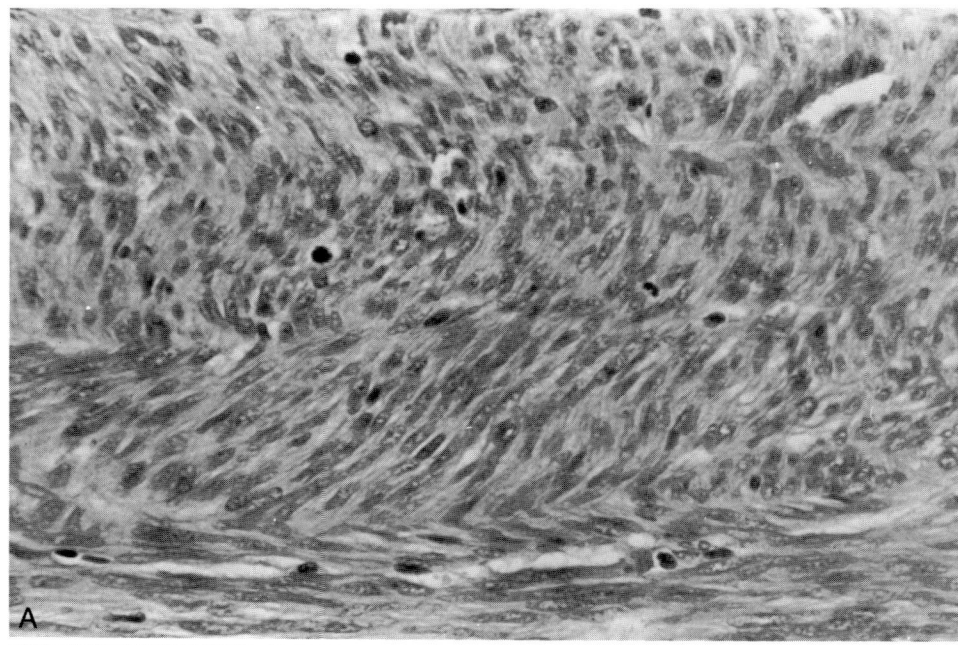
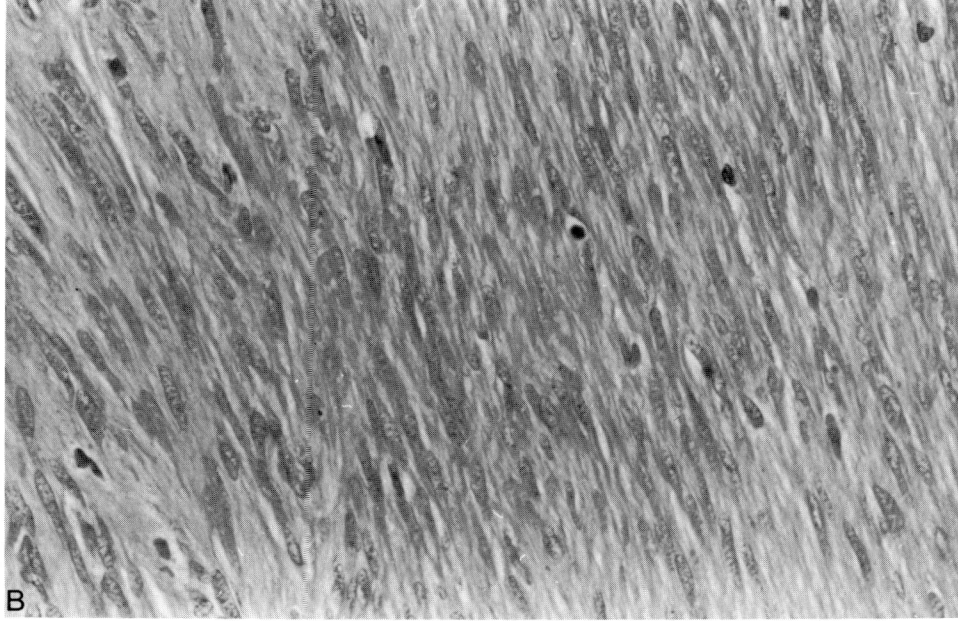

FIGURE 15–39. Comparison of a rectal leiomyosarcoma (A) with tightly packed spindle cells and a leiomyoma (B) with less cellularity. Note the mitoses in A at the left and right center. (×330)

may occur. It is not clear whether this clinical story is a manifestation of the tumor's intrinsic growth capabilities or simply a result of inadequate local excision. Possibly both factors enter in. When they are first observed, these neoplasms are composed of long, slender, uniform spindle cells with dark nuclei (Figure 15–39A). These cells are arranged in small fascicles. Mitotic figures are usually present but in low frequency. The cells are densely packed together, so that the tumors resemble the cellular leiomyomas of the stomach. With each recurrence, the cells tend to become shorter and even more tightly packed, the nuclei become more vesicular rather than dark, mitotic figures become more frequent, and the fascicles become broader and sheetlike. Also, with subsequent recurrences, epithelioid cells are likely to appear, either scattered or in clusters. Occasionally at initial presentation the tumor will have the full-blown malignant features or a biopsy will contain areas of mucosal infiltration, an indication of malignancy. These characteristics suggest that highly cellular spindle cell tumors deep in the rectal wall should be treated in a most aggressive manner at initial presentation. Such treatment may decrease local recurrence, but it may not affect survival.[42,43] Less cellular tumors, presumably the benign counterparts of these progressively worsening sarcomas, also appear in the deep rectal wall and are characterized by their smaller size, circumscription, larger cells, less dense cellularity, and

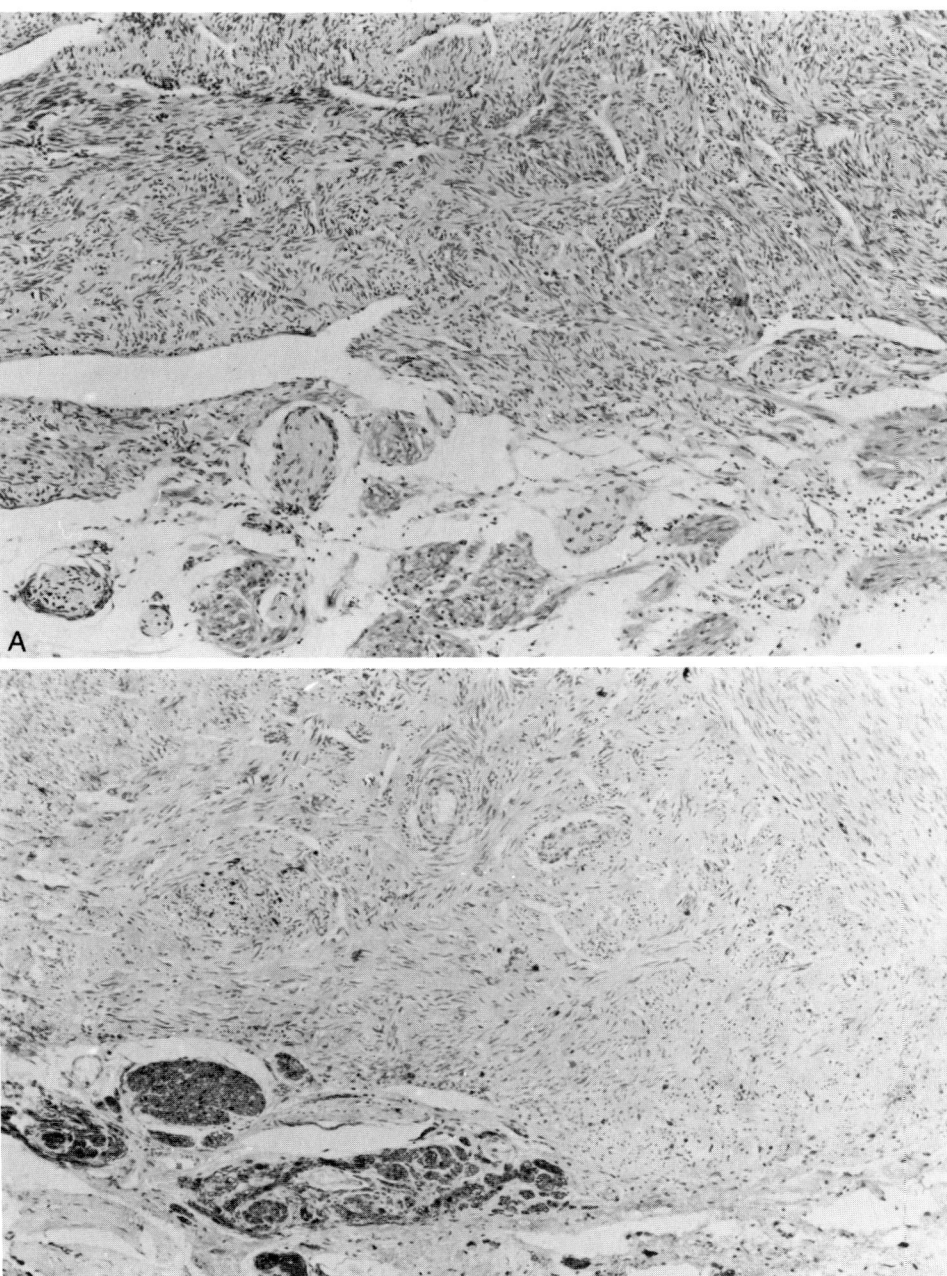

FIGURE 15–40. The tiny stromal tumor of the interface of the myenteric plexus and muscularis propria. *A*, A myenteric nerve at the periphery (lower left corner) is partly surrounded by the tumor, which is situated mainly in the upper half of the field. The darker bundles at the lower edge of the field are muscularis propria. (×83) *B*, This section is stained for S-100 protein, which strongly stains the nerve at the lower left corner but is only positive in scattered cells within the tumor, possibly trapped Schwann cells. The tumor cells otherwise do not contain stainable S-100. (×83)

virtually absent mitotic figures[44] (Figure 15–39B). There is some suggestion that large tumors considered to be leiomyomas of the rectum may recur if they are inadequately excised, but it is not known whether these are leiomyomas or less cellular sarcomas.

Tiny Stromal Tumor of Muscularis Propria/Myenteric Plexus

The practicing surgical pathologist with a heavy case load periodically is sent a tiny nodule for frozen section that the surgeon finds protruding on the mesenteric surface anywhere in the gut, but usually the small bowel or stomach. Often the laparotomy was performed for possible metastatic tumor in the first place. Thus, to the surgeon, this small lump is suspect. Microscopically, this tumor lies within the muscularis propria in the region of the myenteric plexus (Figure 15–40). In some views, both the myenteric nerves and the smooth muscle fibers of the muscularis propria are enveloped by the tumor. The tumor cells may even appear to wrap around nerve twigs. The tumor cells are uniform and spindle-shaped, arranged in short fascicles, and interdigitate with the smooth muscle cells (Figure 15–41). Calcification and sclerosis are common.

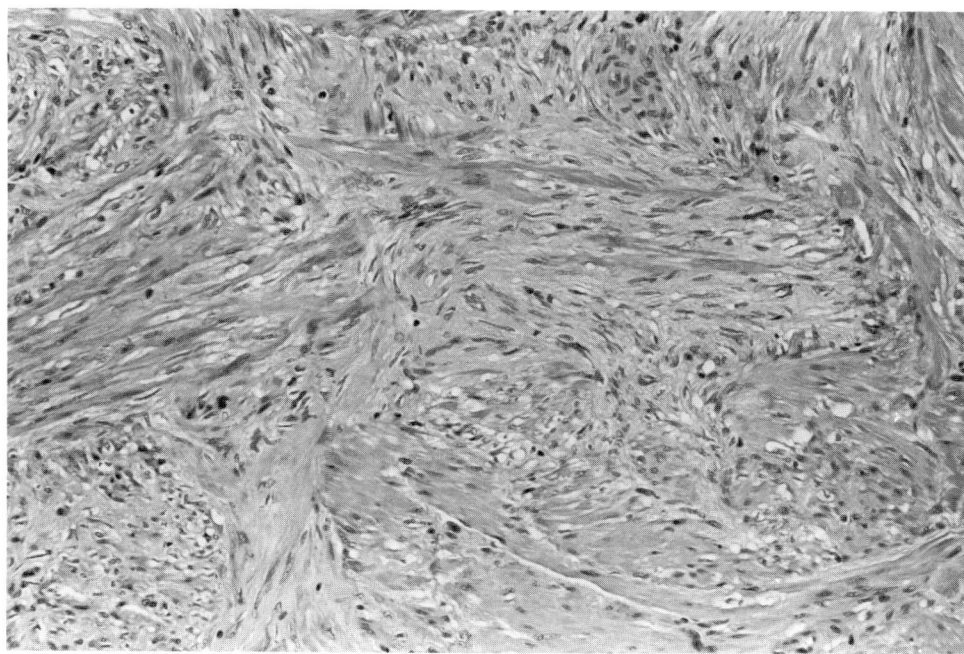

FIGURE 15-41. High-power magnification of the tumor in Figure 15-40. The pale tumor cells interdigitate with the darker-staining smooth-muscle fibers of the muscularis propria. (×330)

These tumors look exactly the same no matter in what site they occur. Immunohistochemically, they are no different from other spindle cell gastrointestinal tract tumors. Occasional cells contain S-100 protein, but most do not. Such positively staining cells may not even be tumor cells but may be trapped myenteric Schwann cells. These proliferations rarely exceed 1 cm in diameter, and they are not malignant. Their major significance is that they constitute a frozen section diagnostic problem.

TUMORS AND TUMOR-LIKE PROLIFERATIONS OF ADIPOSE TISSUE

Lipoma and Liposarcoma

Lipomas have been found in all levels of the gastrointestinal tract; but the colon, especially the right side, seems to be the most common site.[45-49] Grossly, these are circumscribed intramural yellow masses that attenuate the overlying mucosa (Figure 15-42). The larger lesions may be ulcerated and have secondary fibrotic and hemorrhagic changes at the ulcer base. Occasional lipomas are pedunculated, and, as a result, may cause intussusception with intestinal obstruction. Large tumors obviously are more likely to produce symptoms of bleeding, pain, or obstruction than are smaller ones. Rare cases of multiple lipomas occur; and sometimes, especially in the small intestine, these lumps are so numerous that the condition has been called lipomatosis.[50] Many lipomas are discovered as incidental findings during endoscopic procedures. Biopsies, if taken deeply enough, will often yield the characteristic solid sheet of submucosal adipocytes.

Microscopically, these are submucosal masses of rather uniform adipose cells that compress the muscularis mucosae and often cause thinning of the overlying mucosa. In the occasional case which has an ulcer, sclerotic septa may penetrate the tumor from the base of the ulcer; and occasionally there may be associated atypical-appearing granulation tissue with proliferating, somewhat pleomorphic spindle and stellate cells.[51] (Figure 15-43).

Descriptions of gastrointestinal lipomas are especially prevalent in the radiologic literature because of a set of fairly characteristic features, including pliability, accounting for the changing shape of the tumor, and low density, as seen in computed tomographic studies.

A few gastrointestinal liposarcomas have been reported.[52] It is not always clear whether these are really liposarcomas or epithelioid stromal tumors with clear cytoplasm.

Lipomatous Hypertrophy of the Ileocecal Valve

The ileocecal valve is a slender projection of smooth muscle from the inner muscularis propria covered on one side by ileal mucosa, on the other side by colonic mucosa, and on the tip by a variable-sized area of peculiar transitional mucosa with features of both small intestine and colon. Usually, the submucosa on both sides of this muscular projection contains adipose tissue. On occasions, this adipose tissue becomes exces-

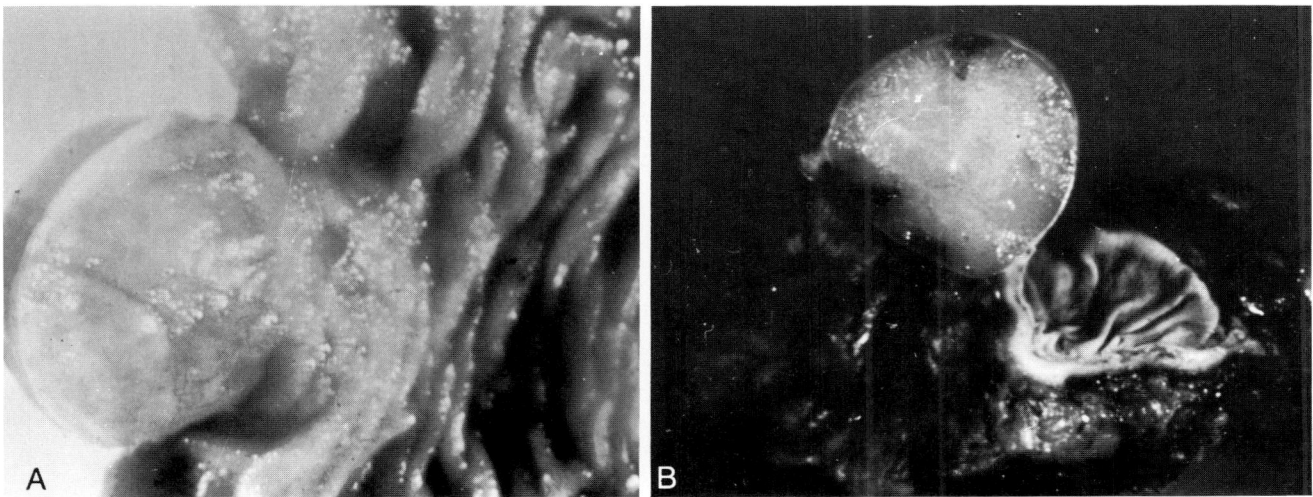

Figure 15-42. Two gross views of submucosal lipomas with the typical circumscribed yellow nodules. *A*, Ileum. *B*, Colon. (Courtesy of Dr. Donald Antonioli, Boston, Mass.)

sive, producing a large, protruding ileocecal valve that grossly resembles the uterine cervix or a set of large pouting yellow lips[53,54] (Figure 15-44).

As the big valve protrudes into the cecal lumen, it can produce a dramatic radiographic filling defect resembling a neoplasm, even a cecal carcinoma; this seems to be the reason for the notoriety of this aberration. Now that colonic barium studies have been largely replaced by colonoscopy, this condition no longer has such importance. The endoscopists seem to recognize it readily. Periodically, an endoscopist will take a biopsy specimen of one of these "lips," which appears microscopically as a chunk of adipose tissue covered by normal mucosa, a picture identical to that in biopsy of a lipoma.

The patients may have nonspecific problems such as constipation or abdominal pain, presumably the reasons for the radiographic or endoscopic studies in the first place, but it does not seem that the large valves cause such symptoms. A few cases of intestinal obstruction or bleeding from an ulcerated valve have been reported, but these are unusual.

No one knows why this excess adipose tissue occurs in these valves. Obesity is not an explanation; more persons with lipomatous hypertrophy are slender than are obese. The fact that patients with this are com-

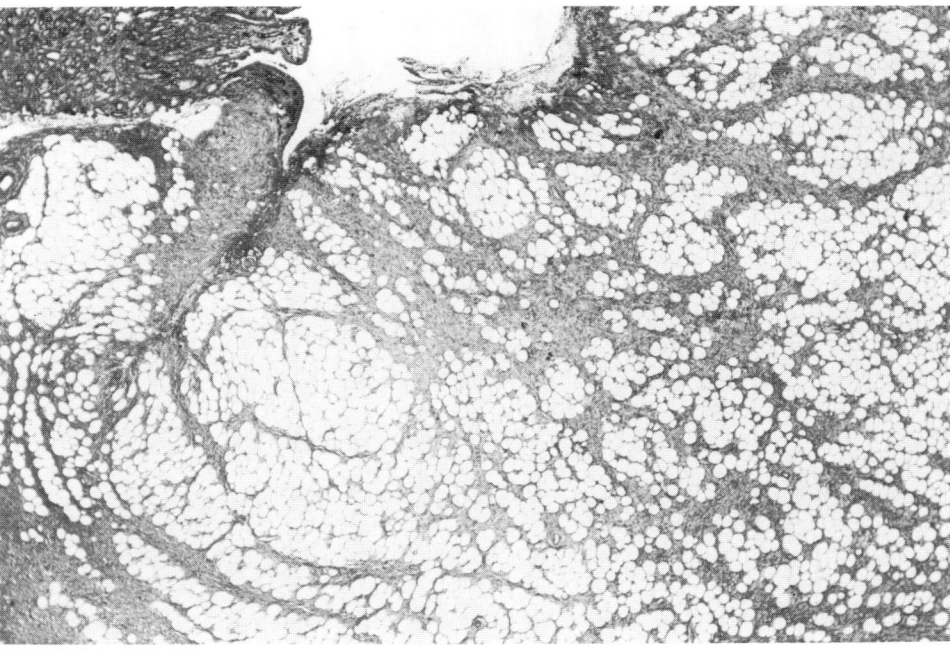

FIGURE 15-43. This ulcerated lipoma of the duodenum is crisscrossed by granulation tissue and fibrous septa radiating from the base of the ulcer. (×13)

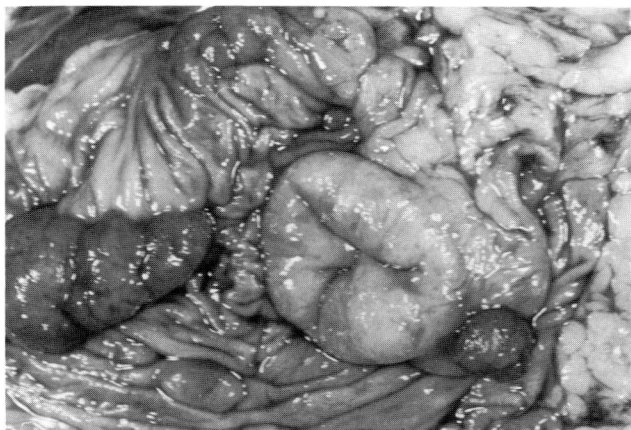

FIGURE 15–44. Lipomatous hypertrophy of the ileocecal valve. The large nodules to the left and right of this huge, pale valve are adenomas of the cecal mucosa. Smaller adenomas are present above and below the valve.

monly middle-aged women may mean that there is a hormonal component. Perhaps they are simply exaggerations of the normal that fall outside of the two–standard deviation level of confidence.

TUMORS AND TUMOR-LIKE PROLIFERATIONS OF VESSELS

Glomus Tumors

The glomus tumor is a benign neoplasm composed of uniform round cells that are ultrastructurally mature smooth muscle cells. In the gut, almost all glomus tumors occur within the stomach, especially the antral region, where they appear grossly as intramural, rather circumscribed, masses.[55-57] Most are about 2 to 2.5 cm across, but occasionally they grow to 4 cm in diameter. Obviously, the larger ones are likely to be ulcerated.

Microscopically, these tumors lie mostly within the muscularis propria, where they form nodules separated by bands of hypertrophic, often collagenized smooth muscle (Figure 15–45). The mucosa is never infiltrated. The tumor cells are monotonous, round cells with central uniform nuclei and pale to clear cytoplasm (Figure 15–46). The cells are arranged in sheets, cords, or clusters, usually intimately applied to the walls of capillaries, some of which may be peculiarly angulated or dilated. Thus, structurally, these tumors look exactly like their counterparts in the skin. The major differential diagnosis for a small intramural round-cell tumor is an epithelioid leiomyoma. Grossly, glomus tumors are so small that they probably never reach the size of metastasizing epithelioid stromal tumors. Histologically, the major differences involve the uniformity of the cells in the glomus tumor, where each cell is almost exactly the same as the one next to it. In contrast, the cells of epithelioid leiomyomas are likely to be much more variable, and they are likely to be much larger. Furthermore, the characteristic perivascular orientation of the glomus cells is only rarely encountered in epithelioid stromal tumors and then only in a few small foci.

Other Vascular Tumors

Angiomas, both of blood vascular and lymphatic types, occur in the gut and look exactly as they do anywhere else in the body. Some have cavernous channels, some have lobulated small-bore capillary channels, some have thicker-walled vessels, and some have

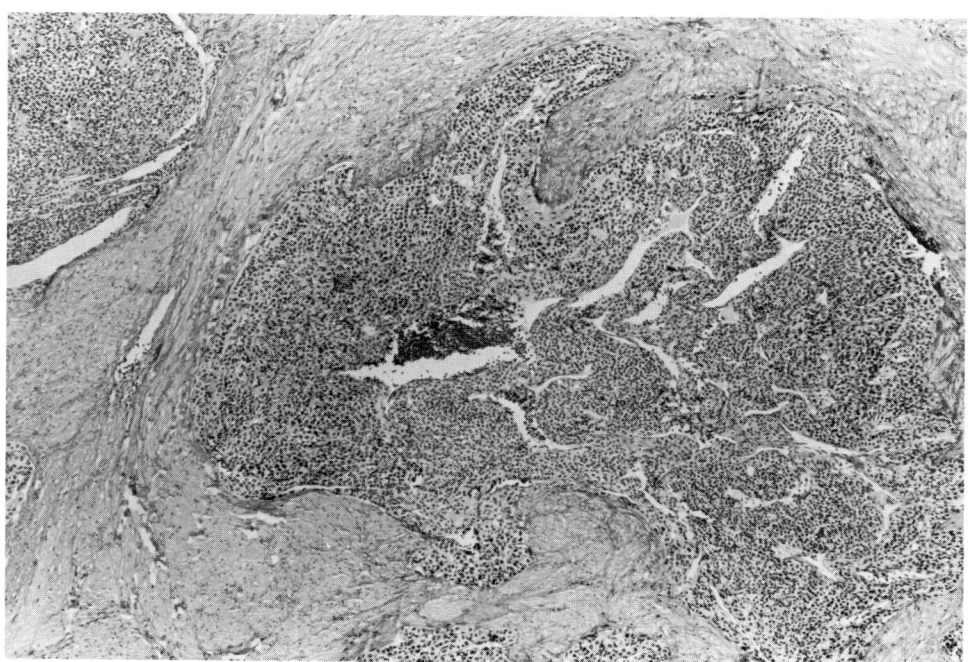

FIGURE 15–45. A gastric glomus tumor. Several nodules of neoplasm are separated by hypertrophic smooth-muscle septa from the muscularis propria. Note the elongated and angulated vascular channels in the nodules. (×53)

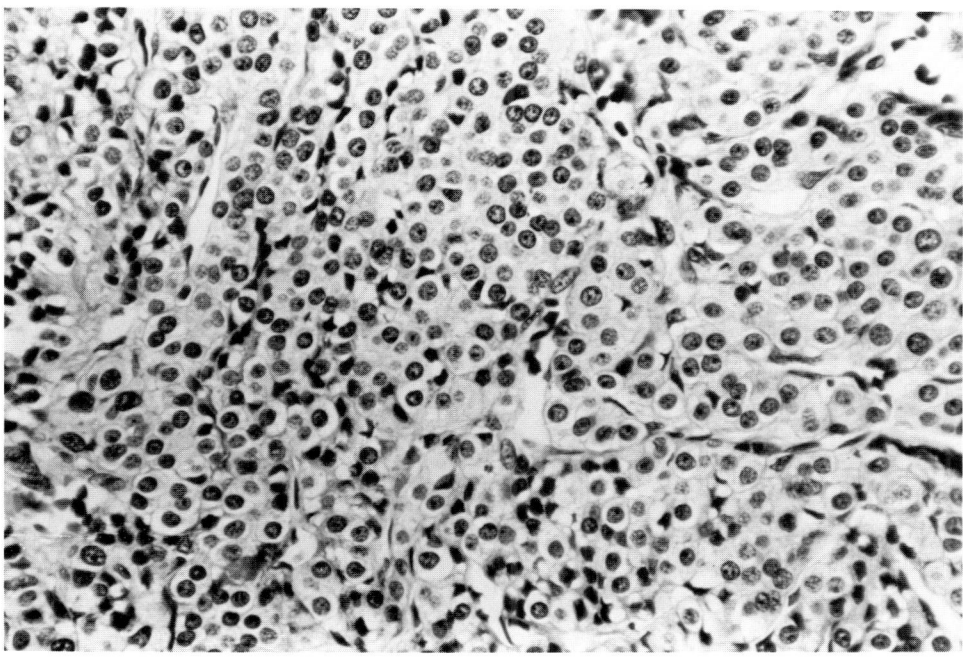

FIGURE 15–46. High-power view of a gastric glomus tumor. The cells are uniform and round and have pale or clear cytoplasm. Compare these cells with the cells of the epithelioid leiomyoma in Figure 15–23 at the same magnification. (×330)

various mixtures of these.[58–61] Some are small, whereas others involve long segments of bowel, especially in the colon. Gastrointestinal angiosarcomas are so rare that meaningful discussion is impossible.

There is an older body of literature describing gastrointestinal hemangiopericytomas, especially those arising in the stomach. It appears that almost all of these were really epithelioid myomas and sarcomas that had prominent perivascular orientation, as described earlier in this chapter. However, a rare, but real, hemangiopericytoma will appear every so often within the gut.[62] Kaposi's sarcoma involving the bowel is increased in patients with AIDS and is discussed in Chapters 12 and 14. For information on other vascular tumors, see Chapter 12.

TUMORS AND TUMOR-LIKE PROLIFERATIONS OF FIBROUS TISSUE

Inflammatory Fibroid Polyps

Inflammatory fibroid polyp (IFP) is the name given collectively to a group of expansile, mainly submucosal lumps in all levels of the gut, which contain a mixture of spindle cells, small vessels, and inflammatory cells.[63–74] Careful analysis of these lesions suggests that they may not be homogeneous as the common name implies.

Inflammatory fibroid polyps occur mainly in two sites, the distal stomach or pylorus and the distal ileum. Rare cases have been reported in the esophagus, colon, more proximal small intestine, and more proximal stomach; but they are too uncommon for any meaningful clinical and pathologic data to have accumulated.

Table 15–1 compares IFPs in the two most common locations. The gastric lesions usually arise immediately proximal to the pyloric sphincter musculature, where they produce sessile lumps, although a few pedunculated tumors have been reported. They are mostly small lesions, with a median size of about 2.5 cm. As a result, most reported cases have occurred either in asymptomatic individuals or in individuals with symptoms not clearly the result of the tumor, such as vague epigastric pain. Thus, most of these lesions have been detected as incidental findings during laparotomies for other reasons. Occasional tumors reach 4 to 5 cm across, and some of them occasionally produce gastric

Table 15–1 COMPARISON BETWEEN INFLAMMATORY FIBROID POLYPS IN STOMACH AND ILEUM

	Stomach	Ileum
Age	Mid sixth decade	Mid sixth decade
Sex	Males slightly greater than females	Males slightly greater than females
Site	Prepyloric	Terminal
Size	75% 3 cm or less	Greater than 2 cm (median, 4+ cm)
Symptoms	None; occasional outlet obstruction if over 2.5 cm	Intestinal obstruction (intussusception)
Lower Border	Submucosa, sharp	Muscularis propria or subserosa, infiltrating
Upper Border	Mucosa, infiltrating	Submucosa, sharp
Microscopic	Perivascular	Loose like granulation tissue
Associations	? Atrophic gastritis ? Pernicious anemia	None

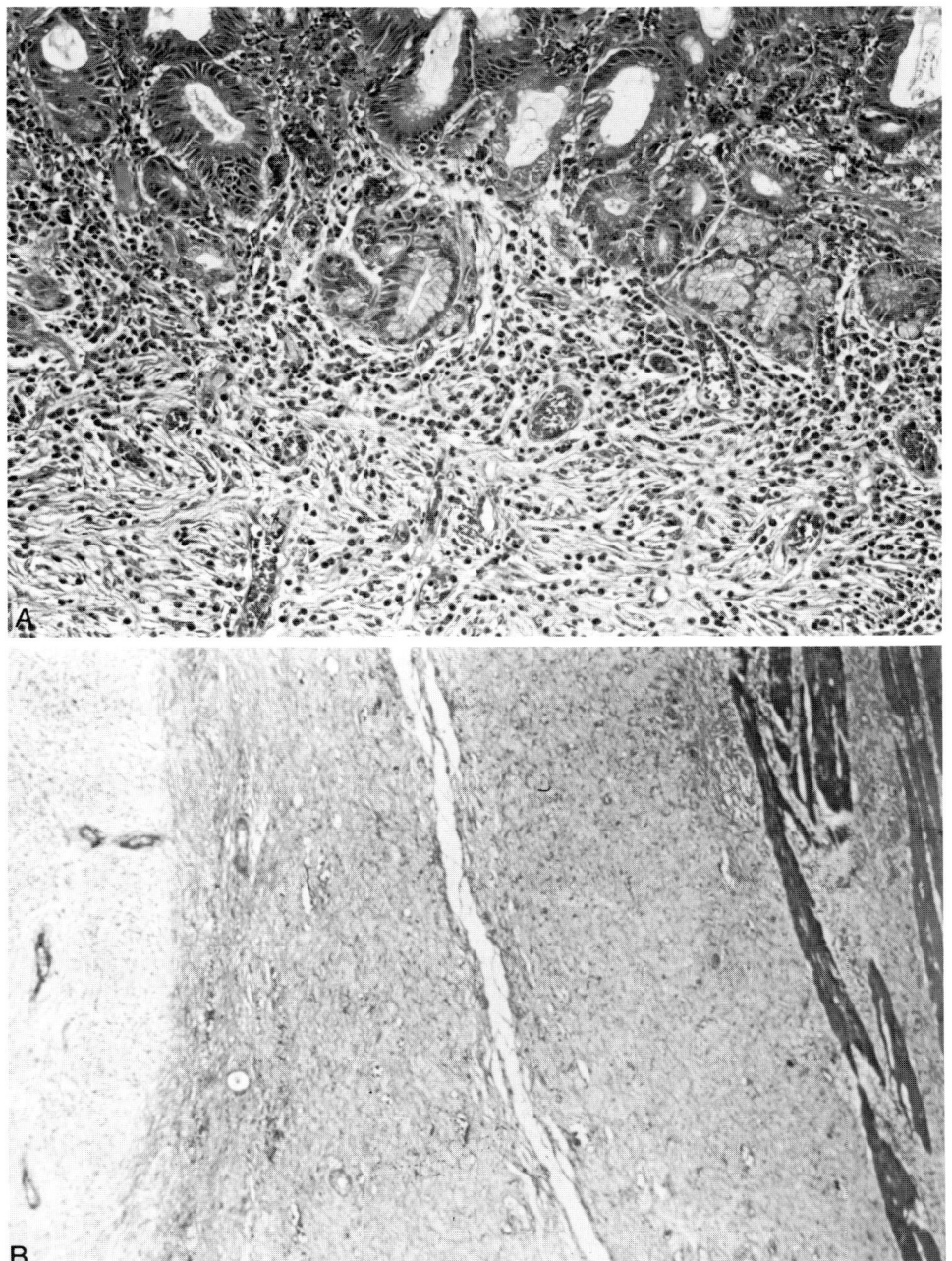

FIGURE 15–47. The gastric inflammatory fibroid polyp. *A*, Involvement of the base of the mucosa by the tumor cells. (×132) *B*, The pale tumor on the left has a sharp lower border in the submucosa (center). The muscularis propria is on the right. (×33)

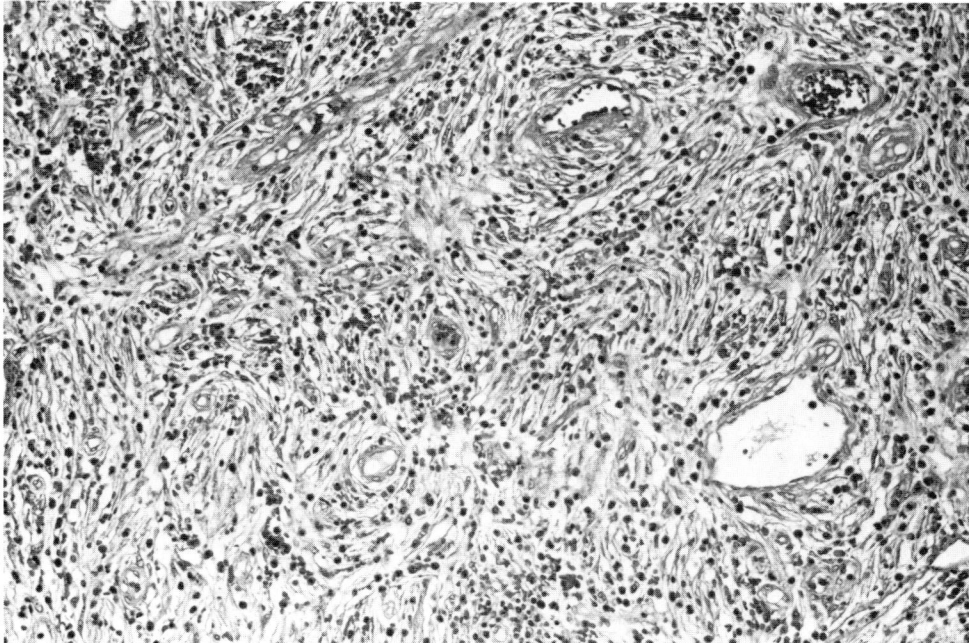

FIGURE 15-48. Gastric IFP. The perivascular orientation of spindle and inflammatory cells. (×132)

outlet obstruction. Some gastric IFPs have overlying ulcers, but it seems that symptoms do not correlate with the presence or absence of an ulcer. There is a hint that IFPs are more common in patients with atrophic gastritis, including those with pernicious anemia.

These gastric tumors tend to fill the superficial submucosa and have a sharp lower border deeper in that layer. Only rarely do they involve the muscularis propria. Superficially, they spread apart or splay the bundles of the muscularis mucosae and infiltrate the base of the mucosa, where they separate the glands (Figure 15-47). In one study, several tumors were described as totally mucosal, suggesting origin in mucosa. These tumors are composed of plump spindle cells and inflammatory cells, usually including many eosinophils; and the spindle cells and eosinophils tend to form concentric layers about small, thin-walled vessels, which usually are seen in cross-sectioned profiles (Figure 15-48).

The terminal-ileal IFPs differ from the gastric lesions. They are larger and are almost all pedunculated (Figure 15-49). As a result, they tend to produce symptoms, most frequently the result of intussusception with intestinal obstruction as the pedunculated tumor forms the leading edge of the internal hernia (Figure 15-50). In a recent report, ileal IFPs were described as being an important cause of small-intestinal obstruction in Malawi in Africa.[75] Possibly, therefore, there is a geographic high-risk area. Furthermore, as a result of these gross characteristics, the ileal polyps are usually extensively ulcerated. The ileal IFPs tend to be transmural, filling the submucosa, replacing the muscularis propria, and often having a large subserosal component as well (Figure 15-51). These tumors look like ex-

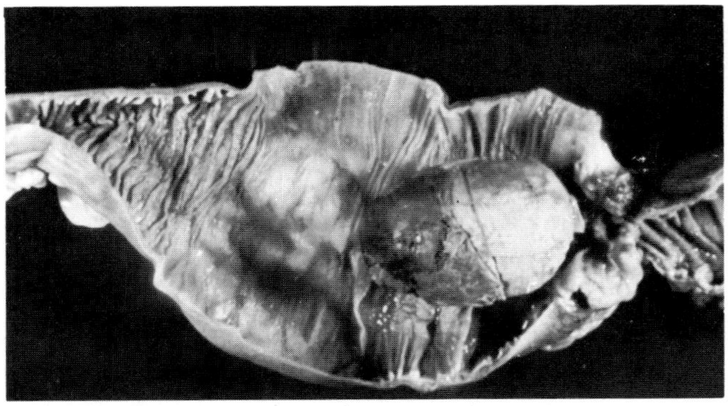

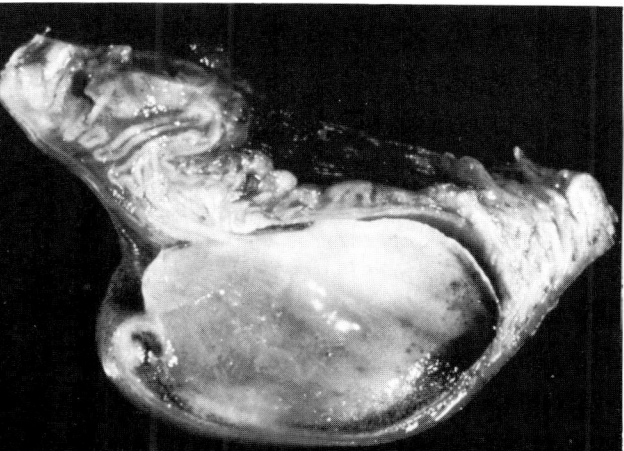

FIGURE 15-49. Ileal IFP. A typical gross polypoid lesion within a dilated segment of bowel.

FIGURE 15-50. This ileal IFP forms the leading edge of an intussusception that is captured in the distal segment of ileum. The cross section of the tumor is pale and glistening. (Courtesy of Dr. Mahendra Ranchod, San Jose, Calif.)

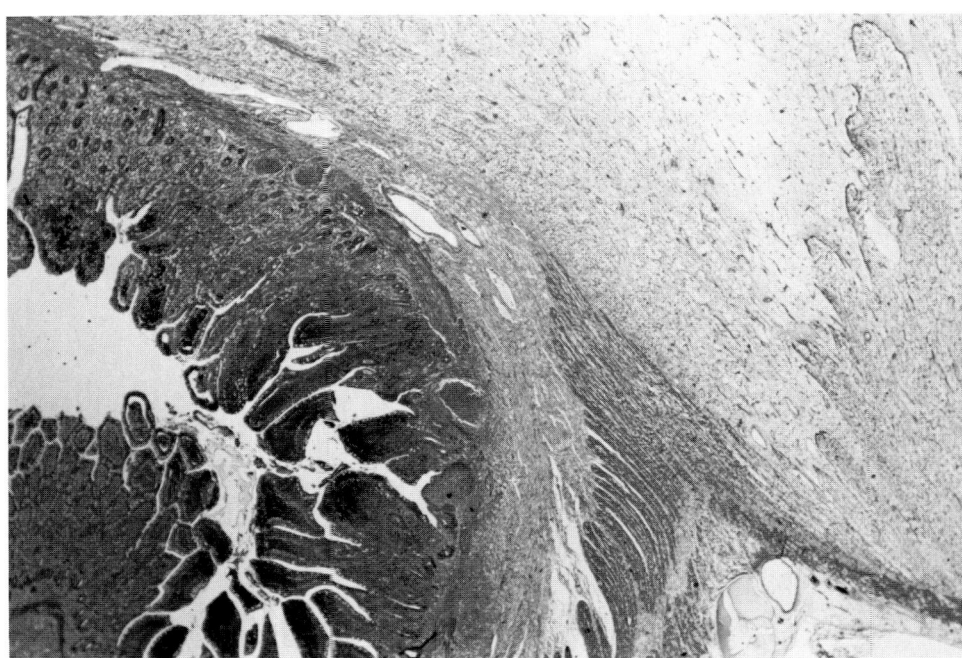

FIGURE 15-51. This ileal IFP fills the submucosa (top) and gradually replaces the muscularis propria (right). (×13)

cessive granulation tissue; and compared with the gastric lesions, they are likely to have more edematous stroma, more elongated than rounded vascular profiles, a cell population likely to be more stellate cells than spindle cells, no prominent perivascular laminations, and an inflammatory cell population more mixed, including plasma cells and lymphocytes as well as eosinophils (Figure 15-52). Occasionally, the ileal IFPs have highly proliferative foci with many mitoses and nuclear hyperchromatism. Such areas may resemble sarcoma superficially.

Peculiarly, the esophageal IFPs usually resemble those in the terminal ileum, whereas those in the colon are likely to look more like those in the stomach.

The histogenesis of these lesions has not been clarified to date. They have been called collectively "inflammatory fibroid polyps," an attempt to indicate that they are not neoplastic, but induced by inflammation. Of course, this implies that there must be some inflammatory stimulus, and none has yet been identified. In ultrastructural studies on the small-intestinal tumors, the stellate and spindle cells have features of fibroblasts and myofibroblasts, a finding that correlates quite well with the granulation tissue appearance.[70,72–74] Ultrastructural and immunohistochemical information on the stomach lesions suggests that the proliferating spindle cells are fibroblasts.[75]

Giant Fibrovascular Polyp of Esophagus

Every so often, a patient presenting with gradually evolving dysphagia will have a long, slender polyp arising from the upper esophagus behind the cricoid cartilage and filling the lumen for various numbers of centimeters, sometimes all the way to the gastric cardia[76] (Figure 15-53). The core of such polyps is composed of a loose stellate and spindle cell proliferation in a myxoid, rather vascular stroma (Figure 15-54). Sometimes adipose tissue cells are mixed as well. These lumps are designated "giant fibrovascular or fibrolipomatous polyps." We do not know what they are, but they seem to be exclusively an esophageal phenomenon. They may be stromal neoplasms or submucosal redundancies or even vascular aberrations. Whatever their essence, they are benign; but they may become huge before they produce symptoms. The major complication is regurgitation of the polyp with impaction on the larynx and asphyxiation. These lesions are so rare that they appear in single case reports. In their detailed book on the pathology of the esophagus, Enterline and Thompson state that they have never seen a case.[77] At the University of Michigan, we had only one case, and that one presented during the writing of this chapter.

TUMORS AND TUMOR-LIKE PROLIFERATIONS OF NERVOUS TISSUE

As mentioned earlier in this chapter, many gut stromal tumors have been reported as some type of nerve sheath tumor, with names such as *neurofibroma, neurilemmoma, schwannoma, neuroma,* or their malignant counterparts. It appears that most of these reports describe tumors that are really identical to those reported as being of smooth muscle differentiation, so that it is unnecessary to describe them again in a separate part of this chapter. Classic gastrointestinal schwannomas

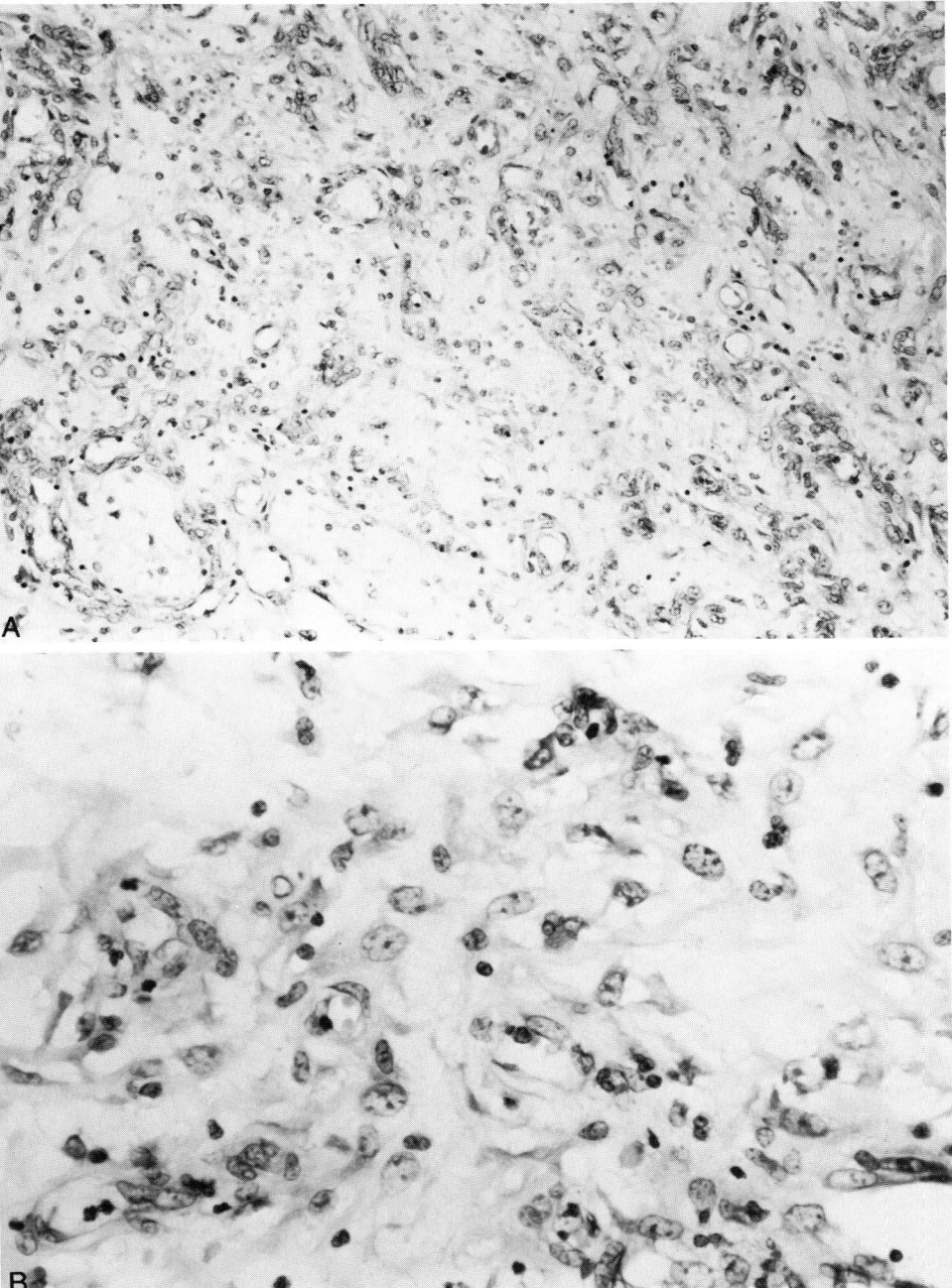

FIGURE 15–52. An ileal IFP. *A*, Loose, edematous, highly vascularized stroma resembling granulation tissue. (×132) *B*, High-power view of the stellate and spindle cells with the superimposed inflammatory cells and the prominent capillaries. (×330)

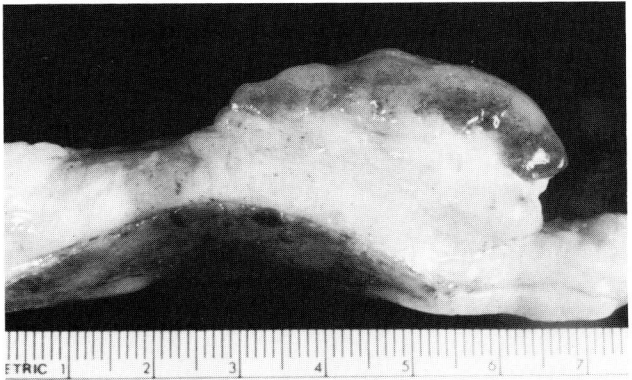

FIGURE 15–53. A giant fibrovascular polyp of the esophagus on cross section. This 9-cm-long structure was attached to the high cervical esophagus by the pedicle on the right.

with capsules, both palisading and microcystic spindle cell proliferation patterns, and typical sclerotic blood vessels and degenerative changes are too rare to be of concern. Nevertheless, there are occasional nerve sheath and nervous tissue tumors that do involve the gastrointestinal tract, three of which are mentioned in more detail, the mural neurofibroma, mucosal and mural ganglioneuromatosis, and granular cell tumors.

Intramural Neurofibroma

It is quite common for patients with von Recklinghausen's multiple neurofibromatosis to have gastrointestinal involvement. Mostly, these manifestations involve the formation of neurofibromas of the plexiform pattern characterized by expansion of nerves by spindle cells and collagen bundles all loosely arranged in a mucopolysaccharide-rich stroma (Figure 15–55). Less commonly, diffuse neurofibromas may be found extending from the submucosa across the muscularis mucosae into the mucosa, where they expand the mucosa and distort the crypts, thereby producing a picture resembling the mucosa in incipient juvenile polyps (Figure 15–56). The occurrence of a typical neurofibroma of the gastrointestinal tract in the absence of von Recklinghausen's disease is too rare. Furthermore, it must be remembered that even in von Recklinghausen's disease, gut stromal tumors of typical or usual type may occur.[17] Malignancies or nerve sheath sarcomas have been reported as arising in the gut in von Recklinghausen's disease, but documentation of their nerve sheath differentiation is uniformly poor.[78]

Ganglioneuroma and Ganglioneuromatosis

Within the alimentary tract, mainly in the colon, occasional proliferations of nerves and their associated Schwann cells and ganglion cells occur in any or all of the plexuses, a process designated as ganglioneuromatosis (Figure 15–57). Although ganglion cells normally do not reside within the gastrointestinal tract mucosa, on occasion such proliferations involve the mucosa, often secondary to submucosal plexus lesions, but sometimes totally confined to mucosa, thereby producing polyps or plaques.[79] In such mucosal lesions, the Schwann cells and neurites extend among the ep-

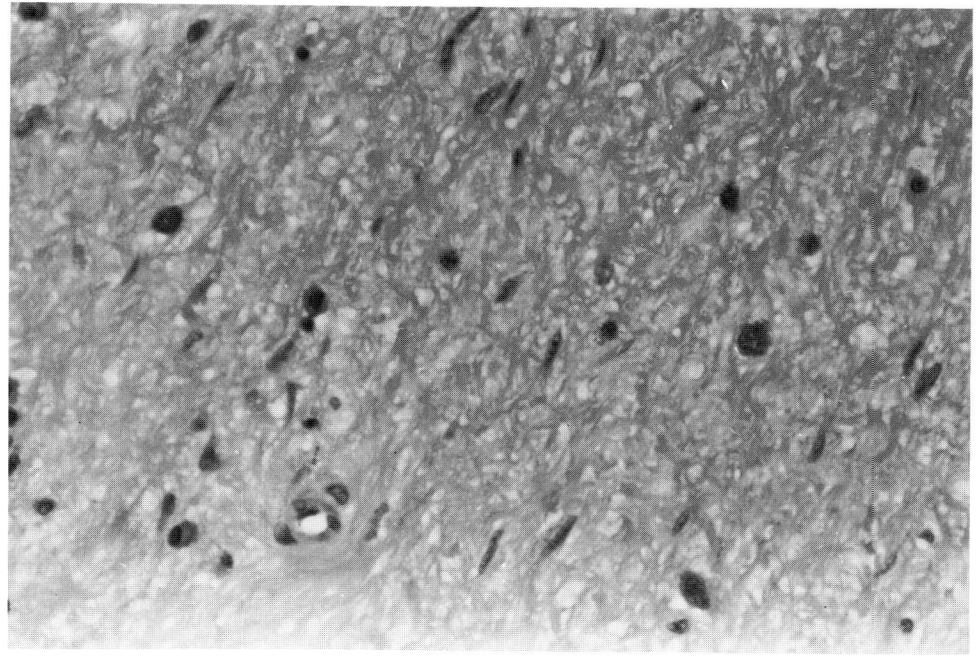

FIGURE 15–54. High-power view of a gastric glomus tumor. The cells are uniform and round and have pale or clear cytoplasm. Compare these cells with the cells of the epithelioid leiomyoma in Figure 15–23 at the same magnification. (×330)

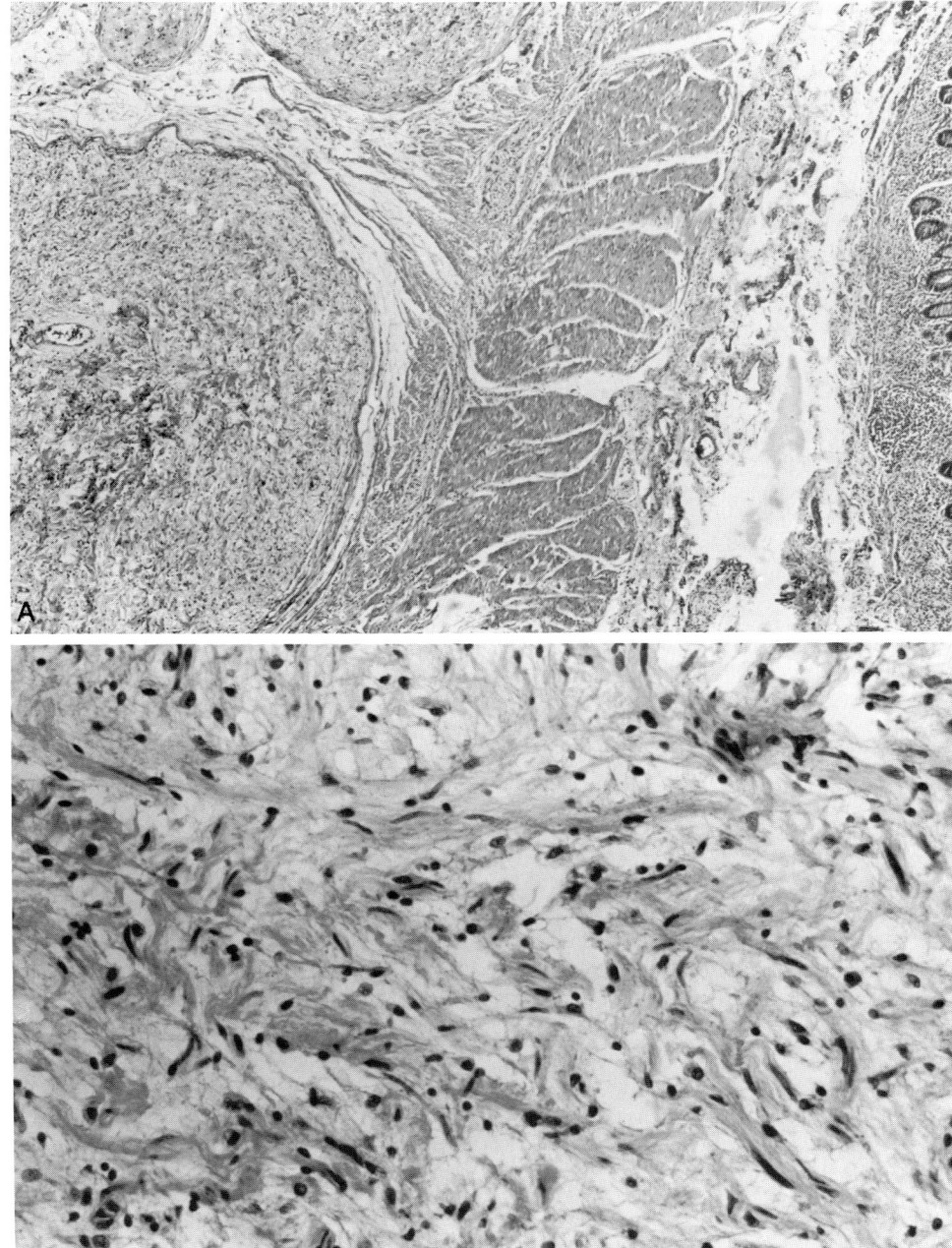

FIGURE 15-55. Plexiform neurofibroma of the small bowel in a patient with von Recklinghausen's disease. *A,* Low-power view of the typical expansion of the nerves in the gut wall, forming nodules. (×33) *B,* High-power view of the loose spindle cells and collagen bundles. (×330)

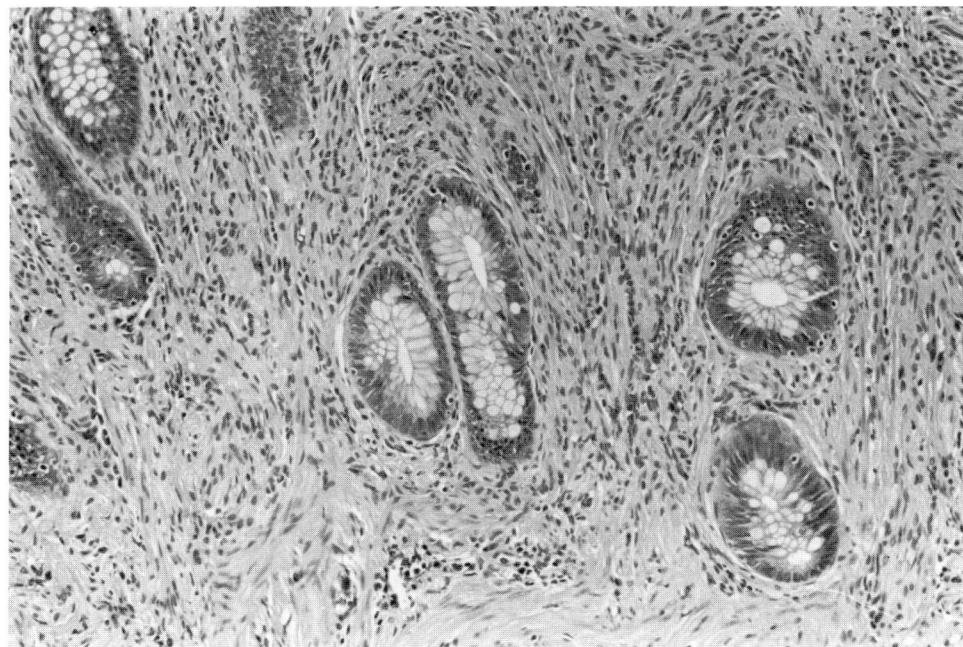

FIGURE 15-56. A diffuse colonic mucosal neurofibroma in a case of von Recklinghausen's disease. The crypts are widely separated by the spindle-cell proliferation. (×132)

ithelial elements, whether glands, pits, or crypts, separating them and often distorting them, which results in branching, dilated, or bizarrely shaped tubules situated in a hypercellular expanded lamina propria. Such distortion resembles that encountered in juvenile polyps. Mixed with the Schwann cells are variable numbers of ganglion cells, sometimes clustered but often isolated, and in occasional lesions very difficult to find. In a few instances, no ganglion cells may be found in the mucosa, but the nerve and Schwann cell proliferations are present, a situation encouraging the use of the designation *neuroma*.

The pattern of bowel wall, including mucosal involvement, has led to a plethora of descriptors, including *"polypoid," "nonpolypoid,"* and *"diffuse" ganglioneuromatosis* and *"solitary ganglioneuroma,"* which seems to be synonymous with *"localized ganglioneuromatosis."* These lesions, whatever their modifications, have been described as common manifestations of multiple endocrine neoplasia (MEN) type IIb syndrome and rarely of von Recklinghausen's disease.[79] Other cases have been reported in which these lesions are associated with multiple juvenile polyps, colonic adenomas, a cecal carcinoma, and Cowden's syndrome, as well as other complex multiorgan disorders.[80-83] They can also occur alone, not as part of a syndrome. Gangliocytic paraganglioma is discussed in Chapter 13.

Granular Cell Tumors

Granular cell tumors of the gastrointestinal tract are exactly like their namesake in the skin or mouth.[84-88] They are intramural nodules that produce sessile lumps when viewed from the mucosal aspect. Granular cell tumors are composed of rather uniform plump spindle or epithelioid cells that contain plentiful coarsely granular eosinophilic cytoplasm. The granules are periodic acid–Schiff (PAS)–positive after diastase predigestion and on electron-microscopic analysis are seen as giant lysosomes filled with a mixture of granular and membranous debris. Also, like their counterparts elsewhere, the cells of the gastrointestinal granular cell tumors stain positively with the antibody to the S-100 protein. The spindle cells are arranged in packets or blunt fascicles. In the gut, granular cell tumors have been found in all sites; but most, by far, arise in the esophagus, where they are likely to be associated with an overlying squamous mucosal alteration that may be hyperplastic, even to the point of pseudoepitheliomatous hyperplasia. In some cases, the epithelium actually may be thinner than normal (Figure 15-58). The cells of the granular cell tumor usually fill the lamina propria and hug the base of this squamous epithelium. Thus, a full-thickness mucosal biopsy is quite likely to pick up the diagnostic cells. In other gastrointestinal sites, the tumorous granular cells create submucosal masses, replace the muscularis mucosae, and extend into the lamina propria. This pattern of mucosal infiltration is common only to the granular cell tumors, diffuse neurofibromas, ganglioneuromatosis, the gastric variants of inflammatory fibroid polyps, and the sarcomas.

In the esophagus, about two thirds occur in the lower part, with the remaining one third split evenly between the upper and the middle parts. The size of the tumor correlates with symptoms, mainly dysphagia or pain. Today tiny granular cell tumors are being found serendipitously during upper endoscopy in asymptomatic patients.

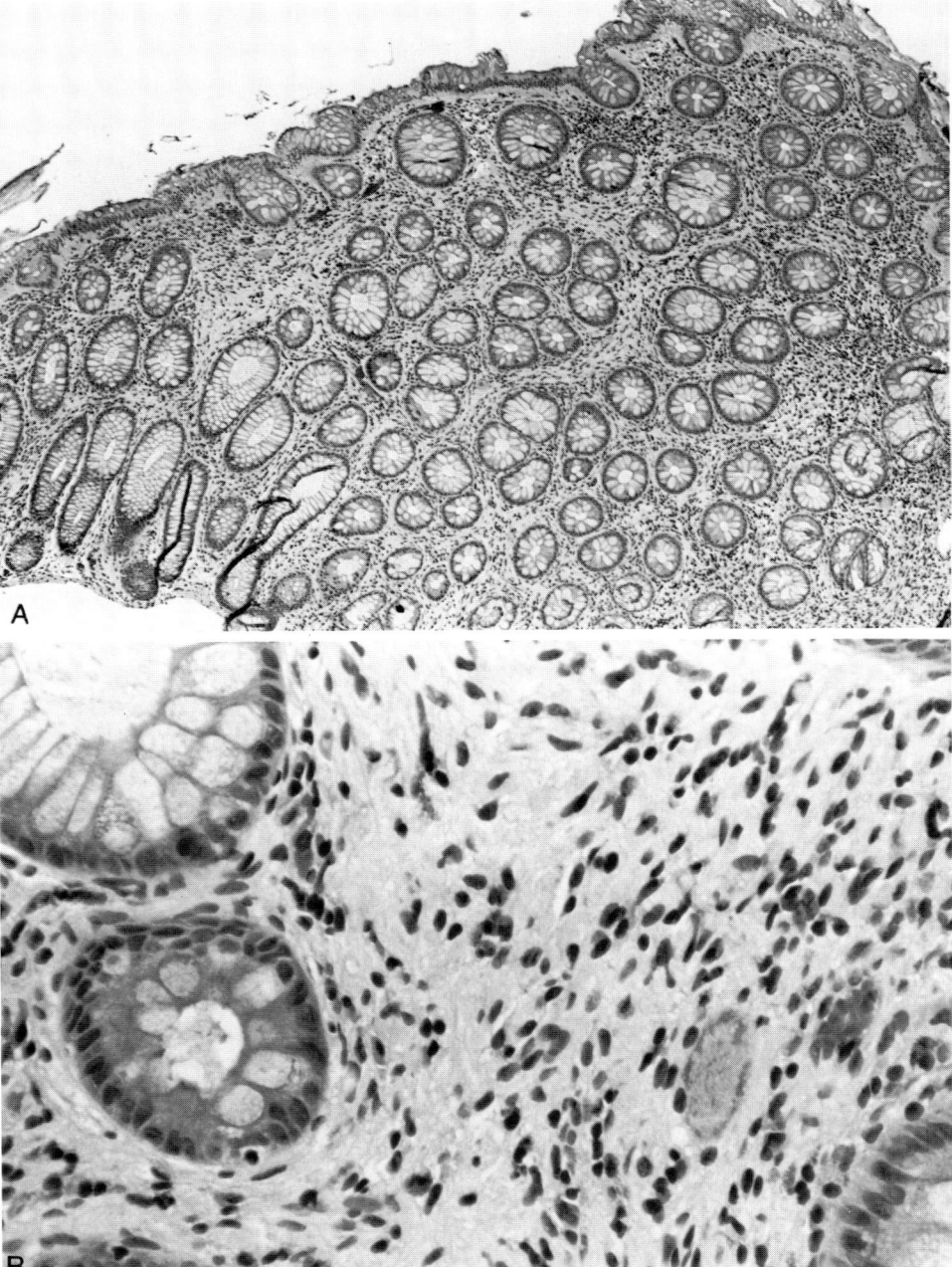

FIGURE 15–57. Ganglioneuromatosis of the colon. *A*, In places, the colonic lamina propria is expanded and the crypts are somewhat distorted. (×53) *B*, High-power view of one of these foci. The lamina propria expansion is due mainly to the spindle cells; but there is a single ganglion cell near the lower right corner, identified by its peripheral Nissl granules. (×330)

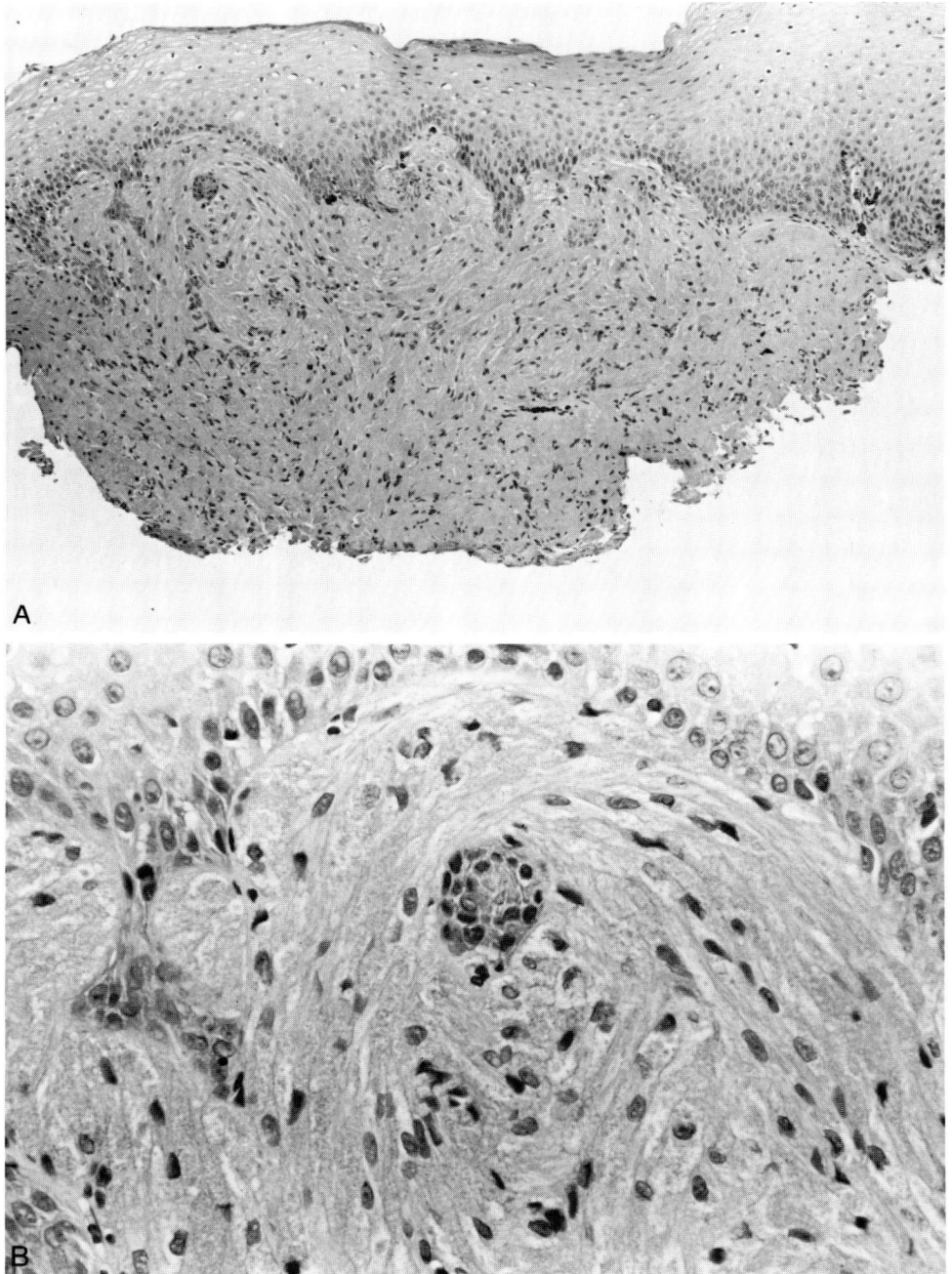

FIGURE 15–58. Granular cell tumor of the esophagus. *A*, Immediately beneath the sawtoothed epithelium is a nodule of spindle cells, the fascicles of which interdigitate with the deeply projecting squamous prongs. (×83) *B*, High-power view of the spindle cells with granular cytoplasm. (×330)

References

1. Nojima T, Gebhardt MC, Mankin HJ, Schiller AL: Extraosseous osteosarcoma presenting with intestinal hemorrhage: Case report and literature review. Hum Pathol 17:85–87, 1986.
2. Stout AP: Tumors of the stomach. Section VI, Fascicle 21. Atlas of Tumor Pathology. Armed Forces Institute of Pathology, Washington, DC, 1953.
3. Golden T, Stout AP: Smooth muscle tumors of the gastrointestinal tract and retroperitoneal tissues. Surg Gynecol Obstet 73:784–810, 1941.
4. Appelman HD: Smooth muscle tumors of the gastrointestinal tract: What we know that Stout didn't know. Am J Surg Pathol 10 (Suppl):83–99, 1986.
5. Brown EF, Banner BF, Gould VE: Differential diagnosis of gastrointestinal schwannomas and leiomyomas: A detailed histologic study with electron microscopic correlation. Lab Invest 50:7A, 1984.
6. Cornog JL Jr: Gastric leiomyoblastoma: A clinical and ultrastructural study. Cancer 34:711–719, 1974.
7. Hajdu SI, Erlandson RA, Paglia MA: Light and electron microscopic studies of a gastric leiomyoblastoma. Arch Pathol 93:36–41, 1972.
8. Knapp RH, Wick MR, Goellner JR: Leiomyoblastomas and their relationship to other smooth-muscle tumors of the gastrointestinal tract. Am J Surg Pathol 8:449–461, 1984.
9. Salazar H, Totten RS: Leiomyoblastoma of the stomach: An ultrastructural study. Cancer 25:176–185, 1970.
10. Weiss RA, Mackay B: Malignant smooth muscle tumors of the gastrointestinal tract. Ultrastruct Pathol 2:231–240, 1981.
11. Welsh RA, Meyer AT: Ultrastructure of gastric leiomyoma. Arch Pathol 87:71–81, 1969.
12. Evans DJ, Lampert JA, Jacobs M: Intermediate filaments in smooth muscle tumors. J Clin Pathol 36:57–61, 1983.
13. Donner L, deLanerolle P, Costa J: Immunoreactivity of paraffin-embedded normal tissues and mesenchymal tumors for smooth muscle myosin. Am J Clin Pathol 80:677–681, 1983.
14. Mazur MT, Clark HB: Gastric stromal tumors: Reappraisal of histogenesis. Am J Surg Pathol 7:507–519, 1983.
15. Pike AM, Lloyd RV, Appelman HD: Differentiation of gut stromal tumors: An immunohistochemical study. Hum Pathol 19:830–834, 1988.
16. Saul SH, Rast ML, Brooks JJ: The immunohistochemistry of gastrointestinal stromal tumors. Am J Surg Pathol 11:464–473, 1987.
17. Schaldenbrand JD, Appelman HD: Solitary solid stromal gastrointestinal tumors in von Recklinghausen's disease with minimal smooth muscle differentiation. Hum Pathol 15:229–232, 1984.
18. Appelman HD: Stromal tumor of the esophagus, stomach and duodenum. In: Appelman HD (ed): Pathology of the Esophagus, Stomach, and Duodenum: Contemporary Issues in Surgical Pathology. New York, Churchill Livingstone, 1984.
19. Carney JA: The triad of gastric epithelioid leiomyosarcoma, functioning extra-adrenal paraganglioma and pulmonary chondroma. Cancer 43:374–382, 1979.
20. Carney JA: The triad of gastric epithelioid leiomyosarcoma, pulmonary chondroma and functioning extra-adrenal paraganglioma: A five-year review. Medicine 62:159–169, 1983.
21. Ranchod M, Kempson RL: Smooth muscle tumors of the gastrointestinal tract and retroperitoneum. Cancer 39:255–262, 1977.
22. Akwari OE, Dozois RR, Weiland LH, Beahrs OH: Leiomyosarcoma of the small and large bowel. Cancer 42:1375–1384, 1978.
23. Shiu MH, Farr GH, Papachristou DN, Hajdu SI: Myosarcomas of the stomach: Natural history, prognostic factors and management. Cancer 49:177–187, 1982.
24. Evans HL: Smooth muscle tumors of the gastrointestinal tract: A study of 56 cases followed for a minimum of 10 years. Cancer 56:2242–2250, 1985.
25. Lindsay PC, Ordonez N, Raaf JH: Gastric leiomyosarcomas: Clinical and pathological review of fifty patients. J Surg Oncol 18:399–421, 1981.
26. Appelman HD, Helwig EB: Gastric epithelioid leiomyoma and leiomyosarcoma (leiomyoblastoma). Cancer 38:708–728, 1976.
27. Seremetis MG, Lyons WS, DeGuzman VC, Peabody JW Jr: Leiomyomata of the eosphagus: An analysis of 838 cases. Cancer 38:2166–2177, 1976.
28. Takubo K, Nakagawa H, Tsuchiya S, et al: Seedling leiomyoma of the esophagus and esophagogastric junction zone. Hum Pathol 12:1006–1010, 1981.
29. Enterline H, Thompson J: Pathology of the Esophagus. New York, Springer-Verlag, 1984, pp 169–171.
30. Fernandas JP, Mascarenhas MJ, daCosta JC, Correia JP: Diffuse leiomyomatosis of the esophagus. Dig Dis 20:684–690, 1975.
31. Heald J, Moussalli H, Hasleton PS: Diffuse leiomyomatosis of the oesophagus. Histopathology 10:755–759, 1986.
32. Kabuto T, Taniguchi K, Iwanaga T, et al: Diffuse leiomyomatosis of the esophagus. Dig Dis Sci 25:388–391, 1980.
33. DeMeester TR, Skinner DB: Polypoid sarcomas of the esophagus: A rare but potentially curable neoplasm. Ann Thorac Surg 20:405–417, 1975.
34. Gaede JT, Postlethwait RW, Shelburne JD, et al: Leiomyosarcomas of the esophagus: Report of two cases, one with associated squamous cell carcinoma. J Thorac Cardiovasc Surg 75:740–746, 1978.
35. Rainer WG, Brus R: Leiomyosarcoma of the esophagus: Review of the literature and report of 3 cases. Surgery 58:343–350, 1965.
36. Vartio T, Nickels J, Hockerstedt K, Scheinin TM: Rhabdomyosarcoma of the oesophagus. Virchows Arch [A] 386:357–361, 1980.
37. Appelman HD, Helwig EB: Cellular leiomyomas of the stomach in 49 patients. Arch Pathol Lab Med 101:373–377, 1977.
38. Martin JF, Bazin P, Feroldi J, Cabanne F: Tumeurs myoides intramurales de l'estomac: Considerations microscopiques à propos de 6 cas. Ann Anat Pathol (Paris) 5:484–497, 1960.
39. Stout AP: Bizarre smooth muscle tumors of the stomach. Cancer 15:400–409, 1962.
40. Appelman HD, Helwig EB: Sarcomas of the stomach. Am J Clin Pathol 67:2–10, 1977.
41. Tang CK, Melamed MR: Leiomyosarcoma of the colon exclusive of the rectum. Am J Gastroenterol 64:376–381, 1975.
42. Walsh TH, Mann CV: Smooth muscle neoplasms of the rectum and anal canal. Br J Surg 71:597–599, 1984.
43. Khalifa AA, Bong WL, Rao VK, Williams MJ: Leiomyosarcoma of the rectum—report of a case and review of the literature. Dis Colon Rectum 29:427–432, 1986.
44. Sasaki K, Gutoh Y, Nakayama Y, et al: Leiomyoma of the rectum. Int Surg 70:149–152, 1985.
45. Wychulis AR, Jackman CJ, Mayo CW: Submucous lipomas of the colon and rectum. Surg Gynecol Obstet 118:337–340, 1964.
46. Peiser J, Ovnat A, Herz A, Hirsch M, Charuzi I: Lipoma of the esophagus. Isr J Med Sci 20:1068–1070, 1984.
47. Agha FP, Dent TL, Fiddian-Green RC, et al: Bleeding lipoma of the upper gastrointestinal tract. Am Surg 51:279–285, 1985.
48. Michowitz M, Lazebnik N, Noy S, Lazebnik R: Lipoma of the colon: A report of 22 cases. Am Surg 51:449–454, 1985.
49. Whetstone MR, Zuckerman MJ, Saltzstein EC, Boman D: CT diagnosis of duodenal lipoma. Am J Gastroenterol 80:251–252, 1985.
50. Climie ARW, Wylin RF: Small-intestinal lipomatosis. Arch Pathol Lab Med 105:40–42, 1981.
51. Snover DC: Atypical lipomas of the colon: Report of two cases with pseudomalignant features. Dis Colon Rectum 27:485–488, 1984.
52. Laky D, Stoica T: Gastric liposarcoma: A case report. Pathol Res Pract 181:112–115, 1986.
53. Boquist L, Bargdahl L, Andersson A: Lipomatosis of the ileocecal valve. Cancer 29:136–140, 1972.
54. Skaane P, Eide TJ, Westgaard T, Gauperaa T: Lipomatosis and true lipomas of the ileocecal valve. ROFO 135:663–668, 1981.
55. Kay S, Callahan WP Jr, Murray MR, et al: Glomus tumors of the stomach. Cancer 4:726–736, 1951.
56. Appelman HD, Helwig EB: Glomus tumors of the stomach. Cancer 23:203–213, 1969.
57. Almagro UA, Schulte WJ, Norback DH, Turcotte JK: Glomus tumor of the stomach: Histologic and ultrastructural features. Am J Clin Pathol 75:415–419, 1981.
58. Okumura T, Tanoue S, Chiba K, Tanaka S: Lobular capillary hemangioma of the esophagus: A case report and review of the literature. Acta Pathol Jpn 33:1303–1308, 1983.

59. Ikeda K, Murayama H, Takano H, et al: Massive intestinal bleeding in hemangiomatosis of the duodenum. Endoscopy 12:306–310, 1980.
60. Kuroda Y, Katoh H, Ohsato K: Cystic lymphangioma of the colon: Report of a case and review of the literature. Dis Colon Rectum 27:679–682, 1984.
61. Mills CS, Lloyd TV, Van Aman ME, Lucas J: Diffuse hemangiomatosis of the colon. J Clin Gastroenterol 7:416–421, 1985.
62. Genter B, Mir K, Strauss R, et al: Hemangiopericytoma of the colon: Report of a case and review of the literature. Dis Colon Rectum 25:149–156, 1982.
63. Vanek J: Gastric submucosal granuloma with eosinophilic infiltration. Am J Pathol 25:397–411, 1949.
64. Helwig EB, Ranier A: Inflammatory fibroid polyps of the stomach. Surg Gynecol Obstet 96:355–367, 1953.
65. Bullock WK, Moran ET: Inflammatory fibroid polyps of the stomach. Cancer 6:488–493, 1953.
66. Salm R: Gastric fibroma with eosinophilic infiltration. Gut 6:85–91, 1965.
67. Samter TG, Alstott DF, Kurlander GJ: Inflammatory fibroid polyps of the gastrointestinal tract: A report of 3 cases, 2 occurring in children. Am J Clin Pathol 45:420–436, 1966.
68. Goldman RL, Friedman NB: Neurogenic nature of so-called inflammatory fibroid polyps of the stomach. Cancer 20:134–143, 1967.
69. LiVolsi VA, Perzin KA: Inflammatory pseudotumors (inflammatory fibrous polyps) of the esophagus. Am J Dig Dis 20:475–481, 1975.
70. Benjamin SP, Hawk WA, Turnbull RB: Fibrous inflammatory polyps of the ileum and cecum. Cancer 39:1300–1305, 1977.
71. Johnstone JM, Morson BC: Inflammatory fibroid polyps of the gastrointestinal tract. Histopathology 2:349–361, 1978.
72. Navas-Palacios JJ, Colina-Ruizdelgado F, Sanchez-Larren MD, Cortes-Carsino J: Inflammatory fibroid polyps of the gastrointestinal tract: An immunohistochemical and electron microscopic study. Cancer 51:1682–1690, 1983.
73. Shimer GR, Helwig EB: Inflammatory fibroid polyps of the intestine. Am J Clin Pathol 81:708–714, 1984.
74. Nkanza NK, King M, Hutt MS: Intussusception due to inflammatory fibroid polyps of the ileum: A report of 12 cases from Africa. Br J Surg 67:271–274, 1980.
75. Ishikura H, Sato F, Naka A, Kodama T, Aizawa M: Inflammatory fibroid polyp of the stomach. Acta Pathol Jpn 36:327–335, 1986.
76. Patel J, Kieffer RW, Martin M, Avant GR: Giant fibrovascular polyp of the esophagus. Gastroenterology 87:953–956, 1984.
77. Enterline H, Thompson J: Pathology of the Esophagus. New York, Springer-Verlag, 1984, pp 172–173.
78. Croker JR, Greenstein RJ: Malignant schwannoma of the stomach in a patient with von Recklinghausen's disease. Histopathol 3:79–85, 1979.
79. Carney JA, Go VLW, Sizemore GW, Hayles AB: Alimentary-tract ganglioneuromatosis: A major component of the syndrome of multiple endocrine neoplasias, type 2b. N Engl J Med 295:1287–1291, 1976.
80. Snover DC, Weigent CE, Sumner HW: Diffuse mucosal ganglioneuromatosis of the colon associated with adenocarcinoma. Am J Clin Pathol 75:225–229, 1981.
81. Mendelsohn G, Diamond MP: Familial ganglioneuromatous polyposis of the large bowel: Report of a family with associated juvenile polyposis. Am J Surg Pathol 8:515–520, 1984.
82. Weidner N, Flanders DJ, Mitros FA: Mucosal ganglioneuromatosis associated with multiple colonic polyps. Am J Surg Pathol 8:779–786, 1984.
83. Lashner BA, Riddell RH, Winans CS: Ganglioneuromatosis of the colon and extensive glycogenic acanthosis in Cowden's disease. Dig Dis Sci 31:213–216, 1986.
84. Schwartz DT, Gaetz HP: Multiple granular cell myoblastomas of the stomach. Am J Clin Pathol 44:453–457, 1965.
85. Calhoun T, Odelowo EOO, Ali S, et al: Granular cell myoblastoma: Another unusual esophageal lesion. J Thorac Cardiovasc Surg 69:472–475, 1975.
86. Johnston J, Helwig EB: Granular cell tumors of the gastrointestinal tract and perianal region: A study of 74 cases. Dig Dis Sci 26:807–816, 1981.
87. Vuyk HD, Snow GB, Tiwari RM, et al: Granular cell tumor of the proximal esophagus: A rare disease. Cancer 55:445–449, 1985.
88. Coutinho DS deS, Soga J, Yoshikawa T, et al: Granular cell tumors of the esophagus: A report of two cases and review of the literature. Am J Gastroenterol 80:758–762, 1985.

CHAPTER 16

Systemic and Miscellaneous Disorders

HARVEY GOLDMAN, M.D.

DISEASES OF OTHER ORGANS AND SYSTEMS
Cardiovascular System
Ischemic Disease
Lymphangiectasia
Respiratory System
Kidneys and Urinary System
Uremia
Secondary Infections
Diseases Common to the Kidneys and Gastrointestinal Tract
Complications of Ureterosigmoidostomy
Hematologic System
Hemorrhagic Disorders
Sickle Cell Anemia
Iron Deficiency Anemia
Megaloblastic Anemia
Polycythemia
Leukemia and Lymphoma
Endocrine System
Thyroid Diseases
Parathyroid Diseases
Adrenal Diseases
Diabetes Mellitus
Reproductive System
Diseases of Contiguous Tissues
Effects of Pregnancy and Exogenous Hormones
Skin and Soft Tissues and Other Systemic Conditions

Skin Diseases
Dermatitis Herpetiformis
Erythema Multiforme
Köhlmeier-Degos Disease
Soft Tissue Diseases
Rheumatoid Arthritis
Reactive Arthritis
Sjögren's Syndrome
Pancreas, Biliary Tract, and Liver
Cystic Fibrosis
Other Pancreatic and Biliary Diseases
Hepatic Diseases
Hemochromatosis

VITAMIN DISORDERS
Fat-Soluble Vitamins
Vitamin K Deficiency
Disorders of Other Fat-Soluble Vitamins
Water-Soluble Vitamins
Pellagra
Disorders of Other Water-Soluble Vitamins

DEPOSITIONS
Conditions That May Simulate Storage Diseases
Lipoprotein Disorders
Tangier Disease
Abetalipoproteinemia
Glycolipid Storage Diseases

Gangliosidosis
Sulfatidosis
Fabry's Disease
Niemann-Pick Disease
Mucolipidosis
Lipid Pigment Disorders
Neuronal Ceroid Lipofuscinosis
Brown Bowel Syndrome
Melanosis Coli
Other Storage Diseases
Wolman's Disease
Mucopolysaccharidosis
Mannosidosis
Cystinosis
Glycogen Storage Disease
Iron Storage Disease
Other Pigment Depositions
Amyloidosis

GRANULOMATOUS DISORDERS
Infections
Crohn's Disease
Foreign Body Granulomas
Isolated Granulomas
Sarcoidosis
Chronic Granulomatous Disease
Malacoplakia
Histiocytosis X
Miscellaneous Granulomatous Conditions

This chapter deals with conditions that are primarily due to diseases of other organs and with systemic disorders that may affect multiple portions of the alimentary tract.[1] Some of these are presented in detail in other parts of the book, and only the salient findings are reviewed here.

DISEASES OF OTHER ORGANS AND SYSTEMS

Nonspecific or constitutional symptoms referable to the gastrointestinal tract are exceedingly common in diseases affecting other organs and tissues in the body.

These include anorexia; nausea; vomiting; abdominal pain, often crampy; and either diarrhea or constipation. These symptoms may herald the onset of the diseases and persist for a variable time. They are also commonly seen in persons in stressful situations.[2] They are thought to be related to stimulation of components of the autonomic nervous system and to the effects of mediators, such as prostaglandins, that are released as part of an inflammatory reaction. In addition, the gastrointestinal tract is a common site for the development of opportunistic infections[3-7] and drug reactions[8-11] that may be attributed to diseases of other organs and their therapies.

Cardiovascular System

Ischemic Disease

The most common effects on the gastrointesinal tract are seen in cases of cardiac failure and of shock and in those with occlusive lesions of the mesenteric vessels, and the lesions range from mucosal necrosis to transmural infarction of the intestines.[12-15] Ischemic damage may also be seen in cases of disseminated intravascular coagulation, where the cause is probably low blood flow rather than obstruction of the small vessels, and in patients with vaculitis, which may be associated with many systemic conditions.[16,17] These subjects are presented in Chapter 12.

Lymphangiectasia

In some patients with sustained high central venous pressure such as may occur in constrictive pericarditis and in valvular lesions of the right side of the heart, the elevated pressure may be transmitted to the mesenteric and intestinal lymphatic system, which may result in marked dilation of the lacteals and a leakage of protein-rich fluid into the gut lumen.[18,19] The jejunal mucosal biopsy is normal except for the diffuse dilation of the lymphatics in the lamina propria, but it is sometimes difficult to distinguish this finding from the effects of a traumatized sample.[20-22] The condition must also be separated from primary lymphangiectasia, which is more common in children and in which the mucosa reveals focal malformations of the small lymphatic vessels. This topic and the overall subject of protein-losing enteropathy is covered in Chapter 29.

Respiratory System

Hypoxemia for whatever reason can facilitate the development of or worsen any ischemic injury of the intestines, and patients with chronic obstructive lung disease have an increased incidence of peptic ulcers of the duodenum.[23] The latter is thought to be mainly related to the appearance of hypercapnia, which results in the stimulation of excess gastric acid secretion.[24]

Some patients with bronchial carcinoid tumors and oat cell carcinomas develop a watery diarrhea, due to the release of serotonin and other ectopic hormones from the tumors, leading to hypermotility of the gut musculature and a reduced transit time.

Kidneys and Urinary System

Uremia

A variety of injuries affecting the gastrointestinal tract are commonly seen in patients with chronic renal disease,[25,26] including those who have received hemodialysis and renal allografts.[27-31] These are noted in about 60% of cases with uremia and include the appearance of mucosal and submucosal hemorrhages, ulcers, and segmental areas of enteritis and colitis. The hemorrhages are frequently multiple, are more often seen in the stomach and duodenum,[31-33] and are thought to be due to bleeding abnormalities such as platelet dysfunction that are present in patients with renal failure; a prominent telangiectasia has been noted in the gastric mucosa in some transplant patients.[34] Multiple small ulcers are also noted in the upper tract and small intestine[35]; whereas they tend to be solitary and larger in the colon, most occurring in the cecum.[36,37] There are probably multiple factors involved in the genesis of the ulcers,[28,32,33,38,39] including damage to the gastric mucosal barrier by urea, resulting in increased back diffusion of acid; secondary hyperparathyroidism, leading to increased acid secretion; and bacterial conversion of the urea in the gut lumen to ammonia, which might be irritating to the intestinal mucosa. Larger areas of hemorrhage and necrosis with variable inflammation may be seen in the intestines, and these lesions most closely resemble ischemic disease.[40-42] Pseudomembranes may also be present, but they tend to be larger than those seen in antibiotic-associated colitis, and a constant pathogen has not been identified in the uremic cases. There is no correlation between the occurrence of these various lesions and the type and duration of the renal disease or the severity of the renal failure.

The clinical presentation is dependent on the type and distribution of the lesions and includes some combination of bleeding, abdominal pain, and diarrhea. Most of the lesions regress upon treatment of the renal failure, but they may persist; complications include marked hemorrhage,[35,39] perforation,[41] and obstruction due to fibrous stricture formation. The histologic features of the uremic lesions are nonspecific, and the diagnosis is dependent on the compatible clinical information and on the exclusion of other causes.

Secondary Infections

Additional problems can develop in patients receiving immunosuppressive therapy for their renal disease or transplant and consist of opportunistic infections of the gut.[43] In the esophagus these are mainly due to herpes and candida[44]; and in the intestine they are due to these agents as well as cytomegalovirus,[45] other fungi,[4] and uncommon parasites such as *Cryptosporidium*[46] and *Strongyloides*.[47] Accordingly, when one encounters an ulcer or inflammatory condition of the intestine in a patient with chronic renal disease, the possible causes are the uremic lesion *per se*, ischemic disease, an opportunistic infection, and a drug effect. Mucosal biopsy can help in such cases in detecting the lesions and identifying the particular infectious agents.[21,22,48-51]

Diseases Common to the Kidneys and Gastrointestinal Tract

Both the kidneys and the gastrointestinal tract are involved in a variety of systemic disorders, and this combination is particularly prominent in those diseases with a vasculitic component[17,52] or with an infiltrative lesion such as amyloidosis.[53] Indeed, in cases where the major lesions are in the kidney, aspiration biopsy of the rectum is often chosen, because it is less traumatic, in looking for evidence of vasculitis[54,55] or amyloid deposits[56] in the submucosal vessels. The more common causes of the vasculitis affecting the smaller vessels of the two organs are lupus erythematosus,[57,58] rheumatoid arthritis,[59,60] and Henoch-Schönlein purpura.[61] In the hemolytic-uremic syndrome, there is often antecedent inflammatory disease of the intestinal tract characterized by the presence of marked edema and hemorrhages in the mucosa and wall.[62-65] These vascular lesions are presented in Chapter 12. An Ig-A type of glomerulonephritis has been noted in some patients with a chronic enteritis such as celiac disease,[66,67] and it is thought that this results from an increased circulation of the immunoglobulin and immune complexes.

Complications of Ureterosigmoidostomy

In infants with exstrophy of the urinary bladder and other obstructive lesions of the cloacogenic area, the ureters were formerly implanted into the sigmoid colon. This results in slight inflammation and crypt hyperplasia of the adjacent colonic mucosa and the occasional formation of small inflammatory polyps, but these changes typically have no clinical significance.[68,69] It has been demonstrated, however, that the colonic mucosa adjacent to the ureteral openings is exceptionally prone to the later development of neoplasms, including adenomas and adenocarcinoma.[69-75] The tumors usually appear in patients between the ages of 15 and 25, and they present either with rectal bleeding or, more often, with signs of ureteral obstruction. The gross and histologic features of the neoplasms are identical to those seen in the colon in general, and the prognosis after surgical resection is dependent on the presence and extent of invasion by the carcinoma. Since recognition of this complication, the procedure of ureterosigmoidostomy has no longer been employed and has been replaced by the creation of an ileal bladder in patients requiring diversion of the urinary system. In those cases in which the ureters are connected to the colon, it is recommended that the patient undergo periodic endoscopic examination with mucosal biopsy for epithelial dysplasia[76,77] (Figure 16-1). In this

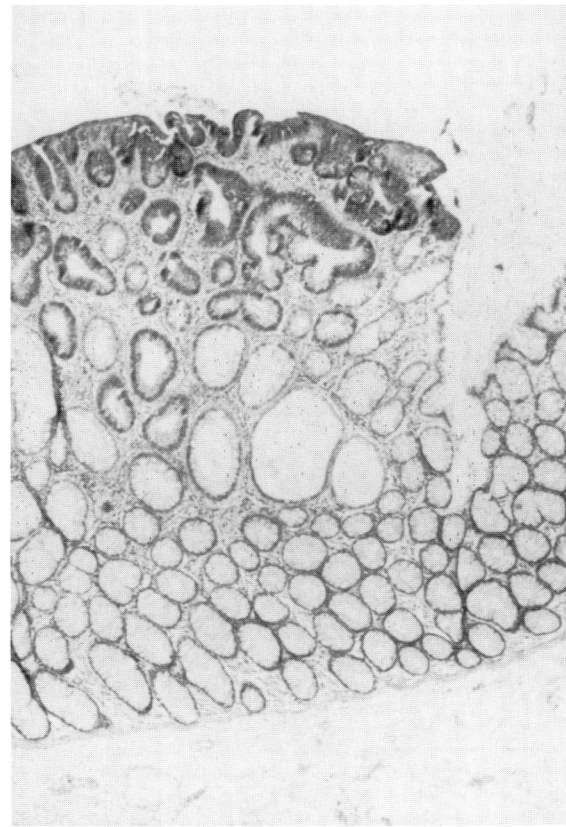

FIGURE 16-1. Colonic mucosal biopsy next to the ureteral orifice in patient with a ureteral implant in the sigmoid colon. There is a superficial focus of adenomatous epithelium (top left and center) representing glandular dysplasia. (H&E, × 100)

regard, we have observed unusual positions of the ureter such as in the transverse colon, and an early radiologic study of the urinary system should be obtained for determination of the exact location of the ureteral implants.

Hematologic System

Hemorrhagic Disorders

Patients with bleeding and coagulation disorders of all causes may have spontaneous hemorrhages in any part of the gastrointestinal tract, and it is estimated that this occurs sometime in the course of about 20% of patients with hemophilia.[1] The lesions in the primary bleeding disorders usually regress promptly, and examples of massive bleeding or obstruction from an intramural hematoma are rare.

Sickle Cell Anemia

Cases of sickle cell disease are prone to the development of ischemic lesions of the intestines,[78,79] which are more commonly located in the watershed area of the distal transverse colon and splenic flexure, and these are thought to result from or to be facilitated by the abnormal sickling and hyperviscosity of the blood. As in other instances of a sickle cell crisis, the intestinal disease is often precipitated by a state of dehydration in the patient. The lesions are usually superficial and respond to medical therapy, consisting of hydration and antibiotics; surgical resection is rarely needed. These effects on the intestine have not been described in other types of hemoglobinopathies.

Iron Deficiency Anemia

The rate of iron absorption is normally controlled by the concentration of protein-bound iron in the surface epithelial cells of the proximal small intestine.[80] In the common causes of iron deficiency anemia due to chronic bleeding or to poor nutrition, there is a reduction in the amount of iron in the surface cells leading to an increased rate of absorption, but this is not accompanied by any structural change at a histologic level. This control mechanism is altered in the abnormal state of primary hemochromatosis, in which iron absorption continues despite the saturated levels in the epithelial cells (see Hepatic Diseases for further details). The Plummer-Vinson syndrome is characterized by the presence of iron deficiency anemia and by squamous-lined webs in the proximal esophagus.[81] This esophagus may be prone to malignant transformation (see Chapter 18).

Megaloblastic Anemia

In the anemias due to deficiencies of folic acid and vitamin B_{12}, there is a characteristic megaloblastic proliferation of all actively growing cells, including not only the immature blood cells but also many of the epithelial cells in the body.[82] This epithelial change can be readily appreciated in the gut, particularly in the stomach and the small intestine.[83-86] Present in the gastric pits and in the intestinal crypts and lower part of the villi are large, rounded cells that contain enlarged and immature-appearing nuclei. These megaloblastic cells are distinguished from ordinary regeneration by the larger size of the nuclei and the relative diminution of the amount of cytoplasm, and from neoplastic cells by the lack of hyperchromasia and pleomorphism. There is also an overall reduction in the number of mitoses. The intestinal villi are often partially blunted in cases of folate deficiency, but it is not completely clear whether this alteration can itself lead to a functional problem or whether it is a sign of an underlying condition such as celiac or tropical sprue that is responsible for the nutrient problem. It is noteworthy, in this regard, that most patients with tropical sprue can be treated simply with folate, such treatment resulting in complete resolution of the histologic lesion as well as the functional effect.[87] This evolution may still reflect the normal healing in a patient who is no longer exposed to the primary cause of the disease (see Chapter 29). These changes in the small intestine are also observed in cases of vitamin B_{12} deficiency due to pernicious anemia and are not associated with clinical problems,[83] which supports the notion that they are of a secondary nature. There are no gross changes or complications that result from the megaloblastic proliferations, whatever the cause; and the lesions promptly regress upon correction of the folate or B_{12} deficiency. The pathology of primary pernicious anemia, which is due to gastritis of corpus mucosa, is covered in Chapter 20.

Polycythemia

In patients with primary polycythemia, thrombosis can occur in the portal and mesenteric veins, leading to hemorrhage and infarction of the intestines.[16] The abnormal clotting is probably related to the hyperviscosity of the blood that may be present in this condition. The lesions typically involve the deeper parts of the wall, including the muscularis propria and the serosal layer; and surgery is ordinarily required. The specific diagnosis is provided by the finding of venous thrombi in the mesenteric or mesocolic tissues that are not in the field of the infarction and by the pertinent clinical information. The features of hemorrhagic infarction of the intestine are otherwise nonspecific and can be seen in the advanced phase of ischemic disease due to reduced flow or occlusion of the arterial system and in other common causes of venous obstruction such as volvulus, hernia, and peritoneal adhesions (see Chapter 12).

Leukemia and Lymphoma

The gastrointestinal tract is commonly affected in cases of leukemia, either directly by the tumor or by the various complications of the disease and its therapy.[88-91] These are more often observed in the more aggressive types of leukemia, including the myelogenous and acute lymphoblastic forms. The tumor infiltrates are usually multifocal, can affect all parts of the alimentary tract, and are often concentrated in the submucosal and mucosal layers. They vary in size from microscopic foci to several centimeters in diameter, and the larger nodules have a soft tan to pale yellow appearance and are frequently associated with a central ulceration on the mucosal aspect. The lesions are often a source of hemorrhage into the lumen, and perforation of the bowel wall can occur when there is extensive necrosis, a circumstance that may be facilitated by treatment of the tumor; obstruction from the tumor itself is uncommon and more often is related to the effects of therapy leading to prominent edema or to fibrosis.

As a result of the leukemic infiltration and destruction of the marrow elements and of the potent therapeutic drugs used, secondary effects appear in many tissues of the body. These frequently involve all parts of the gastrointestinal tract and consist of fresh hemorrhages; toxic injuries,[92,93] which are more often noted in the small intestine (see Chapter 9); and increased infections with the common appearance of opportunistic types[94,95] and with unusual forms such as neutropenic colitis[96] (see Chapter 26). In addition, patients who have received bone marrow transplants may develop a graft-versus-host reaction,[97,98] resulting in inflammation and ulceration of the stomach and small intestine in the acute form[97-101] and more focal lesions of the proximal esophagus[102] and intestines[98,103] in the chronic type (see Chapter 14). Malignant lymphoma can involve the gastrointestinal tract in several forms, including primary tumors,[104,105] which may be solitary or diffuse, the latter more common in the small intestine, where they may cause a malabsorptive state[106,107]; contiguous spread from tumors arising in the mesenteric lymph nodes; and as part of a generalized dissemination.[108] This topic is covered in Chapter 14.

Endocrine System

Many of the effects noted in the gastrointestinal tract as a result of endocrine diseases involve changes in motility. This subject is presented in greater detail in Chapter 11.

Thyroid Diseases

Hyperthyroidism may be associated with hypermotility of the gut,[109-111] resulting in rapid gastric emptying,[112] reduced transit time, and the appearance of watery diarrhea or steatorrhea.[113] There are no constant structural changes in the mucosa and wall of the bowel,[114] and the functional effects are believed to be due to the rapid transit. In contrast, there is often a delay in gastric emptying and a reduced motility in hypothyroidism,[111,115,116] and severe cases may reveal edema and mild inflammation of the intestinal wall.[117] Patients often exhibit marked constipation, and this can favor the development of fecal impactions, megacolon, and rectal prolapse. Malabsorption may also occur and appears to be related to stasis and bacterial proliferation in the small intestine. The intestinal mucosa is usually normal; or there may be patchy inflammation in the jejunum, which is probably related to the excess bacteria.

A chronic atrophic gastritis with reduced acid secretion is seen in some cases of hypothyroidism and of thyroiditis, and these patients frequently have serum antibodies to both thyroglobulin and intrinsic factor.[118] Patients with medullary carcinoma of the thyroid, either isolated or as part of a multiple endocrine adenoma syndrome, may have prominent watery diarrhea.[119] There are no morphologic changes in the intestinal mucosa, and the diarrhea is thought to be due to the release of ectopic hormones from the tumor leading to hypermotility of the gut. In this regard, calcitonin, which is the natural hormone of these tumors, does not have a stimulatory effect on the bowel muscle.

Parathyroid Diseases

Patients with untreated hyperparathyroidism frequently have gastrointestinal symptoms, including nausea and vomiting, abdominal pain, and either diarrhea or constipation.[120-122] The effects are believed to be mainly due to hypercalcemia, which can lead to increased acid secretion, and peptic ulcers of the duodenum are seen in about 15% of cases.[123,124] Ectopic calcifications may also appear, but this is typically a microscopic finding and causes no clinical problem. Patients with hypoparathyroidism may develop malabsorption, which might be due to stagnant bowel. There is also a rare syndrome that includes hypoparathyroidism, Addison's disease, and atrophic gastritis.[125]

Adrenal Diseases

Patients with Addison's disease frequently present with a variety of gastrointestinal symptoms, including anorexia, weight loss, abdominal pain, and diarrhea, causing dehydration.[126] There are rare cases thought to have an immunologic basis, in which inflammatory lesions leading to atrophy are noted in the adrenal cortex and in other endocrine tissues, including the thyroid and parathyroid, and these are frequently associated with an atrophic gastritis.[118,125] Patients with pheochromocytoma often have nonspecific gastrointestinal symptoms. In addition, there are uncommon cases involving severe constipation, leading to megacolon, and enterocolitis that are thought to be due to the vasoconstrictive action of excess circulating catecholamines.[127]

Diabetes Mellitus

Changes in gastrointestinal structure and function are often noted in patients with diabetes mellitus,[128-132] and most are thought to be mediated by damage to the enteric nervous system. There is, however, no close correlation between the appearance of most of these effects and the duration and severity of the diabetes or the presence of a peripheral neuropathy. A decrease in the contractility of the esophageal musculature and a reduced pressure of the lower esophageal sphincter have been observed, but these do not usually have any clinical significance.[133] The stomach can become atonic, which can lead to poor emptying and marked dilation; this condition is seen more often in patients with decompensated disease.[134,135] If this condition is not corrected, there can be pressure damage, resulting in flattening and erosions of the mucosa, thinning of the wall, and potential perforation. The features of chronic gastritis affecting the proximal stomach have been noted in about two thirds of patients with diabetes,[136] and this is associated with reduced acid secretion, a decreased incidence of duodenal peptic ulcers,[137] and frank pernicious anemia in about 5% of cases. Whether the gastric disease is due to an immunologic injury, as in ordinary atrophic gastritis, or is the result of repeated episodes of gastric dilation is not known.

Patients with diabetes also experience periodic episodes of watery diarrhea and abdominal crampy pain.[128-132,138,139] This appears to be more common in young patients with the insulin-dependent form of diabetes; is often associated with other complications, including peripheral neuropathy; and is thought to be due to a motility disturbance. Steatorrhea and other signs of malabsorption can also develop. The possible causes include hypomotility of the small bowel, leading to stasis and bacterial proliferation; associated inflammation or tumor of the exocrine pancreas; and obstruction of the bile duct by gallstones. In addition, it has been suggested that celiac disease is more common in persons with diabetes,[140] but this is not certain. Patchy, nonspecific inflammatory changes have been noted in the small-intestinal mucosa, and these are probably related to the bowel stasis.[141–143] Although abnormalities are not typically seen in the ganglia and nerves of the intestinal wall by ordinary histologic examination, special studies employing silver stains have revealed changes in these neural structures in some cases.[138,144] This subject is covered in Chapter 11.

Reproductive System

Diseases of Contiguous Tissues

Because of its close proximity, lesions of the pelvic organs and tissues can have an impact on the intestinal tract, and the effects are most commonly noted in the sigmoid colon and rectum. Various inflammatory conditions and neoplasms of the uterine adnexa may compress or extend into the wall of the distal intestine, and prostatic carcinoma can directly invade the rectum. This may result in a localized obstruction or bleeding, the latter due either to pressure effects on the mucosa or to actual invasion of this layer by tumor. Mucosal biopsy can help in the determination and typing of the secondary cancers and in their distinction from primary intestinal lesions. It should be noted, however, that the histologic features of some of the pelvic tumors such as the mucinous types in the ovary can be very similar or identical to those of colonic lesions; the separation may depend on the results of immunocytochemical and ultrastructural studies and the gross distribution of the tumor. For example, prostatic carcinomas can usually be identified by the presence of prostate-specific antigen and the prostate fraction of acid phosphatase, and ovarian tumors may lack the characteristic terminal webs that are present in colonic adenocarcinomas. In addition, lesions may develop in the bowel as a result of radiation and drug therapy of genital tract cancers; these effects are described in Chapter 9. Endometriosis commonly affects the intestinal tract, and the lesions are most often present in the serosa and muscularis propria of the sigmoid colon and rectum,[145,146] where they may invoke a prominent fibrous tissue and smooth muscle response; this subject is covered in Chapter 28.

Effects of Pregnancy and Exogenous Hormones

Nausea and vomiting are characteristic symptoms of early pregnancy and are also noted in some patients who are taking exogenous estrogens or oral contraceptives. There are no structural changes in the gastrointestinal tract, and the effects are probably mediated through the nervous system. In addition, heartburn is commonly observed during pregnancy and is thought to be mainly due to the action of the hormones leading to a reduced lower esophageal sphincter pressure.[147] The expansion of the uterus, resulting in an increase of the intra-abdominal pressure, may be a contributing factor in the later stages of pregnancy. There is no evidence for suggesting that pregnancy is the cause of clinically significant peptic esophagitis, although it may worsen a pre-existing condition. Constipation is a frequent problem during the late stage of pregnancy and is related to pressure from the enlarged uterus and/or the ingestion of supplemental calcium medications. After multiple pregnancies with vaginal deliveries, there can develop damage to and weakening of the wall separating the posterior vagina and the rectum. This may lead to protrusion of the rectal wall into the vagina at the time of straining and result in intermittent episodes of constipation and fecal incontinence. There are no constant abnormalities noted in the rectal mucosa, and the prolapse can be readily corrected by surgery. Extensive clinical investigations have not revealed any deleterious effects of pregnancy on the course of patients with ulcerative colitis and Crohn's disease.[148] Other uncommon effects of increased estrogen levels may occur during pregnancy but are more often noted with sustained use of oral contraceptives or other exogenous hormones in older patients; these include the sporadic appearance of intestinal hemorrhages and inflammation[149,150] (see Chapter 9) and the promotion of thromboses.

Skin and Soft Tissues and Other Systemic Conditions

Skin Diseases

A variety of proliferative and bullous conditions of the skin may exceptionally involve the esophagus, usually the upper portion. These include pemphigus,[151] bullous pemphigoid,[152] epidermolysis bullosa,[153–157] and erythema multiforme.[158,159] Similarly, tumors of the epidermis and skin appendages can affect the anal canal and are presented in Chapter 34. Some patients with acrodermatitis enteropathica develop diarrhea in association with nonspecific inflammation of the small-intestinal mucosa [160] and inclusions in the Paneth cells.[161] The condition is thought to be due to zinc deficiency (see Chapter 29).

Dermatitis Herpetiformis

There is a strong association between dermatitis herpetiformis and celiac disease (see Chapter 29), probably due to genetic concordance.[162–164] In about two thirds of patients with the skin condition, abnormalities are noted in the mucosa of the proximal small intestine,[162–167] ranging from patchy blunting of villi to complete loss of villi. Severe cases show signs of malabsorption and respond to a gluten-free diet.[168–171] Most patients with the skin condition have no intestinal problems, however; and a jejunal mucosal biopsy should only be obtained in the symptomatic patients. It has been reported that the skin lesions may also regress on a gluten-free diet,[172] but this has not been firmly established. Recent studies have revealed a variant of dermatitis herpetiformis in which the cutaneous IgA deposition is in the form of a linear band at the epidermal-dermal junction, rather than its usual granular form at the tips of the dermal papillae. This subtype is referred to as linear-IgA bullous dermatosis, and limited studies have shown only minimal abnormalities in jejunal structure and no functional problems in these cases.[173]

Erythema Multiforme

Erythema multiforme is a common skin disorder that is characterized by the presence of multiple small red papules and vesicles and the histologic appearance of lymphocytic infiltrates around small vessels in the upper dermis, together with a variable degree of epidermal necrosis. The disease is called the Stevens-Johnson syndrome when it affects mucosal surfaces such as the lips, oral cavity, and conjunctiva. There may also be rare involvement of the alimentary tract, most cases occcurring in the distal half of the esophagus.[158,159] Present on the surface of the esophageal mucosa are small white patches, ranging in size from 2 to 5 mm in diameter, that resemble monilial infection. Histologic examination reveals a superficial ulceration and intraepithelial inflammation and individual cell necrosis of the adjacent intact squamous epithelium. Lesions have been noted exceptionally in the mucosa of the small and large intestines and reveal foci of crypt epithelial destruction with mononuclear inflammatory cells but a paucity of neutrophils in the lamina propria.[51,174] Patients may present with dysphagia with the esophageal lesion and abdominal pain and bloody diarrhea with intestinal disease. The lesions typically regress, and local complications in the gut have not been observed.

Köhlmeier-Degos Disease

This is a rare disorder characterized by the appearance of multiple vasculitic lesions of the skin, referred to as malignant atrophic papulosis, and subsequent spread to many other tissues of the body.[175-177] Lesions of the intestines have been noted in about 60% of cases and consist of fibrinoid necrosis of small arteries and veins, together with a predominantly lymphocytic infiltrate around the vessels in the early stage and the development of intimal proliferation and organized thrombi in advanced cases. This results in areas of ischemic necrosis and ulceration of the intestine, which often proceeds to perforation of the bowel.

Soft Tissue Diseases

There are several congenital and acquired disorders with primary effects in the connective tissues, such as the Ehlers-Danlos syndrome,[178-179] pseudoxanthoma elasticum,[180,181] Fabry's disease,[182-186] systemic sclerosis,[187-191] mixed connective tissue disease,[192] and visceral myopathies.[192-195] These can damage the musculature of the various parts of the alimentary tract. In particular, involvement with systemic sclerosis is common, and the effects include esophageal dysmotility and injury to the lower esophageal sphincter, which favor the development of peptic esophagitis; stasis of the small intestine, leading to bacterial proliferation and steatorrhea; and the appearance of megacolon.[196,197] All of these connective tissue disorders promote hypomotility and the formation of diverticula,[186,198,199] which is especially prominent in the small intestine. In addition, the gut may uncommonly be affected in systemic cases of myositis[200,201] and some degenerative diseases of the skeletal muscles.[202-203] This subject is covered in Chapter 11. The gut is also a common target organ for the effects of the systemic vasculitides,[17] such as lupus erythematosus[57,58,204,205] and periarteritis nodosum.[206,207] These conditions are discussed in Chapter 12.

Rheumatoid Arthritis

Gastrointestinal abnormalities are observed in about one quarter of the patients with long-standing rheumatoid arthritis, and these are due mostly to the occurrence of a necrotizing vasculitis affecting the medium-sized and small arteries.[59,66,208-212] The vascular lesions are mild and cause no clinical problems in most cases,[213] but they can lead to the development of mucosal hemorrhages, focal ulcers, and exceptionally to larger areas of infarction, mainly of the intestines.[60,201] Because the pathologic features are otherwise nonspecific, the diagnosis is dependent on the clinical information and on the exclusion of other causes of vasculitis. Additional problems may appear that are related to the long-term use of medications, including ulcerations of the stomach and duodenum from aspirin,[214] corticosteroids,[215] and other anti-inflammatory agents,[9] and an enteritis or colitis from gold salts[216-220] (see Chapter 9). Patients with rheumatoid arthritis are also prone to the formation of secondary amyloidosis, and the deposits frequently involve the gastrointestinal tract. Rectal biopsies are often obtained in cases with suspected vasculitis or amyloidosis, and these as well as biopsies from other sites should be of the larger aspiration type to ensure an adequate sample of submucosa.[54,55]

Reactive Arthritis

In some patients presenting with nonspecific arthritis, endoscopy has revealed patchy areas of inflammation and small erosions in the mucosa of the colon and distal ileum that are not associated with drug therapy or with significant intestinal symptoms.[221] Gross lesions were noted in 30% and microscopic alterations of acute and chronic inflammation in 61% of cases of seronegative spondylarthropathy.[222] It was suggested that the gut disease might be the primary event, but its cause is not known. As yet, these cases have not evolved into the classic forms of idiopathic inflammatory bowel disease.

Sjögren's Syndrome

Abnormalities of the alimentary tract are occasionally noted in patients with the Sjögren's syndrome,[223] and the effects are more common in the esophagus and stomach. It is important to separate the changes that are related to the glandular inflammation from those of systemic sclerosis, which may coexist in these patients. There is commonly present an atrophy and chronic inflammation of the esophageal glands; this, together with similar effects in the salivary glands and oral cavity, may lead to dysphagia. Some cases reveal a reduced esophageal mobility, but this is more prominent in patients with systemic sclerosis. An atrophic gastritis with reduced gastric acid secretions and the presence of parietal cell antibodies is observed in most cases of Sjögren's syndrome. Dysfunction of the intestinal muscle and the development of steatorrhea are seen only in patients with associated systemic sclerosis. There are also isolated reports of celiac disease, enteritis and colitis, that are thought to have a vasculitic basis, and of colonic ulcers in patients with the syndrome.

Pancreas, Biliary Tract, and Liver

Cystic Fibrosis

This condition, also referred to as mucoviscidosis, is characterized by the presence of abnormally viscid mucus that causes the obstruction of small ducts, with major effects noted in the bronchi and lungs and in the pancreas.[224] There is a tendency for multiple infections and the development of chronic inflammatory disease, and steatorrhea often appears as a consequence of chronic pancreatitis and maldigestion of lipids. This effect may be enhanced by biliary obstruction, leading to a reduction of bile salts; patients with cystic fibrosis also have an increased incidence of gallstones. Lesions are less commonly noted in other ducts and glands, including the bile ductules in the liver and the intestinal mucosa.

Meconium ileus is a complication noted mainly in newborns and infants and consists of one or more areas of obstruction of the small intestine due to a partially solidified admixture of the thick mucus and fecal contents.[225] The lesions are more common in the distal half of the small intestine, can extend from one to several centimeters in length, and reveal evidence of mucosal damage that is probably due to a pressure effect of the luminal mass. Histologic features include hemorrhage and necrosis of the mucosa, which may slough and be followed by a stage of granulation tissue and the presence of hardened and crystalline fecal material, which frequently evokes a foreign body giant cell reaction. It is probable that superficial lesions limited to the mucosa are capable of complete regression. The ulcers can extend deep into the submucosa and the muscularis propria, however, and be associated with marked fibrosis, leading to permanent stricture formation. Indeed, it is believed that cystic fibrosis may be a major cause of atresias of the jejunum.[226]

A prominence of luminal mucus and enlarged goblet cells may occasionally be seen in older children with the disease, and this can lead to distention and obstruction of narrow regions such as the appendix (see Chapter 33). It had been considered that the size of the goblet mucous cells, as visualized in small-intestinal and colonic mucosal biopsies, might serve as a test for the diagnosis of cystic fibrosis[227,228]; but this has not succeeded because there is too much variability and considerable overlap with specimens obtained from control patients without the disease.[229]

Other Pancreatic and Biliary Diseases

Lipid maldigestion and steatorrhea are commonly seen in cases of long-standing chronic pancreatitis and of pancreatic ductal obstruction due to tumor or calculi. This effect is due simply to the reduced secretion or excretion of the pancreatic enzymes and is associated in very severe cases with maldigestion of proteins and carbohydrates as well. The mucosa of the small intestine is usually normal but may show patchy areas of inflammation, which are probably the result of pooling of the undigested nutrients and secondary bacterial proliferation. Obstruction of the common bile duct for any reason can lead to a reduction in the excretion of bile salts and also favor the development of steatorrhea. The fat maldigestion that occurs in these various disorders can further result in a deficiency of vitamin K and the appearance of fresh hemorrhages in the gastrointestinal tract. A variety of endocrine tumors of the pancreas, including those that produce gastrin, glucagon, and somatostatin, can affect the gastrointestinal tract; this subject is covered in Chapter 13.

Hepatic Diseases

Patients with acute liver disease such as viral hepatitis typically present with nausea, vomiting, and abdominal pain. These represent constitutional symptoms, and there are no alterations observed in the gastrointestinal tract. Disorders associated with chronic cholestasis may develop steatorrhea, which is probably related to a decrease in excretion of the bile salts by the liver. This effect may be seen in any type of cirrhosis but is a more prominent feature in cases of primary biliary cirrhosis. There also appears to be an increased frequency of celiac disease in patients with primary biliary cirrhosis.[230] Hemorrhages in all parts of the gastrointestinal tract, ranging from scattered petechiae to extensive bleeding, are often noted in patients with liver disease. These are seen mainly in cases of acute or chronic disease with extensive hepatic necrosis and are related to a decrease in the synthesis of clotting factors such as prothrombin. A reduction in platelets, which occurs in patients with sustained portal hypertension and hypersplenism and in some patients with circulating antibodies to the thrombocytes, can also contribute to the formation of gut hemorrhages. An increase in

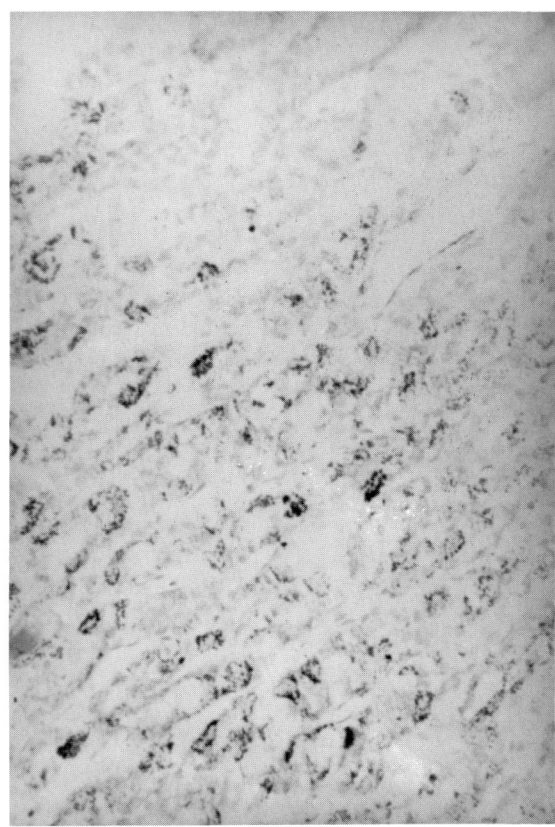

FIGURE 16–2. Gastric corpus mucosa in case of hemochromatosis, showing marked deposition of iron in the parietal cells. (Prussian blue reaction for iron, × 250)

major cause, alcoholism, including esophageal and gastric varices, the Mallory-Weiss tear of the esophagogastric junction, gastritis, and portal venous thrombosis leading to bowel infarction.

Hemochromatosis

In the advanced stage of both the primary and secondary forms of hemochromatosis, iron deposits are noted in the parenchymal cells throughout the body. These are evident in the epithelial cells of the gut and appear to be especially prominent in the parietal cells of the stomach,[231] but they are not associated with any sign of injury (Figure 16–2). There is also no structural change to account for the increased rate of iron absorption by the small intestine in the primary type.[80,232] Hemosiderin deposits are frequently noted within the macrophages in the lamina propria of the normal intestine,[233] and these are increased in patients with hemosiderosis and with the secondary form of hemochromatosis (Figure 16–3).

VITAMIN DISORDERS

Symptoms referable to multiple vitamin deficiencies are often noted in the various malabsorptive disorders.[234] These disorders are covered in Chapter 29.

Fat-Soluble Vitamins

Vitamin K Deficiency

A deficiency in vitamin K for whatever reason leads to a decrease in the formation of prothrombin and other essential clotting factors by the liver, and this can result in the appearance of fresh hemorrhages in all parts of the body.[235] The effects on the gastrointestinal tract are variable and often unpredictable, and the le-

the incidence of duodenal peptic ulcers is observed in patients with cirrhosis, particularly in those who have had a portacaval shunt, and is thought to be due to reduced degradation of gastric secretagogues such as histamine and gastrin. Several other disorders of the gastrointestinal tract are attributed to cirrhosis and its

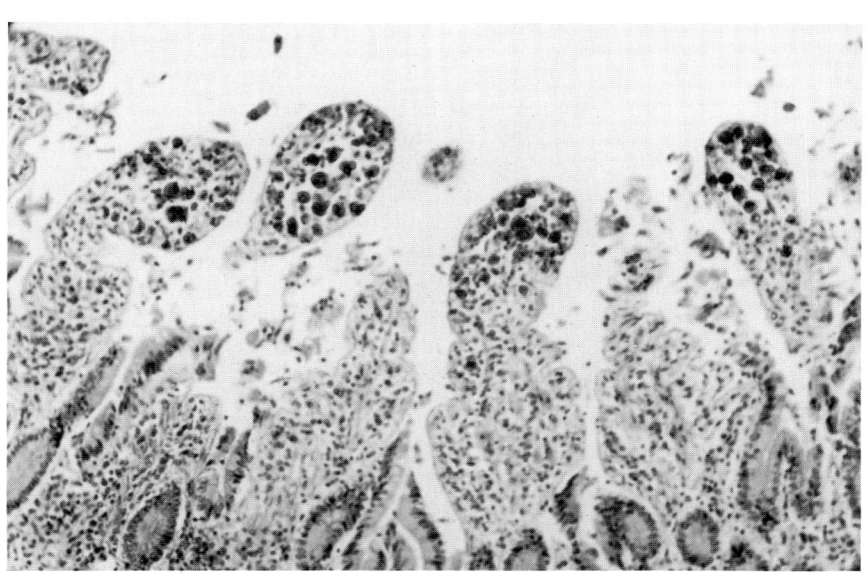

FIGURE 16–3. Jejunal mucosa in case of hemosiderosis. There are numerous clumps of hemosiderin in the macrophages, located within the lamina propria of the villi. (H&E, × 100)

sions can occur in any part of the tract and range from focal petechiae of the mucosal and serosal surfaces to larger areas of hemorrhage with extensive bleeding into the gut lumen. There are no special features to permit their distinction from other causes of spontaneous hemorrhage in the bowel, and the diagnosis relies on the demonstration of a condition that could cause the vitamin depletion and on the exclusion of other causes of hypoprothrombinemia. The hemorrhages typically regress upon correction of the vitamin disorder, and complications such as ulceration, fibrous stricture, and perforation of the bowel are not observed. Residual foci of hemosiderin-filled macrophages may persist in the tissues for a short period of time but eventually disappear; the finding of such macrophages in the lamina propria is not diagnostic, because they may also be seen in normal persons.

Disorders of Other Fat-Soluble Vitamins

It has been suggested that the brown bowel syndrome, which is characterized by the deposition of a lipofuscin type of pigment in the intestinal wall, might be caused by a deficiency in vitamin E, but this has not been clearly established (see Depositions). Deficiencies in vitamins A and D cause no direct effects on the gastrointestinal tract. Hypervitaminosis D may be associated with symptoms that are largely related to the upper tract and that are thought to be due to hypercalcemia and its stimulatory effect on gastric acid secretion.

Water-Soluble Vitamins

Pellagra

This disorder of niacin deficiency is usually due to a decrease in oral intake and is much more prevalent in developing countries. It is also occasionally noted in persons with poor or unusual nutritional habits such as alcoholics, those who follow food fads, and the elderly. The deficiency leads to an interference with the normal renewal of the epithelia in many parts of the body, and the most marked effects are noted in the skin, oral cavity, and intestinal tract.[236] The result is focal ulcers or more extensive and confluent lesions of the small intestine and colon, and patients typically present with abdominal pain and bloody diarrhea. The character of the inflammation is nonspecific, and the intact mucosa of the small intestine may show milder changes in the form of villous shortening and increased inflammatory cells.[237] It is often difficult, however, to distinguish these morphologic features from those due to concurrent intestinal infections, which are also commonly observed in persons from poor societies. Indeed, both conditions may coexist in the same patient. Furthermore, the effects in pellagra may be compounded by the presence of deficiencies of other B vitamins and by the development of secondary infections, which are often due to opportunistic agents. The lesions are shallow and resolve with specific vitamin therapy unless there is associated infection or tropical sprue,[87,238] and local complications are rare. The diagnosis of pellagra is often initially overlooked in Western countries because of its relative rarity and the nonspecific nature of the lesions. It depends on the recognition of other features of the disease, including dermatitis and mental confusion; the exclusion of infections and other known causes of intestinal lesions; and ultimately the response to treatment with niacin.

Disorders of Other Water-Soluble Vitamins

Deficiencies of thiamine, riboflavin, and pyridoxine do not cause direct injury to the gastrointestinal tract but may worsen the intestinal lesions of pellagra. Cases of folic acid and B_{12} deficiency are associated with a megaloblastic proliferation of the epithelial cells that is most prominent in the stomach and small intestine.[83–86] This subject is presented in the section on diseases of the hematologic system. The features of scurvy, due to vitamin C deficiency, include the appearance of hemorrhages and delay in wound healing, but prominent effects in the gastrointestinal tract are rare.

DEPOSITIONS

The term *depositions* is used to signify the presence in the tissues of an excessive amount of a normal or endogenous component of the body or the appearance

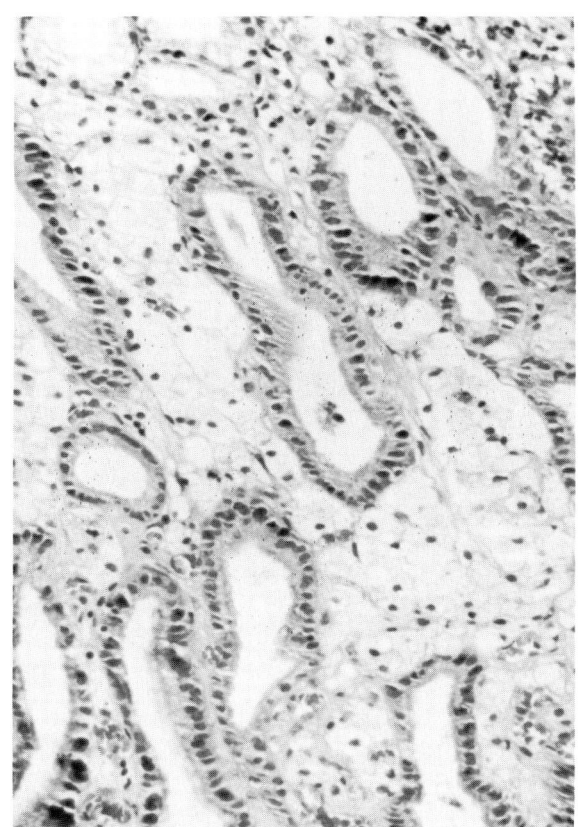

FIGURE 16–4. Gastric xanthoma, showing numerous finely vacuolated (foamy) macrophages within the lamina propria. The epithelium is intact. (H&E, × 250)

of an abnormal or exogenous substance. The diseases involved are often referred to as storage disorders, particularly when they have an hereditary basis. The deposited materials are variable and include examples of proteins, lipids, carbohydrates, minerals, and pigments. Some of these conditions are unique to the gastrointestinal tract, but most can affect many tissues in the body. The deposits may be an incidental finding in the gut; yet this area can serve as an accessible site for their diagnosis, or they may lead to significant disease of the alimentary tract.

Conditions That May Simulate Storage Diseases

In the consideration of a storage disease, it is necessary to exclude more common conditions such as localized xanthomatous reactions[239-241] and clusters of muciphages[49,242] in the lamina propria. Xanthomas or xanthelasmas represent the accumulation of neural lipid and cholesterol within macrophages and are usually visualized grossly as tiny yellow nodules or streaks on the mucosal surface (Figure 16–4). They are thought to be a consequence of mucosal hemorrhage in severe inflammatory diseases and are seen most often in the stomach,[239] particularly the proximal remnant after surgery for peptic ulcer disease, and in the duodenum.[241] Foamy macrophages due to the inclusion of organisms with prominent lipid capsules are also seen in Whipple's disease and in infection with *Mycobacterium avium-intracellulare*[243] (Figure 16–5).

Muciphages are macrophages that contain mucus in their cytoplasm and are observed most frequently in the large intestine.[242] Although it was formerly thought that the appearance of muciphages was a sequela of laxative use or of a prior inflammatory condition, they are seen almost invariably in the lamina propria of normal persons of all ages (Figure 16–6). The vacuoles in muciphages tend to be large and irregularly shaped, and their nature is identified readily by the periodic acid-Schiff (PAS) reaction and other stains for mucus. Exceptionally, the cells of a granular cell tumor (so-called "myoblastoma") may be mistaken for enlarged macrophages. They have a distinctly granular-appear-

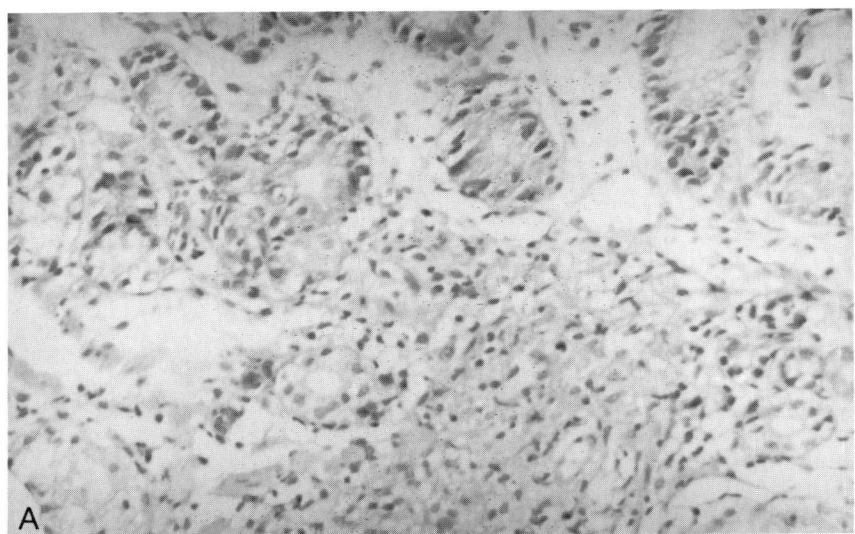
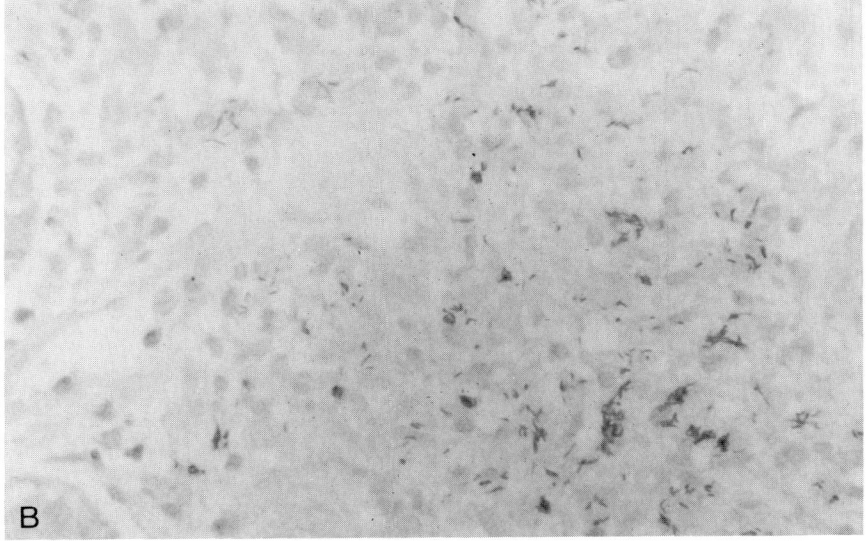

FIGURE 16–5. *A*, Gastric mucosa in case of acquired immunodeficiency syndrome. A collection of enlarged, slightly vacuolated macrophages is present in the lower right portion. (H&E, × 400) *B*, Same tissue as in *A*, showing many acid-fast bacilli (of *Mycobacterium avium* complex), both within macrophages and lying free in the lamina propria. (Ziehl-Nielson stain, × 400)

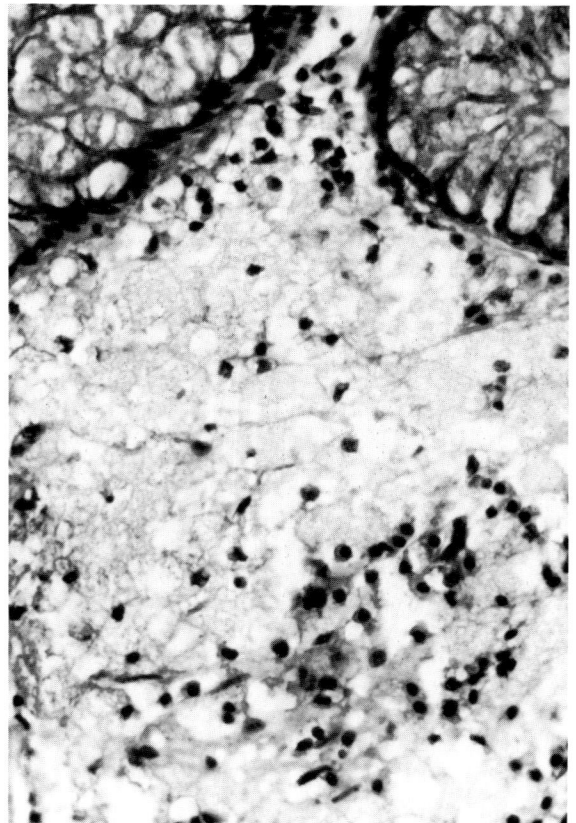

FIGURE 16-6. Colonic mucosa, revealing a large cluster of mucin-filled macrophages (muciphages) in the lamina propria, just beneath the surface epithelium in this example. The cytoplasmic vacuoles are coarser than in those due to lipids. (PAS, × 400)

ing cytoplasm without vacuoles and stain faintly with the PAS reaction. The characteristics of pigmented macrophages are discussed in the section on lipid pigment disorders. In this regard, an increase in macrophages containing a lipofuscin-type pigment in the lamina propria is often present in patients with chronic granulomatous disease; the pigment is restricted to these cells, and there may be other signs of the disease in the form of inflammation and granulomas.

Lipoprotein Disorders

Tangier Disease

This is characterized by a reduction in the serum levels of the high-density alpha-lipoproteins and of cholesterol and by the deposition of cholesterol esters in the phagocytic cells of several organs, including the liver, spleen, bone marrow, lymph nodes, and gut.[244] The patients are able to synthesize the apoproteins in the intestinal epithelium and to form chylomicrons, but there appears to be a defect in its catabolism.[245] The patient may present with hepatosplenomegaly, signs of a peripheral neuropathy, and occasional diarrhea. There is no steatorrhea, because alpha-lipoproteins are not involved in lipid absorption. Lesions are noted in the small intestine and colon and consist of tiny yellow nodules, less than a few millimeters in diameter, on the mucosal surface. Histologic study reveals finely vacuolated, lipid-laden macrophages and some free lipid in the lamina propria.[246,247] Because the identical appearance can be seen in any xanthomatous lesion, the specific diagnosis of Tangier disease depends on the blood lipid findings and the other clinical features. Muciphages are commonly present in the lamina propria of the large intestine in normal persons, and these are readily distinguished by their coarser vacuoles and positive reactions for mucin in the cytoplasm. Lipid-filled macrophages may also be seen in other storage diseases, such as the glycolipid disorders, but these cases usually reveal deposits in other mesenchymal elements and in nerves as well.

Abetalipoproteinemia

This disease is caused by a failure to form beta-lipoproteins, which are required for optimal absorption of lipids in the gut, resulting in their absence in the blood as well as a marked reduction in the levels of triglycerides and a general diminution in other lipids.[248,249] Additional features include the presence of steatorrhea, which usually begins in early childhood; acantholytic red blood cells due to defects in the lipid membrane; and neurologic lesions involving the cerebellum, basal ganglia, retina, and peripheral nerves.[250] The patients are capable of normal intraluminal digestion of lipids, the transport of triglycerides and monoglycerides, and their re-esterification within the absorptive cells of the small intestine. The defect lies in the inability to form normal chylomicrons, and the lipids are not excreted from the epithelial cells into the lymphatics. The structural alterations in the gastrointestinal tract are limited to the small intestine, and most of the information has been based on studies of jejunal mucosal biopsies.[251-253] The villi are of normal dimensions, but there is a striking accumulation of lipid within the covering absorptive cells, and the mucosal lymphatics are collapsed (Figure 16-7). The lipid is seen as rounded vacuoles of irregular size, and their nature can be confirmed by fat stains such as oil red O on nondehydrated histologic sections and by ultrastructural study. The appearance of the villous epithelial cells is similar to that in a normal person after a recent lipid-rich meal, but the biopsies are obtained in fasted patients. There is no evidence of damage to the epithelial cells or of other abnormalities in the mucosa. The diagnosis is determined by the distinctive blood lipid and other clinical features, and small-intestinal biopsy is mostly done for investigative purposes. Since lipid absorption through the portal venous route appears to be unaffected, medium chain triglycerides can be used in the treatment.

Glycolipid Storage Diseases

There are several inherited disorders of lipid and carbohydrate metabolism that are associated with depos-

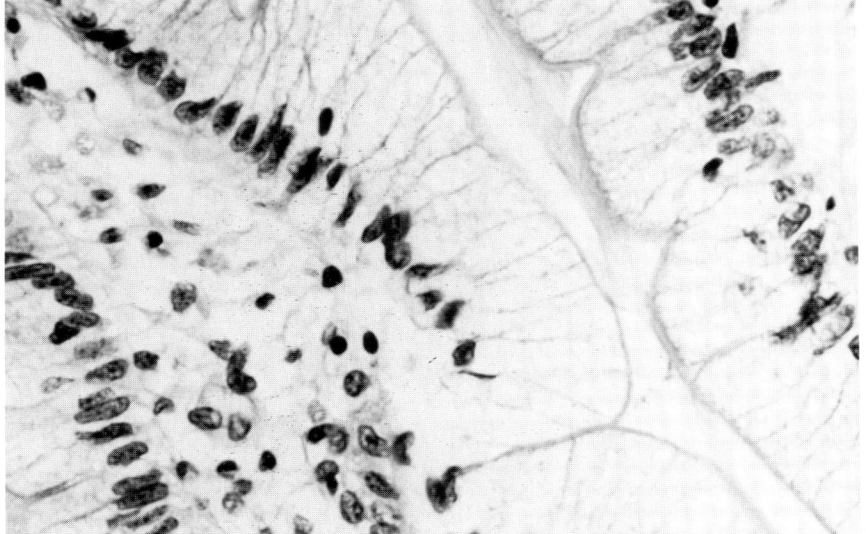

FIGURE 16–7. Jejunal mucosa in case of abetalipoproteinemia. There is a marked clearness of the cytoplasm of the surface absorptive cells due to the presence of many closely packed fine vacuoles, representing the retained triglycerides within these cells. The epithelium is intact, and there is no evidence of degeneration of the absorptive cells. (H&E, × 400)

its of substances in many tissues of the body[254,255]; and the materials are most often localized in the phagocytic cells, other mesenchymal cells, and neurones (Table 16–1). Glycolipid diseases are rare, usually due to deficiencies of lysosomal enzymes, and mostly transmitted as autosomal recessive conditions. Although involvement of the gastrointestinal tract is often present, the lesions are typically small and are usually not productive of local problems in the gut.[256] In the examination of intestinal biopsies of these storage diseases with depositions in the macrophages and nervous tissue elements, the appearance at light microscopy may be relatively nonspecific.[257,258] The macrophages most often reveal a foamy cytoplasm due to the presence of numerous closely packed small vacuoles, and the identification of the specific contents usually requires other techniques such as histochemical and ultrastructural studies.[259] Indeed, because of the nonspecificity of the results obtained with intestinal biopsies, these have been largely supplanted by other procedures for the purpose of the primary diagnosis.[260] Studies of the specific enzyme content of circulating leukocytes and of biopsies of the skin, conjunctiva and skeletal muscles have been employed.[51,261]

Gangliosidosis[262–264]

Prominent lipid deposits have been observed in rectal biopsies from patients with GM gangliosidosis, β-galactosidase-neuraminidase deficiency, Tay-Sachs disease, and Sandhoff's disease. Lipid bodies, both free in the cytoplasm or as membrane-bound cytosomes,

Table 16–1 STORAGE DISEASES OF GASTROINTESTINAL TRACT: NATURE AND LOCALIZATION OF DEPOSITS

		Location of Deposit§			
Disorder	Chemical	*Macrophage*	*Muscle*	*Nerve/Ganglia*	*Other¶*
Glycolipids					
Gangliosidosis*	Ganglioside	0	0	+	+
Metachromatic leukoencephalopathy	Sulfatide	+	0	0	rare
Fabry's disease	Ceramide trihexoside	+	+	+	+
Niemann-Pick	Sphingomyelin	+	+	+	+
I-cell disease	Mucolipid	0	0	rare	+
Lipid pigments					
Melanosis	Lipofuscin	++	0	0	0
Neuronal forms†	Lipofuscin	++	+	rare	+
Brown bowel disease	Lipofuscin	++	++	+	+
Other					
Wolman's disease	Cholesterol ester	+	0	0	0
Mucopolysaccharidosis‡	Heparin and other sulfates	0	0	0	+
Mannosidosis	Oligosaccharides	+	+	+	+
Cystinosis	Cystine	+	0	0	0

*Includes GM_1 and GM_2 (Tay-Sachs and Sandhoff) types.
†Changes most marked in infantile type (Batten's) and rare in adult form (Kufs').
‡Includes Hurler (I), Hunter (II), and Sanfilippo (III) types.
§Present (++ or +), rare, or absent (0).
¶Other mesenchymal elements, including Schwann cells, fibroblasts, and endothelial cells.

are seen in unmyelinated axons, Schwann cells, endothelial cells, fibroblasts, and plasma cells.[259] The cytosomes range in size from 0.3 to 1.0 µm in diameter. There are no lipid deposits in the muscle cells or in the macrophages. The lipid deposition is probably present in other parts of the gastrointestinal tract but is not associated with any clinical problems.

Sulfatidosis

In metachromatic leukoencephalopathy, free lipid bodies without cytosomes are present in the cytoplasm of Schwann cells.[259] The macrophages in the lamina propria may contain inclusions that stain with toluidine blue and other metachromatic stains.[254,257,258] There is usually no involvement of other mesenchymal cells or of axons, and gastrointestinal symptoms are typically absent.

Fabry's Disease

Fabry's disease is a sex-linked lysosomal storage disease affecting males, with major involvement of the skin, kidneys, heart, and nervous system.[182] Mild gastrointestinal symptoms are noted in most patients and male family members and appear to be related to reduced motility.[183,184] Uncommonly, there may develop delayed gastric emptying leading to early satiety and bacterial proliferation in the small intestine, resulting in more marked diarrhea and steatorrhea. It has also been demonstrated that the abnormal deposition can cause weakening of the muscularis propria and favor the formation of small-bowel diverticula.[186] Abundant lipid deposits are noted in many tissue elements of the gut, including macrophages, endothelial cells, smooth muscle, ganglia, axons, and Schwann cells.[185,265] See Chapter 11 for further details.

Niemann-Pick Disease

Lipid bodies are often present in macrophages, other mesenchymal cells, and the ganglia of the gut, but motility problems are only rarely observed.[259,266] The deposits range in size from 0.2 to 1.7 µm in diameter and have a variable appearance, including homogeneous and laminated bodies and those with a central lucency.

Mucolipidosis

Lipid bodies and enlarged lysosomes have been noted in Schwann cells, fibroblasts, and endothelial cells of patients with I-cell disease.[259] There is only rare involvement of axons and no alteration of the ganglia or macrophages. Gastrointestinal disease does not develop.

Lipid Pigment Disorders

Ceroid or lipofuscin pigment represents the undigesible residue of lipid oxidation and peroxidation reactions within the cells. The pigment is not affected by the dehydration procedures and reacts with the Sudan fat stains in paraffin-embedded sections. It also stains with acid-fast stains and with the PAS reaction and has a bright yellow autofluorescence. This substance is often referred to as "wear and tear" pigment and accumulates in the parenchymal cells of the body in direct relation to aging. Scattered macrophages containing lipofuscin pigments are seen in the lamina propria of normal persons.[267,268] Conditions associated with increased deposition of these pigments or with their appearance in abnormal locations have been termed ceroidosis or lipofuscinosis. The presence of increased macrophages containing a lipofuscin-type pigment in the lamina propria has also been noted in cases of chronic granulomatous disease.

Neuronal Ceroid Lipofuscinosis

Neuronal ceroid lipofuscinoses are rare lysosomal storage diseases and include the infantile and juvenile forms of Batten's disease and the adult type of Kufs' disease. They are characterized by the deposition of pigment in many cells of the body, with major involvement of the central nervous system and retina, and the changes are most marked in the infantile type. Because the particular enzyme deficiency is not known, the diagnosis often depends on biopsies, including those of skeletal muscle[261] and the rectum.[269] There is prominent pigment deposition within the macrophages of the lamina propria, which can be readily detected by light microscopy; in comparison with the normal state, the macrophages occur in clusters and the granules appear larger and coarser. Lesser amounts of pigment are seen in the Schwann cells, muscle cells, and endothelial cells. There is only rare involvement of the axons, and the ganglia are uninvolved. Electron microscopy reveals lipid bodies of variable density and configuration and membrane-bound cytosomes that range up to 3.5 µm in diameter. Similar distribution of the pigment but of lesser concentration is noted in the juvenile type, whereas the adult form shows sparse pigment only in the neurons. The cause of the lipofuscin deposition in these disorders is not known, and the structural findings are not entirely specific. Ceroid deposits are seen in macrophages in patients with chronic granulomatous disease and in melanosis coli, and more widespread pigment is noted in the brown bowel syndrome. The diagnoses of Batten's and Kufs' diseases are dependent on the compatible clinical features and are aided by the ultrastructural characteristics. Symptoms referable to the gastrointestinal tract do not occur.

Brown Bowel Syndrome

This is a rare, acquired disorder that is characterized by the marked deposition of ceroid or lipofuscin pigment in the bowel muscle, leading to the appearance of dark brown tissues.[270–273] It is most commonly observed in the small intestine but may affect the stomach and colon and, exceptionally, the entire tract. This condition is typically seen in association with a variety of malabsorptive disorders,[272,274,275] including cystic fibrosis, celiac disease, biliary cirrhosis, biliary atresia, and Crohn's disease, and is thought to be a consequence of vitamin E deficiency.[276] This vitamin, α-tocopherol, is an antioxidant, and it is postulated that its absence may promote an increase in lipid oxidation and the excess formation of the lipofuscin pigment. It is not clear, however, why the bowel condition should be so infrequent in view of the common occurrence of malabsorption of fat-soluble vitamins in the underlying diseases. There are usually no clinical problems that are directly related to the brown bowel, although a decrease in contractibility has been rarely observed. The pigment deposition is most prominent in the smooth muscle cells of the muscularis propria, and lesser amounts are seen in the macrophages, ganglia, nerves, and vessel walls. The staining characteristics are typical for lipofuscin and include positive reactions with Sudan black in dehydrated sections, with acid-fast stains, and with the PAS technique. The pigment exhibits a bright yellow autofluorescence and does not react with stains for iron or other minerals. Ultrastructural studies have revealed that the lipid pigment is concentrated in the perinuclear Golgi region of the muscle cells.[272,277] Enlarged and deformed mitochondria are also noted, and it has been suggested that an alteration in these organelles may be important in the genesis of the pigment lesion.[271,277] A lipofuscin deposition may be seen in macrophages of normal persons and of patients with melanosis coli and chronic granulomatous disease, and more widespread distribution in other mesenchymal cells and nerves is noted in Batten's disease. None of these other conditions reveals the extreme deposition in the muscle, however, which is diagnostic of the brown bowel syndrome.

Melanosis Coli

This is characterized by the presence of a lipofuscin-like pigment in the macrophages of the lamina propria throughout the rectum, colon, and appendix.[278] The condition is described in the section on miscellaneous inflammatory disorders of the colon in Chapter 28.

Other Storage Diseases

Wolman's Disease

Wolman's disease is due to a deficiency in lysosomal acid phosphatase and is characterized by the appearance of increased serum cholesterol and enlargement of the liver and spleen.[279] Deposits of cholesterol esters are located in the lymphoid tissues and phagocytic cells, including the macrophages in the lamina propria of the gastrointestinal tract.[280] There are no lipid deposits in the other mesenchymal cells or neurons in the gut wall, and gastrointestinal symptoms are not present. Similar lesions of cholesterol deposits limited to the macrophages may be seen in localized xanthomatous reactions, which are more common in the stomach, and in Tangier disease; and the diagnosis of Wolman's disease is based on the blood lipid findings and on the determination of the specific enzyme deficiency in leukocytes.

Mucopolysaccharidosis

Deposits of heparin sulfate have been described in rectal biopsies of patients with mucopolysaccharidosis, including the Hurler's, Hunter's, and Sanfilippo's types.[259,281] Membrane-bound vacuoles are noted in fibroblasts, plasma cells, endothelial cells, and occasional Schwann cells; but they appear to be absent in muscle, nerves, ganglia, and macrophages. Most of the vacuoles are vacant, whereas others show a dispersed granular or globular material. There are no gastrointestinal symptoms.

Mannosidosis

Mannosidosis is characterized by the presence of mannose-containing oligosaccharides in the lysosomes of many cells in the body, including nerve cells, muscle cells, fibroblasts, and macrophages. The deposits are in the form of small membrane-bound bodies with fibrillar material or vacuoles with scant granules. There are no specific effects on gut function.

Cystinosis

Alterations have been noted in thin-section electron-microscopic studies of jejunal mucosal biopsies in cystinosis.[282] These include the appearance of angular spaces that conform to the size and shape of cystine crystals within the macrophages and ground substance of the lamina propria and the occasional presence of vacuoles in the absorptive epithelial cells. These alterations do not result in gastrointestinal disease.

Glycogen Storage Disease

There are several forms of glycogen storage disease, with principal involvement of the liver, heart, and skeletal muscles. In the gut, the striated muscle of the upper esophagus is uncommonly affected, leading to poor contractility and dysphagia, and glycogen deposits are rarely noted in the smooth muscles of the intestines.[283]

Iron Storage Disease

Hemochromatosis is presented in the section on hepatic diseases.

Other Pigment Depositions

Pseudomelanin deposition has been noted in the duodenal mucosa and is discussed above and in the section on melanosis coli in Chapter 28. Carbon and other exogenous pigments are occasionally seen in the normal gut mucosa and are especially concentrated in lymphoid nodules.[284,285]

Amyloidosis

Definition and Types. Amyloid in its pure form is a specific fibrous protein and appears as an interlacing network of fibrils with a diameter of 7.5 to 10 nm that can be recognized with certainty by ultrastructural examination.[53] It is coupled in tissues to glycoproteins, which constitute about 10% of the deposits, and this allows for the more rapid and economic identification of the amyloid by special histochemical stains at the light-microscopic level. The most specific of these reactions is that with the Congo red stain, which when viewed with polarized light reveals the characteristic apple-green birefringence of amyloid. The condition of amyloidosis has been traditionally separated into systemic or generalized types, which in turn may be primary or secondary to long-standing inflammatory diseases, a localized form in which the amyloid is limited to a single organ or system, and special categories that are associated with various neoplasms and hereditary diseases.[286,287] The pre-existing inflammatory diseases include chronic infections, rheumatoid arthritis, and Crohn's disease. Despite the identical morphologic features of amyloid in all of these types, there are distinct chemical and antigenic differences that allow for a newer, more exact classification of amyloidosis based on the dominant fibrillar protein.[288,289] Thus, the amyloid is composed of immunoglobulin light chains and referred to as the AL type in primary systemic amyloidosis and in B-cell neoplasms, including multiple myeloma; whereas a different protein called amyloid-associated, or AA, type is seen in the secondary systemic cases and in familial Mediterranean fever. Many of the localized and neuropathic forms contain a prealbumin as the major constituent of the amyloid. Interestingly, the purely localized form of amyloidosis has not been noted in the gastrointestinal tract. Rather, the amyloid occurs as part of the systemic disease; it most commonly affects the small vessels and infrequently is associated with larger infiltrates in the tissues of the gut, leading to local functional problems.

Pathophysiology and Clinical Features. Except for the rarer hereditary forms,[290-292] amyloidosis tends to be more common in middle-aged and older persons, the primary systemic type being more typical in the latter.[293-295] It has been estimated from autopsy studies that amyloid involvement of the gastrointestinal tract is present in over three quarters and possibly in all cases of systemic amyloidosis. In most cases, however, the amyloid deposits are patchy and generally limited to the small vessels, and there are either no symptoms referable to the gut or only rare episodes of bleeding. Clinical problems can develop due to greater and more widespread involvement of the vessels and to the appearance of infiltrates of amyloid in the nervous and muscular tissues.[296-299] These are characterized by (1) more frequent and severe hemorrhages,[300,301] resulting from fragility and rupture of affected vessels; (2) focal ulcers, which are more commonly noted in the stomach[302-304] and colon,[305,306] due probably to localized ischemia as a further consequence of the damaged vessels; and (3) reduced motility from amyloid deposits in the wall.[292,307-309] The motor disturbances have been noted in all parts of the tract and include reduced contractions of the distal esophagus with occasional formation of megaesophagus; prolonged emptying time and outlet obstruction of the stomach; and an increase in the transit time, which may result in dilatation of the intestine. This subject is presented in further detail in Chapter 11. Malabsorption may also develop[310,311] and is due mainly to stasis and bacterial proliferation in the small intestine. The patient's symptoms depend on the particular problem and consist of upper or lower tract bleeding, those of peptic disease, and either diarrhea or constipation.

Pathology. The histologic appearance of amyloid is the same in all forms of amyloidosis. With the standard hematoxylin and eosin (H&E)–stained sections, it presents as a homogeneous pink, hyaline substance that may contain small slitlike spaces due to a cracking of the material during the tissue preparation. Histochemical stains based on attached carbohydrates are employed to distinguish amyloid from other proteins, and these techniques include metachromatic dyes such as toluidine blue and crystal violet, the fluorochrome thioflavin, and most specifically the Congo red stain with polarized light to show the apple-green birefringence. The amyloid also stains faintly with the PAS reaction but is negative with various lipid and mineral stains. The amyloid deposits are most often concentrated in the media of the small arteries and arterioles in any part of the bowel wall, and these are readily detected in biopsy samples that include the submucosa (Figures 16–8 and 16–9). Occasionally noted is a

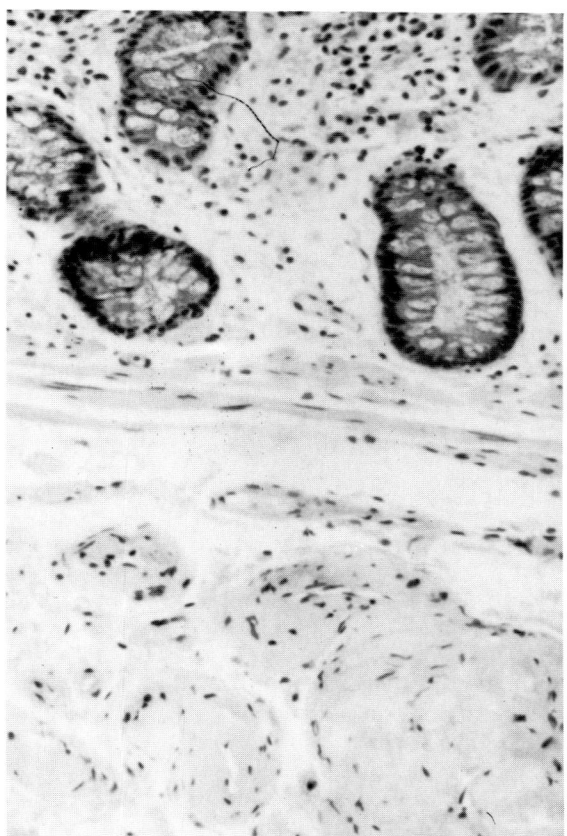

FIGURE 16–8. Rectal mucosa and upper submucosa in a case of systemic amyloidosis. There is a marked hyaline thickening of the media of the small arteries located in the submucosa (bottom), resulting in almost complete obliteration of the vessel lumen. (H&E, × 100)

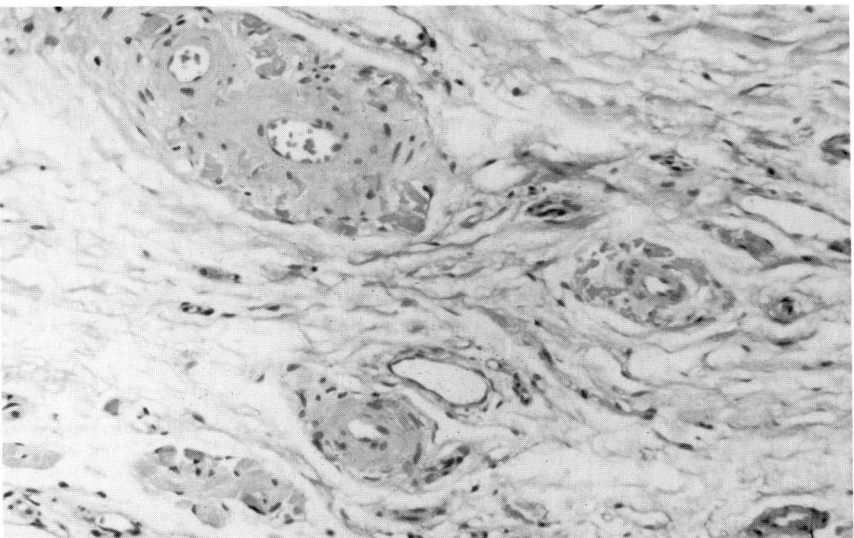

FIGURE 16–9. Colonic submucosa in a case of systemic amyloidosis, showing hyaline thickening of the small vessel media and some free strands outside the vessels. (H&E, × 250)

patchy or diffuse infiltrate in the lamina propria and submucosa that is outside of the vessels, and it is thought that this might be the result of the trauma of the biopsy procedure leading to an escape of amyloid from the vessels.

In patients with motility problems, the amyloid is also observed in the region of the muscularis propria and ganglia, and the infiltrates range in amount from fine strands to extensive replacement of the muscle (Figure 16–10). The severe cases may cause gross alterations in the form of a thickened intestinal wall with a waxy appearance, and nodular masses of amyloid may rarely project into the gut lumen.[312–314] Gross changes are otherwise lacking in most cases of amyloidosis or reveal the effects of complications such as ulcers and dilation; rarely, amyloidosis may develop in a case of Crohn's disease.[315]

Differential Diagnosis. The diagnosis of amyloidosis depends simply on its identification in a biopsy specimen or other tissue sample, ordinarily accomplished by means of special histochemical stains but also by means of ultrastructural examination.[316] The differential is related to the particular location of the amyloid deposits. In the vascular walls the amyloid must be distinguished from the very common changes of arteriosclerosis that also result in the appearance of a pink hyaline thickening of the media. The amyloid infiltrates in the muscle need to be separated from collagen, which is seen in systemic sclerosis and in the later stages of intestinal myopathies. Furthermore, in cases of secondary amyloidosis with mucosal damage, it may be necessary to sort out the effects that are due directly to the amyloid disorder and those of the underlying disease and its therapy.

Mucosal Biopsy. Mucosal biopsy of the rectum is the preferred choice for establishing the diagnosis of systemic amyloidosis, whether primary or secondary, because the rectum is readily accessible and the pro-

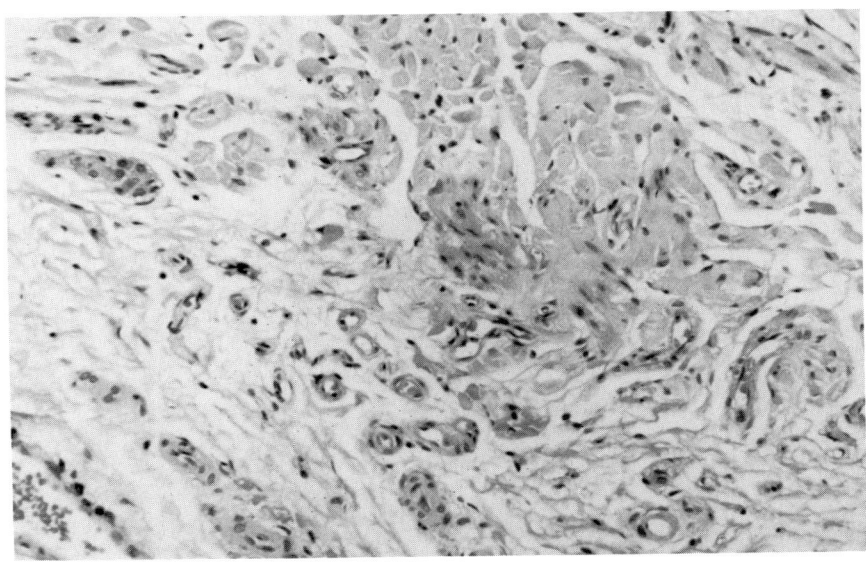

FIGURE 16–10. Colonic muscularis propria in a case of systemic amyloidosis, showing prominent infiltrate of hyaline amyloid material replacing the muscle fibers. (H&E, × 100)

cedure is associated with minimal discomfort and a high rate of detection.[56,311,317-319] This applies to patients who have no clinical problems attributable to the gastrointestinal tract, who represent the majority, and also to those who have suspected amyloid disease in an internal organ such as the liver or kidney. Because the aim of the procedure is obtaining a sample of the arteries, the biopsy must be of the aspiration type to ensure the inclusion of a large portion of submucosa. It has been estimated that in patients with systemic amyloidosis that is not associated with clinically significant gut involvement, amyloid is detected in the rectal biopsy in about 80% to 85% of cases. The deposits in some instances may be minimal and unassociated with any apparent thickening of the arterial walls on standard H&E sections, and it is essential that the special stains be applied in all cases for the highest sensitivity. The question has arisen, however, as to whether the finding of amyloid restricted to the vessel walls in elderly patients can always be considered evidence of significant disease. In this regard, the senile cardiovascular type of amyloidosis is a fairly common condition in such patients and is often asymptomatic. The possibility, therefore, exists that the finding of amyloid in the submucosal vessels of older patients is simply a reflection of aging; this issue has not been resolved. Mucosal biopsy is occasionally performed in a search for amyloid in other parts of the gastrointestinal tract, particularly in patients with signs of mucosal inflammation or ulceration and in those with malabsorption. It is again important that the sample be deep enough to include the submucosal vessels. Positive biopsies have been noted in all parts of the tract, including the stomach[312,320] and the small intestine.[321]

GRANULOMATOUS DISORDERS

There are many conditions of varied etiology that are associated with granulomatous inflammation in the gastrointestinal tract (Table 16–2). This subject has been reviewed by Haggitt.[322] The most common disorders are infections (see Chapter 26) and Crohn's disease (see Chapter 27). Foreign body reactions with granulomas are described in the particular sections on the stomach (Chapter 20), and the intestines (Chapter 28). The present section briefly reviews some of the common disorders and provides details on those diseases that are not covered fully in other parts of the book.

Granulomas are composed of nodular collections of macrophages (or histiocytes) that are often hypertrophied and that may be fused to form multinucleated giant cells. Variable features present in some granulomas include necrosis of the liquefactive, coagulative, or caseous types; other inflammatory cells, including neutrophils, eosinophils, and lymphocytes; signs of repair and fibrosis; and inclusions of all sorts within the macrophages. Also apparent may be the particular causative agent such as a microorganism or foreign material within the granuloma. The granulomas should not be confused with lymphoid nodules, which are composed

Table 16–2 GRANULOMATOUS DISORDERS OF THE GASTROINTESTINAL TRACT

Infections
  Bacterial—*Chlamydia, Yersinia, Mycobacterium* (human, *avium*), *Campylobacter,* syphilis
  Fungal—*Histoplasma, Blastomyces, Cryptococcus,* Phycomycetes
  Helminthic—*Schistosoma, Anisakidae,* other worms

Crohn's disease

Foreign body reactions
  Food, feces, and mucin
  Suture, talc, and starch
  Barium and oils

Miscellaneous
  Isolated granulomas (especially of stomach)
  Sarcoidosis
  Malacoplakia
  Chronic granulomatous disease of childhood
  Histiocytosis X
  Reaction to carcinoma
  Granulomatous vasculitis

Modified from Haggitt RC: Granulomatous diseases of the gastrointestinal tract. In Joachim HL (ed): Pathology of Granulomas. New York, Raven Press, 1983, pp 257–305.

of mature lymphocytes surrounding a germinal center (Figure 16–11). Occasionally noted is an enlargement of the cytoplasm of the germinal center cells, causing them to appear more epithelial; these can be recognized by their restricted location to the center of the lymphoid nodule. Other structures that may be mistaken for granulomas, particularly in tangential sections, include ganglia and nerves, the fibrous sheath around the crypts, and foci of disrupted or hypertrophied muscle cells. Clusters of macrophages containing mucin (muciphages) or lipid substances (foam cells) and isolated giant cells should also be distinguished from well-formed granulomas (see Figures 16–4 and 16–6). Lipogranulomas are observed in lymph nodes and consist of poorly circumscribed collections of lipid vacuoles of variable size both within and between macrophages. They probably result from the drainage of oils and other lipid substances that are absorbed from the bowel or released from fatty areas that are damaged by many diseases, including tumors. The macrophages in lipogranulomas do not typically have an enlarged or epithelial appearance.

Infections

Granulomas are a characteristic feature of tuberculosis, yersinial infections, several fungal diseases (such as histoplasmosis, blastomycosis, cryptococcosis, and phycomycosis), and the parasitic disorders of schistosomiasis and anisakiasis.[322] They may also be seen in some cases of infection due to *Myobacterium avium-intracellulare* in immunosuppressed patients, although the inflammatory reaction is often severely inhibited, resulting only in the presence of small clusters of foamy macrophages in most instances, and in reactions to intestinal worms.[323,324] Granulomas are only rarely

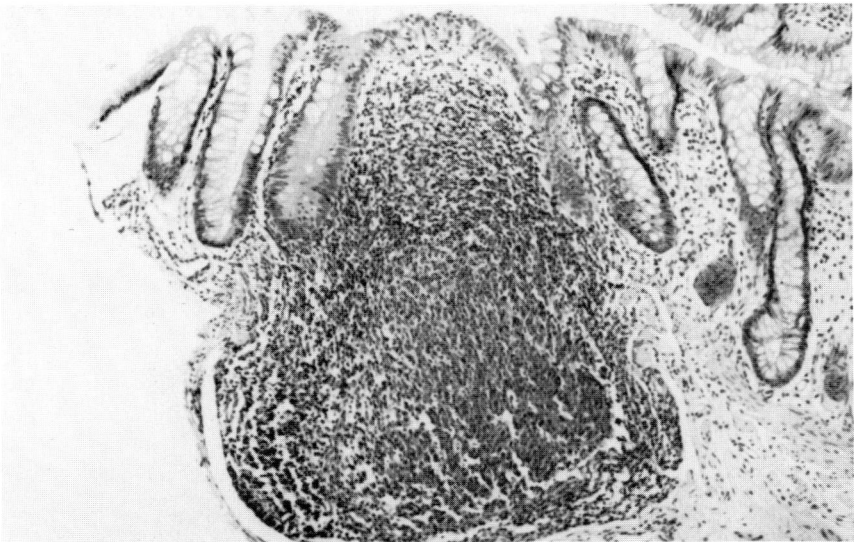

FIGURE 16–11. Lymphoid nodule in the normal colonic mucosa, extending into the upper part of the submucosa (bottom). It contains a well-formed germinal center. (H&E, × 40)

noted in other infections, including lymphogranuloma venereum and related chlamydial infections,[325,326] *Campylobacter* infection of the intestines,[327] and syphilis.[328] Cases of Whipple's disease may occasionally be associated with a granulomatous reaction[329]; the granulomas are usually in lymph nodes but may on occasion be present in the bowel wall. Staining with the PAS reaction is not conclusive, but the organisms can be identified by ultrastructural study or their presence shown by the immunohistochemical demonstration of a typical bacterial antigen profile (see Chapter 29). Malacoplakia is presented subsequently in a separate section.

Crohn's Disease

Granulomas are present in about half of cases of Crohn's disease and may be located in any layer of the bowel wall.[330–332] They are also noted in the regional lymph nodes in about 15% to 20% of cases and uncommonly in distant sites such as the liver. The granulomas are typically devoid of necrosis except when associated with extensive fat necrosis or with foreign material (see Chapter 27 for further details).

Foreign Body Granulomas

The most common reactions are due to fecal material at sites of perforation, to mucin from ruptured crypts, and to suture material; these as well as other foreign body reactions are summarized in Chapter 28.

Isolated Granulomas

The presence of solitary or multiple granulomas without an apparent cause can be occasionally seen in any part of the alimentary tract, usually in the mucosal layer. It is important in these situations to exclude granulomas that are due to ruptured crypts or to foreign materials, and multiple sections of the tissue block may be needed. It follows that the sporadic granuloma could occur in some disease that is not expected to be associated with its presence, such as ulcerative colitis; but this is fortunately a rare event. The finding of a granuloma in the gut must, therefore, always be considered in context with the other morphologic and clinical features of a case. Isolated granulomatous inflammation most often involves the stomach[333–337]; this is described in Chapter 20 (Figure 16–12).

Sarcoidosis

Sarcoidosis is a granulomatous disorder of unknown etiology that most often affects the lungs and hilar lymph nodes.[338–340] There may be involvement of multiple tissues in the body, but it typically spares the gastrointestinal tract, and disease limited to or starting in the gut is extremely rare. Before 1960 there was a tendency to ascribe most cases of granulomas in the tract to sarcoidosis if there was no overt evidence of infection or Crohn's disease. This assignment proved to be incorrect,[334] and the diagnosis of gastrointestinal sarcoidosis now depends on the finding of coexisting disease in a more characteristic location in the body.

Pathology. Most lesions have been described in the stomach and the rectum,[341–348] and there are rare instances of esophageal involvement[349] and of generalized intestinal disease.[350–353] There may be thickened mucosal folds and pyloric obstruction, which can be visualized by radiographic and endoscopic examination; and biopsy reveals multiple granulomas. The granulomas are concentrated in the mucosa and submucosa. They are composed of enlarged or epithelioid macrophages, which often contain laminated calcific inclusions within the cytoplasm. There is frequently an admixture of lymphocytes and eosinophils at the

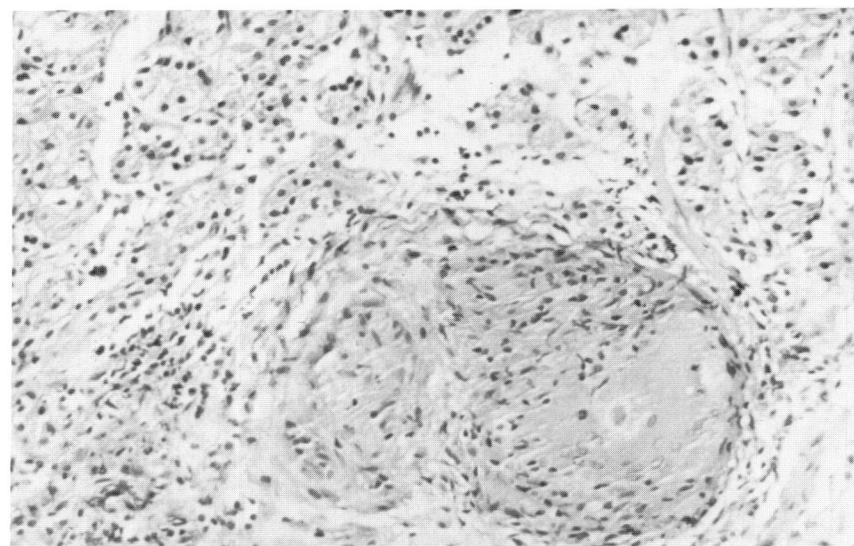

FIGURE 16–12. Gastric antral mucosa in a case of isolated granuloma of the stomach. There are several well-circumscribed granulomas located in the mucosa. (H&E, × 100)

periphery of the granulomas, and there may be some fibrinoid material in the center but no areas of caseous necrosis. The adjacent mucosa may reveal signs of a more diffuse inflammation.

Differential Diagnosis. The diagnosis of gastrointestinal sarcoidosis depends on the thorough exclusion of other causes of granulomatous inflammation and on the presence of the disease in another typical organ system, such as the lung. The disease must be distinguished from infections such as tuberculosis by appropriate stains and cultures and from Crohn's disease, which would reveal other characteristic lesions in the intestines. Within the stomach, isolated granulomatous gastritis must also be considered in cases that lack evidence of systemic disease. It should be stressed that sarcoidosis of the gastrointestinal tract is very rare and that all other causes of granulomas, including local foreign body reactions, must be eliminated.

Chronic Granulomatous Disease

Definition, Etiology, and Clinical Features. This is a rare inherited disorder of phagocytic function characterized by the appearance of multiple and recurrent infections in infants and children.[354,355] The phagocytic leukocytes lack the ability to generate hydrogen peroxide and are unable to eliminate catalase-positive bacteria and fungi. Patients typically have chronic infections with abscesses of many organs, including the skin, lungs, liver, and bones. They often have enlargement of the lymph nodes, liver, and spleen. The diagnosis is established by a negative nitroblue tetrazolium assay and other tests showing reduced bactericidal activity in the leukocytes. Gastrointestinal problems occur in about one quarter of the cases and include gastritis and pyloric obstruction,[356] vitamin B_{12} deficiency with an abnormal Schilling test that is usually not corrected by the addition of intrinsic factor,[357] persistent perineal abscesses, and occasional cases of steatorrhea and of diffuse colitis[358] that may mimic Crohn's disease.

Pathology. The basic pathology of chronic granulomatous disease is the result of pyogenic infections leading to necrosis and abscess formation and the frequent development of granulomas, the latter caused by the inability of the macrophages to catabolize the intracellular microorganisms. Necrotizing lesions with deep ulcers and inflammatory sinus tracts have been noted in the stomach, colon, and perianal region.[354,355] The granulomas in these areas are often sparse and poorly formed, and there is usually a marked infiltrate of eosinophils. Patients with colitis may have multiple ulcers and inflammatory pseudopolyps, simulating Crohn's disease. Interestingly, the responsible microorganisms are typically not detectable in the gut lesions by special stains or cultures. In most patients with chronic granulomatous disease, including those without overt necrotizing lesions in the gastrointestinal tract, additional abnormalities are noted in the intact mucosa, and these can be identified by jejunal and rectocolonic biopsies.[21,22,354] There are clusters of enlarged macrophages, ranging in size from 50 to 100 μm in diameter, within the lamina propria. They contain within their cytoplasm vacuoles and a golden-brown, lipofuscin-like pigment that stains positively with fat stains and the PAS reaction. When marked, the macrophages can extend between and separate the bases of the crypts from the muscularis mucosae, and isolated cells are occasionally noted in the submucosa. Rectal biopsies have also demonstrated the appearance of granulomas, in the absence of cryptitis, and an overall increase in inflammatory cells in the lamina propria and submucosa, including mononuclear cell types, neutrophils, and eosinophils, in about half of the cases studied.

Differential Diagnosis. The diagnosis of chronic granulomatous disease depends ultimately on the

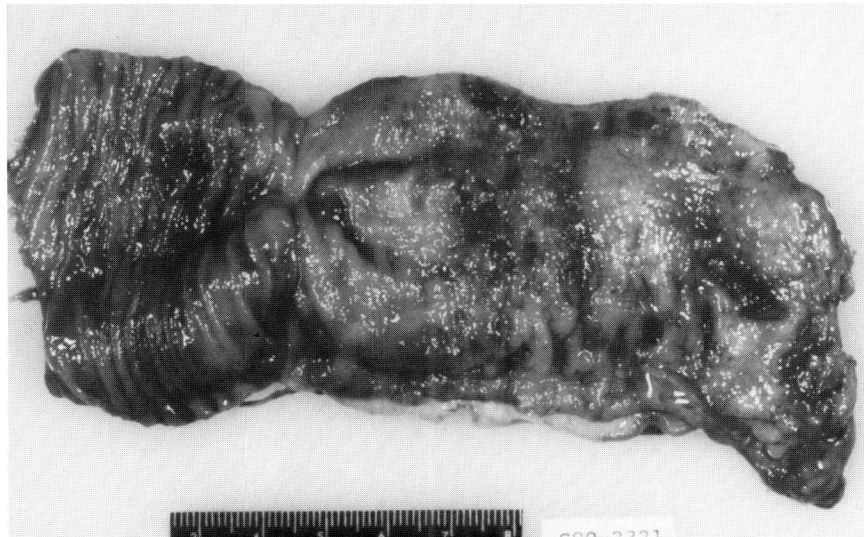

FIGURE 16-13. Malacoplakia of the colon. The mucosal surface is effaced by the presence of numerous soft plaques with central areas of ulceration.

demonstration of the impaired bactericidal action of the macrophages or neutrophilic leukocytes. The inflammatory and ulcerative lesions of the stomach and colon must be distinguished mainly from primary granulomatous infections by appropriate stains and cultures and from Crohn's disease by the lack of necrotizing lesions in other tissues and organs. Primary immunodeficiency disorders may be associated with secondary infections of the gut, but these frequently involve the small intestine and opportunistic agents and are not associated with a granulomatous reaction.[359] Scattered macrophages containing a lipofuscin-like pigment are seen in the colonic mucosa of normal persons and are more abundant in cases of melanosis coli, but they do not form clusters or nodules and are typically very sparse or absent in the small-intestinal mucosa. Although prominent macrophages with lipid pigments are observed in some storage disorders such as Batten's disease and in the brown bowel syndrome, these conditions reveal more widespread depositions in the nerve and muscle cells. There are many other storage diseases and other conditions with lipid-filled macrophages, and these can be distinguished by their absence of PAS-positive pigments (see Depositions). Foamy macrophages containing PAS-positive material are also seen in Whipple's disease and in infection with *Mycobacterium avium-intracellulare*, but they do not reveal refractile pigments in standard histologic sections.

Malacoplakia

Definition, Etiology, and Clinical Features. Malacoplakia is a rare disorder characterized by the development of plaquelike lesions and the distinctive appearance of mineralized inclusions within macrophages.[360,361] It is thought to be due to an acquired defect in the lysosomal function of monocytic-phagocytic cells, resulting in the promotion of infections that are usually due to enteric organisms such as *E. coli*.[362,363] The exact deficiency has not been established, although it has been suggested that the error might be corrected by the use of cholinergic agonists.[364] The disease is most frequently seen in the urinary tract,[365,366] but it may affect almost any tissue in the body.[361] The gastrointestinal tract ranks second in order of distribution,[367] and most cases have been noted in the colon,[368-378] with rare instances in the esophagus, stomach,[362] small intestine, and appendix. The intestinal disease is often associated with extension into the regional lymph nodes, mesentery, and retroperitoneum. In contrast to disease of the urinary tract, which is more common in older women, cases with gut involvement affect both sexes equally and all age groups, including children. Rare associations with other colonic disorders such as ulcerative colitis[375] and carcinoma[378] have been noted. Presenting symptoms have been mainly related to the colonic disease and include fever, bleeding, and the appearance of masses in the bowel and retroperitoneum. The disease persists, and complications such as bowel obstruction, perforation, and fistula formation often develop.

Pathology. The colon is involved in the great majority of the cases, and isolated disease of the upper tract or small intestine is very rare. The early lesions are soft, flat, yellow to tan nodules on the mucosal surface. Scattered small plaques have been noted in the stomach, whereas they tend to coalesce into larger masses or more diffuse lesions in the intestines (Figure 16-13). The intestinal lesions also extend into the wall, where they may promote bowel perforation and fistula formation. The histologic features are distinctive,[363,380-383] revealing masses of enlarged macrophages that contain characteristic inclusions. Present in all of these cells is an abundance of enlarged membrane-bound lysosomes, ranging in size from 1 to 3 μm in diameter, which stain positively with the PAS reaction (Figure 16-14). In addition, many of the macrophages contain

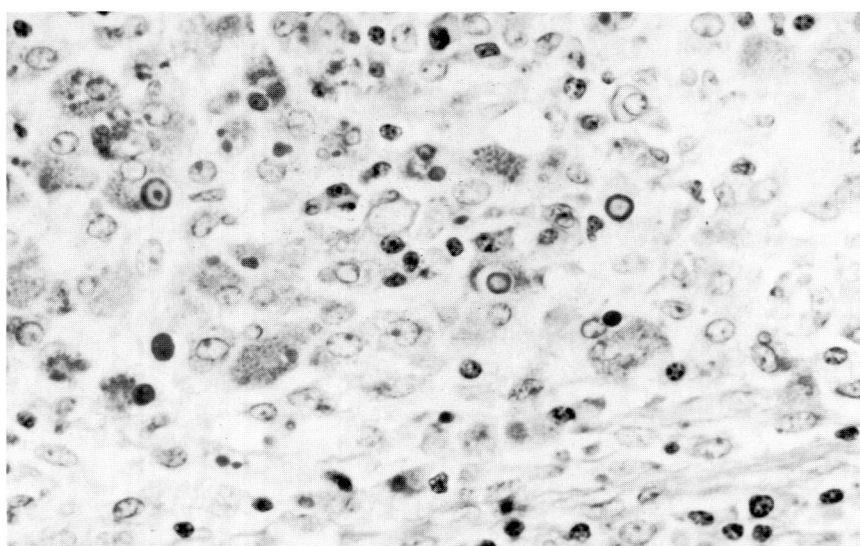

FIGURE 16–14. Malacoplakia of the colon, revealing prominent phagolysosomes within the cytoplasm of the macrophages. (PAS, × 400)

the diagnostic Michaelis-Gutmann bodies, which probably evolve from the mineralization of the lysosomes. These bodies measure 2.5 to 9.5 μm in diameter and are composed of a central matrix of glycolipid material and an outer mineral layer that reacts with stains for iron and calcium (Figure 16–15). Other inflammatory cell types of a nonspecific nature may be present in the tissues adjacent to the masses of macrophages.

Differential Diagnosis. The diagnosis of malacoplakia is based on the finding of masses of macrophages that contain the characteristic Michaelis-Gutmann inclusion bodies within their cytoplasm. Although the disorder may resemble chronic infections, Crohn's disease, and tumors with multiple soft nodules, such as lymphomas, at the clinical or gross level, the distinction can be readily made by microscopic examination. There are many other conditions that are associated with a prominence of macrophages, but none of these have the distinctive mineralized inclusions.

Histiocytosis X

Histiocytosis X is an uncommon condition noted in children that is characterized by the proliferation of histiocytes in several tissues of the body.[384–386] It appears that many of these cells may represent Langerhans cells on the basis of the presence of Birbeck granules by electron-microscopic study and the results of immunocytochemical techniques.[387] Depending on the overall severity and distribution of the lesions, the disease has been divided into three forms: the localized eosinophilic granuloma, the Hand-Schüller-Christian type with prominent depositions, and the disseminated

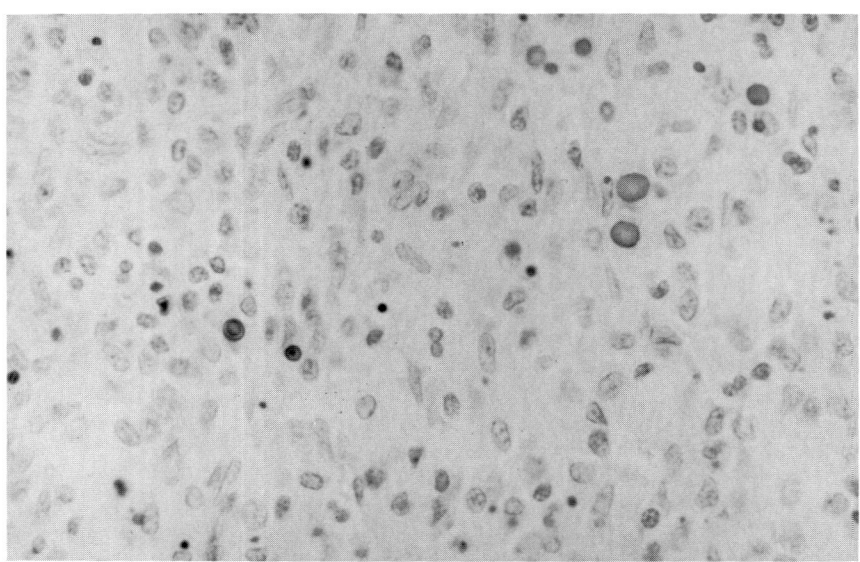

FIGURE 16–15. Malacoplakia of colon. The Michaelis-Guttman inclusions in the macrophages are highlighted by the deposition of iron. This can also be demonstrated with stains for calcium. (Prussian blue reaction for iron, × 400)

Letterer-Siwe form. It has become evident, however, that a sharp demarcation cannot be made between these forms in most cases of histiocytosis X. The term *eosinophilic granuloma* has also been used variably to describe lesions of the gastrointestinal tract that are not related to the histiocytic disorder or even to a granulomatous condition[322]; it has been applied to unusual polyps such as the inflammatory fibroid polyp and to the mural form of eosinophilic gastroenteritis.

Pathology. Within the digestive tract, the histiocytic lesions most commonly affect the major bile ducts and ductules within the portal tracts of the liver, which leads to their destruction and the frequent development of a biliary cirrhosis.[388,389] This may result in reduced bile salt excretion and the appearance of diarrhea and, rarely, steatorrhea. In a personal review of fatal cases of histiocytosis X, small collections of histiocytes were observed in the lamina propria of the small intestine in one half of the patients. This had been noted previously[390] but usually does not have any clinical significance. The histiocytes are arranged in a compact cluster, and they are enlarged and have a finely granular cytoplasm with only rare vacuoles. There is no other inflammation or evidence of damage to the intestinal mucosa. These nodular lesions have also been detected in mucosal biopsies of the stomach[391] and rectum.[392] They should be distinguishable from other conditions with accumulation of macrophages in the lamina propria by the absence of prominent vacuoles or pigments.

Miscellaneous Granulomatous Conditions

Granulomas are occasionally observed in the bowel wall and draining lymph nodes in the vicinity of carcinomas,[322,393] and these possibly occur in response to tumor antigens. They have also been noted rarely in some forms of vasculitis.[394]

References

1. Sack TL, Sleisenger MH: Effects of systemic and extra-intestinal disease on the gut. In Sleisenger MH, Fordtran JS (eds): Gastrointestinal Disease, 4th ed. Philadelphia, WB Saunders Co, 1989, pp 488–528.
2. Lennard-Jones JE: Functional gastrointestinal disorders. N Engl J Med 308:431–435, 1983.
3. Hinnant KL, Rotterdam HZ, Bell ET, Tapper ML: Cytomegalovirus infection of the alimentary tract: A clinicopathological correlation. Am J Gastroenterol 81:944–950, 1986.
4. Rosen PP: Opportunistic fungal infections in patients with neoplastic diseases. Pathol Annu 11:255–315, 1976.
5. Ament ME, Rubin CE: Relation of giardiasis to abnormal intestinal structure and function in gastrointestinal immunodeficiency syndromes. Gastroenterology 62:216–226, 1972.
6. Casemore DP, Sands RL, Curry A: Cryptosporidium species: A "new" human pathogen. J Clin Pathol 38:1321–1336, 1985.
7. Dworkin B, Wormser GP, Rosenthal WS, et al: Gastrointestinal manifestations of the acquired immunodeficiency syndrome: A review of 22 cases. Am J Gastroenterol 80:774–778, 1985.
8. Riddell RH: The gastrointestinal tract. In Riddell RH (ed): Pathology of Drug-Induced and Toxic Diseases. New York, Churchill Livingstone, 1982, pp 515–606.
9. Pemberton RE, Strand LJ: A review of upper gastrointestinal effects of the newer non-steroidal anti-inflammatory agents. Dig Dis Sci 24:53–64, 1979.
10. Fortson WC, Tedesco FJ: Drug-induced colitis: A review. Am J Gastroenterol 79:878–883, 1984.
11. Lewis JH: Gastrointestinal injury due to medicinal agents. Am J Gastroenterol 81:819–834, 1986.
12. Williams LF Jr: Vascular insufficiency of the intestines. Gastroenterology 61:757–777, 1971.
13. Whitehead R: The pathology of ischemia of the intestines. Pathol Annu 11:1–52, 1976.
14. Alschibaja T, Morson BC: Ischemic bowel disease. J Clin Pathol 11:68–77, 1977.
15. Swerdlow SH, Antonioli DA, Goldman H: Intestinal infarction: a new classification. Arch Pathol Lab Med 105:218, 1981.
16. Norris HT: Reexamination of the spectrum of ischemic bowel disease. In Norris HT (ed): Pathology of the Colon, Small Intestine, and Anus. New York, Churchill Livingstone, 1983, pp 109–120.
17. Camilleri M, Pusey CD, Chadwick VS, Rees AJ: Gastrointestinal manifestations of systemic vasculitis. Q J Med 206:141–149, 1983.
18. Nelson DL, Blaese RM, Strober W, et al: Constrictive pericarditis, intestinal lymphangiectasia, and reversible immunologic deficiency. J Pediatr 86:548–554, 1975.
19. Strober W, Cohen LS, Waldmann TA et al: Tricuspid regurgitation. A newly recognized cause of protein-losing enteropathy, lymphocytopenia, and immunologic deficiency. Am J Med 44:482–550, 1968.
20. Asakura H, Miura S, Morashita T, et al: Endoscopic and histopathological study on primary and secondary intestinal lymphangiectasia. Dig Dis Sci 26:312–320, 1981.
21. Perera DR, Weinstein WM, Rubin CE: Small intestinal biopsy. Hum Pathol 6:157–217, 1975.
22. Dobbins WO III: Small bowel biopsy in malabsorptive states. In Norris HT (ed): Pathology of the Colon, Small Intestine, and Anus. New York, Churchill Livingstone, 1983, pp 121–165.
23. Glick DL, Kern F Jr: Peptic ulcer in chronic obstructive bronchopulmonary disease: A prospective clinical study of prevalence. Gastroenterology 47:153–160, 1964.
24. Ellison LT, Ellison RG, Carter CH, et al: The role of hypercapnia and hypoxia in the etiology of peptic ulceration in patients with chronic obstructive pulmonary emphysema. Am Rev Respir Dis 89:909–916, 1964.
25. Jaffe RH, Laing DR: Changes of the digestive tract in uremia: A pathologic anatomic study. Arch Intern Med 53:851–864, 1934.
26. Mason EE: Gastrointestinal lesions occurring in uremia. Ann Intern Med 37:96–105, 1952.
27. Berg B, Groth CG, Magnusson G et al: Gastrointestinal complications in 248 kidney transplant recipients. Scand J Urol Nephrol Suppl 29:19–20, 1975.
28. Meyers WC, Harris N, Stein S, et al: Alimentary tract complications after renal transplantation. Ann Surg 190:535–542, 1979.
29. Archibald SD, Jirsch DW, Bear RA: Gastrointestinal complications of renal transplantation. 2. The colon. Can Med Assoc J 119:1301–1314, 1978.
30. Franzin G, Musola R, Mencarelli R: Morphological changes of the gastroduodenal mucosa in regular dialysis in uremic patients. Histopathology 6:429–437, 1982.
31. Musola R, Franzin G, Mora R, Manfrini C: Prevalence of gastroduodenal lesions in uremic patients undergoing dialysis and after transplantation. Gastrointest Endosc 30:343–346, 1984.
32. Margolis DM, Saylor JL, Geisse G, et al: Upper gastrointestinal disease in chronic renal failure. Arch Intern Med 138:1214–1217, 1978.
33. Tani N, Harasawa S, Suzuki S, et al: Lesions of the upper gastrointestinal tract in patients with chronic renal failure. Gastroenterol Jpn 15:480, 1980.
34. Cunningham JT: Gastric telangiectasias in chronic hemodialysis patients: A report of six cases. Gastroenterology 81:1131–1133, 1981.

35. Shepard AMM, Stewart WK, Wormsley KG: Peptic ulceration in chronic renal failure. Lancet 1:1357–1359, 1973.
36. Sutherland DER, Chan FY, Fouchar E, et al: The bleeding cecal ulcer in transplant patients. Surgery 86:386–398, 1979.
37. Huded F, Posner GL, Tick R: Non-specific ulcer of the colon in a chronic hemodialysis patient. Am J Gastroenterol 77:913–916, 1982.
38. Dinoso VP Jr, Murthy SNS, Saris AL, et al: Gastric and pancreatic function in patients with end-stage renal disease. J Clin Gastroenterol 4:321–324, 1982.
39. Franzin G, Musola R, Mencarelli R: Changes in the mucosa of the stomach and duodenum during immunosuppressive therapy after renal transplantation. Histopathology 6:439–449, 1982.
40. Sawyer OI, Garwin PJ, Codd JE, et al: Colorectal complications of renal allograft transplantation. Arch Surg 113:84–86, 1978.
41. Bischel MD, Reese T, Engel J: Spontaneous perforation of the colon in a hemodialysis patient. Am J Gastroenterol 74:182–184, 1980.
42. Diamond SM, Emmett M, Henrich WL: Bowel infarction as a cause of death in dialysis patients. J Am Med Assoc 256:2545–2547, 1987.
43. Komorowski RA, Cohen EB, Kauffman HM, Adams MB: Gastrointestinal complications in renal transplant recipients. Am J Clin Pathol 86:161–167, 1986.
44. Watts SJ, Alexander LC, Fawcett K, et al: Herpes simplex esophagitis in a renal transplant patient treated with Cyclosporine A: a case report. Am J Gastroenterol 81:185–188, 1986.
45. Franzin G, Muolo A, Griminelli T: Cytomegalovirus inclusions in the gastroduodenal mucosa of patients after renal transplantation. Gut 22:698–701, 1981.
46. Weisburger WR, Hutcheon DF, Yardley JH, et al: Cryptosporidiosis in an immunosuppressed renal transplant recipient with IgA deficiency. Am J Clin Pathol 72:473–478, 1979.
47. Ainley CC, Clarke DG, Timothy AR, Thompson RPH: Strongyloides stercoralis hyperinfection associated with cimetidine in an immunosuppressed patient: Diagnosis by endoscopic biopsy. Gut 27:337–338, 1986.
48. Goldman H, Antonioli DA: Mucosal biopsy of the esophagus, stomach and proximal duodenum. Hum Pathol 13:423–448, 1982.
49. Goldman H, Antonioli DA: Mucosal biopsy of the rectum, colon and distal ileum. Hum Pathol 13:981–1012, 1982.
50. Whitehead R: Mucosal Biopsy of the Gastrointestinal Tract, 3rd Edition. Philadelphia, WB Saunders Co, 1985.
51. Rotterdam H, Sommers SC: Biopsy Diagnosis of the Digestive Tract. New York, Raven Press, 1981.
52. Fauci AS, Haynes BF, Katz P: The spectrum of vasculitis. Clinical, pathologic, immunologic, and therapeutic considerations. Ann Intern Med 89:660–676, 1978.
53. Cohen AS: Amyloidosis. N Engl J Med 277:522–530; 574–583; 628–637, 1967.
54. Schneider RE, Dobbins WO: Suction biopsy of the rectal mucosa for diagnosis of arteritis in rheumatoid arthritis and related diseases. Ann Intern Med 68:561–568, 1968.
55. Tribe CR, Scott DGI, Bacon PA: Rectal biopsy in the diagnosis of systemic vasculitis. J Clin Pathol 34:843–850, 1981.
56. Gafni J, Sohar E: Rectal biopsy for the diagnosis of amyloidosis. Am J Med Sci 240:332–336, 1960.
57. Gore RM, Marn CS, Ujiki GT, et al: Ischemic colitis associated with systemic lupus erythermatosus. Dis Colon Rectum 26:449–451, 1983.
58. Wood ML, Foulds IS, French MA: Protein-losing enteropathy due to systemic lupus erythematosus. Gut 25:1013–1015, 1984.
59. Burt RW, Berenson MM, Samuelson CO, Cathey WJ: Rheumatoid vasculitis of the colon presenting as pancolitis. Dig Dis Sci 28:183–188, 1983.
60. McCurley TL, Collins RD: Intestinal infarction in rheumatoid arthritis: Three cases due to unusual obliterative vascular lesion. Arch Pathol Lab Med 108:125–128, 1984.
61. Morichau-Beauchant M, Touchard G, Maire P, et al: Jejunal IgA and C3 deposition in adult Henoch-Schönlein purpura with severe intestinal manifestations. Gastroenterology 82:1438–1442, 1982.
62. Lieberman E: Hemolytic-uremic syndrome. J Pediatr 80:1–16, 1972.
63. Craner GE, Burdick GE: Acute colitis resembling ulcerative colitis in the hemolytic-uremic syndrome. Am J Dig Dis 21:74–76, 1976.
64. Tochen ML, Campbell JR: Colitis in children with the hemolytic-uremic syndrome. J Pediatr Surg 12:213–219, 1977.
65. Whitington PF, Friedman AL, Chesney RW: Gastrointestinal disease in the hemolytic-uremic syndrome. Gastroenterology 76:728–733, 1979.
66. Helin H, Mastonen J, Reunala T, Pasternack A: IgA nephropathy associated with celiac disease and dermatitis herpetiformis. Arch Pathol Lab Med 107:324–327, 1983.
67. Katz A, Dyck RF, Bear RA: Celiac disease associated with immune complex glomerulonephritis. Clin Nephrol 11:39–44, 1979.
68. Lasser A, Acosta AE: Colonic neoplasms complicating ureterosigmoidostomy. Cancer 35:1218–1222, 1975.
69. Ali MH, Satti MB, Al-Nafussi A: Multiple benign colonic polypi at the site of ureterosigmoidostomy. Cancer 53:1006–1010, 1984.
70. Aldis AS: Carcinoma of colon following transplantation of the ureters, and at the site of the transplantation. Proc Roy Soc Med 54:159–160, 1961.
71. Kille JN, Glick S: Neoplasia complicating ureterosigmoidostomy. Br Med J 4:783–784, 1967.
72. Whitaker RH, Rugle RCB, Dow D: Colonic tumors following ureterosigmoidostomy. Br J Urol 43:562–575, 1971.
73. Recht KA, Belis JA, Kandzari SJ, Milam DF: Ureterosigmoidostomy followed by carcinoma of the colon. Cancer 44:1538–1542, 1979.
74. Ansell ID, Vellacott KD: Colonic polyps complicating ureterosigmoidostomy. Histopathology 4:429–436, 1980.
75. Cipolla R, Garcia RL: Colonic polyps and adenocarcinoma complicating ureterosigmoidostomy: Report of a case. Am J Gastroenterol 79:453–457, 1984.
76. Stewart M, Macrae FA, William CB: Neoplasia and ureterosigmoidostomy: A colonoscopy survey. Br J Surg 69:414–416, 1982.
77. Sterling JR, Uehling DT, Gilchrist KW: Value of colonoscopy after ureterosigmoidostomy. Surgery 96:784–790, 1984.
78. Tomlinson WJ: Abdominal crises in sickle cell anemia: A clinical-pathologic study of eleven cases with a suggested explanation for their causes. Am J Med Sci 209:722–741, 1945.
79. Gage TP, Gagnier JM: Ischemic colitis complicating sickle cell crisis. Gastroenterology 84:171–174, 1983.
80. Astaldi G, Meardi G, Lisino T: The iron content of jejunal mucosa obtained by Crosby's biopsy in haemochromatosis and haemosiderosis. Blood 28:70–82, 1966.
81. Chisholm M, Ardran GM, Callender ST, et al: Iron deficiency and autoimmunity in postcricoid webs. Q J Med 40:421–423, 1971.
82. Graham RM, Rheault MH: Characteristic cellular changes in epithelial cells in pernicious anemia. J Lab Clin Med 43:235–245, 1954.
83. Foroozan P, Trier JS: Mucosa of the small intestine in pernicious anemia. N Engl J Med 277:553–559, 1967.
84. Winawer DR, Sullivan LW, Herbert V, Zamcheck N: Jejunal mucosa in patients with nutritional folate deficiency and megaloblastic anemia. N Engl J Med 272:892–895, 1965.
85. Hermos JA, Adams WM, Liu YK, et al: Mucosa of the small intestine in folate-deficient alcoholics. Ann Intern Med 76:959–965, 1972.
86. Bianchi A, Chipman DW, Dreskin A, et al: Nutritional folic acid deficiency with megaloblastic changes in the small bowel epithelium. N Engl J Med 282:859–861, 1970.
87. Lindenbaum J: Tropical enteropathy. Gastroenterology 64:637–652, 1973.
88. Cornes JS, Jones TG: Leukemic lesions of the gastrointestinal tract. J Clin Pathol 15:305–313, 1962.
89. Prolla JC, Kirsner JB: The gastrointestinal lesions and complications of the leukemias. Ann Intern Med 61:1084–1103, 1964.
90. Fromke VL, Weber LW: Extensive leukemic infiltration of the gastrointestinal tract in chronic lymphosarcoma cell leukemia. Am J Med 56:879–882, 1974.
91. Dewar GJ, Lim CNH, Michalyshyn B: Gastrointestinal complications in patients with acute and chronic leukemia. Can J Surg 24:67–71, 1981.

92. Smith FP, Kisner DL, Widerlite L, et al: Chemotherapeutic alteration of small intestinal morphology and function: A progress report. J Clin Gastroenterol 1:203, 1979.
93. Gwavava NJT, Pinkerton CR, Glasgow JFT, et al: Small bowel enterocyte abnormalities caused by methotrexate treatment in acute lymphoblastic leukaemia of childhood. J Clin Pathol 34:790–795, 1981.
94. Bodey GP: Fungal infections complicating acute leukemia. J Chronic Dis 19:667–687, 1966.
95. Strayer DS, Phillips GB, Barker KH, et al: Gastric cytomegalovirus infection in bone marrow transplant patients: An indication of generalized disease. Cancer 48:1478–1483, 1981.
96. Kies MS, Leudke DW, Boyd FJ, McCue MJ: Neutropenic enterocolitis. Cancer 43:730–734, 1979.
97. Slavin, RE, Woodruff JM: The pathology of bone marrow transplantation. Pathol Annu 9:291–344, 1974.
98. McDonald GB, Shulman HM, Sullivan KM, Spencer GD: Intestinal and hepatic complications of human bone marrow transplantation. Part I. Gastroenterology 90:460–477, 1986.
99. Snover DC, Weisdorf SA, Vercolotti GM, et al: A histopathologic study of gastric and small intestinal graft-versus-host disease following allogeneic bone marrow transplantation. Hum Pathol 16:387–392, 1985.
100. Spencer GD, Shulman HM, Mayerson D, et al: Diffuse intestinal ulceration after marrow transplantation: A clinicopathologic study of 13 patients. Hum Pathol 17:621–633, 1986.
101. Thornung D, Howard JD: Epithelial denudement in the gastrointestinal tracts of two bone marrow transplant recipients. Hum Pathol 17:560–566, 1986.
102. McDonald GB, Sullivan KM, Schuffler MD, et al: Esophageal abnormalities in chronic graft-vs-host disease in humans. Gastroenterology 80:914–921, 1981.
103. Sale GE, Shulman HM, McDonald JB, et al: Gastrointestinal graft-versus-host disease in man: A clinicopathologic study of the rectal biopsy. Am J Surg Pathol 3:291–300, 1979.
104. Lewin KJ, Ranchod M, Dorfman RF: Lymphomas of the gastrointestinal tract: A study of 177 cases presenting with gastrointestinal disease. Cancer 42:693–707, 1978.
105. Isaacson PG, Spencer J, Connolly CE, et al: Malignant histiocytosis of the intestine: A T-cell lymphoma. Lancet 2:688–691, 1985.
106. Eidelman S, Parkins A, Rubin CE: Abdominal lymphoma presenting as malabsorption: A clinicopathologic study of nine cases in Israel, and a review of the literature. Medicine 45:111–137, 1966.
107. Ramot B: Malabsorption due to lymphomatous disease. Ann Rev Med 22:19, 1971.
108. Appelman HD, Hirsch SD, Schnitzer B, Coon WW: Clinicopathologic overview of gastrointestinal lymphomas. Am J Surg Pathol 9(Suppl):71–83, 1985.
109. Shirer JW: Hypermotility of the gastrointestinal tract in hyperthyroidism. Am J Med Sci 186:73–78, 1933.
110. Scarf M: Gastrointestinal manifestations of hyperthyroidism. J Lab Clin Med 21:1253–1258, 1936.
111. Miller LJ, Gorman CA, Go VLW: Gut-thyroid interrelationships. Gastroenterology 75:901–911, 1978.
112. Bock OAA, Witts LJ: Gastric acidity and gastric biopsy in thyrotoxicosis. Br Med J 2:20–24, 1963.
113. Thomas FB, Caldwell JH, Greenberger NJ: Steatorrhea in thyrotoxicosis: Relation to hypermotility and excessive dietary fat. Ann Intern Med 78:669–675, 1973.
114. Hellesen C, Friis T, Larsen E, et al: Small intestinal histology, radiology, and absorption in hyperthyroidism. Scand J Gastroenterol 4:169–175, 1969.
115. Bastenie PA: Paralytic ileus in severe hypothyroidism. Lancet 1:413–416, 1946.
116. Wells I, Smith B, Hinton M: Acute ileus in myxoedema. Br Med J 1:211–212, 1977.
117. Case records of the Massachusetts General Hospital. N Engl J Med 272:1118–1127, 1965.
118. Irvine WJ: The association of atrophic gastritis with autoimmune thyroid disease. Clin Endocrinol Metab 4:351, 1975.
119. Carney JA, Hayles AB: Alimentary tract manifestations of multiple endocrine neoplasia, type 2b. Mayo Clin Proc 52:543, 1977.
120. St. Goar WT: Gastrointestinal symptoms as a clue to the diagnosis of primary hyperparathyroidism. A review of 45 cases. Ann Intern Med 46:102–118, 1957.
121. Eversmann JJ, Farmer RG, Brown CH et al: Gastrointestinal manifestations of hyperparathyroidism. Arch Intern Med 119:605–609, 1967.
122. Gardner EC Jr, Hersh T: Primary hyperparathyroidism and the gastrointestinal tract. South Med J 74:197–199, 1981.
123. Frame B, Haubrich WS: Peptic ulcer and hyperparathyroidism: A survey of 300 ulcer patients. Arch Intern Med 105:536–541, 1960.
124. Linos DA, van Heerden JA, Abboud CF, Edis AJ: Primary hyperparathyroidism and peptic ulcer disease. Arch Surg 113:384–386, 1978.
125. Morse WI, Cochrane WA, Landrigan P et al: Familial hypoparathyroidism with pernicious anemia, steatorrhea and adrenocortical insufficiency. N Engl J Med 264:1021–1026, 1961.
126. Tobin MV, Aldridge SA, Morris AI, et al: Gastrointestinal manifestations of Addison's disease. Am J Gastroenterol 84:1302–1305, 1989.
127. Rosati LA, Augur NA Jr: Ischemic enterocolitis in pheochromocytoma. Gastroenterology 60:581–585, 1971.
128. Katz LA, Spiro HM: Gastrointestinal manifestations of diabetes. N Engl J Med 275:1350–1361, 1966.
129. Goyal RK, Spiro HM: Gastrointestinal manifestations of diabetes mellitus. Med Clin North Am 55:1031–1044, 1971.
130. Scarpello JHB, Sloden GE: Diabetes and the gut. Gut 19:1153–1162, 1978.
131. Taub S, Mariani A, Barkin JS: Gastrointestinal manifestations of diabetes mellitus. Diabetes Care 2:437, 1979.
132. Feldman M, Schiller LR: Disorders of gastrointestinal motility associated with diabetes mellitus. Ann Intern Med 98:378–384, 1983.
133. Hollis JB, Castell DO, Braddon RL: Esophageal function in diabetes mellitus and its relation to peripheral neuropathy. Gastroenterology 73:1098–1102, 1977.
134. Marshak RH, Maklansky D: Diabetic gastropathy. Am J Dig Dis 9:366–370, 1964.
135. Liavag I, Tonjum S: Gastric retention in diabetes mellitus. Acta Chir Scand 137:593, 1971.
136. Angervall L, Dotevall G, Lehmann KE: The gastric mucosa in diabetes mellitus: Functional and histopathological study. Acta Med Scand 169:339–349, 1961.
137. Dotevall G: Incidence of peptic ulcer disease in diabetes mellitus. Acta Med Scand 164:463, 1959.
138. Hensley GT, Soergel P: Neuropathologic findings in diabetic diarrhoea. Arch Pathol 85:587–597, 1968.
139. Malins JM, Mayne N: Diabetic diarrhoea: a study of 13 patients with jejunal biopsy. Diabetes 18:858–866, 1969.
140. Walsh CH, Cooper BT, Wright AD, et al: Diabetes mellitus and coeliac disease: a clinical study. Q J Med 185:89–100, 1978.
141. Berge KG, Sprague RG, Bennet WA: The intestinal tract in diabetic diarrhea: A pathologic study. Diabetes 5:289–294, 1956.
142. Drewes VM, Olsen S: Histological changes in the small bowel in diabetes mellitus: A study of peroral biopsy specimens. Acta Pathol Microbiol Scand 63:478–480, 1965.
143. Riecken EO, Zennek A, Lay A, Menge H: Quantitative study of mucosal structure, enzyme activities and phenylalanine accumulation in jejunal biopsies of patients with early and late onset diabetes. Gut 20:1001–1007, 1979.
144. Smith B: Neuropathology of the eosophagus in diabetes mellitus. J Neurol Neurosurg Psych 37:1151–1154, 1974.
145. Jenkinson EL, Brown WH: Endometriosis: A study of 117 cases with special reference to constricting lesions of the rectum and sigmoid colon. JAMA 122:349–354, 1943.
146. Spjut HJ, Perkins DE: Endometriosis of the sigmoid colon and rectum. AJR 82:1070, 1959.
147. McKay Hart D: Heartburn in pregnancy. J Int Med Res 6(Suppl 1):1–5, 1978.
148. Vender RJ, Spiro HM: Inflammatory bowel disease and pregnancy. J Clin Gastroenterol 4:231–249, 1982.
149. Bernardino ME, Lawson TL: Discrete colonic ulcers associated with oral contraceptives. Am J Dig Dis 21:503–506, 1976.
150. Tedesco FJ, Volpicelli NA, Moore FS: Estrogen- and progesterone-associated colitis: A disorder with clinical and endoscopic features mimicking Crohn's colitis. Gastrointest Endosc 28:247–249, 1982.

151. Eliakim R, Goldin E, Livskin R, Okon E: Esophageal involvement in pemphigus vulgaris. Am J Gastroenterol 83:155–157, 1988.
152. Sharon P, Green ML, Rachmilewitz D: Esophageal involvement in bullous pemphigoid. Gastrointest Endosc 24:122–123, 1978.
153. Nix TE Jr, Christianson HB: Epidermolysis bullosa of the esophagus: Report of two cases and review of the literature. South Med J 58:612–620, 1965.
154. Orlando RC, Bozymski EM, Briggaman RA: Epidermolysis bullosa: gastrointestinal manifestations. Ann Intern Med 81:203–206, 1974.
155. Rabinowitz BN, Coldwell JG, Jegatheson S: Epidermolysis bullosa and gastrointestinal anomalies. J Pediatr 95:488, 1979.
156. Johnston DE, Koehler RE, Balfe DM: Clinical manifestations of epidermolysis bullosa dystrophica. Dig Dis Sci 26:1144–1149, 1981.
157. Agha FP, Francis IR, Ellis CN: Esophageal involvement in epidermolysis bullosa dystrophica: Clinical and roentgenographic manifestations. Gastrointest Radiol 8:111–117, 1983.
158. Zweiban B, Cohen H, Chandrasoma P: Gastrointestinal involvement complicating Stevens-Johnson syndrome. Gastroenterology 91:469–472, 1986.
159. Heer M, Altorfer J, Burger H-R, Wäeti M: Bullous esophageal lesions due to cotrimoxazole: An immune-mediated process? Gastroenterology 88:1954–1957, 1985.
160. Kelly R, Davidson GP, Townley R, Campbell PE: Reversible intestinal mucosal abnormalities in acrodermatitis enteropathica. Arch Dis Child 51:219–222, 1976.
161. Bohane TD, Cutz E, Hamilton JR, Gall DG: Acrodermatitis enteropathica, zinc and the Paneth cell: A case report with family studies. Gastroenterology 73:587–592, 1977.
162. Brow JR, Parker F, Weinstein WM et al: The small intestinal mucosa in dermatitis herpetiformis. I. Severity and distribution of the small intestinal lesion and associated malabsorption. Gastroenterology 60:355–361, 1971.
163. Scott BB, Losowsky MS: Patchiness and duodenal-jejunal variation of the mucosal abnormality in coeliac disease and dermatitis herpetiformis. Gut 17:984–992, 1976.
164. Katz SI, Hall RP III, Lawley TJ, et al: Dermatitis herpetiformis: the skin and the gut. Ann Intern Med 93:857–874, 1980.
165. Marks R, Whittle MW, Beard RJ, et al: Small bowel abnormalities in dermatitis herpetiformis. Br Med J 1:552–555, 1968.
166. Fry L, Seah PP, Harper PG, et al: The small intestine in dermatitis herpetiformis. J Clin Pathol 27:817–824, 1974.
167. Kosnai I, Karpati S, Savilahti E, et al: Gluten challenge in children with dermatitis herpetiformis: A clinical, morphological and immunohistological study. Gut 27:1464–1470, 1986.
168. Weinstein WM, Brow JR, Parker F, et al: The small intestinal mucosa in dermatitis herpetiformis. II. Relationship of the small intestinal lesion to gluten. Gastroenterolgy 60:362–369, 1971.
169. Fry L, Seah PP, Riches DJ, Hoffbrand AV: Clearance of skin lesions in dermatitis herpetiformis after gluten withdrawal. Lancet 1:288–291, 1973.
170. Cooper BT, Mallos E, Trotter MD, Cooke WT: Response of the skin in dermatitis herpetiformis to a gluten-free diet, with reference to jejunal morphology. Gut 19:754–758, 1978.
171. Gawkrodger DJ, Blackwell JN, Gilmour HM, et al: Dermatitis herpetiformis: Diagnosis, diet and demography. Gut 25:151–157, 1984.
172. Leonard J, Haffendon G, Tucker W, et al: Gluten challenge in dermatitis herpetiformis. N Engl J Med 308:816–819, 1983.
173. de Franchis R, Primignani M, Cipolla M, et al: Small bowel involvement in dermatitis herpetiformis and in linear-IgA bullous dermatosis. J Clin Gastroenterol 5:429–436, 1983.
174. Crawford GM, Luikart RH II: Erythema multiforme with colitis. JAMA 140:780–781, 1949.
175. Sidi E, Reinberg A, Spinasse JB, Hinchy M: Lethal cutaneous and gastrointestinal arteriolar thrombosis (malignant atrophying papulosis of Degos). JAMA 174:1170–1173, 1960.
176. Degos R: Malignant atrophic papulosis. Br J Dermatol 100:21–35, 1979.
177. Case records of the Massachusetts General Hospital. N Engl J Med 303:1104–1111, 1980.
178. Bain NH: Ehlers-Danlos syndrome: Case report. Am J Gastroenterol 67:167–170, 1977.
179. Sigurdson E, Stern HS, Houpt J, et al: The Ehlers-Danlos syndrome and colonic perforation: Report of a case and physiologic assessment of underlying motility disorder. Dis Colon Rectum 28:962–966, 1985.
180. Goodman RM, Smith EW, Paton D, et al: Pseudoxanthoma elasticum: A clinical and histopathological study. Medicine 42:297–334, 1963.
181. Cocco AE, Grayer DL, Walker BA, Martyn LJ: The stomach in pseudoxanthoma elasticum. JAMA 210:2381–2382, 1969.
182. Bagdade JD, Parker F, Ways PO, et al: Fabry's disease: A correlative clinical, morphologic and biochemical study. Lab Invest 18:681–688, 1968.
183. Flynn DM, Lake BD, Boothby DB, Young EP: Gut lesions in Fabry's disease without a rash. Arch Dis Child 47:26–33, 1972.
184. Sheth KJ, Werlin SL, Freeman ME, Hodach AE: Gastrointestinal structure and function in Fabry's disease. Am J Gastroenterol 76:246–251, 1981.
185. O'Brien BD, Schnitka TK, McDougall R, et al: Pathophysiologic and ultrastructural basis for intestinal symptoms in Fabry's disease. Gastroenterology 82:957–962, 1982.
186. Friedman LS, Kirkham SE, Thistlethwaite JR, et al: Jejunal diverticulosis with perforation as a complication of Fabry's disease. Gastroenterology 86:558–563, 1984.
187. Goldgraber MB, Kirsner JB: Scleroderma of the gastrointestinal tract: A review. Arch Pathol 64:255–265, 1957.
188. Hoskins LC, Norris HT, Gottlieb LS, Zamcheck N: Functional and morphologic alterations of the gastrointestinal tract in progressive systemic sclerosis (scleroderma). Am J Med 33:459–470, 1962.
189. Peachey RD, Creamer B, Pierce JW: Sclerodermatous involvement of the stomach and the small and large bowel. Gut 10:285–292, 1969.
190. Poirer TJ, Rankin GB: Gastrointestinal manifestations of progressive systemic scleroderma based on a review of 364 cases. Am J Gastroenterol 58:30–44, 1972.
191. Schuffler MD, Beegle RG: Progressive systemic sclerosis of the gastrointestinal tract and hereditary hollow visceral myopathy: Two distinguishable disorders of intestinal smooth muscle. Gastroenterology 77:664–671, 1979.
192. Marshall JB, Kretschmar JM, Gerhardt DC, et al: Gastrointestinal manifestations of mixed connective tissue disease. Gastroenterology 98:1232–1238, 1990.
193. Schuffler MD, Lowe MC, Bill AH: Studies of idiopathic intestinal pseudoobstruction. I. Hereditary hollow visceral myopathy: Clinical and pathological studies. Gastroenterology 73:327–338, 1977.
194. Anuras S, Crane SA, Faulk DL, et al: Intestinal pseudoobstruction. Gastroenterology 74:1318–1324, 1978.
195. Faulk DL, Anuras S, Christensen J: Chronic intestinal pseudoobstruction. Gastroenterology 74:922–931, 1978.
196. Orringer MB, Dabich L, Zarafonetis CJ, et al: Gastroesophageal reflux in esophageal scleroderma: Diagnosis and implications. Ann Thorac Surg 22:120–130, 1976.
197. Cohen S, Laufer I, Snape WJ et al: The gastrointestinal manifestations of scleroderma: Pathogenesis and management. Gastroenterology 79:155–160, 1980.
198. Compton R: Scleroderma with diverticulosis and colonic obstruction. Am J Surg 118:602–606, 1969.
199. Krishnamurthy S, Kelly MM, Rohrmann CA, Schuffler MD: Jejunal diverticulosis: A heterogeneous disorder caused by a variety of abnormalities of smooth muscle or myenteric plexus. Gastroenterology 85:538–547, 1983.
200. Feldman F, Marshak RH: Dermatomyositis with significant involvement of the gastrointestinal tract. Am J Roentgenol 90:746, 1963.
201. Kleckner FS: Dermatomyositis and its manifestations in the gastrointestinal tract. Am J Gastroenterol 53:141–146, 1970.
202. Nowak TV, Ionasescu V, Anuras S: Gastrointestinal manifestations of the muscular dystrophies. Gastroenterology 82:800–810, 1982.
203. Leon SH, Schuffler MD, Kettler M, Rohrmann CA: Chronic intestinal pseudoobstruction as a complication of Duchenne's muscular dystrophy. Gastroenterology 90:455–459, 1986.
204. Brown CH, Shirey EK, Haserick JR: Gastrointestinal manifes-

tations of systemic lupus erythematosus. Gastroenterology 31:649–666, 1956.
205. Hoffman BI, Katz WW: The gastrointestinal manifestations of systemic lupus erythematosus: A review of the literature. Semin Arthritis Rheum 9:237–247, 1980.
206. Wold LE, Bagenstoss AH: Gastrointestinal lesions of periarteritis nodosa. Mayo Clin Proc 24:28–35, 1949.
207. Wood, MK, Read DR, Kraft AR, Barreta TM: A rare cause of ischemic colitis—polyarteritis nodosa. Dis Colon Rectum 22:428, 1979.
208. Adler RH, Norcross BM, Lockie L: Arteritis and infarction of the intestine in rheumatoid arthritis. JAMA 180:921–926, 1962.
209. Bywaters EGL, Scott JT: The natural history of vascular lesions in rheumatoid arthritis. J Chron Dis 16:905–914, 1963.
210. Bienenstock H, Minick CR, Rogoff B: Mesenteric arteritis and intestinal infarction in rheumatoid disease. Arch Intern Med 119:359–364, 1967.
211. Petterson T, Wegelius O, Skrituars B: Gastrointestinal disturbances in patients with severe rheumatoid arthritis. Acta Med Scand 188:139, 1970.
212. Lindsay MK, Tavadia HB, Whyte AS, et al: Acute abdomen in rheumatoid arthritis due to necrotizing arteritis. Br Med J 2:592–593, 1973.
213. Marcolongo R, Bayell PF, Montagnani M: Gastrointestinal involvement in rheumatoid arthritis: A biopsy study. J Rheumatol 6:163–173, 1979.
214. Silvoso GR, Ivey KJ, Butt JH, et al: Incidence of gastric lesions in patients with rheumatic disease on chronic aspirin therapy. Ann Intern Med 91:517–520, 1979.
215. Prillaman WW, Hurst DC, Ball GV, et al: Intestinal complications in rheumatoid arteritis and their relationship to corticosteroid therapy. J Chron Dis 27:475–481, 1974.
216. Stein HB, Urowitz MB: Gold-induced enterocolitis: Case report and literature review. J Rheumatol 3:21–26, 1976.
217. Skolnick BR, Katz LA, Kozower M: Life-threatening enterocolitis after gold salt therapy. J Clin Gastroenterol 1:145–148, 1979.
218. Reinhart WH, Kapeller M, Halter F: Severe pseudomembranous and ulcerative colitis during gold therapy. Endoscopy 15:70–72, 1983.
219. McCormick PA, O'Donoghue D, Lemass B: Gold-induced colitis: Case report and literature review. Irish Med J 78:17–18, 1985.
220. Jackson CW, Haboubi NY, Whorwell PJ, Schofield PF: Gold-induced enterocolitis. Gut 27:452–456, 1986.
221. Cuvelier C, Barbatis C, Mielants H, et al: Histopathology of intestinal inflammation related to reactive arthritis. Gut 28:394–401, 1987.
222. DeVos M, Cuvelier C, Mielants N, et al: Ileocolonoscopy in seronegative spondylarthropathy. Gastroenterology 96:339–344, 1989.
223. Shearn MA: Sjögren's Syndrome. Major Problems in Internal Medicine, Vol II. Philadelphia, WB Saunders Co, 1971, pp 130–135.
224. Park RW, Grand RJ: Gastrointestinal manifestations of cystic fibrosis: A review. Gastroenterology 81:1143–1161, 1981.
225. Jeffrey I, Durrans D, Wells M, Fox H: The pathology of meconium ileus equivalent. J Clin Pathol 36:1292–1297, 1983.
226. Carpenter HM: Pathogenesis of congenital jejunal atresia. Arch Pathol 73:390–396, 1962.
227. Parkins RA, Eidelman S, Rubin CE et al: The diagnosis of cystic fibrosis by rectal suction biopsy. Lancet 2:851–856, 1963.
228. Hage E, Anderson FU: Light and electron microscopic studies of rectal biopsies in cystic fibrosis. Acta Pathol Microbiol Scand 80A:345, 1972.
229. Neutra MR, Grand RJ, Trier JS: Glycoprotein synthesis, transport, and secretion by epithelial cells of human rectal mucosa: Normal and cystic fibrosis. Lab Invest 36:525–546, 1977.
230. Logan RFA, Ferguson A, Finlayson NDC, Weis DG: Primary biliary cirrhosis and celiac disease: An association? Lancet 1:230–233, 1978.
231. Conte D, Velio P, Brunelli L, et al: Stainable iron in gastric and duodenal mucosa of primary hemochromatosis patients and alcoholics. Am J Gastroenterol 82:237–240, 1987.
232. Powell LW, Campbell CB, Wilson E: Intestinal mucosal uptake of iron and iron retention in idiopathic haemochromatosis as evidence for a mucosal abnormality. Gut 11:727–731, 1970.
233. Steckman M, Bozymski EM: Hemosiderosis of the duodenum. Gastrointest Endosc 29:326–327, 1983.
234. Robbins SL, Cotran RS, Kumar V: Pathologic Basis of Disease, 3rd ed. Philadelphia, WB Saunders Co, 1984, pp 399–429.
235. Ansell JE, et al: The spectrum of vitamin K deficiency. JAMA 238:40–42, 1977.
236. Spivak JL, Jackson DL: Pellagra: An analysis of 18 patients and review of the literature. Johns Hopkins Med J 140:295–309, 1977.
237. Mehta SK, Kaur S, Avastni G, et al: Small intestinal deficiency in pellagra. Am J Clin Nutr 25:545–549, 1972.
238. Cook GC: Etiology and pathogenesis of postinfective tropical malabsorption (tropical sprue). Lancet 1:721–723, 1984.
239. Domellof L, Ericksson S, Helander HF, et al: Lipid islands in the gastric mucosa after resection for benign ulcer disease. Gastroenterology 72:14–18, 1977.
240. Drude RB, Balart LA, Herrington JP, et al: Gastric xanthoma: Histological similarity to signet ring cell carcinoma. J Clin Gastroenterol 4:217–221, 1982.
241. Coletta U, Stargill BC: Isolated xanthomatosis of the small bowel. Hum Pathol 16:422–424, 1985.
242. Azzopardi JG, Evans DJ: Mucoprotein-containing histiocytes (muciphages) in the rectum. J Clin Pathol 19:368–374, 1966.
243. Roth RI, Owen RZ, Keren DF, Volberding PA: Intestinal infection with Mycobacterium avium in acquired immune deficiency syndrome (AIDS): Histological and clinical comparison with Whipple's disease. Dig Dis Sci 30:497–504, 1985.
244. Herbert PN, Forte T, Heinen RJ, Fredrickson DS: Tangier disease. N Engl J Med 299:519–521, 1978.
245. Glickman RM, Green PHR, Less RS, Tall A: Apolipoprotein A-I synthesis in normal intestinal mucosa and in Tangier disease. N Engl J Med 299:1424–1427, 1978.
246. Bale PM, Clifton-Bligh P, Benjamin BNP, Whyte HM: Pathology of Tangier disease. J Clin Pathol 24:609–616, 1971.
247. Ferrans VJ, Fredrickson DS: The pathology of Tangier disease: A light and electron microscopic study. Am J Pathol 78:101, 1975.
248. Isselbacher KJ, Scheig R, Plotkin GR, Caulfield JB: Congenital beta-lipoprotein deficiency: A hereditary disorder involving a defect in the absorption and transport of lipids. Medicine 43:347–361, 1964.
249. Gotto A, Levy R, John K, et al: On the protein defect in a-beta-lipoproteinemia. N Engl J Med 284:813–818, 1971.
250. Kayden HJ: Abetalipoproteinemia. Annu Rev Med 23:285–296, 1972.
251. Dobbins WO III: An ultrastructural study of the intestinal mucosa in congenital Abetalipoprotein deficiency with particular emphasis upon the intestinal absorptive cell. Gastroenterology 50:195–210, 1966.
252. Greenwood N: The jejunal mucosa in two cases of A-beta-lipoproteinemia. Am J Gastroenterol 65:160–162, 1976.
253. Delpre G, Kadish U, Glantz I: Endoscopic assessment in abetalipoproteinemia (Bassen-Kornzweig syndrome). Endoscopy 10:59–62, 1978.
254. Landing BH, Silverman FN, Craig JM, et al: Familial neurovisceral lipidosis. Am J Dis Child 108:503–522, 1964.
255. Brady RO: The genetic mismanagement of complex lipid metabolism. Bull NY Acad Med 47:173–182, 1971.
256. Adachi M, Volk BW, Schneck L, Torii J: Fine structure of the myenteric plexus in various lipidoses. Arch Pathol 87:228–241, 1969.
257. Bodian M, Lake BD: The rectal approach to neuropathology. Br J Surg 50:702–714, 1963.
258. Den Tandt WR, Vio PMA, Eggermont E: Intestinal biopsy in lysosomal storage disease (letter). Lancet 2:1149, 1974.
259. Yamano T, Shimada M, Okada S, et al: Ultrastructural study of biopsy specimens of rectal mucosa: Its use in neuronal storage diseases. Arch Pathol Lab Med 106:673–677, 1982.
260. Brett EM, Lake BD: Reassessment of rectal approach to neuropathology in childhood: Review of 307 biopsies over 11 years. Arch Dis Child 50:753, 1975.
261. Carpenter S, Karpati G: Lysosomal storage in human skeletal muscle. Hum Pathol 17:683–703, 1986.

262. Schneck L, Volk BW, Saifer A: The gangliosidoses. Am J Med 46:245–263, 1969.
263. O'Brien JS: Generalized gangliosidosis. Handbook Clin Neurol 10:462–483, 1970.
264. Volk BW, Adachi M, Schneck L: The gangliosidoses. Hum Pathol 6:555–569, 1975.
265. Rowe JW, Gilliam JI, Warthin TA: Intestinal manifestations of Fabry's disease. Ann Intern Med 81:628–631, 1974.
266. Dinari G, Rosenbach Y, Grunebaum M, et al: Gastrointestinal manifestations of Niemann-Pick disease. Enzyme 25:407–412, 1980.
267. Ansanelli V Jr, Lane N: Lipochrome ("ceroid") pigmentation of the small intestine. Ann Surg 146:117–123, 1957.
268. Fox B: Lipofuscinosis of the gastrointestinal tract in man. J Clin Pathol 20:806–813, 1967.
269. Rapola J, Santavuori P, Savilahti E: Suction biopsy of rectal mucosa in the diagnosis of infantile and juvenile types of neuronal ceroid lipofuscinoses. Hum Pathol 15:352–360, 1984.
270. Toffler AH, Hukill PB, Spiro HM: Brown-bowel syndrome. Ann Intern Med 58:872–877, 1963.
271. Foster CS: The brown bowel syndrome: A possible smooth muscle mitochondrial myopathy? Histopathology 3:1–17, 1979.
272. Gallagher RL: Intestinal ceroid deposition—"Brown bowel syndrome": A light and electron microscopic study. Virchows Arch Pathol Anat 389:145–151, 1980.
273. Hosler JP, Kimmel KK, Moeller DD: The "brown bowel syndrome": A case report. Am J Gastroenterol 77:854–855, 1982.
274. Papp JP, Farmer RG, Hawk WA: Ceroid deposition of the small intestine associated with regional enteritis. Cleve Clin Q 30:189–194, 1969.
275. Lambert JR, Luk SC, Pritzker KPH: Brown bowel syndrome in Crohn's disease. Arch Pathol Lab Med 104:201–205, 1980.
276. Bauman MB, Di Mase JD, Oshi F, Senior JR: Brown bowel and skeletal myopathy associated with vitamin E depletion in pancreatic insufficiency. Gastroenterology 54:93–100, 1968.
277. Horn T, Svendsen LB, Johansen A, Backer O: Brown bowel syndrome. Ultrastruct Pathol 8:357–361, 1985.
278. Wittoesch JH, Jackman RJ, MacDonald JR: Melanosis coli: General review and study of 887 cases. Dis Colon Rectum 1:172–180, 1958.
279. Lough J, Fawcett J, Wiegensberg B: Wolman's disease: An electron microscopic, histochemical and biochemical study. Arch Pathol 89:103–110, 1970.
280. Partin JC, Schubert WK: Small intestinal mucosa in cholesterol ester storage disease: A light and electron microscope study. Gastroenterology 57:542–558, 1969.
281. Dorfman A, Matalon R: The mucopolysaccharidoses: A review. Proc Natl Acad Sci 73:630–637, 1976.
282. Morecki R, Paunier L, Hamilton JR: Intestinal mucosa in cystinosis. Arch Pathol 86:297–307, 1968.
283. Sidbury JB Jr, Heick HM: Glycogen storage diseases: A review with emphasis on gastrointestinal manifestations. South Med J 61:915–922, 1968.
284. Shephard NA, Crocker PR, Smith AP, Levison DA: Exogenous pigment in Peyer's patches. Hum Pathol 18:50–54, 1987.
285. Urbanski SJ, Arsenault L, Green FHY, Haber G: Pigment resembling atmospheric dust in Peyer's patches. Modern Pathol 2:222–226, 1989.
286. Wright JR, Calkins E: Clinical-pathologic differentiation of common amyloid syndromes. Medicine 60:429–448, 1981.
287. Kyle RA, Bayrd ED: Amyloidosis: Review of 236 cases. Medicine 54:271–299, 1975.
288. Cohen AS: An update of clinical, pathologic and biochemical aspects of amyloidosis. Int J Dermatol 20:515, 1981.
289. Glenner GG: Amyloid deposits and amyloidosis: the beta-fibrilloses. N Engl J Med 302:1283–1292, 1333–1343, 1980.
290. Gafni J, Sohar E, Heller H: The inherited amyloidoses. Lancet 1:71, 1964.
291. Mordechai R, Sohar E: Intestinal malabsorption: First manifestation of amyloidosis in familial Mediterranean fever. Gastroenterology 66:446–449, 1974.
292. Steen LE, Oberg L: Familial amyloidosis with polyneuropathy: Roentgenological and gastroscopic appearance of gastrointestinal involvement. Am J Gastroenterol 78:417–420, 1980.
293. Golden A: Primary systemic amyloidosis of the alimentary tract. Arch Intern Med 75:413–416, 1945.
294. Brody IA, Westlake PT, Laster L: Causes of intestinal symptoms in primary amyloidosis. Arch Intern Med 113:512–518, 1964.
295. Chernenkoff RM, Costopoulos LB, Bain GO: Gastrointestinal manifestations of primary amyloidosis. Can Med Assoc J 106:567–569, 1972.
296. Gilat T, Spiro HM: Amyloidosis and the gut. Am J Dig Dis 13:619–633, 1968.
297. Gilat T, Revach M, Sohar E: Deposition of amyloid in the gastrointestinal tract. Gut 10:98–104, 1969.
298. Monteiro JG: The digestive system in familial amyloidotic polyneuropathy. Am J Gastroenterol 60:47–59, 1973.
299. Kumar SS, Appavu SS, Abcarion H, Barreta T: Amyloidosis of the colon: Report of a case and review of the literature. Dis Colon Rectum 26:541–544, 1983.
300. Jarnum S: Gastrointestinal hemorrhage and protein loss in primary amyloidosis. Gut 6:14–18, 1965.
301. Levy DJ, Franklin GO, Rosenthal WS: Gastrointestinal bleeding and amyloidosis. Am J Gastroenterol 77:422–426, 1982.
302. Brom B, Bunk S, Marks IN: Ischemic colitis, gastric ulceration, and malabsorption in a case of primary amyloidosis. Gastroenterology 57:319–323, 1969.
303. Yamada M, Hatakeyama S, Tsukagoshi H: Gastrointestinal amyloid deposition in AL (primary or myeloma-associated) and AA (secondary) amyloidosis: Diagnostic value of a gastric biopsy. Hum Pathol 16:1206–1211, 1985.
304. Walley VM: Amyloid deposition in a gastric arteriovenous malformation. Arch Pathol Lab Med 110:69–71, 1986.
305. Perarnau JM, Raabe JJ, Courrier A, et al: A rare etiology of ischemic colitis—amyloid colitis. Endoscopy 14:107–109, 1982.
306. Vernon SE: Amyloid colitis. Dis Colon Rectum 25:728–730, 1982.
307. Legge DA, Wollaeger EE, Carlson HC: Intestinal pseudoobstruction in systemic amyloidosis. Gut 11:764–767, 1970.
308. Battle WM, Rubin MR, Cohen S, Snope WJ JR: Gastrointestinal motility dysfunction in amyloidosis. N Engl J Med 301:24–25, 1979.
309. Wald A, Kichler J, Mendelow H: Amyloidosis and chronic intestinal pseudoobstruction. Dig Dis Sci 26:462–465, 1981.
310. Herskovic T, Bartholomew LG, Green PA: Amyloidosis and malabsorption syndrome. Arch Int Med 114:629–633, 1964.
311. Schmidt H, Fruehmorgan P, Riemann JF, et al: Mucosal suggillations in the colon in secondary amyloidosis. Endoscopy 13:181–183, 1981.
312. Hunter AM, Campbell IW, Borsey DDG, Macaulay RAA: Protein-losing enteropathy due to gastrointestinal amyloidosis. Postgrad Med J 55:822, 1979.
313. Johnson DH, Guthrie TH, Tedesco FJ, et al: Amyloidosis masquerading as inflammatory bowel disease with a mass lesion, simulating malignancy. Am J Gastroenterol 77:141–145, 1982.
314. Jensen K, Raynor S, Rose SG et al: Amyloid tumors of the gastrointestinal tract: A report of two cases and review of the literature. Am J Gastroenterol 80:784–786, 1985.
315. Fitchen JH: Amyloidosis in granulomatous ileocolitis. N Engl J Med 292:352–353, 1975.
316. Shousha S, Lowdell CP, Bull TB, Parkins RA: Secondary amyloidosis of the gastrointestinal tract: An electron microscopic study. Hum Pathol 16:596–601, 1985.
317. Fentum PH, Turnberg LA, Wormsley KG: Biopsy of the rectum as an aid to the diagnosis of amyloidosis. Br Med J 1:364, 1962.
318. Kyle A, Spencer RJ, Dahlin DC: Value of rectal biopsy in the diagnosis of primary systemic amyloidosis. Am J Med Sci 251:501–506, 1966.
319. Coughlin GP, Remer RG, Grant AK: Endoscopic diagnosis of amyloidosis. Gastrointest Endosc 26:154, 1980.
320. Ohno F, Numata Y, Yamano T, et al: Gastroscopic biopsy of the stomach for the diagnosis of amyloidosis. Gastroenterol Jpn 17:415–421, 1982.
321. Green PA, Higgins JA, Brown AL Jr, et al: Amyloidosis: Appraisal of intubation biopsy of the small intestine in diagnosis. Gastroenterology 41:452–456, 1961.
322. Haggitt RC: Granulomatous diseases of the gastrointestinal tract. In Ioachim HL (ed): Pathology of Granulomas. New York, Raven Press, 1983, pp 257–305.

323. Kojima Y, Sakuma H, Izumi R et al: A case of granuloma of the ascending colon due to penetration of *Trichuris trichiura*. Gastroenterol Jpn 16:193–196, 1981.
324. Vafai M, Mohit P: Granuloma of the anal canal due to *Enterobius vermicularis*: Report of a case. Dis Colon Rectum 26:349–350, 1983.
325. Geller SA, Zimmerman MJ, Cohen A: Rectal biopsy in early *lymphogranuloma venereum* proctitis. Am J Gastroenterol 74:433–435, 1980.
326. Quinn TC, Goodell SE, Mhrtichion E, et al: *Chlamydia trachomatis* proctitis. N Engl J Med 305:195–200, 1981.
327. Surawicz CM, Belic L: Rectal biopsy helps to distinguish acute self-limited colitis from idiopathic inflammatory bowel disease. Gastroenterology 86:104–113, 1984.
328. Surawicz CM, Goodell SE, Quinn TC, et al: Spectrum of rectal biopsy abnormalities in homosexual men with intestinal symptoms. Gastroenterology 91:651–659, 1986.
329. Cho C, Linscheer WG, Hirschkorn MA, Ashutosh K: Sarcoid-like granuloma as an early manifestation of Whipple's disease. Gastroenterology 87:941–947, 1984.
330. Chambers TJ, Morson BC: The granuloma in Crohn's disease. Gut 20:269–274, 1979.
331. Surawicz CM, Meisel JL, Ylvisaker T, et al: Rectal biopsy in the diagnosis of Crohn's disease: Value of multiple biopsies and serial sectioning. Gastroenterology 80:66–71, 1981.
332. Petri M, Poulson SS, Christensen K, Jarnum S: The incidence of granulomas in serial sections of rectal biopsies from patients with Crohn's disease. Acta Pathol Microbiol Immunol Scand 90:145–147, 1982.
333. Goldgraber MB, Kirsner JB, Baskin HF: Nonspecific granulomatous disease of the stomach: A clinical pathological study. Arch Intern Med 102:10–24, 1958.
334. Fahimi HD, Deren JJ, Gottleib LS, et al: Isolated granulomatous gastritis. Gastroenterology 45:161–175, 1963.
335. Khan MH, Lam R, Tamoney HJ: Isolated granulomatous gastritis. Am J Gastroenterol 71:90–94, 1979.
336. Schinella RA, Ackert J: Isolated granulomatous disease of the stomach: report of three cases presenting as incidental findings in gastrectomy specimens. Am J Gastroenterol 72:30–35, 1979.
337. Weinstock JV: Idiopathic isolated granulomatous gastritis: Spontaneous resolution without surgical intervention. Dig Dis Sci 25:233–235, 1980.
338. Longcope WT, Freiman DG: A study of sarcoidosis: Based on a combined investigation of 160 cases including 30 autopsies from the Johns Hopkins Hospital and Massachusetts General Hospital. Medicine 31:1–132, 1952.
339. Israel HL, Stones M: Sarcoidosis: clinical observations on 160 cases. Arch Intern Med 102:766–776, 1958.
340. James DG, Neville E, Siltzbach LE, et al: A worldwide review of sarcoidosis. Ann NY Acad Sci 278:321–334, 1976.
341. Scott NM, Smith VM, Cox PA, Palmer ED: Sarcoid and sarcoid-like granulomas of the stomach. Arch Intern Med 92:741–749, 1953.
342. Wadina GS, Melamed A: Gastric granuloma (sarcoidosis?). Am J Gastroenterol 45:11–21, 1966.
343. Gould SR, Handley AJ, Barnardo DE: Rectal involvement and gastric involvement in a case of sarcoidosis. Gut 14:971–973, 1973.
344. Berens DL, Montes M: Gastric sarcoidosis. NY State J Med 75:1290–1293, 1975.
345. Konda J, Ruth M, Sassaris M et al: Sarcoidosis of the stomach and rectum. Am J Gastroenterol 73:516, 1980.
346. Tobi M, Kobrin I, Ariel I: Rectal involvement in sarcoidosis. Dis Colon Rectum 25:491–493, 1982.
347. Tinker MA, Viswanathan B, Laufer H, Margolis IB: Acute appendicitis and pernicious anemia as complications of gastrointestinal sarcoidosis. Am J Gastroenterol 79:868–872, 1984.
348. Chinitz MA, Brandt LJ, Frank MS et al: Symptomatic sarcoidosis of the stomach. Dig Dis Sci 30:682–688, 1985.
349. Polachek AA, Matre WJ: Gastrointestinal sarcoidosis: report of a case involving the esophagus. Am J Dig Dis 9:429–433, 1964.
350. MacFarlane DA: Intestinal sarcoidosis. Br J Surg 4:639–642, 1955.
351. Popovic OS, Brkic S, Bojic P et al: Sarcoidosis and protein losing enteropathy. Gastroenterology 78:119–125, 1980.
352. Rauf A, Davis P, Levendoglu H: Sarcoidosis of the small intestine. Am J Gastroenterol 83:187–189, 1988.
353. Sprague R, Harper P, McClain S, et al: Disseminated gastrointestinal sarcoidosis: Case report and review of the literature. Gastroenterology 87:421–425, 1984.
354. Ament ME, Ochs HD: Gastrointestinal manifestations of chronic granulomatous disease. N Engl J Med 288:382–387, 1973.
355. Werlin SL, Chusid MJ, Caya J, et al: Colitis in chronic granulomatous disease. Gastroenterology 82:328–331, 1981.
356. Griscom NT, Kirkpatrick JA, Girdany JA, et al: Gastric antral narrowing in chronic granulomatous disease of childhood. Pediatrics 54:456–460, 1974.
357. Harris BH, Boles ET: Intestinal lesions in chronic granulomatous disease of childhood. J Pediatr Surg 5:955–956, 1973.
358. Sty JR, Chusid MJ, Babbitt DP, et al: Involvement of the colon in chronic granulomatous disease of childhood. Radiology 132:618, 1979.
359. Ament ME, Ochs HD, Davis SD: Structure and function of the gastrointestinal tract in primary immunodeficiency syndromes: A study of 39 patients. Medicine 52:227–248, 1973.
360. Damjanov I, Katz SM: Malakoplakia. Pathol Annu 16:103, 1981.
361. McClure J: Malakoplakia. J Pathol 140:275–330, 1983.
362. Yunis EJ, Estevez JM, Pinson GJ, et al: Malakoplakia: Discussion of pathogenesis and report of three cases including one of fatal gastric and colonic involvement. Arch Pathol 83:180–187, 1967.
363. Lewin KJ, Fair WR, Steibigel RT, et al: Clinical and laboratory studies into the pathogenesis of malakoplakia. J Clin Pathol 29:354–363, 1976.
364. Abdou NI, NaPombejara C, Sagawa A, et al: Malakoplakia: Evidence for monocyte lysosomal abnormality correctable by cholinergic agonist in vitro and in vivo. N Engl J Med 297:1413–1418, 1977.
365. Nation EF: Malakoplakia of the urinary tract. J Urol 76:576, 1956.
366. Melicow MM: Malakoplakia. J Urol 78:33–40, 1957.
367. Ranchod M, Kahn LB: Malakoplakia of the gastrointestinal tract. Arch Pathol 94:90–97, 1972.
368. Gonzalez-Angulo A, Corral E, Garcia-Torres R, et al: Malakoplakia of the colon. Gastroenterology 48:383–387, 1965.
369. Terner MY, Lattes R: Malakoplakia of colon and retroperitoneum. Am J Clin Pathol 44:20–31, 1965.
370. Finlay-Jones MB, Blackwell JB, Papadimitriou JM: Malakoplakia of the colon. Am J Clin Pathol 50:320–329, 1968.
371. Joyeuse R, Lott JV, Mihaelis M, Gumucio CC: Malakoplakia of the colon and rectum: Report of a case and review of the literature. Surgery 81:189–192, 1971.
372. DiSilvio TV, Bartlett EF: Malakoplakia of the colon. Arch Pathol 92:167–171, 1971.
373. Dockerty MB: Primary malakoplakia of the colon. Mayo Clin Proc 47:114–116, 1972.
374. De LaGarza T, Nunez-Rasilla V, Alegre-Palafox R, Albores-Saavedra J: Malakoplakia of the colon. Dis Colon Rectum 16:216–233, 1973.
375. MacKay EH: Malakoplakia in ulcerative colitis. Arch Pathol Lab Med 102:140–145, 1978.
376. Miranda D, Vuletin JC, Kauffman SL: Disseminated histiocytosis and intestinal malakoplakia. Arch Pathol Lab Med 103:302–308. 1979.
377. McClure J: Malakoplakia of the gastrointestinal tract. Postgrad Med J 57:95–103, 1981.
378. Moran CA, West B, Schwartz IS: Malacoplakia of the colon in association with colonic adenocarcinoma. Am J Gastroenterol 84:1580–1582, 1989.
379. Nakabayashi H, Ito T, Izutsu K et al: Malakoplakia of the stomach: Report of a case and review of the literature. Arch Pathol Lab Med 102:136–139, 1978.
380. Lewin KJ, Harell GS, Lee AS, et al: Malakoplakia: an electron microscopic study: Demonstration of bacilliform organisms in malakoplakic macrophages. Gastroenterology 66:28–45, 1974.
381. Chaudhry AP, Saigal KP, Intengan M, Nickerson PA: Malakoplakia of the large intestine found incidentally at necropsy:

Light and electron microscopic features. Dis Colon Rectum 22:73–81, 1979.
382. McClure J, Cameron CHS, Garrett R: The ultrastructural features of malakoplakia. J Pathol Bacteriol 134:13–25, 1981.
383. Stevens S, McClure J: The histochemical features of the Michaelis-Gutmann body and a consideration of the pathophysiological mechanisms of its formation. J Pathol 137:119–127, 1982.
384. Newton WA Jr, Hamoudi AB: Histiocytosis: A histologic classification and clinical correlation. Perspect Pediatr Pathol 1:251, 1973.
385. Lahey ME: Histiocytosis X—an analysis of prognostic factors. J Pediatr 87:184–189, 1975.
386. Oberman HA: Idiopathic histiocytosis: A clinicopathologic study of 49 cases and review of the literature. Pediatrics 28:307–327, 1981.
387. Mierau GW, Favara BE, Brenman JM: Electron microscopy of histiocytes. Ultrastruct Pathol 3:137–142, 1982.
388. Parker JW, Lichtenstein L: Severe hepatic involvement in chronic disseminated histiocytosis X. Am J Clin Pathol 40:624–632, 1963.
389. Landing BH, Wells TR, Reed GB, Narayen MS: Diseases of the bile ducts in children. In Gall EA, Mostofi FK (eds): The Liver. Baltimore, Williams & Wilkins, 1973, pp 503–509.
390. Keeling JW, Harris JT: Intestinal malabsorption in infants with histiocytosis X. Arch Dis Child 48:350–354, 1973.
391. Iwofuchi M, Watanabe H, Shiratsuka M: Primary benign histiocytosis of the stomach: A report of a case showing spontaneous remission after 5½ years. Am J Surg Pathol 14:489–496, 1990.
392. Lee RG, Braziel RM, Stenzel P: Gastrointestinal involvement in Langerhans cell histiocytosis (Histiocytosis X): Diagnosis by rectal biopsy. Modern Pathol 3:154–157, 1990.
393. Gregorie HB, Otherson H, Moore MP: The significance of sarcoid-like lesions in association with malignant neoplasms. Am J Surg 104:577–586, 1962.
394. Churg J, Strauss L: Allergic granulomatosis, allergic angiitis and periarteritis nodosa. Am J Pathol 27:277–301, 1951.

PART 3

ESOPHAGUS

CHAPTER 17

Esophagitis

STANLEY R. HAMILTON, M.D.

PATHOLOGIC FINDINGS

NORMAL HISTOLOGIC VARIANTS
Glycogenic Acanthosis
Ectopic Sebaceous Glands
Melanocytic Proliferation

ESOPHAGITIS DUE TO INFECTIOUS AGENTS
Fungal Esophagitis
Opportunistic Fungal Esophagitis
Candidal Esophagitis
Aspergillus and *Phycomycetes* Esophagitis
Pathogenic Fungal Esophagitis
Viral Esophagitis
Herpes Esophagitis
Cytomegalovirus Esophagitis
Esophagitis Associated with Varicella, Rubella, and Variola
Esophagitis Due to HIV and Epstein-Barr Virus
Human Papillomavirus Infection of the Esophagus
Bacterial Esophagitis
Opportunistic Bacterial Esophagitis
Mycobacterial Esophagitis
Actinomyces Israeli Esophagitis
Miscellaneous Bacterial Esophagitis

Spirochetal (Syphilitic) Esophagitis
Parasitic Esophagitis

ESOPHAGEAL INJURY DUE TO EXOGENOUS CHEMICALS
Lye, Acids, Detergents, and Other Household Products
Drug Contact
Sclerotherapy for Esophageal Varices
Chemotherapeutic Agents

ESOPHAGEAL TRAUMA

ESOPHAGEAL INJURY DUE TO PHYSICAL AGENTS
Radiation Esophagitis
Thermal Injury

HIATAL HERNIA
Sliding Hiatal Hernia
Paraesophageal Hernia
Other Diaphragmatic Hernias

GASTROESOPHAGEAL REFLUX
Low-Grade Changes
High-Grade Changes
Barrett's Esophagus
Histopathologic Features
Ultrastructural Studies

Histopathologic Diagnosis
Differential Diagnosis
Dysplasia and Adenocarcinoma in Barrett's Mucosa
Biopsies for Monitoring Barrett's Mucosa

MOTOR AND RELATED DISORDERS OF THE ESOPHAGUS
Achalasia
Rings and Webs
Diverticula

ESOPHAGEAL INVOLVEMENT BY SYSTEMIC DISEASES
Collagen Vascular–Connective Tissue Diseases
Crohn's Disease
Behçet's Disease
Eosinophilic Gastroenteritis and Esophagitis
Dermatologic Diseases
Sarcoidosis
Immunodeficiency
Graft-versus-Host Disease
Amyloidosis

CONCLUDING COMMENTS

The esophagus is involved by a wide variety of inflammatory and other nonneoplastic disorders. Pathologists are often involved in the diagnosis of esophagitis in examining specimens from endoscopic biopsy, surgical resection, and autopsy. Pathologic recognition of the specific cause of esophagitis is often difficult, and the situation is confounded by the relatively common occurrence of multifactorial esophagitis. This chapter emphasizes the pathologic findings that are helpful in differential diagnosis.

PATHOLOGIC FINDINGS

Esophagitis means inflammation of the esophagus and connotes the presence of inflammatory cells, since

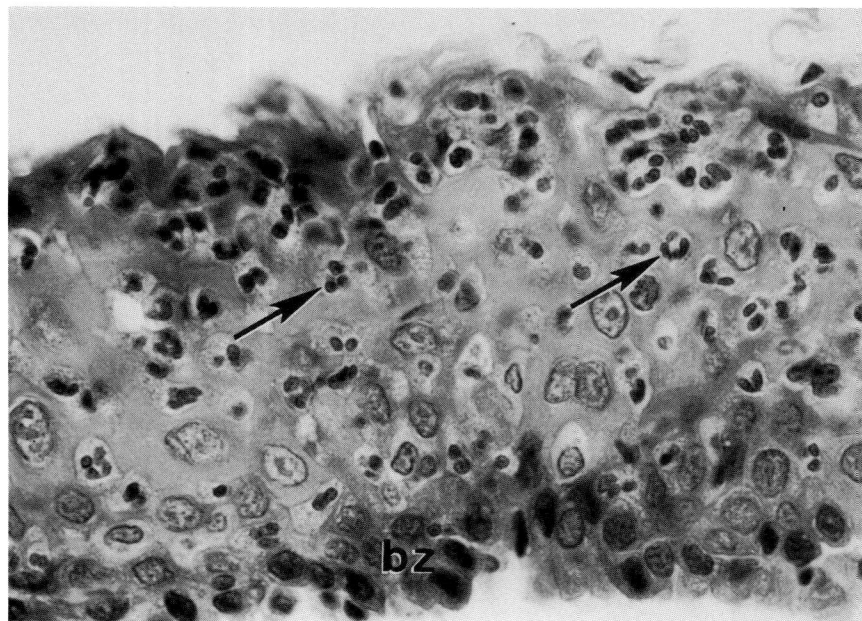

FIGURE 17-1. Active esophagitis. The squamous epithelium is heavily infiltrated by neutrophils (arrows) and thinned because of erosion of the superficial layers. The basal zone (bz) is reactive with hyperchromatic nuclei, and the epithelium is immature, as manifested by enlarged nuclei with prominent nucleoli in the prickle cell layer.

these are easily recognized by light microscopy. Esophagitis has numerous causes, only a few of which involve diagnostic histopathologic findings. Evidence of severe injury in the form of erosion and ulceration is sometimes present in patients with esophagitis, and any injury is usually followed by a stereotyped repair process with similar histopathologic findings regardless of the cause.

Active esophagitis is characterized by infiltration of the squamous epithelium by polymorphonuclear leukocytes, usually neutrophils (Figure 17-1). In addition, accompanying findings include congestion with dilated blood vessels ("vascular lakes") in the lamina propria and epithelial edema characterized by enlargement and clearing of cells and of the spaces between them. The repair process consists in part of epithelial proliferation. The histopathologic findings in this reactive epithelial response to injury include thickening of the basal zone with increased mitotic figures; elongation and increased numbers of lamina propria papillae; and the presence at the luminal surface of immature ovoid squamous epithelial cells with enlarged nuclei. These features represent *reactive epithelial changes* (Figure 17-2).

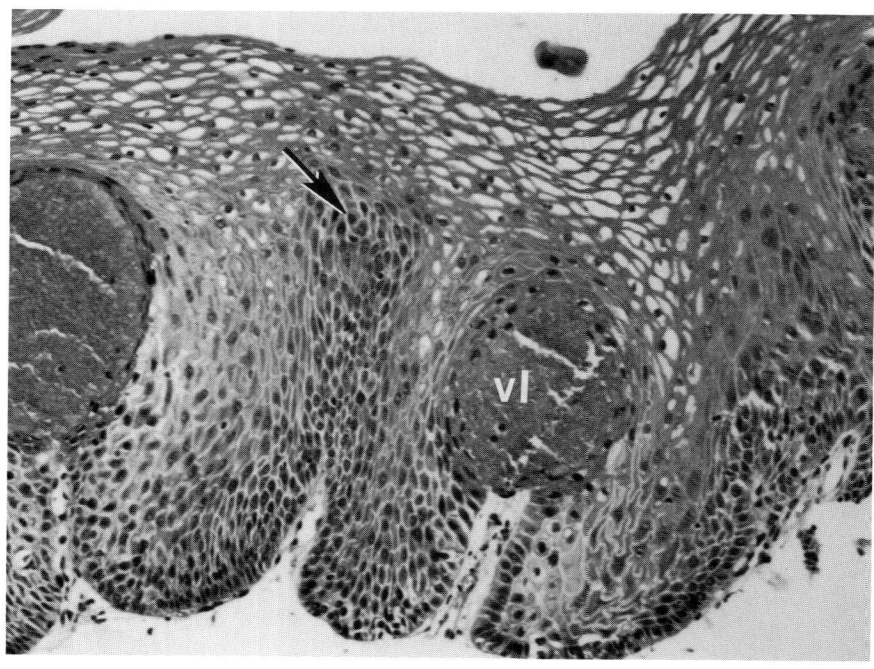

FIGURE 17-2. Reactive epithelial changes and vascular lakes in esophageal squamous epithelium. The vascular papillae (arrow) are elongated, extending approximately three fourths of the thickness of the epithelium. Vascular lakes (vl) are formed by dilated vascular papillae with congestion. The basal zone (which can be delineated by the absence of staining with periodic acid–Schiff [PAS] stain) is of normal thickness in this example.

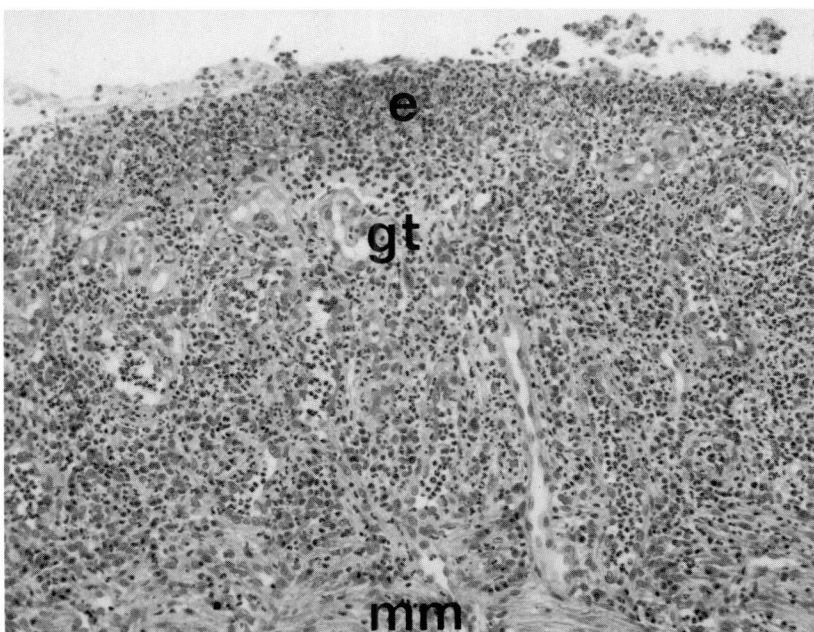

FIGURE 17–3. Active chronic ulcer of the esophagus. Luminal fibrinoinflammatory exudate (e) overlies inflamed granulation tissue (gt) which occupies the region of the lamina propria on the luminal side of the muscularis mucosae (mm). An ulcer in the esophagus has full-thickness loss of the squamous epithelium but does not necessarily extend into the muscularis mucosae, in contrast to other regions of the gastrointestinal tract, because of the layer of lamina propria connective tissue between the epithelium and smooth muscle.

Chronic esophagitis cannot be defined well pathologically because of ambiguity in the term *chronic*. On the one hand, lymphocytes and plasma cells, generally regarded as chronic inflammatory cells, are a common histopathologic finding in the lamina propria. Chronic inflammation can persist long after active esophagitis and its clinical symptoms have resolved and therefore may relate poorly to the patient's clinical status. In this situation, application by the pathologist of the term *chronic esophagitis* seems inappropriate to the patient's resolved symptoms. On the other hand, active esophagitis can persist clinically and become chronic in the temporal sense, but biopsies may continue to show predominantly acute inflammation, particularly in the epithelium. Again, in this situation, use by the pathologist of *chronic esophagitis* does not portray accurately the clinical circumstances with ongoing acute injury. Because of these ambiguities, the term should probably not be used for pathologic findings without qualification. Clinical chronic esophagitis connotes recurrent or persistent disease and is usually associated with reflux esophagitis; it can include histologic findings of Barrett's esophagus and/or peptic stricture (see below).

With severe injury in active esophagitis, epithelial destruction can occur. *Erosion* refers to less than full-thickness destruction of the epithelium such that the superficial layers are absent but the deeper layers, including the basal zone, remain (see Figure 17–1). The deeper layers of the epithelium commonly show active inflammation with neutrophils, and luminal fibroinflammatory exudate is frequently present. If sufficient time has elapsed between onset of injury and time of tissue sampling, reactive epithelial changes accompany erosion.

An *ulcer* results from severe injury and is characterized by complete loss of the epithelium (Figure 17–3). After ulceration, the lamina propria or even deeper layers of the esophageal wall are exposed to the luminal contents. In an *acute ulcer* of recent occurrence, the base consists of necrotic tissue and debris with active inflammation and exudate. With time, the repair processes characterized by epithelial regeneration and growth of granulation tissue into the base, with fibrosis and scarring, occur. Continuation of injury along with the repair processes results in an *active chronic ulcer* (see Figure 17–3). Re-epithelization is manifested by a layer of immature epithelial cells migrating from the periphery of the ulcer. When a layer of epithelium covers the ulcer but the mucosa has not been reconstituted, the term *healing ulcer* can be applied. Completion of mucosa reconstitution results in a *healed ulcer*, but reactive epithelial changes may persist for some time.

The importance of these definitions of active esophagitis, erosion, and ulcer relates to the complications of esophagitis. Generally, severe hemorrhage, perforation, and stricture formation occur as a result of ulceration. Hemorrhage and perforation are produced by the ulceration itself, whereas stricture formation results from the deposition of scar tissue as part of the repair process. Thus, recognition of the early stages of injury in endoscopic biopsy specimens may lead to therapy, which can prevent the development of ulceration, whatever the cause of the injury, and its complications.

NORMAL HISTOLOGIC VARIANTS

Glycogenic Acanthosis

Glycogenic acanthosis appears as white mucosal plaques. Specimens showing prominent glycogenic ac-

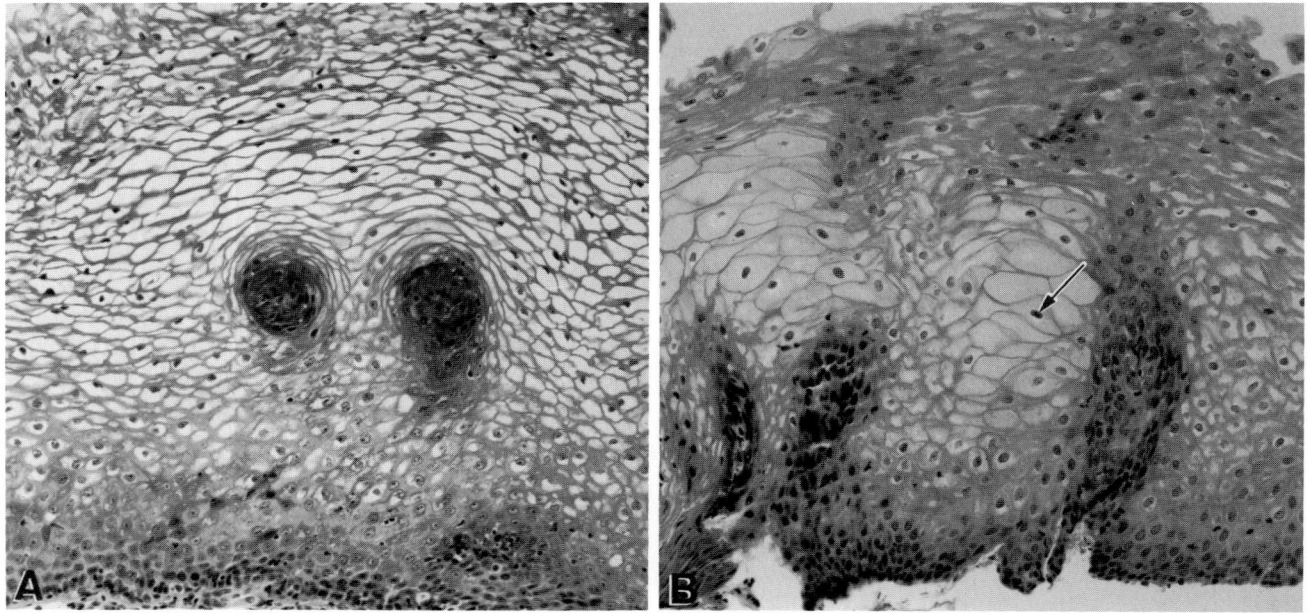

FIGURE 17–4. Glycogenic acanthosis and balloon cells in esophageal squamous epithelium. A, Glycogenic acanthosis has thickened squamous epithelium with increased numbers of enlarged cells characterized by clear ctyoplasm that contains glycogen (demonstrable by PAS stain). B, Balloon cells are enlarged squamous epithelial cells with translucent cytoplasm due to the presence of plasma proteins, which signify increased cellular permeability related to injury. The plasma proteins can be demonstrated by immunohistochemical methods. The cytoplasm of balloon cells stains poorly with PAS stain, in contrast to glycogenic acanthosis. The nuclei are often pyknotic (arrow). The squamous epithelium with balloon cells is usually of normal thickness. (Same magnification as A.)

anthosis (Figure 17–4A) are frequently submitted as "leukoplakia." The plaques are formed of large clusters of enlarged clear cells grouped together in the upper layers of the thickened squamous epithelium. The cells contain abundant glycogen, much of which is removed during histologic processing, which results in the clear appearance unless fixative to preserve glycogen (e.g., Carnoy's fluid) or frozen section is used. The reason for the development of clusters of such cells is unknown.

"Balloon cells" are enlarged squamous epithelial cells that resemble the cells of glycogenic acanthosis but have translucent, rather than clear, cytoplasm in hematoxylin and eosin (H&E)–stained sections (Figure 17–4B). Balloon cells can be seen to contain plasma proteins when examined by immunohistochemical methodology and appear to develop as a result of increased permeability of the cell membrane, attributable to injury. The nuclei are often pyknotic. Balloon cells can be found in the middle or superficial layers of the squamous epithelium, depending upon the nature of the epithelial injury: with chronic gastroesophageal reflux, the balloon cells are typically in the middle layers, whereas with infectious esophagitis and acute chemical injury the balloon cells are usually superficial. Balloon cells can be distinguished easily from glycogenic acanthosis by absence of the periodic acid–Schiff (PAS) staining characteristics of glycogen.

Ectopic Sebaceous Glands

Ectopic sebaceous glands in the lamina propria have been found to produce endoscopically visible nodules. The histopathologic appearance of the glands themselves is similar to that in the skin.

Melanocytic Proliferation

Melanocytes are present in the basal layer of the squamous epithelium. In occasional patients, melanocytic proliferation occurs with melanocytes in all layers of the epithelium, as well as melanin-containing macrophages in the lamina propria. This melanocytic proliferation is seen grossly or endoscopically as a small pigmented area, most commonly in the mid esophagus.

ESOPHAGITIS DUE TO INFECTIOUS AGENTS

The esophagus is affected by infectious agents of a number of types (Table 17–1). The various agents have various portals of entry into the esophagus; they may enter through the mucosal surface, via the vascular and lymphatic systems, or by direct extension from adjacent mediastinal structures. The site of esophageal infection is influenced both by characteristics of the agent and host factors. Although the organisms are presented individually here, it should be kept in mind that in many patients with infective esophagitis there is more than one agent identifiable by microbiologic and histopathologic methods; these cases represent mixed infections. This is particularly important in immunocompromised patients, including those with

Table 17-1 USUAL LOCALIZATIONS OF INFECTIOUS AGENTS IN THE ESOPHAGUS

Agent	Lumen Only	Squamous Epithelium	Ulcer Bed and/or Mural Structures
Fungi			
Opportunistic fungi		X	X
Candida			
Aspergillus			
Phycomycetes			
Pathogenic fungi			X
Histoplasma			
Blastomyces			
Sporothrix			
Paracoccidioides			
Viruses			
Herpes virus, viral exanthems		X	
Human immunodeficiency virus			
Epstein-Barr virus			
Human papilloma virus			
Cytomegalovirus			X
Bacteria			
Opportunistic bacteria		X	X
Tuberculous and nontuberculous mycobacteria			X
Miscellaneous bacteria	X	X	X
Spirochetes			
Treponema pallidum			X
Parasites			
Ascaris	X		
Amoeba			X
Echinococcus			X
Cysticercus			
Trichinella			
Filaria			

human immunodeficiency virus (HIV) infection and acquired immunodeficiency syndrome (AIDS).

Fungal Esophagitis

Fungal infections of the esophagus can be considered in two categories: those caused by organisms with little inherent pathogenicity but occurring with underlying abnormality in the host (opportunistic fungi) and those caused by organisms with inherent pathogenicity (pathogenic fungi). The opportunistic fungal infections are by far the more commonly encountered.

Opportunistic Fungal Esophagitis

Candidal Esophagitis (Figures 17-5 to 17-9)

Candidal (monilial) esophagitis is usually due to *Candida albicans* or occasionally *Candida tropicalis* or *krusei*. *Candida (Torulopsis) globrata*, which has distinguishing histopathologic characteristics (see Figure 17-9), also produces esophagitis in rare cases.

Candidal esophagitis is usually an opportunistic infection that occurs in association with some abnormality in the host. The systemic conditions favoring the development of candidiasis in general and esophageal candidiasis in particular include medication with broad-spectrum antibacterial antibiotics, systemic steroids, cytotoxic chemotherapy for cancer, immune suppression after organ transplantation, AIDS, postoperative state, and low birth weight. Local esophageal injury further promotes the fungal infection.

The yeasts are commensal inhabitants of the gastrointestinal tract, including the mouth and oropharynx, in a sizable percentage of persons. The organisms appear to reach the esophagus by being swallowed, but clinically evident oral thrush is absent in many patients with candidal esophagitis. Pre-existing abnormality in the esophageal mucosal surface predisposes to the infection.

The clinical spectrum of candidal esophagitis has been categorized into acute, subacute, and chronic forms. Acute candidal esophagitis is the most commonly encountered form. This form typically occurs in the lower esophagus of compromised patients and is of sudden onset. With progression of the infection into the esophageal wall, the acute form may lead to disseminated candidiasis. Rare examples of perforation have been reported. Esophageal stenosis may result from spasm, mucosal edema, and a thick pseudomembrane composed of *Candida*, accumulated squamous epithelial debris, and fibrinoinflammatory exudate (see Figure 17-5). Local treatment of acute candidal esophagitis often results in resolution with no sequelae. Occasional patients, however, develop an esophageal stricture late in the course, probably due to fibrosis resulting from previous extension of the infectious and inflammatory process into the esophageal wall or submucosal glands.

Subacute candidal esophagitis is uncommon. This form seems to occur as indolent, often asymptomatic, infection in patients who are not apparently compromised. The subacute form is usually first recognized when the patient presents with complaints resulting from an esophageal stricture and/or intramural pseudodiverticulosis. The strictures are most common in the upper esophagus and are said to be more pliant than

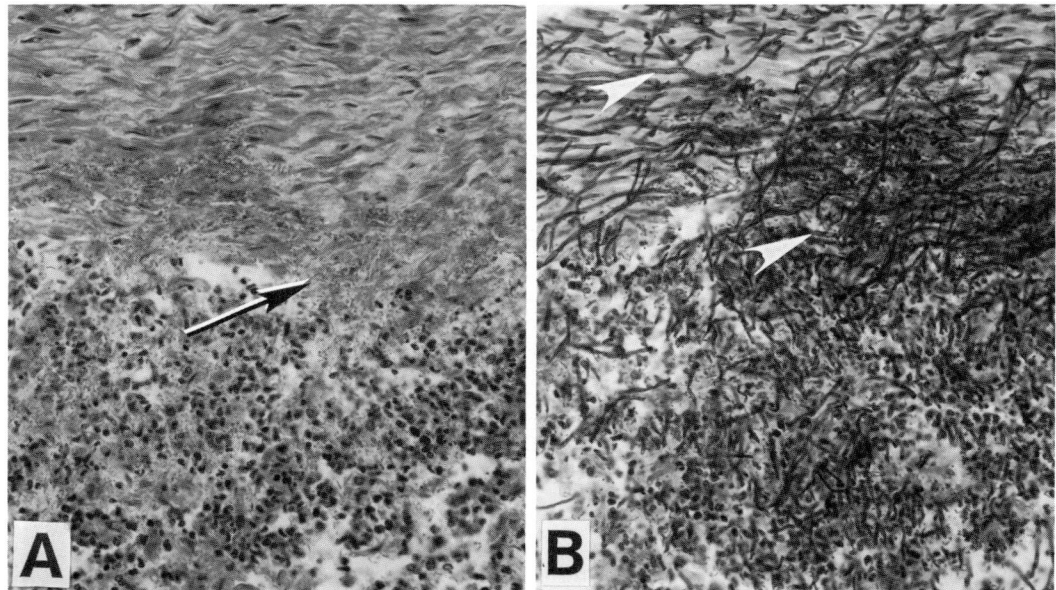

FIGURE 17–5. Candidal esophagitis. *A*, With hematoxylin and eosin stain, layers of accumulated squamous epithelial debris with numerous bacteria (arrow) and inflammatory cells are obvious, but the *Candida* organisms are difficult to visualize. *B*, With PAS stain of the same tissue fragment as shown in A, large numbers of candidal pseudohyphae (arrowhead) are evident throughout the tissue. (Same magnification as *A*.)

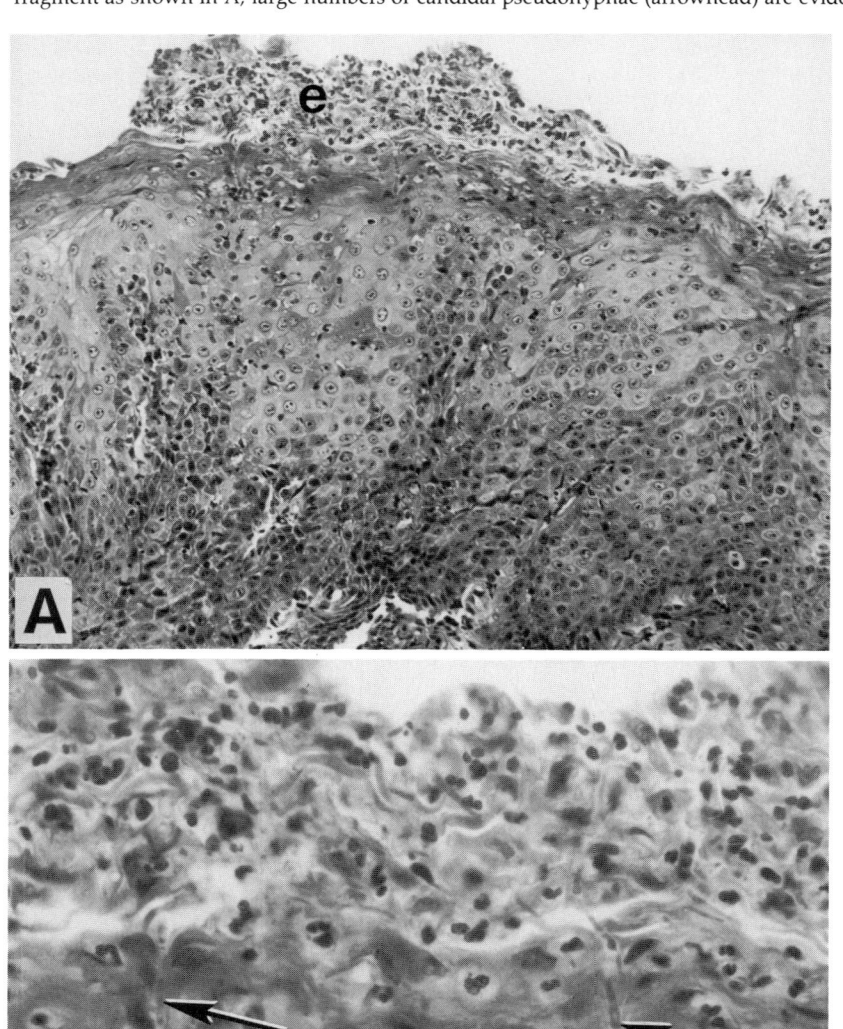

FIGURE 17–6. Candidal esophagitis. *A*, Reactive squamous epithelium with intraepithelial neutrophils and luminal fibrinoinflammatory exudate (e) containing *Candida* are present. *B*, *Candida* pseudohyphae (arrows) extend into the superficial layers of the squamous epithelium beneath the exudate.

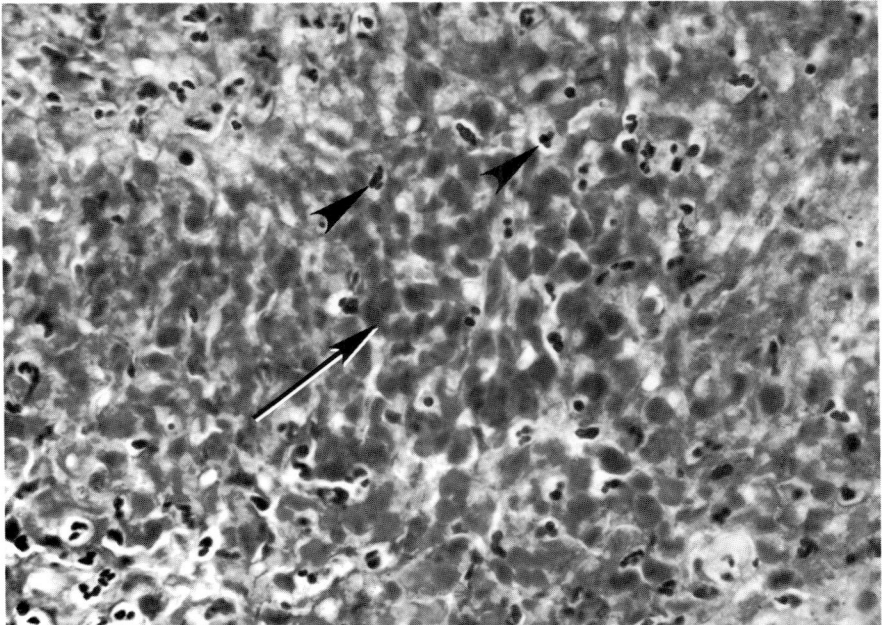

FIGURE 17–7. Candidal esophagitis with characteristic "mummified" necrotic tissue. The outlines of necrotic squamous epithelial cells are evident (arrow) and contrast with intact neutrophils (arrowheads). Although no *Candida* organisms are identified in this field, they were evident in an adjoining area of the tissue. This histopathologic appearance should lead to a careful search for *Candida* with the use of a stain for fungi.

strictures due to other causes. Intramural pseudodiverticulosis, as the name implies, is recognized on barium contrast studies by the presence of what appear to be multiple small diverticula within the wall of the esophagus. Autopsy cases of intramural pseudodiverticulosis show *Candida* involving the ducts of submucosal glands with hyperplasia of the squamous epithelium. Obstruction, dilatation, inflammation, and destruction of the glands result, producing outpouchings communicating with the esophageal lumen, which are filled by barium and produce the characteristic radiographic appearance. The association among the occurrence in the upper esophagus of large numbers of submucosal glands, *Candida*-related strictures, and intramural pseudodiverticulosis has suggested a pathogenetic relationship to some authors. Disseminated candidiasis rarely results from subacute candidal esophagitis.

Chronic candidal esophagitis is rare. This form generally occurs with chronic mucocutaneous candidiasis associated with a variety of cell-mediated immunologic deficits. Granulomatous inflammation in response to *Candida* sometimes occurs in this form. Fibrous esophageal strictures may occur, but esophageal narrowing

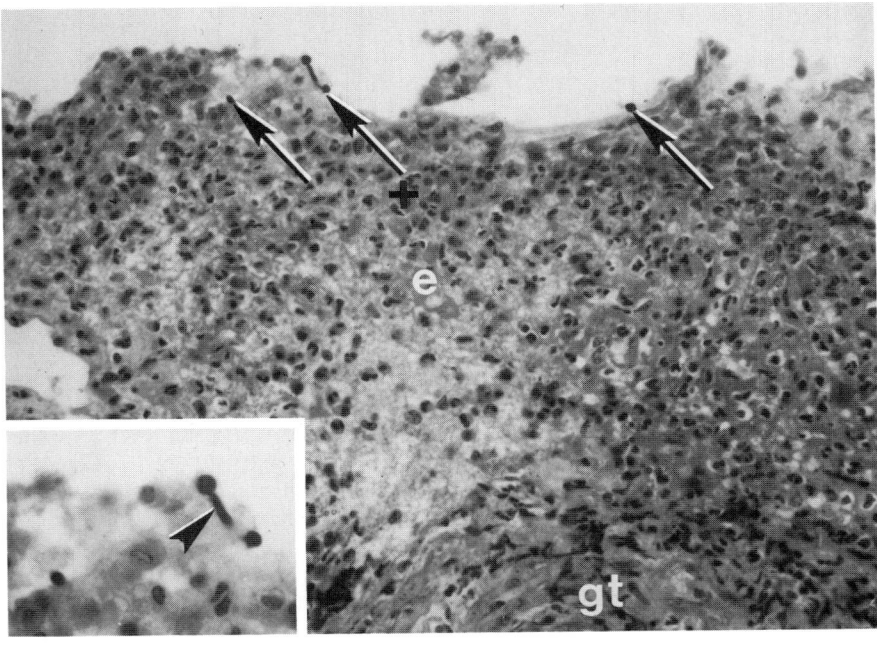

FIGURE 17–8. Candidal colonization of esophageal ulcer. The fibrinoinflammatory exudate (e) overlying inflamed granulation tissue (gt) contains scattered yeast forms of *Candida* (arrows) in this PAS-stained section. The inset shows the area indicated by the plus (+) sign, where pseudohyphal formation (arrowhead) is evident in one *Candida* yeast.

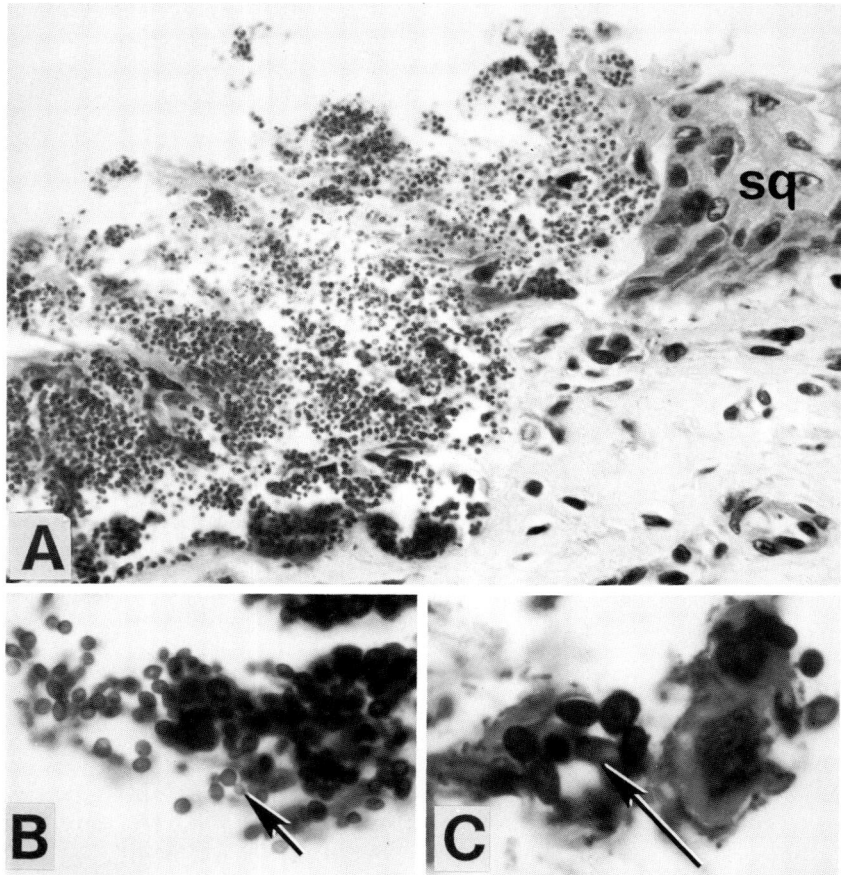

FIGURE 17–9. Esophagitis due to *Candida (Torulopsis) globrata*. *A*, Small, round yeasts characteristic of *C. globrata* extend through the squamous epithelium (sq) into the lamina propria. No inflammatory response is evident because of marked neutropenia induced by cytotoxic chemotherapy in the patient. *B*, High-power view of *C. globrata*. Budding of one yeast is evident (arrow). *C*, *Candida albicans* at the same magnification as *B*, illustrating larger size, ovoid shape, and the presence of pseudohyphae (arrow), which are not evident in *C. globrata*.

due to inflammation and spasm are more common. Disseminated candidiasis resulting from chronic candidal esophagitis is uncommon.

The histopathologic features of candidal esophagitis have great variability (see Figures 17–5 to 17–9). *Candida* may appear as budding yeast forms or pseudohyphae; they may be few or numerous. The esophageal tissue may show necrosis, ulceration, erosion, or intact epithelium. The severity of inflammatory response is also variable, depending upon patient capabilities. The yeast and pseudohyphae may invade the esophageal tissue to variable depths, or the organisms may show no evidence of invasion.

Candida organisms are basophilic in H&E-stained sections. Even when numerous, the organisms are difficult to visualize in the midst of inflammatory exudate and debris. As a result, routine use of a stain for fungi (PAS, which may be conveniently included in combination with alcian blue, pH 2.5, or methenamine silver) is recommended, particularly when inflammation is identified (see Figure 17–5). The yeast forms of *C. albicans, tropicalis,* and *krusei* are oval. Buds frequently extend from the yeast cells (blastospores) and may elongate to produce nonseptate pseudohyphae under conditions that inhibit cell division but not growth. The pseudohyphae may grow to striking lengths and interdigitate to form large clumps of organisms. The pseudohyphal form of the organism usually occurs in invaded tissue, although yeast forms can also invade. With colonization and invasion, the proportion of the organisms in the pseudohyphal form increases with the age of the lesion.

C. albicans, tropicalis and *krusei* cannot be differentiated in histopathologic sections; *C. albicans* is most common. *C. (Torulopsis) globrata,* however, is smaller than the other species and tends to occur as large masses of round, budding yeast without pseudohyphae (see Figure 17–9). *Candida* organisms are usually accompanied by numerous bacteria. Sometimes histopathologic evidence of other fungi (Figure 17–10) or of viral esophagitis (Figure 17–11) is also found (see the next section and Viral Esophagitis). Occasionally, the squamous epithelium is intact, with *Candida* in a mass along the luminal surface (see Figure 17–6). Pseudohyphae often extend into the superficial layers of the epithelium, which shows active inflammation and reactive epithelial changes. The pseudohyphae appear to anchor the fungal mass, which may be quite thick because of the presence of accumulated layers of squamous epithelial debris. Erosion of the invaded epithelium is sometimes present. More commonly, complete epithelial loss with ulceration is present, manifested by fibrinoinflammatory exudate containing neutrophils, necrotic debris, and inflamed granulation tissue. The exudate in the base of an ulcer often contains budding yeast without pseudohyphae or evidence of tissue in-

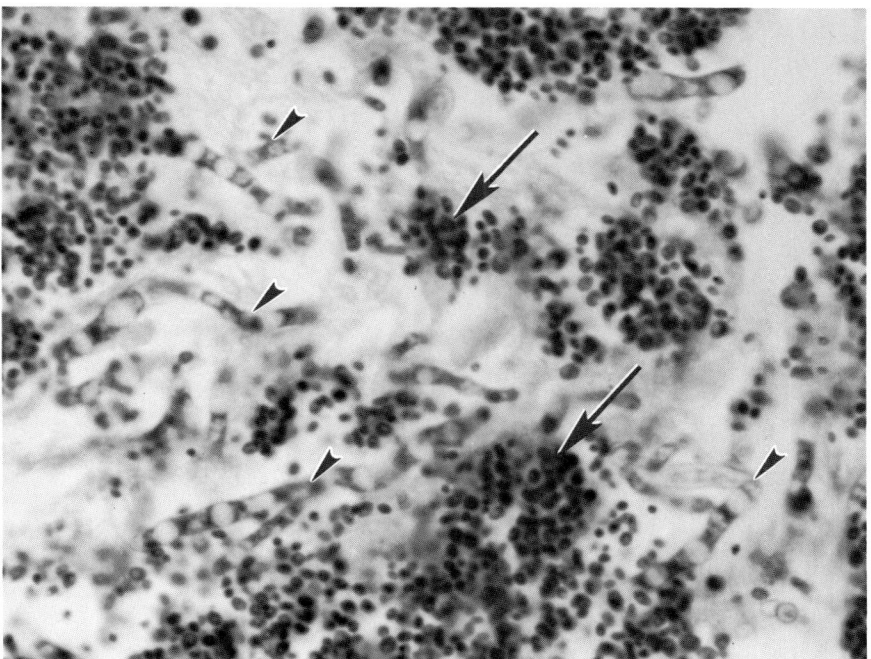

FIGURE 17-10. Mixed fungal esophagitis. *Candida (Torulopsis) glabrata* (arrows) and *Aspergillus* (arrowheads) in necrotic tissue from esophageal biopsy of a patient receiving intensive cytotoxic chemotherapy.

vasion (see Figure 17-8). Large fungal masses are sometimes attached to the ulcer base. The presence of "mummified" necrotic tissue with intact inflammatory cells (see Figure 17-7) should heighten the suspicion of *Candida*; staining of additional sections is recommended if the organisms are not demonstrated on initial examination of specimens containing necrotic tissue with this appearance.

From a clinical and therapeutic standpoint, a fact of major importance concerning candidal esophagitis is that it may serve as a portal of entry for disseminated candidiasis. Biopsy histopathology plays a role in assessing the risk of dissemination, along with the clinical characteristics of the patient, and may influence the decision to undertake systemic as opposed to local antifungal therapy. For this reason, in addition to the diagnosis of *Candida* esophagitis, a biopsy report should provide the clinician with an indication of the numbers of fungi, their morphologic form (e.g., yeast or pseudohyphae), the nature of the specimen in which the

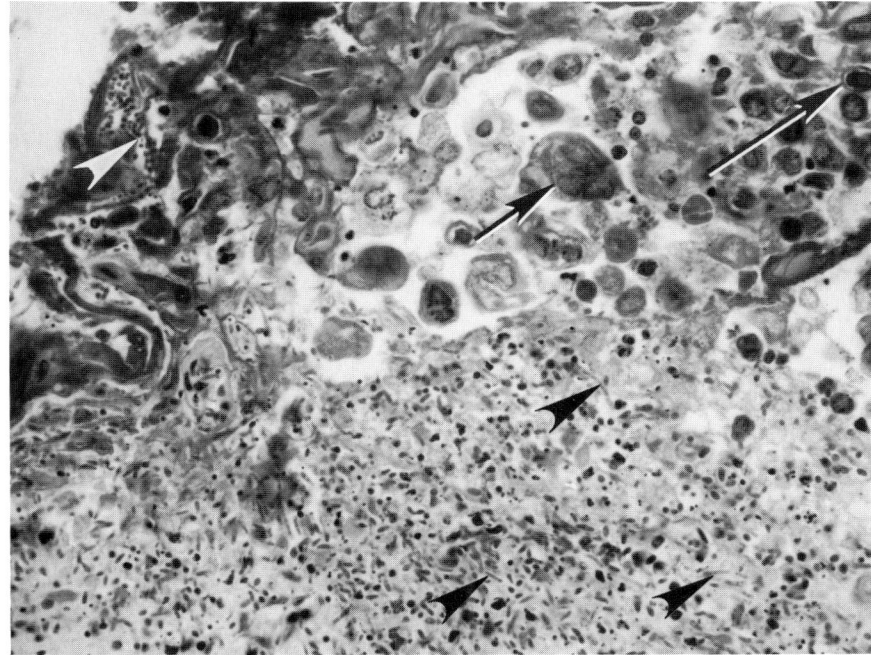

FIGURE 17-11. Mixed fungal and viral esophagitis. Candidal esophagitis is evident with budding yeast (white arrowhead) in squamous epithelium and pseudohyphae (black arrowheads) in lamina propria beneath squamous epithelium with herpes inclusions (arrows). The characteristic inclusions have a peri-inclusion halo (long arrow) in some cells and occur in multinucleated epithelial giant cells (short arrow).

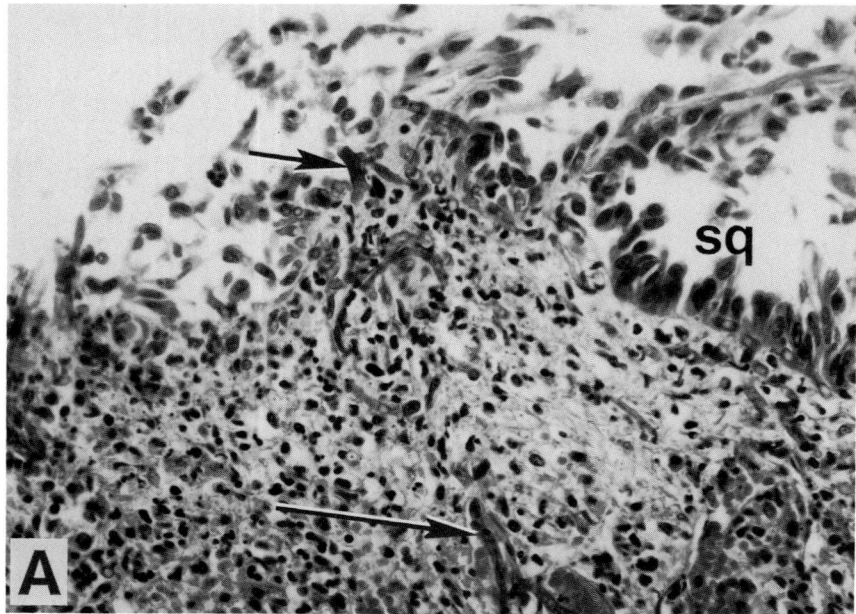
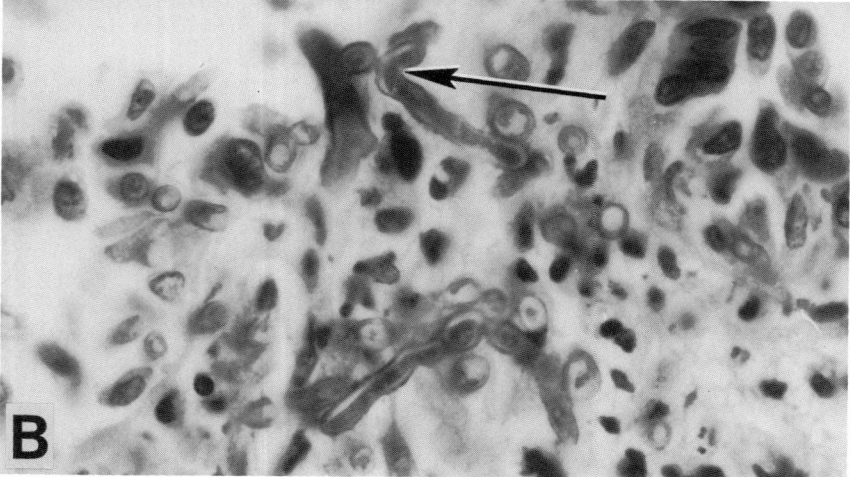

FIGURE 17–12. *Aspergillus* esophagitis. *A,* Characteristic dichotomously branching septate hyphae (short arrow) of *Aspergillus* infiltrate degenerating squamous epithelium (sq) and the lamina propria with blood vessel invasion (long arrow). *B,* High-power view of the area indicated by the short arrow in *A.* Dichotomous branching (arrow) is evident.

organisms are located (e.g., exudate or tissue), the severity of the inflammatory response, and the depth of invasion if present. However, the significance of *Candida* is often unclear, because colonization may occur after other forms of esophageal injury, e.g., gastroesophageal reflux. Furthermore, the problem of sampling affects assessment of invasion in biopsy specimens. Biopsies are sometimes taken after therapy for candidal esophagitis for assessment of efficacy.

Aspergillus *and Phycomycetes Esophagitis*
(see Figure 17–10; Figure 17–12)

Aspergillus esophagitis and Phycomycetes esophagitis are two rare forms of opportunistic esophagitis caused by unrelated organisms. They are considered together because of the similarities of the clinical and pathologic features. *Aspergillus* infections may be caused by any one of several species, including *A. fumigatus, A. niger,* and *A. flavus.* Phycomycetes (mucormycosis) infection includes fungi from the genera *Absidia, Rhizopus,* and *Mucor.* Esophageal infections with these organisms are essentially limited to severely compromised hosts. Esophageal infection appears to result from either direct mucosal involvement from the lumen after swallowing of inhaled organisms or involvement of the esophageal wall after extension from contiguous structures, or after blood-borne dissemination. Esophageal infection is usually associated with involvement of other portions of the gastrointestinal tract or widely disseminated disease.

Aspergillus in tissue is characterized by septate hyphae with dichotomous branching that produces acute angles (see Figures 17–10 and 17–12). Phycomycetes show broad irregular nonseptate hyphae with obtuse to right-angle branches. Both types of organisms may be difficult to identify in H&E-stained sections but stain well with methenamine silver. Fungal cultures permit specification.

Both types of organisms have a predilection for blood vessel invasion (see Figure 17–12). Arterial involvement produces thrombosis and infarction with coagulative necrosis. The presence of infarcted tissue in the esophagus of an immunocompromised patient, therefore, should lead to a careful search for these types of organisms. The organisms may also be found in ulcerated tissue. Because infections with *Aspergillus* and Phycomycetes occur in severely compromised patients, inflammatory response is often minimal. Additional infectious agents may also be present (see Figure 17–10).

Pathogenic Fungal Esophagitis

Pathogenic fungi reported to involve the esophagus include *Histoplasma capsulatum, Blastomyces dermatitidis* (North American blastomycosis), *Sporothrix schenckii,* and *Paracoccidioides brasiliensis* (South American blastomycosis), but esophageal infection by pathogenic fungi is rare. For example, in an autopsy series of 120 cases of disseminated histoplasmosis, esophageal involvement was found in only two patients, but other series have provided prevalences of up to 13%.

Esophageal infection by pathogenic fungi generally occurs in apparently normal individuals during the course of disseminated disease. Disseminated infections with pathogenic fungi can also occur in immunocompromised hosts exposed in endemic areas. The primary site from which esophageal involvement occurs is usually the lungs, and both direct extension and hematogenous spread to the esophagus are possible. Primary esophageal involvement by pathogenic fungi has not been demonstrated convincingly. Patients generally have extrinsic compression, stricture, mass, or ulceration of the esophagus. Organisms cannot be demonstrated in endoscopic biopsy specimens unless mucosal involvement is present.

Histoplasmal esophagitis usually develops by extension from involved subcarinal lymph nodes. Intracellular yeasts in histiocytes occur in granulomatous inflammation, and active inflammation with neutrophils is sometimes present. In H&E-stained sections, the yeasts appear small, with an artifactual clear area between the cell wall and retracted cytoplasm, which was misinterpreted as a capsule (hence, "*capsulatum*"). PAS and methenamine silver stain the cell wall and demonstrate the true size of the yeast. Biopsy diagnosis of histoplasmal esophagitis depends upon demonstration of the organisms in the base of ulcerated areas. Culture is important because of the problem of sampling.

Blastomycotic esophagitis has been reported to have histopathologic features similar to those in the skin, a squamous-lined surface that is commonly affected in disseminated disease. The squamous epithelium often shows pseudoepitheliomatous hyperplasia. The yeasts are large and usually extracellular. The cytoplasm is retracted from the capsule. Acute inflammation, necrosis, and granulomatous inflammation are common; but the organisms are often difficult to find. As a result, culture is important in diagnosis.

Viral Esophagitis

Viruses which infect the esophagus are included in Table 17–1.

Herpes Esophagitis (see Figure 17–11; Figures 17–13 to 17–15)

This form of viral esophagitis is generally due to herpes simplex virus type I (except in neonates). The portal of entry is uncertain, but swallowing of infected saliva has been suggested. The virus can be harbored in the salivary glands, and some patients have herpetic gingivostomatitis as a possible source.

Herpes esophagitis is usually an opportunistic infection, although occasional cases occur in patients without apparent underlying disease. Infections with other pathogens and of other organs are commonly associated with herpetic esophagitis. The major clinical importance of herpetic ulcers lies often in their being a portal of entry for bacteria and fungi (see Figure 17–11), and individual epithelial cells have been shown to have dual infection with herpesvirus and *Candida.* Herpes esophagitis is often asymptomatic such that antemortem diagnosis was uncommon in the past; in some patients, however, odynophagia or dysphagia leads to endoscopic investigation, including biopsy and/or cytology. Strictures rarely develop.

Esophageal involvement is common in disseminated herpes simplex virus infection in neonates. Because the infection is usually acquired intrapartum, most cases are due to type 2 virus. If the neonate survives, esophageal stenosis is common.

Herpes infection of the esophagus usually results in ulcer formation. Specimens properly taken from the edges and base of the ulcer show both squamous epithelium and fibroinflammatory exudate containing neutrophils (see Figure 17–13). Granulation tissue is typically absent because of the acute nature of the ulcers. The epithelium contains the histopathologic evidence of herpetic infection in the form of smudgy "ground-glass" eosinophilic to amphophilic intranuclear inclusions. The inclusions show a range of morphologic features (see Figure 17–14), some filling the nucleus to the nuclear membrane (Cowdry type B) and others having a halo-like clear area between them and the chromatin clumped against the nuclear membrane (Cowdry type A). The epithelial cells that contain inclusions are sometimes enlarged and multinucleated. Loss of cohesion of the infected cells with hyalinization of the cytoplasm is often seen. The inclusion-bearing epithelial cells are usually confined to the area immediately adjacent to the ulcer (see Figure 17–13). In rare cases, herpes can be identified in the connective tissue bed of an esophageal ulcer. Occasionally, inclusions are found in biopsies of intact epithelium or endoscop-

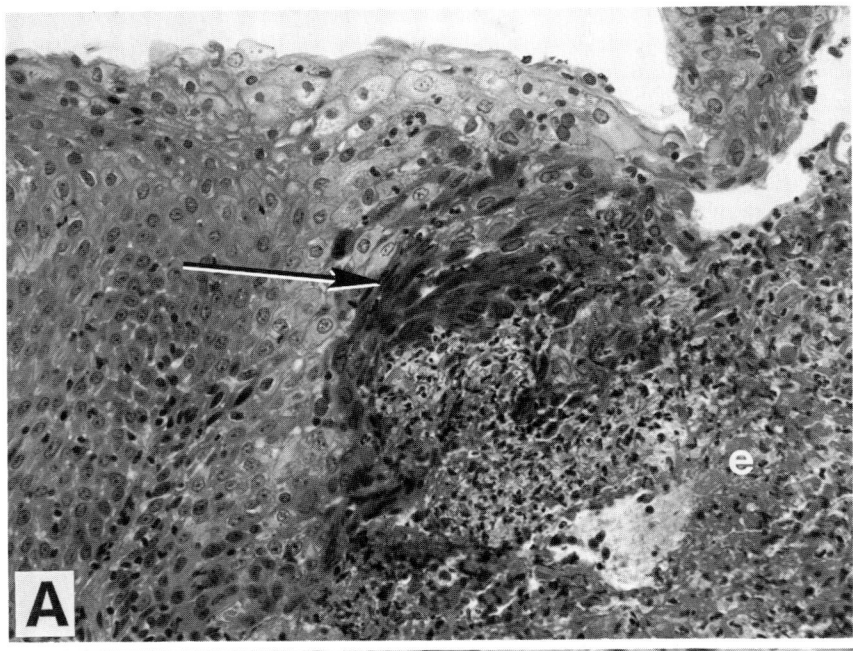
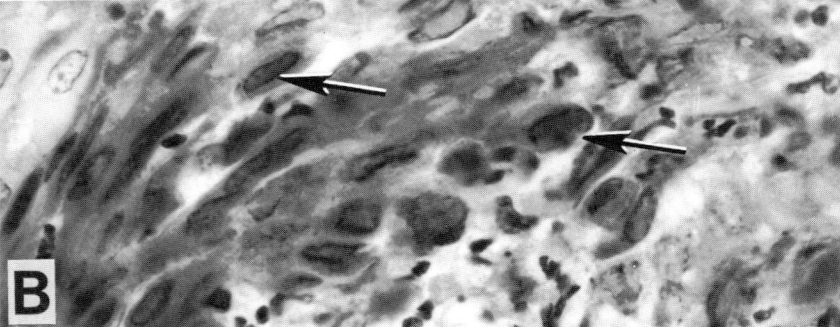

FIGURE 17–13. Herpetic esophagitis. *A*, Acute erosion with luminal fibrinoinflammatory exudate (e) has herpetic inclusions characteristically located in the squamous epithelial cells at the periphery (arrow). *B*, High-power view of area indicated by the arrow in *A*. Typical herpes inclusions are evident in squamous epithelial cells (arrows).

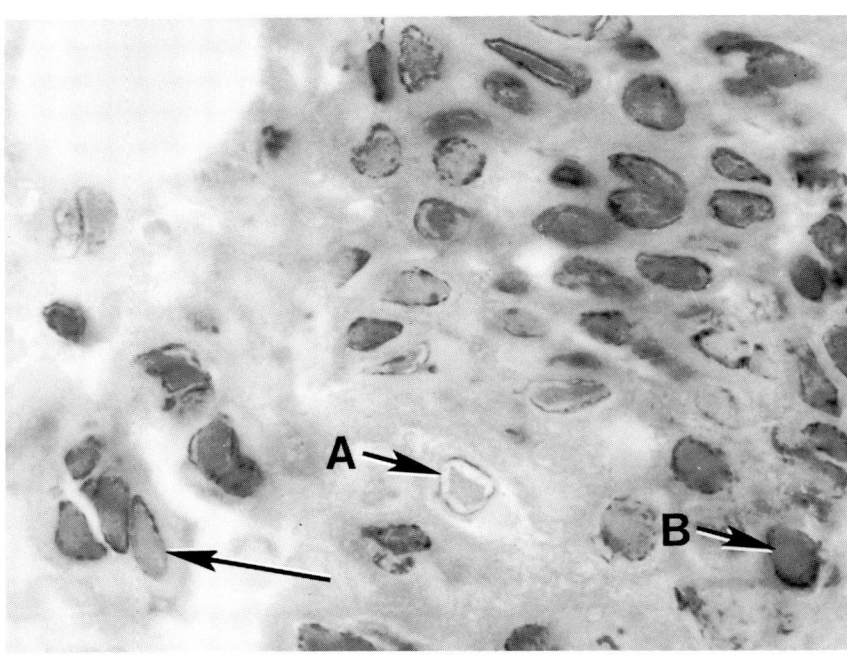

FIGURE 17–14. Herpetic esophagitis. The range in the appearance of herpetic inclusions in squamous epithelium is evident. Cowdry type A (arrow labeled A) and Cowdry type B (arrow labeled B) are illustrated along with a multinucleated epithelial giant cell (long arrow) with inclusions.

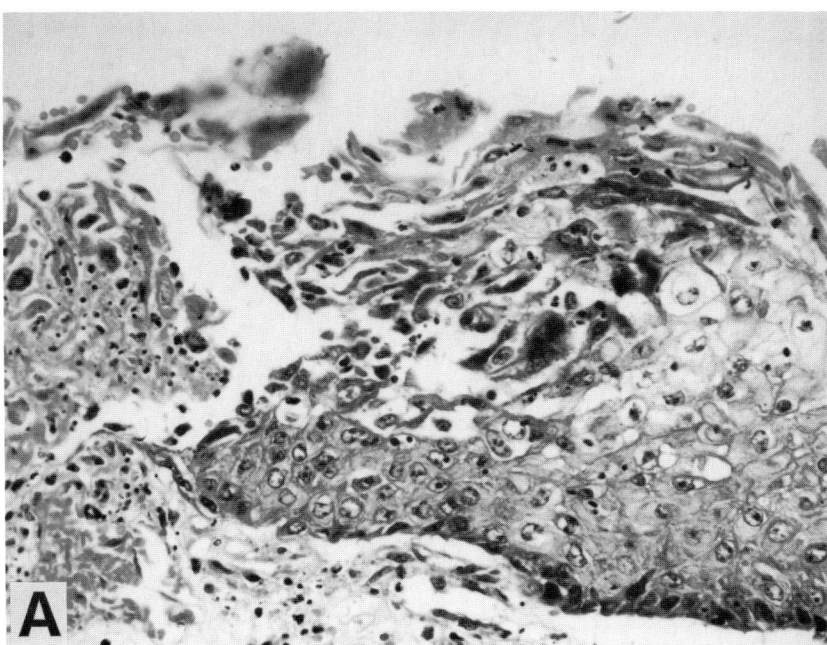

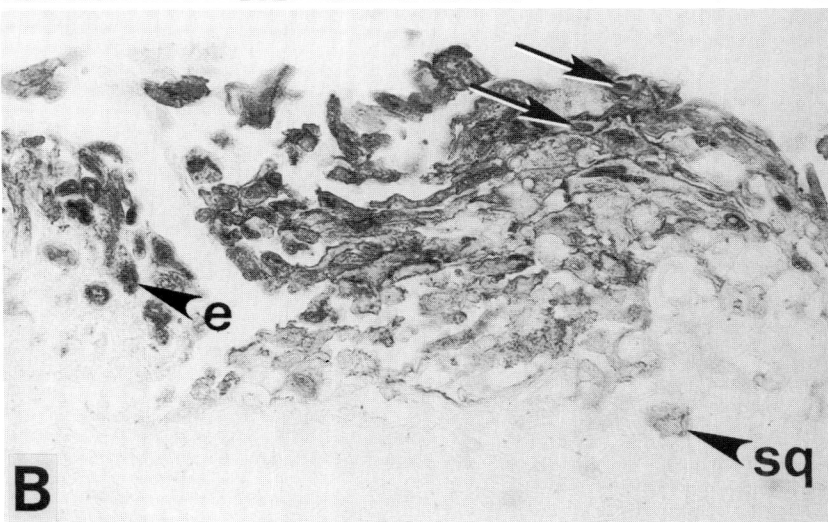

FIGURE 17-15. Herpetic esophagitis. *A*, H&E-stained section demonstrates degenerating squamous epithelium with ill-defined viral inclusions. *B*, Immunoperoxidase stain for herpes simplex virus antigens in serial section adjoining section shown in *A*. Antigen is evident in necrotic cellular debris in the fibrinoinflammatory exudate (e) and the cytoplasm of squamous epithelial cells without inclusions (sq), as well as in intranuclear inclusions themselves (arrows).

ically visible intraepithelial vesicles, which appear to represent preulcerative lesions. When epithelial virus inclusions are identified, the differential diagnosis includes the other types of viral infections that involve squamous epithelium, particularly varicella (see Table 17–1 and the following section).

Immunohistochemical studies using specific antiherpes simplex virus type 1 and 2 antibodies can be used to confirm herpetic esophagitis (see Figure 17–15). In addition, immunohistochemical studies demonstrate that herpetic antigens are present in epithelial cells that do not have recognizable inclusions. This finding supports the observation that inclusion formation occurs relatively late in the development of the infection. As a result, occasional cases of herpetic esophagitis may not be recognizable histopathologically because inclusions are absent, but more commonly this situation results from the problem of sampling.

Histopathologic diagnosis depends upon the detection of characteristic inclusions. Specimens, therefore, must include squamous epithelium from the periphery of the ulcer for the inclusions to be found, as described above (see Table 17–1). Because of the problem of sampling, multiple specimens, brush cytology, and viral cultures can increase the likelihood of diagnosis. Since herpetic ulcers serve as portals of entry for other organisms, particularly candida (see Figure 17–11), stains for fungi should be used routinely in assessment of biopsy specimens with herpetic esophagitis. Viral and fungal cultures and smears taken at the time of endoscopy are also helpful. Bacteria are often identifiable in herpetic ulcers, which can serve as the portal of entry for bacterial infections; but the significance of bacteria is difficult to determine because simple colonization can occur.

Cytomegalovirus Esophagitis (Figure 17–16)

As was the case for herpes esophagitis, cytomegalovirus (CMV) infection of the esophagus is generally an opportunistic infection. CMV esophagitis generally occurs along with generalized CMV infection. The portal of entry is uncertain but may be through viremia with localization in areas of previous esophageal injury, as well as from infected saliva in the esophageal lumen. CMV appears to be a secondary infecting agent in many cases, and its role in producing primary esophageal injury is often open to question. Systemic and esophageal infections with other organisms frequently accompany CMV esophagitis. Antemortem diagnosis usually results from endoscopy and biopsy of an immunocompromised patient with odynophagia or dysphagia.

Ulceration is the usual finding in CMV esophagitis. Specimens of the ulcer base generally show fibrinoinflammatory exudate containing neutrophils and inflamed granulation tissue with characteristic inclusions. The enlarged cells in capillary walls that show inclusions often bulge into the vessel lumen, but the infected cells may be pericytes as well as endothelial cells. Smooth muscle cells of the muscularis mucosae and fibrocytes in connective tissue also appear to be involved in some cases (see Figure 17–16). In addition to being enlarged (cytomegaly), the affected cells have an enlarged nucleus, often with a purple inclusion surrounded by a clear halo, resulting in an "owl's eye" appearance. Cytoplasmic inclusions are often evident. The cells with distinctive inclusions are characteristic of CMV infection, but other enlarged cells in the specimen frequently contain only rudimentary inclusions. In some cases, fully developed inclusions may not be found despite a careful search. Immunohistochemistry with anti-CMV antibodies is especially helpful in such cases. The epithelium in biopsies from the periphery of the ulcer shows reactive changes and sometimes active inflammation, but not inclusions (see Table 17–1).

Histopathologic diagnosis depends upon the detection of characteristic inclusions. In contrast to herpetic esophagitis, in which the inclusions are usually in the epithelium at the periphery of the ulcer, CMV inclusions are found in the ulcer base as described above. Properly taken specimens, therefore, must include samples of both the base and the periphery of an ulcer. Because infected cells that have not yet formed an inclusion cannot always be distinguished confidently from reactive cells in ulcers with other causes, viral cultures and immunohistochemical studies for CMV can be helpful. Specimens with CMV should be evaluated for histopathologic evidence of other organisms, especially herpesvirus and *Candida* in patients with AIDS.

Esophagitis Associated with Varicella, Rubella, and Variola

Clinical involvement of the esophagus by the viral exanthem varicella has been reported, and autopsy histopathology indicates that the esophageal lesions are similar to those in the squamous epithelium of the skin. Early abnormalities include degeneration of the basal zone of the epithelium, characterized by swelling with rarefaction and vacuolization of the cytoplasm. In larger lesions, the basal layer separates from the lamina propria. Acidophilic nuclear inclusions, cytoplasmic inclusions, and occasional giant epithelial cells are also seen.

Involvement of the esophagus in congenital rubella has also been reported. Multinucleated squamous epithelial cells with intranuclear inclusions were present, but the reported case is subject to criticism because the electron-microscopic features of the viral particles were different from those of the usual rubella.

Esophageal involvement by variola (smallpox) is now of only historical interest.

Esophagitis due to HIV and Epstein-Barr Virus

Aphthous ulcers have been found in patients with HIV-1 infection, and viral particles have been identified by electron microscopy of the lesions. As a consequence, HIV-1 infection of the esophagus with ulceration has been suggested to occur during the early phases of HIV infection and seroconversion. A recent report of five patients with HIV-1 infection suggested that Epstein-Barr virus can also infect the squamous epithelium of the esophagus and contribute to esophageal ulceration in patients with AIDS. Esophageal symptoms, especially dysphagia, are common in patients with AIDS. Esophageal abnormalities in such patients can be due to a variety of causes, including infections by *Candida*, herpesvirus, and CMV.

Human Papillomavirus Infection of the Esophagus

Squamous papillomas with koilocytic change occur rarely. Confirmation of human papillomavirus can be obtained by immunohistochemistry or *in situ* hybridization.

Bacterial Esophagitis

Bacteria are often present in specimens with histopathologic evidence of ulceration, but usually represent secondary infectious agents, either alone (Figure 17–17) or with fungi or viruses. Bacterial colonization of the esophageal epithelium can also occur with obstruction due to a variety of causes (Figure 17–18). Primary bacterial infections appear to be rare in the antibiotic era, except in severely compromised hosts, but can be an occult source of bacteremia.

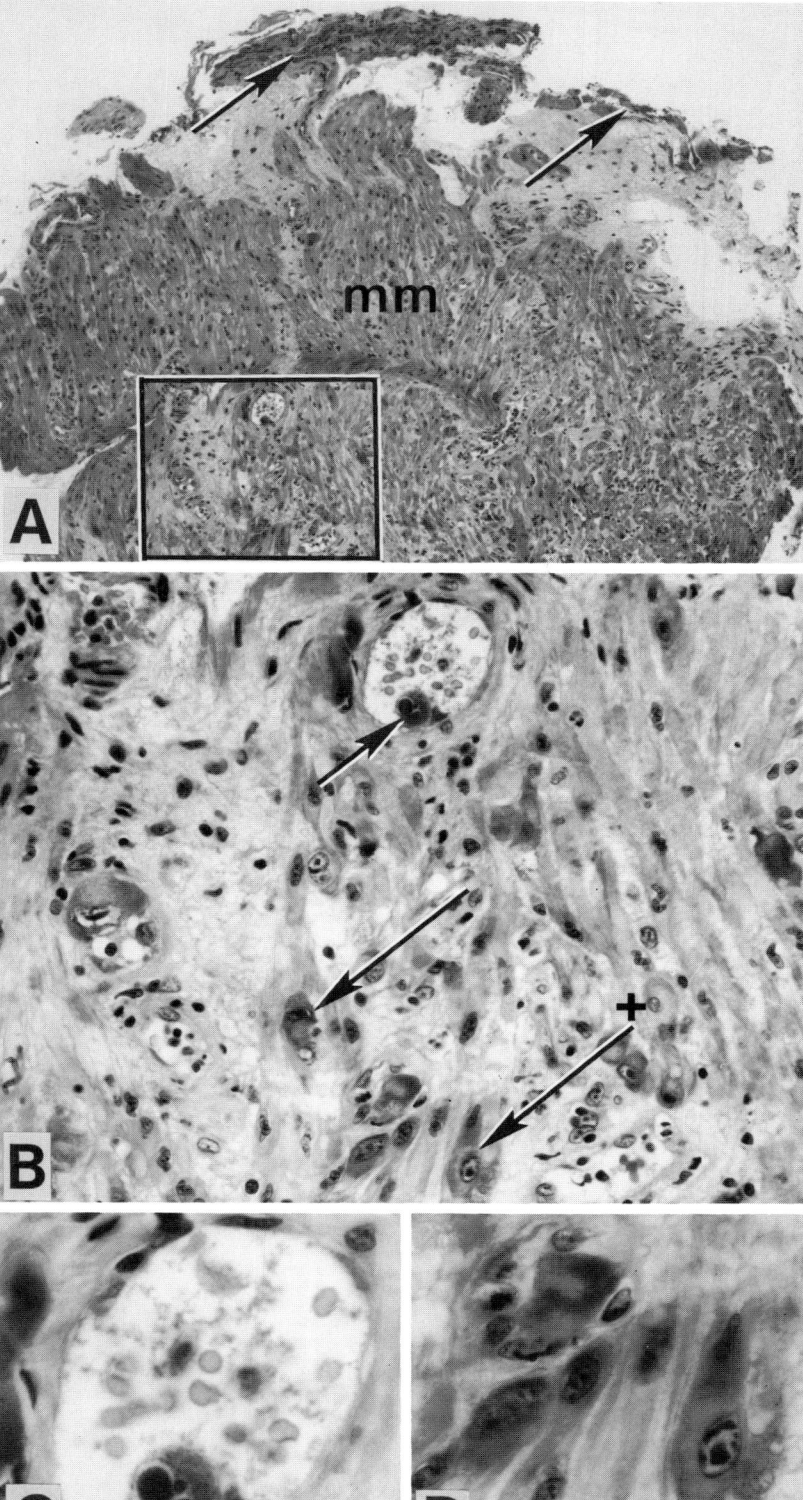

FIGURE 17–16. Cytomegaloviral (CMV) esophagitis. *A*, Acute ulcer with necrotic debris (arrows) extends into muscularis mucosae (mm). See *B* for a high-power view of the area enclosed by the box. *B*, Characteristic inclusions of cytomegalovirus are present in the lumen of capillaries (short arrow) and smooth muscle cells (long arrows). *C*, High-power view of the area indicated by the short arrow in *B*. The CMV inclusion involves an endothelial cell. *D*, High-power view of the area indicated by the long arrow with a plus (+) sign in *B*. An early CMV inclusion is evident in a smooth muscle cell.

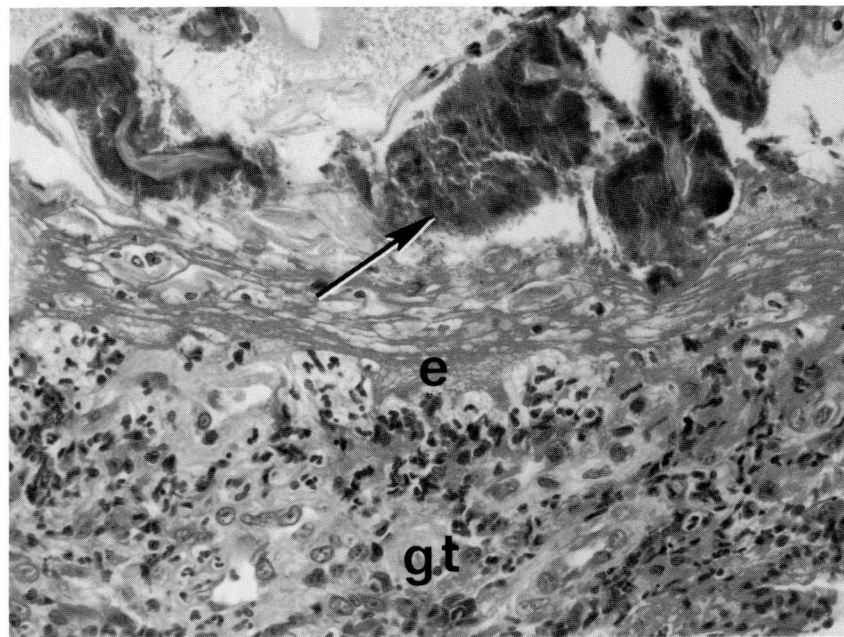

FIGURE 17-17. Bacterial colonization of esophageal ulcer. An active chronic ulcer with inflamed granulation tissue (gt) and luminal fibrinoinflammatory exudate (e) contains bacterial colonies (arrow) in the luminal debris.

Opportunistic Bacterial Esophagitis

Great attention has been focused on opportunistic fungal and viral esophagitis in severely compromised patients. However, bacteria are primary pathogens in opportunistic esophageal infections, accounting for about 10% to 15% of cases of infective esophagitis. Esophagitis due to a single species of bacteria and to mixed bacterial flora have been described. Implicated bacteria include a wide variety of gram-positive and gram-negative organisms, but bacterial esophagitis with bacteremia is usually due to gram-positive bacteria. Antecedent esophageal injury probably contributes to the pathogenesis of the esophageal infection.

Opportunistic bacterial esophagitis is characterized histopathologically by numerous bacteria extending into the lamina propria and involving blood vessels with necrosis of the squamous epithelium (Figure 17–19). The absence of inflammation in the face of numerous organisms is a striking feature caused by gran-

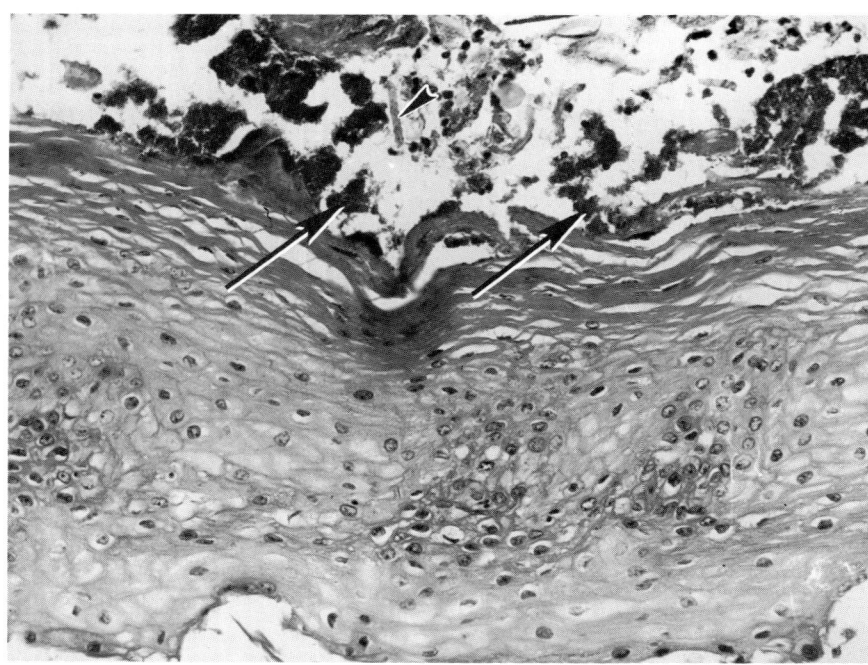

FIGURE 17-18. Bacterial colonization of esophageal epithelium in a patient with esophageal obstruction due to external compression. Numerous bacteria (arrows) are present on the luminal surface, but with no evidence of inflammatory response. The luminal debris also contains food material (arrowhead).

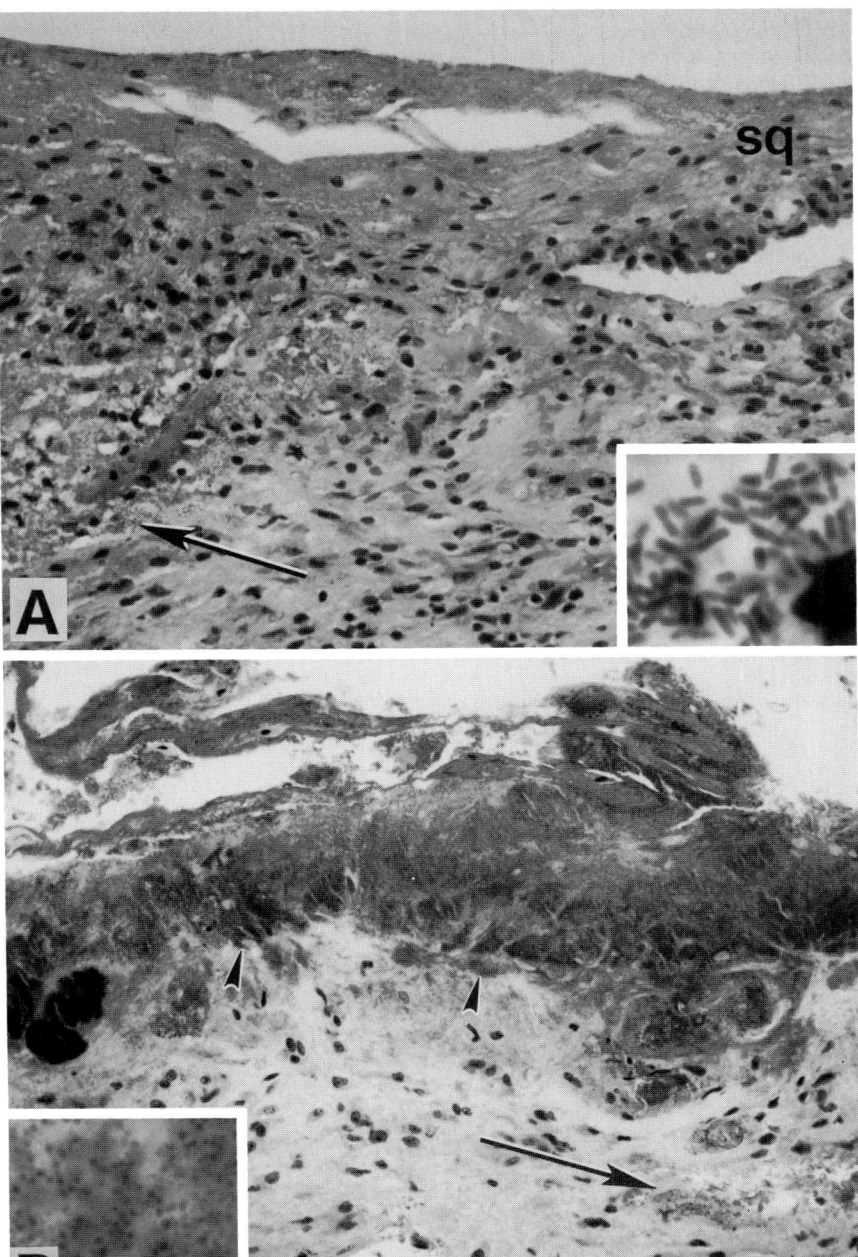

FIGURE 17–19. Opportunistic bacterial esophagitis. A, Escherichia coli esophagitis. Necrotic squamous epithelium (sq) contains numerous bacteria, which extend into the lamina propria (arrow). The *inset* demonstrates the bacilli at high magnification. Tissue Gram staining showed gram-negative bacilli, and the patient's blood cultures were positive for *E. coli*, which indicated bacteremic bacterial esophagitis. No inflammatory response to the infection is evident because of the patient's profound neutropenia, resulting from cytotoxic chemotherapy. B, Streptococcal esophagitis. Extensive erosion of the squamous epithelium is evident with a large mass of bacteria (arrowheads) involving the lamina propria. Blood vessels (arrow) contain bacteria. The *inset* shows small cocci, which were gram-positive on tissue Gram stain. No inflammatory response to the infection is evident.

ulocytopenia in some patients, but acute inflammation may be present in nonneutropenic patients.

Mycobacterial Esophagitis

Mycobacterium tuberculosis infection involving the esophagus is rare. Portals of entry include direct extension from tuberculous pharyngitis; direct extension from mediastinal lymph nodes or the vertebral column; and the vascular system in disseminated (miliary) tuberculosis. Mucosal involvement as a primary site or due to swallowing of infected sputum is very rare (only 25 of 16,489 autopsy patients in one series). Endoscopically, esophageal tuberculosis may be characterized by ulceration or a mass lesion. Complications include obstruction and tracheobronchial fistula.

Specimens may show the range of histopathologic findings in tuberculosis, including nonspecific inflammation as well as caseating granulomas with epithelioid histiocytes and multinucleated giant cells. The differential diagnosis includes other causes of esophagitis as well as other diseases characterized by granulomas. Identification of acid-fast bacilli in histopathologic sections or culture of *M. tuberculosis* from the esophagus results in correct diagnosis. In cases without mucosal involvement, however, biopsy specimens are unable to

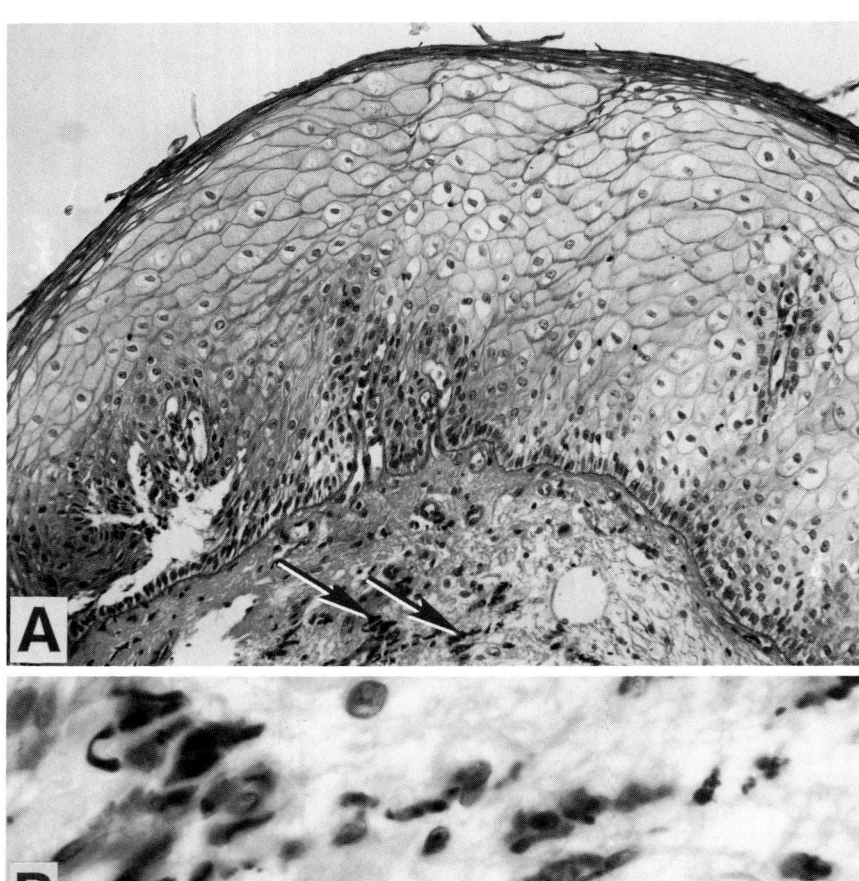

FIGURE 17–20. Whipple's disease involving the esophagus. *A*, PAS staining shows characteristic PAS-positive granules in histiocytes in the lamina propria (arrows). *B*, High-power view of the area indicated by the arrows in *A*. PAS-positive granules are identical to those found in the small intestinal biopsy specimen of the patient.

show histopathologic evidence of the underlying tuberculosis because of the shallow depth of the specimens.

Myobacterium avium-intracellulare occasionally involves the esophagus in patients with AIDS.

Actinomyces Israeli Esophagitis

Actinomyces organisms are anaerobic gram-positive bacteria that are frequently normal flora in the oronasopharynx, including the gingiva and tonsils. Both primary and secondary infections of the esophagus by *Actinomyces* have been reported. Primary mucosal involvement may result from swallowing of a foreign body, which produces injury to the epithelium and allows entry of the organism. Invasion into the esophageal wall can then occur, with formation of sinus tracts and abscesses, particularly in the upper esophagus. Secondary involvement of the esophagus occurs by extension from hilar lymph nodes and the vertebral column or by hematogenous dissemination.

Diagnosis depends upon recognition of "sulfur granules," the small yellow bodies representing colonies of the organisms, or histopathologic identification of the intertwined thin, branching filaments. The filaments at the periphery of the colonies are club-shaped, with an enlargement at the end. Fibrinoinflammatory exudate with neutrophils usually surrounds the colonies, and granulation tissue representing the fistula tract may also be present. Differential diagnosis includes colonies of other bacteria in tissue (botryomycosis) and the Splendore-Hoeppli phenomenon (bacterial colonies surrounded by eosinophilic material). *Actinomyces* may appear in esophageal specimens as a contaminant, probably from the oronasopharynx; careful consideration should precede a diagnosis of esophageal involvement by the organism.

Miscellaneous Bacterial Esophagitis

Historically, esophageal infections have been identified with *Corynebacterium diphtheriae*, *Salmonella typhosa* and *Shigella*. A case of esophageal infection by *Lactobacillus acidophilus* has been reported, although the clinical setting and features of the infection resembled candidal esophagitis. Whipple's disease can involve the esophagus (Figure 17–20).

Spirochetal (Syphilitic) Esophagitis

Clinically evident *Treponema pallidum* infection involving the esophagus is extremely rare (two cases in 7000 patients in one series). When it does occur, it is generally in the acquired, rather than the congenital, form of syphilis. Primary lesions (chancres) of the esophagus are unusual. Secondary lesions occur in the esophagus as part of the generalized involvement but are rarely identified because the skin lesions usually dominate the clinical findings. The secondary lesions are superficial and usually heal. Tertiary lesions in the esophagus are uncommon but are more likely to undergo biopsy because they are manifested clinically. Four main types of lesions have been described: ulcers due to ischemia resulting from endarteritis; active syphilitic lesions that have extended directly into the esophagus from adjacent organs or lymph nodes; submucosa gummas, which may enlarge and rupture into the esophageal lumen; strictures due to scarring that resulted from healing of the first three types of lesions.

Specimens may show a range of findings, from necrosis in gummas, which is indistinguishable from caseous necrosis of tuberculosis, to intact squamous epithelium, with characteristic vasculitis in the lamina propria and submucosa. As in syphilis involving other body sites, the vasculitis shows a prominent perivascular accumulation of plasma cells. The lumen of an affected artery is often obliterated (hence "endarteritis"). Spirochetes may be demonstrable in primary and secondary lesions with silver impregnation techniques, such as the Dieterle stain; tertiary lesions lack spirochetes. Therefore, diagnosis of syphilis involving the esophagus usually depends upon the presence of the characteristic vasculitis in the setting of a compatible clinical and serologic picture, rather than demonstration of spirochetes in specimens, because the tertiary lesions are most commonly encountered.

Parasitic Esophagitis

Esophageal involvement by parasitic infections is extremely uncommon in developed countries. The most common parasitic involvement is by Chagas' disease, which produces reactive changes in the squamous epithelium as a consequence of stasis after denervation. *Ascaris* passes through the lumen of the esophagus as part of its life cycle. (Maggots can also be identified in the lumen.) Mucosal involvement by amebiasis can occur. The esophageal wall can be affected by *Echinococcus, Cysticercus, Trichinella,* and *Filaria.*

ESOPHAGEAL INJURY DUE TO EXOGENOUS CHEMICALS

Lye, Acids, Detergents, and Other Household Products

Ingestion of lye, acids, or nonphosphate detergents, either accidentally or as a suicide attempt, often produces dramatic injury to the esophagus. Although endoscopy is often performed for assessment of the severity of injury, biopsies are rarely done. In the occasional case in which biopsy has been performed, the specimens usually show only hemorrhagic, necrotic tissue and fibrinoinflammatory exudate, representing the effects of the chemical and the inflammatory response to the injury. If the patient survives, evidence of repair processes, including granulation tissue and regenerating epithelium, can be found in biopsy specimens. Autopsy specimens may show a range of findings that depend on the time course until the patient's death. Surgical specimens most commonly result from resection of strictures, which are characterized by transmural scarring, often with ongoing ulceration even years after the initial injury. The lye-injured esophagus is associated with increased risk of squamous carcinoma. Less serious esophageal injury (Figure 17-21) can result from ingestion of a variety of

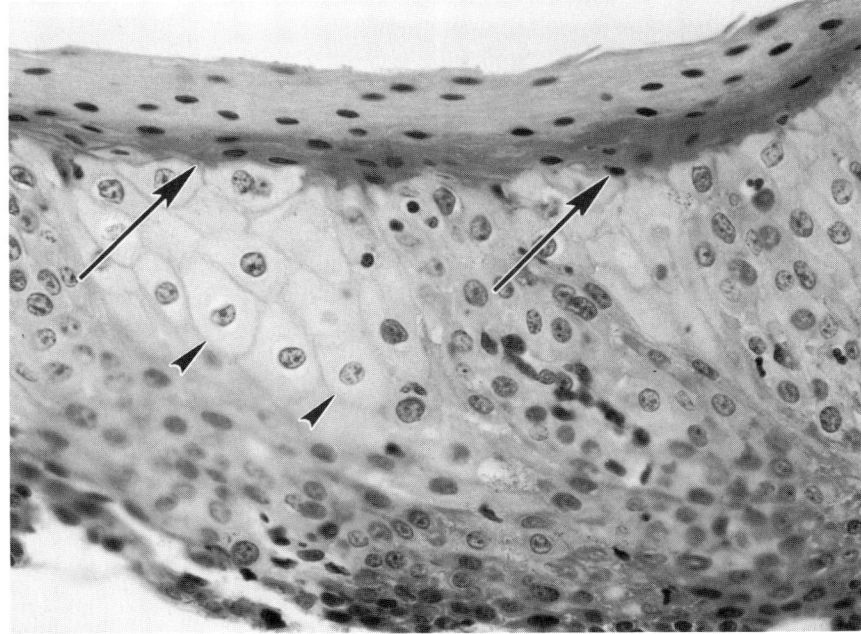

FIGURE 17-21. Lysol injury to esophageal epithelium. Esophageal biopsy specimen taken 4 hours after Lysol ingestion by a child shows bandlike fixation of the superficial layers of the squamous epithelium (arrows) with hyperchromatic nuclei and balloon cells (arrowheads) in the subjacent layers. Only a few neutrophils are evident.

household products. The nature and severity of the injury depend upon the chemical constituents.

Drug Contact

Esophageal ulceration and/or inflammation have been reported with a large number of drugs (Table 17–2). Direct contact with the mucosa is the usual mechanism of injury. Delay in esophageal passage of tablets is common in normal individuals at recumbency, particularly the elderly; ingestion of medications just before lying down or with small fluid volume increases the risk of slow passage. Patients with structural abnormalities of the esophagus are at particular risk. Extrinsic compression associated with left atrial enlargement from mitral valve disease and intrinsic structural abnormalities such as a neoplasm, stricture, and hiatal hernia are predisposing factors. Motility abnormalities with increased lower esophageal sphincter pressure (e.g., achalasia) and abnormal peristalsis (e.g., scleroderma and diffuse esophageal spasm) may also delay passage of medication.

The formulation of the drug is an important factor in esophageal injury: large tablets, capsules, and tablets with hygroscopic agents to accelerate disintegration are more likely to remain in the esophagus and release the contained drug. The chemical nature of the drug affects the potential for injury when the drug is released: the ulcerogenic nature of potassium chloride is well known, whereas dissolved doxycyline HCl, tetracycline HCl, and ferrous sulfate have acidic pH, and emepronium bromide is basic. Hyperosmolality and heat generated during dissolving may also play a role in injury. Stricture formation and death due to perforation or hemorrhage may occur as complications of drug-induced injury; these complications have been reported most commonly with slow-release potassium chloride tablets. Specimens of drug-induced esophageal injury usually show findings of nonspecific ulceration and/or esophagitis. However, Kayexalate in sorbitol occasionally causes local coagulative necrosis of the mucosa; the crystals have a characteristic appearance in H&E-stained sections (Figure 17–22) and are PAS-positive and acid-fast, which allows recognition of the cause of the injury.

With some drugs, esophagitis is attributed to mechanisms other than direct contact with the esophageal mucosa. These mechanisms include immunologic or allergic injury, cytotoxic effects (see Chemotherapeutic Agents), and induction of gastroesophageal reflux by production of lower esophageal sphincter dysfunction (see Gastroesophageal Reflux).

Sclerotherapy for Esophageal Varices

Injection of esophageal varices with a sclerosing solution under visualization through an esophagoscope was described in 1939. In recent years, interest has

Table 17–2 DRUGS ASSOCIATED WITH ESOPHAGITIS AND ULCERATION

Antibiotics
   Doxycycline
   Tetracycline hydrochloride
   Oxytetracycline
   Minocycline hydrochloride
   Clindamycin phosphate
   Lincomycin hydrochloride
   Trimethoprim-sulfamethoxazole
   Erythromycin
   Chloramphenicol
   Tinadazole
   Phenoxymethyl penicillin
   Apocillin
Anti-inflammatory and related drugs
   Aspirin and aspirin-containing combination products
   *Indomethacin
   Ibuprofen
   Piroxicam
   Phenylbutazone
   Prednisone and prednisolone
   Diphenhydramine hydrochloride
   Cromolyn inhalant
   Theophylline
Cardiovascular drugs
   *Quinidine
   *Alprenolol
   *Potassium chloride tablets
Chemotherapeutic agents
   Fluorouracil
   Cytosine arabinoside
   Estramustine phosphate
Nutritional supplements
   Ferrous sulfate and
   ferrous succinate
   Ascorbic acid
   Multivitamin tablets
Miscellaneous
   Emepronium bromide
   Cimetidine
   Chloral hydrate
   Cocaine
   Phenytoin
   Kayexalate
   Acetaminophen

*Associated with severe ulceration, perforation, or stricture.

again developed with the use of fiberoptic instruments. The findings in the esophagus after sclerotherapy have been described in a number of autopsy series. Necrosis with inflammation, hemorrhage, granulation tissue, and scarring are seen, the features influenced by the time since injection and the severity of the injury (Figure 17–23). Morrhuate can be identified histopathologically (see Figure 17–23).

Chemotherapeutic Agents

Esophageal mucosal injury can result from the effects of various systemic chemotherapeutic agents. The basal zone of the squamous epithelium sometimes is atypical owing to cytotoxic effects on the proliferative zone (Figure 17–24).

Further details on chemical and drug injuries of the esophagus are provided in Chapter 9.

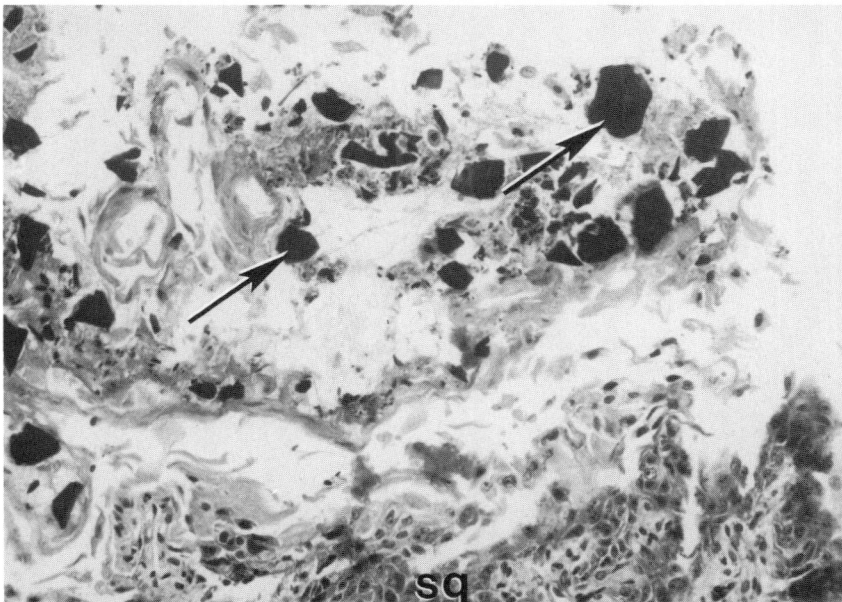

FIGURE 17-22. Esophagitis due to Kayexalate in sorbitol. Necrosis of the superficial layers of the squamous epithelium (sq) is present in areas containing characteristic crystals of Kayexalate (arrows).

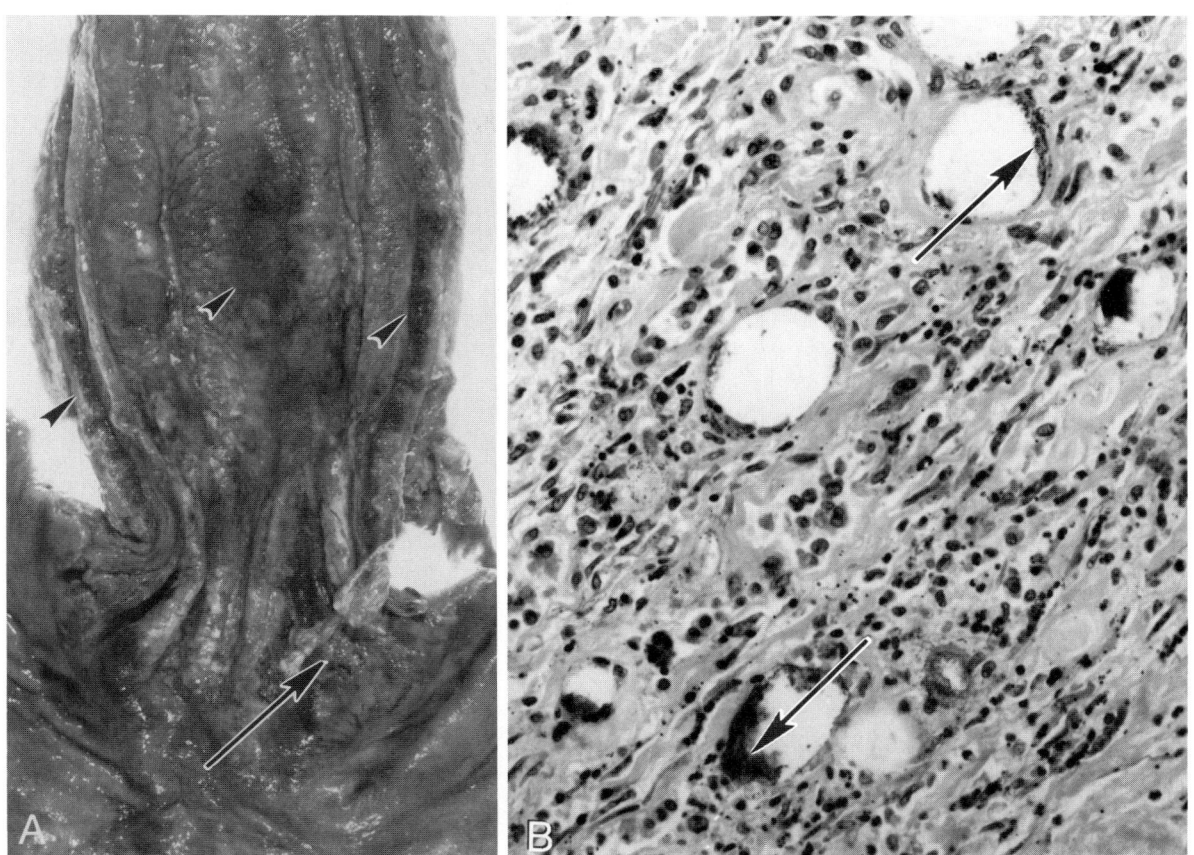

FIGURE 17-23. Esophageal perforation after sclerotherapy for esophageal varices. *A*, Transmural necrosis (arrow) is present with mural hemorrhage involving the entire distal esophagus (arrowheads). *B*, Morrhuate sclerosing agent in tissue. The morrhuate (arrows) appears golden brown and is often associated with vacuoles.

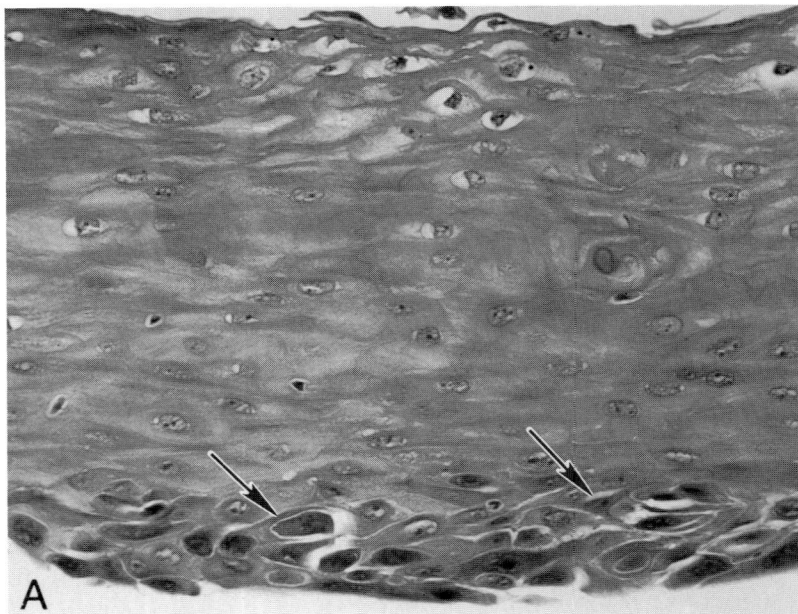
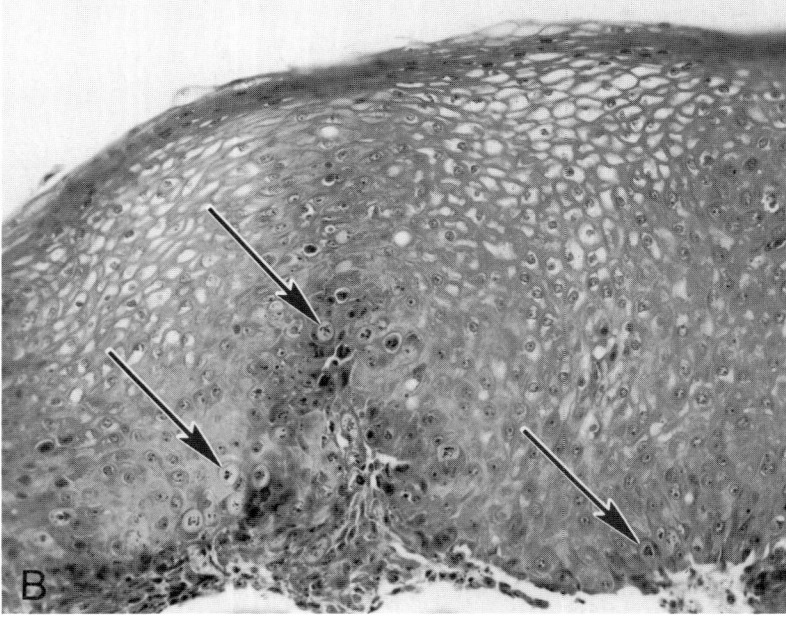

FIGURE 17–24. Chemotherapy effects in esophageal epithelium. *A,* In this example from a patient receiving combination chemotherapy, the basal zone (arrows) shows nuclear abnormalities due to the effects of cytotoxic drugs. Epithelial maturation is abnormal with ovoid immature nuclei at the luminal surface. *B,* In this example from a patient receiving Taxol, many epithelial cells in the basal zone are in mitotic arrest (arrows), as also occurs with colchicine. Wide dispersion of nuclear material is a characteristic finding.

ESOPHAGEAL TRAUMA

External trauma to the esophagus may occur with both blunt and penetrating trauma to the neck and thorax. Internal trauma can result from swallowed foreign bodies, including food and bezoars; from vomiting; and from iatrogenic injury by instruments, catheters, and tubes. Luminal hemorrhage is common, and rupture with perforation into the mediastinum may occur. Mallory-Weiss tears and hematomas at the gastroesophageal junction region may develop after emesis or aborted sneezes. Spontaneous hematomas also occur, most often proximally or at multiple sites, in patients with acquired or congenital coagulopathies.

These types of lesions are most commonly encountered by the pathologist at autopsy. Endoscopy is often performed in these clinical settings, but biopsies are rarely done. In one report, the biopsy specimen of a Mallory-Weiss tear showed necrosis, hemorrhage, and inflammation. Hematomas may be mistaken for tumors on radiographic and endoscopic examination, and a biopsy specimen in one report showed blood clot with attenuated squamous epithelium. Esophageal injury due to nasogastric intubation has most commonly been due to gastroesophageal reflux from interference with lower esophageal sphincter function, rather than direct mucosal injury, since the advent of soft tubes (see Gastroesophageal Reflux). Foreign body reactions,

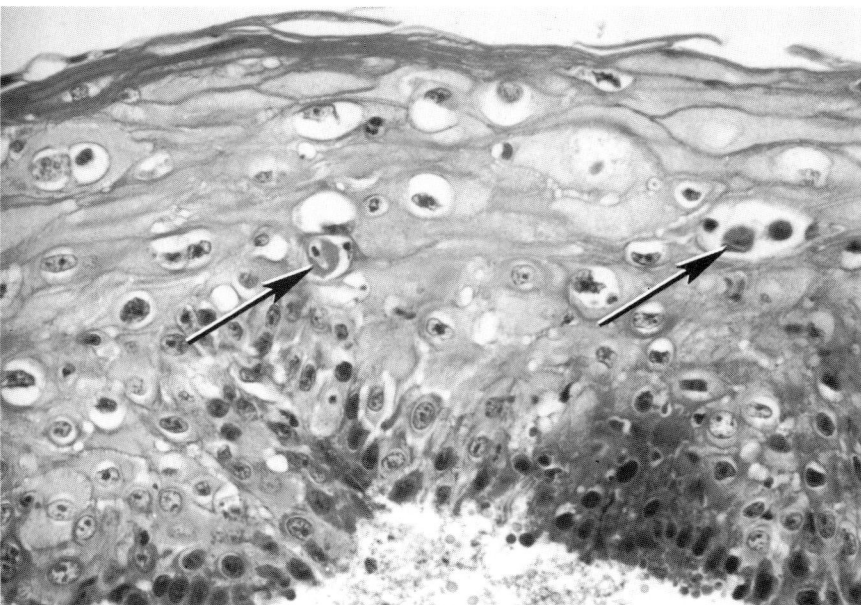

FIGURE 17-25. Acute radiation esophagitis. Esophageal biopsy taken during the third week of radiotherapy for mediastinal lymphoma shows degenerating epithelial cells with formation of acidophilic bodies (arrows) and reactive epithelial changes.

including multinucleated giant cells, can occur if foreign material is introduced into the mucosa.

ESOPHAGEAL INJURY DUE TO PHYSICAL AGENTS

Radiation Esophagitis

The esophagus is often exposed to radiation during radiotherapy for tumors of the lung, mediastinum, or vertebral column. Radiation injury and recovery are influenced by the type of radiotherapy, the dose, the time course of administration, and a variety of patient-related factors. The spectrum of injury may range from mild degenerative changes in dividing cells and temporary hyperemia to total necrosis of the esophageal wall. Similarly, repair processes may be rapid and complete or incomplete with nonhealing ulcers and scarring. The tolerated dose of radiation is said to be about 6000 rads, given at a rate of 1000 rads per week; strictures rarely occur at this dose, but chemotherapy with adriamycin appears to reduce tolerance. The components of the esophageal wall show varying degrees of radiosensitivity and resistance: the squamous epithelium and blood vessels are relatively radiosensitive, whereas smooth muscle of the muscularis mucosae and muscularis propria and fibrous connective tissue are relatively radioresistant. Within the squamous epithelium of the mucosal surface and ducts of submucosal glands, the basal zone, with its proliferating cells, is more sensitive than the superficial layers, composed of differentiated postmitotic cells. Radiation esophagitis can be classified into acute and chronic forms on the basis of the time course and pathogenetic mechanisms involved.

Acute radiation esophagitis occurs during the first few weeks after therapy due to the direct injurious effects of the radiation. The epithelium and blood vessels are the main sites of the abnormalities in the acute phase (Figure 17-25). *Chronic radiadtion esophagitis* occurs weeks to months after irradiation; chronic fibrovascular lesions predominate, leading to ongoing ischemic necrosis, scarring, and impaired epithelial cell proliferation.

Although patients are often symptomatic during acute radiation esophagitis, biopsies are rarely obtained. In the first few days after radiotherapy, the squamous epithelium shows degenerative changes, focal necrosis, and decreased mitotic figures in the basal zone. Blood vessels are dilated and congested and have swollen endothelial cells. Lamina propria and submucosal connective tissue show edema and scattered inflammatory cells. In the second week, necrosis and thinning of the epithelium is more marked, often with some sloughing of debris and exudate into the lumen to produce erosions with pseudomembranes. In the third and fourth weeks, the epithelial necrosis is accompanied by regeneration (see Figure 17-25). Also, the submucosa shows chronic inflammation and increased numbers of fibroblasts.

Biopsies are sometimes taken in patients with chronic radiation esophagitis. As radiation esophagitis enters the chronic phase, the epithelium may show either hyperplasia with parakeratosis or atrophy. Atypical cells are sometimes seen in the basal zone. The lamina propria and submucosa show progressive fibrosis, sometimes with a homogeneous hyalinized appearance and atypical fibroblasts. The fibrosis leads to stricture formation in some patients. Inflammatory cell infiltration, usually consisting of lymphocytes and plasma cells, is typically mild. In addition, telangiectatic capillaries and thick-walled hyalinized arterioles, sometimes with intimal foam cells and luminal narrowing, may be identified. Endothelial cells are enlarged and bizarre. Chronic ulcers with nonspecific inflamed granulation tissue may develop as a result of vascular insufficiency. Hemosiderin may be seen as a result of previous hemorrhage. When submucosal glands are included in the specimen, atrophy, fibrosis, and squamous metaplasia may be seen.

The most important aspect of pathologic diagnosis of radiation esophagitis is the clinical history of previous radiotherapy. The histopathologic findings described above provide pathologic confirmation and an objective assessment of the severity of injury within the limitations of sampling. In addition, the specimen should be examined carefully for evidence of complicating factors such as superinfecting bacteria, fungi, and viruses, as well as recurrent or residual tumor.

Additional information on radiation esophagitis is in Chapter 9.

Thermal Injury

Heat injury to the esophageal mucosa can occur from ingestion of excessively hot food or beverages. Microwaved food has been reported to lead to such injury because of uneven heat distribution; there may be extremely high temperatures in the center of some food items, which can be swallowed because of their cooler exterior. Cold injury to the esophagus is unusual.

HIATAL HERNIA
(Si-Chun Ming, M.D.)

In hiatal hernia, the upper portion of the stomach (rarely, the entire stomach, a segment of the colon, or the spleen) evaginates through the widened esophageal hiatus of the diaphragm into the thorax. It is a relatively common condition: on routine barium examination it was found in 0.8% to 2.9% of adults. When intra-abdominal pressure was increased during examination, the prevalence increased to 2.1% to 11.8%, and lying in the prone position also increased the occurrence of hiatal hernia. In symptomatic patients subjected to endoscopic or manometric examination, hiatal hernia was found in 16% to 22%. There is, however, wide geographic variation. Hiatal hernia is common in Western countries and uncommon in Africa: barium examination of symptomatic Nigerians revealed hiatal hernia in only 0.39%. Western dietary habits are thought to be responsible for the difference in frequency. The prevalence of hiatal hernia increases with age. It is, however, well recognized in infants and children, with a reported prevalence of 0.62% in children undergoing barium examination.

The cause of hiatal hernia is unknown. It is likely to be environmental rather than genetic. Structurally, there is separation of the diaphragmatic crura and widening of the space between the crura and the esophageal wall. There are two major types of hiatal hernia: axial, or sliding, and nonaxial, or paraesophageal. Rarely, extensive scarring of the esophagus may result in retraction of the esophagus and herniation of the gastric cardia.

Sliding Hiatal Hernia

The sliding hiatal hernia is by far the more common, constituting about 95% of the cases. About 60% of sliding hiatal hernias are less than 3 cm in diameter, and only 14% are more than 5 cm in diameter, according to the study by Pridie. Rare instances of herniation of the entire stomach have been reported. The herniated portion of the stomach can usually be reduced back into the abdominal cavity. The small asymptomatic hernias are merely anatomic phenomena and have no clinical significance. Most commonly the symptoms are related to accompanying reflux esophagitis rather than to the hernia itself.

The relationship between the sliding hiatal hernia and reflux esophagitis is complex and controversial. It is evident that these two conditions often coexist but are not totally dependent on each other. Berstad et al. reported that 63% of the patients with reflux esophagitis had hiatal hernia, while only 8% of patients without reflux esophagitis had it. Conversely, 42% of patients with hiatal hernia had no esophagitis. Low pressure of the lower esophageal sphincter (LES) and a short intra-abdominal segment of LES contribute to cardial incompetence and result in gastroesophageal reflux. In the presence of hiatal hernia, the acidic fluid trapped in the hernia enters the esophagus when the LES is relaxed, accounting for delayed esophageal clearance and contributing to subsequent esophagitis. (Reflux esophagitis is discussed in detail below.)

In addition to peptic esophagitis, the herniated stomach may become ulcerated, causing bleeding and perforation. Bleeding can also occur from incarcerated mucosal folds of the herniated stomach. In one report, ulceration caused aortogastric fistula. A large hernia may become incarcerated, causing obstruction: Haas et al. reported volvulus of the stomach in 21 of 138 surgically treated cases. Additional complications associated with hiatal hernia include diffuse esophageal spasm, carcinoma in the gastric cardia, cardiac arrhythmia, fibrosis of the lung, Mallory-Weiss syndrome, and intussusception of esophagus into the hernia. Rarely, rectal bleeding has been reported to occur from the colon that herniates through the diaphragmatic hiatus. Coincidental lesions with hiatal hernia include Zenker's diverticulum, colonic diverticulosis, and gallstones.

Paraesophageal Hernia

Paraesophageal hernia constitutes about 5% of hiatal hernia cases. It is not age-related. The LES is not affected and there is no reflux esophagitis, unless a sliding hernia coexists. The herniated portion of the stomach is usually along the greater curvature. Other organs such as the small bowel, the colon, and the spleen may also enter the paraesophageal hernia. Paraesophageal hernias may be caused by previous surgery in the region of the diaphragmatic hiatus, including operations for sliding hernia: 13% of cases at the Lahey Clinic in Boston had an iatrogenic cause.

Complications of paraesophageal hernia are serious and may be fatal. They include bleeding from ulcer, obstruction, volvulus, incarceration, and strangulation of the herniated stomach. In one case the ulcer penetrated into the right ventricle of the heart, causing massive bleeding. Because of the seriousness of the complications, early surgical repair of paraesophageal hernia has been advocated.

Other Diaphragmatic Hernias

Hernias may develop at sites away from the esophageal hiatus. The congenital ones may be symptomatic at birth and can be diagnosed *in utero* by sonography. They are usually located posterolaterally, involving the foramen of Bochdalek, or retrosternally, involving the foramen of Morgagni. These and other congenital diaphragmatic hernias are discussed in detail in Chapter 8. Respiratory problems are prominent in these patients because of hypoplasia of the lung in the presence of a large intrathoracic mass of abdominal organs or because of aspiration of regurgitated materials. Extracorporeal membrane oxygenation has been beneficial to these patients. Hernia may also be caused by traumatic injury to the diaphragm.

GASTROESOPHAGEAL REFLUX

Reflux esophagitis refers in general to esophageal inflammation resulting from gastroesophageal reflux, which is the regurgitation of gastric contents into the esophagus. However, reflux of intestinal contents after total gastrectomy with esophagojejunostomy can also produce reflux esophagitis. The specific clinical, endoscopic, radiologic, and pathologic definitions of *reflux esophagitis* are strikingly different. For example, the endoscopic definition refers to the presence of visible reddening of the mucosal surface, due to prominent blood vessels. On the other hand, *-itis* to the pathologist generally connotes the presence of inflammatory cells. The endoscopist is often unable to identify those patients with acute inflammatory cell infiltration of the epithelium, representing more severe injury, from those without active inflammation. As a result of the potential for confusion based on disparate definitions of *reflux esophagitis*, the phrase *changes due to gastroesophageal reflux* is used in this chapter for discussion of the histopathologic findings.

Persistent gastroesophageal reflux results from loss of effective antireflux mechanisms. These mechanisms appear to include anatomic factors at the gastroesophageal junction and diaphragmatic hiatus, but intrinsic lower esophageal sphincter tone is of cardinal importance. The specific sphincter abnormalities leading to gastroesophageal reflux are the subject of considerable investigation. In occasional patients, esophageal intubation, involvement of the muscularis propria by scleroderma, or a tumor at the esophagogastric junction can result in reflux. Persistent vomiting, sometimes on a psychogenic basis, can be considered as an extreme form of reflux. Reflux esophagitis is often part of a spectrum of upper gastrointestinal tract peptic disease, accompanied by gastritis and duodenitis.

Of particular importance is that *gastroesophageal reflux* and *reflux esophagitis* are not synonymous, because "physiologic" reflux occurs in normal individuals. The development of esophagitis as a consequence of reflux depends on (1) the volume of refluxed gastric fluid, which is affected by gastric secretion, gastric emptying, and duodenogastric reflux; (2) the potency of the reflux material, which can include biliary and pancreatic secretions following duodenogastric reflux as well as hydrochloric acid and pepsin produced by the gastric epithelium; (3) the efficiency of esophageal clearing of refluxed material by gravity, peristalsis, saliva, and normal esophageal sphincter relaxation with deglutition, because the efficiency of clearing in turn determines contact time with the mucosa; and (4) the resistance of the esophageal squamous epithelium.

At the cellular level, reflux-induced squamous epithelial injury may be due to damage to mucopolysaccharide intercellular cement and resultant back-diffusion of hydrogen ions, which leads to further damage. Increased cellular desquamation and increased epithelial cell turnover appear to occur in response to injury; if the severity of the injury exceeds the repair processes, inflammatory cell infiltration of the epithelium or even erosion and ulceration can result.

Categorization of reflux changes into "acute" and "chronic" based upon the histopathologic character of the inflammatory cell infiltrate and epithelial changes is best avoided because of the discordance between the histopathologic terminology and the time course of the process in the patient. For example, a biopsy diagnosis of "acute esophagitis" due to the presence of neutrophils in the specimen is inappropriate in a patient with months or years of reflux esophagitis. On the other hand, the pathogenesis of peptic complications of gastroesophageal reflux can be used as a basis for classification of the histopathologic changes into *high-grade* and *low-grade* types. Peptic strictures and Barrett's esophagus result from mucosal ulceration with loss of squamous epithelium and subsequent repair processes, i.e., deposition of scar tissue in the case of stricture, and re-epithelization with columnar epithelium in the case of Barrett's esophagus (see Barrett's Esophagus). Furthermore, frank ulceration is often preceded by epithelial erosion with less than full-thickness destruction. Therefore, *high-grade changes due to gastroesophageal reflux* are characterized histopathologically by evidence of epithelial injury and destruction, usually accompanied by active inflammation, including neutrophils. These findings indicate severe insult to the esophageal mucosa. Less severe epithelial injury without histopathologic evidence of destruction or active inflammation but with reactive epithelial changes occurs in *low-grade changes due to gastroesophageal reflux*. However, in using this classification, it should be kept in mind that in addition to the peptic complications, gas-

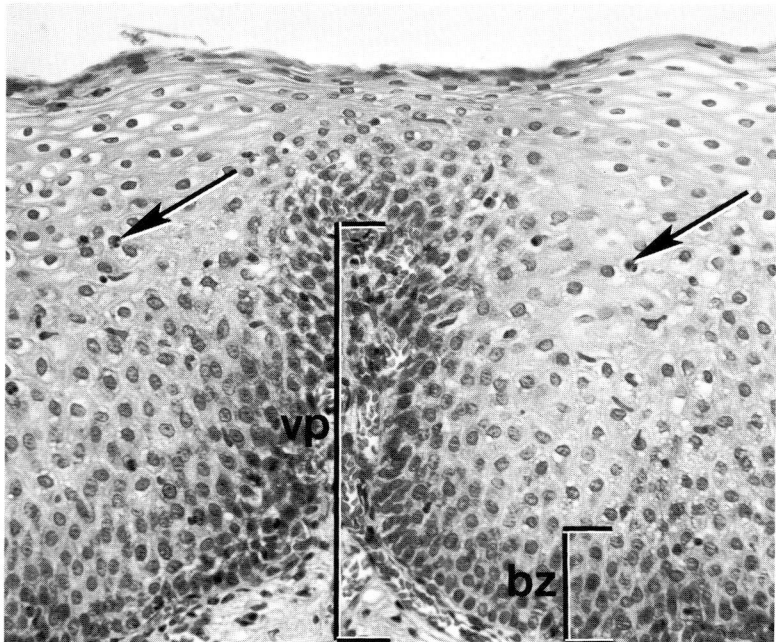

FIGURE 17–26. Low-grade changes due to gastroesophageal reflux. The esophageal epithelium in this biopsy taken about 3 cm above the esophagogastric junction has elongated vascular papillae (vp) and widened basal zone (bz). Scattered intraepithelial eosinophils (arrows) are also present.

troesophageal reflux has received attention with regard to a possible role in the pathogenesis of asthma and sudden infant death syndrome. Aspiration pneumonia may occur as a complication. As a result, the severity of the histopathologic findings may not be related to the severity or the gravity of the clinical picture.

The histopathologic changes due to gastroesophageal reflux present a wide spectrum of findings, ranging from subtle reactive epithelial changes to active esophagitis, peptic erosion, and ulcer. The histopathologic changes have been described in both capsule and endoscopic biopsy specimens in studies attempting to delineate clinically significant reflux or to correlate endoscopic findings in reflux esophagitis.

Low-Grade Changes

These reactive epithelial changes have received a great deal of attention in the literature since Ishmail-Beigi et al. described in 1970 "basal cell hyperplasia of the squamous epithelium" and "location of the papillae close to the epithelial surface" as "the histological consequences of gastroesophageal reflux." Their criteria in well-oriented capsule biopsies taken about 2 cm above the manometrically demonstrated lower esophageal sphincter were (1) the basal zone comprising more than 15% of the total thickness of the epithelium and (2) papillae extending more than two thirds of the distance to the surface (Figure 17–26). Additional features of low-grade changes due to gastroesophageal reflux described by other authors include vascularization of the epithelium with dilated vessels ("lakes") at the tops of the papillae (see Figure 17–2), increased numbers of papillae, loss of the longitudinal orientation of the surface epithelial cells due to the presence of ovoid immature cells at the surface, increased mitotic figures and incorporation of tritiated thymidine in the basal zone, and "balloon cells," i.e., enlarged translucent squamous epithelial cells that contain plasma proteins (see Figure 17–4B). Except for balloon cells and vascular lakes, these features are morphologic consequences of increased epithelial proliferation resulting from relatively mild injury induced by reflux. By contrast, balloon cells are the result of epithelial injury with increased permeability of the cell membrane and usually occur in the midzone of the squamous epithelium in patients with chronic gastroesophageal reflux. Vascular lakes are equivalent to congestion and represent the vascular phase of the inflammatory process. The epithelial changes of reflux esophagitis are summarized in Table 17–3. The changes are similar to

Table 17–3 EPITHELIAL CHANGES OF REFLUX ESOPHAGITIS

Histopathologic Feature	Pathogenetic Mechanism
Erosion/ulcer	Severe epithelial injury
Balloon cells	Epithelial injury
Vascular dilatation ("lakes") in papillae	Vascular phase of inflammatory response
Polymorphonuclear leukocytes (neutrophils/eosinophils)	Leukocytic phase of inflammatory response
Elongation of vascular papillae	Epithelial proliferation
Increased numbers of vascular papillae	Epithelial proliferation
Immature epithelial cells at luminal surface	Epithelial proliferation
Widening of basal zone of epithelium	Epithelial proliferation
Increased mitotic figures in epithelium	Epithelial proliferation

those induced by injury to squamous epithelium of other body sites, e.g., skin.

Very rare intraepithelial polymorphonuclear leukocytes may be seen as part of the spectrum of low-grade changes due to gastroesophageal reflux. The presence of more than a very few in a biopsy specimen should lead to classification of the reflux changes as high-grade, especially if the epithelium shows injury or prominent reactive changes. Intraepithelial eosinophils (see Figure 17–26) have been reported to be an indicator of delayed acid clearance after reflux, even in the absence of reactive epithelial changes. In the lamina propria, chronic inflammation with lymphocytes, eosinophils, plasma cells, and lymphoid aggregates and fibrosis may be found; but the relationship of these findings to reflux-induced injury is uncertain.

The ultrastructural features of the squamous epithelium in reflux esophagitis have been described. Intracellular findings included edema, mitochondrial damage, membrane whorls, dilatation of the endoplasmic reticulum and Golgi apparatus, reduced membrane-coated granules, and occurrence of keratohyaline and parakeratotic granules. Intercellular spaces were enlarged and contained particulate debris with neutral mucosubstances. When cells were present in the intercellular spaces, they were usually lymphocytes, but neutrophils were found occasionally. The epithelial basement membranes showed areas of thickening, thinning, and interruption; and anchoring fibrils were increased.

High-Grade Changes

A range of features can be seen. Active esophagitis is characterized by active inflammation and epithelial injury (see Figure 17–1). Neutrophils usually predominate in the active inflammation when epithelial injury is severe and may be seen in both the epithelium and lamina propria. In occasional cases, the heavy polymorphonuclear infiltrate consists of eosinophils producing the histopathologic finding of "eosinophilic esophagitis" (Table 17–4). The factors determining the predominant cell type in the infiltrate are unknown. Lymphocytes in intercellular spaces of the epithelium sometimes have elongated nuclei and must be distinguished from polymorphonuclear leukocytes (Figure 17–27). Intercellular lymphocytes are sometimes numerous but even then do not appear to indicate high-grade esophageal mucosal injury. Epithelial injury is manifested by edema, which appears as widened intercellular spaces; and loss of epithelial cell cohesion is sometimes evident. Epithelial cell necrosis is usually not a prominent feature, even with intense polymorphonuclear leukocytic infiltration. Reactive epithelial findings usually accompany active inflammation.

Epithelial destruction can take the form of erosion, acute ulcer, or active chronic ulcer (see Figure 17–3). Luminal fibrinoinflammatory exudate often occurs on the surface of adjacent epithelium as well as in the eroded area and ulcer crater itself. The presence of ex-

Table 17–4 DIFFERENTIAL DIAGNOSES OF EOSINOPHILIC INFILTRATION OF ESOPHAGEAL EPITHELIUM

Acid-peptic reflux
Alkaline reflux
Infectious esophagitis
Eosinophilic gastroenteritis
Drug injury
Allergic esophagitis
Idiopathic eosinophilic esophagitis

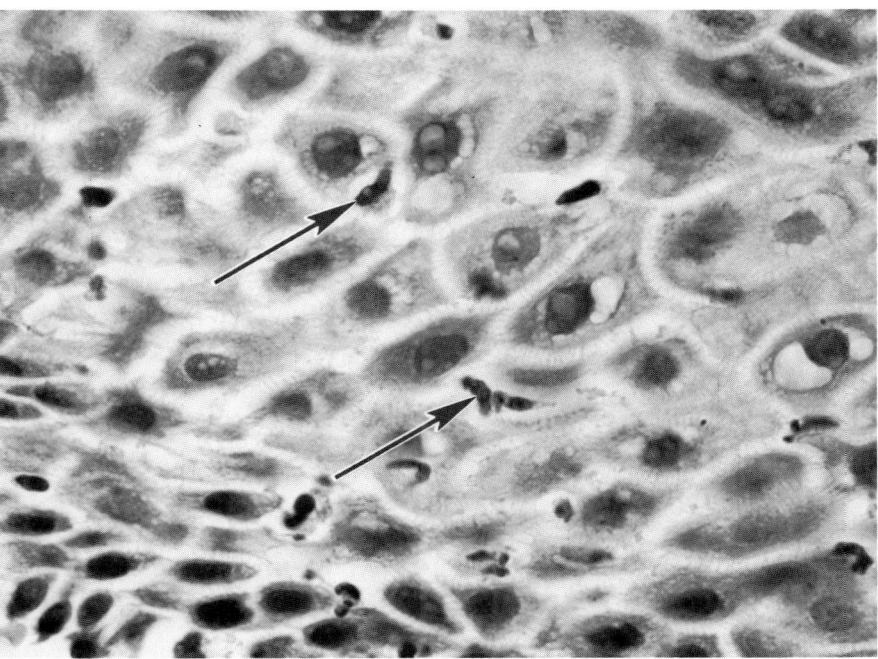

FIGURE 17–27. Lymphocytes in intercellular spaces of esophageal squamous epithelium. The "squiggly" nuclei and absence of cytoplasm containing granules help to distinguish lymphocytes from eosinophils and neutrophils.

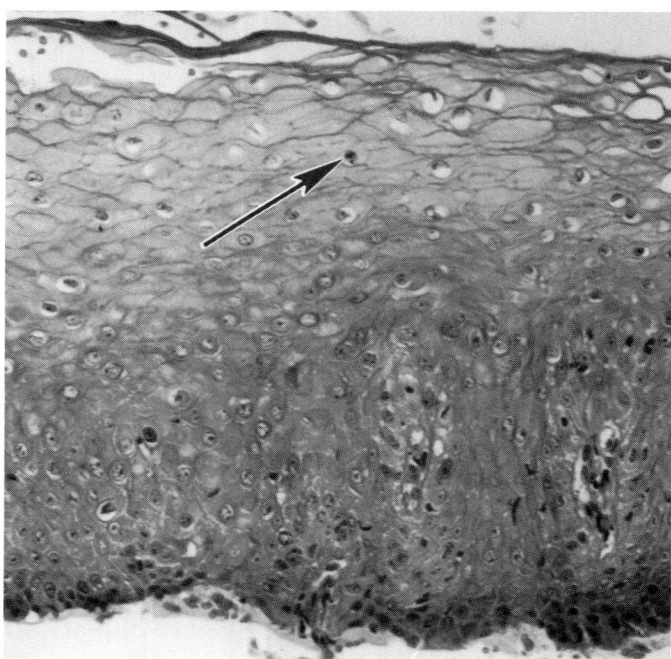

FIGURE 17–28. Epithelial changes due to alkaline reflux. In this patient with total gastrectomy and esophagojejunal anastomosis, the squamous epithelium contains scattered intraepithelial eosinophils (arrow) and has reactive epithelial changes indistinguishable from those of acid reflux.

udate in specimens often provides evidence of erosion or an ulcer when tissue fragments showing epithelial destruction are not included. This finding can be especially helpful in biopsy specimens because of the problem of sampling. The depth of ulceration can often be determined relative to the muscularis mucosae or muscularis propria, including that in biopsy specimens from the ulcer base. Inflammatory polyps with granulation tissue and reactive epithelial changes sometimes occur. In extreme cases, septa may bridge the esophageal lumen, leading to a "double-barreled" appearance. Aortoesophageal fistula has also been reported as a consequence of reflux.

The utility of esophageal biopsies in the evaluation of cases of suspected gastroesophageal reflux and reflux esophagitis is controversial. Some authors have reported that esophageal biopsy is an excellent diagnostic tool in this clinical setting, whereas others have not supported these claims. Interpretation of inflammation and reactive epithelial changes as evidence of reflux esophagitis is complicated by several factors. First, the changes are etiologically nonspecific, occurring in response to esophageal epithelial injury of *any* etiology as part of the body's stereotyped inflammatory and reparative processes. For example, the abnormalities can occur as a consequence of alkaline reflux (Figure 17–28) as well as acid reflux, which is the usual clinical situation. From the morphologic perspective, the histopathologic features are sometimes discordant: elongated vascular tufts may occur without basal zone thickening, and balloon cells indicating injury may be seen in the absence of reactive epithelial changes (Figure 17–29). Second, squamous epithelium with reactive changes is normally distributed in the distal few centimeters of esophagus, probably as a result of "physiologic" gastroesophageal reflux. Thus, interpretation of reactive epithelium as evidence of abnormality depends heavily upon the site of the biopsy specimens relative to the lower esophageal sphincter. The endoscopist, therefore, plays a key role when choosing the level of the biopsy. Furthermore, at a given level the histopathologic findings often have a nonuniform, patchy distribution around the circumference of the esophagus. Sampling, therefore, plays an important role in the biopsy findings, and the endoscopist should

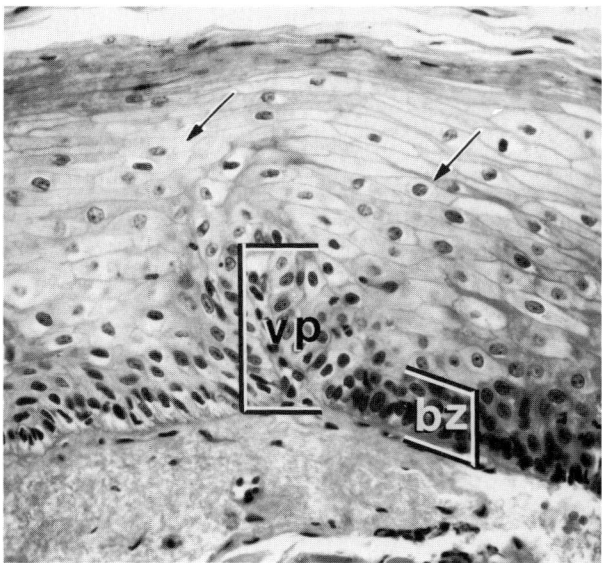

FIGURE 17–29. Disparity between evidence of epithelial injury and reactive changes in a patient with reflux esophagitis. Numerous balloon cells are present in the middle layers of the squamous epithelium (arrows), but the vascular papillae (vp) and basal zone (bz) are of normal size.

take multiple biopsies to reduce the problem of sampling. Third, histopathologic assessment itself is affected by the type of biopsy specimen and the histologic techniques used for embedding and sectioning. Some authors have insisted that only capsule biopsies are suitable for evaluation of reflux changes, whereas others have found endoscopic biopsies to be satisfactory. Endoscopic biopsy specimens are obtained far more often in current practice and appear to be interpretable *if* numerous step sections are cut through the specimen. With this approach, some portion of the biopsy specimen will usually be sufficiently well-oriented for interpretation of length of vascular papillae and width of basal zone. Furthermore, dilatation of vessels in the papillae and increased numbers of papillae can be assessed even in poorly oriented specimens; papillae appear to be increased in number when they overlap on a line perpendicular to the basal layer in *en face* sections. The final point regarding histopathologic assessment is intra- and inter-observer variation. Most studies have addressed this factor only superficially. One study directed at this problem, however, found intra- and inter-observer disagreement on two separate interpretations of the same specimen of 20%, even when assessment was limited to "normal" versus "abnormal."

The histopathologic features that occur as a consequence of gastroesophageal reflux-associated changes are an important aspect of the pathophysiology of reflux esophagitis. Their usefulness as a diagnostic test, however, depends upon their clinical utility. Several studies under carefully controlled conditions have given esophageal biopsy high marks as a diagnostic test for gastroesophageal reflux. Furthermore, in one study with 24-hour esophageal pH monitoring of a large number of patients, the degree of exposure of the distal esophageal mucosa to gastric acid was highly correlated with length of papillae and thickness of the basal zone. On the other hand, the correlation coefficients were only .275 to .333, and wide scatter is evident in the graphs comparing the histopathologic features in each biopsy specimen with acid exposure. These results do not bode well for esophageal biopsy as a robust diagnostic test for reflux in individual patients because of poor predictive values.

In patients with gastroesophageal reflux, problems of specificity, topography of findings, specimen type, histologic processing, observer variation, and clinical correlation enter into the interpretation of esophageal biopsy specimens. Appropriate use of biopsy is determined by the goal of the endoscopist in taking the specimens. Histopathologic evidence of esophagitis and reactive epithelial changes can have a large number of causes. Some have specific features that do permit identification of the cause (e.g., infectious esophagitis with morphologic evidence of the organisms). Biopsy cannot be used in the primary diagnosis of reflux esophagitis, but it is helpful in identifying esophagitis due to other causes or due to other factors complicating reflux. In a patient with documented reflux, biopsy to evaluate the severity of the mucosal injury is inappropriate. Endoscopic examination with biopsy is best for identification of active esophagitis, erosion, or ulcer. Biopsies are also especially helpful in calling attention to patients in whom the histopathologic findings are more severe than was suggested by the endoscopic appearance. High-grade changes of gastroesophageal reflux lead to aggressive management to prevent the peptic complications of esophageal stricture and Barrett's esophagus in addition to relieving symptoms. After antireflux therapy, follow-up biopsies for determining the objective response are appropriate.

Barrett's Esophagus

Barrett's esophagus is the eponym applied to the columnar epithelium-lined lower esophagus which is acquired as a complication of chronic gastroesophageal reflux. The precise prevalence of Barrett's esophagus is unknown, but one autopsy study found 376 cases per 100,000 population. Many affected persons are asymptomatic, however. The prevalence in patients who undergo upper gastrointestinal tract endoscopy and biopsy is about 1% to 2%, and among patients with symptoms of gastroesophageal reflux who undergo endoscopy and biopsy, the prevalence is about 10%.

The clinical importance of Barrett's esophagus is enhanced by its predisposition to malignancy. Adenocarcinoma in Barrett's esophagus accounts for the majority of adenocarcinomas of the esophagogastric junction and esophagus. Many of the patients are not known to have Barrett's esophagus until they present with the complicating adenocarcinoma. Among patients with recognized Barrett's esophagus, about 10% have or eventually develop adenocarcinoma, and the risk is about 40 times that of the general population. However, the incidence in follow-up studies of patients with Barrett's esophagus is low: only about 1/200 to 1/400 patient-years of follow-up.

The publication by N. R. Barrett in 1950 first called attention to the columnar epithelium–lined lower esophagus, although cases had been identified earlier. Much of the confusion about the entity resulted from failure to appreciate the reflux-related etiology and pathogenesis, beginning with Barrett himself: he described the columnar-lined structure as intrathoracic stomach due to congenitally short esophagus. After the columnar-lined region was demonstrated to be esophagus, Barrett proposed that the epithelium was congenital embryonic epithelium. The available evidence now indicates that Barrett's esophagus is generally acquired as a consequence of chronic gastroesophageal reflux and reflux esophagitis, although a congenital origin is still proposed in a few cases.

Evidence cited as favoring gastroesophageal reflux as the cause of Barrett's esophagus includes endoscopic observations with sequential biopsies showing upward migration of columnar-lined mucosa over time with continuing reflux; acquisition of Barrett's mucosa with onset of gastroesophageal reflux after esophagogastrostomy following partial esophagogastrectomy; experimental studies in animal models demonstrating healing of denuded esophagus with columnar-lined mucosa in the setting of reflux; failure to identify Barrett's esophagus in extensive autopsy studies of stillborns and neonates; and the absence from Barrett's epithelium of gastrin-containing cells, which are present in congenital gastric heterotopia in Meckel's diverticulum and gastric duplication (although gastrin and gastrin-containing cells have been identified in Barrett's mucosa in other studies). Ethanol abuse and acid secretion from parietal cells in Barrett's mucosa have been suggested to play a role in etiology. Barrett's esophagus has also been reported to be acquired after total gastrectomy, which indicates that reflux of gastric contents is not necessarily required.

The pathogenesis of Barrett's esophagus has been the subject of speculation by many authors. Direct metaplasia of squamous epithelium into columnar epithelium has little good evidence to support it. On the other hand, destruction of acid-, pepsin-, and bile-sensitive squamous-lined mucosa by chronic gastroesophageal reflux followed by re-epithelization with more resistant columnar epithelium is supported by both clinical and experimental evidence. The "cell of origin" of the columnar epithelium has been debated in the literature. Migration of columnar cells from esophageal cardiac glands has been suggested on histologic grounds. However, migration of undifferentiated columnar progenitor cells from adjacent gastric and Barrett's mucosa into an ulcerated area, followed by their differentiation to columnar epithelial cells of various types is more consistent with the usual mechanisms of mucosal healing. Migration of squamous progenitor cells from the adjacent squamous epithelium probably occurs simultaneously, but in the abnormal milieu of ongoing reflux-induced injury, the columnar progenitor cells may have selective advantage. Totipotentiality of the undifferentiated cells is also a possible explanation, in that the cells may differentiate into either columnar or squamous cells, depending upon the milieu. Proliferation of connective tissue cells occurs to form lamina propria of the Barrett mucosa. Over time, intestinalization appears to occur in the columnar epithelium, which is often initially gastric in type.

Whatever the precise mechanism, Barrett's mucosa is metaplastic columnar-lined mucosa that has replaced the original squamous-lined mucosa and provides greater resistance to the effects of gastroesophageal reflux and can undergo further metaplasia to intestinal-type differentiation. Differences among patients in severity and location of reflux-induced injury and in the characteristics of the repair process probably influence the mucosal remodeling. The dynamic nature of this pathogenetic process in turn may account for the variability of Barrett's esophagus, including the topography of Barrett's mucosa; the variable association with ulcer, stricture, and esophagitis; and the variable histopathologic features of the Barrett mucosa (see below).

Barrett's esophagus is best considered as a morphologic (and therefore endoscopic and surgical) syndrome with a variety of possible components (Figure 17–30). The *sine qua non* is columnar epithelium-lined lower

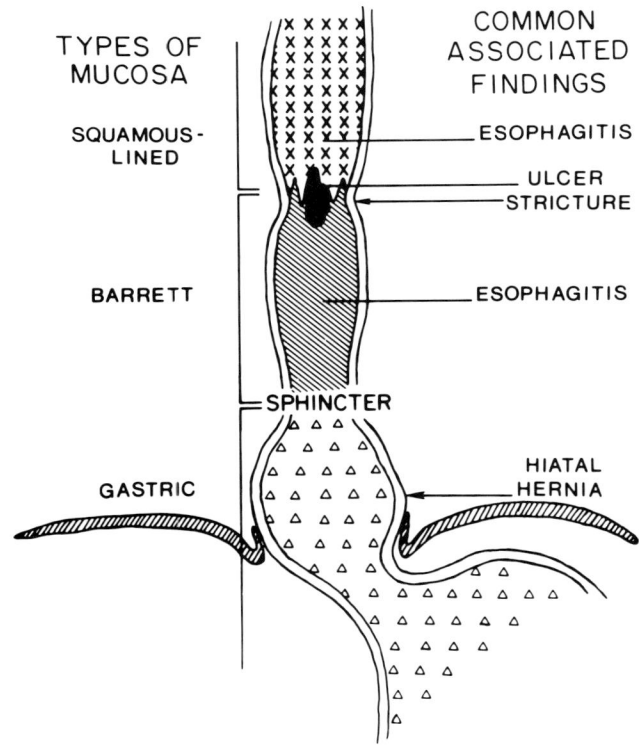

FIGURE 17–30. Diagrammatic representation of Barrett's esophagus. The columnar-lined mucosa acquired secondary to gastroesophageal reflux extends from the lower esophageal sphincter zone into the esophagus for variable distances. Other findings associated with Barrett's mucosa include ulcer, stricture, reflux esophagitis in both squamous-lined mucosa and Barrett's mucosa, and hiatal hernia.

esophagus. By definition, the squamocolumnar junction on the mucosal surface is located above the anatomic esophagogastric junction. Barrett's mucosa can have a wide variety of topographic appearances. Classically, Barrett's mucosa appears as a circumferential sheet resembling gastric mucosa without rugae that extends for variable distances into the esophagus above the lower esophageal sphincter zone. However, tongues, fingers, or even islands of Barrett's mucosa involving only portions of the esophageal circumference occur frequently. Regardless of the topography, some portion of the Barrett mucosa generally occurs in continuity with the true gastric mucosa below it (although one exceptional case with Barrett's mucosa in continuity with heterotopic gastric mucosa in the mid esophagus has been reported). Islands of squamous-lined mucosa often remain within the columnar-lined region, attesting to the esophageal location.

The variable components of the Barrett syndrome are peptic ulcer, stricture, reflux esophagitis, and hiatal hernia. The Barrett ulcer is commonly seen at the squamocolumnar junction at the uppermost extent of the Barrett mucosa, but ulcers also occur within the columnar-lined region, sometimes in association with squamous-lined remnants. The Barrett stricture typically occurs at the uppermost extent of the Barrett mucosa, as a sequela of deep ulceration at that site. Occasion-

Table 17-5 HISTOPATHOLOGIC CLASSIFICATION OF BARRETT'S MUCOSA

Category	Typical Macroscopic Configuration	Predominant Glandular Epithelial Cells	Predominant Surface Epithelial Cells	Evidence of Intestinal Differentiation
Distinctive-type	Villous structures and cryptlike glands	Columnar mucous	Goblet interspersed among columnar mucous	Goblet cells Absorptive cells Paneth cells (variable)
Cardiac-type	Glands with deep pits	Columnar mucous	Columnar mucous	Absent
Fundic-type	Glands with shallow pits	Parietal, chief	Columnar mucous	Absent
Indeterminate-type	Variable	Variable	Variable	Variable

ally more than one stricture is seen, presumably as a result of more than one area of ulceration or repeated episodes. Spasm of the muscularis propria may sometimes produce radiographic or endoscopic evidence of a stricture that will not be present on pathologic examination.

Reflux esophagitis can involve the squamous-lined mucosa above the uppermost extent of the Barrett mucosa as well as the columnar-lined mucosa itself. This finding represents the consequence of ongoing reflux of gastric contents into the esophagus (see discussion of reflux esophagitis). Hiatal hernia, characterized by extension of stomach through the diaphragmatic hiatus into the thoracic cavity, may be subtle or obvious. A key aspect of the diagnosis of Barrett's esophagus is recognition that the columnar-lined esophagus may be associated with none, some, or all of the other components of the morphologic Barrett syndrome.

Histopathologic Features

A bewildering array of terminology for Barrett's mucosa has been used in the literature because of the wide spectrum of histopathologic features that can be seen. The types of cells identified in the epithelium of Barrett's mucosa include gastric-type columnar mucus-containing cells, which stain, with PAS and sometimes with alcian blue, pH 2.5 (AB), and mucicarmine; intestinal-type goblet cells, which stain with PAS, AB, and mucicarmine; columnar epithelial cells with a brush border and no mucus vacuoles, similar to small-intestinal absorptive epithelial cells; Paneth cells, with their characteristic eosinophilic cytoplasmic granules; parietal and chief cells; and neuroendocrine cells, which can be argyrophil, argentaffin, and enterochromaffin, and which contain various hormones as noted by immunohistochemistry, including somatostatin, serotonin, substance P, enkephalin, and gastrin. The cell types identified by light microscopy in Barrett's epithelium thus include various constituents of normal gastric and small-intestinal epithelium.

The macroscopic architecture of Barrett's mucosa can include glands with deep and shallow pits, as in gastric mucosa, and villous structures resembling small-intestinal mucosa. The lamina propria of all types of Barrett's mucosa can show varying severity of congestion, edema, acute and chronic inflammation, and fibrosis. These findings appear to be related to ongoing reflux-induced injury. Acute inflammation involving the epithelium is often accompanied by reactive epithelial changes that can be misinterpreted as dysplasia. Chronic inflammatory cells in the lamina propria may include plasma cells, lymphocytes, and eosinophils with scattered histiocytes and mast cells.

A variety of mucosa histopathology can be seen in any one patient, forming a mosaic or zonal arrangement of mucosal types. Barrett's mucosa also shows wide variation in histopathologic appearance among patients. Although it has shortcomings due to the arbitrary pigeonholing of specimens representing a continuum of findings, the classification shown in Table 17-5 can be used for Barrett's mucosa.

Distinctive-type Barrett's mucosa has a villiform configuration and cryptlike glands (Figures 17-31A). The villous structures vary widely in appearance, and the glands vary in number. The glands are often contiguous with the muscularis mucosae, and no intervening connective tissue is present in many examples. This contrasts with the findings in the usual squamous-lined esophageal mucosa and appears to be a manifestation of previous ulceration of the lamina propria with epithelial regeneration directly on the smooth muscle. The glands may show cystic dilatation, particularly with active inflammation of the epithelium resulting in gland abscesses.

The epithelium of the villous structures and glands is usually composed in large part of columnar mucous cells with PAS-staining gastric-type mucin. Goblet cells which stain with PAS, AB, and mucicarmine are both interspersed among and contiguous with the columnar mucous cells (Figure 17-31B). This distinctive epithelial morphologic appearance with interspersed goblet cells is identical to that of incomplete intestinal metaplasia of gastric mucosa but contrasts with that of complete intestinal metaplasia, in which the columnar mucous cells are inapparent in intestinalized glands by light microscopy. The characteristic interspersed goblet cells allow histopathologic recognition of distinctive-type Barrett's mucosa. The proportion of goblet cells varies widely, and absorptive cells also accompany the goblet cells. In some examples, the intestinalized cells dominate the epithelial morphology. Paneth cells may

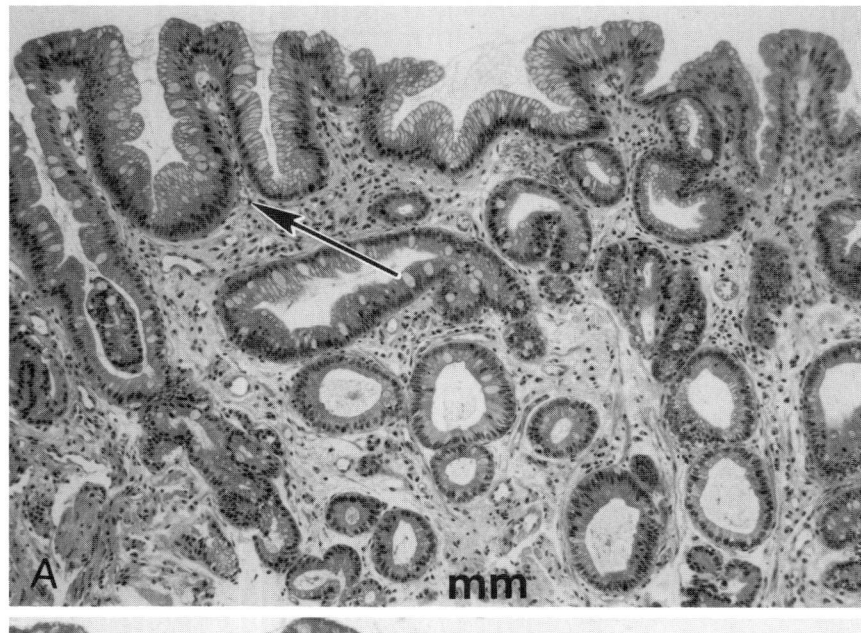
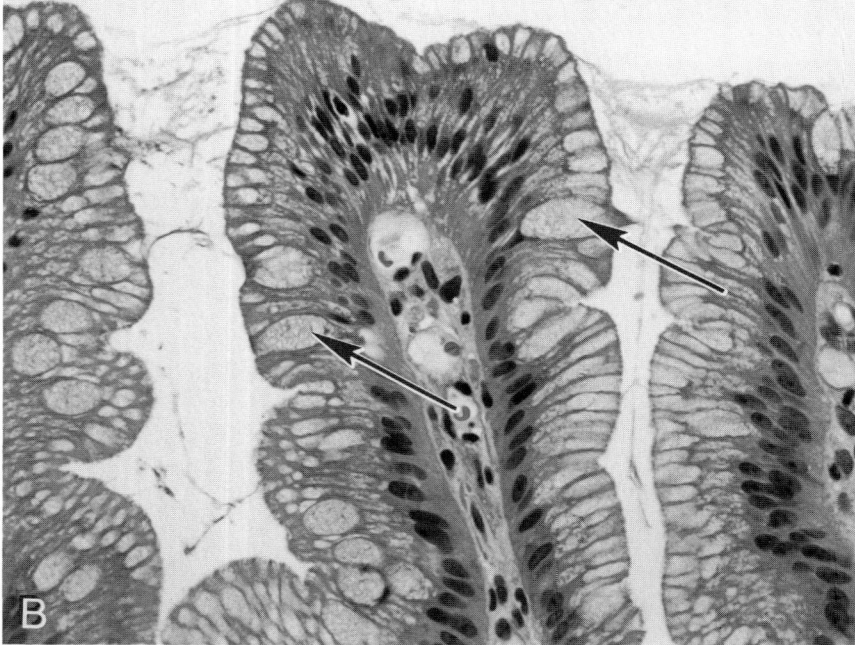

FIGURE 17–31. Barrett's mucosa of the distinctive type. *A*, Villiform architecture (arrow) with subjacent glands is evident. The glands adjoin the muscularis mucosae (mm). *B*, High-power view of the area indicated by the arrow in *A*. The distinctive-type epithelium is characterized by goblet cells (arrows) interspersed among columnar mucous cells.

be seen, usually in association with numerous goblet cells, small-intestinal–type columnar absorptive cells, and relatively few columnar mucous cells; these findings appear to represent advanced intestinalization. Plump columnar cells with prominent mucin vacuoles that resemble goblet cells in H&E-stained sections but do not stain with AB are seen in some cases. An array of argyrophil, argentaffin, and enterochromaffin cells is present; these endocrine cells are most numerous in the glands. A few parietal and chief cells may be scattered through the epithelium of the glands. The distinctive-type Barrett mucosa is present in the majority of adult patients with Barrett's esophagus but is less frequent in children, providing evidence for the occurrence of intestinalization over time.

Cardiac-type Barrett's mucosa, as the name implies, resembles gastric cardiac mucosa (Figure 17–32). This type of Barrett's mucosa sometimes contains deep pits, which may produce a villiform configuration. Mucus-containing epithelial cells are the predominant cell type in both surface and glandular epithelium. Endocrine cells are present, and scattered parietal and chief cells can occur. Goblet cells are very few in number and if present are widely scattered, although intestinal-type mucin staining with AB or mucicarmine can be seen in columnar mucous cells (the precise border between

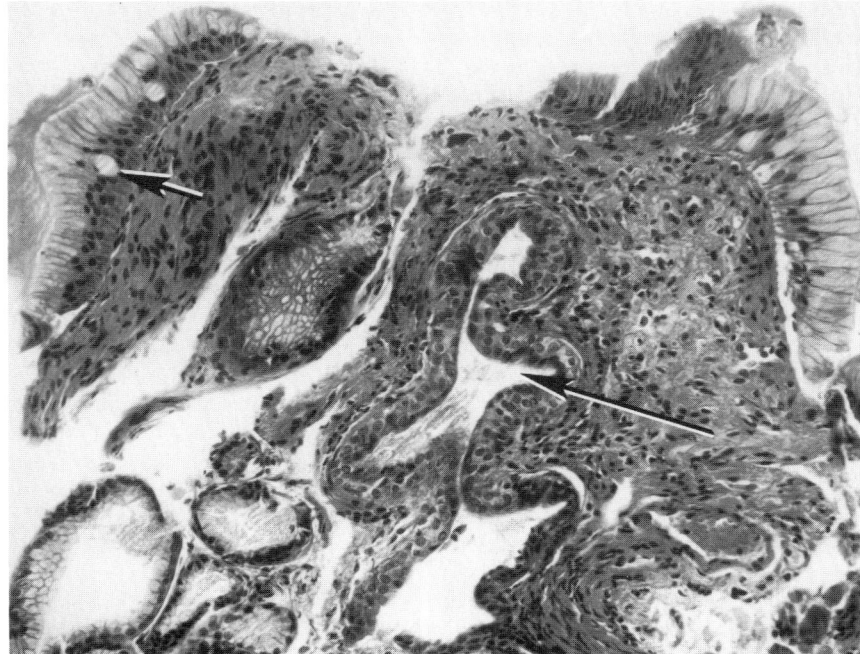

FIGURE 17-32. Cardiac-type Barrett's mucosa. The cardiac-type epithelium is composed of columnar mucous cells, some of which have distended vacuoles (short arrow). The mucosal architecture is abnormal, with fibrosis and chronic inflammation in the lamina propria. The squamous-lined duct (long arrow) of an esophageal submucosal gland localizes the specimen to the esophagus.

distinctive-type and cardiac-type Barrett's mucosa is arbitrary). Cardiac-type Barrett's mucosa usually differs from normal gastric cardiac mucosa in having glandular distortion, edema, and chronic inflammation.

Fundic-type Barrett's mucosa appears to be the least common form. Again as the name implies, the mucosa resembles gastric fundic mucosa in having shallow pits lined by mucus-containing columnar cells and a heavy complement of parietal and chief cells in the glands. Like cardiac-type Barrett's mucosa, the fundic-type mucosa often lacks a completely normal configuration, showing distorted or short glands and a villiform surface. Endocrine cells are present. Intestinal differentiation is absent.

A zonal distribution of Barrett's mucosa has been suggested in some patients: When zonal, the distinctive-type mucosa occurs most proximally, the fundic-type most distally, and the cardiac-type mucosa interposed between the other two. However, other studies of resection specimens, rather than biopsy specimens with their inherent sampling problem, found a mosaic distribution of the various types of mucosa.

The category of *indeterminate-type Barrett's mucosa* is provided because of the wide spectrum of histopathologic features; peculiar configurations and types of epithelium are found in some patients. As a result, a particular specimen may not meet precisely the criteria of the first three categories. For example, foci of complete intestinal differentiation manifested by goblet cells and small-intestinal columnar cells without interspersed columnar mucous cells sometimes occur in Barrett's mucosa that would otherwise be classified as cardiac-type or fundic-type. In other cases, small-intestinal–type mucin that stains strongly with AB occurs in columnar mucous cells in the absence of recognizable goblet cells. Since the characteristic pattern of goblet cells interspersed with columnar mucous cells is absent, categorization as distinctive-type does not seem justified, although some authors accept this criterion. Biopsy sampling often plays a role in these troublesome cases, because specimens from other areas of the Barrett mucosa may show the usual distinctive-type, cardiac-type, or fundic-type mucosa. The presence of dysplasia can also lead to classification of Barrett mucosa as indeterminate type by obscuring the characteristics of the antecedent columnar epithelium.

Ultrastructural Studies

Transmission electron-microscopic studies of the epithelial and endocrine cells in Barrett's mucosa have been reported. The findings confirm those of light microscopy. Scanning electron-microscopic studies produce spectacular views of the mucosal and epithelial surfaces.

Histopathologic Diagnosis

The diagnosis of Barrett's esophagus is as much a matter of specimen site as histopathologic findings in the specimen. The pathologist examining a surgical resection specimen or autopsy specimen can identify the location of a tissue sample submitted for histology. In addition, histopathologic landmarks in the esophageal wall are available to aid in localization (e.g., esophageal submucosal glands, twisting of the muscle fibers of the muscularis propria in the lower esophageal sphincter zone). For biopsy specimens, however, the pathologist is dependent on the endoscopist for the site from which the specimen is taken. Mural structures are rarely accessible to mucosal biopsy. In the proper setting, mucosa with the histopathologic features of gastric cardiac or fundic mucosa represents cardiac-type or fundic-type Barrett's mucosa, respectively, if the specimen was taken above the anatomic esophagogastric junction. Such is not the case if the biopsy was taken from the gastric cardia or a hiatal hernia pouch. Ideally, interpretation of biopsy specimens requires demonstration of the lower esophageal sphincter zone, preferably by manometry, and documentation by the endoscopist of the topography and location of the suspected columnar-lined areas, including the biopsy sites. Diagrammatic documentation by the endoscopist is particularly helpful when biopsies will be taken during serial follow-up endoscopies for monitoring effects of therapy and development of dysplasia (see below). Some clinical situations make diagnosis difficult. The presence of a stricture at the upper extent of the Barrett mucosa may prohibit further advancement of the endoscope so that directed biopsies can be obtained. Patients with a short segment of Barrett's mucosa in the region of the esophagogastric junction pose the greatest problem in diagnosis. The definition of Barrett's esophagus as columnar-lined lower esophagus acquired secondary to chronic gastroesophageal reflux does not translate easily into diagnostic criteria because the acquired pathogenesis is not often evident in the histopathologic findings.

The *criteria for diagnosis of Barrett's esophagus* include histopathologic findings, specimen localization, and topography of the columnar-lined mucosa. The histopathologic findings are (1) the presence of distinctive-type Barrett's mucosa or (2) demonstration of other columnar-lined mucosa with histopathologic features appropriate for Barrett's mucosa (Table 17-5). Also needed are (1) endoscopic localization of the biopsy site to the esophagus and (2) endoscopic demonstration of at least a portion of the columnar-lined mucosa in continuity with gastric mucosa (see Differential Diagnosis).

Distinctive-type Barrett's mucosa in an esophageal biopsy specimen is usually diagnostic of Barrett's esophagus. In the absence of distinctive-type mucosa, appropriate histopathologic findings include the presence of any of the other types of Barrett's mucosa, including cardiac-type and fundic-type. However, in this situation endoscopic localization of the biopsy sites to the esophagus is also needed, preferably with manometric demonstration of the lower esophageal sphincter zone, which is almost never done except in research settings. Occasionally, biopsy specimens can be localized to the esophagus on the histopathologic basis of esophageal submucosal glands (not cardiac glands) with their characteristic AB-staining epithelium or their squamous-lined ducts beneath the columnar-lined mucosa in the specimen (see Figure 17-32). The ducts alone are sometimes seen in the mucosa. Also, when circumferential biopsies are taken at the same level of the esophagus, the presence of squamous-lined mucosa along with another specimen showing presumed Barrett's mucosa at the same level increases confidence that the biopsy specimens were from esophagus originally lined by squamous epithelium. If gastric biopsies accompany the esophageal biopsies, the finding of intestinal differentiation in the candidate esophageal columnar-lined mucosa in the absence of gastric mucosal intestinalization provides circumstantial histopathologic evidence favoring Barrett's mucosa. Finally, endoscopic demonstration of at least part of the columnar-lined mucosa in continuity with gastric mucosa favors Barrett's esophagus rather than gastric heterotopia.

Additional circumstantial evidence for Barrett's esophagus, which may be absent in some cases, includes demonstration of gastroesophageal reflux, demonstration of ulceration and/or a stricture at the upper extent of the columnar-lined mucosa, evidence of reflux esophagitis in the squamous-lined mucosa above the columnar-lined region, and the presence of a hiatal hernia (see Figure 17-30).

Some authors require the presence of 2 or 3 cm of cardiac-type or fundic-type mucosa for a diagnosis of Barrett's esophagus. These numeric definitions do not permit recognition of short-segment Barrett's esophagus unless distinctive-type mucosa is present. Such definitions are not applicable in pediatric patients, who often lack distinctive-type mucosa and have a much shorter esophagus than do adults.

Differential Diagnosis

As discussed above, the distinctive-type Barrett mucosa in an esophageal specimen is essentially diagnostic of Barrett's esophagus. Other types of columnar epithelium-lined mucosa in specimens of the esophagus can represent the following:

1. *True gastric cardiac or fundic mucosa.* In this situation, the specimen was usually obtained from a hiatal hernia pouch that was mistaken for esophagus by the endoscopist or pathologist. For this reason, manometric localization of the lower esophageal sphincter zone is highly desirable in evaluating patients for Barrett's esophagus but rarely done. This type of mucosa cannot be differentiated reliably from Barrett's mucosa of the cardiac or fundic type by histopathology alone.

2. *Embryonic ciliated cell rests.* These rests represent remnants of the columnar epithelium which lines the embryonic esophagus until about the seventh fetal month, when replacement by squamous epithelium typically is completed. Such rests are incidental findings, usually in the upper esophagus of young children. Cilia can be identified on the luminal surface of the columnar epithelial cells, and the epithelium is simplistic, with only occasional well-formed glands. This type of epithelium is not seen in Barrett's esophagus.

3. *Tracheobronchial remnants.* Esophageal strictures due to tracheobronchial remnants in the lower esophagus occur rarely (Figure 17-33). The surface epithelium sometimes shows pseudostratified ciliated columnar epithelium of the type present in the respiratory tract, and the remnants often contain cartilage. This type of mucosa is not seen in Barrett's esophagus. In

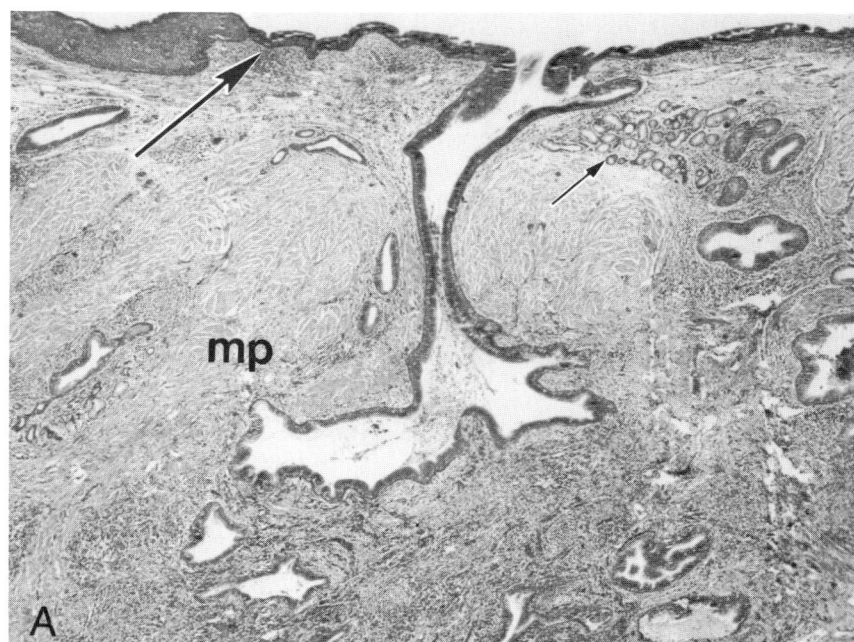

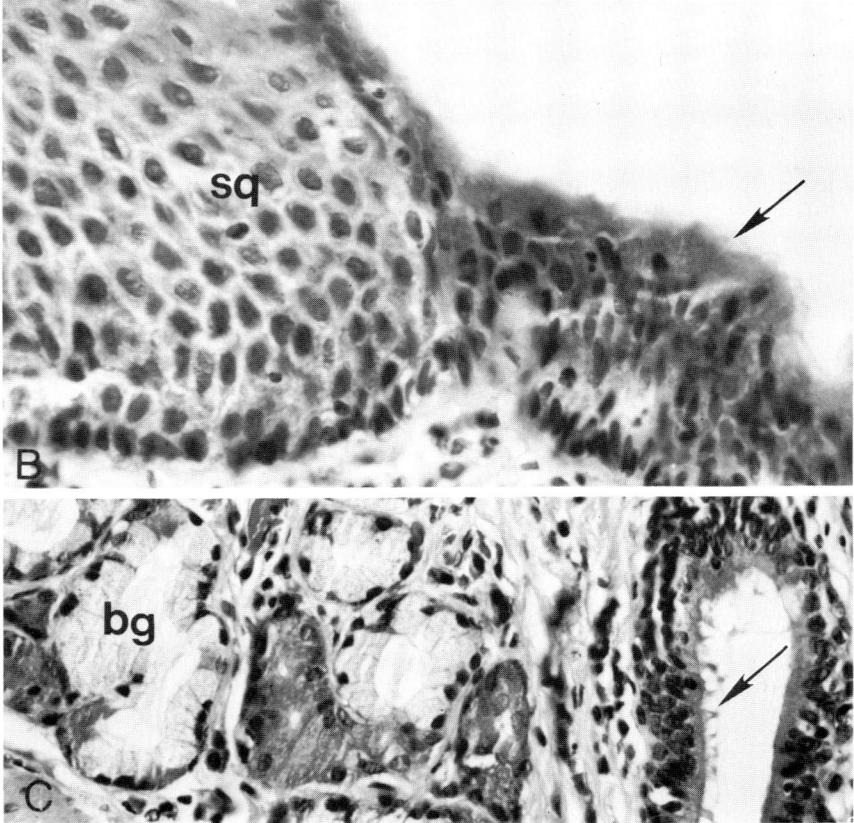

FIGURE 17–33. Tracheobronchial remnant that presented as a distal esophageal stricture in an adult. *A*, Ciliated respiratory epithelium is present on the esophageal luminal surface (large arrow) and lines cystic spaces, which extend through the muscularis propria (mp) into periesophageal soft tissue. Bronchial glands (small arrow) accompany the respiratory epithelium-lined structures. Islands of cartilage were present in other areas. *B*, Junction of squamous epithelium (sq) and respiratory epithelium on the esophageal luminal surface in area indicated by large arrow in upper panel. Cilia (arrow) are evident on the apical surface of the respiratory epithelium. *C*, Bronchial glands (bg) accompany respiratory epithelium-lined structures with ciliated epithelium (arrow).

many cases, squamous epithelium overlies the remnants which are located deep in the wall and are not obtainable by biopsy.

4. *Gastric heterotopia (ectopia).* Gastric epithelium or mucosa can occur in the esophagus, presumably as a result of misplacement or abnormal differentiation during embryonic development. Small foci of columnar epithelium may be interspersed in the squamous epithelium, particularly in the upper esophagus. Heterotopic mucosa can be composed of fundic-, transitional-, or antral-type glands. Peptic ulceration and adenocarcinoma can be complications of gastric het-

erotopia, further confusing the distinction from Barrett's esophagus. The endoscopic demonstration of columnar-lined mucosa in continuity with gastric mucosa provides evidence favoring Barrett's esophagus, although islands of true Barrett's mucosa may be formed during the ongoing process of injury and repair in the esophagus. Interpretation of findings in the esophagogastric junction region is also complicated by the common occurrence of esophageal cardiac glands, which can be interspersed with the squamous epithelium.

The pathologist's diagnosis for biopsy specimens with columnar-lined mucosa said to be from the esophagus must take into account the endoscopist's observations. The biopsy report should indicate the type of columnar-lined mucosa and whether or not dysplasia is present or suspected if the specimen is thought to represent Barrett's mucosa (see next section). Biopsy specimens showing the distinctive type of Barrett mucosa can be reported as such, e.g., "Barrett's mucosa of the distinctive type. Negative for dysplasia." Specimens with cardiac- or fundic-type mucosa can be reported for interpretation in light of other clinical evidence, e.g., "Cardiac-type mucosa consistent with Barrett's mucosa if the specimen was obtained from the esophagus. Negative for dysplasia." Specimens showing mucosa of other types can be reported descriptively.

Dysplasia and Adenocarcinoma in Barrett's Mucosa

The association between adenocarcinoma and Barrett's esophagus (Figure 17–34) is now well recognized as a result of numerous case reports and a series which have been published. Barrett's esophagus can be termed a *premalignant condition,* i.e., a clinical state which increases the risk of cancer. The factors producing the high risk are not as yet known; white men constitute the vast majority of patients with Barrett's carcinoma, in contrast to squamous carcinoma of the esophagus, in which nonwhites predominate. The possible role of alcohol and tobacco as in squamous carcinoma of the esophagus has been raised. In many patients, adenocarcinoma arising in Barrett's esophagus is accompanied by dysplasia (esophageal columnar intraepithelial neoplasia) in the surrounding Barrett mucosa. Sequential biopsy specimens have demonstrated development of adenocarcinoma in some reported patients who were initially found to have dysplasia alone. As a result, a dysplasia-carcinoma sequence is evident in Barrett's mucosa, as occurs generally in carcinogenesis involving epithelial surfaces. The natural history of dysplasia remains to be defined precisely, but based upon the few available reported patients the dysplasia-adenocarcinoma sequence appears to occur over a few years. In addition to adenocarcinoma, squamous carcinoma of the esophagus has been reported in patients with Barrett's esophagus.

As used here, *dysplasia* indicates a *neoplastic abnormality.* Dysplasia in Barrett's mucosa is characterized histopathologically by abnormalities in mucosal archi-

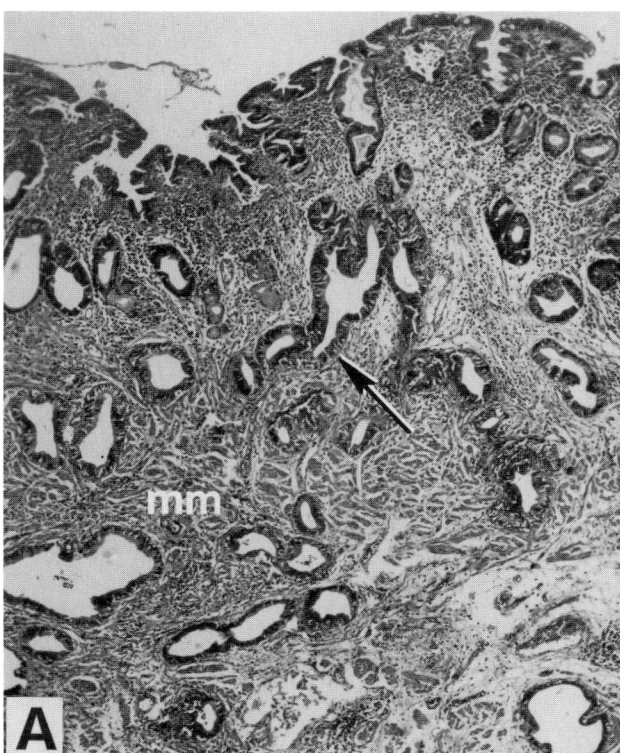

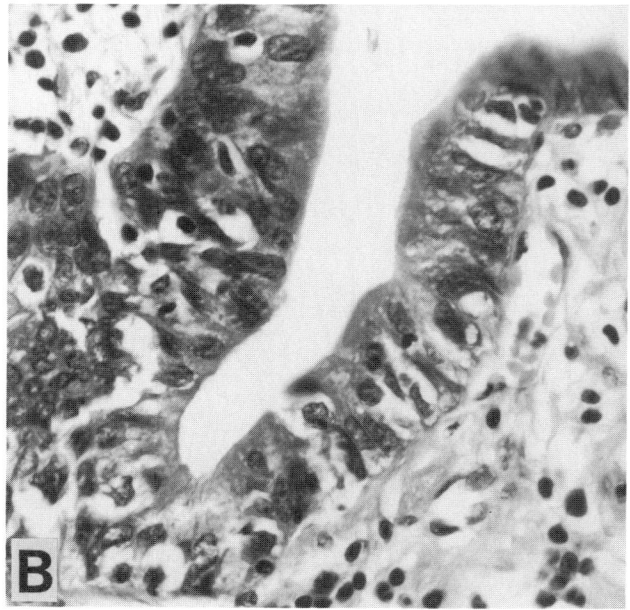

FIGURE 17–34. Adenocarcinoma arising in Barrett's esophagus. *A,* Adenocarcinoma infiltrates the muscularis mucosae (mm) and the submucosa. The overlying Barrett's mucosa has distorted glands (arrow) lined by dysplastic epithelium that appear to give rise to the submucosal invasion and may represent intramucosal adenocarcinoma. *B,* High-power view of the gland indicated by the arrow in *A*. The epithelium is hypercellular, with stratified, cytologically atypical, irregular nuclei with loss of polarity.

tecture, in epithelial characteristics, and in epithelial cell cytology (Figures 17–35 to 17–39). The presence of proliferated or bizarrely shaped glands and villiform structures is common in dysplastic Barrett's mucosa,

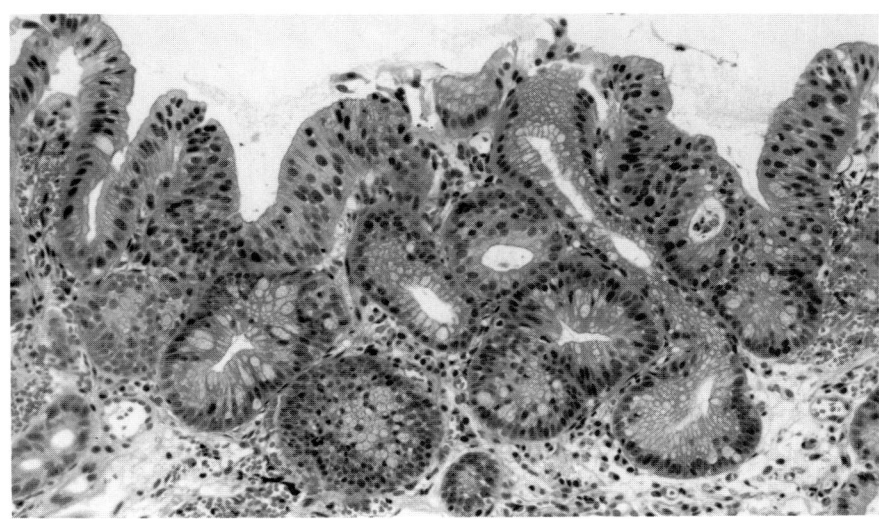

FIGURE 17-35. Low-grade epithelial dysplasia (esophageal columnar intra-epithelial neoplasia) in Barrett's mucosa of the distinctive type. The villous structures are blunt and short, and there is proliferation of glands, which are in close proximity to each other. The epithelium is mildly hypercellular, with full-thickness stratification of small and relatively uniform nuclei characterized by mild pleomorphism and loss of polarity. Mucous vacuoles are evident in the cytoplasm of the dysplastic epithelial cells.

which resembles adenomas of other sites in the gastrointestinal tract. The epithelium is hypercellular, with stratified, enlarged, irregular, pleomorphic nuclei showing loss of polarity, hyperchromatism with abnormal distribution of chromatin, and prominent nucleoli. Epithelial differentiation is also abnormal, because cytoplasmic mucin is generally decreased in amount and when present, often occurs in relatively apical vacuoles of relatively uniform size. This appearance contrasts with that of the prominent mucin in columnar cells and goblet cells of Barrett's mucosa without dysplasia. The architectural and epithelial features often produce an adenomatous appearance of dysplastic Barrett's mucosa. In other cases, the dysplasia has vesicular nuclei without prominent hypercellularity and stratification. The features of Barrett's dysplasia are similar in many respects to dysplasia in gastric mucosa (see also Chapters 19, 20, and 25). The type of dysplastic Barrett's mucosa, i.e., distinctive or cardiac, is often difficult to determine because of the replacement of the antecedent epithelium and therefore is sometimes of indeterminate type.

Histopathologic assessment of dysplasia in Barrett's mucosa is complicated by the occurrence of nonneoplastic reactive epithelial changes (Figure 17–40). Reactive changes are often associated with active inflammation, due to persistent gastroesophageal reflux with reflux esophagitis involving the Barrett mucosa. The problem of distinguishing the effects of inflammation from dysplasia is similar to that encountered with in-

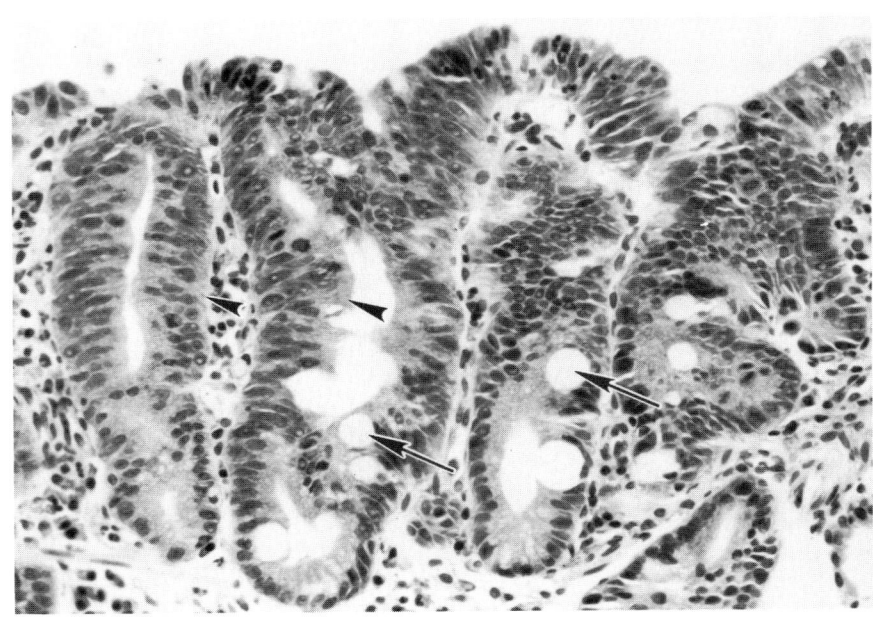

FIGURE 17-36. Intermediate-grade epithelial dysplasia (esophageal columnar intraepithelial neoplasia) in Barrett's mucosa of the distinctive type. The mucosal architecture is characterized by relatively uniform glands with no villous structures. The dysplastic epithelium is hypercellular with full-thickness stratification (arrowheads) of moderately pleomorphic nuclei. Goblet cells (arrows) remain in the epithelium.

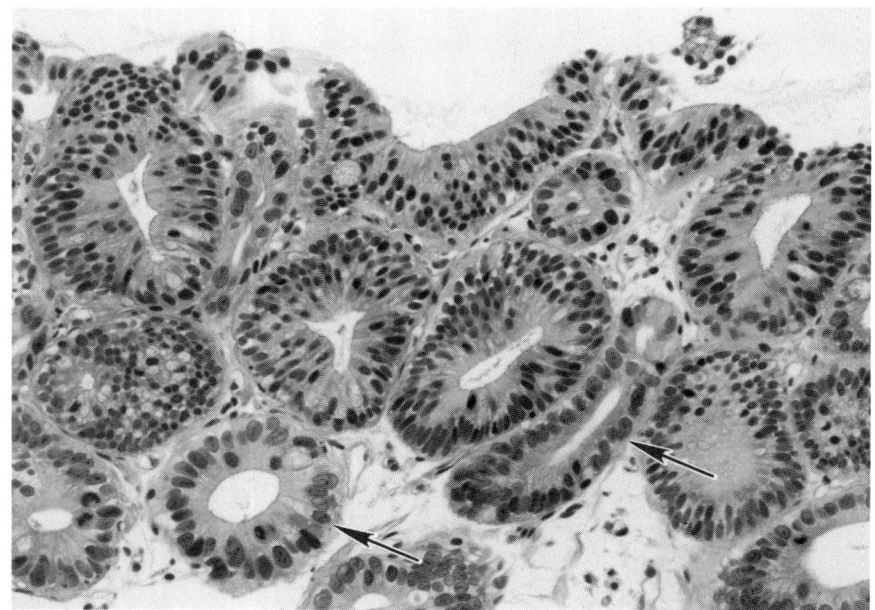

FIGURE 17–37. Intermediate-grade dysplasia (esophageal columnar intra-epithelial neoplasia) in Barrett's mucosa of the distinctive type. The mucosal architecture is characterized by glandular proliferation. The dysplastic epithelium is moderately hypercellular, with full-thickness stratification of relatively uniform small nuclei except in some glands, where nuclear enlargement with prominent nucleoli is evident (arrows). Epithelial mucin content is markedly reduced.

flammatory bowel disease. Therefore, the terminology for classification of colonic biopsy specimens developed by the Inflammatory Bowel Disease-Dysplasia Morphology Study Group (see Chapter 27) is also useful for specimens of Barrett's mucosa. Specimens are classified as "negative for dysplasia," "indefinite for dysplasia," or "positive for dysplasia." The "negative for dysplasia" category includes those specimens with reactive epithelial changes associated with active inflammation. "Indefinite for dysplasia" is applied to specimens about which there is uncertainty as to whether the epithelial abnormalities represent reactive changes or dysplasia. Uncertainty can arise from the nature of the histopathologic abnormalities or technical problems with specimen processing, such as poor orientation. The "indefinite" category is particularly useful in allowing pathologists to express simultaneously their concern and uncertainty about the nature of the epithelial abnormalities, thereby heightening endoscopists' awareness of the need for additional evaluation. The "indefinite" category can be subdivided into "probably negative," "unknown (no choice)," and "probably positive" to allow expression of the degree of concern, although intra- and interobserver variation may hinder the utility of this subdivision. Specimens with unequivocal dysplasia are categorized as "low-grade," "intermediate-grade," or "high-grade" on the basis of the severity of the abnormalities and their reported relationship to invasive adenocarcinoma (some authors use only two grades, low and high, to attempt to improve upon reproducibility of classification).

The histopathologic criteria for classifying biopsy

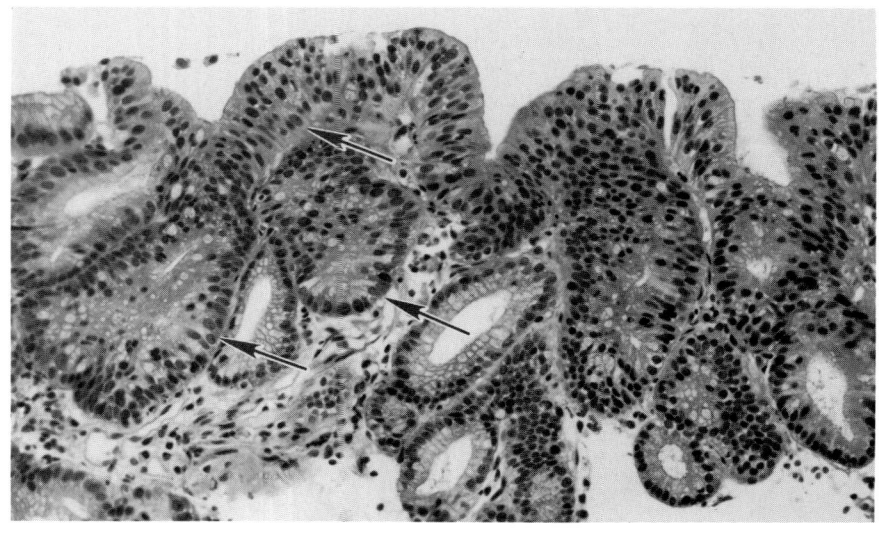

FIGURE 17–38. High-grade dysplasia (esophageal columnar intraepithelial neoplasia) in Barrett's mucosa of the distinctive type. The mucosal architecture shows blunt villi with proliferated glands. The epithelium is markedly hypercellular with full-thickness stratification of hyperchromatic nuclei. Enlarged nuclei with prominent nucleoli are present in some areas (arrows), including the surface epithelium. Epithelial mucin content is reduced.

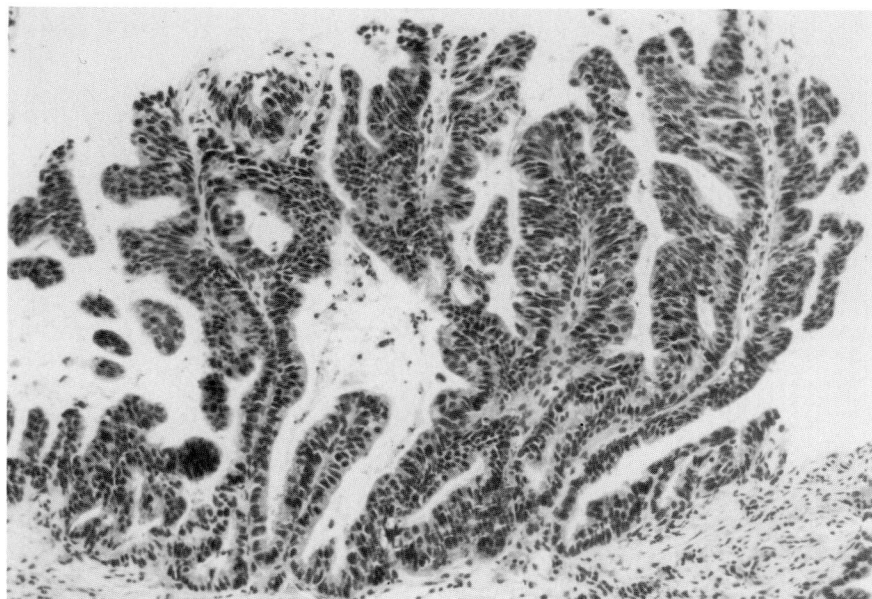

FIGURE 17-39. High-grade epithelial dysplasia (esophageal columnar intraepithelial neoplasia) in Barrett's mucosa of indeterminate type. Bizarre villiform and papillary structures are lined by markedly hypercellular epithelium with full-thickness stratification of small, hyperchromatic and pleomorphic nuclei.

specimens as "indefinite" or "positive" often require interpretation of epithelial abnormalities in the context of active inflammation. If an ulcer, erosion, or more than a few neutrophils are present in the Barrett mucosa, careful consideration should precede classification of a biopsy specimen as positive. The criteria for separating high-grade, intermediate-grade, and low-grade dysplasia are also arbitrary but include severity of mucosal architectural disturbance, epithelial cellularity, and extent of stratification of nuclei, along with loss of polarity, prominent nuclear enlargement, irregularity, pleomorphism, hyperchromatism, and nucleolar enlargement. The implications of the categories for patient management are discussed below (see Biopsies for Monitoring Barrett's Mucosa). The presence of mucosal invasion (intramucosal adenocarcinoma) can be difficult to distinguish from high-grade dysplasia. Such invasion (Figure 17-41) mandates consideration of therapeutic, rather than prophylactic, esophagectomy.

Various methods have been applied to attempt to improve upon dysplasia as evidence of neoplastic

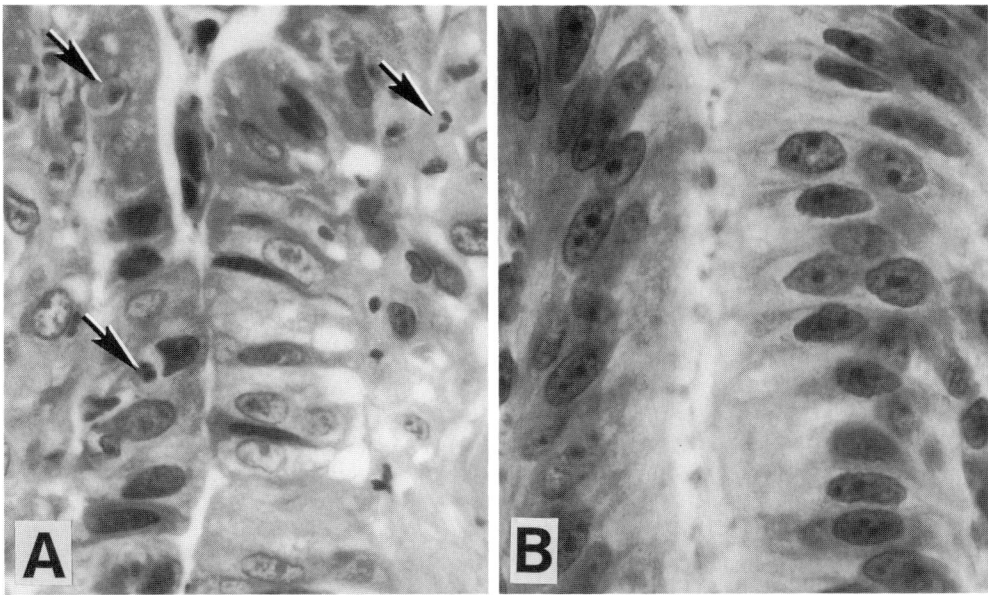

FIGURE 17-40. Comparison of reactive and dysplastic Barrett's epithelium. *A,* Reactive epithelium. In this example, adjoining an active chronic ulcer in distinctive-type Barrett's mucosa, the striking abnormalities include full-thickness stratification of vesicular nuclei with prominent nucleoli. Polymorphonuclear leukocytes (arrows) are present. *B,* High-grade dysplasia in Barrett's mucosa of indeterminate type. The enlarged nuclei have striking cytologic abnormalities, including hyperchromatism and irregular, multiple nucleoli. (Same magnification as *A.*)

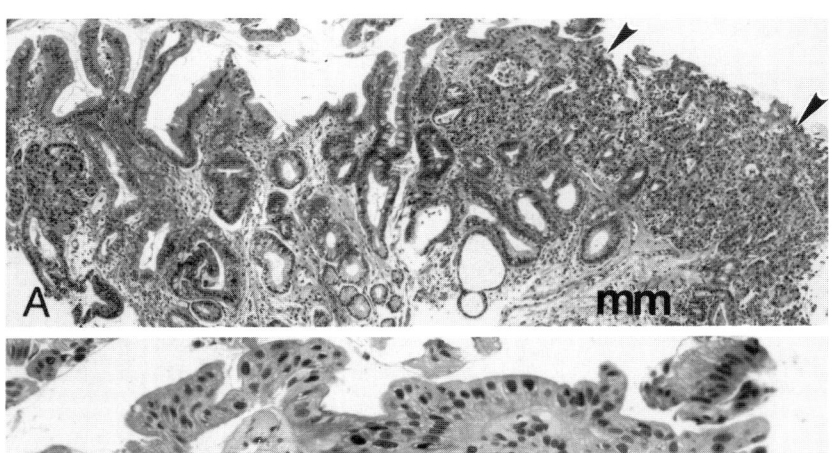
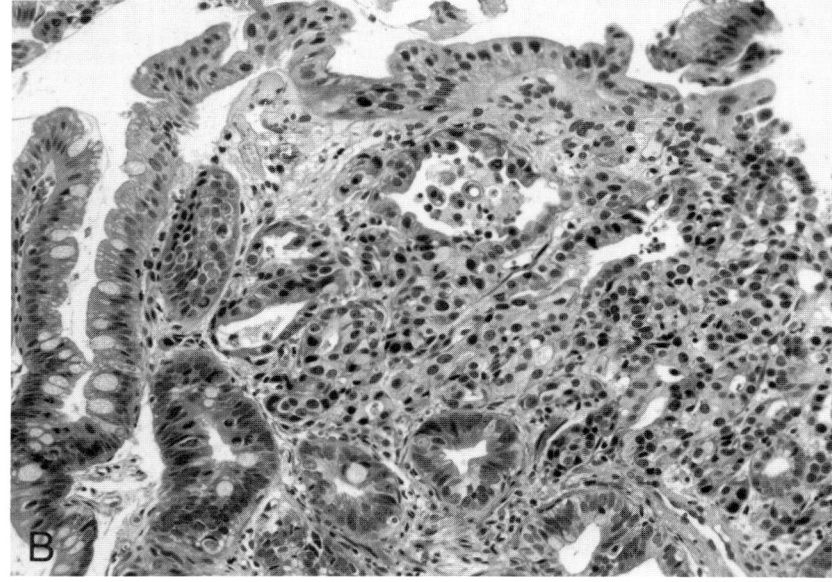

FIGURE 17–41. Adenocarcinoma invading lamina propria of distinctive-type Barrett's mucosa. A, This esophageal biopsy specimen shows obliteration of Barrett's glands by infiltrating adenocarcinoma (arrowheads) which does not breach the muscularis mucosae (mm) and is confined to the lamina propria. B, High-power view of intramucosal adenocarcinoma. The glandular architecture of the Barrett mucosa is replaced by the infiltrating glands of the adenocarcinoma involving the lamina propria.

change in Barrett's mucosa. These methods include markers of epithelial proliferation, histochemical and immunohistochemical studies of epithelial mucin and carcinoembryonic antigen expression, assay for ornithine decarboxylase (ODC, the rate-limiting enzyme in polyamine biosynthesis), and flow cytometry and image analysis for altered total DNA content in nuclei. DNA aneuploidy and ODC activity are currently the most promising markers in the hands of some investigators.

Additional discussion of dysplasia and carcinoma in Barrett's esophagus is presented in Chapter 19.

Biopsies for Monitoring Barrett's Mucosa

Two major types of complications occur in patients with Barrett's esophagus:

1. Peptic complications of ulceration, including resultant hemorrhage, penetration into mediastinal structures, stricture formation, and continued upward extension of Barrett's mucosa.
2. Neoplastic complication of development of dysplasia and adenocarcinoma (see previous discussion). After the diagnosis of Barrett's esophagus is made, endoscopic biopsies are often obtained to monitor the effects of antireflux therapy and development of neoplasia.

With effective antireflux therapy, active inflammation, erosion, and ulceration in Barrett's mucosa as well as in the squamous-lined mucosa above it decrease in severity. Biopsy evaluation of the squamous-lined region is important after therapy, as diminishing epithelial injury in the esophagus above Barrett mucosa may prevent further upward extension. Regression of Barrett's mucosa and replacement by squamous-lined mucosa after antireflux surgery or after medical antireflux therapy, including use of a drug that improves lower esophageal sphincter function, has been reported but appears to be uncommon. Documentation of cases of such regression, however, is strongly dependent upon localizing the biopsies to the same level of the esophagus on different occasions. Surgical manipulation of the esophagus complicates assessment of the biopsy site because of possible changes in distances from the incisors. Thus, interpretation of the obtaining of columnar-lined mucosa on one occasion and squamous-lined mucosa at a later endoscopy as evidence of regression requires caution.

Although controversial, surveillance for dysplasia and adenocarcinoma is now generally regarded as part of management of patients with Barrett's esophagus. In most patients without surveillance, adenocarcinoma arising in Barrett's esophagus is advanced at the time of presentation, and survival is poor. The hope of improved outcome rests on early detection and prevention of the columnar epithelial dysplasia–adenocarcinoma sequence. As a result, yearly surveillance endoscopy is often recommended on an empiric basis for patients known to have Barrett's esophagus. The decision to undertake surveillance should be made only when the patient's overall physical condition would permit a "prophylactic" esophagectomy to remove Barrett's esophagus with premalignancy or early malignancy. If the patient is not a candidate for treatment because of other medical problems, surveillance is pointless. Patients should continue surveillance even if they are on antireflux therapy and asymptomatic, because there is little evidence for lessening of the neoplastic predilection of Barrett's mucosa by successful therapy. The overall impact of surveillance on the incidence of and mortality from adenocarcinoma arising in Barrett's esophagus remains to be assessed. In our series and others, a sizable minority of Barrett patients with adenocarcinoma would not have been included in a surveillance program: these patients were recognized to have Barrett's esophagus only after they presented with adenocarcinoma arising in it. Such patients did not have a previous history of symptomatic gastroesophageal reflux or reflux esophagitis to bring them to medical attention. Such patients cannot benefit from even an optimal surveillance program. On the other hand, the few patients in whom dysplasia and adenocarcinoma have developed during surveillance have a good outcome if esophagectomy is performed successfully. Surveillance of the large bowel is also a consideration because of several reports indicating increased prevalence of colorectal adenomas and carcinomas in patients with Barrett's esophagus.

In the evaluation of dysplasia, cytology specimens obtained by brushing as well as multiple biopsy specimens appear to be useful in sampling large surface areas of Barrett's mucosa. Invasive adenocarcinoma may develop in Barrett's mucosa with dysplasia, which is less severe than carcinoma *in situ;* and invasion may be difficult to recognize owing to the shallowness of biopsy specimens and the tendency of carcinoma to "drop off" beneath an area of dysplasia (see Figure 17–34). As a result, confirmed high-grade dysplasia in a patient's biopsy specimens should raise the question of "prophylactic" esophagectomy, because about one third to one half of patients with biopsy diagnosis of high-grade dysplasia will be found to have adenocarcinoma in their esophagectomy specimen. The occurrence of synchronous adenocarcinoma and dysplasia is more frequent in patients who are found to have dysplasia when the diagnosis of Barrett's esophagus is first made (prevalent cases of dysplasia) than in those in whom dysplasia develops under surveillance (incident cases of dysplasia). Expected operative morbidity and mortality in the particular patient under consideration in the hands of the clinicians managing the patient are the major determinants of outcome.

MOTOR AND RELATED DISORDERS OF THE ESOPHAGUS

Achalasia

This condition is characterized by two defects: First, the lower esophageal sphincter provides an impediment to flow due to spasm and/or failure of relaxation; second, the lower two thirds of the esophagus, representing the portion with smooth muscle, shows failure of normal peristalsis with contraction but no progressive peristalsis. A large number of studies have investigated the neuropathologic changes in the esophageal wall in achalasia. Reported abnormalities include decreased or absent ganglion cells in the myenteric plexus and the presence in ganglion cells of Lewy bodies of the type seen in the brain of patients with Parkinson's disease. Dilatation of the mid and upper esophagus and hypertrophy of the muscularis propria (Figure 17–42) are attributable to the functional obstruction in the distal esophagus. Findings related to previous therapy may be seen: some patients develop reflux esophagitis after dilatation (see Figure 17–42).

Endoscopic biopsies in patients with presumed achalasia may be performed at the time of initial evaluation because of the possibility of tumor in the esophagogastric junction region as the cause of the clinical picture. In addition, patients with achalasia appear to have an increased incidence of squamous carcinoma of the esophagus, and biopsies are sometimes taken for the evaluation of dysplasia (see Chapter 18). Specimens show the effects of chronic stasis on the esophageal mucosa (Figure 17–43), as also occurs with Chagas' disease and above strictures with various causes. Reactive epithelial changes and balloon cells, sometimes with active inflammation, may be present. Food material, *Candida,* and bacteria are sometimes seen on the luminal surface. The mucosal surface may have a corrugated appearance, with a pearly white color; and squamous papillomas have been reported. In longstanding cases, cornification and keratinization of the surface epithelial layers may be present.

Rings and Webs

Constrictions of the esophageal lumen may be found at any level of the esophagus. The constrictions may be formed by mucosal rings, which do not involve the muscularis propria; by muscular or contractile rings; by ringlike peptic strictures; and by benign tumors. Upper esophageal webs may be found in patients without or with anemia, the latter referred to as Paterson-Kelly or Plummer-Vinson syndrome. The histopathologic findings in such webs include reactive epithelial changes with proliferation of the basal zone, elongation of vascular papillae, and parakeratosis, along with chronic inflammation, fibrosis, and hemosiderin deposition in the lamina propria. The nature of lower esophageal rings and webs is a matter of unresolved controversy,

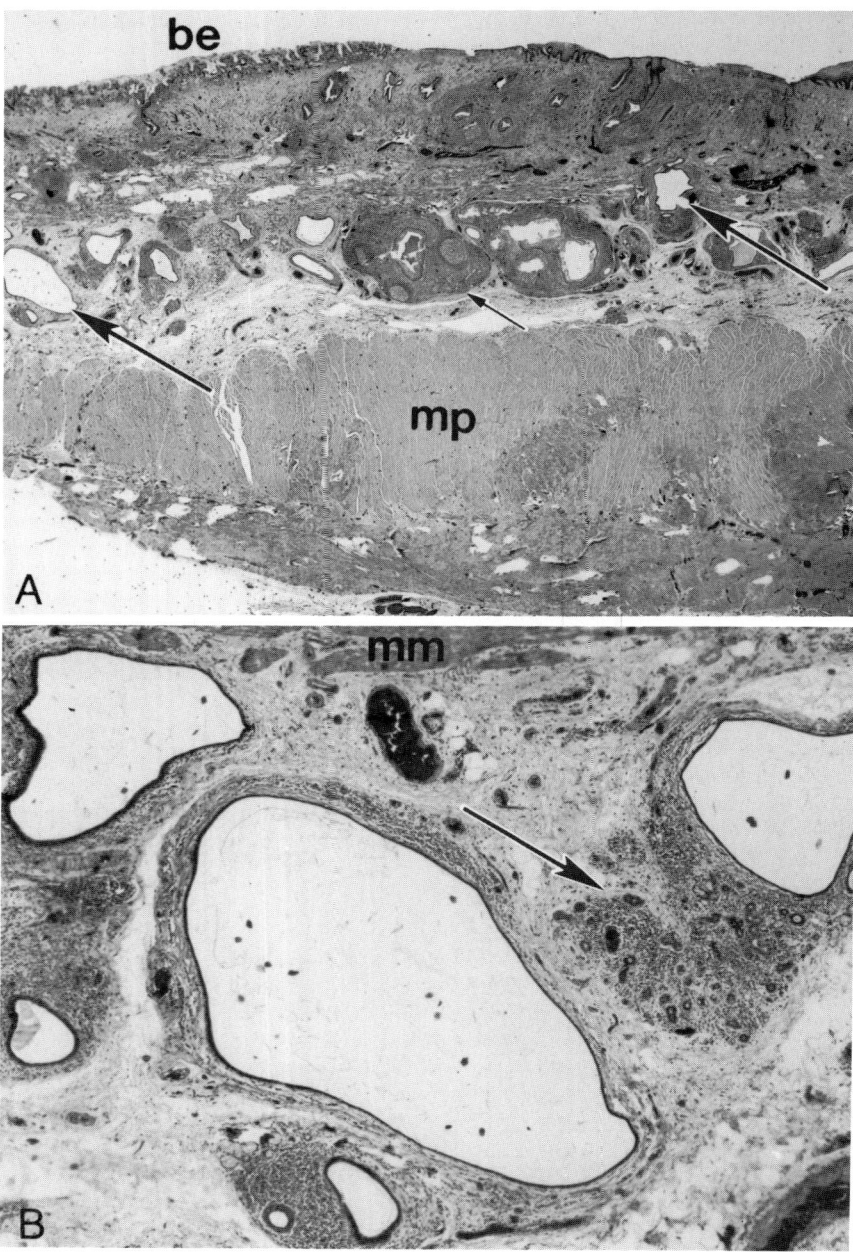

FIGURE 17–42. Achalasia with Barrett's esophagus secondary to gastroesophageal reflux resulting from dilatation procedures and with intramural pseudodiverticulosis. *A,* Hypertrophy of the muscularis propria (mp) is evident. The Barrett esophagus (be) has cardiac-type and distinctive-type mucosa. Esophageal intramural pseudodiverticulosis is manifested by cystic dilatation of submucosal gland ducts (large arrow), some of which have surrounding lymphoid tissue (small arrow). *B,* Higher-power view of intramural pseudodiverticulosis. Dilatation of the squamous-lined ducts of the esophageal submucosal glands deep to the muscularis mucosae (mm) is accompanied by atrophy of the glands (arrow).

probably due to the variability of the pathologic findings. The "Schatzki ring" (Figure 17–44) is reported by some authors to be located at the squamocolumnar junction; others have found the ring to be located within squamous-lined esophagus. Webs can be acquired as a result of severe esophageal injury from gastroesophageal reflux, radiation, lye-induced injury, and graft-versus-host disease.

Diverticula

Traction and pulsion diverticula occur in the esophagus. Intramural pseudodiverticulosis results from cystic dilatation of the ducts of esophageal submucosal glands (see Figure 17–42) due to obstruction, which can result from candidiasis and other etiologies. Additional information is provided in Chapter 30.

ESOPHAGEAL INVOLVEMENT BY SYSTEMIC DISEASES

Collagen Vascular–Connective Tissue Diseases

Esophageal motor abnormalities are a well-recognized feature of collagen vascular–connective tissue disease, particularly progressive systemic sclerosis (scleroderma), but also mixed connective tissue disease,

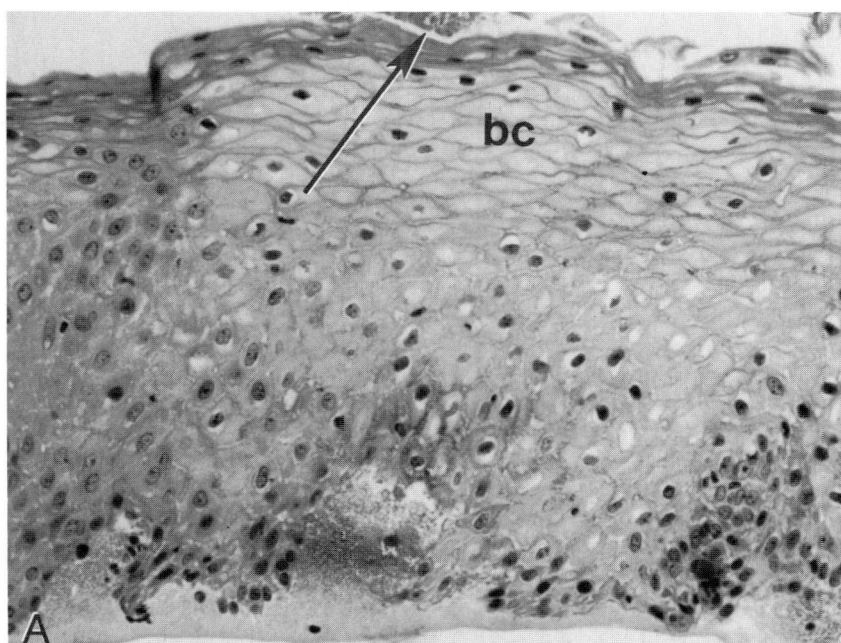
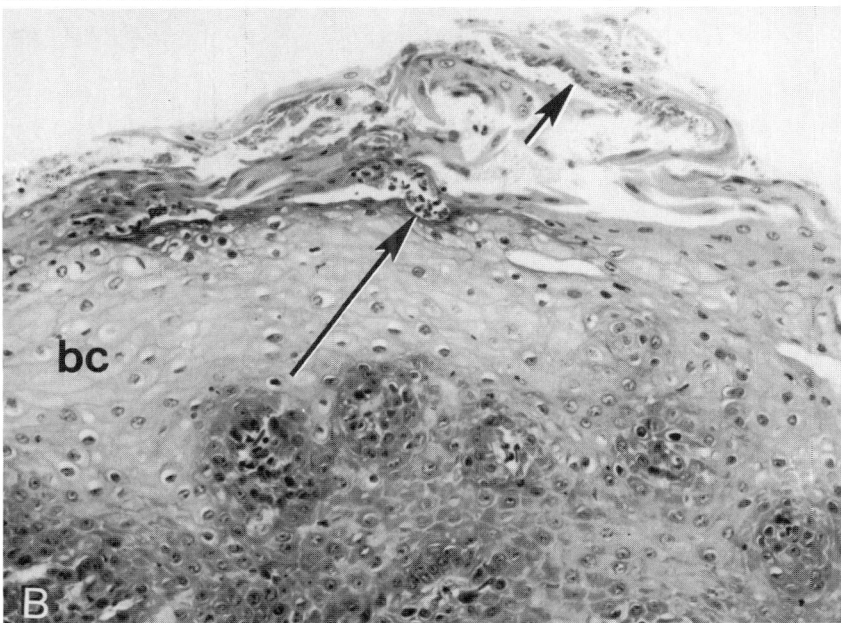

FIGURE 17–43. Squamous epithelial findings in achalasia. Food material (arrow in *A*) and bacterial colonies (short arrow in *B*) are present on the luminal surface. Polymorphonuclear leukocytes (long arrow in *B*) accompany the bacterial colonization. Balloon cells (bc) are present in the upper layers of the epithelium in both examples, along with reactive epithelial changes.

systemic lupus erythematosus, rheumatoid arthritis, dermatomyositis, and Sjögren's syndrome. Fibrous replacement of the outer layer of the muscularis propria is the characteristic finding in scleroderma. Ulcers and strictures can occur as primary manifestations of the diseases, particularly rheumatoid arthritis, ankylosing spondylitis, and Sjögren's syndrome, as well as secondary to gastroesophageal reflux associated with abnormal lower esophageal sphincter function. The pathologic findings in the ulcers and strictures are usually etiologically nonspecific. However, in occasional cases, arteritis may be demonstrable. See Chapter 16 for further details.

Crohn's Disease

The etiology of Crohn's disease is unknown at the present time, but generalized mucosal abnormality of the gastrointestinal tract is a well-recognized characteristic of the disease. Occasional patients have clinically evident esophageal involvement. Most have obvious Crohn's disease elsewhere, but some with only "regional esophagitis" have been reported. Crohn's disease involving the esophagus generally shows the pathologic features found in other sites: discrete ulceration, fistulas, strictures, and transmural inflammation. Certain recognition is dependent upon the finding of a

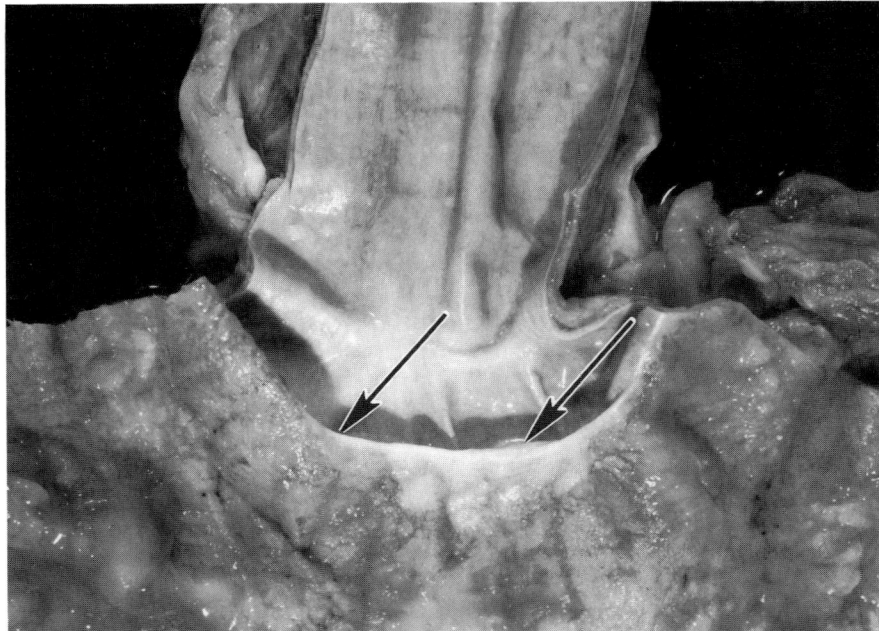

FIGURE 17–44. Lower esophageal ring. The shelflike circumferential ring (arrows) involves the esophagogastric junction and lower esophagus in this autopsy specimen, which was fixed before opening. Histopathology showed that the ring was formed of protruding mucosa and submucosa but not muscularis propria.

characteristic noncaseating epithelioid cell granuloma in the appropriate clinical setting (Table 17–6).

A wide range of pathologic abnormalities is seen in biopsy specimens, including nonspecific ulcers and active inflammation as well as characteristic granulomas, sometimes with multinucleated giant cells in the lamina propria or submucosa if it is included. Aphthoid ulcers have been reported, but biopsy specimens showed only intact squamous epithelium with acute inflammation. In one unusual case, Crohn's disease of the esophagus occurred along with Barrett's esophagus.

Crohn's disease manifested by nonspecific ulceration or acute and chronic mucosal inflammation is difficult to identify because of the occurrence of so many other causes of esophagitis with similar or nonspecific findings that can also occur in patients who have Crohn's disease (see outline at beginning of chapter). Furthermore, the shallow depth of both endoscopic and capsule biopsies precludes the specimen showing the characteristic abnormalities in the deep layers of the esophageal wall, which are important criteria for recognition of Crohn's disease, especially in unusual sites.

The chances of identifying a granuloma in specimens of Crohn's disease are affected by many factors, including the occurrence of the granulomatous form of Crohn's disease in the patient; the site, number, and size of the granulomas; the site, number, and size of the histopathologic specimens; the number of slides prepared; and the diligence with which the slides are examined. The differential diagnosis of granulomatous esophagitis (see Table 17–6) must be considered in patients thought to have Crohn's disease involving the esophagus. See Chapter 27 for further details.

Behçet's Disease

Recurrent ulcers of the mouth and genitalia associated with uveitis or iridocyclitis constitute Behçet's disease. Differentiation from Crohn's disease is problematic. Esophageal ulcers occur in occasional patients but show only nonspecific inflammation and ulcer. Disordered esophageal motility has also been reported in association with a normal mucosal surface. See Chapter 28 for further details.

Eosinophilic Gastroenteritis and Esophagitis

Esophageal involvement by eosinophilic gastroenteritis has been reported; the findings included the presence of eosinophils in any layer of the esophageal wall. Mucosal involvement is accompanied by reactive epithelial changes of basal zone proliferation and elongated vascular papillae. Of note in this regard, "eosinophilic esophagitis" is most commonly due to gastroesophageal reflux with eosinophilic involvement of only the mucosa (see Table 17–4). Allergic esophagitis in the absence of eosinophilic gastroenteritis also occurs and involves the mucosa. Eosinophilic inflammation of the esophagus can be associated with drug injury.

Table 17–6 DIFFERENTIAL DIAGNOSIS OF GRANULOMATOUS ESOPHAGITIS

Tuberculosis
Histoplasmosis
Blastomycosis
Foreign body reaction
Crohn's disease
Sarcoidosis

ESOPHAGITIS

Table 17-7 DERMATOLOGIC DISEASE AFFECTING THE ESOPHAGUS

Bullous dermatoses
   Epidermolysis bullosa of the autosomal recessive dystrophic, acquired, and letalis types
   Pemphigus vulgaris
   Bullous pemphigoid
   Benign mucous membrane pemphigoid
   Familial benign chronic pemphigus
   Darier's disease (keratosis follicularis)
   Angina bullosa haemorrhagica
   Hailey-Hailey disease
Toxic epidermal necrolysis
Stevens-Johnson syndrome
Acanthosis nigricans
Tylosis (keratosis palmaris et plantaris)
Lichen sclerosis

Dermatologic Diseases

Because the esophagus and skin both have squamous epithelium, it is not surprising that a variety of dermatologic diseases affect the esophagus (Table 17-7). In many patients, esophageal involvement accompanies skin disease, but in occasional instances only the esophagus is affected. The findings generally resemble those in the skin (see Chapter 16.) In tylosis, there is an increased incidence of esophageal carcinoma.

Sarcoidosis

The etiology of sarcoidosis is unknown at the present time. External compression of the esophagus by enlarged mediastinal lymph nodes as well as intrinsic involvement of the esophageal wall have been reported as causes of symptoms in occasional patients. With intrinsic involvement, the characteristic noncaseating epithelioid cell granulomas can occur in the lamina propria and submucosa, where they are detectable by biopsy, as well as in the deeper layers of the esophageal wall. The differential diagnosis of esophageal granulomas is presented in Table 17-6. See also Chapter 16.

Immunodeficiency

In addition to the variety of infectious agents which can affect the esophagus in immunocompromised patients, nonspecific ulcers have also been described.

Graft-versus-Host Disease

Esophageal squamous epithelium, like that in the skin and mucous membranes, is a target (Figures 17-45 and 17-46). Biopsies are sometimes performed for differential diagnosis of esophageal symptoms, partic-

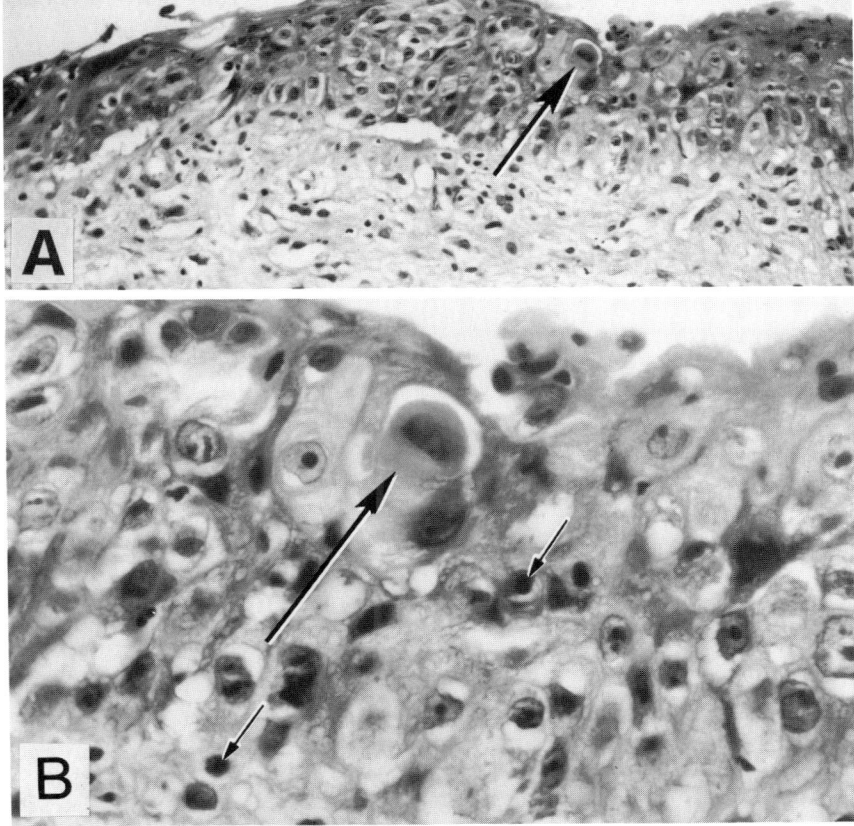

FIGURE 17-45. Graft-versus-host disease involving the esophagus 18 days after allogeneic bone marrow transplant. *A*, The squamous epithelium is thin, with focal detachment from the lamina propria and scattered dyskaryotic cells (arrow). *B*, High-power view of the area indicated by the arrow in *A*. The dyskaryotic cell (large arrow) has dense cytoplasm and nuclear degeneration. The epithelium is immature, with ovoid cells containing prominent nucleoli subjacent to the luminal surface. Lymphocytes (small arrows) representing infiltrating donor cells are present in the epithelium.

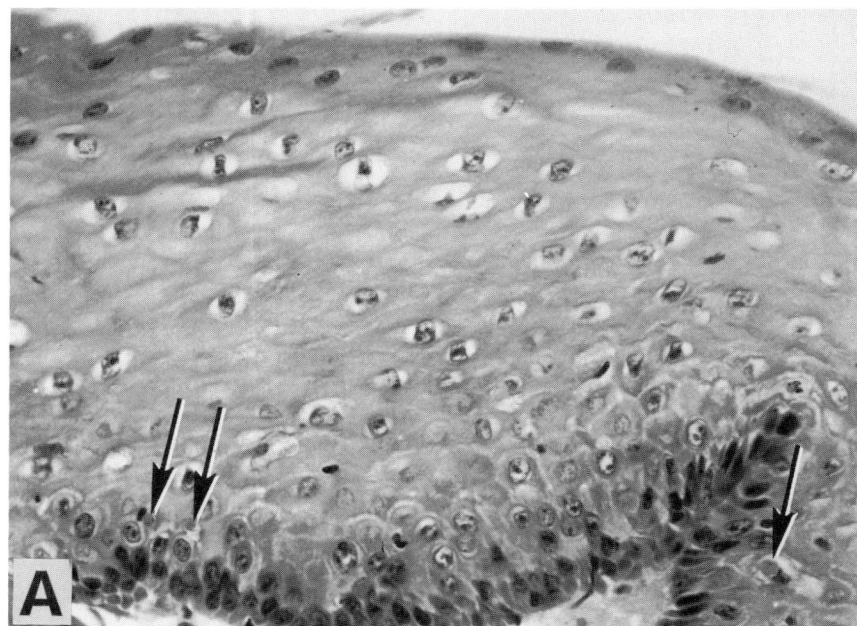
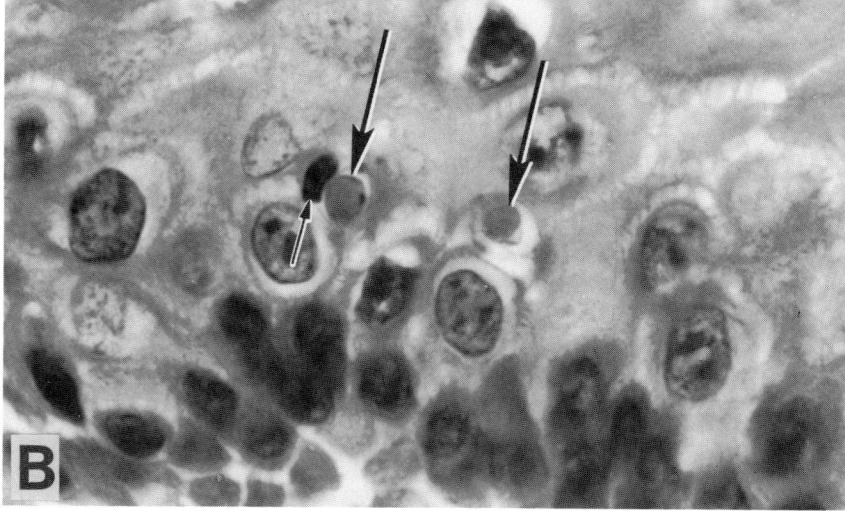

FIGURE 17–46. Mild graft-versus-host disease involving the esophagus 60 days after allogeneic bone marrow transplant. A, Epithelial maturation is abnormal, with immature cells at the luminal surface and hyperchromatic nuclei in the basal zone. Degenerating squamous epithelial cells (arrows) are present immediately above the basal zone. B, High-power view of the area indicated by the two arrows in A. The degenerating epithelial cells (large arrows) are accompanied by a satellite donor lymphocyte (small arrow).

ularly those caused by infectious agents. See Chapter 14 for further details.

Amyloidosis

Esophageal involvement by amyloid is uncommon in patients with amyloidosis. Deposition in blood vessels, muscularis mucosae, and lamina propria connective tissue may occur (Figure 17–47). Additional information is provided in Chapters 11 and 16.

CONCLUDING COMMENTS

By far the most common esophageal inflammatory disease encountered by most pathologists is reflux esophagitis. The proliferation of fiberoptic endoscopes and the widespread favorable publicity among endoscopists for the utility of esophageal biopsy in the evaluation of patients with reflux symptoms assures the numeric superiority of reflux esophagitis for the foreseeable future. Follow-up of patients with treated reflux esophagitis and Barrett's esophagus will also continue to provide many specimens. Although the histopathologic features in reflux esophagitis are etiologically nonspecific, other forms of esophagitis do have characteristic findings. Most notable are the various forms of infective esophagitis in which morphologic evidence of the causative organism(s) may be identifiable. The emergence of AIDS in addition to immunosuppressive therapies for transplantation and neoplasia as conditions in which patients commonly have esophageal symptoms also focuses attention on infective esophagitis. Nonetheless, the pathologic

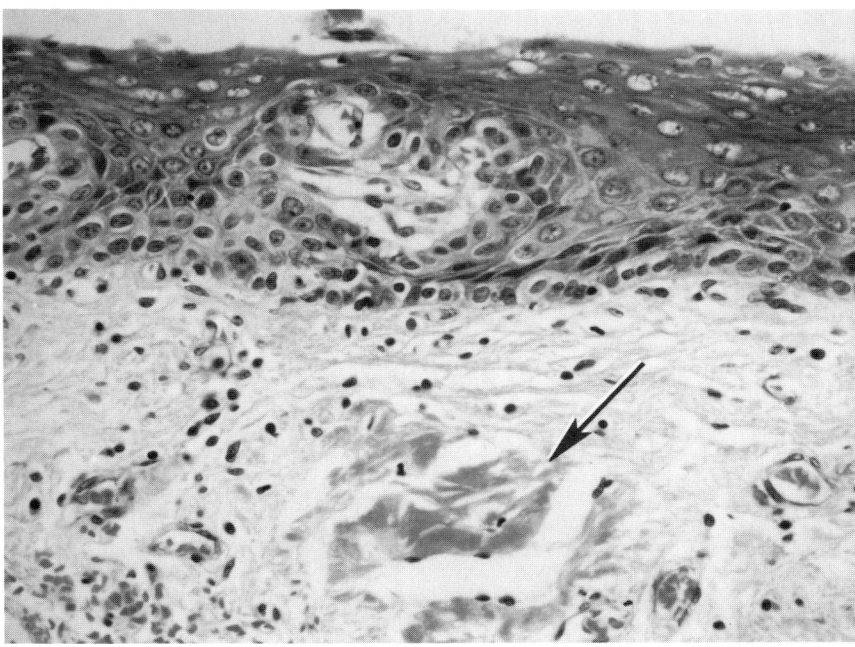

FIGURE 17–47. Secondary amyloidosis involving the esophagus. Amyloid (arrow) is present in the wall of a vein in the lamina propria.

characteristics of esophageal inflammation rarely establish its cause. As a result, the clinical history is likely to remain the key element for interpretation of esophagitis in specimens from biopsy, resection, and autopsy.

Additional Reading

General Topics

Appelman HD (ed): Pathology of the Esophagus, Stomach and Duodenum. New York, Churchill Livingstone, 1984.
Castell DO, Johnson LF (eds): Esophageal Function in Health and Disease. New York, Elsevier, 1983.
Enterline H, Thompson J: Pathology of the Esophagus. New York, Springer-Verlag, 1984.
Hill LD (ed): The Esophagus: Medical and Surgical Management. Philadelphia, WB Saunders, 1988.
Postlethwait RW: Surgery of the Esophagus. Norwalk, Conn, Appleton-Century-Crofts, 1986.

Pathologic Findings

Dalgaard JB: Oesophago-gastro-duodenal ulcerations encountered at autopsy. Acta Path Microbiol Scand 41:1, 1957.
Goldenberg SP, Wain SL, Marignani P: Acute necrotizing esophagitis. Gastroenterology 98:493, 1990.
Patton RB, Sommers SC: The histopathology of infarction and other ulcerative diseases of the esophagus. Am J Clin Pathol 33:516, 1960.
Tilestrom W: Esophageal ulcerations. Am J Med Sci 132:240, 1906.

Normal Morphologic Features

Al Yassin TM, Toner PG: Fine structure of squamous epithelium and submucosal glands of human oesophagus. J Anat 123:705, 1977.
Denardi FG, Riddell RH: The normal esophagus. Am J Surg Pathol 15:296, 1991.
Geboes K, De Wolf-Peeters C, Rutgeerts P, Janssens J, Vantrappen G, Desmet V: Lymphocytes and Langerhans cells in the human oesophageal epithelium. Virchows Arch [A] 401:45, 1983.
Hopwood D, Logan KR, Bouchier IAD: The electron microscopy of the normal human oesophageal epithelium. Virchows Arch [B] 26:345, 1978.
Robinson KM, Maistry L, Evers P: Surface features of normal and neoplastic human esophageal cells *in vivo* and *in vitro*. Scan Electron Microsc II:213, 1981.

Glycogenic Acanthosis

Bender MD, Allison J, Cuartos F: Glycogenic acanthosis of the esophagus: A form of benign epithelial hyperplasia. Gastroenterology 65:373, 1973.
Glick SN, Teplick SK, Goldstein J, et al: Glycogenic acanthosis of the esophagus. AJR 139:683, 1982.
Stern Z, Sharon P, Ligumsky M: Glycogenic acanthosis of the esophagus: a benign but confusing endoscopic lesion. Am J Gastroenterol 74:261, 1980.

Ectopic Sebaceous Glands

Ramkrishnan T, Brinker JE: Ectopic sebaceous glands in the esophagus. Gastrointest Endosc 24:293, 1978.
Zak FG, Lawson W: Sebaceous glands in the esophagus. Arch Dermatol 112:1153, 1976.

Melanocytic Proliferation

Ohashi K, Kato Y, Kanno J, Kasuga T: Melanocytes and melanosis of the oesophagus in Japanese subjects: Analysis of factors affecting their increase. Virchows Arch [A] 417:137, 1990.
Sharma SS, Venkateswaran S, Chacko A, Mathan M: Melanosis of the esophagus. An endoscopic, histochemical, and ultrastructural study. Gastroenterology 100:13–16, 1991.
Tateishi R, Taniguchi H, Wada A, et al: Argyrophil cells and melanocytes in esophageal mucosa. Arch Pathol 98:87, 1974.

Fungal Esophagitis—*Candida*

Brown JW, McKee WM: Acute monilial esophagitis occurring without underlying disease in young male. Dig Dis 17:85, 1972.
Dutta SK, Al-Ibrahim MS: Immunological studies in acute pseudomembranous esophageal candidiasis. Gastroenterology 75:292, 1978.
Gefter WB, Laufer I, Edells S, Gohel VK: Candidiasis in the obstructed esophagus. Radiology 138:25, 1981.
Goff JS: Infectious causes of esophagitis. Ann Rev Med 39:163, 1988.
Gonzales-Crussi F, Iung OS: Esophageal moniliasis as a cause of death. Am J Surg 109:634, 1965.
Ho C, Cullen JB, Gray RR: An unusual manifestation of esophageal moniliasis. Radiology 123:287, 1977.

Kelvin FM, Clark WM, Thompson WM, Hauck T: Chronic oesophageal stricture due to moniliasis. Br J Radiol 51:826, 1978.

Knoke M, Bernhardt H: Endoscopic aspects of mycosis in the upper digestive tract. Endoscopy 12:295, 1980.

Kodsi BE, Wickremesinghe PC, Kozinn PJ, et al: Candida esophagitis: A prospective study of 27 cases. Gastroenterology 71:715, 1976.

Jones JM, Glass NR, Belzer FO: Fatal Candida esophagitis in two diabetics after renal transplantation. Arch Surg 117:499, 1982.

Lefkowitz M, Elsa LJ, Levine RJ: Candida infection complicating peptic esophageal ulcer: Infection in an aortic esophageal fistula. Arch Intern Med 113:672, 1964.

Mathieson R, Dutta SK: Candida esophagitis. Dig Dis Sci 28:365, 1983.

Orringer MB, Sloan H: Monilial esophagitis: An increasingly frequent cause of esophageal stenosis? Ann Thorac Surg 26:364, 1978.

Ott DJ, Gelfand DW: Esophageal stricture secondary to candidiasis. Gastrointest Radiol 2:323, 1978.

Prolla JL, Kirsner JB: Gastrointestinal lesions and complications of leukemias. Ann Intern Med 61:1084, 1964.

Quie PG, Chilgren RA: Acute disseminated and chronic mucocutaneous candidiasis. Semin Hematol 8:227, 1971.

Ratton J, Hallak A, Rozen P, et al: Esophageal monilioma and mucosal bridge. Gastrointest Endosc 28:114, 1982.

Runfeld W, Jenkins D, Scott BB: Unsuspected gastroesophageal candidiasis: An endoscopic study. Gut 21:A895, 1980.

Scott BB, Jenkins D: Gastro-oesophageal candidiasis. Gut 23:137, 1982.

Sheft DJ, Shrago G: Esophageal moniliasis: Spectrum of disease. J Am Med Assoc 213:1859, 1970.

Tytgat GN, Surachno S, Groot WP, Schellekens PT: A case of chronic oropharyngo-esophageal candidiasis with immunological deficiency. Gastroenterology 72:536, 1977.

Walsh TJ, Hamilton SR, Belitsos N: Esophageal candidiasis: Managing an increasingly prevalent infection. Postgrad Med 84:193–205, 1988.

Fungal Esophagitis—*Torulopsis*

Bentlif PS, Wiedermann B: Esophagitis caused by Torulopsis globrata: Case report. Am J Gastroenterol 71:395, 1979.

Grimley PM, Wright LD, Jennings AE: Torulopsis globrata infection in man. Am J Clin Pathol 43:216, 1965.

Fungal Esophagitis—*Aspergillus* and *Phycomycetes*

Baker RD: Mucormycosis (opportunistic phycomycosis). In Baker RD (ed): The Pathologic Anatomy of Mycosis: Human Infection with Fungi, Actinomycetes and Algae. New York, Springer-Verlag, 1971, p 894.

Heffernan AGA, Asper SP: Insidious fungal disease: A clinicopathologic study of secondary aspergillosis. Bull Johns Hopkins Hosp 118:10, 1966.

Hutter RVP: Phycomycetous infection (mucormycosis) in cancer patients: A complication of therapy. Cancer 12:330, 1959.

McBride RA, Corson JM, Dammin JJ: Mucormycosis: Two cases of disseminated disease with cultural identification: Review of literature. Am J Med 28:832, 1960.

Whiteway DE and Virata RL: Mucormycosis. Arch Intern Med 139:944, 1979.

Young RC, Bennett JE, Vogel CL, et al: Aspergillosis: The spectrum of the disease in 98 patients. Medicine 49:147, 1970.

Fungal Esophagitis—Histoplasmosis

Coss KC, Wheat LJ, Conces DJ, et al: Esophageal fistula complicating mediastinal histoplasmosis: Response to amphotericin B. Am J Med 83:343, 1987.

Dines DE, Payne WS, Bernatz PE, Pairolero PC: Mediastinal granuloma and fibrosing mediastinitis. Chest 75:320, 1979.

Goodwin RA, Loyd JE, Des Prez RM: Histoplasmosis in normal hosts. Medicine (Baltimore) 60:231, 1981.

Jenkins DW, Fisk DW, Byrd RB: Mediastinal histoplasmosis with esophageal abscess: Two case reports. Gastroenterology 70:109, 1976.

Miller DP, Everett ED: Gastrointestinal histoplasmosis. J Clin Gastroenterol 1:233, 1979.

Fungal Esophagitis—Other Pathogenic Fungi

Angulo A, Pollak L: Paracoccidioidomycosis. In Baker RD (ed): The Pathologic Anatomy of Mycoses: Human Infection with Fungi, Actinomycetes and Algae. New York, Springer-Verlag, 1971, p 547.

Khandekar A, Moser D, Fidler WJ: Blastomycosis of the esophagus. Ann Thorac Surg 30:71, 1979.

Kunkel WM, Jr, Weed LA, McDonald JR, Claggett OT: Collective review: North American blastomycosis—Gilchrist's disease: Clinicopathologic study of ninety cases. Int Abstr Surg 99:1, 1954.

Ziliotta A Jr, Kunzle JE, Takeda FA: Paracoccidioidomycosis of the esophagus: Report of a case. Rev Inst Med Trop Sao Paulo 22:261, 1980.

Viral Esophagitis—Herpes

Bastian JF, Kaufman IA: Herpes simplex esophagitis in a healthy 10-year-old boy. J Pediatr 100:426, 1982.

Buss DH, Schary M: Herpes virus infection of the esophagus and other visceral organs in adults. Am J Med 66:457, 1979.

Clocuh YPA, Hansen W: Herpes esophagitis: Cytological diagnosis of a rare viral disease. Dtsch Med Wochenschr 106:25, 1981.

Depew WT, Prentice RSA, Beck IT, et al: Herpes simplex ulcerative esophagitis in a healthy subject. Am J Gastroenterol 68:381, 1977.

Fishbein PF, Tuthill R, Kressel H, Friedman H, Snape WJ: Herpes simplex esophagitis: A cause of upper-gastrointestinal bleeding. Dig Dis Sci 24:540, 1974.

Howilder W, Goldbert HI: Gastroesophageal involvement in herpes simplex. Gastroenterology 70:775, 1976.

Lasser A: Herpes simplex virus esophagitis. Acta Cytol 21:301, 1977.

Lightdale CJ, Wolf DJ, Marcucci RA, Salyer WR: Herpetic esophagitis in patients with cancer: Antemortem diagnosis by brush cytology. Cancer 39:223, 1977.

McKay JS, Day DW: Herpes simplex oesophagitis. Histopathology 7:409, 1983.

Meyers C, Durkin MG, Love L: Radiographic findings in herpetic esophagitis. Radiology 119:21, 1976.

Mirra SS, Bryan JA, Butz WC, Miles ML: Concomitant herpes-monilial esophagitis: Case report with ultrastructural study. Hum Pathol 13:760, 1982.

Muller SA, Herrmann EC, Winkelmann RK: Herpes simplex infections in hematologic malignancies. Am J Med 52:102, 1972.

Nash G, Ross JW: Herpetic esophagitis: A common cause of esophageal ulceration. Hum Pathol 5:339, 1974.

Owensby LC, Stammer JL: Esophagitis associated with Herpes simplex infection in an immunocompetent host. Gastroenterology 74:1305, 1978.

Solammadevi SV, Patwardhan R: Herpes esophagitis. Am J Gastroenterol 77:48, 1982.

Weiden PL, Schuffler MD: Herpes esophagitis complicating Hodgkin's disease. Cancer 33:1100, 1974.

White CL III, Hamilton SR: Immunoperoxidase localization of viral antigens in Herpes esophagitis. (Abstract) Lab Invest 48:92A, 1983.

Viral Esophagitis—Cytomegalovirus

Allen JI, Silvis SE, Summer HW, McClain CJ: Cytomegalic inclusion disease diagnosed endoscopically. Dig Dis Sci 26:133, 1981.

Freeman HJ, Schnitzka TK, Pierce JRA, Weinstein WM: Cytomegalovirus infection of the gastrointestinal tract in a patient with late onset immunodeficiency syndrome. Gastroenterology 73:1397, 1977.

Henson D: Cytomegalovirus inclusion bodies in the gastrointestinal tract. Arch Pathol 93:477, 1972.

St. Onge G, Bezahler GH: Giant esophageal ulcer associated with cytomegalovirus. Gastroenterology 83:127, 1982.

Toghill PJ, McGaughey M: Cytomegalovirus esophagitis. Br Med J 2:294, 1972.

Wilcox CM, Diehl DL, Cello JP, Margaretten W, Jacobson MA: Cytomegalovirus esophagitis in patients with AIDS: A clinical, endoscopic, and pathologic correlation. Ann Intern Med 113:589, 1990.

Viral Esophagitis—Viral Exanthems

Bardhan KD: Cimetidine in "chicken pox oesophagitis." Br Med J 1:370, 1978.

Chatty EM, Tomeh MO, Mercer RD, Osborne DO: Congenital rubella syndrome with viral esophagitis. An electron microscopic study. Cleve Clin Q 38:73, 1971.
Johnson HN: Visceral lesions associated with varicella. Arch Pathol 30:292, 1940.

Esophagitis Due to HIV and Related Viruses

Adkins MS, Raccuia JS, Acinapura AJ: Esophageal perforation in a patient with acquired immunodeficiency syndrome. Ann Thorac Surg 50:299, 1990.
Bach MC, Valenti AJ, Howell DA, Smith TJ: Odynophagia from aphthous ulcers of the pharynx and esophagus in the acquired immunodeficiency syndrome (AIDS). Ann Intern Med 109:338, 1988.
Bartewlsman JFWM, Lang JMA, van Leeuwen R, et al: Acute primary HIV esophagitis. Endoscopy 22:184, 1990.
Connolly GM, Hawkins D, Harcourt-Webster JN, et al: Oesophageal symptoms, their causes, treatment, and prognosis in patients with the acquired immunodeficiency syndrome. Gut 30:1033, 1989.
Kitchen VS, Helbert M, Francis ND, et al: Epstein-Barr virus associated oesophageal ulcers in AIDS. Gut 31:1223, 1990.
Lafeuillade A, Mazzerbo F, Aubert L, et al: Corticosteroid-responsive giant oesophageal ulcer in AIDS. Presse Medicale 19:1725, 1990.
Rabeneck L, Boyko WJ, McLean DM, et al: Unusual esophageal ulcers containing enveloped viruslike particles in homosexual men. Gastroenterology 90:1882, 1986.
Rabeneck L, Popovic M, Gartner S: Acute HIV infection presenting with painful swallowing and esophageal ulcers. JAMA 263:2318, 1990.
Schechter M, Pannain VLN, deOliveira AV: Papovavirus-associated esophageal ulceration in a patient with AIDS. AIDS 5:238, 1991.

Papillomavirus Infection of the Esophagus

Williamson AL, Jaskiesicz K, Gunning A: The detection of human papillomavirus in oesophageal lesions. Anticancer Res 11:263, 1991.

Opportunistic Bacterial Esophagitis

Walsh TJ, Belitsos NJ, Hamilton SR: Bacterial esophagitis in immunocompromised patients. Arch Intern Med 146:1345, 1986.

Mycobacterial Esophagitis

Dow CJ: Oesophageal tuberculosis: Four cases. Gut 22:234, 1981.
Eng J, Sabanathan S: Tuberculosis of the esophagus. Digest Dis Sci 36:536, 1991.
Ito Y, Kobayashi S, Kasugai T: Tuberculosis of the esophagus. Am J Gastroenterol 65:454, 1976.
Milnes JP, Holmes GKT: Recurrent oesophageal stricture due to tuberculosis. Br Med J 286:1977, 1983.
Montes I, Larson E, Haiderer O: Tuberculosis strictures of the esophagus. Chest 60:194, 1971.
Pradhan SA, Mehta AR: Tuberculosis of the esophagus. A case report. Ind J Cancer 13:383, 1976.
Schneider R: Tuberculous esophagitis. Gastrointest Radiol 1:143, 1976.
Scully RE, Galdabini JJ, McNeely BU: Case records of the Massachusetts General Hospital. Weekly clinicopathological exercises. N Engl J Med 296:384, 1977.
Wigley FM, Murray HW, Mann RB: Unusual manifestation of tuberculosis: TE fistula. Am J Med 60:310, 1976.

Actinomycetic and Other Bacterial Esophagitis

Mann NS, Borkar BB, Mann SK: Phlegmonous esophagitis associated with epiphrenic diverticulum. Am J Gastroenterol 70:510, 1978.
McManus JPA, Webb JN: A yeast-like infection of the esophagus caused by Lactobacillus acidophilus. Gastroenterology 68:583–586, 1975.
Vinson PP and Sutherland CG: Esophagobronchial fistula resulting from actinomycosis: Report of a case. Radiology 6:63, 1978.

Spirochetal Esophagitis

Hudson TR, Head JR: Syphilis of the esophagus. J Thorac Surg 20:216, 1950.
Stone J, Freidberg SA: Obstructive syphilitic esophagitis. J Am Med Assoc 177:711, 1961.

Parasitic Esophagitis

Zucoloto S, Derezende JM: Mucosal alterations in human chronic chagasic esophagopathy. Digestion 47:138, 1990.

Esophageal Injury Due to Exogenous Chemicals

Abramson AL: Corrosive injury of the esophagus: Result of ingesting some denture cleanser tablets and powder. Arch Otolaryngol 104:514, 1978.
Anyanwu CH, Okonkwo PO: Oesophageal strictures induced by herbal preparation. Trans R Soc Trop Med Hyg 75:864, 1981.
Burrington JD: Clinitest burns of the esophagus. Ann Thorac Surg 20:400, 1975.
Dafoe CS, Ross CA: Acute corrosive esophagitis. Thorax 24:291, 1969.
Lee JR, Simonowitz D, Block GE: Corrosive injury of the stomach and esophagus by non-phosphate detergents. Proc Inst Med Chic 29:8, 1972.
Lovejoy FH Jr: Corrosive injury of the esophagus in children: Failure of corticosteroid treatment reemphasizes prevention. N Engl J Med 323:668, 1990.
Mansson I: Diagnosis of acute corrosive lesions of the oesophagus. J Laryngol Otol 92:499, 1978.
Oakes DD, Shenck JP, Mark JBD: Lye ingestion. Clinical patterns and therapeutic implications. J Thorac Cardiovasc Surg 83:194, 1982.
Osterberg RE, Bierbower GW, Seabaugh VM, et al: Potential biological hazards of commercially available cleansers for dentures. J Toxicol Environ Health 3:969, 1977.
Poelman JR, Hausman RH, Holtsma HFW: Endoscopy in lye burns of oesophagus and stomach. Endoscopy 9:172, 1977.
Potter JL: Acute zinc chloride ingestion in a young child. Ann Emerg Med 10:267, 1981.
Symbas PN, Vlasis SE, Hatcher CR Jr: Esophagitis secondary to ingestion of caustic material. Ann Thorac Surg 36:73, 1983.
Widmer F, Aeberhard P: Acid and alkali corrosion of esophagus, stomach and duodenum. Schweiz Med Wochenschr 112:742, 1982.

Drug Contact—Reviews

Bonavina L, DeMeester TR, McChesney L, et al: Drug-induced esophageal strictures. Ann Surg 206:173, 1987.
Collins FJ, Matthews HR, Baker SE, Strakova JM: Drug-induced oesophageal injury. Br Med J 1:1673, 1979.
Doman DB, Ginsberg AL: The hazard of drug-induced esophagitis. Hosp Pract 16:17, 1981.
Eichenberger P, Blum AL: Drug-induced esophageal lesions. Acta Endosc 10:273, 1980.
Kikendall JW, Friedman AC, Oyewole MA, et al: Pill-induced esophageal injury: Case reports and review of the medical literature. Dig Dis Sci 28:174, 1983.
Mason SJ, O'Meara TF: Drug-induced esophagitis. J Clin Gastroenterol 3:115, 1981.
McCord GS, Clouse RE: Pill-induced esophageal strictures: Clinical features and risk factors for development. Am J Med 88:512, 1990.
Perry PA, Dean BS, Krenzelok EP: Drug-induced esophageal injury. J Toxicol Clin Toxicol 27:281, 1989.

Drug Contact—Emepronium

Barrison IG, Tremby PW, Kane SP: Oesophageal ulceration due to emepronium bromide. Endoscopy 12:197, 1980.
Fellows IW, Ogilvie AL, Atkinson M: Oesophageal stricture associated with emepronium bromide therapy. Postgrad Med J 58:43, 1982.
Hillman LL, Scobie BA, Pomare EW, Austad WI: Acute esophagitis due to emepronium bromide. NZ Med J 93:4, 1981.
Kenwright S, Norris ADC: Oesophageal ulceration due to emepronium bromide. Lancet 1:548, 1977.
Tobias R, Cullis S, Kottler RE, et al: Emepronium bromide-induced oesophagitis: Case reports. S Afr Med J 61:368, 1982.

Drug Contact—Potassium

Lambert JR, Newman A: Ulceration and strictures of the esophagus due to oral potassium chloride (slow release tablet) therapy. Am J Gastroenterol 73:508, 1980.
McCall AJ: Slow-K ulceration of oesophagus with aneurysmal left atrium. Br Med J 3:230, 1975.
Peters JL: Benign oesophageal stricture following oral potassium chloride therapy. Br J Surg 63:698, 1976.

Drug Contact—Antibiotics

Bjarnsson I, Bjornsson S: Oesophageal ulcers: An adverse reaction to co-trimoxazole. Acta Med Scand 209:431, 1981.
Channer KS, Hollanders D: Tetracycline-induced oesophageal ulceration. Br Med J 282:1359, 1981.
Cummin ARC, Hangartner JRW: Oesophago-atrial fistula—A side effect of tetracycline. J Roy Soc Med 83:745, 1990.
Delpre G, Kadish U, Stahl B: Induction of esophageal injuries by doxycycline and other pills: A frequent but preventable occurrence. Dig Dis Sci 34:797, 1989.
Finet L, Saleme R, Delcenserie R, Dupas JL: Esophageal ulceration association with ingestion of dextropropoxyphene-paracetamol tablets. Gastroenterol Clin Biol 14:1033, 1990.
Lehair P, Bigard MA, Cain P: Acute erosion of the esophagus due to granudoxy. Gastroenterol Clin Biol 15:91, 1991.
Levine MS: Giant esophageal ulcer due to Clinoril. AJR 156:955, 1991.
Sutton DR, Gasnold JK: Oesophageal ulceration due to clindamycin. Br Med J 1:1598, 1977.
Winckler K: Tetracycline ulcers of the oesophagus: Endoscopy, histology and roentgenology in 2 cases, and review of the literature. Endoscopy 13:225, 1981.

Drug Contact—Miscellaneous Drugs

Abbarah TR, Fredell JE, Ellens GB: Ulceration by oral ferrous sulfate. JAMA 236:2320, 1976.
Bataille C, Soumagne D, Loly J, Brassinne A: Esophageal ulceration due to indomethacin. Digestion 24:66, 1982.
Bohane TD, Perrault J, Fowler RS: Oesophagitis and oesophageal obstruction from quinidine tablets in association with left atrial enlargement: A case report. Aust Paediatr J 14:191, 1978.
Heller SR, Fellows IW, Ogilvie AL, Atkinson M: Non-steroidal anti-inflammatory drugs and benign oesophageal stricture. Br Med J 285:167, 1982.
Kharasch S, Vinci R, Reece R: Esophagitis, epiglottitis, and cocaine alkaloid (crack)—Accidental poisoning or child abuse? Pediatrics 86:117, 1990.
Lamouliatte H, Plane D, Quinton A: Ulcere oesophagien apres prise orale de bromure de pinaverium. Gastroenterol Clin Biol 5:812, 1981.
McLean D: Drug-induced oesophageal ulceration. Br Med J 282:6280, 1981.
Santucci L, Patoia L, Fiorucci S, et al: Oesophageal lesions during treatment with piroxicam. Br Med J 300:1018, 1990.
Seidner DL, Roberts IM, Smith MS: Esophageal obstruction after ingestion of a fiber-containing diet pill. Gastroenterology 99:1820, 1990.
Walta DC, Giddens JD, Johnson LF, Kelley JL, Waugh DF: Localized proximal esophagitis secondary to ascorbic acid ingestion and esophageal motor disorder. Gastroenterology 70:766, 1976.
Wiholm BE: Oesophageal injury associated with pivmecillinam tablets. Eur J Clin Pharmacol 37:605, 1989.

Sclerotherapy

Ayres SJ, Goff JS, Warren GH: Endoscopic sclerotherapy for bleeding esophageal varices: Effects and complications. Ann Intern Med 98:900, 1983.
Evans DMD, Jones DB, Cleary BK, Smith PM: Oesophageal varices treated by sclerotherapy: A histopathologic study. Gut 23:615, 1982.
Helpap B, Bollweg L: Morphological changes in the terminal oesophagus with varices, following sclerosis of the wall. Endoscopy 13:229, 1981.
Ponce J, Froufe A, de la Morena E, et al: Morphometric study of the esophageal mucosa in patients with variceal bleeding. Hepatology 1:641, 1981.

Chemotherapeutic Agents

Greco FA, Breveton HD, Kent H, et al: Adriamycin and enhanced radiation reaction in normal esophagus and skin. Ann Intern Med 85:294, 1976.
Horwich A, Lokich JJ, Bloomer WP: Doxorubicin, radiotherapy, and oesophageal stricture. Lancet 2:561, 1975.
Hruban RH, Yardley JH, Donehower RC, Boitnott JK: Epithelial necrosis in the gastrointestinal tract associated with polymerized microtubule accumulation and mitotic arrest. Cancer 63:72, 1989.
Slavin RE, Dias MP, Saral R: Cytosine arabinoside induced gastrointestinal toxic alterations in sequential chemotherapeutic protocols. Cancer 42:1747, 1978.

Esophageal Trauma

Appleton DS, Sandrasagra FA, Flower CD: Perforated esophagus: review of twenty-eight consecutive cases. Clin Radiol 30:493, 1979.
Brewer LA, Carter R, Mulder GA, Stiles QR: Options in the management of perforations of the esophagus. Am J Surg 152:62, 1986.
Crysdale WS, Sendi KS, Yoo J: Esophageal foreign bodies in children—15 year review of 484 cases. Ann Otol Rhinol Laryngol 100:320, 1991.
Farivar M: Bee sting of the esophagus. N Engl J Med 305:1020, 1981.
Foley MJ, Ghagremani GG, Rogers LF: Reappraisal of contrast media used to detect upper gastrointestinal perforations: comparison to ionic water-soluble media with barium sulfate. Radiology 144:231, 1982.
Han SY, McElvein RB, Aldrete JS, Tishler JM: Perforation of the esophagus: Correlation of site and cause with plain film findings. AJR 145:537, 1985.
Hunter TB, Protell RL, Horsley WW: Food laceration of the esophagus. AJR 140:503, 1983.
Kerr WF: "Spontaneous" intramural rupture and "spontaneous" intramural haematoma of the oesophagus. Thorax 36:74, 1981.
Meislin H, Kobernick M: Corn chip laceration of the esophagus and evaluation of suspected esophageal perforation. Ann Emerg Med 12:455, 1983.
Nadi P, Ong GB: Foreign body in the esophagus: A review of 2394 cases. Br J Surg 65:5, 1978.
Oldenburger D, Gundlach WJ: Intramural esophageal hematoma in a hemophiliac: An unusual cause of gastrointestinal bleeding. JAMA 237:800, 1977.
Shay SS, Berendson RA, Johnson LF: Esophageal hematoma: Four new cases, a review, and proposed etiology. Dig Dis Sci 26:1019, 1981.
Steadman C, Kerlin P, Crimmins F, et al: Spontaneous intramural rupture of the oesophagus. Gut 31:845, 1990.
Stratemeier PH: Massive esophageal hemorrhage in leukemia. Am J Roentgenol 129:1106, 1977.
Szanto I, Kiss J: Oesophagus bezoar diagnosed and removed endoscopically. Endoscopy 8:206, 1976.
Zenone EA, Trotman BW: Boerhaave's syndrome: Spontaneous formation of an esophageal-bronchial fistula. JAMA 238:2048–2049, 1977.

Radiation Esophagitis

Berthrong M, Fajardo LF: Radiation injury in surgical pathology. Part II. Alimentary tract. Am J Surg Pathol 5:153, 1981.
Goldstein HM, Rogers LF, Fletcher GH, Dodd GD: Radiological manifestations of radiation-induced injury to the normal upper gastrointestinal tract. Radiology 117:135, 1975.
Lepke RA, Libshitz HI: Radiation-induced injury of the esophagus. Radiology 148:375, 1983.
Papazian A, Capron JP, Ducroix JP, et al: Mucosal bridges of the upper esophagus after radiotherapy for Hodgkin's disease. Gastroenterology 84:1028, 1983.
Yang ZY, Hu YH, Gu XZ: Non-cancerous ulcer in the esophagus after radiotherapy for esophageal carcinoma: A report of 27 patients. Radiother Oncol 19:121, 1990.

Thermal Injury

Lieberman DA, Keefee EB: Esophageal burn and the microwave oven. Ann Intern Med 97:137, 1982.

Stevens AE, Dove GA: Oesophageal cast: Oesophagitis. Lancet 2:1279, 1980.

Grana L, Ablin RJ, Goldman S, Milhouse E: Freezing of the esophagus: Histological changes and immunological response. Int Surg 66:295, 1981.

Hiatal Hernia

Arima T, Igarashi M, Shiraishi M, Nakamura T: Hiatal herniation of the colon in an infant. Int Surg 73:196, 1988.

Axelrod FB, Maayan C, Hazzi C, et al: Bradycardia associated with hiatal hernia and gastroesophageal reflux relieved by surgery. Am J Gastroenterol 82:159, 1987.

Barrett NR: Hiatus hernia: A review of some controversial points. Br J Surg 42:231, 1954.

Bassey OO, Eyo EE, Akinhanmi GA: Incidence of hiatus hernia and gastro-oesophageal reflux in 1030 prospective barium meal examinations in adult Nigerians. Thorax 32:356, 1977.

Berstad A, Weberg R, Froyshov LI, et al: Relationship of hiatus hernia to reflux oesophagitis: A prospective study of coincidence, using endoscopy. Scand J Gastroenterol 21:55, 1986.

Borrie J, Shaw JH: Hiatal hernia co-existing with oesophagogastric malignancy. N Z Med J 92:47, 1980.

Bozzuto TM: Intermittent obstruction of an incarcerated hiatal hernia with a total thoracic stomach. Am J Emerg Med 8:388, 1990.

Burkitt DP: Hiatus hernia: Is it preventable? Am J Clin Nutr 34:428, 1981.

Carre IJ, Froggatt P: Oesophageal hiatus hernia in three generations of one family. Gut 11:51, 1970.

Cathcart RS III, Gregorie HB Jr, Holmes SL: Nonreflux complications of hiatal hernia. Am Surg 53:320, 1987.

Dunn DB, Quick G: Incarcerated paraesophageal hernia. Am J Emerg Med 8:36, 1990.

Gage-White L: Incidence of Zenker's diverticulum with hiatus hernia. Laryngoscope 98:527, 1988.

Ghahremani GG, Collins PA: Esophago-gastric invagination in patients with sliding hiatus hernia. Gastrointest Radiol 1:253, 1976.

Haas O, Rat P, Christophe M, et al: Surgical results of intrathoracic gastric volvulus complicating hiatal hernia. Br J Surg 77:1379, 1990.

Heiss K, Manning P, Oldham KT, et al: Reversal of mortality for congenital diaphragmatic hernia with ECMO. Ann Surg 209:225, 1989.

Jonsell G: The incidence of sliding hiatal hernias in patients with gastroesophageal reflux requiring operation. Acta Chir Scand 149:63, 1983.

Kielhofner MA, Schnell G, Schubert TT, Kebede-Daniels D: Aortogastric fistula from hiatal hernia ulcer: A cause of massive upper gastrointestinal bleeding. J Clin Gastroenterol 9:697, 1987.

Laforet EG: Acute hemorrhagic incarceration of prolapsed gastric mucosa. Gastroenterology 70:589, 1976.

Mayer DA, Gray GF, Teixidor HS, Thorbjarnarson B: Carcinoma of the gastric cardia and hiatal hernia. J Thorac Cardiovasc Surg 71:592, 1976.

Mellet JS, Cilliers PH: Penetration of a gastric ulcer into the right ventricle: A complication of para-oesophageal hiatus hernia. South Afr Med J 72:44, 1987.

Mittal RK, Lange RC, McCallum RW: Identification and mechanism of delayed esophageal acid clearance in subjects with hiatus hernia. Gastroenterology 92:130, 1987.

Pridie RB: Incidence and coincidence of hiatus hernia. Gut 7:188, 1966.

Riggs W Jr: The incidence of hiatal hernia in infants and children: Results of a survey of members of the Society of Pediatric Radiology. Radiology 120:451, 1976.

Salling N, Falensteen AM, Larsen LG: Non-traumatic perforation of gastric ulcer in a hiatal hernia to the pericardium. Acta Med Scand 213:225, 1983.

Sato H, Takase S, Takada A: The association of esophageal hiatus hernia with Mallory-Weiss syndrome. Gastroenterol Jpn 24:233, 1989.

Sebayel MI, Qasabi QO, Katugampola W, Ahmed I: Traumatic diaphragmatic hernia: Review of 15 cases. Br J Accident Surg 20:94, 1989.

Gastroesophageal Reflux

Ariagno RL, Guilleminault C, Baldwin R: Movement and gastroesophageal reflux in awake term infants with near miss SIDS, unrelated to apnea. J Pediatr 100:894, 1982.

Behar J: Reflux esophagitis. Arch Intern Med 136:560, 1976.

Behar J, Sheahan DG: Histologic abnormalities in reflux esophagitis. Arch Pathol 99:387, 1975.

Bennett JR: Etiology, pathogenesis, and clinical manifestations of gastro-oesophageal reflux disease. Scand J Gastroenterol 23(S146):67, 1988.

Bhan I, Leape LL, Ramenofsky ML: Histologic features of esophageal biopsies from children with gastroesophageal reflux. Lab Invest 46:2, 1982.

Black DD, Haggitt RC, Orenstein SR, Whitington PF: Esophagitis in infants. Morphometric histological diagnosis and correlation with measures of gastroesophageal reflux. Gastroenterology 98:1408, 1990.

Brand DL, Eastwood IR, Martin D, et al: Esophageal symptoms, manometry and histology before and after antireflux surgery: A long-term follow-up study. Gastroenterology 76:1393, 1979.

Brown LF, Goldman H, Antonioli DA: Intraepithelial eosinophils in endoscopic biopsies of adults with reflux esophagitis. Am J Surg Pathol 8:899, 1984.

Castell DO, Wu WC, Ott DJ (eds): Gastro-oesophageal Reflux Disease—Pathogenesis, Diagnosis, Therapy. Mount Kisco, NY, Futura Publishing Co, 1985.

Christiansen T, Funch-Jensen P, Jacobsen NO, Thommesen P: Radiologic quantitation of gastro-oesophageal reflux: Correlation between height of food stimulated gastro-oesophageal reflux and level of histologic changes in reflux oesophagitis. Acta Radiol 28:731, 1987.

Cronen P, Snow N, Nightingale D: Aortoesophageal fistula secondary to reflux esophagitis. Ann Thorac Surg 33:78, 1982.

Curci M, Dibbins A: Gastroesophageal reflux in children: An underrated disease. Am J Surg 143:413, 1982.

Darling DB, McCauley RGK, Leape LL, Ramenofsky ML: The child with peptic esophagitis: A correlation of radiologic signs with esophageal pathology. Radiology 145:673, 1982.

DeMeester TR, Bonavina L, Iascone C, et al: Chronic respiratory symptoms and occult gastroesophageal reflux: A prospective clinical study and results of surgical therapy. Ann Surg 211:337, 1990.

Dent J, Holloway RH, Toouli J, Dodds WJ: Mechanisms of lower oesophageal sphincter incompetence in patients with symptomatic gastroesophageal reflux. Gut 29:1020, 1988.

Dodds WJ, Dent J, Hogan WJ, et al: Mechanisms of gastroesophageal reflux in patients with reflux esophagitis. N Engl J Med 307:1547, 1982.

Eastwood GL: Histologic changes in gastroesophageal reflux. J Clin Gastroenterol 8 (Suppl 1), 1986.

Eller JL, Zoter FMH, Zuck TF, Brott W: Inflammatory polyp: A complication in esophagus lined by columnar epithelium. Radiology 98:145, 1971.

Eriksen CA, Sadek SA, Cranford C, et al: Reflux oesophagitis and oesophageal transit: Evidence for a primary oesophageal motor disorder. Gut 29:448, 1988.

Fink SM, Barwick KW, Winchenbach CL, et al: Reassessment of esophageal histology in normal subjects: A comparison of suction and endoscopic techniques. J Clin Gastroenterol 5:177, 1983.

Fisher RS, Cohen S: Gastroesophageal reflux. Med Clin N Am 62:3, 1978.

Fisher RS, Roberts GS, Grabowski CJ, Cohen S: Altered lower esophageal sphincter function during early pregnancy. Gastroenterology 74:1233, 1978.

Funch-Jensen P, Cock K, Christensen LA, et al: Microscopic appearance of the esophageal mucosa in a consecutive series of patients submitted to upper endoscopy: Correlation with gastro-esophageal

reflux symptoms and macroscopic findings. Scand J Gastroenterol 21:65, 1986.
Gaultier CL: Interference between gastroesophageal reflux and sleep in near miss SIDS. Clin Rev Allergy 8:395, 1990.
Geboes K, Desmet V, Vantrappen G, Mebis J: Vascular changes in the esophageal mucosa: an early histologic sign of esophagitis. Gastrointestinal Endoscopy 26:29, 1980.
Gillison EW, Nyhus LM, Bombeck CT: The significance of bile in reflux esophagitis. Surg Gynecol Obstet 134:419, 1972.
Goodall RJR, Faris JE, Cooper DN, et al: Relationship between asthma and gastro-esophageal reflux. Thorax 36:116, 1981.
Heading RC: Epidemiology of oesophageal reflux disease. Scand J Gastroenterology 24 Suppl. 168:33, 1989.
Herbst JJ, Book LS, Bray PF: Gastroesophageal reflux in the "near miss" sudden infant death syndrome. J Pediatr 92:73, 1978.
Herbst JM, Johnson DG, Oliveros MA: Gastroesophageal reflux with protein-losing entropathy and finger clubbing. Am J Dis Child 130:1256, 1976.
Herbst JJ, Meyers WF: Gastroesophageal reflux in children. Adv Pediatr 28:159, 1981.
Himal HS: Alkaline gastritis and alkaline esophagitis: A review. Can J Surg 20:403, 1977.
Hopwood D, Bateson MC, Milne G, Bouchier IAD: Fffects of bile acids and hydrogen ion on the fine structure of oesophageal epithelium. Gut 22:306, 1981.
Ismail-Beigi F, Pope CE II: Distribution of the histological changes of gastroesophageal reflux in the distal esophagus of man. Gastroenterology 66:1109, 1974.
Jamieson GG, Duranceau A: Gastroesophageal Reflux. Philadelphia, WB Saunders, 1988.
Janisch HD, von Kleist D, Hampel KE: Intraepithelial eosinophils in esophageal reflux. Gastroenterology 85:785, 1983.
Jessurun J, Yardley JH, Giardiello FM, Hamilton SR: Intracytoplasmic plasma proteins in distended esophageal squamous cells (balloon cells). Modern Pathol 1:175, 1988.
Johnson DG, Jolley SG: Gastroesophageal reflux in infants and children. Recognition and treatment. Surg Clin North Am 61:1101, 1983.
Jones TB, Heller RM, Kirchner SG, Greene HL: Inflammatory esophagogastric polyp in children. AJR 133:314, 1979.
Kaufman JE, Kaye MD: Induction of gastroesophageal reflux by alcohol. Gut 19:336, 1978.
Kaye MD: Postprandial gastro-oesophageal reflux in healthy people. Gut 18:709, 1977.
Knuff TE, Benjamin SB, Worsham F, et al: Histologic evaluation of chronic gastroesophageal reflux. An evaluation of biopsy methods and diagnostic criteria. Dig Dis Sci 29:194, 1984.
Kraus BB, Sinclair JW, Castel DO: Gastroesophageal reflux in runners—characteristics and treatment. Ann Intern Med 112:429, 1990.
Leape LL, Holder TM, Franklin JD, et al: Respiratory arrest in infants secondary to gastroesophageal reflux. Pediatrics 60:924, 1977.
Livstone EM, Sheahan DG, Behar J: Studies of esophageal epithelial cell proliferation in patients with reflux esophagitis. Gastroenterology 73:1315, 1977.
Mansfield LE: Interactions, associations, and relationships between the lungs and the esophagus. Clin Rev Allergy 8:381, 1990.
Marshall JB, Kretschmar JM, Diazarias AA: Gastroesophageal reflux as a pathogenic factor in the development of symptomatic lower esophageal rings. Arch Intern Med 150:1669, 1990.
Matikamen M, Loatikainen T, Kalima T, Kivilaakso E: Bile acid composition and esophagitis after total gastrectomy. Am J Surg 143:196, 1982.
Mihaus AA, Slaughter RL, Goldman LM, Hirschowitz BI: Double lumen esophagus due to reflux esophagitis with fibrous septum formation. Gastroenterology 71:136, 1976.
Nielson DW, Heldt GP, Tooley WH: Stridor and gastroesophageal reflux in infants. Pediatrics 85:1034, 1990.
Nothmann BJ, Wright JR, Shuster MM: In vitro vital staining as an aid to identification of esophagogastric mucosal junction in man. Am J Dig Dis 17:919, 1972.
O'Sullivan GC, DeMeester TR, Joelsson BE, et al: Interaction of lower esophageal sphincter pressure and length of sphincter in the abdomen as determinants of gastroesophageal competence. Am J Surg 14:40, 1982.

Pellegrini CA, DeMeester TR, Wernly TA, et al: Alkaline gastroesophageal reflux. Am J Surg 135:177, 1978.
Phaosawasdi K, Mayer E, Tolin R, et al: Comparative effects of alcohol on the lower esophageal (LES) and pyloric (PS) sphincters. Gastroenterology 74:1078, 1978.
Pope CE: Respiratory complications of gastro-oesophageal reflux. Scand J Gastroenterol 24(Suppl 168):67, 1989.
Rabin MS, Bremmer CG, Botha JR: The reflux gastroesophageal polyp. Am J Gastroenterol 73:451, 1980.
Raymond JI, Khan AH, Cain LR, Ramin JE: Multiple esophagogastric fistulas resulting from reflux esophagitis. Am J Gastroenterol 73:430, 1980.
Reinig JW: Esophagopericardial fistula in a scleroderma patient with peptic esophagitis. Arch Intern Med 143:1486, 1983.
Richardson JD, Kuhns JG, Richardson RL, Polk HC Jr: Properly conducted fundoplication reverses histologic evidence of esophagitis. Ann Surg 197:763, 1983.
Shoenut JP, Wieler JA, Micflikier AB, Teskey JM: Esophageal reflux before and after isolated myotomy for achalasia. Surgery 108:876–879, 1990.
Shub MD, Ulshen MH, Hargrove CB, et al: Esophagitis: A frequent consequence of gastroesophageal reflux in infancy. J Pediatr 107:881, 1985.
Snyder RW, Dumas PR, Kolts BE: Esophagoatrial fistula with previous pericarditis complicating esophageal ulceration: report of two cases and review of the literature. Chest 98:679, 1990.
Sonnenberg A, Lepsien G, Muller-Lissner SA, Koelz HR: When is esophagitis healed? Esophageal endoscopy, histology and function before and after cimetidine treatment. Dig Dis Sci 27:297, 1982.
Tummala V, Barwick KW, Sontag SJ, et al: The significance of intraepithelial eosinophils in the histologic diagnosis of gastroesophageal reflux. Am J Clin Pathol 87:43, 1987.
Tytgat GNJ, Nio CY, Schotborgh RH: Reflux esophagitis. Scand J Gastro 25:1, 1990.
Van Thiel DH, Gavaler JS, Jushi SN: Heartburn of pregnancy. Gastroenterology 72:666, 1977.
Van Thiel DH, Gavaler JS, Strumple J: Lower esophageal sphincter pressure in women using sequential oral contraceptives. Gastroenterology 71:232, 1976.
Zaninotto G, DeMeester TR, Schweizer W, et al: The lower esophageal sphincter in health and disease. Am J Surg 155:104, 1988.

Barrett's Esophagus

Allan NK, Weitzner S, Scott L, Khalil KG: Adenocarcinoma arising in Barrett's esophagus with synchronous squamous cell carcinoma of the esophagus. Southern Med J 79:1036, 1986.
Altorki NK, Sunagawa M, Little AG, Skinner DB: High-grade dysplasia in the columnar-lined esophagus. Am J Surg 161:97, 1991.
Atkinson M: Barrett's oesophagus—to screen or not to screen? Gut 30:2, 1989.
Banner BF, Memoli VA, Warren WH, Gould VE: Carcinoma with multi-directional differentiation arising in Barrett's esophagus. Ultrastruct Pathol 4:205, 1983.
Barrett NR: Chronic peptic ulcer of the oesophagus and 'oesophagitis'. Br J Surg 38:175, 1950.
Barrett NR: The lower esophagus lined by columnar epithelium. Surgery 41:881, 1957.
Berenson MM, Herbst JJ, Freston JW: Enzyme and ultrastructural characteristics of esophageal columnar epithelium. Am J Dig Dis 19:895, 1974.
Blot WJ, Devesa SS, Kneller RW, Fraumeni JF: Rising incidence of adenocarcinoma of the esophagus and gastric cardia. JAMA 265:1287, 1991.
Brand DL, Ylvisaker JT, Gelfand M, Pope CE II: Regression of columnar esophageal (Barrett's) epithelium after anti-reflux surgery. N Engl J Med 302:844, 1980.
Bremner CG: Barrett's oesophagus. Br J Surg 76:995, 1989.
Burke AP, Sobin LH, Shekitka KM, Helwig EB: Dysplasia of the stomach and Barrett esophagus: a follow-up study. Mod Pathol 4:336, 1991.
Burke AP, Sobin LH, Shekitka KM, Avallone FA: Correlation of nucleolar organizer region and glandular dysplasia of the stomach and esophagus. Mod Pathol 3:357, 1990.

Cameron AJ, Ott BJ, Payne WS: The incidence of adenocarcinoma in columnar-lined Barrett's esophagus. N Engl J Med 313:857, 1985.
Cameron AJ, Payne WS: Barrett's esophagus occurring as a complication of scleroderma. Mayo Clin Proc 53:612, 1978.
Cameron AJ, Zinsmeister AR, Ballard DJ, Carney JA: Prevalence of columnar-lined (Barrett's) esophagus. Gastroenterology 99:918, 1990.
Cooper JE, Spitz L, Wilkins BM: Barrett's esophagus in children: a histologic and histochemical study of 11 cases. J Pediatr Surg 22:191, 1987.
Dahms BB, Rothstein FC: Barrett's esophagus in children: A consequence of chronic gastroesophageal reflux. Gastroenterology 86:318, 1984.
DeBaecque C, Potet F, Molas G, et al: Superficial adenocarcinoma of the oesophagus arising in Barrett's mucosa with dysplasia: A clinicopathological study of 12 patients. Histopathology 16:213, 1990.
DeMeester TR, Atwood SEA, Smyrk TC, et al: Surgical therapy in Barrett's esophagus. Ann Surg 212:528, 1990.
Fennerty MB, Sampliner RE, Way D, et al: Discordance between flow cytometric abnormalities and dysplasia in Barrett's esophagus. Gastroenterology 97:815, 1989.
Feurle GE, Helmstaedter V, Buehring A, et al: Distinct immunohistochemical findings in columnar epithelium of esophageal inlet patch and of Barrett esophagus. Dig Dis Sci 35:86, 1990.
Garewal H, Meltzer P, Trent J, et al: Epidermal growth factor receptor overexpression and trisomy-7 in a case of Barrett's esophagus. Dig Dis Sci 35:1115, 1990.
Garewal HS, Sampliner R, Liu Y, Trent JM: Chromosomal rearrangements in Barrett's esophagus. Cancer Genet Cytogenet 42:281, 1989.
Garewal HS, Sampliner R, Gerner E, et al: Ornithine decarboxylase activity in Barrett's esophagus: A potential marker for dysplasia. Gastroenterology 94:819, 1988.
Garewal HS, Sampliner RE, Fennerty MB: Flow cytometry in Barrett's esophagus. What have we learned so far? Dig Dis Sci 36:548, 1991.
Goldsmith MF: Regression of Barrett's esophagus seen after surgical intervention. Arch Intern Med 144:1117, 1984.
Gottfried MR, McClave SA, Boyce HW: Incomplete intestinal metaplasia in the diagnosis of columnar lined esophagus (Barrett's esophagus). Am J Clin Pathol 92:741, 1989.
Griffin M, Sweeney EC: The relationship of endocrine cells, dysplasia and carcinoembryonic antigen in Barrett's mucosa to adenocarcinoma of the oesophagus. Histopathology 11:53, 1987.
Haggitt RC, Reid BJ, Rabinovitch PS, Rubin CE: Barrett's esophagus: Correlation between mucin histochemistry, flow cytometry, and histologic diagnosis for predicting increased cancer risk. Am J Pathol 131:53, 1988.
Hague AK, Merkel M: Total columnar-lined esophagus—a case for congenital origin? Arch Pathol Lab Med 105:546, 1981.
Hameeteman W, Tytgat GN, Houthoff HJ, van den Twell JG: Barrett's esophagus: Development of dysplasia and adenocarcinoma. Gastroenterology 96:1249, 1989.
Hamilton SR, Pathogenesis of columnar cell-lined (Barrett's) esophagus. In Spechler SJ, Goyal RK (eds). Barrett's Esophagus: Pathophysiology, Diagnosis and Management. New York, Elsevier, 1985, p 29.
Hamilton SR: Adenocarcinoma in Barrett's oesophagus. In Whitehead R (ed): Oesophageal and Gastrointestinal Pathology. Churchill Livingstone, 1989. p 683.
Hamilton SR, Hutcheon DF, Ravich WJ, et al: Adenocarcinoma in Barrett esophagus after elimination of gastroesophageal reflux. Gastroenterology 86:356, 1984.
Hamilton SR, Smith RRL, Cameron JL: Prevalence and characteristics of Barrett esophagus in patients with adenocarcinoma of the esophagus or esophagogastric junction. Hum Pathol 19:942, 1988.
Hamilton SR, Smith RRL: Carcinoembryonic antigen (CEA) in Barrett esophagus and associated adenocarcinoma: an immunohistochemical study. (Abstract.) Gastroenterology 88:1411, 1985
Hamilton SR, Smith RRL: The relationship between columnar epithelial dysplasia and invasive adenocarcinoma arising in Barrett esophagus. Am J Clin Pathol 87:301, 1987.
Hamilton SR, Yardley JH: Regeneration of cardiac type mucosa and acquisition of Barrett mucosa after esophagogastrostomy. Gastroenterology 72:669, 1977.

James PD, Atkinson M: Value of DNA image cytometry in the prediction of malignant changes in Barrett's oesophagus. Gut 30:899, 1989.
Jauregui HO, Davessar K, Hale JH, et al: Mucin histochemistry of intestinal metaplasia in Barrett's esophagus. Modern Pathol 1:188, 1988.
Kalish RJ, Clancy PE, Orringer MB, Appelman HD: Clinical, epidemiologic, and morphologic comparison between adenocarcinomas arising in Barrett's esophageal mucosa and in the gastric cardia. Gastroenterology 86:461, 1984.
Kortan P, Warren RE, Gardner J: Barrett's esophagus in 6 patients with surgically treated achalasia. J Clin Gastroenterol 3:557, 1981.
Lee RG: Mucins in Barrett's esophagus: A histochemical study. Am J Clin Pathol 81:500, 1984.
Levi F. Ollyo J-B, LaVecchia C, et al: The consumption of tobacco, alcohol and the risk of adenocarcinoma in Barrett's esophagus. Int J Cancer 45:852, 1990.
Levine DS, Reid BJ, Haggitt RC, et al: Correlation of ultrastructural aberrations with dysplasia and flow cytometric abnormalities in Barrett's epithelium. Gastroenterology 96:355, 1989.
Levine DS, Rubin CE, Reid BJ, Haggitt RC: Specialized metaplastic columnar epithelium in Barrett's esophagus. A comparative transmission electron microscopic study. Lab Invest 60:418, 1989.
Mangla JC: Barrett's epithelium: Regression or no regression? N Engl J Med 303:529, 1980.
McDonald GB, Brand DL, Thorning DR: Multiple adenomatous neoplasms arising in columnar-lined (Barrett's) esophagus. Gastroenterology 72:1317, 1977.
Meyer W, Vollmar F, Bar W: Barrett-esophagus following total gastrectomy. A contribution to its pathogenesis. Endoscopy 11:121, 1979.
Mills LR, Schuman BM, Assad RT, et al: Scanning electron microscopy of dysplastic Barrett's epithelium. Mod Pathol 2:112, 1989.
Naef AP, Savary M, Ozzello L: Columnar-lined lower esophagus: An acquired lesion with malignant predisposition: Report on 140 cases of Barrett's esophagus with 12 adenocarcinomas. J Thorac Cardiovasc Surg 70:826, 1975.
Ozzello L, Savary M, Roethlisberger B: Columnar mucosa of the distal esophagus in patients with gastroesophageal reflux. Pathol Annu 1:41, 1977.
Parrilla P, Ortiz A, de Haro LFM, et al: Evaluation of the magnitude of gastro-oesophageal reflux in Barrett's esophagus. Gut 31:964, 1990.
Paull A, Trier JS, Dalton MD, et al: The histologic spectrum of Barrett's esophagus. N Engl J Med 295:476, 1976.
Paull G, Yardley JH: Gastric and esophageal Campylobacter pylori in patients with Barrett's esophagus. Gastroenterology 95:216, 1988.
Penchmaur M, Potet F, Goldfain D: Mucin histochemistry of the columnar epithelium of the oesophagus (Barrett's oesophagus): A prospective biopsy study. J Clin Pathol 37:607, 1984.
Postlethwait RW, Musser AW: Changes in esophagus in one thousand autopsy specimens. J Thorac Cardiovasc Surg 68:953, 1974.
Qualman SJ, Murray RD, McClung HJ, Lucas J: Intestinal metaplasia is age related in Barrett's esophagus. Arch Pathol Lab Med 114:1236, 1990.
Ransom JM, Patel GJ, Clift SA, et al: Extended and limited types of Barrett's esophagus in the adult. Ann Thorac Surg 33:19, 1982.
Reid BJ, Haggitt RC, Rubin CE, et al: Observer variation in the diagnosis of dysplasia in Barrett's esophagus. Hum Pathol 19:166, 1988.
Reid BJ, Weinstein WM, Lewin KJ, et al: Endoscopic biopsy can detect high-grade dysplasia or early adenocarcinoma in Barrett's esophagus without grossly recognizable neoplastic lesions. Gastroenterology 94:81, 1988.
Resano CH, Cabrera N, Cueto DG, et al: Double early epidermoid carcinoma of the esophagus in columnar epithelium. Endoscopy 17:73, 1985.
Riddell RH: Dysplasia and regression in Barrett's epithelium. In Spechler SJ, Goyal RK (eds): Barrett's Esophagus: Pathophysiology, Diagnosis and Management. New York, Elsevier, 1985, p 143.
Robey SS, Hamilton SR, Gupta PK, Erozan YS: Diagnostic value of

cytopathology in Barrett esophagus and associated carcinoma. Am J Clin Pathol 89:493, 1988.

Rosenberg JC, Budev H, Edwards RC, et al: Analysis of adenocarcinoma in Barrett's esophagus utilizing a staging system. Cancer 55:1353, 1985.

Rosengard AM, Hamilton SR: Squamous carcinoma of the esophagus in patients with Barrett esophagus. Modern Pathol 2:2, 1989.

Rothery GA, Patterson JE, Stoddard DJ, Day DW: Histological and histochemical changes in the columnar lined (Barrett's) oesophagus. Gut 27:1062, 1986.

Sampliner RE, Garewal HS, Fennerty MB, Aickin M: Lack of impact of therapy on extent of Barrett's esophagus in 67 patients. Dig Dis Sci 35:93, 1990.

Sarr MG, Hamilton SR, Marrone GC, Cameron JL: Barrett's esophagus: Its prevalence and association with adenocarcinoma in patients with symptoms of gastro-esophageal reflux. Am J Surg 149:187, 1985.

Sartori S, Nielson I, Indelli M, et al: Barrett esophagus after chemotherapy with cyclophosphamide, methotrexate, and 5-fluorouracil (CMF): An iatrogenic injury. Ann Intern Med 114:210, 1991.

Schreiber DS, Apstein M, Hermos JA: Paneth cells in Barrett's esophagus. Gastroenterology 74:1302, 1978.

Smith RRL, Hamilton SR, Boitnott JK, Rogers EL: The spectrum of carcinoma arising in Barrett's esophagus: A clinicopathologic study of 26 patients. Am J Surg Pathol 8:563, 1984.

Snyder JD, Goldman H: Barrett's esophagus in children and young adults: Frequent association with mental retardation Dig Dis Sci 35:1185, 1990.

Spechler SJ: Endoscopic surveillance for patients with Barrett esophagus: Does the cancer risk justify the practice? Ann Intern Med 106:902, 1987.

Spechler SJ, Goyal RK (eds): Barrett's Esophagus: Pathophysiology, Diagnosis and Management. New York, Elsevier, 1985.

Spechler SJ, Goyal RK: Barrett's esophagus. N Engl J Med 315:362, 1986.

Spechler SJ, Schimmel EM, Dalton JW, et al: Barrett's epithelium complicating lye ingestion with sparing of the distal esophagus. Gastroenterology 81:580, 1981.

Streitz JM Jr, Ellis FH Jr, Gibb SP, et al: Adenocarcinoma in Barrett's esophagus: A clinicopathologic study of 65 cases. Ann Surg 213:122, 1991.

Talley NJ, Cameron AJ, Shorter RG, et al: Campylobacter pylori and Barrett's esophagus. Mayo Clin Proc 63:1176, 1988.

Thompson JJ, Zinssen KR, Enterline HT: Barrett's metaplasia and adenocarcinoma of the esophagus and gastroesophageal junction. Hum Pathol 14:42, 1983.

van der Veen AH, Dees J, Blankenstein JD, van Blankenstein M: Adenocarcinoma in Barrett's oesophagus: an overrated risk. Gut 30:14, 1989.

Wang HH, Antonioli DA, Goldman H: Comparative features of esophageal and gastric adenocarcinomas: Recent changes in type and frequency. Hum Pathol 17:482, 1986.

Waring JP, Legrand J, Chinichian A, Sanowski RA: Duodenogastric reflux in patients with Barrett's esophagus. Dig Dis Sci 35:759, 1990.

Weil RJ: Esophagectomy for Barrett's esophagus. Ann Thorac Surg 50:858, 1990.

Williamson WA, Ellis H Jr, Gibb SP, et al: Effect of antireflux operation on Barrett's mucosa. Ann Thorac Surg 49:537, 1990.

Zwas F, Shields HM, Doos WG, et al: Scanning electron microscopy of Barrett's epithelium and its correlation with light microscopy and mucin stains. Gastroenterology 90:1932, 1986.

Differential Diagnosis of Barrett's Esophagus

Christensen WN, Sternberg SS: Adenocarcinoma of the upper esophagus arising in ectopic gastric mucosa. Am J Surg Pathol 11:397, 1987.

Flejou JF, Potet F, Molas G, et al: Campylobacter-like organisms in heterotopic gastric mucosa of the upper oesophagus. J Clin Pathol 43:961, 1990.

Ibrahim NBN, Sandry RJ: Congenital oesophageal stenosis caused by tracheobronchial strictures in the oesophageal wall. Thorax 36:465, 1981.

Jabbari M, Goresky CA, Laugh J: The inlet patch: heterotopic gastric mucosa in the upper esophagus. Gastroenterology 89:352, 1985.

Nishina T, Tsuchida Y, Saito S: Congenital esophageal stenosis due to tracheobronchial remnants and its associated anomalies. J Pediatr Surg 16:190, 1981.

Raeburn C: Columnar ciliated epithelium in the adult esophagus. J Pathol Bacteriol 63:157, 1951.

Sneed WF, LaGarde DC, Kosutt MS, Arensman RM: Esophageal stenosis due to cartilaginous tracheobronchial remnants. J Pediatr Surg 14:786, 1979.

Achalasia

Adams CWH, Brain RHF, Trounce JR: Ganglion cells in achalasia of the cardia. Virchows Arch [B] 372:75, 1976.

Ferguson TB, Woodbury JD, Roper CL, Burford TH: Giant muscular hypertrophy of the esophagus. Ann Thorac Surg 8:209, 1969.

Gilles M, Nicks R, Skyring A: Clinical manometric, and pathologic studies in diffuse oesophageal spasm. Br Med J 2:527, 1967.

Katz SJ, Lieberman A, Hechtman HB: Spontaneous perforation of the esophagus associated with smooth muscle hypertrophy. Am J Surg 127:328, 1974.

Kreczy A, Gassner J, Mikuz G: Idiopathic hypertrophy of the oesophagus in children: A case report and review of the literature. Virchows Arch [A]: 417:81, 1990.

Marshall JB, Diaz-Arias AA, Bochna GS, Vogele KA: Achalasia due to diffuse esophageal leiomyomatosis and inherited as an autosomal dominant disorder: Report of a family study. Gastroenterology 98:1358, 1990.

Qualman SJ, Haupt HM, Yang P, Hamilton SR: Esophageal Lewy bodies associated with ganglion cell loss in achalasia: Similarity to Parkinson's disease. Gastroenterology 87:848, 1984.

Saba DE, Vargas-Cortes DF: Idiopathic muscular hypertrophy of the esophagus. Postmortem incidental findings in six cases and review of the literature. Chest 73:28, 1978.

Smith B: The neurological lesion in achalasia of the cardia. Gut 11:388, 1970.

Rings and Webs

Bretagne JF, Ramee MP, Gosselin M, Gastard J: Esophageal keratosis associated with peptic stricture. Gastroenterol Clin Biol 6:869, 1982.

Eckardt VF, Adami B, Hucker H, Leeder H: The esophagogastric junction in patients with asymptomatic lower esophageal mucosal webs. Gastroenterology 79:1426, 1980.

Entwistle CC, Jacobs A: Histological findings in the Paterson-Kelly syndrome. J Clin Pathol 18:408, 1965.

Goyal RK, Glancy JJ, Spiro HM: Lower esophageal ring. N Engl J Med 282:1298, 1970.

Hendrix TR: Schatzki ring, epithelial junction, and hiatal hernia—an unresolved controversy. Gastroenterology 79:584, 1980.

Janisch HD, Eckardt VF: Histological abnormalities in patients with multiple esophageal webs. Dig Dis Sci 27:503, 1982.

Lesser PB, Moyer P, Andrews PJ, Dreyfuss JR: Upper oesophageal ring. Ann Intern Med 88:657, 1978.

Marshall JB, Kretschmar JM, Diazarias AA: Gastroesophageal reflux as a pathogenic factor in the development of symptomatic lower esophageal rings. Arch Intern Med 150:1669, 1990.

Schatzki R, Gary JE: Dysphagia due to a diaphragm-like localized narrowing in the lower esophagus ("lower esophageal ring"). Am J Roentgenol 20:91, 1953.

Shifleet DW, Gilliam JH, Wu WC, et al: Multiple esophageal webs. Gastroenterology 77:556, 1979.

Intramural Pseudodiverticulosis

Bruhlmann WF, Zollikoten CL, Maranta E, et al: Intramural pseudodiverticulosis of the esophagus: Report of seven cases and literature review. Gastrointest Radiol 6:199, 1981.

Evans PR: Oesophageal intramural pseudodiverticulosis—always benign. Aust NZ J Med 21:58, 1991.

Farman J, Rosen Y, Dallemand S, et al: Esophagitis cystica: Lower esophageal retention cysts. Am J Roentgenol 128:495, 1977.
Piazza M, Palma PD: Polycystic "dystrophy" of the esophagus. Am J Clin Pathol 67:307, 1977.
Troupiz RH: Intramural esophageal diverticulosis and moniliasis: Possible association. AJR 104:613, 1968.
Voirol W, Welsh RA, Genet EF: Esophagitis cystica. Am J Gastroenterol 59:446, 1973.

Collagen Vascular–Connective Tissue Diseases

Bretagne JF, Launois B, Ferrand B, Gastard J: Rheumatoid stricture of the esophagus. Gastroenterol Clin Biol 6:709, 1982.
Burkert K, Berges N, Borchard F, et al: Osophagus stenose bei Sjögren-Syndrom. Med Klin 75:192, 1980.
Gutierrez F, Valenzuela JE, Ehresmann GR, et al: Esophageal dysfunction in patients with mixed connective tissue diseases and systemic lupus erythematosus. Dig Dis Sci 27:592, 1982.
Kleckner FS: Dermatomyositis and its manifestations in the gastrointestinal tract. Am J Gastroenterol 53:141, 1970.
Nishikai M, Asaba G, Homma M: Rheumatoid esophageal disease. Am J Gastroenterol 67:29, 1977.
Orringer MB, Dabick L, Zarafonetis CJD, Sloan H: Gastroesophageal reflux in esophageal scleroderma: Diagnosis and implications. Ann Thorac Surg 22:120, 1976.
Ramirez-Mata M, Pina-ancira FF, Alarcon-Segovia D: Abnormal esophageal motility in primary Sjogren's syndrome. J Rheumatol 31:63, 1976.
Russell ML, Friesen D, Henderson RD, Hanna WM: Ultrastructure of the esophagus in scleroderma. Arthritis Rheum 25:1117, 1982.
Weihrauch TR, Korting GW, Ewe K, Vogt G: Esophageal dysfunction and its pathogenesis in progressive systemic sclerosis. Klin Wochenschr 56:963, 1978.

Crohn's Disease

Bianco L, Sategna-Guidetti C, Colombatti G, Peyre S: Crohn's disease of the upper gastro-intestinal tract: Case report and review of the literature. Panminerva Med 23:11, 1981.
Gobel V, Long BW, Richter G: Aphthous ulcers in the esophagus with Crohn colitis. Am J Roentgenol 137:72, 1982.
Lee CS, Mangla JC, Lee SSC: Crohn's disease in Barrett's esophagus. Am J Gastroenterol 69:646, 1978.
LiVolsi VA, Jaretzki A: Granulomatous esophagitis: A case of Crohn's disease limited to the esophagus. Gastroenterology 64:313, 1973.
Madden JL, Ravid JM, Haddad JR: Regional esophagitis: Specific entity simulating Crohn's disease. Ann Surg 170:351, 1969.
Miller LJ, Thistle JL, Payne WS, et al: Crohn's disease involving the esophagus and colon: Case report. Mayo Clin Proc 52:35, 1977.
Werthamer S, Zak FG, Milailos P, Amaral L: Granulomatous esophagitis (Crohn's disease) associated with granulomatous enterocolitis. NY State J Med 76:938, 1976.
Woodtli W, Buhler H, Seefeld U, et al: Findings in the upper gastrointestinal tract in Crohn's disease. Schweiz Med Wochenschr 113:709, 1983.

Behçet's Syndrome

Chajek T, Fainaru M: Behçet's disease: Report of 41 cases. Medicine (Baltimore) 54:179, 1975.
Lebwohl O, Forde KA, Berdon WE, Morrison S: Ulcerative esophagitis and colitis in a pediatric patient with Behçet's syndrome. Response to steroid therapy. Am J Gastroenterol 68:550, 1977.
Lorenzetti ME, Forbes IJ, Robertsthomson IC: Oesophageal and ileal ulceration in Behçet's disease. J Gastroenterol Hepatol 5:714, 1990.
Parkin JV, Wight DGD: Behçet's disease and the alimentary tract. Postgrad Med J 51:260, 1975.

Eosinophilic Esophagitis

Dobbins JW, Sheahan DG, Behar J: Eosinophilic gastroenteritis with esophageal involvement. Gastroenterology 72:1312, 1977.
Lee RG: Marked eosinophilia in esophageal mucosal biopsies. Am J Surg Pathol 9:475, 1985.
Munch R, Kuhlmann U, Makek M, et al: Eosinophilic esophagitis, a rare form of eosinophilic gastroenteritis. Schweiz Med Wochenschr 112:731, 1982.

Dermatologic Diseases

Dickens CM, Hastletine D, Walton S, Bennett JR: The oesophagus in lichen planus: An endoscopic study. Br Med J 300:84, 1990.
Gnanapragasam A: Oesophageal involvement in epidermolysis bullosa. J Larnygol Otol 91:271, 1977.
Guedon C, Kuffer R, Thomine E, et al: Esophageal lichen sclerosus associated with local stenosis. Gastroenterol Clin Biol 6:1049, 1980.
Hillemeier C, Touloukian R, McCallum R, Gryboski J: Esophageal web: A previously unrealized complication of epidermolysis bullosa. Pediatrics 67:678, 1981.
Howel-Evans W, McConnel RB, Clarke CA, Shephard PM: Carcinoma of the oesophagus with keratosis palmaris et plantaris(tylosis): A study of two families. Q J Med 27:413, 1958.
Itai Y, Kogure T, Okuyama Y, Akiyama H: Radiological manifestations of esophageal involvement in acanthosis nigricans. Br J Radiol 49:592, 1976.
Johnston DE, Koehler RE, Balte DM: Clinical manifestations of epidermolysis bullosa dystrophica. Dig Dis Sci 26:1144, 1981.
Kahn D, Hutchinson E: Esophageal involvement in familial benign chronic pemphigus. Arch Dermatol 109:718, 1974.
Kaplan RP, Touloukian J, Ahmed AR, Newcomber VD: Esophagitis dissecans superficialis associated with pemphigus vulgaris. J Am Assoc Dermatol 4:682, 1981.
Larregue M, Katz M, Gasquet C, et al: Cocolisatius oesophagiennes de la dyscleratose folliculaire, maladie de Darier: Description radiologique: A propos de 4 cas. Ann Med Interne (Paris) 128:487, 1977.
Manier JW, Kaplan AP: Polydysplastic epidermolysis bullosa with esophageal stricture: Report of a case. Gastrointest Endosc 19:19, 1972.
Mignon FC, Laroche L, Revuz J, et al: L'association acanthosis nigricans-papillomatase oesophagienne diffuse. Nouv Presse Med 4:2507, 1975.
Munyer TP, Margulis AR: Tylosis. AJR 136:1026, 1981.
Pearson RW: Epidermolysis bullosa hereditaria lethalis. Arch Dermatol 109:349, 1974.
Renner WR, Johnson JF, Lichtenstein JE, Kirks DR: Esophageal inflammation and stricture—complication of chronic granulomatous disease of childhood. Radiology 178:189, 1991.
Stewart MI, Woodley DT, Briggaman RA: Epidermolysis bullosa acquisita and associated symptomatic esophageal webs. Arch Dermatol 127:373, 1991.
Trattner A, Lurie R, Leiser A, David M, et al: Esophageal involvement in pemphigus vulgaris: A clinical, histologic, and immunopathologic study. J Am Acad Dermatol 24:233, 1991.
Warren RB, Warner TFCS, Gilbert EF, Pellet JR: Acquired double-barrel esophagus in epidermolysis bullosa dystrophica. Thorax 35:472, 1980.
Wood DR, Patterson JB, Orlando RC: Pemphigus vulgaris of the esophagus. Ann Intern Med 96:189, 1982.

Sarcoidosis

Cook DM, Dines DE: Sarcoidosis: Report of a case presenting as dysphagia. Chest 57:84, 1970.
Davies RJ: Dysphagia, abdominal pain and sarcoid granulomata. Br Med J 3:564, 1972.
Weisner PJ, Kleinman MS, Coadeomi JJ: Sarcoidosis of the esophagus. Am J Dig Dis 16:943, 1971.

Graft-Versus-Host Disease

McDonald GB, Sullivan KM, Schuffler MD, et al: Esophageal abnormality in chronic graft-versus-host disease in humans. Gastroenterology 80:914, 1981.
Slavin RE, Woodruff JM: The pathology of bone marrow transplantation. In Sommers SC (ed): Pathology Annual. New York, Appleton-Century-Crofts, 1974, p 312.

Amyloid

Busuttil A, More IAR, Jones DG: Amyloid deposits in the trachea and esophagus: Ultrastructural confirmation. Laryngoscope 86:850, 1976.

Heitzman EJ, Heitzman GC, Elliott CF: Primary esophageal amyloidosis: Report of a case with bleeding, perforation, and survival following resection. Arch Intern Med 109:595, 1962.

Kyle RA, Bayrd ED: Amyloidosis: Review of 236 cases. Medicine 54:271, 1975.

Miller RH: Amyloid disease—an unusual cause of megalo-oesophagus. S Afr Med J 43:1202, 1969.

Solanke TF, Olurin, EO, Nwakonobi F, Udeozo IOK: Primary amyloid tumour of the oesophagus treated by colon transplant. Br J Surg 54:943, 1967.

CHAPTER 18

Squamous Cell Carcinoma of the Esophagus

FU-SHENG LIU, M.D.
QI-LU WANG, M.D.

EPIDEMIOLOGY
Age Distribution
Sex Distribution
Geographic Distribution
Mass Surveys in China
Migrant Studies
Incidence in the Fowl in China

ETIOLOGY
Dietary Factors
Trace Elements
Dietary Habits in High-Risk Regions in China
Nitrosamines
Alcohol Consumption and Smoking
Genetic Factors

ASSOCIATED CONDITIONS AND PRECANCEROUS LESIONS
Associated Conditions
Chronic Esophagitis
Achalasia
Benign Stricture
Hiatal Hernia
Plummer-Vinson Syndrome
Diverticulum
Celiac Disease
Precancerous Lesions
Squamous Papilloma
Dysplasia of Squamous Epithelium
Histologic Study
Cytologic Classification
Follow-up Study

PATHOLOGY
Location
Early Esophageal Carcinoma
Gross Types
Histologic Types
Advanced Esophageal Carcinoma
Variants of Squamous Cell Carcinoma
Verrucous Carcinoma
Spindle Cell Carcinoma (Carcinosarcoma)
Staging
Spread and Metastasis
Pathologic Factors Affecting Prognosis

CLINICOPATHOLOGIC CORRELATION
Clinical Presentation and Diagnosis
Complications and Causes of Death
Treatment
Surgical Resection
Radiation Therapy
Postirradiation Pathologic Changes
Factors Affecting Morphologic Changes
Radiation-Induced Tissue Changes
Grading of Radiation-Induced Pathologic Changes

The esophagus is normally lined by a squamous epithelium. It is therefore not surprising that squamous cell carcinoma is the most common malignant epithelial neoplasm in the esophagus. It is a tumor long associated with alcohol consumption and other dietary habits. In this regard, epidemiologic studies, first in southern Africa, then in Iran, and more recently in northern China, have yielded much valuable information, even though the specific etiologic agent or agents have not yet been identified.

Squamous cell carcinoma of the esophagus carries a very grave prognosis. It is often diagnosed at a late stage, and its location in the chest makes complete eradication of the lesion difficult. The early stage of the tumor was once poorly understood. Studies in China have remedied this situation to a great extent, in documenting the pathologic features of early esophageal cancer and precancerous lesions. These advances have affected the clinical management and the survival rates of the patients.

EPIDEMIOLOGY

Age Distribution

Carcinoma of the esophagus is largely a disease of late middle and old age. It is rare in patients under 30 years of age, and the incidence gradually increases with advancing age. Postlethwait and Sealy[1] reviewed 9244 cases from the literature and found that 2755 of the patients (29.8%) were 50 to 59 years of age and 3121 (33.8%) were 60 to 69 years of age. Li and colleagues[2] analyzed 1831 patients with esophageal cancer from three provinces in northern China and found the highest incidence in those 50 to 59 (618 cases, or 33.8%) and 60 to 69 (593 cases, or 32.4%) years of age.

Sex Distribution

Carcinoma of the esophagus is more common in men than in women, but the reported male/female ratio in the literature varies. Kiviranta[3] surveyed data for more than 12,000 patients from various countries and found that the disease always occurred more often in men; ratios ranged from 2:1 to 20:1. In the materials collected from the literature, Postlethwait and Sealy found reports of 10,519 male patients and 4,044 female patients, a ratio of 2.6:1.[1]

A similar situation has been demonstrated in China. According to Li and colleagues,[2] the male/female ratio varies from 1.3:1 to 2.7:1 in different regions. An epidemiologic investigation[4] in an area of northern China covering a population of 50 million showed that the ratio averaged beween 1.6:1 and 1:1 and that the higher the mortality in a locality, the lower the ratio.

Geographic Distribution

The rate of death from esophageal cancer varies greatly in different countries and regions. Data obtained by the World Health Organization and published in 1977[5] showed that the mortality rate, standardized to the world population, was highest in both sexes in China. Puerto Rico ranked second, and Singapore ranked third (Figure 18–1). Cumulative mortality up to 74 years of age was 4.05% for Chinese men and 1.96% for Chinese women. The incidence in Chinese men is double that of men in Singapore, and mortality in Chinese women is three times as high as that in Puerto Rican women.

In the United States, the estimated number of cases of esophageal cancer for 1989 was 10,100, and the estimated number of deaths was 9400, approximately 3.8 per 100,000 population.[6] The mortality rate has remained essentially stable since 1930. It has been noted, however, that death rates in both sexes in the black population have increased so that they are nearly three times those in the white population.[7] An increase in the incidence rates in blacks was also noted in parts of South Africa.[8]

In China,[5] deaths due to cancer of the esophagus constitute 26.46% of all cancer deaths in men and 19.74% in women. Among all cancers, it ranks second in mortality only to cancer of the stomach. The districts

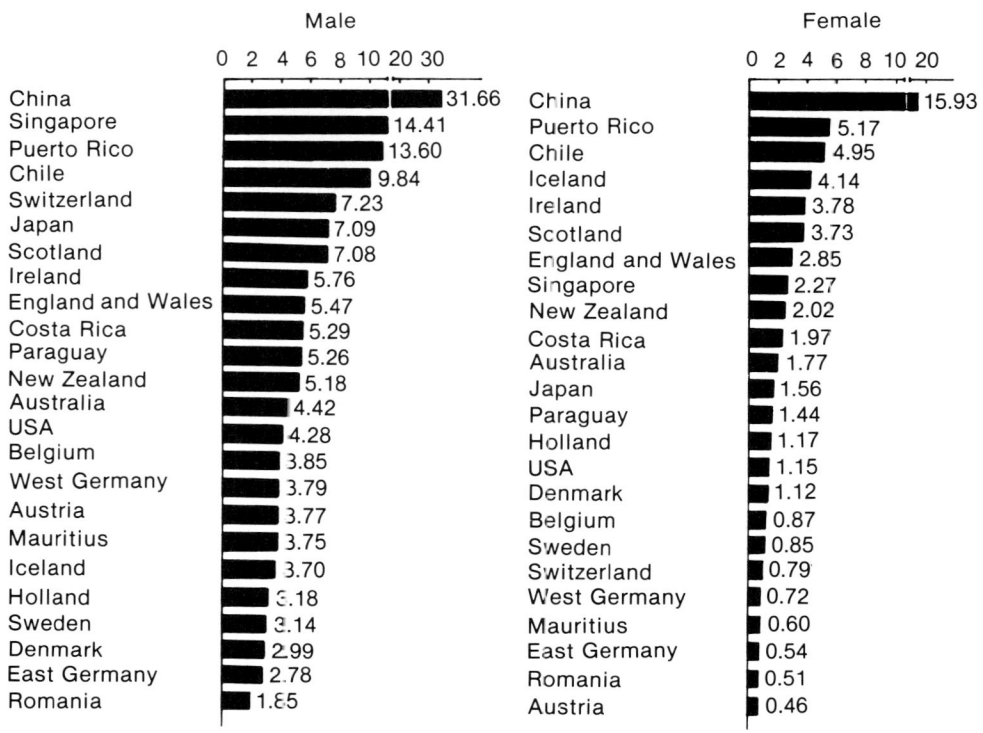

FIGURE 18–1. Age-adjusted mortality for esophageal cancer in selected countries. (From Liu BQ, Li B: Epidemiology of carcinoma of the esophagus in China. In Huang GJ, Wu YK (eds): Carcinoma of the Esophagus and Gastric Cardia. Berlin, Springer-Verlag, 1984, p 4.)

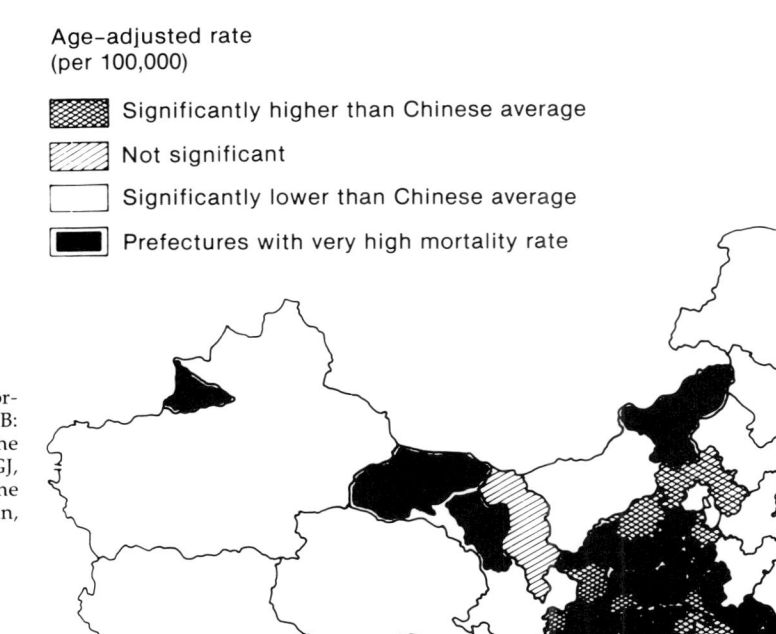

FIGURE 18–2. Distribution of mortality in China. (From Liu BQ, Li B: Epidemiology of carcinoma of the esophagus in China. In Huang GJ, Wu YK (eds): Carcinoma of the Esophagus and Gastric Cardia. Berlin, Springer-Verlag, 1984, p 10.)

with a mortality rate from esophageal cancer higher than the national average make up a hand-shaped zone extending from the east coastal region to Sichuan Province in the west. The northern part of the zone extends to the suburbs of Beijing, and its southern area includes the region south of Yangtze River. Additional high-risk areas are along the southeast coastline and in parts of Xinjiang autonomous regions in the northwest (Figure 18–2). The region with the highest risk in China is Lin County (Linxian) in Henan Province, where the adjusted mortality rates for esophageal cancer are in men 161.3 and in women 102.9 per 100,000.[9] It is striking that in Fanxian, about 100 miles away, the corresponding mortality rates are only 26.54 and 7.49. Marked differences in the incidence rates within a short distance also exist in other regions. The endemic nature of the disease indicates a strong influence of environmental, rather than genetic factors.

Mass Surveys in China

Mass surveys for esophageal cancer have been carried out in Linxian since 1959 with the aid of cytologic examination involving a flexible catheter with an inflatable balloon attached to the distal end to collect the specimen. The apparatus (Figure 18–3) is a double-lumen or single-lumen tube made of rubber or plastic. It is 65 cm long and 0.25 cm in diameter. The inflatable balloon is about 5 cm long and 2.5 cm in diameter and is covered with a cotton mesh net. In the double-lumen tube, the proximal end is divided into two tubes, one for air injection and the other for suction.

The examination is performed on fasting persons with an empty stomach. After the balloon passes the gastric cardia, it is inflated with about 30 ml of air.

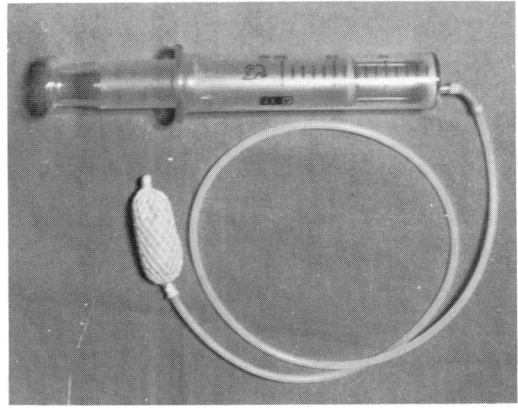

FIGURE 18–3. Balloon catheter with a syringe.

When the tube is being pulled back, it is slightly deflated so that the balloon can be pulled back into the esophagus. When it reaches the 20-cm mark from the mouth, it is deflated completely and withdrawn. In general, the balloon cytologic examination is very safe, easy to control, and effective in both mass surveys and clinical usage. Through this technique, many early esophageal cancers have been found.[10] It is also effective in the detection and follow-up of dysplasia in the esophagus and gastric cardia.

Migrant Studies

Several studies reported differences in the site-specific cancer risks between the native and foreign-born populations in the United States.[11] Similar observations have been made in other countries. In the United States, the incidence of esophageal cancer among blacks exceeds that among whites, and the incidence among Chinese immigrants is higher than among native-born Chinese. In China, from 1967 to 1969, about 60,000 people migrated from Xichuan County, a high-risk region, of Henan Province, to the low-risk regions of Zhongxiang and Jinmen counties, of Hubei Province. The death rates of esophageal cancer in the native-born in Zhongxiang and Jinmen were 15.39/100,000 and 7.13/100,000, respectively. Ten years after migration, the migrant people in these regions continued to have death rates of 75.81/100,000 and 98.30/100,000, which is 5 to 13 times higher than that of the local people. Thus the carcinogenic influence has a long-lasting effect.

Incidence in the Fowl in China

In the high-risk area of human esophageal cancer in China, esophageal cancer has also been found in the domestic fowl.[12] Tumors in the chicken are found mainly in the pharynx and the upper part of the esophagus; 58.6% occur in the latter. The largest lesion ever found had a diameter of more than 5 cm. The tumors can be classified into cauliflower, nodular, and infiltrating types (Figure 18–4), and 96.6% of the lesions are squamous cell carcinomas. The incidence of these

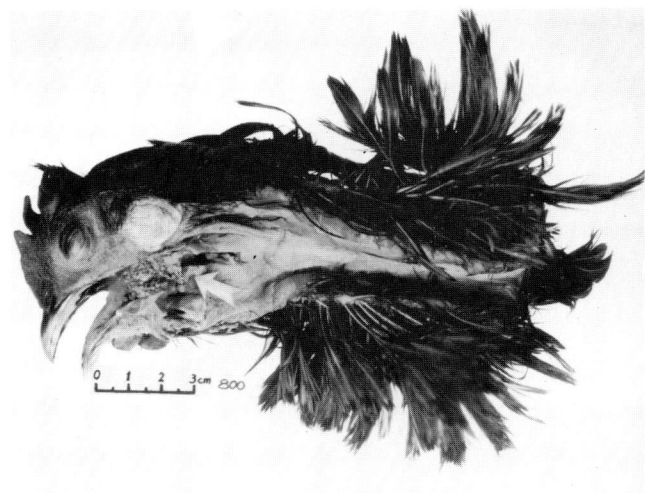

FIGURE 18–4. Cauliflower-shaped carcinoma (arrow) of the esophagus in a chicken.

tumors in the high-risk area of Linxian and that in the low-risk area of Fanxian are 175.8 and 18.9 per 100,000, respectively, figures that are comparable to those in man in these regions (Table 18–1).

ETIOLOGY

Studies in the high-risk areas, such as the eastern coastal regions of the Caspian Sea in Iran and in Linxian, in China, have suggested that dietary, environmental, and endogenous factors are etiologically important in esophageal cancer.

Dietary Factors

In the high-risk areas of esophageal cancer, poor dietary conditions may play an important role. There is often a low intake of vitamins A and C, riboflavin, animal protein, fat, and fresh vegetables and fruit. Some persons have symptoms of riboflavin deficiency, such as cheilosis, glossitis, and a burning sensation of the tongue. Zheng and associates[13] studied the urinary ex-

Table 18–1 PREVALENCE OF PHARYNGEAL AND ESOPHAGEAL CARCINOMAS IN DOMESTIC FOWL FROM LINXIAN (HIGH RISK) AND FANXIAN (LOW RISK), HENAN PROVINCE, CHINA

Age Years	Linxian			Fanxian		
	No. of Chickens	No. of Cancers	Prevalence (per 100,000)	No. of Chickens	No. of Cancers	Prevalence (per 100,000)
0	3,460	0	0	3,911	0	0
2	11,563	6	52	6,087	2	32
5	2,617	20	764	518	0	0
7	941	6	638	62	0	0
10	193	1	518	10	0	0
Total	18,774	33	175.8	10,588	2	18.9

From Liu BQ, Li B: Epidemiology of carcinoma of the esophagus in China. In Huang GJ, Wu YK (eds): Carcinoma of the Esophagus and Gastric Cardia. Berlin, Springer-Verlag, 1984, p 21.)

cretion of a test dose (5 mg) of riboflavin in peasants of Linxian. Most of the peasants tested excreted less than 1 mg of riboflavin in the urine over a 4-hour period, which indicated inadequate intake of riboflavin. In an experiment with rats, riboflavin deficiency increased the incidence of esophageal cancer induced by methylbenzylnitrosamine and shortened the latent period of the development of cancer.[14]

Trace Elements

The role of trace elements has also been investigated in China. Trace elements such as molybdenum, zinc, copper, magnesium, manganese, and cobalt are low in the drinking water of high-risk areas. However, Plummer-Vinson syndrome, an iron deficiency disease, was not seen in Linxian. Burrell and coauthors[15] reported a relative deficiency of molybdenum, copper, zinc, and magnesium in the soil of Transki, South Africa, where the incidence of esophageal cancer was high. Nemenko and colleagues[16] reported a low content of molybdenum in Guryer areas of Kazakhstan, in the Soviet Union. In the high-risk areas in China the levels of molybdenum and zinc in foodstuffs are low.[17] Experimentally dietary zinc deficiency induces parakeratosis in the esophagus of rats.[18]

Dietary Habits in High-Risk Regions in China

Pickled vegetables are eaten daily in several areas with high incidence of esophageal cancer in China. Many species of fungi have been found in pickled vegetables, particularly *Geotrichum candidum* and *Fusarium moniliforme*. Extracts of Linxian pickles induced hyperplasia of the esophageal epithelium as well as papilloma of the forestomach in mice.[19] *In vitro* testing showed the presence of mutagenic and carcinogenic substances in the pickled vegetable extracts.[20,21] Furthermore, fungal infection is common in the esophagus in Linxian. Xia[22] examined 155 biopsy specimens of human esophagus, including 30 cases of early cancer and adenocarcinoma of cardia from Linxian and other areas, and found fungal infection, especially *Candida albicans,* in the hyperplastic epithelium in 30% and in the cancerous tissue in 15% of the biopsy specimens.

Nitrosamines

It is known that N-nitroso compounds induce esophageal cancer in experimental animals. Some nitrosamines have been used as model substances for the induction of esophageal cancer in animals. In such studies, the sequence of epithelial hyperplasia, dysplasia, and carcinoma *in situ* has been observed.[23] In Linxian, although the level of N-nitroso compounds in food is less than 10 parts per billion, their precursors—nitrates, nitrites, and secondary amines—are widely distributed in the food and the environment. Under the acidic conditions in the stomach, N-nitroso compounds can be easily formed and become the main endogenous source of these carcinogens.[20]

Alcohol Consumption and Smoking

Alcohol consumption and smoking have been implicated in causing esophageal cancer in Europe and North America,[24] probably because of carcinogenic substances in them.[25] However, they are not significant factors in some high-risk areas, such as Iran and China.

Genetic Factors

Genetic factors in esophageal carcinogenesis are implicated by the finding of familial aggregations of esophageal cancer, as noted in China.[26] It is possible, however, that shared environmental, rather than genetic, factors may be in play. On the other hand, a study in Iran revealed a high incidence of esophageal carcinoma in the blood relatives but not in the relatives by marriage.[27] Genetic factors are clearly involved in families with familial tylosis in whose members esophageal cancer is common.[28] Additional information is given in Chapter 6.

ASSOCIATED CONDITIONS AND PRECANCEROUS LESIONS

Associated Conditions

Chronic Esophagitis

Chronic esophagitis is a common disease. It is usually very difficult to find the cause. Endoscopy and esophagoscopic biopsies performed in the high-risk regions of Iran and China have revealed an incidence of chronic esophagitis that is unusually high in comparison with that in the low-risk population.[29] Dysplasia was present in a small number of the biopsy specimens.

Achalasia

There is much evidence that achalasia is a precancerous lesion. Ellis[30] reported seven cases of esophageal cancer among 24 autopsies performed on achalasia patients. However, the reported incidences vary. In a report by Chuong and coauthors,[31] none of the achalasia patients reviewed or followed had esophageal cancer.

Benign Stricture

Benign esophageal stricture is uncommon. In a mass survey for esophageal cancer in Linxian, China, among 16,000 people examined with cytologic and radiologic methods, six cases of benign stricture of the esophagus were found, which is a rather high incidence. None of the patients had esophageal cancer, however. In adults, benign stricture usually develops after ingestion of caustic chemicals in childhood. The incidence of esophageal carcinoma in such cases varied from 0% to 4%. In one large series, carcinoma was present in 12 of 846 patients, mostly in the midesophagus.[32]

Hiatal Hernia

Hiatal hernia is common. It is often associated with reflux esophagitis.[33] In 1959, Adler and Rodriquez[34] found carcinoma in 21 of 814 hernia patients: 12 in the stomach and 9 in the esophagus. Among the esophageal cancers, seven were squamous cell carcinoma and two were adenocarcinomas. A similar observation was made recently in patients with squamous cell carcinoma of the distal esophagus, in whom hiatal hernia and reflux esophagitis appeared to be associated factors.[35] There have been many reports of adenocarcinoma in the lower esophagus lined with columnar epithelium in patients with hiatal hernia and reflux esophagitis. Detailed descriptions of these conditions are given in Chapters 17 and 19.

Plummer-Vinson Syndrome

A considerable number of patients suffering from Plummer-Vinson syndrome for many years develop carcinoma in the hypopharynx or esophagus, particularly at the postcricoid region. The relatively high incidence of esophageal cancer in Swedish women has been explained on this basis.[36]

Diverticulum

Although there are sporadic cases of reports of carcinoma in the pharyngoesophageal diverticulum,[37] there is no evidence that they are etiologically related.

Celiac Disease

The incidence of lymphoma and gastrointestinal cancer is increased in patients with celiac disease. Most of the gastrointestinal carcinomas are in the esophagus.[38]

Precancerous Lesions

Squamous Papilloma

In animal experiments, esophageal carcinoma sometimes develops from the papilloma.[23] Papilloma of the esophagus in man is uncommon. Although a number of cases have been reported, most of them are based on gross appearance at endoscopy. The sizes range from a few millimeters to 2 cm. A few of them are multiple. It usually occurs in the lower third of the esophagus. Most of the patients have other disorders such as hiatal hernia and peptic ulcer. Colina and associates[39] reviewed 20 cases, including 3 of their own. In our institute, only 1 papilloma was found among 1100 esophagectomy specimens. Papillomas of the distal esophagus are not associated with malignant change. Larger squamous papillomas have in rare instances been observed in the upper esophagus, usually in conjunction with similar lesions in the trachea and bronchi. These lesions may be associated with the development of cancer.

Dysplasia of Squamous Epithelium

Histologic Study

Dysplasia in the squamous epithelium adjacent to an esophageal carcinoma is present in most cases.[40,41] Histologically, the dysplastic lesions are usually categorized into mild, moderate, and severe grades. Severe dysplasia is most potentially malignant. Among 150 cases of early esophageal cancer that we studied,[42] simple hyperplasia in the adjacent mucosa occurred in 142 patients (94.7%), dysplasia or atypical hyperplasia (Figure 18–5) in 100 (66.7%), and epithelial atrophy in 8 (5.3%). Most lesions were contiguous with the main tumors, but in 34 cases they were 0.3 to 7.5 cm apart. Carcinoma *in situ* was present in 84 cases. It was the

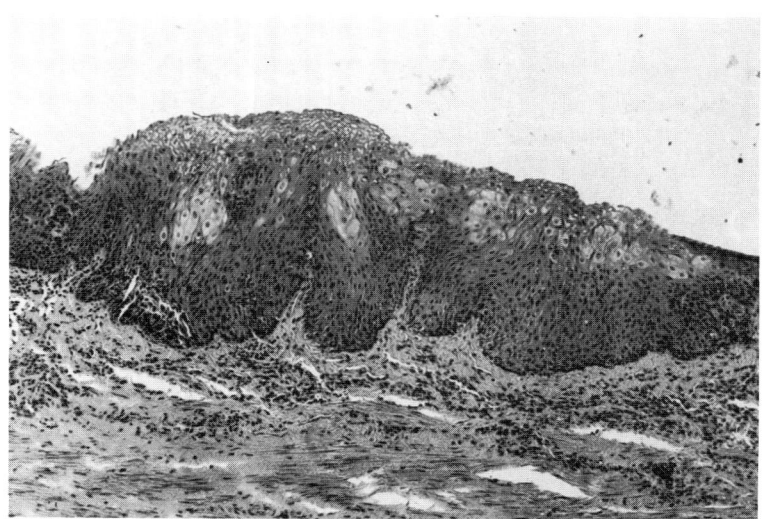

FIGURE 18–5. Atypical hyperplasia (mild dysplasia) of the esophageal mucosa. (× 100)

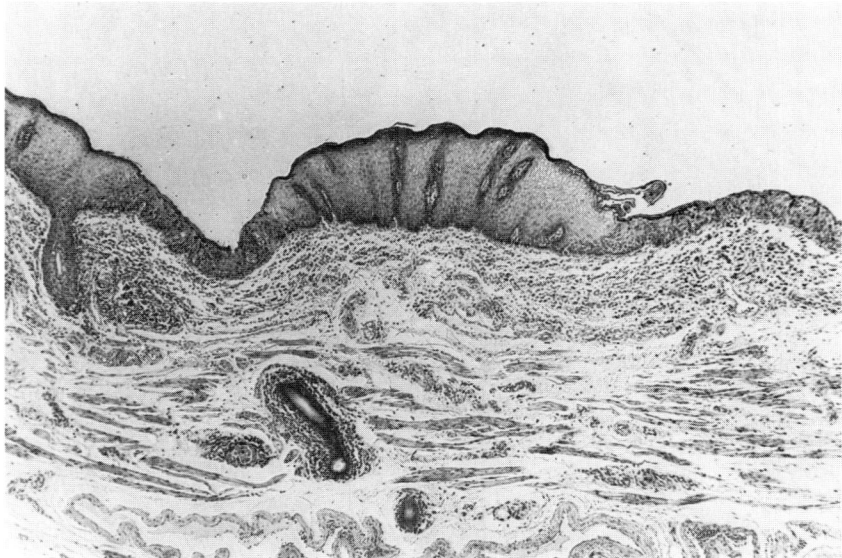

FIGURE 18–6. Multicentric carcinoma *in situ* in the mucosa adjacent to an advanced invasive squamous cell carcinoma of the esophagus. (× 40)

only form of carcinoma in 48 cases. In 36 other cases, it accompanied early invasive cancer. Carcinoma *in situ* is sometimes multicentric (Figure 18–6). These changes in the epithelium adjacent to a carcinoma probably represent stages of cancer development from simple hyperplasia through dysplasia to carcinoma *in situ*.

Hurlimann and Gardiol[43] described two types of high-grade dysplasia. One type was located deep in the epithelium. The cells had a pagetoid appearance and contained keratin of low molecular weight. The other type involved the whole thickness of the epithelium and contained keratin of the type present in the stratified epithelium. The former type was associated with undifferentiated carcinoma, whereas the latter type was related to differentiated squamous cell carcinoma.

Cytologic Classification

Dysplastic as well as cancer cells are readily recognized by cytologic examination, a method used extensively in mass surveys of esophageal cancer in China. According to Shen,[10] the epithelial cells of the esophageal mucosa seen in the cytologic smear are classified into five grades:

Grade I: Normal. The exfoliated cells of the esophagus in the normal situation are chiefly intermediate cells. Parabasal cells are rarely exfoliated, and basal cells usually are not.

Grade II: Mild dysplasia. There is a mild degree of hyperchromasia of the cells. The chromatin content of the nucleus is two to three times greater than in normal cells of the same layer. The chromatin granules are fine, and the nuclear membrane is not thickened.

Grade III: Severe dysplasia. The size of the nuclei in the dysplastic cells is three or more times larger than that in normal cells. Hyperchromasia is prominent. The chromatin granules become coarse but are fairly uniform. The nuclear membrane is slightly thickened but regular.

Grade IV: Near carcinoma. The nuclei are five or more times greater in size than those in the normal cell of the same layer. The nuclear membrane is thickened but still regular.

Grade V: Carcinoma. The diameter of the nucleus exceeds one third of the total diameter of the cell. The malignant features of the nuclei are very evident.

Additional discussions on the cytologic features of esophageal epithelial cells are presented in Chapter 4.

Follow-up Study

Severe dysplasia is the major precancerous lesion of the esophagus. Cytologic studies have indicated, however, that dysplasia is an unstable condition. In a series of over 500 patients with severe dysplasia with a follow-up period of up to 5 years, about 40% regressed to mild dysplasia or normal epithelium, about 20% progressed to cancer, and 20% remained unchanged. Shu and co-workers[44] followed 530 cases of severe dysplasia of the esophageal epithelium. During a follow-up period of 1 to 12 years, 79 patients (14.9%) developed cancer. In another group of 530 patients with mild esophageal hyperplasia who were followed for the same period of time, five cases of cancer (0.94%) were found. In a third group of patients who had only normal epithelial cells and were followed for 1 to 5 years, no carcinoma of esophagus developed. Thus, although reversible, severe dysplasia of the epithelium must be carefully followed so that carcinoma can be detected at an early stage.

PATHOLOGY

Location

In most reports, esophageal cancer is found most commonly in the mid third of the esophagus in about half of cases.[45] Similar results have been found in

Table 18–2 RELATIONSHIP BETWEEN GROSS MORPHOLOGIC AND HISTOLOGIC FEATURES IN EARLY ESOPHAGEAL CARCINOMA

Histologic Features	Gross Pathologic Features					
	Occult	Erosive	Plaque	Papillary	Total	%
Intraepithelial	11	22	14	1	48	32.0
Intramucosal	0	20	35	4	59	39.3
Submucosal	0	8	28	7	43	28.7
Total	11	50	77	12	150	100.0

China.[46] A method combining balloon cytology with esophagoscopy and x-ray examination has been used in diagnosing esophageal cancer in high-incidence areas in China. The site distribution is more likely to be accurate by this method. In a group of 3633 cases from Linxian Hospital,[47] the tumor was in the upper third of the esophagus in 426 (11.7%), the middle third in 2301 (63.3%), and the lower third in 906 (24.9%).

Early Esophageal Carcinoma

Esophageal carcinomas are often discovered late. The pathologic features of the early lesions have been known only since the 1960s, largely because of data accumulated in China.[42,48–50] An early esophageal carcinoma is defined as a tumor that has not extended beyond the submucosa and has not metastasized.

Gross Types

Four types of early esophageal carcinoma can be distinguished grossly: occult, erosive, plaque, and papillary. Their relative frequencies are listed in Table 18–2.

Occult Type. The mucosa in the cancerous area has the same thickness as the normal mucosa. In the fresh specimen, the diseased mucosa appears pink and congested. In the fixed specimen, the lesion is hardly perceptible to the naked eye (Figure 18–7). Early esophageal cancer of this type is rarely seen in the surgically resected specimens.

Erosive Type. The lesion is slightly depressed or mildly eroded. It has a maplike configuration with irregular margins that are sharply demarcated from the normal mucosa (Figure 18–8). The eroded area is finely granular, with occasional islets of normal mucosa. Superficial defects of the mucosa may be seen on the cut surface. This type is seen quite often among surgically resected specimens.

Plaque Type. The lesion is slightly elevated and has a coarse, granular surface that may show small areas of erosion (Figure 18–9). After fixation, the mucosa becomes pale, and both longitudinal and transverse rugae are interrupted. The lesion is often extensive and in some cases involves the whole circumference. On the cut surface the mucosa is markedly thickened in the region of the lesion. Most lesions of this type are located within the lamina propria, but in some cases the submucosa is involved. Most early esophageal carcinomas removed by surgery are of this type.

Papillary Type. The lesion presents as a papillary or polypoid protrusion, usually 1 to 3 cm in diameter (Figure 18–10). There is a clear demarcation between the edge of the lesion and the surrounding normal mucosa. On occasion, erosions covered with inflammatory exudate are present on the surface. On the cut surface the lesion protrudes toward the esophageal lumen and infiltrates the wall. Early esophageal cancer of this type is rare.

Liu and colleagues[42] analyzed 150 surgical specimens of early esophageal carcinoma. The lesions were

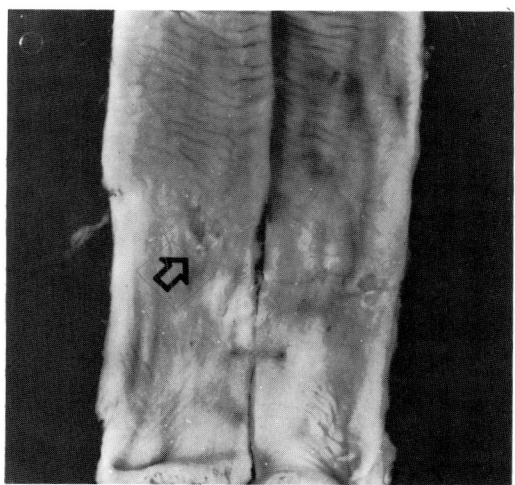

FIGURE 18–7. Early esophageal cancer, occult type. The lesion (arrow) is small, and its boundary is indistinct.

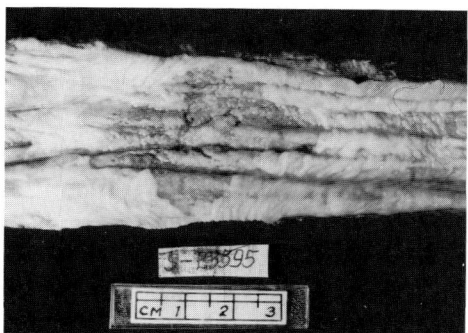

FIGURE 18–8. Early esophageal cancer, erosive type. The lesion is maplike, with irregular margins.

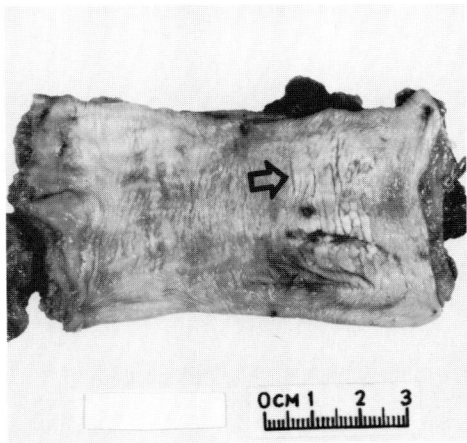

FIGURE 18-9. Early esophageal cancer, plaque type. The lesion (arrow) is slightly elevated and swollen, with a coarse, granular surface.

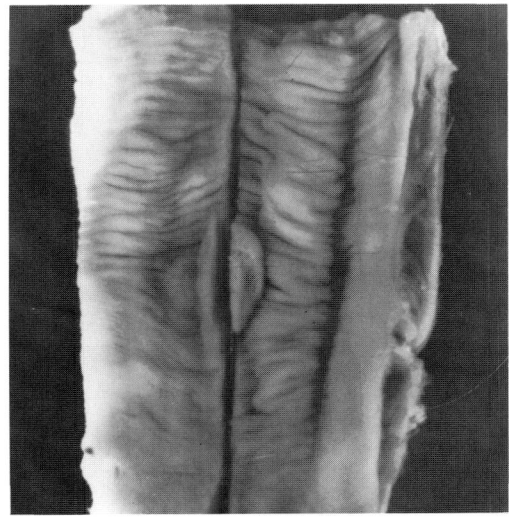

FIGURE 18-10. Early esophageal cancer, papillary type. The lesion presents as a small papillary mass protruding from the surface of the esophageal mucosa.

in the middle and lower portions of the esophagus in 148 cases (98.7%) and in the upper portion in only two cases (1.3%). The smallest tumor was 0.4 cm in diameter; the largest, 8.5 cm. Of the 11 occult lesions, nine were less than 1 cm in diameter, whereas most lesions of the other types were larger, ranging from 1 to 4 cm. Sugimachi and associates found 42 early cases among 370 esophageal carcinomas (11.4%).[51] Lymph node metastasis was present in six cases with submucosal lesions. Five patients died of recurrences.

Histologic Types

Histologically, the early esophageal carcinomas are classified into intraepithelial, intramucosal, and submucosal types. Their frequencies are shown in Table 18-2.

Intraepithelial Carcinoma (Carcinoma *in Situ*). These cancer cells occupy the entire thickness of esophageal epithelium, but the basement membrane remains intact (Figure 18-11). This type was seen in 48 of 150 cases (32.0%) studied by Liu and colleagues.[42] Glandular ducts were involved in 11 cases. According to the degree of differentiation and morphology of the cancer cells, subdivision into large-cell and small-cell carcinoma *in situ* can be made. In the large-cell type, the carcinomatous mucosa is thickened, and the cancer cells are large and well differentiated but evidently pleomorphic and arranged irregularly. Mitosis is frequently observed. This type of lesion is commonly seen in the plaque and papillary carcinomas. In the small-cell type, the cancerous mucosa is thin, and cancer cells are poorly differentiated, small, round, or spindle-shaped and contain scanty cytoplasm. The nuclei are hyperchromatic, and instances of mitosis are numerous. This type of lesion is often seen in the erosive carcinoma.

Intramucosal Carcinoma. This carcinoma develops when small groups of cancer cells escape from an in-

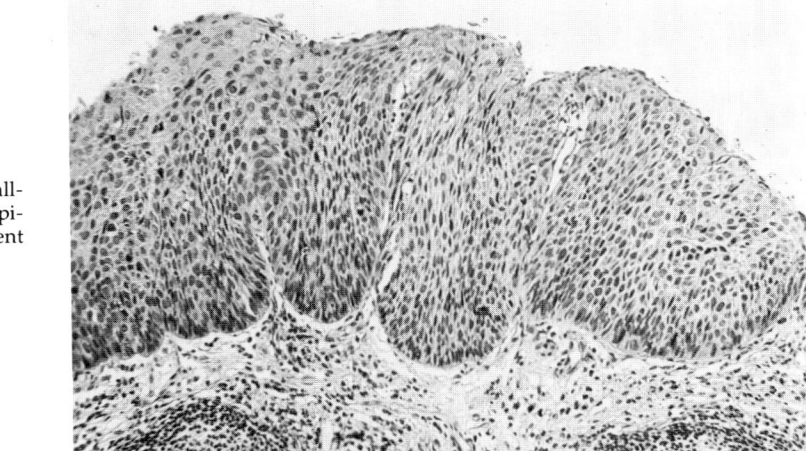

FIGURE 18-11. Squamous cell carcinoma *in situ*, small-cell type, of the esophagus. The entire thickness of epithelium is occupied by tumor cells, but the basement membrane is intact. ($\times$ 50)

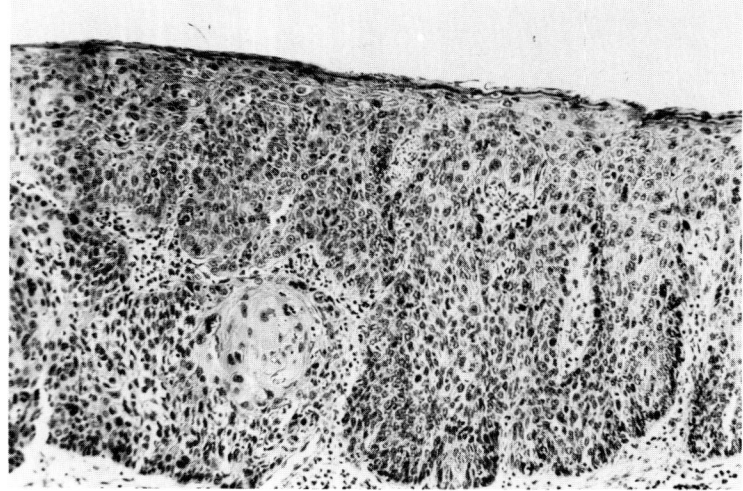

FIGURE 18-12. Intramucosal carcinoma of the esophagus. Groups of tumor cells have penetrated into the lamina propria. (× 150)

traepithelial carcinoma, penetrate the basement membrane, and infiltrate the lamina propria of the esophagus (Figure 18-12). The area of invasion is small and usually difficult to detect with the naked eye. It was seen in 59 cases (39.3%).[42]

Submucosal Carcinoma. In this type, the cancer cells have penetrated through the muscularis mucosa into the submucosa but have not reached the muscularis proper, and there are no metastases into the regional lymph nodes. This lesion is rather large, the area of invasion is wide, and there is an inflammatory reaction of variable degree around the lesion. It was seen in 43 cases (28.7%).[42]

The stroma beneath the early esophageal carcinoma shows varying degrees of chronic inflammation. Similar inflammatory reaction, but of different proportion, can often be observed in the lamina propria beneath the epithelium adjacent to the carcinoma.

Advanced Esophageal Carcinoma

Advanced carcinomas of the esophagus are usually nodular lesions with varying degrees of ulceration. Palmer[52] suggested that most esophageal cancers can be classified readily into four groups: polypoid, fungating, ulcerative, and infiltrating. This classification is similar to that proposed by Ming[45] except that the polypoid tumor is not listed separately in the latter because such a tumor without ulceration is extremely rare.

On the basis of the experience accumulated in China since 1960, researchers have formulated a classification of esophageal carcinoma that is as valuable clinically as it is pathologically.[53-56] We classified the advanced lesions into medullary, fungating, ulcerative, scirrhous, and intraluminal types.

Medullary Type. This type of cancer usually involves the whole thickness of the esophageal wall and most or all of its circumference (Figure 18-13). The involved segment is markedly thickened. The edges of the tumor are raised, and there is ulceration of varying depth on the surface of the solid tumor mass. The cut surface of the cancer is gray to white and has a homogeneous appearance. Under a microscope, the cancer cells appear to be arranged in clumps and sheets with various degrees of differentiation and with moderate or scanty connective tissue and a mild inflammatory reaction.

Fungating Type. This type of cancer is usually oval and protrudes into the lumen of the esophagus like a flat mushroom (Figure 18-14). The edges are well defined and raised. In most cases, the cancer does not involve the entire circumference of the esophagus. The cut surface shows that the cancer may infiltrate the whole thickness of the esophageal wall but seldom involves neighboring structures. Under a microscope, the cancer cells appear to be arranged in large patches with a moderate inflammatory reaction and connective tissue proliferation.

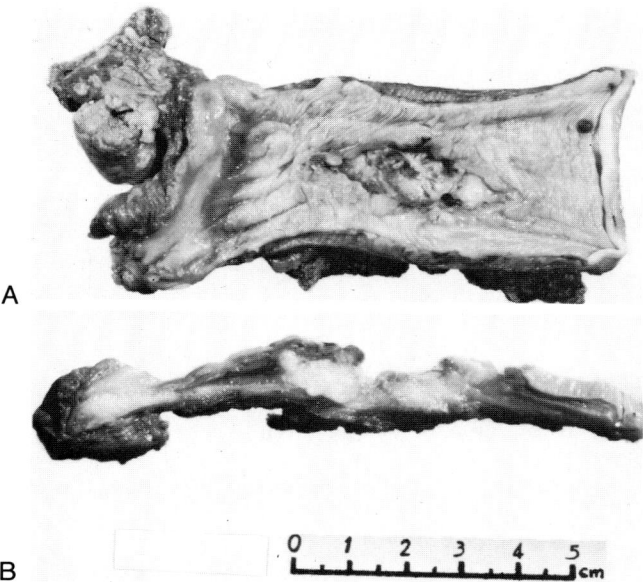

FIGURE 18-13. Esophageal carcinoma, medullary type. A, The edges of the tumor are raised, and an ulceration is present on the surface. B, The cut surface shows that the segment of esophageal wall occupied by the carcinoma is markedly thickened, with an ulceration in the center.

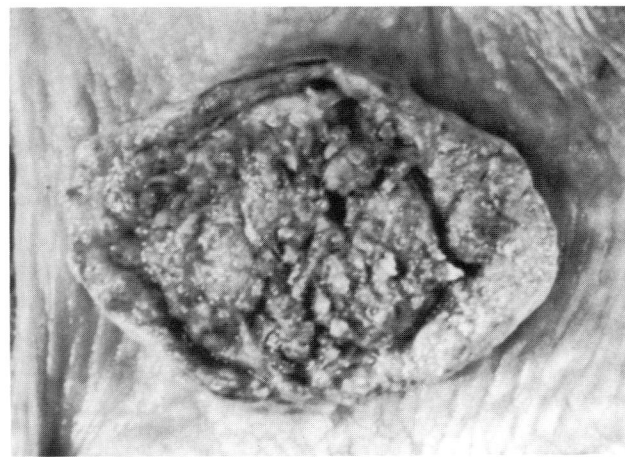

FIGURE 18-14. Esophageal carcinoma, fungating type. The tumor is oval and like a flat mushroom, protruding into the lumen of the esophagus.

Ulcerative Type. The lesion presents as an undermining ulcer and usually involves only a portion of the circumference of the esophagus (Figure 18-15). The edges of the ulcer may be slightly raised above the surface of the surrounding mucosa. The base penetrates deep into the muscular layer of the esophagus, often invading the periesophageal fibrous tissue and sometimes causing perforation of the esophagus. The surface of the ulcer may be covered with an abundant inflammatory exudate. Under a microscope, the cancer cells show a moderate degree of differentiation with relatively prominent inflammatory infiltration and connective tissue proliferation.

Scirrhous (Stenosing) Type. This type of cancer forms a short tubular structure that causes stenosis or

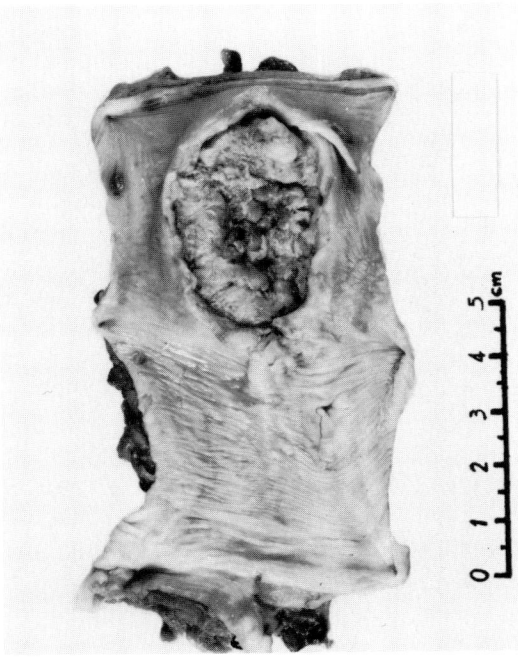

FIGURE 18-15. Esophageal carcinoma, ulcerative type. The lesion presents as a deeply penetrating ulcer.

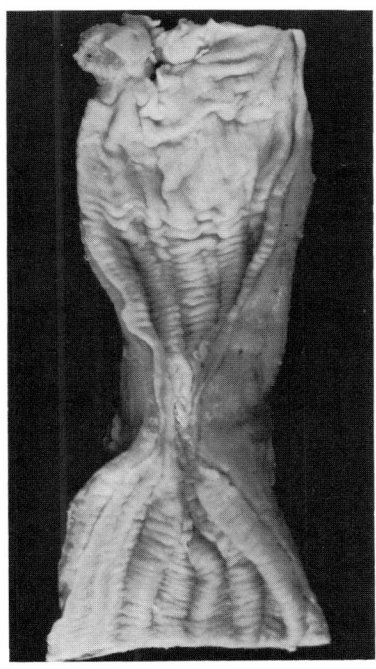

FIGURE 18-16. Esophageal carcinoma, scirrhous type. The tumor forms a short, tubular stenosis of the esophagus.

obstruction of the esophagus (Figure 18-16). The lesion almost always involves the whole circumference of the organ. The cancerous tissue infiltrates and gradually merges with the esophageal wall. After fixation, the mucosal surface shows prominent radiating rugae. Usually there is no ulceration, or only a few erosions. The stenosis is characteristically concentric and symmetric with marked dilatation about the lesion. The cut surface of the cancer shows dense tumor tissue mingled with fibrous tissue. Under a microscope, the cancer cells appear to be arranged in irregular strands with abundant connective tissue proliferation, deeply infiltrating the muscular layer of the esophagus and sometimes spreading beyond the normal boundary of the organ.

Intraluminal (Polypoid) Type. The oval or round mass of this type of tumor protrudes into the markedly dilated lumen of the esophagus (Figure 18-17). The

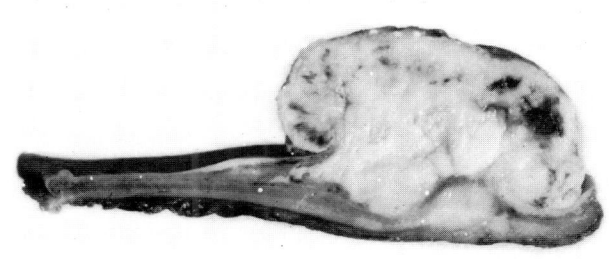

FIGURE 18-17. Esophageal carcinoma, intraluminar type. Cut surface shows an oval mass of tumor protruding into the lumen of the esophagus.

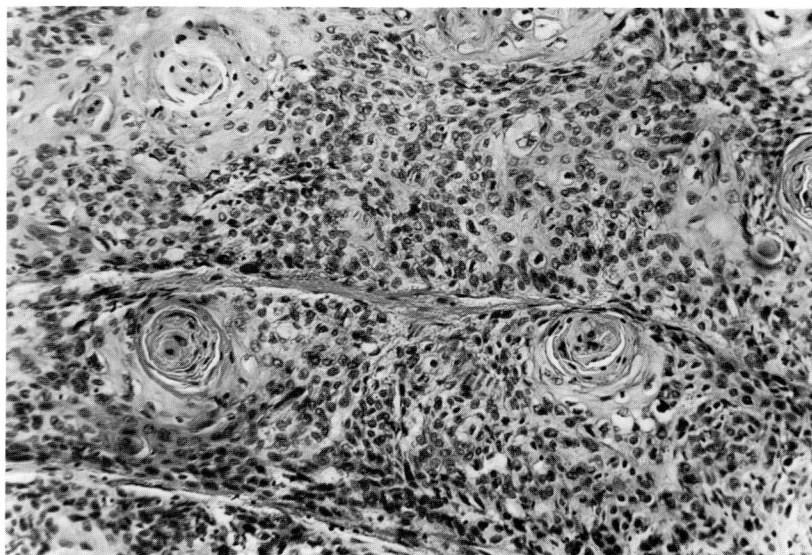

FIGURE 18-18. Grade I squamous cell carcinoma of the esophagus. The tumor cells with numerous pearl formations can be seen. (× 180)

base is usually broad, and there is often an erosion or a shallow, irregular ulceration on the surface of the tumor. Most of the cancer cells are poorly to moderately differentiated, with indistinct keratinization and intercellular bridges. The tumor sometimes infiltrates only a portion of the muscular layer. There are usually numerous blood vessels with only a mild inflammatory reaction in the stroma. Tumor emboli are often seen in both blood and lymph vessels. The gross appearance of this type is similar to that of carcinosarcoma. Histologically, however, they can be easily distinguished.

Huang and co-workers[56] found 27 intraluminal cases (about 2% of the total) among the esophageal carcinomas surgically resected between 1970 and 1980 in our institute. Twenty-three of the patients were male and only four were female. Histologically, there were 24 cases of squamous cell carcinoma, two of adenocarcinoma, and one of adenoacanthoma.

Sun and Wu[46] analyzed 444 surgical specimens of advanced esophageal carcinoma: 252 (56.8%) were medullary, 82 (18.5%) fungating, 59 (13.3%) ulcerative, 38 (8.6%) scirrhous, and 13 (2.9%) miscellaneous. In another analysis of the gross types of 397 surgical specimens,[57] there were 242 (61.0%) medullary, 48 (12.1%) fungating, 50 (12.6%) ulcerative, 22 (5.5%) scirrhous, 13 (3.3%) intraluminal, and 22 (5.5%) miscellaneous cases.

None of these types seem to have a predilection for any particular site. About half of the medullary carcinomas are more than 5 cm long, whereas most of the ulcerative and scirrhous types are shorter than 5 cm. Marked dysplasia is often observed in the scirrhous type, but ulcerative and fungating types are usually accompanied by only mild to moderate dysplasia. Scirrhous and medullary types have usually infiltrated the entire thickness of the esophageal wall by the time they are diagnosed, but the fungating type often infiltrates only part of the muscular layer. Patients who have the fungating and ulcerative types have a somewhat better prognosis than patients with other types.

In intraluminal carcinomas, the resectability rate is high, but long-term results are often poor.

The histologic morphology of the advanced carcinoma varies, depending on the degree of differentiation. A three-grade classification has been widely adopted in China. Its basic criteria are as follows:

Grade I: The cancer cells are well differentiated, large, polygonal, or round, with evident keratinization and intercellular bridges (Figure 18-18). Mitoses are not frequent.

Grade II: The cancer cells are rather large; of moderate differentiation; and round, oval, or polygonal, with a certain amount of pleomorphism. There may be moderate keratinization or a few epithelial pearls. Mitoses are often seen. Intercellular bridges usually can be found.

Grade III: Most of the tumor cells are spindle-shaped, ovoid, or irregular. They are small and have scanty cytoplasm (Figure 18-19). Mitoses are frequent. There is no keratinization or intercellular bridges. The lesion can still be recognized as squamous cell carcinoma and can be distinguished from undifferentiated carcinoma.

This three-grade classification is easy to apply. Liu[57] analyzed 417 resected specimens of squamous cell carcinoma of the esophagus and found the proportions of grades I, II, and III to be 26.1%, 65.3%, and 8.6%, respectively. Chen and Lin[58] studied 500 cases and found the proportions to be 24.4%, 64.8%, and 10.8%.

Variants of Squamous Cell Carcinoma

Verrucous Carcinoma

Verrucous carcinoma is rare in the esophagus. Agha and co-workers found only eight cases in the English literature.[59] It is characterized by an exophytic growth with a papillary surface. Histologically, the papillary

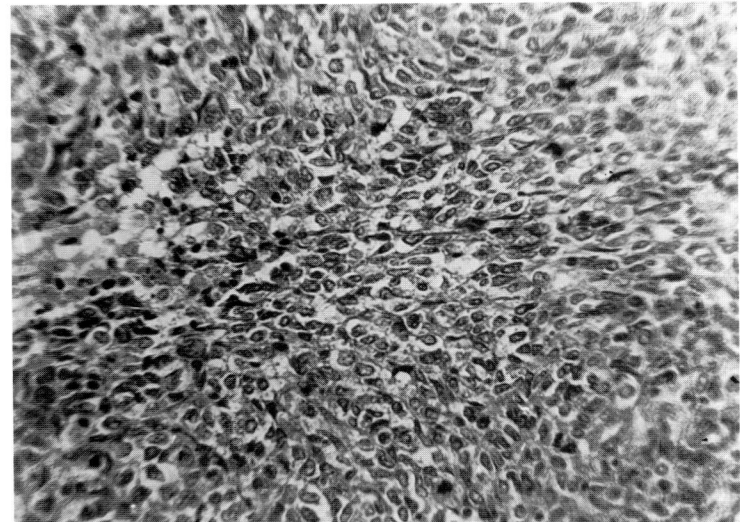

FIGURE 18-19. Grade III carcinoma of the esophagus. (× 100)

fronds are composed of moderately differentiated squamous cells supported by a core of delicate fibrous stroma.[45] The tumor grows and invades slowly, and metastasis is uncommon.[60,61]

Spindle Cell Carcinoma (Carcinosarcoma)

In this tumor some cells assume a spindle shape. Focal spindle cell components are not uncommon in an otherwise typical squamous tumor. In rare instances, the spindle cells constitute the major portion of the tumor. Such a tumor has been called carcinosarcoma or pseudosarcoma. As a result of electron-microscopic and immunohistochemical findings, it is now generally agreed that the "sarcomatous" cells are in fact squamous cells. Thus, the carcinosarcoma has been called polypoid carcinoma because the majority of these tumors are exophytic polypoid masses.[62] Liu and Zhang reviewed nine such cases.[63] Most of these tumors are large and polypoid, with a rather long and slender pedicle. The surface either is smooth and intact or has only scattered small and shallow ulcers (Figure 18-20). The cut surface is like fish flesh. Under a microscope, the tumor appears to be composed mainly of spindle cells, whereas the ordinary squamous cells often appear only as a preinvasive lesion and may be found only at the base of the mass or in the mucosa adjacent to the pedicle. This tumor is further discussed in Chapter 19.

Staging

Clinicopathologic staging of esophageal cancer is very important in planning treatment and in evaluating treatment results.

The TNM Staging System of the American Joint Committee on Cancer.[64] This system is based on the features of the primary tumor (T), the extent of lymph node involvement (N), and the presence or absence of distant metastasis (M). Postsurgical resection–pathologic (pTNM) staging is based on the pathologic features of the resected specimen and on data available at the time of surgery. The system is summarized in Table 18-3.

The Clinicopathologic Staging System Used in China.[65] This system was established in 1979. The clinical staging of esophageal cancer in China is based on clinical and roentgenographic findings. When pathologic findings are available, the staging is based chiefly on the extent of tumor invasion and metastases. In the latter situation, when the tumor is confined to the mucosa (carcinoma *in situ*), it is in stage 0. When the tumor has invaded submucosa, it is in stage I. When the tumor has invaded superficial muscularis propria, it is stage II. In stages 0, I, and II, there is no lymph node metastasis. When the cancer has invaded the lymph node, it is classified as stage III. When distal metastasis is present, it is stage IV. In this system, the esophageal carcinoma of stage 0 or I is "early"; stage II or III, "intermediate"; and stage IV, "late." In late cases there are often severe complications. Of 976

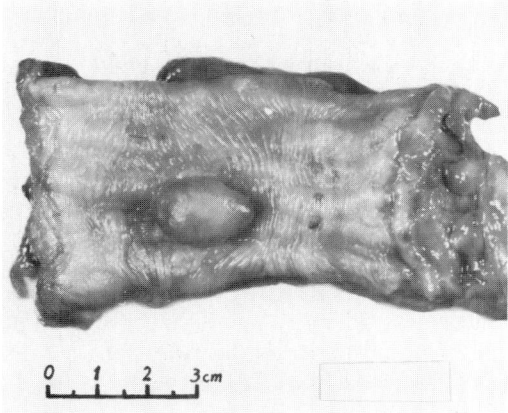

FIGURE 18-20. Carcinosarcoma of the esophagus. The tumor is polypoid, and the surface is smooth.

Table 18-3 TNM CLASSIFICATION OF ESOPHAGEAL CANCER BY THE AMERICAN JOINT COMMITTEE ON CANCER[64]

Stage	Primary Tumor (T)*	Lymph Nodes (N)†	Distant Metastasis (M)‡
0	T_{is}	N_0	M_0
I	T_1	N_0	M_0
IIA	T_2	N_0	M_0
	T_3	N_0	M_0
IIB	T_1	N_1	M_0
	T_2	N_1	M_0
III	T_3	N_1	M_0
	T_4	Any N	M_0
IV	Any T	Any N	M_1

*T_{is}, carcinoma in situ; T_1, invasion of lamina propria or submucosa; T_2, invasion of muscularis propria; T_3, invasion of adventitia; T_4, invasion of adjacent structures.
†N_0, no metastases; N_1, regional lymph node metastasis.
‡M_0, distant metastasis absent; M_1, distant metastasis present.

cases reported by Huang and coauthors,[66] the representative percentages of cases in stages I through IV were 0.6, 22.3, 72.4, and 4.6.

Spread and Metastasis

Squamous esophageal carcinomas spread and metastasize basically in the following four ways.

Intramural Spread. Esophageal carcinoma may spread vertically by deep infiltration into the esophageal wall and the surrounding tissue or horizontally along the plane of the muscular layer to form nodules imitating separate primary tumors. Such secondary lesions may be 5 to 6 cm from the parent tumor. Some authors have stated that some cases of carcinoma *in situ* in which the carcinomatous cells in the basal layer of the epithelium adjacent to the principal tumor end abruptly when they meet the normal epithelium may be the result of this type of tumor spread.[41]

Soga and colleagues[67] applied the term *superficial spreading type* to the carcinomas showing intramucosal extension of the tumor 20 mm or more beyond the main lesion. The incidence was 6.1%. Metastasis to the lymph node was high in these tumors, in half of the early cases and in all of the advanced cases.

Contiguous Involvement of Neighboring Organs. Esophageal cancers very often invade neighboring organs by contiguous extension. Depending on the location of the tumor, various organs may be involved with different frequency. Thus, carcinoma in the upper segment of the esophagus may invade the larynx, the trachea, and the soft tissues of the neck. Tumors of the middle part may invade the bronchi and lung; erode and perforate the aorta, causing fatal hemorrhage; or involve the thoracic duct, the azygos vein, or the hila of the lungs. Tumors of the lower segment may involve the pericardium, diaphragm, and gastric cardia. Fistulous tracts may form along the cancerous tissue and cause fatal infectious inflammation in the mediastinum or the lung.

Lymphatic Spread. The tumor may penetrate into the lymphatic vessels in the submucosa or deeper layers of the esophageal wall. Spread by means of the lymphatics occurs frequently and early in esophageal carcinoma. However, in a small number of patients metastasis is absent even in the late stage of the disease. Most metastatic lesions are limited to the intrathoracic lymph nodes, but it should be pointed out that "jumping" metastasis to the neck or abdominal lymph nodes without intrathoracic involvement has been observed in as many as 24% of cases.[68,69] It is probable, however, that hidden microscopic metastasis may be revealed by meticulous microscopic examination of the intrathoracic nodes. The reported frequency of lymph node metastasis varies, depending on the stage of the disease. In our own experience dealing with surgically resected specimens, metastasis was present in 42% of the cases. In the 2440 autopsy cases compiled by Postlethwait and Sealy,[1] lymph node metastasis was present in 1648 (67%). The most commonly involved nodes, in decreasing frequency, were mediastinal, abdominal, paratracheal, paraesophageal, cervical, and supraclavicular.

Hematogeneous Metastasis. Distant metastases are common at autopsy. The most commonly involved organs are the liver and the lung, each in about 20% to 30% of cases.[45,70,71] However, in our own materials, 26 of 41 autopsy cases had no distant metastasis.[72]

Pathologic Factors Affecting Prognosis

Stage. The stage of esophageal cancer at the time of diagnosis has the most significant prognostic value. In an analysis of 522 cases treated with resection,[57] the 3- and 5-year survival rates in the group of patients with cancer infiltrating only a portion of the muscular layer of the esophagus (stage II) were 45.5% and 40.4%, respectively; whereas in the group with cancer penetrating beyond the esophageal wall (stage III), the rates were 31.8% and 24.4%. Huang and coauthors[66] reported the results of surgical treatment for esophageal carcinoma; the 5-year survival rates of pTNM stages I, II, III, and IV cases were 83.3% (5/6), 46.3% (101/218), 26.4% (187/707), and 6.7% (3/45), respectively. The 5-year survival rates of patients with early esophageal carcinoma are much better than those of patients with advanced invasive carcinoma; Endo and coauthors[73] reported a 64% survival rate (18/28); Huang and associates,[50] 85.9%; and Liu and colleagues,[42] 85.5% (59/69).

The presence or absence of lymph node metastases clearly affects the course and prognosis of the disease. The 5-year survival rate of patients without lymph node metastases is about three times that of patients with lymph node metastases.[66,73]

Location. One important mode of tumor spread is contiguous involvement of neighboring organs. It is evident that the nature of the organ so invaded would influence the curability of the lesion. This situation is unique for the esophageal cancer. For instance, carcinoma of the midthoracic esophagus may penetrate into trachea and lung to produce a fistula and persistent infection or may invade and rupture the aorta to cause fatal bleeding. Furthermore, the nature of neighboring organs may influence the feasibility of intensive radiotherapy.

Growth Pattern. Sun and Wu[74] found that of 56 cases with a sheetlike growth pattern, 35 survived longer than 5 years and 21 died within 2 years after surgery and that of 44 patients with thin strand growth pattern, 29 died within 2 years and only 15 survived for 5 years. Furthermore, in patients who died within 2 years, the periphery of the tumor often showed wide infiltration; whereas in patients living longer than 5 years, the periphery of the tumor tissue showed degeneration.

Size. Some data indicate that the smaller the cancer is, the better the prognosis.[75] The differences among cases with tumors larger than 6 cm are small, however.[73,75] Huang and coauthors[66] found that patients with tumors smaller than 3 cm had a 5-year survival rate of 48%, whereas that of patients with larger tumors was only 28.9%.

Histologic Grade. Opinions on the relationship between histologic grade and prognosis vary widely among authors. Wu and coworkers[76] found the 5-year survival rates in grades I, II, and III were 40% (6/15), 20.5% (8/39), and 20% (3/15), respectively, and claimed that a definite relationship existed. Liu[57] reported that in a series of 417 cases, the corresponding rates were 38.2% (34/89), 23.7% (54/228), and 33.3% (9/27). Nick and associates[77] and Younghusband and Aluwihare[78] found no significant influence of grading of tumors on survival time. Giuli and Gignoux[79] reported that undifferentiated or poorly differentiated squamous cell carcinoma paradoxically had a somewhat better long-term prognosis than the well-differentiated tumors. These results suggest that one may expect a better prognosis for well-differentiated tumors, but the relationship between the degrees of differentiation and prognosis is not consistent.

Stromal Reaction. Younghusband and Aluwihare[78] noted that the host immune reactions against the tumor, such as sinus histiocytosis and follicular hyperplasia in the lymph nodes and lymphocytic infiltration in the tumor, had a favorable influence on the survival of the patient.

Ploidy of Carcinoma Cells. Measurement of DNA content by flow cytometry showed that about 70% of esophageal carcinomas were aneuploid.[80,81] Yu and associates found that the aneuploid tumors were poorly differentiated and in the advanced stage and had more lymph node metastases and invasion than the euploid tumors.[80] A similar view was expressed by others.[82] On the other hand, Ruol and colleagues[81] found no such relationship and that the slightly better survival rate of euploid tumors was not statistically significant.

CLINICOPATHOLOGIC CORRELATION

Clinical Presentation and Diagnosis

The symptoms of early esophageal cancer are mild in the majority of patients and usually related to deglutition. They consist of retrosternal discomfort or pain and a sense of friction, burning, or slow passage of the food. The diagnosis of early cancer is based chiefly on exfoliative cytology and x-ray examination, rather than specific symptoms. There is usually a period of several years of vague symptoms before diagnosis by cytologic examination. In the later stage most patients have varying degrees of dysphagia. Dysphagia is intermittent at first, when the patient swallows solid or coarse food. Several weeks later, it becomes persistent; then the patient prefers liquid food. The dysphagia is related to the pathologic type of the tumor and the level of its location. In late cases, the patient has extreme cachexia and dehydration. Other symptoms depend on the extent of tumor invasion and the types of organs secondarily involved.

Complications and Causes of Death

Serious complications often occur in patients with esophageal carcinoma. In an autopsy analysis of 41 cases,[72] pneumonia and lung abscess were present in 28, chronic pleuritis and emphysema in 27, hydrothorax in 14, hydropericardium in 7, mediastinitis in 6, empyema in 6, ascites in 4, splenic abscess in 2, pulmonary thrombosis in 1, and subacute endocarditis in 1. Esophageal fistulas communicating with neighboring organs were found in 24 patients and anastomotic leakage in 3. In 13 cases, the fistulas involved the aorta (Figure 18–21). Palmer[52] summarized six reports of a total of 630 cases of esophageal carcinoma and found perforation in 152 cases, affecting the tracheobronchial tree in 112.

Most patients with untreated esophageal carcinoma die eventually of serious complications; some, of cachexia.[83] Infection in the neighboring organs, particularly the lung, is a common cause of death, as noted previously.

Several reports have been published on fatal hemorrhage caused by esophageal cancer. Airenga[84] reported 4 cases and reviewed 99 others from the literature. Aortoesophageal fistula was the cause of fatal

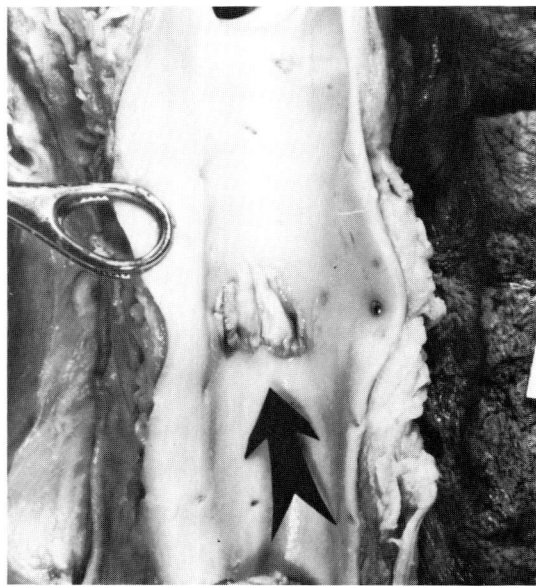

FIGURE 18–21. Perforation of aorta caused by invasion from metastatic esophageal cancer in the mediastinal lymph node.

hemorrhage in 78 of these cases. There were 13 such cases in our own materials.[72] Possible reasons for aortic rupture include radiation injury, infection, and thrombosis of the vasa vasorum leading to necrosis of the aortic wall.[85–88] Liu[72] found severe lesions in the intima, media, and adventitia at the perforation site of the irradiated aorta, but not in the nonperforated tissue. All authors have noted that the tumor cells infiltrate only the aortic adventitia, never invading the media and intima. It is probable that the cancerous adhesion of the esophagus to aortic adventitia, the inflammatory reaction and the vasculitis of vasa vasorum in the adventitia, rather than radiation damage alone, lead to severe ischemia of the aortic wall, which can no longer withstand the high pressure of blood from inside and eventually ruptures.

Treatment

Surgical Resection

In China, the first successful esophageal resection was performed in 1940. Extensive clinical experience has been accumulated. Since the use of cytologic examinations in mass surveys, many early esophageal cancers have been found. At the Linxian Hospital, the 5-year postoperative survival rate for early cancer patients was more than 85% and for patients with relatively late cancer, 44%. The 5-year survival rate for early cancer after radiotherapy alone was 61%. Thus, radical resection is most effective for the early cases.

Radiation Therapy

For the late cases, the combination of preoperative irradiation and surgery is now well accepted. The advanced cases, particularly if the tumor has metastasized to other organs or distant lymph nodes when first seen in the clinic, are not suitable for operation but can be treated by radiotherapy. Among 9104 patients admitted for the treatment of esophageal cancer from 1958 to 1980 at our institute, only 1798 (19.8%) were operated upon: 947 by surgery alone, 692 by preoperative irradiation and surgery, and 159 by surgery and postoperative irradiation. Of the other patients, 6501 (71.4%) were treated by irradiation alone and 805 (8.8%) by chemotherapy. The 5-year survival rate after treatment with combined preoperative radiotherapy and surgery was 31.6%.[89] Although the 5-year survival rate was only 8.4% after radiotherapy alone in the late advanced cases, the radiotherapy lengthened the lives of some patients.[90] Chemotherapy alone was not effective.

Postirradiation Pathologic Changes

Because many patients are treated with radiotherapy, knowledge of tissue changes following irradiation is important for assessment of the effectiveness of the treatment.

Factors Affecting Morphologic Changes

The postirradiation morphology of esophageal carcinoma may be influenced by a number of factors. For example, external and intracavitary irradiation may have disparate effects, and different dose levels may cause different morphologic changes. Undifferentiated carcinomas are markedly radiosensitive; squamous cell carcinomas, moderately so; and adenocarcinoma, relatively resistant. As a rule, the less differentiated the tumor cells, the more sensitive is the tumor to irradiation. Tumor tissue with a rich blood supply reacts more sensitively to irradiation. The morphologic changes are also more pronounced in specimens taken some time subsequent to irradiation than in those taken shortly afterward. The main tumor in the invasive carcinoma of the esophagus is more sensitive to external irradiation than the *in situ* and superficial carcinoma in the adjacent area.

Radiation-Induced Tissue Changes

The reaction of esophageal carcinoma to irradiation consists of three consecutive but overlapping stages.[91] In the initial stage of tissue injury, the major features are degeneration and necrosis of tumor cells. The second stage of removal of necrotic tissue is characterized mainly by granulation tissue formation, inflammatory infiltration, and the presence of foreign body giant cells. The final stage of repair is marked mainly by the presence of granulation tissue, fibroblastic proliferation, and scar formation.

Radiation changes in the tumor cells occur in both the nuclei and the cytoplasm. Acute irradiation at high dosage often causes necrosis of tumor cells. The nuclei are ruptured and cell debris is scattered in the tumor matrix. However, repeated irradiation at low doses may cause a series of changes of different degrees. The cells are swollen and irregular. The structure of the nucleus becomes indistinct and later becomes transparent and resembles a bull's-eye. The chromatin becomes coarse, unevenly distributed, and, later, aggregate near the nuclear envelope. Sometimes the nucleoli disappear. In the cytoplasm acidophilic bodies may be noted. Cytoplasmic vacuoles are often present in which may be found Sudan-III–positive or mucinous material. In more severely damaged tumor tissue, the cells may be pyknotic, swollen, or balloon-like. Large clusters of keratinized material may be present. Mononuclear and multinucleate bizarre tumor cells can frequently be observed.

In China, some patients were treated with intraluminal radiotherapy with ^{60}Co. A number of patients had resection of the tumor-bearing portion after irradiation. Liu and Lin[92] have studied 29 such specimens. Grossly, the tumors revealed characteristic annular ulceration. The surface was grayish white to grayish yellow and frequently covered with a pseudomembrane, the border was distinct, hyperemic, and edematous. In 7 cases, however, the tumor was rather large, and there was no annular ulceration. Microscopically, all 29 cases showed degeneration and necrosis of tumor cells and a certain stromal reaction. The degree of degenerative changes varied in different layers of the esophageal wall. The most remarkable changes of tumor cells were seen in the mucosa and submucosa. In five patients, four of whom had early cancer, no viable carcinoma could be detected, indicating that intraluminal irradiation was effective in the treatment of the early lesion.

Grading of Radiation-Induced Pathologic Changes

After analyzing 250 resected specimens of preoperatively irradiated esophageal carcinoma, Liu[57] classified the radiation changes into three grades (grade II and III reactions are associated with a better prognosis):

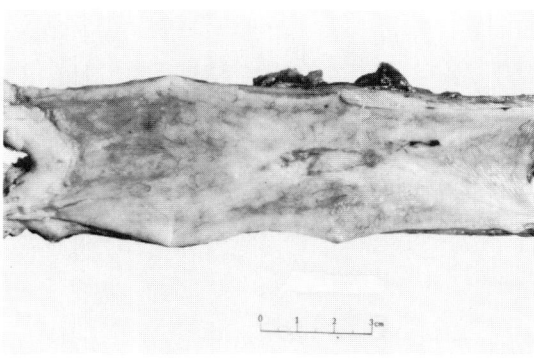

FIGURE 18–22. Squamous cell carcinoma of the esophagus after radiotherapy. The postradiation reaction was grade II. The tumor size had been reduced considerably.

Grade I: Mild reaction. Grossly, tumor size remains the same or decreases only slightly. Microscopically, only a portion of the tumor cells are degenerated, many others remaining intact. Inflammatory infiltration is not pronounced.

Grade II: Moderate reaction. Grossly, tumor size is greatly reduced and tumor contours are blurred (Figure 18–22). The ulceration becomes shallow and may disappear. On the cut surface, the tumor tissue is grayish red or brownish red, and the border is obscured. Microscopically, the majority of tumor cells have disappeared and the remaining degenerated tumor cells are surrounded by fibrous tissue, keratin, cholesterol crystals, and calcification (Figure 18–23). Foreign body giant cells and neutrophils can be observed in the tumor matrix, and capillaries are abundant. Late in this stage, inflammatory infiltration may be reduced, and fibrous tissue proliferates.

Grade III: Marked reaction. Grossly, no obvious tumor is seen, but occasionally a small, shallow ulceration may be present (Figure 18–24). On the cut surface, the esophageal wall is thin, and its structure is obscured. Microscopically, no tumor cells can be found.

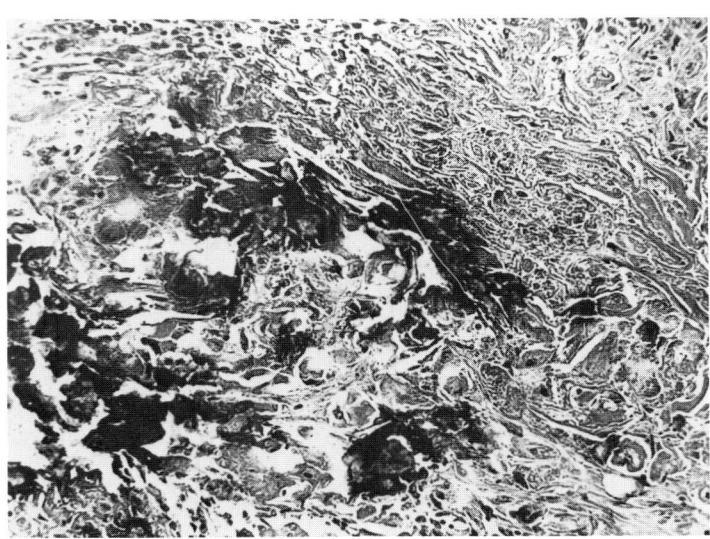

FIGURE 18–23. Squamous cell carcinoma of the esophagus after irradiation. Calcification can be seen in the midst of keratinized material. ($\times$ 200)

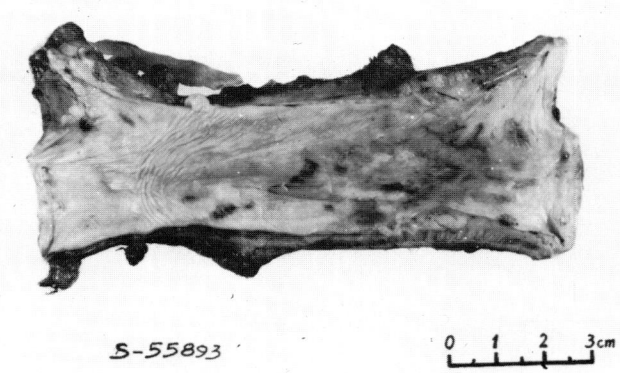

FIGURE 18-24. Squamous cell carcinoma of the esophagus, radiation reaction grade III. Grossly, no obvious tumor or ulceration can be seen.

There is fibrosis or scar formation in the tumor bed, and the surface is lined by a thin layer of squamous epithelium.

The degree of tissue reaction is proportional to the radiation dose.[89] Among Liu's 250 cases mentioned above,[57] all 22 tumors irradiated with less than 1500 rads showed grade I changes. Of the 41 lesions receiving over 5000 rads, 20 showed grade III alterations, and 15 had grade II changes. The 5-year survival rate is 22.3% for grade I changes, 32.4% for grade II, and 37.8% for grade III. The findings indicate that the long-term survival of patients with esophageal cancer may be improved by preoperative radiotherapy.[93]

References

1. Postlethwait RW, Sealy WC: Surgery of the Esophagus. New York, Appleton-Century-Crofts, 1979, p 348.
2. Li KH, Kao JC, Wu YK: A survey of the prevalence of carcinoma of the esophagus in North China. In The Chinese Academy of Medical Sciences (ed): Selected Papers on Cancer Research. Shanghai, Shanghai Scientific and Technical Publishers, 1962, p 215.
3. Kiviranta UK: Carcinoma of the esophagus: Its incidence, age and sex distribution and prognosis in Finland. Acta Otolaryngol 42:73-88, 1952.
4. The Coordinating Group for Research on the Etiology of Esophageal Cancer in North China: The epidemiology and etiology of esophageal cancer in North China: A preliminary report. Chin Med J 1:167-183, 1975.
5. Liu BQ, Li B: Epidemiology of carcinoma of the esophagus in China. In Huang GJ, Wu YK (eds): Carcinoma of the Esophagus and Gastric Cardia. Berlin, Springer-Verlag, 1984, p 4.
6. Silverberg E, Lubera JA: Cancer statistics, 1989. CA 39:3-20, 1989.
7. Garfinkel L, Poindexter CE, Silverberg E: Cancer in black Americans. CA 30:39-44, 1980.
8. Mannell A, Murray W: Oesophageal cancer in South Africa: A review of 1926 cases. Cancer 64:2604-2608, 1989.
9. Cancer Prevention and Treatment Research Center of the Ministry of Health: Research investigation on the mortality from malignant tumors in China [in Chinese]. Beijing, People's Health Press, 1979, p 96.
10. Shen Q: Diagnostic cytology and early detection. In Huang CJ, Wu YK (eds): Carcinoma of the Esophagus and Gastric Cardia. Berlin, Springer-Verlag, 1984, p 157.
11. King H, Huensel W: Cancer mortality among foreign and native-born Chinese in the United States. J Chron Dis 26:623-646, 1973.
12. Department of Pathology, Cancer Institute, Chinese Academy of Medical Sciences: Epidemiology and pathology of cancer of the pharynx and esophagus in the chicken [in Chinese]. Cancer Res Prev Treat (Beijing) 3:6-12, 1976.
13. Zheng SF, Qin QS, Li AL, Liu XF: A study on urinary excretion of test-dose riboflavin in peasants of Linxian County [in Chinese]. Chin J Prev Treat 15:300, 1981.
14. Lin PZ: Effect of riboflavin deficiency and high dose of vitamin C on tumor development in the esophagus and liver in rats. Chung Hua Chung Liu Tsa Chih 7:171-174, 1985.
15. Burrell RJW, Roach WA, Shadwell A: Esophageal cancer in the Bantu of the Transkei associated with mineral deficiency in garden plants. J Natl Cancer Inst 36:201-209, 1966.
16. Nemenko BA, Moldakuloba MM, Zorina SN: Esophageal cancer incidence in Guryer Province depending on mineral water content [in Russian]. Vopr Onkol 9:75-76, 1976.
17. Department of Chemical Etiology and Carcinogenesis, Cancer Institute, Chinese Academy of Medical Sciences: Analysis of molybdenum in serum, urine and hair samples of the inhabitants in high and low-incidence areas of esophageal cancer [in Chinese]. Cancer Res Prev Treat (Beijing) 4:19-25, 1978.
18. Follis RH Jr, Day HG, McCullum EV: Histological studies of rats fed a diet extremely low in zinc. J Nutr 22:223-237, 1941.
19. Li MH, Lu SH, Ji C, et al: Experimental studies on the carcinogenicity of fungus-contaminated food from Linxian County. Proc 10th Int Symp Princes Takamatsu Cancer Res Fund, Tokyo, 1980, pp 139-148.
20. Li MX, Cheng SJ: Etiology of carcinoma of the esophagus. In Huang GJ, Wu YK (eds): Carcinoma of the Esophagus and Gastric Cardia. Berlin, Springer-Verlag, 1984, p 40.
21. Cheng SJ, Ziang YZ, Li MH, Lo HZ: A mutagenic metabolite produced by Fusarium moniliforme isolated from Linxian County, China. Carcinogenesis 6:903-905, 1985.
22. Xia QJ: Carcinogenesis in the esophagus. In Huang, GJ, Wu YK (eds): Carcinoma of the Esophagus and Gastric Cardia. Berlin, Springer-Verlag, 1984, p 54.
23. Ming SC: Precancerous states of the esophagus and stomach. In Carter RL (ed): Precancerous States. London, Oxford University Press, 1984, p 192.
24. Tuyas AJ, Pequignot G, Gignoux M, Valla A: Cancers of the digestive tract, alcohol and tobacco. Int J Cancer 30:9-11, 1982.
25. Tuyas AJ, Gricuite LL: Carcinogenic substances in alcoholic beverage. Excerpta Med Int Congr Ser 484:130, 1980.
26. Ackerman LV, Weinstein IB, Kaplan HS: Cancer of the esophagus. In Kaplan HS, Tsuchitani PJ (eds): Cancer in China. New York, Alan R. Liss, 1978, pp 111-136.
27. Ghadirian P: Familial history of esophageal cancer. Cancer 58:2112-2116, 1985.
28. Harper PS, Harper RMJ, Howell-Evans AW: Carcinoma of the esophagus with tylosis. Quart J Med 38:317-333, 1970.
29. Monuz N, Crespi M, Grassi A, et al: Precursor lesions of esophageal cancer in high risk populations in Iran and China. Lancet 1:876-879, 1982.
30. Ellis FG: The aetiology and treatment of achalasia of the cardia. Ann Roy Coll Surg Engl 30:155-182, 1962.
31. Chuong JJ, DuBovik S, McCallum RW: Achalasia as a risk factor for esophageal carcinoma: A reappraisal. Dig Dis Sci 29:1105-1108, 1984.
32. Hoplins RA, Postlethwait RW: Caustic burns and carcinoma of the esophagus. Ann Surg 194:146-148, 1981.
33. Wright RS, Hurwitz AL: Relationships of hiatal hernia to endoscopically proven reflux esophagitis. Dig Dis Sci 24:311-313, 1979.
34. Adler RH, Rodriquez J: The association of hiatus hernia and gastroesophageal malignancy. J Thorac Cardiovasc Surg 37:553-569, 1959.
35. Kuylenstierna R, Munck-Wikland E: Esophagitis and cancer of the esophagus. Cancer 56:837-839, 1985.
36. Wynder EL, Hultberg S, Jacobsson F, Bross IJ: Environmental factors in cancer of the upper alimentary tract: A Swedish study with special reference to Plummer-Vinson (Paterson-Kelly) syndrome. Cancer 10:470-487, 1957.
37. Wychulis AR, Gunnlaugsson GH, Claggett OT: Carcinoma oc-

curring in pharyngoesophageal diverticulum: Report of three cases. Surgery 66:976–979, 1969.
38. Holmes GKT, Stokes PL, Sorahan TM, et al: Coeliac disease, gluten-free diet and malignancy. Gut 17:612–619, 1976.
39. Colina F, Solis JA, Munoz MT: Squamous papilloma of the esophagus. Am J Gastroenterol 74:410–414, 1980.
40. Liu FS, Zhou CN: Pathology of carcinoma of the esophagus. In Huang GJ, Wu YK (eds): Carcinoma of the Esophagus and Gastric Cardia. Berlin, Springer-Verlag, 1984, p 89.
41. Ming SC: Tumors of the esophagus and stomach, Series 2, Supplement. Washington, DC, Armed Forces Institute of Pathology, 1985, pp S2–S8.
42. Liu FS, Li L, Qu SL: Clinical and pathological characteristics of early esophageal cancer. Clin Oncol 1:539–557, 1982.
43. Hurlimann J, Gardiol D: Immunohistochemistry of dysplasias and carcinomas of the esophageal epithelium. Pathol Res Pract 184:567–576, 1989.
44. Shu YJ, Yuan XQ, Jin SP: Further investigation of the relationship between dysplasia and cancer of the esophagus [in Chinese]. Chin Med J 1:39–41, 1981.
45. Ming SC: Tumors of the esophagus and stomach, Series 2. Washington, DC, Armed Forces Institute of Pathology, 1973, pp 29–43.
46. Sun SQ, Wu X: Pathology of carcinoma of the esophagus. In Wu YK, Huang GJ (eds): Carcinoma of the Esophagus and Gastric Cardia [in Chinese]. Shanghai, Shanghai Scientific and Technical Publishers, 1965, p 35.
47. Liu FS: Pathology of the esophageal cancer [in Chinese]. Cancer Res Prev Treat (Beijing) 3:74–83, 1976.
48. The Coordinating Group for Cancer Research of Henen Province and Linxian County Hospital: The early diagnosis of esophageal cancer [in Chinese]. Beijing, People's Medical Publishing House, 1973, p 70.
49. The Coordinating Group for Research on Esophageal Carcinoma, Chinese Academy of Medical Sciences in Henen Province: Early detection of carcinoma of the esophagus [in Chinese]. Natl Med J China 53:451–453, 1973.
50. Huang GJ, Shao LF, Zhang DW: Diagnosis and surgical treatment of early esophageal carcinoma. Chin Med J 94:229–232, 1981.
51. Sugimachi K, Ohno S, Matsuda H, et al: Clinicopathologic study of early stage esophageal carcinoma. Br J Surg 76:759–763, 1989.
52. Palmer ED: The Esophagus and Its Diseases. London, Cassell, 1952, p 375.
53. Wu YK, Liu Y, Hu MH: The classification of types of carcinoma of the esophagus [in Chinese]. Natl Med J China 76:213–228, 1958.
54. Sun SQ, Yu PL, Tang J: A study on the incidence rate, sex and age distribution and classification of esophageal cancer [in Chinese]. Chin J Pathol 6:81–87, 1960.
55. Wu X, Liu YE, Liu YW, Wu YK: Pathological types of squamous cell carcinoma of esophagus. In The Chinese Academy of Medical Sciences (ed): Selected Papers on Cancer Research. Shanghai, Shanghai Scientific and Technical Publishers, 1962, p 163.
56. Huang GJ, Gu XZ, Liu FS, Wang ZY: Further studies on the separate entity of intraluminal type of esophageal carcinoma [in Chinese]. Chin J Oncol 3:110–112, 1981.
57. Liu FS: Pathological study of 858 cases of esophageal cancer [in Chinese]. Cancer Res Prev Treat (Beijing) 4:273–277, 1977.
58. Chen YY, Lin QX: A clinico-pathological analysis of 500 cases of esophageal cancer from Quanzhou area, Fujian Province [in Chinese]. Tianjin Med J Sect Oncol 2:118–119, 1964.
59. Agha FP, Weatherbee L, Sams JS: Verrucous carcinoma of the esophagus. Am J Gastroenterol 79:844–849, 1984.
60. Minielly JA, Harrison EG, Fontana FS, Payne WS: Verrucous squamous cell carcinoma of the esophagus. Cancer 20:2078–2087, 1967.
61. Meyerowitz BR, Shea LT: The natural history of squamous verrucose carcinoma of the esophagus. J Thorac Cardiovasc Surg 61:646–649, 1971.
62. Kuhajda FP, Sun TT, Mendelsohn G: Polypoid squamous carcinoma of the esophagus: A case report with immunostaining for keratin. Am J Surg Pathol 7:495–499, 1983.
63. Liu FS, Zhang DW: A report of nine cases of the esophageal carcinosarcoma [in Chinese]. Chin J Oncol 2:78–81, 1980.
64. Beahrs OH, Henson DE, Hutter RVP, Myers MH: Manual for Staging of Cancer, 3rd ed. Philadelphia, JB Lippincott, 1983, pp 63–67.
65. Huang GJ, Wu YK: Clinical diagnosis. In Huang GJ, Wu YK (eds): Carcinoma of the Esophagus and Gastric Cardia. Berlin, Springer-Verlag, 1984, p 244.
66. Huang GJ, Zhang DW, Wang GQ, et al: Surgical treatment of carcinoma of the esophagus: Report of 1647 cases. Chin Med J 94:305–307, 1981.
67. Soga J, Tanaka O, Sasaki K, et al: Superficial spreading type carcinoma of the esophagus. Cancer 50:1641–1645, 1980.
68. Sannohe Y, Hiratsuke R, Doki K: Lymph node metastasis in cancer of the thoracic esophagus. Am J Surg 14:216–218, 1981.
69. Hiroko IDE, Endo M, Hani WF: Lymph node metastasis of carcinoma of the thoracic esophagus [in Japanese]. Operation 28:1355–1364, 1974.
70. Yamashita N: A statistical analysis concerning the routes of dissemination of cancer of the esophagus based on the autopsy record [in Japanese with English abstract]. J Jpn Soc Cancer Ther 14:1146–1149, 1979.
71. Dormanns E: Das Oesphaguscarcinom: Ergebnisse der unter Mitarbeit von 39 pathologischen Instituten Deutschlands durchgeführten Erhebung über das Oesophaguscarcinom (1925–1933). Z Krebsforsch 49:86–108, 1939.
72. Liu FS: Autoptic analysis of 41 cases of esophageal cancer [in Chinese with English abstract]. Natl Med J China 60:218–222, 1980.
73. Endo M, Kinoshita Y, Yamada A, et al: The present state of surgical treatment of thoracic esophageal cancer [in Japanese with English abstract]. J Jpn Bronchoesophag Soc 31:199–205, 1980.
74. Sun SQ, Wu X: Factors influencing the prognosis of patients with squamous cell carcinoma of the esophagus: Correlation of the morphology of 100 surgical specimens and the postoperative life span [in Chinese with English abstract]. Chin J Oncol 2:119–124, 1980.
75. Miller C: Carcinoma of thoracic esophagus and cardia: A review of 405 cases. Br J Surg 49:507–522, 1962.
76. Wu YK, Huang KC, Chang W: Remote results of resection of squamous cell carcinoma of the esophagus. In The Chinese Academy of Medical Sciences (ed): Selected Papers on Cancer Research. Shanghai, Shanghai Scientific and Technical Publishers, 1962, p 194.
77. Nick R, Green D, McClathchie G: A clinicopathological study of some factors influencing survival in cancer of the esophagus: A survey of ten years experience. Aust N Z J Surg 43:3–13, 1973.
78. Younghusband JD, Aluwihare APR: Carcinoma of the oesophagus: Factors influencing survival. Br J Surg 57:422–430, 1970.
79. Giuli K, Gignoux M: Treatment of carcinoma of the esophagus: retrospective study of 2400 patients. Ann Surg 192:44–52, 1980.
80. Yu JM, Yang LH, Guo-Qian, et al: Flow cytometric analysis DNA content in esophageal carcinoma: Correlation with histologic and clinical features. Cancer 64:80–82, 1989.
81. Ruol A, Segalin A, Panozzo M, et al: Flow cytometric DNA analysis of squamous cell carcinoma of the esophagus. Cancer 65:1185–1188, 1990.
82. Kuwano H, Sugimachi K: DNA analysis and prognosis of digestive tract cancers. Semin Surg Oncol 6:28–35, 1990.
83. Kato T, Koike N, Niibe H, Murakami Y: Treatment of cancer of the esophagus by radiation, Part 2: Recurrence and cause of death [in Japanese with English abstract]. Nippon Acta Radiol 35:321–327, 1975.
84. Airenga DP: Fatal hemorrhage complicating carcinoma of the esophagus. Am J Gastroenterol 65:422–426, 1976.
85. Marcial-Rojas RA, Castro JR: Irradiation injury to the elastic arteries in the course of treatment for neoplastic disease. Ann Otol Rhinol Laryngol 71:945–958, 1962.
86. Soreide O, Janssen CW Jr, Kvan G, Hartveit F: Aorto-oesophageal fistula complicating carcinoma of the esophagus: Review of the literature and report of a case following irradiation and cytostatic therapy. Scand J Thorac Cardiovasc Surg 10:79–84, 1976.
87. Postoloff AV, Cannon WM: Genesis of aortic perforation secondary to carcinoma of the esophagus: Report of investigation in two cases. Arch Pathol 41:533–539, 1946.
88. Poon TP, Kanshepolsky J, Tchertkoff V: Rupture of the aorta due to radiation injury. JAMA 205:875–878, 1968.

89. Wu YK, Huang GJ: Surgical treatment. In Huang GJ, Wu YK (eds): Carcinoma of the Esophagus and Gastric Cardia. Berlin, Springer-Verlag, 1984, p 276.
90. Gu XZ: Radiotherapy for carcinoma of the esophagus. In Huang GJ, Wu YK (eds): Carcinoma of the Esophagus and Gastric Cardia. Berlin, Springer-Verlag, 1984, p 270.
91. Liu FS: Pathological studies of esophageal cancer [in Chinese with English abstract]. Chin J Oncol 2:146–149, 1980.
92. Liu FS, Lin H: Morphological change after intracavitary radiotherapy of esophageal cancer [in Chinese]. Tianjin Med J Sect Oncl 2:63–64, 1979.
93. Huang GJ, Gu XZ, Zhang RG, et al: Combined preoperative irradiation and surgery in esophageal carcinoma: Report of 408 cases. Chin Med J 94:73–76, 1981.

CHAPTER 19

Adenocarcinoma and Other Epithelial Tumors of the Esophagus

SI-CHUN MING, M.D.

ADENOCARCINOMA
Adenocarcinoma in Barrett's Esophagus
Prevalence and Incidence
Etiology and Risk Factors
Dysplasia of Barrett's Epithelium
Intestinal Metaplasia in Barrett's Epithelium
Adenoma
Pathology of Barrett's Adenocarcinoma
Location
Gross Morphology
Microscopic Features
Clinicopathologic Correlation
Comparison and Differentiation of Barrett's Adenocarcinoma and Adenocarcinoma of the Gastric Cardia
Adenocarcinomas Not Associated with Barrett's Epithelium

ADENOACANTHOMA, ADENOSQUAMOUS CARCINOMA, MUCOEPIDERMOID CARCINOMA, AND ADENOID CYSTIC CARCINOMA

CARCINOSARCOMA

CARCINOID AND SMALL-CELL CARCINOMA

MALIGNANT MELANOMA

CHORIOCARCINOMA

SECONDARY AND METASTATIC TUMORS

BENIGN TUMORS AND TUMOR-LIKE LESIONS
Squamous Cell Papilloma
Adenoma
Polyps
Cysts

During early fetal life, the esophagus is lined by columnar cells. Squamous cells begin to appear in the fourteenth week of fetal life, spreading from the middle of the esophagus to both ends. Residual columnar cells and glands may persist into childhood and even adult life, particularly at the upper end. The incidence of such occurrence was reported to be 11.8% in children[1] and 4% in adults.[2,3]

Although residual columnar cells may be present in the distal esophagus, attention has been focused on the columnar epithelium associated with hiatal hernia and reflux of gastric juice into the esophagus. This columnar epithelium has distinct histologic compositions. It resembles the mucosa found in the stomach. It may be made of cardiac (junctional), fundic, or intestinalized (specialized[4]) epithelium, often in combination. This type of epithelium is known as Barrett's epithelium because it was described in detail by Barrett, beginning in 1950.[5,6] A full account of Barrett's epithelium is presented in Chapter 17.

The esophagus has its own glands, which are submucosal, with ducts penetrating through the squamous epithelium into the lumen of the esophagus. These esophageal glands are developed in late fetal life and in early postpartum periods. They resemble minor salivary glands and are composed mainly of mucous cells and occasionally of serous cells. These three types of columnar and glandular epithelium are potential sources of adenocarcinoma in the esophagus that seem to have become increasingly common in recent years, either because of an increased incidence of Barrett's epithelium or because of increased awareness and better diagnostic criteria. An additional potential origin of adenocarcinoma in the esophagus is the totipotential cells of the esophageal epithelium. Such basally located cells are not clearly delineated, but circumstances sug-

Table 19–1 TYPE AND ORIGIN OF EPITHELIAL TUMORS OF ESOPHAGUS

Tumor Type	Origin
Malignant Tumors	
Squamous cell carcinoma	
Ordinary squamous cell carcinoma	Squamous epithelium
Verrucous carcinoma	Squamous epithelium
Spindle squamous cell carcinoma	Squamous epithelium
Adenosquamous carcinoma	Squamous cell with metaplasia
Carcinosarcoma	Totipotential cell
Adenocarcinoma	
Ordinary adenocarcinoma	Columnar epithelium
Adenoacanthoma	Columnar cell with metaplasia
Mucoepidermoid carcinoma	Esophageal gland duct
Adenoid cystic carcinoma	Esophageal gland duct
Choriocarcinoma	Germ cell rest
Oat cell carcinoma and carcinoid	Kulchitsky or totipotential cell
Malignant melanoma	Melanocytes
Benign tumors	
Squamous cell papilloma	Squamous epithelium
Adenoma	Columnar epithelium

gest that some epithelial tumors other than ordinary squamous cell carcinoma may have developed from the totipotential cells of normal squamous epithelium. Totipotential cells may be also responsible for columnar cell metaplasia in the Barrett esophagus.

The types of epithelial tumors of the esophagus and their possible cell of origin are summarized in Table 19–1.

ADENOCARCINOMA

Adenocarcinomas involving the esophagus usually occur at the lower portion. The general consensus used to be that such tumors were gastric in origin and invaded the esophagus secondarily. This concept has been drastically modified in the recent years, particularly since the late 1970s. It is clear now that many adenocarcinomas of the lower esophagus are primary tumors originating in Barrett's epithelium.

Adenocarcinomas of esophageal gland or duct origin are rare. These tumors have distinctive features. Most adenocarcinomas of the esophagus are ordinary glandular carcinomas similar in histologic appearance to those seen in the stomach or intestines. Although it is possible that some ordinary adenocarcinomas of the esophagus may have originated from the esophageal gland, there have been no reports documenting tumors of gland origin, such as pleomorphic adenoma and acinic cell carcinoma, which are known to occur in the salivary glands.

The reported incidences and locations of the adenocarcinomas are listed in Table 19–2. Among all carcinomas involving the esophagus, on average 10.9% are adenocarcinomas, 2.5% are primary adenocarcinomas of the esophagus, and 1.7% are confirmed Barrett's adenocarcinomas. Thus about two thirds to three fourths of adenocarcinomas are secondary, mainly due to extension from a gastric tumor. In contrast to these reports, Wang and associates reported 12 adenocarcinomas among 35 esophageal carcinomas (34%).[16] Eleven of the adenocarcinomas were associated with Barrett's epithelium. In contrast, there were only nine carcinomas involving the esophagogastric junction.

The origin of a minority of primary esophageal adenocarcinoma could not be ascertained in Barrett's epithelium. However, this possibility remains likely. In fact, nearly all the primary adenocarcinomas of the esophagus had been found to be related to the Barrett's epithelium in recent reports.[13,16]

Adenocarcinoma in Barrett's Esophagus

Barrett originally thought that the esophagus with columnar epithelium lining its lower portion was a congenitally short esophagus if one defined the esophagus as an organ lined by squamous epithelium. Subsequent studies gave much evidence to support that Barrett's epithelium is acquired and is located in the esophagus, not in the stomach.[17] Furthermore, clinical follow-up studies[18,19] and experiments in dogs[20] indicate a cephalid extension of the columnar epithelium from the cardiac end of the stomach. Thus the Barrett epithelium has been considered to have grown from the gastric cardia into the lower esophagus to replace the squamous epithelium destroyed by reflux esophagitis. If this is the only source of Barrett's epithelium, it has to be invariably connected with the gastric mucosa. Yet it is common to see isolated patches of Barrett's epithelium surrounded by squamous cells.[21] A metaplastic origin of the columnar epithelium could easily explain such an occurrence that the columnar epithelium occurs *de novo* from the residual epithelial cells in a denuded region through a metaplastic process.[17,22] This possibility is supported by an experiment in dogs showing the development of columnar epithelium in an area disconnected from the gastric mucosa where the squamous mucosa had been stripped off.[23] The metaplastic origin of the epithelium may explain its unique histologic composition, quite different from that of the adjacent gastric cardia, and the high incidence of malignant transformation in this abnormal tissue. In this regard, the congenitally present gastric epithelium can readily be differentiated from the Barrett epithelium in most instances because the former is usually composed of well-developed fundic glands, whereas in the latter, the fundic glands are uncommon and, if present, appear atrophic.

Because the incidence of carcinoma in Barrett's epithelium is much higher than that in the gastric mucosa, it is important to ascertain the nature of the epithelium, particularly in the bioptic specimen. The marker structures for the esophageal origin of the tissue are squamous epithelium, submucosal esophageal glands and their ducts, and, if present, the bilayer structure of the esophageal muscularis propria and adventitial tissue instead of serosa. One should also take into consideration the opinions of the endoscopist, who has a reli-

Table 19-2 ADENOCARCINOMA OF THE ESOPHAGUS: INCIDENCE AND LOCATION

	Reference and Year Reported									
	7 1955	8 1966	9 1968	10 1974	11 1979	12 1980	13 1983	14 1984	15 1985	
Location (in number of cases)										Total
Total carcinoma	603	1312	558	275	350	1002	594	89		4783
Adenocarcinoma	60		101	20		69		25	67	342
Cardia involved			85	15		17		8	55	180
Esophagus only	5	10	16	5	13	52	19	17	12	149
Upper esophagus					1	2	1			4
Mid esophagus				3	2	5	8			18
Lower esophagus				2	10	45	10			67
Barrett's carcinoma		1	6				19	17	12	55
Incidence (in percentages)										Average
Among all carcinomas										
Adenocarcinoma	10.0%		18.1%	7.3%		6.9%		28.1%		10.9%
Primary adenocarcinoma	0.8%	0.8%	2.9%	1.8%	3.7%	5.2%	3.2%			2.5%
Barrett's carcinoma		0.1%	1.1%				3.2%	19.1%		1.7%
Among adenocarcinomas										
Primary adenocarcinoma	8.3%		15.8%	25.0%		75.4%		19.1%	17.9%	31.3%
Barrett's carcinoma			6.0%					68.0%	17.9%	18.1%
Among primary adenocarcinomas										
Barrett's carcinoma		10%	37.5%				100%	100%	100%	74.3%

able view of the origin of the biopsied specimen during esophagoscopy. Furthermore, Barrett's epithelium has three main histologic patterns: cardiac, fundic, and specialized.[4] The last type of epithelium is composed of goblet cells that secrete intestinal-type acidic mucins and intervening cells that may be absorptive cells or mucous cells, particularly the latter. The intestinalized epithelium is distinctive (Figure 19-1) and is present in most cases.[24,25] In general, intestinal metaplasia is not common in the cardiac mucosa. It is even less likely to have incomplete metaplasia with mucous columnar cells interposing between the goblet cells. Because Barrett's epithelium is a glandular epithelium, carcinomas originating in it are adenocarcinomas. However, a few carcinomas have been squamous cell carcinomas.[26,27] Squamous cell carcinoma may also develop in the squamous epithelium above Barrett's epithelium.[28]

Prevalence and Incidence

The incidence of adenocarcinoma in Barrett's epithelium has not yet been determined, because the incidence of Barrett's epithelium itself is unknown. Naef and colleagues[29] reported the latter incidence of 3.5% in patients with hiatal hernia and reflux and 11.4% in reflux esophagitis. In recent reports by Winters and coworkers[30] and Schnell and associates,[24] they were 12.4% and 13%, respectively, in patients with reflux

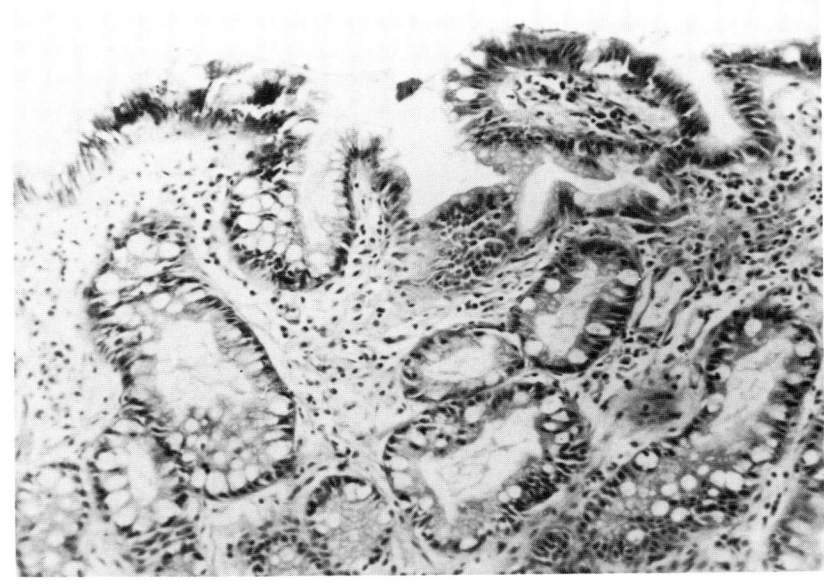

FIGURE 19-1. Barrett's epithelium, showing incomplete intestinal metaplasia with goblet cells and varying numbers of intervening columnar mucous cells. At the right there are more inflammatory cells, and the glands are slightly hyperplastic. ($\times$ 150)

symptoms. Because the occurrence of Barrett's epithelium is not directly related to the severity of reflux symptoms,[30,31] the incidence of Barrett's epithelium is likely to be much higher and the prevalence of carcinoma in Barrett's epithelium lower than those reported.

The reported prevalence rate of carcinoma in Barrett's epithelium in 17 reports reviewed varied from 0%[4,18,32,33] to 46.5%.[34] The average was 13.6% among 994 patients.[4,17,18,29,32–44] In six reports, a prevalence of 8% to 15% was given.[17,29,38,40–42] There were a few follow-up studies in which carcinoma appeared in an average of 2.4% of cases after a follow-up period of up to 20 years.[39,40,44,45] The incidence of carcinoma in Barrett's esophagus is almost 30-fold to 40-fold of that in the general population.[40,46,47] However, Bremner did not encounter any carcinoma in follow-up of his cases of up to 11 years.[35] In another report, only one carcinoma developed in 170 patient years.[47] Thus the probability of carcinoma is much higher at the time of initial diagnosis of Barrett's epithelium than in later years, after the presence of Barrett's epithelium has been established.

These data indicate that Barrett's epithelium is a high-risk condition for carcinomatous change. At the time of initial diagnosis, one tenth of the patients may already have a carcinoma in it. Although the incidence of carcinoma in the follow-up years is low, it is still much higher than the incidence of esophageal carcinoma in the general population.

Etiology and Risk Factors

The cause of carcinoma in Barrett's epithelium is unknown. Chronic gastroesophageal reflux is usually present. However, successful antireflux therapy does not prevent the development of carcinoma.[48,49] A smoking and drinking history is commonly noted but not constant.[34,50,51] Associated diseases in patients with Barrett's carcinoma include achalasia,[52,53] scleroderma,[22,54,55] and Zollinger-Ellison syndrome,[56] all of which were accompanied by esophagitis. In the case of scleroderma, however, long-term follow-up study did not show any significant increase of esophageal carcinoma.[54,55]

In contrast to the lack of information on the possible etiologic factors, a number of local tissue changes have been implicated in the development of carcinoma in Barrett's epithelium. These local risk factors include the degree of epithelial dysplasia, the nature of metaplastic changes in the columnar epithelium, and the presence of adenoma. Although carcinoma may be more common in extensive than in limited columnar epithelium,[38] the size of the columnar epithelium surrounding the carcinoma is markedly variable and may be absent, possibly overgrown by the neoplastic tissue.

Dysplasia of Barrett's Epithelium

Dysplastic changes of the mucosa commonly coexist with the adenocarcinoma,[14,21,22,34,49,50,52,57–60] in all cases in some reports.[22,50,59] In our own cases, dysplasia was present in 7 of 16 carcinoma cases; in addition, adenomatous lesions were present in 5 others.[60] Thus dysplasia is a marker for an existing carcinoma; surgical resection of the involved esophagus has been advocated.[21,50,53,57,61]

Dysplastic changes usually occur in the intestinalized epithelium of Barrett's esophagus.[21,22,34,58,62] Dysplasia has been divided into low and high grades; the latter include moderate and severe dysplasia, as well as carcinoma *in situ,* included by some authors.[34,59] The criteria are based on the degree of differentiation, maturation, and pleomorphism of the cells and architectural arrangement of the cells and the glands. Because the structure of Barrett's epithelium resembles that of the gastric mucosa, the same criteria for dysplasia may be applied to both (see Chapter 25). Briefly, the low-grade or mild dysplasia (Figure 19–2) shows decreased mucus secretion, crowding of slender columnar cells

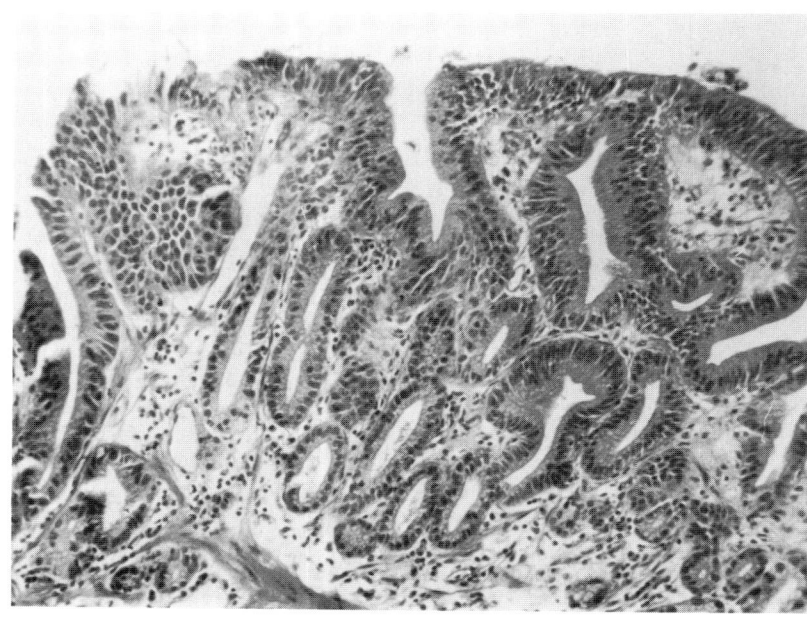

FIGURE 19–2. Barrett's epithelium, showing mild dysplasia of foveolar-type epithelium with low columnar cells, decreased mucus secretion, and pseudostratification. The nuclei are oval to slender. Their size is relatively uniform. (× 150)

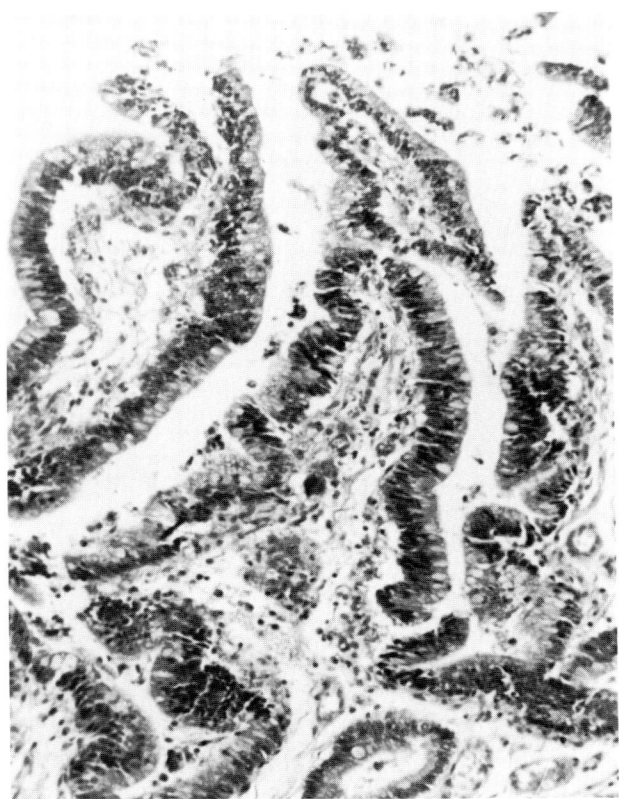

FIGURE 19-3. Barrett's epithelium showing moderate dysplasia of intestinalized epithelium. There is prominent pseudostratification and reduction of mucus vacuoles. The surface region has a papillary appearance. (× 140)

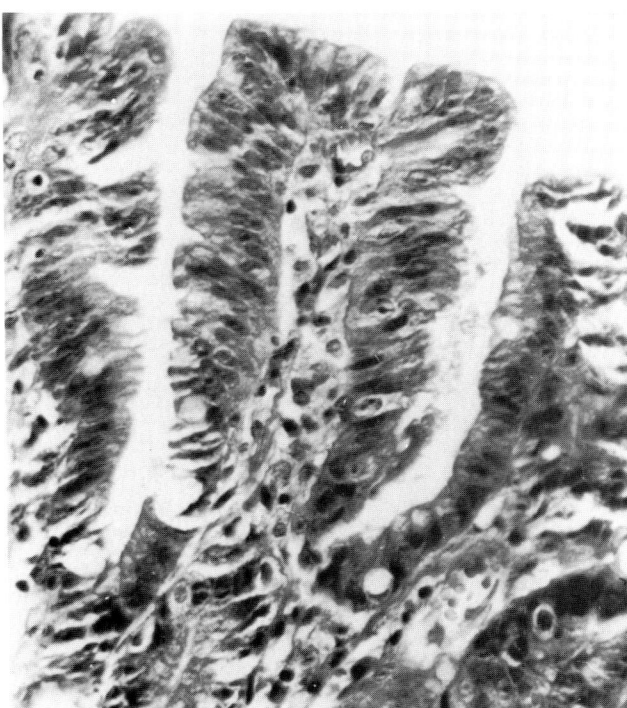

FIGURE 19-4. Barrett's epithelium, showing severe dysplasia of intestinalized epithelium. There is pseudostratification, reduction of mucus secretion, plump nuclei, and pleomorphism. (× 240)

with pseudostratified nuclei, and occasional mitosis. There is no or only mild pleomorphism. The glands retain the normal contour but may be enlarged. The high-grade dysplasia (Figures 19-3 and 19-4) shows moderate pleomorphism, plump cells, marked reduction of mucus secretion, and frequent mitosis. The glands may show budding, branching, crowding, and intraluminal infolding. In carcinoma in situ the cells are plump and large, pleomorphism is prominent, mitosis is frequent, and the glands may be distorted. Flow cytometry provides data on ploidy of the dysplastic cells and is a useful adjuvant for the evaluation of the degree of dysplasia.[63,64] Ultrastructurally, the aneuploid or polypoid cells show depletion and alteration of organelles for mucus production, dilated rough endoplasmic reticulum, and accumulation of glycogen.[65]

From Barrett's esophagus, carcinoma may evolve through the stages of intestinal metaplasia, dysplasia, preinvasive stage of intraglandular carcinoma (so-called carcinoma in situ) and, finally, invasive carcinoma. However, there is no evidence at the present time that this evolution is inevitable, even for the high-grade dysplasia. Furthermore, it is not known what frequency or duration is necessary for the highly dysplastic epithelium to become malignant. The question of natural history of dysplasia can be solved by prospective follow-up studies. Such studies on the dysplastic gastric epithelium, which the dysplastic Barrett's epithelium closely resembles, suggest that the dysplastic process is reversible and is not necessarily neoplastic, whereas the adenoma is neoplastic and does not revert to normal. The gastric dysplasia is discussed in detail in Chapter 25.

Long-term follow-up studies on the dysplastic Barrett's esophagus are few at the present time. Lee reported a follow-up on six patients of up to 29 months.[57] Four patients had high-grade dysplasia and subsequently had esophagectomy. Three of the four esophagi had invasive carcinoma, through the wall in two. The remaining esophagus had an adenoma. Two patients with low-grade dysplasia developed no clinical evidence of carcinoma. The advanced stage of the carcinoma in such a short follow-up period merely reaffirms that dysplasia is a marker and an indicator for a coexisting carcinoma. A similar report was given by Skinner and coauthors, who found carcinoma in two out of three esophagi that showed dysplasia only in the previous biopsies.[34] Reid and co-workers reported the findings of seven esophagi, four resected for high-grade dysplasia in the biopsy and three for carcinoma in situ.[66] The former four esophagi again showed only high-grade dysplasia, and one patient died postoperatively. The latter group of three esophagi showed in situ carcinoma in two and submucosal carcinoma in one. The development of carcinoma in association with high-grade dysplasia also was reported by others.[62,67] These reports indicate that the probability of carcinoma coexisting with high-grade dysplasia is high, and a careful search for the carcinoma must be taken immediately. If the carcinoma is not found by intensive search, the choice of long-term follow-up in short, regular intervals versus esophagectomy should be bal-

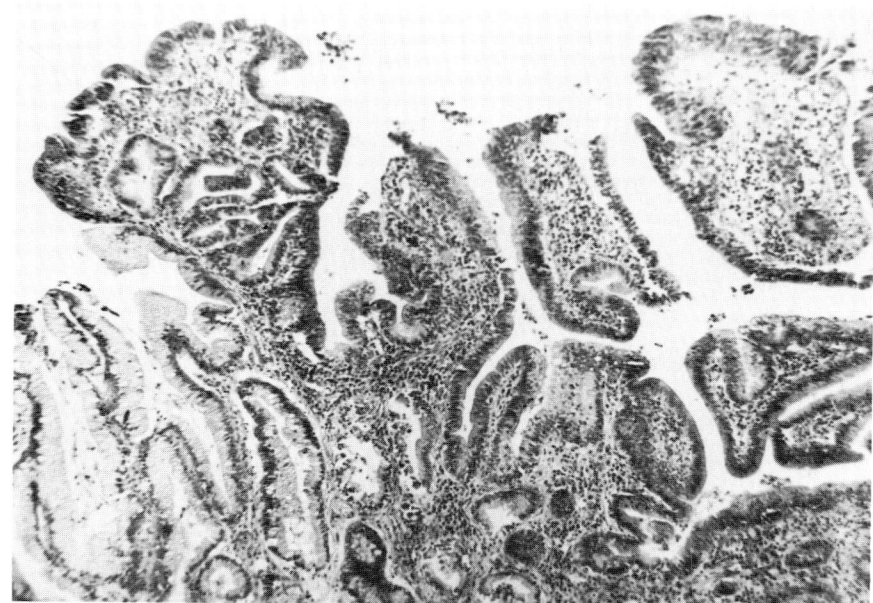

FIGURE 19-5. Papillary adenoma of Barrett's esophagus. The nonneoplastic Barrett's epithelium is shown at the left. ($\times$ 60)

anced against the possibility of grave complications of the operation. The diagnosis of low-grade dysplasia appears to have less ominous importance. Its progression to high-grade dysplasia and carcinoma has not been documented. It should be regularly followed up nevertheless.

Intestinal Metaplasia in Barrett's Epithelium

The specialized epithelium of Barrett's epithelium appears identical to the intestinalized gastric epithelium,[68] particularly the incomplete type. It is characterized by the presence of goblet cells, interspersed by either absorptive cells (complete form of intestinal metaplasia) or mucous columnar cells (incomplete form of intestinal metaplasia). Paneth cells are absent in the latter but also rare in the former. The goblet cells secrete acid mucin, as in the intestines. The mucoprotein in the columnar cells may be neutral as in the normal stomach, low-acidic (sialated) as in the small intestine, or high-acidic (sulfated) as in the colon. The sulfomucin-secreting incomplete metaplasia is seen commonly in the carcinomatous but not the benign Barrett's esophagus,[68] a situation similar to that found in the stomach. Furthermore, dysplasia most frequently has been found to involve the intestinal-type epithelium.

Adenoma

Dysplastic epithelium may be adenomatous.[34] The term *adenoma* is used here to denote an unequivocal

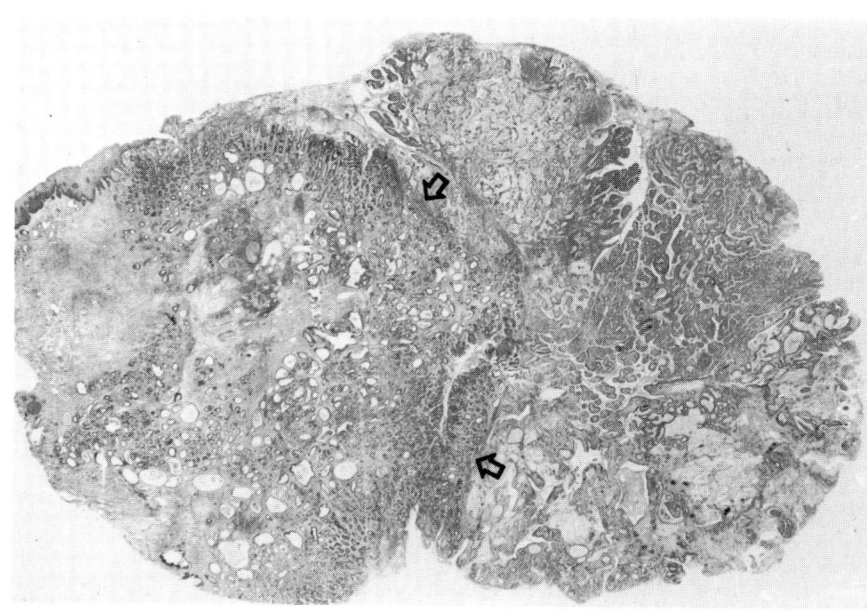

FIGURE 19-6. A scanning view of a nodular tumor. The right half is a moderately differentiated adenocarcinoma. The left half is an adenoma. The arrows indicate their interface. ($\times$ 75)

Gross Morphology

The early Barrett's carcinomas are usually flat, but some may be polypoid and large, measuring up to 4.5 cm.[53] The majority of the tumors are advanced at the time of diagnosis and have invaded through the esophageal wall into the adventitia. The features stated in three reports are shown in Table 19-3. Most tumors are flat and ulcerated (Figure 19-8), and about one third are polypoid or fungating (Figure 19-9). Diffusely infiltrative lesions in the form of linitis plastica[73] and grossly papillary lesions[74] are rare (Figure 19-10). The size of the tumors varies and can be up to 10 cm in diameter. Two separate carcinomas may be present in the same esophagus.[13,59]

Microscopic Features

The microscopic features of Barrett's carcinoma are similar to those of gastric carcinoma. Most tumors are well-differentiated or moderately differentiated adenocarcinomas (Figures 19-11 and 19-12). The diffusely infiltrative carcinoma in one of our patients was a signet-ring cell carcinoma (Figure 19-13). Signet-ring cells had occasionally been reported by others.[73,75,76] The tumor infiltration may be by single glands (Figure 19-14). Vascular and perineural invasion may be present (Figure 19-15). The amount of mucus in the tumor varies. Occasional tumors have mucus pools. In general, the mucin is present in the lumen of the tumorous glands, but intracellular mucus goblets are few and scattered. Lymph node metastasis occurs in about three quarters of cases, even if the tumor involves only mucosa or submucosa. The growth pattern of the tumor is nearly equally divided between expanding and infiltrative types. In terms of Lauren's classification used for gastric carcinoma[77] (a detailed explanation is given in Chapter 25), 11 of our 16 cases were of intestinal type, 3 were diffuse type, and 2 were unclassified. Other tumors occurring in Barrett's epithelium include squamous cell carcinoma,[26,27] adenosquamous carcinoma,

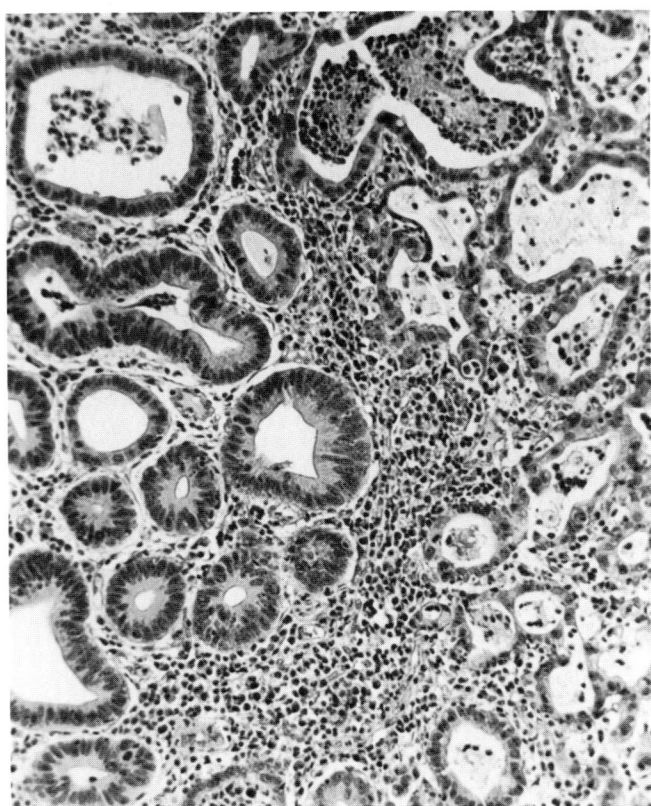

FIGURE 19-7. High magnification of the interface shown in Figure 19-6. The adenoma is on the left and adenocarcinoma on the right. The latter is mucus-secreting. (× 150)

benign neoplasia. It is characterized by and differentiated from the dysplastic lesion by its localized nature with sharp demarcation from the surrounding tissue (Figure 19-5). Using this criterion, we found five cases of adenoma in continuity with adenocarcinoma among 16 carcinomatous Barrett's esophagi.[60] One of them occupied half of a nodule, the other half being an invasive adenocarcinoma (Figures 19-6 and 19-7). A similar case was reported by Stillman and Selwyn.[69] Thompson and associates reported, among eight carcinomatous cases, two adenomas with *in situ* carcinomatous change in them.[22] One of the adenomas resembled the villous adenoma of colon, with invasive carcinoma in it. A case of multiple villous and adenomatous nodules with focal carcinoma was reported by MacDonald and colleagues.[70] These cases identified adenoma as a potential source of malignancy in Barrett's esophagus.

Pathology of Barrett's Adenocarcinoma

Location

Adenocarcinoma arising in Barrett's epithelium occurs mostly at the distal portion of the esophagus and often invades the adjacent cardia of the stomach.[29] Occasional carcinomas occur in the midesophagus.[14,49,71] In one report, the carcinoma developed in the cervical esophagus in a patient with a long history of gastric reflux and extensive Barrett's epithelium.[72]

Table 19-3 ADENOCARCINOMA OF BARRETT'S ESOPHAGUS

	Reference		
	60	13	59
No. cases	16	19	26
Male/female	16/0	15/4	19/7
Mean age	58	60	57
Gross			
Ulcerated/flat	10	X	17
Fungating/polypoid	5	X	9
Diffusely infiltrative	1	1	0
Multiple carcinoma	0	6	4
Size (cm)*	1-10.5	2-8.5	0.6-9
Extension to			
Submucosa	3†	3	1
Muscle coat	2†	2	2
Adventitia	11†	14	23

X, not stated.
*Maximal dimensions.
†One case in each group had no lymph node involvement.

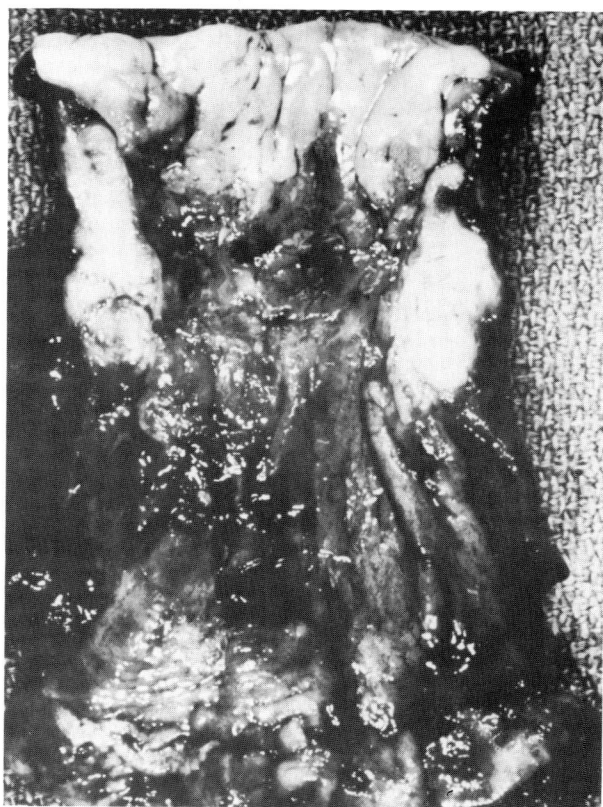

FIGURE 19–8. Gross appearance of an ulcerative Barrett's carcinoma. Its lower end is about 2.5 cm above the cardiac orifice. The tumor was a well-differentiated adenocarcinoma, measured 2.5 cm long and 1 cm thick, and involved 5 of the 6 cm of circumference of the esophagus. The congested Barrett's epithelium extended from the distal esophagus to the tumor region.

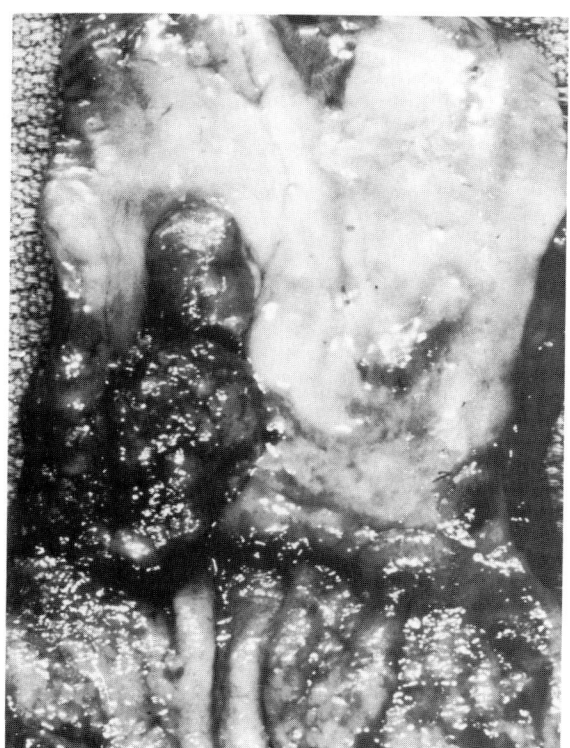

FIGURE 19–9. Gross appearance of a congested nodular Barrett's carcinoma, measuring 4.5 by 2.0 by 0.7 cm high. The surface of its lower two thirds was hemorrhagic and eroded. Barrett's epithelium was present in small patches to the left of the tumor.

and adenocarcinoid.[59] The occurrence of these latter tumors supports the view that Barrett's epithelium arises from totipotential cells.

The esophageal epithelium adjacent to the carcinoma shows varying degrees of reflux esophagitis. The size of residual Barrett's epithelium is variable and may be absent,[22] presumably replaced by the tumor cells. Dysplasia, sometimes together with *in situ* carcinomatous change, is present in most—even all—cases.[22,50,59] In occasional cases, Barrett's adenocarcinoma coexists with a separate squamous cell carcinoma in the squamous epithelium of the same esophagus.[59,78,79]

Benign Barrett's epithelium has many specialized cells, including cells secreting various types of muco-

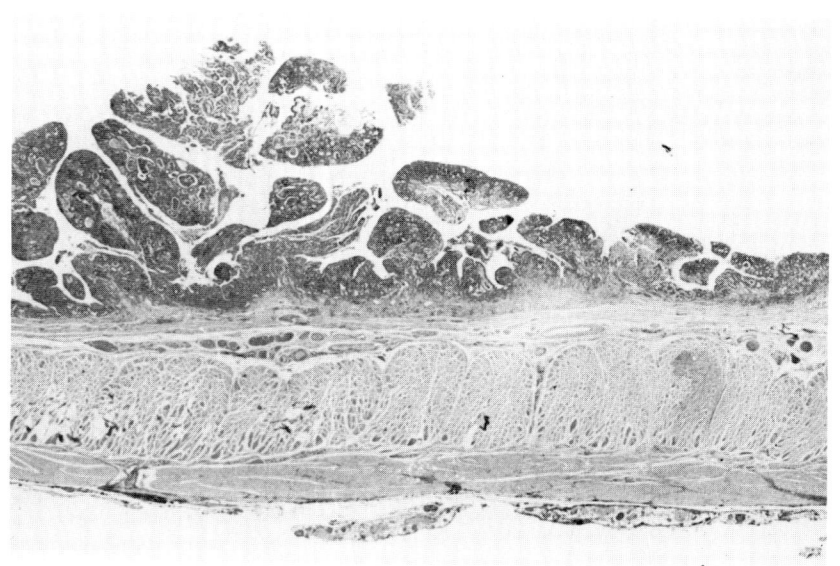

FIGURE 19–10. A scanning view of a papillary Barrett's carcinoma. The tumor is limited to the mucosa in this section. The two-layer structure of muscularis propria of the esophagus is clearly shown. ($\times$ 5.5)

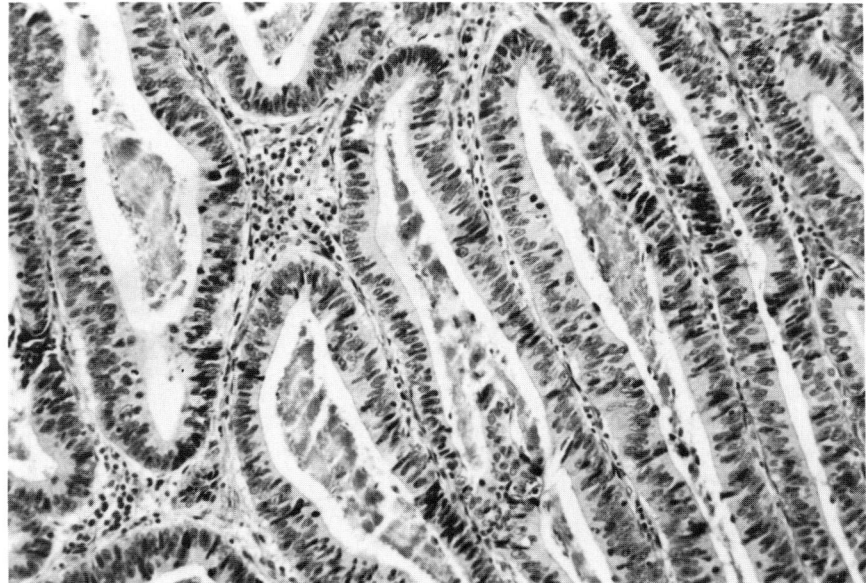

FIGURE 19-11. A well-differentiated adenocarcinoma of Barrett's esophagus. (× 150)

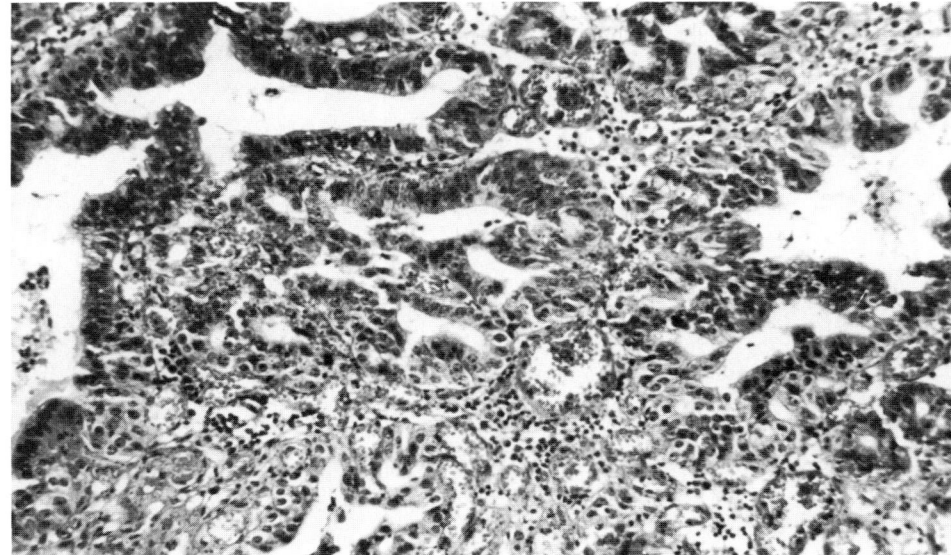

FIGURE 19-12. A moderately to poorly differentiated adenocarcinoma of Barrett's esophagus. (× 150)

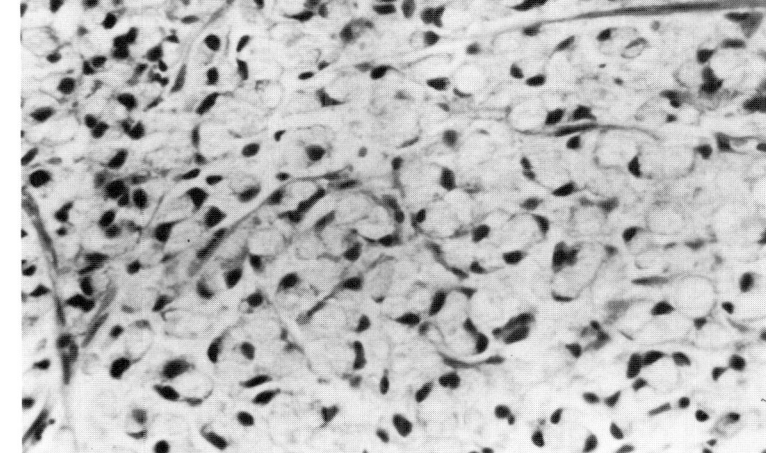

FIGURE 19-13. A signet-ring cell carcinoma of Barrett's esophagus. (× 240)

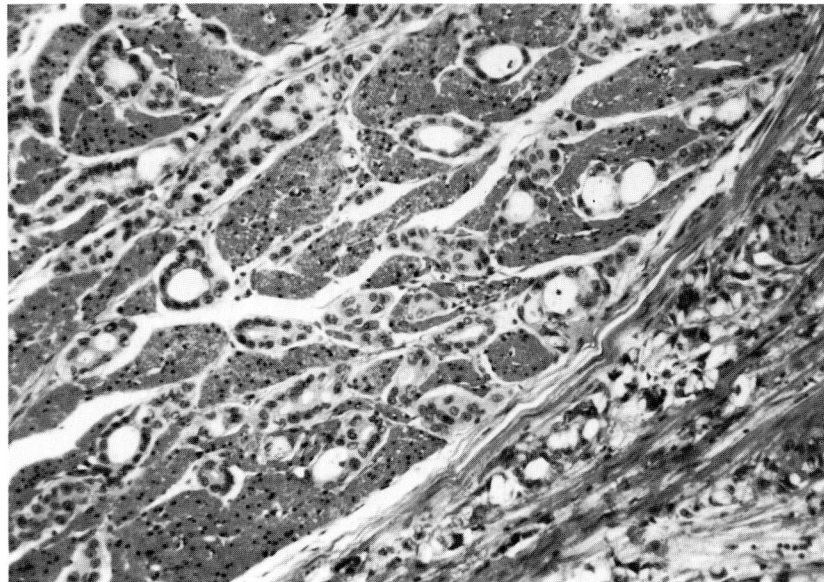

FIGURE 19–14. An infiltrative type of well-differentiated adenocarcinoma, showing infiltration of muscularis propria by individual glands. Signet-ring carcinoma cells are present in the right lower corner. (× 150)

protein, chief cells, parietal cells, Paneth cells, and endocrine cells.[4,11,17,22] Similarly, Barrett's adenocarcinoma cells have also been found to secrete different types of mucin, with prominent sulfomucin in many cases. Hormones, including gastrin, bombesin, substance P, somatostatin, and serotonin, have been found in some tumors.[80]

Clinicopathologic Correlation

Barrett's esophagus is more common in men than in women. Male domination is heightened in carcinoma cases.[31,34,59,81] In our series, all 16 patients were men (see Table 19–3). The mean age in the late sixth decade of life is similar in both benign and malignant cases.[59,81] In some reports, the cancer patients were slightly older.[34,82] In any case, the mean age is lower than that of patients with gastric carcinoma.[59] Racially, whites are more frequently affected than blacks, even in hospitals where black populations are high.[34,59] The prominent symptoms are dysphagia and symptoms of gastric reflux.[13,59,81,82] However, the reflux symptoms have been found in a relatively low percentage of cases[46,51,82] and have been of shorter duration than in nonmalignant patients.[42] Other symptoms include weight loss, bleeding, fatigue, chest pain, and vomiting.[13] One patient had osteoarthropathy that disappeared after the resection of Barrett's carcinoma.[80]

The prognosis of Barrett's carcinoma is poor except in early cases.[13,50,71,83] Poor survival, early recurrence,

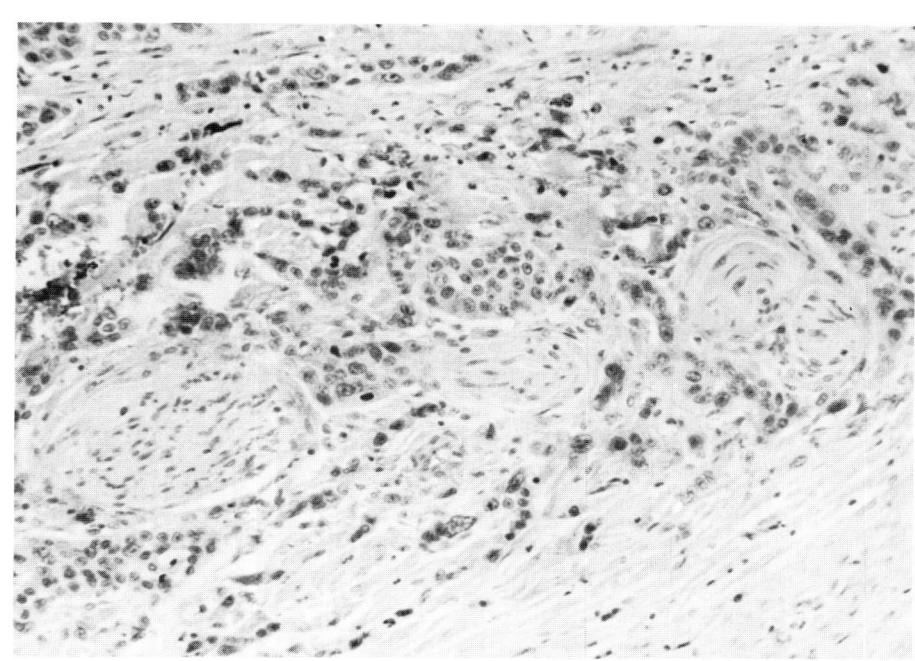

FIGURE 19–15. An infiltrative type of poorly differentiated adenocarcinoma, showing perineural invasion. (× 200)

and risk of lymph node metastasis have been shown to be related to the ploidy of the tumor cells.[84] Two of our 16 patients had no lymph node metastasis and survived 5 and 13 years, respectively. Three other patients with lymph node involvement lived without tumor for more than 4 years. Others have also noted that Barrett's carcinoma patients may have better survival rates than patients with squamous cell carcinoma of the esophagus,[85] and that the survival period may be long.[49] Many reports, however, gave a poor prognosis, similar to that of esophageal carcinoma in general.[31,59] The survival rates given by Sanfey and colleagues[51] were 34% at 2 years and 14.8% at 5 years. The mean survival of curatively resected cases reported by Witt and associates was only 12 months.[13] It is clear that early diagnosis results in better prognosis. In this regard, cytologic examination supplementing the biopsy diagnosis and close surveillance of cases with dysplasia are useful tools for bringing about the early diagnosis. The question of routine, systematic surveillance of Barrett's esophagus by endoscopy and biopsy has been debated. Some investigators believed that it was not indicated because the incidence of malignancy appeared to be not as high as previously reported.[40,47]

Comparison and Differentiation of Barrett's Adenocarcinoma and Adenocarcinoma of the Gastric Cardia

The vast majority of Barrett's adenocarcinomas occur in the distal segment of the esophagus and may extend into the gastric cardia. Conversely, adenocarcinoma of cardia may extend into the esophagus. There is no barrier to carcinomatous invasion at the esophagogastric junction. Furthermore, the histologic features of these carcinomas are essentially the same. It is therefore extremely difficult to differentiate them on the basis of pathologic features alone. The basis for differentiation is circumstantial, relying on factors such as the location of the center of the tumor and the presence or absence of histologic landmarks of the respective organs. The latter include the submucosal esophageal gland, the well-defined, two-layer structure of esophageal muscularis propria, the location of diaphragm insertion, and the absence of serosa on the esophageal exterior. Obviously, these features cannot be applied to a biopsy specimen. In some cases, the specialized, incompletely intestinalized epithelium gives a reasonably reliable clue to the esophageal location of the lesion.

The misgivings of this difficulty are diminished somewhat by the observation that adenocarcinomas of the distal esophagus, esophagogastric junction, and gastric cardia share many common features pathologically and epidemiologically and that they may form an entity distinct from squamous carcinoma of the esophagus and adenocarcinoma of the distal stomach.[15,16,22,86] These common features include younger age (sixth versus seventh decade), male domination, high incidence of smoking and alcohol consumption, symptom complexes related to hiatal hernia and reflux esophagitis, and the low incidence of signet-ring cell carcinoma. It should be noted that squamous cell carcinoma can also occur at the esophagogastric junction. Its incidence is only about one tenth of that of adenocarcinomas of the cardia.[87,88] The prognosis of squamous cell carcinoma in this location is better than that of adenocarcinoma.[87,89]

Adenocarcinoma Not Associated with Barrett's Epithelium

Adenocarcinoma of the lower esophagus may have arisen in Barrett's epithelium even if the benign epithelium is not present in the microscopic sections examined. The carcinoma may have destroyed it. The use of a dissecting microscope has been helpful in the search for any minute focus of Barrett's epithelium.[22]

When the adenocarcinoma is located in the middle[12,37,72,90-93] or upper[11,12,94-96] esophagus, it is often associated with the gastric type of epithelium or superficial glands. The former usually contain parietal or chief cells. These types of epithelium and glands are considered to be congenital remnants or ectopic tissue. However, Barrett's metaplasia may on occasion be diffuse and give rise to a carcinoma in the upper esophagus.[72] In any case, the clinical and pathologic features of adenocarcinoma in the proximal regions of the esophagus do not have distinctive features.

ADENOACANTHOMA, ADENOSQUAMOUS CARCINOMA, MUCOEPIDERMOID CARCINOMA, AND ADENOID CYSTIC CARCINOMA

Adenoacanthoma and adenosquamous carcinoma are characterized by the presence of both squamous and glandular cells. An adenoacanthoma is an adenocarcinoma with focal squamous metaplasia (Figure 19-16). An adenoacanthoma was found in Barrett's epithelium by Smith and co-workers.[59] Squamous cells found in another Barrett adenocarcinoma were reported by Banner and associates.[80] Such occurrences are rare. Conversely, an adenosquamous carcinoma is basically a squamous cell carcinoma in which there are occasional glandular components. This combination occurred in 23 of 195 squamous cell carcinomas reviewed by Kuwano and colleagues.[97] They suggested that such tumors might have arisen from the esophageal glands or ducts in addition to the squamous epithelium. Alternatively, the tumor cells may have originated from the totipotential cells of the squamous epithelium.

Mucoepidermoid carcinoma is also composed of both squamous and glandular cells. It should be distinguished from adenoacanthoma, although in some reports the term *adenoacanthoma* has been applied to tumors that are probably mucoepidermoid tumors.[8,98] The mucoepidermoid carcinoma is rare. Only nine cases had been reported up to 1978.[99,100] It originates from the excretory ducts of the submucosal esophageal glands.[99,101] One case was reported to have arisen in a

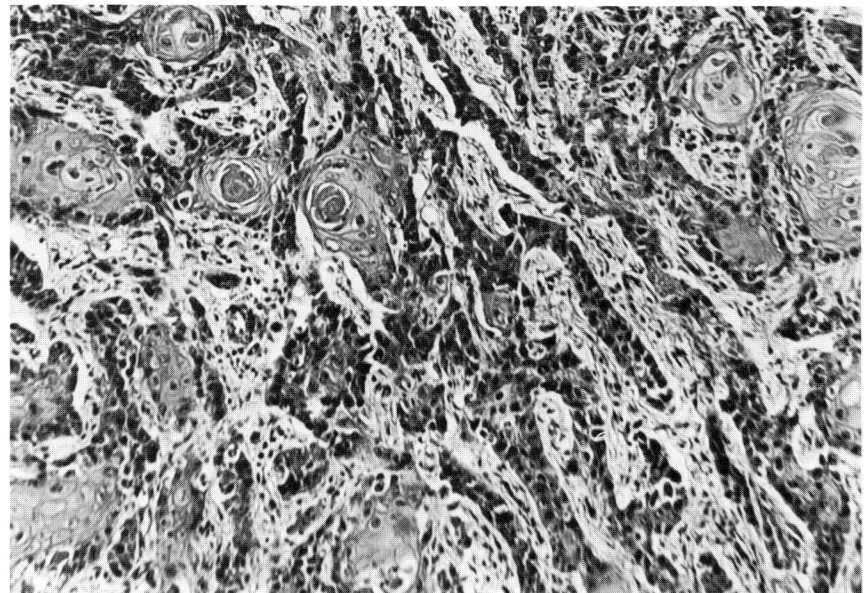

FIGURE 19–16. An adenoacanthoma of the esophagus, showing squamous metaplasia of a poorly differentiated tubular adenocarcinoma. (× 200)

Barrett esophagus.[102] As in similar tumors in the salivary gland, the squamous and mucous cells in esophageal mucoepidermoid tumors are intimately intermingled, although their relative numbers vary. As seen by electron microscopy, some cells contain both keratin and secretory granules.[99] As seen by light microscopy, squamous cells show intercellular bridges, keratin, and occasional pearl formation. The mucous cells have intracellular mucin droplets. There may be large cystic areas containing extracellular secretion. Smaller intermediate cells are also present. The tumor can occur anywhere in the esophagus, but most reported tumors were in the lower or mid portion. It is located primarily in the submucosa, and the overlying mucosa may remain intact,[100,103] creating a diagnostic problem for radiologic and endoscopic visualization. Clinically, the patients are mostly men and in the seventh decade. Although most tumors are resectable, metastasis is common and the prognosis is poor.[103,104]

Adenoid cystic carcinoma, also known as cylindroma, is another tumor that originates from the esophageal gland.[97,105–107] It is also rare. Petursson reviewed 44 cases reported in the literature up to 1986.[108] It is located primarily in the submucosa but may become ulcerated or polypoid.[104] In the latter situation, it has a smooth surface and an intact covering epithelium.[106,109] Histologically, it is composed of well-defined islands of tumor cells with a cribriform pattern and many cystic spaces. When studied by electron microscopy, the cysts contain replicated basement membrane and are lined by epithelial cells.[107] Myoepithelial cells are also present. Some tumors have a basiloid appearance.[110] In spite of the histologic similarity between the esophageal tumor and similar tumor of the major salivary gland, which is a relatively indolent tumor, the esophageal tumors tend to have widespread metastasis and a low survival rate.[103,108,109] Clinically, the tumors occur about equally in men and women. Most patients are in the seventh decade. The tumors are found mostly in the middle third of the esophagus.

CARCINOSARCOMA

Carcinosarcomas are polypoid tumors characterized by the presence of both polyhedral carcinomatous and sarcoma-like spindle cells in the same tumor[111] (Figure 19–17). The carcinomatous elements are usually superficial, whereas the spindle cells are deep-seated. There is a varying degree of intermingling of the cell types. In the metastatic lesion, usually both components are present. When the carcinoma is limited to the surface region near the tumor pedicle or base without intermingling with the deeper spindle cells, the tumor has been called a pseudosarcoma.[112] This concept was enhanced by the observation that the metastatic lesion from such a tumor contained only the carcinomatous cells.[112] The distinction between carcinosarcoma and pseudosarcoma is no longer considered valid because metastasis of spindle cells from the "pseudosarcoma" has been reported.[113,114] Thus the term *pseudosarcoma* is a misnomer and should be avoided.

The carcinoma cells in these lesions are of squamous type, and intraepithelial malignancy is commonly present. The origin of spindle cells has been extensively investigated. When studied by electron microscopy, the spindle cells often have desmosomes and tonofilaments.[115–117] When immunohistochemically stained, they are seen to contain keratin.[118–120] Thus the spindle cells are actually squamous cells. Conversely, there is also evidence that at least in some carcinosarcomas, the spindle cells are truly fibroblasts,[113] containing intracellular collagen,[115] intermediate filaments, and vimentin.[120,121] Cartilaginous and osseous elements may be

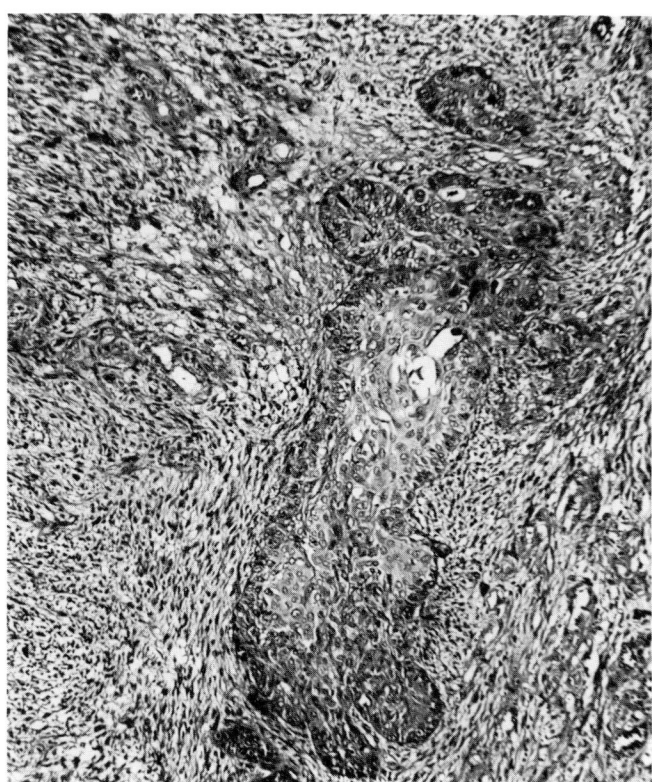

FIGURE 19-17. A so-called carcinosarcoma of the esophagus, showing a patch of squamous cell component surrounded by spindle cells. (× 90)

present. In view of these findings, it may be concluded that carcinosarcoma of the esophagus is a variant of squamous cell carcinoma in which most of the spindle tumor cells are modified squamous cells and some are metaplastic mesenchymal cells. Study of DNA contents of the tumor[122] revealed that aneuploidy was found more often in the squamous cells than in the spindle cells, suggesting a possible explanation for more frequent lymphatic metastasis by the former.

Because nearly all carcinosarcomas are polypoid, the term *polypoid carcinoma* has been proposed for these tumors.[114,119] However, not all polypoid carcinomas are carcinosarcomas. In fact, only a small number are. Among 22 large polypoid carcinomas of the esophagus reviewed at the Armed Forces Institute of Pathology, 15 were spindle cell carcinomas, 2 carcinosarcomas, 3 squamous cell carcinomas, and 2 oat cell carcinomas.[121] Polypoid ordinary squamous cell carcinoma is apparently not as rare in China as in the United States (see Chapter 18).

Carcinosarcomas of the esophagus have a characteristic gross appearance. They are nearly all polypoid, occasionally with a narrow stalk. Grossly ulcerative and infiltrative tumors are rare.[104] When diagnosed, they are often large, up to 12 cm in diameter.[111] The lumen of the esophagus is distended but may not be obstructed, and the symptoms come late. The depth of tumor invasion varies. If invasion is superficial, the prognosis is favorable.[123] In most cases, however, there are deep invasion and lymph node metastasis, and the survival rate is similar to that of ordinary squamous cell carcinoma.[124,125] Sex and age distribution of the patients and the location of the tumor are also similar to those for squamous cell carcinoma. Additional features of carcinosarcoma of the esophagus are discussed in Chapter 18.

CARCINOID AND SMALL-CELL CARCINOMA

Carcinoids are rare in the esophagus. Of six cases reported up to 1980, one was apparently an invasion from the stomach.[126] Four were in the distal esophagus,[127-130] and one was in the upper esophagus.[131] The last tumor had mucus-producing adenocarcinoma admixed with the carcinoid tissue. The carcinoid is composed of uniform cells in sheets and trabeculae (Figure 19-18). The tumor may give positive argentaffin and argyrophil stains.[130,131] One tumor had adrenocorticotropic hormone (ACTH) activity.[129] One reported carcinoid in the upper esophagus had areas of adenocarcinoma secreting mucin.[131]

A related endocrine cell tumor in the esophagus is the small-cell (oat cell) carcinoma, which is composed of small cells with hyperchromatic nuclei and scanty cytoplasm (Figure 19-19). It is identical to the oat cell carcinoma of the lung histologically, ultrastructurally, and in staining characteristics. The tumor is usually argyrophilic, but only rarely argentaffinic.[71,132-135] Neurosecretory granules are seen by electron microscopy.[133,135-137] Some cells also have tonofilaments.[130] ACTH activity is often present,[129,133,135,136,138] but Cushing's syndrome has not been reported. Calcitonin was present in some tumors.[135] One case with inappropriate antidiuretic hormone syndrome and another case with hypercalcemia have been reported.[139]

Oat cell carcinoma of the esophagus was first recognized by McKeown.[140] He reported two cases. The tumors in both cases were ulcerated. Histologically, one was composed purely of oat cells, but the other had a mixture of squamous and oat cells. Since then many cases have been reported. In 1989, McFadden and colleagues found 129 cases in the world literature.[141] The reported incidences among all carcinomas of the esophagus varied from 0.05% to 7.6%.[134,139,142] In 1984, Doherty and associates reviewed 66 cases and reported 6 additional cases.[139] They noted that about two thirds of the tumors were pure oat cell carcinomas. The other tumors often had squamous carcinoma cells, less commonly adenocarcinoma and, rarely, carcinoid differentiation. Combination of oat cells and other cell types prompted some investigators to raise the possibility of tumor origin from the totipotential cells in the squamous epithelium,[135,136] in addition to the argyrophilic cells that were found in 14 of 50 esophagi by Tateishi and co-workers.[143] In one case, an aberrant columnar epithelium was the site of presumed origin.[140]

Small-cell carcinoma has also been called *argyrophil*

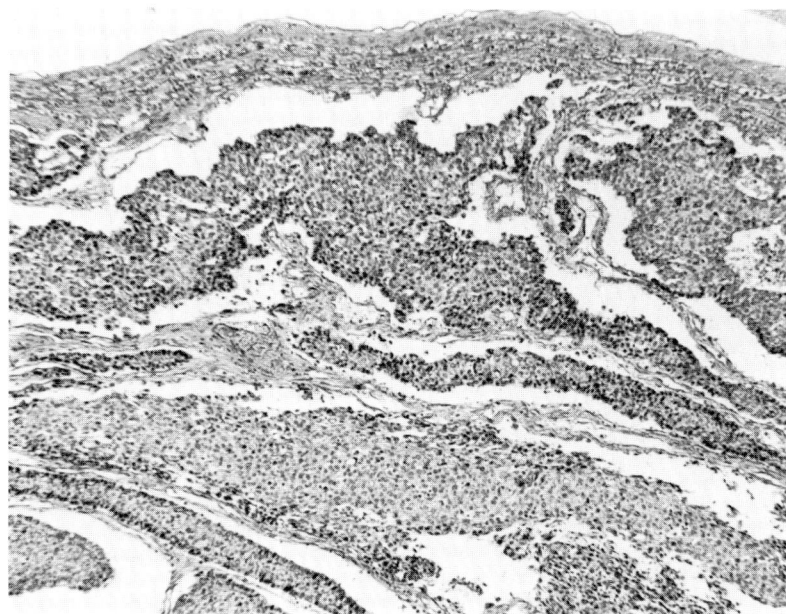

FIGURE 19–18. A carcinoid of the esophagus showing sheets of uniform tumor cells with hyperchromatic cells at the periphery.

cell carcinoma.[133] It has been suggested that a small-cell carcinoma showing negative argyrophil reaction and neurosecretory granules should be called non–oat cell type.[144,145] Because they can also coexist with squamous cell carcinoma, an origin in the squamous epithelium or duct of esophageal gland was proposed for the non–oat cell type of small-cell carcinoma.[144] Clinically, there is no difference between the oat cell type and non–oat cell type. They occur mainly in the sixth and seventh decades in both sexes. The tumor is usually fungating or ulcerated. Polypoid form is rare.[121,135] It may be multiple.[146] The size varies from 2.5 to 14.5 cm.[134] The most common location is in the distal portion of the esophagus. The prognosis is poor even when the primary growth is limited.[134,138,139,141,142] Multidrug chemotherapy may offer temporary remission.[146,147]

MALIGNANT MELANOMA

Primary malignant melanoma of the esophagus is rare and accounts for about 0.1% of esophageal malignant tumors.[148] Its existence was in doubt until the demonstration of melanoytes in the normal esophageal epithelium in 2.5% to 8% of cases by Fontana's silver stain and in 11.5% by dopa reaction.[143,149] In association with primary melanoma, there is a marked increase in the number of melanocytes in some cases, re-

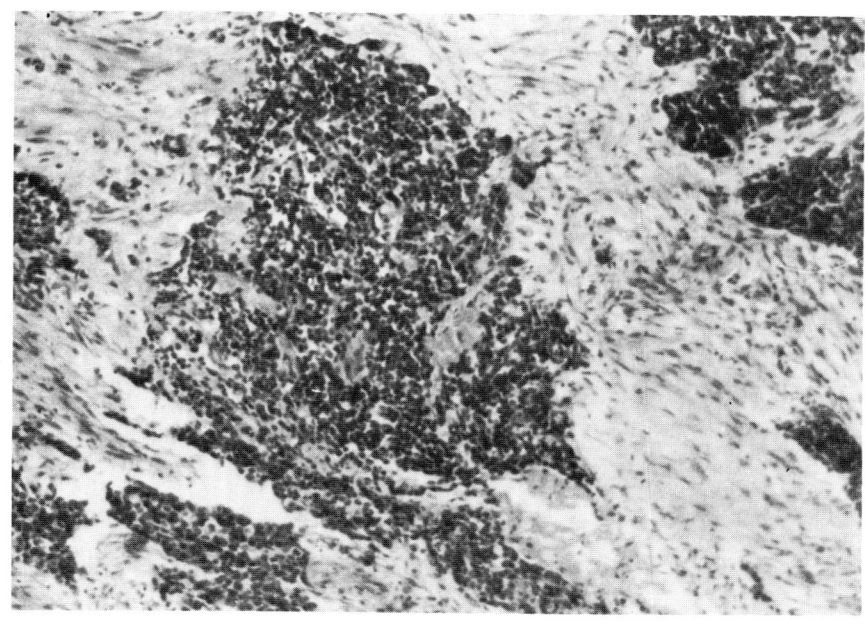

FIGURE 19–19. A small-cell (oat cell) carcinoma of the esophagus. The tumor cells are markedly hyperchromatic, and the cytoplasm is scanty and hardly visible at this magnification. ($\times$ 120)

sulting in extensive brown pigmentation of the esophageal mucosa beyond the tumor, even the entire esophagus.[150-152] Junctional changes with melanoma cells at the interface of the covering squamous epithelium and lamina propria are commonly present.[150,153-155] In some reports, there is a prominent lentiginous growth pattern.[150,152,154] The presence of junctional change is taken as the conclusive evidence of the primary nature of the melanoma and should be searched for. If the junctional change is absent, the primary nature of the tumor can only be ascertained by exclusion of any other possible sources. Melanoma that metastasizes to the esophagus is rare, however, in contrast to that which metastasizes to the stomach and intestines, which has a relatively high incidence.[156]

Primary malignant melanoma is located most frequently in the lower esophagus; it rarely appears in the upper portion.[148,157,158] It is nearly always a polypoid lesion,[104,156] often with a smooth surface.[154] Dark pigmentation may be striking.[148,157,158] Like other polypoid tumors, the melanoma at the time of diagnosis is often quite large. One patient had multiple nodules.[159] Histologically, the tumor is characterized by marked cellularity, frequent mitoses, and presence of melanin pigments. Electron microscopy reveals many melanosomes and premelanosomes. Clinically, there is a 2:1 male/female ratio.[158] One patient was a 7-year-old boy,[160] and another male patient was 31.[161] The other reported patients were in the sixth and seventh decades. Lymphatic metastasis is common.[158] Prognosis is poor; the 5-year survival rate is only 4.2%.[148,158] Radiotherapy and chemotherapy may be beneficial.[154,158,162]

CHORIOCARCINOMA

Trillo and associates reported a large choriocarcinoma of the lower esophagus with metastasis in a 40-year-old woman.[163] Autopsy revealed cyto- and syncytiotrophoblasts. Two other reported cases had gonadotropin secretion. One was a widespread choriocarcinoma with an ulcerative primary lesion in the esophagus.[164] The tumor contained a focus of well-differentiated adenocarcinoma. In the other case, an undifferentiated carcinoma, possibly of squamous cell origin, was present in addition to the choriocarcinoma.[165]

SECONDARY AND METASTATIC TUMORS

About 3% of all carcinoma cases metastasize to the esophagus.[166] The esophagus may be invaded directly by malignant tumors in the mediastinal lymph nodes, which may have primary lesions such as lymphoma or metastatic tumors. Carcinomas of the upper stomach and hypopharynx may extend into the contiguous esophagus. Tumors of these organs can also metastasize to the esophageal wall via the lymphatics. Thus, Antler and co-workers found esophageal involvement in 33 of 423 cases of lung carcinoma at autopsy, 14 by direct invasion.[167] Majima and associates found that 65% of carcinomas of the upper stomach showed esophageal invasion, mostly by submucosal lymphatics.[168] Carcinoma of the breast metastasizes to the esophagus via lymphatics and intercostal vessels, sometimes causing dysphagia and esophageal stenosis.[169-172] In most cases, dysphagia was caused by external compression by involved nodes.[171] Such complications may occur several years after the diagnosis of carcinoma in the breast.[169,170] The hematogenous route appears to be operating in the case of metastatic melanoma to the esophagus.

The metastatic tumors of the esophagus are generally external to the intact mucosa. An intraluminal mass or a large ulceration is exceedingly rare unless the esophageal lesion is in continuity with the primary tumor. The exception is the metastatic melanoma in the esophagus, which, like the primary melanoma, may form a large pigmented polypoid mass.[173,174] This is the reason the junctional melanomatous change must be searched for in identifying the primary nature of a melanomatous lesion in the esophagus.

BENIGN TUMORS AND TUMOR-LIKE LESIONS

Benign tumors of the esophagus are mostly mesenchymal in origin and are presented in Chapter 15. Epithelial benign tumors, namely, squamous cell papilloma and adenoma, are rare. Among 522 benign esophageal tumors reported by Schmidt and coauthors[175] and Plachta,[176] there were only 14 papillomas and 5 adenomas, in contrast to 283 leiomyomas, 110 polyps, and 59 cysts.

Squamous Cell Papilloma

Squamous cell papilloma is a sessile lesion. Its papillae are composed of a central core of connective tissue covered with hyperplastic squamous cells in an orderly arrangement and without dysplastic changes.[177] Its incidence at endoscopy is only 0.04%.[176,179] The distal esophagus is the usual site. Most of them are only a few millimeters in size,[178,180] although large ones of up to 6 cm in the greatest dimension have been reported.[181,182] The majority of papillomas are single.[179] In one report, a 6-year-old girl had multiple papillomas in the hypopharynx and the entire length of the esophagus, which regressed spontaneously in 2 years.[183] Another report was of a 2½-year-old boy with multiple esophageal papillomas. His mother had vulvar condyloma at the time the child was born.[184] These cases suggest a possible viral origin of papillomas. By immunohistochemical study, human papillomavirus antigen was demonstrated in one case.[185] Other investigators, however, did not find the virus in the lesion.[179] In experimental animals, esophageal papilloma could be produced by carcinogens and were precancerous.[186] Papillomas in man have not shown any evidence of malignant potential.[178]

Adenoma

Adenomas of the esophagus were reported recently in Barrett's esophagus.[57,60–71] They are described previously in this chapter. Earlier reports showing normal-appearing glands may not be true adenomas.[177] Adenomas of the submucosal esophageal gland have not been reported.

Polyps

Polyps of the esophagus are composed of mesenchymal tissue and are covered by intact squamous epithelium. The mesenchymal tissue may be fibrous, vascular, adipose, or a combination, and the polyp is named accordingly, such as *fibrovascular polyp*[187–189] and *pedunculated lipoma*.[190,191] They can be quite large and may produce a dramatic clinical presentation, such as regurgitation of the polyp, causing asphyxiation and even death.[187,191] Inflammatory polyps have also been reported.[192,193] In one case, there was prominent eosinophilic infiltration.[194] Other benign mesenchymal tumors, such as leiomyoma and granular cell tumor, are discussed in Chapter 15.

Cysts

Isolated retention cysts formed by dilated ducts of the esophageal glands are relatively common.[195] They are submucosal and occur more often in the lower esophagus than elsewhere. They may form a dome-shaped bulge but are usually small and asymptomatic.

Duplication cysts of developmental origin are primarily extramural and connect with the esophagus only partially or not at all. These cysts may be lined by esophageal, bronchial, or gastric epithelium. Rarely, the cyst is located intramurally within the esophageal wall.[196] Its lining epithelium is commonly ciliated. Congenital cysts are discussed in Chapter 8.

References

1. Rector LE, Connerley ML: Aberrant mucosa in the esophagus in infants and in children. Arch Pathol 31:1285–1294, 1941.
2. Ottenjann R, Kunert H, Kuhner W, Seib HJ: Magenschleimhaut Inselnim zervikalen Osophagus. Ihre potentielle pathogenetische Beutung. Dtsch Med Wochenschr 108:246–249, 1983.
3. Jabbari M, Goresky CA, Lough J, et al: The inlet patch: Heterotopic gastric mucosa in the upper esophagus. Gastroenterology 89:352–356, 1985.
4. Paull A, Trier JS, Dalton MD, et al: The histologic spectrum of Barrett's esophagus. N Engl J Med 295:476–480, 1976.
5. Barrett NR: Chronic peptic ulcer of the oesophagus and esophagitis. Br J Surg 38:175–182, 1950.
6. Barrett NR: The lower esophagus lined by columnar epithelium. Surgery 41:881–894, 1957.
7. Puestow CB, Gillesby WJ, Guynn VL: Cancer of the esophagus. Arch Surg 70:662–671, 1955.
8. Raphal HA, Ellis FH Jr, Dockerty MD: Primary adenocarcinoma of the esophagus: 18 year review and review of literature. Ann Surg 164:785–796, 1966.
9. Lortat-Jacob JL, Maillard CH, Richard F, et al: Primary esophageal adenocarcinoma: Report of 16 cases. Surgery 64:535–543, 1968.
10. Hankins JR, Cole FN, Attar S, et al: Adenocarcinoma involving the esophagus. J Thorac Cardiovasc Surg 68:148–158, 1974.
11. Bosch A, Frias Z, Caldwell WL: Adenocarcinoma of the esophagus. Cancer 43:1557–1561, 1979.
12. Cederqvist C, Zielsen J, Berthelsen A, Hansen HS: Adenocarcinoma of the esophagus. Acta Chir Scand 146:411–415, 1980.
13. Witt TR, Bains MS, Zaman MB: Adenocarcinoma in Barrett's esophagus. J Thorac Cardiovasc Surg 85:337–345, 1983.
14. Levine MS, Caroline D, Thompson JJ, et al: Adenocarcinoma of the esophagus: Relationship to Barrett mucosa. Radiology 150:305–309, 1984.
15. Morstyn G, Thomas RJ, Ma J, et al: Similarity between adenocarcinoma (AC) arising in Barrett's esophagus (BE) and AC arising at the cardioesophageal junction (CEJ). (Abstract) Proc Annu Meet Am Assoc Cancer Res 26:147, 1985.
16. Wang HH, Antoniolli DA, Goldman H: Comparative features of esophageal and gastric adenocarcinoma: Recent changes in type and frequency. Hum Pathol 17:482–487, 1986.
17. Ozzello L, Savary M, Rooethlisberger B: Columnar mucosa of the distal esophagus in patients with gastroesophageal reflux. Pathol Annu 12:41–86, 1977.
18. Borrie J, Goldwater L: Columnar cell-lined esophagus: Assessment of etiology and treatment. A 22 year experience. J Thorac Cardiovasc Surg 71:825–834, 1976.
19. Halvorsen JF, Semb BK: The Barrett syndrome (the columnar-lined lower esophagus): An acquired condition secondary to reflux esophagitis. A case report with discussion of pathogenesis. Acta Chir Scand 141:683–687, 1975.
20. Bremner CG, Lynch VP, Ellis FH Jr.: Barrett's esophagus: Congenital or acquired? An experimental study of esophageal mucosal regeneration in the dog. Surgery 68:209–216, 1970.
21. Saubier EC, Gouillat C, Samaniego C, et al: Adenocarcinoma in columnar lined Barrett's esophagus. Analysis of 13 esophagectomies. Am J Surg 150:365–369, 1985.
22. Thompson JJ, Zinsser KR, Enterline HT: Barrett's metaplasia and adenocarcinoma of the esophagus and gastroesophageal junction. Hum Pathol 14:42–61, 1983.
23. Gillen P, West AB, Keeling P, Hennessy TPJ: Barrett's oesophagus: A pathophysiological study. (Abstract) Proceedings International Esophageal Week, Munich, 1986, p 90.
24. Schnell T, Sontag S, Wanner J: Endoscopic screening for Barrett's esophagus (BE), esophageal adenocarcinoma (AdCA) and other mucosal changes in ambulatory subjects with symptomatic gastroesophageal reflux (GER). (Abstract) Gastroenterology 88:1576, 1985.
25. Zwas F, Schields HM, Doos WG, et al: Scanning electron microscopy of Barrett's epithelium and its correlation with light microscopy and mucin stains. Gastroenterology 90:1932–1941, 1986.
26. Tamura H, Schulman SA: Barrett type esophagus associated with squamous carcinoma. Chest 59:330–332, 1971.
27. Resano CH, Cabrera N, Gonzalez-Cueto D, et al: Double early epidermoid carcinoma of the esophagus in columnar epithelium. Endoscopy 17:73–75, 1985.
28. Rosengard AM, Hamilton SR: Squamous carcinoma of the esophagus in patients with Barrett esophagus. Mod Pathol 2:2–7, 1989.
29. Naef AP, Savary M, Ozzello L: Columnar lined lower esophagus: An acquired lesion with malignant predisposition. Report on 140 cases of Barrett's esophagus with 12 adenocarcinomas. J Thorac Cardiovasc Surg 70:826–834, 1975.
30. Winters C Jr, Spyrling TJ, Chobanian SJ, et al: Barrett's esophagus. A prevalent, occult complication of gastroesophageal reflux disease. Gastroenterology 92:118–124, 1987.
31. Spechler SJ, Goyal RK: Barrettt's esophagus. N Engl J Med 315:362–371, 1986.
32. Johnston JH: Gastric lined esophagus associated with rings and stenosis. Ann Surg 173:641–648, 1971.
33. Burgess JN, Payne WS, Andersen HA, et al: Barrett esophagus. The columnar epithelial lined lower esophagus. Proc Mayo Clin 46:728–734, 1971.
34. Skinner DB, Walther BC, Riddell RH, et al: Barrett's esophagus. Comparison of benign and malignant cases. Ann Surg 198:554–566, 1983.

35. Bremner CG: Benign stricture of the esophagus. Curr Probl Surg 19:401–489, 1982.
36. Messian RA, Hermos JA, Robbins AH, et al: Barrett's esophagus: Clinical review of 26 cases. Am J Gastroenterol 69:458–466, 1978.
37. Radigan LR, Glover JL, Shipley FE, Shoemaker RE: Barrett esophagus. Arch Surg 112:486–490, 1977.
38. Ramson JM, Patel GK, Clift SA, et al: Extended and limited types of Barrett's esophagus in the adult. Ann Thorac Surg 33:19–27, 1982.
39. Cameron AJ, Ott BJ, Patne WS: The incidence of adenocarcinoma in columnar-lined (Barrett's) esophagus. N Engl J Med 313:857–859, 1985.
40. Spechler SJ, Robbins AH, Rubins HB, et al: Adenocarcinoma in Barrett's esophagus. An overrated risk? Gastroenterology 87:927–933, 1984.
41. Stemmer EA, Adams WE: The incidence of carcinoma at the esophagogastric junction in short esophagus. Arch Surg 81:771–780, 1960.
42. Sarr MG, Hamilton SR, Marrone GC, Cameron JL: Barrett's esophagus: Its prevalence and association with adenocarcinoma in patients with symptoms of gastroesophageal reflux. Am J Surg 149:187–193, 1985.
43. Starnes VA, Adkins RB, Ballinger JF, Sawyers JL: Barrett's esophagus. A surgical entity. Arch Surg 119:563–567, 1984.
44. Sprung DJ, Ellis FH Jr, Gibb SP: Incidence of adenocarcinoma in Barrett's esophagus. (Abstract) Am J Gastroenterol 79:817, 1984.
45. Hawe A, Payne WS, Weiland LH, Fontana RS: Adenocarcinoma in the columnar epithelial lined lower (Barrett) oesophagus. Thorax 28:511–514, 1973.
46. Skinner DB: The columnar lined esophagus and adenocarcinoma. Ann Thorac Surg 40:321–322, 1985.
47. Van der Veen AH, Dees J, et al: Adenocarcinoma in Barrett's oesophagus: An overrated risk. Gut 30:14–18, 1989.
48. Hamilton SR, Hutcheon DF, Ravich WJ, et al: Adenocarcinoma in Barrett's esophagus after elimination of gastroesophageal reflux. Gastroenterology 86:356–360, 1984.
49. Haggitt RC, Tryzelaar J, Ellis FH, Colcher H: Adenocarcinoma complicating columnar epithelium lined (Barrett's) esophagus. Am J Clin Pathol 70:1–5, 1978.
50. Rosenberg JC, Budev H, Edwards RC, et al: Analysis of adenocarcinoma in Barrett's esophagus utilizing a staging system. Cancer 55:1353–1360, 1985.
51. Sanfey H, Hamilton SR, Smith RR, Cameron JL: Carcinoma arising in Barrett's esophagus. Surg Gynecol Obstet 161:570–574, 1985.
52. Feczko PJ, Ma CK, Halpert RD, Batra SK: Barrett's metaplasia and dysplasia in postmyotomy achalasia patients. Am J Gastroenterol 78:265–268, 1983.
53. Levine MS, Dillon EC, Saul SH, Laufer I: Early esophageal cancer. AJR 146:507–512, 1986.
54. Segel MC, Campbell WL, Medsger TA Jr, Roumm AD: Systemic sclerosis (scleroderma) and esophageal adenocarcinoma: Is increased patient screening necessary? Gastroenterology 89:485–488, 1985.
55. Katzka DA, Reynolds JC, Saul SH, et al: Barrett's metaplasia and adenocarcinoma of the esophagus in scleroderma. Am J Med 82:46–52, 1987.
56. Symonds DA, Ramsey HE: Adenocarcinoma arising in Barrett's esophagus with Zollinger-Ellison syndrome. Am J Clin Pathol 73:823–826, 1980.
57. Lee RG: Dysplasia in Barrett's esophagus. A clinicopathologic study of six patients. Am J Surg Pathol 9:845–852, 1985.
58. Schmidt HG, Riddell RH, Walther B, et al: Dysplasia in Barrett's esophagus. J Cancer Res Clin Oncol 110:145–152, 1985.
59. Smith RRL, Hamilton SR, Boitnott JK, Rogers EL: The Spectrum of carcinoma arising in Barrett's esophagus. A clinicopathologic study of 26 patients. Am J Surg Pathol 8:563–573, 1984.
60. Ming SC: Tumors of the Esophagus and Stomach. Supplement. Fascicle 7. Second series. Atlas of Tumor Pathology. Armed Forces Institute of Pathology, Washington, DC, 1985, pp S9–S17.
61. Dent J: Approaches to oesophageal columnar metaplasia (Barrett's oesophagus). Scand J Gastroenterol Suppl 168:60–66, 1989.
62. Hameeteman W, Tytgat GN, Houthoff HJ, van den Tweel JG: Barrett's esophagus: Development of dysplasia and adenocarcinoma. Gastroenterology 96:1249–1256, 1989.
63. Reid BJ, Haggitt RC, Rubin CE, Rabinovitch PS: Flow cytometry complements histology in detecting patients at risk for Barrett's adenocarcinoma. (Asbtract) Gastroenterology 90:1600, 1986.
64. James PD, Atkinson M: Value of DNA image cytometry in the prediction of malignant change in Barrett's oesophagus. Gut 30:899–905, 1989.
65. Levine DS, Reid BJ, Haggitt RC, et al: Correlation of ultrastructural aberrations with dysplasia and low cytometric abnormalities in Barrett's epithelium. Gastroenterology 96:355–367, 1989.
66. Reid BJ, Lewin K, VanDeventer G, et al: Barrett's esophagus: High grade dysplasia and intramucosal carcinoma detected by endoscopic biopsy surveillance. (Abstract) Gastroenterology 90:1601, 1986.
67. Ovaska J, Miettinen M, Kivilaakso E: Adenocarcinoma arising in Barrett's esophagus. Dig Dis Sci 34:1336–1339, 1989.
68. Jass JR: Mucin histochemistry of the columnar epithelium of oesophagus: A retrospective study. J Clin Pathol 34:866–870, 1981.
69. Stillman AE, Selwyn JI: Primary adenocarcinoma of the esophagus arising in a columnar lined esophagus. Am J Dig Dis 20:577–582, 1975.
70. McDonald GB, Brand DL, Thorning DR: Multiple adenomatous neoplasms arising in columnar-lined (Barrett's) esophagus. Gastroenterology 72:1317–1321, 1977.
71. Jernstrom P, Brewer LA III: Primary adenocarcinoma of the mid-esophagus arising in ectopic gastric mucosa with associated hiatal hernia and reflux esophagitis (Dawson's syndrome). Cancer 26:1343–1348, 1970.
72. Goodwin WJ Jr, Larson DL, Sajjad SM: Adenocarcinoma of the cervical esophagus in a patient with extensive columnar cell-lined (Barrett's) esophagus. Otolaryngol Head Neck Surg 91:446–449, 1983.
73. Chejfec G, Jablokow VR, Gould VE: Linitis plastica carcinoma of the esophagus. Cancer 51:2139–3143, 1983.
74. Ming SC, Bullough PG: Coexisting adenocarcinomas of the esophagus and of the esophagogastric junction. Am J Dig Dis 8:439–443, 1963.
75. Berenson MM, Riddell RH, Skinner DB, Freston JW: Malignant transformation of esophageal columnar epithelium. Cancer 41:554–561, 1978.
76. Nakamura T, Tohyama H, Nagamachi Y: "Barrett's esophagus" adenocarcinoma: A case report. Jpn J Surg 10:137–141, 1981.
77. Lauren P: The two histological main types of gastric carcinoma: Diffuse and so-called intestinal type carcinoma. Acta Pathol Microbiol Scand 64:31–49, 1965.
78. Allan NK, Weitzner S, Scott L, Kahlil KG: Adenocarcinoma arising in Barrett's esophagus with synchronous squamous cell carcinoma of the esophagus. South Med J 79:1036–1039, 1986.
79. Sheahan DG, Berman MA: Barrett's mucosa with multiple carcinomas of the esophagus and oral cavity. J Clin Gastroenterol 8:103–107, 1986.
80. Banner BF, Memoli VA, Warren WH, Gould VE: Carcinoma with multidirectional differentiation arising in Barrett's esophagus. Ultrastruct Pathol 4:205–217, 1983.
81. Sjogren RW, Johnson LF: Barrett's esophagus: A review. Am J Med 74:313–321, 1983.
82. Harle IA, Finley RJ, Belsheim M, et al: Management of adenocarcinoma in a columnar lined esophagus. Ann Thorac Surg 40:330–335, 1985.
83. Belladonna JA, Hajdu SI, Bains MS, Winawer SJ: Adenocarcinoma in-situ of Barrett's esophagus diagnosed by endoscopic cytology. N Engl J Med 291:895–896, 1974.
84. Schneeberger AL, Finley RJ, Troster M, et al: The prognostic significance of tumor ploidy and pathology in adenocarcinoma of the esophagogastric junction. Cancer 65:1206–1210, 1990.
85. Mangla JC: Barrett's esophagus: An old entity rediscovered. J Clin Gastroenterol 3:347–56, 1981.
86. MacDonald WC: Clinical and pathologic features of adenocarcinoma of the gastric cardia. Cancer 29:724–732, 1972.
87. Gunnlaugsson GH, Wychulis AR, Roland C, Ellis FH Jr: Analysis of the records of 1657 patients with carcinoma of the

esophagus and cardia of the stomach. Surg Gynecol Obstet 130:997–1005, 1970.
88. Webb JN, Busuttil A: Adenocarcinoma of the esophagus and of the esophagogastric junction. Br J Surg 65:475–479, 1978.
89. Ellis FH Jr, Jackson RC, Krueger JT Jr, et al: Carcinoma of the esophagus and cardia. Result of the treatment. N Engl J Med 260:351–358, 1959.
90. Armstrong RA, Blalock JB, Carrera GM: Adenocarcinoma of the middle third of the esophagus arising from ectopic gastric mucosa. J Thorac Surg 37:398–403, 1959.
91. Dawson JL: Adenocarcinoma of the middle oesophagus arising in an oesophagus lined by gastric (parietal) epithelium. Br J Surg 51:940–942, 1964.
92. Morson BC, Belcher JR: Adenocarcinoma of the oesophagus and ectopic gastric mucosa. Br J Cancer 6:127–130, 1952.
93. Shimazu H, Kobori O, Shoji M, et al: Superficial carcioma of the esophagus. Gastroenterol Jpn 18:409–416, 1983.
94. Carrie A: Adenocarcinoma of the upper end of the oesophagus arising from ectopic gastric epithelium. Br J Surg 37:474, 1939–1940.
95. Davis WM, Goodwin MN Jr, Black HC Jr, Hawk JC: Polypoid adenocarcinoma of the cervical esophagus. Arch Pathol 88:367–370, 1969.
96. Hewlett AB: The superficial glands of the esophagus. J Exp Med 5:319–331, 1900–1901.
97. Kuwano H, Ueo H, Sugimachi K, et al: Glandular or mucus secreting components in squamous cell carcinoma of the esophagus. Cancer 56:514–518, 1985.
98. McPeak E, Arons WL: Adenoacanthoma of the esophagus. A report of one case with consideration of the tumor's resemblance to so-called salivary gland tumor. Arch Pathol 44:385–390, 1947.
99. Woodard BH, Shelburne JD, Vollmer RT, Postlethwait RW: Mucoepidermoid carcinoma of the esophagus: a case report. Hum Pathol 9:352–354, 1978.
100. Osamura RY, Sato S, Miwa M, Miwa T: Mucoepidermoid carcinoma of the esophagus. Report of an unoperated autopsy case and review of literature. Am J Gastroenterol 69:467–470, 1978.
101. Matsufuji H, Kuwano H, Ueo H, et al: Mucoepidermoid carcinoma of the esophagus—a case report. Jpn J Surg 15:5–9, 1985.
102. Pascal RR, Clearfield HR: Mucoepidermoid (adenosquamous) carcinoma arising in Barrett's esophagus. Dig Dis Sci 32:428–432, 1987.
103. Bell-Thomson J, Haggitt RC, Ellis FH Jr: Mucoepidermoid and adenoid cystic carcinomas of the esophagus. J Thorac Cardiovasc Surg 79:438–446, 1979.
104. Postlethwait RW: Malignant tumors other than squamous cell carcinoma. In Surgery of the Esophagus, 2nd ed. Norwalk, Conn, Appleton-Century-Crofts, 1986, pp 443–467.
105. Azzopardi JG, Menzies T. Primary oesophageal adenocarcinoma: Confirmation of its existence by the finding of mucous gland tumors. Br J Surg 49:497–506, 1962.
106. Kabuto T, Taniguchi K, Iwanaga T, et al. Primary adenoid cystic carcinoma of the esophagus: Report of a case. Cancer 43:2452–2456, 1979.
107. Sweeney EC, Cooney T: Adenoid cystic carcinoma of the esophagus: A light and electron microscopic study. Cancer 45:1516–1525, 1980.
108. Petursson SR: Adenoid cystic carcinoma of the esophagus. Complete response to combination chemotherapy. Cancer 15:1464–1467, 1986.
109. Kormano MJ, Yrjana J: Radiology of uncommon esophageal neoplasms. Eur J Radiol 1:51–56, 1981.
110. Epstein JI, Sears DL, Tucker RS, Eagan JW Jr: Carcinoma of the esophagus with adenoid cystic differentiation. Cancer 53:1131–1136, 1984.
111. Stout AP, Humphrey GH II, Rottenberg LA: A case of carcinosarcoma of the esophagus. AJR, 61:461–469, 1949.
112. Lane N: Pseudosarcoma (polypoid sarcoma-like masses) associated with squamous cell carcinoma of the mouth, fauces and larynx. Report of 10 cases. Cancer 10:19–41, 1957.
113. Martin MR, Kahn LB: So-called pseudosarcoma of the esophagus: Nodal metastases of the spindle cell element. Arch Pathol Lab Med 101:604–609, 1977.
114. Osamura RY, Shimamura K, Hata J, et al: Polypoid carcinoma of the esophagus. A unifying term for "carcinosarcoma" and "pseudosarcoma." Am J Surg Pathol 2:202–208, 1978.
115. Battifora H: Spindle cell carcinoma. Cancer 37:2275–2282, 1976.
116. Agha FP, Keren DF: Spindle cell squamous carcinoma of the esophagus: a tumor with biphasic morphology. AJR 145:541–545, 1985.
117. Takubo K, Tsuchiya S, Nakagawa H, et al: Psendosarcoma of the esophagus. Hum Pathol 13:503–505, 1983.
118. Hanada M, Nakano K, Ii Y, Yamashita H: Carcinosarcoma of the esophagus with osseous and cartilagenous production. A combined study of keratin immunohistochemistry and electron microscopy. Acta Pathol Jpn 34:669–678, 1984.
119. Kuhajda FP, Sun TT, Mendelsohn G: Polypoid squamous carcinoma of the esophagus. A case report with immunostaining for keratin. Am J Surg Pathol 7:495–499, 1983.
120. Gal AA, Martin SE, Kernen JA, Patterson MJ: Spindle cell carcinoma of the esophagus. An immunohistochemical study. Cancer 60:2244–2250, 1987.
121. Ooi A, Kawahara E, Okada Y, et al: Carcinosarcoma of the esophagus. An immunohistochemical and electron microscopic study. Acta Pathol Jpn 36:151–159, 1986.
122. Linder J, Radio SJ, Wooldridge V, Roggli V: Quantitative DNA analysis of polypoid esophageal and laryngeal neoplasms. (Abstract) Lab Invest 58:55A, 1988.
123. DeMeester TR, Skinner DJ: Polypoid sarcomas of the esophagus. A rare but potentially curable neoplasm. Ann Thorac Surg 20:405–417, 1975.
124. Hinderleider CD, Aguam AS, Wilder JR: Carcinosarcoma of the esophagus: A case report and review of the literature. Int Surg 64:13–19, 1979.
125. Nichols, T Yokoo H, Craig RM, Shields TW: Pseudosarcoma of the esophagus. Three new cases and review of the literature. Am J Gastroenterol 72:615–622, 1979.
126. Brodman HR, Pai BN: Malignant carcinoid of the stomach and distal esophagus. Review of the literature and a case report. Am J Dig Dis 13:677–681, 1968.
127. Brenner S, Heimlich H, Widman M: Carcinoid of esophagus. NY State J Med 69:1337–1339, 1969.
128. Cook MG, Eubesi V, Betts CM: Oat cell carcinoma of the esophagus. A recently recognized entity. J Clin Pathol 29:1068–1073, 1976.
129. Imura H, Matsukura S, Yamamoto H, et al: Studies on ectopic ACTH producing tumors: II. Clinical and biochemical features of 30 cases. Cancer 35:1430–1437, 1975.
130. Younghusband JD, Aluwihare APR: Carcinoma of the oesophagus: Factors influencing survival. Br J Surg 57:422–439, 1970.
131. Chong FK, Graham JH, Madoff IM: Mucin-producing carcinoid ("composite tumor") of upper third of esophagus: A variant of carcinoid tumor. Cancer 44:1853–1859, 1979.
132. Reid HA, Richardson WW, Corrin B: Oat Cell carcinoma of esophagus. Cancer 45:2342–2347, 1980.
133. Tateishi R, Taniguchi K, Horai T, et al: Argyrophil cell carcinoma (apudoma) of the esophagus. A histopathologic entity. Virchows Arch [A] 371:283–294, 1976.
134. Briggs JC, Ibrahim NBN: Oat cell carcinoma of the oesophagus: A clinico-pathological study of 23 cases. Histopathology 7:261–277, 1983.
135. Mori M, Matsukuma A, Adachi Y, et al: Small cell carcinoma of the esophagus. Cancer 63:564–573, 1989.
136. Ho KJ, Herrera GA, Jones JM, Alexander CB: Small cell carcinoma of the esophagus: Evidence for a unified histogenesis. Hum Pathol 15:460–468, 1984.
137. Horai T, Kobayshi A, Tateishi R, et al: A cytologic study on small cell carcinoma of the esophagus. Cancer 41:1890–1896, 1978.
138. Imai T, Sannohe Y, Okano H: Oat cell carcinoma (apudoma) of the esophagus: A case report. Cancer 41:358–364, 1978.
139. Doherty MA, McIntyre M, Arnott SJ: Oat cell carcinoma of esophagus: A report of six British patients with a review of the literature. Int J Radiat Oncol Biol Phys 10:147–152, 1984.
140. McKeown F: Oat cell carcinoma of the oesophagus. J Pathol 64:889–891, 1952.
141. McFadden DW, Rudnicki M, Talamini MA: Primary small cell carcinoma of the esophagus. Ann Thorac Surg 47:477–480, 1989.

142. Nichols GL, Kelsen DP: Small cell carcinoma of the esophagus. The Memorial Hospital experience 1970 to 1987. Cancer 64:1531–1533, 1989.
143. Tateishi R, Taniguchi H, Wada A, et al: Argyrophil cells and melanocytes in esophageal mucosa. Arch Pathol 98:87–89, 1974.
144. Kishida H, Sodemoto Y, Ushigome S, et al: Non-oat cell small cell carcinoma of the esophagus. Report of a case with ultrastructural observation. Acta Pathol Jpn 33:403–413, 1983.
145. Sato T, Mukai M, Ando N, et al: Small cell carcinoma (non-oat cell type) of the esophagus concomitant with invasive squamous cell carcinoma and carcinoma in situ. A case report. Cancer 57:328–332, 1986.
146. Rosenthal SN, Lemkin JA: Multiple small cell carcinomas of the esophagus. Cancer 51:1944–1946, 1983.
147. Kelsen DP, Weston E, Kurtz R, et al: Small cell carcinoma of the esophagus: Treatment by chemotherapy alone. Cancer 45:1558–1561, 1980.
148. Chalkiadakis G, Wihlm JM, Morand G, et al: Primary malignant melanoma of the esophagus. Ann Thorac Surg 39:472–475, 1985.
149. De la Pava S, Nigogosyan G, Pickren JW, Cabrera A: Melanosis of the esophagus. Cancer 16:48–50, 1963.
150. Takubo K, Kanda Y, Ishii M, et al: Primary malignant melanoma of the esophagus. Hum Pathol 14:727–730, 1983.
151. Kreuser ED: Primary malignant melanoma of the esophagus. Virchows Arch [A] 385:49–59, 1979.
152. Piccone VA, Klopstock R, LeVeen HH, Sika J: Primary malignant melanoma of the esophagus associated with melanosis of the entire esophagus. First case report. J Thorac Cardiovasc Surg 59:864–870, 1970.
153. Aldovini D, Detassis C, Piscioli F: Primary malignant melanoma of the esophagus. Brush cytology and histogenesis. Acta Cytol 27:65–68, 1983.
154. Ludwig ME, Shaw R, De Suto-Nagy G: Primary malignant melanoma of the esophagus. Cancer 48:2528–2534, 1981.
155. Isaacs JL, Quirke P: Two cases of primary malignant melanoma of the oesophagus. Clin Radiol 39:455–457, 1988.
156. Beardmolr GL, Davies NC, McLeod R, et al: Malignant melanoma in Queensland: A study of 219 deaths. Aust J Dermatol 10:158–168, 1969.
157. Mills SE, Cooper PH: Malignant melanoma of the digestive system. Pathol Annu 18:1–26, 1983.
158. Sabanathan S, Eng J, Pradhan GN: Primary malignant melanoma of the esophagus. Am J Gastroenterol 84:1475–1481, 1989.
159. Assor D, Santa Cruz D: Multifocal malignant melanoma of the esophagus. South Med J 72:1009–1012, 1979.
160. Basque GJ, Boline JE, Holyoke JB: Malignant melanoma of the esophagus: First reported case in a child. Am J Clin Pathol 53:609–611, 1970.
161. Boulafendis D, Damiani M, Sie E, et al: Primary malignant melanoma of the esophagus in a young adult. Am J Gastroenterol 80:417–420, 1985.
162. Jawalekar K, Tretter P: Primary malignant melanoma of the esophagus: Report of two cases. J Surg Oncol 12:19–25, 1979.
163. Trillo A, Accettullo LM, Yeiter TL: Choriocarcinoma of the esophagus: Histologic and cytologic findings. A case report. Acta Cytol 23:69–74, 1979.
164. McKechnie JC, Fechner RE: Choriocarcinoma and adenocarcinoma of the esophagus with gonadotropin secretion. Cancer 27:694–702, 1971.
165. Sasano N, Abe S, Satake O: Choriocarcinoma mimicry of an esophageal carcinoma with urinary gonadotropic activities. Tohoku J Exp Med 100:153–163, 1970.
166. Abrams HL, Spiro R, Goldstein N: Metastases in carcinoma. Analysis of 1000 autopsied cases. Cancer 3:74–85, 1950.
167. Antler AS, Ough Y, Pitchumoni CS, et al: Gastrointestinal metastases from malignant tumors of the lungs. Cancer 49:170–172, 1982.
168. Majima S, Yamaguchi I, Hoshida K, et al: Esophageal extension of carcinoma of the stomach. Tohoku J Exp Med 83:237–244, 1964.
169. Anderson MF, Harell GS: Secondary esophageal tumors. AJR 135:1243–1246, 1980.
170. Holyokw ED, Nemoto T, Dao TL: Esophageal metastases and dysphagia in patients with carcinoma of the breast. J Surg Oncol 1:97–107, 1979.
171. Laforet EG, Kondi ES: Postmastectomy dysphagia. Am J Surg 121:368–372, 1971.
172. Polk HC, Camp FA, Walker AW: Dysphagia and esophageal stenosis. Manifestation of metastatic mammary carcinoma. Cancer 20:2002–2007, 1967.
173. Butler ML, Van Heertum RL, Teplick SK: Metastatic malignant melanoma of the esophagus: A case report. Gastroenterology 69:1334–1337, 1975.
174. Wood CB, Wood RA: Metastatic malignant melanoma of the esophagus. Am J Dig Dis 20:786–789, 1975.
175. Schmidt HW, Claggett OT, Harrison EG Jr: Benign tumors and cysts of the esophagus. J Thorac Cardiovasc Surg 41:717–732, 1961.
176. Plachta A: Benign tumors of the esophagus. Review of literature and report of 99 cases. Am J Gastroenterol 38:639–652, 1962.
177. Ming SC: Tumors of the esophagus and stomach. Fascicle 7, Second series. Atlas of Tumor Pathology, Armed Forces Institute of Pathology, Washington, DC, 1973, pp 22–23.
178. Fernandez-Rodriguez CM, Badia-Figuerola N, Ruiz del Arbol L, et al: Squamous papilloma of the esophagus: Report of six cases with long-term follow-up in four patients. Am J Gastroenterol 81:1059–1062, 1986.
179. Colina F, Solis JA, Munoz MT: Squamous papilloma of the esophagus. A report of three cases and review of the literature. Am J Gastroenterol 74:410–414, 1980.
180. Javdan P, Pitman ER: Squamous papilloma of esophagus. Dig Dis Sci 29:317–320, 1984.
181. Walker JH: Giant papilloma of the thoracic esophagus. AJR 131:519–520, 1978.
182. Lombardi JP, Tang D, Yhre OA: Squamous cell papilloma of the esophagus: A case report and review of the literature. Int Surg 65:459–461, 1980.
183. Frootko NJ, Rogers JH: Oesophageal papillomata in the child. J Laryngol Otol 92:822–824, 1978.
184. Nuwayhid NS, Ballard ET, Cotton R: Esophageal papillomatosis: Case report. Ann Otol Rhinol Laryngol 86:623–626, 1977.
185. Syrjanen K, Pyrhonen S, Aukee S, Soskela E: Squamous cell papilloma of the esophagus: A tumour probably caused by human papilloma virus (HPV). Diagn Histopathol 5:291–296, 1982.
186. Napalkov NP, Pozharisski KM: Morphogenesis of experimental tumors of the esophagus. J Natl Cancer Inst 42:927–940, 1969.
187. Ming SC: Tumors of the esophagus and stomach. Fascicle 7. Second series. Atlas of Tumor Pathology. Armed Forces Institute of Pathology, Washington, DC, 1973, p 68.
188. Vrabec DP, Colley AT: Giant intraluminal polyps of the esophagus. Ann Otol Rhinol Laryngol. 92:344–348, 1983.
189. Patel J, Kieffer RW, Martin M, Avant GR: Giant fibrovascular polyp of the esophagus. Gastroeterology 87:953–956, 1984.
190. Peiser J, Ovnat A, Herz A, et al: Lipoma of the esophagus. Isr J Med Sci 20:1068–1070, 1984.
191. Zonderland HM, Ginai AZ: Lipoma of the esophagus. Diagn Imag Clin Med 53:265–268, 1984.
192. Eller JL, Ziter FMH, Zuck TF, Brott W: Inflammatory polyp: A complication in esophagus lined by columnar epithelium. Radiology 98:145–146, 1971.
193. LiVolsi VA, Perzin KH: Inflammatory pseudotumors (inflammatory fibrous polyps) of the esophagus. A clinicopathologic study. Am J Dig Dis 20:475–481, 1975.
194. Leand PM, Murray GF, Zuidema GD, Shelley WM: Obstructing esophageal polyp with eosinophilic infiltration. So-called eosinophilic granuloma. Am J Surg 116:93–96, 1968.
195. Ming SC: Tumors of the esophagus and stomach. Second series. Atlas of Tumor Pathology, Fascicle 7. Washington, DC, Armed Forces Institute of Pathology, 1973, pp 19–22.
196. Akiyama S, Sakamoto M, Imaizuimi M, et al: Esophageal cyst: A case report and review of the literature. Jpn J Surg 10:338–342, 1980.

PART 4

STOMACH

CHAPTER 20

Gastritis

HARVEY GOLDMAN, M.D.

ACUTE GASTRITIS

CHRONIC GASTRITIS
Types
General Pathologic Features
Chronic Antral Gastritis
Chronic Fundic Gastritis
Postgastrectomy Gastritis
Chronic Erosive Gastritis
Chronic Hypertrophic Gastritis
Complications
Xanthoma
Epithelial Polyps
Dysplasia and Adenocarcinoma
Carcinoid Tumors

CORROSIVE GASTRITIS

INFECTIONS OF THE STOMACH
Viral Infections
Bacterial Infections
Helicobacter Pylori Infection

Acute Phlegmonous Gastritis
Acute Emphysematous Gastritis
Tuberculosis
Mycobacterium Avium-intracellulare Infection
Actinomycosis
Syphilis
Fungal Infections
Candidiasis
Histoplasmosis
Mucormycosis (Phycomycosis)
Parasitic Infections
Anisakiasis
Other Helminthic Infections

MISCELLANEOUS CONDITIONS OF THE STOMACH
Mallory-Weiss Syndrome
Gastritis Due to Physical and Chemical Agents
Radiation Effects and Damage
Gastric Freezing

Eosinophilic Gastritis
Gastritis Associated with Motor and Mechanical Disorders
Congenital Pyloric Stenosis
Diverticula of the Stomach
Bezoars
Gastric Atony
Gastritis Associated with Vascular Diseases
Gastric Antral Vascular Ectasia
Other Vascular Lesions
Granulomatous Diseases of the Stomach
Crohn's Disease of the Stomach
Isolated Granulomatous Gastritis
Gastritis Cystica Profunda
Other Conditions

MUCOSAL BIOPSY

This chapter concentrates on the inflammatory conditions that principally involve or are limited to the stomach. Gastritis can also occur in many other disorders affecting the gut, as a primary or secondary event, and these are covered in other parts of the book and will be reviewed briefly here.

Definitions and Disease Location. Unless otherwise qualified, the term *gastritis* denotes an inflammatory lesion that primarily begins in the gastric mucosa. Cases of gastritis have been further divided into acute and chronic forms on the basis of temporal relations and the clinical course.[1] Acute gastritis is characterized by sudden onset, a relatively uniform set of clinical and pathologic features, and a rapid resolution following

elimination of the causative agent. In chronic gastritis, the onset is often more insidious, and the clinical course typically is protracted and occasioned by the appearance of remissions and relapses. Furthermore, cases of chronic gastritis seem to include multiple entities, and both the clinical and pathologic features are more variable.[2] The terms *acute gastritis* and *chronic gastritis* should not be related solely to the histologic findings (such as the presence of neutrophils to signify acute disease), because this may obscure the use of the terms in defining the disorders on the basis of their duration. When a patient with chronic gastritis has a relapse or recurrence, there will be acute inflammation in the mucosa in the form of a variable amount of necro-

Table 20-1. CLASSIFICATION OF GASTRITIS*

Toxic chemicals and drugs
    Acute gastritis
    Chronic antral gastritis
    Postgastrectomy gastritis
    Corrosive gastritis
Immunologic injury
    Chronic fundic gastritis
Infections
    Chronic antral gastritis
    Other
Allergic disease
Radiation
Vascular diseases
    Stress gastritis and ulcer
    Gastric antral vascular ectasia
    Ischemic disease (rare)
Motor and mechanical disorders
    Obstruction, diverticula, bezoars, atony
Granulomatous conditions
    Crohn's disease
    Isolated granulomatous gastritis
    Foreign body reactions and infections
    Rare: sarcoidosis, chronic granulomatous disease
Miscellaneous
    Uremia, amyloidosis, graft-versus-host disease
    Pseudolymphoma

*Gastritis may be primary and limited to the stomach, associated with disease in other parts of the gut, or secondary to other conditions affecting the stomach. Based on the severity of the lesions, the primary disorders can be further divided into nonerosive and erosive forms.

sis and a neutrophilic reaction, but it is preferable to refer to this as active gastritis or chronic active gastritis rather than acute gastritis.

There is a rough correlation between the cause of the gastritis and the primary or dominant location of the lesion in the stomach.[3] Thus, gastritis that is due to toxic substances such as ethanol and anti-inflammatory drugs or to *Helicobacter pylori* infection is concentrated in the antral mucosa, whereas lesions that result from immunologic damage begin in the gastric corpus and fundus. With increased duration of disease, however, the two types of chronic gastritis may overlap in their locations. Many of the less common disorders, including other infections, allergic gastritis, and the granulomatous diseases, show more major effects in the gastric antrum. Some of the conditions, such as antral gastritis and stress ulceration, are frequently associated with similar lesions in the proximal duodenal mucosa; this is probably related to the same etiologic factors and to hyperacidity acting on the contiguous tissues.

Classification of Gastritis. The preferred classification of gastritis is based mainly on its etiology and pathogenesis, but also includes categories that relate to the expected duration of the disease, its initial localization in the stomach, and special morphologic features (Table 20-1). This listing encompasses cases in which the gastritis is the primary or sole lesion in the gut (such as the common forms of acute toxic gastritis and the various types of chronic gastritis) and those in which the gastric inflammation is often associated with lesions in other parts of the gut (e.g., allergic and infectious diseases) or occur as a secondary event to mechanical and vascular conditions.

ACUTE GASTRITIS

Acute gastritis is a self-limited condition that is typically confined to the antral region and characterized by a nonspecific acute inflammatory reaction in the mucosa with a variable degree of hemorrhage, necrosis, and erosions.[4] Based on the presence of the latter features, descriptive terms such as *acute hemorrhagic gastritis* and *acute nonerosive* versus *erosive gastritis* have been employed, and these phrases relate mainly to the severity of the lesions rather than to the particular etiology.[5]

Because most cases of acute gastritis are due to the ingestion of toxic substances such as ethanol and drugs or to the reflux of bile salts, this condition has also been referred to as acute toxic (or chemical or drug) gastritis.[6] This subject, particularly the aspects dealing with its pathogenesis, is partially covered in Chapter 9.

Etiology and Pathogenesis. As noted above, the majority of cases of acute gastritis are due to the intake of ethanol[7-10] and the anti-inflammatory drugs such as aspirin[11-13] and the various nonsteroidal agents.[6,14,15] In cases lacking such a history, it is thought that the injury results from the reflux of bile salts through an incompetent pyloric sphincter into the gastric antrum,[16-20] although this circumstance is usually not documented in an individual patient. All of these substances are lipid soluble, and it is believed that they dissolve in the cytomembranes of the surface mucous cells in the antrum. This damages the mucosal barrier and facilitates the increased back-diffusion of hydrogen ions into the mucosa.[21,22] Multiple factors appear to be involved in the mucosal destruction, including a direct damage to the surface layer of mucous cells, a reduction in the protective prostaglandins that are made in these cells,[23,24] and a vasoconstrictive effect by the acid on the small vessels in the underlying lamina propria; see Chapter 9 for further details.

The presence of *H. pylori* has been noted in association with cases of chronic active gastritis (see below). Although rare instances of acute gastritis have been observed after the ingestion of the bacterium,[25] there is as yet no evidence to incriminate this organism as a cause of the usual cases of acute toxic gastritis.

Clinical Features. Patients with acute gastritis typically present with the abrupt onset of upper abdominal pain of a burning quality and nausea and vomiting, and the diagnosis is usually established by the clinical history.[4] Overt hematemesis is noted in the more severe cases, and endoscopic examination is often performed in such patients to separate the erosive and nonerosive forms and to distinguish gastritis from other causes of upper tract hemorrhage, such as bleeding varices, a Mallory-Weiss tear, or a chronic peptic ulcer.[26,27] The lesion of acute gastritis is usually too superficial to be appreciated by radiographic study of the stomach.

The great majority of patients respond promptly to the elimination of any toxic agents and to medications that reduce gastric acidity. Exceptionally, surgical resection or angiographic injection of vasoconstrictive substances may be required in cases with uncontrolled

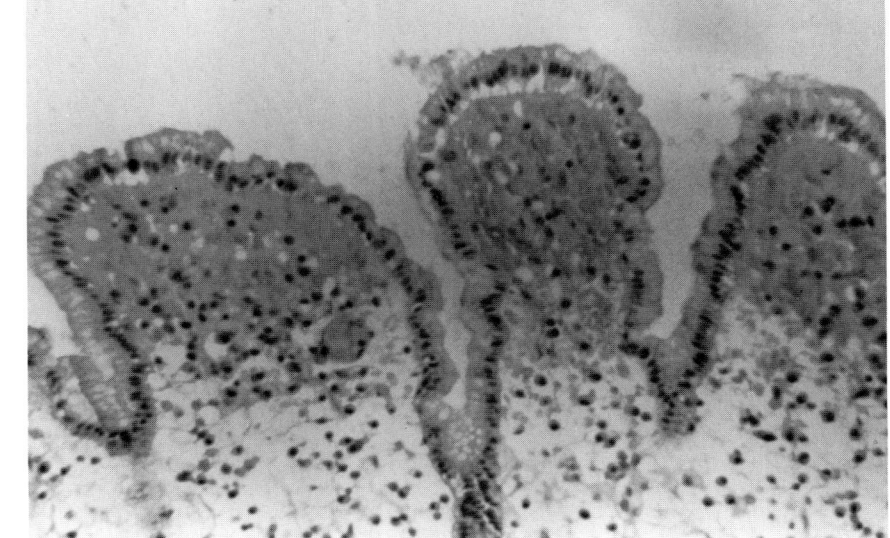

FIGURE 20-1. Gastric mucosal biopsy, showing fresh hemorrhages in the superficial part of the lamina propria. The surface and pit mucous cells are intact, and there is no neutrophilic reaction. Although such changes can be seen in the earliest phase of an acute gastritis, they can also be the result of the endoscopic procedure alone. (H&E, × 310)

hemorrhage. Most patients recover completely without sequelae, but acute gastritis can recur, and it is possible that some cases of chronic antral gastritis develop following repeated exposure to toxic substances.

Pathology. Most of the information has been obtained from the endoscopic appearances and mucosal biopsy samples,[5,10,26-28] because resection of tissue in acute gastritis is rarely needed. At a macroscopic level, the milder cases show some combination of edema, erythema, scattered petechiae, and friability of the mucosal surface. The more marked examples are associated with greater hemorrhage, ranging from multiple streaks to diffuse involvement of the mucosa, and the appearance of superficial erosions. As noted above, such cases have been termed acute hemorrhagic or acute erosive gastritis. The lesions are ordinarily limited to the antrum but may extend in the severe cases to involve the lower part of the gastric corpus. In cases due to the ingestion of alcohol and drugs, there may be an associated duodenitis (see Chapter 28). The endoscopic study serves to identify the gastritis and/or duodenitis and to exclude a chronic peptic ulcer in these areas.

The histologic features of acute gastritis are ordinarily confined to the mucosal layer and are entirely nonspecific. The earliest lesions, established by investigative studies in animals and humans, reveal only edema, congestion, and patchy hemorrhages in the upper part of the lamina propria;[29] and it is impossible to distinguish these features from the potential traumatic effects of the endoscopic procedure (Figure 20-1). Most cases of acute gastritis due to bile reflux exhibit such minor alterations.[19] More certain features of acute gastritis include damage to the surface and foveolar (pit) mucous cells and the presence of neutrophils in the lamina propria and in the epithelial layer (Figures 20-2, 20-3). The milder lesions are limited to the upper third or half of the mucosa and are frequently associ-

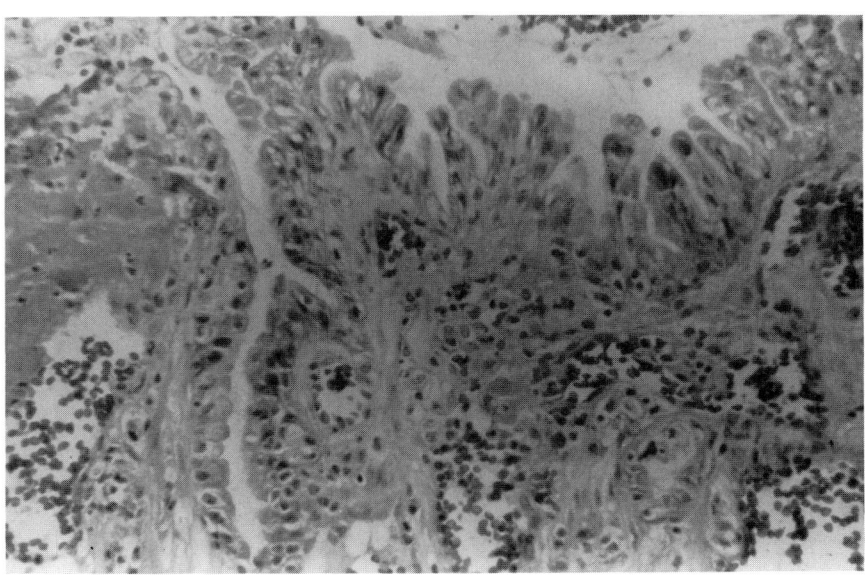

FIGURE 20-2. Gastric antral mucosal biopsy, showing features of acute gastritis, including damage of the surface and pit mucous cell, marked congestion of the lamina propria, and slight neutrophilic infiltrate (upper left). (H&E, × 100)

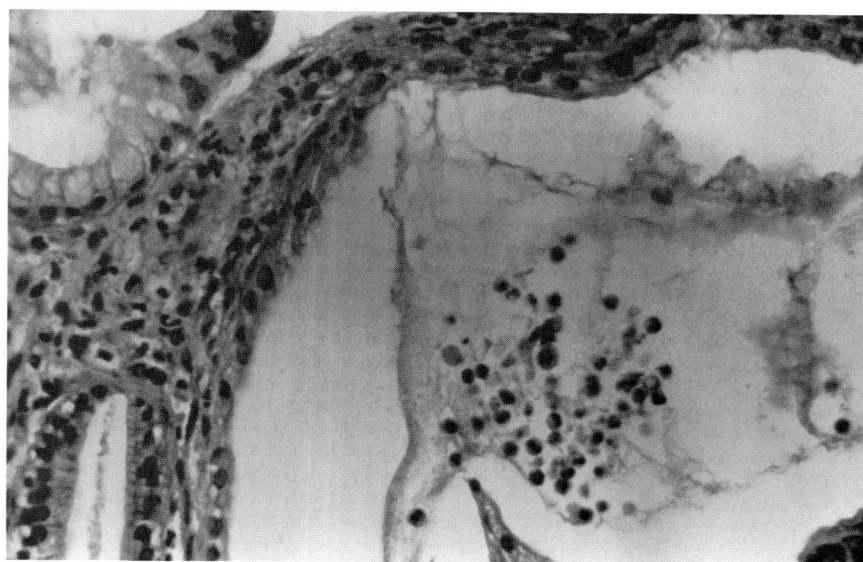

FIGURE 20–3. Gastric mucosal biopsy with acute gastritis. There is prominent dilatation of the gastric pit, damage to the epithelial cells, and a cluster of neutrophils in the lumen. (H&E, × 500)

ated with focal dilatation of the gastric pits. The underlying pyloric glands are usually not involved. In the more extensive cases, there is greater hemorrhage and necrosis leading to the formation of patchy erosions, which represent superficial ulcers that are limited to the mucosal layer. There may also be vascular congestion but usually no inflammation in the submucosa in the severe cases. It should be remembered that small numbers of mononuclear inflammatory cells and occasional eosinophils are present in the lamina propria of the normal gastric antrum,[30] especially in adults; and these are not conspicuously increased in cases of acute gastritis. Indeed, if an increase of such cells is encountered, it should raise the possibility of alternative causes or the presence of an underlying chronic gastritis.

The healing phase of acute gastritis is characterized by a reduction in the congestion and neutrophilic reaction and by the appearance of regenerative epithelium. The gastric pits are transiently elongated and contain scattered mitoses (Figure 20–4). Ultimately, there is a complete return to the normal mucosal structure in most cases. After repeated attacks of acute gastritis, however, it is possible that some cases evolve into a chronic gastritis, as described below.

Differential Diagnosis. Because the morphologic features of acute (toxic) gastritis are nonspecific, the diagnosis is dependent on the clinical history and on the exclusion of a discrete ulcer or of other inflammatory disorders (such as infections, allergic disease, and chronic active gastritis) that may affect the stomach. Localized ulcers of an acute or chronic type can be readily discerned by endoscopic and radiographic examinations. Mucosal biopsy samples are often obtained at the edge of the ulcers for excluding malignancy, and these samples usually reveal a prominent degree of mucosal inflammation, especially in cases of chronic peptic ulcers. It is important, in these instances,

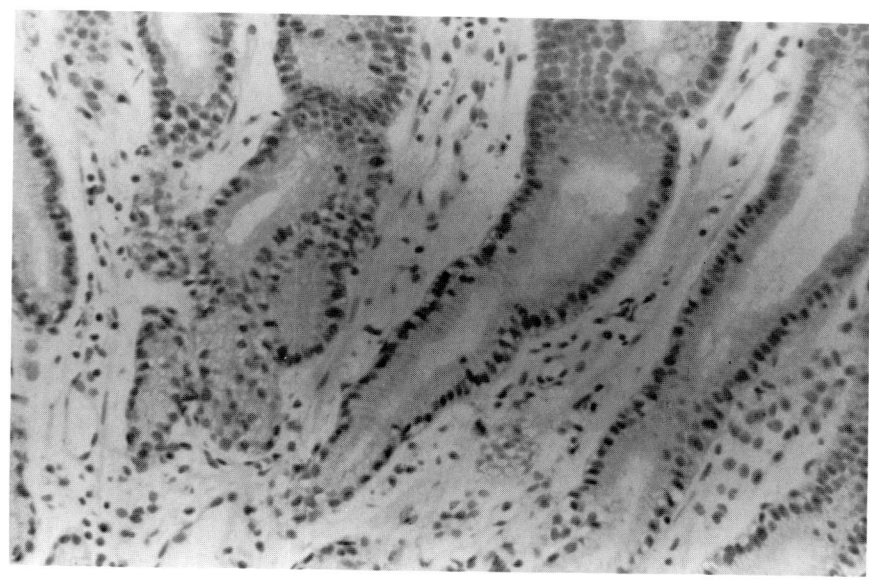

FIGURE 20–4. Gastric antral mucosal biopsy of the healing phase of acute gastritis. There is a prominent lengthening of the foveolae due to regeneration, with mitoses evident in the center and little inflammation. (H&E, × 130)

to appreciate that the inflammation is a component of the peptic ulcer disease and not an independent sign of an acute gastritis. Accordingly, it is preferable that the pathologic report in such cases simply record that acute and/or chronic inflammation is present and avoid the diagnostic terms *acute gastritis* and *chronic gastritis*. Although this may seem to be simply semantic quibbling, it is helpful to the clinician because it eliminates the confusion caused by a mixing of histologic and clinical diagnostic terms.

In about one half of cases of acute drug-induced ulcer, such as those due to salicylates, there is only minimal or no inflammation in the adjacent mucosa, and this information can occasionally be of assistance in establishing the cause of a gastric ulcer.[31,32] Patients with acute stress ulceration are usually much sicker and frequently reveal multiple ulcers in the stomach and duodenum, and this diagnosis is typically established by recognition of the underlying clinical condition that has precipitated the development of the stress lesions.

A nonspecific inflammatory reaction is noted in most infectious lesions of the stomach, but their nature is suspected or revealed by the identification of the microorganisms, cellular inclusions, or a granulomatous response. Furthermore, many patients with gastric infections present with a history of immunodeficiency, as discussed below. Antral involvement is common in allergic gastroenteritis, and this lesion is ordinarily distinguished from acute gastritis by noting the abundant eosinophilic reaction (see Chapter 10). Occasional cases of acute toxic gastritis, however, reveal a localized prominence of mucosal eosinophils; and this may cause difficulty in the evaluation of biopsy samples. It is a help that the peripheral blood eosinophil count is commonly elevated in cases of allergic disease, whereas it is normal in acute toxic gastritis.

The same etiologic agents are involved in most cases of acute gastritis and chronic active antral gastritis, and both conditions reveal epithelial destruction and neutrophils in the mucosa. Aside from the clinical history, which may disclose the duration of the disorder, the chronic form will show, in addition, an increase in the number of mononuclear inflammatory cells in the lamina propria, a variable atrophy of the pyloric glands, and the frequent presence of intestinal metaplasia.

CHRONIC GASTRITIS

Types

In contrast to acute gastritis, cases of chronic gastritis are characterized by greater variation in cause, location of the disease in the stomach, and clinical features. The major types of chronic gastritis are listed in Table 20–2. The two most common forms are separated by their different causes and primary sites of injury into chronic fundic gastritis and chronic antral gastritis; these have been called, respectively, type A and type B chronic gastritis.[3] Other types of chronic gastritis relate to a particular pathogenesis, such as the gastritis that de-

Table 20–2. MAJOR TYPES OF CHRONIC GASTRITIS

Chronic antral gastritis
Chronic fundic gastritis
Postgastrectomy gastritis
Chronic erosive gastritis
Chronic hypertrophic gastritis
Chronic infections

velops in patients that have had a distal gastric resection and gastrojejunostomy, or to cases with a prominence of certain morphologic features, including multiple erosions (chronic erosive gastritis) or hypertrophy of the surface and foveolar area (chronic hypertrophic gastritis).

General Pathologic Features

Independent of the particular type of chronic gastritis, many of the histologic alterations observed are similar and differ mainly in their extent (Table 20–3).

Features of Chronic Disease. Common features that signify the chronic nature of the lesion include the presence of increased numbers of mononuclear inflammatory cells (macrophages, lymphocytes, and plasma cells) and occasionally of eosinophils in the lamina propria (Figure 20–5); a progressive destruction of the specialized glands that contain parietal and chief cells in the fundus and corpus or of the pyloric glands in the antrum, which causes thinning of the mucosal layer in the late stages of the disease; and the appearance of intestinal metaplasia in all parts of the stomach and of pyloric (also called pseudopyloric) metaplasia in place of the lost glands in the proximal stomach.[2,33–38] More variable features seen in chronic gastritis are an increase in the indigenous endocrine cells and a hyperplasia of the foveolar mucous cells, and the latter may result in the formation of localized polyps or of a diffuse hypertrophy of the mucosal surface. The lesion of chronic gastritis is confined to the mucosal layer; there may be submucosal congestion during active gastritis, but the rest of the gastric wall is otherwise unaffected.

Features of Active Disease. Active disease, often corresponding to a clinical relapse, can be superimposed on any type of chronic gastritis and is character-

Table 20–3. HISTOLOGIC FEATURES OF CHRONIC GASTRITIS

Signs of chronic disease
  Increased mononuclear inflammatory cells and eosinophils in lamina propria, with occasional prominence of lymphoid nodules
  Loss of specialized glands
  Intestinal and pyloric gland metaplasia
  Variable hyperplasia of surface-foveolar mucous cells
  Early increase and late decrease of indigenous endocrine cells
Signs of active disease
  Epithelial cell degeneration and regeneration, with variable erosions
  Neutrophilic reaction in lamina propria and epithelial layer

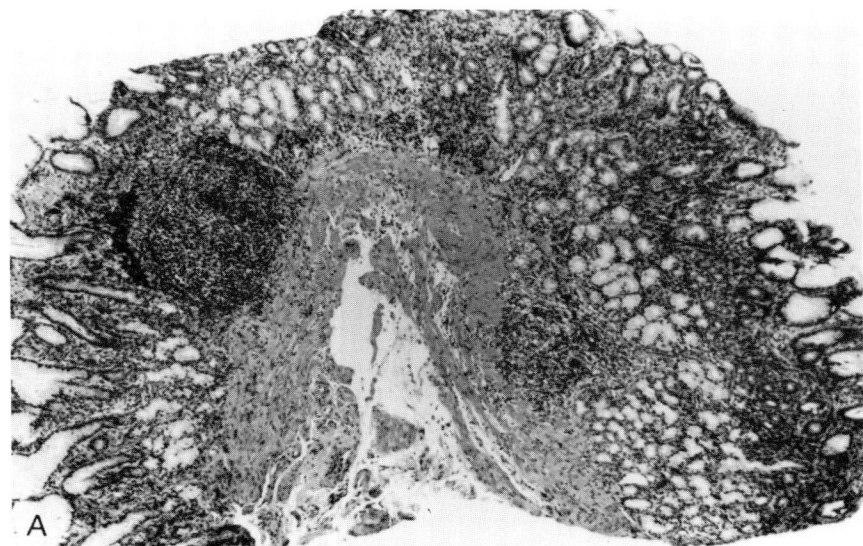

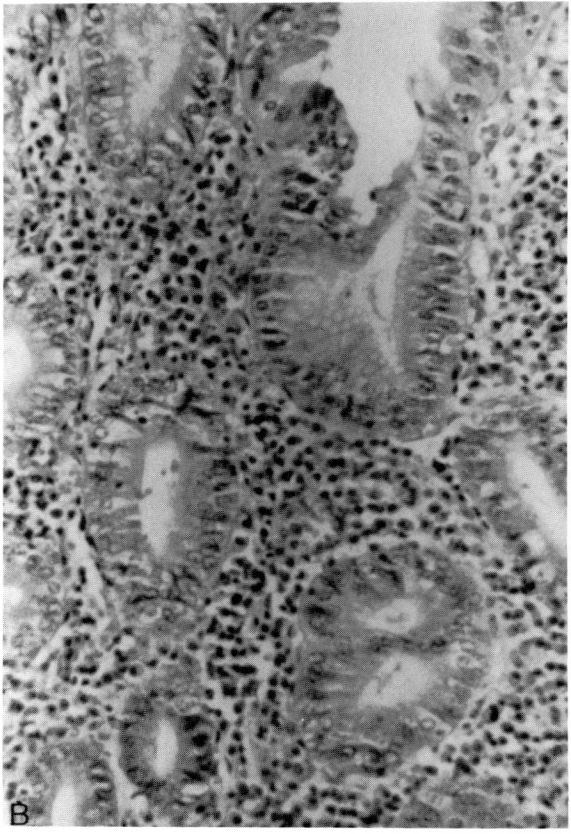

FIGURE 20–5. *A*, Gastric antral mucosal biopsy with chronic gastritis. There is a marked infiltrate of mononuclear inflammatory cells in the lamina propria, with lymphoid nodules adjacent to and extending into the muscularis mucosae. There is a variable loss of pyloric glands (left and top). (H&E, × 32) *B*, Gastric mucosal biopsy with chronic gastritis. There is a marked increase of mononuclear inflammatory cells in the lamina propria, regeneration of the gastric pits, and focal infiltrates of mononuclear cells in the epithelial layer. Contrast with acute gastritis in Figures 20–2 and 20–4. (H&E, × 100)

ized by the presence of degeneration and regeneration of the epithelial cells and a neutrophilic reaction in the lamina propria and epithelial area (Figure 20–6). These features alone are indistinguishable from those seen in acute gastritis and also include vascular congestion and dilation of the gastric pits, which may contain clusters of neutrophils. The surface is usually intact; but superficial erosions can appear in the more severe cases, especially in those affecting the antrum, and can exceptionally be the dominant feature (see secton on chronic erosive gastritis). The active lesions always involve the surface and foveolar regions, and they extend to the underlying mucosal glands in the advanced cases. Depending on whether or not there is the presence of necrosis and acute inflammation, the cases can be categorized as chronic active gastritis or chronic inactive gastritis. As mentioned earlier, it is best not to use the term *acute gastritis* in this setting, so that there will be no confusion with the separate clinical entity of acute toxic gastritis.

Special Features and Terms. A variety of additional terms have been employed to indicate the extent of the

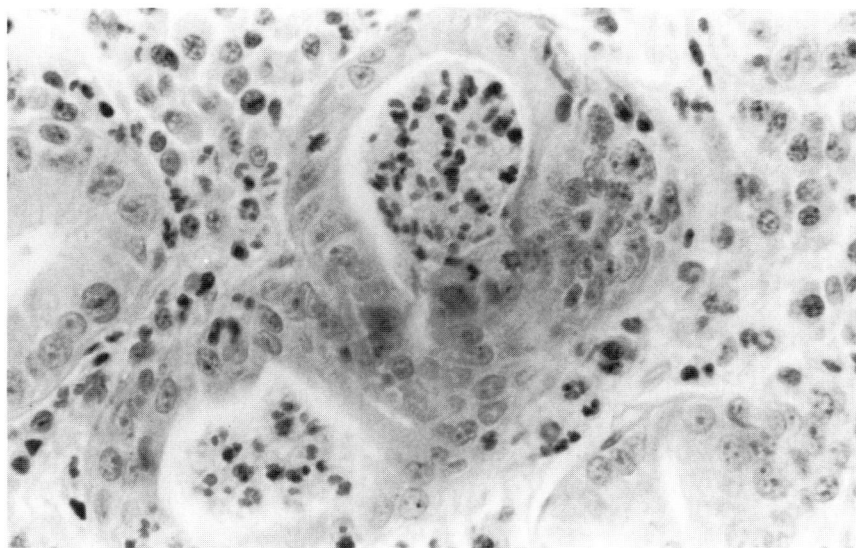

FIGURE 20-6. Gastric mucosal biopsy with chronic active gastritis. Many neutrophils are present in the lumens of the gastric pits and in the lamina propria. The epithelial nuclei show features of regeneration, characterized by enlargement, a stippled chromatin pattern, and prominent nucleoli. (H&E, × 100)

chronic gastritis in the mucosa, special morphologic features, and functional disturbances (Table 20-4). In the early stage of chronic gastritis, whether in the antrum or the corpus-fundus, the inflammation is limited to the surface and gastric pit region. The underlying mucosal glands are either intact or mildly affected, and this lesion is referred to as *chronic superficial gastritis*.[39,40] The mild lesion may persist or eventually extend, usually over a period of several years, to a stage characterized by progressive destruction of the mucosal glands, which is called *chronic atrophic gastritis.* Some of the atrophic cases are associated with a prominent proliferation of lymphoid nodules in the mucosa, termed chronic follicular gastritis, but this feature appears to be just a histologic variation and not a sign of a separate entity. Other cases show complete loss of the specialized mucosal glands but little or no inflammation and have been called *gastric atrophy.* Although it is not usually possible to establish the sequence of histologic stages in an individual patient, it is generally believed that the state of gastric atrophy is a final sequela of a chronic atrophic gastritis.[41] The atrophic effect is typically more pronounced in cases involving the fundus-corpus and may eventually lead to the functional disorder of primary pernicious anemia.

Intestinal Metaplasia. A common and striking histologic feature of all types of chronic gastritis is the presence of intestinal cells and glands in the gastric mucosa.[42-44] This metaplasia is seen in the majority of cases, both in the antrum and in the corpus, and appears to increase in quantity in direct relation to the duration of the disease. The amount of intestinal metaplasia in chronic gastritis varies considerably from scattered foci to extensive replacement of large parts of the gastric mucosa. In the early or milder cases, the lesion tends to be in the foveolar region in the upper part of the mucosa and may involve only one to a few pits. It is often focal and merges with the gastric mucous cells on the surface or in the foveolae. The advanced cases of metaplasia are more frequently associated with the atrophic forms of chronic gastritis and reveal larger and deeper areas that may extend to the mucosal base and occupy the entire mucosal thickness.

Intestinal metaplasia has been extensively investigated, and there are detailed descriptions of its ultrastructure,[45-47] enzymatic content,[48,49] and mucin histochemical characteristics.[50-53] There appear to be two major forms of intestinal metaplasia (complete and incomplete), based in part on a similarity in structure and function to the normal mucosa of the small intestine and of the colon (Table 20-5).[54-56] In type I (or com-

Table 20-4. STAGES OF CHRONIC GASTRITIS

Category	Inflammation	Specialized Glands
Chronic superficial gastritis	Limited to foveolar region or upper gland area	Intact or mild decrease
Chronic atrophic gastritis*	Involves full thickness of mucosa	Marked decrease to complete loss
Gastric atrophy*	None or minimal	Complete loss

*Pernicious anemia occurs in cases of chronic atrophic gastritis and gastric atrophy involving the corpus-fundic region.

Table 20-5. MAJOR TYPES OF INTESTINAL METAPLASIA

Feature	Type I (Complete)	Type IIB (Incomplete)
Absorptive cells	Many	Absent
Paneth cells	Present	Rare
Goblet mucous cells	Few	Many
Foveolar mucous cells	Rare	Many
Stains for		
Sialomucins	Positive	Positive
Sulfomucins	Negative	Positive
Strong association with carcinoma	No	Yes

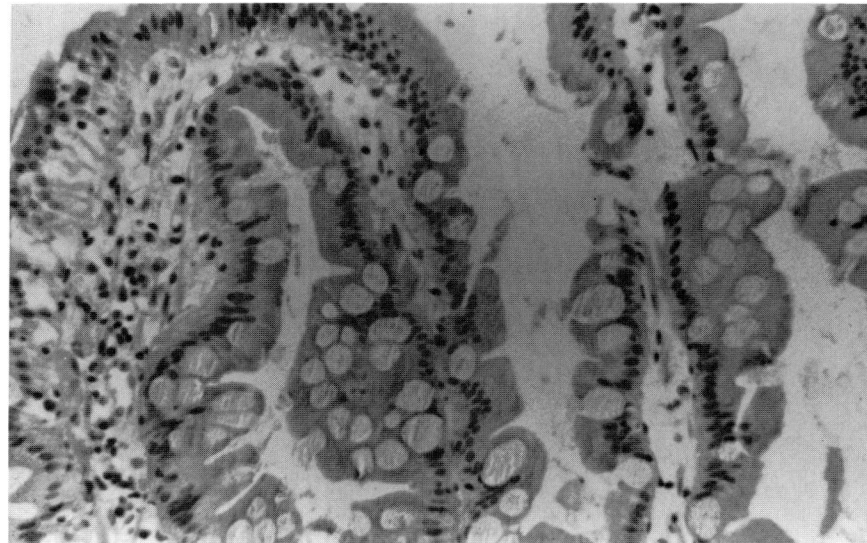

FIGURE 20–7. Gastric mucosa with example of the complete (small-intestinal) form of intestinal metaplasia. There are numerous goblet-type mucous cells and absorptive cells, and a villus-like structure is present on the right. (H&E, × 130)

plete) intestinal metaplasia, the lesion most resembles the small intestine and reveals numerous columnar absorptive cells; relatively fewer goblet mucous cells, which contain mildly acidic mucins such as sialomucin; a variable number of Paneth cells, which tend to be concentrated at the base of the glands; and an occasional villous surface, which is usually poorly formed (Figure 20–7). The absorptive cells have a fully developed brush border that contains alkaline phosphatase, β-glucuronidase, and other enzymatic markers of this region; and studies have shown that the cells are capable of lipid absorption.[57,58] In contrast, type IIB (or incomplete) intestinal metaplasia consists of a mixture of gastric foveolar and colonic-type goblet mucous cells (Figure 20–8). Both types of mucous cells contain highly acidic mucins such as sulfomucin as well as sialomucin, the mucosal surface is generally flat, and there are no fully developed absorptive cells and only rare Paneth cells.[54–56] Type IIA intestinal metaplasia appears to be a variant of type IIB, in which the goblet cells have sulfomucins but the foveolar cells contain mainly sialomucins. Some investigators have substituted the term *type II* for *IIA* and *typeIII* for *IIB*.[53] Intestinal-type endocrine cells are also present in the various forms of metaplasia.[59]

The areas of intestinal metaplasia are readily seen in the gastric mucosa by the ordinary hematoxylin and eosin (H&E) preparation and can be enhanced by the use of mucin stains (Figure 20–9).[50–53] Many mucin stains have been studied, and commonly used are the periodic acid-Schiff (PAS) reaction for neutral glycoproteins, alcian blue at pH 2.5 for sialomucins and other slightly acidic mucosubstances, and alcian blue at pH 1.0 and metachromatic stains for the strongly acidic

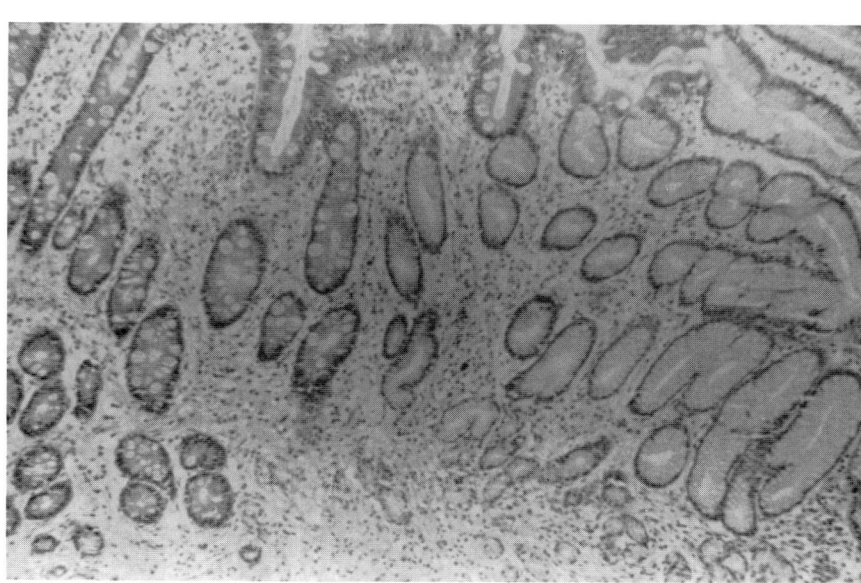

FIGURE 20–8. Gastric antral mucosa revealing foveolar hyperplasia on the right and the incomplete (colonic) form of intestinal metaplasia on the left. Compared with Figure 20–7, the metaplastic area shows more mucous cells and no villous configuration. (H&E, × 80)

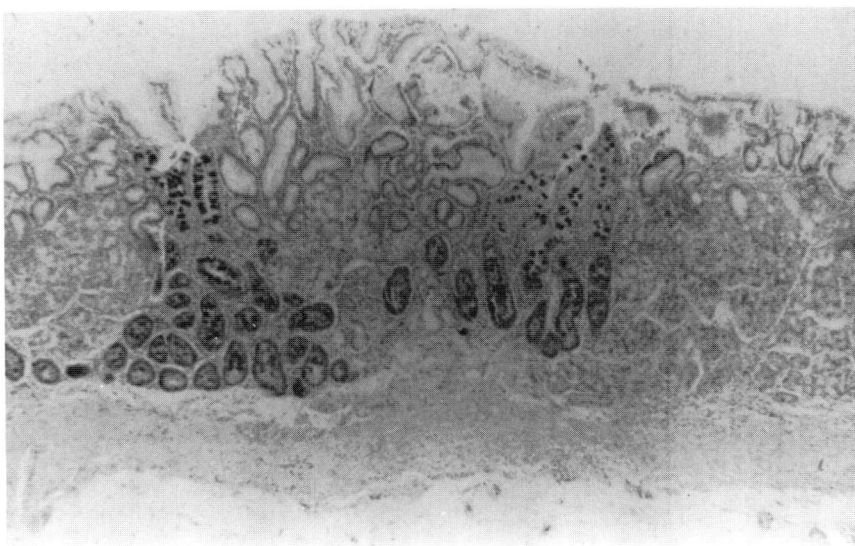

FIGURE 20-9. Gastric corpus mucosa with two foci of intestinal metaplasia, highlighted by a special stain for acidic mucins. (Alcian blue at pH 2.5, × 32)

mucins. The high iron diamine stain appears to be most specific for the identification of sulfomucins.[60,61] In the normal stomach, the surface and foveolar mucous cells are columnar in shape, and the mucin vacuoles are relatively small and concentrated at the luminal end of the cells. The mucin stains strongly with the PAS reaction and is negative for acid substances, except for a faint staining with alcian blue at pH 2.5 in the lower part of the gastric pits in the proximal stomach. This alcian blue positivity is occasionally increased in the foveolar cells in cases of gastritis but is never as intense as in areas of intestinal metaplasia. The goblet mucous cells of the normal intestines and of the metaplasia are identical in appearance, showing a bulging of the lateral membranes due to the presence of many large mucin vacuoles that fill the cytoplasm and that extrude from the surface. The goblet mucus stains faintly with the PAS reaction, strongly with alcian blue at pH 2.5 in the normal small intestine and type I metaplasia, and strongly with alcian blue at both pH 2.5 and 1.0 as well as with the high iron diamine in the normal colon and type IIB metaplasia.

Although there has been an effort to strictly categorize the various types of intestinal metaplasia, it should be stressed that there really is a spectrum with considerable heterogeneity.[51,54] This is evident in the admixture noted in type IIA metaplasia; in the finding of contiguous, columnar-shaped foveolar cells that stain strongly for acid mucins; and in the occasional identification of cells that seem to share both neutral and acidic vacuoles within their cytoplasm.[45]

The importance of the finding of intestinal metaplasia in the stomach is that it helps to identify a case of chronic gastritis. Furthermore, because the incidence of gastric carcinoma is increased in patients with long-standing gastritis and many of the tumors are composed of intestinal-type glands,[62,63] it was formerly considered that the metaplasia might be a necessary precursor lesion of the tumor. It is now generally accepted, however, that this is not the case and that the metaplasia is simply one of the signs of the underlying inflammatory condition.[64] There remains debate over whether the presence of the metaplasia can define a subgroup of patients with chronic gastritis who are especially prone to the development of carcinoma. Metaplasia overall is too ubiquitous a lesion, but recent studies have shown that malignant tumors of the stomach are more often associated with type IIB, the incomplete form of intestinal metaplasia.[65-72] It is probable, however, that this form of metaplasia will also be too common to serve as a useful marker for surveillance, but prospective studies are needed to settle this issue. Chapter 25 provides further details about the structure and significance of intestinal metaplasia.

Chronic Antral Gastritis

Chronic antral gastritis is the type B or environmental form of chronic gastritis that is thought to be caused by toxic substances, and probably by certain bacteria, and in which the lesion is largely confined to the antral mucosa. The prevalence increases with age, and practically all persons over age 40 have some degree of chronic inflammatory changes in the antrum. Only a small number, however, have more active and extensive disease with atrophy and have a clinical disturbance.

Etiology and Pathogenesis. It was formerly thought that most cases of chronic antral gastritis resulted from repeated episodes of acute injury due to ethanol[8,73] and drugs[6,10-15] or to reflux of bile salts into the stomach,[16-20,74,75] but these circumstances are often not documented. These agents act by damaging the membranes of the surface mucous cells, rendering them more permeable to back-diffusion of acid; further details are provided above in the section Acute Gastritis and in Chapter 9. Also incriminated has been the in-

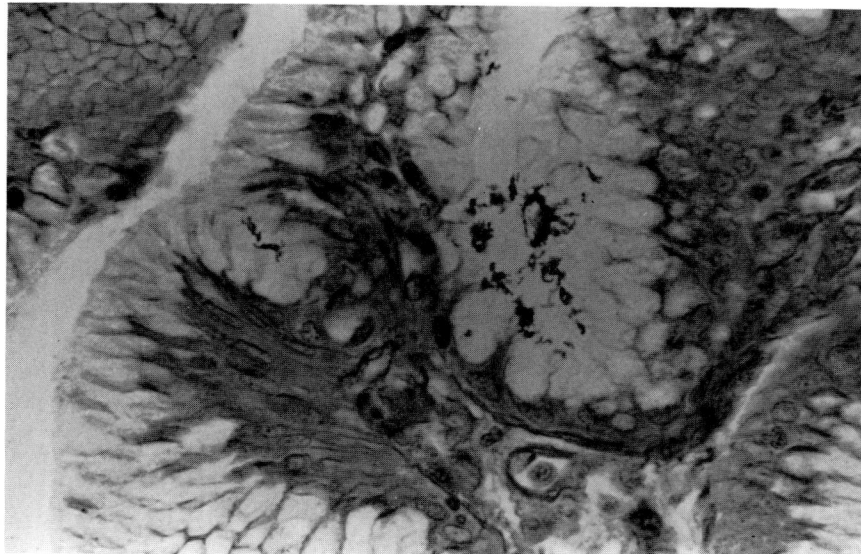

FIGURE 20-10. Gastric pit containing numerous *Helicobacter pylori* microorganisms, in a case of chronic active gastritis. (Dieterle silver, × 500)

gestion of a great deal of spicy foods[76] and smoked products, especially in countries in which such diets are a customary practice.

Role of *Helicobacter* Organisms. Although bacteria have long been noted in the gastric lumen,[77] it has recently been demonstrated that one particular organism, *H. pylori*, is more constantly seen in active cases of chronic antral gastritis.[38,78-88] This agent was formerly referred to as a *Campylobacter*-like organism and also called *C. pyloridis* and *C. pylori*. It can be readily detected by histologic examination of mucosal biopsies, by culture of gastric mucosal tissue, and by a specific serologic test.[79,87,89,90] Furthermore, the organisms are rich in urease, which can be measured in the mucosa[91] and which also can serve as the basis for a noninvasive breath test.[92] Radioactively labeled urea is ingested and the quantity of tagged-carbon dioxide is measured in the expired air. The *Helicobacter* organisms can be seen in regular H&E preparations and are enhanced by a variety of stains, including Gram's, Giemsa, and especially silver stains of the Warthin-Starry type (Figures 20-10 and 20-11).[93,94] They have a spiral shape, measure about 3.5 μm in length and 0.5 μm in width, and are selectively located on the surface and in the lumina of the gastric pits.[95] The organisms can be destroyed by the gastric acid but survive by attaching to the surface cells beneath the mucous layer. By ultrastructural examination, there appears to be a partial envelopment of the organisms by the surface membranes, similar to the adherence of some forms of *Escherichia coli* in the intestines.[96-98]

The gastric microorganisms are found in about 65% to 75% of patients with chronic antral gastritis who have active disease and in only 5% or less of those with inactive disease or a normal mucosa. They are also noted in asymptomatic persons who have histologic evidence of active gastritis; the prevalence increases with age.[99] Interestingly, the bacteria are seen in the antrum of over three quarters of the patients with chronic peptic ulcers of the stomach and duodenum, and it is thought that the common factor is the presence of chronic active gastritis, which so often accompanies the ulcer disease. The bacteria are less often found in the gastric corpus-fundus and in the duodenal mucosa and then typically when the patient has an active antral gastritis;[38,100] in the duodenum, they have

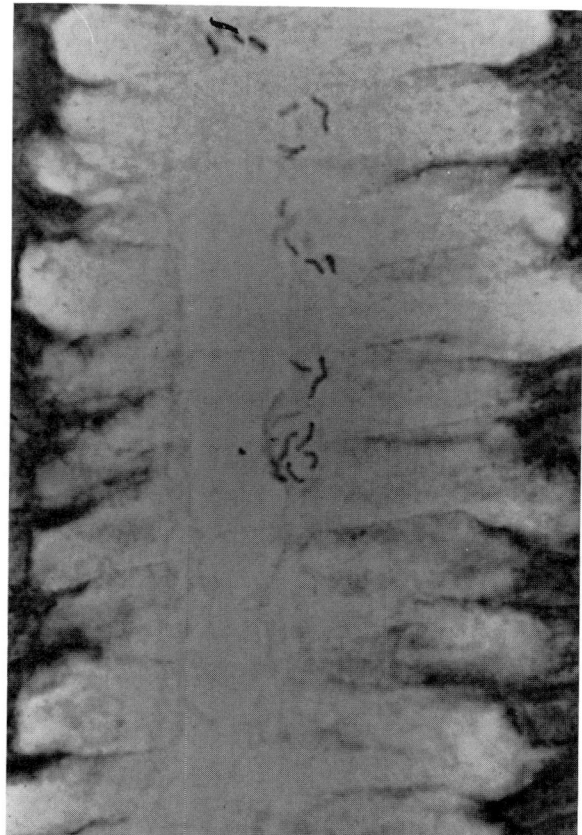

FIGURE 20-11. Higher magnification of a gastric pit, showing several *Helicobacter pylori* bacteria in close apposition to the surfaces of the foveolar mucous cells. (Dieterle silver, × 800)

been seen only in areas of gastric mucous cell metaplasia, suggesting that a specific receptor present in such cells may be needed for the attachment of the organism to the cell surface. The organisms have also been noted in the esophagus in some patients with Barrett's esophagus, but only in cases that have associated active gastritis and bacteria in the gastric antrum,[101] and in areas of heterotopic gastric mucosa.[102]

The appearance of H. pylori in the gastric antrum correlates best with the presence of active disease, and several studies have shown a loss of both symptoms and organisms after treatment with antimicrobial drugs, including a variety of antibiotics and bismuth-containing compounds.[103] Furthermore, there have been a few recorded cases of ingestion of the organisms, either accidental[104] or by intent,[25,85] leading to a gastritis with histologic confirmation of the presence of the bacteria and active inflammation in the mucosa. Nevertheless, it has not as yet been conclusively established that H. pylori is the primary agent responsible for the development of most cases of chronic antral gastritis.[105] An alternative explanation is that the bacterium is a secondary invader that thrives in the inflammatory environment. Even if this is the situation, however, it remains possible that the organism can foster an episode of active inflammation and thus contribute to the appearance of clinical disease and the overall progression of the disorder. Further large-scale studies will be needed to resolve this important issue.

Role of Other Bacteria. Other bacteria have been noted in the gastric antrum, and some may represent saprophytes. One organism, measuring about 5 to 6 μm in length and more tightly spiralled than H. pylori, has been seen uncommonly in cases of chronic active antral gastritis and could represent another causative agent.[106-108] It is gram-negative and usually detected in antral smears rather than in the histologic sections. The bacterium has not been completely identified; larger studies, including response to therapy, are awaited.

Clinical Features. The clinical aspects of chronic antral gastritis are mainly related to the episodes of active disease and are generally similar to those seen in patients with acute toxic gastritis.[4,5,105] There is typically a sudden onset of abdominal pain and vomiting, with bleeding in the severe cases, and a fairly rapid resolution following elimination of any toxic agents (such as ethanol and drugs) and the use of medications to reduce the effects of gastric acidity. This subject is covered more fully in the earlier section on acute gastritis. As previously noted, the majority of patients with chronic active gastritis affecting the antrum harbor H. pylori in the gastric mucosa, and initial clinical trials with antimicrobial agents have resulted in a diminution or complete clearing of symptoms in most cases.

There does not appear to be any specific functional effect that can be attributed to the loss of pyloric glands in the later or atrophic stage of the disease. However, the atrophy is occasionally associated with a reduction in the antral endocrine cells, including those that produce gastrin, and this can result in decreased acid secretion and hypochlorhydria. It is probable that the back diffusion of acid that occurs during active disease also contributes to the low concentration of acid in the gastric lumen.

Pathology. The common features of chronic gastritis and of active disease are described earlier in the section on general pathologic features.[2,33-38] In the early stages, the alterations are largely confined to the gastric pit region in the upper mucosa and consist mainly of an increase in the amount of mononuclear inflammation in the lamina propria and a variable degree of foveolar hyperplasia (see Figure 20-5). With advancement of the disease, there is extension of the inflammation into the lower part of the mucosa, a partial loss of the pyloric glands and the endocrine cells that are located in this region, and a progressive replacement of the mucosa by intestinal metaplasia (see Figure 20-7). As a result of the inflammation and the variable types of glands, the mucosal surface, which is ordinarily fairly smooth in the normal antrum, develops a more granular appearance.[110] Occasionally, there is persistence of the foveolar hyperplasia, leading to the formation of localized hyperplastic polyps or to a more diffuse thickening of the mucosal surface.[111] The normal antral mucosa contains a prominent amount of fibromuscular stroma in its lamina propria, and this tissue may show focal areas of either destruction or condensation.

The active phase of chronic antral gastritis is characterized by the additional presence of acute inflammation and variable necrosis (see Figure 20-6); this typically starts in the pit region and extends to the lower mucosa in the severe cases. It appears that areas of intestinal metaplasia are infrequently involved with the active inflammation, which suggests that the metaplastic tissue may be resistant to the action of the injurious agents. As noted above, clusters of H. pylori are often present on the surface and in the lumina of the superficial gastric pits at the time of active disease, whereas they are usually absent during the inactive phase of chronic gastritis. The bacteria are typically seen in association with the gastric mucous cells and less often with the intestinal cells.

It is not known whether the progression of the chronic gastritis to the atrophic stage is continuous or the result of recurrent episodes of active disease. In the late stages of chronic antral gastritis, the disease often extends into the junctional area and the lower part of the gastric corpus. However, the uppermost region of the stomach, including the cardia and the fundus, is ordinarily spared, and there are no functional effects from this spread.

Differential Diagnosis. The majority of adults, and probably all persons over 40 years of age, reveal patchy areas of chronic inflammation and intestinal metaplasia in the gastric antrum; this finding alone is not usually associated with clinical problems. In contrast, the lesions are more diffuse in patients with chronic gastritis. Because the histologic features of chronic antral gastritis are relatively nonspecific, the diagnosis is dependent on a compatible clinical history and on the exclusion of other inflammatory disorders that preferentially involve the antrum. The condition is distinguished from acute gastritis by the history of repeated episodes and by the finding of signs of chronic inflammation in the gastric mucosa. Cases of chronic peptic ulcer invariably have chronic inflammation in the adjacent intact mucosa, but the ulcers can be readily visualized by gross endoscopic and radiographic examinations. Other inflammatory disorders reveal more characteristic features, such as the presence of microorganisms or granulomas in other infections and a prominent eosinophilic reaction in allergic disease. See the earlier section on acute gastritis for further details regarding the differential diagnosis of active gastritis.

Chronic Fundic Gastritis

Chronic fundic gastritis corresponds to the type A form of chronic gastritis, in which the lesion typically occurs in older persons; primarily affects the fundic and corpus mucosa; and is believed to result from an immunologic injury.[112-114] As with other forms of chronic gastritis, there appear to be stages or degrees of severity, ranging from superficial mucosal inflammation to complete atrophy of the specialized glands.[39,40] In long-standing cases, there is often spread of the inflammatory lesions into the antral region. Indeed, because the prevalence of chronic antral gastritis is fairly high, the two forms of chronic fundic and of chronic antral gastritis may coexist in the same patient.

Etiology and Pathogenesis. It is generally accepted that cases of chronic fundic gastritis occurring in adults are a consequence of continuous immunologic damage of the mucosa.[114-117] Over half of the patients have antibodies to components of parietal cells and intrinsic factor in the serum and gastric fluid.[118,119] There is also a common association with other diseases that are thought to have an immunologic basis, including thyroiditis and hypothyroidism, diabetes mellitus, adrenal insufficiency, Sjögren's disease, and myasthenia gravis; and patients frequently have shared autoantibodies to the various tissues.[120] The exact mechanism of the injury in the stomach is not known. Despite the presence of the gastric antibodies, it is not proven that they are responsible for the initiation or even the perpetuation of the disorder; rather, the release of the antibodies could be simply secondary to the tissue damage. Furthermore, the character of the inflammatory cells in the gastric mucosa, dominated by the presence of lymphocytes and other mononuclear cells, suggests instead that a cellular type of immunologic injury may be involved. Whatever the mechanism, the effects in the gastric mucosa are clear, and there develops over the course of several years a progressive destruction of the specialized glands containing the parietal (oxyntic) and chief cells throughout the corpus and fundic region.

There is a rare juvenile form of primary pernicious anemia, and its cause is not known.[121] Interestingly, despite the same functional effect, only some cases reveal an atrophic mucosa, whereas others show preservation of the specialized glands, which suggests that multiple factors or causes may be involved, including a biochemical blockage of the secretory process or its products.

Clinical Features. The clinical effects are due to the loss of the cells in the specialized glands of the corpus-fundic region and become evident only in the advanced or atrophic stage of the disease.[122-124] The damage to the chief cells leads to a reduction in the class of pepsinogens, but this causes no functional deficit, because there are many more proteolytic enzymes normally excreted by the pancreas. More major effects result from the loss of parietal cells, leading to achlorhydria, and particularly of the intrinsic factor that is located in its cellular membranes. The latter is required for the optimal absorption of vitamin B_{12} in the ileum following binding of the intrinsic factor to the ingested vitamin, and the loss of the factor ultimately results in the development of primary pernicious anemia. The effects of the reduced acid secretion are less striking. There will be reduced activation of the pepsinogens to pepsins, but this is not important because of the alternative supply of pancreatic enzymes. Although the loss of gastric acid may permit the survival of more ingested microorganisms, theoretically favoring the appearance of more infections in the stomach and intestines, this is not a major problem unless the patient's immune system is otherwise compromised. The achlorhydria also causes a sustained stimulation of the gastrin-producing endocrine cells in the antrum,[125] resulting in hypergastrinemia and, rarely, in the appearance of multiple hyperplastic nodules of endocrine cells and carcinoid tumors in the antrum.

The adult cases typically are seen in older persons, usually over 60 years of age in the atrophic stage of the disease, with the appearance of a megaloblastic anemia. The anemia is often severe, and the diagnosis is dependent on the findings of achlorhydria, both basal and stimulated, and of an abnormal Schilling test, which is corrected by the addition of intrinsic factor. Gastric biopsy samples are not ordinarily obtained for the diagnosis, because small samples may not be representative of the entire corpus-fundic region, and the functional tests are more specific. Unlike antral gastritis, the early stage of the fundic disease is not punctuated by episodes of clinically evident active gastritis. It has been noted that in less advanced cases, when there is still preservation of some of the specialized glands, the lesion may be inhibited or arrested by the use of corticosteroid hormones.[126] The anemia responds fully to treatment by injection of vitamin B_{12}, but patients are at some increased risk for the development of polyps and carcinoma of the stomach,[127-129] as discussed later.

Pathology. The common alterations of chronic gastritis are described earlier in the section on general pathologic features.[2,33-38] In the early stage of the disorder, called chronic superficial gastritis, there are increased mononuclear inflammatory cells in the upper part of the lamina propria, beneath the surface epithelium and between the gastric pits (Figure 20-12). Damage to the superficial mucous epithelial cells and the acute inflammatory reaction are usually patchy and slight. As the disease advances, typically over many years, there are extension of the mononuclear and acute inflammatory reactions into the lower part of the

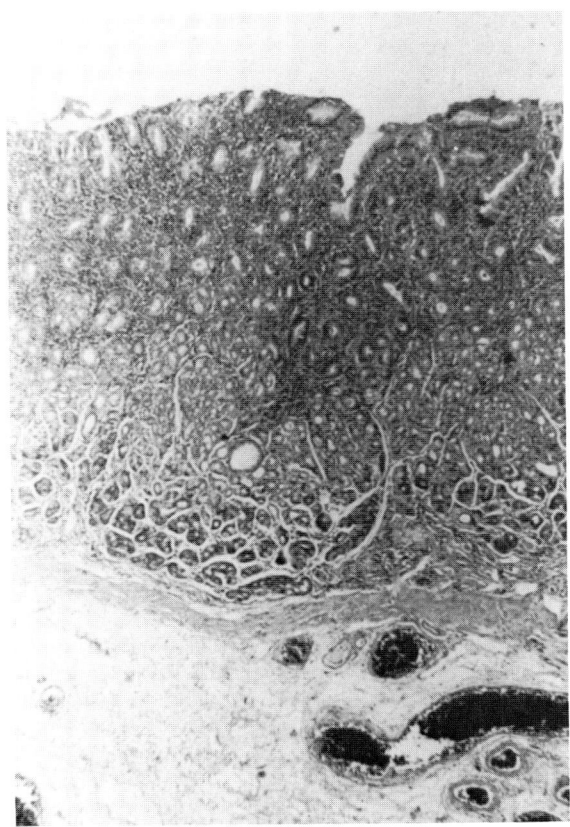

FIGURE 20-12. Gastric corpus mucosa with superficial chronic gastritis. There is a dense infiltrate of mononuclear inflammatory cells that is limited to the upper half of the mucosa. The lower half of the mucosa and submucosa (bottom) are not involved. (H&E, × 13)

mucosa and a progressive destruction of the specialized glands throughout the corpus-fundic region (Figure 20-13). Over time, the mucosa becomes replaced by a mixture of areas of foveolar hyperplasia and intestinal metaplasia (see Figure 20-8); there is also often a prominent pyloric gland metaplasia in the basal part. The disorder is referred to as chronic atropic gastritis at this stage; some cases with complete loss of the specialized glands have minimal inflammation, and these have been called gastric atrophy but probably represent the end stage of the same disorder.

The disease is limited to the mucosa; there is commonly vascular congestion in the submucosa but no other abnormalities of the gastric wall. The mucosa is usually thinner than it normally is, and this causes a decrease in the size and number of the rugae and enhanced visualization of the submucosal vessels on gross examination (Figure 20-14).[110] Alternatively, some cases reveal greater foveolar hyperplasia, leading to the formation of multiple hyperplastic polyps (Figure 20-15) or, exceptionally, to a diffuse hypertrophy of the mucosa.[130-132]

The findings in the gastric antrum in cases of chronic fundic gastritis are variable.[133] In most patients, there are only patchy areas of chronic inflammation with intestinal metaplasia, equivalent in degree to what is seen in normal adult persons. The pyloric glands in the antrum are intact, and there is often seen a hyperplasia of the endocrine cells,[134] including those producing gastrin, that is thought to result from the sustained stimulation by the low gastric acid concentration in the lumen (Figure 20-16). This occasionally leads to the formation of multiple small nodules of endocrine cells and carcinoid tumors in the antrum. In some cases of chronic fundic gastritis, in contrast, the antral mucosa reveals more widespread inflammatory changes with atrophy; it is not usually known whether this represents an extension of the fundic disease into the antrum or a coexistence of the two forms of chronic fundic and chronic antral gastritis in the same patient. The incidence of *H. pylori* in the antrum is low, even in cases with active inflammation.[135]

Differential Diagnosis. In the late atrophic stage of chronic fundic gastritis with the appearance of the megaloblastic anemia, the diagnosis is readily deter-

FIGURE 20-13. Gastric corpus mucosa in case of chronic atrophic gastritis with primary pernicious anemia. There is a thinning of the mucosa and a complete loss of the specialized gastric glands. The mucosa has been replaced by intestinal glands on the left and by pyloric glands at the right, representing metaplasia. The submucosa (bottom) is not affected. (H&E, × 32)

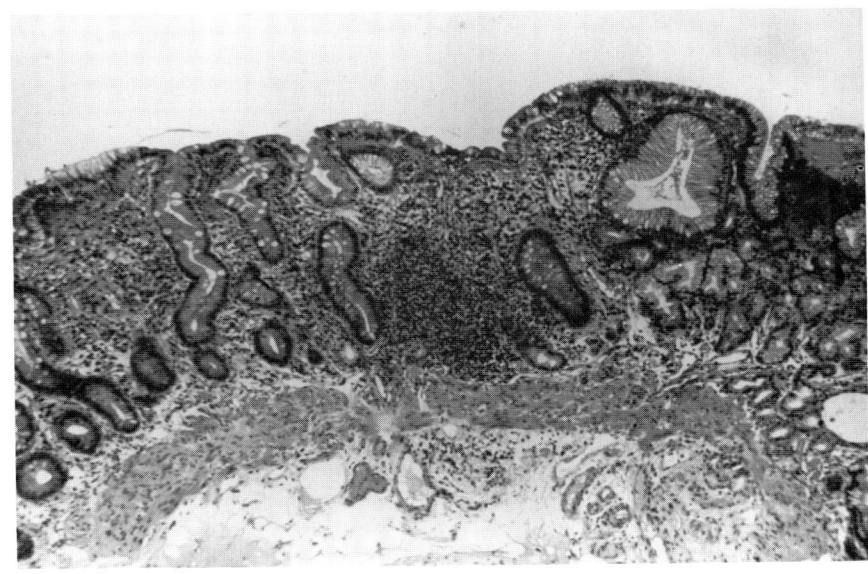

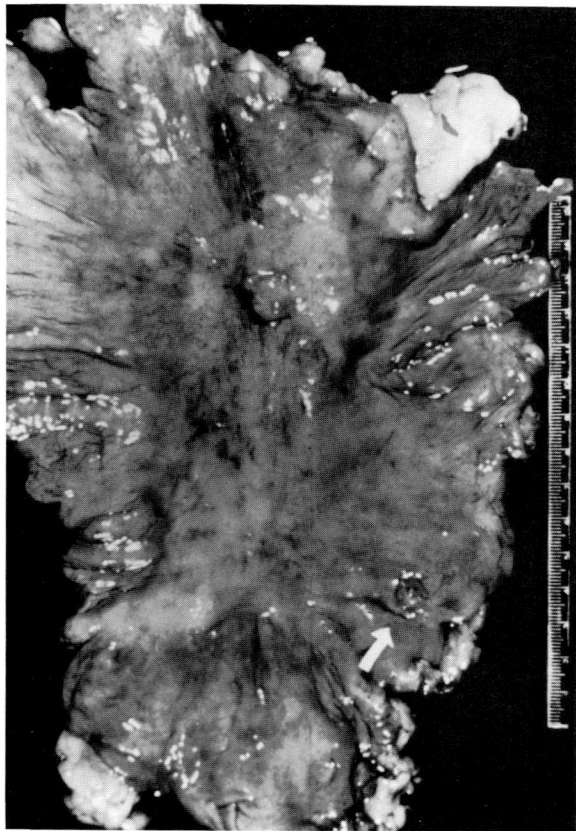

FIGURE 20–14. Segment of stomach with contiguous duodenum (bottom) in a case of atrophic gastritis and pernicious anemia, showing absence of rugae. There are two small hyperplastic polyps, one at the arrow and one to the top of the center.

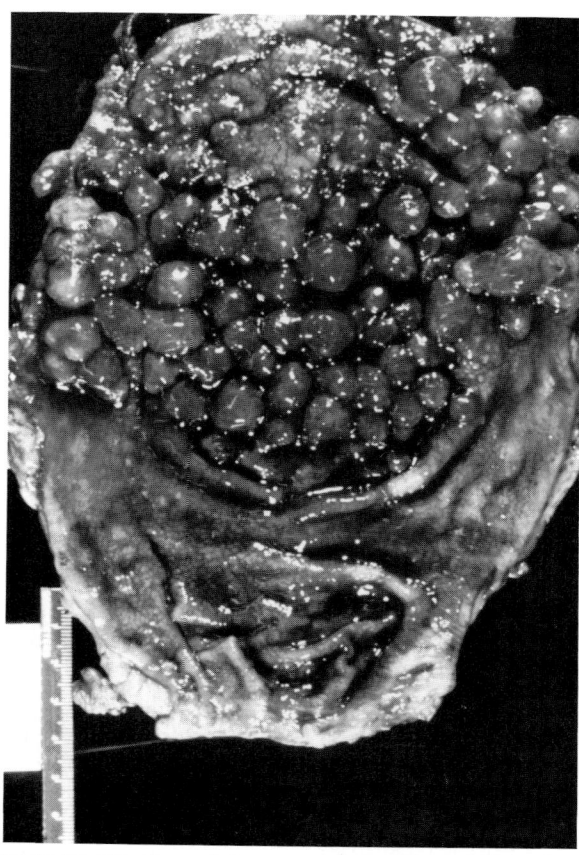

FIGURE 20–15. Stomach in a case of atrophic gastritis and pernicious anemia revealing a large conglomerate of hyperplastic polyps in the corpus region (top).

mined by the functional tests of gastric acid secretion and of vitamin B_{12} absorption. If only the histologic features are considered, the differential is also limited because most inflammatory disorders of the stomach (such as acute gastritis, chronic peptic ulcers, infections, and allergic disease) primarily affect the antrum. Superficial chronic inflammation, usually very mild and associated with only rare foci of acute inflammation and of intestinal metaplasia, may be occasionally seen in older persons and in the late stage of chronic

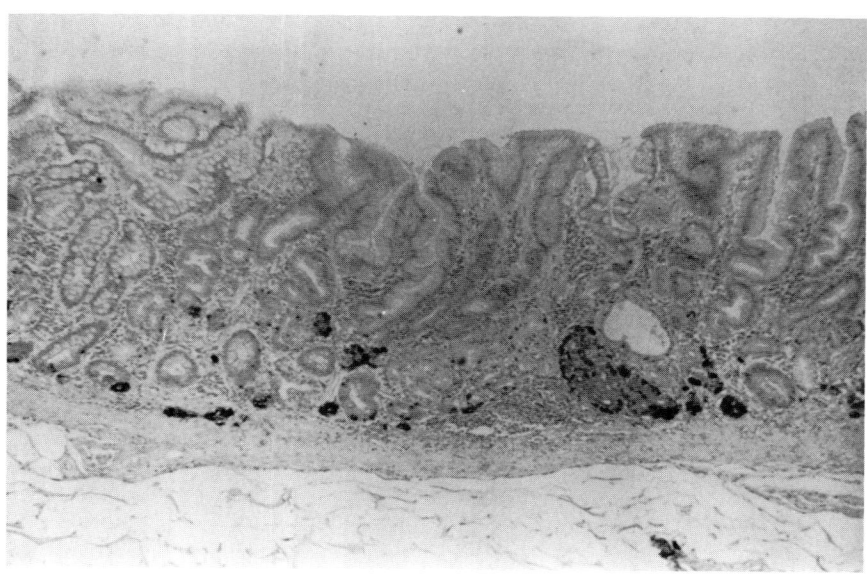

FIGURE 20–16. Gastric antral mucosa in a case of atrophic corpus gastritis and pernicious anemia. A special stain reveals an increase in the number of endocrine cells, which stain dark, with a large nest (microcarcinoid) in the lower right basal portion of the mucosa. The submucosa is at the bottom. (Chromogranin, × 32)

antral gastritis. Localized areas of atrophy of the corpus mucosa may occur, overlying mural tumors and adjacent to rare helminthic infections. In the case of the development of mucosal polyps (see Figure 20–15), it is necessary to distinguish the common hyperplastic (or regenerative) type from adenomas and carcinomas, and this is readily accomplished by biopsy examination. When there is a diffuse foveolar cell hyperplasia resulting in enlarged rugae and an overall thickening of the mucosal surface, the differential diagnosis includes consideration of tumor infiltration, both of carcinoma and of lymphoma, and Ménétrier's disease.[136] The latter in its pure form shows an isolated hyperplasia of the surface-foveolar mucous cells, resulting in marked lengthening of the gastric pits, and only minimal or no inflammation; the underlying specialized glands are not affected.

Postgastrectomy Gastritis

Etiology and Clinical Features. Inflammation of the gastric corpus mucosa invariably occurs after excision or bypass of the pyloric sphincter.[137,138] It is seen in patients who have had an antral gastrectomy and either a gastrojejunostomy (Billroth II) or a gastroduodenostomy (Billroth I); it is also seen after only a gastrojejunostomy. The antrectomy is most often performed for the treatment of chronic peptic ulcers of either the stomach or the duodenum. The gastritis is thought to result from the constant reflux of bile salts through the open stoma, resulting in damage to the membranes of the surface epithelial cells, which allows an increased back-diffusion of acid into the mucosa.[139] Alternatively, because the resected antra are usually inflamed, the subsequent appearance of gastritis in the proximal stomach may simply represent an extension of the underlying inflammatory condition to this area.

Although in all patients who have undergone these operative procedures histologic alterations develop, clinically apparent disease is noted in only about 10%.[124,140,141] The features are those that would be expected in any case of active gastritis and include intermittent episodes of upper abdominal burning pain and hemorrhage in the more severe examples. Treatment is essentially medical and consists of the use of agents that reduce or neutralize gastric acid and that bind to the bile salts. The disorder of bile-induced gastritis must be distinguished from other conditions that can occur in patients who have had an antral resection, including the dumping syndrome and a bacterial proliferation state resulting from an enlarged afferent loop of jejunum.

Pathology. The inflammatory lesion begins in the corpus mucosa just adjacent to the anastomotic stoma and may spread with time to affect much of the proximal stomach.[138,142–144] The features are generally similar to those seen in chronic fundic gastritis and include the presence of mononuclear inflammatory cells and a loss of the specialized corpus glands, which are replaced by pyloric glands. There is often a more prominent degree of acute inflammation and a focal cystic dilation of the gastric pits (Figure 20–17). Interestingly, intestinal metaplasia is observed in fewer than half of the cases and is rarely a dominant feature. The atrophy of the specialized corpus glands is typically patchy in the early stage but may become confluent with increased duration; a complete loss of the glands in the corpus and fundus with the development of pernicious anemia has only rarely been recorded. As with other types of chronic gastritis, in some cases there is a prominent degree of foveolar cell hyperplasia, resulting in the formation of hyperplastic polyps or, rarely, a diffuse mucosal hypertrophy.[145–147] This proliferation may be especially prominent at the stoma and associated with the extension of mature glands into the underlying submucosa, representing a localized form of gastritis cystica profunda; the lesion can simulate carcinoma and is described further in the following section on gastritis cystica. Other late effects, including the

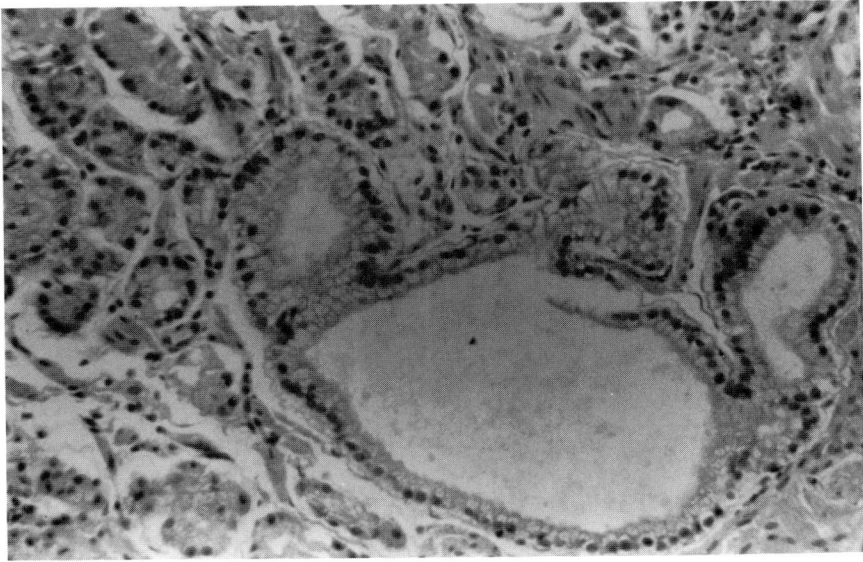

FIGURE 20–17. Gastric corpus mucosa in case of postgastrectomy gastritis, showing pyloric gland metaplasia with cystic glands. (H&E, × 130)

predisposition to dysplasia and carcinoma, are discussed in the section on complications of chronic gastritis.

Differential Diagnosis. The diagnosis of gastritis following distal gastric resection or bypass is promptly suggested by the clinical history, but further studies are needed to exclude other causes of the recurrent pain and bleeding. Radiographic and endoscopic procedures, with biopsy if needed, are employed for detection of a recurrent peptic ulcer, which is typically on the intestinal side of the anastomosis; for evaluation of any mass lesions; and for identification of other causes of inflammation and hemorrhage in the upper alimentary tract. The histologic features of the gastritis are essentially nonspecific; but the findings of prominent cystic dilation of the gastric pits, the preservation of small clusters of parietal and chief cells, and a relative paucity of intestinal metaplasia may help in distinguishing the postgastrectomy type from other forms of chronic gastritis affecting the corpus.

Chronic Erosive Gastritis

Chronic erosive gastritis is a form of chronic active gastritis in which the mucosal surface is markedly deformed by the presence of alternating areas of erosions and small polyps.[148-151] The condition has also been called varioliform gastritis. There is typically a diffuse involvement of the fundic-corpus region and more variable effects in the antrum. This mucosal appearance may simulate a tumor on radiographic and endoscopic examination and may even cause difficulty in biopsy interpretation. The condition is possible a subset of chronic gastritis and separately designated because of the special gross features and the potential confusion with carcinoma.

Histologic study reveals multiple erosions, usually a marked acute and chronic inflammatory cell reaction that extends into and dilates the underlying glandular lumina, and pseudopolyp formation of the adjacent intact mucosa (Figure 20–18). The polypoid areas show a prominent regeneration of the gastric foveolae, which become irregular in size and shape; this appearance, together with the cystic glands, can resemble that of early gastric carcinoma affecting the mucosa. The nuclei of the regenerating epithelial cells are enlarged and have prominent nucleoli but, in contrast to those of tumor cells, are generally regular in size and shape and lack prominent hyperchromatism (Figure 20–19); also, there is usually more abundant cytoplasm in the regenerative cells. Another helpful feature is that the mucosa in chronic erosive gastritis, when it affects the corpus region, reveals partial preservation of the parietal and chief cells lining the inflamed and dilated glands, whereas these specialized cells are generally absent in tumor glands (Figure 20–20).

The diagnosis of chronic erosive gastritis is based on the gross appearance of the lesion and on documentation by histologic examination of its inflammatory nature. Cases of acute toxic gastritis and of stress ulceration may reveal multiple erosions and regenerative glands, but the lesions are usually limited to or dominant in the antrum in acute gastritis; in both conditions, prominent polyp formation and chronic inflammation are absent. As noted earlier, erosions and hyperplastic polyps can be seen in standard cases of chronic antral gastritis and chronic fundic gastritis; the designation of chronic erosive gastritis may be dependent on simply the presence of both features to a marked degree.

Lymphocytic Gastritis. It has been noted in cases of chronic erosive (varioliform) gastritis that there is a marked increase in the number of lymphocytes within the epithelial layer lining the gastric surface and foveolae, particularly in those cases affecting the corpus region.[152] Conversely, of all cases designated by biopsy as showing this lymphocytic gastritis, about 20% did not exhibit the gross thickening of the mucosa, which suggests that the lymphocytic infiltrate may represent

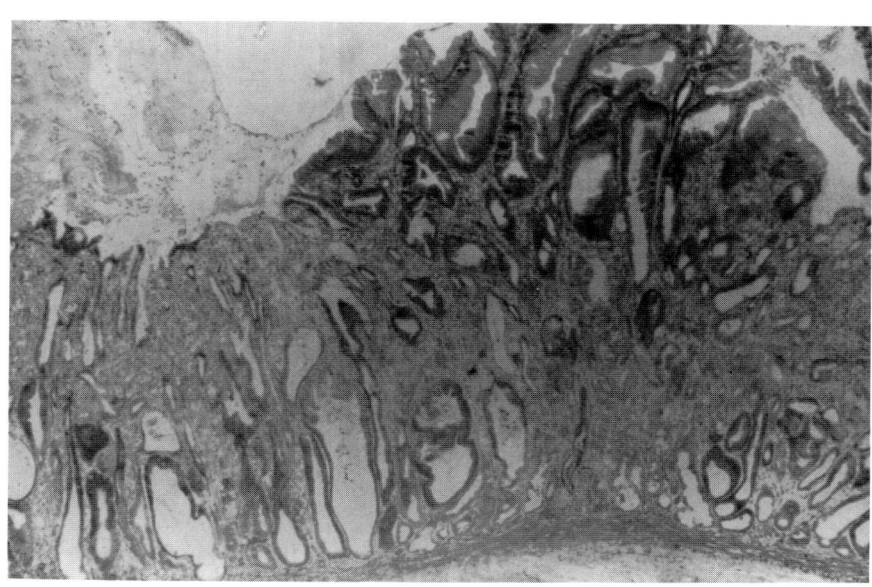

FIGURE 20–18. Gastric mucosa in case of chronic erosive (varioliform) gastritis. Present are alternating areas of erosion (left) and foveolar hyperplasia (right). The submucosa is at the bottom. (H&E, × 80)

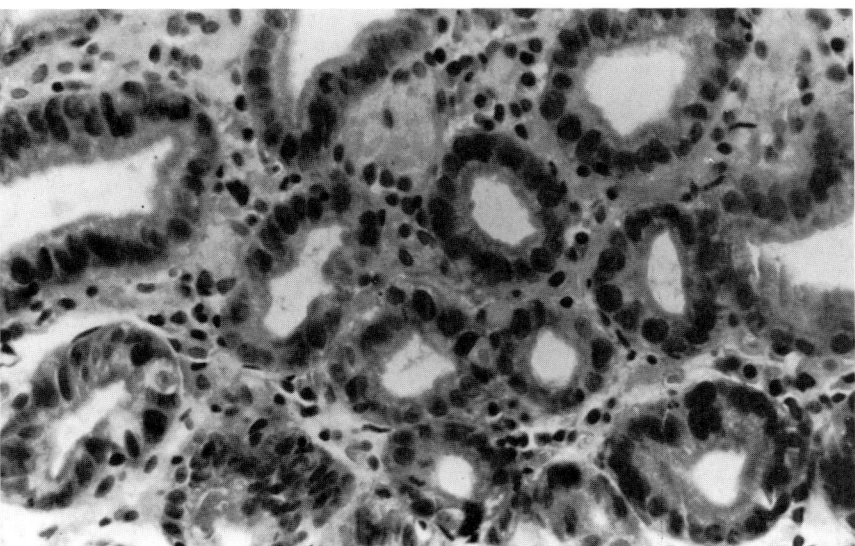

FIGURE 20–19. Gastric foveolae in a case of chronic erosive gastritis, showing marked regeneration. The epithelial nuclei are enlarged but are mostly round and fairly regular in size and shape. Contrast with the dysplastic epithelium in Figure 20–21. (H&E, × 310)

an early or precursor lesion. Similar lymphocytic lesions that are limited to the antrum appear to be less specific, because they have been seen in otherwise ordinary cases of chronic antral gastritis, including those associated with H. pylori infection.[153] Interestingly, an equivalent degree of increased lymphocytes has been observed in the gastric surface-foveolar epithelium in about half of a series of cases of celiac sprue[154]; it is probable that the presence of the lymphocytic infiltrate is a nonspecific marker of a variety of immunologically directed disorders. There does not appear to be any association between celiac disease and the fully developed gross lesion of chronic erosive gastritis.

Chronic Hypertrophic Gastritis

Chronic hypertrophic gastritis is a variant form of chronic gastritis in which there is a prominent degree of hyperplasia of the surface and foveolar mucous cells, resulting in marked and often diffuse hypertrophy of the involved segment of mucosa.[111,130–132] It can be seen in cases of both chronic antral and chronic fundic gastritis, and the reason for the pronounced hyperplasia in these instances is not known. Some details are provided in the earlier sections on general pathologic features and differential diagnosis of chronic fundic gastritis, and the subject is covered more fully in Chapter 22, on mucosal hypertrophy and hyperplasia of the stomach.

Complications

There are certain conditions of the stomach that occur more frequently in patients with the various types of chronic gastritis. Some of the lesions are a direct consequence of the inflammatory process, such as

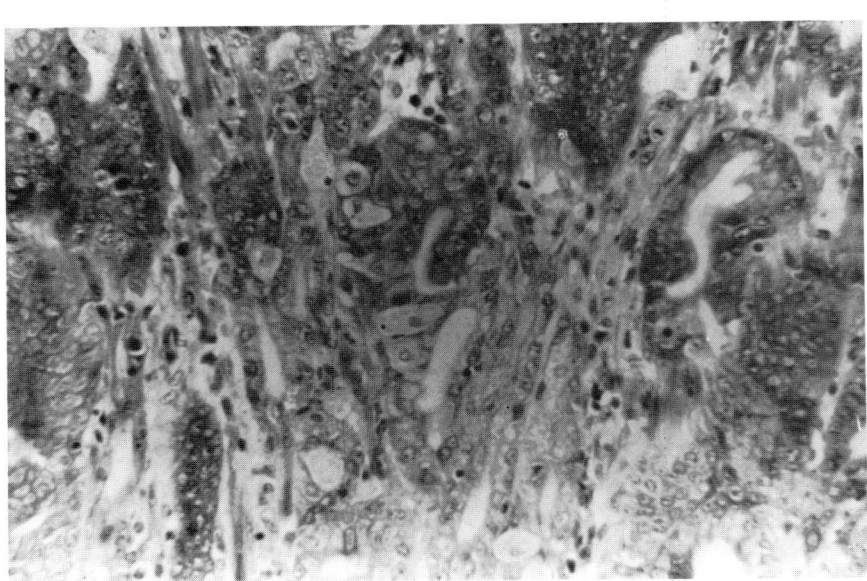

FIGURE 20–20. Gastric mucosa in a case of chronic erosive gastritis. There is irregularity of the regenerating glands (top). Scattered throughout are intact parietal cells, which appear polygonal and have pale cytoplasm and central nuclei. (H&E, × 200)

xanthomas and hyperplastic (or regenerative) polyps; whereas others relate to an increased propensity of the chronically inflamed mucosa to develop neoplasms, including adenomas, carcinomas, and carcinoid tumors. Chronic inflammation of the antral mucosa is also noted in patients with chronic peptic ulcers of the antrum, and the inflammatory lesion may be a necessary factor for the ulcer formation in this region; this topic is covered in Chapter 21, on peptic ulcer disease.

Xanthoma

Xanthomas are slightly raised, yellow nodules on the mucosal surface and typically measure only a few millimeters in diameter.[155–159] The lesions are sessile, may be single or multiple, and are more often noted in the corpus-fundic region. The nodules are composed of a core of numerous, finely vacuolated macrophages that contain lipids within the lamina propria and are covered by normal or slightly hyperplastic epithelium (see Chapter 16, Figure 16-4). They are confined to the mucosa, and there is usually no conspicuous inflammation in the lesion. Although xanthomas occasionally may be seen in a noninflamed stomach, they are much more frequently noted in cases of chronic gastritis, particularly in the postgastrectomy form.[160,161] It is thought that the lesion results from prior episodes of mucosal hemorrhage and that the lipids are derived from the destroyed blood cells. The natural course is not known, but it is probable that the nodules can spontaneously resolve.

The diagnosis of xanthoma is ordinarily made on regular H&E preparations; staining for fat, which would require frozen sections, is neither available nor needed. Lesions that might be confused with xanthomas include clusters of macrophages containing mucin (muciphages) and granular cell tumors within the gastric mucosa. Muciphages are infrequently noted in the stomach, in contrast to colonic mucosa, and they contain larger and more irregular cytoplasmic vacuoles that stain strongly with the PAS reaction (see Chapter 16, Figure 16-6). The cells of a granular cell tumor ("myoblastoma") have a distinct granular cytoplasm that stains weakly with the PAS reaction. Although signet-ring cell carcinomas may present with sheets of cells in the lamina propria, particularly in biopsy specimens, they contain mucus, and their nature is readily discerned by the highly irregular and hyperchromatic nuclei. Some granulomas, especially those due to foreign bodies or to *Mycobacterium avium-intracellulare*, may contain enlarged and vacuolated macrophages; but the lesions are much smaller, circumscribed, and usually associated with giant cells and other inflammatory cells. Rarer causes of macrophage accumulations in the mucosa include chronic granulomatous disease of childhood, which reveals cytoplasmic pigment, and malakoplakia, which has characteristic inclusions.

Epithelial Polyps

As noted above, some cases of chronic gastritis, of both antral and fundic types, are associated with foveolar cell hyperplasia, and this can result in the formation of localized hyperplastic (regenerative) polyps.[145–147] They appear to be more common in the proximal stomach and have been found in up to 10% of patients with chronic fundic gastritis in the atrophic stage and of the postgastrectomy cases.[162] The polyps are usually small, sessile, and have a smooth or coarsely lobular surface.[163,164] They are frequently multiple and, exceptionally, may present with a large conglomerate of lesions that effaces the mucosal surface (see Figure 20-15). Hyperplastic polyps are composed of a core of edematous and inflamed lamina propria and contain a variable number of pyloric glands and a variable amount of hyperplastic or actively regenerative foveolar epithelium; intestinal metaplasia may be present but usually is not a prominent feature. The polypoid lesions are analogous to the inflammatory pseudopolyps that are seen in cases of chronic colitis; these and other epithelial polyps of the stomach are described more fully in Chapter 23.

Although fundic gland polyps, consisting of intact fundic mucosa with focal cystic dilation of the pits and glands, have been noted in cases of chronic gastritis, it is not established that they are more frequent in these conditions. Adenomas of the stomach, representing benign neoplasms of the gastric epithelium, are generally rare but appear to be more common in patients with chronic gastritis; they have been noted in 1% of cases in some series of postgastrectomy gastritis.[162] Compared with hyperplastic polyps, the adenomas are typically larger, have a more papillary surface contour, and contain dysplastic epithelium of the foveolar or intestinal metaplastic types. They also may contain foci of adenocarcinoma.

Dysplasia and Adenocarcinoma

It is generally accepted that patients with the atrophic forms of chronic gastritis are at increased risk for the development of gastric adenocarcinoma after a latent period of about 10 years.[165] The prevalence in different geographic regions varies widely, however, and is probably related to the baseline frequency of such tumors in each country. In areas with a high rate of gastric carcinoma, follow-up studies of patients with gastric atrophy and pernicious anemia have revealed an eight- to tenfold increase of tumors after 10 to 15 years of known disease.[127–129,166,167] Similarly, an increased frequency of carcinoma in the order of 1% to 5% has been noted in the proximal stomach (referred to as stump carcinoma) 10 to 15 years after an antral resection.[162,168–179] Again, the enhanced risk has been well documented in countries that have a high *de novo* rate of carcinoma, such as Scandinavia and England, whereas it has not been clearly established in the United States.[180–182] The stump tumors typically occur in the mucosa just proximal to the anastomosis where the inflammation is the greatest. It has been suggested that the risk of tumor is greater in patients who have had a Billroth II operation and that the rate is related in part to the reason for the previous resection. Thus more tumors are seen in patients 10 to 15 years after

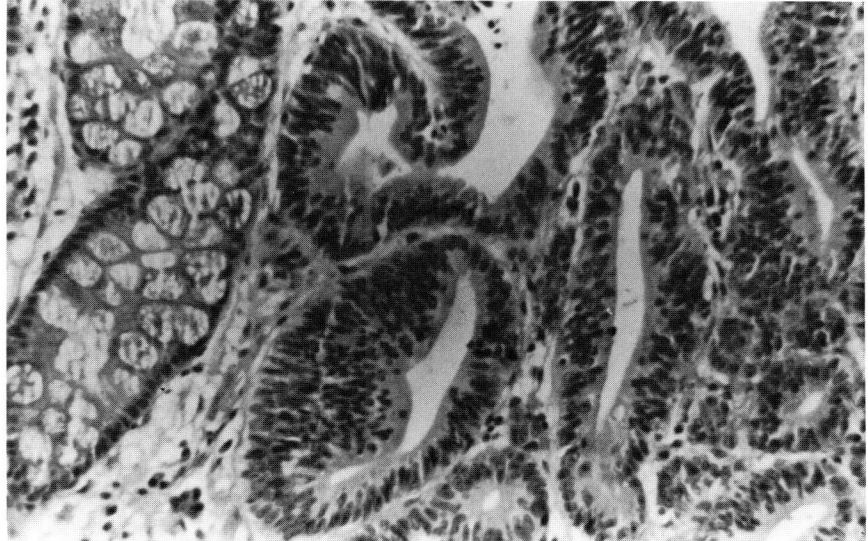

FIGURE 20-21. Gastric mucosa revealing glandular dysplasia (center and right). Compared with regeneration (Figure 20-19), the dysplastic epithelium shows more variation in size and shape, prominent pallisading, and hyperchromatism of the nuclei. A gland with nondysplastic intestinal metaplasia is at the left. (H&E, × 200)

antrectomy for duodenal ulcer disease, whereas the rate after 15 to 20 or more years is greater in those who underwent resection of gastric ulcers.

Cases of gastric adenocarcinoma of the intestinal type that show gland formation are often associated with the finding of glandular dysplasia of the adjacent nontumorous mucosa (Figure 20-21).[183] Histologic evidence of dysplasia has also been observed in the flat mucosa in advance of the formation of overt carcinoma in patients with pernicious anemia[127-129] and those with postgastrectomy gastritis.[162,173,184-188] This finding has served as the basis for use of endoscopic and mucosal biopsy surveillance in high-risk patients.[189] It appears that the detection of a severe or high-grade dysplasia correlates best with tumor development,[190-193] but the clinical application of the finding of biopsy evidence of dysplasia in the absence of apparent carcinoma is not settled. Furthermore, it is not known whether the identification of dysplasia will prove more useful than the search for gross features of early and minute gastric carcinomas.[165,194-196] This subject of dysplasia and carcinoma is covered more completely in Chapter 25.

Carcinoid Tumors

An increase in cases of endocrine cell hyperplasia[133,134,197] and carcinoid tumors[198-205] of the antrum has been noted in patients with chronic atrophic gastritis involving the corpus and fundus. This is believed to be due to the reduced or absent gastric secretion, resulting in a loss of the normal negative feedback and a sustained stimulation of the antral endocrine cells. The tumors are usually multiple. Most are tiny, ranging from microscopic foci to tumors that are a few millimeters in diameter (see Figure 20-16); lesions larger than a centimeter are rarely observed. The antral endocrine cells may contain and secrete a variety of polypeptide hormones, and the tumors are especially rich in gastrin and serotonin derived, respectively, from the G cells and enterochromaffin-like (ECL) cells. Functional problems from the excess hormonal secretion are occasionally noted and include effects on the peripheral vasculature and on gastrointestinal motility. See Chapter 13, Disorders of Endocrine System, for further details.

CORROSIVE GASTRITIS

Etiology and Clinical Features. Corrosive gastritis is due to the ingestion of highly toxic chemicals, including strong alkaline, acid, and fixative solutions.[206-208] The compounds most often involved are sodium hydroxide (lye); sulfuric, nitric, and hydrochloric acids; and formaldehyde. Cases appear after the accidental intake of these substances, which are present in many household cleaning products, or represent a suicidal effort. The degree of damage is dependent on the amount and concentration of the toxic material, and the injury may be lessened if the stomach contains food, which would cover and protect part of the mucosal surface. Although alkali exert their greatest effect on the esophageal squamous mucosa, they can also damage the stomach. As a result of pylorospasm, there is typically no injury of the duodenum.

The patients present promptly with intense oropharyngeal and midepigastric pain. There is also hemorrhage in the acute cases, peritonitis if there is deep mural necrosis, and signs of obstruction in those who later develop strictures. Initial medical therapy is of a supportive type, and surgical resection is required in cases with protracted hemorrhage, peritonitis, and obstruction.[209]

Pathology. The dominant effect is in the antral region, and the lesions resemble those seen in ischemic disease of the bowel. Milder cases reveal patchy or diffuse hemorrhagic necrosis of the mucosal layer, which heals with just minor fibrosis in the submucosa. The more marked examples have greater necrosis that extends into the gastric wall, and this can lead to perforation, peritonitis, and potential fatality. There is reactive inflammation of a nonspecific nature, and in cases with deep necrosis marked fibrosis and stricture of the pyloric area often develop. The diagnosis is provided by the clinical history, and additional studies are ordinarily not required. Endoscopy is sometimes employed for gauging the extent of injury or identifying the presence of a stricture.[208,210]

INFECTIONS OF THE STOMACH

Infections of the stomach are listed in Table 20–6. Infections are much less common in the stomach, compared with the intestinal tract, probably because of the high concentration of hydrochloric acid. Interestingly, however, patients who develop atrophic fundic gastritis and achlorhydria do not have a marked increase in gastric infections, which suggests that additional factors are operative in this protection. Like in other parts of the gut, the stomach can also be involved in opportunistic infections, which typically occur in debilitated and immunocompromised patients and in patients with extensive necrosis due to other underlying conditions.[211]

Viral Infections

Although the term *gastroenteritis* is often used clinically to refer to cases of transient viral infections of the gut, such as those due to the Norwalk agent and other enteroviruses, the histologic lesions are limited to the small intestinal mucosa, and the stomach is spared in these cases.[212] After an investigative study employing gastroscopy, several previously normal persons developed gastritis and hypochlorhydria that lasted for several weeks. It was postulated that the cause might be viral contamination of the endoscopes. It has subsequently been shown, however, that these cases probably were due to infection with *H. pylori*.[104]

Herpesvirus. Infection with the herpes simplex viruses typically favors the squamous cell–lined mucosa of the esophagus and anal canal,[213] and effects on the tissues with glandular mucosa are rare. Cases in the stomach have been noted only in immunodeficient patients and are usually associated with more widespread herpetic infection in the body.[214,215] The lesions are similar in appearance to herpesvirus infection elsewhere and reveal multiple vesicles on the mucosal surface that proceed to small erosions. The diagnosis is determined by the finding of the typical intranuclear inclusion within the mucous epithelial cells; the multinucleated giant cells that are characteristically seen in infections of the squamous epithelium are rarely present. Little is known of the natural course of the gastric infection, and the clinical behavior is dependent on the underlying disorder.

Cytomegalovirus. The virus has been increasingly demonstrated in the gastric and duodenal mucosa in patients who are immunocompromised.[211,216–223] It has been noted in cases of the acquired immunodeficiency syndrome (AIDS) and in patients receiving immunosuppressive drugs for renal transplants and other inflammatory conditions.[224,225] There may be involvement of the intact mucosa or a previously ulcerated area.[217,219] The characteristic features are the presence of the typical red intranuclear and large intracytoplasmic inclusions within the covering epithelial cells as well as the endothelial cells and other mesenchymal cells in the lamina propria or in the granulation tissue beneath an ulcer (Figure 20–22). As with the finding of cytomegalovirus elsewhere in the body, it is not known whether the virus can initiate the tissue injury or is a secondary invader in an area of prior inflammation and necrosis. The virus could serve to sustain or enhance the tissue destruction, and it has been suggested that a positive culture of the tissue, or possibly a rise in its serologic titer, is seen in such cases.

Bacterial Infections

Bacteria are often noted over areas of necrosis and tumors in the stomach, and they are also commonly seen in cases of stress ulceration due to extensive body burns. It is thought that the organisms are saprophytes and that they do not contribute to the tissue injury.

Helicobacter Pylori Infection

H. pylori organisms are found in the gastric antrum in two thirds to three quarters of patients with chronic active gastritis and chronic peptic ulcers of the stomach and duodenum, but it has not yet been established whether the organisms are the primary cause of the inflammation or serve as promoting factors. This subject was covered previously in the section Chronic Antral Gastritis.

Table 20–6. INFECTIONS OF THE STOMACH*

Viral
  Herpes simplex virus† infection
  Cytomegalovirus† infection
Bacterial
  Helicobacter pylori infection in chronic antral gastritis
  Pyogenic infection in phlegmonous and emphysematous gastritis
  Tuberculosis
  Mycobacterium avium-intracellulare† infection
  Actinomyces infection
  Syphilis
Fungal
  Candida (Monilia)† infection
  Histoplasma infection
  Mucor (Phycomycetes)† infection
Protozoan
  Cryptosporidia† infection
  Giardia infection (in fluid)
Helminthic
  Anisakis infection
  Strongyloides infection†
  Rare: infection with *Schistosoma*, *Ascaris*, flukes

*Infection may be limited to stomach, associated with lesions in other regions of the gut, or part of a systemic spread.
†Usually present in immunocompromised or severely debilitated patients.

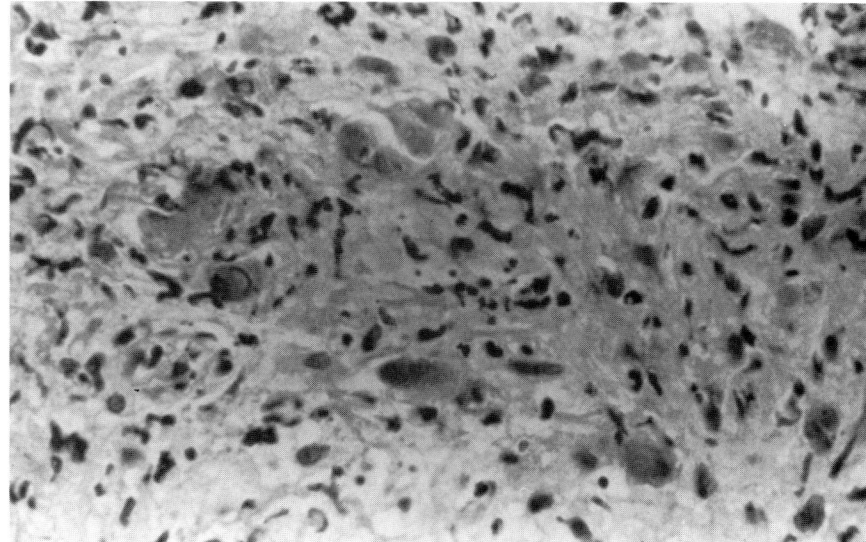

FIGURE 20–22. Base of a gastric ulcer, showing effects of cytomegalovirus in the mesenchymal elements. There are large intranuclear and intracytoplasmic inclusions. (H&E, × 500)

Acute Phlegmonous Gastritis

Acute phlegmonous gastritis is a rare condition characterized by the presence of extensive and often transmural necrosis associated with intense suppuration.[226-230] It is usually caused by infection with hemolytic streptococci; other organisms observed have included pneumococci, staphylococci, and coliform bacteria. It is seen more often in older persons, particularly those with general debility, with septicemia, or in shock. The patients present with pain, hematemesis, and signs of acute abdomen; antibiotic therapy alone is insufficient, and early gastric resection is required so that death can be avoided. Examination of the stomach usually reveals diffuse involvement with a deep red to purple color, prominent mural thickening, and pockets of pus that ooze from the submucosa and peritoneal surface. Histologic features include marked necrosis of all parts of the gastric wall, sloughing of the mucosa, many neutrophils and microorganisms, and thrombosis of the small blood vessels. Possibly because of the general looseness of the tissue, the inflammatory and thrombotic features are often best visualized in the submucosal layer. Unless resected, the cases develop gastric perforation and generalized peritonitis. The diagnosis is suggested by the presence of the bacteria together with the very marked acute inflammatory reaction and is confirmed by culture of the gastric tissue. Ordinary ischemic disease is rarely noted in the stomach and would not reveal as prominent an inflammatory reaction. The inflammatory lesions in the common disorders of acute gastritis and chronic gastritis are limited to the mucosa, and peptic ulcers are localized conditions.

Acute Emphysematous Gastritis

Acute emphysematous gastritis is probably a variant of phlegmonous gastritis, in which the responsible microorganisms are gas-forming and most cases are caused by *Clostridium welchii*.[231] It is more often noted in patients with malignant tumors of the stomach and in those that have had prior corrosive damage. The morphologic features are similar to those of the phlegmonous cases except for the addition of gas-filled spaces of variable size in the gastric wall, and these areas can be identified by radiographic examination. The diagnosis is provided by the distinctive features and culture of the gastric tissue. Postmortem tissues may reveal extensive autolysis and gas-filled spaces due to the secondary invasion and proliferation of enteric bacteria, but there is no inflammation. Pneumatosis is ordinarily confined to the intestines, and the spaces lack bacteria and neutrophils. Other conditions that may be associated with the appearance of spaces in the gastric wall include gastritis cystica profunda and mucinous carcinoma, but the mucinous nature of the contents and lining of epithelial cells in these conditions is evident.

Tuberculosis

Gastrointestinal tuberculosis is uncommon in Western countries; most cases affect the ileocecal region, and there is only rare involvement of the stomach.[232-235] Practically all cases in the United States result from primary pulmonary infection, either as part of a systemic spread or by the swallowing of infective material that has been coughed up into the oral cavity. The gastric lesions have a predilection for the antral-pyloric region and are often associated with contiguous disease of the duodenum. Some cases show deep ulceration with occasional fissure formation, whereas others reveal marked thickening and folds of the antral mucosa. The patients typically present with signs of gastric outlet obstruction, and the radiographic and endoscopic appearances may simulate malignancy. Histologic examination is characteristic, showing numerous granulomas in all layers of the gastric wall. There may or may not be necrosis in the granulomas, and the diagnosis is secured by the demonstration of tubercle bacilli on acid-fast staining and by culture of the gastric tissue. The stains are more often positive in cases with caseating granulomas. The inflammation around the ulcers and fissures is otherwise nonspecific, and a fibrous stricture can develop in the late cases. Medical therapy is sufficient in most cases, with surgery reserved for those with permanent obstruction, and the overall prognosis is dependent on the extent of infection in the body.

The differential diagnosis at the clinical and macroscopic levels includes tumors, which are usually confined to the stomach but, exceptionally, may extend across the pyloric sphincter, and ordinary peptic ulcer disease, which typically presents with a more localized lesion and lacks fissures. The distinction from Crohn's disease may be more difficult, because both disorders affect the same areas of the gut and may be associated with mural fissures and a granulomatous reaction. Of help is the fact that granulomas are present in only one half of cases of Crohn's disease and never reveal necrosis unless associated with foreign material, whereas they are always present in tuberculosis and frequently show caseation. Ultimately, the distinction is made by finding the organism in stains or culture. Other granulomatous disorders that can affect the stomac are described in the sections that follow, and include sarcoidosis; foreign body reactions; infections due to *M. avium-intracellulare*, syphilis, and histoplasmosis; and isolated granulomatous gastritis. In most of these conditions, there is much less tissue destruction, and the granulomas are rarely of the caseating type.

Mycobacterium Avium-Intracellulare Infection

Mycobacterium avium-intracellulare infection (MAI) has been recently described in humans and occurs exclusively in patients with AIDS or other immunocompromised conditions.[211,236] The infection can involve multiple tissues of the body, including the liver and all portions of the gastrointestinal tract from the esophagus to the rectum. There is usually concomitant involvement of the stomach and duodenum, and the lesions are concentrated in the mucosal layer, revealing small clusters of enlarged macrophages or poorly formed granulomas without necrosis in the lamina propria (see Chapter 16, Figure 16–5). Acid-fast stains demonstrate abundant organisms both within the macrophages and lying free in the stroma, and cultures are not ordinarily required. Because the macrophages may vary considerably in amount and even can be absent in a single tissue section, it is generally recommended that acid-fast stains be routinely used in gut mucosal biopsies in all patients with AIDS. There is usually no acute or other inflammatory reaction and a lack of tissue necrosis in the MAI infections of the stomach. However, additional opportunistic infections are frequently present in the gut and other body tissues, and the overall prognosis is dire.

Actinomycosis

Actinomycosis is an uncommon bacterial infection of the gut due to *Actinomyces israelii*, and the lesions are most often noted in the terminal ileum, cecum, and appendix.[237] The responsible organisms are filamentous, gram-positive anaerobic bacteria that normally reside in the oral cavity, especially in the tonsillar region, and they have a typical gross appearance consisting of tiny, yellow "sulfur granules." Infection of the stomach is very rare and is usually located in the antral region.[237–239] It is characterized by persistent ulceration with occasional fistulas and a thickened wall that resembles a tumor and requires resection. The histologic features are distinctive, revealing a chronic abscess in the gastric wall with marked neutrophilia and numerous bacterial colonies, and the diagnosis is afforded by these findings and culture of the exudate.

Syphilis

Some patients with early secondary syphilis have inflammatory lesions of a nonspecific nature in gastric and colonic mucosa.[240–242] The mucosa reveals acute and chronic inflammatory cells, occasional small erosions, and numerous *Treponema pallidum* spirochetes by the Warthin-Starry silver stain or the acridine orange fluorochrome stain; granulomas are not present in these cases. These patients often lack any gastrointestinal symptoms, however; and the mucosal findings are mainly observed in investigative studies. Both the gut and the cutaneous lesions resolve following specific antibiotic therapy. More rarely, symptomatic cases of gastric syphilis occur in the late secondary and tertiary stages of the disease.[243–246] Patients present with signs of gastritis or obstruction, and the clinical suspicion, based on the gross appearance of a thickened gastric wall, is usually of a tumor. The characteristic morphologic features are an expansion of the submucosal layer by inflammation and fibrosis and the presence of an obliterative endarteritis. There is usually also acute and chronic inflammation of the mucosa, which can lead to enlarged folds,[247] and hypertrophy of the muscularis propria; the overall gross appearance can resemble linitis plastica. Granulomatous lesions or gummas rarely are observed. Because the histologic features are not absolutely specific, a high level of suspicion for the infection is needed. The diagnosis is provided by the finding of spirochetes in the tissue, either in the inflamed mucosa or in the area of the involved submucosal vessels, and by positive serologic tests.

The differential diagnosis is fairly limited and includes tumors at the gross level and conditions that are associated with prominent fibrosis, such as radiation damage and systemic sclerosis. An equivalent degree of submucosal fibrosis and vascular changes can be seen in the late stages after radiation; there also may be atypical mesenchymal cells and pronounced ectasia of the small vessels in the mucosa. In systemic sclerosis, the fibrosis is not limited to the submucosa, but extends throughout the muscularis propria. The ordinary cases of chronic gastritis lack the mural findings, and patients with peptic ulcers or with Crohn's disease have more localized lesions.

Fungal Infections

The fungi act as opportunistic agents and typically appear in debilitated or immunocompromised patients and in areas of prior necrosis.[248,249]

Candidiasis

Fungal elements of *Candida albicans* are frequently noted overlying the base of chronic peptic ulcers of the stomach (Figure 20–23), and it has been suggested that the fungi enhance the degree of necrosis and that these cases have protracted disease and deeper ulcers with more perforations.[250,251] Other studies, however, have noted the fungi but failed to show any correlation with the amount of necrosis and the clinical course, and this issue is not completely resolved.[252,253] It has also been postulated that the number of organisms might be increased in the stomach of patients who are receiving potent medications such as H_2-blockers to reduce gastric acidity, but there have not been adequate control studies, and the deleterious effects from the presence of the fungi in these cases have not been substantiated.

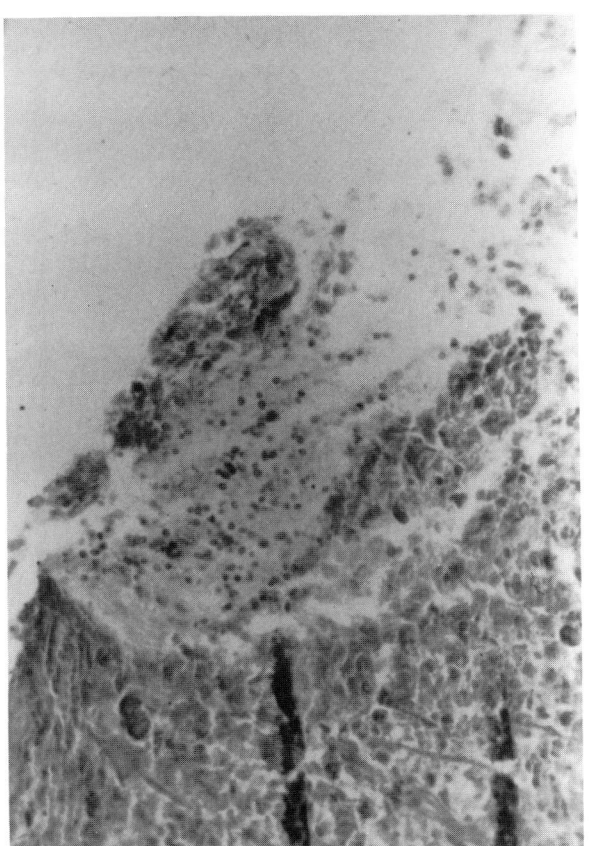

FIGURE 20–23. Surface of chronic peptic ulcer of stomach, showing necrotic material and a large number of fungal spores on the top (center). (Gridley, × 200)

Primary and secondary monilial infections definitely have been noted in the stomach and appear to be confined to patients with severe debility or an immunodeficiency condition.[254–258] Such infections are more common in the esophagus[259] but can affect any part of the gut, and multiple sites can be involved in an individual case. The lesions appear as multiple plaques or ulcers of the mucosa in any part of the stomach. There is variable inflammation of a nonspecific nature, and the diagnosis is secured by the demonstration of the characteristic slender pseudohyphae in biopsy samples or scrapings of the mucosal lesions; cultures are ordinarily not needed. The infection can respond to specific antifungal therapy, but other types of infections may be present, and the overall prognosis relates to the underlying condition.

Histoplasmosis

There are rare examples of systemic spread of histoplasmosis to the gut.[260–263] The disease most often is noted in the intestines but can, on rare occasions, affect the stomach. The lesions appear as single or multiple areas of ulceration and contain numerous granulomas, which are usually noncaseating. The organisms of *Histoplasma capsulatum* grow as spores in the body, are typically small and located within the macrophage or giant-cell cytoplasm in the granulomas, and are best demonstrated by silver stains. The differential diagnosis includes other granulomatous conditions of the stomach that may be associated with tissue destruction, principally tuberculosis and Crohn's disease.

Mucormycosis (Phycomycosis)

Mucormycosis is infection due to the Mucor agents, which are part of the Mucoraceae family, in the Phycometes class. Gastric infection is rare, seen only in severely debilitated or immunocompromised patients, and appears to be more prevalent in tropical regions.[264–267] The lesions can affect any part of the stomach and show extensive hemorrhage, necrosis, and thrombosed vessels; they may extend deep into the gastric wall, resulting in perforation. The inflammatory reaction is nonspecific and lacks granulomas, and the specific diagnosis is provided by the identification of the fungi. The organisms are relatively large hyphae that are nonseptate and have short branches; they can be seen in regular H&E preparations and are enhanced by silver stains and the PAS reaction.

Parasitic Infections

Protozoan infections do not ordinarily occur in the stomach. In patients with achlorhydria due to atrophic gastritis who are undergoing endoscopic examination, *Giardia lamblia* has been occasionally noted in the cytologic smears but does not cause gastric lesions. In patients with AIDS cryptosporidial infection of the small intestines can develop, and the organism may also be occasionally found in the stomach.[268] Similarly, helminthic infestations typically occur in the intestines and only rarely affect the stomach.

Anisakiasis

Anisakiasis results from the ingestion of the larvae of the small nematode, *Anisakis,* and is most frequent in countries such as Japan in which the population consumes large amounts of raw fish.[269-271] The disorder has been noted in the United States and typically causes a chronic lesion in the distal ileum that can resemble Crohn's disease. Infection in the stomach is less common and may be associated with the acute onset of pain just a few hours after the ingestion of the larvae. Endoscopic examination at this early stage may reveal mucosal swelling and inflammation as well as the organism, which has burrowed into the mucosa but is still partially in the lumen. Most cases resolve spontaneously, but in some there is persistence, with the development of necrosis and a poorly formed granulomatous reaction containing large numbers of eosinophils. The inflammation can extend into the gastric wall, causing a deep ulcer or a mass lesion and necessitating resection in some cases. The differential diagnosis includes other lesions that can be associated with prominent necrosis and an eosinophilic reaction, such as Crohn's disease and the rare mural form of eosinophilic gastroenteritis; the specific diagnosis of anisakiasis depends on the finding of worm fragments in the lesion.

Other Helminthic Infections

There have been rare cases reported of helminthic involvement of the stomach due to *Strongyloides stercoralis,*[272,273] which is typically seen in immunocompromised hosts, and to *Schistosoma mansoni.*[124] There is usually ulceration of the mucosa and a prominent inflammatory reaction, with many eosinophils and occasional granulomas. The diagnosis requires the identification of the specific ova in the tissues or the stools. *Ascaris*[274,275] and various flukes have also been noted rarely in the stomach.

MISCELLANEOUS CONDITIONS OF THE STOMACH

Mallory-Weiss Syndrome

Etiology and Clinical Features. The Mallory-Weiss lesion is a longitudinal tear of the mucosa at the esophagocardiac junction that is believed to be a consequence of severe retching.[276-278] It is more commonly observed in alcoholics, presumably because they frequently experience episodes of toxic gastritis that lead to severe vomiting, and the patients typically present with heartburn or midepigastric pain and hematemesis. Upper tract endoscopy is ordinarily performed for sorting out the various causes of hemorrhage in such patients, which include severe gastritis and ruptured esophageal or gastric varices as well as the Mallory-Weiss tear. Medical therapy, consisting of the elimination of any toxic substances from the diet and the reduction or neutralization of gastric acid, is usually sufficient, and balloon tamponade or surgery is reserved for patients with prolonged hemorrhage and impending perforation.

Pathology. The Mallory-Weiss lesion is characteristic. It is a longitudinal laceration of the mucosa that straddles the cardioesophageal junction (Figure 20-24), usually single, and measures less than a centimeter in length. The term *syndrome* has been used because some cases, possibly representing an earlier stage of the condition, show only prominent mucosal hemorrhage in this area, without the tear. The typical lesion extends into the deep part of the submucosa and is associated with marked hemorrhage from the torn vessels and later with a nonspecific acute inflammatory reaction. Healing is usually prompt and may be associated with a slight degree of submucosal fibrosis, but without stricture formation. Complications are uncommon and include persistence of the lesion, which can develop into a larger ulcer with greater hemorrhage, and penetration of the tear into the deeper parts of the wall, leading to perforation.

The differential diagnosis is limited and consists of ulcerating lesions of the junctional area, which can be seen in severe cases of reflux esophagitis and in the mucosa overlying an early carcinoma or a mural mass such as a leiomyoma of the lower esophageal and gas-

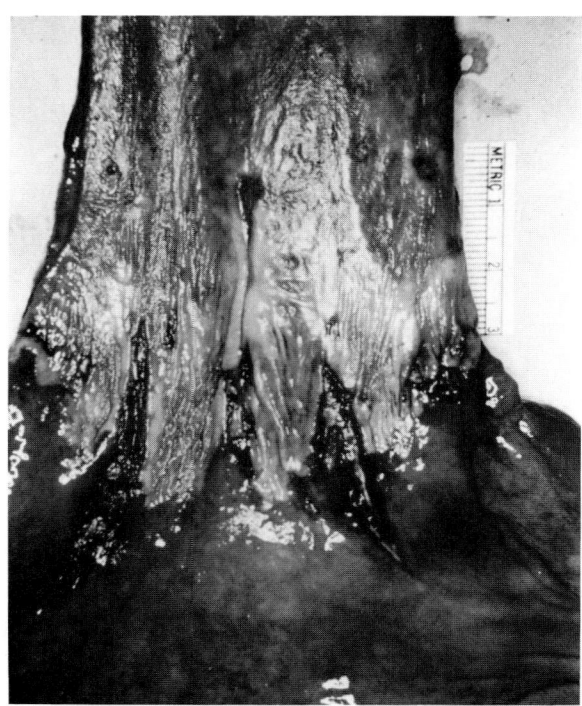

FIGURE 20-24. Segment of esophagus (top) and stomach in a case of Mallory-Weiss syndrome. There are several longitudinal tears of the mucosa straddling the esophagocardiac junction.

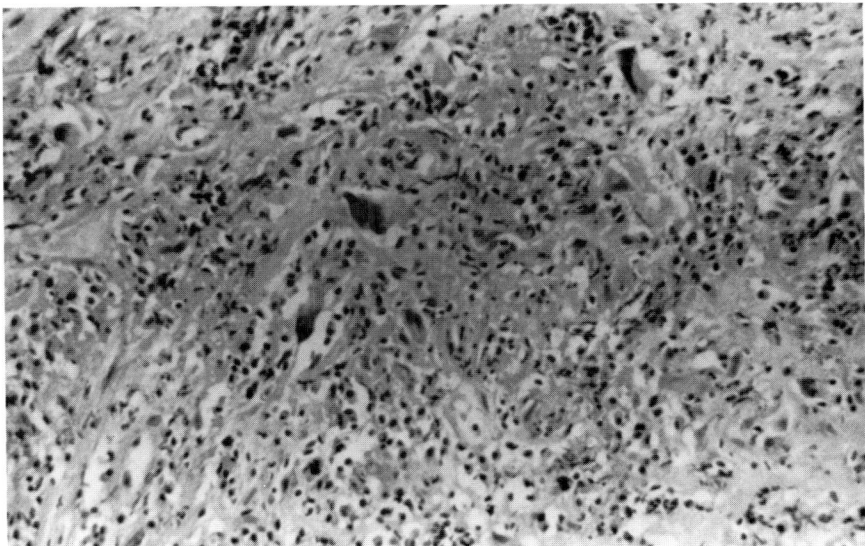

FIGURE 20-25. Gastric tissue in case of radiation-induced injury. There is marked fibrosis and the presence of enlarged atypical nuclei in the mesenchymal cells. (H&E, × 200)

tric cardiac regions. In all of these conditions, the ulcerated area is often larger and less constantly located right at the junction, and the typical clinical history of severe vomiting and retching is usually absent.

Gastritis Due to Physical and Chemical Agents. This subject is detailed in the previous sections Acute Gastritis and Chronic Antral Gastritis and in Chapter 9. The major points related to the action of physical agents on the stomach are provided here.

Radiation Effects and Damage

Patients with severe peptic ulcer disease who are poor surgical candidates have occasionally received gastric irradiation in an attempt to reduce the number of parietal cells.[279,280] The dose is in the order of 1500 rads and the gastric injury is typically confined to the mucosa, revealing patchy or confluent areas of active gastritis and a partial reduction of the specialized glands in the corpus-fundic region. There are usually no other distinctive histologic features or the development of complications. The patient may experience mild abdominal pain, and the gastritis can be readily seen by endoscopy and biopsy. Because the inflammatory features are entirely nonspecific, the cause of the gastritis in these cases and its distinction from the other common forms of active gastritis are dependent on the clinical information.

More extensive gastric damage can occur when radiation doses of 4500 rads or more are applied, alone or in conjunction with chemotherapy, for the treatment of tumors of the stomach or contiguous tissues.[281–283] In the acute phase, there is prominent edema and inflammation of the mucosa and submucosa with the development of focal erosions and sloughing of the mucosal layer, and a transient obstruction from the swelling may ensue in the cardia or pyloric regions.[284] These superficial lesions usually subside without sequelae over a period of a few weeks. In some cases, there is a persistence or recurrence of the gastric damage with the formation of deeper ulcers that are more often in the antrum and may simulate a chronic peptic ulcer. These lesions can develop months to years after the initial radiation exposure and are thought to be mediated by damage to the vessels in the gastric wall and perigastric tissues.

The histologic findings noted in this later (subacute or chronic) phase of radiation disease include nonspecific findings such as necrosis and inflammatory cells and the more distinctive features associated with radiation[283]—a marked amount of granulation tissue and fibrosis in the submucosa that appears to be in excess of that expected from the ulcer extent; the presence of atypical fibroblasts and endothelial cells with enlarged and variably hyperchromatic nuclei (Figure 20–25); and vascular changes consisting of any combination of an active endarteritis, thrombosis, intimal thickening, and fibrotic occlusion. Endoscopy and mucosal biopsy are often performed in these cases to distinguish among radiation- or drug-induced lesions, opportunistic infections, and recurrent tumor. The diagnosis of radiation effects and disease of the stomach may be suggested by the histologic features but is also dependent on the clinical history and on the exclusion of the other conditions.

Gastric Freezing

In an attempt to reduce acid secretion, iced solutions formerly were instilled into the gastric lumen.[285–287] This resulted in a patchy or diffuse hemorrhagic necrosis of the mucosa and a variable but transient fall in the gastric acid concentration. It was never established whether the decreased acid was due to a reversible loss of the parietal cells or to an exaggerated back-diffusion of acid through the inflamed mucosa. There was prompt healing of the mucosa without sustained benefit to the patients, and this procedure is no longer employed.

Eosinophilic Gastritis

There are two major types of eosinophilic gastroenteritis,[288] a mucosal form, which has an allergic basis and has also been called allergic gastroenteritis,[289] and a rare mural form.[290] The stomach is often affected in both conditions. Indeed, the antral mucosa is so often involved in the allergic cases that mucosal biopsy of this area is recommended to help establish the diagnosis.[291] This topic is presented in Chapter 10.

Gastritis Associated with Motor and Mechanical Disorders

This subject is primarily covered in Chapter 11, and the secondary inflammatory changes that may complicate some of the conditions are highlighted here.

Congenital Pyloric Stenosis

Infants with congenital pyloric stenosis may develop a nonspecific inflammation of the gastric mucosa as a result of obstruction and distention of the gastric lumen. After the diagnosis and surgical therapy, the mucosa reverts to normal, and there are no complications. In some infants with allergic gastritis there can develop marked swelling and obstruction of the distal antrum, and this must be distinguished from the congenital type of pyloric obstruction.[292] See Chapters 8 and 10 for further details about the congenital and allergic diseases.

Diverticula of the Stomach

There are two major types of diverticula noted in the stomach.[293–295] The more common pulsion form is usually located on the posterior wall of the proximal stomach near the cardia, and is thought to be due to a localized congenital weakness of the wall in that area. There may be some mild chronic inflammation in the diverticular mucosa, but the patients are typically without symptoms; exceptionally, there may develop a blockage of the diverticulum that leads to greater and active inflammation and requires surgical excision. The other type of diverticulum is found in the antrum in conjunction with a deep penetrating peptic ulcer or tumor and is invariably inflamed.

Bezoars

Bezoars include a variety of plant products, hair, foods such as partially diagnosed citrus fruits, collections of drug capsules, fungal balls, and other foreign objects that might be ingested or accidentally retained after an endoscopic procedure.[296–298] The development of a large mass from the bezoar and its retention in the stomach are favored by poor digestion and are seen more often in edentulous patients and in those that have had a partial gastrectomy.[298–300] Gastric inflammation usually results from the impaction of these objects on the mucosal surface, which can lead to inflammation, ulceration, and occasionally perforation. An obstruction resulting in gastric dilatation and secondary mucosal damage may also occur.

Gastric Atony

A prominent dilatation of the stomach can be observed in patients with various endocrine diseases and motor disorders such as systemic sclerosis, and the lesion is more frequent and may be especially pronounced in cases of diabetes mellitus. An abdominal mass can be appreciated by physical examination and confirmed by a radiographic test. If the lesion is not decompressed, the elevated pressure can cause a hemorrhagic necrosis and inflammation of the mucosa and gastric wall, with the potential for perforation.

Gastritis Associated with Vascular Diseases

Necrosis and variable inflammation can result from diseases of the major vessels and microcirculation of the stomach. Causes include ordinary ischemic disease[301,302] and volvulus, which are very uncommon in the stomach, vasculitis, and atheromatous[303,304] and foreign body emboli; these conditions are detailed in Chapter 12. The acute, stress-induced lesions are also believed to have a vascular basis and are presented in Chapter 21. As a result of the portal hypertension, large gastric varices commonly develop, and these cases are sometimes associated with a more widespread small-vessel ectasia and inflammation in the mucosa.[305–307] Localized gastric ulcers with marked epithelial atypia have been noted in some patients who have received instillation of chemotherapeutic agents into the hepatic arteries for the treatment of hepatic tumors.[308,309]

Gastric Antral Vascular Ectasia

Gastric antral vascular ectasia is a form of gastritis characterized by the presence of both inflammatory and vascular components in the mucosa.[310–314] Most cases occur in older women, and the patients typically present with chronic bleeding and iron deficiency anemia. The lesion is localized to the antral region, and gross endoscopic examination reveals prominent longitudinal folds that have striking red streaks; this appearance has been likened to the rind of a watermelon and called the "watermelon stomach." The histologic features in the mucosa are distinctive, revealing not only acute and chronic inflammatory cells and small foci of intestinal metaplasia but also an apparent increase in the amount of fibromuscular stroma and numerous dilated blood vessels, many of which contain recent and organizing thrombi. There is congestion of the submucosal vessels but no evidence of a vascular malformation based on angiographic and morphologic examinations. The enlarged mucosal folds result from a hypertrophy of the surface-foveolar mucous cells, and these areas also contain the prominent stroma and ectatic vessels. Some cases show a thickening of the muscularis propria and/or a prolapse of the hypertrophied folds into the duodenum. Medical therapy consisting of oral iron and transfusions is insufficient, and antral resection is ultimately required and is curative.

The diagnosis of gastric antral vascular ectasia is based on the typical endoscopic and bioptic appearances of the mucosa together with a compatible clinical history. The more common cases of chronic antral gastritis may contain an enhanced amount of fibromuscular stroma in the lamina propria but do not show as many dilated blood vessels and lack the thrombi. Other conditions that can be associated with prominent mucosal thickening and the appearance of folds in the antral region are cases of gastritis due to allergic and granulomatous diseases and infiltrative tumors, all of which have distinguishing histologic features. In Ménétrier's disease, the large folds are confined to the corpus-fundic region.

Other Vascular Lesions

Considering the clinical aspects of recurrent hemorrhage, the differential diagnosis of ectasia would also include vascular malformations. In gastric angiodysplasia, there is an arteriovenous aneurysm or malformation that is primarily located in the submucosa[315–318]; the lesions are often multiple, found in any part of the stomach, and identified by angiographic study. Arterial aneurysms, known also as Dieulafoy's disease, occur more often in younger patients, are usually present in the proximal stomach, and cause a localized ulceration.[319–322] In these vascular lesions, the episodes of hemorrhage are often massive and demand early surgery.

Granulomatous Diseases of the Stomach

The major granulomatous disorders affecting the stomach are sarcoidosis, Crohn's disease, infections, foreign body reactions, and isolated disease.[323,324] These conditions generally involve the antral region and are often associated with prominent mucosal and mural thickening that can simulate the gross appearance of a malignancy. The patients typically present with signs of gastritis and/or pyloric obstruction, and the diagnosis of a granulomatous lesion is provided by mucosal biopsy examination.

Gastric infections that commonly contain distinct granulomas include tuberculosis and histoplasmosis, but we are currently seeing many more cases due to *Mycobacterium avium-intracellulare* in immunocompromised patients; these diseases were presented earlier in the section on infections of the stomach. Foreign body granulomas may result from a variety of substances, such as suture material, talc, or starch, which may be introduced during a surgical procedure; barium from a radiographic study; extravasated mucus in inflammatory and neoplastic conditions; and, surprisingly, even cereal products.[324–327] The foreign body lesions are usually small, and they can be multiple and located in any part of the gastric wall, from the mucosal to the serosal layers. It is now appreciated that sarcoidosis only rarely involves the stomach or other regions of the alimentary tract, and its diagnosis depends on the finding of concomitant disease in a more characteristic location, such as the lungs and hilar lymph nodes. Chapter 16, on systemic and miscellaneous disorders, and Chapter 28, on other inflammatory disorders of intestines, give further details about foreign body reactions and sarcoidosis, as well as the rare effects of malakoplakia and chronic granulomatous disease of childhood in the stomach, and provide general discussion of granulomatous disorders affecting the gut.

Crohn's Disease of the Stomach

In patients with established Crohn's disease of the distal small intestine and the colon, microscopic alterations are noted in the gastric mucosa in about one quarter to one half of the cases.[328,329] These changes are detected in mucosal biopsy samples and consist of patchy areas of active gastritis and granulomas. Patients typically lack any symptoms referable to the gastritis, and the finding of these features does not predict that they will develop clinically significant disease in this area.

Uncommonly, cases of Crohn's disease of the intestine are associated with more major evidence of gastric involvement, characterized by the presence of single or multiple ulcers that are concentrated in the antrum and of deep mural fissures.[330–332] Granulomas without necrosis are seen in about one half of the cases (see Chapter 27, Figure 27–45). There is also often involvement of the contiguous duodenum, and patients experience pain, bleeding, and signs of pyloric obstruction. Exceptionally, the stomach is secondarily affected by a fistula that extends from a diseased area of intestine; in such cases, the gastric inflammation is minimal and confined to the area of the fistulous opening. Isolated Crohn's disease of the stomach is extremely rare, and one should be wary of making this diagnosis until there is demonstration of intestinal disease.

The diagnosis of Crohn's disease of the stomach, alone or in conjunction with duodenal disease, is ordinarily suggested by the clinical history of known intestinal involvement and by the radiographic features and is supported by the finding of granulomas in biopsy samples of the inflamed areas. In the common cases of chronic peptic disease, the ulcers are typically single, and there are no fissures or granulomas. The morphologic features of Crohn's disease may be identical to those seen in gastric or gastroduodenal tuberculosis, and the distinction is dependent on the clinical history and, if needed, on culture of the lesion. The granulomas in tuberculosis may or may not show caseation, and positive stains for the tubercle bacilli are generally positive only in the cases with caseation. In isolated granulomatous gastritis, there is usually no ulceration, and the duodenum is not affected. Chapter 27 on Crohn's disease provides additional details.

Isolated Granulomatous Gastritis

Isolated granulomatous gastritis is an uncommon disorder of unknown cause that is characterized by the presence of a granulomatous inflammation of the gastric antrum.[333-337] It appears to be limited to the stomach and is not associated with disease in other parts of the gut or body tissues. Most cases occur in older persons, and patients typically present with signs of gastritis and/or pyloric obstruction. There is often a thickening of the gastric mucosa and wall, and the radiographic and gross endoscopic findings raise the suspicion of a tumor. Histologic study reveals numerous noncaseating granulomas that are concentrated in the mucosa (Figure 20-26), neutrophils and increased mononuclear inflammatory cells in the intervening lamina propria, and a variable amount of hyperplasia of the surface-foveolar mucous cells (see Chapter 16, Figure 16-12). There is typically no ulceration. Additional radiographic studies of the lungs and intestines are performed to exclude more generalized granulomatous diseases. Considering the rarity of granulomatous infection in this area, culture of the gastric lesion is usually not done. The disease is self-limited and resolves after a period of several weeks to months, without the development of a chronic gastritis or other sequelae. Although corticosteroid therapy has been occasionally used, most cases require only symptomatic relief.

The diagnosis of isolated granulomatous gastritis depends on the finding of granulomas without necrosis in a mucosal biopsy sample of the antrum, on the absence of more destructive lesions such as ulcers and fissures, on negative stains for microorganisms, and on the exclusion of the other granulomatous diseases that can affect the stomach. Patients with sarcoidosis or with Crohn's disease are more often younger and reveal lesions in other, more characteristic sites. Furthermore, cases of Crohn's disease may disclose ulcers or mural fissures and involvement of the duodenum. Any of the common diseases of the antrum, such as chronic antral gastritis and chronic peptic ulcer, may contain a rare granuloma that is probably of the foreign body type. Perhaps the most difficult diagnosis to distinguish is a case of gastric tuberculosis that has no apparent disease in the lungs and other parts of the gut, and in which the granulomas are noncaseating and stain negatively for microorganisms. Accordingly, gastric tissue is obtained by repeat biopsy for specific culture in situations where the patient seems unusually ill, has any other suspicious feature (such as a history of pulmonary disease, a positive tuberculin skin test, or exposure to a tuberculous patient), or fails to improve.

Gastritis Cystica Profunda

Gastritis cystica profunda is a rare condition in which mature glandular epithelium extends into the tissues beneath the muscularis mucosae.[338-341] It is analogous to similar conditions affecting the small and large intestines that are called, respectively, enteritis and colitis cystica profunda. The gastric lesion seems to be much less common and is usually seen in association with an inflammatory lesion of the mucosa, such as in cases of chronic gastritis. It has been experimentally produced in rodents by high doses of salicylates, but there is no evidence to incriminate these or any other drugs in the human cases. The glands typically extend into the upper part of the submucosa and rarely into the deeper parts of the gastric wall (Figure 20-27). They are usually composed of cystic pyloric glands, which may show slight inflammation and signs of regeneration but no dysplasia of the epithelium (Figure 20-28). The cystic change in the glands is also often noted in the mucosa. The natural course of these lesions is not known.

The most pronounced examples of this lesion have been noted in the region of the gastric stoma in patients who have had a gastroenterostomy.[338] There is frequently associated a prominent, polypoid hyperplasia of the mucosal foveolar cells, resulting in a mass lesion; this must be distinguished from carcinoma, which can also develop in the gastric stump of such patients.[162,168-179] Indeed, the actual coexistence of gastritis cystica and adenocarcinoma has been noted,[342,343] and surgical resection is required in such cases.

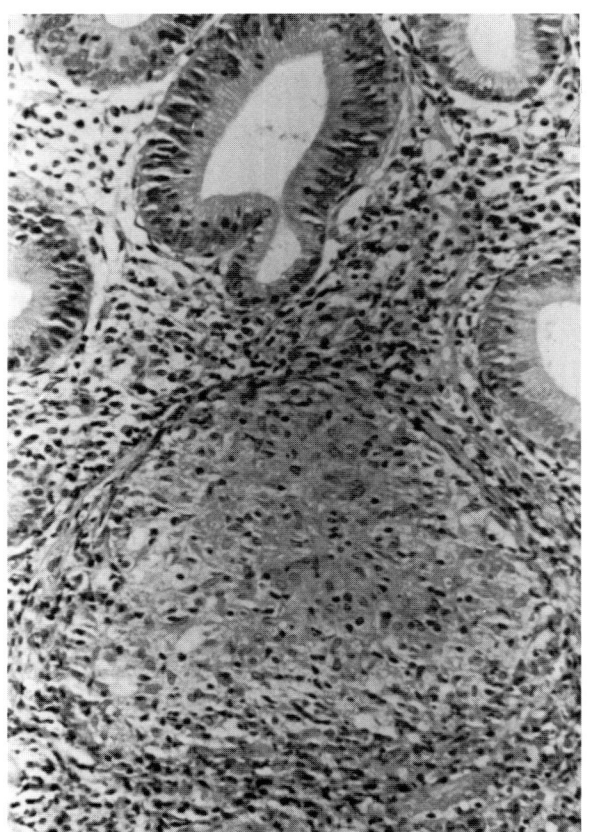

FIGURE 20-26. Gastric antral mucosa in a case of isolated granulomatous gastritis. There is a well-formed granuloma without necrosis in the lamina propria (bottom). (H&E, × 200)

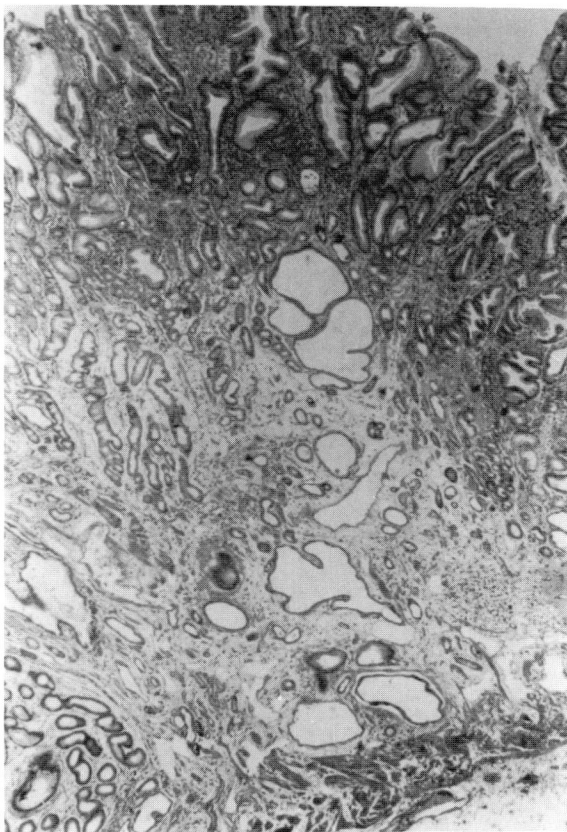

FIGURE 20–27. Gastric corpus mucosa in a case of gastritis cystica profunda, with the luminal surface at the top and a small fragment of muscularis mucosae at the bottom on the right. This occurred in the proximal gastric remnant near the stoma after a distal gastric resection. There is a marked expansion of the mucosa, due mainly to foveolar hyperplasia; many of the glands are cystic. There is also edema and inflammation of the lamina propria and an absence of the specialized corpus glands. (H&E, × 13)

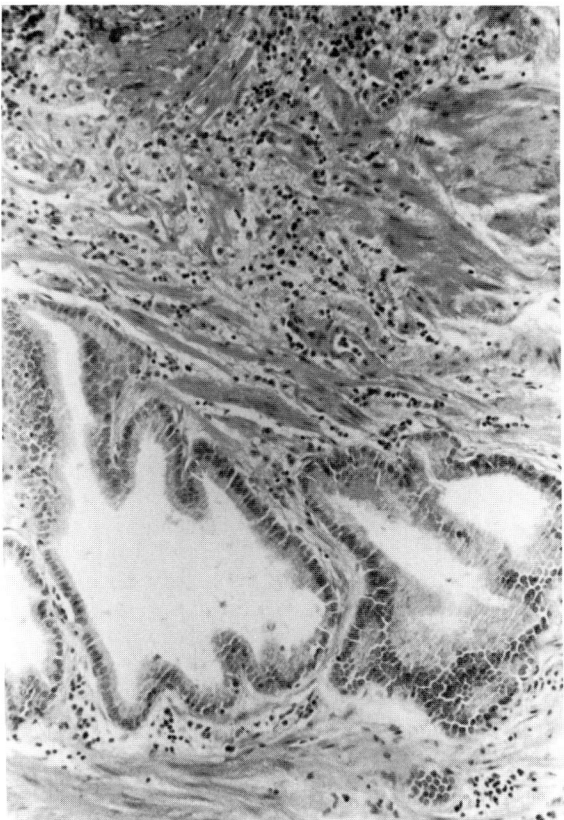

FIGURE 20–28. Gastric corpus mucosa in a case of gastritis cystica profunda. Cystic glands containing mature foveolar epithelium are present, as are associated mononuclear inflammatory cells, in the region of the disrupted muscularis mucosae (fragments, upper right and bottom). Contrast with the dysplastic epithelium in Figure 20–21. (H&E, × 200)

The diagnosis of gastritis cystica is based on the identification of normal or regenerative epithelium in the misplaced glands, in contrast to the expected dysplasia and prominent stroma in an invasive carcinoma. Cases of hamartomatous polyps in the Peutz-Jeghers syndrome may show extension of mature glands into the gastric wall but would be associated with multiple polyps and greater involvement of the small intestine. Other conditions, such as some foreign body reactions, emphysematous gastritis, and postmortem autolysis, can produce irregular spaces in the submucosa that may vaguely resemble dilated glandular lumina; such spaces, however, are readily distinguished by their lack of mucin and epithelial cell lining.

Other Conditions

Xanthoma (or xanthelasma) of the stomach was presented previously in the section on complications of chronic gastritis, and the topics of pseudolymphoma[344] and graft-versus-host disease[345] are included in Chapter 14, on disorders of the lymphoid system. The inflammatory effects of uremia[346,347] and of amyloidosis,[348] as well as of other metabolic and endocrine disorders that can affect the stomach, are detailed in Chapter 16.

There has been a report of a single case of chronic active gastritis in a child, in which a gastric biopsy revealed pronounced fibrosis in the upper and midportions of the mucosa.[349] This was termed "collagenous gastritis," but there appears to be no relationship between this case and collagenous sprue or collagenous colitis. The cause of the gastritis and the significance of the collagen deposition are not known.

MUCOSAL BIOPSY

Endoscopy and mucosal biopsy of the stomach increasingly are being performed in the evaluation of patients with gastritis and gastric ulcers.[33–37,236,350–352] These biopsies can assist in the diagnosis of gastritis and its various forms, in the monitoring of cases following therapy, and in the detection of complications. The technical aspects and overall discussion of the endoscopic procedure are presented in Chapter 3.

There is a relatively poor correlation between the gross endoscopic appearances and the histologic findings in cases of acute and of active chronic gastritis, particularly in those that lack overt erosions.[28,29,353] Accordingly, if an endoscopic study is done in a patient with suspected gastritis but reveals only nonerosive changes such as patchy erythema or small hemorrhages of the mucosa, biopsy samples should be obtained for a search for more certain evidence of inflammation. Cases of both acute toxic gastritis and of the active phase of a chronic gastritis reveal some mixture of necrosis, a neutrophilic reaction, and regenerative glands; and H. pylori can be readily detected. Biopsy can also assist in establishing chronic disease by showing some combination of a marked increase of mononuclear cells in the lamina propria, a loss of the specialized glands, and the appearance of intestinal metaplasia. Biopsy is less helpful in establishing the stage of chronic disease, whether superficial or atrophic, because there can be considerable variation in the degree of histologic damage in the various biopsy samples. Even if multiple tissue samples are obtained, the results are usually still not as sensitive or reliable as the results of functional tests in the determination of the atrophic stage, especially in cases of the fundic type.

Mucosal biopsy of the stomach may suggest or provide support for the diagnosis of some of the less common causes of gastritis, such as other infections, allergic disease, and granulomatous conditions. Involvement of the gastric antrum is noted in practically all cases of allergic gastroenteritis, revealing a prominent infiltrate of eosinophils; mucosal biopsy of this area is recommended in the evaluation of such cases. Patients with long-standing chronic gastritis have an increased risk for the development of gastric tumors, and surveillance endoscopy with mucosal biopsy is often performed, especially in countries with a relatively high baseline incidence of carcinoma. These biopsies serve to distinguish between hyperplastic (regenerative) polyps and adenomas and to identify areas of dysplasia and early gastric carcinoma.

References

1. Palmer ED: Gastritis: A reevaluation. Medicine 33:199, 1954.
2. Owen DA: Gastritis and duodenitis. In Appelman HD (ed): Pathology of the Esophagus, Stomach, and Duodenum. London, Churchill Livingstone, 1984, pp 37–77.
3. Strickland RG, Mackay IR: A reappraisal of the nature and significance of chronic atrophic gastritis. Am J Dig Dis 18:426, 1973.
4. Dagredi AE, Lee ER, Bosco DL, et al: The clinical spectrum of hemorrhagic erosive gastritis. Am J Gastroenterol 60:30, 1973.
5. Weinstein WM: The diagnosis and classification of gastritis and duodenitis. J Clin Gastroenterol 3(Suppl 1):7–16, 1981.
6. Cooke AR: Drug damage to the gastroduodenum. In Sleisenger MH, Fordtran JS (eds): Gastrointestinal Disease, 2nd ed. Philadelphia, WB Saunders, 1978, pp 807–826.
7. Wynn-Williams A: Effects of alcohol on gastric mucosa. Br Med J 1:256, 1956.
8. Gottfried EB, Korsten MA, Lieber CS: Alcohol-induced gastric and duodenal lesions in man. Am J Gastroenterol 70:587–592, 1978.
9. Valencia-Parparcen J: Alcoholic gastritis. Clin Gastroenterol 10:389, 1981.
10. Laine L, Weinstein WM: Histology of alcoholic hemorrhagic "gastritis": A prospective evaluation. Gastroenterology 94:1254–1262, 1988.
11. Kuiper DH, Overholt BF, Fall DJ, et al: Gastroscopic findings and fecal blood loss following aspirin administration. Am J Dig Dis 14:761, 1969.
12. Langman MJS: Epidemiological evidence for the association of aspirin and acute gastrointestinal bleeding. Gut 11:627, 1970.
13. Metzger WH, McAdam L, Bluestone R, Guth PH: Acute gastric mucosal injury during continuous or interrupted aspirin ingestion in humans. Am J Dig Dis 21:963–968, 1976.
14. McIntyre RL, Irani MS, Piris J: Histological study of the effects of three anti-inflammatory preparations on the gastric mucosa. J Clin Pathol 34:836, 1981.
15. Graham DY, Smith JL: Gastroduodenal complications of chronic NSAID therapy. Am J Gastroenterol 83:1081–1084, 1988.
16. Brooks WS, Wenger J, Hersh T: Bile reflux gastritis: Analysis of fasting and postprandial gastric aspirates. Am J Gastroenterol 64:286–291, 1975.
17. Mann NS: Bile-induced acute erosive gastritis. Its prevention by antacid, cholestyramine, and prostaglandin E_2. Am J Dig Dis 21:89–92, 1976.
18. Meshkinpour H, Marks JW, Schoenfield LJ, et al: Reflux gastritis syndrome: Mechanism of symptoms. Gastroenterology 79:1283, 1980.
19. Dixon MF, O'Connor HJ, Axon ATR, et al: Reflux gastritis: A distinct histopathological entity? J Clin Pathol 39:524–530, 1986.
20. Niemela S, Kaittunen T, Heikkila J, Lehtola J: Characteristics of bile gastritis. Scand J Gastroenterol 22:345–354, 1987.
21. Davenport HW: Back diffusion of acid through the gastric mucosa and its physiological consequences. In Glass GBJ (ed): Progress in Gastroenterology. Vol 2. New York, Grune & Stratton, 1970.
22. Smith BM: Permeability of the human gastric mucosa: Alteration by acetylsalicylic acid and ethanol. N Engl J Med 285:216, 1971.
23. Robert A: Cytoprotection by prostaglandins. Gastroenterology 77:761, 1979.
24. Miller TA, Jacobson ED: Gastrointestinal cytoprotection by prostaglandins: Progress report. Gut 20:75, 1979.
25. Marshall BJ, Armstrong JA, McGechie DB, Glancy RJ: An attempt to fulfill Koch's postulates for pyloric Campylobacter. Med J Aust 142:436–439, 1985.
26. Myren J, Serck-Hanssen A: The gastroscopic diagnosis of gastritis with particular reference to mucosal reddening and mucus covering. Scand J Gastroenterol 9:457–462, 1974.
27. Burbage EJ, French SW, Tarder G, et al: Correlation between gross and histologic findings in the postoperative stomach. Gastrointest Endosc 25:3, 1979.
28. Elta GH, Appelman HD, Behler EM, et al: A study of the correlation between endoscopic and histological diagnoses in gastroduodenitis. Am J Gastroenterol 82:749–753, 1987.
29. Laine L, Weinstein WM: Subepithelial hemorrhages and erosions of human stomach. Dig Dis Sci 33:490–503, 1988.
30. Kreunig J, Bosman FT, Kuiper G, et al: Gastric and duodenal mucosa in "healthy" individuals: An endoscopic and histological study of 50 volunteers. J Clin Pathol 31:69, 1978.
31. McDonald WC: Correlation of mucosal histology and aspirin intake in chronic gastric ulcer. Gastroenterology 65:381, 1973.
32. Hamilton SR, Yardley JH: Endoscopic biopsy diagnosis of aspirin-associated chronic gastric ulcers. (Abstract) Gastroenterology 78:1178, 1980.
33. Matteran RA: A biopsy study of chronic gastritis and gastric atrophy. J Pathol Bacteriol 63:389, 1951.
34. Joske RA, Finckh ES, Wood IJ: Gastric biopsy: A study of 1000 consecutive successful gastric biopsies. Q J Med 24:269–294, 1955.
35. MacDonald WC, Rubin CE: Gastric biopsy—a critical evaluation. Gastroenterology 53:143–170, 1967.
36. Whitehead SC, Truelove SC, Gear MWL: The histological diagnosis of chronic gastritis in fiberoptic gastroscope biopsy specimens. J Clin Pathol 25:1, 1972.
37. Owen DA: The diagnosis and significance of gastritis. Pathol Annu 14:247, 1979.
38. Yardley JH: Pathology of chronic gastritis and duodenitis. In Goldman H, Appelman HD, Kaufman N (eds): Gastrointestinal Pathology. Baltimore, Williams & Wilkins, 1990, pp 69–143.
39. Siurala M, Salmi HJ: Long-term follow-up of subjects with superficial gastritis or a normal gastric mucosa. Scand J Gastroenterol 6:459–463, 1971.

40. Ihamaki T, Sankkonen M, Siurala M: Long term observation of subjects with normal mucosa and superficial gastritis: Results of 23–27 years follow-up examinations. Scand J Gastroenterol 13:771, 1978.
41. Cheli R, Giacosa A: Chronic atrophic gastritis and gastric mucosal atrophy—one and same. Gastrointest Endosc 29:23–25, 1983.
42. Morson BC, Intestinal metaplasia of the gastric mucosa. Br J Cancer 9:365–376, 1955.
43. Stemmermann G, Hayashi T: Intestinal metaplasia of the gastric mucosa: A gross and microscopic study of its distribution in various disease states. J Natl Cancer Inst 41:627–634, 1968.
44. Shousha S, Barrison IG, El-Sayeed W, et al: A study of incidence and relationship of intestinal metaplasia of gastric antrum and gastric metaplasia of duodenum in patients with non-ulcer dyspepsia. Dig Dis Sci 29:311–316, 1984.
45. Goldman H, Ming SC: Fine structure of intestinal metaplasia and adenocarcinoma of the human stomach. Lab Invest 18:203, 1968.
46. Chiao S-F, Weisberg H: Ultrastructure of the gastric mucosa in patients with atrophic gastritis and pernicious anaemia. Gastroenterology 59:36, 1970.
47. Stockton M, McCall I: Comparative electron microscopic features of normal, intermediate and metaplastic pyloric epithelium. Histopathology 7:859–871, 1983.
48. Planteydt HT, Willighagen RGJ: Enzyme histochemistry of the human stomach with special reference to intestinal metaplasia. J Pathol Bacteriol 80:713–722, 1960.
49. Matsukura N, Suzuki K, Kawachi T, et al: Distribution of marker enzymes and mucin in intestinal metaplasia of the stomach and relation of complete and incomplete types of metaplasia to minute gastric cancer. J Natl Cancer Inst 65:231–236, 1980.
50. Lev R: The mucin histochemistry of normal and neoplastic gastric mucosa. Lab Invest 14:2080, 1965.
51. Goldman H, Ming SC: Mucins in normal and metaplastic gastrointestinal epithelium: Histochemical distribution. Arch Pathol 85:580, 1968.
52. Gad A: A histochemical study of human alimentary tract mucosubstances in health and disease: II. Inflammatory conditions. Br J Cancer 23:64, 1969.
53. Jass JR, Filipe MI: The mucin profiles of normal gastric mucosa, intestinal metaplasia and its variants and gastric carcinoma. Histochem J 13:931–939, 1981.
54. Iida F, Murata F, Nagata T: Histochemical studies of mucosubstances in metaplastic epithelium of the stomach with special reference to the development of intestinal metaplasia. Histochemistry 56:229–237, 1978.
55. Teglbjaerg PS, Nielson HO: "Small intestinal type" and "colonic type" intestinal metaplasia of the human stomach. Acta Pathol Microbiol Scand [A] 86:351, 1978.
56. Segura DI, Montero C: Histochemical characterization of different types of intestinal metaplasia in gastric mucosa. Cancer 52:498–503, 1983.
57. Rubin W, Ross LL, Jeffries GH, Sleisenger MH: Some physiologic properties of heterotopic intestinal epithelium. Lab Invest 16:813, 1967.
58. Siurala M, Tarpila S: Absorptive function of intestinal metaplasia of the stomach. Scand J Gastroenterol 3:75, 1968.
59. Bordi C, Ravazzola M: Endocrine cells in the intestinal metaplasia of gastric mucosa. Am J Pathol 90:391–395, 1979.
60. Spicer SS: Diamine methods for differentiating mucosubstances histochemically. J Histochem Cytochem 13:211–234, 1965.
61. Filipe MI, Potet F, Bogomoletz WV, et al: Incomplete sulphomucin-secreting intestinal metaplasia for gastric cancer. Preliminary data from a prospective study from three centres. Gut 26:1319–1326, 1985.
62. Morson BC: Carcinoma arising from areas of intestinal metaplasia in the gastric mucosa. Br J Cancer 9:377–385, 1955.
63. Lauren P: The two histological main types of gastric carcinoma: Diffuse and so-called intestinal type carcinoma. An attempt at a histoclinical classification. Acta Pathol Microbiol Scand 64:31–49, 1965.
64. Ming SC, Goldman H, Freiman DG: Intestinal metaplasia and histogenesis of carcinoma in human stomach: Light and electron microscopic study. Cancer 20:1418, 1967.
65. Jass JR, Filipe MI: A variant of intestinal metaplasia associated with gastric carcinoma: A histochemical study. Histopathology 3:191–199, 1979.
66. Sipponen P, Seppala K, Varis K, et al: Intestinal metaplasia with colonic-type sulphomucins in the gastric mucosa; its association with gastric carcinoma. Acta Pathol Microbiol Scand [A] 88:217–224, 1980.
67. Jass JR, Filipe MI: Sulphamucins and precancerous lesions of the human stomach. Histopathology 4:271, 1980.
68. Iida F, Kusama J: Gastric carcinoma and intestinal metaplasia. Significance of types of intestinal metaplasia upon development of gastric carcinoma. Cancer 50:2854–2858, 1982.
69. Sipponen P, Kekki M, Siuralla M: Atrophic chronic gastritis and intestinal metaplasia in gastric carcinoma. Comparison with representative population sample. Cancer 52:1062–1068, 1983.
70. Lei D-N, Yu J-Y: Types of mucosal metaplasia in relation to the histogenesis of gastric carcinoma. Arch Pathol Lab Med 108:220–224, 1984.
71. Turoni H, Lurie B, Chaimoff CH, Kessler E: The diagnostic significance of sulfated acid mucin content in gastric intestinal metaplasia with early gastric cancer. Am J Gastroenterol 81:343–345, 1986.
72. Huang C-B, Xu J, Huang J-F, Meng X-Y: Sulphomucin colonic type intestinal metaplasia and carcinoma in the stomach. A histochemical study of 115 cases obtained by biopsy. Cancer 57:1370–1375, 1986.
73. Parl FF, Lev R, Thomas E, et al: Histologic and morphometric study of chronic gastritis in alcoholic patients. Hum Pathol 40:45, 1979.
74. Cheli R, Giacosa A, Molinari F: Chronic atrophic gastritis and duodenogastric reflux. Scand J Gastroenterol 16(Suppl 67):125, 1981.
75. Emmanouilidis A, Nicolopoulou-Stamati P, Manousos O: The histologic pattern of bile gastritis. Gastrointest Endosc 30:179–182, 1984.
76. Myes BM, Smith JL, Graham DY: Effect of red pepper and black pepper on the stomach. Am J Gastroenterol 82:211–214, 1987.
77. Steer HW: Ultrastructure of cell migration through the gastric epithelium and its relationship to bacteria. J Clin Pathol 28:639–646, 1975.
78. Warren JR, Marshall BJ: Unidentified curved bacilli on gastric epithelium in active chronic gastritis. Lancet 1:1273, 1983.
79. Jones DM, Lessells AM, Eldridge J: Campylobacter-like organisms in the gastric mucosa: Culture, histological and serological studies. J Clin Pathol 37:1002, 1984.
80. Marshall BJ, McGechie DB, Rogers PA, Glancy RJ: Pyloric Campylobacter infection and gastroduodenal disease. Med J Aust 142:439–444, 1985.
81. Johnston BJ, Reed PI, Ali MH: Campylobacter-like organisms in duodenal and antral endoscopic biopsies: Relationship to inflammation. Gut 27:1132–1137, 1986.
82. Rathbone BJ, Wyatt JI, Heatley RV: Campylobacter pyloridis—a new factor in peptic ulcer disease. Gut 27:635–641, 1986.
83. Taylor DE, Hargreaves JA, Lai-King NG, et al: Isolation and characterization of Campylobacter pyloridis from gastric biopsies. Am J Clin Pathol 87:49–54, 1987.
84. Hazell SL, Hennessy WB, Borody TJ, et al: Campylobacter pyloridis gastritis: II. Distribution of bacteria and associated inflammation in the gastroduodenal environment. Am J Gastroenterol 82:297–301, 1987.
85. Morris A, Nicholson G: Ingestion of Campylobacter pyloridis causes gastritis and raised fasting gastric pH. Am J Gastroenterol 82:192–199, 1987.
86. Drumna B, Sherman P, Cutz E, Karmali M: Association of Campylobacter pylori on the gastric mucosa with antral gastritis in children. N Engl J Med 316:1557–1561, 1987.
87. Blaser MJ: Gastric Campylobacter-like organisms, gastritis, and peptic ulcer disease. Gastroenterology 93:371–383, 1987.
88. Pettross CW, Appelman HD, Cohen H, et al: Prevalence of Campylobacter pylori and association with antral mucosal histology in subjects with and without upper gastrointestinal symptoms. Dig Dis Sci 33:649–653, 1988.
89. Barbosa AJA, Queiroz DMR, Mender EN, et al: Immunocytochemical identification of Campylobacter pylori in gastritis and correlation with culture. Arch Pathol Lab Med 112:523–525, 1988.

90. Rathbone BJ, Wyatt JI, Worsley BW, et al: Systemic and local antibody responses to gastric *Campylobacter pyloridis* in non-ulcer dyspepsia. Gut 27:642–647, 1986.
91. Hazell SL, Borody TJ, Gal A, Lee A: *Campylobacter pyloridis* gastritis: I. Detection of urease as a marker of bacterial colonization and gastritis. Am J Gastroenterol 82:292–296, 1987.
92. Graham DY, Klein PD, Evans DJ Jr, et al: *Campylobacter pylori* detected noninvasively by the ^{13}C-urea breath test. Lancet 1:1174–1177, 1987.
93. Montgomery EA, Martin DF, Peura DA: Rapid diagnosis of Campylobacter pylori by Gram stain. Am J Clin Pathol 90:606–609, 1988.
94. Nichols L, Sughayer M, Eichelberger K, et al: Campylobacter pylori gastritis: Clinical features, histology, Gram stain, urease and culture results. Am J Clin Pathol (In press).
95. Rollason TP, Stone J, Rhodes JM: Spiral organisms in endoscopic biopsies of the human stomach. J Clin Pathol 37:23–26, 1984.
96. Price AB, Levi J, Dolby JM, et al: *Campylobacter pyloridis* in peptic ulcer disease: Microbiology, pathology, and scanning electron microscopy. Gut 26:1183–1188, 1985.
97. Tricottet V, Bruneval P, Vire O, Camilleri JP: *Campylobacter*-like organisms and surface epithelium abnormalities in active, chronic gastritis in humans: an ultrastructural study. Ultrastuct Pathol 10:113–122, 1986.
98. Chen XG, Correa P, Offerhaus J, et al: Ultrastructure of the gastric mucosa harboring *Campylobacter*-like organisms. Am J Clin Pathol 86:575–582, 1986.
99. Dooley CP, Cohen H, Fitzgibbons PL, et al: Prevalence of Helicobacter pylori infection and histologic gastritis in asymptomatic persons. N Engl J Med 321:1562–1566, 1989.
100. Frierson HF, Caldwell SH, Marshall BJ: Duodenal biopsy findings for patients with non-ulcer dyspepsia with or without Campylobacter pylori gastritis. Mod Pathol 3:271–276, 1990.
101. Paull G, Yardley JH: Gastric and esophageal Campylobacter pylori in patients with Barrett's esophagus. Gastroenterology 95:216–218, 1988.
102. Dye KR, Marshall BJ, Frierson HF, et al: Campylobacter pylori colonizing heterotopic gastric tissue in the rectum. Am J Clin Pathol 93:144–147, 1990.
103. McNulty CAM, Gearty JC, Crump B, et al: *Campylobacter pyloridis* and associated gastritis. Investigator-blind, placebo-controlled trial of bismuth salicylate and erythromycin ethylsuccinate. Br Med J 293:645–649, 1986.
104. Graham DY, Alpert LC, Smith JL, Yoshimura HH: Iatrogenic Campylobacter pylori infection as a cause of epidemic achlorhydria. Am J Gastroenterol 83:974–980, 1988.
105. Bartlett JG: Campylobacter pylori: Fact or fancy? (Editorial) Gastroenterology 94:229–232, 1988.
106. McNulty CAM, Dent JC, Curry A, et al: New spiral bacterium in gastric mucosa. J Clin Pathol 42:585–591, 1989.
107. Morris A, Ali MR, Thomsen L, Hollis B: Tightly spiral shaped bacteria in the human stomach: Another cause of active chronic gastritis? Gut 31:139–143, 1990.
108. Fischer R, Samiach W, Schwenke E: "Gastrospirillum hominis": Another four cases (Letter) Lancet 1:59, 1990.
109. Greenlaw R, Sheahan DG, DeLuca V, et al: Gastroduodenitis: A broader concept of peptic ulcer disease. Dig Dis Sci 25:660, 1980.
110. Meshkinpour H, Orlando RA, Arguello JF, et al: Significance of endoscopically visible blood vessels as an index of atrophic gastritis. Am J Gastroenterol 71:376, 1979.
111. Stamp GWH, Palmer K, Misiewicz JJ: Antral hypertrophic gastritis: A rare cause of iron deficiency. J Clin Pathol 38:390–392, 1985.
112. Strickland RG, Bhatal PS, Korman MG, et al: Serum gastrin and the antral mucosa in atrophic gastritis. Br Med J 4:451, 1971.
113. Lambert R: Chronic gastritis: A critical study of the progressive atrophy of the gastric mucosa. Digestion 7:83, 1972.
114. Glass GBJ, Pitchumoni CS: Atrophic gastritis. Hum Pathol 6:219, 1975.
115. Edwards FC, Coghill NF: Aetiological factors in chronic atrophic gastritis. Br Med J 2:1409, 1966.
116. Chisholm M: Immunology of gastritis. Clin Gastroenterol 5:419, 1976.
117. Glass GBJ: Immunology of atrophic gastritis. N Y State J Med 77:1697–1706, 1977.
118. Coghill NF, Doniach D, Roitt IM, et al: Autoantibodies in simple atrophic gastritis. Gut 6:48, 1965.
119. Wright R, Whitehead R, Wangel AG, et al: Autoantibodies and microscopic appearance of gastric mucosa. Lancet 1:618–621, 1966.
120. Doniach D, Roitt IM, Taylor KB: Autoimmune phenomena in pernicious anaemia. Serologic overlap with thyroiditis, thyrotoxicosis, and systemic lupus erythematosus. Br Med J 1:1374, 1963.
121. Lillibridge CA, Brandborg LL, Rubin CE: Childhood pernicious anaemia: Gastrointestinal secretory histological and electron microscopic aspects. Gastroenterology 52:792, 1967.
122. Wynn-Williams A, Coghill NF, Edwards F: The gastric mucosa in pernicious anaemia: Biopsy studies. Br J Haematol 4:457, 1958.
123. Irvine WJ, Cullen DR, Mawhinney H: Natural history of autoimmune achlorhydric atrophic gastritis: a 1–15 year follow-up study. Lancet 2:482–485, 1974.
124. Weinstein WM: Gastritis. In Sleisenger MH, Fordtran JS (eds): Gastrointestinal Disease, 4th ed. Philadelphia, WB Saunders, 1989, pp 792–813.
125. McGuigan JE, Trudeau WL: Serum gastrin concentrations in pernicious anaemia. N Engl J Med 282:358–361, 1970.
126. Jeffries GH, Todd JE, Sleisenger MH: The effect of prednisolone on gastric mucosal histology, gastric secretion, and vitamin B_{12} absorption in patients with pernicious anemia. J Clin Invest 45:803, 1966.
127. Siurala M, Varis K, Wiljasalo M: Studies of patients with atrophic gastritis: A 10–15 year follow-up. Scand J Gastroenterol 1:40, 1966.
128. Cheli R, Santi L, Ciancamerla G, Canciani G: A clinical and statistical follow-up study of atrophic gastritis. Am J Dig Dis 18:1061–1066, 1973.
129. Siurala M, Lehtola J, Thamaki T: Atrophic gastritis and its sequelae: Results of 19–23 years of follow-up examinations. Scand J Gastroenterol 9:441–446, 1974.
130. Churid EL, Hirsch RL, Colcher H: Spectrum of hypertrophic gastropy: Giant rugal folds, polyposis and carcinoma of the stomach. Case report and review of the literature. Arch Intern Med 114:621, 1964.
131. Schindler R: Gastric carcinoma and gastritis, with reference to coexistence of carcinoma and chronic hypertrophic glandular gastritis. Am J Dig Dis 10:607, 1965.
132. Overholt BF, Jeffries GH: Hypertrophic hypersecretory protein-losing gastropathy. Gastroenterology 58:80–87, 1970.
133. Lewin KJ, Dowling F, Wright JP, et al: Gastric morphology and serum gastrin levels in pernicious anemia. Gut 17:551, 1976.
134. Rubin W: A fine structural characterization of the proliferated endocrine cells in atrophic gastric mucosa. Am J Pathol 70:109, 1973.
135. Flejou JF, Bahame P, Smith AC, et al: Pernicious anemia and Campylobacter like organisms: Is the gastric antrum resistant to colonization? Gut 30:60–64, 1989.
136. Scharschmidt BF: The natural history of hypertrophic gastropathy (Ménétrier's disease). Am J Med 63:644, 1977.
137. Simon L, Figus AI, Bajtai A: Chronic gastritis following resection of the stomach. Am J Gastroenterol 60:477, 1973.
138. Sauktonen M, Sipponen, P, Varis K, et al: Morphological and dynamic behavior of the gastric mucosa after partial gastrectomy with special reference to the gastroenterostomy area. Hepatogastroenterology 27:48, 1980.
139. Bechi P, Amorosi A, Mazzanti R, et al: Gastric histology and fasting bile reflux after partial gastrectomy. Gastroenterology 93:335–343, 1987.
140. Aukee S, Krohn K: Occurrence and progression of gastritis in patients operated on for peptic ulcer. Scand J Gastroenterol 7:541, 1972.
141. Hoare AM, Jones EL, Alexander-Williams J, Hawkins CF: Symptomatic significance of gastric mucosal changes after surgery for peptic ulcer. Gut 18:295, 1977.
142. Skinner JM, Heenan PJ, Whitehead R: Atrophic gastritis in gastrectomy specimens. Br J Surg 62:23–25, 1975.
143. Geboes K, Rutgeerts P, Broeckaert L, et al: Histologic appear-

ances of endoscopic gastric mucosal biopsies 10–20 years after partial gastrectomy. Ann Surg 192:179, 1980.
144. Pickford IR, Craven JL, Hall R, et al: Endoscopic examination of the gastric remnant 31–39 years after subtotal gastrectomy for peptic ulcer. Gut 25:393–397, 1984.
145. Elsborg L, Andersen D, Myhre-Jensen O, Bastrup-Madsen P: Gastric mucosal polyps in pernicious anaemia. Scand J Gastroenterol 12:49–52, 1977.
146. Joffe N, Goldman H, Antonioli DA: Recurring hyperplastic gastric polyps following subtotal gastrectomy. Am J Roentgenol 130:301, 1978.
147. Stemmermann GN, Hayashi T: Hyperplastic polyps of the gastric mucosa adjacent to gastroenterostomy stomas. Am J Clin Pathol 71:341, 1979.
148. Clarke AC, Lee SP, Nicholson GI. Gastritis varioliformis. Am J Gastroenterol 68:599–602, 1977.
149. Lambert R, Andre C, Moulinier B, Bugnon B: Diffuse varioliform gastritis. Digestion 17:159–167, 1978.
150. Green PHR, Gold RP, Marboe CC, et al: Chronic erosive gastritis: Clinical, diagnostic and pathological features in nine patients. Am J Gastroenterol 77:543–547, 1982.
151. Elta GH, Fawaz KA, Dayal Y, et al: Chronic erosive gastritis—a recently recognized disorder. Dig Dis Sci 28:7–12, 1983.
152. Haot J, Jouret A, Willette M, et al: Lymphocytic gastritis—prospective study of its relationship with varioliform gastritis. Gut 31:282–285, 1990.
153. Dixon MF, Wyatt JI, Burke DA, Rathbone BJ: Lymphocytic gastritis—Relationship to Campylobacter pylori infection. J Pathol 154:125–132, 1988.
154. Wolber R, Owen D, DelBuono L, et al: Lymphocytic gastritis in patients with celiac sprue or spruelike intestinal disease. Gastroenterology 98:310–315, 1990.
155. Kimura K: Gastric xanthelasmas. Arch Pathol 87:110–117, 1969.
156. Javdan P, Pitman ER, Schwartz IS: Gastric xanthelasma: Endoscopic recognition. Gastroenterology 67:1006–1010, 1974.
157. Mast A, Elewaut A, Mortier G, et al: Gastric xanthoma. Am J Gastroenterol 65:311–317, 1976.
158. Drude RB, Balart LA, Herrington JP, et al: Gastric xanthoma: Histological similarity to signet ring cell carcinoma. J Clin Gastroenterol 4:217–221, 1982.
159. Kunze KC, Baum RA, Nasrallah SM: Gastric xanthoma. Gastrointest Endosc 33:114–115, 1987.
160. Domellof L, Ericksson S, Helander HF, et al: Lipid islands in the gastric mucosa after resection for benign ulcer disease. Gastroenterology 72:14, 1977.
161. Terruzzi V, Minoli G, Butti GC, Rossini A: Gastric lipid islands in the gastric stump and in non-operated stomach. Endoscopy 12:58–62, 1980.
162. Klugman HJ, Wohlgemuth B: Results of endoscopic and bioptical examinations in the stump stomach after resection. Billroth II. Z Gesamte Inn Med 36:208–215, 1981.
163. Ming SC, Goldman H: Gastric polyps: A histogenetic classification and its relation to carcinoma. Cancer 18:721, 1965.
164. Tomasulo J: Gastric polyps: Histologic types and their relationship to gastric carcinoma. Cancer 27:1346, 1971.
165. Antonioli DA: Gastric carcinoma and its precursors. In: Goldman H, Appelman HD, Kaufman N (eds): Gastrointestinal Pathology. Baltimore, Williams & Wilkins, 1990, pp 144–180.
166. Mosbeck J, Videbaek A: Mortality from and risk of gastric carcinoma among patients with pernicious anemia. Br Med J 2:390, 1950.
167. Elsborg L, Mosbeck J: Pernicious anemia as a risk factor in gastric cancer. Acta Med Scand 206:315, 1979.
168. Kobayashi S, Prolla JD, Kirsner JB: Late gastric carcinoma developing after surgery for benign condition. Dig Dis Sci 15:905–912, 1970.
169. Stalsberg H, Taksdal S: Stomach cancer following gastric surgery for benign conditions. Lancet 2:1175–1177, 1971.
170. Saegesser F, James D: Cancer of the gastric stump after partial gastrectomy (Billroth II principle) for ulcer. Cancer 19:1150, 1972.
171. Hammar E: The localization of precancerous changes and carcinoma after previous gastric operation for benign conditions. Acta Pathol Microbiol Scand [A] 84:495, 1976.
172. Schrumpf E, Serck-Hanssen A, Stadaar J, et al: Mucosal changes in the gastric stump 20 to 25 years after partial gastrectomy. Lancet 2:467, 1977.
173. Domellof L, Eriksson S, Janunger KG: Carcinoma and possible precancerous change of the gastric stump after Billroth II resection. Gastroenterology 73:462, 1977.
174. Savage A, Jones S: Histological appearances of the gastric mucosa 15 to 27 years after partial gastrectomy. J Clin Pathol 32:179, 1979.
175. Giarelli L, Melato M, Stanta G, et al: Gastric resection: A cause of high frequency of gastric carcinoma. Cancer 52:1113–1116, 1983.
176. Schuman BM, Waldbaum JR, Hitz SW: Carcinoma of the gastric remnant in a U.S. population. Gastrointest Endosc 30:71–73, 1984.
177. Caygill CPJ, Kirkham JS, Hill MJ, Northfield TC: Mortality from gastric cancer following gastric surgery for peptic ulcer. Lancet 1:929–931, 1986.
178. Viste A, Opheim P, Thunald J, et al: Risk of carcinoma following gastric operations for benign disease: A historical cohort study of 3470 patients. Lancet 2:502–505, 1986.
179. Pointner R, Schwab G, Konigsrainer A, et al: Early cancer of the gastric remnant. Gut 29:298–301, 1988.
180. Schafer LW, Larson DE, Melton J, et al: The risk of gastric carcinoma after surgical treatment for benign ulcer disease. A population-based study in Olmsted County, Minnesota. N Engl J Med 309:1210–1213, 1983.
181. Logan RFA, Langman MJS: Screening for gastric cancer after gastric surgery. Lancet 2:667–669, 1983.
182. Sandler RS, Johnson MD, Holland KL: Risk of stomach cancer after gastric surgery for benign conditions: A case-control study. Dig Dis Sci 29:703–708, 1984.
183. Cuello C, Correa P, Zarama G, et al: Histopathology of gastric dysplasia. Am J Surg Pathol 3:491–500, 1979.
184. Janunger K-G, Domellof L: Gastric polyps and precancerous mucosal changes after partial gastrectomy. Acta Chir Scand 144:293, 1978.
185. Borchard F, Mittelstaedt A, Kieker R: Incidence of epithelial dysplasia after partial gastric resection. Pathol Res Pract 164:282–293, 1979.
186. Farrands PA, Blake JRS, Ansell ID, et al: Endoscopic review of patients who have had gastric surgery. Br Med J 286:755–758, 1983.
187. Graem N, Fischer AB, Beck H: Dysplasia and carcinoma in the Billroth II resected stomach 27–35 years post-operatively. Acta Pathol Microbiol Scand 92:185–188, 1984.
188. Offerhaus G, Volstadt J, Huibregtse K, Tytgat GNJ: Endoscopic screening for malignancy in the gastric remnant: The clinical significance of dysplasia in gastric mucosa. J Clin Pathol 37:748–754, 1984.
189. Saraga E-P, Gardial D, Costa J: Gastric dysplasia: A histological follow-up study. Am J Surg Pathol 11:788–796, 1987.
190. Morson BC, Sobin LH, Grundmann E, et al: Precancerous conditions and epithelial dysplasia of the stomach. J Clin Pathol 33:231–240, 1980.
191. Ming S-C, Bajtai A, Correa, P, et al: Gastric dysplasia: Significance and pathologic criteria. Cancer 54:1794–1801, 1984.
192. del Corral MJM, Pardo-Mindon FJ, Razquin S, Ojeda C: Risk of cancer in patients with gastric dysplasia. Follow-up study of 67 patients. Cancer 65:2078–2085, 1990.
193. de Dombal FT, Price AB, Thompson H, et al: The British Society of Gastroenterology early gastric cancer/dysplasia survey: An interim report. Gut 31:115–120, 1990.
194. Hirota T, Itabashi M, Suzuki K, et al: Clinicopathologic study of minute and small early gastric cancers. Pathol Annu 15:1, 1980.
195. Qizilbash A: Early gastric carcinoma. Arch Pathol Lab Med 101:610, 1977.
196. Green PHR, O'Toole KM, Weinberg LM, et al: Early gastric cancer. Gastroenterology 81:247–256, 1981.
197. Polak JM, Hoffbrand AV, Reed PI, et al: Qualitative and quantitative studies of antral and fundic G cells in pernicious anemia. Scand J Gastroenterol 8:361, 1973.
198. Black WC, Haffner HE: Diffuse hyperplasia of gastric argyrophil cells and multiple carcinoid tumors: An historical and ultrastructural study. Cancer 21:1080–1099, 1968.

199. Harris AI, Greenberg H: Pernicious anemia and the development of carcinoid tumors of the stomach. JAMA 239:1160, 1978.
200. Russo A, Buffa R, Grasso G, et al: Gastric gastrinoma and diffuse G cell hyperplasia associated with chronic atrophic gastritis: Endoscopic detection and removal. Digestion 20:416, 1980.
201. Goldman H, French S, Burbige E: Kulchitsky cell hyperplasia and multiple metastasizing carcinoids of the stomach. Cancer 47:2620, 1981.
202. Hodges JR, Isaacson P, Wright R: Diffuse enterochromaffin-like (ECL) cell hyperplasia and multiple gastric carcinoids: a complication of pernicious anemia. Gut 22:237–241, 1981.
203. Borch K, Renvall H, Ludberg G: Gastric endocrine cell hyperplasia and carcinoid tumors in pernicious anemia. Gastroenterology 88:638–648, 1985.
204. Muller J, Kirchner T, Muller-Hermelink HK: Gastric endocrine cell hyperplasia and carcinoid tumors in atrophic gastritis type A. Am J Surg Pathol 11:909–917, 1987.
205. Itsuno M, Watanabe H, Iwafuchi M, et al: Multiple carcinoids and endocrine cell micronests in type A gastritis: Their morphology, histogenesis, and natural history. Cancer 63:881–890, 1989.
206. Citron B, Pincus I, Geokas M, Haverback B: Chemical trauma of the esophagus and stomach. Surg Clin North Am 48:1303, 1968.
207. Allen R, Thoshinsky M, Stallone R, Hunt R: Corrosive injuries of the stomach. Arch Surg 100:409, 1970.
208. Lowe JE, Graham DY, Bolsaubin EV Jr, Lanza FL: Corrosive injury to the stomach: The natural history and role of fiberoptic endoscopy. Am J Surg 137:803–806, 1979.
209. Marks I, Bank S, Werbeloff M, et al: The natural history of corrosive gastritis. Am J Dig Dis 8:509, 1963.
210. Sugawa C, Mullins RJ, Lucas CE, Leibold WC: The value of early endoscopy following caustic ingestion. Surg Gynecol Obstet 153:553–556, 1981.
211. Dworkin B, Wormser GP, Rosenthal WS, et al: Gastrointestinal manifestations of the acquired immunodeficiency syndrome: A review of 22 cases. Am J Gastroenterol 80:774–778, 1985.
212. Wilderlite L, Trier JS, Blacklow NR, Schrieber DS: Structure of the gastric mucosa in acute infectious nonbacterial gastroenteritis. Gastroenterology 68:425, 1975.
213. Nash G, Ross J: Herpetic esophagitis: A common cause of esophageal ulceration. Hum Pathol 5:339, 1974.
214. Howiler W, Goldberg HI: Gastroesophageal involvement in herpes simplex. Gastroenterology 70:775, 1976.
215. Sperling HV, Reed WG: Herpetic gastritis. Am J Dig Dis 22:1034, 1977.
216. Freeman HJ, Shnitka TK, Piercey JRA, et al: Cytomegalovirus infection of the gastrointestinal tract in a patient with late onset immunodeficiency syndrome. Gastroenterology 73:1397, 1977.
217. Campbell DA, Piercey JRA, Shnitka TK, et al: Cytomegalovirus-associated gastric ulcer. Gastroenterology 72:533–535, 1977.
218. Allen JI, Silvis SE, Summer HW, et al: Cytomegalic inclusion disease diagnosed endoscopically. Dig Dis Sci 26:133, 1981.
219. Andrade JS, Bambirra EA, Lima GF, et al: Gastric cytomegalic inclusion bodies diagnosed by histologic examination of endoscopic biopsies in patients with gastric ulcer. Am J Clin Pathol 79:493–496, 1983.
220. Knapp AB, Horst DA, Eliopoulos G, et al: Widespread cytomegalovirus gastroenterocolitis in a patient with acquired immunodeficiency syndrome. Gastroenterology 85:1399–1402, 1983.
221. Gertler SL, Pressman J, Price P, et al: Gastrointestinal cytomegalovirus infection in a homosexual man with severe acquired immunodeficiency syndrome. Gastroenterology 85:1403–1406, 1983.
222. Freedman SL, Wright TL, Altman DF: Gastrointestinal Kaposi's sarcoma in patients with acquired immunodeficiency syndrome: Endoscopic and autopsy findings. Gastroenterology 89:102–108, 1985.
223. Hinnant KL, Rotterdam HZ, Bell ET, et al: Cytomegalovirus infection of the alimentary tract: A clinicopathological correlation. Am J Gastroenterol 81:944–950, 1986.
224. Franzin G, Muolo A, Griminelli T: Cytomegalovirus inclusions in the gastroduodenal mucosa of patients after renal transplantation. Gut 22:698–701, 1981.
225. Strayer DS, Phillips GB, Barker KH, et al: Gastric cytomegalovirus infection in bone marrow transplant patients. Cancer 48:1478–1483, 1981.
226. Palmer ED: The morphologic consequences of acute exogenous (staphylococcic) gastroenteritis on the gastric mucosa. Gastroenterology 19:462–475, 1951.
227. Gonzalez-Crussi F, Hackett RL: Phlegmonous gastritis. Arch Surg 93:990–995, 1966.
228. Nevin NC, Eakins D, Clarke SD, Carson DJL: Acute phlegmonous gastritis. Br J Surg 56:268–270, 1969.
229. Miller AI, Smith M, Rogers AI: Phlegmonous gastritis. Gastroenterology 68:231, 1975.
230. Nicholson BW, Maull KI, Scher LA: Phlegmonous gastritis: Clinical presentation and surgical management. South Med J 73:875, 1980.
231. Gonzalez L, Schowengerdt C, Skinner H, Lynch P: Emphysematous gastritis. Surg Gynecol Obstet 116:79, 1963.
232. Palmer ED: Tuberculosis of the stomach and the stomach in tuberculosis: A review with particular reference to gross pathology and gastroscopic diagnosis. Am Rev Tuberc 61:116–130, 1950.
233. Chazan B, Aitchison J: Gastric tuberculosis. Br Med J 2:1288, 1960.
234. Misra RC, Agarwal SK, Prakash P, et al: Gastric tuberculosis. Endoscopy 14:235–237, 1982.
235. Subei I, Attar B, Schmitt G, Levendoglu H: Primary gastric tuberculosis: A case report and literature review. Am J Gastroenterol 82:769–772, 1983.
236. Rotterdam H: Contributions of gastrointestinal biopsy to an understanding of gastrointestinal disease. Am J Gastroenterol 78:140–148, 1983.
237. Berardi RS: Abdominal actinomycosis. Surg Gynecol Obstet 149:257, 1979.
238. Wilson E: Abdominal actinomycosis with special reference to the stomach. Br J Surg 49:266, 1962.
239. Van Olmen G, Larmuseau MF, Geboes K, et al: Primary gastric actinomycosis: A case report and review of the literature. Am J Gastroenterol 79:512–516, 1984.
240. Mitchell R, Bralow S: Acute erosive gastritis due to early syphilis. Ann Intern Med 61:933, 1964.
241. Butz WC, Watts JC, Rosales-Quintana S, et al: Erosive gastritis as a manifestation of secondary syphilis. Am J Clin Pathol 63:895, 1975.
242. Besses C, Sans-Sabrofen J, Badia X, et al: Ulceroinfiltrative syphilitic gastropathy: Silver stain diagnosis from biopsy specimen. Am J Gastroenterol 82:773–774, 1987.
243. Palmer ED: Syphilis of the stomach and the stomach in syphilis: A review of the literature with particular reference to gross pathology and gastroscopic diagnosis. Am J Syph Gonorrh Vener Dis 33:481–496, 1949.
244. Cooley R, Childers J: Acquired symphilis of the stomach. Gastroenterology 39:201, 1960.
245. Reisman TN, Leverett FL, Hudson JR, Kalser MH: Syphilitic gastropathy. Am J Dig Dis 20:588–593, 1975.
246. Beckman JW, Schuman BM: Antral gastritis and ulceration in a patient with secondary syphilis. Gastrointest Endosc 32:353–356, 1986.
247. Morin ME, Tan A: Diffuse enlargement of gastric folds as a manifestation of secondary syphilis. Am J Gastroenterol 74:170–172, 1980.
248. Smith JMB: Mycoses of the alimentary tract: Progress report. Gut 10:1035, 1969.
249. Eras P, Goldstein MJ, Sherlock P: Candida infection of the gastrointestinal tract. Medicine 51:367, 1972.
250. Katzenstein ALA, Maksen J: Candidal infection of gastric ulcers: histology, incidence and clinical significance. Am J Clin Pathol 71:137, 1979.
251. Peters M, Weiner J, Whelan G: Fungal infection associated with gastroduodenal ulceration: Endoscopic and pathologic appearances. Gastroenterology 78:350, 1980.
252. Gotlieb-Jensen K, Andersen J: Occurrence of Candida in gastric ulcers. Significance for the healing process. Gastroenterology 85:535–537, 1983.

253. Loffeld RJ, Loffeld BC, Arends JW, et al: Fungal colonization of gastric ulcers. Am J Gastroenterol 83:730–733, 1988.
254. Nelson R, Bruni M, Goldstein M: Primary gastric candidiasis in uncompromised subjects. Gastrointest Endosc 22:92, 1975.
255. Gillespie PE, Green PH, Barrett PJ, et al: Gastric candidiasis. Med J Aust 1:228, 1978.
256. Minoli G, Terruzzi V, Rossini A: Gastroduodenal candidiasis occurring without underlying diseases (primary gastroduodenal candidiasis). Endoscopy 1:18–22, 1979.
257. Scott BB, Jenkins D: Gastro-oesophageal candidiasis. Gut 23:137–139, 1982.
258. Young JA, Elias E: Gastro-oesophageal candidiasis: Diagnosis by brush cytology. J Clin Pathol 38:293–296, 1985.
259. Kodsi BE, Wickremesinghe PC, Kozinin PJ, et al: Candida esophagitis: A prospective study of 27 cases. Gastroenterology 71:715, 1976.
260. Pinkerton H, Iverson L: Histoplasmosis: Three fatal cases with disseminated sarcoid-like lesions. Arch Intern Med 90:456–467, 1952
261. Nudelman H, Rakatansky H: Gastric histoplasmosis—a case report. JAMA 195:44, 1966.
262. Fisher JR, Sanowski RA: Disseminated histoplasmosis producing hypertrophic gastric folds. Dig Dis Sci 23:282, 1978.
263. Miller DP, Everett ED: Gastrointestinal histoplasmosis. J Clin Gastroenterol 1:233, 1979.
264. Kahn LB: Gastric mucormycosis: A report of a case with a review of the literature. S Afr Med J 37:1265–1269, 1963.
265. Deal WB, Johnson JE III: Gastric phycomycosis: Report of a case and review of the literature. Gastroenterology 57:579, 1969.
266. Lawson H, Schmaman A: Gastric phycomycosis. Br J Surg 61:743, 1974.
267. Lyon DT, Schubert TT, Mantia AG, Kaplan MH: Phycomycosis of the gastrointestinal tract. Am J Gastroenterol 72:379–391, 1979.
268. Garone MA, Winston BJ, Lewin JH: Cryptosporidiosis of the stomach. Am J Gastroenterol 81:465–470, 1986.
269. Asami K, Watanuki T, Sakai H, et al: Two cases of stomach granuloma caused by Anisakis-like larval nematodes in Japan. Am J Trop Med Hyg 14:119, 1965.
270. Watt IA, McLean NR, Girdwood RWA, et al: Eosinophilic gastroenteritis associated with a larval anisakine nematode. Lancet 2:893–894, 1979.
271. Hsiu J-G, Gomsey AJ, Ives CE, et al: Gastric anisakiasis: Report of a case with clinical, endoscopic, and histological findings. Am J Gastroenterol 81:1185–1187, 1986.
272. Scowden EB, Schaffner W, Stone WJ: Overwhelming strongyloidiasis. An unappreciated opportunistic infection. Medicine 57:527, 1978.
273. Ainley CC, Clarke DG, Timothy AR, Thompson RPH: *Strongyloides stercoralis* hyperinfection associated with cimetidine in an immunosuppressed patient: Diagnosis by endoscopic biopsy. Gut 27:337–338, 1986.
274. Jacob GS, Al Nakib B, Al Ruwaih A: Ascariasis producing upper gastrointestinal hemorrhage. Endoscopy 15:67, 1983.
275. Choudhuri G, Saha SS, Tandon RK: Gastric ascariasis. Am J Gastroenterol 81:788–790, 1986.
276. Mallory GK, Weiss S: Hemorrhages from lacerations of the cardiac orifice of the stomach due to vomiting. Am J Med Sci 178:506, 1929.
277. Knauer CM: Mallory-Weiss syndrome. Gastroenterolygy 71:5, 1976.
278. Graham DY, Schwartz SJ: The spectrum of the Mallory-Weiss tear. Medicine 57:307, 1978.
279. Levin E, Clayman CB, Palmer WL, Kirsner JB: Observations on the value of gastric irradiation in the treatment of duodenal ulcer. Gastroenterology 32:42, 1957.
280. Clayman CB, Palmer WL, Kirsner JB: Gastric irradiation in the treatment of peptic ulcer. Gastroenterology 55:403, 1968.
281. Wood IJ, Ralston M, Kurrle GR: Irradiation injury to gastrointestinal tract: clinical features, management and pathogenesis. Australas Ann Med 12:143, 1963.
282. Novak JM, Collins JT, Donowitz M, et al: Effects of radiation on the human gastrointestinal tract. J Clin Gastroenterol 1:9, 1979.
283. Berthrong M, Fajardo LF: Radiation injury in surgical pathology: II. Alimentary tract. Am J Surg Pathol 5:153, 1981.
284. Goldgraber MB, Rubin CE, Palmer WL, et al: The early gastric response to irradiation, a serial biopsy study. Gastroenterology 27:1–20, 1954.
285. McIlrath DC, Hallenbeck GA: Review of gastric freezing. JAMA 190:715, 1964.
286. Barner HB, Collins CH, Jones TI, Garlick TB: Morphology of human stomach after therapeutic freezing. Arch Surg 90:358, 1965.
287. Perry GT, Dunphy JV, Fruin RC, Littman A: Gastric freezing for duodenal ulcer. A double blind study. Gastroenterology 47:6, 1964.
288. Klein NC, Hargrove RL, Sleisenger MH, et al: Eosinophilic gastroenteritis. Medicine 40:299, 1970.
289. Goldman H, Proujansky R: Allergic proctitis and gastroenteritis in children: Clinical and mucosal biopsy features in 53 cases. Am J Surg Pathol 10:75–86, 1986.
290. Johnstone JM, Morson BC: Eosinophilic gastroenteritis. Histopathology 2:335–348, 1978.
291. Katz AJ, Goldman H, Grand RJ: Gastric mucosal biopsy in eosinophilic (allergic) gastroenteritis. Gastroenterology 73:705, 1977.
292. Snyder JD, Rosenblum N, Wershil B, et al: Pyloric stenosis and eosinophilic gastroenteritis in infants. J Pediatr Gastroenterol Nutr 6:543–547, 1987.
293. Gile JF: Diverticula of the stomach. N Engl J Med 204:268–269, 1931.
294. Palmer E: Gastric diverticula, a collective review. Int Abstr Surg 92:417, 1951.
295. Eras P, Beranbaum S: Gastric diverticula: Congenital and acquired. Am J Gastroenterol 57:120, 1972.
296. Kadian RS, Rose JF, Mann NS: Gastric bezoars—spontaneous resolution. Am J Gastroenterol 70:79–80, 1978.
297. Holloway W, Lee S, Nicholson G: The composition and dissolution of phytobezoars. Arch Pathol Lab Med 104:159, 1980.
298. Raffin SB: Bezoars. In Sleisenger MH, Fordtran JS (eds): Gastrointestinal Disease, 4th ed. Philadelphia, WB Saunders, 1989, pp 741–745.
299. Cain GD, Moore P, Patterson M: Bezoar—a complication of postgastrectomy state. Am J Dig Dis 13:801–809, 1968.
300. Goldstein HM, Cohen LE, Hagen RO, Wells RF: Gastric bezoars: A frequent complication in the postoperative ulcer patient. Radiology 107:341–344, 1973.
301. Force T, MacDonald D, Eade OE, et al: Ischemic gastritis and duodenitis. Dig Dis Sci 25:307, 1980.
302. Cherry RD, Jabbari M, Goresky CA, et al: Chronic mesenteric vascular insufficiency with gastric ulceration. Gastroenterology 91:1548–1552, 1986.
303. Taylor NS, Gueft B, Lebowich RJ: Atheromatous embolization: A cause of gastric ulcers and small bowel necrosis. Gastroenterology 47:97, 1964.
304. Romano TJ, Graham SM, Chuong J, et al: Bleeding colonic ulcers secondary to atheromatous microemboli after left heart catheterization. J Clin Gastroenterol 10:693–698, 1988.
305. McCormack TT, Sims J, Eyre-Brook I, et al: Gastric lesions in portal hypertension: Inflammatory gastritis or congestive gastropathy? Gut 26:1226–1232, 1985.
306. Quintero E, Pique JM, Bombi JA, et al: Gastric mucosal vascular ectasias causing bleeding in cirrhosis: A distinct entity associated with hypergastrinemia and low serum levels of pepsinogen I. Gastroenterology 93:1054–1061, 1987.
307. Tarnowski AS, Sarfeh IJ, Stochura J, et al. Microvascular abnormalities of the portal hypertensive gastric mucosa. Hepatology 8:1488–1494, 1988.
308. Petras RE, Hart WR, Bukowski RM: Gastric epithelial atypia associated with hepatic arterial infusion chemotherapy: Its distinction from early gastric carcinoma. Cancer 56:745–750, 1985.
309. Jewell LD, Fields AL, Murray CJW, Thomson ABR: Erosive gastroduodenitis with marked epithelial atypia after hepatic infusion chemotherapy. Am J Gastroenterol 80:421–424, 1985.
310. Jabbari M, Cherry R, Lough JO, et al: Gastric antral vascular ectasia: The watermelon stomach. Gastroenterology 87:1165–1170, 1984.

311. Lee FI, Costello F, Flanagan N, Vasudero KS: Diffuse antral vascular ectasia. Gastrointest Endosc 30:87–90, 1984.
312. Kruger R, Ryan ME, Dickson KB, Nunez JF: Diffuse vascular ectasia of the gastric antrum. Am J Gastroenterol 82:421–426, 1987.
313. Suit PF, Petras RE, Bauer TW, Petrini JL: Gastric antral vascular ectasia: A histologic and morphometric study. (Abstract) Lab Invest 56:77A, 1987.
314. Ma CK, Behrle KM, Rosenberg BF, et al: Gastric antral vascular ectasia: The watermelon stomach. Surg Pathol 1:231–239, 1988.
315. Richter RM: Massive gastric hemorrhage from submucosal arterial malformation. Am J Gastroenterol 64:324–326, 1975.
316. Sherman L, Shenoy SS, Satchidanand SK, et al: Arteriovenous malformation of the stomach. Am J Gastroenterol 72:160–164, 1979.
317. Ona FV, Ahluwalia M: Endoscopic appearance of gastric angiodysplasia in hereditary hemorrhagic telangiectasia. Am J Gastroenterol 73:148–149, 1980.
318. Gunnlaugsson O: Angiodysplasia of the stomach and duodenum. Gastrointest Endosc 31:251–254, 1985.
319. Jules GL, Labitzke HG, Lamb R, Allen R: The pathogenesis of Dieulafoy's gastric erosion. Am J Gastroenterol 79:195–200, 1984.
320. Sarles HE Jr, Schenkein JP, Hecht RM, et al: Dieulafoy's ulcer: A rare cause of massive gastric hemorrhage in an 11-year-old girl. Case report and literature review. Am J Gastroenterol 79:930–932, 1984.
321. Van Zanten SJOV, Bartelsman JFWM, Schipper ME, Tytgat GNJ: Recurrent massive haematemesis from Dieulafoy vascular malformations—a review of 101 cases. Gut 27:213–222, 1986.
322. Mikó TL, Thomazy VA: The caliber persistent artery of the stomach: A unifying approach to gastric aneurysm, Dieulafoy's lesion, and submucosal arterial malformation. Hum Pathol 19:914–921, 1988.
323. Present D, Lindner A, Janowitz H: Granulomatous disease of the gastrointestinal tract. Ann Rev Med 17:243, 1966.
324. Haggitt RC: Granulomatous diseases of the gastrointestinal tract. In Iochim HL (ed): Pathology of Granulomas. New York, Raven Press, 1983, pp 257–305.
325. Belleza NA, Lowman RM: Suture granuloma of the stomach following total colectomy. Radiology 127:84, 1978.
326. Harned RK, Anderson JC, Owen DR: Suture granuloma of the stomach following splenectomy. Am J Gastroenterol 72:302–305, 1979.
327. Morson BC, Dawson IMP: Gastrointestinal Pathology, 2nd ed. London, Blackwell Scientific, 1979, pp 113–114.
328. Rutgeerts P, Onette E, Vantrappen G, et al: Crohn's disease of the stomach and duodenum: A clinical study with emphasis on the value of endoscopy and endoscopic biopsies. Endoscopy 12:288, 1980.
329. Korelitz BI, Waye JD, Kreuning J, et al: Crohn's disease in endoscopic biopsies of the gastric antrum and duodenum. Am J Gastroenterol 76:103–109, 1981.
330. Pryse-Davies J: Gastro-duodenal Crohn's disease. J Clin Pathol 17:90, 1964.
331. Fielding JF, Toye DKM, Beton DC, et al: Crohn's disease of the stomach and duodenum. Gut 11:1001, 1970.
332. Haggitt RC, Meissner WA: Crohn's disease of the upper gastrointestinal tract. Am J Clin Pathol 59:613–622, 1973.
333. Fahimi HD, Deren JJ, Gottleib LS, et al: Isolated granulomatous gastritis. Gastroenterology 45:161, 1963.
334. Khan MH, Lam R, Tamoney HJ: Isolated granulomatous gastritis. Am J Gastroenterol 71:90, 1979.
335. Schinella RA, Ackert J: Isolated granulomatous disease of the stomach: Report of 3 cases presenting as incidental findings in gastrectomy specimens. Am J Gastroenterol 72:30–35, 1979.
336. Brown KM, Kass M, Wilson R: Isolated granulomatous gastritis. Treatment with corticosteroids. J Clin Gastroenterol 9:442–446, 1987.
337. Grimaste VV, Janowitz HD, Waye JD: Granulomatous gastritis: A case report and review of the literature. Am J Gastroenterol 84:1315–1318, 1989.
338. Littler ER, Gleibermann E: Gastritis cystica polyposa (gastric mucosal prolapse at gastroenterostomy site, with cystic and infiltrative epithelial hyperplasia). Cancer 29:205, 1972.
339. Honore LH, Lewis AS, Ohara KE: Gastritic glandularis et cystica profunda: Report of 3 cases with discussion of etiology and pathogenesis. Dig Dis Sci 24:48–52, 1979.
340. Franzen G, Novelli P: Gastritis cystica profunda. Histopathology 5:535–547, 1981.
341. Fonde EC, Rodning CB: Gastritis cystica profunda. Am J Gastroenterol 81:459–464, 1986.
342. Qizilbash AH: Gastritis cystica and carcinoma arising in old gastrojejunostomy stomach. Can Med Assoc J 112:1432–1433, 1975.
343. Bogomoletz WV, Potet F, Barge J, et al: Pathological features and mucin histochemistry of primary gastric stump carcinoma associated with gastritis cystica polyposa. A study of six cases. Am J Surg Pathol 9:401–410, 1985.
344. Brooks JJ, Enterline HT: Gastric pseudolymphoma. Its three subtypes and relation to lymphoma. Cancer 51:476–486, 1983.
345. Snover DC, Weisdorf SA, Vercolotti GM, et al: A histopathologic study of gastric and small intestinal graft-versus-host disease following allogeneic bone marrow transplantation. Hum Pathol 16:387–392, 1985.
346. Franzin G, Musola R, Mencarelli R: Morphological changes of the gastroduodenal mucosa in regular dialysis uraemic patients. Histopathology 6:429, 1982.
347. Musola R, Franzin G, Mora R, Manfrini C: Prevalence of gastroduodenal lesions in uremic patients undergoing dialysis and after renal transplantation. Gastrointest Endosc 30:343–346, 1984.
348. Yamada M, Hatakeyama S, Tsukagoshi H: Gastrointestinal amyloid deposition in AL (primary or myeloma-associated) and AA (secondary) amyloidosis: Diagnostic value of a gastric biopsy. Hum Pathol 16:1206–1211, 1985.
349. Calletti RB, Trainer TD: Collagenous gastritis. Gastroenterology 97:1552–1555, 1989.
350. Goldman H, Antonioli DA: Mucosal biopsy of the esophagus, stomach, and proximal duodenum. Hum Pathol 13:423–448, 1982.
351. Rotterdam H, Sommers SC: Biopsy Diagnosis of the Digestive Tract. New York, Raven Press, 1981, pp 45–164.
352. Whitehead R: Mucosal Biopsy of the Gastrointestinal Tract, 3rd ed. Philadelphia, WB Saunders, 1985, pp 31–64.
353. Fung WP, Papadimitriou JM, Matz LR: Endoscopic, histologic and ultrastructural correlations in chronic gastritis. Am J Gastroenterol 71:269–279, 1979.

CHAPTER 21

Stress Ulcer and Chronic Peptic Ulcer Disease

HARVEY GOLDMAN, M.D.

STRESS ULCER
Definition, Etiology, and Pathogenesis
Clinical Features
Pathology
Differential Diagnosis

CHRONIC PEPTIC ULCER DISEASE
Definition
Epidemiology
Etiology and Pathogenesis

Review of Normal Gastric Secretion
General Factors
Role of *Helicobacter Pylori*
Duodenal Ulcer
Gastric Ulcer
Clinical Features
Pathology
Location of Disease
Gross Features
Histologic Features
Examination of the Surgical Specimen
Differential Diagnosis

Complications
Medical
Surgical
Relation of Ulcer to Gastric Carcinoma
Other Ulcer Conditions
Esophagus
Gastric Heterotopia
Stomal Ulcers
Retained Antrum
Zollinger-Ellison Syndrome

MUCOSAL BIOPSY

Practically all causes of mucosal inflammation can lead to localized areas of destruction, and the sloughing of the necrotic mucosa results in the appearance of erosions or ulcers. An erosion represents a tissue deficit that is shallow and limited to the mucosa, whereas an ulcer crater extends into the submucosa or deeper parts of the gut wall. This chapter deals with the disorders of acute stress-produced ulcers and of chronic peptic ulcer disease, both of which are dominantly located in the stomach and duodenum. Details of other inflammatory conditions of these areas that can cause secondary ulcers are contained mainly in Chapters 9, 20, and 28.

STRESS ULCER

Definition, Etiology, and Pathogenesis

This condition is characterized by the appearance of acute erosions or ulcers of the stomach and duodenum in patients who are severely ill as a result of a variety of physical stresses, including trauma, burns, increased intercranial pressure, and sepsis.[1-4] The lesions in burn cases are also called Curling's ulcer,[5-7] and those associated with cranial damage are called Cushing's ulcer.[8,9] It is believed that the common pathogenetic factor is mucosal ischemia, due to overt shock or to the release and circulation of vasoconstrictive substances, and that the reduced blood flow, together with the indigenous acid in the gastric lumen, accounts for the mucosal injury.[1,10] Hyperacidity is noted only in the cases with increased intracranial pressure, whether due to trauma or to a brain tumor, and is mediated by the vagus nerves, because it can be suppressed by anticholinergic drugs. Most cases of stress ulcer have normal or reduced gastric acid, but the presence of some acid in the lumen is a prerequisite for the formation of the erosions and ulcers.[11-13] The reduced mucosal blood flow can lead to damage of the surface and foveolar mucous cells, favoring the back-diffusion of acid and the loss of cytoprotective substances such as prostaglandins, and to a delay in renewal of these cells.

There are numerous experimental models of stress

ulcers in animals induced by restraint, exertion, burns, and traumatic or hemorrhagic shock.[14-16] As in the human disease, the presence of gastric acid in the lumen is needed for the full development of the lesion, because the effect of the stress can be ameliorated or eliminated by the prior use of agents that inhibit or neutralize acid secretion. This is the basis for the prophylactic use of antacids and H_2-blockers in high-risk patients, as discussed later.

Clinical Features

The dominant clinical findings relate to the underlying traumatic and septic conditions, and patients often present with signs of shock, respiratory or renal failure, and jaundice.[2-4,17,18] With the appearance of the stress ulcers, there is the added potential for gastrointestinal hemorrhage, which may prove life-threatening in these fragile patients.[17-20] The bleeding varies in amount and typically has an abrupt onset without prior signs of gastric distress. Rarely, there is deep penetration or perforation of the ulcer, leading to peritonitis. The clinical diagnosis of the stress ulcers is readily determined by gross endoscopic examination, and the lesions are usually too superficial to be detected by ordinary radiographic studies.

Following the successful use of modern techniques to sustain patients with severe trauma and shock, an increase in the frequency of stress ulcers was observed in the surgical intensive care units, leading to significant hemorrhage in about 10% of the cases.[1,3,18] To combat this complication, the prophylactic use of antacids or other acid-neutralizing agents in high-risk patients has become standard and has resulted in a marked decline in the number of cases with prominent hemorrhage and in the overall mortality from stress ulcer.[21-23] It has been noted, however, that the sustained use of H_2-blockers such as cimetidine can promote the growth of coliform organisms and the development of pneumonia, particularly in patients receiving artificial ventilation for long periods.

The treatment of patients with established stress ulcers consists of correcting the underlying promoting condition, especially shock, and of neutralizing the acid or inhibiting the gastric secretions.[24,25] The latter also helps to deter the hemorrhage, because coagulation is optimal at a neutral pH and pepsins interfere with platelet agglutination. In cases with uncontrolled bleeding, angiographic injections of vasopressin, gel foam, or preformed clots are attempted, and a surgical resection or devascularization procedure ultimately may be required.[4,20,26,27]

Pathology

Gross Features. The primary lesions noted in stressed patients are confined to the mucosa of the stomach and proximal duodenum (Figure 21-1) and consist of a spectrum of alterations, ranging from patchy hemorrhages to discrete erosions and ulcers.[28] They may be single or multiple and most often are concentrated in the corpus and fundus of the stomach (Figure 21-2), in contrast to the antral localization of chronic peptic ulcers and of the erosive cases of acute or chronic gastritis due to ethanol and drugs. The lesions are typically small, most less than 1 cm in diameter; are elliptical or circular in shape; and have sharply defined margins. Interestingly, the early lesions noted in the experimental models in animals, such as those due to restraint or exertion, often have a linear configuration, but this is not characteristic of the human cases. The ulcers are typically shallow and have a red base; rarely, there may be a deeper penetration into the wall or a perforation with exudate on the peritoneal surface.

Histologic Features. The stress-induced erosions and ulcers are of an acute nature.[14,28] The earliest lesion, which is best visualized in experimental animals,

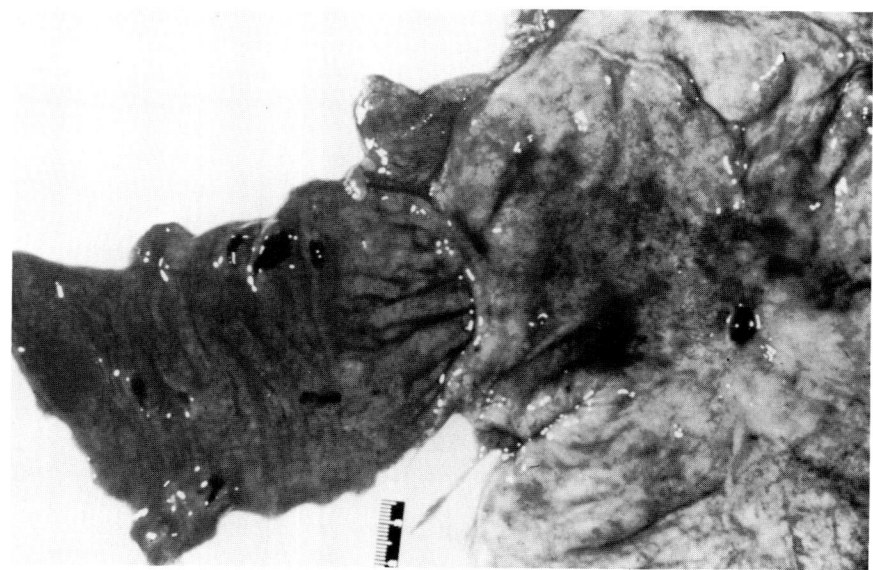

FIGURE 21-1. Acute stress ulcers. Multiple, small hemorrhagic ulcers are noted in the duodenum (left) and a single ulcer, together with diffuse mucosal congestion and hemorrhage in the gastric antral mucosa (right).

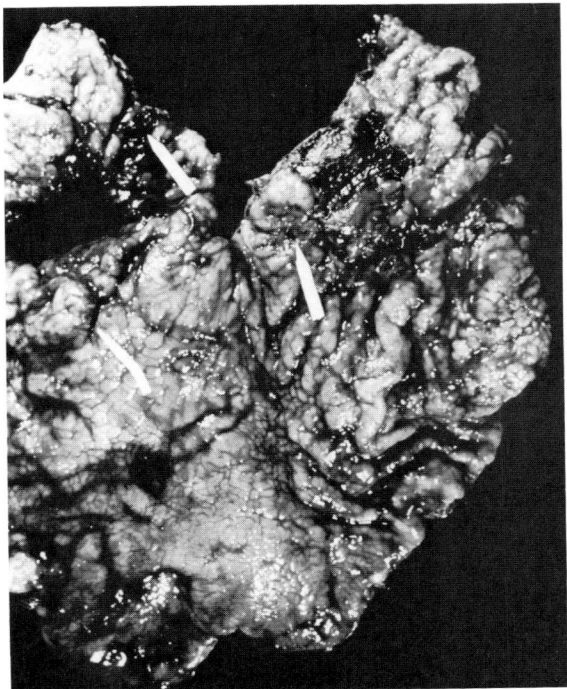

FIGURE 21-2. Gastrectomy specimen, with the duodenal portion at bottom. Multiple ulcers (arrows) are seen in the gastric corpus and a larger one in the upper right portion.

consists of a localized area of hemorrhage and necrosis without inflammation that is limited to the mucosa and has the appearance of an acute ischemic infarction (Figure 21-3).[16] This is followed by sloughing of the necrotic tissue, resulting in the ulcer crater, and a marked acute inflammatory reaction, consisting of congested vessels and many neutrophils, in the adjacent intact mucosa and in the underlying submucosa (Figure 21-4). The deeper parts of the wall are unaffected unless there is a perforation. With healing, the eroded area is replaced by regenerating glands, and this can result in the transient presence of a slight depression of the mucosal surface (Figure 21-5).[17] Because the ulcer is superficial, there is usually no significant granulation tissue or fibrosis, and the stress lesions typically heal without any sequelae and do not recur in the absence of the underlying stress condition. There are ordinarily no signs of chronic inflammation in the ulcer or the surrounding mucosa.

Differential Diagnosis

The diagnosis of stress ulcer is promptly suggested by the appearance of upper gastrointestinal hemorrhage in a severely ill patient. Endoscopy is often performed for confirmation and to exclude other causes of bleeding, and biopsy is not needed if the typical lesions are observed. Acute erosions and ulcers can be seen in the more severe cases of acute gastritis and of chronic gastritis due to toxic agents such as ethanol, drugs, and bile reflux; but these lesions are typically confined to the antral region and are usually associated with more widespread inflammation. Although some studies have included these examples of toxic or chemical gastritis in a broad list of stress conditions that can cause acute ulceration of the stomach and duodenum, this lumping should be avoided because the lesions seen in association with severe bodily injury have a different pathogenesis and generally more aggressive behavior.

Chronic peptic ulcers are readily distinguished from acute stress ulcer by their limited localization to the antrum or the first part of the duodenum. They are usually single and reveal evidence of chronic inflammation and scarring in the ulcer and in the adjacent mucosa.

CHRONIC PEPTIC ULCER DISEASE

The following general sections deal with the features of peptic ulcer disease in the common sites of the antrum and duodenum, and the characteristics of the dis-

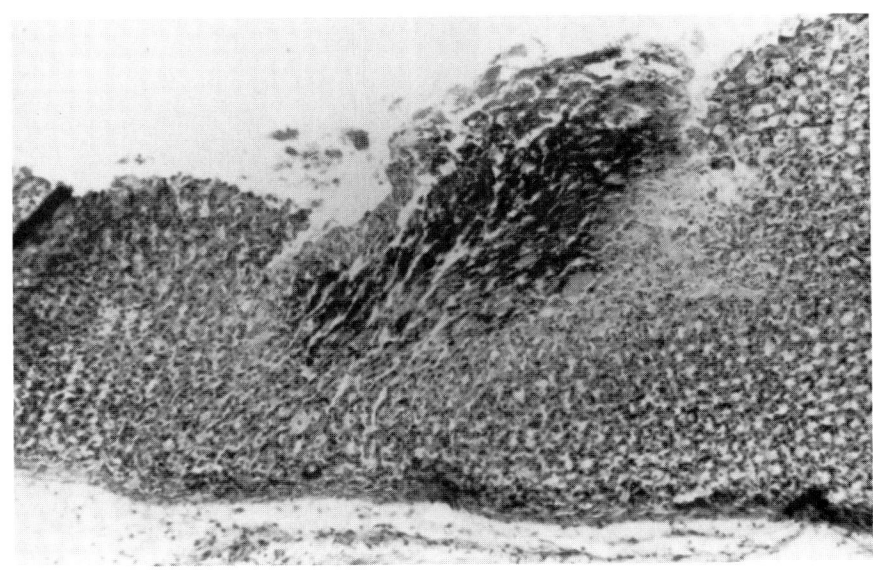

FIGURE 21-3. Gastric corpus mucosa from a rodent following restraint-induced stress. The submucosa is at the bottom. There is a sharply localized area of hemorrhage and necrosis involving the superficial half of the mucosa. (H&E, × 80)

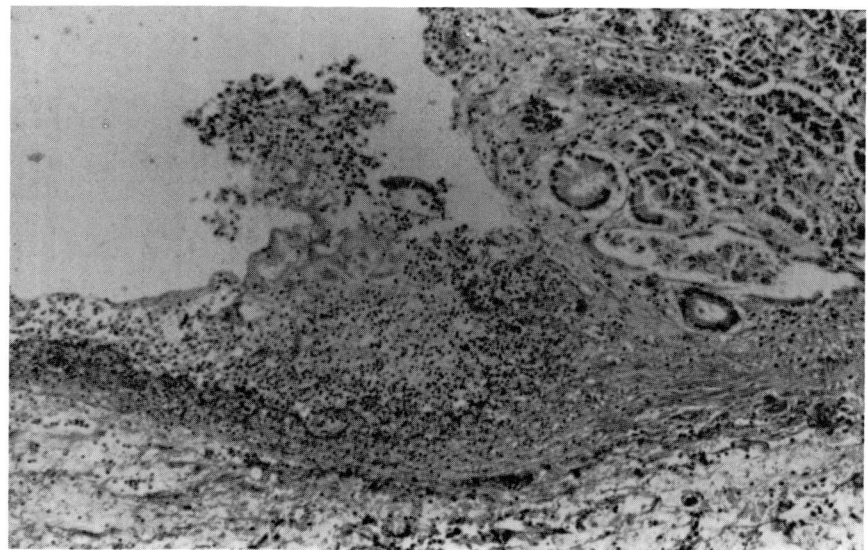

FIGURE 21–4. Acute stress ulcer of the stomach, with a portion of intact mucosa at top right. There is mucosal destruction, with marked neutrophilic reaction. The underlying submucosa (at bottom) shows congestion and slight inflammatory infiltrate but no fibrosis. Contrast with Figures 21–10 and 21–11, examples of chronic peptic ulcers. (H&E, × 100)

ease in the other locations of the gut are presented at the end.

Definition

A peptic ulcer is a localized ulcerating lesion of the gut, usually present in the stomach or the duodenum, that is due in part to the action of gastric acid and pepsin. In most conditions, however, the gastric secretions are not the primary cause of the injury, but rather are a necessary factor in its development. The term *acute peptic ulcer* is rarely used in an unqualified fashion because it embraces a variety of disorders of different causes, including acute stress lesions and ulcers due to toxic chemicals and drugs.[29] Stress ulcers are discussed in the section above, and the chemical and drug lesions are discussed in Chapter 9.

Chronic peptic ulcer disease is a common disorder of unknown primary cause that is characterized by the recurrent appearance of ulcers that are usually solitary and most often in the antrum and in the first part of the duodenum.[30–33] Because the same etiologic factors are involved in the genesis of inflammatory lesions in these areas, the patients may encounter a spectrum of pathologic effects, ranging from gastritis or duodenitis to overt ulceration.[34]

Epidemiology

Chronic peptic ulcer disease is more common in whites[35] and in persons living in highly industrialized nations,[36] and it has been established that over 10 million people are affected in the United States. Duodenal ulcer disease is about three times more common than

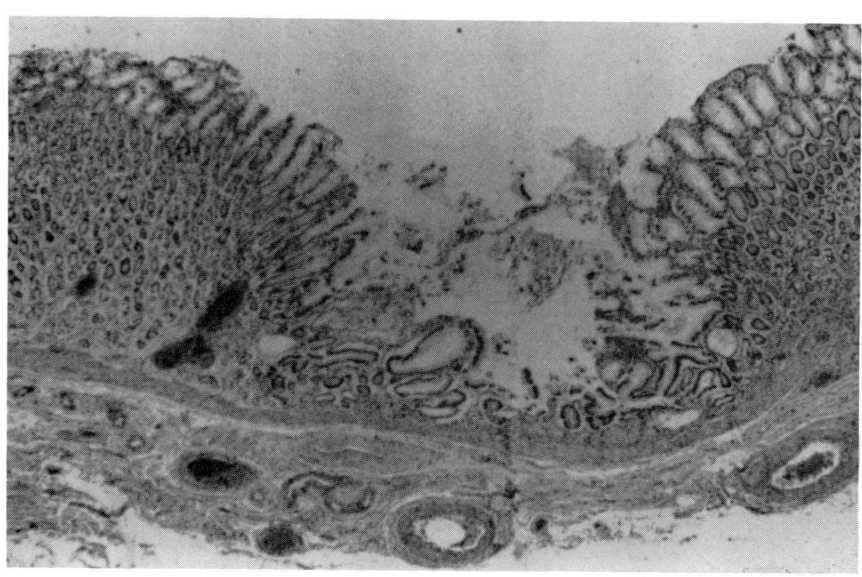

FIGURE 21–5. Healing stress ulcer of the stomach, showing mucosal loss and regenerative glands at base of mucosa. The underlying muscularis mucosae and submucosa (at bottom) are intact, without evidence of chronic features such as fibrosis. (H&E, × 80)

gastric ulcers but has shown a decline over the past two decades.[37] Males are more often affected than females, with ratios of 4:1 or higher in duodenal ulcer and 1.5 to 2:1 in gastric cases. Duodenal ulcers affect persons of all ages, including children and young adults; whereas gastric ulcers are more frequently noted in patients over age 40. The disease is more common in persons who smoke cigarettes,[38] but it is difficult to sort out this component from the general lifestyle of the patients.[39,40] There does not appear to be any constant relationship to dietary factors.

Etiology and Pathogenesis

Review of Normal Gastric Secretion

Hydrochloric acid is produced in the parietal (or oxyntic) cells and the class of pepsinogens in the chief cells that are located in the specialized glands of the fundic and corpus mucosa. The major physiologic stimuli for gastric secretion are the vagus nerves and the gastrin-producing endocrine cells (G cells) that are concentrated amidst the pyloric glands in the antral mucosa. The parietal cells also respond to other agents such as histamine, and their function is dependent on an adequate mucosal blood supply. In the first or cerebral phase of gastric secretion, the vagi act both directly on the parietal cells and indirectly by stimulation of the G cells. This is followed by the second or gastric phase, characterized by antral distention and greater stimulation of the gastrin cells. The final or intestinal phase depends on the release of other hormones, such as enterogastrone and somatostatin, that inhibit and curtail the gastric secretions. The pepsinogens are converted to the active pepsins, which are proteolytic enzymes by their low pH. After the ingestion of a solid meal, the pyloric sphincter remains closed, and the major function of the stomach is the churning and physical disruption of the nutrients as well as the secretion of the gastric fluid; the pylorus opens in response to sensors in its mucosa when the solution becomes isotonic. The gastric acid is partially diluted by the alkaline secretions from the antral pyloric and duodenal Brunner's glands and ultimately is neutralized by the biliary and pancreatic secretions in the small intestine. Chapter 2 provides further details.

General Factors

There have been extensive investigations of the factors involved in the etiology of chronic peptic ulcer disease, and the reader is referred to the reviews on this subject for more details.[30–33,41–43] The two most important factors are the amount of gastric acid[43] and the mucosal resistance.[44,45] In order for a peptic ulcer to develop, some gastric acid must be present, but an increase in gastric secretions is only regularly seen in some cases of duodenal ulcers and in conditions with hypergastrinemia, such as the Zollinger-Ellison syndrome. Mucosal resistance is dependent on numerous components,[44,45] including adequate blood supply, normal renewal and differentiation of the surface epithelial cells, and the production of the mucous coat that covers the surface[46] and possibly of other protective agents such as prostaglandins.[13] A higher rate of peptic ulcers, especially of the duodenum, has been noted in persons with blood group type O and in those who do not secrete the blood group substances into the gastrointestinal tract.[47,48]

An increase in duodenal ulcer incidence is also seen in first-degree relatives of patients, and a genetic basis is suggested by the finding of a higher frequency of concordance of ulcer disease in monozygotic than that in dizygotic twins.[49] Further support for a genetic predisposition comes from the observations of more ulcers in persons with an elevated level of serum pepsinogen type I[50] and possibly in those with the HLA-B5 and HLA-B12 phenotypes.[32,51] Additional information on the role of genetic factors in the development of peptic ulcer disease is provided in Chapter 6.

Psychologic factors have also been incriminated, because emotional stress can lead to vagal stimulation and an increase in the gastric secretion of acid and pepsin.[39,40,52,53] One has the image of the harassed executive popping pills to abort the ulcer symptoms. It appears that such stresses are not the primary cause of peptic ulcer disease, but that they can serve as promoting or precipitating factors. Other conditions that can facilitate the development of peptic ulcers are listed in Table 21–1 and include chronic pulmonary and renal diseases, hyperparathyroidism, hepatic cirrhosis, and systemic mastocytosis.[54–58] Most of these disorders act by enhancing gastric acid secretion and are further discussed in Chapter 16. There are a large variety of noxious chemicals and drugs such as ethanol, salicylates, corticosteroids, indomethacin, and other nonsteroidal agents that can cause an acute gastritis or an ulcer but also can activate a chronic peptic ulcer.[59–66] It is probable that these agents operate by further damaging the mucosa and reducing its resistance; they are detailed in Chapter 9.

Role of *Helicobacter pylori*

These bacteria (formerly called *Campylobacter pylori*) are observed in the gastric antral mucosa in three quarters or more of cases of chronic peptic ulcer affecting either the stomach or the duodenum.[67–70] They are

Table 21–1. CONDITIONS ASSOCIATED WITH CHRONIC PEPTIC ULCERS

Promoting conditions
    Chronic pulmonary disease
    Chronic renal failure
    Hepatic cirrhosis
    Hyperparathyroidism
    Multiple endocrine neoplasia, type I
    Systemic mastocytosis
Precipitating factors
    Analgesics
    Anti-inflammatory drugs
    Ethanol and smoking
    Psychologic stress

only found in the duodenum in areas of gastric mucous cell metaplasia. The organisms are also regularly seen in patients with chronic active gastritis involving the antrum who do not have ulcers (see Chapter 20, Figures 20–10 and 20–11). It has been proposed that the bacteria may be the cause of both the gastritis and the reduced mucosal resistance that leads to ulcer formation in the stomach.[71,72] The relationship to duodenal ulcer is less clear, when one considers that there are fewer bacteria and less inflammation in this area and that hyperacidity is often present in these cases. It remains possible that the colonization is a secondary event or that the organisms can add to the mucosal injury to promote the ulcer formation. It is noteworthy that healing of peptic ulcers of either the stomach or the duodenum is often facilitated by specific antimicrobial treatment and elimination of the bacteria.[73] See Chronic Antral Gastritis in Chapter 20 for further details about these bacteria and their possible relationship to gastric diseases.

Duodenal Ulcer

Many patients with duodenal peptic ulcer have demonstrable hyperacidity, either when fasting or after stimulation with a test meal, and it is thought that this is the dominant factor in the development of ulcer disease in this area.[41,43] It is probable that the small-intestinal epithelium is innately less resistant than the gastric mucosa to the effects of the acid and pepsin, and this would explain the preferential localization of the ulcer in the mucosa that is just distal to the pylorus in the first part of the duodenum. This area would be the first to be exposed to the acid-pepsin load, whereas beyond this region there would be neutralization by the biliary and pancreatic secretions. It has also been suggested that patients with duodenal ulcers have more rapid gastric emptying, which would promote the delivery of high acid concentrations into the duodenum.[74] It is noteworthy that the site of peptic ulcers is similar in other situations; the recurrent stomal ulcer is typically in the jejunum just beyond the anastomosis, and ulcers that develop in association with gastric heterotopia (such as in a Meckel's diverticulum) are also in the immediately adjacent small-intestinal mucosa. In contrast, in cases of Zollinger-Ellison syndrome, there is so much acid secretion that ulcers may be observed throughout the duodenum and even in the jejunum.

Some patients with duodenal ulcer disease have an associated peptic duodenitis, and the same etiologic factors may be involved in the initiation and precipitation of the two disorders. The amount of inflammation is usually less than that seen in cases of gastric ulcer, however; and there is no strong evidence to indicate that factors other than acid and pepsin are commonly operative in reducing the resistance of the duodenal mucosa in the usual case of duodenal ulcer.

Gastric Ulcer

In cases of gastric peptic ulcer, in contrast to duodenal disease, the relative importance of the two major factors of acid amount and mucosal resistance is reversed. There is typically a normal or reduced concentration of gastric acid, and prior mucosal injury from other causes appears to be a prerequisite for the development of the gastric ulcer.[75] Practically all patients have evidence of diffuse inflammation of the surrounding mucosa[76–78] indicative of a chronic antral gastritis that can be caused by *H. pylori* or by a variety of toxic substances, such as ethanol, drugs, and bile reflux.[63,79–83] These chemical agents act by damaging the membranes of the surface epithelial cells in the antrum, rendering them more permeable to back-diffusion of acid;[75,84,85] this would explain why some patients have a reduced acid concentration in the gastric lumen. There is also no increase in the gastric secretions of acid and pepsin in most cases. About 10% of the patients have ulcers in both the antrum and duodenum, and these cases more often reveal hyperacidity; in some there is initially a duodenal ulcer with pyloric obstruction that leads to gastric antral distention, stimulation of the gastrin-producing cells, and increased acid production.[86]

As noted above, *H. pylori* organisms are also commonly present in the antral mucosa, and the question of whether these bacteria cause or contribute to the gastritis and ulcer formation is as yet not settled. Also unresolved are why only a small fraction of cases of chronic antral gastritis proceed to formation of ulcers and why the ulcers are typically solitary and recur in the same location. Many of the antral ulcers are located at the junction with the corpus mucosa, suggesting that this area may be exposed to a higher concentration of gastric secretions. Because patients with gastric ulcers are often older, it has been suggested that degenerative vascular disease of the local arteries may be an added factor in determining the occurrence and site of the lesion.

Clinical Features

Patients with peptic ulcers typically present with episodes of epigastric burning pain that are related to times of acid secretion and to the absence of food in the stomach.[87–89] Thus the pain usually occurs 1 to 2 hours after a meal or at night, when the stomach has acid but is relatively empty of solid contents. Although the interval between eating and the appearance of pain may be shorter in cases of gastric ulcer, compared with duodenal lesions, there is considerable overlap. Some of the episodes are precipitated by the ingestion of a drug or an emotional crisis, but more often there is no special antecedent history. Other symptoms include occasional nausea, vomiting, and bleeding; these are generally present in more severe cases and are discussed in the section on complications. The disease is characterized by periods of resolution or remission and repeated recurrences or relapses, and the patient is never completely cured. The patient may also experience milder attacks without overt ulceration that are thought to be due to the underlying or associated mucosal inflammation, referred to as antral gastritis and peptic duodenitis.

The presence and particular location of the peptic ulcer are ordinarily determined by radiographic study. Endoscopic examination with biopsy and cytology are often added in the evaluation of gastric ulcers, particularly in older patients and in cases that do not heal promptly, to distinguish the ulcer from a malignant tumor. Acid secretory studies, both basal and stimulated by histamine or pentagastrin, and serum gastrin levels are also obtained in uncertain or unusual cases.[43,90,91] The standard medical treatment of peptic ulcer disease involves the use of a large variety of antacid compounds, H_2-blocking agents, and other protective drugs, and the resolution of the ulcer is monitored by radiographic and/or endoscopic procedures.[32,33,92,93] In addition, the value of antibiotics and bismuth compounds in eradicating *H. pylori* is being extensively tested. The use of a bland diet may help to alleviate the symptoms but does not by itself promote healing of the ulcer, and there is no evidence to support the use of the medications in the prevention of recurrences. Surgery is reserved for intractable disease and other complications and for cases of persistent gastric ulcer that cannot be distinguished from malignancy; the various procedures are presented later in the section on complications.

Pathology

Despite differences in the etiology and pathogenesis of peptic ulcers involving the stomach, duodenum, and other locations, the morphologic features are the same.[94-96]

Location of Disease

About 75% of cases of chronic peptic ulcer occur in the pyloric region and the first portion of the duodenum, and 20% occur in the gastric antrum (Table 21-2). The antral cases are more often noted in the junctional area next to the corpus mucosa and along the lesser curvature but can involve any part.[97-99] The corpus-fundic region of the stomach is typically spared, in contrast to tumors that can occur in this area. Other sites are the lower esophagus in cases of reflux esophagitis, recurrent stomal ulcers following gastric resection, ulcers that can occur in association with foci of gastric heterotopia, and more widespread lesions of the duodenum and jejunum in the Zollinger-Ellison syndrome; these are discussed later in the section on other conditions.

Table 21-2. LOCATION OF CHRONIC PEPTIC ULCERS

Common disease	
First part of duodenum	(70%-75%)
Gastric antrum	(20%-25%)
Other conditions	
Distal esophagus in reflux esophagitis	
Jejunum in recurrent stomal ulcer following antral resection	
Distal duodenum and jejunum in Zollinger-Ellison syndrome	
Meckel's diverticulum, ileum, and rectum in cases of gastric heterotopia	

Gross Features

Ulcers of either the duodenum (Figure 21-6) or the stomach (Figures 21-7 and 21-8) are commonly single and vary markedly in size from one to several centimeters in diameter. Rarely, the gastric lesions can be 10 cm in diameter or larger and are referred to as giant ulcers.[100,101] Multiple ulcers, usually only two in number, are seen in about 10% of cases. These are usually present in the stomach, or there is one in the stomach and one in the duodenum.[102,103] The lesions are sharply demarcated, and the mucosal edges have a regular contour. Although the margins appear flat on gross examination of specimens, a uniform elevation due to edema is commonly appreciated by radiography and endoscopy. The surrounding mucosa, particularly in

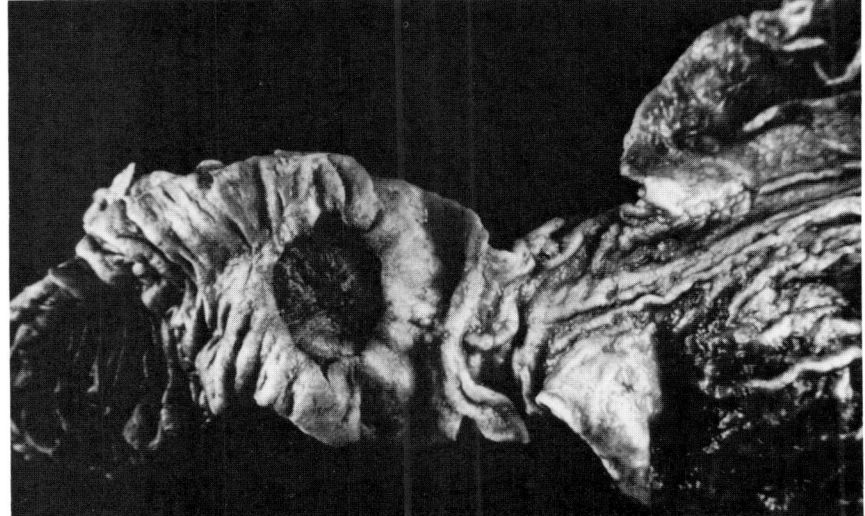

FIGURE 21-6. Segment of the stomach (right) and duodenum, revealing a large chronic peptic ulcer in the first portion of the duodenum. Note sharp demarcation of ulcer edges.

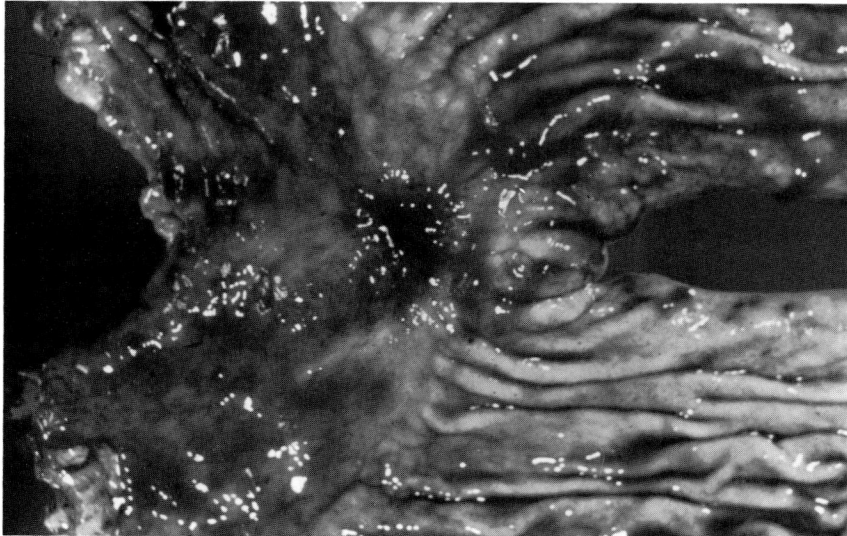

FIGURE 21-7. Segment of the stomach with the corpus at right. There is a small chronic peptic ulcer of the gastric antrum at the junction with the corpus.

cases of gastric ulcer, often has a granular appearance that is due to the presence of the associated diffuse mucosal inflammation. The serosal surface is either normal or shows adhesions or puckering in cases of deep ulcers. When the ulcers extend through the wall, they can penetrate a variety of neighboring structures, such as the pancreas, spleen, biliary tract, liver, and colon.[104-108] The features of the other complications, including hemorrhage, perforation, and obstruction, are presented in a later section. With healing there can be a prominence of the mucosal folds that radiate from the lesion (Figure 21-9),[109] and the deeper ulcers that extend into the muscularis propria may cause a weakening of the wall leading to the formation of a localized diverticulum.

Histologic Features

The features of chronic peptic ulcers are entirely nonspecific and consist of those of the active disease, the reparative process, and scarring from previous episodes. The ulcers extend at least into the submucosa and often into the muscularis propria (Figure 21-10). In the active lesions there are zones of necrosis, neutrophilic reaction, granulation tissue, and fibrosis that extend from the mucosal surface into the wall (Figures 21-11 and 21-12). The surrounding intact mucosa of the gastric ulcers is always inflamed and reveals acute and chronic inflammatory cells and variable amounts of intestinal metaplasia.[76-78,110] There are also numerous small bacteria, representing *H. pylori*, on the surface and in the lumina of the superficial gastric pits in most gastric cases (see Figures 20-10 and 20-11 in Chapter 20).[67,68,111] The gastric epithelium in the surface and foveolar region shows the effects of degeneration and regeneration (Figure 21-13), and it is important that this change not be confused with dysplasia; the distinction may be particularly difficult in the small and often distorted mucosal biopsy samples. The epithelial cell nuclei are enlarged and have a central nucleolus, but they are typically regular in size and shape and lack hyperchromatism.

The appearance of the mucosa around a duodenal ulcer is more variable. There is usually less inflammation; and *H. pylori* is rarely observed, and only in areas of gastric mucous-cell metaplasia.[70] There is less concern about the regenerative epithelium in the duodenum because carcinoma does not ordinarily occur in this area, and mucosal biopsies are not routinely obtained. Other bacteria are frequently noted in the necrotic area of large ulcers of both the stomach and the duodenum, but they are thought to represent saprophytes that do not affect the lesion. Candida organisms are also occasionally seen (see Figure 20-23 in Chapter 20), and it has been suggested that they contribute to

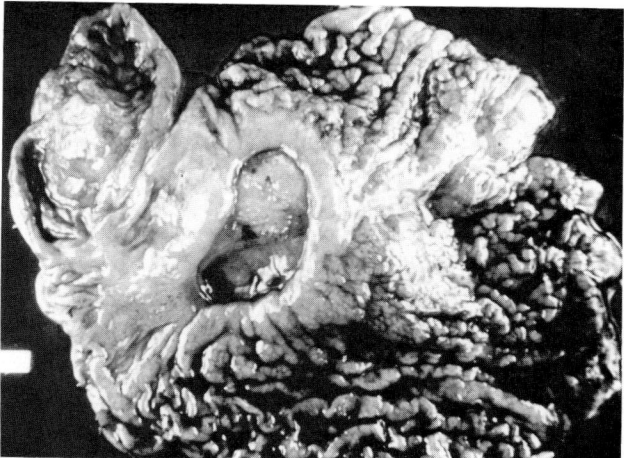

FIGURE 21-8. Segment of the stomach with the contiguous duodenum (upper left), showing a large chronic peptic ulcer of the antrum. The rugae near the ulcer are irregular, but the ulcer edges appear uniform and sharply demarcated. The tissue at the ulcer base represents granulation tissue.

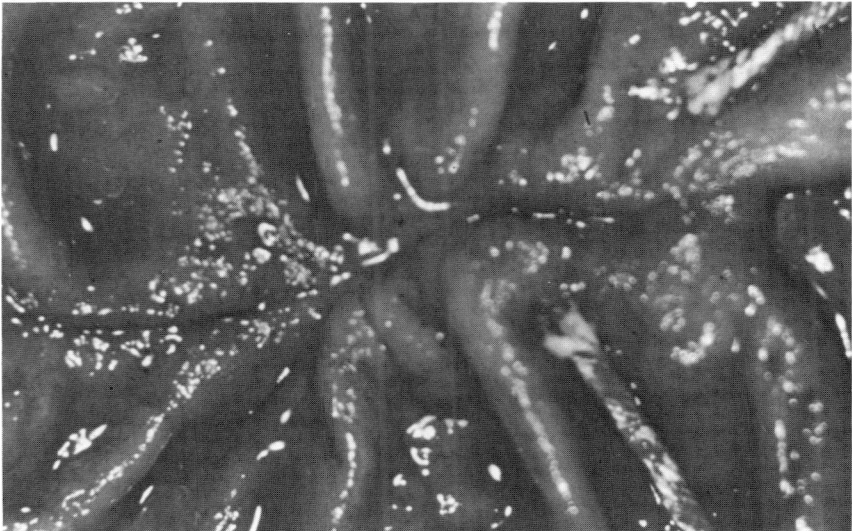

FIGURE 21-9. Healed chronic peptic ulcer of the stomach, revealing irregular and enlarged rugae that appear to radiate from the lesion.

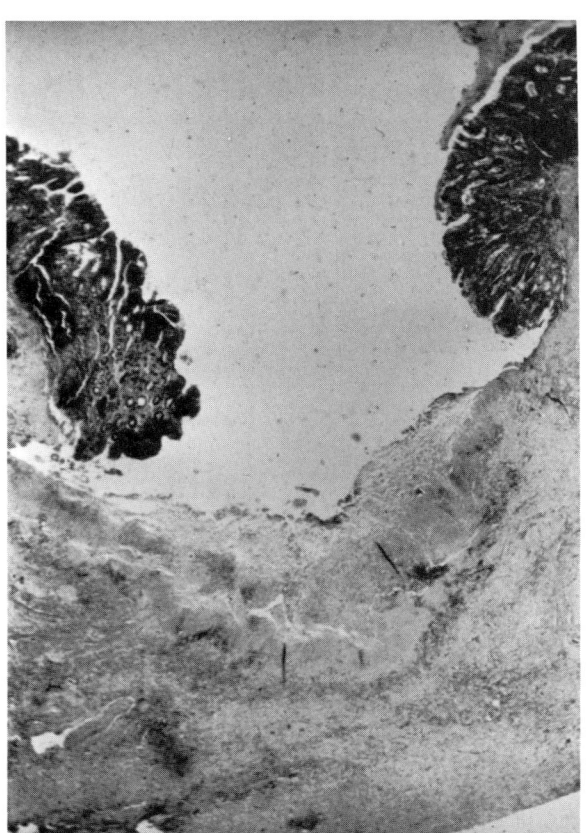

FIGURE 21-10. Chronic active peptic ulcer of the stomach, showing an ulcer crater extending into the submucosa and intact, inflamed mucosa at the edges. The ulcer base is composed of necrotic tissue and fibrosis, the latter serving as evidence of chronic disease. Contrast with Figure 21-4, an example of an acute stress ulcer. (H&E, × 13)

the necrosis, resulting in a greater chance of perforation and an overall worse prognosis.[112,113] Other studies have failed to confirm these results, however, and the issue is not completely resolved.[114,115] Additional variable features include the presence of eroded vessels, giant cells, or poorly formed granulomas that probably represent a reaction to entrapped foreign material, and rarely abundant eosinophils without an apparent cause (see Chapter 10, Figure 10-2). Furthermore, an increase in the number of the antral G cells is noted in some of the cases of duodenal ulcer[116,117] (see Chapter 13).

With healing of the lesion, there is less necrosis, more abundant granulation tissue and fibrosis, and a transient hyperplasia of the surface-foveolar mucous cells. The fibrosis replaces the normal structures of the submucosa and muscularis propria (see Figure 21-11), and its amount relates to the overall size and depth of the lesion. The blood vessels at the bottom of the lesion often show a patchy inflammation and a fibrous thickening of the intima that is especially pronounced in the fibrotic areas, and it is thought that these changes are of a secondary nature.

Examination of the Surgical Specimen

Gastric antral resection is commonly performed in cases of chronic peptic ulcers of both the stomach and the duodenum, either for removal of a gastric lesion or for excision of the area containing the gastrin-producing endocrine cells. It is generally recommended that the specimen be opened along the greater curvature, unless there is a lesion in this area, and that measurements be routinely obtained of the circumferences of the proximal and distal margins and of the length of the stomach along the lesser and greater curvatures. The distal end should be inspected for identification of the pyloric sphincter; when normal, this appears as a thickened area of musculature with a slight elevation

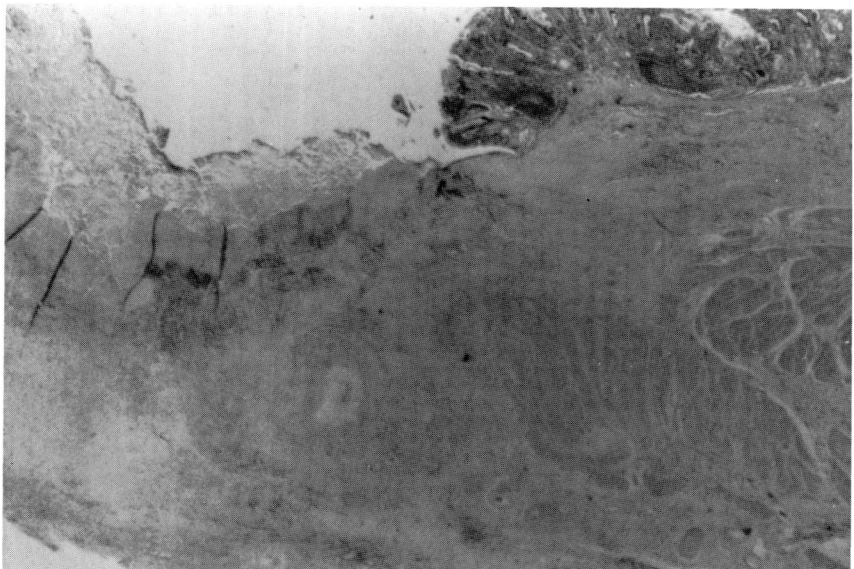

FIGURE 21-11. Chronic active ulcer of the stomach, showing ulceration and necrosis extending into the submucosa and extensive fibrosis of the underlying muscularis (lower left). A vessel is noted in the center, and intact mucosa and muscularis propria can be seen at the right. (H&E, × 16)

of the mucosal surface that then slopes sharply into the duodenum. Sections should be taken from any lesions that are observed, from random areas of the antrum for determination of the presence and extent of any gastritis, and from the resection margins for confirmation that the antrum has been completely excised. In particular, sections should be obtained for identification of duodenal mucosa at the distal end and the gastric corpus type of mucosa at the proximal end; these findings should be included in the pathology report.

Differential Diagnosis

General Aspects. The diagnosis of a chronic peptic ulcer is determined in most cases by the typical location of the lesion, together with the characteristic clinical and radiographic features. The differential diagnosis includes a variety of inflammatory lesions that can develop ulcers in the stomach and duodenum. In most infections the ulcers are multiple and relatively shallow, and the diagnosis is supplied by the characteristic histology or culture. Ulcers can be caused directly by chemicals and drugs; aside from the history, there is often a paucity of inflammation in the adjacent mucosa, which helps to identify these as acute lesions.[118,119] Crohn's disease can, exceptionally, present with a large ulcer of the stomach or duodenum; and the distinction is dependent on the finding of other characteristic features such as fissures and granulomas or disease in other parts of the intestine.

Duodenal Ulcer. Carcinoma is rare in the duodenum and is usually located beyond the first portion, particularly in the region of the papilla of Vater. Stress

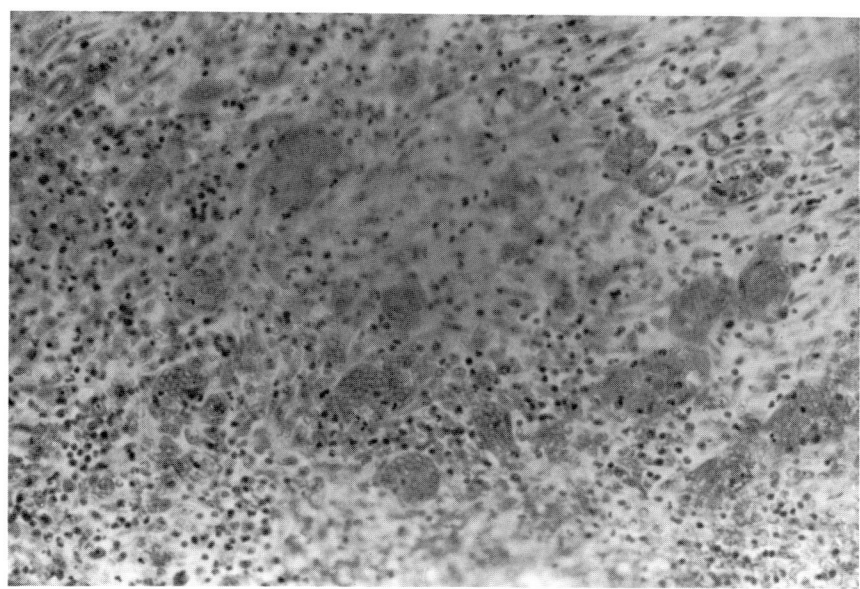

FIGURE 21-12. Base of chronic active peptic ulcer, revealing prominent granulation tissue. (H&E, × 200)

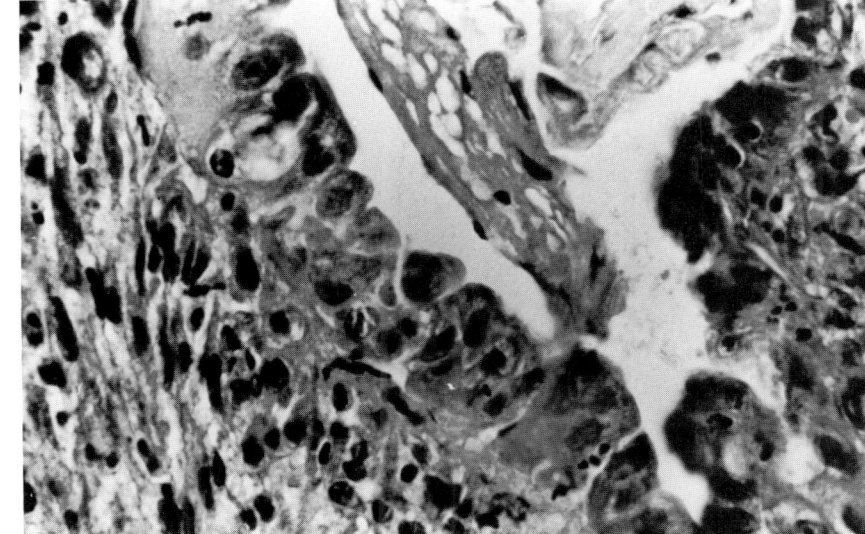

FIGURE 21–13. Edge of chronic active peptic ulcer of the stomach. There are signs of marked degeneration and regeneration of the surface and foveolar (pit) epithelia. Although enlarged, the epithelial nuclei tend to be regular in size and shape, and the cells have abundant cytoplasm. Contrast with the example of dysplastic epithelium seen in Figure 20–21 in Chapter 20. (H&E, × 500) (From Goldman H, Antonioli DA: Mucosal biopsy of the esophagus, stomach, and proximal duodenum. Hum Pathol 13:423, 1982.)

ulcers are acute lesions that tend to be multiple and shallow, and they present in patients with severe bodily trauma or shock. Peptic ulcer and peptic duodenitis share the same cause and clinical features, and the distinction is based simply on whether an ulcer can be grossly identified. As noted above, these two conditions are parts of a spectrum of peptic disease of the duodenum and probably differ only in severity; see the section on duodenitis in Chapter 28 for further details.

Gastric Ulcer. The principal distinction to be made in a case of a gastric ulcer is between a benign peptic lesion and a malignant tumor,[120–125] usually an adenocarcinoma but also a malignant lymphoma. Carcinomas can occur in any part of the stomach, whereas peptic ulcers are limited to the antral region. Although carcinomas are less often at the lesser curvature, where most peptic ulcers occur, there is considerable overlap; investigation of any persistent ulcer of the stomach is required. Size alone is not a helpful criterion because peptic ulcers can be very large,[100,101] whereas early gastric carcinoma can be small and totally mimic a benign ulcer in appearance.[125–127] When estimates are made on the basis of gross radiographic or endoscopic examination regarding whether an ulcerated lesion is benign or malignant, there is an erroneous impression in over a quarter of the cases (Figure 21–14). Accordingly, histologic study is mandatory; and it has been observed that the taking of at least four biopsy samples, including one from the center of the lesion, together with brush cytology should make the distinction in practically all cases.[128–132] There is a greater problem in the detection of malignant lymphoma and its distinction from marked inflammation (or pseudolymphoma) and from carcinoma, and a resection is often needed to re-

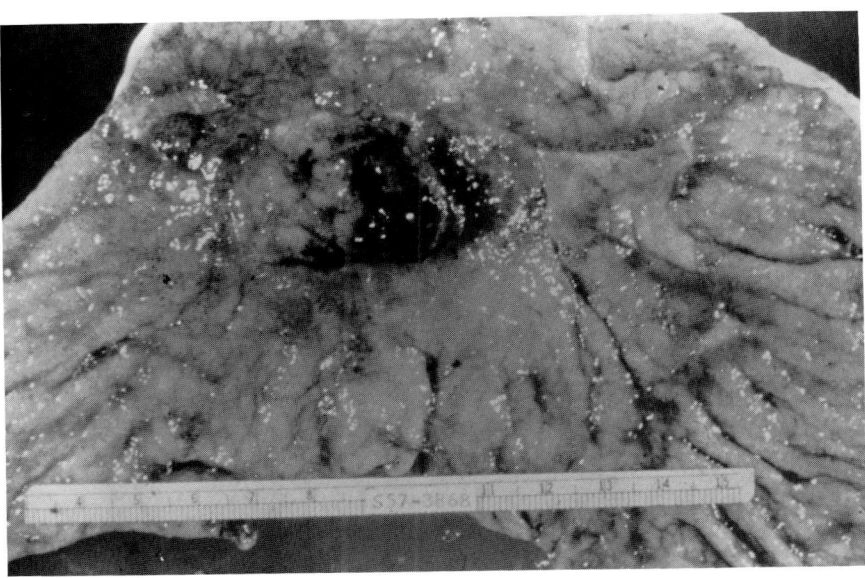

FIGURE 21–14. Segment of the stomach, revealing a large ulcer in the antrum that proved to be a carcinoma. Compare with Figures 21–7 and 21–8.

solve the issue. Chapter 14, on lymphoma, and Chapter 25, on gastric adenocarcinoma, provide further details.

Erosions of the gastric antral mucosa can occur in cases of acute toxic gastritis and of chronic antral gastritis and are readily distinguished by their multiple and shallow nature. Stress ulcers that are associated with severe bodily trauma or shock are often multiple and typically in the fundic-corpus region.

Complications

Medical

Major complications that are directly related to the peptic ulcer disease are commonly seen and include hemorrhage, penetration into contiguous tissues, perforation, and obstruction[133] (Table 21-3). Although most patients experience some slight bleeding, a massive hemorrhage requiring several units of replacement blood is observed at some time in the course of about 10% of the cases (Figure 21-15). This is typically associated with a deep ulcer and erosion of one or more large vessels.[134,135] When a relatively small ulcer is noted together with a single, large bleeding artery, the possibility of a vascular malformation such as Dieulafoy's lesion of the stomach should be considered; this is more common in young adults and is usually located in the proximal stomach.[136,137]

A free perforation into the peritoneal cavity is seen in about 5% to 10% of hospitalized patients and results from the extension of an ulcer through the anterior wall of the stomach or duodenum (Figure 21-16).[138,139] It is associated with the presence of a purulent exudate on the serosal surface (Figure 21-17), and patients typically present with signs of an acute abdomen and require immediate surgery to avoid fatality. When an ulcer extends through the posterior wall, there is commonly a penetration into the pancreas[104,140] and, less often, into other neighboring organs such as the spleen (Figure 21-18), biliary tract, liver, and colon.[105-108] Such lesions are noted in about 15% of gastric ulcers and 25% of duodenal lesions, leading to greater pain and signs of an acute pancreatitis or a fistula. Gastric outlet obstruction can result from either edema or fibrosis around an ulcer in the pyloric channel or duodenum (Figure 21-19), and permanent effects are observed in about 5% of cases.[141,142]

Surgical

Surgery is required for the treatment of patients with chronic peptic ulcer who have intractable disease that has not responded to medical therapy; for any of the complications of uncontrolled hemorrhage, perforation, penetration, or fibrotic obstruction; and for lesions that cannot be adequately distinguished from malignancy.[133,143,144] The three main types of operations are a

Table 21-3. COMPLICATIONS OF CHRONIC PEPTIC ULCER DISEASE

Medical
    Intractable disease
    Hemorrhage
    Perforation
    Penetration of adjacent organs
    Obstruction

Surgical
    Recurrent stomal ulcer
    Retained antrum
    Postgastrectomy gastritis
    Dumping syndrome
    Afferent loop syndrome

Gastric adenocarcinoma
    Antrum related to associated chronic antral gastritis
    Proximal stomach (stump) following antral resection

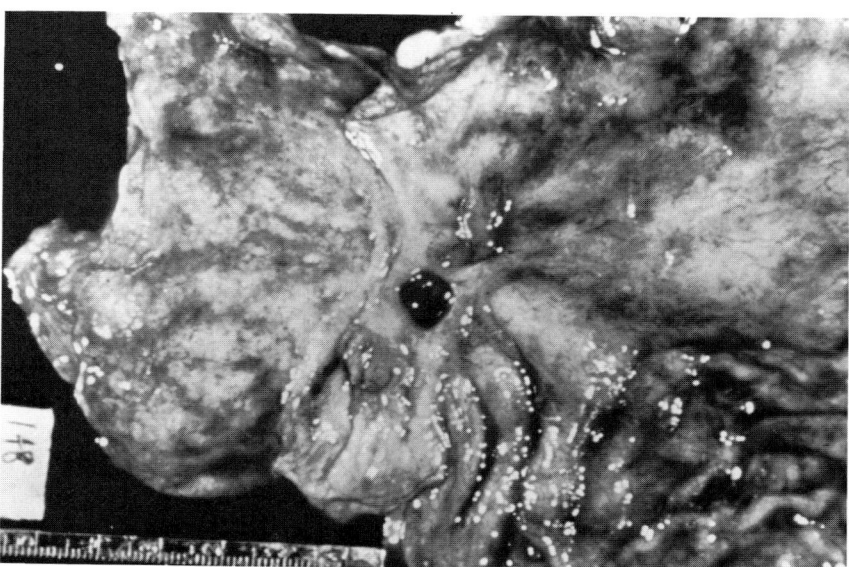

FIGURE 21-15. Segment of the stomach with the contiguous duodenum at the left. There is a discrete chronic peptic ulcer of the lower antrum that is hemorrhagic. Despite the relatively small size of the ulcer, there was massive hemorrhage requiring resection.

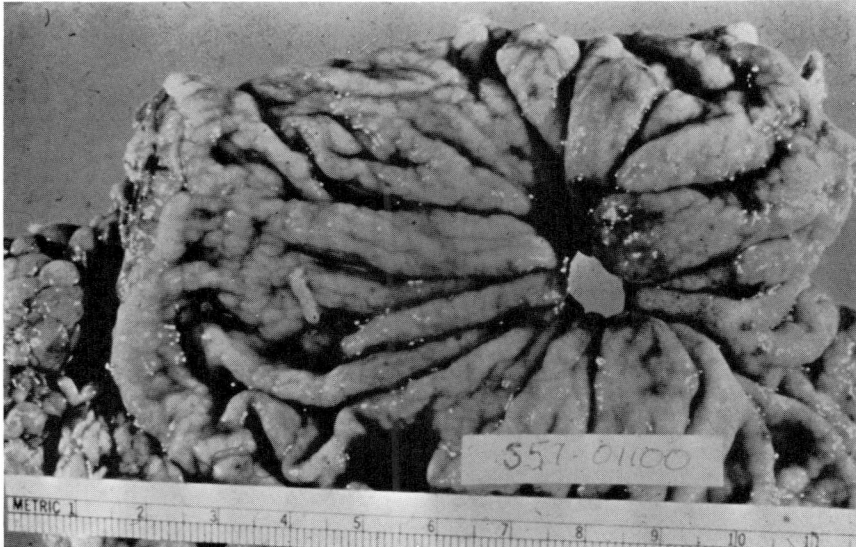

FIGURE 12–16. Segment of the stomach with a transmural perforation of a chronic peptic ulcer. A portion of the ulcer can be seen next to the perforation, and the rugae radiate from the lesion, indicative of chronicity.

resection of a gastric lesion, the correction of a particular complication (e.g., an omental patch over a site of perforation or a bypass gastrojejunostomy for pyloric obstruction), and a procedure to reduce gastric acid secretion. The latter is most often done in cases of duodenal ulcer and consists, at least, of a vagotomy (truncal, selective, or highly selective aimed at just the innervation of the parietal cell area) together with a drainage procedure such as a pyloroplasty. Alternatively, an antrectomy or large subtotal resection is performed to eliminate the gastrin-producing endocrine cells, and the proximal stomach is connected either to the duodenum (Billroth I) or to a loop of proximal jejunum (Billroth II).

As a general rule, the more extensive operations with gastric resection are associated with less recurrence of ulcer disease but with a greater chance of other complications from the surgery.[145] Thus recurrent ulcers are observed in about 10% of cases after a vagotomy but in only a few percent after a subtotal gastrectomy. The ulcers occur in the part of the small intestine, either the duodenum or the jejunum, that is immediately adjacent to the stomach (Figure 21–20). Patients with a gastric resection regularly develop a gastritis of the residual stomach that is thought to be due mainly to the constant reflux of bile salts through the stoma, and this is productive of pain and mild bleeding in about 10% of cases[146]; see the section on postgastrectomy gastritis in Chapter 20 for further details. Other complications that can appear in patients who have had a gastric resection include the dumping syndrome[147] and a maldigestive disorder.[148,149] The former is caused by the

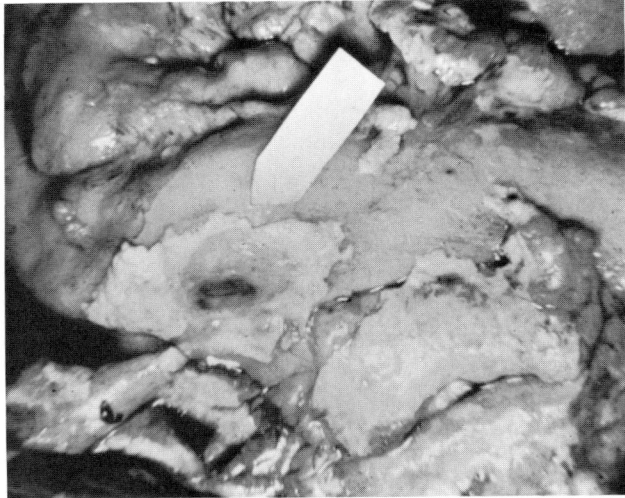

FIGURE 21–17. Peritoneal surface of the stomach, revealing a perforated chronic peptic ulcer surrounded by inflammatory exudate (arrow).

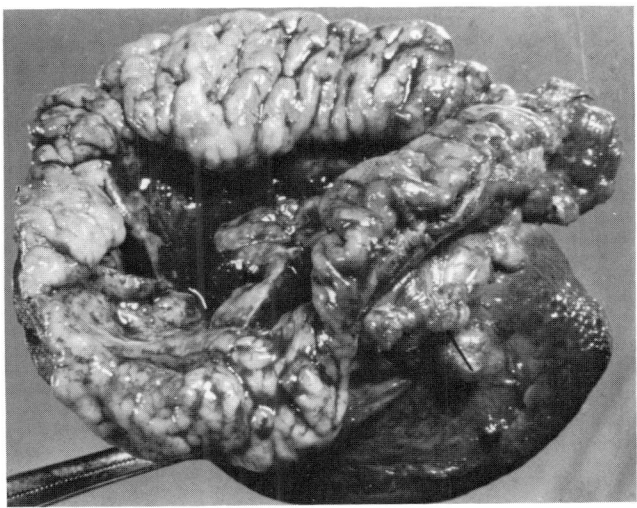

FIGURE 21–18. Large chronic peptic ulcer of the stomach that penetrated the spleen (external surface of the spleen, lower right).

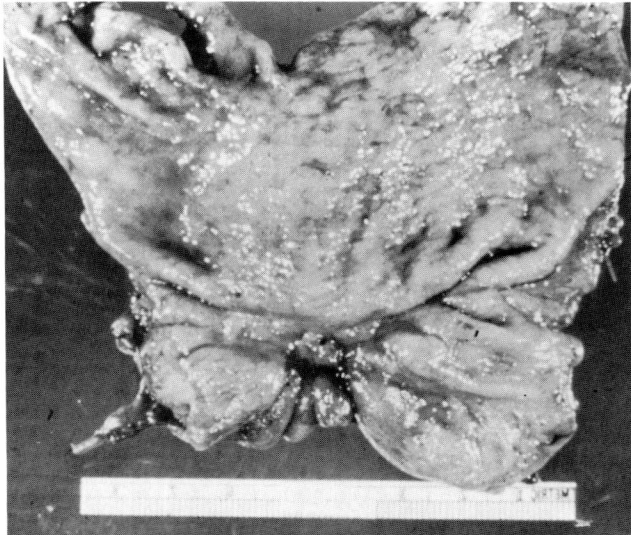

FIGURE 21–19. Segment of the distal stomach, showing a chronic active peptic ulcer and contraction of pyloric region (bottom).

rapid passage of a hyperosmolar meal into the jejunum and results in pain and diarrhea. A mild degree of steatorrhea is noted in most patients and is probably due to poor dilution and mixing of the meal with the biliary and pancreatic sections; this is usually just seen in the chemical analysis of the stool and is uncommonly productive of symptomatic disease. In the afferent loop syndrome, there is a bacterial overgrowth in the static small bowel segment proximal to the stoma, and this can lead to bile salt deconjugation and a greater amount of maldigestion and clinically evident steatorrhea.

Relation of Ulcer to Gastric Carcinoma

It was formerly thought that adenocarcinoma could develop in a benign peptic ulcer lesion as a late complication, but this appears to be a rare event.[150,151] Rather, cases of peptic ulcer disease are invariably associated with a more diffuse chronic gastritis in the surrounding antral mucosa, and it is the latter condition that has a greater frequency of cancer development. Thus patients with chronic peptic ulcers of the stomach do have a slightly higher incidence of gastric carcinoma, but the tumors can occur in any part of the stomach and not preferentially in the area of the prior ulcer. This does not appear to be a major problem in the United States, however; and surveillance studies are not in use.

A similar situation exists in patients who have had an antral resection and gastroduodenostomy or gastrojejunostomy for the treatment of peptic ulcers of either the stomach or the duodenum. As noted above, these patients regularly develop a chronic gastritis in the proximal stomach and experience an increased risk for the formation of adenomas, dysplasia, and adenocarcinoma[152–154]; see the section on complications of chronic gastritis in Chapter 20 and also Chapter 25, on gastric adenocarcinoma, for further details.

It should also be noted that some cases of gastric carcinoma present with a relatively small lesion and a secondary ulcer that can mimic the appearance of a benign ulcer (see Figure 21–14).[125,127] Indeed, medical therapy can result in partial or, exceptionally, complete healing of the ulcerated area; the need for close observation and biopsy of any suspicious or unusual gastric ulcer lesion is therefore stressed.

Other Ulcer Conditions

Esophagus

Ulcers as well as mucosal inflammation are frequently seen in patients with reflux esophagitis, either of the primary type or in various motor disturbances such as systemic sclerosis. Reflux disease is a common condition that is due mainly to an incompetence of the lower esophageal sphincter, allowing for the excess reflux and retention of acid and pepsin in the lower esophagus, and this subject is covered in Chapter 17.

Gastric Heterotopia

Foci of well-formed gastric corpus-fundic mucosa have been observed in many parts of the gut, including the upper esophagus, duodenum, rectum, Meckel's diverticulum, and duplication cysts[155–159]; these are described in Chapter 28. The cells of the specialized gastric glands in these ectopic lesions are functional and produce acid and pepsin, but whether an ulcer develops is dependent on other local factors. Thus, ulceration has only rarely been noted in the esophageal lesions,[160] presumably because there is rapid transit from this area, and has not been described in the duodenal lesions, where there is prompt neutralization of the acid by the abundant biliary and pancreatic secretions.

In contrast, peptic ulcers can occur in areas of gastric heterotopia affecting the rectum[161,162] or Meckel's diverticulum,[163,164] because these regions are relatively static, allowing time for the acid and pepsin to act. The ulcers typically occur in the area of intestine that is immediately adjacent to the ectopic gastric mucosa. In Meckel's lesion, the ulcer is usually in the diverticulum but may on occasion be located in the contiguous ileum when there is a diffuse heterotopia of the diverticular mucosa. The lesions can result in massive hemorrhage or in a perforation of the diverticulum, and this condition is a major consideration in the differential diagnosis in children who present with colonic bleeding or peritonitis. The original gastric foci can be obliterated by the secondary inflammation, as evidenced by its finding in only one half of resected diverticula. Rectal involvement is rare, and the patients typically have deep ulcers and complex fistulas that can penetrate the perineum (see Chapter 28).

Stomal Ulcers

Stomal ulcers are recurrent lesions in patients who have had a gastric resection for the treatment of peptic

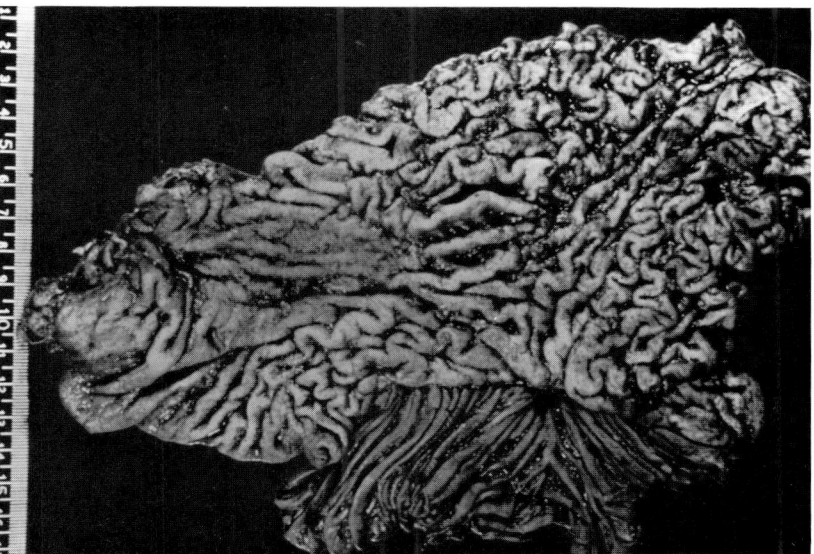

FIGURE 21–20. Segment of the stomach (top) and the jejunum connected by a side-to-side anastomosis following a Billroth II procedure. There is a small recurrent chronic peptic ulcer in the jejunum just next to the anastomosis.

ulcer disease of either the stomach or the duodenum[165]; see the previous section on surgical complications for further details. The ulcers are usually small and are regularly located in the small intestine that is immediately contiguous to the residual stomach at the anastomosis, either in the duodenum after a Billroth I operation or in the jejunum after a Billroth II resection (Figure 21–20). The patients typically present with pain or bleeding,[166] and radiographic and endoscopic studies are performed to distinguish recurrent peptic ulcer disease from the postgastrectomy type of gastritis and from other complications of surgery. Because recurrent ulcer following a gastric resection is relatively uncommon, a particular provocative condition should be sought, such as the ingestion of a toxic chemical or drug, a retained distal antrum, the Zollinger-Ellison syndrome, or an imperfectly constructed anastomosis.

Retained Antrum

This is a rare circumstance that can occur in a patient who has a Billroth II operation when a part of the distal antrum and pyloric sphincter is not excised. It is more likely to happen if there has been a pyloric channel or duodenal ulcer with marked scarring that results in the obliteration of the normal configuration of the pyloric sphincter. Because the retained portion of the antrum is a blind sac that is attached only to the duodenum and is not exposed to any acid formed in the proximal stomach, there is maximum stimulation of the antral G cells, resulting in hypergastrinemia and recurrent stomal ulcers.[167] A similar problem does not regularly develop if a part of the proximal antrum is retained, because this is in contact with the gastric corpus and acid; nevertheless, if too much antrum remains, the original operation can be ineffective. It is therefore important that the resection margins of any gastrectomy specimen be routinely examined, as noted above. The diagnosis of a retained distal antrum is provided by serum gastrin and radiographic studies, and it is promptly corrected by surgical excision.

Zollinger-Ellison Syndrome

The Zollinger-Ellison syndrome is an uncommon disorder that probably accounts for less than 1% of the cases of peptic ulcer disease. It is characterized by the presence of an autonomous source of gastrin leading to parietal cell hyperplasia, sustained hyperacidity, and multiple refractory ulcers of the stomach and small intestine.[168–171] The syndrome is due most often to a pancreatic islet cell tumor or "gastrinoma" (75% to 80% of cases), a diffuse islet cell hyperplasia (10%), or a tumor in the duodenal wall (5% to 10%)[172–174]; rare sources include gastrinomas of the stomach, jejunum, liver, ovary, and parathyroid and a diffuse G-cell hyperplasia in the gastric antrum. About 25% of the pancreatic tumors are associated with the multiple endocrine neoplasm type I syndrome,[175,176] which includes pituitary chromophobe adenomas and parathyroid hyperplasia; and two thirds are malignant. The basal gastric acid level is regularly elevated and often approaches the stimulated level; and there is a marked increase in the serum gastrin, which is further stimulated by infusions of secretin and calcium.[177,178] These substances ordinarily suppress the gastrin level in persons without the syndrome.

There is a great expansion of the number of parietal cells, which may be three to five times the norm, with extension of the parietal cells into the gastric pit region (Figures 21–21 and 21–22). This usually results in a gross enlargement of the gastric rugae that can be appreciated by radiographic and endoscopic studies (Figure 21–23).[169,170,173] In contrast to ordinary peptic ulcer disease, the ulcers in Zollinger-Ellison syndrome are more often multiple (about 25% of cases) and occur in unusual sites such as the distal duodenum in 15% and the jejunum in 10%; there are often additional areas of

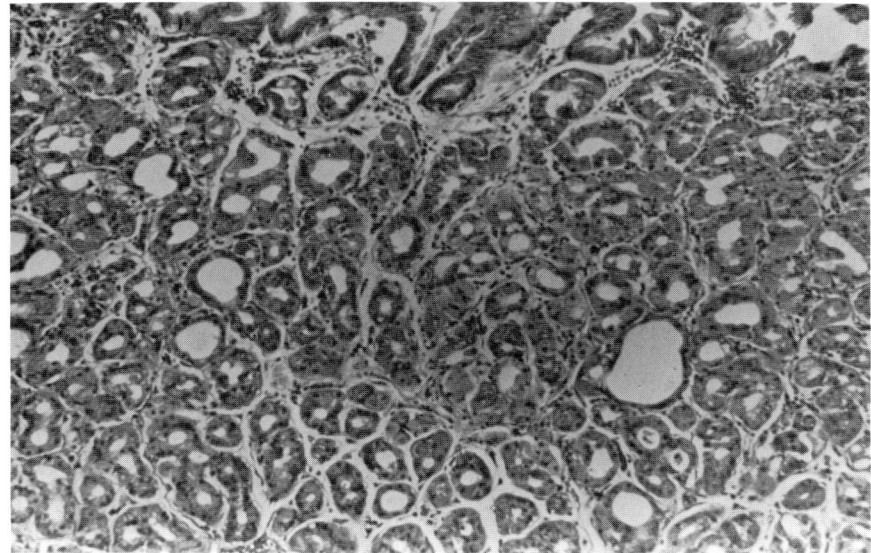

FIGURE 21–21. Gastric corpus mucosa in a case of Zollinger-Ellison syndrome. There is a marked hyperplasia of the parietal cells that extends into the neck and foveolar region (top). (H&E, × 80)

inflammation and superficial erosions in the intervening small-intestinal mucosa.[179] Other consequences of the high gastric acid and fluid volume include the appearance of diarrhea and, occasionally, steatorrhea due to the dilution and inactivation of the bile salts.[179,180]

The diagnosis of the syndrome is usually apparent from the constellation of radiographic and chemical findings.[171,181] Marked elevations of the serum gastrin can also be seen in patients with chronic fundic gastritis and pernicious anemia, a retained gastric antrum, and exceptionally in cases of renal insufficiency or massive intestinal resection. Rugal hypertrophy may be a normal variant and is observed in cases of Ménétrier's disease and tumors. Treatment consists of the removal of any benign tumors, which constitute only a minority of the cases, and is mainly directed at reducing the acid secretion by the use of H_2-blocking drugs or, if needed, by gastrectomy.[171,182,183] Even though patients often have a malignant tumor, these are usually indolent, and most of the morbidity and early fatality is related to the ulcers. See Chapter 13, on endocrine disorders, and Chapter 22, on mucosal hyperplasia of the stomach, for further details.

MUCOSAL BIOPSY

The general techniques and uses of endoscopy and biopsy are covered in Chapter 3. These procedures are commonly employed in patients with gastric and duodenal ulcers in recognition of the lesions, in distinguishing cases of erosive gastritis or duodenitis and acute ulcers from chronic peptic ulcer disease, in monitoring the course following therapy, and in detecting

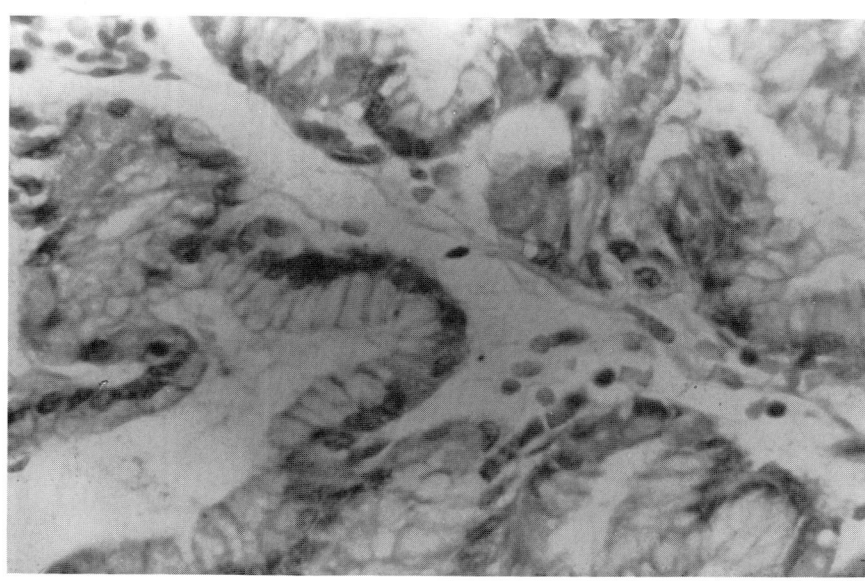

FIGURE 21–22. Gastric corpus mucosa in a case of Zollinger-Ellison syndrome, revealing presence of several parietal cells (round granular cells with central nuclei) in the foveolar (pit) region. (H&E, × 500)

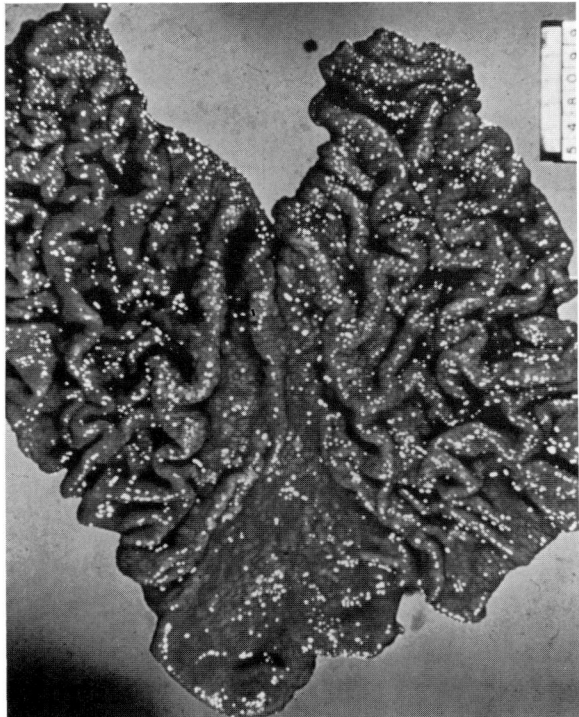

FIGURE 21-23. Stomach in a case of the Zollinger-Ellison syndrome, showing marked enlargement of the rugae.

complications.[132,184,185] Endoscopy is generally more sensitive than radiography in the finding of small ulcers, especially if they are relatively shallow. Biopsy of an ulcer edge can sometimes indicate that the lesion is an acute one, such as that due to a drug.[118,119] There is a lack of inflammation in one half of the acute cases, whereas there is always a prominent inflammation in the mucosa next to a chronic peptic ulcer. The most important use of endoscopy is in distinguishing a benign peptic ulcer from a malignant tumor,[128-132,186,187] either a carcinoma or a lymphoma in the stomach.

References

1. Skillman JJ, Silen W: Stress ulcers. Lancet 2:1303, 1972.
2. Eiseman B, Heyman RL: Stress ulcers—a continuing challenge. N Engl J Med 282:372, 1970.
3. Moody FG, Cheung LY, Simons MA, et al: Stress and the acute gastric mucosal lesion. Am J Dig Dis 21:148, 1976.
4. Skillman JJ, Silen W: Stress ulceration in the acutely ill. Annu Rev Med 27:9, 1976.
5. Pruitt BA, Foley FD, Moncrief JA: Curling's ulcer: Clinicopathologic study of 323 cases. Ann Surg 172:523, 1970.
6. Czaja AJ, McAlhany JC, Pruitt BA: Acute gastroduodenal disease after thermal injury: An endoscopic evaluation of incidence and natural history. N Engl J Med 291:925, 1974.
7. Pruitt BA, Goodwin CW: Stress ulcer disease in the burned patient. World J Surg 5:209, 1981.
8. Cushing H: Peptic ulcers and the interbrain. Surg Gynecol Obstet 55:1, 1932.
9. Kamada T, Fusamoto J, Kawano S, et al: Gastrointestinal bleeding following head injury: A clinical study of 433 cases. J Trauma 17:44, 1977.
10. McClelland RN, Shires GT, Pager M: Gastric secretory and splanchnic blood flow in man following severe trauma and hemorrhagic shock. Am J Surg 121:134, 1971.
11. Fischer RP, Jelense S, Fulton RL: The maintenance of gastric mucosal barrier during the early erosive gastritis component of stress ulceration. Surgery 80:40, 1976.
12. Kivilaakso E, Silen W: Pathogenesis of experimental gastric-mucosal injury. N Engl J Med 301:364-369, 1979.
13. Robert A: Cytoprotection by prostaglandins. Gastroenterology 77:761, 1979.
14. Robert A, Kauffman GL: Stress ulcers, erosions and gastric mucosal injury. In Sleisenger MH, Fordtran JS (eds): Gastrointestinal Disease, 4th ed. Philadelphia, WB Saunders, 1989, pp 772-792.
15. Brodie DA, Hanson HM: A study of the factors involved in the production of gastric ulcers by the restraint technique. Gastroenterology 38:353, 1960.
16. Goldman H, Rosoff CB: Pathogenesis of acute gastric stress ulcer. Am J Pathol 52:227, 1968.
17. Skillman JJ, Bushnell LS, Goldman H, et al: Respiratory failure, hypotension, sepsis and jaundice: A clinical syndrome associated with lethal hemorrhage from acute stress ulceration of the stomach. Am J Surg 117:523, 1969.
18. Lucas CF: Stress ulceration: The clinical problem. World J Surg 5:139, 1981.
19. Flowers RS, Kyle K, Hoerr SO: Post-operative hemorrhage from stress ulceration of the stomach and duodenum. Am J Surg 119:632-639, 1970.
20. Lucas CE, Sugawa C, Riddle J, et al: Natural history and surgical dilemma of "stress" gastric bleeding. Arch Surg 102:266, 1971.
21. Hastings PR, Skillman JJ, Bushnell LS, et al: Antacid titration in the prevention of acute gastrointestinal bleeding: A controlled randomized trial of 100 critically ill patients. N Engl J Med 298:1041, 1978.
22. Menguy R: The prophylaxis of stress ulceration. N Engl J Med 302:461, 1980.
23. Priebe HJ, Skillman JJ: Methods of prophylaxis in stress ulcer disease. World J Surg 5:223, 1981.
24. Simonian SJ, Curtis LE: Treatment of hemorrhagic gastritis by antacid. Ann Surg 184:429, 1976.
25. Cheung LY: Treatment of established stress ulcer disease. World J Surg 5:235, 1981.
26. Cody HS, Wichern WA: Choice of operation for acute gastric mucosal hemorrhage: Report of 36 cases and literature review. Am J Surg 135:322, 1977.
27. Hubert JP, Kernan PD, Welch JS, et al: The surgical management of bleeding stress ulcers. Ann Surg 191:672, 1980.
28. Lev R: "Stress" ulcers following war wounds in Vietnam: A morphologic and histochemical study. Lab Invest 25:471, 1971.
29. Cooke AR: Drug damage to the gastroduodenum. In Sleisenger MH, Fordtran JS (eds): Gastrointestinal Disease, 2nd ed. Philadelphia, WB Saunders, 1978, pp 807-826.
30. Bynum TE, Hartsuck J, Jacobson ED: Gastric ulcer. Gastroenterology 62:1052, 1972.
31. Grossman MI, Isenberg JI, Walsh JH: Peptic diseases. Gastroenterology 69:1071, 1975.
32. Soll AH: Duodenal ulcer and drug therapy. In Sleisenger MH, Fordtran JS (eds): Gastrointestinal Disease, 4th ed. Philadelphia, WB Saunders, 1989, pp 814-879.
33. Richardson CT: Gastric ulcer. In Sleisenger MH, Fordtran JS (eds): Gastrointestinal Disease, 4th ed. Philadelphia, WB Saunders, 1989, pp 879-909.
34. Owen DA: Gastritis and duodenitis. In Appleman HD (ed): Pathology of the Esophagus, Stomach, and Duodenum. London, Churchill-Livingston, 1984, pp 37-77.
35. Kurata JH, Haile BH: Racial difference in peptic ulcer disease: Fact or myth. Gastroenterology 83:166, 1982.
36. Langman MJS: Changing patterns in the epidemiology of peptic ulcer. Clin Gastroenterol 2:219, 1973.
37. Mendeloff AI: What has been happening to duodenal ulcer? Gastroenterology 67:1020, 1974.
38. Friedman GD, Siegelaub AB, Seltzer CC: Cigarettes, alcohol, coffee and peptic ulcer. N Engl J Med 290:469, 1974.
39. Thomas J, Grieg M, Piper DW: Chronic gastric ulcer and life events. Gastroenterology 78:905, 1980.

40. Piper DW, McIntosh JH, Ariotti DE, et al: Life events and chronic duodenal ulcer: A case control study. Gut 22:1011, 1981.
41. Wormsley KG: The pathophysiology of duodenal ulceration. Gut 15:59, 1974.
42. Ippoliti A, Walsh J: Newer concept in the pathogenesis of peptic ulcer disease. Surg Clin North Am 56:1479, 1976.
43. Grossman MI: Abnormalities of acid secretion in patients with duodenal ulcers. Gastroenterology 75:524, 1978.
44. Cooke AR: The role of the mucosal barrier in drug-induced gastric ulceration and erosions. Am J Dig Dis 21:155, 1976.
45. Guth PH: Pathogenesis of gastric mucosal injury. Annu Rev Med 33:183, 1982.
46. Menguy, R: Gastric mucus and the gastric mucous barrier. Am J Surg 117:806, 1969.
47. Daintree-Johnson H, Love AHG, Rogers NC, et al: Gastric ulcers, blood groups and acid secretion. Gut 5:402, 1964.
48. Johnson HD: Gastric ulcer: Classification, blood group characteristics, secretion patterns and pathogenesis. Ann Surg 162:996, 1965.
49. Eberhard G: The personality and peptic ulcer. Preliminary report of a twin study. Acta Psychiatr Scand 203:131, 1968.
50. Rotter JI, Rimoin DL, Gursky JM, et al: HLA-B5 associated with duodenal ulcer. Gastroenterology 73:438, 1977.
51. Ellis A, Woodrow JC: HLA and duodenal ulcer. Gut 20:760, 1979.
52. Alp MH, Court JH, Grant AK: Personality pattern and emotional stress in the genesis of gastric ulcer. Gut 11:773, 1970.
53. Feldman EJ, Elashoff JD, Samloff IM, et al: Psychologic stress and duodenal ulcer. N Engl J Med 302:1206, 1980.
54. Langman MJS, Cooke AR: Gastric and duodenal ulcer and their associated diseases. Lancet 1:680–683, 1976.
55. Archibald SD, Jirsch DW, Bear RA: A. Gastrointestinal complications of renal transplantation. 1. The upper gastrointestinal tract. Can Med Assoc J 119:1291, 1978.
56. Kirsner JB: The parathyroids and peptic ulcer. Gastroenterology 34:145, 1958.
57. Kirk AP, Dooley JS, Hunt RH: Peptic ulceration in patients with chronic liver disease. Dig Dis Sci 25:756, 1980.
58. Amman RW, Vetter D, Deyhle P, et al: Gastrointestinal involvement in systemic mastocytosis. Gut 17:107, 1976.
59. Kirsner JB: Drug-induced peptic ulcer. Ann Intern Med 47:666, 1957.
60. Douglas RA, Johnston ED: Aspirin and chronic gastric ulcer. Med J Aust 2:893, 1961.
61. Levy M: Aspirin use in patients with major upper gastrointestinal bleeding and peptic ulcer disease. N Engl J Med 290:1158, 1974.
62. Silvoso GR, Ivey KJ, Butt JH, et al: Incidence of gastric lesions in patients with rheumatic disease on chronic aspirin therapy. Ann Intern Med 91:517, 1979.
63. Piper DW, McIntosh JH, Ariotti DE, et al: Analgesic ingestion and chronic peptic ulcer. Gastroenterology 80:427, 1981.
64. Conn HO, Blitzer BL: Nonassociation of adrenocorticosteroid therapy and peptic ulcer. N Engl J Med 294:473, 1976.
65. Pemberton RE, Strand LJ: A review of upper gastrointestinal effects of the newer nonsteroidal anti-inflammatory agents. Dig Dis Sci 24:53–64, 1979.
66. Armstrong CP, Blower AL: Non-steroidal anti-inflammatory drugs and life threatening complications of peptic ulceration. Gut 28:527–532, 1987.
67. Price AB, Levi J, Dolby JM, et al: *Campylobacter pyloridis* in peptic ulcer disease: Microbiology, pathology, and scanning electron microscopy. Gut 26:1183–1188, 1985.
68. Johnston BJ, Reed PI, Ali MH: Campylobacter-like organisms in duodenal and antral endoscopic biopsies: Relationship to inflammation. Gut 27:1132–1137, 1986.
69. Andersen LP, Holck S, Poolsen CO, et al: *Campylobacter pyloridis* in peptic ulcer disease. I. Gastric and duodenal infection caused by *C. pyloridis*: Histopathologic and microbiologic findings. Scand J Gastroenterol 22:219–224, 1987.
70. Blaser MJ: Gastric *Campylobacter*-like organisms, gastritis, and peptic ulcer disease. Gastroenterology 93:371–383, 1987.
71. Rathbone BJ, Wyatt JI, Heatley RV: *Campylobacter pyloridis*—a new factor in peptic ulcer disease. Gut 27:635–641, 1986.
72. Marshall BJ: Peptic ulcer: An infectious disease? Hosp Pract 22:69–78, 1987.
73. Rauws EAJ, Tytgat GNJ: Cure of duodenal ulcer associated with eradication of Helicobacter pylori. Lancet 1:1233–1235, 1990.
74. Lam SK, Isenberg JI, Grossman MI, et al: Rapic gastric emptying in duodenal ulcer patients. Dig Dis Sci 27:598, 1982.
75. Rhodes J: Etiology of gastric ulcer. Gastroenterology 63:171, 1972.
76. Mackay IR, Hislop IG: Chronic gastritis and gastric ulcer. Gut 7:228–233, 1966.
77. Gear MWL, Truelove SC, Whitehead R: Gastric ulcer and gastritis. Gut 12:639–645, 1971.
78. Trier JS: Morphology of the gastric mucosa in patients with ulcer disease. Am J Dig Dis 21:138–140, 1976.
79. Flint FJ, Grech P: Pyloric regurgitation and gastric ulcer. Gut 11:735–737, 1970.
80. Delaney JP, Cheng JWB, Butler BA, Ritchie WP: Gastric ulcer and regurgitation gastritis. Gut 11:715–729, 1970.
81. Fisher RS, Cohen S: Pyloric-sphincter dysfunction in patients with gastric ulcer. N Engl J Med 288:273, 1973.
82. Rovelstad RA: The incompetent pyloric sphincter: Bile and mucosal ulceration. Am J Dig Dis 21:165, 1976.
83. Thomas WEG: Duodeno-gastric reflux: A common factor in pathogenesis of gastric and duodenal ulcer. Lancet 2:1166, 1980.
84. Davenport HW: Back diffusion of acid through the gastric mucosa and its physiological consequences. In Glass GBJ (ed): Progress in Gastroenterology. Vol 2. New York, Grune & Stratton, 1970.
85. Overholt B, Pollard H: Acid diffusion into the human gastric mucosa. Gastroenterology 54:182, 1968.
86. Dragstedt LR, Woodward ER: Gastric stasis: A cause of gastric ulcer. Scand J Gastroenterol 5:243, 1970.
87. Smith FH, Jordan SM: Gastric ulcer: A study of 600 cases. Gastroenterology 11:575, 1948.
88. Chapman ML: Peptic ulcer: A medical perspective. Med Clin North Am 62:39, 1978.
89. Misiewicz JJ: Peptic ulceration and its correlation with symptoms. Clin Gastroenterol 7:571, 1978.
90. Wesdorp RIC, Fisher JE: Plasma-gastrin and acid secretion in patients with peptic ulceration. Lancet 2:857–860, 1974.
91. Walsh JH, Lam SK: Physiology and pathology of gastrin. Clin Gastroenterol 9:567, 1980.
92. Peterson WL, Studevant RAL, Frankl HD, et al: Healing of duodenal ulcer with an antacid regimen. N Engl J Med 297:341–345, 1977.
93. Isenberg JI, Peterson WL, Elashoff JD, et al: Healing of benign gastric ulcer with low-dose antacid or cimetidine: A double-blind, randomized, placebo-controlled trial. N Engl J Med 308:1319–1324, 1983.
94. Karsner HT: The pathology of peptic ulcer of the stomach. JAMA 85:1376, 1925.
95. Magnus HA: The pathology of peptic ulceration. Postgrad Med J 30:131, 1954.
96. Shimazu H, Koniski T, Yamogishi T, et al: A histopathological study on pyloric ulcer. Gastroenterol Jpn 15:362, 1980.
97. Oi M, Oshida K, Sugimura S: The location of gastric ulcer. Gastroenterology 36:45–56, 1959.
98. Kimura K: Chronological transition of the fundic-pyloric border determined by stepwise biopsy of the lesser and greater curvatures of the stomach. Gastroenterology 63:584, 1972.
99. Thomas J, Greig M, McIntosh J, et al: The location of chronic gastric ulcer. Digestion 20:79, 1980.
100. Jennings DA, Richardson JE: Giant lesser curve gastric ulcers. Lancet 2:343, 1954.
101. Lumsden K, MacLarnon JC, Dawson J: Giant duodenal ulcer. Gut 11:592, 1970.
102. Boyle JD: Multiple gastric ulcers. Gastroenterology 61:628, 1971.
103. Bonnevie O: Gastric and duodenal ulcers in the same patients. Scand J Gastroenterol 10:657, 1975.
104. Ross JR, Reaves LE: Syndrome of posterior penetrating-ulcer. Med Clin North Am 50:461, 1966.

105. Joffe N, Antonioli DA: Penetration into spleen by benign gastric ulcer. Clin Radiol 32:177, 1981.
106. Sarr MG, Shepard AJ, Zuidema GD: Choledochoduodenal fistula: An unusual complication of duodenal ulcer disease. Am J Surg 141:736, 1981.
107. Guerrieri C, Waxman M: Hepatic tissue in gastroscopic biopsy: Evidence of hepatic penetration by peptic ulcer. Am J Gastroenterol 82:890–893, 1987.
108. Cody JH, DiVincenti FC, Cowick DR, Mahanes JR: Gastrocolic and Gastrojejunocolic fistulae: Report of twelve cases and review of the literature. Ann Surg 181:376, 1975.
109. Mori K, Shinya H, Wolff WI: Polypoid reparative mucosal proliferation at the site of a healed gastric ulcer: Sequential gastroscopic, radiological and histological observations. Gastroenterology 61:523, 1971.
110. Oohara T, Tohma H, Aono G, et al: Intestinal metaplasia of the regenerative epithelia in 549 gastric ulcers. Hum Pathol 14:1066–1071, 1983.
111. Steer HW: The gastro-duodenal epithelium in peptic ulceration. J Pathol 146:355–362, 1985.
112. Katzenstein ALA, Maksen J: Candidal infection of gastric ulcers: Histology, incidence and clinical significance. Am J Clin Pathol 71:137, 1979.
113. Peters M, Weiner J, Whelan G: Fungal infection associated with gastroduodenal ulceration: Endoscopic and pathologic appearance. Gastroenterology 78:350, 1980.
114. Gotlieb-Jensen K, Andersen J: Occurrence of Candida in gastric ulcers: Significance for the healing process. Gastroenterology 85:535–537, 1983.
115. Loffeld RJ, Loffeld BC, Arends JW, et al: Fungal colonization of gastric ulcers. Am J Gastroenterol 83:730–733, 1988.
116. Ganguli PC: Antral gastrin-cell hyperplasia in peptic ulcer disease. Lancet 1:583, 1974.
117. Takahashi T, Shimazu H, Yamagishi T, Tani M: G-cell populations in resected stomachs from gastric and duodenal ulcer patients. Gastroenterology 78:498–504, 1980.
118. McDonald WC: Correlation of mucosal histology and aspirin intake in chronic gastric ulcer. Gastroenterology 65:381, 1973.
119. Hamilton ST, Yardley JH: Endoscopic biopsy diagnosis of aspirin-associated chronic gastric ulcers. (Abstract) Gastroenterology 78:1178, 1980.
120. Salupere VP: Gastric biopsy in peptic ulcer: A follow-up study. Scand J Gastroenterol 4:537–543, 1969.
121. Gear MWL, Truelove SC, Williams DG, et al: Gastric cancer simulating benign gastric ulcer. Br J Surg 56:739, 1969.
122. Montgomery RD, Richardson BP: Gastric ulcer and cancer. Q J Med 44:591, 1975.
123. Dekker W, Tytgat GN: Diagnostic accuracy of fiberendoscopy in the detection of upper intestinal malignancy: A follow-up analysis. Gastroenterology 73:710, 1977.
124. Mountford RA, Brown P, Salmon PR, et al: Gastric cancer detection in gastric ulcer disease. Gut 21:9–17, 1980.
125. Podolsky I, Storms PR, Richardson CT, et al: Gastric adenocarcinoma masquerading endoscopically as benign gastric ulcer: A five-year experience. Dig Dis Sci 33:1057–1063, 1988.
126. Hirota T, Itabashi N, Suzuki K, et al: Clinicopathologic study of minute and small early gastric cancer. Pathol Annu 15:1, 1980.
127. Green PHR, O'Toole KM, Weinberg LM, et al: Early gastric cancer. Gastroenterology 81:247, 1981.
128. Witzel L, Halter F, Gretillat PA, et al: Evaluation of specific value of endoscopic biopsies and brush cytology for malignancies of the esophagus and stomach. Gut 27:375, 1976.
129. Halter F, Witzel L, Gretillat PA, et al: Diagnostic value of biopsy, guided lavage, and brush cytology in esophagogastroscopy. Am J Dig Dis 22:129–131, 1977.
130. Qizilbash AH, Casteli M, Kowalski MA, et al: Endoscopic brush cytology and biopsy in the diagnosis of cancer of the upper gastrointestinal tract. Acta Cytol 24:313, 1980.
131. Graham DY, Schwartz JT, Cain GD, et al: Prospective evaluation of biopsy number in the diagnosis of esophageal and gastric carcinoma. Gastroenterology 82:228, 1982.
132. Goldman H, Antonioli DA: Mucosal biopsy of the esophagus, stomach, and proximal duodenum. Hum Pathol 13:423–448, 1982.
133. Graham DY: Complications of peptic ulcer disease and indications for surgery. In Sleisenger MH, Fordtran JS (eds): Gastrointestinal Disease, 4th ed. Philadelphia, WB Saunders, 1989, pp 925–938.
134. Chinn AB, Weckesser EC: Acute hemorrhage from peptic ulceration: An analysis of 322 cases. Ann Intern Med 34:339, 1951.
135. Cotten PB, Rosenberg MT, Waldram RPL: Early endoscopy of esophagus, stomach, and duodenal bulb in patients with hematemesis and melena. Br Med J 2:1505, 1973.
136. Van Zanten SJOV, Bartelsman JFWM, Schipper ME, Tytgat GNJ: Recurrent massive haematemesis from Dieulafoy vascular malformations: A review of 101 cases. Gut 27:213–222, 1986.
137. Miko TL, Thomazy VA: The caliber persistent artery of the stomach: A unifying approach to gastric aneurysm, Dieulafoy's lesion, and submucosal arterial malformation. Hum Pathol 19:914–921, 1988.
138. Rees JR, Thorlyarnasson B: Perforated gastric ulcer. Am J Surg 126:93, 1973.
139. Sawyers JL, Herrington JL Jr, Mulherin JL, et al: Acute perforated duodenal ulcer. Arch Surg 110:527, 1975.
140. Norris JR, Haubrich WS: The incidence and clinical features of penetration in peptic ulceration. JAMA 178:386, 1961.
141. Kozell DD, Meyer KA: Obstructing gastroduodenal ulcer, symptoms and signs. Arch Surg 89:491, 1964.
142. Kreel L, Ellis H: Pyloric stenosis in adults: A clinical and radiological study of 100 consecutive patients. Gut 6:253, 1965.
143. Pheils MT, Mayday GB, Gillett DJ, Dunn RM: Surgery for benign gastric ulcer. Med J Aust 1:56, 1970.
144. Scott JW, Sawyers JL, Gobbel WG Jr, Harrington JL Jr: Definitive surgical treatment in duodenal ulcer disease. Curr Probl Surg 10:3, 1968.
145. Price WE, Grizzle JE, Postlethwait RW, et al: Results of operation for duodenal ulcer. Surg Gynecol Obstet 131:233, 1970.
146. Meshkinpour H, Marks JW, Schoenfield LJ, Bonnoris GG: Reflux gastritis syndrome: Mechanism of symptoms. Gastroenterology 79:1283, 1980.
147. Tabaquchali S: The pathophysiological role of small intestinal flora. Scand J Gastroenterol (Suppl 6) 5:139, 1970.
148. Lundh G: Intestinal digestion and absorption after gastrectomy. Acta Chir Scand (Suppl) 231:1, 1958.
149. Brooke-Cowden GL, Braasch JW, Gibb SO, et al: Postgastrectomy syndromes. Am J Surg 131:464, 1976.
150. Ellis J, Kingston RD, Brookes VS, Waterhouse JAH: Gastric carcinoma and previous peptic ulceration. Br J Surg 66:117, 1979.
151. Papachriston DN, Agnanti N, Fortner JG: Gastric carcinoma after treatment of ulcer. Am J Surg 139:193, 1980.
152. Domellof L, Erickson S, Janunger KG: Carcinoma and possible precancerous changes of the gastric stump after Billroth II resection. Gastroenterology 73:462, 1977.
153. Offerhaus GJA, Stodt J, Huibregtse K, et al: The mucosa of the gastric remnant harboring malignancy: Histologic findings in the biopsy specimens of 504 asymptomatic patients 15 to 46 years after partial gastrectomy with emphasis on nonmalignant lesions. Cancer 64:698–703, 1989.
154. Lundegardh G, Adami H-O, Helmich C, et al: Stomach Cancer after partial gastrectomy for benign ulcer disease. N Engl J Med 319:195–200, 1988.
155. Jabbori M, Goesky CA, Lough J, et al: The inlet patch: Heterotopic gastric mucosa in the upper esophagus. Gastroenterology 89:352–356, 1985.
156. Franzin G, Musola R, Negri A, et al: Heterotopic gastric (fundic) mucosa in the duodenum. Endoscopy 14:166–167, 1982.
157. Wolff M: Heterotopic gastric epithelium in the rectum: A report of three new cases with a review of 87 cases of gastric heterotopia in the alimentary canal. Am J Clin Pathol 55:604–616, 1971.
158. Seagram CG, Louch RE, Stephens CA, Wentworth P: Meckel's diverticulum: A 10-year review of 218 cases. Can J Surg 11:369–373, 1968.
159. Bower RJ, Seiber WK, Kiesewetter WB: Alimentary tract duplications in children. Ann Surg 188:669–674, 1978.
160. Truong LD, Stroebein JR, McKechnie JC: Gastric heterotopia of the proximal esophagus: A report of four cases detected by endoscopy and review of the literature. Am J Gastroenterol 81:1162–1166, 1986.

161. Debas HT, Chaum H, Thomson FB, et al: Functioning heterotopic oxyntic mucosa in the rectum. Gastroenterol Clin Biol 7:39–42, 1983.
162. Kaloni BP, Vaezzadeh K, Sieber WK: Gastric heterotopia in rectum complicated by rectovesical fistula. Dig Dis Sci 28:378–380, 1983.
163. Case record of the Massachusetts General Hospital. N Engl J Med 302:958–962, 1980.
164. Meguid M, Erakis AJ: Complications of Meckel's diverticulum in infants. Surg Gynecol Obstet 139:541–544, 1974.
165. Printen KJ, Scott D, Mason EE: Stomal ulcers after gastric bypass. Arch Surg 115:525, 1980.
166. Hunt PS, Dowling J, Korman M, Hansky J: Bleeding stomal ulceration. Aust J Surg 49:15, 1979.
167. Webster MW, Barnes EL, Stremple JF: Serum gastrin levels in the differential diagnosis of recurrent peptic ulceration due to retained gastric antrum. Am J Surg 135:248, 1978.
168. Zollinger RM, Ellison EH: Primary ulcerations of jejunum associated with islet cell tumors of pancreas. Ann Surg 142:709–728, 1955.
169. Ellison EH, Wilson SD: The Zollinger-Ellison syndrome: Reappraisal and evaluation of 260 registered cases. Ann Surg 160:512, 1964.
170. Isenberg JI, Walsh JH, Grossman NI: Zollinger-Ellison syndrome. Gastroenterology 65:140–165, 1973.
171. Wolfe MM, Jensen RT: Zollinger-Ellison syndrome: Current concepts in diagnosis and management. N Engl J Med 317:1200–1209, 1987.
172. Greider MH, Rosai J, McGuigan JE: The human pancreatic islet cells and their tumors. II. Ulcerogenic and diarrheogenic tumors. Cancer 33:1423, 1974.
173. Creutzfeldt W, Arnold R, Creutzfeldt C, et al: Pathomorphologic, biochemical and diagnostic aspects of gastrinomas (Zollinger-Ellison syndrome). Hum Pathol 6:47, 1975.
174. Solcia E, Capella C, Buffa R, et al: Pathology of the Zollinger-Ellison syndrome. In Fenoglio CM (eds): Progress in Surgical Pathology. Vol 1. New York, Masson, 1980, pp 119–133.
175. Ballard HS, Frame B, Hartsock RJ: Familial multiple endocrine adenoma-peptic ulcer complex. Medicine 43:481, 1964.
176. Craven DE, Goodman AD, Carter JH: Familial multiple endocrine adenomatosis: Multiple endocrine neoplasiam type I. Arch Intern Med 129:567, 1972.
177. McGuigan JE, Wolfe MM: Secretin injection test in the diagnosis of gastrinoma. Gastroenterology 79:1324, 1980.
178. DeVeney CW, DeVeney KS, Jaffe BM, et al: Use of calcium and secretin in the diagnosis of gastrinoma (Zollinger-Ellison syndrome). Ann Intern Med 87:680, 1977.
179. Mansbach CM, Wilkins RM, Dobbins WO, Taylor MP: Intestinal mucosal function and structure in the steatorrhea of Zollinger-Ellison syndrome. Arch Intern Med 121:487, 1968.
180. Shimoda SS, Saunder DR, Rubin CE: The Zollinger-Ellison syndrome with steatorrhea: Mechanisms of fat and vitamin B-12 malabsorption. Gastroenterology 55:705, 1968.
181. Straus E, Yalow RS: Differential diagosis in hyperchlorhydric hypergastrinemia. Gastroenterology 66:867, 1974.
182. Bonfils S, Mignon M, Gratton H: Cimetidine treatment of acute and chronic Zollinger-Ellison syndrome. World J Surg 3:597, 1979.
183. McCarthy DM: The place of surgery in the Zollinger-Ellison syndrome. N Engl J Med 302:1344, 1980.
184. Rotterdam H, Sommers SC: Biopsy Diagnosis of the Digestive Tract. New York, Raven Press, 1981, pp 45–164.
185. Whitehead R: Mucosal Biopsy of the Gastrointestinal Tract, 3rd ed. Philadelphia, WB Saunders, 1985, pp 31–64.
186. Kobayashi S, Prolla JC, Kirsner JB: Brushing cytology of the esophagus and stomach under direct vision by fiberscopes. Acta Cytol 14:223, 1970.
187. Hanson JT, Thorenson C, Morrissey JF: Brush cytology in the diagnosis of upper gastrointestinal malignancy. Gastrointest Endosc 26:33, 1980.

CHAPTER 22

Mucosal Hypertrophy and Hyperplasia of the Stomach

HARVEY GOLDMAN, M.D.

FOCAL MUCOSAL HYPERTROPHY OF THE STOMACH
Polyps
Inflammatory Lesions
Heterotopic Pancreatic Tissue

DIFFUSE MUCOSAL HYPERTROPHY OF THE STOMACH
Zollinger-Ellison Syndrome

Definition, Etiology, and Pathogenesis
Clinical Features
Pathologic Features
Diagnosis and Differential Diagnosis
Ménétrier's Disease
Definition, Etiology, and Pathogenesis
Clinical Features
Pathologic Features
Diagnosis and Differential Diagnosis
Relation to Carcinoma

Childhood Cases
Other Types of Hypertrophic, Hypersecretory Gastropathy
Cases Without Protein Loss
Cases With Protein Loss
Inflammatory and Neoplastic Conditions
Inflammatory Disorders
Tumors

A localized or diffuse thickening or hypertrophy of the gastric mucosa can result from a discrete hyperplasia of one or more of the epithelial elements of the mucosa or from inflammatory and tumor infiltrates. The epithelia that may be involved include the surface-foveolar (pit) mucous cells, the specialized parietal and chief cells of the corpus-fundus, the pyloric glands, and various combinations. The lesions can be focal, multifocal, or diffuse; the latter are usually concentrated in a particular region such as the corpus (e.g., Zollinger-Ellison syndrome and Ménétrier's disease) or the antrum (most inflammatory lesions) or are present throughout the stomach (most tumors).

Depending on the location and extent of the mucosal hypertrophy, the lesions are visualized as polyps, as an enlargement of the rugae, or as some other deformity of the mucosal surface. Clinical features relate to the complications of polyps, to the presence of hypersecretory states, or to the effects of any underlying inflammatory or neoplastic disease. Most of the conditions resulting in mucosal hypertrophy are discussed in other parts of the book, principally in Chapter 20, on gastritis, Chapter 21, on peptic ulcer disease, and Chapter 23, on gastric polyps. The salient features of these disorders as well as complete descriptions of the remaining conditions are presented here.

FOCAL MUCOSAL HYPERTROPHY OF THE STOMACH

The principle causes of a focal or multifocal thickening of the gastric mucosa are polyps, the localized effects of inflammation and repair, and the presence of heterotopic (ectopic) tissues (Table 22–1).

Polyps

Gastric polyps are described in detail in Chapter 23 and include lesions of an inflammatory, hyperplastic (regenerative), hamartomatous, or neoplastic nature. The nonneoplastic polyps represent localized expansions of the mucosa and are usually composed of hyperplastic epithelial elements, mainly the surface-foveolar mucous cells and pyloric glands, together with

Table 22–1. CAUSES OF FOCAL MUCOSAL HYPERTROPHY OF THE STOMACH

Polyps
    Inflammatory
    Hamartomatous
    Hyperplastic
    Neoplastic
Inflammatory lesions
    Edema
    Regeneration
Heterotopic tissue

varying amounts of edema, inflammatory cells, and proliferating stromal cells of the lamina propria.[1-3] Less common lesions noted are fundic gland polyps,[4] which contain specialized corpus epithelial cells with prominent cystic change, and benign lymphoid polyps due to localized areas of marked lymphoid hyperplasia.[5] The polyps are usually single but can be multiple and occasionally confluent in appearance (see Chapter 20, Figure 20–15). Multiple gastric polyps of varying types are also encountered in the several polyposis syndromes, including familial adenomatous polyposis coli, generalized juvenile polyposis, the Peutz-Jeghers syndrome, and the Cronkhite-Canada syndrome.[6-9]

Inflammatory Lesions

Commonly noted in the stomach are localized mucosal thickenings due to inflammatory edema and regenerative tissue. These are most often observed adjacent to ulcers and appear as a uniform elevation of the mucosa or as deformed folds (see Chapter 21, Figure 21–9). Mucosal biopsies are frequently obtained from such areas to confirm the inflammatory nature of the lesions and to exclude other more significant lesions, such as neoplasms.

Heterotopic Pancreatic Tissue

Ectopic foci of mature pancreatic tissue may be observed in the stomach, usually in the distal portion, or in the duodenum.[10-13] The gastric implants consist of the pancreatic elements alone or in combination with varying amounts of bile ductular epithelium and smooth muscle. When there is an especially prominent amount of muscle tissue present, the lesions have also been called adenomyomatous harmartomas and adenomyomas, but there are probably variants of the heterotopic process.[14] The lesions are usually small and confined to the gastric wall but may occasionally enlarge and extend into the mucosal region (Figure 22–1). They may be visualized at endoscopic examination as slightly raised, often umbilicated nodules,[15] although biopsy samples are usually too superficial for detection of the heterotopic glandular tissue. The umbilication represents the outlet of an exocrine duct. These are further described in Chapter 8.

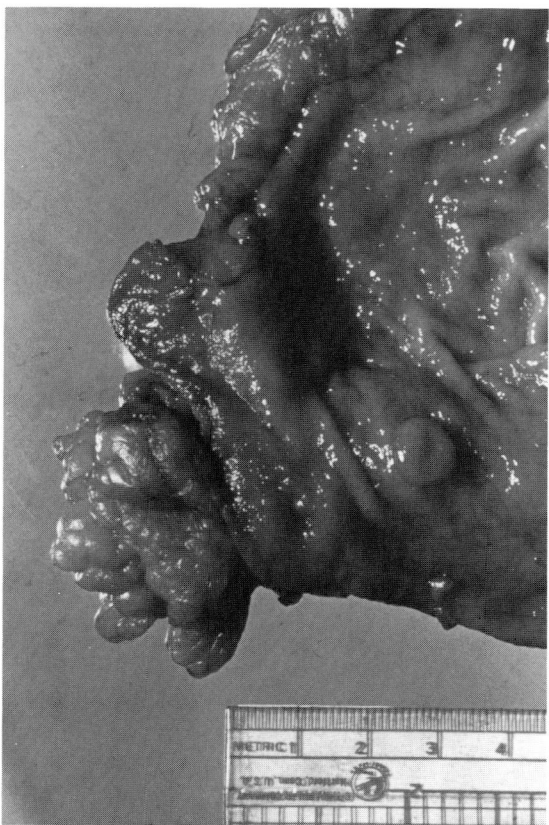

FIGURE 22–1. Heterotopic pancreatic tissue in the stomach. Photograph is of the lower part of the gastric antrum, with the pylorus and rim of contiguous duodenum at the left. There is a localized, polypoid swelling (bottom) of the mucosa due to the presence of the ectopic pancreatic tissue. A fine umbilication is noted on the surface, representing the outlet of a pancreatic duct. (Courtesy of Dr. Karoly Balogh, New England Deaconess Hospital, Boston, Massachusetts.)

DIFFUSE MUCOSAL HYPERTROPHY OF THE STOMACH

The causes of diffuse thickening or hypertrophy of the gastric mucosa, involving a major portion such as the corpus or antrum or the entire stomach, are listed in Table 22–2. It should be stressed that one of the principal causes, perhaps the most common one, of enlarged gastric folds or rugae is simply a variation of the normal size.[16-18] Rugae are limited to the gastric fundus and corpus region and are composed of both mucosal and submucosal tissues. Their enlargement can be readily appreciated by radiographic and gross endoscopic examination, and the diagnosis of a normal variation is dependent on noting that the rugae are simply enlarged but not deformed in any way and on excluding any associated inflammation or hypersecretory state.

More significant causes of diffuse mucosal hypertrophy in the stomach include hyperplasia of the parietal cells (Zollinger-Ellison syndrome), the surface-foveolar mucous cells (Ménétrier's disease), or some combination (other forms of hypertrophic gastropathy).[14,19] These must be distinguished from a variety of inflam-

Table 22–2. CAUSES OF DIFFUSE MUCOSAL HYPERTROPHY OF THE STOMACH

Normal variation
Zollinger-Ellison syndrome
Ménétrier's disease
Hypertrophic, hypersecretory gastropathy (other rare types)
Inflammatory disorders
    Tuberculosis, syphilis, and sarcoidosis
    Isolated granulomatous gastritis
    Allergic gastroenteritis
    Lymphocytic gastritis
    Gastritis cystica polyposa and profunda
Tumors
    Lymphoma
    Carcinoma

matory and neoplastic conditions that can also infiltrate and expand the mucosal region.

Zollinger-Ellison Syndrome

This condition is detailed in Chapter 13, on endocrine disorders, and in Chapter 21, on peptic ulcers, and briefly summarized here.

Definition, Etiology, and Pathogenesis

The components of the syndrome include an autonomous source of gastrin, a maximal stimulation and hyperplasia of the gastric parietal cells, and the presence of uncontrolled peptic ulcer disease and occasionally maldigestion.[20–22] Over 90% of the cases are due to islet cell hyperplasia or tumors ("gastrinomas") of the pancreas, usually malignant but slowly growing;[23,24] other causes include tumors in the duodenal wall and rarely in the jejunum and a diffuse hyperplasia of the antral G cells.[25,26]

Clinical Features

There is massive and continuous hypersecretion of gastric acid, resulting in multiple erosions and ulcers of the stomach, all parts of the duodenum, and even the jejunum. Because of the great amount of acid and fluid produced, there may result an inadequate dilution of the acid by the biliary secretions and an inactivation of the primary bile salts, leading to diarrhea and maldigestion of fats. The diagnosis is usually secured by the detection of excess gastrin in the blood, made worse by calcium infusions, and by noting that the basal and stimulated acid outputs are equivalent.[27] Treatment consists of the removal of any resectable tumors and of the use of H_2-blocking agents, with gastric resection reserved for intractable cases.[28]

Pathologic Features

The gastric effects of the Zollinger-Ellison syndrome are described in Chapter 21 and include the presence of regularly enlarged rugae (see Figure 21–23) due to a marked hyperplasia of the parietal cells in the fundus-

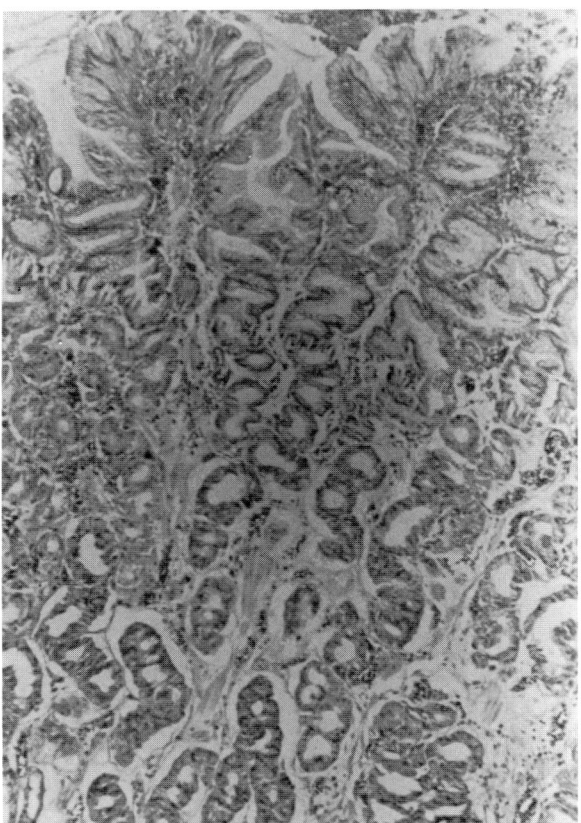

FIGURE 22–2. Gastric corpus mucosa in a case of the Zollinger-Ellison syndrome, with the surface at the top. There is a marked expansion of the mucosa due to a hyperplasia of the parietal cells, which extend into the foveolar region. Most of the gastric glands are dilated, reflecting the increased secretion of the parietal cells. There is a mild edema of the lamina propria but no significant increase in inflammatory cells. (H&E, × 80)

corpus region (Figures 22–2 and 21–21).[26] Many of the gastric glands are cystic due to the acid hypersecretion (Figure 22–3). The hyperplastic parietal cells are also noted in the foveolar region (Figure 21–22), which can be appreciated in endoscopic biopsies, but this feature is not specific for the syndrome.[18] Although the deeper, aspiration type of mucosal biopsy can be used for counting and documenting the parietal cell hyperplasia, other functional studies are more typically used for the diagnosis. Within the corpus region, there is no associated inflammation and no hyperplasia of the surface-foveolar mucous cells. Multiple mucosal erosions and ulcers, with acute and chronic inflammatory features, are observed within the antrum, all parts of the duodenum, and occasionally the jejunum. These features, together with the complication of peptic ulcer disease, are discussed in detail in Chapter 21. The characteristics of cases due to hyperplasia of the antral G cells are provided in Chapter 13.

Diagnosis and Differential Diagnosis

The diagnosis of the Zollinger-Ellison syndrome is suspected in any patient with multiple or intractable

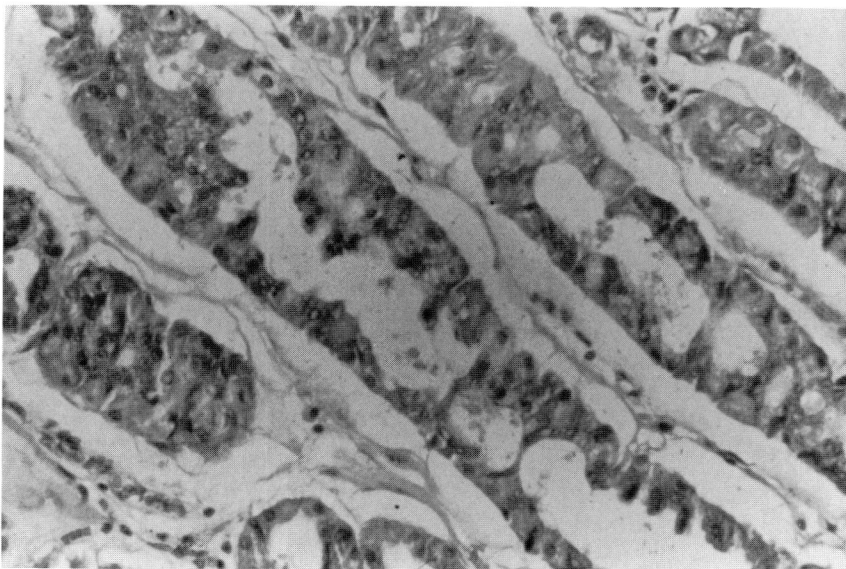

FIGURE 22-3. Gastric corpus glands in the Zollinger-Ellison syndrome; same case as in Figure 22-2, revealing the dilation of the glands and edema of the lamina propria. (H&E, × 200)

peptic ulcer disease and confirmed by documentation of maximal acid production and hypergastrinemia. Angiographic studies are typically needed to identify the presence and extent of the underlying tumor. The pathologic features in the gastric corpus are distinctive. Other causes of diffuse mucosal thickening in this area include Ménétrier's disease, which reveals a hyperplasia of the surface-foveolar mucous cells; lymphocytic (varioliform) gastritis, showing marked inflammation; and infiltration by tumor. The rarer forms of hypertrophic gastropathy, described below, may show hyperplasia of both the mucous cells and the specialized glands and are not associated with a gastrinoma.

Ménétrier's Disease

Definition, Etiology, and Pathogenesis

Ménétrier's disease, originally described in 1888,[29] is a relatively rare disorder characterized by a diffuse hyperplasia of the surface-foveolar mucous cells of the stomach.[30-34] It is usually limited to the corpus-fundic region, but may occasionally extend into parts of the antrum.[35] The causes and pathogenesis are not known, although a frequent association with prior respiratory infections has been noted in childhood cases. The disease is associated with normal or reduced gastric acid and with protein loss from the mucosa, resulting in hypoalbuminemia.[30,36,37] The reduced gastric acid noted may be due in part to dilution by the mucous secretions or to loss of the parietal cells secondary to expansion of the foveolar cells; this issue has not been satisfactorily decided.

A major problem in the understanding of Ménétrier's disease relates to the poor or uncertain documentation of the essential features in many of the reported cases.[19,38,39] There has been a tendency to consider all cases with giant folds in the proximal stomach, usually excepting cases of Zollinger-Ellison, as potential examples of Ménétrier's disease without further consideration of the histologic and functional features. This has resulted in the inclusion of many cases that are probably examples of more ordinary chronic gastritis;[40,41] indeed, the alleged association of carcinoma with Ménétrier's disease may be related instead to this confusion with other cases of chronic gastritis. The certain cases of Ménétrier's disease require the documentation of foveolar hyperplasia without marked inflammation, the lack of increased acid production, and evidence of protein loss from the mucosa.[19]

Clinical Features

Most cases are seen in adults 30 to 60 years of age, and 75% are in men. Familial cases have been recorded rarely.[42] Patients present with epigastric pain, weight loss, and diarrhea; and there is evidence of peripheral edema in many of the cases. Further studies reveal marked enlargement of the gastric rugae, protein loss in the gut from the hyperplastic mucous cells, and hypoalbuminemia causing the edema. Other causes of hypoalbuminemia, such as renal diseases, and other sources of the protein loss in the gut must be excluded. Medical treatment is mainly limited to albumin replacement and other maintenance of adequate nutrition. Some cases regress spontaneously,[43,44] but surgical resection is often required for persistent cases in adults to eliminate the lesion.[45,46]

Pathologic Features

The essential pathologic feature is a marked hyperplasia of the foveolar (pit) mucous cells.[14,18,19,37,47,48] The foveolae are greatly elongated, often tortuous and cystic in appearance, and composed mainly of mature mucous cells with little evidence of active regenerative

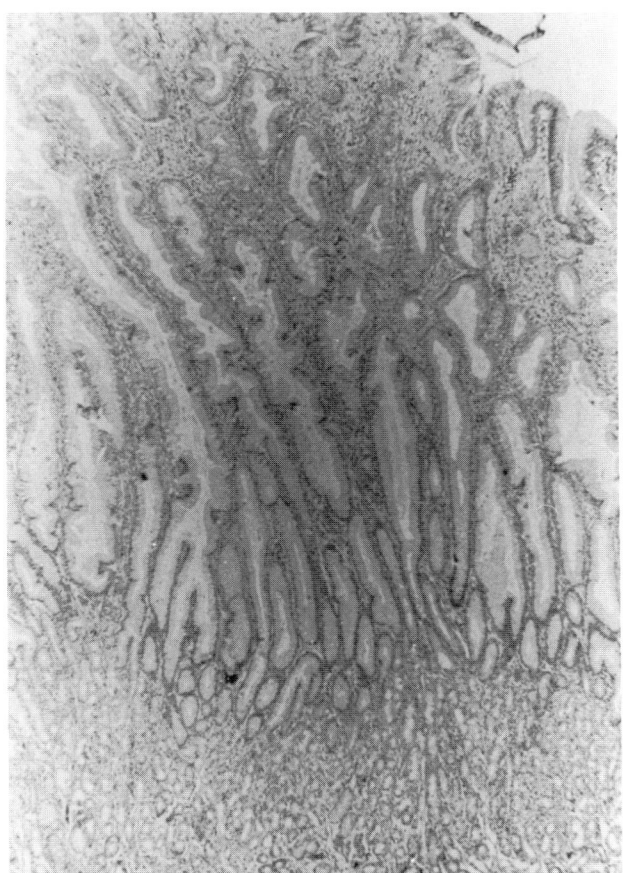

FIGURE 22-4. Gastric corpus mucosa in a case of Ménétrier's disease. There is a marked hyperplasia of the gastric foveolae (pits), with slight inflammation in the lamina propria, resulting in a thickening (hypertrophy) of the gastric mucosa. The normal corpus glands are at the bottom. The foveolar region represents about two thirds of the mucosal thickness in this sample, in contrast to the normal gastric body, where the foveolae occupy only about 20%. (H&E, × 13) (Courtesy of Dr. Donald Antonioli, Beth Israel Hospital, Boston, Massachusetts.)

cells or mitoses (Figures 22-4 to 22-6). There are no ulcerations, the number of inflammatory cells in the epithelial layer and lamina propria is typically slight, and intestinal metaplasia is uncommon. The lesion is dominantly present in the corpus region, and the quantity of underlying parietal and chief cells is either normal or moderately reduced. A marked or complete loss of the specialized corpus glands, such as occurs in cases of chronic atrophic gastritis, is not observed. The foveolar mucous cells can be accented with mucin stains such as the periodic acid–Schiff (PAS) reaction, revealing an intense staining throughout the cytoplasm (Figure 22-7). In contrast, the neutral mucin granules are typically concentrated in the upper portions of the cells in the normal stomach.

At a gross level, the rugae are irregularly enlarged and often associated with polypoid areas that are very cystic and ooze mucus from the cut surface (Figure 22-8). Mucosal biopsies can readily identify the foveolar hyperplasia and serve also to exclude other causes of enlarged rugae such as inflammatory lesions and tumors.[18,49,50] Considering the limited size of the mucosal biopsy, the sample may consist almost entirely of the hyperplastic foveolae in contrast to a biopsy of a normal or inflamed mucosa, which would contain a substantial component of the specialized glands (see Figure 22-5); in such cases, the biopsy may offer the first suggestion that the patient has Ménétrier's disease. There are no abnormalities of the rest of the gastric wall and no association with other protein-losing disorders of the gut. Contrary to some earlier reports, there is usually no associated dysplasia or carcinoma in the lesions.

Diagnosis and Differential Diagnosis

As noted above, the diagnosis of definite cases of Ménétrier's disease requires the demonstration of enlarged gastric rugae due principally to a hyperplasia of

FIGURE 22-5. Gastric corpus mucosal biopsy in a case of Ménétrier's disease, showing a marked hyperplasia of the foveolar mucous cells without significant inflammation. A small portion of the specialized glands is present at the lower left. (H&E, × 80) (From Goldman H, Antonioli DA: Mucosal biopsy of the esophagus, stomach, and proximal duodenum. Hum Pathol 13:423–448, 1982.)

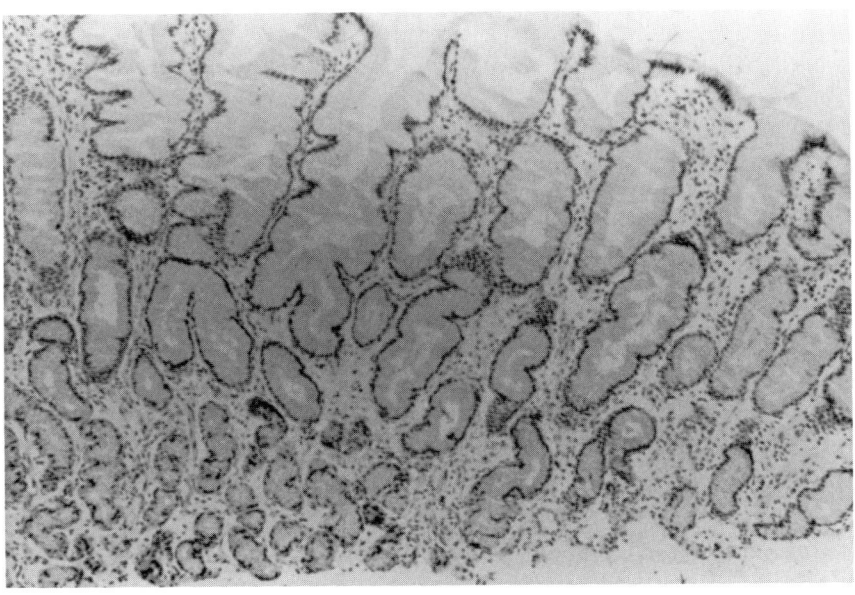

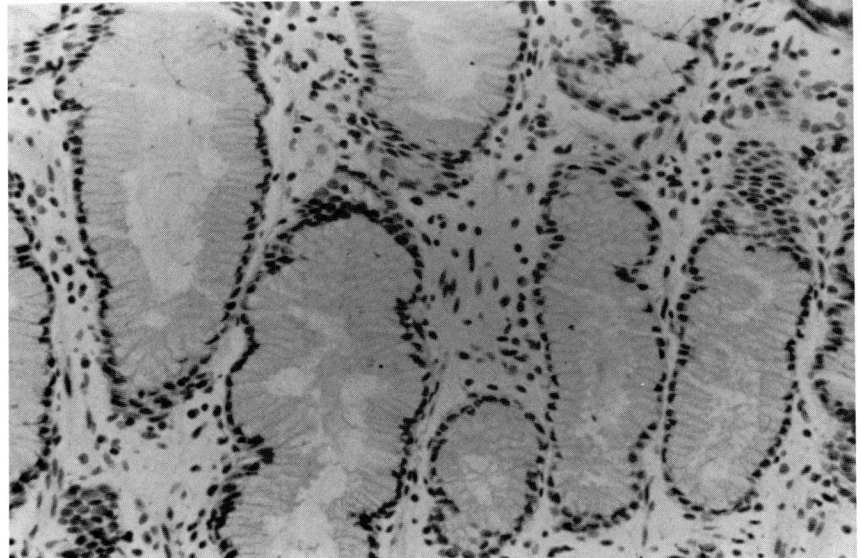

FIGURE 22–6. Gastric corpus mucosal biopsy in Ménétrier's disease; same case as Figure 22–5, showing the hyperplastic and enlarged foveolar cells whose cytoplasm is filled with mucus. The nuclei are limited to the basal region of the cells and show no signs of active regeneration. There is mild edema and a small number of mononuclear inflammatory cells in the lamina propria but no inflammation in the epithelial layer. (H&E, × 200)

the foveolar mucous cells in the proximal part of the stomach; that is, not associated with significant inflammation; the absence of hyperplasia of other epithelial elements such as parietal cells and excess acid production; and evidence of protein loss from the mucosa, leading to reduced serum albumin. It is probable that in both the early phase and the healing phase of the disease, the morphologic features can exist without significant functional effects. Unfortunately, the clinical course in most cases of Ménétrier's disease in adults is unpredictable.

Histologic confirmation is needed for assurance of the correct diagnosis and exclusion of other causes of giant folds in the proximal part of the stomach. There is acid hypersecretion and no hyperplasia of the foveolar mucous cells or protein loss in the classic Zollinger-Ellison syndrome, and considerable inflammation is noted in cases of lymphocytic gastritis and other forms of chronic gastritis. The rarer types of hypertrophic gastropathy reveal hyperplasia of both the mucous cells and the specialized glands. Tumors such as large villous adenomas, carcinomas, and lymphomas can present with gross configurations simulating enlarged mucosal folds and be associated exceptionally with protein loss; these are ultimately distinguished by histologic examination.

Problems can arise in the interpretation of the small endoscopic biopsy specimens. Because these are limited in number and size, one must carefully correlate the histologic findings with the overall gross appearance of the mucosa and the functional features. Biopsies may reveal a localized area of foveolar hyperplasia that overlies a more ominous tumor lesion or that is a part of the healing phase of an inflammatory condition. The latter is more of a problem in the antrum, where most inflammatory disorders are concentrated. Such areas of foveolar hyperplasia are usually not composed entirely of mature mucous cells, as seen in Ménétrier's disease. There is typically the presence of many mitoses and regenerating cells with enlarged nuclei and reduced cytoplasm. In selected cases, the larger aspiration and snare biopsies might be considered; these permit evaluation of a greater depth of the mucosa and can help to exclude an underlying tumor.[50]

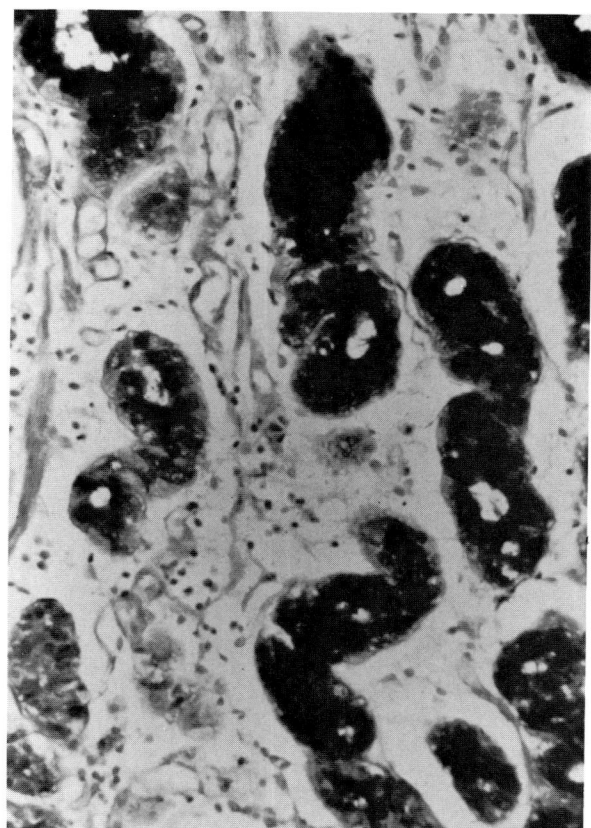

FIGURE 22–7. Gastric corpus mucosal biopsy in Ménétrier's disease; same case as Figures 22–4 and 22–5, revealing intense staining for neutral mucin in the foveolar cells. There is staining of the entire cytoplasm, in contrast to normal foveolar cells, which show the mucin limited to the upper part of the cells. (PAS, × 100)

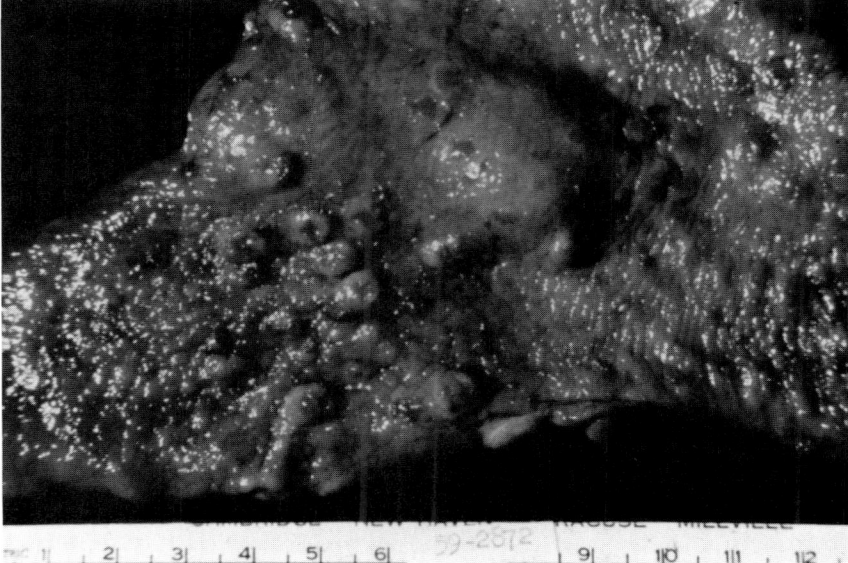

FIGURE 22–8. Stomach in a case of Ménétrier's disease, with a portion of the antrum on the left. There is an irregular thickening of the corpus mucosa with numerous polypoid areas, extending to the junction with the antrum. The normal gastric rugae are not seen. (Courtesy of Dr. Karoly Balogh, New England Deaconess Hospital, Boston, Massachusetts.)

Relation to Carcinoma

Over the years, there have been many isolated reports claiming a link between Ménétrier's disease and the development of carcinoma in adult patients, similar to that noted with chronic atrophic gastritis and pernicious anemia.[31,34,51] The documentation has been generally poor, however, and it is probable that most of these cases instead represent examples of the more common forms of chronic gastritis or situations with newly developed inflammation and repair that is secondary to the tumor. This disclaimer is supported by the frequent presence of significant inflammation in the lesions and by the lack of a defined, long-term course before the tumor development. The issue is not completely settled, but it seems unlikely that carcinoma is an important complication of Ménétrier's disease.[19]

Childhood Cases of Ménétrier's Disease

There is often an antecedent history of a respiratory infection and a peripheral blood eosinophilia, but the exact cause and pathogenesis are not established. Compared with the cases in adults, those in children are self-limited and regress spontaneously after several weeks, and there is no need for surgical excision.[52–56] There are no recurrences and no association with carcinoma. The major concern in differential diagnosis is allergic gastroenteritis, which may have enlarged gastric folds and protein loss.[57] In the allergic condition, however, the lesion is typically in the gastric antrum, there is often evidence of blood loss and anemia, and an increase of eosinophils is noted in the tissue (see Chapter 10).[58]

Other Types of Hypertrophic, Hypersecretory Gastropathy

There are other, very rare disorders, characterized by a variable hyperplasia of the foveolar mucous cells and the parietal cells.[19] Their cause and pathogenesis are not known. It is possible that some cases represent variants of the Zollinger-Ellison syndrome and Ménétrier's disease.

Cases Without Protein Loss

Cases without protein loss reveal a focal and nodular thickening of the corpus mucosa due mainly to a hyperplasia of the parietal cells, acid hypersecretion, and multiple peptic ulcers of the gastric antrum and duodenum.[59–61] There is usually no significant hyperplasia of the surface-foveolar mucous cells. These cases most closely resemble those with the Zollinger-Ellison syndrome but lack a demonstrable source of autonomous G cells and hypergastrinemia. Nevertheless, they may represent a milder form of the syndrome with a more focal hyperplasia of the parietal cell mass. Further studies are needed.

Cases with Protein Loss

The few cases with protein loss reported exhibit a hyperplasia of the foveolar mucous cells and a protein loss from the stomach. In contrast to typical Ménétrier's disease, there is also a variable expansion of the parietal cells, acid hypersecretion, and development of peptic ulcers.[62,63]

Inflammatory and Neoplastic Conditions

Inflammatory Disorders

A large variety of specific inflammatory conditions can be associated with gastric mucosal thickening, either localized or diffuse. These mainly affect the antrum and include infections such as tuberculosis and syphilis, eosinophilic (allergic) gastroenteritis, isolated granulomatous gastritis, chronic granulomatous dis-

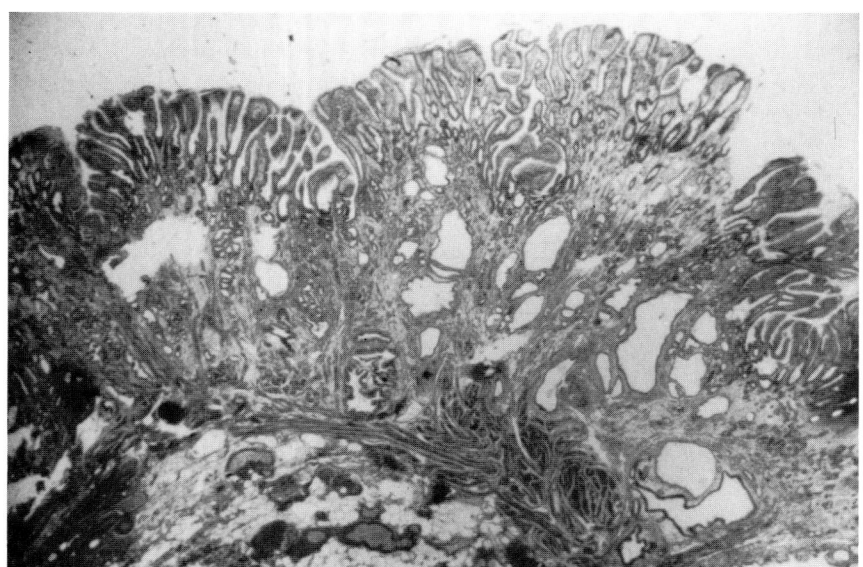

FIGURE 22–9. Gastric corpus in a case of gastritis cystica polyposa, with small portion of submucosa at bottom. This developed in the proximal stomach remnant following a subtotal resection of the distal stomach. There is a marked regeneration and hyperplasia of the gastric foveolae, some of which are cystic, a considerable loss of the specialized corpus glands, and associated inflammation in the lamina propria. (H&E, × 31)

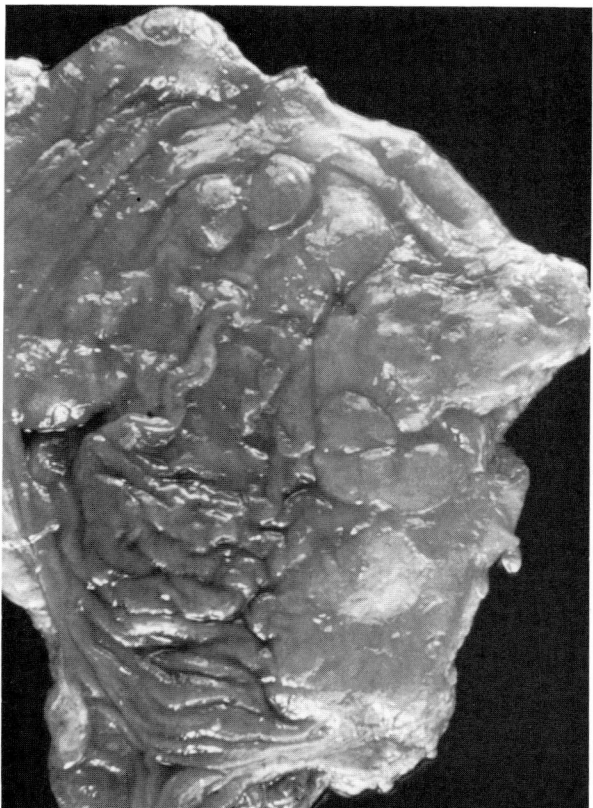

FIGURE 22–10. Stomach in a case of diffuse lymphoma, with the antral region at the bottom. There is a marked thickening and deformity of the mucosa surface throughout the stomach due to the tumor infiltration and associated edema. The normal gastric rugae are not seen.

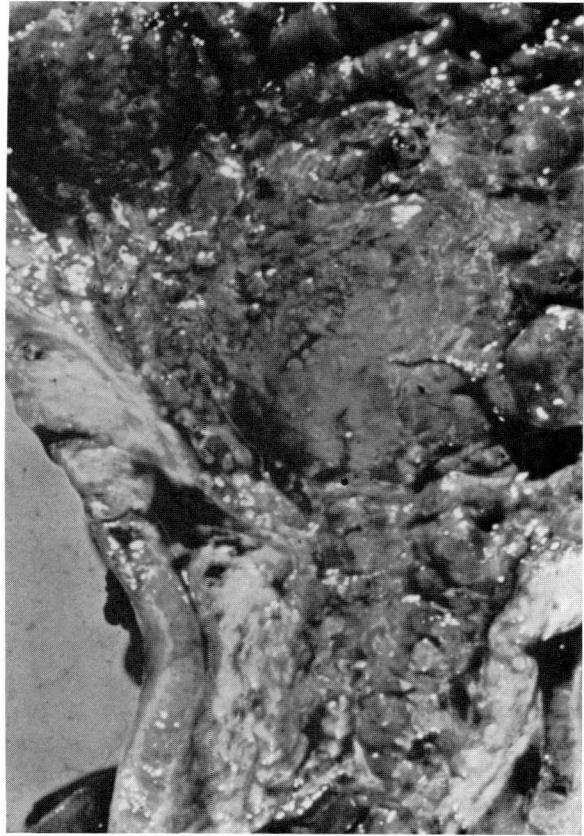

FIGURE 22–11. Stomach in a case of diffuse adenocarcinoma of the linitis plastica type, with the antral region at the bottom. In addition to the mural expansion, there is a marked thickening of the mucosa and nodular irregularity of its surface. Some remnants of gastric rugae are seen at the top.

ease, and sarcoidosis.[64-69] The mucosal hypertrophy can be marked, leading to pyloric obstruction and requiring biopsy to exclude tumors. Furthermore, in any case of the more ordinary forms of chronic antral gastritis or chronic fundic gastritis areas of polypoid or diffuse foveolar hyperplasia can develop.[70] These inflammatory disorders are typically distinguished from the syndromes described above by the presence of significant inflammation.

Lymphocytic gastritis (also termed varioliform gastritis and chronic erosive gastritis) exhibits a prominent mucosal hypertrophy of either the proximal part of the stomach or the entire stomach.[71-75] The cases can occasionally be a cause of protein loss[76] and are recognized by the heavy inflammatory infiltrate, particularly of lymphocytes in the epithelial layer, and by the alternating areas of erosions and mucosal thickenings (see Chapter 20, Figure 20–18). A marked degree of mucosal thickening is noted in cases of gastritis cystica polyposa and gastritis cystica profunda[77-80]; the former reveals cystic glands in the mucosa (Figure 22–9), whereas the latter also contains dilated glands in the submucosa. These lesions may be diffuse or more localized, and they are especially prominent next to gastrojejunostomy stomas (see Chapter 20, Figure 20–27). The allergic disorders are described in Chapter 10, and the other inflammatory conditions in Chapter 20.

Tumors

Although most neoplasms of the stomach present as solitary masses, they can occasionally be more widespread and lead to a diffuse mucosal thickening characterized by aberrant folds. These are most often seen with lymphomas (Figure 22–10), with primary carcinomas of the linitis plastica type (Figure 22–11), and rarely with metastatic tumors (see Chapter 14, on lymphomas, and Chapter 25, on gastric carcinoma).

References

1. Ming SC, Goldman H: Gastric polyps: A histogenetic classification and its relation to carcinoma. Cancer 18:721, 1965.
2. Tomasulo J: Gastric polyps: Histologic types and their relationship to gastric carcinoma. Cancer 27:1346, 1971.
3. Stemmermann GN, Hayashi T: Hyperplastic polyps of the gastric mucosa adjacent to gastroenterostomy stomas. Am J Clin Pathol 71:341, 1979.
4. Lee RG, Burt RW: The histopathology of fundic gland polyps of the stomach. Am J Clin Pathol 86:498–503, 1986.
5. Ranchod M, Lewin KJ, Dorfman RF: Lymphoid hyperplasia of the gastro-intestinal tract: A study of 26 cases and review of the literature. Am J Surg Pathol 2:383–400, 1978.
6. Watanabe H, Enjoji M, Yao T, et al: Gastric lesions in familial adenomatous polyposis coli: Their incidence and histological analysis. Hum Pathol 9:269, 1978.
7. Sachatello CR, Pickren JW, Grace JT: Generalized juvenile gastrointestinal polyposis. Gastroenterology 58:669, 1970.
8. Williams GT, Bussey HJR, Morson BC: Hamartomatous polyps in Peutz-Jeghers syndrome. N Engl J Med 299:101, 1978.
9. Burke AP, Sobin LH: The pathology of Cronkhite-Canada polyps: A comparison to juvenile polyposis. Am J Surg Pathol 13:940–946, 1989.
10. Taylor AL: The epithelial heterotopias of the alimentary tract. J Pathol Bacteriol 30:375–380, 1944.
11. Branch CD, Gross RE: Aberrant pancreatic tissue in GI tract. Surg Gynecol Obstet 82:527, 1946.
12. Barbosa JC, Dockerty MB, Waugh JM: Pancreatic heterotopia: Review of literature and report of 41 authenticated surgical cases, of which 25 were clinically significant. Surg Gynecol Obstet 85:527–542, 1946.
13. Kaneda M, Yano T, Yamamoto T, et al: Ectopic pancreas on the stomach presenting as an inflammatory abdominal mass. Am J Gastroenterol 84:663–666, 1989.
14. Ming SC: Tumors of the esophagus and stomach. In Atlas of Tumor Pathology, 2nd series, fascicle 7. Washington, DC, Armed Forces Institute of Pathology, 1973.
15. Caberwal D, Kogan SJ, Levitt SB: Ectopic pancreas presenting as an umbilical mass. J Pediatr Surg 593–595, 1977.
16. Reeder MM, Olmstead WW, Cooper PH: Large gastric folds, local or widespread. JAMA 230:273, 1974.
17. Press AJ: Practical significance of gastric rugal folds. AJR 125:172, 1975.
18. Goldman H, Antonioli DA: Mucosal biopsy of the esophagus, stomach, and proximal duodenum. Hum Pathol 13:423–448, 1982.
19. Appelman HD: Localized and extensive expansions of the gastric mucosa: Mucosal polyps and giant folds. In Appelman HD (ed): Pathology of the Esophagus, Stomach, and Duodenum. New York, Churchill Livingstone, 1984, pp 79–119.
20. Zollinger RM, Ellison EH: Primary ulcerations of jejunum associated with islet cell tumors of pancreas. Ann Surg 142:709–728, 1955.
21. Ellison EH, Wilson SD: The Zollinger-Ellison syndrome: Reappraisal and evaluation of 260 registered cases. Ann Surg 160:512, 1964.
22. Isenberg JI, Walsh JH, Grossman MI: Zollinger-Ellison syndrome. Gastroenterology 65:140–165, 1973.
23. Greider MH, Rosai J, McGuigan JE: The human pancreatic islet cells and their tumors: II. Ulcerogenic and diarrheogenic tumors. Cancer 33:1423, 1974.
24. Creutzfeldt W, Arnold R, Creutzfeldt C, et al: Pathomorphologic, biochemical and diagnostic aspects of gastrinomas (Zollinger-Ellison syndrome). Hum Pathol 6:47, 1975.
25. Gangul PC: Antral gastrin-cell hyperplasia in peptic ulcer disease. Lancet 1:583, 1974.
26. Solcia E, Capella C, Buffa R, et al: Pathology of the Zollinger-Ellison syndrome. In Fenoglio CM, Wolff M (eds): Progress in Surgical Pathology. Vol 1. New York, Masson, 1980, pp 119–133.
27. Wolfe MM, Jensen RT: Zollinger-Ellison syndrome: Current concepts in diagnosis and management. N Engl J Med 317:1200–1209, 1987.
28. McCarthy DM: The place of surgery in the Zollinger-Ellison syndrome. N Engl J Med 302:1344, 1980.
29. Ménétrier P: Des polyadenomes gastriques et de leurs rapports avec le cancer de l'estomac. Arch Physiol Norm Pathol 1:32–55, 236–262, 1888.
30. Chokas WV, Connor DH, Innes RC: Giant hypertrophy of the gastric mucosa, hypoproteinemia and edema (Ménétrier's disease). Am J Med 27:125–131, 1959.
31. Scharschmidt BF: The natural history of hypertrophic gastropathy (Ménétrier's disease): Report of a case with 16 year follow-up and review of 120 cases from the literature. Am J Med 63:644, 1977.
32. Davis JM, Gray GF, Thorbjarnarson B: Ménétrier's disease: A clinicopathologic study of six cases. Ann Surg 185:456, 1977.
33. Fieber SS, Rickert RR: Hyperplastic gastropathy. Analysis of 50 selected cases from 1955–1980. Am J Gastroenterol 76:321, 1981.
34. Cooper BT, Chadwick VS: Ménétrier's disease. In Baron JH, Moody RG (eds): Gastroenterology. I. Foregut. London, Butterworths, 1981.
35. Olmsted WW, Cooper PH, Madewell JE: Involvement of the gastric antrum in Ménétrier's disease. AJR 76:524, 1976.
36. Smith RL, Powell DW: Prolonged treatment of Ménétrier's disease with an oral anticholinergic drug. Gastroenterology 74:903, 1978.
37. Kelly DG, Miller LJ, Malagelada J-R, et al: Giant hypertrophic gastropathy (Ménétrier's disease): Pharmacologic effects on pro-

tein leakage and mucosal ultrastructure. Gastroenterology 83:581–589, 1982.
38. Riegel N, DelVecchio A, Gillson VH: Ménétrier's disease: A case report and brief literature review. Am J Gastroenterol 53:264, 1953.
39. Palmer ED: What Ménétrier really said. Gastrointest Endosc 15:83, 1968.
40. Frank BW, Kern F Jr: Ménétrier's disease: Spontaneous metamorphosis of giant hypertrophy of the gastric mucosa to atrophic gastritis. Gastroenterology 53:953, 1967.
41. Berenson MM, Sannella J, Freston JW: Ménétrier's disease: Serial morphological, secretory, and serological observations. Gastroenterology 70:257, 1976.
42. Larsen B, Tarp V, Kristensen E: Familial giant hypertrophic gastritis (Ménétrier's disease). Gut 28:1517–1521, 1987.
43. Lesser PB, Falchuk KR, Singer M, Isselbocher KJ: Ménétrier's disease: Report of a case with transient and reversible findings. Gastroenterology 68:1598–1601, 1975.
44. Walker FB IV: Spontaneous remission in hypertrophic gastropathy (Ménétrier's disease). South Med J 74:1273, 1981.
45. Scott HW Jr, Shull HJ, Law DH IV, et al: Surgical management of Ménétrier's disease with protein-losing gastropathy. Ann Surg 181:765, 1975.
46. Gold BM, Meyers MA: Progression of Ménétrier's disease with postoperative gastrojejunal intussusception. Gastroenterology 73:583, 1977.
47. Kenney FD, Dockerty MB, Waugh JM: Giant hypertrophy of gastric mucosa: A clinical and pathological study. Cancer 7:671, 1954.
48. Butz WC: Giant hypertrophic gastritis: A report of fourteen cases. Gastroenterology 39:183, 1960.
49. Bjork JT, Geenen JE, Komorowski RA, et al: Ménétrier's disease diagnosed by electrosurgical snare biopsy. JAMA 238:1755, 1977.
50. Komorowski RA, Caya JG, Geenen JE: The morphologic spectrum of large gastric folds: Utility of the snare biopsy. Gastrointest Endosc 32:190–192, 1986.
51. Morson BC, Sobin LH, Grundmann E, et al: Precancerous conditions and epithelial dysplasia in the stomach. J Clin Pathol 33:711–721, 1980.
52. Sandberg DH: Hypertrophic gastropathy (Ménétrier's disease) in childhood. J Pediatr 78:866, 1971.
53. Chouraqui JP, Roy CC, Brochu P, et al: Ménétrier's disease in children: Report of a patient and review of sixteen other cases. Gastroenterology 80:1042, 1981.
54. Stillman AE, Sieber O, Manthei U, et al: Transient protein-losing enteropathy and enlarged gastric rugae in childhood. Am J Dis Child 135:29, 1981.
55. Kraut JR, Powell R, Hruby MA, Lloyd-Still JD: Ménétrier's disease in childhood: Report of two cases and a review of the literature. J Pediatr Surg 16:707–711, 1981.
56. Baker A, Volberg F, Summer T, Moran R: Childhood Ménétrier's disease: Four new cases and discussion of the literature. Gastrointest Radiol 11:131–134, 1986.
57. Teele RL, Katz AJ, Goldman H, et al: The radiographic features of eosinophilic gastroenteritis (allergic gastroenteropathy) of childhood. Am J Radiol 132:575, 1979.
58. Goldman H, Proujansky R: Allergic proctitis and gastroenteritis in children: Clinical and mucosal biopsy features in 53 cases. Am J Surg Pathol 10:75–86, 1986.
59. Schindler R: On hypertrophic glandular gastritis, hypertrophic gastropathy, and parietal cell mass. Gastroenterology 45:77, 1963.
60. Stempien SJ, Dagradi AE, Reingold IM, et al: Hypertrophic hypersecretory gastropathy: Analysis of 15 cases and a review of the pertinent literature. Am J Dig Dis 9:471, 1964.
61. Tann DTD, Stempien SJ, Dagradi AE: The clinical spectrum of hypertrophic hypersecretory gastropathy: Report of 50 patients. Gastrointest Endosc 18:69, 1971.
62. Brooks AM, Isenberg J, Goldstein H: Giant thickening of the gastric mucosa with acid hypersecretion and protein-losing gastropathy. Gastroenterology 58:73, 1970.
63. Overholt BF, Jeffries GH: Hypertrophic, hypersecretory protein-losing gastropathy. Gastroenterology 58:80, 1970.
64. Subei I, Attar B, Schmitt G, Levendoglu H: Primary gastric tuberculosis: A case report and literature review. Am J Gastroenterol 82:769–772, 1987.
65. Besses C, Sans-Sabrofen J, Badia X, et al: Ulceroinfiltrative syphilitic gastropathy: Silver stain diagnosis from biopsy specimen. Am J Gastroenterol 82:773–774, 1987.
66. Katz AJ, Goldman H, Grand RJ: Gastric mucosal biopsy in eosinophilic (allergic) gastroenteritis. Gastroenterology 73:705, 1977.
67. Khan MH, Lam R, Tamoney HJ: Isolated granulomatous gastritis. Am J Gastroenterol 71:90, 1979.
68. Ament ME, Ochs HD: Gastrointestinal manifestations of chronic granulomatous disease. N Engl J Med 288:382, 1973.
69. Chinitz MA, Brandt LJ, Frank MS, et al: Symptomatic sarcoidosis of the stomach. Dig Dis Sci 30:682–688, 1985.
70. Stamp GWH, Palmer K, Misiewicz JJ: Antral hypertrophic gastritis: A rare cause of iron deficiency. J Clin Pathol 38:390–392, 1985.
71. Clarke AC, Lee SP, Nicholson GI: Gastritis varioliformis. Am J Gastroenterol 68:599–602, 1977.
72. Lambert R, Andre C, Moulinier B, Bugnon B: Diffuse varioliform gastritis. Digestion 17:159–167, 1978.
73. Green PHR, Gold RP, Marboe CC, et al: Chronic erosive gastritis: Clinical, diagnostic and pathological features in nine patients. Am J Gastroenterol 77:543–547, 1982.
74. Elta GH, Fawaz KA, Dayal Y, et al: Chronic erosive gastritis—a recently recognized disorder. Dig Dis Sci 28:7–12, 1983.
75. Haot J, Jouret A, Willette M, et al: Lymphocytic gastritis—prospective study of its relationship with varioliform gastritis. Gut 31:282–285, 1990.
76. Crampton JR, Hunter JO, Neale G, Wight DGD: Chronic lymphocytic gastritis and protein losing gastropathy. Gut 30:71–74, 1989.
77. Littler ER, Gleibermann E: Gastritis cystica polyposa (gastric mucosal prolapse at gastroenterostomy site, with cystic and infiltrative epithelial hyperplasia). Cancer 29:205, 1972.
78. Honore LH, Lewis AS, Ohara KE: Gastritic glandularis et cystica profunda: Report of 3 cases with discussion of etiology and pathogenesis. Dig Dis Sci 24:48–52, 1979.
79. Franzen G, Novelli P: Gastritis cystica profunda. Histopathology 5:535–547, 1981.
80. Fonde EC, Rodning CB: Gastritis cystica profunda. Am J Gastroenterol 81:459–464, 1986.

CHAPTER 23

Epithelial Polyps of the Stomach

SI-CHUN MING, M.D.

DEFINITION AND INCIDENCE	Incidence Histogenesis	**HAMARTOMATOUS POLYP** Peutz-Jeghers Syndrome
CLINICAL ASPECTS	Subtypes and Pathology Flat Adenoma	Juvenile Polyposis Syndrome Fundic Gland Polyp
HISTOLOGIC DIAGNOSIS AND TISSUE SAMPLING	Papillary (Villous) Adenoma Malignancy and Adenoma	Foveolar Polyp **INFLAMMATORY POLYP**
HISTORICAL REVIEW	**HYPERPLASTIC (REGENERATIVE) POLYP**	**HETEROTOPIC POLYP**
HISTOLOGIC CLASSIFICATION	Histogenesis and Various Forms Pathology	Heterotopic Pancreas Brunner's Gland Hyperplasia
ADENOMAS	Malignant Potential	Adenomyoma

DEFINITION AND INCIDENCE

A polyp is a nodular lesion that protrudes above the mucosal surface of the stomach into the lumen. Such a lesion can be neoplastic as well as nonneoplastic and implies no tissue or cellular composition. Its nature can be determined only by histologic examination. When the histologic composition is known, the term *polyp* is usually applied to a lesion with prominent epithelial components. The relative frequency of benign polypoid lesions is listed in Table 23–1.[1] Excluded from this table are the lesions caused by diffuse mucosal hyperplasia.

Gastric polyps are not common. Their incidence among autopsies and by radiologic survey is about 0.4%.[2] In a mass survey in Japan, gastric polyps were found in 0.23%.[3] In recent years, gastroscopy has been widely used. The incidence of gastric polyps found at endoscopy is higher, about 3% to 5%.[4-6] Among the tumors, polyps used to account for 3.1% of all gastric tumors and 41% of benign tumors.[1] The frequency has increased to about 90% of benign tumors in patients who have undergone endoscopy.[4] The incidence of gastric polyps is high in certain conditions: 22% to 37% in pernicious anemia[7,8]; 6% in chronic atrophic gastritis[9]; and 4% to 20% in the gastric stump after partial gastrectomy, depending on postresection duration.[10,11] Carcinoma often coexists with polyps in the same stomach.[2,12] Morson found polyps in 44% of consecutively resected carcinomatous stomachs.[13]

CLINICAL ASPECTS

The polyps can be classified according to the location of the bulk of the lesion in relation to the wall of the stomach into intraluminal and intramural types. Such a distinction is clinically relevant. The intraluminal polyp is usually a mucosal lesion, which may bleed if its surface is eroded, or obstruct if it is large and located near the orifices of the stomach. The intramural lesion is usually submucosal and is asymptomatic if small. When it is large, the covering mucosa may become ulcerated and bleed. A large intramural mass may also be obstructive if strategically located. Other symptoms are usually vague and infrequent; they include epigastric discomfort, anorexia, and dyspepsia.

Table 23-1. BENIGN POLYPOID LESIONS OF THE STOMACH IN ORDER OF FREQUENCY

Type of Lesion	Total Number	%
Epithelial polyp	252	40.9
Leiomyoma	230	37.3
Inflammatory polyp	29	4.7
Heterotopic tissue	25	4.1
Lipoma	21	3.4
Neurogenic tumor	19	3.1
Vascular tumor	13	2.1
Eosinophilic granuloma	12	1.9
Fibroma	9	1.5
Miscellaneous lesions	6	1.0
Total	616	100.0

Modified from Ming SC: Tumors of the Esophagus and Stomach. In Atlas of Tumor Pathology, Second Series, Fascicle 7. Armed Forces Institute of Pathology, Washington, DC, 1973, p 99.

HISTOLOGIC DIAGNOSIS AND TISSUE SAMPLING

In order to establish a correct diagnosis and to render a proper treatment, one must make a histologic diagnosis on the basis of biopsied tissue. This was dramatically illustrated by Niv and Bat, who found that nearly one half of 99 polyps seen in 13,500 gastroscopies turned out to be either normal or inflammatory in the biopsy.[14] The interpretation of the biopsy sample also requires care. A mucosal or superficial biopsy of the polyp will not reveal the nature of a submucosally located intramural lesion. Even for the mucosal or intraluminal lesion, a superficial biopsy may not be diagnostic, because the histologic features of different types of lesions may be similar in focal areas. For instance, the hyperplastic, juvenile, and inflammatory polyps all have elongated and dilated foveolae and interstitial inflammation. A definite diagnosis may not be possible unless the entire lesion is examined. Seifert and Elster compared the diagnoses of biopsied and excised tissues of the same polyps and noted that discrepancies were present in 53 of 75 polyps; significant inadequacy of the biopsied specimen was noted in 20 of these 53 polyps.[15] Furthermore, an excisional biopsy is clearly necessary for evaluation of possible malignant change within the polyp.

HISTORICAL REVIEW

The first report of a gastric polyp was said to be made by Amatus Lusitanus in 1557 (cited by Marshak and Feldman[16]). Morgagni was said to have described a pedunculated polyp near the pylorus in 1761, and Cruveilhier in 1835 mentioned that the polyp might cause obstruction or become malignant (cited by Spriggs[17]). It was not until 1888, however, that the formation process and the malignant transformation of the gastric polyp were described and illustrated in detail by Ménétrier.[18] Ménétrier gave the name *polyadenoma* to multiple polyps in the stomach and classified them into two categories: polypoid polyadenomas (*polyadenomes polypeux*) and clothlike polyadenomas (*polyadenomes en nappe*). The basic pathologic features were those of glandular hyperplasia, which in the former was localized in the form of sessile or pedunculated polyps and in the latter was extensive, forming large mucosal folds resembling ruffled cloth or cerebral convolutions that could be either localized or diffuse. Ménétrier described two cases of carcinoma of the stomach with metastasis to the liver. One was an ulcerated carcinoma accompanied by multiple polypoid polyadenomas, and the other was a diffusely infiltrating carcinoma with large mucosal folds. The latter condition of clothlike polyadenoma is now known as Ménétrier's disease and is described in detail in Chapter 22. It is rare, and its malignant potential is uncertain, although there are reports of this effect.[19] The malignant potential of polypoid polyadenoma is a controversial topic.

Ménétrier's *polyadenomes polypeux* are hyperplastic polyps that are not neoplastic, according to the current understanding of the disease. His case 6 showed an ulcerated carcinoma in a stomach with multiple polyps. A similar case was reported by Mills.[20] These are cases of association between polyp and carcinoma but not a developmental continuum. However, some authors used the presence of a separate carcinoma as evidence of the malignant potential of the polyp,[21-23] and the reported incidence of carcinoma in the stomach with polyps was as high as 51%.[22] There were also reports of malignant change in the polyp. The incidences varied from 0% to 29%.[21,24-29] These results are difficult to interpret because neither the histologic nature of the polyp nor the criteria for malignancy were always described. Some authors relied instead on the size and the number of the polyps as indicators of malignant potential. Predictably, the results varied greatly.[2]

The first significant effort in the histologic classification of gastric polyps was made by Rieniets and Broders in 1945 and 1946.[30] In a series of publications, they divided gastric polyps into 18 different types in two basic forms. One form was called adenoma, made of hyperplastic glands and tubules. The other form was called papillary adenoma. These forms correspond to the current terms *hyperplastic polyp* and *adenoma*. Rieniets and Broders recognized the high incidence of malignant transformation in the papillary adenomas. Malignant change in such a lesion was reported as early as 1917 by Finney and Friedenwald, who reported two cases of papilloma; in one case, a follow-up biopsy revealed malignancy.[31] In 1951, Walk reviewed 51 reported and 2 new cases of villous tumors of the stomach.[32] There were 67 tumors, with malignancy in 40 (60%). Additional case reports confirmed malignant change in villous adenomas of the stomach.[33-35]

It had become apparent by the early 1960s that the significance of gastric polyps lay in their malignant potential, that the malignant potential was not uniform among the polyps, and that the polyps might be histologically heterogeneous. In 1965, Ming and Goldman recognized two basic forms of gastric polyps: one was composed of normal-appearing cells lining elongated and hyperplastic foveolae and pyloric-type glands; the other contained glands made of atypical cells similar to those in a colonic adenoma.[36] The former type was given the name *regenerative polyp*, implying a reparative nature; the latter was called *adenomatous polyp*, with the same pathologic implication as the adenomatous polyp of the colon. These two types have, in addition to cytologic differences, different gross morphologic features and strikingly different malignant potential: there is essentially no malignant potential in the former and high malignant potential in the latter. Since then, these basic concepts have remained correct. Minor modifications have been made, however. For instance, a more commonly used name for the regenerative polyp is *hyperplastic polyp*, as proposed by Tomasulo,[37] because the cause of this polyp is unknown, although the reparative nature of the polyp remains most likely. Another modification is the recognition of a flat form of adenoma, in contrast to the papillovillous type.[2] The flat adenoma was first reported in Japan as a form of atypical epithelium[38] or borderline lesion.[39] It is relatively common in Japan and rare in the United States. The third modification is the realization that the stomach and other parts of the upper gastrointestinal tract are frequently affected in the genetically controlled polyposis syndromes, which primarily affect the colon. Gastric polyps are common in patients with Gardner's syndrome, or familial polyposis coli,[40] and juvenile polyposis.[41] Similarly, the stomach is often involved in the nonhereditary Cronkhite-Canada syndrome.[42]

HISTOLOGIC CLASSIFICATION OF EPITHELIAL POLYPS

Classification of the epithelial polyps of the stomach is best when based on the histologic and cytologic features of the lesion. Table 23–2 lists the major subtypes of the polyps. The benign neoplastic polyps are composed of immature and dysplastic cells similar to those present in the colonic adenoma. On the basis of the architectural pattern, the cytologic appearances of component cells, and the known biologic potentials, the adenomas are subdivided into flat and papillary (villous) types. Rarely, dysplastic or adenomatous lesions are present in the hyperplastic polyp. Some malignant epithelial tumors, namely, carcinoma and carcinoid, may appear polypoid. They can be either primary or secondary. The latter type is usually submucosal. The nonneoplastic polyps are composed of normal-appearing epithelial structures and cells, together with varying amounts of similarly normal-appearing mesenchymal tissue. The most common subtype is the hyperplastic polyp. Hyperplastic foveolae and pyloric-type glands are the dominant structures. Hamartomatous polyps are composed of tissues that are normal for the site, including both the epithelial and mesenchymal elements. The inflammatory polyps are made largely of inflammatory cells. The heterotopic polyps are choristomas containing tissues of neighboring organs not present in the normal stomach. Finally, the polyp may be composed of nodules of normal mucosa surrounded by atrophic tissue.

Table 23-2. HISTOLOGIC CLASSIFICATION OF EPITHELIAL GASTRIC POLYPS

Neoplastic polyp
  Benign: Adenoma
    Flat (tubular) adenoma
    Papillary (villous) adenoma
  Malignant
    Primary polypoid carcinoma and carcinoid
    Secondary tumors
Nonneoplastic polyp
  Hyperplastic polyp
    Polypoid foveolar hyperplasia
    Hyperplastic (regenerative) polyp
    Hyperplastic polyp with dysplastic (adenomatous) lesion
  Hamartomatous polyp
    Peutz-Jeghers polyp
    Juvenile polyp
    Fundic gland polyp
    Foveolar polyp
  Inflammatory polyp
    Inflammatory (retention) polyp
    Polyp in Cronkhite-Canada syndrome
  Heterotopic polyp
    Ectopic pancreatic tissue
    Ectopic Brunner gland hyperplasia
    Adenomyoma
Nodular mucosal remnants

There are other classifications of gastric polyps. They are compared in Table 23–3. The classification proposed by Elster[43] is popular in Europe. It introduces the concept of foveolar hyperplasia as a separate entity. Endoscopically, this lesion is small and sessile. It is common at the region of healing ulcer or erosion and areas adjacent to carcinoma. In the larger lesion, the hyperplastic foveolae expand and elongate toward the mucosal base, where the glands proper remain largely unchanged. This type of polyp was given the name *hyperplasiogenous polyp* by Elster to indicate organ specificity and to distinguish it from the hyperplastic polyp of the colon. When the glands proper become hyperplastic and increased in number, the polyp takes on an adenomatous appearance. Elster considered this type of polyp a well-differentiated adenoma. Such polyps have also been called hyperplastic adenomatous polyps.[44,45] In the recent classification, all of these forms are considered merely variants of hyperplastic polyp.[2] Rarely, part of the hyperplastic polyp contains atypical glands identical to those of a true adenoma.[46] Such a polyp is considered to have mixed adenomatous and nonneoplastic hyperplastic components,[47] and the adenomatous elements may be precancerous.[46,48] Nakamura and Nakano divided gastric polyps into four types.[49] Type I is an eroded sessile polyp with foveolar hyperplasia; type II corresponds to the usual hyperplastic polyp. Type III is the flat adenoma, and type IV is the papillary adenoma.

In 1955, Morson called attention to the fact that some gastric polyps are composed of intestinal epithelium.[13] He noted that three of five such polyps under-

Table 23-3. COMPARISON OF CLASSIFICATIONS OF HYPERPLASTIC AND ADENOMATOUS GASTRIC POLYPS

Authors	Nonneoplastic Polyp			Neoplastic Polyp		
Ming[2,46,48]	——————Hyperplastic (regenerative) polyp——————			——————Adenoma——————		
	Polypoid foveolar hyperplasia	——————Hyperplastic polyp——————		Adenomatous lesion in hyperplastic polyp	Flat adenoma	Papillary (villous) adenoma
Elster[43]	Focal foveolar hyperplasia	Hyperplasiogenous polyp	Adenoma with high differentiation		Borderline lesion, protruded	Adenoma with moderate differentiation
Koch et al[45]	Polypoid foveolar hyperplasia	Hyperplastic polyp	Hyperplastic adenomatous polyp	Adenomatous villous polyp		Villous polyp
Snover[47]	Foveolar hyperplasia	——————Hyperplastic polyp——————		Mixed adenomatous hyperplastic polyp		Adenomatous, villoglandular, villous polyp
Nakamura and Nakano[49]	Type II polyp	——————Type I polyp——————			Type III polyp	Type IV polyp
Kozuka et al[50,51]	——————Hyperplastic (gastric type) polyp——————			Hyperplastic polyp with adenoma	Adenomatous (metaplastic) polyp	
Goldman and Appelman[52]	——————Polyp without atypical hyperplasia——————			——————Polyp with atypical hyperplasia——————		

Not included: foveolar adenoma[47] and antral foveolar polyp.[52] These do not have counterparts in other classifications.

went malignant change, whereas seven polyps with gastric epithelium did not. A similar view was held by Kozuka and colleagues, who also divided gastric polyps into gastric and metaplastic types.[50] Malignant change was present in 42% of the latter, less than 1% of the former, and 10% of polyps with mixed epithelia. The metaplastic polyps are mostly adenomas and the gastric polyps are hyperplastic polyps.[51] Goldman and Appelman classified gastric polyps according to the presence or absence of atypical hyperplasia.[52] All polyps that underwent malignant change had atypical hyperplasia. In addition, they described a form of antral polyp composed of compact foveolar cells and called it the antral foveolar polyp. A similar lesion called foveolar adenoma was described by Snover.[47] However, this lesion was located in the body of the stomach. Snover also documented seven polyps with mixed adenomatous and hyperplastic features.

ADENOMAS

Incidence

Adenomas of the stomach are not common. Among epithelial gastric polyps, the incidence of adenoma is 8% to 10%.[5,36,47,53,54] High incidences of 15.5% and 25% were reported by Stamm and associates[55] and Tomasulo,[37] respectively. The adenomas occur mainly in the early seventh decade of life, with an average age at 62.6 years.[56] Its incidence increases with age, being only 0.1% in the third decade and rising to 3.7% in the ninth decade.[57] Men are more affected than women, with a ratio of about 2:1. The preferred location is the distal portion of the stomach, particularly the antrum.[36–38]

Histogenesis

Adenoma of the stomach resembles adenoma of the colon in its histologic appearance. It is composed of immature cells with varying degrees of dysplasia. Most cells are tall, columnar cells without specific markers. It is not uncommon, however, that a distinct, although often short and coarse, striated border is present on the luminal surface of the cells, indicating an intestinal character. Other intestinal features include goblet cells and Paneth cells. Argentaffin cells may be present also.[36,37,58] The mucin in the adenoma is often acidic,[59] secreted by the normal intestines but not the normal stomach. Furthermore, the mucosa surrounding the adenoma usually shows atrophic gastritis with prominent intestinal metaplasia, including the incomplete type.[13,36] These features suggest a relationship between gastric adenoma and intestinal metaplasia, and the term *metaplastic polyp* has been applied to the adenoma.[50] However, the relationship between adenoma and incomplete intestinal metaplasia is uncertain, because Paneth cells and striated borders are not features of incomplete metaplasia.[59,60]

The adenomas by definition are noninvasive. Nevertheless, they show horizontal spread of the neoplastic cells within the confines of the epithelium, resulting in a sharp demarcation between the adenoma and the neighboring nonneoplastic epithelium.

Subtypes and Pathology

The World Health Organization (WHO) histologic typing divides the gastric adenomas into tubular, tubulovillous (papillotubular), and villous (papillary) types.[61] These histologic patterns are reflected by two

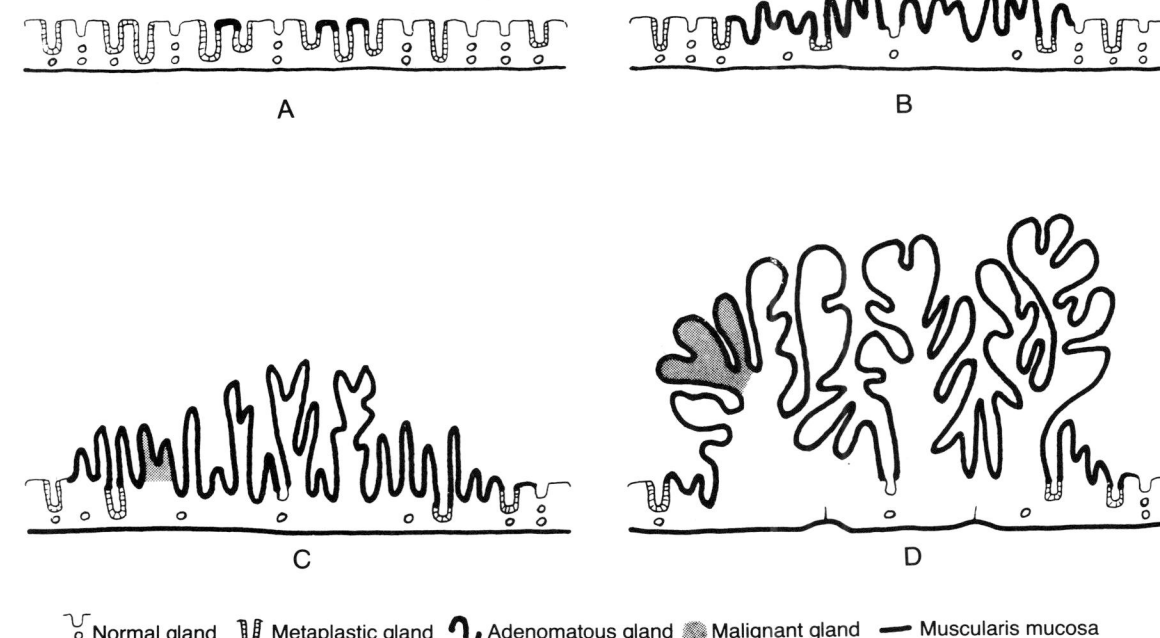

FIGURE 23–1. Schematic presentation of the subtypes of gastric adenoma. A, Adenoma develops in the superficial epithelium in a metaplastic mucosa. B, Flat (tubular) adenoma. The adenoma shows a horizontal growth and occupies the upper layer of the mucosa. Nonneoplastic gastric tissue remains in the deep region. C, Villous or papillotubular adenoma. The adenoma shows a vertical as well as horizontal growth with villous projections. D, Papillary adenoma. The adenoma shows a balanced horizontal and vertical growth. Deep crevices separate the adenoma into nodular partitions. Malignant change may occur in any area, more frequently in the elevated lesions. (From Ming SC: Tumors of the Esophagus and Stomach. Supplement. In Atlas of Tumor Pathology, Second Series, Fascicle 7. Armed Forces Institute of Pathology, Washington, DC, 1985, p S24.)

gross forms, namely, flat and papillary. The former includes the tubular adenoma, and the latter includes the papillotubular and papillary (villous) histologic types. These two types are schematically represented in Figure 23–1. The adenomas are usually solitary lesions. In Watanabe's series[58] of 75 cases, single adenomas were seen in 50 patients, two adenomas in 19 patients, three adenomas in 5 patients, and five adenomas in 1 patient. There is no evidence that the individual adenomas are multicellular in origin, but they may be seen in discontinuous patches in the histologic sections.

Flat Adenoma

Flat adenoma of the stomach is called tubular adenoma by the WHO classification.[61] It is the most common form of adenoma in the stomach. The flat adenoma is usually a slightly elevated lesion with an irregular but flat surface or takes on varying degrees of nodularity (Figure 23–2). It is also known as a IIa-like lesion,[56] because its gross shape resembles the raised type IIa early carcinoma of the stomach (see Chapter 24). Occasional lesions may be smooth surfaced, even with the surface of the surrounding mucosa (IIb-like lesion).[56,57] Recently, a grossly depressed form (IIc-like lesion) has been reported.[62] The protruded ones (I-like) may be sessile (Is-like) or pedunculated (Ip-like). The respective frequencies of these types among 213 flat adenomas analyzed by Hirota at the National Cancer Center Research Institute, Tokyo, Japan (T. Hirota, personal communication), were as follows: Is-like type, 9.4%; Ip-like type, 0.9%; IIa-like type, 68.1%; IIb-like type, 13.6%; IIc-like type, 5.2%; and combined IIa and IIc-like lesions, 2.8%. The flat adenomas are usually small, averaging 1 cm in diameter. Over 80% of them are less than 2 cm in diameter.[56]

The histologic features of flat adenoma are unique. Although the cells in other adenomas, including those in the colon, extend to the entire thickness of the mucosa, the gastric flat adenoma, particularly the IIa-like type, usually occupies only the upper one third to one half of the gastric mucosa and maintains a two-layer structure (Figure 23–3A and B). The depressed adenomas usually occupy the whole thickness of the mucosa.

In flat adenomas, the cells are slender and compact, and the rows of nuclei form a picket-fence appearance along the base of the cells (Figure 23–3C). Pleomorphism and mitosis are not evident. The lack of aggressive growth is correlated with the relative absence of active cell proliferation, as compared with the cells in the papillary adenoma. Electron microscopy reveals features resembling the intestinal-type carcinoma with sparse microvilli, reduced endoplasmic reticulum and mucin granules, and the presence of blebs on the apical surface. These features were taken as indicative of the neoplastic nature of the lesion and a tendency to malignancy.[63] The deep glands are cytologically normal, although cystic dilatation and metaplastic changes are common. The dilatation of the deep glands is probably due to interruption of the excretory upper portion of

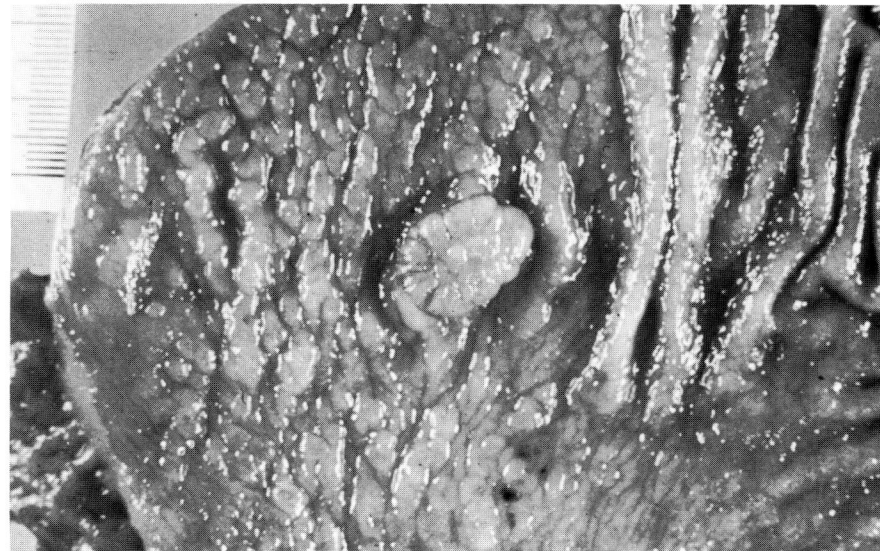

FIGURE 23–2. Flat adenoma, gross morphology. The adenoma is a IIa-like lesion. It is raised slightly above the mucosal surface. (Courtesy of Dr. T. Hirota, National Cancer Center Research Institute, Tokyo, Japan.)

the glands by the adenomatous tissue. The two-layer architecture and relative indolence of the immature epithelial cells are hallmarks distinguishing the flat adenoma from the papillary adenoma.

The intermediate position of the flat adenoma, in terms of the size and shape, between the normal mucosa and the papillary (villous) adenoma suggests the possibility that flat adenomas are the earlier lesions of the latter. However, follow-up studies have not confirmed this view. Most flat adenomas appear stationary. Kamiya and co-workers followed 85 lesions in 74 patients for 6 months to 12 years, and only 8 showed gross changes: 4 became smaller and 4 others larger.[57] None disappeared.

In spite of the lack of growth, the flat adenoma is clearly neoplastic, as evidenced by the cellular atypism and a relatively high incidence of malignant change, about 10%, within the lesion. Conversely, it has been equated with the dysplastic epithelium. Sugano and coauthors were among the first to call attention to this lesion. They called it simply "atypical epithelium"[38] Nagayo was instrumental in devising a five-group grading system from normal (group 1) to cancer (group 5) for the evaluation of the gastric mucosa in the biopsies.[39] The group 3 lesion is called a borderline lesion, and the flat adenoma was used to illustrate this lesion. Thus the flat adenoma and dysplasia have unfortunately been taken by some to be synonymous. They must be distinguished. The flat adenoma is characterized by a relative uniformity in its composition of immature cells lining the branching and interrelated network of tubules.[64] It is a sharply delineated lesion, and the atypical cells end abruptly when they meet the normal neighboring cells (Figure 23–4). These features are common to other adenomas in the digestive tract. In contrast, the common dysplastic epithelium exhibits a reactive process in a labile state. The degree of dysplasia fluctuates from area to area and in various times. The change is gradual, and the mucosa as a whole is usually atrophic, although the shortened glands are actively proliferating. Details of dysplastic changes in the gastric mucosa are described in Chapter 25.

Papillary (Villous) Adenoma

Papillary adenomas of the stomach are nodular lesions with a papillary contour and deep crevices. (Figures 23–5 and 23–6). They are either sessile or broad-based. On radiologic examination, barium trapped in the crevices gives a soap-bubble appearance. They are soft, velvety, and freely mobile. Fixation to the deep tissue indicates carcinomatous change with invasion. The size varies. A size as large as 15 cm in the greatest dimension has been reported.[33,34] The average size is 4 cm.[32,36] They are located more commonly in the antrum than elsewhere.

The papillary or villous pattern is histologically evident; (Figures 23–7 and 23–8). The predominant cells are columnar cells, some of which have striated borders (Figure 23–9). Goblet cells (Figure 23–10) and, rarely, Paneth cells are present. Sulfomucin as well as sialomucin are often present, although some have reported negative results for sulfomucin.[65] Adenomas with malignant change are positive for carcinoembryonic antigen.[65] There are also cells containing gastrin, somatostatin, and glicentin.[66] The cells in papillary adenomas are typically dysplastic. In contrast to the relative uniformity of cells in flat adenomas, pleomorphism and mitoses are common in papillary adenomas. The neoplastic cells end abruptly at the junction with the neighboring epithelium, which often exhibits prominent intestinal metaplasia (Figure 23–11).

Rarely, the villous adenoma appears to be composed of gastric epithelial cells. Among 144 adenomas in Hirota's series, 6 (4.2%) were the gastric type, 3 (2.1%) had mixed gastric and intestinal cells, and the rest were the intestinal type.[56]

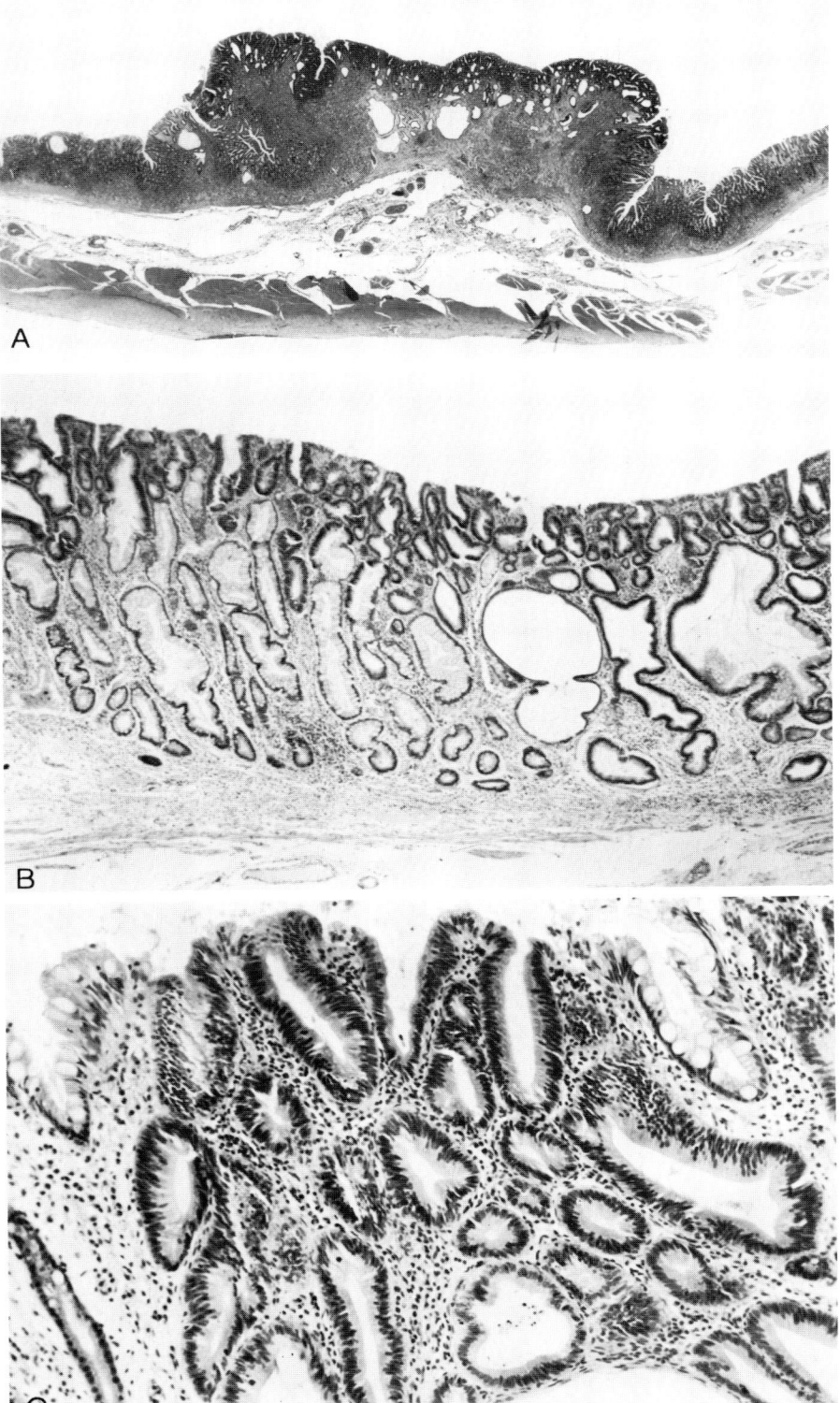

FIGURE 23–3. Flat adenoma, histologic appearance. *A*, Scanning view of the lesion shown in Figure 23–2. The adenomatous tissue occupies the upper third of the mucosa. The deep glands are dilated. *B*, Higher magnification to show the two-tier appearance. The glands at left show intestinal metaplasia. (× 80) *C*, The adenomatous glands are lined by compact columnar cells. The slender nuclei are basally located. The adjacent mucosa shows intestinal metaplasia. (× 200)

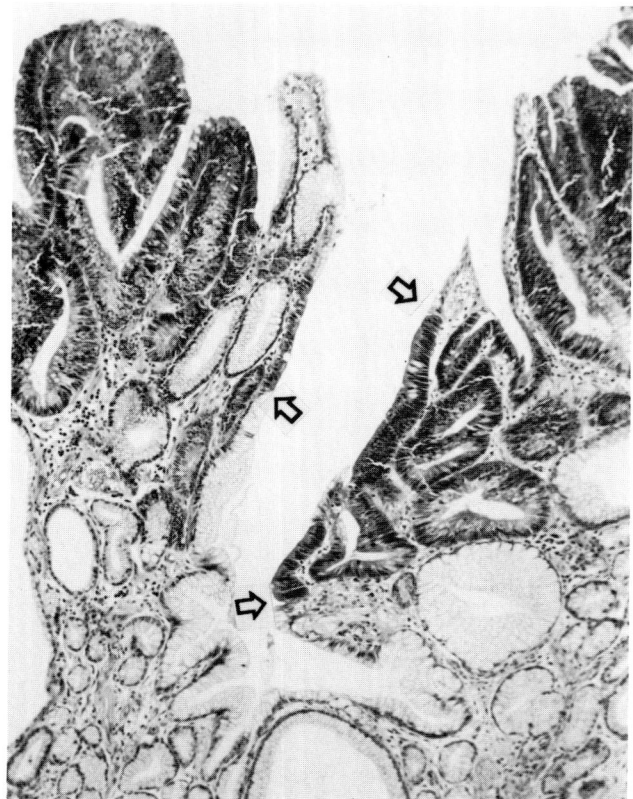

FIGURE 23–4. Flat adenoma. The transitions between the compact columnar cells of the adenoma and the neighboring normal foveolar cells (arrows) are abrupt. (× 80)

Malignancy and Adenoma

Gastric adenomas, like the adenomas of the colon, have a high incidence of malignant transformation, particularly in the papillary or villous lesions. Review

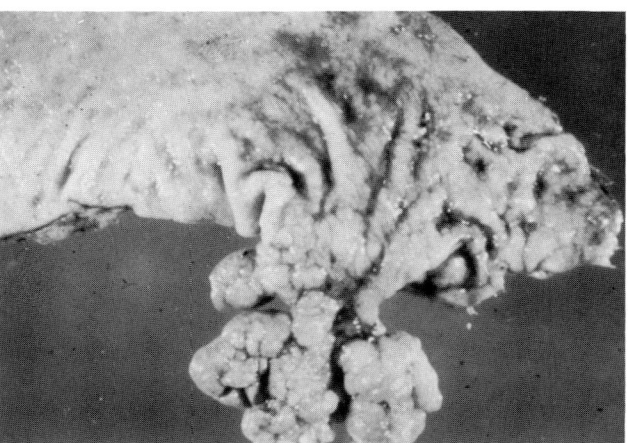

FIGURE 23–5. Papillary adenoma. The papillary nodules are partitioned by deep crevices. The base is broad, and the adenomatous tissue extends to the adjacent mucosa. (From Ming SC: Tumors of the Esophagus and Stomach. In Atlas of Tumor Pathology, Second Series, Fascicle 7. Armed Forces Institute of Pathology, Washington, DC, 1973, p 124.)

of reports up to 1972 revealed malignancy in 41% of the adenomas, with a range of 6% to 75%.[2] The lower incidences of 6% and 18% were found in the flat adenomas.[38,67] Recent reports have shown similar findings (see Table 23–4). Malignant change was present in 34% of adenomas, with a range of 5% to 76%.[5,6,47,49,50,53,56,62,68] Again, the flat adenomas have lower incidence of malignant change. The rate of malignant change in flat adenoma increases with the grade of dysplasia, the papillary pattern, and the size of the lesion.[56] Furthermore, independent coexisting carcinomas are common (see Figure 23–6). In Hirota and associates' series of 121 cases, early carcinoma was present in 55 cases and advanced cancer in 29 cases.[56]

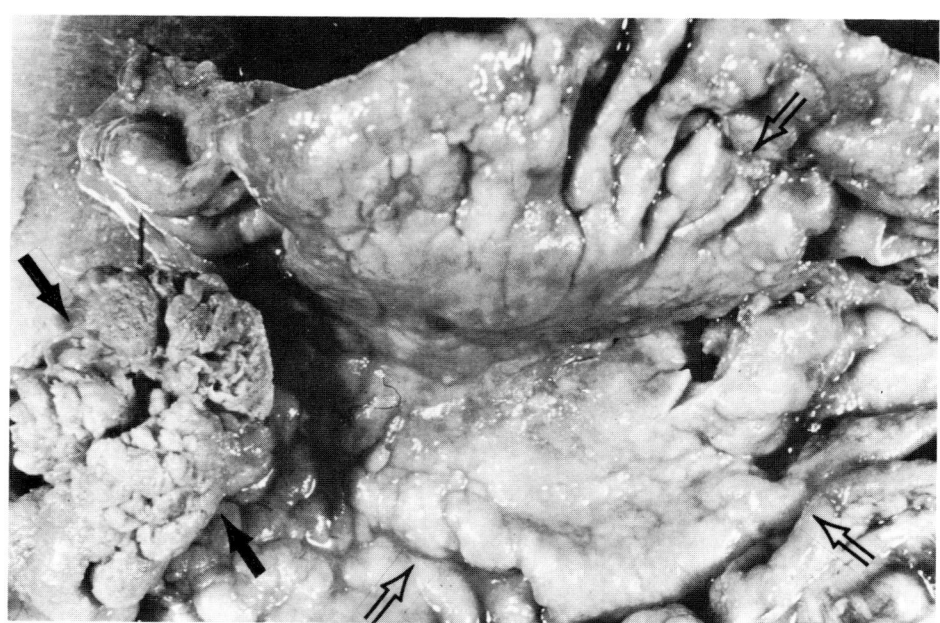

FIGURE 23–6. Papillary adenoma. The nodular adenoma (solid arrows) is shown on the left. The plaquelike thickening of the stomach wall (open arrows) was an infiltrative carcinoma. (From Ming SC. Tumors of the Esophagus and Stomach. In Atlas of Tumor Pathology, Second Series, Fascicle 7. Armed Forces Institute of Pathology, Washington, DC, 1973, p 124.)

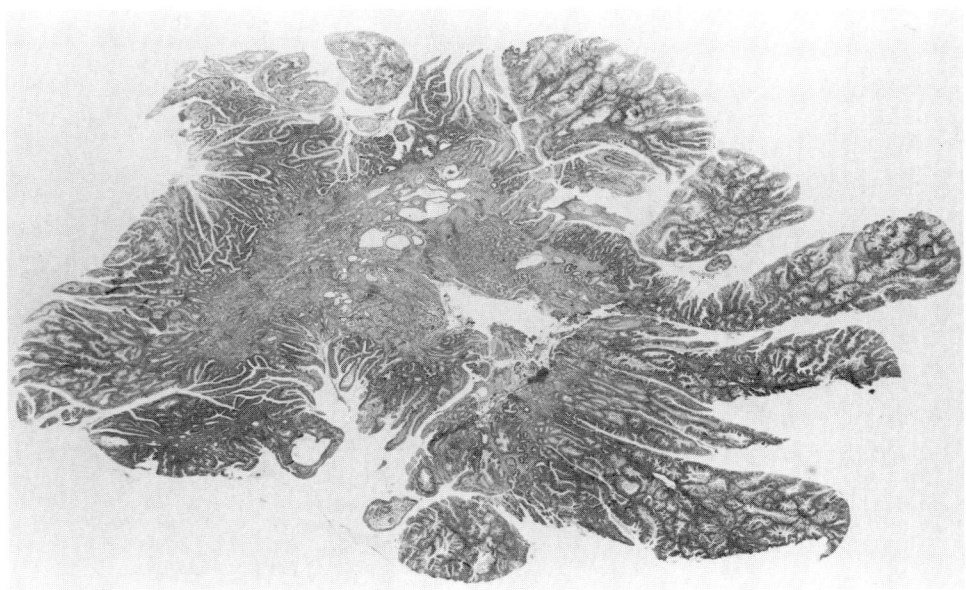

FIGURE 23–7. Papillary adenoma. This scanning histologic view of the adenoma in Figure 23–5 shows papillary lobulation of the lesion with focal areas of villous formation. (× 10) (A lower magnification is shown in Ming SC: The classification and significance of gastric polyps. In Yardley JH, Morson BM (eds): The Gastrointestinal Tract. Baltimore, Williams & Wilkins, 1977, p 149. Reproduced with permission.)

However, only 1 of 29 patients reported by Laxen and colleagues had gastric cancer outside the adenoma.[5]

There have been a few follow-up studies. Laxen and colleagues reported new polyps in 6 of 14 cases within 5 years,[5] and carcinomas in 3 cases in 15 years.[69] Sugano and associates noted no change of the "atypical epithelium" in a 2-year follow-up study.[38] Kamiya and co-workers followed 85 adenomas, mostly of the flat type, in 74 patients for 6 months to 12 years; carcinoma developed in 9 adenomas.[57] They also noted a gross change of size in 8 and a shift of the degree of dysplasia in 12. Thus, a close relationship between adenoma and carcinoma exists, even for the relatively indolent flat adenoma.

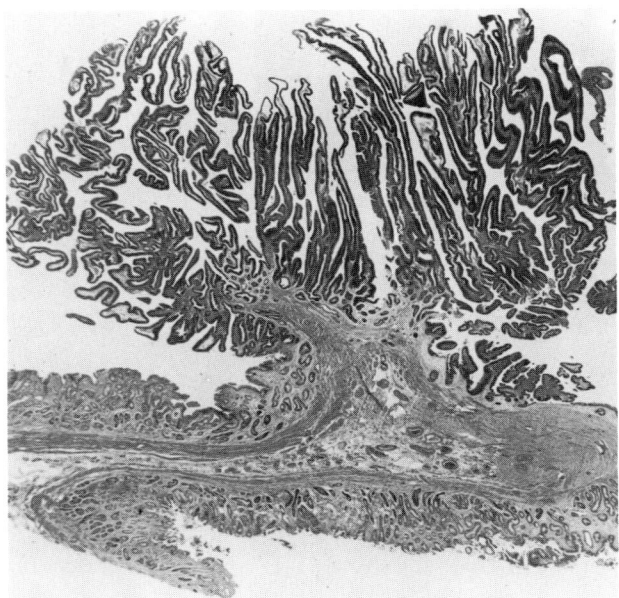

FIGURE 23–8. Villous adenoma. This scanning histologic view shows long slender villous fronds. (× 11)

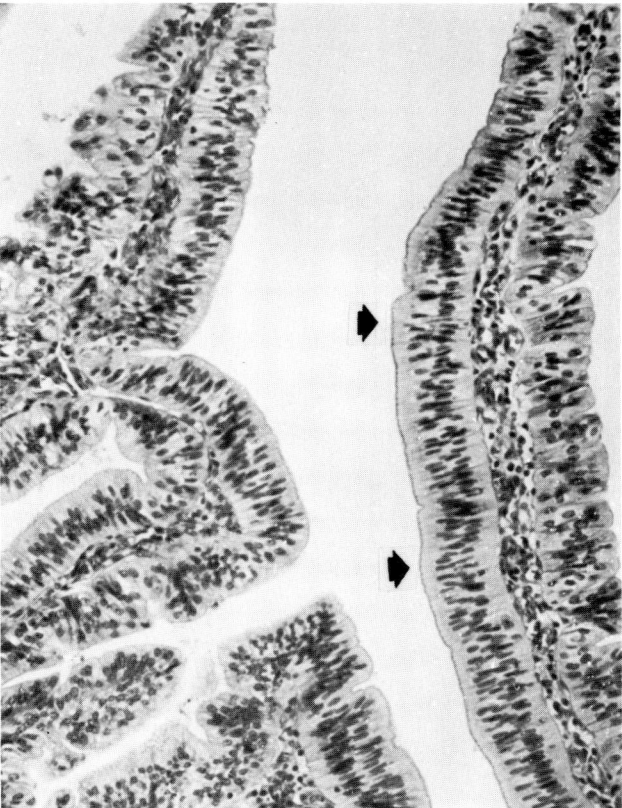

FIGURE 23–9. Villous adenoma. The cells lining the right side of the glandular crevice show a distinct striated border on their luminal surface (arrows). The cells to the left of the crevice have a faintly stained and thinner apical border. The nuclei are pseudostratified and centrally seated. There is no mucous secretion. (× 300)

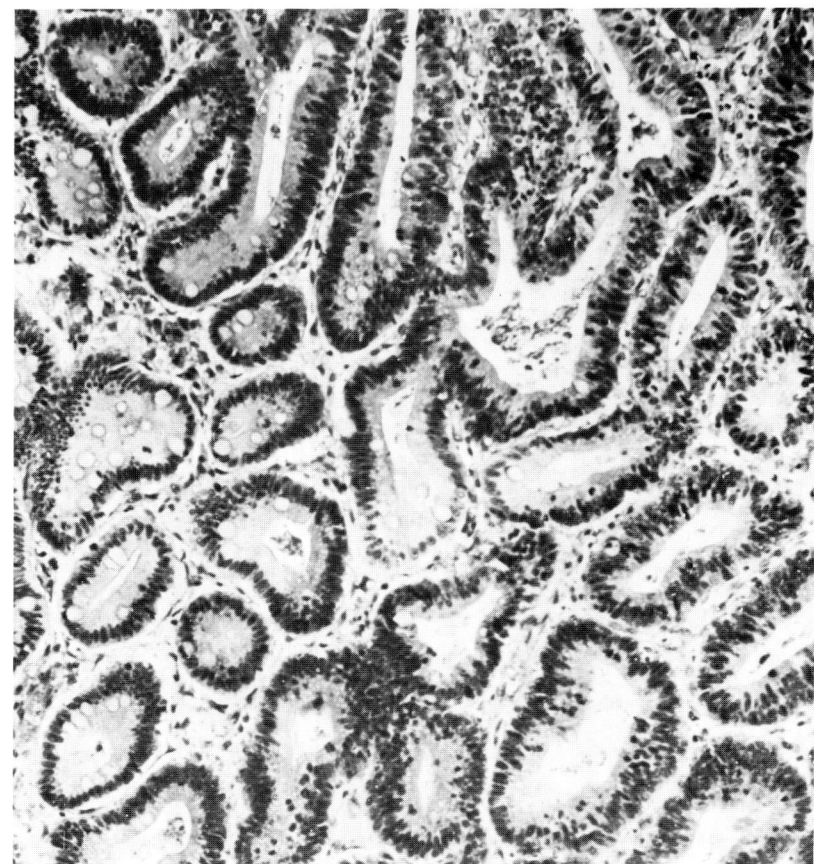

FIGURE 23-10. Papillary adenoma. Goblet cells are present in the differentiated glands. The less-differentiated cells are markedly pseudostratified. (× 200)

FIGURE 23-11. Papillary adenoma. The nonneoplastic mucosa below the adenomatous tissue shows intestinal metaplasia. Goblet cells are evident. (× 140)

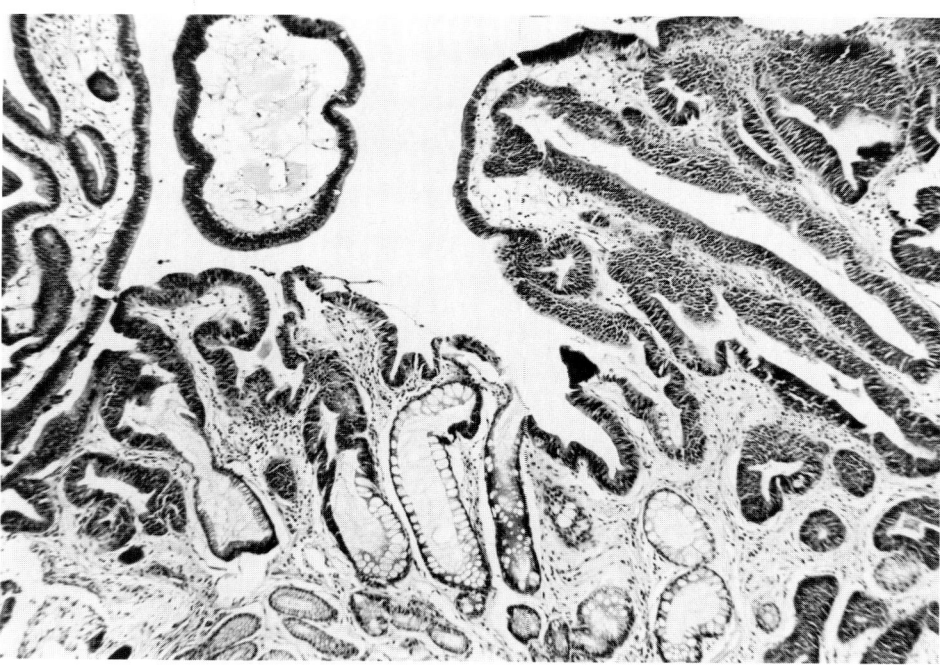

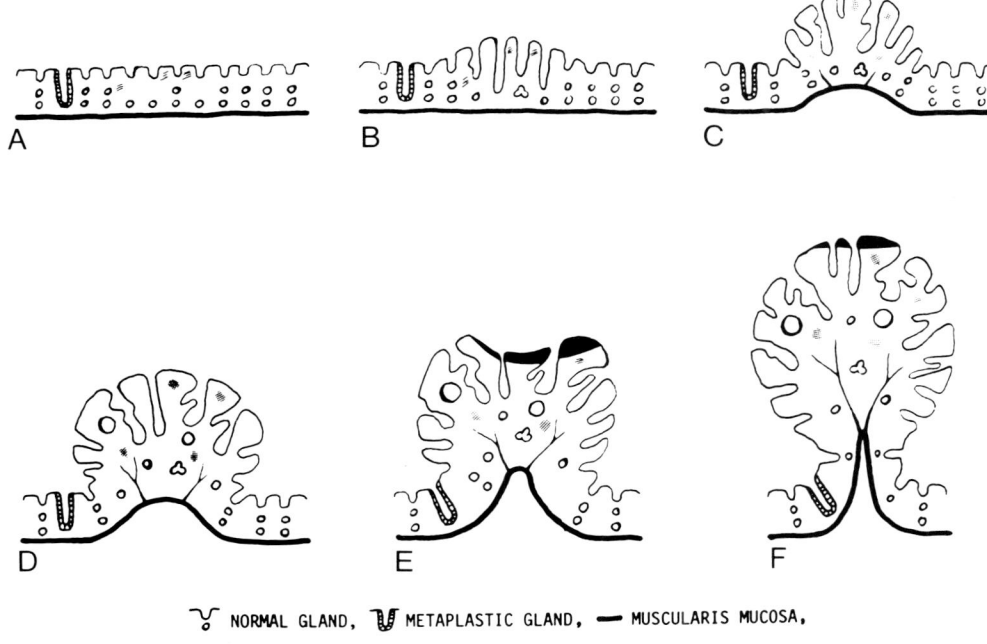

FIGURE 23–12. Schematic presentation of various forms of hyperplastic polyp. A, The mucosa in which the hyperplastic polyp arises usually shows focal chronic inflammation and mild atrophy. Intestinal metaplasia is mild or absent. B and C, Polypoid foveolar hyperplasia resulting from elongation of the hyperplastic foveolae. D, Dome-shaped sessile polyp with branching and cystic foveolae and pyloric glands at the base. E, Sessile polyp with erosion and acute inflammation at the top. F, Well-formed polyp with a short pedicle. (From Ming SC: Tumors of the Esophagus and Stomach. Supplement. In Atlas of Tumor Pathology, Second Series, Fascicle 7. Armed Forces Institute of Pathology, Washington, DC, 1985, p S24.)

HYPERPLASTIC (REGENERATIVE) POLYP

Histogenesis and Various Forms

The hyperplastic polyp is composed, for the most part, of markedly elongated and hyperplastic foveolae of the gastric glands. Figure 23–12 illustrates various forms of the hyperplastic polyp. The hyperplasia usually occurs in a chronically inflamed mucosa with a mild degree of atrophy (Figure 23–12A). The small polyps are sessile, hemispherical lesions in the form of polypoid foveolar hyperplasia (Figure 23–12B and C). The number of foveolae does not appear increased. Further enlargement of the polyp (Figure 23–12D–F) appears to be the result of branching and dilatation of the hyperplastic foveolae. The newly formed foveolae are not connected with the deep glands, which are almost entirely of the pyloric type. In some cases, the deep glands are increased in number. In general, they contribute little to the size of the polyp. Secondary surface erosion is common (Figure 23–12E). In most cases, the erosion and acute inflammation destroy the glands and reduce their number. A reparative response to the erosion with secondary hyperplasia of the surrounding glands as suggested by Nakamura and Nakano's type II polyp[49] is not common. However, active regeneration with immature cells and presence of mitosis may accompany the erosion. A well-developed hyperplastic polyp is a distinct oval lesion (Figure 23–12F). This scheme of the development of hyperplastic polyp proposes that the polyp is the result of excessive and apparently unchecked regenerative growth of the normal proliferative zone of the gastric epithelium, that is, the deep foveola and the neck region of the glands. Support of this proposal is found in the reports of polyp formation in the region of healed ulcer,[70] at the stomach side of the gastroenterostomy stoma,[10,11,71,72] and in stomachs with gastritis and pernicious anemia.[7,9,73] The incidence of hyperplastic polyps is particularly high in the gastric remnant after partial gastrectomy. Polyps were present in 20% of patients whose stomachs had been resected more than 20 years previously.[71] Koga and coauthors found local hyperplastic changes in 66% of the resected specimens of postgastrectomy stump.[72] Enterogastric reflux is common in these patients, but its role in polyp formation is not certain. The immediate stimulus for the formation of the polyp has not been determined. Finally, hyperplastic polyps may enlarge, shrink, or disappear.[5,7,57,74,75]

Pathology

Hyperplastic polyps are generally small lesions with a smooth domelike or olive shape (Figure 23–13). Erosion may occur at the top. The average size is 1 cm, and most are under 1.5 cm in diameter.[2] However, large

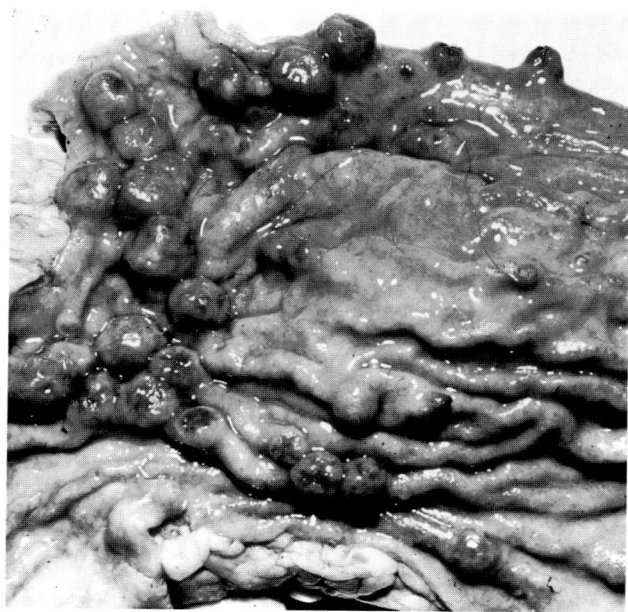

FIGURE 23–13. Hyperplastic polyp. The size of the polyps was relatively uniform, about 1 cm in diameter. Several polyps had an eroded top. (From Ming SC: The classification and significance of gastric polyps. In Yardley JH, Morson BM (eds): The Gastrointestinal Tract. Baltimore, Williams & Wilkins, 1977, p 149. Reproduced with permission.)

polyps up to 12 cm in diameter have been reported.[6] The large ones may have a papillary appearance similar to that of a papillary adenoma.[76] Most of the polyps are sessile, but some may have a long pedicle. The number of patients with a single polyp is nearly equal to that of patients with multiple polyps. The multiple polyps generally appear uniform in shape and size. When the polyps number more than 50, the term *hyperplastic polyposis* is applied.[4] Such cases are rare. Hyperplastic polyps are randomly distributed, with a slight prevalence in the antrum. In the body of the stomach, the hyperplastic polyp typically sits on the rugal fold.[44]

Histologically, the hyperplastic polyp is composed principally of dilated, elongated, and branching foveolae. The hyperplastic foveolae are lined by either normal-appearing mucous cells or hypertrophic cells with abundant cytoplasm. The cells in some glands have eosinophilic cytoplasm, hyperchromatic nuclei, and nucleoli. These "pinky ducts" were thought to be newly formed and to participate in the polypoid expansion of the lesion.[77] The hyperplastic cells are crowded, and intraglandular infolding is common (Figure 23–14). There is no pseudostratification, however, and the nuclei remain basally located. Mitotic activities are rare except in the surface area, where active proliferation

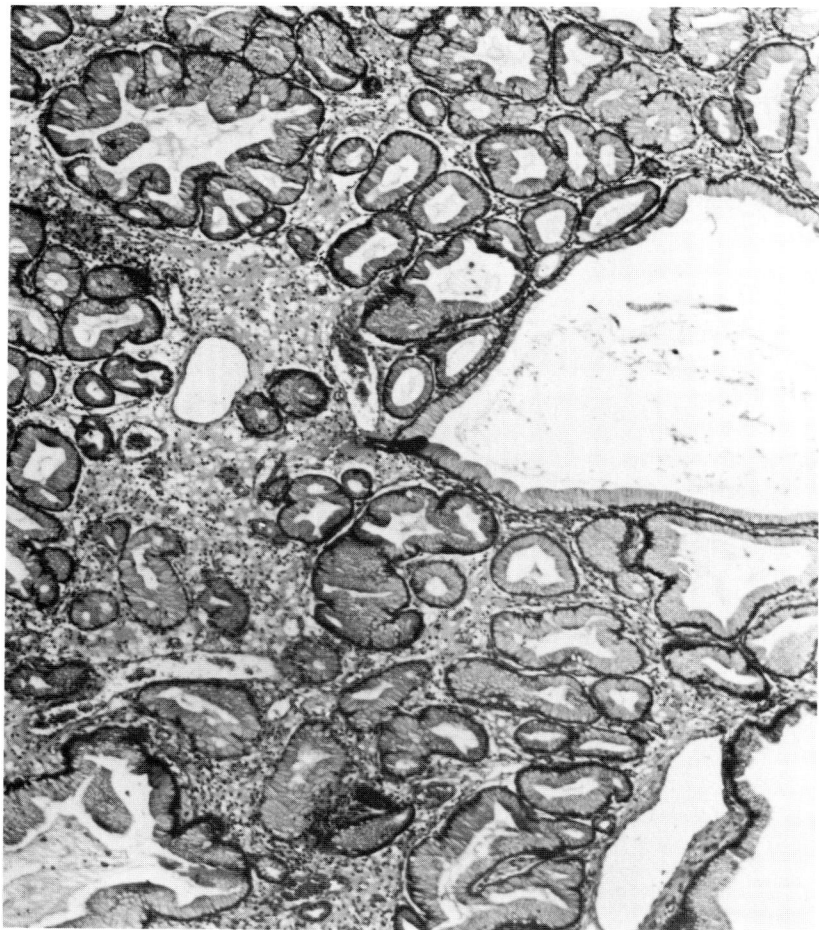

FIGURE 23–14. Hyperplastic polyp. The polyp is composed of many hyperplastic and dilated foveolae. The tall columnar cells have basally located nuclei. The stroma is chronically inflamed and edematous. ($\times$ 140)

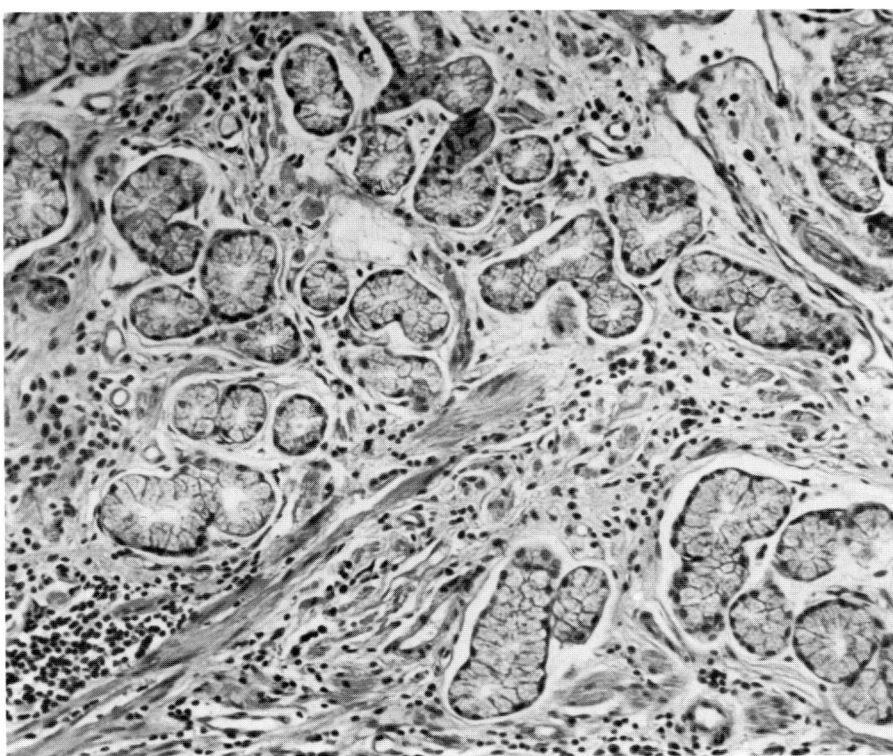

FIGURE 23-15. Hyperplastic polyp. Normal-appearing pyloric-type glands are separated by inflamed stromal tissue and thin bundles of muscle cells. (× 200)

may be present in response to erosion and acute inflammation. The histologic appearance of cellular normality is reflected by DNA measurements showing a diploid pattern and the labeling index with ^{3}H-thymidine identical to that of the normal mucosa.[78]

The deep glands are of pyloric type even when the polyp is located in the fundic mucosa, apparently a result of pseudopyloric metaplasia. In the small polyps, the number of these glands is the same as that in the surrounding mucosa. At this stage, the lesion is called by the descriptive name *polypoid foveolar hyperplasia.* This subtype of hyperplastic polyp is a useful clinical entity.[45] It is applied to the small mucosal elevation commonly seen endoscopically but essentially normal histologically, except for foveolar hyperplasia and moderate superficial chronic gastritis. In some clinics, this entity is the most common form of hyperplastic polyp.[45] In the well-formed polyp, the number of pyloric glands varies. In some, the presence of many glands gives the polyp a superficial resemblance to an adenoma, and the term *hyperplastic adenomatous polyp* is applied.[43,45] The morphology of the deep glands is, however, normal; and there is no cellular atypia (Figure 23-15). In reality, the glands represent merely another component in the hyperplastic process of the polyp.

The lamina propria in the hyperplastic polyp shows varying degrees of chronic inflammation and edema, most prominent in the superficial region (see Figure 23-14). Nodular collections of lymphocytes are common, occasionally with germinal centers. The surface area of the polyp may show erosion and acute inflammation accompanied by granulation tissue formation, prominent vascularity, and telangiectasia. In the loose connective stromal tissue, bundles of smooth muscle cells are often present, extending from their origin in the muscularis mucosae into the deep portions of the polyp (see Figure 23-15). The muscle bundles are slender and taper off toward the upper portion of the polyp and usually do not reach the surface region.

Rarely, dysplastic or adenomatous tissue is present in the hyperplastic polyp, admixed with hyperplastic foveolae (Figure 23-16). The dysplastic immature cells may resemble either foveolar cells or metaplastic cells. Because the overall configuration and the majority of the tissue in such a polyp are identical to those of hyperplastic polyp, the adenomatous change is considered to be secondary[48,79] and the term *dysplastic (adenomatous) hyperplastic polyp* has been applied to it.[48] Snover gave the name *mixed adenomatous-hyperplastic polyp* and placed it in the category of adenoma.[47] He found 7 such cases among 182, one of which had *in situ* carcinoma in it.

Another unusual anomaly in the hyperplastic polyp is the presence of globoid signet-ring–like cells in the dilated foveolae (Figure 23-17). These cells are large and secrete sialomucin. The nuclei are compressed against the cell membrane and are irregularly oriented. A similar lesion occurring in a flat gastric mucosa has been called globoid dysplasia and is considered to be the precursor of signet-ring cell carcinoma (see Chapter 25). The significance of this change in the polyp is not clear.

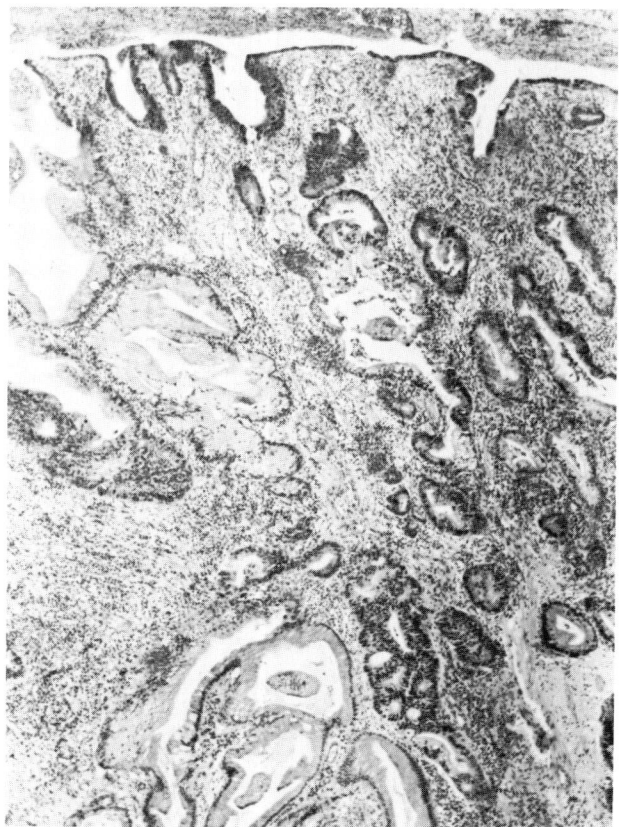

FIGURE 23–16. Hyperplastic polyp with dysplastic changes. Hyperplastic and dilated foveolae are shown at the left upper and lower center. Other glands show varying degrees of dysplasia with hyperchromatic and pseudostratified cells. (× 80) (Courtesy of Dr. I. Kline, Lankenau Hospital, Philadelphia, Pa.)

Malignant Potential

None of the regenerative polyps studied by Ming and Goldman[36] showed cellular atypism or malignant transformation. Since then, it has been generally accepted that the hyperplastic (regenerative) polyp had no malignant potential. There had been sporadic reports to the contrary, however. The incidence is low, averaging 1% among reported cases and 2% among polyps in a previous review.[2] More recently, malignant change within the polyp has been repeatedly reported (Table 23–4). However, the incidence remains low, 1.0% of polyps and 1.7% of cases on average. The incidence of coexisting carcinoma away from the polyp is lower in the recent than in the earlier reports, 7.4% and 22%, respectively. The malignancy within the polyp has been illustrated in several reports,[2,53,80–82] which leaves no doubt of its occurrence (Figure 23–18). The much higher rate of carcinomatous change outside the polyp emphasizes the importance of careful evaluation of the entire stomach when the polyp is present. In addition, Laxen and associates found three carcinomas in association with, but none within, the inflammatory polyps among 130 cases,[5] indicating the unstable state of gastric mucosa in that situation also.

A few follow-up studies on the hyperplastic polyp have been reported. In Laxén's series of 147 patients whose cases were followed for up to 15.5 years, carcinoma developed in 3 cases outside the polyp and in none in the polyp.[69] Kawai and colleagues followed 110 polyps for up to 15 years; carcinoma developed in 1 at 3 years.[83] In none of 974 polyps followed for 6 months to 11 years by Yamagata and Hisamichi did carcinoma develop.[84] So far, metastasis and death from malignant change in a hyperplastic polyp has not been reported.

The mechanism of malignant transformation in the hyperplastic polyp is unknown. Kozuka and co-workers emphasized metaplastic change and reported a malignant incidence of 11% when metaplasia is present, in contrast to 2% when it is absent.[50] Ming stressed the importance of dysplastic or adenomatous change in the polyp.[46] This concept was supported by the following observations. Snover reported malignant change in 1 of 7 mixed adenomatous-hyperplastic polyps, in contrast to 1 in 127 hyperplastic polyps.[47] The malignant polyp reported by Ghazi and coauthors was in the adenomatous area of a 6-cm polyp.[6] Dysplastic changes

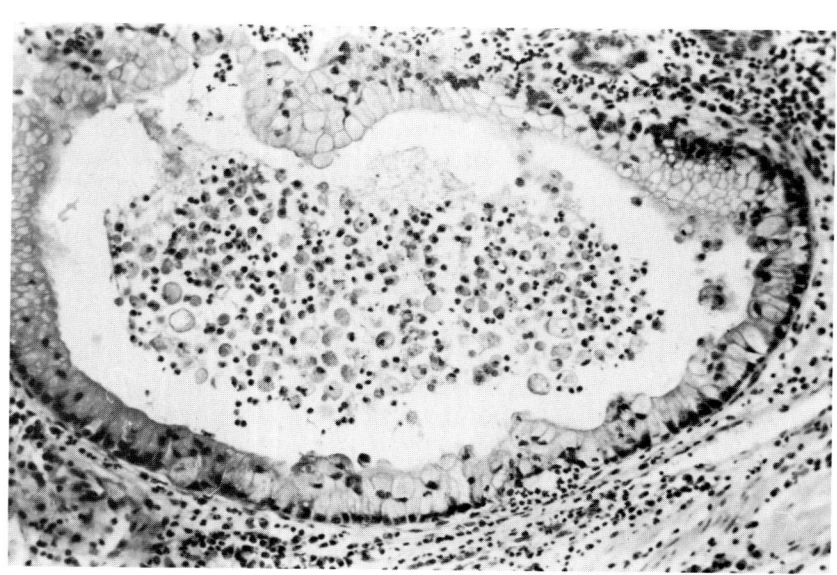

FIGURE 23–17. Hyperplastic polyp showing globoid cells in a dilated foveola. These cells are oval, bulging with acidic mucin, and the nuclei are compressed against the cell membrane, as in the signet-ring cells. Some cells are free in the lumen, admixed with inflammatory cells. (× 200)

Table 23-4. REPORTED FREQUENCY OF MALIGNANT CHANGE IN AND COEXISTING CARCINOMA OUTSIDE THE GASTRIC POLYP AT THE TIME OF DIAGNOSIS OF THE POLYP

Reference		Malignant Change in Polyp		Coexisting Carcinoma Outside Polyp	
No.	Year	*Adenoma*	*Hyperplastic Polyp*	*Adenoma*	*Hyperplastic Polyp*
2	1946–1972	41% (150/362)*	2.0% (4/204)*	48% (52/108)*	—
		19% (11/57)†	1.0% (3/293)†	42% (52/123)†	22% (46/208)†
5	1982	35% (10/29)†	2.0% (4/198)†**	3.4% (1/29)†	4.5% (9/198)†**
6	1984	13% (8/60)*	0.4% (1/270)*	—	—
47	1985	27% (4/15)†	0.8% (1/127)†	27% (4/15)†	12% (15/127)†
49	1985	5.9% (4/68)*‡	0.4% (2/504)*	—	—
		33% (13/39)*‖	—	—	—
50	1977	—	0.8% (2/237)*	—	—
53	1986	76% (63/83)*‖	1.3% (7/530)*	—	—
56	1984	14% (15/107)*‡	—	70% (84/121)††	—
		36% (12/33)*§	—	—	—
		75% (3/4)*‖	—	—	—
62	1988	5% (2/40)*¶	—	—	—
67	1981	17% (2/12)*	0.0% (0/28)*	—	—
79	1987	—	2.1% (10/477)*‖	—	—
82	1979	—	0.4% (5/1210)*	—	—
83	1985	—	4.5% (3/67)*	—	—
Subtotal		30% (120/406)*	0.7% (20/2845)*	—	—
		32% (14/44)†	2.2% (8/367)†	54% (89/165)†	7.4% (24/325)†
Total		34% (272/808)*	1.0% (34/3526)*	48% (52/108)*	—
		25% (25/101)†	1.7% (11/660)†	49% (141/288)†	13% (70/533)†

*Number of polyps.
†Number of cases.
‡Flat adenoma.
§Papillotubular adenoma.
‖Papillary adenoma.
¶Depressed adenoma.
**Hyperplastic polyp and polypoid foveolar hyperplasia.
††55 early and 29 advanced gastric carcinomas.

in the polyp were also noted by Hattori,[85] Koch and colleagues,[45] and Daibo and associates.[79] Hattori[85] found them in 11 of 67 polyps, 9 in the gastric epithelium and 2 in the intestinalized epithelium. Carcinomas were present in three polyps. Two carcinomas were of gastric type, and one was intestinal. The high frequency of involvement of the gastric type of cell may be expected because this is the dominant type of cell in the hyperplastic polyp. Laxén and associates noticed the increasing average age of patients with different types of polyps—58 years for patients with inflammatory polyp, 60 years for foveolar hyperplasia, 64 years for hyperplastic polyp, and 72 years for adenomas—which suggests a chronologic order for the development of these lesions.[5] Kozuka and co-workers held a similar view and proposed a histogenetic sequence from gastritis to carcinoma through the stages of hyperplastic polyp and adenoma.[51]

HAMARTOMATOUS POLYP

The hamartomatous polyps are tumor-like nodules composed of tissues normally present in the location, usually in a disorganized arrangement. Because the stomach has many different types of cells, the composition of hamartomatous polyps is not uniform. They occur most commonly in the hereditary gastrointestinal polyposis syndromes, namely, the Peutz-Jeghers syndrome, Gardner's syndrome and related familial polyposis coli, and juvenile polyposis. The genetic aspects of these conditions are discussed in Chapter 6. In these syndromes, the polyps are located more commonly and in larger numbers in the intestines than in the stomach. The morphologic characteristics and other features of the intestinal polyps are described in Chapter 31. The gastric polyps in these syndromes are described here. It should be realized that the gastric and intestinal polyps in the same disease may be of different types and that even if the polyps belong to the same basic type, there are specific features distinguishing the polyps in different syndromes. For instance, whereas the intestinal polyps in Gardner's syndrome and familial polyposis coli are mostly adenomas, the most common form of gastric polyp in these syndromes is hamartomatous, involving mainly the fundic mucosa. Although the polyps in Peutz-Jeghers syndrome and those in juvenile polyposis are both hamartomatous, they have different histologic characteristics. Finally, the hamartomatous polyps may be seen in patients without other characteristics of the syndromes.

Peutz-Jeghers Syndrome

Peutz-Jeghers syndrome has two components: polyps in the gastrointestinal tract and mucocutaneous pigmentation. The polyps in the Peutz-Jeghers syndrome are prototypes of the hamartomatous polyp.

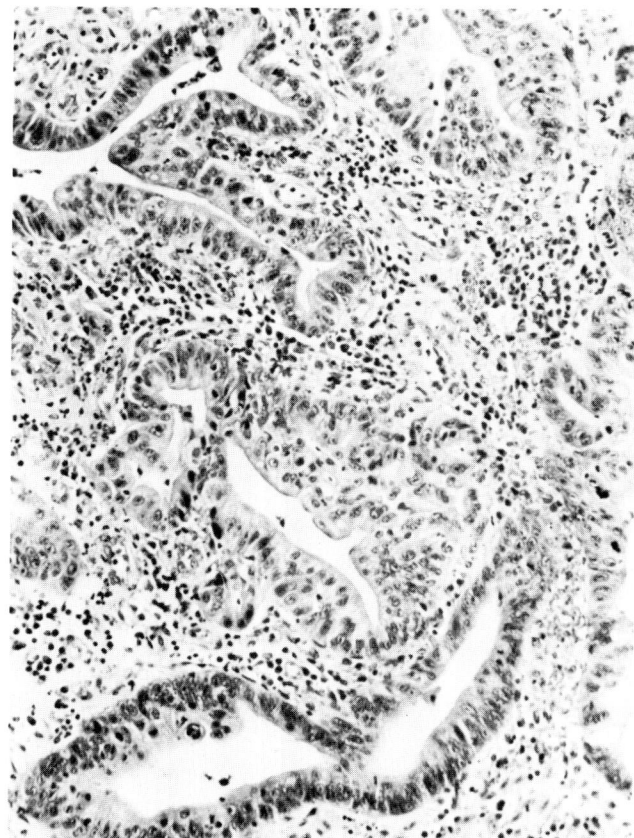

FIGURE 23–18. Carcinomatous lesion in the hyperplastic polyp with dysplastic changes shown in Figure 23–16. (Courtesy of Dr. I. Kline, Lankenau Hospital, Philadelphia, Pa.) (× 200)

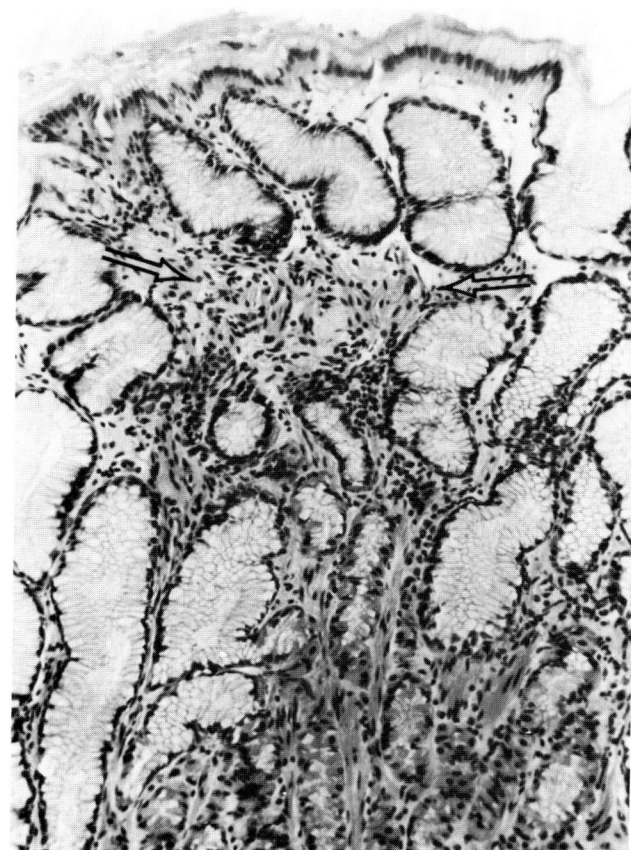

FIGURE 23–19. Peutz-Jeghers polyp. The foveolae are hyperplastic, but the fundic glands are normal. They are separated by thin bundles of muscle cells, some of which are near the mucosal surface (arrows). There is no inflammation. (× 200) (From Ming SC: The classification and significance of gastric polyps. In Yardley JH, Morson BM (eds): The Gastrointestinal Tract. Baltimore, Williams & Wilkins, 1977, p 149. Reproduced with permission.)

They occur most commonly in the small intestines. Gastric polyps are present in 25% to 49% of patients.[86–88] Most of them are small, less than 1 cm in diameter. They are rarely large enough to cause symptoms. Microscopically, the polyps show prominent foveolar hyperplasia and varying amounts of deep glands, the type of which corresponds to the location of the polyp (Figure 23–19). Smooth muscle bundles of variable thickness extend from muscularis mucosae into the polyp, occasionally up to the surface area. Irregularity of muscle thickness may also be present in the media of blood vessels. All the cells appear normal. There is no inflammation in the lamina propria. These features distinguish the hamartomatous Peutz-Jeghers polyp from other types of gastric polyp.

A few patients with Peutz-Jeghers syndrome may have only pigmentation or only polyposis.[86,89] Conversely, hamartomatous polyps of the Peutz-Jeghers type without pigmentation or a familial history have also been reported.[90–92] In two such cases, reported by Katz and associates, polyps measured 5 by 11 and 4 by 6 cm, respectively, and caused obstruction and bleeding.[92]

The possibility of malignant change in the Peutz-Jeghers polyp has been a controversial issue. The high incidence of carcinoma in the early reports was apparently due to the misinterpretation of the intermingling of glandular tissue with muscle bundles as evidence of cancerous invasion.[86,93,94] When those cases were excluded, Reid recognized malignant change in 2% to 3% of cases.[93] It is interesting to note that such epithelial misplacement was not seen in the gastric polyps in a large review.[95] The carcinoma, like the polyp, occurs more commonly in the intestines[87]; but its location in the stomach and duodenum is disproportionally high.[93] The development of carcinoma in the patients with Peutz-Jeghers syndrome has been amply documented and illustrated not only in the stomach[88,96–100] but also in other organs such as breasts, ovary, lung, and others.[88,101] The role of the polyp in the carcinogenesis has remained unsettled.[102] In most cases, the carcinoma was large and the polyps small. Actual demonstration of carcinoma in the polyp is rarely accomplished. In the case of the colon, the carcinoma may have developed in the adenomatous, rather than hamartomatous, polyp. In the small bowel, adenomatous change in a malignant hamartomatous polyp has also been reported.[103] Cochet and coauthors reported dysplastic changes in the polyp in association with a gastric carcinoma in the son and a duodenal carcinoma in the mother.[99]

Peutz-Jeghers syndrome becomes manifest early in life. The diagnosis is made in the first three decades. Peutz-Jeghers patients who also have carcinoma are young, as compared with those with cancer in the general population. Dodds and associates gave an average age of 27 years for patients with gastric carcinoma, 38 years for duodenal carcinoma, and 41 years for colonic carcinoma.[87]

Table 23-5. SUBTYPES OF JUVENILE POLYPS

	Location of Polyps	Familial History
Solitary juvenile polyp[104]	Colorectum	Absent
Juvenile polyposis coli[105]	Colorectum, few in small bowel	Present in 40%
Juvenile gastrointestinal polyposis[106]	Stomach to rectum	Present
Familial juvenile polyposis of stomach[107]	Stomach	Present

Juvenile Polyposis Syndrome

Juvenile polyps are characterized grossly by a smooth surface and histologically by many dilated glands filled with mucus and an inflamed stroma.[104] Because this type of polyp occurs mostly in the children, it has been given the name *juvenile polyp*. It is now a pathologic entity, and the term has been applied to any polyp with similar histologic features, regardless of the age of the patient at the time of diagnosis. There are four types of clinical presentation, as shown in Table 23-5. The most common presentation is an isolated polyp in the rectum or colon of the children.[104] In juvenile polyposis coli, there are numerous polyps in the colon and a few in the small intestines.[105] A familial history is present in less than one half of cases. The stomach is involved in juvenile gastrointestinal polyposis, which may occur in infants and young children as well as adults.[41,106-108] One patient was a 63-year-old woman.[106] The infantile type has a recessive genetic pattern of transmission, whereas the one involving older persons has dominant genetic transmission.[109] As the patient grew older, the number of new polyps decreased.[110] There have also been cases of juvenile polyposis limited to the stomach.[107,111] These syndromes may be related. Stemper and colleagues studied a kindred in which 21 members had gastrointestinal lesions; there were polyps only in 10, carcinoma only in 6, and both in 5.[112] Polyps were present in the colon and rectum only in 7 cases, the colon and stomach in 2, the stomach only in 1, and the rectum and jejunum in 1. The number of polyps varied from one to many. An example of gastric lesions is shown in Figure 23-20. The patient had numerous small polyps and one large juvenile polyp in the stomach. In the colon were many juvenile polyps and an adenoma.

The cause of an isolated juvenile polyp is unknown. Some pathologists favor inflammation as the cause, because of the presence of many inflammatory cells and retention of mucus in the dilated glands.[104] Thus, juvenile polyps have also been called inflammatory or retention polyps. Morson, conversely, pointing out the similarity of the stromal tissue in the polyp and the lamina propria of the normal colon, considered juvenile polyps hamartomatous.[113] The detection of juvenile polyposis in infancy[106,109] and the hyperplastic changes without retention cysts or inflammation in the early lesions[106] favor the theory of the hamartomatous nature of the juvenile polyp, at least in the case of hereditary syndromes.

The juvenile polyps in the stomach are composed of hyperplastic foveolae and an edematous stroma with

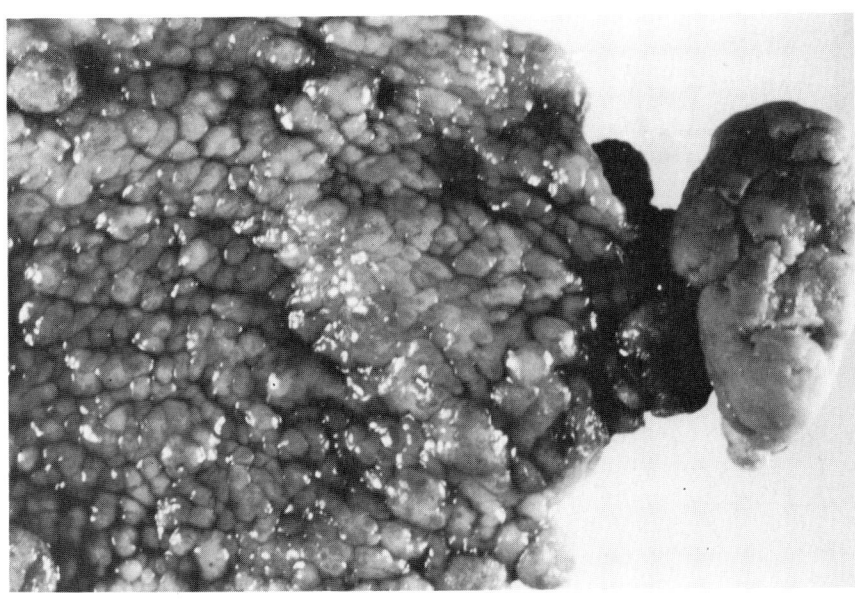

FIGURE 23-20. Juvenile gastrointestinal polyposis. The stomach mucosa was studded with numerous small polyps of uniform size except for one large polyp shown on the right. The polyps were composed of dilated foveolae and edematous stroma with chronic inflammation. The large polyp measured 5 by 3 by 2 cm and had focal malignant change, shown in Figure 23-22. The patient had numerous juvenile polyps and one adenoma in the colon, which was resected 4 years before gastrectomy. There were neither ectodermal changes nor a familial history of polyposis. (Courtesy of Dr. Arthur Aufdeheide, St. Luke's Hospital, Duluth, Minn.)

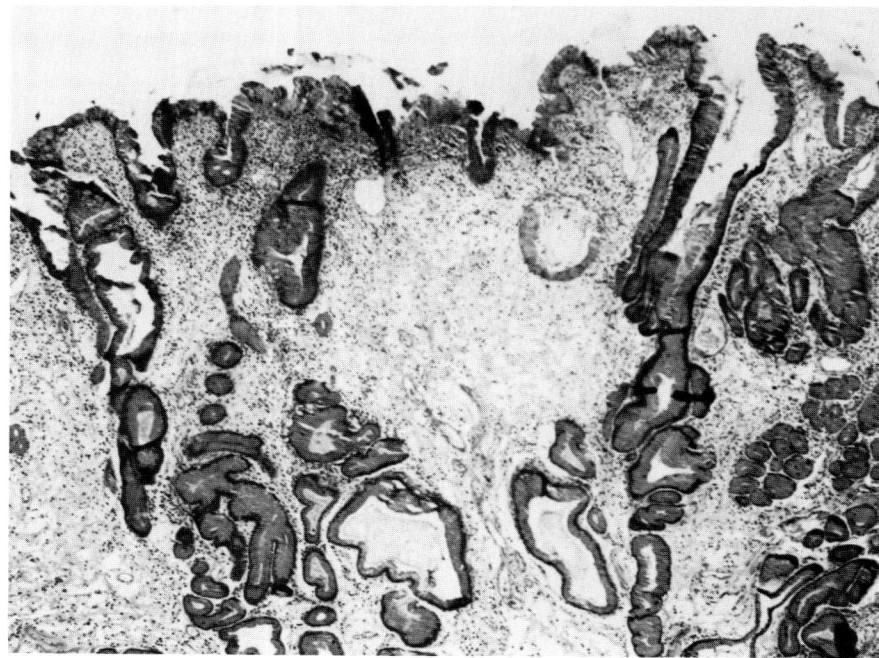

FIGURE 23–21. Juvenile gastrointestinal polyposis. Photomicrograph of one of the small polyps shown in Figure 23-20, showing dilated glands and edematous and inflamed stroma. (× 80) (Courtesy of Dr. Arthur Aufdeheide, St. Luke's Hospital, Duluth, Minn.)

inflammatory cells (Figure 23–21). This composition closely resembles the common hyperplastic polyp of the stomach. Another type of polyp that requires differentiation is the polyp in the Cronkhite-Canada syndrome. The latter is an inflammatory polyp with retention cysts. Distinguishing between these three types of polyps is difficult. A definitive diagnosis requires knowledge of the clinical background of the patient, factors such as age, symptoms, and distribution and number of polyps.

Carcinomas develop occasionally in patients with juvenile polyposis, as well as in family members who do not have the polyp.[112] Most carcinomas have been found in the colon, and a few have been found in the stomach. Carcinomas in the colon may have developed independently in the adenomatous lesion that occurs either coincidentally or as a secondary change within the juvenile polyp.[41,108,114] The relationship between the gastric polyp and the carcinoma is not clear. In one report, there was dysplasia in the gastric polyps.[108] In another report, a 13-year-old girl was found to have hyperplastic polyps in the stomach and juvenile, Peutz-Jeghers, and adenomatous polyps in the colon.[115] The polyps were apparently formed *de novo*, because there were no intermediate types. Figure 23–22 shows carcinomatous tissue in the dysplastic area of a large, lobulated juvenile polyp in the stomach shown in Figure 23–20.

Fundic Gland Polyp

The fundic gland polyp, also known as fundic gland hyperplasia, occurs in the oxyntic mucosa of the stomach. It is composed of normal-appearing fundic glands with parietal and chief cells in increased numbers. In one report, muscle cells were also present in a single polyp.[116] Many of the glands are cystically dilated, tortuous, or budding[4,117]; therefore, such polyps have been simply called *glandular cysts*.[118,119] The fundic gland polyp was first described in detail by Watanabe and coworkers in 6 of 22 patients with familial polyposis coli.[40] They appeared as numerous small sessile polyps less than 5 mm in diameter. Subsequently, fundic gland polyps have been found in patients with Gardner's syndrome[120,121] and patients with polyposis coli.[115,122–125] Histochemical studies revealed that the fundic gland polyps secrete O-acylated sialic acid,[124] glucagon, and glicentin,[126] which are normally present only in the fetal stomach. Histologically, however, the constituent cells of the polyp appear normal. Furthermore, the polyp may regress and disappear,[47,119–127] which suggests that these lesions may not be hamartomatous.

Fundic gland polyps are also found in persons without colonic polyposis,[47,90,128,129] probably even more commonly in nonpolyposis patients.[114,128] Eidt and Stolte[119] reviewed 1500 cases; 596 patients were examined for colonic lesions. Familial adenomatosis coli or Gardner's syndrome was present in only 21 cases, simple adenomas in 66, adenocarcinomas in 21, and other types of polyps in 50. The remaining 438 patients had clinically normal colon.

The stomach in familial polyposis coli patients may also contain adenomas, which are more common in the pyloric than in the fundic mucosa; carcinoma; and carcinoids.[40,123,125,130–133]

Foveolar Polyp

In 1972, Goldman and Appelman described 11 antral foveolar polyps in eight patients.[52] The polyps were composed of tightly packed, arborized foveolae lined

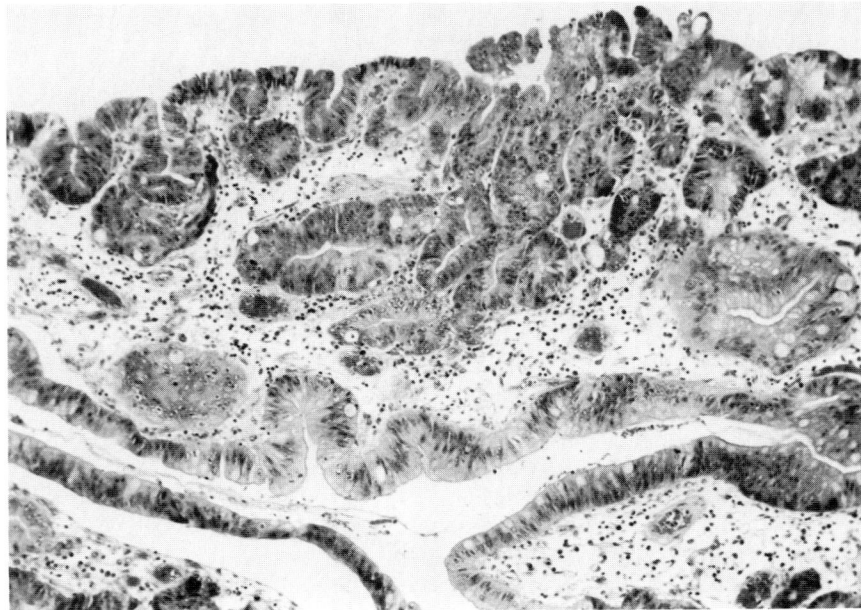

FIGURE 23-22. Juvenile gastrointestinal polyposis. Photomicrograph of the large gastric juvenile polyp in Figure 23-20. A focus of carcinoma is shown in the surface region. The gland beneath it shows intestinal metaplasia and dysplastic changes. (× 300) (Courtesy of Dr. Arthur Aufdeheide, St. Luke's Hospital, Duluth, Minn.)

by normal-appearing tall mucous cells that contained only neutral glycoprotein. The stroma was delicate, and there was no inflammation. Mild metaplasia was present in one third of the polyps, and about one fourth were larger than 2 cm. Carcinoma of the stomach and colon was present in one case each. An 8-cm polyp of this type was described by Snover.[47] The polyp was located in the body of the stomach and was called foveolar adenoma. These polyps are probably hamartomatous. They can be readily distinguished from hyperplastic polyps and polypoid foveolar hyperplasia by the lack of stromal inflammation and cystic dilatation.

INFLAMMATORY POLYP

The inflammatory polyp accounts for one third of gastric polyp cases in Laxén's series.[5] None of the polyps showed malignant change, but gastric carcinoma outside the polyp was present in 3 of 130 cases.

Inflammatory polyps are heterogeneous and encompass several entities. A polyp made of inflammatory granulation tissue can be properly called an *inflammatory pseudopolyp* because there is loss or even absence of glandular tissue. A special form of inflammatory polyp known as an *inflammatory fibroid polyp* is described in Chapter 15. It occurs most commonly in the stomach. Another example of inflammatory polyp of interest is the eosinophilic granuloma, which is discussed in Chapter 20.

Inflammatory polyps with prominent cystic glands may be called *retention polyps*, because the dilated glands are filled with retained mucus. Such a polyp is rare in the stomach. None was listed among 182 polyps collected by Snover.[47] Retention polyps resemble hyperplastic polyps on the one hand and juvenile polyps of genetic influence on the other. Histologically, the differentiation is difficult. The characteristics of the retention polyp are markedly edematous and inflamed stroma, the much-dilated foveolae, and the usually absent deep glands proper. The polyps in the Cronkhite-Canada syndrome are of this type. This syndrome is characterized by diffuse gastrointestinal polyposis and ectodermal changes. In this syndrome, polyps are common in the stomach. In one case, there was polyposis in the stomach and duodenum but not in the colon.[42] The gastric polyps are 0.5 to 1.5 cm in diameter. They either are long and fingerlike[134] or resemble a hydatid mole.[42,135] Carcinoma was reported in the stomach in two cases;[136] the cancer was not in the polyp. Additional discussion of the Cronkhite-Canada syndrome is presented in Chapter 31.

HETEROTOPIC POLYP

Heterotopic tissues from the neighboring pancreas and duodenum may occur in the stomach as polyps.

Heterotopic Pancreas

The heterotopic pancreas occurs in the intestines as well as in the stomach. Among 543 cases reviewed by Busard and Walters, 276 were in the intestine, 149 in the stomach, and 30 in Meckel's diverticulum.[137] Lai and Tompkins reported a case in a duplicated stomach.[138] The heterotopic polyps account for 4% of polypoid lesions in the stomach (see Table 23-1). The prepyloric region is a favored site in the stomach.[139] In the case reported by DeBord and associates, there were two lesions, one in the antrum and the other at the esophagogastric junction.[140] Heterotopic pancreas is primarily a submucosal lesion. The nipple-like lesion has a dimpled center corresponding to the excretory duct. However, many lesions are polypoid and some are ulcerated.[138,139] The symptoms correlate with the size of the lesion and the extent of mucosal involvement.[141] Bleeding is a common manifestation. Rarely, the lesion looks malignant,[142] but actual malignant change is rare.[143,144] Histologically, the heterotopic tissue is composed mainly of exocrine glands and ducts. Islet cells are present in varying amounts.[145] There was a report of a case of Zollinger-Ellison syndrome due to a non-β islet cell tumor in the heterotopic pancreas.[146]

Brunner's Gland Hyperplasia

Polypoid lesions consisting of Brunner's glands have been called adenomas because of the tightly packed glands. In reality, there is only hyperplasia, and the glands are normal. The lesion occurs mainly in the duodenum and only rarely in the stomach, always in the prepyloric region,[147,148] where it may be obstructive. Whether it is a hamartoma or simple hyperplasia is not clear, although the stationary appearance favors the former.

Adenomyoma

There is a rare gastric lesion related to the above entities known as adenomyoma or adenomyosis, composed of a mixture of ducts lined by columnar cells and bundles of smooth muscle in a haphazard arrangement.[149-152] Pancreatic tissue and Brunner's glands are often present. Most of the lesions are less than 2 cm and some are up to 5 cm in diameter. In one case, excessive mucus secretion caused pseudomyxoma peritonei.[152]

References

1. Ming SC: Tumors of the esophagus and stomach. In Atlas of Tumor Pathology, 2nd series, fascicle 7. Washington, DC, Armed Forces Institute of Pathology, 1973, pp 99–101.
2. Ming SC: The classification and significance of gastric polyps. In Yardley JH, Morson BM (eds): The Gastrointestinal Tract. Baltimore, Williams & Wilkins, 1977, pp 149–175.
3. Ueno K, Oshiba S, Yamagata S, et al: Histo-clinical classification and follow-up study of gastric polyp. Tohoku J Exp Med 118 (Suppl):23–38, 1976.
4. Rösch W: Epidemiology, pathogenesis, diagnosis, treatment of benign gastric tumours. Front Gastrointest Res 6:167–184, 1980.
5. Laxén F, Sipponen P, Ihamaki T, et al: Gastric polyps; their morphological and endoscopical characteristics and relation to gastric carcinoma. Acta Pathol Microbiol Scand [A] 90:221–228, 1982.
6. Ghazi A, Ferstenberg H, Shinya H: Endoscopic gastroduodenal polypectomy. Ann Surg 200:175–180, 1984.
7. Elsborg L, Andersen D, Myhere-Jensen O, Bastrup-Madsen P: Gastric mucosal polyps in pernicious anaemia. Scand J Gastroenterol 12:49–52, 1977.
8. Stockbrugger RW, Menon GG, Beilby JO, et al: Gastroscopic screening in 80 patients with pernicious anaemia. Gut 24:1141–1147, 1983.
9. Siurala M: Gastritis, its fate and sequelae. Ann Clin Res 13:111–113, 1981.
10. Janunger K, Domellof L: Gastric polyps and precancerous mucosal changes after partial gastrectomy. Acta Chir Scand 144:293–298, 1978.
11. Ovaska JT, Ekfors TO, Havia TV, Kujari HP: Endoscopic follow-up after resection for gastric or duodenal ulcer. Acta Chir Scand 152:289–295, 1986.
12. Seifert E, Gail K, Weismuller J: Gastric polypectomy. Long-term results (survey of 23 centres in Germany). Endoscopy 15:8–11, 1983.
13. Morson BC: Gastric polyps composed of intestinal epithelium. Br J Cancer 9:550–557, 1955.
14. Niv Y, Bat L: Gastric polyps—a clinical study. Isr J Med Sci 21:841–844, 1985.
15. Seifert E, Elster K: Gastric polypectomy. Am J Gastroenterol 63:451–456, 1975.
16. Marshak RH, Feldman F: Gastric polyps. Am J Dig Dis 10:909–935, 1965.
17. Spriggs EI: Polyps of the stomach and polypoid gastritis. Q J Med 12:1–60, 1943.
18. Ménétrier P: Des polyadenomes gastriques et de leurs rapport avec le cancer de l'estomac. Arch Physiol Norm Pathol 1:32–55, 236–262, 1888.
19. Williams SM, Harned RK, Settles RH: Adenocarcinoma of the stomach in association with Ménétrier's disease. Gastrointest Radiol 3:387–390, 1978.
20. Mills GP: Multiple polypi of the stomach (Gastritis polyposa): With the report of a case. Br J Surg 10:226–231, 1922.
21. Eklof O: Benign tumours of the stomach and duodenum. A clinical and roentgenographic study with special reference to adenomatous polyps and the relation to malignancy. Acta Chir Scand Suppl 291:1–57, 1962.
22. Lawrence JC: Gastrointestinal polyps: Statistical study of malignancy incidence. Am J Surg 31:499–505, 1936.
23. Pearl FL, Brunn H: Multiple gastric polyposis: A supplementary report of 41 cases, including 3 personal cases. Surg Gynecol Obstet 76:257–281, 1943.
24. Carey JB, Hay LJ: Gastric polyps. Gastroenterology 10:102–107, 1948.
25. Plachta A, Speer FD: Gastric polyps and their relationship to carcinoma of the stomach: Review of literature and report of 65 cases. Am J Gastroenterol 28:160–175, 1957.
26. Berg JM: Histological aspects of the relation between gastric adenomatous polyps and gastric cancer. Cancer 11:1149–1155, 1958.
27. Kiefer ED, Christiansen PA: Benign tumors of the stomach and duodenum. Med Clin North Am 40:381–389, 1956.
28. Rosato F, Noto JA: Gastric polyps. Am J Surg 111:647–650, 1966.
29. McNeer G, Joly DJ, Berg JW: The significance of adenomatous polyps. In McNeer G, Pack GT (eds): Neoplasm of the Stomach Philadelphia, JB Lippincott, 1967, pp 56–80.
30. Rieniets JH, Broders AC: Gastric adenomas: A pathologic study. West J Surg Obstet Gynecol 53:163–170, 1945; 54:21–39, 1946.
31. Finney JMT, Friedenwald J: Gastric polyposis. Am J Med Sci 154:683–689, 1917.
32. Walk L: Villous tumors of the stomach: Clinical review and report of 2 cases. Arch Intern Med 87:560–569, 1951.
33. Meltzer AD, Ostrum BJ, Isard HJ: Villous tumors of the stomach and duodenum. Radiology 87:511–513, 1966.
34. Shauffer IA, O'Conner SJ: Villous tumor of the stomach. Radiology 86:734–735, 1966.
35. Ross RJ: Villous adenoma of the stomach. JAMA 195:583–584, 1966.
36. Ming SC, Goldman H: Gastric polyps: A histogenetic classification and its relation to carcinoma. Cancer 18:721–726, 1965.
37. Tomasulo J: Gastric polyps; histologic types and their relationship to gastric carcinoma. Cancer 27:1346–1355, 1971.
38. Sugano H, Nakamura K, Takagi K: An atypical epithelium of the stomach: A clinicopathological entity. Gann Monogr Cancer Res 11:257–269, 1971.
39. Nagayo T: Histological diagnosis of biopsied gastric mucosa with special reference to that of borderline lesions. Gann Monogr Cancer Res 11:245–256, 1971.

40. Watanabe H, Enjoji M, Yao T, Ohsato K: Gastric lesions in familial adenomatosis coli: Their incidence and histological analysis. Hum Pathol 9:269–283, 1978.
41. Beacham DH, Shields HM, Raffensperger EC, Enterline HT: Juvenile and adenomatous gastrointestinal polyposis. Am J Dig Dis 23:1137–1143, 1978.
42. Kindblom LG, Angervall L, Santesson B, Selander S: Cronkhite-Canada syndrome. Case report. Cancer 39:2651–2657, 1977.
43. Elster K: Histologic classification of gastric polyps. Curr Top Pathol 65:77–93, 1976.
44. Ming SC: Tumors of the esophagus and stomach. In Atlas of Tumor Pathology, 2nd series, fascicle 7. Washington, DC, Armed Forces Institute of Pathology, 1973, pp 124–143.
45. Koch HK, Lesch R, Cremer M, Oehlert W: Polyp and polypoid foveolar hyperplasia in gastric biopsy specimens and their precancerous prevalence. Front Gastrointest Res 4:183–191, 1979.
46. Ming SC: Tumors of the esophagus and stomach (supplement). In Atlas of Tumor Pathology, 2nd series, fascicle 7. Washington, DC, Armed Forces Institute of Pathology, 1985, pp S24–S32.
47. Snover DC: Benign epithelial polyps of the stomach. Pathol Annu 20:303–329, 1985.
48. Ming SC: Malignant potential of epithelial polyps of the stomach. In Ming SC (ed): Precursors of Gastric Cancer. New York, Praeger, 1984, pp 219–231.
49. Nakamura T, Nakano G: Histopathological classification and malignant change in gastric polyps. J Clin Pathol 38:754–764, 1985.
50. Kozuka S, Masamoto K, Suzuki S, et al: Histogenetic types and size of polypoid lesion of the stomach, with special reference to cancerous changes. Gann 68:267–274, 1977.
51. Kozuka S: Gastric polyps. In Filipe MI, Jass JR (eds): Gastric Carcinoma. London, Churchill Livingston, 1986, pp 132–151.
52. Goldman DS, Appelman HD: Gastric mucosal polyps. Am J Clin Pathol 58:434–444, 1972.
53. Nagayo T: Histogenesis and Precursors of Human Gastric Cancer. New York, Springer-Verlag, 1986, pp 103–111.
54. Harju E: Gastric polyposis and malignancy. Br J Surg 73:532–533, 1986.
55. Stamm B, Sulser H, Stahlberger-Bucher R: Pathology of gastric mucosa polyps. Schweiz Med Wochenschr 115:1120–1127, 1985.
56. Hirota T, Okada T, Itabashi M, Kitaoka H: Histogenesis of human gastric cancer—with special reference to the significance of adenoma as a precancerous lesion. In Ming SC (ed): Precursors of Gastric Cancer. New York, Praeger, 1984, pp 233–252.
57. Kamiya T, Morishita T, Asakura H, et al: Long term follow-up on gastric adenoma and its relation to gastric protruded carcinoma. Cancer 50:2493–2503, 1982.
58. Watanabe H: Argentaffin cells in adenoma of the stomach. Cancer 30:1267–1274, 1972.
59. Jass JR, Filipe MI: Sulphomucins and precancerous lesions of the human stomach. Histopathology 4:271–279, 1980.
60. Ming SC: Intestinal metaplasia: Its heterogeneous nature and significance. In Ming SC (ed): Precursors of Gastric Cancer. New York, Praeger, 1984, pp 141–153.
61. Watanabe H, Jass JR, Sobin LH: WHO histological typing of oesophageal and gastric tumours, 2nd ed. New York Springer-Verlag, 1990, pp 19–20.
62. Nakamura K, Sagakuchi H, Enjoji M: Depressed adenoma of the stomach. Cancer 62:2197–2202, 1988.
63. Riemann JF, Schmidt H, Hermanek P: On the ultrastructure of the gastric "borderline lesion." J Cancer Res Clin Oncol 105:285–291, 1983.
64. Takahashi T, Iwama N. Atypical glands in gastric adenoma. Three-dimensional architecture compared with carcinomatous and metaplastic glands. Virchows Arch [A] 403:135–148, 1984.
65. Inaba S, Tanaka T, Okanoue T, et al: Villous tumor of the stomach associated with adenocarcinomas: A histochemical study of mucosubstances. Jpn J Clin Oncol 14:691–698, 1984.
66. Ito H, Yokozaki H, Hata J, et al: Glicentin-containing cells in intestinal metaplasia, adenoma and carcinoma of the stomach. Virchows Arch [A] 404:17–29, 1984.
67. Nakamura T: Pathohistologische Einteilung der Magenpolypen mit spezifischer Betrachtung ihrer malignen Entartung. Chirurg 41:122–130, 1970.
68. ReMine SG, Hughes RW Jr, Weiland LH: Endoscopic gastric polypectomies. Mayo Clin Proc 56:371–375, 1981.
69. Laxén F: Gastric carcinoma and pernicious anaemia in long-term endoscopic follow-up of subjects with gastric polyps. Scand J Gastroenterol 19:535–540, 1984.
70. Mori K, Shinya H, Wolff WI: Polypoid reparative mucosal proliferation at the site of a healed gastric ulcer: Sequential gastroscopic, radiological and histological observation. Gastroenterology 61:523–529, 1971.
71. Stemmermann GN, Hayashi T: Hyperplastic polyps of the gastric mucosa adjacent to gastroenterostomy stomas. Am J Clin Pathol 71:341–345, 1979.
72. Koga S, Watanabe H, Enjoji M: Stomal polypoid hypertrophic gastritis: A polypoid gastric lesion at gastroenterostomy site. Cancer 43:647–657, 1979.
73. Ihamaki T, Kekki M, Sipponen P, Siurala M: The sequelae and course of chronic gastritis during a 30 to 34 year bioptic follow-up study. Scand J Gastroenterol 20:485–491, 1985.
74. Mizuno H, Kobayashi S, Kasugai T: Endoscopic follow-up of gastric polyps. Gastrointest Endosc 21:112–115, 1975.
75. Tsukamoto Y, Nishitani H, Oshiumi Y, Okawa T: Spontaneous disappearance of gastric polyps: Report of four cases. AJR 129:893–897, 1977.
76. Mukada T, Kashiwagura J, Itasaka K, et al: Giant hyperplasiogenous polyp of the stomach simulating malignant polyp. Tohoku J Exp Med 142:125–130, 1984.
77. Muto T, Oota K: Polypogenesis of gastric mucosa. Gann 61:435–442, 1970.
78. Petrova AS, Subrichina GN, Tschistjakova OV, et al: Flow cytometry, cytomorphology, histology and autoradiography in human gastric hyperplastic polyps and the surrounding mucosa. Oncology 39:308–313, 1982.
79. Daibo M, Itabashi M, Hirota T: Malignant transformation of gastric hyperplastic polyps. Am J Gastroenterol 82:1016–1025, 1987.
80. Remmele W, Kolb EF: Malignant transformation of hyperplasiogenic polyps of the stomach case report. Endoscopy 10:63–65, 1978.
81. Papp JP, Joseph JI: Adenocarcinoma occurring in a hyperplastic gastric polyp. Removal by electrosurgical polypectomy. Gastrointest Endosc 23:38–39, 1976.
82. Mockel W: Hyperplasiogenic gastric polyps and stomach cancer. Endoscopic findings of early stomach cancer in 3 out of 42 biopsies of hyperplasiogenic polyps. Fortschr Med 102:635–638, 1984.
83. Kawai K, Kizu M, Miyaoka T: Epidemiology and pathogenesis of gastric cancer. Front Gastrointest Res 6:71–86, 1980.
84. Yamagata S, Hisamichi S: Precancerous lesions of the stomach. World J Surg 3:671–673, 1979.
85. Hattori T: Morphological range of hyperplastic polyps and carcinomas arising in hyperplastic polyps of the stomach. J Clin Pathol 38:622–630, 1985.
86. Bartholomew LG, Moore CE, Dahlin D, Waugh JM: Intestinal polyposis associated with mucocutaneous pigmentation. Surg Gynecol Obstet 115:1–11, 1962.
87. Dodds WJ, Schulte WJ, Hensley GT, Hogan WJ: Peutz-Jeghers syndrome and gastrointestinal malignancy. AJR 115:374–377, 1972.
88. Utsunomiya J, Gocho H, Miyanaga T, et al: Peutz-Jeghers syndrome: Its natural course and management. Johns Hopkins Med J 136:71–82, 1975.
89. Erbe RW: Inherited gastrointestinal polyposis syndromes. N Engl J Med 294:1101–1104, 1976.
90. Tatsuta M, Okuda S, Tamura H, Taniguschi H: Gastric hamartomatous polyps in the absence of familial polyposis coli. Cancer 45:818–823, 1980.
91. Briccoli A, Guarasci N, Pezcoller C, et al: Stomach polyps: Clinical and therapeutic considerations. Minerva Chir 36:905–928, 1981.
92. Katz LB, Tenembaum MM, Kreel I: Gastric hamartomatous polyps in the absence of familial polyposis: Report of two cases. Mt Sinai J Med (NY) 49:426–429, 1982.

93. Reid JD: Intestinal carcinoma in the Peutz-Jeghers syndrome. JAMA 229:833–834, 1974.
94. Bolwell JS, James PD: Peutz-Jeghers syndrome with pseudoinvasion of hamartomatous polyps and multiple epithelial neoplasms. Histopathology 3:39–50, 1979.
95. Shepherd NA, Bussey HJR, Jass JR: Epithelial misplacement in Peutz-Jeghers polyps: A diagnostic pitfall. Am J Surg Pathol 11:743–749, 1987.
96. Horn RC Jr, Payne WA, Fine G: The Peutz-Jeghers syndrome (gastrointestinal polyposis with mucocutaneous pigmentation): Report of a case terminating with disseminated gastrointestinal cancer. Arch Pathol 76:29–37, 1963.
97. Achord JL, Proctor HD: Malignant degeneration and metastasis in Peutz-Jeghers syndrome. Arch Intern Med 111:498–502, 1963.
98. Payson BA, Moumgis B: Metastasizing carcinoma of the stomach in Peutz-Jeghers syndrome. Ann Surg 165:145–151, 1967.
99. Cochet B, Carrol J, Desbeillets L, Widgren S: Peutz-Jeghers syndrome associated with gastrointestinal carcinoma. Gut 20:169–175, 1979.
100. Halbert RE: Peutz-Jeghers syndrome with metastasizing gastric adenocarcinoma: Report of a case. Arch Pathol Lab Med 106:517–520, 1982.
101. Trau H, Schewach-Millet M, Fisher BK, Tsur H: Peutz-Jeghers syndrome and bilateral breast carcinoma. Cancer 50:788–792, 1982.
102. Linos DA, Dozois RR, Dahlin DC, Bartholomew LG: Does Peutz-Jeghers syndrome predispose to gastrointestinal malignancy? A later look. Arch Surg 116:1182–1184, 1981.
103. Perzin KH, Bridge MF: Adenomatous and carcinomatous changes in hamartomatous polyps of the small intestine (Peutz-Jeghers syndrome): Report of a case and review of the literature. Cancer 49:971–983, 1982.
104. Roth SI, Helwig EB: Juvenile polyps of the colon and rectum. Cancer 16:468–479, 1963.
105. Veale AMO, McCall I, Bussey HJR, Morson BC: Juvenile polyposis coli. J Med Genet 3:5–16, 1966.
106. Sachatello CR, Pickren JW, Grace JT Jr: Generalized juvenile gastrointestinal polyposis: A hereditary syndrome. Gastroenterology 58:699–708, 1979.
107. Watanabe A, Nagashima H, Motoi M, Ogawa K: Familial juvenile polyposis of the stomach. Gastroenterology. 77:148–151, 1979.
108. Goodman ZD, Yardley JH, Milligan FD: Pathogenesis of colonic polyps in multiple juvenile polyposis: Report of a case associated with gastric polyps and carcinoma of the rectum. Cancer 43:1906–1913, 1979.
109. Sachatello CR, Griffin WO Jr: Hereditary polypoid diseases of the gastrointestinal tract: A working classification. Am J Surg 129:198–203, 1975.
110. Ray JE, Heald RJ: Growing up with juvenile gastrointestinal polyposis. Report of a case. Dis Colon Rectum 14:368–380, 1971.
111. Dos Santos JG, de Magalhaes J: Familial gastric polyposis. A new entity. J Genet Hum 28:293–297, 1980.
112. Stemper TJ, Kent TH, Summers RW: Juvenile polyposis and gastrointestinal carcinoma: A study of a kindred. Ann Intern Med 83:639–646, 1975.
113. Morson BC: Some peculiarities in the histology of intestinal polyps. Dis Colon Rectum 5:337–344, 1962.
114. Grigioni WF, Alampi G, Martinelli G, Piccoluga A: Atypical juvenile polyposis. Histopathology 5:361–376, 1981.
115. Weill-Bousson M, Fischer D, Reyd P, et al: Complex recto-colic adenomatous and hamartomatous polyposis with hyperplastic gastric polyps in a 13-year-old girl. Gastroenterol Clin Biol 8:621–626, 1984.
116. Hanada M, Takami M, Hirata K, et al: Hyperplastic fundic gland polyp of the stomach. Acta Pathol Jpn 33:1269–1277, 1983.
117. Lee RG, Burt RW: The histopathology of fundic gland polyps of the stomach. Am J Clin Pathol 86:498–503, 1986.
118. Elster K, Eidt H, Ottenjann R, et al: Drusenkorperzysten, eine polypoide lasion der Magenschleimhaut. Dtsch Med Wochenschr 6:183–187, 1977.
119. Eidt S, Stolte M: Gastric glandular cysts: Investigations into their genesis and relationship to colorectal epithelial tumors. Z Gastroenterol 27:212–217, 1989.
120. Burt RW, Berenson MM, Lee RG, et al: Upper gastrointestinal polyps in Gardner's syndrome. Gastroenterology 86:295–301, 1984.
121. Tonelli F, Nardi F, Bechi P, et al: Extracolonic polyps in familial polyposis coli and Gardner's syndrome. Dis Colon Rectum 28:664–668, 1985.
122. Bulow S, Lauritsen KB, Johansen A, et al: Gastroduodenal polyps in familial polyposis coli. Dis Colon Rectum 28:90–93, 1985.
123. Ranzi T, Castagnone D, Velio P, et al: Gastric and duodenal polyps in familial polyposis coli. Gut 22:363–367, 1981.
124. Nishiura M, Hirota T, Itabashi M, et al: A clinical and histopathological study of gastric polyps in familial polyposis coli. Am J Gastroenterol 79:98–103, 1984.
125. Jarvinen H, Nyberg M, Peltokallio P: Upper gastrointestinal tract polyps in familial adenomatosis. Gut 24:333–339, 1983.
126. Hara M, Tsutsumi Y, Watanabe K, et al: Solitary gastric polyps in the fundic gland area: A histochemical study. Acta Pathol Jpn 35:831–840, 1985.
127. Iida M, Yao T, Watanabe H, et al: Spontaneous disappearance of fundic gland polyposis: Report of three cases. Gastroenterology 79:725–728, 1980.
128. Sipponen P, Laxen F, Seppala K: Cystic 'hamartomatous' gastric polyps: A disorder of oxyntic glands. Histopathology 7:729–737, 1983.
129. Choi HY, Cooper HS, Sorokin JJ, Gordon SJ: Fundic gland polyposis: Is it a specific lesion related to familial polyposis of the colon? Lab Invest 50:10A–11A, 1984.
130. Utsunomiya J, Maki T, Iwama T, et al: Gastric lesion of familial polyposis coli. Cancer 34:745–754, 1974.
131. Shemesh E, Bat L: A prospective evaluation of the upper gastrointestinal tract and periampullary region in patients with Gardner syndrome. Am J Gastroenterol 80:825–827, 1985.
132. Coffey RJ Jr, Knight CD Jr, Van Heerden JA, Weiland LH: Gastric adenocarcinoma complicating Gardner's syndrome in a North American Woman. Gastroenterology 88:1263–1266, 1985.
133. Lindberg B, Koch NG: A family with atypical colonic polyposis and gastric cancer: A three decade follow up. Cancer 35:255–259, 1975.
134. Jarnum S, Jenson H: Diffuse gastrointestinal polyposis with ectodermal changes: A case with severe malabsorption and enteric loss of plasma proteins and electrolytes. Gastroenterology 50:107–118, 1966.
135. Manousos O, Webster CU: Diffuse gastrointestinal polyposis with ectodermal changes. Gut 7:375–379, 1966.
136. Sagara K, Fujiyama S, Kamuro Y, et al: Cronkhite-Canada syndrome associated with gastric cancer: Report of a case. Gastroenterol Jpn 18:260–266, 1983.
137. Busard JM, Walters W: Heterotopic pancreatic tissue. Arch Surg 60:674–682, 1950.
138. Lai EC, Tompkins RK: Heterotopic pancreas. Review of a 26 year experience. Am J Surg 151:697–700, 1986.
139. Yamagiwa H, Ishihara A, Sekoguchi T, Matsuzaki O: Heterotopic pancreas in surgically resected stomach. Gastroenterol Jpn 12:380–386, 1977.
140. Debord JR, Majarakis JD, Myhus LM: An unusual case of heterotopic pancreas of the stomach. Am J Surg 141:269–273, 1981.
141. Armstrong CP, King PM, Dixon JM, Macleod IB: The clinical significance of heterotopic pancreas in the gastrointestinal tract. Br J Surg 68:384–387, 1981.
142. Beccaria A, Beccaria E, Oliaro A, et al: Aberrant pancreas in gastric site. Minerva Med 68:1441–1446, 1977.
143. Goldfarb WB, Bennett D, Monafo W: Carcinoma in heterotopic gastric pancreas. Ann Surg 158:56–58, 1963.
144. Hickman DM, Frey CF, Carson JW: Adenocarcinoma arising in gastric heterotopic pancreas. West J Med 135:57–62, 1981.
145. Tomita T, Kanabe S: Islet tissue in the heterotopic pancreas. Arch Pathol Lab Med 107:469–472, 1983.
146. San Juan F, Treiger M, Silvestre W, et al: Zollinger-Ellison syndrome: Presentation of a case of non-beta-cell adenoma in a

147. Williams AW, Michie W: Adenomatosis of the stomach of Brunner gland type. Br J Surg 45:259–263, 1957.
148. Johnson CD, Bynum TE: Brunner gland heterotopia presenting as gastric antral polyps. Gastrointest Endosc 22:210–211, 1976.
149. Goldberg HI, Margulis AR: Adenomyoma of the stomach. AJR 96:382–387, 1966.
150. Stewart TW Jr, Mills LR: Adenomyoma of the stomach. South Med J 77:1337–1338, 1984.
151. Lasser A, Koufman WB: Adenomyoma of the stomach. Am J Dig Dis 22:965–969, 1977.
152. Ng WC, Yeoh SC, Joseph VT, Ong BH: Adenomyoma of the pylorus presenting as intestinal obstruction with pseudomyxoma peritonei: A case report. Ann Acad Med Singapore 10:562–565, 1981.

heterotopic pancreas with duodeno-jejunal peptic ulceration. Hospital (Rio de Janiero) 67:1148–1160, 1965.

CHAPTER 24

Early Gastric Carcinoma

TERUYUKI HIROTA, M.D.
SI-CHUN MING, M.D.

HISTORY

PROGRESS IN CLINICAL DIAGNOSIS

AGE AND SEX OF PATIENTS

DEFINITIONS

PATHOLOGY
Location and Frequency of the Tumor
Macroscopic Features
Macroscopic Classification
Prevalence and Chronologic Changes of Macroscopic Types
Size

Histologic Features and Classification
Common Types of Early Gastric Carcinoma
Papillary Adenocarcinoma
Tubular Adenocarcinoma
Poorly Differentiated Adenocarcinoma
Signet-ring Cell Adenocarcinoma
Mucinous Adenocarcinoma
Special Types of Early Gastric Carcinoma
Adenosquamous Carcinoma
Squamous Cell Carcinoma
Carcinoid Tumor
Undifferentiated Carcinoma
Other Types
Frequency of Histologic Types
Ulceration in Early Gastric Cancer

Frequency of Ulceration
Relation of Ulceration to Submucosal Invasion
Multiple Occurrence of Early Gastric Cancer
Metastasis to Lymph Nodes

NATURAL HISTORY
Histogenesis
Growth Pattern
Growth Rate

PRECANCEROUS LESIONS

RECURRENCE OF CANCER AFTER SURGERY AND PROGNOSIS

Gastric carcinoma is one of the leading causes of cancer death in the world. The geographic distribution of its incidence rates varies greatly. Japan has one of the highest rates, 54.6 per 100,000 in the male population and 25.0 per 100,000 in the female population during the period from 1984 to 1986,[1] whereas the corresponding rates for the United States were 7.0 and 3.4, among the lowest in the world. Because gastric cancer causes the highest mortality in Japan in both sexes, great efforts were placed on early diagnosis and treatment. As a result, many early gastric cancers have been detected, greatly improving the overall cure rate. In addition, study of the early stages of the tumor helps to elucidate its pathogenesis and precursors. In spite of extensive reporting on all aspects of early gastric cancer from Japan, however, the percentage of early cases remains low in many other countries, including the United States. The discussion of early gastric cancer in this chapter is based primarily on the experience in Japan.

HISTORY

Verse was credited as the first to describe early cancer of the stomach as an entity.[2,3] In 1903, he reported seven cases of *Schleimhautcarcinome* with carcinoma involving the mucosa and submucosa.[4] Subsequently, such a tumor has been reported variously as carcinoma *in situ*,[5] carcinoma of superficial spreading type,[6] superficial carcinoma,[7-9] superficial erosive cancer,[10] and surface carcinoma.[11] It was not until 1962, however, that the concept of early gastric cancer was firmly established. In that year, the macroscopic classification of early gastric cancer was presented by the Japanese Gastroenterological Endoscopy Society.[12-14] Since

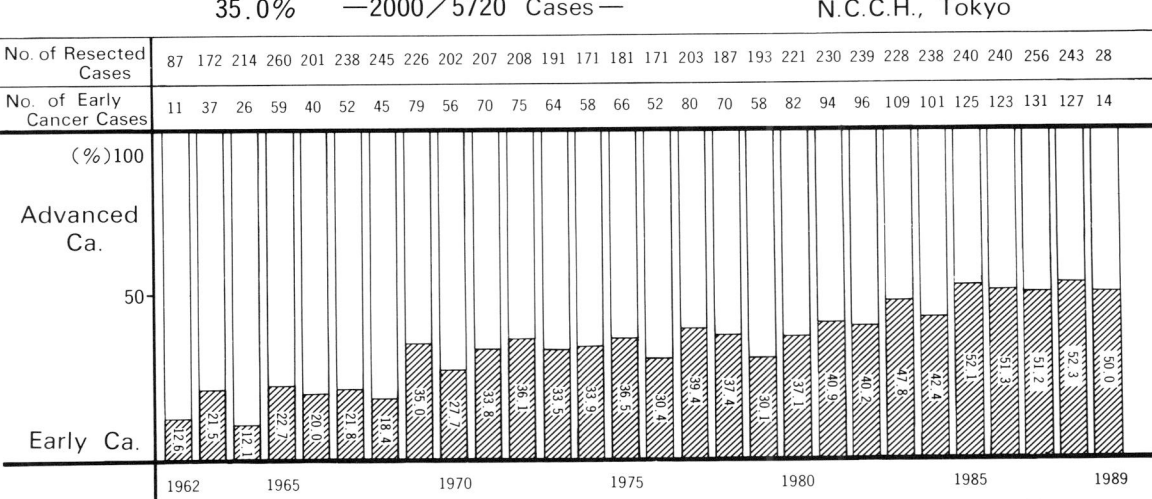

FIGURE 24–1. Chronologic trend in the percentage of early cancer among all patients with gastric carcinoma operated on at the National Cancer Center Hospital in Tokyo, Japan.

then, combined study meetings of clinicians and pathologists have been held periodically in Japan. As a result, remarkable progress has been made in diagnostic methods for early gastric cancer, especially in radiologic and endoscopic studies based on morphologic features. These methods have been extensively applied to mass health surveillance, resulting in life-saving early detection and surgical therapy for gastric cancer. Currently, even detection of a malignant lesion measuring less than 5 mm is not very difficult.

Except in certain institutions, however, the number of advanced cases of gastric cancer far exceeded those of early gastric cancer. During the 24 years from its opening to December 1985, 5009 patients with gastric cancer were treated surgically at the National Cancer Center in Tokyo. Early gastric cancer was found in 1627 (32%); advanced gastric cancer was found in the remaining 68%. The Japan Gastric Cancer Registry, started in 1962 by the Gastric Cancer Study Group, now has 29,902 cases on file.

At the National Cancer Center Hospital, there has been a steady increase in the percentage of early cases among surgically treated gastric cancers through the years, so that now 50% of the cases are in the early stage (Figure 24–1), with a corresponding increase in the overall survival rate for gastric cancer. Similar results have been seen in other Japanese institutions.[2,15] In Europe and the United States it was not until the early 1970s that the term *early gastric cancer* was employed in various reports, and the percentage of early cases among the diagnosed gastric carcinomas remained low, around 10%.[3,16,17] All of these reports, however, were based on a small number of cases. Of 87 cases reported by Elster and associates[18] in Germany, the peak age was in the fifth decade. Otherwise, there was no significant difference between the German and Japanese cases. Green and co-workers,[19] in the United States, reported 69 early cases among a total of 549 gastric cancers, an incidence of 13%. They have noted an increase in the incidence in recent years and a 5-year survival rate of 97%.

PROGRESS IN CLINICAL DIAGNOSIS

Radiologic diagnostic methods have contributed significantly to the detection of early gastric cancer; the accomplishments of Shirakabe and Ichikawa[15,20,21] in the application of the double-contrast method should be especially highly regarded. They produced images that were almost identical to the macroscopic appearance of the surgically removed stomach.

The remarkable contribution of endoscopic examination is also widely recognized. Gastrocameras and endoscopes with camera attachments at the tip, as well as histologic diagnosis using gastric biopsy specimens obtained with a fibergastroscope, were developed and further advanced the potential of gastric endoscopy. For the detection of gastric carcinomas measuring less than 1 cm, the contribution of endoscopy is especially important; indeed, endoscopy has become almost indispensable in the diagnosis of malignancy. Histologic examination of the gastric biopsy specimen is now included in the routine work of pathologists, who are now direct participants in the early diagnosis of gastric cancer. Correct preoperative diagnosis is now possible in 95% to 98% of cases, based on histologic findings in the biopsy specimens.

AGE AND SEX OF PATIENTS

Although the age of patients undergoing surgery for early gastric cancer had been reported to be predominantly in the fifth decade,[18] our data indicate a peak in the seventh decade, with a male-to-female ratio of approximately 2:1 (Figure 24–2). This ratio is nearly constant in world mortality statistics, regardless of the

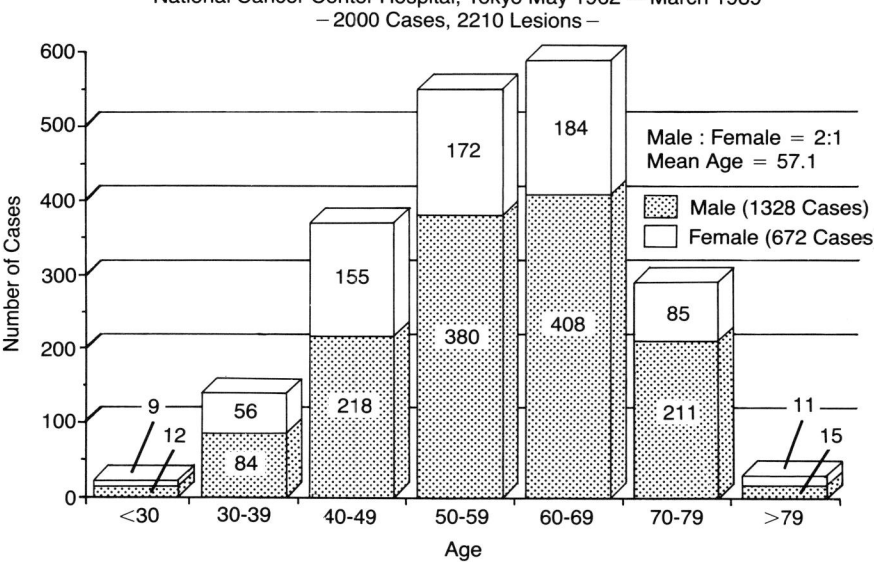

FIGURE 24-2. Age and sex distribution of patients with early gastric cancer at the National Cancer Center Hospital in Tokyo, Japan.

prevalence of gastric cancer in each country. There is a wide age distribution, and early gastric cancer is seen as early as the late teens. A slight increase of patients over 60 years of age since early 1970s has been noted.[22] The polypoid lesions are common in the old, whereas the large depressed and ulcerated lesions are common in young patients.[2] There is a female predominance until the fourth decade. Men predominate in the forties and fifties, and a peak is reached in the sixties for both men and women. Among surgical cases, little male-to-female difference was noted in a small number of patients in their eighties. Among patients with advanced age, however, a considerable number were not operated on; and so these data may not reflect the true prevalence rate.

DEFINITIONS

Early gastric cancer is defined as a primary carcinoma of the stomach with carcinomatous infiltration limited to the mucosa and submucosal layer (Figure 24-3), regardless of the presence or absence of lymph node metastases.[12-14] Discussions concerning the presence or absence of lymph node metastases were subsequently carried out. Based on the opinions of internists participating in the diagnosis, a decision was made not to take the presence or absence of metastases into consideration. The word *early* here indicates the possibility of complete surgical resection and does not imply a time dimension. Although the presence or absence of lymph node metastases and prognosis are intimately related, preoperative diagnostic procedures are incapable of identifying these metastases. Even if metastases are found, those with positive metastases represent less than 9% of the whole series of early gastric cancers. Adequate regional lymphadenectomy has resulted in a 5-year survival rate higher than 95%, an excellent prognosis.

PATHOLOGY

Location and Frequency of Tumor

The stomach is divided into the upper (C, for corpus), middle (M), and lower (A, for antrum) thirds along the long axis.[12] Along the transverse axis, the anterior and posterior walls, the greater and lesser curvatures, and the whole circumference are distinguished.

At the National Cancer Center Hospital in Tokyo, the occurrence of early gastric cancer in the M region is the highest (56.3%), followed by the A and C regions (Figure 24-4), especially in the group with ulcer within the cancer. In the whole series of patients subjected to surgery for gastric cancer in the Japan Registry, including advanced cases, occurrence in the pyloric portion or A region is the highest (44.6%), followed by location in the M region (39.3%) and the C region (16.1%). In-

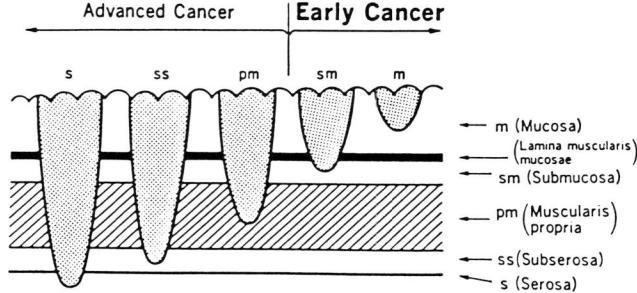

FIGURE 24-3. Definition of early and advanced gastric cancers according to the level of cancerous invasion in the gastric wall.

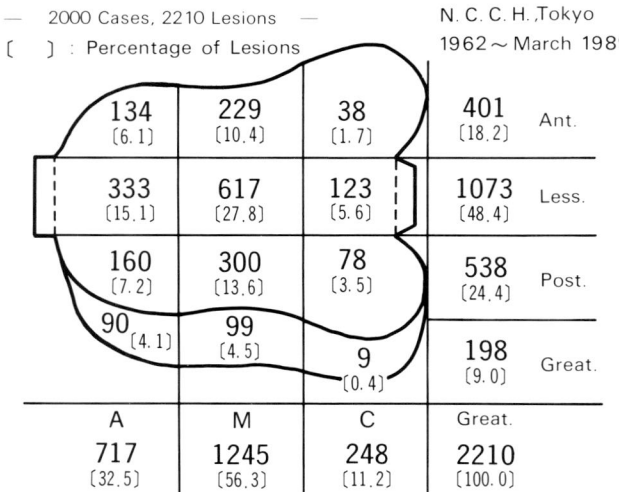

FIGURE 24-4. Location of early gastric cancer at the National Cancer Center Hospital in Tokyo, Japan. A, distal third; M, middle third; C, proximal third; Ant., anterior wall; Less., lesser curvature; Post., posterior wall; Great., greater curvature.

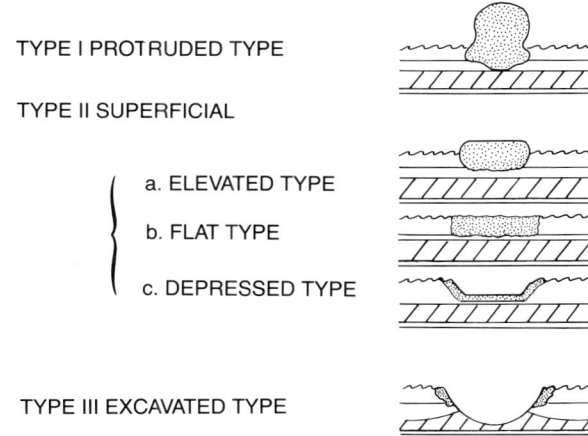

FIGURE 24-5. Macroscopic classification of early gastric cancer. Basic types.

stead of representing the true regional incidence, these data probably reflect multiple factors, including the rate of detection and feasibility of surgical resection.

Early gastric cancer occurs most frequently on the lesser curvature (48.4%), followed by the posterior wall (24.4%), anterior wall (18.2%), and greater curvature (9.0%) (see Figure 24-4). A considerable difference is found in comparison with advanced cancers, probably because of the difference in the rate of detection.

Macroscopic Features

Macroscopic Classification

Borrmann's classification of gastric carcinoma according to gross morphologic features is widely accepted.[23] It separates the tumors into four types: type I for polypoid tumors, type II for fungating tumors, type III for ulcerated tumors, and type IV for diffusely infiltrating tumors. These gross types are applied to advanced carcinomas. The early gastric cancer is not included but has been classified as Borrmann's type O in the recent years.[2]

The macroscopic classification of early gastric cancer is shown in Figure 24-5 and includes type I (protruding type), type II (superficial type), and type III (excavated type).

Type I tumor is a nodular lesion that often shows an irregular surface with crevices between the papillary projections (Figure 24-6).

Type II lesions are further subdivided into type IIa (superficial elevated type), with a slight elevation of the lesion approximately twice the thickness of mucosa to 5 mm; type IIb (superficial flat type), with the level of the lesion approximately the same as the surrounding mucosa; and type IIc (superficial depressed type), with a shallow depression.

Type IIc cancer is the most frequent and most important lesion in clinical diagnosis (Table 24-1). In this type, the erosive surface of the carcinoma is slightly lower than the surrounding mucosa. It varies in size (Figure 24-7 to 24-11). Nagayo[24] subdivided type IIc lesions into two types: a IIc′ type, well-demarcated and less than 3 cm in diameter, and a IIc″ type, poorly demarcated and larger than 3 cm in diameter. The larger one has also been called superficial spreading type.[6]

The tips of the mucosal folds converging at the type IIc lesion show characteristic pen-tip–like narrowing, i.e., narrowing with indentation and an abrupt border (see Figures 24-7 to 24-10). The depressed surface of the type IIc lesion is characterized as follows: (1) Unlike the surrounding mucosa, it is flattened (see Figure 24-7) and occasionally accompanied by granular changes of various sizes (see Figure 24-8). (2) Within the depressed area, an ulcer scar or an open ulcer may be present, which may be shallow (see Figure 24-7) or deep (see Figure 24-8). (3) There is a disappearance of the glistening surface. (4) There are color tone changes.

Type III cancer shows a deep, ulcer-like excavation surrounded by a narrow rim of carcinomatous tissue along the ulcer border. This lesion may resemble a benign ulcer. A pure type III lesion is rare, with a frequency rate less than 1% (see Table 24-1).

A combined type of early gastric cancer indicates the coexistence of more than two of the basic macroscopic types in a single lesion (Figure 24-12). Discussions are still in progress as to which type should be designated first. In general, the type occupying the larger area is written first, regardless of the histogenesis. For example, when ulceration beyond the muscularis mucosa is found within a type IIc lesion and the ulcer is more conspicuous than the IIc lesion, this combined lesion is called type III + type IIc (Figure 24-13). When elevation and excavation coexist, opinions may be divided between calling it type IIa + type IIc or type IIc + type IIa (Figure 24-14), but these designations make little

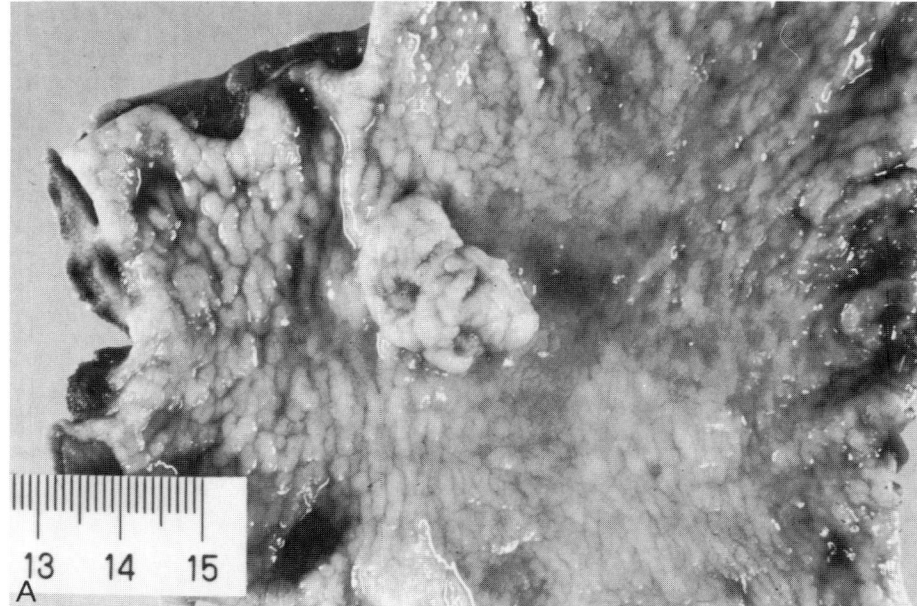
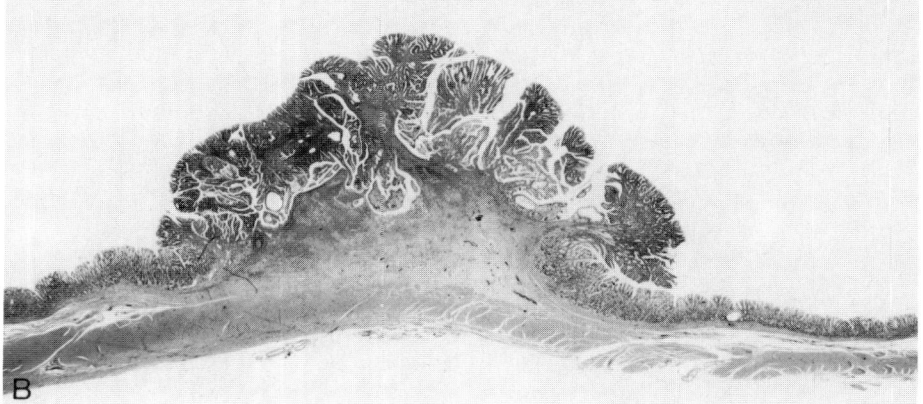

FIGURE 24-6. Protruded type I early gastric carcinoma. A, Gross morphology. B, Microscopic morphology. The tumor is papillary. There is focal infiltration into the submucosa.

Table 24-1. MACROSCOPIC TYPES OF EARLY GASTRIC CANCER*

Macroscopic Type	Lesions	%	Groups (%)
I	150	6.8	
IIa	190	8.6	A (23.8)
IIa + IIc	186	8.4	
IIb	72	3.3	B (3.3)
IIc	1337	60.5	
IIc + III	155	7.0	
IIc + IIa	53	2.4	C (72.9)
III	14	0.6	
III + IIc	53	2.4	
Total	2210	100	(100)

*National Cancer Center Hospital, Tokyo, May 1962 to March 1989 (2000 cases, 2210 lesions).
A, predominantly protruded or elevated lesions; B, flat lesions; C, predominantly depressed or excavated lesions.

difference as to the rate of lymph node metastasis or prognosis, according to our statistical data. As described above, attempts were made to avoid terminology associated with pre-existing concepts for the definition, classification, and designation; and abstract expressions were employed instead.

The gross types can be combined into three groups according to the dominating features: A, protruded or elevated lesions; B, flat lesions; and C, depressed or excavated lesions. Their frequencies are listed in Table 24-1.

Prevalence and Chronologic Changes of Macroscopic Types

The prevalence of macroscopic types of early gastric cancer varies somewhat among institutions. In the Japanese national statistics, type IIc was seen most frequently (33.8%), followed by type IIc + type III (23.4%), type I (9.7%), type IIa (9%), and type IIa + type IIc (6.5%). In our data, type IIc also was found most frequently (60.5%) (see Table 24-1). Of 1252

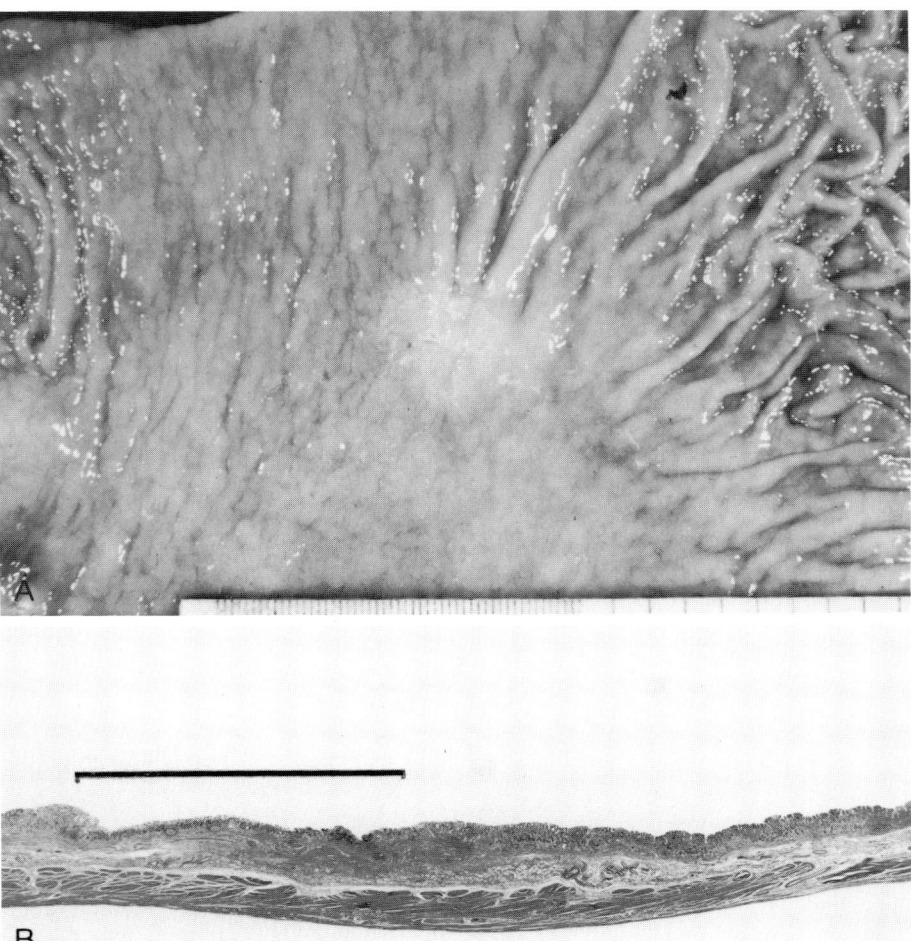

FIGURE 24–7. Shallowly depressed type IIc early gastric carcinoma. A, Gross morphology. B, Scanning view of the microscopic morphology. There is fibrosis in the submucosa. The line marks the extent of the tumor.

cases studied by Nagayo,[2] type IIc" was the most frequent (41.9%), followed by III (22.6%), IIc' (19.3%), IIa (8.1%), I (6.2%), and IIb (1.9%). In contrast, among cases studied by Johansen,[3] 13.3% of the tumors were type IIb.

The distribution of macroscopic types has changed during the past 25 years. Initially, the depressed type accounted for 68.0%, with a recent increase to 75.3%. The frequency of elevated type is decreasing. Among the depressed types, the relatively shallow type IIc lesion (see Figures 24–7 and 24–9) has become predominant. The type III lesion has virtually disappeared since 1974.[22]

Size

In the early 1960s, 86% of early gastric cancers were larger than 2 cm. Smaller lesions have been increasingly diagnosed in recent years (Figure 24–15), reflecting the progress in diagnostic methods. The small cancer (less than 10 mm in size) and particularly the minute cancer (less than 5 mm in size) are important, not only in their potential for a total cure but also in their contribution to the understanding of premalignant lesions.[25] Type IIb lesions constitute 58.3% of the tumors less than 5 mm in diameter and 0% of tumors larger than 5 mm,[15] which indicates that as the tumor grows larger, the originally flat lesion becomes either protruding or depressed.

Histologic Features and Classification

The classifications proposed by Lauren[26] and the World Health Organization (WHO)[27] are often used. In the former, gastric carcinomas of the ordinary type are separated into intestinal and diffuse types. In the latter, the traditional histologic classifications are used (see below). Gastric carcinomas have also been classified according to growth patterns into expanding and infiltrative types.[28] In Japan, gastric carcinomas are often classified into differentiated and undifferentiated types.[29] The differentiated adenocarcinomas in this classification include well-differentiated to moderately differentiated glandular adenocarcinomas. The undifferentiated carcinomas show little or no glandular formation but include such differentiated tumors as signet-ring cell carcinoma and mucinous adenocarcinoma, as well as poorly differentiated adenocarcinoma and undifferentiated solid tumors. The intestinal, ex-

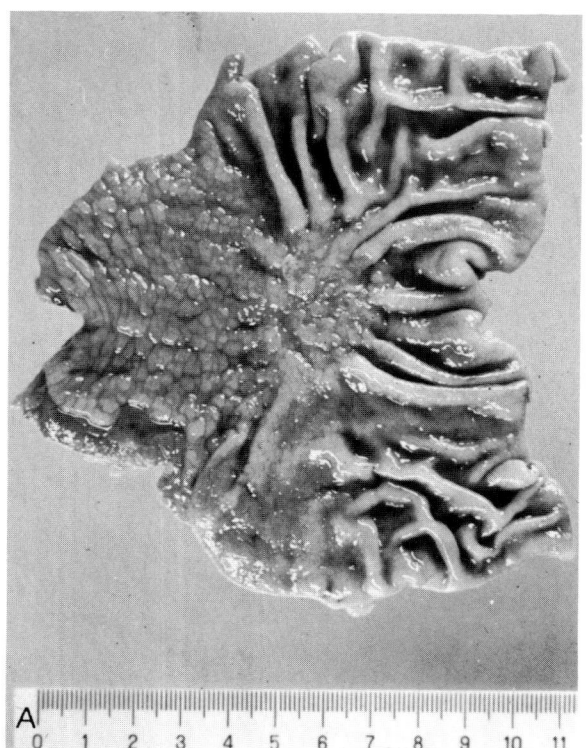

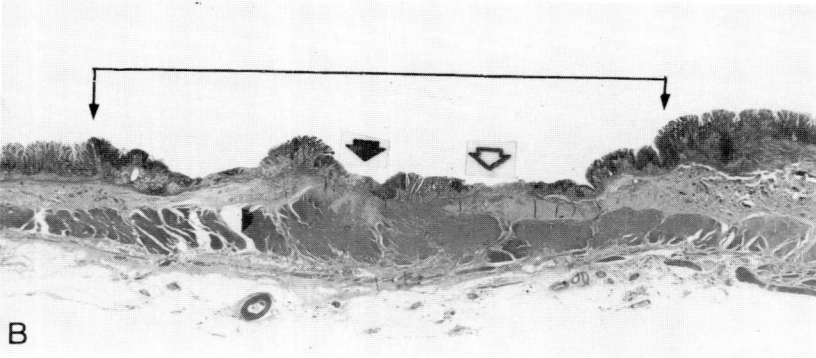

FIGURE 24–8. Deeply depressed type IIc early gastric carcinoma. *A*, Gross morphology. *B*, Scanning view of the microscopic morphology. Both open ulcer (open arrow) and scar tissue (closed arrow) are present in the submucosa. The line marks the extent of the tumor.

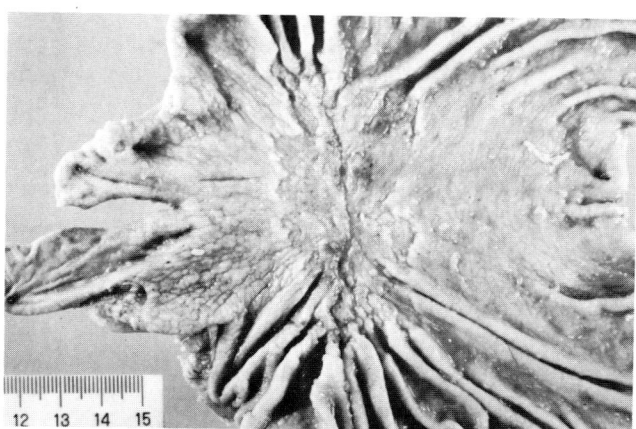

FIGURE 24–9. Typical depressed type IIc early gastric carcinoma.

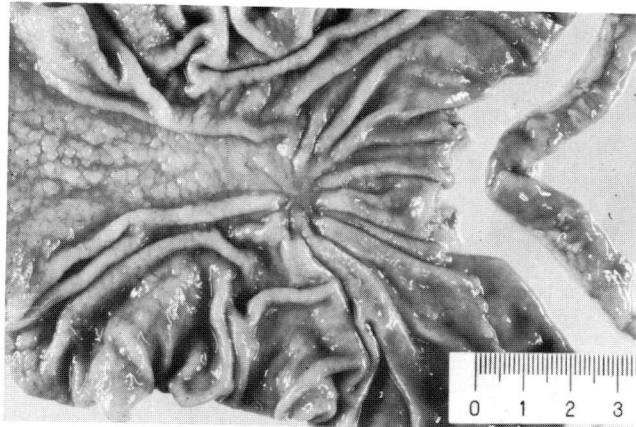

FIGURE 24–10. Small type IIc early gastric carcinoma with ulceration.

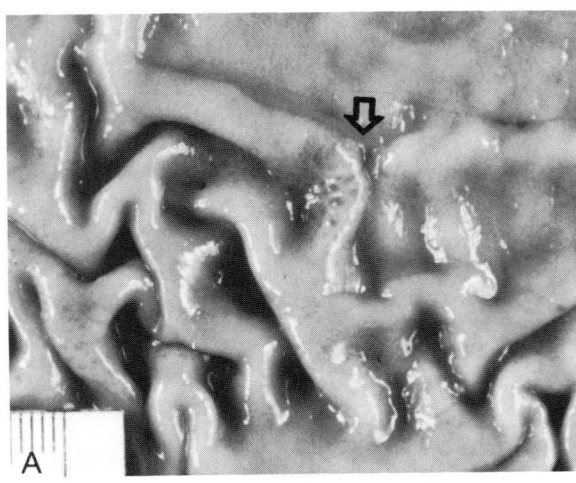
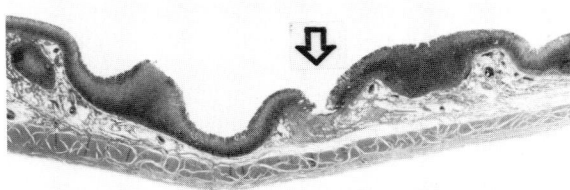
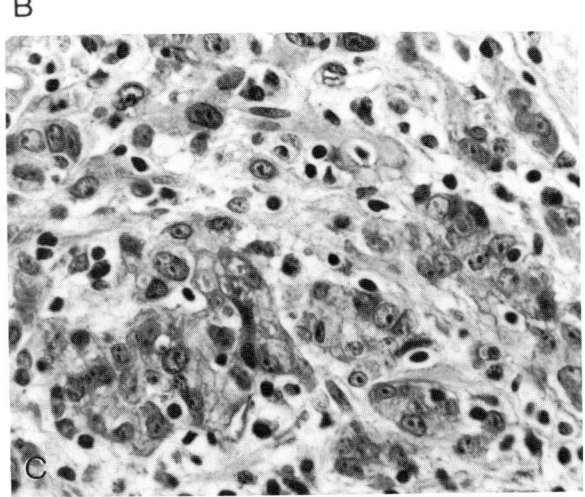

FIGURE 24–11. Minute type IIc early gastric carcinoma. *A*, Gross morphology. *B*, Scanning view of microscopic morphology. *C*, High magnification of the tumor showing poorly differentiated cells. Arrows point at the depressed cancer.

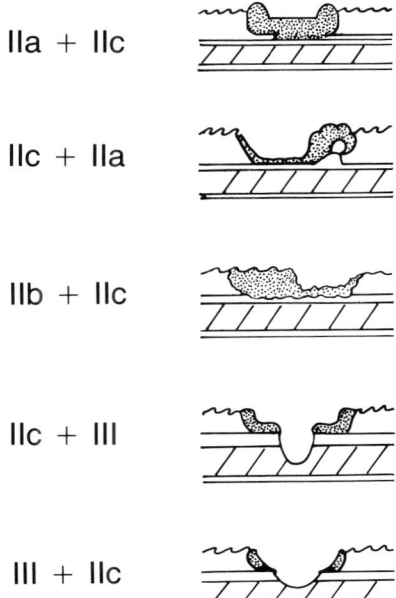

FIGURE 24–12. Macroscopic classification of early gastric cancer. Combined types.

Common Types of Early Gastric Carcinoma

The frequency of these histologic types are listed in Table 24–2.

Papillary Adenocarcinoma

Cuboidal to high cylindrical-shaped carcinoma cells proliferate along the narrow bands of interstitial tissue running in an arborizing pattern (see Figure 24–6B; Figure 24–16). This kind of carcinoma is frequently well developed, with preservation of the axial property of tumor cells. The nuclei are nearly round or irregular in contour, with abundant nucleoplasm and a coarse chromatin pattern.

Tubular Adenocarcinoma

Glandular formation is distinct. Depending on the degree of glandular lumen formation, this type is fur-

panding, and differentiated carcinomas share much similarity, and the diffuse, infiltrative, and undifferentiated carcinomas explained above form another group with similar features.

The Subcommittee for Histological Classification of the Gastric Cancer Study Group in Japan has developed a classification that considers the relative frequency of the tumor as well as the histologic features. This classification, listed in detail below, is similar to the WHO typing.[27] Further discussion on histologic classification of gastric carcinoma is presented in Chapter 25.

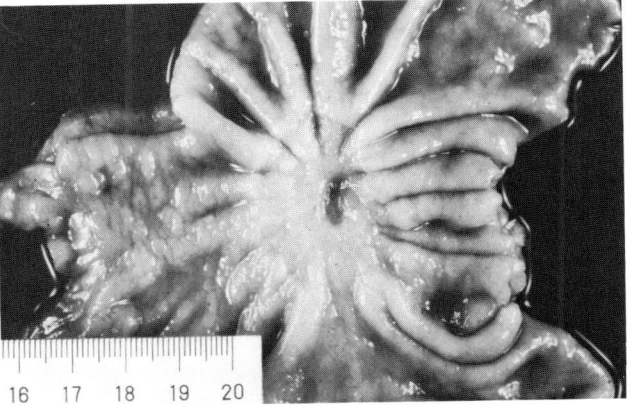

FIGURE 24–13. Combined type IIc and III early gastric cancer.

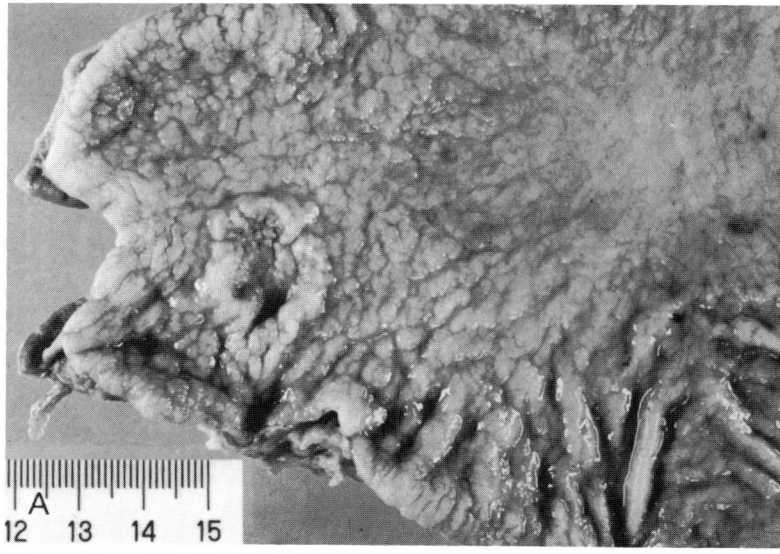

FIGURE 24–14. Combined type IIa and IIc early gastric cancer. *A*, Gross morphology. *B*, Scanning photomicrograph showing elevated margins and the depressed center of the lesion. The line marks the extent of the tumor.

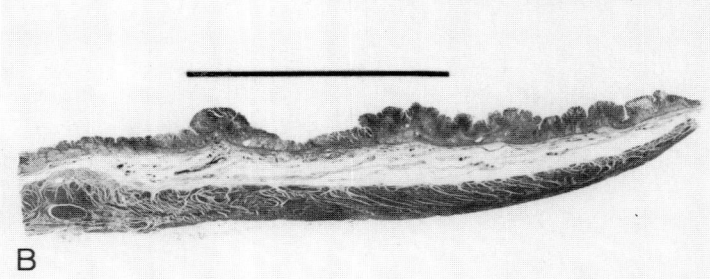

ther divided into well-differentiated and moderately differentiated subtypes. The well-differentiated type is defined as an adenocarcinoma with a distinct glandular structure without complex arborization, despite mild variations in size and irregularity in the glandular structures (see Figure 24–16). Carcinoma cells are frequently high cylindrical to cuboidal, arranged in a single layer. The nuclei are arranged evenly along the base of the cells, with occasional pseudostratification. The nuclei are irregular in shape, with thickening of the nuclear margin, abundant karyoplasm, and a coarse chromatin pattern.

In the moderately differentiated type of tubular adenocarcinoma, the glandular structures are irregular, complex, or incomplete (Figure 24–17). In this type of adenocarcinoma, in addition to the expected marked structural atypia, the axial property of the tumor cell is irregular, with occasional pseudostratification. The nuclei of the tumor cells appear nearly round or irregular in shape, with abundant karyoplasm and a coarse internal structure.

Poorly Differentiated Adenocarcinoma

In this histologic type, the carcinoma consists of solid medullary structures of various sizes with an occasional cordlike arrangement. The individual carcinoma

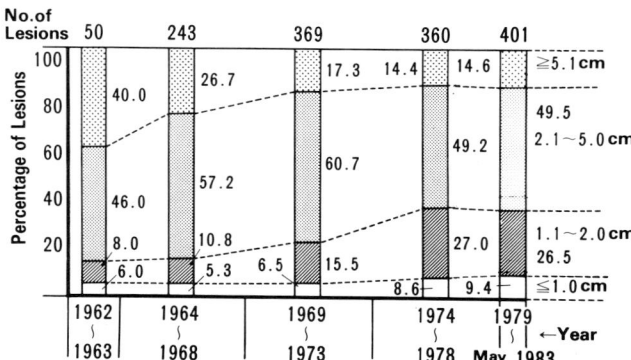

FIGURE 24–15. Chronologic trend in the size of early gastric cancer, in percentage of the lesions, at the National Cancer Center Hospital in Tokyo, Japan.

Table 24–2. HISTOLOGIC TYPES OF EARLY GASTRIC CANCER*

Histologic Type	Lesions	%
Papillary adenocarcinoma	165	7.5
Tubular adenocarcinoma	1152	52.0
Poorly differentiated adenocarcinoma	300	13.6
Signet-ring cell carcinoma	576	26.1
Mucinous adenocarcinoma	17	0.8
Total	2210	100

*National Cancer Center Hospital, Tokyo, May 1962 to March 1989 (2000 cases, 2210 lesions).

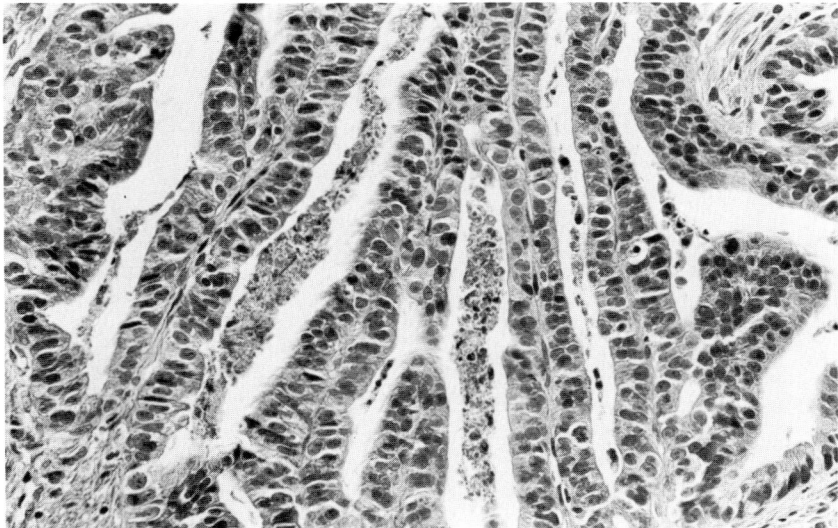

FIGURE 24–16. Well-differentiated tubular early gastric carcinoma, showing a focally papillary pattern.

cells may form small, alveolus-like structures surrounded by relatively coarse intercellular connective tissue (Figure 24–18). Microglandular structure is seen only in a small number of areas. Mucus may be demonstrated in the cytoplasm of tumor cells, but the amount of mucus is usually scanty. The nuclei of the tumor cells vary in size and are nearly round or irregular, with abundant karyoplasm. Numerous mitotic figures are commonly found. This type of carcinoma shows a strong tendency to diffuse infiltration.

Signet-ring Cell Adenocarcinoma

Within the cytoplasm of the tumor cells, a large number of mucous granules are present. The nuclei are irregular, crescent-shaped, and pushed to one side (Figure 24–19). The name of this carcinoma refers to the shape, which resembles a ring with a signet. A small alveolar or cordlike arrangement is noted, occasionally with a solid appearance. In many cases, individual cells proliferate in an isolated fashion, with a strong tendency to diffuse infiltration.

Mucinous Adenocarcinoma

In this type, the carcinoma cells float within mucus pools, exhibiting nodular patterns of various sizes, or line the internal wall of the interstitium surrounding the mucus pools. Some of the carcinoma cells show a signet-ring–like appearance, and others appear cylindrical, with a tubular or papillary arrangement. Thus, this type of carcinoma is a variant of either signet-ring cell carcinoma or glandular adenocarcinoma with abundant mucus secretion. It should be understood that all adenocarcinomas of the stomach secrete mucin, but the amount varies. To qualify for the term of mu-

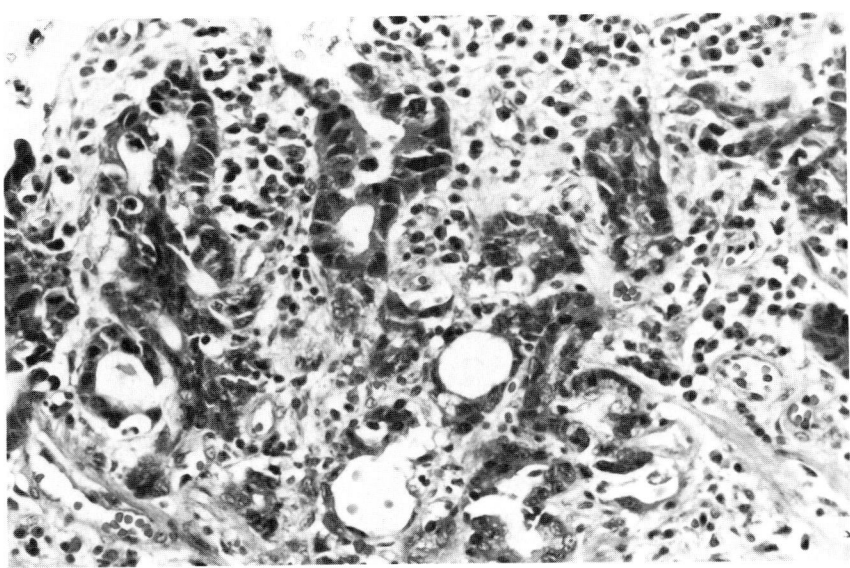

FIGURE 24–17. Type IIc early gastric carcinoma showing a moderately differentiated tubular pattern.

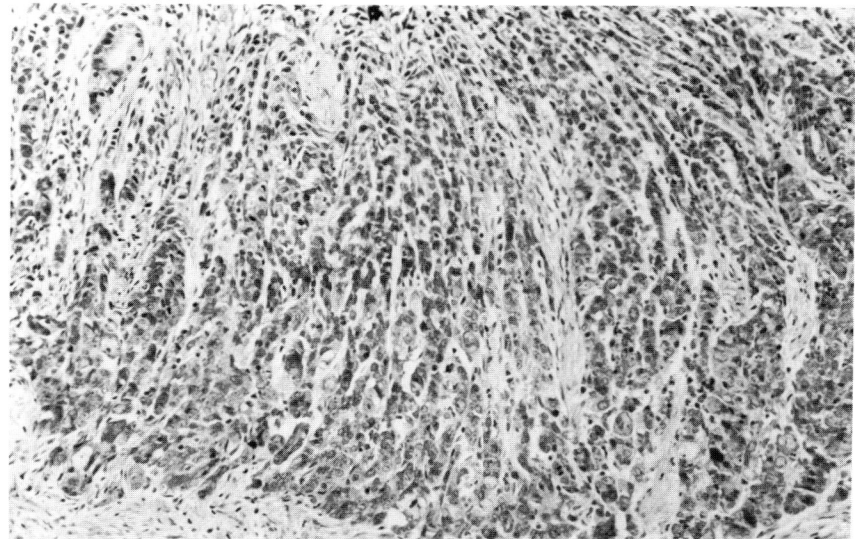

FIGURE 24-18. Type IIc early gastric carcinoma shown in Figure 24-8, showing poorly differentiated histologic features.

cinous carcinoma, the total amount of mucin must exceed 50% or more of total tumor volume.

Special Types of Early Gastric Carcinoma

Adenosquamous Carcinoma

Within a single lesion, a mixed picture of adenocarcinoma and squamous cell carcinoma is seen in approximately equal amounts, with one element occupying at least one third. When a very small area of squamous metaplasia is found within the lesion of adenocarcinoma, the lesion is not classified in this category, and only the description of metaplasia is added to the main diagnosis of adenocarcinoma.

Squamous Cell Carcinoma

The carcinoma cells overlap in a multilayered structure as in the squamous cell epithelium, with a tendency to lamellar arrangement toward the open surface of the tumor or in the center of tumor patches. There are varying degrees of keratinization. The squamous cell carcinoma is rare in the stomach. When it occurs in the cardiac region, it may be an extension of an esophageal carcinoma.

Carcinoid Tumor

The main portion of the tumor frequently occupies the submucosal layer, rather than the mucosa. The tumor cells have abundant cytoplasm, with nearly round and relatively small nuclei filled with homogeneous karyoplasm. The structure of this tumor appears alveolar, cordlike, ribbonlike, or lacelike, occasionally with the formation of rosettes or glandular lumen. Argyrophilic and argentaffin reactions and neurosecretory granules under electron microscopy are useful in the differential diagnosis. Carcinoid is described in detail in Chapter 13.

Undifferentiated Carcinoma

This kind of tumor lacks any specific picture of differentiation, structurally or functionally. It is therefore not possible to establish the origin from the point of view of histogenesis. It should be noted that the undifferentiated carcinoma in this classification is not the same as the undifferentiated carcinoma in the Japanese classification mentioned at the beginning of this section. The latter includes the poorly differentiated as well as some of the differentiated carcinomas described in this section.

Other Types

Choriocarcinoma or malignant chorioepithelioma with syncytio- and cytotrophoblastic cells in varying numbers may occur in the stomach. This type of car-

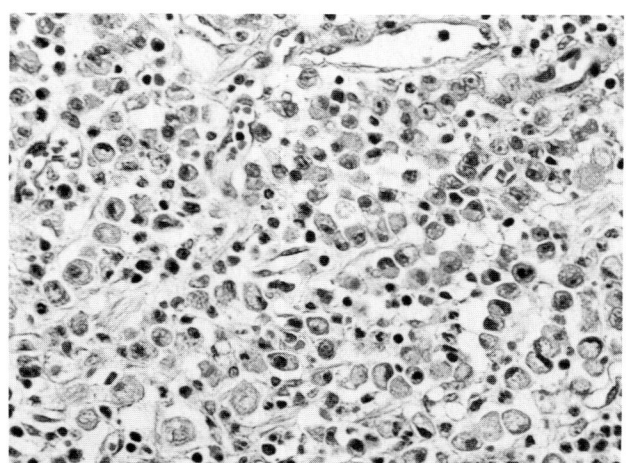

FIGURE 24-19. An early gastric carcinoma, showing signet-ring-shaped cancer cells.

cinoma is frequently accompanied by foci of ordinary adenocarcinoma. An early small-cell carcinoma has been reported.[30] Finally, advanced carcinomas may simulate the early lesions.[31]

Frequency of Histologic Types

Among early gastric cancers diagnosed at the National Cancer Center Hospital in Tokyo, the differentiated type of glandular adenocarcinoma accounts for 56.5%, and the poorly differentiated and undifferentiated carcinomas, for 43.5%. In gastric cancer as a whole, including advanced gastric cancer, papillary adenocarcinoma and tubular adenocarcinoma account for 43.7%, and poorly differentiated adenocarcinomas and signet-ring cell carcinomas account for the majority (56.3%). Signet-ring cell carcinoma accounts for 29.6% of early gastric cancer, but only 22.7% of advanced gastric cancer. The frequency of poorly differentiated adenocarcinoma, conversely, was 11.7% in early cancer and much higher (29.5%) in the advanced cancer. Mucinous adenocarcinoma is rare and is located mainly in the submucosal or deeper layer, so that it accounts for only 0.8% of early gastric cancer; its frequency in advanced gastric cancer is 5.2%.

Ulceration in Early Gastric Cancer

Frequency of Ulceration

Secondary ulcer formation frequently takes place within the early carcinoma. This was found in about 65.4% of the whole group of early gastric cancer and in 80% of patients below the age of 65. Ulceration was less frequent in elderly patients (69.2%). The frequency of ulceration and/or ulcer scar had decreased from 93.5% in 1962 to 71.9% in 1983.[22] According to the classification of Murakami,[32] which expresses four levels of depth of ulceration from Ul-I to Ul-IV, ulcers in the early cancer appear most commonly at the level of Ul-II (involving the submucosa). Formation of an ulcer scar is the main cause of the convergence of mucosal folds toward the carcinomatous lesion.

Relation of Ulceration to Submucosal Invasion

At the National Cancer Center Hospital, a large number of early carcinomas with submucosal invasion was found in the group with ulceration (360 of 529 cases, or 68.1%), but the prevalence rate of submucosal invasion was not much different for the tumors without ulceration (416 cases) and those with ulceration (786 cases), 40.6% and 45.8%, respectively. The prevalence rate of submucosal infiltration reversed in carcinomas larger than 3 cm. The presence of an ulcer, therefore, appears to participate in the development of submucosal invasion in type IIc carcinoma measuring less than 3 cm, whereas in carcinomas larger than 3 cm, pronounced submucosal invasion was found in the absence of ulceration.

Multiple Occurrence of Early Gastric Cancer

Multiple tumors were found in about 8.3% of 500 cases at the National Cancer Center Hospital. In 77% of these, two lesions coexisted in the stomach. Coexistence of three lesions was found in 20% and more than four lesions in 3%. In patients over 65 years of age, the rate of multiple tumors was 13%, twice that of the group under 65 years of age. The background gastric mucosa giving rise to multiple gastric carcinomas frequently revealed extensive intestinal metaplasia. Among 77 specimens studied by Johansen,[3] 8 had two or three early cancers, 6 had one early and one advanced cancers, and 1 had two early and one advanced cancers.

Metastasis to Lymph Nodes

Even in cases of early gastric cancer, lymph node metastases may occur, with a frequency ranging from 0% to 17% in intramucosal carcinomas and 13% to 30% in submucosal carcinomas in Japan.[33] The corresponding ranges in Europe were 1.5% to 7% and 4% to 12.3%, respectively. At the National Cancer Center Hospital, lymph node metastases were seen in 2.1% of cases with tumor limited to the mucosa and in 13.9% of cases with submucosal invasion. The respective percentages in another report from Japan were 4% and 19%.[34] The rate of lymph node metastasis was related to the size of the primary tumor: 4% in tumors less than 1 cm in diameter and 18% in tumors larger than 4 cm.[34] The metastasis from mucosal cancer was limited to the primary regional nodes, but the submucosal cancers may spread to the secondary or tertiary nodes.[35] The frequency of metastases to lymph nodes also varied, depending on the presence or absence of ulceration in the carcinoma. Among cases with tumor limited to the mucosa, metastases were found in 0% of cases without ulceration and in 2% to 3% of cases with ulceration. In cases with submucosal penetration, conversely, lymph node metastases were found in 23.3% of patients without ulceration and in 20% to 30% of those with ulceration.

NATURAL HISTORY

Histogenesis

Histologic examination of early gastric cancer, particularly the minute lesions, allows the opportunity to evaluate the background mucosa from which the early cancerous lesion arises. Such studies revealed that the glandular differentiated carcinoma was associated with intestinal metaplasia, whereas the nonglandular carcinoma arose from the gastric mucosa.[36] By serial-step sections, Hattori noted that carcinoma, metaplasia, and dysplasia all began at the neck region of the glands, where regeneration of the epithelium normally occurred, and concluded that these cellular abnormalities were coincidental lesions.[37] Similar cellular origin from the gland neck was demonstrated for the signet-ring cell carcinoma by Grundmann.[38]

Growth Pattern

Early gastric carcinomas have been classified by Kodama and colleagues according to growth patterns revealed by the appearances on the cross section.[39] Based on the size of the tumor and the amount of submucosal involvement, the early gastric cancers were classified into superficial spreading (super type, 44.9%), small mucosal (36.5%), penetrating (Pen type, 17.4%), and mixed (1.2%) types. The Pen-type tumors were subdivided into A and B types, showing expanding and infiltrative form of submucosal growth, respectively. The importance of this observation lies in the finding that Pen A-type tumors were mostly elevated and had higher rates of lymphatic permeation and lymph node metastasis than other types. Venous permeation was observed only in the Pen A-type tumors. The 10-year survival rate was 65% for Pen A-type tumors and 87% to 100% for other types. DNA measurements showed high ploidy of Pen A tumors and low ploidy of other tumors.[40]

Growth Rate

The growth rate of early gastric cancer appears slow, as judged by many years of clinical symptoms and the large size of some of the tumors.[41] Fugita noted that the clinical doubling time for early gastric cancer ranged from 18 to 108 months, 2 to 3 years on average.[42] He estimated that the early cancer stage might last 14 to 21 years. The growth rate accelerated in the advanced tumor, with doubling time shortened to 2 to 10 months. Tsukuma and associates followed 43 cases of unresected early gastric cancer for 6 to 88 months; the tumor became advanced in 27 cases and remained in the early phase in 16.[43] The long early phase of gastric carcinoma may be one reason for the high yield of early cancer cases detected by mass surveillance programs, aside from advanced diagnostic methods.

PRECANCEROUS LESIONS

The precancerous state of clinical conditions with a high expectancy of cancer development should be distinguished from a precancerous lesion, defined as a pathologic entity showing distinct histopathologic abnormalities and a significantly high frequency of malignant transformation. Many studies indicate that chronic gastritis accompanied by intestinal metaplasia is the most important precancerous lesion. The metaplastic process accompanying the cancerous lesion is often incomplete.[37]

Among the elevated precancerous lesions, adenoma is the most important,[44] followed by hyperplastic polyp and verrucous gastritis. Chronic gastric ulcer, regarded

Precancerous Lesion	No. of Cases	%
Hyperplastic polyp	10	0.53
Adenoma	47	2.47
Chronic ulcer	13	0.68
Atrophic gastritis	1802	94.84
Verrucous gastritis	26	1.37
Stomach remnant	2	0.11
Aberrant pancreas	0	0
Total	1900	100 %

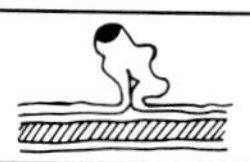

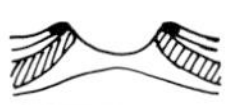

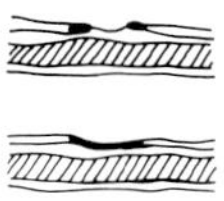

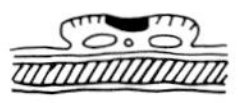

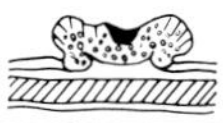

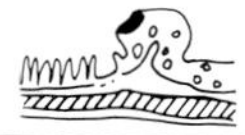

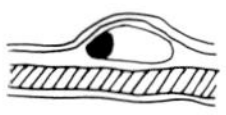

1900 Cases — N.C.C.R.I., Tokyo ~ April 1988

FIGURE 24–20. Incidence of early gastric cancer arising in various precancerous lesions diagnosed at the National Cancer Center Hospital in Tokyo, Japan. Solid black areas depict carcinomatous lesions.

as an important precancerous lesion in the past, has been shown to be of very low significance.[45] The gastric remnant following partial resection and the stomach of patients with pernicious anemia are thought to represent precancerous states. Figure 24–20 shows the frequency of various conditions found in association with early gastric carcinoma.

RECURRENCE OF CANCER AFTER SURGERY AND PROGNOSIS

The rate of recurrence of early gastric cancer 5 years postoperatively is around 3% in cases of intramucosal carcinoma. In cases of submucosal carcinoma, it is as high as 8% to 9%. The recurrence rates 10 years postoperatively may be as high as 10% to 22% in patients with submucosal carcinoma and 8% to 14% in those with intramucosal tumor. Early recurrence generally occurs in cases of submucosal cancer, whereas late recurrence is common in mucosal tumor. Papillary and differentiated adenocarcinomas frequently show hepatic metastases, whereas other types of carcinoma more often have local recurrence.

The postoperative survival rate in patients with early gastric cancer was calculated by means of the actuarial survival rate method. The 5-year survival rate was reported to be 95%, and the 10-year survival rate, 91%, indicating excellent results. When cases with penetration into the mucosa or submucosa were distinguished, almost 100% of patients with carcinoma limited to the mucosa survived for 5 years, whereas only 83% of patients with submucosal penetration survived for 5 years. Prognosis is also influenced by other pathologic factors. Data obtained so far, especially with multifactorial analysis, indicate the influence of lymph node metastases. The histologic type of the tumor has little importance in prognosis.

References

1. Silverberg E, Boring CC, Squires TS: Cancer statistics, 1990. CA 40:9–26, 1990.
2. Nagayo T: Histogenesis and Precursors of Human Gastric Cancer. Berlin, Springer-Verlag, 1986.
3. Johansen A: Early Gastric Cancer. Bispebjerg Hospital, Copenhagen, Denmark, 1981.
4. Verse M: Die Histogenese der Schleimhautcarcinome. Leipzig, 1903.
5. Mallory TB: Carcinoma in situ of the stomach and its bearing on the histogenesis of malignant ulcers. Arch Pathol 30:348–362, 1940.
6. Stout AP: Superficial spreading type of carcinoma of the stomach. Arch Surg 44:651–657, 1942.
7. Konjetzny GE: The superficial cancer of the gastric mucosa. Am J Dig Dis 20:91–96, 1953.
8. Freisen G, Dockerty M, ReMine W: Superficial carcinoma of the stomach. Surgery 51:300–312, 1962.
9. Ming S-C: Classification of gastric carcinoma. In Filipe MI, Jass JR (eds): Gastric Carcinoma. London, Churchill Livingston, 1986, pp 197–216.
10. Ewing J: The beginnings of gastric cancer. Am J Surg 31:204–205, 1936.
11. Mason MK: Surface carcinoma of the stomach. Gut 6:185–193, 1965.
12. Japanese Research Society for Gastric Cancer. The general rules for the gastric cancer study in surgery and pathology. Jpn J Surg 11:127–145, 1981.
13. Kuru M: Atlas of Early Carcinoma of the Stomach. Tokyo, Nakayama-Shoten, 1967.
14. Murakami T: Pathomorphological diagnosis. Definition and gross classification of early gastric cancer. Gann Monogr Cancer Res 11:53–55, 1971.
15. Kurihara M, Keiichi K, Shirakabe H: Diagnosis of small early gastric cancer by x-ray, endoscopy and biopsy. Cancer Detect Prev 4:377–383, 1981.
16. Curtis RE, Kennedy BJ, Myers MH, Hankey BF: Evaluation of AJC stomach cancer staging using the SEER population. Semin Oncol 12:21–31, 1985.
17. Wanke M, Schwan H: Pathology of gastric cancer. World J Surg 3:675–684, 1979.
18. Elster K, Kolaczek F, Shimamoto K, Freitag H: Early gastric cancer—experience in Germany. Endoscopy 7:5–10, 1975.
19. Green PHR, O'Toole KM, Slonim D, et al: Increasing incidence and excellent survival of patients with early gastric cancer: Experience in a United States medical center. Am J Med 85:658–661, 1988.
20. Shirakabe H: Double Contrast Studies of the Stomach. Tokyo, Bunkoda, 1971.
21. Shirakabe H, Ichikawa H, Kumakura K, et al: Atlas of X-ray Diagnosis of Early Gastric Cancer. Tokyo, Igaku Shoin, 1966.
22. Hirota T, Itabashi M, Daibo M, et al: Chronological changes in the morphological features of early gastric cancer, especially recent changes in macroscopic findings. Jpn J Clin Oncol 14:181–199, 1984.
23. Borrmann R: Geshwelste des Magens und Duodenums. In Henke F, Lubarsch O (eds): Handbuch der Spezieller Pathologischen Anatomie und Histologie. Vol 4. Berlin, Springer, 1926, p 865.
24. Nagayo T: Mode of origin of gastric mucosal cancer with special reference to that of "superficial spreading type." Gann Monogr Cancer Res 3:113–121, 1966.
25. Hirota T, Itabashi M, Suzuki K, Yoshida S: Clinical study of minute and small early gastric cancer. Histogenesis of gastric cancer. Pathol Annu 15:1–19, 1980.
26. Lauren P: The two histological main types of gastric carcinoma. Diffuse and so-called intestinal type carcinoma. An attempt at histoclinical classification. Acta Path Microbiol Scand 64:31–49, 1965.
27. Watanabe H, Jass JR, Sabin LH: Histological Typing of Oesophageal and Gastric Tumours. World Health Organization International Histological Classification of Tumours. Berlin, Springer-Verlag, 1989, pp 20–26.
28. Ming SC: Gastric carcinoma: A pathobiological classification. Cancer 39:2475–2485, 1977.
29. Nakamura K: Histogenesis of the Gastric Cancer and Its Clinical Application. Tsukura International Center, Ibaraki, Japan, 1983.
30. Fukuda T, Onishi Y, Nishimaki T, et al: Early gastric cancer of the small cell type. Am J Gastroenterol 83:1176–1179, 1988.
31. Mori M, Adachi Y, Nakamura K, et al: Advanced gastric carcinoma simulating early gastric carcinoma. Cancer 65:1033–1040, 1990.
32. Murakami T: Histogenesis of gastric cancer. Gan Chiryo No Shimpo 2:1–11, 1960.
33. Bogomoletz WV: Early gastric cancer. Am J Surg Pathol 8:381–391, 1984.
34. Fukutomi H, Sakite T: Analysis of early gastric cancer cases collected from major hospitals and institutes in Japan. Jpn J Clin Oncol 14:169–179, 1984.
35. Murakami T: Early cancer of the stomach. World J Surg 3:685–692, 1979.
36. Nakamura K, Sugano H: Microcarcinoma of the stomach measuring less than 5 mm in the largest diameter and its histogenesis. Prog Clin Biol Res 132D:107–116, 1983.
37. Hattori T: Development of adenocarcinoma in the stomach. Cancer 57:1528–1534, 1986.
38. Grundmann E: Histologic types and possible initial stages in early gastric carcinoma. Beitr Pathol Bd 154:256–280, 1975.
39. Kodama Y, Inokuchi K, Soejima K, et al: Growth patterns and prognosis in early gastric carcinoma. Superficially spreading and penetrating growth types. Cancer 51:320–326, 1983.
40. Inokuchi K: Early gastric cancer viewed from its growth patterns. Surg Annu 18:111–128, 1986.
41. Okabe H: Growth of early gastric cancer. Clinical study of growth and invasive patterns of early gastric cancer. Its position in the natural history of gastric cancer. Gann Monogr Cancer Res 11:67–79, 1971.
42. Fujita S: Natural history of human gastric carcinoma in terms of their genesis and progression. Asian Med J 26:787–805, 1983.
43. Tsukuma H, Mishima T, Oshima A: Prospective study of "early" gastric cancer. Int J Cancer 31:421–426, 1983.
44. Hirota T, Okada T, Itabashi M, Kitaoka H: Histogenesis of human gastric cancer—with special reference to the significance of adenoma as a precancerous lesion. In Ming SC (ed): Precursors of Gastric Cancer. New York, Praeger, 1984, pp 233–252.
45. Ming SC: Relationship between gastric carcinoma and chronic gastric ulcer. In Ming SC (ed): Precursors of Gastric Cancer. New York, Praeger, 1984, pp 265–272.

CHAPTER 25

Adenocarcinoma and Other Malignant Epithelial Tumors of the Stomach

SI-CHUN MING, M.D.

FREQUENCY AND CELL TYPES OF GASTRIC TUMORS

CLINICAL MANIFESTATIONS AND DIFFERENTIAL DIAGNOSIS OF GASTRIC TUMORS

ADENOCARCINOMA
Epidemiology and Etiology
Precursors
Precancerous Conditions
Epithelial Polyps
Chronic Atrophic Gastritis
Intestinal Metaplasia
Chronic Gastric Ulcer
Gastric Remnants
Hyperplastic Gastropathy
Other Conditions
Precancerous Lesion: Epithelial Dysplasia

Experimental Gastric Carcinogenesis
Natural History
Pathology
Location and Size
Gross Morphology
Histologic Composition and Variants
Epithelial Elements
Stromal Elements
Spread of Gastric Carcinoma
Marker Substances
Histologic Classifications
World Health Organization (WHO) Typing
Lauren's Classification
Ming's Classification
Other Classifications
TNM Staging
Clinical Aspects
Sex and Age
Clinical Presentations and Diagnosis
Treatment and Prognosis

ADENOCARCINOMA OF THE GASTRIC CARDIA AND ESOPHAGOGASTRIC JUNCTION

SQUAMOUS CELL CARCINOMA, ADENOSQUAMOUS CARCINOMA, AND MUCOEPIDERMOID CARCINOMA

TERATOMA AND CHORIOCARCINOMA

CARCINOSARCOMA

SMALL-CELL CARCINOMA

MULTIPLE PRIMARY AND METASTATIC TUMORS

FREQUENCY AND CELL TYPES OF GASTRIC TUMORS

Many tumors of different tissue origin can occur in the stomach. The gastric tumors, like those in the other parts of the gastrointestinal tract, are dominated by tumors of epithelial origin. Among the epithelial tumors, most are malignant[1] (Table 25–1). This situation is distinctly different from that in the colon, but is analogous to that in the esophagus as well as the lung. All of these organs are derived from the foregut. There is probably an etiologic implication in this phenomenon. While organ specificity is a possibility, the nature of carcinogenic exposure is also a likely factor, as suggested by the experimental models for gastric carcinogenesis: the most effective carcinogens used for stomach experiments are direct-acting ones, whereas procarcinogens requiring metabolic activation are equally effective in colonic carcinogenesis.[2]

The benign epithelial tumors, namely, adenomas and polyps, are presented in Chapter 23. Whereas the nonneoplastic polyps are composed primarily of fove-

Table 25-1 RELATIVE FREQUENCY OF TUMORS OF THE STOMACH

Tumor Type	No. of Cases	%
Malignant tumors	4199	93.0
Carcinoma	3970	87.9
Lymphoma	136	3.0
Leiomyosarcoma	77	1.7
Carcinoid	11	0.3
Others	5	0.1
Benign tumors	315	7.0
Polyps	140	3.1
Leiomyoma	92	2.0
Others	83	1.9
Total	4514	100.0

Modified from Ming SC: Tumors of the Esophagus and Stomach. In Atlas of Tumor Pathology, Second Series, Fascicle 7. Armed Forces Institute of Pathology, Washington, DC, 1973, p 82.

olar mucous cells of the normal stomach, the adenomas are composed of cells of the intestinal type, such as goblet cells, absorptive cells, and in some lesions Paneth cells and intestinal endocrine cells.[3] The adenomas composed of gastric cells are rare.[4] Intestinal features are also common in the carcinomas. In contrast to the adenomas, however, many carcinomas contain cells of the gastric type. In addition, there may be endocrine cells and, less commonly, the squamous cells.[5] Thus, the composition of carcinomas of the stomach reflects the complexity of cell types seen in the normal and metaplastic stomach. The former cell types include, in addition to the surface and foveolar mucous cells,[6] pyloric gland cells[5] and parietal cells[7]; and the latter, in addition to goblet and absorptive cells, include Paneth cells[8] and endocrine cells of the intestinal type, such as cells secreting glicentin.[9] The gastric carcinomas can be made up of more different types of cells than any other tumor in the body.

The presence of cells of the intestinal type clearly links the development of gastric carcinoma with intestinal metaplasia. In the recent years the metaplastic glands have been found to be much more complex than previously considered. The basic question of whether metaplasia is a precancerous lesion or a paracancerous lesion remains, however. The best postulation at present is that both possibilities exist, depending in part on the nature of the metaplastic glands and in part on the nature of carcinogenic inducement.

Gastric carcinomas are linked to more precancerous conditions than any other tumor. In addition to intestinal metaplasia, these include chronic gastritis, chronic ulcers, adenomas and polyps, Ménétrier's disease and other hyperplastic gastropathies, and stomach remnant following partial gastrectomy and gastroenterostomy. At the cellular level, the immediate stage prior to the development of carcinoma appears to be severe dysplasia in most, but not all, cases.

Next to carcinoma, the most frequent tumor in the stomach is the smooth muscle cell tumor, which is presented in Chapter 15. In this case, the benign tumor is far more frequent than the malignant. In this regard, the stomach is the primary site for the epithelioid form of muscle cell tumor, which is intermediate in its behavior between the usual leiomyoma and leiomyosarcoma composed of the spindle-shaped muscle cells. The muscle cell tumors, being submucosal, are ordinarily asymptomatic until they are large enough to cause pressure symptoms or become ulcerated and bleed. The incidence, therefore, has varied in different reports. The frequency shown in Table 25-1 is that of symptomatic tumors. The incidence increases markedly when an effort is made to search for small lesions, to as high as 50% of all stomachs examined.[10] The third most frequent tumor in the stomach is the lymphoma. This is interesting because the stomach, unlike the intestines, is not a principal lymphoid organ. The mucosal stroma is devoid of lymphocytic cells in the fetal and neonatal stomach. With increasing age, however, lymphocytes and plasma cells become constant and are invariably present in the adult stomach, presumably the result of mucosal injury. The depth of lymphoid infiltration is related to age, as shown by the long-term follow-up study of Siurala and his colleagues.[11] Lymphomas usually occur in elderly patients. Other gastric tumors are rare.

CLINICAL MANIFESTATIONS AND DIFFERENTIAL DIAGNOSIS OF GASTRIC TUMORS

The stomach is a voluminous organ. Its large chamber allows the tumor to grow to a large size before its effects become clinically evident. The small caliber of the esophagus and small intestine can be obliterated by a relatively small tumor; obstruction is neither an early nor a common manifestation of the gastric tumors, unless they occur at the portal of entry or exit. The symptoms are usually nonspecific and vague. Epigastric discomfort and dyspepsia are common, partly the result of tumor-associated conditions such as gastritis. Ulcerated lesions may bleed and cause anemia. Anemia may also be caused by gastritis. Weight loss is seen in patients with advanced malignant tumors. These clinical manifestations are nonspecific, and the diagnosis often depends on direct visualization of the lesion by either radiologic imaging or endoscopic studies. Even with such examinations, the nature of the lesion may not be determined until a histologic examination is performed.

Special difficulties may be encountered in specific situations. For instance, an early gastric carcinoma may be grossly invisible, and an ulcerated carcinoma may be indistinguishable from a benign ulcer. In such cases, the tissue that undergoes biopsy may not be representative of the malignant lesions. Multiple biopsies, therefore, are often necessary. Another procedure is the cytologic examination, which can be helpful in screening and in follow-up studies. Detailed discussions of endoscopic and cytologic studies are presented in Chapters 3 and 4, respectively.

ADENOCARCINOMA

Carcinoma is the most important and the most common tumor of the stomach (see Table 25-1). Nearly all gastric carcinomas are adenocarcinomas. Thus, adenocarcinoma is the main focus of concern in dealing with gastric cancers.

Epidemiology and Etiology

The mortality rate of gastric carcinoma has a wide geographic variation (Figure 25-1).[12] Variations are also common within the same country. Epidemiologic studies comparing high-risk with low-risk regions give some insight into possible etiologic factors for gastric carcinoma. Additional information has been obtained by time trend studies, which showed a steady decline in the mortality rate in most countries.[13,14] The decline for the white male population in the United States has been most striking (Figure 25-2).[13,15] In 1990, the estimated number of new cases of gastric cancer in the United States was 23,000, and the estimated number of deaths, 13,700.[15]

The causes of geographic variation and the decline in incidence are unknown, but recent epidemiologic studies have suggested certain possibilities related to one type of gastric carcinoma known as the intestinal type in Lauren's classification, which is explained in the section on histologic classifications. It was noted that this type of carcinoma was more prevalent in high-risk regions than low-risk regions[16,17] and that its decline in incidence accounts for the decline of gastric cancer incidence in general.[18,19] Others, however, did not confirm such findings.[20-22]

The etiology of gastric carcinoma is unknown. A number of systemic and local risk factors have been

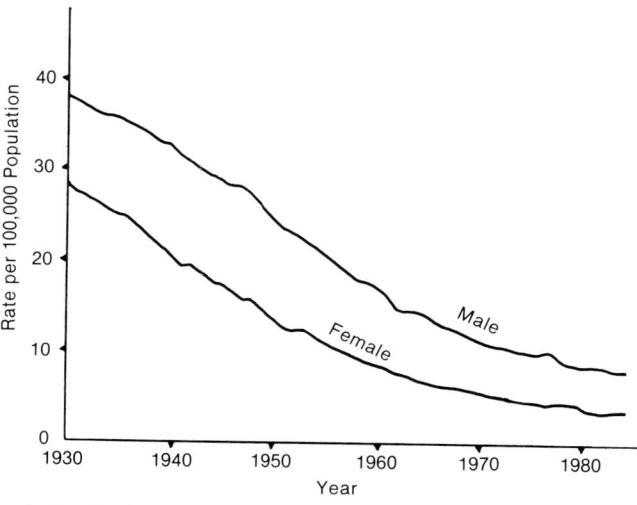

FIGURE 25-2. Decline of the gastric cancer death rate in the United States by sex. Data from Silverberg E, Lubera J: Cancer statistics, 1987. CA 37:2-19, 1987.

identified, however. The latter factors are described below as precursor lesions.

The incidence of gastric carcinoma is known to be higher in persons with blood type A and persons with pernicious anemia.[23,24] These findings suggest some weak genetic influences. The most important factors appear to be environmental, as shown by migrant studies. When people moved from a high-risk region to a low-risk region, the incidence of gastric carcinoma decreased.[13,25,26] The decrease is more pronounced in the second than in the first generation,[27,28] which suggests a lasting effect of carcinogenic exposure in the early life, also indicated by the observation of a prevalence of chronic atrophic gastritis and intestinal metaplasia, known precursor lesions, in a younger population in the high-risk area.[29] Among the environmental factors, dietary factors have been credited for the decline in gastric cancer mortality.[29-31] Starchy, pickled, smoked, and salted foods are risk factors; whereas fresh fruit, vegetables, and vitamins C and E are beneficiary.[32] The importance of salt was emphasized by several investigators[32-34] and denied by others.[35-37] Experiments on rats showed that salt caused gastric mucosal damage, which then enhanced cell proliferation and carcinogen-induced carcinogenesis.[38]

Soybean products are commonly eaten in Asia, where the incidence of gastric carcinoma is high. Soybean sauce mixed with sodium nitrite *in vitro* was found to be mutagenic.[39] However, the concentration of sodium nitrite necessary for the reaction was above the physiologic state in humans.[40] On the other hand, soybean paste (miso), soybean curd (tofu) and soya milk inhibited nitrosamine formation from sodium nitrite *in vitro*.[41] Furthermore, the frequency of soybean paste soup intake was inversely related to the gastric cancer mortality rate in Japan.[42] Other possible risk factors include red wine,[43,44] asbestos,[45,46] and radiation.[47]

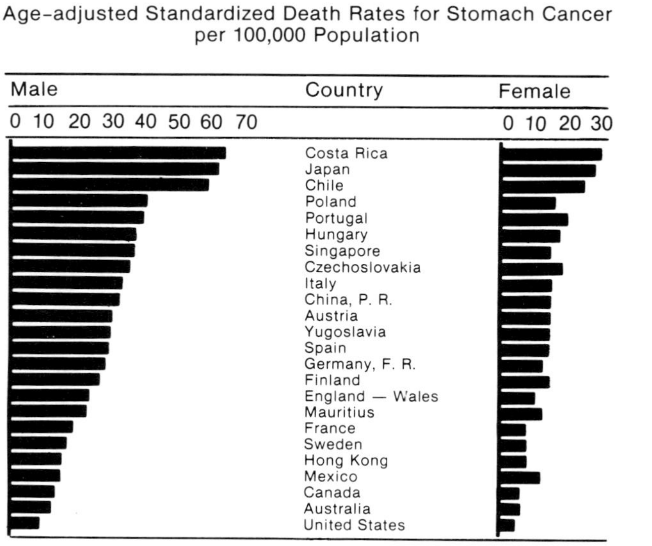

Age-adjusted Standardized Death Rates for Stomach Cancer per 100,000 Population

FIGURE 25-1. Mortality rates for gastric cancer in various countries.

Source of data: 1986 World Health Organization Statistics, based on European standard population, except data on China, which are based on world standard population.

The responsible carcinogens for the human gastric cancer have not been identified. They are suspected of being N-nitroso compounds. Because atrophic gastritis is commonly associated with gastric cancer, a hypothesis for the *in vivo* formation of these compounds has been proposed as follows[26]: atrophic gastritis causes a decrease in the acidity of gastric juice, making possible overgrowth of bacteria, which convert nitrates to nitrites and catalyze *in vivo* N-nitrosation.[48] Evidence supporting this hypothesis is found in several ways. In Columbia, nitrate content in the well water and urinary nitrate excretion in the population are higher in the high-risk area than in the low-risk area.[29] Another source of nitrate and nitrite is the saliva, the results in which appear to be variable.[29,49] The gastric juice pH, which increases in chronic strophic gastritis, is positively related to the level of nitrite and nitrate–reducing bacteria and the concentration of N-nitroso compounds in the juice.[50–52] The gastric juice in high-risk patients is mutagenic.[53,54] The carcinogenic nitroso compounds so formed are probably nitrosamines.[49] Their formation can be blocked by vitamins C and E.[55,56] These data show possible mechanisms of gastric carcinogenesis and point to possible ways of primary prevention by reducing conditions favoring the generation of carcinogens, on the one hand, and inhibition of carcinogen formation with dietary modifications, on the other.

Precursors

As long ago as 1929, Hurst[57] recognized chronic atrophic gastritis, peptic ulcer, adenoma, and polyps as precursors of gastric carcinoma. Since then, intestinal metaplasia, hyperplastic gastropathy, and gastric remnants after partial gastrectomy have also been associated with increased incidence of gastric cancer. The precancerous potential of these conditions is recognized primarily by clinical association with gastric cancer, whereas the pathologic lesions from which carcinoma arises had largely been unknown until recently, when dysplasia of the epithelial cells was recognized as the fundamental premalignant lesion in all of these conditions.

The precursors of gastric carcinoma have been separated into two major categories: precancerous conditions and precancerous lesions.[58] The precancerous conditions are clinical conditions in which there is an increased risk of gastric carcinoma. In the majority of patients with these conditions carcinoma does not develop. The precancerous lesions are pathologic changes from which the carcinoma eventually evolves. It is believed that the development of gastric carcinoma in precancerous conditions is preceded by the occurrence of a precancerous lesion, i.e., dysplasia.

Precancerous Conditions
Epithelial Polyps

The epithelial polyps are classified into five major categories: hyperplastic polyp, adenoma, hamartomatous polyp, inflammatory polyp, and heterotopic polyp. Inflammatory polyps have no malignant potential. Carcinoma may develop very rarely in the hamartomatous polyp and heterotopic pancreatic tissue. Hyperplastic polyp and adenoma, particularly the former, are much more common than the other types of polyps. There was great confusion in the past with regard to their malignant potential. It is now generally accepted that the adenoma is a true neoplasm and that carcinoma develops in it in about 40% of cases. On the other hand, the hyperplastic polyp is probably the result of excessive regeneration following inflammation, and carcinomatous change occurs in it in less than 2% of cases. When carcinoma does develop in the hyperplastic polyp, it involves the dysplastic glands. Detailed discussion of malignant change in gastric polyps is presented in Chapter 23.

Chronic Atrophic Gastritis

Chronic atrophic gastritis is a common condition. It is fully discussed in Chapter 20.

Among the precursor lesions, chronic atrophic gastritis is the most important. Nagayo[59] estimated that it was the precursor of 80% of gastric carcinomas in Japan. Its incidence increases with advanced age, and it is seen mainly in the elderly population. In the high-risk areas for gastric cancer, however, it is commonly present in the young people as well.[29] Based on epidemiologic data, Correa[60] proposed that chronic gastritis had three patterns, probably caused by separate etiologic factors: the *autoimmune* type, involving acid-secreting mucosa; the *hypersecretory* type, involving the pyloric mucosa; and the *environmental* type, involving multiple areas at random but more prominently the fundopyloric junctional zone. Cancer develops more frequently in the first and last types. The significance of chronic atrophic gastritis is demonstrated clearly by Siurala's follow-up studies[11]: Among 116 patients followed for 19 to 23 years, carcinoma developed in 10% and polyp in 6% of the patients. Among 261 controls, carcinoma developed in only 0.6%, and polyp in none. Intestinal metaplasia and dysplasia were much more common in the former group. These lesions are common also in patients with pernicious anemia, in whom chronic atrophic gastritis is a constant feature.[61] The relative risk of developing gastric carcinoma in patients with severe chronic atrophic gastritis in the Finnish population was 18.1 in the antrum and 4.6 in the body of the stomach.[62]

The atrophic gastric mucosa often shows intestinal metaplasia, but the extent of metaplasia varies greatly. With or without intestinal metaplasia, there is an increased proliferative activity in the mucosa, resulting in the presence of relatively immature cells in the glands.[63] In the metaplastic areas, cell proliferation is more evident in the lower portion of the glands; whereas in the nonmetaplastic mucosa, the superficial and foveolar cells are affected. As discussed above, hypochlorhydria secondary to mucosal atrophy creates an altered environment in the stomach in which N-nitrosation may occur, initiating the carcinogenic events.

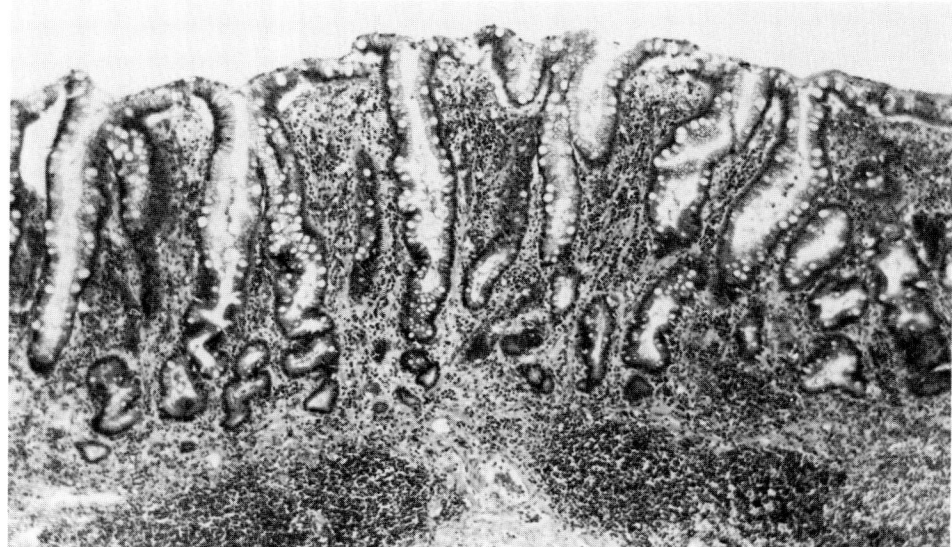

FIGURE 25-3. Complete type of intestinal metaplasia, showing intestinal type crypts lined with goblet cells and absorptive cells. There is severe chronic gastritis with lymphocytic infiltrates extending into the submucosa. (× 55)

The carcinoma that develops in chronic atrophic gastritis is usually the intestinal type, which has been related to intestinal metaplasia.

Intestinal Metaplasia

The surface and foveolae of the normal gastric mucosa are lined by a continuous layer of columnar mucous cells secreting neutral glycoproteins, whereas the goblet cells of the intestines are interspersed by absorptive cells and secrete acidic mucins, which are mainly sialomucins in the small intestines and sulfomucins in the colon. The sialomucins can be further separated into N- and O-acetylated types. These mucins can be easily identified by simple staining procedures such as periodic acid–Schiff reaction (PAS) for all mucoproteins, alcian blue for acidic mucins,[64] periodate-borohydride/potassium hydroxide/PAS for O-acetylated sialomucin[65] and high iron diamine for sulfomucin.[66] The absorptive cells in the small intestine have well-formed microvilli which carry alkaline phosphatase and digestive enzymes such as disaccharidases and peptidases, some of which can be demonstrated in the gross specimen.[67] The absorptive cells in the colon, on the other hand, have only short and sparse microvilli, lacking many enzymes. In intestinal metaplasia, the gastric mucosa is transformed into an intestinal type of mucosa with complex and heterogeneous features.

Intestinal metaplasia begins in the neck region, which is the proliferative zone of the normal gastric gland. In completely developed metaplasia, the gastric mucosa assumes the appearance of small-intestinal mucosa but without villi (Figure 25–3). The glands are lined by absorptive, goblet, Paneth, and endocrine cells. Early ultrastructural and histochemical studies confirmed that these cells were identical to those of the small intestine.[69] In incompletely developed metaplasia, instead of absorptive cells, the columnar cells between the goblet cells are mucous cells resembling foveolar cells[69] (Figure 25–4). The mucus in the goblet cells contains both sialomucin and sulfomucin.[54] The former is more prominent in incomplete metaplasia; the latter, in complete metaplasia (Figure 25–5). The mucus in the columnar cells of incompletely metaplastic glands may be neutral mucoproteins, sialomucin, or sulfomucin.

The concept of different types of metaplasia has been greatly expanded. Matsukura et al.[70] divided intestinal metaplasia into complete and incomplete types as follows: The complete type was composed of the small-intestinal type of glands, whereas the incomplete type had no Paneth cells, lacked certain enzymes, and

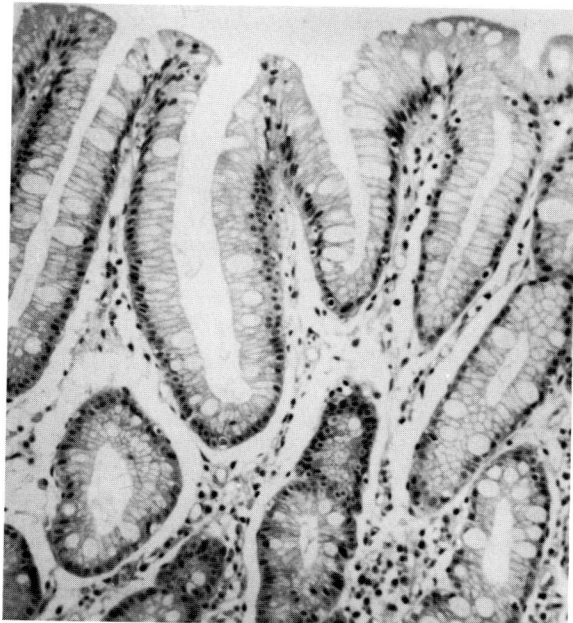

FIGURE 25-4. Incomplete type of intestinal metaplasia, showing glands lined with goblet cells and mucous columnar cells. The latter resemble normal foveolar cells but may secrete acidic intestinal mucins instead of neutral mucoproteins. (× 120)

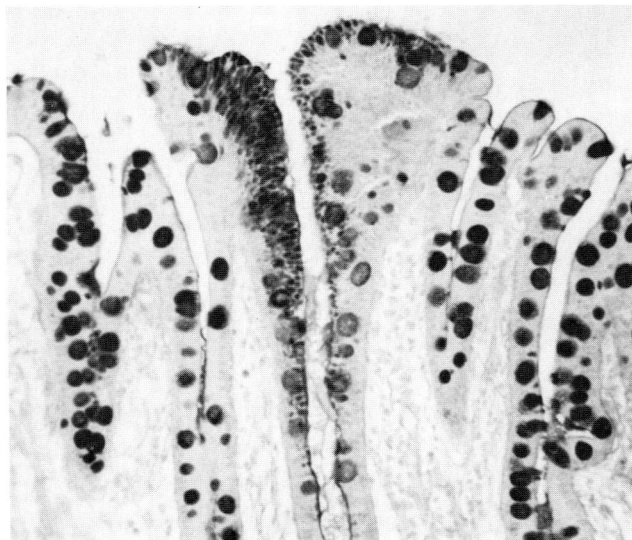

FIGURE 25-5. Intestinal metaplasia with the incomplete type at the center and the complete type at the sides. The tissue is stained with high iron diamine (HID) and alcian blue at pH 2.5 (AB). The goblet cells in complete metaplasia contain sulfomucin, which is stained by HID and shown as black. The goblet cells in incomplete metaplasia contain sialomucin, which is stained by AB and shown as lighter gray. The mucous columnar cells have both types of mucin. (× 200)

secreted sulfomucin. Based on the staining intensity for O-acetylated sialomucin, Teglbjaerg and Nielsen[65] divided intestinal metaplasia into small-intestinal and colonic types. Segura and Montero,[71] however, noted that O-acetylated sialomucin was present also in parts of the small intestine. Jass and Filipe[72] also divided intestinal metaplasia into complete (type I) and incomplete (type II) types, on the basis of the presence of absorptive cells in the former and mucus-secreting columnar cells in the latter. The incomplete type was further divided into A and B subtypes, on the basis of the type of mucin in the columnar cells: nonsulfated mucin in A and sulfated mucin in B. These types were subsequently renamed types I, II, and III.[73] Thus, by a comparison of the composite cells, mucin secretions, and enzyme patterns of the metaplastic mucosa with those of the normal mucosa, the metaplastic processes have been classified into several types (Table 25-2).[68]

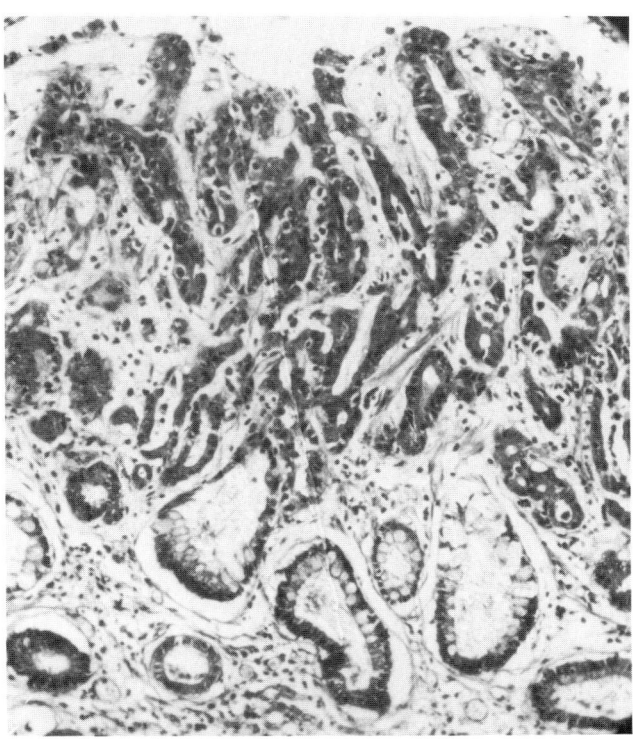

FIGURE 25-6. Superficial adenocarcinoma lies above the benign metaplastic glands. (× 150)

Positive immunohistochemical staining for carcinoembryonic antigen (CEA) has been found in the colonic type of metaplastic glands but not in the small-intestinal type of glands.[74,75] We found only a weak staining in occasional glands, in both the absorptive cells of completely metaplastic mucosa and the columnar cells of the incompletely metaplastic mucosa.

The precancerous nature of intestinal metaplasia is suggested by the observation that carcinoma often occurs in the area of intestinal metaplasia (Figure 25-6). The sulfomucin-secreting and colonic types of metaplasia were said to be related to the intestinal or expanding type of gastric carcinoma by association.[59,76-78] Follow-up studies of type III metaplasia, however, did not show an increased risk of gastric carcinoma.[79,80] In-

Table 25-2 MAJOR DIFFERENCES AMONG SUBTYPES OF INTESTINAL METAPLASIA

	Complete Type		Incomplete Type		
Feature	Small-Intestinal	Colonic	Gastric	Small-Intestinal	Colonic
Goblet cells	+	+	+	+	+
Mucous columnar cells	−	−	+	+	+
Paneth cells	+	−	−	−	−
Absorptive cells	+	+	−	−	−
Striated borders	+	−	−	−	−
Mucoproteins*	Sialomucin	Sulfomucin	Neutral	Sialomucin	Sulfomucin
Microvillar enzymes	+	±	−	−	−

*The mucoproteins indicated are in the goblet cells in the complete type and in the columnar cells in the incomplete type of metaplasia.
+, present; −, absent; ±, some may be present.

testinal metaplasia has been produced in experimental animals by treatments with carcinogens[81,82] and radiation,[83] but its relationship with carcinoma has been inconsistent, and it is not a required precancerous lesion.[83,84] Thus, type III and colonic intestinal metaplasia may be paracancerous, rather than precancerous, lesions.[85,86] In any case, the complete small-intestinal type of metaplasia is so common that its precancerous potential is probably negligible.

Chronic Gastric Ulcer

Chronic gastric ulcers have been considered precancerous lesions in many reports, particularly in the older literature. The term *ulcer-cancer* was introduced by Hauser[87] in 1926 and has since been applied to carcinoma that was thought to have arisen in a chronic gastric ulcer. It is defined as a carcinoma located at the margin but not the base of an unquestionably chronic ulcer.[88] The ulcer-cancer is, therefore, probably an early cancer. However, many reports have included both early and advanced cases.

With the advance in endoscopic diagnosis, there have been many reports of early gastric cancer, mostly from Japan. In the earlier reports, about 70% of cancer cases were said to have had pre-existing ulcers.[89] Recently the importance of the chronic ulcer as a precancerous lesion has been downgraded. There was apparently a steady decrease in the incidence of deeply ulcerated (type III) early gastric cancer in Japan, and cases fulfilling the criteria of ulcer-cancer disappeared.[59] In the meantime, Sakita et al.[90] reported that the malignant ulcer might heal, markedly in 18% to 25% of cases, which invalidated the long-held view that an ulcer that healed was benign and that a carcinoma found in a healing ulcer originated in a benign ulcer. Conversely, carcinomas have been found in stomachs resected for clinically benign ulcer. The reported incidence of this observation is about 2%.[91,92] Nearly one-half of such patients had ulcer symptoms for less than 3 years.[93] Similarly, Farinati et al.[94] found 10 carcinomas in 144 ulcers on follow-up endoscopic biopsies, 9 within 1 year and 1 at 41 months after the original diagnosis. In view of the slow growth of early gastric carcinoma,[89] the relatively short history of the ulcer in such reports indicates that the carcinoma predated the ulcer.

The incidence of carcinoma in long follow-up studies has been low. A 5-year study by Rollag and Jacobsen[96] revealed that in none of 78 ulcer patients did carcinoma develop. In patients who were followed for 9 or more years, the incidence was 2.2%.[97] The slightly higher than expected incidence of gastric cancer in such patients was found to be not statistically significant.[98] Furthermore, the carcinoma might not be in the ulcer. Montgomery and Richardson reported that two of three gastric carcinomas that developed in 160 patients were outside the ulcer.[99] The lack of an increased cancer incidence in ulcer patients was also found in a large autopsy survey.[100] In view of these considerations, it seems reasonable to accept Mallory's postulation that ulceration might destroy an intramu-

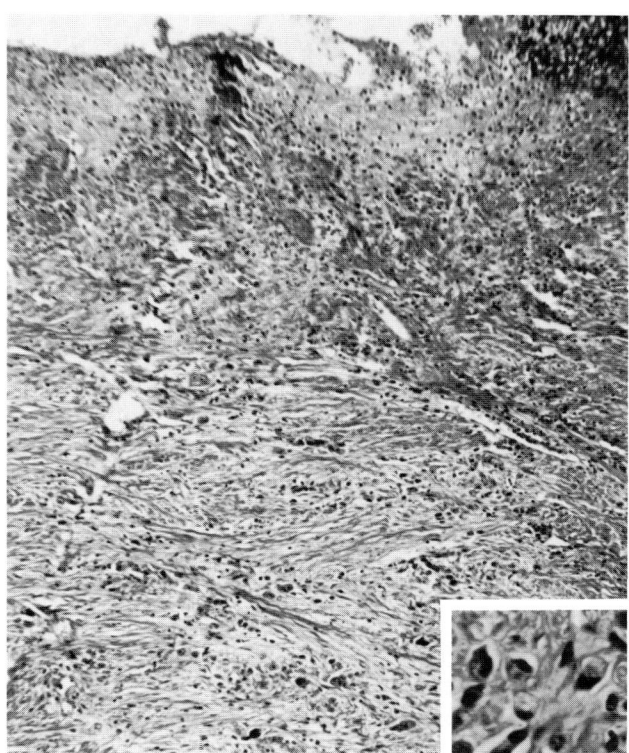

FIGURE 25–7. The base of a chronic peptic ulcer, showing infiltration of individual tumor cells (infiltrative type of carcinoma) in the scar tissue. ($\times$ 90) *Inset*, signet-ring cells in the fibrous tissue. ($\times$ 300)

cosal carcinoma, leaving cancer at the margin but not the base of the ulcer.[101]

Pathologically, evidence for the malignant transformation in a chronic ulcer is found in the fact that the ulcer-associated carcinomas have a unique histologic pattern, namely, a much higher incidence of infiltrative cancer than in the nonulcerated carcinomas, in both early[84,102] and advanced[76] cancers (Figure 25–7). Experimentally, chronically ulcerated gastric mucosa is more susceptible to experimental carcinogenic stimulation than nonulcerated mucosa.[103] This also applies to experimental duodenal ulcers.[104]

There is no question that cancer may develop in a chronic ulcer, but the incidence is not significantly higher than expected. From the data cited above, the incidence of cancer developing in a chronic ulcer of more than 5 years' duration is around 0.5% to 2%, and the incidence of cancer in a stomach resected for clinically benign ulcer is about 2%. More importantly, the malignant ulcer is often misdiagnosed as benign.[105] This situation emphasizes the need to obtain multiple endoscopic biopsies from the ulcer margins in order to achieve a correct diagnosis.

Gastric Remnants

A high incidence of carcinoma in gastric remnants following partial gastrectomy has been repeatedly reported.[106–108] The reported incidence varies from 0% to 7.8% and is usually 2%.[106] In the autopsied cases the incidence was 11.3% in one series[109] and only 0.2% in another.[110] The latter was only one-fifth of the expected rate. Similarly, Schafer et al.[111] found two carcinomas among 338 gastrectomized patients, against the expected number of 2.6. The variation is apparently related in part to the time factor. The incidence increases as the postoperative period lengthens.[108] This factor is in turn influenced by the age of the patient at the time of gastrectomy: the younger the age at the time of gastrectomy, the longer the operation-carcinoma interval.[106] The type of gastrectomy procedure and the nature of the preoperative disease are not factors, although most reports deal with the Billroth II operation on patients with duodenal ulcers.

The carcinoma usually develops more than 10 years after the initial operation. The tumor is often located at the stoma but may be located elsewhere in the stomach. The types of carcinoma are about equally divided between intestinal and diffuse.[112] The gastric remnants commonly show gastritis, cystic glands, intestinal metaplasia, and dysplasia.[106,113] Polyps may also occur, usually of the hyperplastic type. The degree of dysplasia is in general mild, unless accompanied by carcinoma.[107] Dysplasia may regress.[106] Severe dysplasia probably plays an important role in carcinogenesis, and its progression toward carcinoma has been reported.[114]

The lack of sphincteric function at the gastroenterostomy stoma with consequent reflux of bile-containing intestinal contents into the stomach has been cited as a cause of mucosal abnormalities and malignant change in the stomach.[111] This view is supported by the finding that the severity of intestinal metaplasia and dysplasia in the stomach stump correlates with the gastric pH.[115] Experimentally, gastrojejunostomy increases chemically induced cancer in the rat stomach.[110]

Hyperplastic Gastropathy

Gastric mucosa may become thickened in a variety of conditions. A detailed discussion is presented in Chapter 22. When the mucosal hypertrophy is due to epithelial hyperplasia, it usually falls into three categories[117]: glandular hyperplasia with hyperacidity, as in Zollinger-Ellison syndrome; mucous cell hyperplasia with protein loss, as in Ménétrier's disease; and hyperplasia of mixed type, which is often asymptomatic. In the last situation, there is an increase of all glandular elements, which appear normal. The fundic mucosa is involved in all three conditions. The chronic hypertrophic glandular gastritis of Schindler[118] probably also belongs to the last group. Carcinoma is sometimes present in such a stomach. The patients tend to be young and female,[117,118] and the carcinoma is often diffusely infiltrative. It has been postulated that fundic mucosal hyperplasia may be caused by endocrine substances secreted by the tumor cells.[119]

The stomach in Zollinger-Ellison syndrome is not known to have an increased incidence of carcinoma. In Ménétrier's disease there is hyperplasia of mucus-secreting foveolar cells, whereas the deep glands are normal or more commonly atrophic. Carcinoma may de-

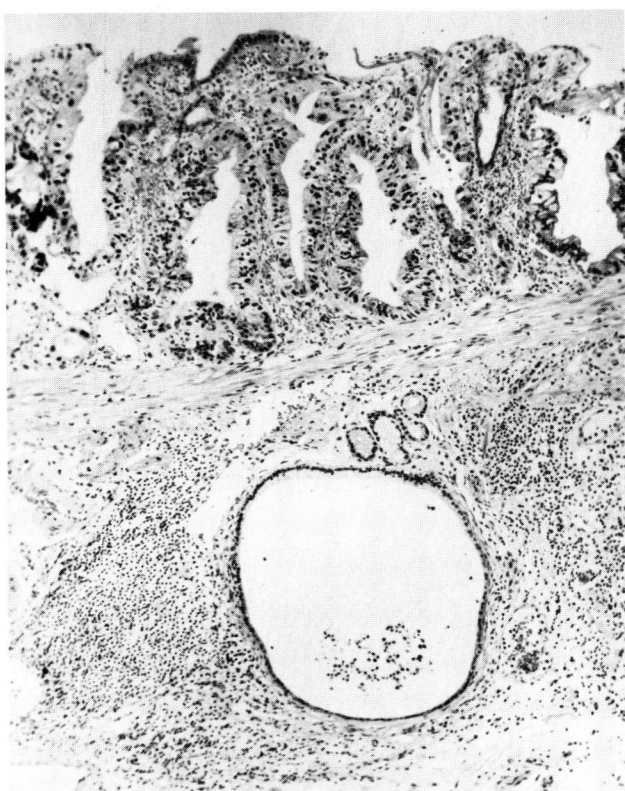

FIGURE 25-8. Submucosal glands, one cystic, underneath an intramucosal adenocarcinoma. (× 120)

velop in such a stomach, as first described by Ménétrier.[120] Ménétrier's disease is rare. Martin collected 214 cases in the literature and found the frequency of malignant change to be 5% to 6%.[121] In the case reported by Wood et al.,[122] the carcinoma was located in grossly unremarkable antrum, whereas the mucosa of the body and fundus of the stomach was grossly hypertrophic. In a personally examined case, an early carcinoma was found in a small atrophic area in otherwise hyperplastic mucosa.

Other Conditions

Intramucosal cysts may be present in the normal-appearing gastric mucosa away from a carcinoma. The incidence and the number of the cysts are higher in high-risk countries than in low-risk countries.[123] The cystic glands are of gastric type when associated with diffuse carcinoma and of intestinal type when associated with intestinal-type cancer.[124] Submucosal cystic glands also may accompany carcinoma, particularly underneath the early carcinoma[125,126] (Figure 25-8). Finally, carcinoma may complicate gastric schistosomiasis, as reported from China.[127]

Precancerous Lesion: Epithelial Dysplasia

In only a small percentage of patients who have one of the conditions discussed above does gastric carcinoma develop. In fact, the premalignant nature of some of these conditions has been disputed. The only precancerous lesion in which adenocarcinoma occurs with certainty is adenoma, and adenomas are composed of dysplastic cells. Epithelial dysplasia also plays an important role in malignant change in other conditions. Thus, dysplasia has become the target of many investigations in the recent years.

Broadly defined, *dysplasia* simply means "abnormal growth" and has been applied to many conditions that have no relation to malignancy. In pathology and cytology, however, the term has become synonymous with *premalignancy*. In this circumstance, *dysplasia* can be defined as "an abnormal state of the tissue characterized by pronounced cellular and structural alterations and showing a propensity to malignant transformation."[128] In the stomach, dysplasia can occur in the metaplastic gland as well as the nonmetaplastic gland.[129]

Studies of gastric dysplasia include DNA and morphometric measurements, cell kinetic studies, and searches for marker substances. The dysplastic cells have increased DNA and, when severe, polyploidy and occasionally aneuploidy.[130-132] The nuclear area is enlarged,[132,133] and the cell cycle is lengthened, but the cell life span is shortened.[130] Carcinoembryonic antigen and oncogenic product are present in the dysplastic cells.[75,134] These studies indicate that in extreme cases, the dysplastic cells resemble malignant cells and may in fact be malignant already.

For the clinical evaluation, light-microscopic examination remains the most useful. With this method, several grading systems have been reported.[58,129,135-138] One popular system uses the descriptive terms *mild*, *moderate*, and *severe*.[58] Cuello et al.[136] classified dysplasia into hyperplastic and adenomatous types, both of which terms were applied to the metaplastic mucosa. Jass' classification[138] was similar: *type I* was applied to adenomatous lesions, and *type II*, to incompletely metaplastic and nonadenomatous mucosa.

The fundamental histologic feature of dysplasia is excessive cell proliferation resulting in an increased number of immature cells. Thus, dysplasia overlaps reparative regeneration at one end of the spectrum and carcinoma at the other end. On occasion, it is difficult, even impossible, to clearly differentiate them. For practicality, the following categories might be used for classifying immature gastric epithelium in order of increasing abnormality.[128]

Simple (Regenerative) Hyperplasia (Figure 25–9). The mucosa maintains the normal configuration, and the cells are regular and uniform and mature normally toward the mucosal surface. Simple hyperplasia is represented by the regenerating epithelium at the border of an ulcer or in an area of active inflammation.

Severe Hyperplasia (Figure 25–10). The immature cells are exuberant and disorganized. They vary slightly in size and shape and are pseudostratified. Normal maturation is still evident at the mucosal surface, which may be elevated because of the increased number of cells. Severe hyperplasia may be seen at the ulcer border, in chronic atrophic gastritis and occasionally the hyperplastic polyp. It may be present also in the mucosa surrounding a carcinoma or an adenoma.

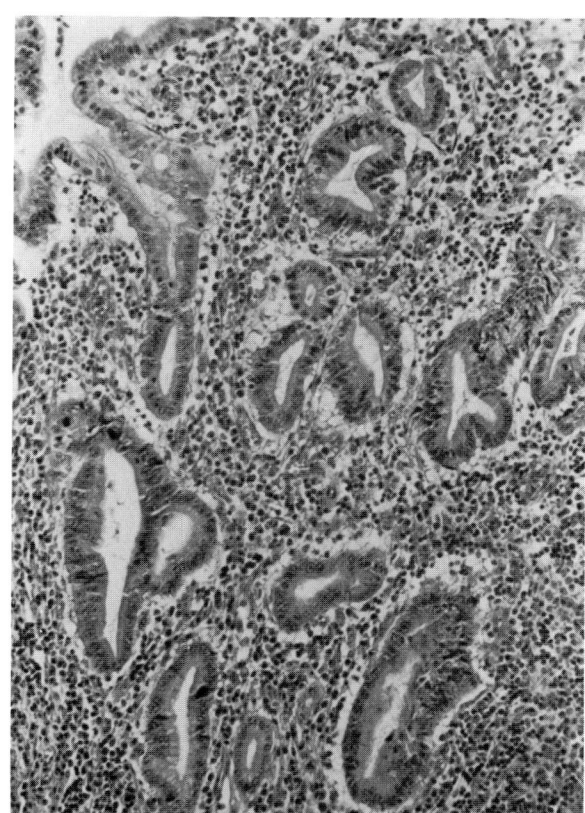

FIGURE 25–9. Simple hyperplasia of gastric glands at the margin of a chronic ulcer. The epithelial cells are immature and slightly pseudostratified. Intracellular mucin is reduced. The nuclei remain basally located. The lamina propria is heavily infiltrated by chronic inflammatory cells. ($\times$ 180)

This condition is intermediate between simple hyperplasia and dysplasia and has also been classified as *mild dysplasia*. It corresponds to the condition of indefinite dysplasia in the colon. The term *severe hyperplasia* is chosen because there is no evidence that this change is premalignant.

Dysplasia (Figures 25–11 and 25–12). The proliferating and immature cells are abnormal, showing mild pleomorphism, variation in size and shape, increased nuclear/cytoplasmic ratio, and poor cellular differentiation. Pseudostratification, nucleoli, and mitosis are common, but giant nuclei and abnormal mitosis are absent. In addition, there may be architectural derangements with budding, branching, and crowding of the glands. Dysplasia may be qualified as moderate or severe or low-grade or high-grade, as in the colon.

Because dysplasia is typically present in the adenoma, a decision must be made as to whether the dysplastic lesion is an adenoma or not. The distinction is important because the adenoma is treated by excision. If the lesion is not an adenoma, regular follow-up examinations may be more appropriate. The differentiating features in favor of an adenoma are (1) a circumscribed and grossly visible lesion, (2) no or minimal inflammation in the stroma, and, (3) relatively uniform cellular features. The dysplastic lesion in other conditons is detectable only microscopically and shows gradations of abnormality.

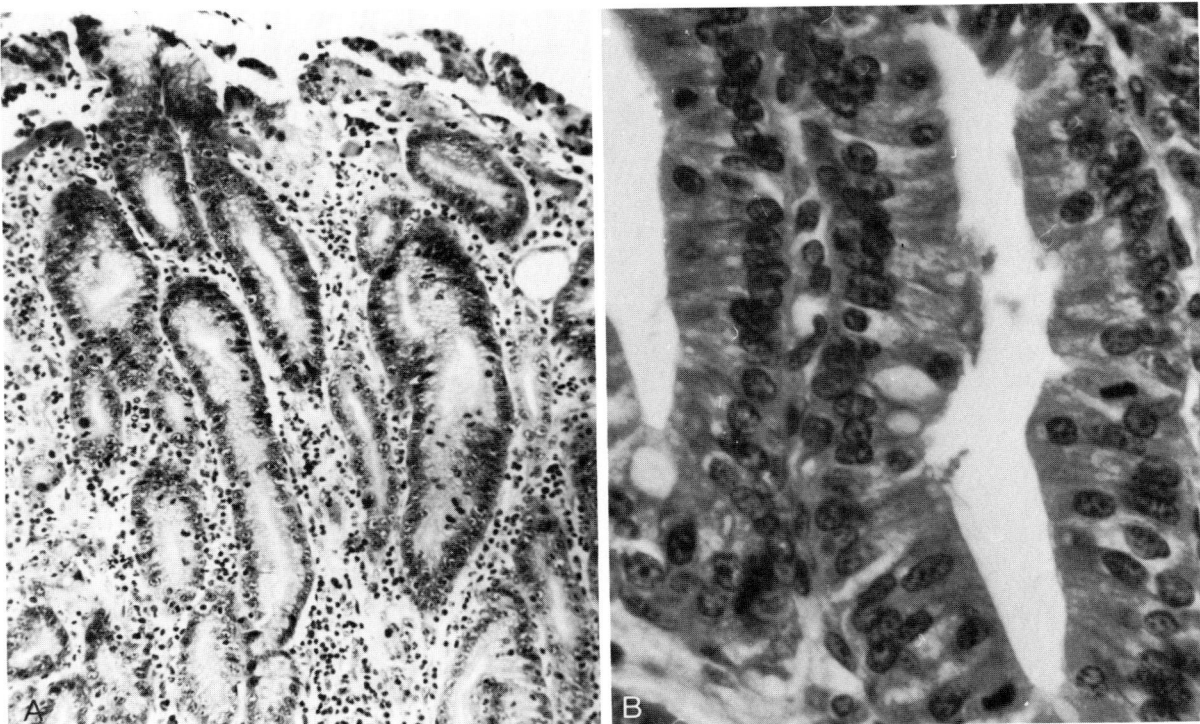

FIGURE 25–10. Severe hyperplasia. A, The gastric glands are slightly irregular. The cells are immature, with many mitotic figures. (× 150) B, Hyperplastic glands showing reduced mucus secretion and mild pseudostratification. The basally located nuclei are uniform in size and shape. There are no nucleoli. Mitoses are present. (× 480)

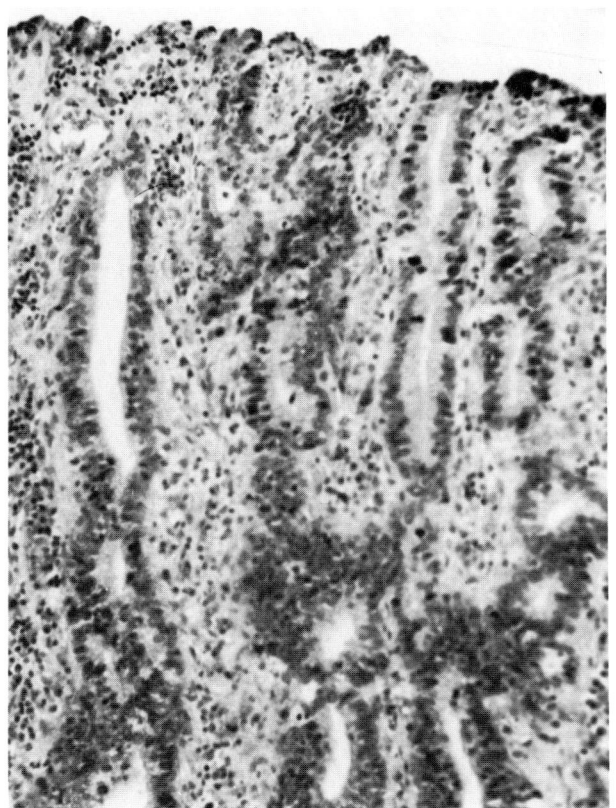

FIGURE 25–11. Severe dysplasia showing irregular branching glands with prominent pseudostratification in some. The cells are short and slightly pleomorphic. There is no mucus secretion. (× 150)

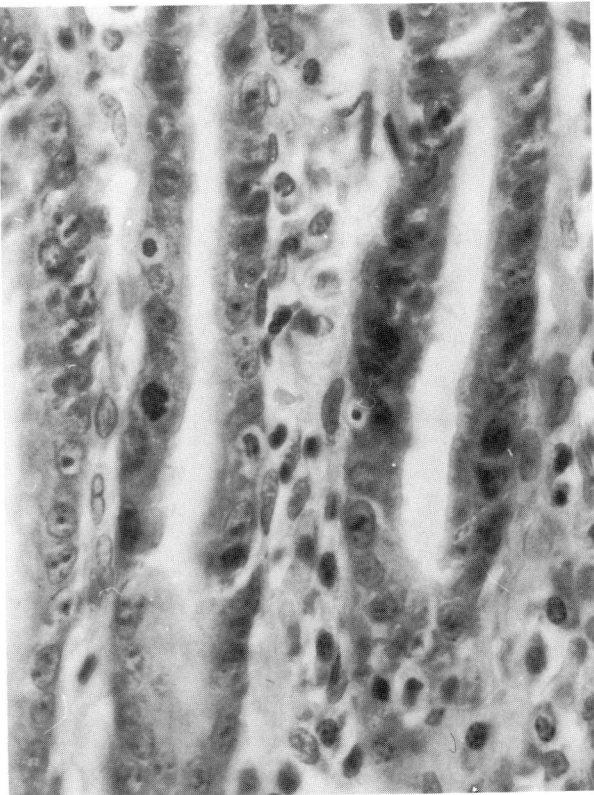

FIGURE 25–12. Severely dysplastic glands with immature cells. The cells are short and devoid of mucus secretion. The nuclei are large and slightly pleomorphic. The nucleoli are prominent. Mitosis is present. (× 480)

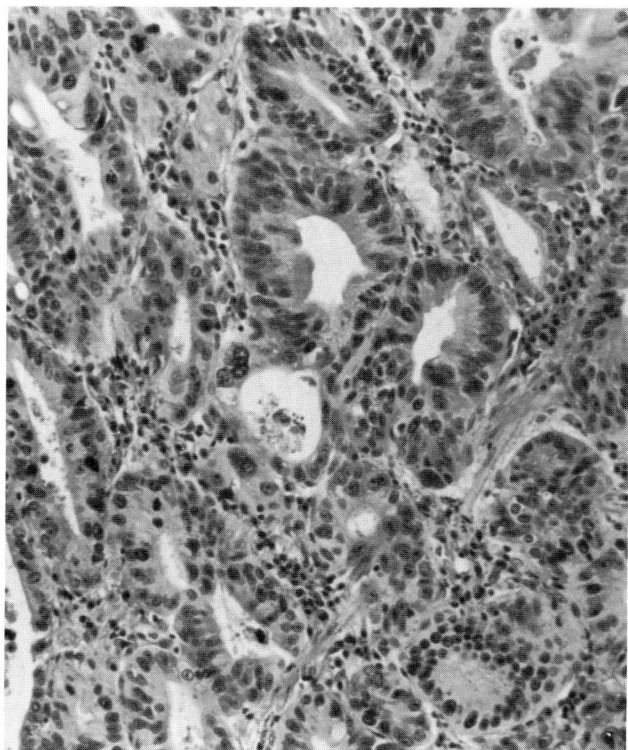

FIGURE 25–13. Possibly carcinomatous glands showing marked pseudostratification, moderate pleomorphism and no mucus secretion. The glands are crowded, but there is no stromal invasion. Definite carcinoma is present in another area. (× 200)

Possible Cancer (Figure 25–13). This term is applied to a lesion with abnormalities so severe that it is difficult to decide whether it is dysplasia or carcinoma *in situ*. The most disturbing feature is usually the prominent pleomorphism. This term should be used only as a temporary measure, and a definitive diagnosis should be made as soon as possible by repeat biopsy. The feature to look for is evidence of stromal invasion (Figure 25–14). Unlike the stratified squamous epithelium and adenomas of the digestive tract, carcinoma *in situ* alone is a rare finding in the stomach. Its existence has even been questioned.[139] It is usually accompanied by invasive lesions in the neighboring tissue. Thus search for stromal invasion will help to clarify a doubtful lesion.

Evidence of the precancerous nature of dysplastic gastric epithelium has been found in two aspects: a high grade of dysplasia is more common in the cancerous stomach than in the benign stomach,[129,140] and carcinoma may develop in the dysplastic stomach. Prospective studies implicate only the severely dysplastic tissue as precancerous.[114,130,141,142] Even in such cases, malignancy usually occurs after years of persisting dysplasia.[130] Conversely, dysplasia may regress, more frequently in the mild and moderate cases than in the severe cases.[130,141,143–145]

In a symposium on the significance of gastric dysplasia, held in 1988,[144] several investigative centers reported the finding of gastric carcinoma, in a total of 99 cases, after the diagnosis of dysplasia in the initial biopsies. The combined incidence of malignancy was 54% in cases of severe dysplasia and 9% in cases of moderate dysplasia. All but one carcinoma were discovered within 2 years of the diagnosis of dysplasia. In a recent report,[145] the respective incidences of malignancy were 31% and 5%. The majority of carcinomas were found within 1 year of the diagnosis of dysplasia. Most of the tumors were early, and the prognosis was good. In view of these data, gastric dysplasia may be considered paracancerous, rather than precancerous. Long-term follow-up studies are still needed to clarify the precancerous nature of gastric dysplasia.

In terms of management, the question of gastrectomy has been raised. Some investigators take the view

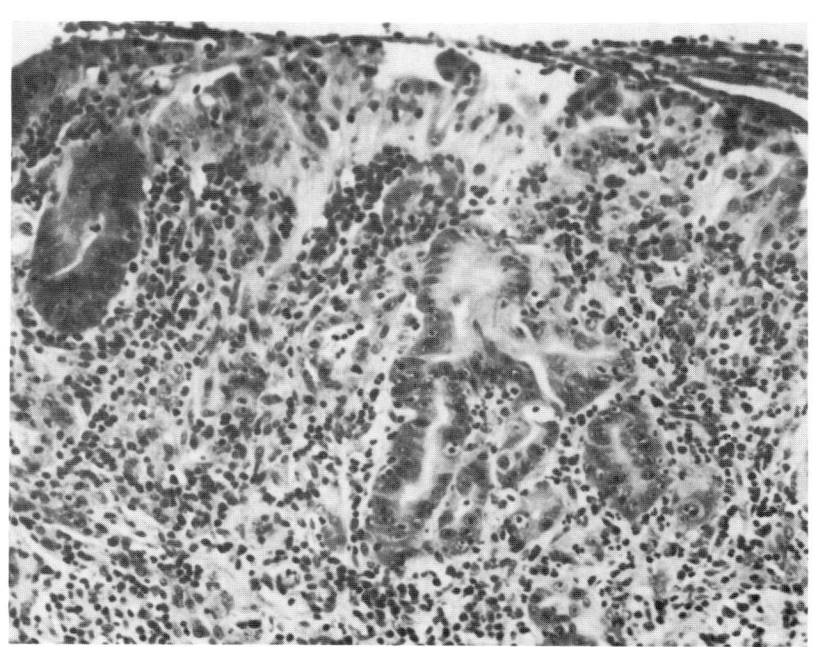

FIGURE 25–14. Small focus of superficial carcinoma with stromal invasion in an area of dysplasia. (× 120)

that the dysplastic tissue is neoplastic[75] and should be treated by gastrectomy, because the colonic lesion is often treated by colectomy. However, the situation surrounding gastric dysplasia is somewhat different from that in the colon, where dysplasia occurs almost exclusively in association with a long-standing debilitating ailment of inflammatory bowel disease, the treatment of which includes colectomy even in the absence of dysplastic lesions. In the stomach, the dysplastic changes in general are multifocal, with unpredictable location. The dysplasia is asymptomatic, and it may regress. The most commonly associated disease is chronic atrophic gastritis, which is not a surgically treatable disease. A conservative approach to gastric dysplasia with follow-up examinations may be appropriate in most cases.[143] More importantly, efforts must be made to search for a coexisting carcinoma because of its frequency, particularly if the dysplasia is severe or of high grade. In high-risk cases, a diligent search at relatively short intervals may reveal a malignant focus only weeks or months later. Surgical resection is clearly indicated in such cases. Because most carcinomas so discovered are early, they are highly curable.[144,145] If no carcinoma is present, a regular follow-up should be continued on patients with high-grade dysplasia.

Dysplasia is found to be closely associated with and is considered a likely premalignant forerunner of the expanding or intestinal type of cancer.[129,137] This type of cancer accounts for two thirds of gastric carcinomas. Dysplasia does not play a prominent role in the development of the infiltrative or diffuse type of gastric cancer. The precancerous lesion of the latter remains uncertain. There are indications, however, that the infiltrative carcinoma may arise from the neck mucous cells[137] or cells with globoid dysplasia.[132]

In *globoid dysplasia* the foveolar cells take on a globoid appearance because the cytoplasm is engorged with excessive amounts of acidic mucin.[130,132] The eccentric nuclei are compressed, and the cells resemble the signet-ring cancer cells (Figure 25–15). The presence of acidic mucin indicates that it is a form of incomplete intestinal metaplasia. The polarity of the cells is disturbed, so that they pile up on each other and their nuclei are abnormally located. Although the globoid dysplasia may be seen in a cancerous stomach, it may also be present in hyperplastic polyps.

Experimental Gastric Carcinogenesis

Adenocarcinoma of the stomach has been induced by radiation and a variety of chemical carcinogens. Since Sugimura et al.[147] used N-methyl-N'-nitro-N-nitrosoguanidine (MNNG) to produce adenomas, adenocarcinomas, and other tumors in the gastrointestinal tract in the rat in the late 1960s, the use of MNNG has become the standard in animal models of gastric carcinogenesis, mostly in rats. Susceptibility to MNNG is genetically controlled. Wistar and ACI rats are susceptible, but Buffalo rats are resistant. The resistance is carried by the F_1 offspring, indicating the dominant character of this trait.[148] The induced carcinoma resem-

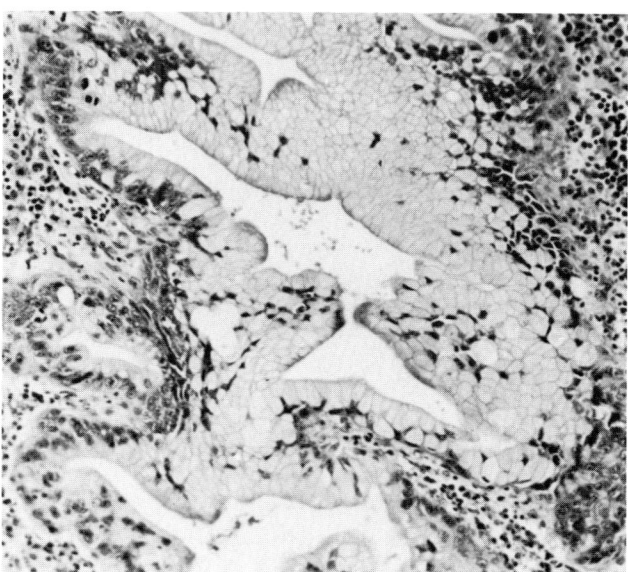

FIGURE 25–15. Globoid dysplasia of the foveolar cells, which are distended by a large globule of mucus compressing the nuclei to the cell membrane. The polarity is lost, and the cells are haphazardly oriented. ($\times$ 200)

bles the human gastric carcinoma. It is mostly well differentiated in rats. In dogs, signet-ring cells are common.[81,149] Electron microscopy reveals both gastric and intestinal types of cells, as well as squamous cells.[84,150] The tumors do not have pepsinogen 1, and the mucosal level of pepsinogen 1 reduces markedly in the precancerous period.[151,152] The ethyl (ENNG) and propyl (PNNG) derivatives of MNNG are less tumorigenic. PNNG has been used in rats.[151,153] ENNG is commonly used in dogs (Figure 25–16). A lower dose of ENNG produces mainly signet-ring cell carcinomas, whereas a higher dose induces glandular adenocarcinomas.[154] The induced signet-ring cell carcinoma may remain intramucosal for several years.[155]

The MNNG-induced adenocarcinomas develop through the stages of superficial erosion, atrophy, and increasing degrees of dysplasia.[135,156] Intestinal metaplasia, generally of the complete type, is common in the rats, but the frequency varies.[83] Change of mucin secretion to acidic type occurs before the morphologic changes of metaplasia occur.[157] In the dog and the monkey, intestinal metaplasia is rare or absent.[149,158] On the other hand, PNNG induces metaplasia more frequently than carcinoma.[153] These observations, together with the finding that the carcinoma cells are capable of differentiating into many cell types, as mentioned above, indicate that intestinal metaplasia is not an important precancerous lesion in experimental gastric carcinogenesis.

Natural History

The development and subsequent course of gastric adenocarcinoma go through several stages. The etiology of human gastric cancer is unknown, and whether

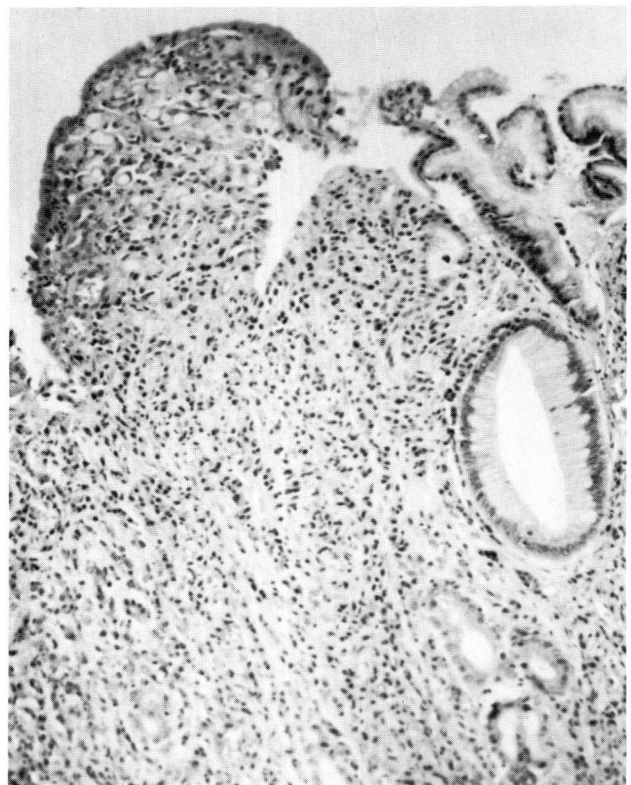

FIGURE 25-16. An infiltrative carcinoma without gland formation was induced in a dog with ENNG. There is neither intestinal metaplasia nor dysplasia in the adjacent mucosa. (× 120) (Courtesy of Dr. Wang Rui-nien, Professor of Pathology, Shanghai Second Medical University, Shanghai, People's Republic of China.)

the precancerous conditions are an integral part of the carcinogenic process or merely change the susceptibility of the tissue to carcinogenesis has not been determined. In any case, it has been postulated that exposure to carcinogens, in high-risk regions, probably occurs during early life,[30] but carcinoma begins after a long latent period of many years. It may develop in either metaplastic or gastric epithelium. In many, but not all, instances, dysplasia appears to be an intermediate step before carcinogenesis.

Since the gastric carcinomas are often diagnosed at the advanced stage, it may be assumed that they are fast-growing tumors. Actually, cell proliferation is slower in gastric cancer than in normal gastric mucosa, the cell cycle time being three times longer in the tumor.[159] On the other hand, the mean cell life span is shortened from 8 to 20 days in the normal mucosa to 1 day in the carcinoma.[130] Combination of these two phenomena results in the slow growth of the gastric carcinoma. It is estimated that it takes 1 to 4 years before the tumor is clinically recognized as an early gastric carcinoma (EGC).[95,160] EGCs also grow slowly, with a doubling time of 2 to 3 years,[160] and may remain superficial for several years.[160,161] These tumors may be large, more than 10 cm in diameter; and the patient usually has a long history of gastric symptoms.[162] Once the tumor penetrates the muscularis proper and beyond, it becomes an advanced gastric carcinoma (AGC). AGCs grow faster than EGCs, with an average doubling time of 2 to 10 months; the doubling time of the metastatic tumor is 0.6 to 2 months.[160] There is increasing DNA polyploidy and aneuploidy as the tumor advances and metastasizes,[163] indicating progressive mutation of the tumor.

Gastric carcinomas have different modes of growth. Some carcinomas grow in a coherent fashion and form large masses (expanding type of growth). Others invade by individual cells or isolated glands (infiltrative type of growth). These variations in the invasion pattern become manifest early and persist throughout the course of the disease. Thus, they are intrinsic biologic characteristics of the cancer cells. The metastasis may be by either venous or lymphatic routes, resulting in different organ involvement and variation in the clinical course and curability of the cancer. The terminal outcome varies from patient to patient. Many factors are involved, as discussed in the section on prognosis.

Pathology

Location and Size

Gastric carcinomas may occur anywhere in the stomach. About one half of them involve the pyloric mucosa; one quarter, the fundic mucosa, and another quarter, both areas.[76,117] In reports on the recent cases, the cardia was involved in 27% of cases,[164] and there was a decrease of antral carcinomas.[165]

The size of gastric carcinoma at the time of diagnosis varies. Most EGCs are 1 to 2 cm in diameter.[98] The AGCs are larger: nearly one half of the tumors are 6 cm or more in diameter, and one seventh are larger than 10 cm.[117] Multiple carcinomas may be present in the same stomach.[166]

Gross Morphology

Grossly, adenocarcinomas of the stomach can be divided, according to a modified Borrmann's classification,[167] into five types[117]:

1. Superficial carcinoma (type 0 carcinoma, early carcinoma)
2. Polypoid carcinoma (Borrmann's type 1 carcinoma)
3. Fungating carcinoma (Borrmann's type 2 carcinoma)
4. Ulcerated carcinoma (Borrmann's type 3 carcinoma)
5. Diffusely infiltrative carcinoma (Borrmann's type 4 carcinoma, linitis plastica carcinoma)

The relative frequency of each type in our materials is 6% for the superficial, 7% for the polypoid, 25% for the ulcerated, 36% for the fungating, and 26% for the diffuse type.[76]

The superficial carcinoma (Figure 25-17) was not in Borrmann's classification but has been called type 0 carcinoma.[168] It involves only the mucosa or mucosa and submucosa and thus is the same as the early carcinoma, and the Japanese classification of EGC is adopted for the subtypes (see Chapter 24). In Japan,

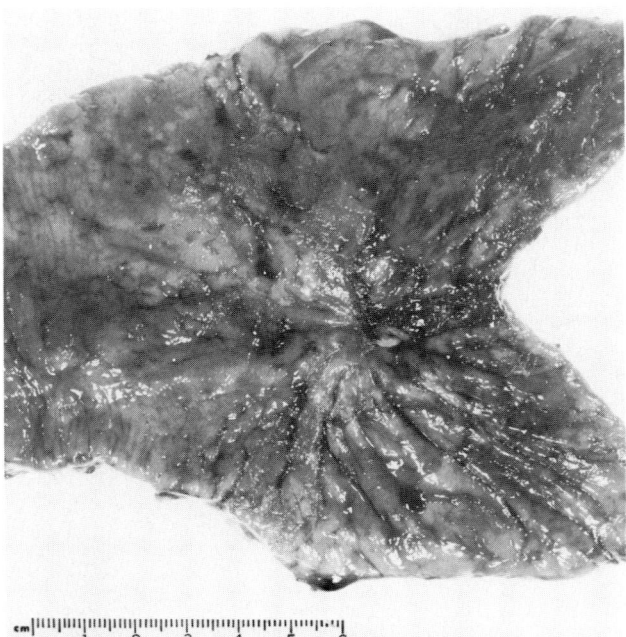

FIGURE 25-17. Superficial (early) carcinoma. The lesion is in a 2-by 3-cm area at the lesser curvature near the proximal resection margin. The surface is congested and slightly depressed. (From Ming SC: Tumors of the Esophagus and Stomach. In Atlas of Tumor Pathology, Second Series, Fascicle 7. Armed Forces Institute of Pathology, Washington, DC, 1973, p 164.)

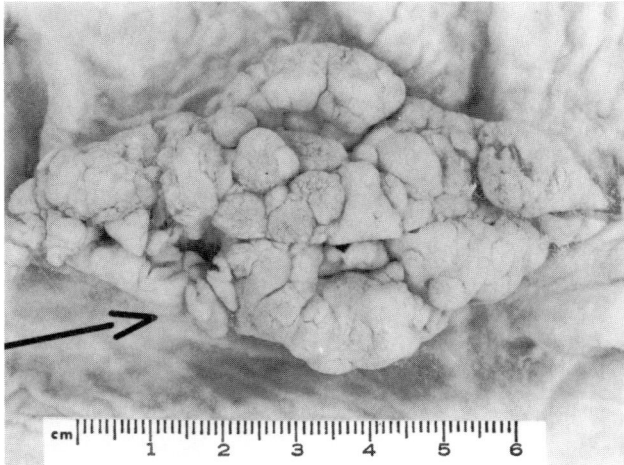

FIGURE 25-18. Polypoid carcinoma. It is lobulated but not ulcerated. (From Ming SC: Tumors of the Esophagus and Stomach. In Atlas of Tumor Pathology, Second Series, Fascicle 7. Armed Forces Institute of Pathology, Washington, DC, 1973, p 166.)

about one third to nearly one half of the resected carcinomas were EGCs.[169,170] In other countries, the incidence remains about 10% or lower.[171,172] Because these tumors may persist for years and may have metastases, the descriptive term *superficial carcinoma* is more appropriate than the term *early carcinoma*. When the tumor is widely spread out, the term *superficial spreading carcinoma* may be applied.[173] The significance of recognizing the superficial carcinoma is that it allows early treatment. Surgical resection of this cancer results in cure in about 94% to 100% of cases.[169,170] A detailed discussion of early gastric carcinoma is presented in Chapter 24.

The polypoid carcinoma (Figure 25-18) is a nodular tumor without gross ulceration. The base is usually broad. The fungating carcinoma (Figure 25-19) is also a nodular tumor, but with a large ulcer at the dome. The bottom of ulcer crater rests on the tumor mass and is above the level of the stomach wall. The ulcerated carcinoma (Figures 25-20 and 25-21) is an excavated tumor, with a penetrating ulcer base and an inconspicuous or only slightly elevated tumor mass at the periphery of the ulcer. It differs from the type III early carcinoma by the presence of tumor cells at the base as well as the margins of the ulcer. When the tumor tissue is limited in amount and location, the lesion may resemble a benign ulcer. In most instances, careful inspection will distinguish a malignant ulcer from a benign ulcer without too much difficulty (Table 25-3). When the gross evidence of malignancy is absent, it is important that sections for microscopic examination include all sides of the ulcer margins. In endoscopic diagnosis, multiple biopsies may be necessary for misdiagnosis to be avoided.

The diffusely infiltrative carcinoma (Figure 25-22) thickens the stomach wall without forming a mass or becoming deeply ulcerated. It may involve the whole stomach or a portion of it. The thick, stiff gastric wall has elicited the term *linitis plastica* for describing this type of tumor. The tumor is commonly accompanied by prominent fibrosis and is therefore also called scirrhous carcinoma.

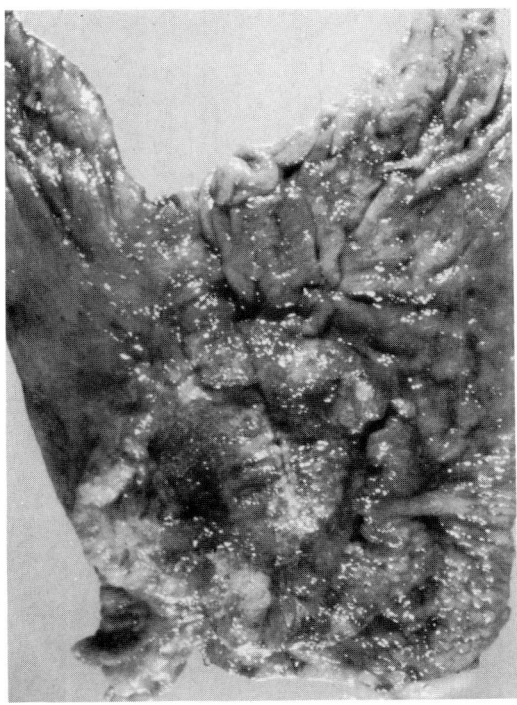

FIGURE 25-19. Fungating carcinoma in the antrum of the stomach. The tumor is raised, and there is a large ulcer on the surface.

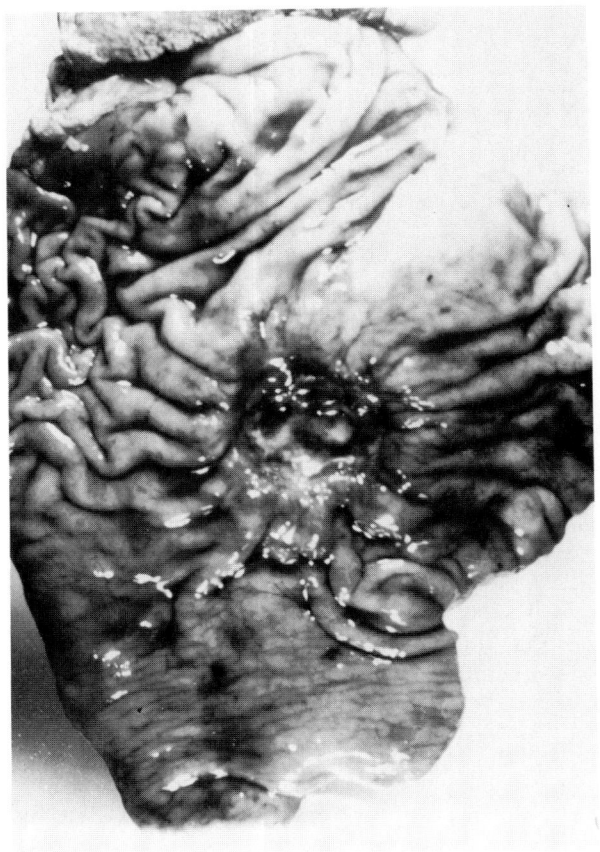

FIGURE 25-20. Ulcerated carcinoma in the distal portion of the body of the stomach. The ulcer base is shaggy and hemorrhagic. Mucosal folds are present at the ulcer margin, except the distal region, where the mucosa slopes into the ulcer base. (From Ming SC: Tumors of the Esophagus and Stomach. In Atlas of Tumor Pathology, Second Series, Fascicle 7. Armed Forces Institute of Pathology, Washington, DC, 1973, p 167.)

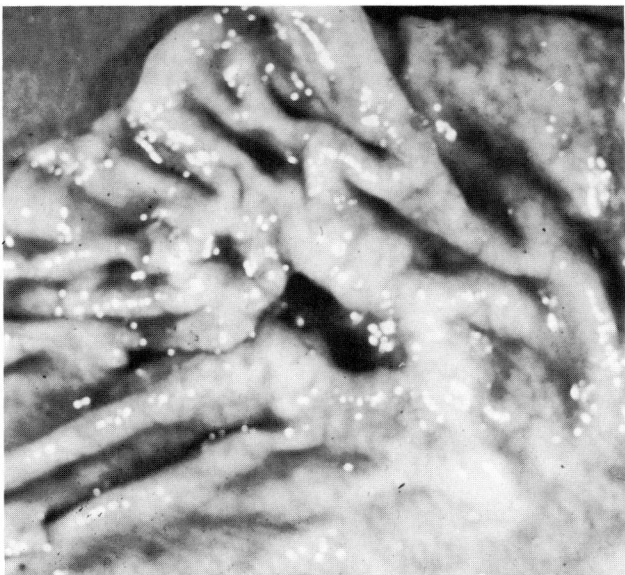

FIGURE 25-21. Ulcerated carcinoma. The deep ulcer is surrounded by a slightly raised wall. Microscopically, the tumor is a signet-ring–cell carcinoma.

Histologic Composition and Variants

Epithelial Elements

The histologic features of gastric adenocarcinoma are complex. The tumor shows varying degrees of differentiation at two levels, architectural and cellular. At the architectural level, a well-differentiated carcinoma is made of well-formed tubular glands (Figure 25-23). Papillary projections may be present in the dilated glandular spaces (Figure 25-24). A poorly differentiated carcinoma has only scattered or no glandular structures. The tumor cells may aggregate to form ribbons or masses (Figure 25-25) or may be individually scattered (Figure 25-26). At the cellular level, a well-differentiated carcinoma is composed of mature functioning cells such as the mucus-secreting goblet cells (Figure 25-27), signet-ring cells (Figure 25-28), and absorptive cells with striated borders (Figure 25-29). A poorly differentiated carcinoma has primitive nonfunctioning cells. These two aspects of differentiation often do not appear together. Many cells in the glandular carcinoma appear immature under the electron microscope, whereas the signet-ring cells are fully functional even though they do not form glands. In principle, cell differentiation is used in judging the degree of differentiation of the tumor. Thus, the signet-ring cell carcinoma is a well-differentiated tumor, and a poorly dif-

Table 25-3 DIFFERENTIATION BETWEEN BENIGN PEPTIC ULCER AND MALIGNANT ULCER (ULCERATED CARCINOMA WITHOUT FORMING MASS)

	Benign Ulcer	Ulcerated Cancer
Ulcer border	Sharp	Fuzzy
Ulcer size	Small	Variable
Ulcer base	Clean, pearly	Necrotic, hemorrhagic
Tissue at base	Pale, rubbery	Granular, gritty
Ulcer depth	Deep into muscularis or beyond	Variable
Mucosa around ulcer	Soft and mobile	Firm and fixed
	Congested, swollen	Pale, solid
Location	Antrum, lesser curvature	Antrum and others
Perforation or massive bleeding	Relatively common	Uncommon
Age of patient	Middle-aged	Old

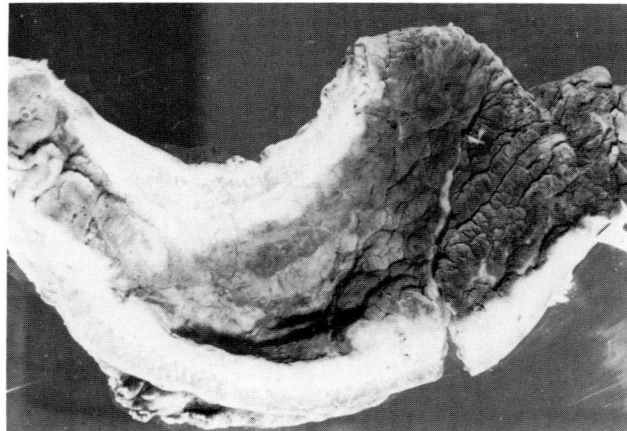

FIGURE 25–22. Diffusely infiltrative carcinoma (linitis plastica). The tumor involves the entire stomach. White scirrhous tumor tissue infiltrates the whole thickness of the gastric wall. (From Ming SC: Tumors of the Esophagus and Stomach. In Atlas of Tumor Pathology, Second Series, Fascicle 7. Armed Forces Institute of Pathology, Washington, DC, 1973, p 176.)

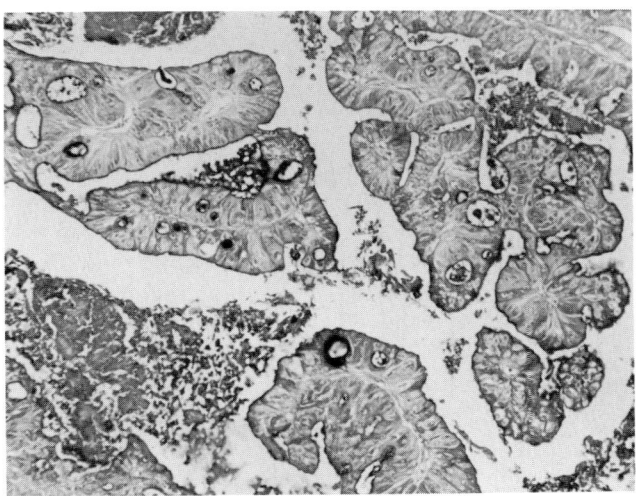

FIGURE 25–24. Papillary fronds in a large cystic area of a carcinoma. The tissue is stained by the periodic acid–Schiff method, which shows black mucus in the tumor tissue and on the surface of the fronds. (× 120)

ferentiated carcinoma may be solid and medullary or scattered and scirrhous.

Many types of cells have been identified in the gastric carcinoma by the histologic and cytologic appearance under the light microscope, by the secretory products as determined by histochemical and immunohistochemical techniques, and by the ultrastructural details under the electron microscope. Many cells are poorly differentiated or undifferentiated.[5] Among the differentiated cells, mucous cells are common. The majority of the mucous cells in glandular carcinoma are goblet cells that secrete intestinal acidic mucins.[5,64,117,174,175] In the diffusely infiltrative carcinoma, the mucous cells often assume the shape of the signet ring. Most of the signet-ring cells are also goblet cells.[117,174,176] The others, however, secrete only neutral glycoprotein, and thus resemble the foveolar or pyloric gland cells (Figure 25–30).[5,6,117,174,177] The gastric type of mucous cells are rare in the glandular carcinoma. Intracellular cysts are occasionally present in the tumor cells.[178] The cysts contain mucous granules and are lined by microvilli.

The non-mucous tumor cells in the tumor are mostly intestinal absorptive cells, having a distinct striated border made of well-formed microvilli[69,174] and containing digestive enzymes.[179] Additional cell types identified include pyloric gland cells,[5,174] endocrine cells,[9,119,180,181] Paneth cells,[8,182,183] parietal cells,[7,184,185] pepsinogen-secreting cells,[186,187] chief cells,[5] and squamous cells.[5] Hepatoid cells have also been reported.[188]

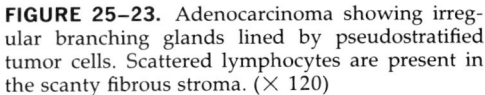

FIGURE 25–23. Adenocarcinoma showing irregular branching glands lined by pseudostratified tumor cells. Scattered lymphocytes are present in the scanty fibrous stroma. (× 120)

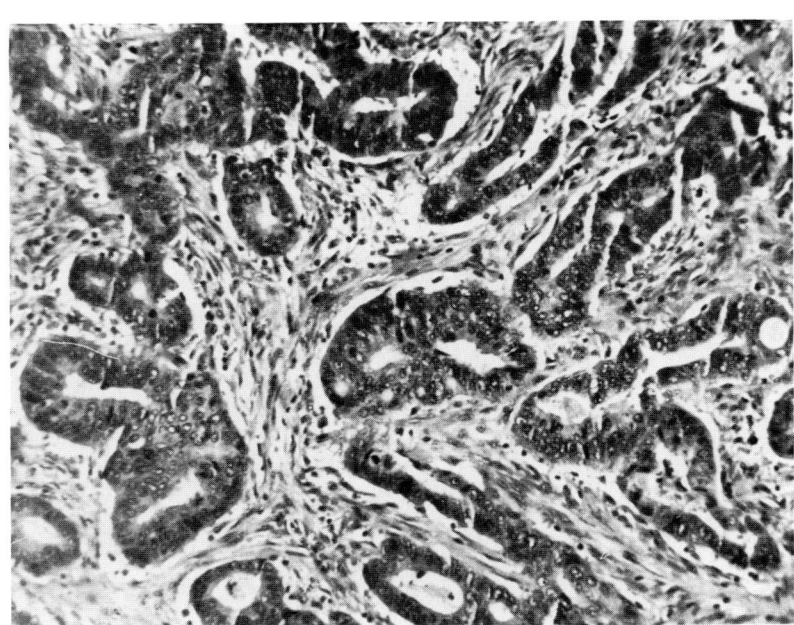

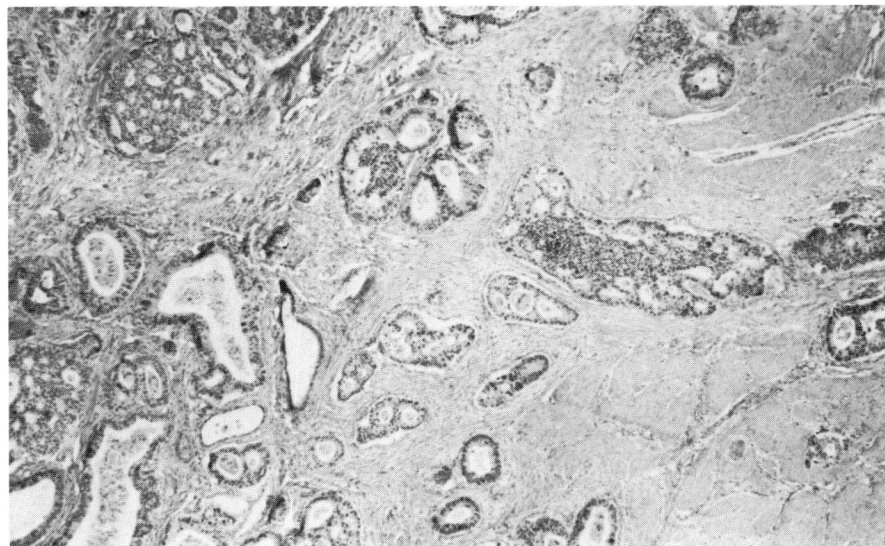

FIGURE 25-25. Expanding type adenocarcinoma, showing glandular tumor tissue forming tubules and masses. (× 65)

The argyrophil cells are sometimes abundant in the solid carcinomas[189] and the diffusely infiltrating carcinomas.[181] The solid carcinomas constitute about 6% of gastric carcinomas and are composed of sheets or masses of poorly differentiated or undifferentiated cells. Murayama et al.[189] examined 20 such tumors under the electron microscope. Mucous cells were present in 12 cases, neurosecretary cells in 5 cases, and both types of cells in 3 cases.

It is evident that the gastric adenocarcinomas are capable of differentiating into many types of cells that may or may not be indigenous to the normal stomach. Different types of cells are often present in the same tumor. Occasionally a specific cell type dominates and is seen as a unique clinicopathologic entity. Such variant tumors include parietal cell carcinoma, hepatoid carcinoma, mixed carcinoid and carcinoma, and Paneth cell carcinoma.

Parietal cell carcinoma was first described by Capella et al.[7] The number of parietal cells in the tumor may vary.[184] These cells form poorly cohesive sheets resembling lymphoma.[185] The identity of the cells is made by electron microscopy. The patients are elderly men. There are no specific symptoms.

Hepatoid carcinoma[188,190] contains a mixture of hepatocellular carcinoma and adenocarcinoma. The former cells are capable of secreting albumin, α-fetoprotein, α_1-antitrypsin, α_1-antichymotrypsin, and occasionally bile,[188,191] with increased serum levels of α-fetoprotein.[191] Most tumors are fungating but may be ulcerated. Metastasis to the liver is common.[188]

Mixed carcinoid and carcinoma may be either a combined tumor with admixed endocrine and exocrine cells or a composite tumor with separate groups of cell types. The endocrine cells secrete a variety of hormones.[192] Detailed information on these tumors is pre-

FIGURE 25-26. Infiltrative type of carcinoma, showing individual largely undifferentiated tumor cells between fascicles of muscle cells. A few cells have mucous globules in the cytoplasm. A moderate amount of fibrous tissue accompanies the tumor cells. (× 200)

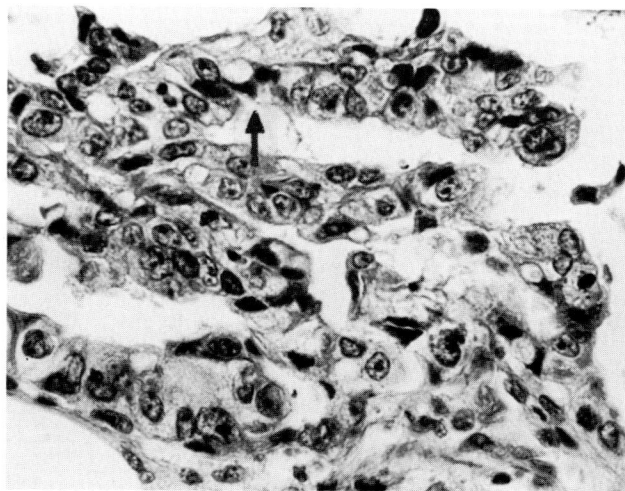

FIGURE 25-27. Moderately differentiated adenocarcinoma, showing the presence of goblet cells, one of which is marked by an arrow. (× 480)

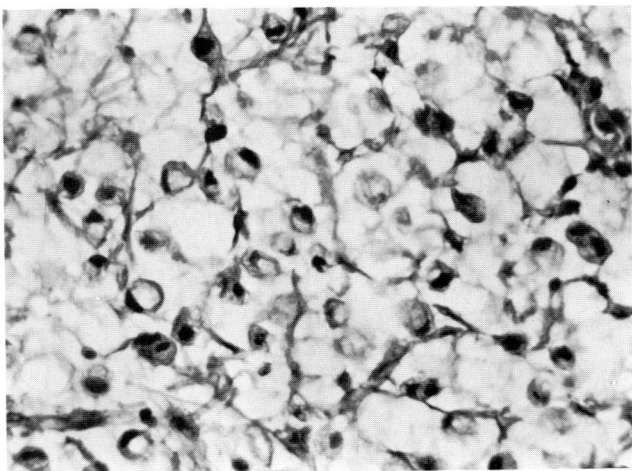

FIGURE 25-28. Signet-ring carcinoma cells with eccentric flattened nuclei and large globules of intracytoplasmic mucin. (× 300)

sented in Chapter 13. In a recent report, the tumor was accompanied by multiple separate carcinoids in the fundic mucosa in a woman with nonantral gastric atrophy.[193]

Paneth cell carcinoma[183] is very rare. Only four cases have been reported. The cells are identified by electron microscopy and by the demonstration of lysozyme in the cells. There are no unusual clinical or gross morphologic features.

Stromal Elements

The stroma of many gastric carcinomas has distinctive features. Lymphocytic infiltration is prominent in some glandular and solid carcinomas.[76] The latter has been given the name *carcinoma with lymphoid stroma*[194–196] (Figure 25-31). These tumors are found in 3.8% of gastric carcinomas.[196] The cells are arranged in trabecular or alveolar pattern and show differentiation toward pyloric glands. Interleukin-1 (IL-1) was demonstrated in many tumor cells. T lymphocytes were present in and around tumor cell nests, but B cells were clustered in lymphoid follicles. It has been postulated that T cells with IL-1 receptors might be induced by IL-1 or related substances released from the tumor cells.[196]

Desmoplastic reaction is prominent in the infiltrative carcinomas.[76,197] The term *scirrhous carcinoma* is applied to such a tumor. The fibrous tissue is grossly evident. The scattered tumor cells may be signet-ring cells or poorly differentiated. Procollagen I has been demonstrated in such tumors[198] and some cell lines[199] but not the medullary carcinomas.[198] The latter are conspicuously devoid of desmoplastic tissue. Furthermore, transforming growth factor β from tumor cells may stimulate both tumor cells and fibroblasts to produce collagen.[199]

Spread of Gastric Carcinoma

In contrast to the carcinomas of stratified squamous epithelium, the gastric carcinomas break through the basement membrane and invade the lamina propria early in the course of the disease,[200] and the stage of *in situ* carcinoma is rarely observed.[139] From the mucosal stroma the tumor cells infiltrate along the blood vessels through muscularis mucosae into the submucosa, in which the cells proliferate to form a balloon-like expansion.[201] As the tumor penetrates the serosa, it may involve a neighboring organ or seed the peritoneal lining. The latter is more common in nonglandular than

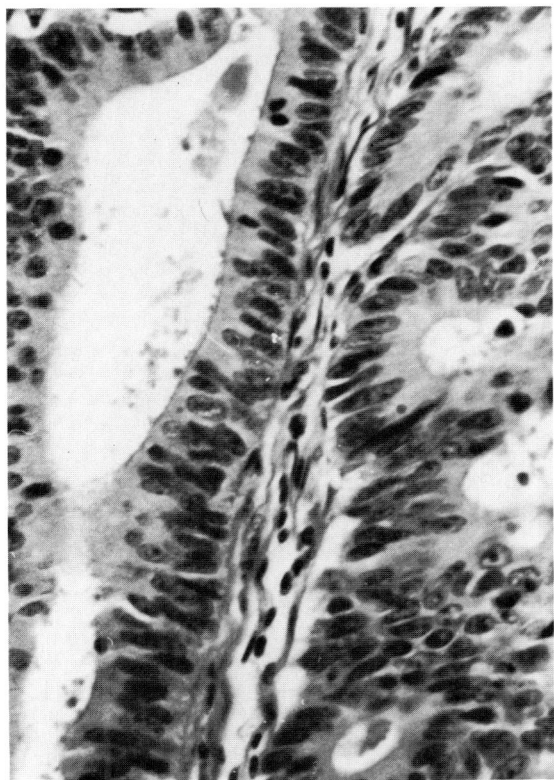

FIGURE 25-29. Well-differentiated adenocarcinoma, showing a striated border on the luminal surface of the tumor cells. (× 375)

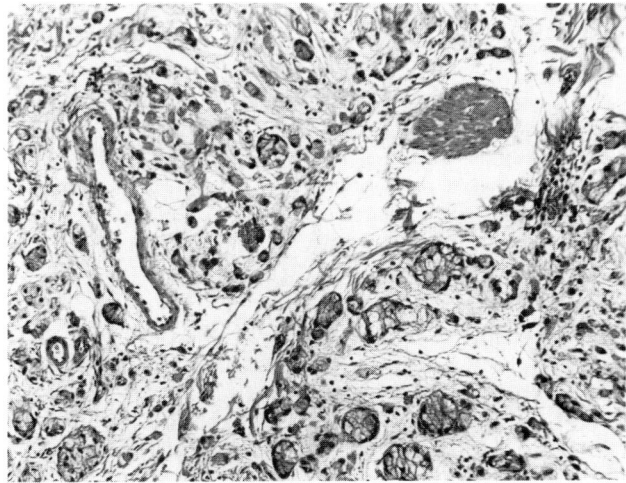

FIGURE 25-30. Infiltrative carcinoma, showing pyloric-type glands and signet-ring cells. (× 110)

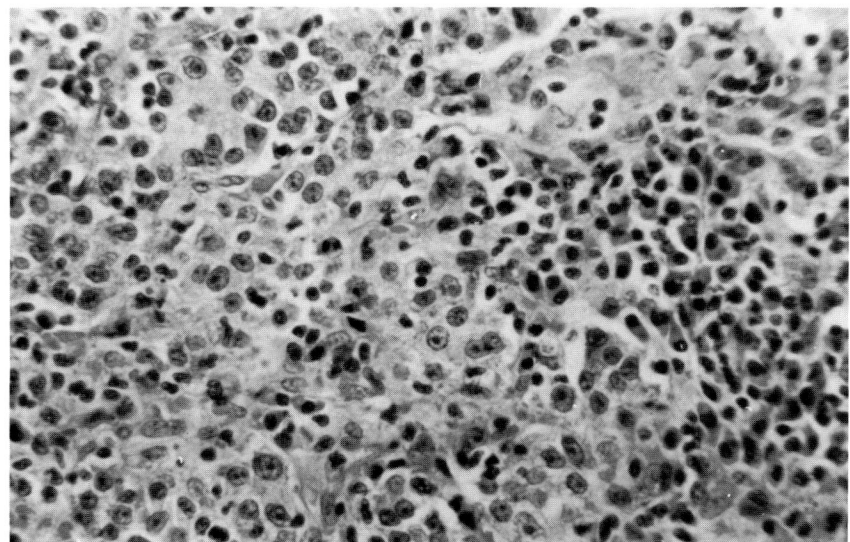

FIGURE 25-31. Carcinoma with lymphoid stroma. Many lymphocytes and plasma cells mingle with undifferentiated carcinoma cells. (× 150)

in glandular carcinomas.[202] A tumor of the upper stomach may extend directly into the esophagus. In fact, the majority of adenocarcinomas at the lower esophagus originate in the stomach (see Chapter 19). At the pyloric end, involvement of the duodenum is usually subserosal and only rarely in the submucosa or mucosa.

Lymphatic permeation may occur in the deep mucosa,[203] and lymph node metastasis is present in 2% to 11% of mucosal carcinomas.[169,204,205] As the tumor invades deeper tissue, the incidence of lymph node involvement increases. Blood vessel invasion begins in the submucosa.[200] By these vascular channels, the tumor cells spread to distant organs. The liver and the lung are most frequently involved. Hematogenous spread to the ovary occurs more frequently in signet-ring cell carcinoma than in glandular carcinoma. Such an ovarian tumor is known as Krukenberg's tumor. The stomach is the site of the primary tumor in 70% of these tumors.[206]

Marker Substances

Because the gastric carcinomas are composed of gastric as well as intestinal cells, many types of mucins,[64,65,72,207,208] enzymes,[181,187,209-213] and hormones[181,214,215] related to these cells have been found in the carcinoma. The neutral mucus, being specific for the gastric mucous cells, is useful in identifying the gastric origin of secondary tumors.[216] Other markers demonstrated by immunohistochemical methods are listed in Table 25-4.

The carcinoembryonic antigen (CEA) is a commonly tested oncofetal antigen and has been demonstrated in the tumor as well as the dysplastic and metaplastic tissue.[74,218,263] CEA is usually present in the luminal cell membrane of glandular tumor cells and in the cytoplasm of signet-ring cells. The serum level of CEA has been used in evaluating clinical cases. Janssen and Orjasaeter[227] noted that it paralleled the stage of the tumor. Its value for postoperative follow-up was questionable, however, because the serum level remained high in most patients. Another possible application of tumor markers is in screening of high-risk populations. The fetal sulfoglycoprotein antigen (FSA) was used in a mass survey.[236] Positive results were obtained in about 9% of persons tested, of whom only 1% had carcinoma. Several oncogenes and their protein products, particularly the *ras* gene and p21,[240,241,244,245] have been demonstrated in the gastric carcinoma. A detailed discussion of oncogene studies is presented in Chapter 6.

Table 25-4 MARKER SUBSTANCES IN GASTRIC ADENOCARCINOMA

Albumin[188,217]
α-fetoprotein[188,214,217-220]
$α_1$-antitrypsin and $α_1$-antichymotrypsin[188,217,221]
Blood group antigens[222-225]
CA 19-9[219,225]
Calcitonin[226]
Carcinoembryonic antigen[214,218,219,222,227,228]
Carcinoplacental alkaline phosphatase[229]
Epidermal growth factors and receptors[119,230-232]
Sex hormones and receptors[233-235]
Ferritin[218]
Fetal sulfoglycoprotein[236]
Glucocorticoid receptor[237]
Human chorionic gonadotropin β subunit[214,217,218,238]
Human placental lactogen[218]
Interleukin 1[196]
Lectin-binding glycoproteins[239]
Lysozyme[8,182]
Oncogens and their products[134,240-246]
Pepsinogens[187,211,212]
Polyamines[247]
Pregnancy-specific β glycoproteins[218]
Procollagens[198,199]
Proliferative cell nuclear antigen[248]
Transferrin[217,218]
Transforming growth factor[199]
Tumor-associated glycoprotein[249]
Tumor-derived colon-specific antigen[218]
DNA ploidy[250-262]

Gastric carcinomas have been studied for their DNA content and ploidy patterns. In general, 60% to 70% of gastric carcinomas are aneuploid.[250,251] The glandular tumors more frequently are aneuploid, whereas the nonglandular diffusely infiltrative carcinomas are mostly diploid.[252–254] It has been noted that the intramucosal signet-ring cells are nearly always diploid, and the aneuploid cell population is found only focally in the deeply invasive portions of the tumor.[255,256] This finding correlates well with the slow rate of growth at the early stage of such tumors in both men and animals.[155,160] The polyploid and aneuploid carcinomas show deeper invasion and more lymph node metastases than diploid tumors and tumors with homogeneous ploidy.[163,251,257,258] They also have a worse prognosis.[163,250,257–260] However, the difference may not be statistically significant[251] and may apply only to the intestinal type carcinoma.[261] The ploidy patterns in the primary and recurrent tumors are consistent.[262]

Histologic Classifications

The histologic composition of gastric carcinoma varies from case to case and from area to area within a case. As a result, several histologic classifications have been proposed, each with a specific purpose.

World Health Organization (WHO) Typing

The World Health Organization classifies the gastric adenocarcinomas into four types: papillary, tubular, mucinous, and signet-ring cell.[264] They are further graded as well-differentiated, moderately differentiated, and poorly differentiated. The undifferentiated carcinoma is classified as a separate entity. The tubular carcinomas are most common. The mucinous carcinoma is also called mucoid or colloid carcinoma. It is characterized by abundant extracellular mucus, which is grossly visible and comprises at least 50% of the total volume of the tumor mass. About 10% of the gastric carcinomas are of this type.[265] Floating in the mucus pool are fragmented tumor gland or individual signet-ring cells. The mucinous carcinoma is therefore a subtype of either the glandular carcinoma or the signet-ring cell carcinoma.

This classification is highly reproducible,[266] and the terms are familiar to all pathologists. It is useful for routine pathologic diagnosis of gastric carcinoma. However, it should be kept in mind that the histologic pattern of gastric carcinoma often varies, so that the diagnosis is based on the dominant pattern and is accurate only for the materials examined.

Lauren's Classification

Lauren[267] divided the gastric carcinomas into two types: intestinal and diffuse, with a relative frequency of 53% and 33%, respectively. The remaining 14% of carcinomas did not fit into these patterns and were unclassified. The intestinal type carcinoma was so named because it has features resembling a differentiated colonic carcinoma (see Figures 25–23, 25–27, and 25–29). The diffuse type is characterized by diffuse infiltration of tumor cells individually or in small nests (see Figure 25–26; Figure 25–32). Clinically, the intestinal type carcinoma has been found to be more common in older male patients, whereas the diffuse carcinoma is more common in younger female patients. The intestinal types have a higher survival rate than the diffuse types.[268]

This classification is reasonably reproducible.[266] In spite of apparent histologic differences, however, electron microscopy and mucin histochemistry have

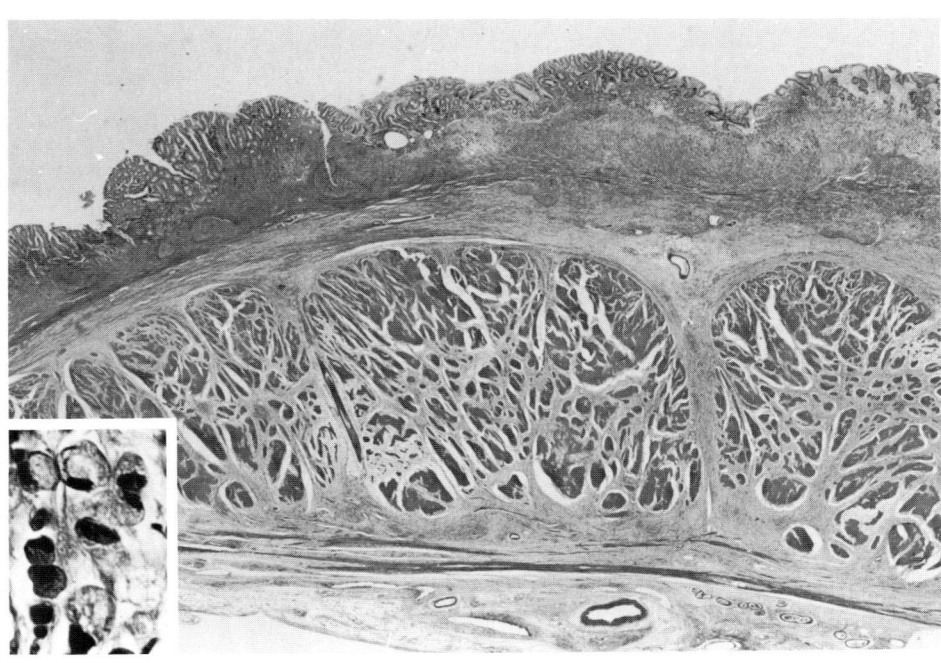
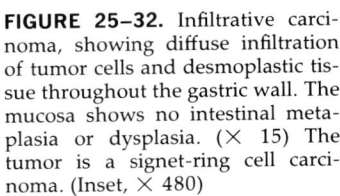

FIGURE 25–32. Infiltrative carcinoma, showing diffuse infiltration of tumor cells and desmoplastic tissue throughout the gastric wall. The mucosa shows no intestinal metaplasia or dysplasia. (× 15) The tumor is a signet-ring cell carcinoma. (Inset, × 480)

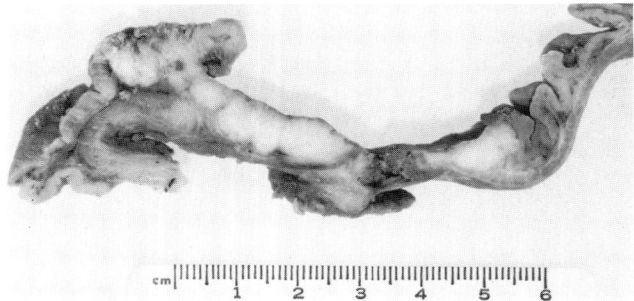

FIGURE 25–33. Cross section of an expanding carcinoma, showing the circumscribed tumor tissue involving the muscular layer. (From Ming SC: Tumors of the Esophagus and Stomach. In Atlas of Tumor Pathology, Second Series, Fascicle 7. Armed Forces Institute of Pathology, Washington, DC, 1973, p 171.)

revealed characteristics of intestinal cells such as well-developed microvilli and acidic mucin in both intestinal and diffuse types.[174,175] On the other hand, only the intestinal type of carcinoma is associated with chronic atrophic gastritis, severe intestinal metaplasia, and dysplasia in the neighboring mucosa.

Lauren's classification has been used in many epidemiologic studies.[17–19,27] The intestinal type of carcinoma is prevalent in high-risk countries.[17] The decline in gastric cancer incidence in many countries has been attributed by some investigators[19] to a decline in the incidence of the intestinal type of carcinoma.

Ming's Classification

Based on the patterns of tumor growth and invasiveness, the gastric carcinomas are divided into expanding and infiltrative types.[76] The expanding carcinoma grows by expansion into nodules or masses, often with a sharply defined periphery compressing the neighboring tissue (see Figure 25–25; Figure 25–33). The infiltrative carcinoma shows infiltration by individual cells (see Figure 25–26) or small glands (see Figure 25–30; Figure 25–34). Their relative frequencies are 67% and 33%, respectively. Both types of carcinoma show varying degrees of cell maturation and differentiation. Large glands, however, are present only in the expanding type. Under the electron microscope, the tumor cells in expanding carcinoma show well-developed desmosomes, which are usually absent in the infiltrative carcinoma even when the cells are in close contact.[269] Lymphocytic infiltration is heavy in the expanding carcinoma, and the desmoplastic response is prominent in the infiltrative carcinoma. The expanding carcinoma is often associated with chronic atrophic gastritis, prominent intestinal metaplasia, and dysplasia. These changes are either mild or absent in the stomach with infiltrative carcinoma.

The microscopic patterns of tumor growth are reflected in the gross appearance of the tumor. The expanding carcinoma shows sharply demarcated tumor mass (see Figure 25–33), whereas the infiltrative carcinoma has indistinct tumor boundaries and does not form gross masses (see Figure 25–22). These features correlate well with the gross morphologic types of the tumor: the expanding carcinomas are polypoid or fungating, and the infiltrative carcinomas are diffusely infiltrative. The ulcerated carcinomas are equally divided between the two types. Thus, this classification can be adopted for clinical use and at the time of surgical exploration. Because the classification is based on the growth pattern of the tumor, it has an important prognostic value. The survival rate of patients with expanding carcinoma has been found to be double that of patients with infiltrative carcinoma.[76,270,271]

There are similarities between Ming's and Lauren's classifications. Carcinomas of the intestinal type are mostly expanding carcinomas, and carcinomas of the diffuse type are infiltrative carcinomas. The solid carcinoma, unclassified by Lauren, is an expanding carcinoma. Conversely, an intestinal type of tumor that is

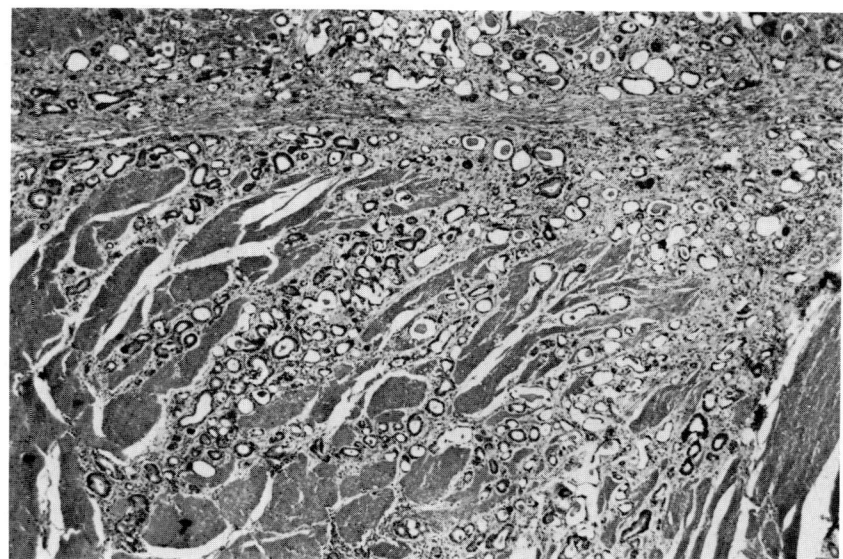

FIGURE 25–34. Infiltrative carcinoma showing infiltration of the muscularis propria by individual small glands. (× 50)

composed of small glands and infiltrated diffusely without mass formation is an infiltrative carcinoma.

Other Classifications

Nakamura[272] simply divided the gastric cancers into differentiated and undifferentiated types, using gland formation as the indicator for differential diagnosis. Thus, the well-differentiated signet-ring cell carcinomas are often put into the category of undifferentiated tumor. Jass[273] separated gastric carcinomas into gastric and intestinal types based on a point system for various histologic features. Mulligan[274] divided gastric carcinomas into mucous cell (46.7%), pylorocardiac gland cell (29.7%), and intestinal cell types (23.6%). This classification was made without the benefit of histochemistry and electron microscopy. Using these techniques, the gastric cancers show many intestinal-type cells[5,69,175] and few pyloric gland cells.[175,176] Finally, the Japanese Research Society for Gastric Cancer[168] designed a comprehensive list of rules for the study of gastric cancer, taking into consideration histologic features as well as clinical observations.

TNM Staging

The American Joint Committee on Cancer (AJCC) developed a staging system based on the extent of tumor invasion (T), the status of lymph node involvement (N), and distant metastasis (M), called TNM staging. It has been periodically revised so that the stages would correlate closely with the survival rate. The system published in 1988[275] is summarized below:

Stage 0:   Tis, N0, M0
Stage IA: T1, N0, M0
      IB: T1, N1, M0; or T2, N0, M0
Stage II: T1, N2, M0; or T2, N1, M0; or T3, N0, M0
Stage IIIA: T2, N2, M0; or T3, N1, M0; or T4, N0, M0
      IIIB: T3, N2, M0; or T4, N1, M0
Stage IV: T4, N2, M0; or Any T, Any N, M1

The terms are defined as follows: Tis, carcinoma *in situ*; T1, carcinoma invading the lamina propria or the submucosa (equivalent to EGC); T2, carcinoma extending into the muscularis proper or the subserosa; T3, carcinoma penetrating the serosa without invading the adjacent structures; T4, carcinoma invading the adjacent structures; N0, no regional lymph node metastasis; N1, metastasis in the perigastric nodes within 3 cm of the primary tumor; N2, metastasis in the perigastric nodes more than 3 cm from the primary tumor or in nodes along the adjacent major arteries; M0, no distant metastasis; M1, distant metastasis. It should be noted that pure *in situ* gastric carcinoma is rare and stage 0 patients have not been listed in the reported series of cases.

Curtis et al.[171] modified an earlier version of the AJCC system and grouped the gastric carcinomas into stages I, IIA, IIB, III, and IV. Stage I corresponded roughly to IA in the current system, IIA to IB, and IIB to II. Among 2132 cases analyzed by them, there were 158 cases (7.4%) in stage I, 208 (9.8%) in stage IIA, 266 (12.5%) in stage IIB, 789 (37%) in stage III, and 711 (33.3%) in stage IV. The relative survival rates at 4 years for these groups were, respectively, 87%, 71%, 35%, 19%, and 3%.

Clinical Aspects

Sex and Age

Gastric carcinomas occur mainly in the old, with a peak in the seventh decade.[76] The infiltrative carcinoma tends to occur more often in younger patients. The male-to-female ratio is about 1.5:1. The ratio is 2:1 for expanding carcinoma and 1:1 for infiltrative carcinoma.[76] A similar sex difference is seen between intestinal and diffuse carcinomas.[267] In about 2% of cases, the carcinoma occurs in the young people, under the age of 35 years, with a reversed male-to-female ratio of 1:2.9.[276] The tumors in the young patients are often diffusely infiltrating and large, and the prognosis is poor.[276,277] Of 37 cases in young patients reported by Bloss et al.,[278] 28 had linitis plastica or poorly differentiated carcinoma, and only 2 patients survived 5 years. The prognosis is better for tumors with endocrine cells than for tumors without them.[214]

Clinical Presentations and Diagnosis

The symptoms of gastric carcinoma are not specific, mainly epigastric pain and discomfort, weight loss, anemia, and those of pre-existing precancerous conditions. Occult blood in the stool is common, but massive bleeding is rare.[279] Unusual presentations include free perforation of the stomach,[280] hypoglycemia,[281] granulocytosis,[282] pneumatosis cystoides,[283] thrombocytopenic purpura and immune complex diseases,[284] microangiopathy,[285] and hepatic failure due to intrasinusoidal metastasis.[286] The duration of symptoms is generally short, less than 1 year, although the tumor at the time of diagnosis is quite large and advanced.

The clinical diagnosis of gastric carcinoma can be readily made by radiologic examination or endoscopic biopsy with 90% accuracy in nearly all cases. The rate of correct diagnosis reaches 97% when both methods are applied.[287] According to one study, the major reasons for false-negative diagnosis with biopsy are an inadequate number of biopsy specimens (less than seven) and misdiagnosis by the pathologist when the number of positive biopsy specimens was three or less.[288] Conversely, a false-positive diagnosis may be made because of misinterpretation of abnormal but benign cells in the specimen.[289] For lesions that are not grossly evident, such as early carcinoma and ulcerated carcinoma and those found in follow-up examinations in cases of severe dysplasia, a liberal number of biopsy specimens may be required for achievement of a high rate of correct diagnosis. In such cases, cytologic study can be very helpful.[290] A full discussion of the endoscopic and cytologic examinations is presented in Chapters 3 and 4, respectively.

The differential diagnosis of primary gastric tumors involves mainly the distinction between the primary lymphoma of the stomach and the solid undifferentiated gastric carcinoma of the expanding type. Features favoring carcinoma are pleomorphism of tumor cells, circumscription of tumor nodules, the presence of markers of epithelial tumors such as mucin and CEA, a desmoplastic response in the stroma, the polyclonal and heterogeneous nature of lymphoid cells in the tumor, and precancerous lesions in the adjacent mucosa.

The primary nature of a gastric carcinoma is usually evident. Occasionally it has to be differentiated from a metastatic tumor. Metastatic tumors in the stomach are rare. They are usually small and submucosally located, covered by an intact mucosa. When a pancreatic or esophageal adenocarcinoma extends into the stomach, the differentiation between it and the primary tumor may be difficult and at times impossible. The decision is based primarily on the location of the bulk of the tumor and the presence of precursor lesions in the surrounding mucosa.

Treatment and Prognosis

Surgical resection of the tumor remains the treatment of choice. However, many cases are diagnosed in the advanced stage, and curable resection is possible in only 30% to 50% of cases.[165,291] The results of treatment are poor: the overall 5-year survival rate is around 10%[292,293]; that in patients with curable resection, about 24% to 35%.[165,291,292] Only 3% of the unresected patients have survived for 4 years[171] and none for 5 years.[291] Because lymph node metastasis adversely affects the survival rate, an aggressive approach to lymphadenectomy as practiced in Japan improves the prognosis. Soga et al.[205] reported a 5-year survival rate in the curably resected cases of 50.6% for all tumors and 38.3% for advanced cases. The situation has changed little in the United States.[294] Additional radiotherapy and chemotherapy have not significantly increased the survival rate,[292-295] although such therapy may prolong remission.[296,297] The hope for cure lies in early diagnosis. The 5-year survival rate for early cancer after resection is 94% to 100%.[169,170] The 10-year survival rate for EGC without lymph node metastasis is also 94% and for that with lymph node metastasis is 53%.[298] In Japan, mass survey has resulted in the discovery of many early cancers. About 52% of survey cases had early cancers, and the 5- and 10-year survival rates of these cases were, respectively, 80% and 78.8%; whereas the corresponding rates among the outpatient group were 56.2% and 55.1%.[299] The combination of early diagnosis and extended surgical resection has contributed to the overall improvement of survival rates for gastric cancer in Japan.[300] The importance of the stage of the tumor at the time of the initial diagnosis as a prognostic factor is also shown in the report of Curtis et al.,[171] cited above. The poor survival of gastric cancer patients in the United States and other countries coincides with a low percentage of early cases, about 10% or less.[171,172,301]

The next important prognostic factor is the biologic behavior of the tumor as manifested in the growth patterns.[76,271,302,303] The survival rate of the expanding carcinoma is nearly double that of the infiltrative carcinoma, independent of other features of the tumor.[270,304,305] Similarly, the prognosis for the intestinal type of carcinoma is better than that for the diffuse carcinoma,[267,268,271] a difference that is partly related to lymphatic involvement.[270,304] Related to these observations is the extent of serosal and peritoneal involvement,[306,307] which is common in the infiltrative carcinoma.[307] Furthermore, the percentage of signet-ring cells in the tumor is inversely related to the survival rate.[308] Heavy infiltration of lymphoid and Langerhans cells in the tumor stroma is a favorable prognostic sign.[194,195,309,310] So is the presence of parietal cells,[184,185,311] endocrine cells,[214] and oncogene c-myc product p62.[312] Unfavorable indicators are the presence of epidermal growth factor and receptor,[230,232] CEA,[313] human chorionic gonadotropin (hCG),[314] lysozyme,[8] estrogen receptor,[234] and heterogenous ploidy of the tumor cells.[257-260] Prognosis is poor for tumors at the cardia,[171,259,260,315] but other locations have no effect. Factors with questionable effects include the grade of tumor differentiation[316,317] and the size of tumor.[302,315] Factors that appear to be not significant include the sex, age, and race; the duration of the symptoms; and the WHO histologic type of the tumor.[302,317]

ADENOCARCINOMA OF THE GASTRIC CARDIA AND ESOPHAGOGASTRIC JUNCTION

The gastric cardia is a small region, normally about 2 cm in length from the esophagogastric junction. This junction offers no barrier to tumor penetration from either the esophagus or the stomach. When a tumor is located in this area, therefore, it is difficult to determine its site of origin unless the tumor is small. It had been assumed in the past that an adenocarcinoma at this region was gastric, even if the esophagus was involved. This situation has changed since the recognition of Barrett's carcinoma as a distinct entity. Many such tumors are now considered esophageal in origin. Regardless of the question of the site of origin, adenocarcinomas at these locations have similar clinicopathologic features.[318,319] These aspects are discussed in Chapter 19.

Clinically there is a male dominance, with a male-to-female ratio of 3:1 to 7:1.[319,320] The peak age is in the sixth decade; the patients are younger than those with carcinoma elsewhere in the stomach.[319,321] A history of smoking and alcohol intake is common.[318] Pathologically, about half of the carcinomas are of the infiltrative type; but the incidence of signet-ring cell tumor is relatively low.[319]

The pathologic features of cardiac carcinoma appear to be changing. Antonioli and Goldman[164] reported an increase in the incidence of cardiac carcinoma, from

0% to 27% of all gastric carcinomas, in their materials. There were also an increase in the number of signet-ring cells, a decreased male-to-female ratio, and an increase in the age of the patients. Similar observations were made by others in Japan[322] and the United Kingdom.[323] Most early cardiac carcinomas are elevated.[324] Of 500 advanced carcinomas analyzed in China,[325] 16% were fungating, 36.4% were ulcerated with raised margins, 28% were ulcerated and infiltrative, and 19.2% were diffusely infiltrative. Histologically, most tumors are well differentiated, and about one tenth are mucinous.[324,325] In 8% of the tumors, there are well-differentiated glands resembling hyperplastic cardiac glands.[325] The cardiac carcinomas often invade the esophagus, in 57% of cases in one study.[326] The prognosis is poor,[171,315] coinciding with a high number of aneuploid tumors.[259,260] The overall postresection survival rate is 19.2% at 5 years and 8.5% at 10 years.[325] The survival rate is lower in patients with esophageal involvement than it is in those without.[326]

SQUAMOUS CELL CARCINOMA, ADENOSQUAMOUS CARCINOMA, AND MUCOEPIDERMOID CARCINOMA

Squamous cells have been identified by electron microscopy in human gastric carcinomas as well as experimental carcinomas in rats.[5,150] They are rarely prominent enough to justify the diagnosis of adenosquamous carcinoma, however. Pure squamous cell carcinoma is even rarer. Mori et al.[327] found 16 adenosquamous carcinomas (0.3%) and 4 squamous cell carcinomas (0.8%) among 5000 resected gastric carcinomas. The incidence reported by others varies from 0.04%[328] to 3.4%,[329] with most around 0.2%.[330,331] Adenosquamous carcinoma has also been called adenoacanthoma.[332]

The tumors may occur anywhere in the stomach, but more than half occur in the antrum. One pure squamous cell carcinoma occurred in a gastric stump.[333] Most tumors are large and ulcerated. Diffusely infiltrative lesions are uncommon. Histologically, the adenosquamous carcinomas are composed of elements of adenocarcinoma and squamous cells, separately or intermingled (Figure 25–35). The glandular components have features of the intestinal type of carcinoma, and the adjacent mucosa shows gastritis and the colonic type of intestinal metaplasia.[334] Mori et al. studied 28 cases.[335] In 16 the adenocarcinoma was differentiated, and in 12 it was undifferentiated. The biologic behavior of these tumors in terms of their gross form, depth of invasion, mode of vascular permeation, and prognosis corresponded with that of similarly classified adenocarcinomas without squamous differentiation. The squamous cell carcinomas are moderately differentiated, with keratinization and pearl formation. With re-examination with multiple sections, Mori et al. found minute areas of adenocarcinoma in 3 of 4 tumors originally diagnosed as pure squamous cell carcinomas.[327] Earlier, Straus et al. had expressed the view that whether the tumor was squamous or adenosquamous depended on the number of sections examined.[328]

Histogenesis of these tumors is uncertain, but reported cases suggest the following possibilities: invasion or metastasis from carcinomas in the neighboring organs, particularly the esophagus; squamous differentiation from totipotential stem cells; squamous metaplasia of adenocarcinoma; and malignant change in pre-existing squamous mucosa, either ectopic or metaplastic.

Invasion of the gastric cardia by an esophageal squamous cell carcinoma can usually be determined by the gross appearance; and the metastasis, often from a midesophageal tumor,[336] is submucosal. Rarely, a large cardiac tumor may be the result of metastasis from a small esophageal tumor.[337] Some reported tumors have been accompanied by benign squamous epithelium in

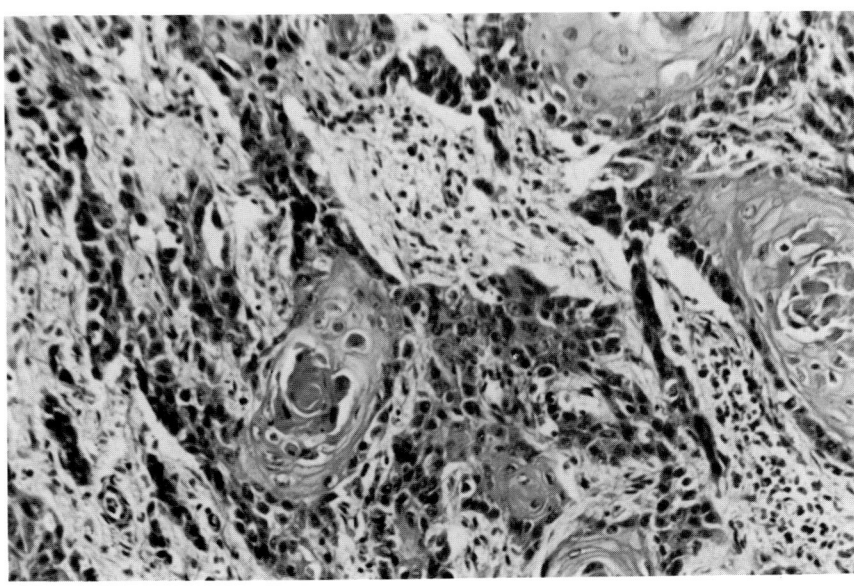

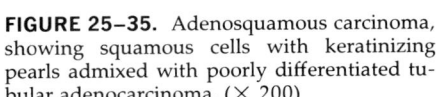

FIGURE 25–35. Adenosquamous carcinoma, showing squamous cells with keratinizing pearls admixed with poorly differentiated tubular adenocarcinoma. (× 200)

the gastric mucosa, which suggests that the tumor originated from the pre-existing squamous cells. When there is a history of injury to the stomach mucosa, the squamous epithelium may be presumed metaplastic[330,338]; without such a history, it may be considered congenital heterotopia.[339] In most cases, there is no benign squamous mucosa. In these cases, whether the squamous cells in the tumor are metaplastic cells of adenocarcinoma or derived from totipotential stem cells is difficult to assess. The former possibility probably applies to the adenosquamous carcinoma, in view of the focal nature of the squamous cells and that the biologic behavior of the tumor is guided by the glandular component. The latter possibility is likely for the pure squamous cell carcinoma. The presence of both tonofilaments and mucous granules in the same cell[340] supports either view. The finding of argentaffin and argyrophil cells as well as glandular and squamous cells in a small-cell carcinoma[341] indicates that the stem cells of the gastric mucosa are capable of differentiating along several lines.

Clinically, there is a male dominance, with a male-to-female ratio of 2:1 to 5:1.[330,332,334,335] The patients' age varied from 29 to 88,[330] and many were under 40 years of age.[334,335] The symptoms and signs are the same as those of the other gastric cancers. The prognosis is poor, and long-term survival is exceptional.[332,335]

Mucoepidermoid carcinoma is another tumor with both glandular and squamous cells. Szogi[342] found 21 cases in the literature and reported another case, postulating the origin from ectopic pancreatic tissue. Recently Hayashi et al.[343] reported another case showing tumor cells in continuity with ectopic submucosal glands.

TERATOMA AND CHORIOCARCINOMA

Teratomas and choriocarcinomas are rare in the stomach. Teratoma was first reported in 1922 by Eusterman and Senty,[344] who reported two cases of dermoid cysts in the stomach, one weighing 1000 gm, in an 8-year-old boy, and the other measuring 6 cm in the greatest dimension, in a 31-year-old man. By 1981, Cairo et al.[345] reviewed 51 cases; only 2 were in females. The majority of the tumors occur in infants, who present with an abdominal mass, sometimes bleeding, and occasionally obstruction. Pathologically, the tumors are large and may project either into the stomach or outward into the abdominal cavity. Tissues of all three germ layers are present, including teeth.[345,346] Teratomas are benign and curable by resection.[347]

Choriocarcinomas are malignant, characterized by the presence of syncytiotrophoblast and cytotrophoblast, which secrete hCG.[348-351] The serum level of hCG may be elevated[282-285] and serve as a marker for prognosis.[351] Immunohistochemical studies reveal that both alpha and beta subunits of hCG are secreted by the tumor[352] and that the secretion is more abundant in the syncytiotrophoblast than the cytotrophoblast.[349,353] Human placental lactogen and pregnancy-specific glycoprotein have also been found in the cytotrophoblast.[350] Clinically, a male patient may have gynecomastia.[348] It should be pointed out that hCG is commonly present in the gastric adenocarcinoma cells.[217,218,238] Among 124 carcinomas analyzed by Fukayama et al.,[352] hCG-α was present in 39, hCG-β in 63, and both in 26 tumors. Alpha subunits were present in papillary and tubular tumors and normal gastric epithelium, and beta subunits were present in microtubular and mucocellular tumors and rarely the normal cells. In four tumors, both units were present synchronously. In one choriocarcinoma similarly studied, synchronous occurrence of both units was present.

Choriocarcinoma often occurs together with adenocarcinoma. Of 47 cases analyzed by Garcia and Ghali,[353] 28 showed both adenocarcinoma and choriocarcinoma in the primary tumor, 13 showed only choriocarcinoma, and 6 showed adenocarcinoma in the stomach and choriocarcinoma in the metastasis. In one case only a focus of intramucosal carcinoma was found. Thus, the adenocarcinoma component might have been missed in a pure choriocarcinoma, a situation similar to that in the squamous cell carcinoma of the stomach. In one case, yolk sac tumor tissue with positive α_1-antitrypsin was also present in the tumor.[353] These histologic and immunohistologic findings support the view that choriocarcinoma originates from the totipotential cell by retrodifferentiation.

CARCINOSARCOMA

Carcinosarcoma of the stomach is composed in part of adenocarcinoma and in part of spindle-cell sarcoma in varying degrees of intermingling and admixture (Figure 25-36). When two tumor components are in contact only at the interface, the tumor is a collision tumor formed by two separate tumors. In a composite tumor, two elements are largely separated but mixed irregularly in some portions, probably the result of separate growth from different cell lines within the same tumor. A combination tumor has evenly mixed components, suggesting differentiation of the same cell line along separate pathways. Of 24 cases of carcinosarcoma of the stomach analyzed by Tanimura and Furuta,[354] 9 were thought to be collision tumors, 7 combination tumors, 6 composite tumors, and 2 of uncertain type.

By immunohistochemical study,[355] the epithelial tumor cells showed positive reaction for cytokeratin, CEA, and epithelial membrane antigen. The spindle tumor cells were positive for vimentin, desmin, and, focally, cytokeratin as well. Thus, the sarcomatous tissue probably derived from the carcinoma cells. The tumor reported by Kumagai et al.[356] was mostly sarcomatous, with teratomatous areas in addition to papillary adenocarcinoma. The sarcomatous tissue may show cartilaginous[357] or smooth muscle[358] differentiation.

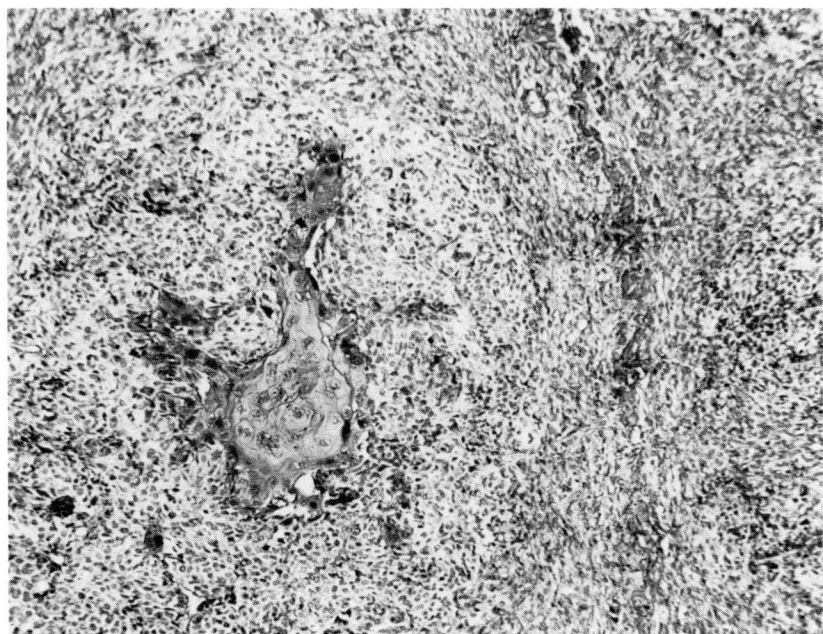

FIGURE 25-36. Carcinosarcoma, showing a patch of squamous cells surrounded by sarcomatous tissue. (From Ming SC: Tumors of the Esophagus and Stomach. In Atlas of Tumor Pathology, Second Series, Fascicle 7. Armed Forces Institute of Pathology, Washington, DC, 1973, p 252.)

SMALL-CELL CARCINOMA

Small-cell carcinoma rarely occurs in the stomach. Only eight cases have been reported.[359] It presents as an ulcerated mass and is composed of small cells with hyperchromatic nuclei and scanty cytoplasm (Figure 25-37), similar to those seen in small-cell carcinoma of the lung. Foci of adenocarcinoma or squamous cell differentiation were present in one half of the reported tumors. In one case, there were three independent foci of adenocarcinomas in the same stomach.[360] The tumor cells contain neurosecretory granules and show positive reactions for chromogranin and nonspecific enolase and negative reactions for CEA and epithelial membrane antigen.[359] The prognosis is poor. Most patients die within 1 year after diagnosis.

MULTIPLE PRIMARY AND METASTATIC TUMORS

Multiple primary adenocarcinomas have been found in 5% to 14% of resected stomachs.[361,362] The incidence of multiplicity is 8.4% among the early gastric cancers and 4.7% among the advanced cancers.[166] It has been suggested that the large early carcinomas might be formed by the collision of multiple small lesions.[362] It is possible that some of the advanced tumors may also be formed by coalition of separate tumors. The presence of separate small early carcinomas in the cancerous stomach is often missed at routine endoscopy. The diagnosis can be improved with the use of the Congo red–methylene blue test during examination.[363]

Two percent of patients with gastric carcinoma have malignant lesions in the other organs, synchronously in about one third of the cases.[364] One half of the lesions were in other segments of the digestive tract. It is not clear, however, whether the incidence of a second tumor is higher or not than that in the general population.[364-367]

Tumors of the neighboring organs, such as the esophagus, pancreas, and transverse colon, may extend directly into the stomach. Metastasis to the stomach is uncommon. It was found in about 0.2% of autopsy subjects.[368] The majority of the metastatic tumors were carcinomas. The primary site of the tumors was the lung in about one half of the cases.[369] Other relatively common primary tumors were carcinomas of pancreas, esophagus, colon, and breast and melanomas of the skin.[368,369] The metastatic lesions in the stomach are primarily submucosal. The large ones may

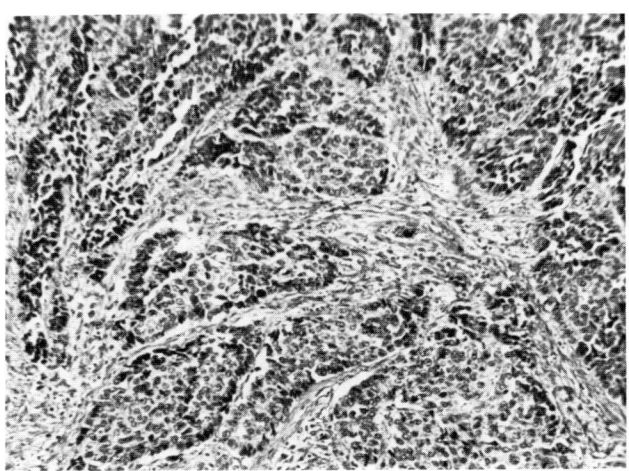

FIGURE 25-37. Small-cell carcinoma showing groups of small tumor cells with dark nuclei and scanty cytoplasm. (× 120)

become polypoid, with an ulcerated crater resembling a volcano, and cause bleeding, pain, or obstruction.[369]

Metastasis from esophageal carcinoma to the gastric cardia was found in 5.6% of cases, mainly by intramural spread.[370] The incidence of metastasis to the gastrointestinal tract from breast carcinoma is 8% to 15%,[368] sometimes resulting in a diffuse thickening of the gastric wall, as in linitis plastica.[371,372] The metastatic lesion in the stomach from cutaneous melanoma may become ulcerated and cause massive bleeding.[373,374]

References

1. Ming SC: Tumors of the esophagus and stomach. In Atlas of Tumor Pathology, 2nd series, fascicle 7. Washington, DC, Armed Forces Institute of Pathology, 1973, p 82.
2. Ming SC, Yu PL: Histogenesis of experimental colonic carcinogenesis. Front Gastrointest Res (In press).
3. Ito H, Yokozaki H, Ito M, Tahara E: Papillary adenoma of the stomach: Pathologic and immunohistochemical study. Arch Pathol Lab Med 113:1030–1034, 1989.
4. Hirota T, Okada T, Itabashi M, Kitaoka H: Histogenesis of human gastric cancer—with special reference to the significance of adenoma as a precancerous lesion. In Ming SC (ed): Precursors of Gastric Cancer. New York, Praeger, 1984, pp 233–252.
5. Sasano N, Nakamura K, Arai M, Akazaki K: Ultrastructural cell patterns in human gastric carcinoma compared with non-neoplastic gastric mucosa: Histogenetic analysis of carcinoma by mucin histochemistry. J Natl Cancer Inst 43:783–802, 1969.
6. Fiocca R, Villani L, Tenti P, et al: The foveolar cell component of gastric cancer. Hum Pathol 21:260–270, 1990.
7. Capella C, Frigerio B, Cornaggia M, et al: Gastric parietal cell carcinoma—a newly recognized entity: Light microscopic and ultrastructural features. Histopathology 8:813–824, 1984.
8. Tahara E, Ito H, Shimamoto F, et al: Lysozyme in human gastric carcinoma: A retrospective immunohistochemical study. Histopathology 6:409–421, 1982.
9. Ito H, Yokozaki H, Hata J, et al: Glicentin-containing cells in intestinal metaplasia, adenoma and carcinoma of the stomach. Virchows Arch [A] 404:17–29, 1984.
10. Meissner WA: Leiomyoma of the stomach. Arch Pathol 38:207–209, 1944.
11. Siurala M: Gastritis, its fate and sequelae. Ann Clin Res 13:111–113, 1981.
12. World Health Organization Statistics 1986: Age standardized death rates for selected causes, by sex, latest available year. World Health Organization, Geneva, 1986, pp 630–637.
13. Campbell H: Cancer mortality in Europe: Site-specific patterns and trends—1955 to 1974. World Health Stat Q 33:241–280, 1980.
14. Aoki K, Tominaga S, Kuroishi T: Age-adjusted death rates for cancer by site in 50 countries. Gann Monogr Cancer Res 26:251–274, 1981.
15. Silverberg E, Boring CC, Squires TS: Cancer statistics, 1990. CA 40:9–26, 1990.
16. Haas JF, Schottenfeld D: Epidemiology of gastric cancer. In Lipkin M, Good RA (ed): Gastrointestinal Tract Cancer. New York, Plenum, 1978, p 173.
17. Munoz N, Correa P, Cuello C, Dugue E: Histologic type of gastric carcinoma in high and low-risk areas. Int J Cancer 3:809–818, 1968.
18. Correa P, Sasano N, Stemmerman GN, Haenszel W: Pathology of gastric carcinoma in Japanese populations: Comparisons between Iiyagi prefecture, Japan and Hawaii. J Natl Cancer Inst 51:1449–1459, 1973.
19. Munoz N, Asvall J: Time trends of intestinal and diffuse types of gastric cancer in Norway. Int J Cancer 8:144–157, 1971.
20. Kubo T: Histological appearance of gastric carcinoma in high and low mortality countries: Comparison between Kyushu, Japan and Minnesota, USA. Cancer 28:726–34, 1971.
21. Whitehead R, Skinner JM, Heenan PJ: Incidence of carcinoma of stomach and tumor type. Br J Cancer 30:370–372, 1974.
22. Wang R: Pathologic comparison between gastric carcinoma and lesions in peri-cancerous mucosa from two districts with different mortality rates in Gansu Province. [In Chinese.] Chung Hua Chung Liu Tsa Chih 11:187–190, 1989.
23. Hanai A, Fujimoto I: Time trends in cancer incidence in Osaka. Gan To Kagaku Ryoho 11:367–376, 1984.
24. Hoskins LC, Loux HA, Britten A, Zamcheck N: Distribution of ABO blood groups in patients with pernicious anemia: Gastric carcinoma associated with pernicious anemia. N Engl J Med 273:633–637, 1965.
25. Haenszel W, Kurihara M, Locke FB, et al: Stomach cancer in Japan. J Natl Cancer Inst 56:265–274, 1976.
26. Correa P, Haenszel W, Tannenbaum S: Epidemiology of gastric carcinoma: Review and future prospects. Natl Cancer Inst Monogr 62:129–134, 1982.
27. McMichael AJ, McCall MG, Hartshorne JM, Woodings TL: Patterns of gastrointestinal cancer in European migrants to Australia: The role of dietary change. Intl J Cancer 25:431–437, 1980.
28. Locke FB, King H: Cancer Mortality Risk Among Japanese in the United States. J Natl Cancer Inst 65:1149–1156, 1980.
29. Cuello C, Correa P, Haenszel W, et al: Gastric cancer in Colombia. I. Cancer risk and suspect environmental agents. J Natl Cancer Inst 57:1015–1020, 1976.
30. Haenszel W, Correa P: Developments in the epidemiology of stomach cancer over the past decade. Cancer Res 35:3452–3459, 1975.
31. Tominaga S: Decreasing trend of stomach cancer in Japan. Jpn J Cancer Res 78:1–10, 1987.
32. Weisburger JH, Horn CL: Human and laboratory studies on the causes and prevention of gastrointestinal cancer. Scand J Gastroenterol Suppl 104:15–26, 1985.
33. Hirayama T: Epidemiology of stomach cancer in Japan with special reference to the strategy for primary prevention. Jpn J Clin Oncol 14:159–168, 1984.
34. Joossens JV, Geboers J: Nutrition and gastric cancer. Proc Nutr Soc 40:37–46, 1981.
35. Lu JB, Qin YM: Correlation between high salt intake and mortality rates for oesophageal and gastric cancers in Henan Province, China. Int J Epidemiol 16:171–176, 1987.
36. Whelton PK, Goldblatt P: An investigation of the relationship between stomach cancer and cerebrovascular disease: Evidence for and against the salt hypothesis. Am J Epidemiol 115:418–427, 1982.
37. Kono S, Ikeda M, Ogata M: Salt and geographical mortality of gastric cancer and stroke in Japan. J Epidemiol Community Health 37:43–46, 1983.
38. Charnley G, Tannenbaum SR: Flow cytometric analysis of the effect of sodium chloride on gastric cancer risk in the rat. Cancer Res 45:5608–5616, 1985.
39. Lin JY, Wang HI, Yeh YC: The mutagenicity of soy bean sauce. Food Cosmet Toxicol 17:329–331, 1979.
40. Nagahara A, Ohshita K, Nasuno S: Relation of nitrite concentration to mutagen formation in soy sauce. Food Chem Toxicol 24:13–15, 1986.
41. Kurechi T, Kikugawa K, Fukuda S, Hasunuma M: Inhibition of N-nitrosamine formation by soya products. Food Cosmet Toxicol 19:425–428, 1981.
42. Hirayama T: Relationship of soybean paste soup intake to gastric cancer risk. Nutr Cancer 3:223–233, 1982.
43. Hoey J, Montvernay C, Lambert R: Wine and tobacco: Risk factors for gastric cancer in France. Am J Epidemiol 113:668–674, 1981.
44. Bull P, Yanez L, Nervi F: Mutagenic substances in red and white wine in Chile, a high risk area for gastric cancer. Mutat Res 187:113–117, 1987.
45. Enterline PE, Hartley J, Henderson V: Asbestos and cancer: A cohort followed up to death. Br J Ind Med 44:396–401, 1987.
46. Kogan FM, Vanchugova NN, Frasch VN: Possibility of inducing glandular stomach cancer in rats exposed to asbestos. Br J Ind Med 44:682–686, 1987.
47. Land CE: Temporal distributions of risk for radiation-induced cancers. J Chronic Dis 40(Suppl 2):45S–57S, 1987.

48. Leach SA, Thompson M, Hill M: Bacterially catalysed N-nitrosation reactions and their relative importance in the human stomach. Carcinogenesis 8:1907–1912, 1987.
49. Mirvish SS: The etiology of gastric cancer: Intragastric nitrosamide formation and other theories. J Natl Cancer Inst 71:629–647, 1983.
50. Reed PI, Smith PLR, Haines K, et al: Gastric juice N-nitrosamines in health and gastroduodenal disease. Lancet 2:550–552, 1981.
51. Schlag P, Bockler R, Peter M: Nitrite and nitrosamines in gastric juice: Risk factors for gastric cancer? Scand J Gastroenterol 17:145–150, 1982.
52. Tannenbaum SR, Moran D, Falchuk KR, et al: Nitrite stability and nitrosation potential in human gastric juice. Cancer Lett 14:131–136, 1981.
53. Montes G, Cuello C, Gordillo G, et al: Mutagenic activity of gastric juice. Cancer Lett 7:307–312, 1979.
54. Morris DL, Youngs D, Muscroft TJ, et al: Mutagenicity in gastric juice. Gut 25:723–727, 1984.
55. Mirvish SS: Effects of vitamins C and E on N-nitroso compound formation, carcinogenesis and cancer. Cancer 58(Suppl):1842–1850, 1986.
56. Weisburger JH, Marquardt H, Mower HF, et al: Inhibition of carcinogenesis: Vitamin C and the prevention of gastric cancer. Prev Med 9:352–361, 1980.
57. Hurst AF: Precursors of carcinoma of the stomach. Lancet 2:1023–1028, 1929.
58. Morson BC, Sobin LH, Grundmann E, et al: Precancerous conditions and epithelial dysplasia in the stomach. J Clin Pathol 33:711–721, 1980.
59. Nagayo T: Precursors of human gastric cancer: Their frequencies and histological characteristics. In Farber E, Kawachi T, Nagayo T, et al (eds): Pathophysiology of Carcinogenesis in Digestive Organs. Tokyo, Tokyo University Press, 1977, pp 151–161.
60. Correa P: Chronic gastritis as a cancer precursor. Scand J Gastroenterol Suppl 104:131–136, 1985.
61. Stockbrugger RW, Menon GG, Beilby JO, et al: Gastroscopic screening in 80 patients with pernicious anaemia. Gut 24:1141–1147, 1983.
62. Sipponen P, Kekki M, Haapakoski J, et al: Gastric cancer risk in chronic atrophic gastritis: Statistical calculation of cross-sectional data. Int J Cancer 35:173–177, 1985.
63. Lipkin M, Correa P, Mikol YB, et al: Proliferative and antigenic modifications in human epithelial cells in chronic atrophic gastritis. J Natl Cancer Inst 75:613–619, 1985.
64. Goldman H, Ming SC: Mucins in normal and neoplastic gastrointestinal epithelium. Histochemical distribution. Arch Pathol 85:580–586, 1968.
65. Teglbjaerg PS, Nielsen HO: "Small intestinal type" and "colonic type" intestinal metaplasia of the human stomach and their relationship to the histogenetic types of gastric adenocarcinoma. Acta Pathol Microbiol Scand 86A:351–355, 1978.
66. Spicer SS: Diamine methods for differentiating mucosubstances histochemically. J Histochem 13:211–234, 1965.
67. Stemmermann GN, Hyashi T: Intestinal metaplasia of the gastric mucosa: A gross and microscopic study of its distribution in various disease states. J Natl Cancer Inst 41:627–634, 1968.
68. Ming SC: Intestinal metaplasia: Its heterogeneous nature and significance. In Ming SC (ed): Precursors of Gastric Cancer. New York, Praeger, 1984, pp 219–231.
69. Goldman H, Ming SC: Fine structure of intestinal metaplasia and adenocarcinoma of the human stomach. Lab Invest 18:203–210, 1968.
70. Matsukura N, Suzuki K, Kawachi T, et al: Distribution of marker enzymes and mucin in intestinal metaplasia in human stomach and relation of complete and incomplete types of intestinal metaplasia to minute gastric carcinomas. J Natl Cancer Inst 65:231–240, 1980.
71. Segura DI, Montero C: Histochemical characterization of different types of intestinal metaplasia in gastric mucosa. Cancer 82:498–503, 1983.
72. Jass JR, Filipe MI: The mucin profile of normal gastric mucosa, intestinal metaplasia and its variants and gastric carcinoma. Histochem J 13:931–939, 1981.
73. Filipe MI, Potet F, Bogomoletz WV, et al: Incomplete sulphomucin-secreting intestinal metaplasia for gastric cancer. Preliminary data from a prospective study from three centres. Gut 26:1319–1326, 1985.
74. Nielsen K, Teglbjaerg PS: On the occurrence of carcinoembryonic antigen (CEA) in different types of intestinal metaplasia of the human stomach. Tumour Biol 5:313–320, 1984.
75. Jass JR, Strudley I, Faludy J: Histochemistry of epithelial metaplasia and dysplasia in human stomach and colorectum. Scand J Gastroenterol [Suppl] 104:109–130, 1984.
76. Ming SC: Gastric carcinoma: A pathobiological classification. Cancer 39:2475–2485, 1977.
77. Correa P, Cuello E, Duque E: Carcinoma and intestinal metaplasia of the stomach in Colombian migrants. J Natl Cancer Inst 44:297–306, 1970.
78. Hirota T, Okada T, Itabashi M, et al: Significance of intestinal metaplasia as a precancerous condition of the stomach. In Ming SC (ed): Precursors of Gastric Cancer. New York, Praeger, 1984, pp 179–193.
79. Ectors N, Dixon MF: The prognostic value of sulphomucin positive intestinal metaplasia in the development of gastric cancer. Histopathology 10:1271–1277, 1986.
80. Ramesar KC, Sanders DS, Hopwood D: Limited value of type III intestinal metaplasia in predicting risk of gastric carcinoma. J Clin Pathol 40:1287–1290, 1987.
81. Saito T, Sasaki O, Tamada R, et al: Sequential studies of development of gastric carcinoma in dogs induced by N-methyl-N'-nitro-N-nitrosoguanidine. Cancer 42:1246–1254, 1978.
82. Tatematsu M, Furihata C, Katsuyama T, et al: Independent induction of intestinal metaplasia and gastric cancer in rats treated with N-methyl-N'-nitro-N-nitrosoguanidine. Cancer Res 43:1335–1341, 1983.
83. Watanabe H, Ito A: Relationship between gastric tumorigenesis and intestinal metaplasia in rats given X-radiation and/or N-methyl-N'-nitro-N-nitrosoguanidine. J Natl Cancer Inst 76:865–870, 1986.
84. Kobori O, Gedigk P, Totovic V: Adenomatous changes and adenocarcinoma of glandular stomach in Wistar rats induced by N-methyl-N'-nitro-N-nitrosoguanidine: An electron microscopic and histochemical study. Virchows Arch [A] 373:37–54, 1977.
85. Ming SC, Goldman H, Freiman DG: Intestinal metaplasia and histogenesis of carcinoma in human stomach: Light and electron microscopic study. Cancer 20:1418–1429, 1967.
86. Hattori T: Development of adenocarcinomas in the stomach. Cancer 57:1528–1534, 1986.
87. Hauser G: Die peptische Schädigungen des Magens, des Duodenums und der Speiseröhre und der peptische postoperative Jejunalgeschwür. In Henke F, Lubarsch O (eds): Handbuch der Spezieller Pathologischen Anatomie und Histologie. Berlin, Springer, 1926, pp 339–811.
88. Newcomb WD: The relationship between peptic ulceration and gastric carcinoma. Br J Surg 20:279–308, 1933.
89. Sano R: Pathological analysis of 300 cases of early gastric cancer with special reference to cancer associated with ulcer. Gann Monogr Cancer Res 11:81–89, 1971.
90. Sakita T, Oguro Y, Takasu S, et al: Observations on the healing of ulcerations in early gastric cancer: The life cycle of the malignant ulcer. Gastroenterology 60:835–844, 1971.
91. Yamagata S, Hisamichi S: Precancerous lesions of the stomach. World J Surg 3:671–673, 1979.
92. Haukland HH, Johnson JA, Eide JT: Carcinoma diagnosed in excised gastric ulcers. Acta Chir Scand 147:439–443, 1981.
93. Majima S, Yamaguchi I, Teshima T, Karube K: On malignant change of gastric ulcer. Tohoku J Exp Med 86:255–276, 1965.
94. Farinati F, Cardin F, Di Mario F, et al: Early and advanced gastric cancer during follow-up of apparently benign gastric ulcer: Significance of the presence of epithelial dysplasia. J Surg Oncol 36:263–267, 1987.
95. Fugita S, Hattori T: Cell proliferation, differentiation and migration in the gastric mucosa: A study on the background of carcinogenesis. In Farber E, Kawachi T, Nagayo T, et al (eds): Pathophysiology of Carcinogenesis in Digestive Organs. Tokyo, Tokyo University Press, 1977, pp 21–36.
96. Rollag A, Jacobsen CD: Gastric ulcer and risk of cancer: A five year follow-up study. Acta Med Scand 216:105–109, 1984.

97. Kawai K, Kizu M, Miyaoka T: Epidemiology and pathogenesis of gastric cancer. Front Gastrointest Res 6:71–86, 1980.
98. Hirohata T: Mortality from gastric cancer and other causes after medical or surgical treatment of gastric ulcer. J Natl Cancer Inst 41:895–908, 1968.
99. Montgomery RD, Richardson BP: Gastric ulcer and cancer. Q J Med 44:591–599, 1975.
100. Hole DJ, Quigley EM, Gillis CR, Watkinson G: Peptic ulcer and cancer: An examination of the relationship between chronic peptic ulcer and gastric carcinoma. Scand J Gastroenterol 22:17–23, 1987.
101. Mallory TB: Carcinoma in situ of the stomach and its bearing on the histogenesis of malignant ulcers. Arch Pathol 30:348–362, 1940.
102. Hirota T, Itabashi M, Suzuki K, Yoshida S: Clinical study of minute and small early gastric cancer: Histogenesis of gastric cancer. Pathol Annu 15:1–19, 1980.
103. Takahashi M, Shirai T, Gukushima S, et al: Effects of fundic ulcers induced by iodoacetamid on development of gastric tumors in rats treated with N-methyl-N'-nitro-N-nitrosoguanidine. Gann 67:47–54, 1975.
104. Jang JJ, Furukawa F, Hasegawa R, et al: Enhancing effect of cysteamine hydrochloride on the development of gastroduodenal tumors induced by N-methyl-N'-nitro-N-nitrosoguanidine in F344 rats. Jpn J Cancer Res 78:571–576, 1987.
105. O'Brien MJ, Burakoff R, Robbins EA: Early gastric cancer: Clinicopathologic study. Am J Med 78:195–202, 1985.
106. Gad A: Carcinoma of the resected stomach. In Ming SC (ed): Precursors of Gastric Cancer. New York, Praeger, 1984, pp 287–313.
107. Schrumpf E, Serck-Hanssen A, Stadaas J, et al: Mucosal changes in the gastric stump, 20–25 years after partial gastrectomy. Lancet 2:467–469, 1977.
108. Graem N, Fischer AB, Beck H: Dysplasia and carcinoma in the Billroth II resected stomach 27 to 35 years postoperatively. Acta Pathol Microbiol Immunol Scand [A] 92:185–188, 1984.
109. Dittrich S, Theuring F: Das Karzinom im operierten Magen—eine autoptische Studie. Zentralbl Allg Pathol 130:211–216, 1985.
110. Tokudome S, Kono S, Ikeda M, et al: A prospective study on primary gastric stump cancer following partial gastrectomy for benign gastroduodenal diseases. Cancer Res 44:2208–2212, 1984.
111. Schafer LW, Larson DE, Melton J III, et al: The risk of gastric carcinoma after surgical treatment of benign ulcer diseases. N Engl J Med 309:1210–1213, 1983.
112. Hammar E: The localization of precancerous changes and carcinoma after previous gastric operation for a benign condition. Acta Pathol Microbiol Scand [A] 84:495–507, 1976.
113. Savage A, Jones S: Histological appearances of the gastric mucosa, 15–27 years after partial gastrectomy. J Clin Pathol 32:179–186, 1979.
114. Offerhaus GJ, Huibregtse K, de Boer J, et al: The operated stomach: A premalignant condition? A prospective endoscopic follow-up study. Scand J Gastroenterol 19:521–524, 1984.
115. Watt PC, Sloan JM, Spencer A, Kennedy TL: Histology of the postoperative stomach before and after diversion of bile. Br Med J [Clin Res] 287:1410–1412, 1983.
116. Houghton, PW, Mortensen NJ, Williamson RC: Effect of duodenogastric reflux on gastric mucosal proliferation after gastric surgery. Br J Surg 74(4):288–291, 1987.
117. Ming SC: Tumors of the esophagus and stomach. In Atlas of Tumor Pathology, 2nd series, fascicle 7. Washington, DC, Armed Forces of Pathology, 1973, pp 144–206.
118. Schindler R: Gastric carcinoma and gastritis: With reference to coexistence of carcinoma and chronic hypertrophic glandular gastritis. Am J Dig Dis 10:607–624, 1965.
119. Stamm B, Saremaslani P: Coincidence of fundic glandular hyperplasia and carcinoma of the stomach. Cancer 63:354–359, 1989.
120. Ménétrier P: Des polyadenomas gastriques et de leurs rapports avec le cancer de l'estomac. Arch Physiol Norm Pathol 1:32–55, 1988.
121. Martin ED. Frequency and evolution of precancerous and dysplastic lesions in the stomach. Excerpta Medica International Congress Series 555:225–230, 1981.
122. Wood MG, Bates C, Brown RC, Losowsky MS: Intramucosal carcinoma of the gastric antrum complicating Ménétrier's disease. J Clin Pathol 36:1071–1075, 1983.
123. Rubio CA, Kato Y, Sugano H, Hirota T: The intramucosal cysts of the stomach. VII. A pathway of gastric carcinogenesis? J Surg Oncol 32:214–219, 1986.
124. Zhu FG, Deng XJ, Cheng NJ: Intramucosal cysts in gastric mucosa adjacent to carcinoma and peptic ulcer: A histochemical study. Histopathology 11:631–638, 1987.
125. Pillay I, Petrelli M: Diffuse cystic glandular malformation of the stomach associated with adenocarcinoma. Cancer 38:915–920, 1976.
126. Iwanaga T, Koyama H, Takahashi Y, et al: Diffuse submucosal cysts and carcinoma of the stomach. Cancer 36:606–614, 1975.
127. Zhou XX: Relationship between gastric schistosomiasis and gastric cancer, chronic gastric ulcer and chronic gastritis: Pathological analysis of 79 cases. [In Chinese.] Chung Hua Ping Li Hsueh Tsa Chih 15:62–64, 1986.
128. Ming SC, Bajtai A, Correa P, et al: Gastric dysplasia. Significance and pathologic criteria. Cancer 54:1794–1801, 1984.
129. Ming SC: Dysplasia of gastric epithelium. Front Gastrointest Res 4:164–172, 1979.
130. Oehlert W: Preneoplastic lesions of the stomach. In Ming SC (ed): Precursors of Gastric Cancer. New York, Praeger, 1984, pp 73–82.
131. Macartney JC, Camplejohn RS: DNA flow cytometry of histological material from dysplastic lesions of human gastric mucosa. J Pathol 150:113–118, 1986.
132. Borchard F: Precancerous conditions and lesions of the stomach. In Rugge M, Arslan-Pagnini C, DiMario F (eds): Carcinoma gastrico e lesioni precancerose dello stomaco. Milan, Edizioni Unicopi, 1986, pp 175–210.
133. Jarvis LR, Whitehead R: Morphometric analysis of gastric dysplasia. J Pathol 147:133–138, 1985.
134. Ohuchi N, Hand PH, Merlo G, et al: Enhanced expression of c-Ha-ras p21 in human stomach adenocarcinomas defined by immunoassays using monoclonal antibodies and in situ hybridization. Cancer Res 47:1413–1420, 1987.
135. Nagayo T: Histological diagnosis of biopsied gastric mucosae with special reference to that of borderline lesions. Gann Monogr Cancer Res 11:245–256, 1971.
136. Cuello C, Correa P, Zarama G, et al: Histopathology of gastric dysplasia: Correlations with gastric juice chemistry. Am J Surg Pathol 3:491–500, 1979.
137. Grundmann E, Schlake W: Histology of possible precancerous stages in the stomach. In Herfarth Ch, Schlag P (eds): Gastric Cancer. Berlin, Springer-Verlag, 1979, pp 72–82.
138. Jass JR: A classification of gastric dysplasia. Histopathology 7:181–193, 1983.
139. Kraus B, Cain H: Is there a carcinoma in-situ of gastric mucosa? Pathol Res Pract 164:342–355, 1979.
140. Meister H, Holubarsch Ch, Haferkamp O, et al: Gastritis, intestinal metaplasia and dysplasia versus benign ulcer in stomach and duodenum and gastric carcinoma: A histotopographical study. Pathol Res Pract 164:259–269, 1979.
141. Saraga EP, Gardiol D, Costa J: Gastric dysplasia: A histological follow-up study. Am J Surg Pathol 11:788–796, 1987.
142. Camilleri JP, Potet F, Amat C, Molas G: Gastric mucosal dysplasia: Preliminary results of a prospective study of patients followed for periods up to six years. In Ming SC (ed): Precursors of Gastric Cancer. New York, Praeger, 1984, pp 83–92.
143. Andersson AP, Lauritsen KB, West F, Johansen A: Dysplasia in gastric mucosa: Prognostic significance. Acta Chir Scand 153:29–31, 1987.
144. Ming SC: Significance of epithelial dysplasia in the esophagus and stomach. Endoscopy 21:38S–49S, 1989.
145. Coma del Corral MJ, Pardo-Mindau FJ, Razquin S, Ojeda C: Risk of cancer in patients with gastric dysplasia: Follow-up study of 67 patients. Cancer 65:2078–2085, 1990.
146. Zampi GA, Amorosi A, Bianchi S: Gastric dysplasia: Precancerous or paracancerous lesion? Endoscopy 21:43S–44S, 1989.
147. Sugimura T, Fujimura S, Baba T: Tumor production in the glandular stomach and alimentary tract of the rat by N-methyl-N'-nitro-N-nitrosoguanidine. Cancer Res 30:455–465, 1970.
148. Ohgaki H, Kawachi T, Matsukura N, et al: Genetic control of susceptibility of rats to gastric carcinoma. Cancer Res 43:3663–3667, 1983.
149. Shimosato Y, Tanaka N, Kogure K, et al: Histopathology of tu-

mors of canine alimentary tract produced by N-methyl-N'-nitro-N-nitrosoguanidine, with particular reference to gastric carcinomas. J Natl Cancer Inst 47:1053–1070, 1971.
150. Uchida Y, Roessner A, Schlake W, et al: Development of tumors in the glandular stomach of rats after oral administration of carcinogens. II. Different cell types in antral carcinoma as revealed by electron microscopy. Z Krebsforsch 87:213–28, 1976.
151. Furihata C, Kawachi T, Sasajima K, et al: Experimental stomach carcinogenes. Eur J Cancer [Suppl] 1:31–37, 1978.
152. Tatematsu M, Furihata C, Katsuyama T, et al: Immunohistochemical demonstration of pyloric gland-type cells with low-pepsinogen isozyme 1 in preneoplastic and neoplastic tissues of rat stomachs treated with N-methyl-N'-nitro-N-nitrosoguanidine. J Natl Cancer Inst 78:771–777, 1987.
153. Wang CX, Williams GM: Comparison of stomach cancer induced in rats by N-methyl-N'-nitro-N-nitrosoguanidine or N-propyl-N'-nitro-N-nitrosoguanidine. Cancer Lett 34:173–185, 1987.
154. Sunagawa M, Takeshita K, Nakajima A, et al: Duration of ENNG administration and its effect on histological differentiation of experimental gastric cancer. Br J Cancer 52:771–779, 1985.
155. Szentirmay Z, Ohgaki H, Maruyama K, et al: Early gastric cancer induced by N-ethyl-N'-nitro-N-nitrosoguanidine in a cynomolgus monkey six years after initial diagnosis of the lesion. Jpn J Cancer Res 81:6–9, 1990.
156. Kunze E, Schauer A, Eder M, Seefeldt C: Early sequential lesions during development of experimental gastric cancer with special reference to dysplasias. J Cancer Res Clin Oncol 95:247–264, 1979.
157. Tsiftsis D, Jass JR, Filipe MI, Wastell C: Altered patterns of mucin secretion in precancerous lesions induced in the glandular part of the stomach by the carcinogen N-methyl-N'-nitro-N-nitrosoguanidine. Invest Cell Pathol 3:399–408, 1980.
158. Ohgaki H, Hasegawa H, Kusama K, et al: Induction of gastric carcinomas in nonhuman primates by N-ethyl-N'-nitro-N-nitrosoguanidine. J Natl Cancer Inst 77:179–186, 1986.
159. Clarkson B, Ota T, Okhita T, O'Conner A: Kinetics of proliferation of cancer cells in neoplastic effusions in man. Cancer 18:1189–1213, 1965.
160. Fujita S: Natural history of human gastric carcinoma in terms of their genesis and progression. Asian Med J 26:787–805, 1983.
161. Tsukuma H, Mishima T, Oshima A: Prospective study of "early" gastric cancer. Int J Cancer 31:421–426, 1983.
162. Okabe H: Growth of early gastric cancer: Clinical study of growth and invasive patterns of early gastric cancer: Its position in the natural history of gastric cancer. Gann Monogr Cancer Res 11:67–79, 1971.
163. Korenaga D, Okamura T, Saito A, et al: DNA ploidy is closely linked to tumor invasion, lymph node metastasis, and prognosis in clinical gastric cancer. Cancer 62:309–313, 1988.
164. Antonioli DA, Goldman H: Changes in the location and type of gastric adenocarcinoma. Cancer 50:775–781, 1982.
165. Meyers WC, Damiano RJ Jr, Rotolo FS, Postlethwait RW: Adenocarcinoma of the stomach: Changing patterns over the last 4 decades. Ann Surg 205:1–8, 1987.
166. Marrano D, Viti G, Grigioni W, Marra A: Synchronous and metachronous cancer of the stomach. Eur J Surg Oncol 13:493–498, 1987.
167. Borrmann R: Geshwelste des Magens und Duodenums. In Henke F, Lubarsch O (eds): Handbuch der Spezieller Pathologischen Anatomie und Histologie. Vol 4. Berlin, Springer, 1926, p 865.
168. Japanese Research Society for Gastric Cancer: The general rules for the gastric cancer study in surgery and pathology. Jpn J Surg 11:127–145, 1981.
169. Ohta H, Noguchi Y, Takagi K, et al: Early gastric carcinoma with special reference to macroscopic classification. Cancer 60:1099–1106, 1987.
170. Yamazaki H, Oshima A, Murakami R, et al: A long-term follow-up study of patients with gastric cancer detected by mass screening. Cancer 63:613–617, 1989.
171. Curtis RE, Kennedy BJ, Myers MH, Hankey BF: Evaluation of AJC stomach cancer staging using the SEER population. Semin Oncol 12:21–31, 1985.
172. Wanke M, Schwan H: Pathology of gastric cancer. World J Surg 3:675–684, 1979.
173. Stout AP: Superficial spreading type of carcinoma of the stomach. Arch Surg 44:651–657, 1942.
174. Fiocca R, Villani L, Tenti P, et al: Characterization of four main cell types in gastric cancer: Foveolar, mucopeptic, intestinal columnar and goblet cells: An histologic, histochemical and ultrastructural study of "early" and "advanced" tumours. Pathol Res Pract 182:308–325, 1987.
175. Nevalainen TJ, Jarvi OH: Ultrastructure of intestinal and diffuse carcinoma. J Pathol 122:129–136, 1977.
176. Yamashiro K, Suzuki H, Nagayo T: Electron microscopic study of signet-ring cells in diffuse carcinoma of the stomach. Virchows Arch [A] 374:275–284, 1977.
177. Sugihara H, Hattori T, Fukuda M, Fujita S: Cell proliferation and differentiation in intramucosal and advanced signet ring cell carcinomas of the human stomach. Virchows Arch [A] 411(2):117–127, 1987.
178. Nevalainen TJ, Jarvi OH: Intracellular cysts in gastric carcinoma. Acta Pathol Microbiol Scand [A] 84:517–522, 1976.
179. Kobori O, Oota K: Mucous substance and enzyme histochemistry of non-neoplastic and neoplastic gastric epithelium in man. Acta Pathol Jpn 24:119–130, 1974.
180. Soga J, Tazawa K, Aizawa O, et al: Argentaffin cell adenocarcinoma of the stomach: An atypical carcinoid? Cancer 28:999–1003, 1971.
181. Tahara E, Ito H, Nakagami K, et al: Scirrhous argyrophil cell carcinoma of the stomach with multiple production of polypeptide hormones, amine, CEA, lysozyme, and HCG. Cancer 49:1904–1915, 1982.
182. Capella C, Cornaggia M, Usellini L, et al: Neoplastic cells containing lysozyme in gastric carcinomas. Pathology 16:87–92, 1984.
183. Kazzaz BA, Eulderink F: Paneth cell-rich carcinoma of the stomach. Histopathology 15:303–305, 1989.
184. Byrne D, Holley MP, Cuschieri A: Parietal cell carcinoma of the stomach: Association with long-term survival after curative resection. Br J Cancer 58:85–87, 1988.
185. Robey-Cafferty SS, Ro JY, McKee EG: Gastric parietal cell carcinoma with an unusual, lymphoma-like histologic appearance: Report of a case. Mod Pathol 2:536–540, 1989.
186. Reid WA, Thompson WD, Kay J: Pepsinogen in gastric carcinoma cells. J Clin Pathol 36:137–139, 1983.
187. Stemmermann GN, Samloff IM, Hayashi T: Pepsinogens I and II in carcinoma of the stomach: An immunohistochemical study. Appl Pathol 3:159–163, 1985.
188. Ishikura H, Kirimoto K, Shamoto M, et al: Hepatoid adenocarcinomas of the stomach: An analysis of seven cases. Cancer 58:119–126, 1986.
189. Murayama H, Imai T, Kikuchi M: Solid carcinomas of the stomach: A combined histochemical, light and electron microscopic study. Cancer 51:1673–1681, 1983.
190. Matias-Guiu X, Guix M: Hepatoid gastric adenocarcinoma. Pathol Res Pract 185:397–400, 1989.
191. Ishikura H, Aizawa M: Hepatoid adenocarcinoma of the stomach. Lab Invest 56:33A, 1987.
192. Tahara E: Endocrine tumors of the gastrointestinal tract: Classification, function and biological behavior. In Watanabe S, Wolff M, Sommers SC (eds): Digestive Disease Pathology. Vol 1. Philadelphia, Field & Wood, 1988, pp 121–147.
193. Caruso ML, Pilato FP, D'Adda T, et al: Composite carcinoid-adenocarcinoma of the stomach associated with multiple gastric carcinoids and nonantral gastric atrophy. Cancer 64:1534–1539, 1989.
194. Watanabe H, Enjoji M, Imai T: Gastric carcinoma with lymphoid stroma: Its morphologic characteristics and prognostic correlation. Cancer 38:232–243, 1976.
195. Okamura T, Kodama Y, Kamegawa T, et al: Gastric carcinoma with lymphoid stroma: Correlation to reactive hyperplasia in regional lymph nodes and prognosis. Jpn J Surg 13:177–183, 1983.
196. Lertprasertsuke N, Tsutsumi Y: Gastric carcinoma with lymphoid stroma: Analysis using mucin histochemistry and immunohistochemistry. Virchows Arch [A] 414:231–241, 1989.
197. Nagai Y, Sunada H, Sano J, et al: Biochemical and immunohistochemical studies on the scirrhous carcinoma of human stomach. Ann NY Acad Sci 460:321–332, 1985.

198. Niitsu Y, Ito N, Kohda K, et al: Immunohistochemical identification of type I procollagen in tumour cells of scirrhous adenocarcinoma of the stomach. Br J Cancer 57:79–82, 1988.
199. Yoshida K, Yokozaki H, Nimoto M, et al: Expression of TGF-β and procollagen type I and type III in human gastric carcinomas. Int J Cancer 44:394–398, 1989.
200. Schade RKO: The borderline between benign and malignant lesions in the stomach. In Grundmann E, Grunze H, Witte S (eds): Early Gastric Cancer: Current Status of Diagnosis. Berlin, Springer-Verlag, 1974, pp 45–53.
201. Sakuma A, Ouchi A, Sugawara T, Sato T: Histologic infiltrating pattern of gastric microcarcinoma by means of serial sections. Cancer 55:1087–1092, 1985.
202. Esaki Y, Hirayama R, Hirokawa K: A comparison of patterns of metastasis in gastric cancer by histologic type and age. Cancer 65:2086–2090, 1990.
203. Lehnert T, Erlandson RA, Decosse JJ: Lymph and blood capillaries of the human gastric mucosa: A morphologic basis for metastasis in early gastric carcinoma. Gastroenterology 89:939–950, 1989.
204. Korenaga D, Haraguchi M, Tsujitani S, et al: Clinicopathological features of mucosal carcinoma of the stomach with lymph node metastasis in eleven patients. Br J Surg 73:431–433, 1986.
205. Soga J, Kobayashi K, Saito J, et al: The role of lymphadenectomy in curative surgery for gastric cancer. World J Surg 3:701–708, 1979.
206. Yakushiji M, Tazaki T, Nishimura H, Kato T: Krukenberg tumors of the ovary: A clinicopathologic analysis of 112 cases. Nippon Sanka Fujinka Gakkai Zasshi 39:479–485, 1987.
207. Nardelli J, Loridon Rosa B, Bara J, Burtin P: Fetal gastric and small intestine pattern of intestinal mucus antigens in human gastric carcinomas. Cancer Res 44:4157–4163, 1984.
208. Filipe MI, Barbatis C, Sandey A, Ma J: Expression of intestinal mucin antigens in the gastric epithelium and its relationship with malignancy. Hum Pathol 19:19–26, 1988.
209. Planteydt HT, Willighagen RGJ: Enzyme histochemistry of the human stomach with special reference to intestinal metaplasia. J Pathol Bacteriol 80:713–722, 1960.
210. Klein NC, Sleisenger MH, Weser E: Disaccharideses, leucine aminopeptidase and glucose uptake in intestinalized gastric mucosa and in gastric carcinoma. Gastroenterol 55:61–67, 1968.
211. Osborn M, Mazzoleni G, Santini D, et al: Villin, intestinal brush border hydrolases and keratin polypeptides in intestinal metaplasia and gastric cancer: An immunohistologic study emphasizing the different degrees of intestinal and gastric differentiation in signet ring cell carcinomas. Virchows Arch [A] 413:303–312, 1988.
212. Busby-Earle RM, Williams AR, Piris J: Pepsinogens in gastric carcinomas. Hum Pathol 17:1031–1035, 1986.
213. Fiocca R, Cornaggia M, Villani L, et al: Expression of pepsinogen II in gastric cancer: Its relationship to local invasion and lymph node metastasis. Cancer 61:956–962, 1988.
214. Radi MJ, Fenoglio-Preiser CM, Bartow SA, et al: Gastric carcinoma in the young: A clinicopathological and immunohistochemical study. Am J Gastroenterol 81:747–756, 1986.
215. Ito H, Hata J, Oda N, et al: Serotonin in tubular adenomas, adenocarcinomas and endocrine tumours of the stomach: An immunohistochemical study. Virchows Arch [A] 410:239–245, 1986.
216. Cook HC: Neutral mucin content of gastric carcinomas as a diagnostic aid in the identification of secondary deposits. Histopathology 6:591–599, 1982.
217. Kodama T, Kameya T, Hirota T, et al: Production of alpha-fetoprotein, normal serum proteins, and human chorionic gonadotropin in stomach cancer: Histologic and immunohistochemical analyses of 35 cases. Cancer 48:1647–1655, 1981.
218. Skinner JM, Whitehead R: Tumor markers in carcinoma and in premalignant states of the stomach in humans. Eur J Cancer [Clin Oncol] 180:227–235, 1982.
219. Jalanko H, Kuusela P, Roberts P, et al: Comparison of a new tumour marker, CA 19-9, with alpha-fetoprotein and carcinoembryonic antigen in patients with upper gastrointestinal diseases. J Clin Pathol 37:218–222, 1984.
220. Ooi A, Nakanishi I, Sakamoto N, et al: Alpha-fetoprotein (AFP)-producing gastric carcinoma: Is it hepatoid differentiation? Cancer 65:1741–1747, 1990.
221. Tahara E, Ito H, Taniyama K, et al: Alpha$_1$-antitrypsin, alpha$_1$-antichymotrypsin, and alpha$_2$-macroglobulin in human gastric carcinomas: A retrospective immunohistochemical study. Hum Pathol 15:957–964, 1984.
222. Denk H, Tappeiner G, Davidovitss A, et al: Carcinoembryonic antigen and blood group substances in carcinomas of the stomach and colon. J Natl Cancer Inst 53:933–942, 1974.
223. Finan PJ, Wight DG, Lennox ES, et al: Human blood group isoantigen expression on normal and malignant gastric epithelium studied with anti-A and anti-B monoclonal antibodies. J Natl Cancer Inst 70:679–685, 1983.
224. Sakamoto S, Watanabe T, Tokumaru T, et al: Expression of Lewis^a, Lewis^b, Lewis^x, Lewis^y, sialyl-Lewis^a, and sialyl-Lewis^x blood group antigens in human gastric carcinoma and in normal gastric tissue. Cancer Res 49:745–752, 1989.
225. Sipponen P, Lindgren J: Sialylated Lewis determinant CA 19-9 in benign and malignant gastric tissue. Acta Pathol Microbiol Immunol Scand [A] 94:305–311, 1986.
226. Ito H, Hata J, Yokozaki H, Tahara E: Calcitonin in human gastric mucosa and carcinoma. J Cancer Res Clin Oncol 112:50–56, 1986.
227. Janssen CW Jr, Orjasaeter H: Carcinoembryonic antigen in patients with gastric carcinoma. Eur J Surg Oncol 12:19–23, 1986.
228. Barillari P, Aurello P, De Angelis R, et al: Tissue CEA as prognostic indicator in a series of 31 cases of gastric cancer. Ital J Surg Sci 18:237–241, 1988.
229. Skinner JM, Whitehead R: Carcinoplacental alkaline phosphatase in malignant and premalignant conditions of the human digestive tract. Virchows Arch [A] 394:109–118, 1981.
230. Tahara E, Sumiyoshi H, Hata J, et al: Human epidermal growth factor in gastric carcinoma as a biologic marker of high malignancy. Jpn J Cancer Res 77:145–152, 1986.
231. Sakai K, Mori S, Kawamoto T, et al: Expression of epidermal growth factor receptors on human gastric epithelia and gastric carcinomas. J Natl Cancer Inst 77:1047–1052, 1986.
232. Yonemura Y, Sugiyama K, Fujimura T, et al: Epidermal growth factor receptor status and S-phase fractions in gastric carcinoma. Oncology 46:158–161, 1989.
233. Uehara Y, Takahashi T, Kojima O, et al: Peroxidase-antiperoxidase staining for estrogen and progesterone in scirrhous type of gastric cancer: Possible existence of the estrogen receptor. Jpn J Surg 16:245–249, 1986.
234. Yokozaki H, Takekura N, Takanashi A, et al: Estrogen receptors in gastric adenocarcinoma: A retrospective immunohistochemical analysis. Virchows Arch [A] 413:297–302, 1988.
235. Wu CW, Chi CW, Chang TJ, et al: Sex hormone receptors in gastric cancer. Cancer 65:1396–1400, 1990.
236. Hakkinen IPT, Heinonen R, Inberg MV, et al: Clinicopathological study of gastric cancers and precancerous states detected by fetal sulfoglycoprotein antigen screening. Cancer Res 40:4308–4312, 1980.
237. Wu CW, Wang SR, Chang TJ, et al: Content of glucocorticoid receptor and arginase in gastric cancer and normal gastric mucosal tissues. Cancer 64:2552–2556, 1989.
238. Manabe T, Adachi M, Hirao K: Human chorionic gonadotropin in normal, inflammatory, and carcinomatous gastric tissue. Gastroenterology 89:1319–1325, 1985.
239. Macartney JC: Lectin histochemistry of galactose and N-acetylgalactosamine glycoconjugates in normal gastric mucosa and gastric cancer and the relationship with ABO and secretor status. J Pathol 150:135–144, 1986.
240. Fujita K, Ohuchi N, Yao T, et al: Frequent overexpression, but not activation by point mutation, of ras genes in primary human gastric cancers. Gastroenterol 93:1339–1345, 1987.
241. Deng GR, Lu YY, Chen SM, et al: Activated c-Ha-ras oncogene with a guanine to thymine transversion at the twelfth codon in a human stomach cancer cell line. Cancer Res 47:3195–3198, 1987.
242. Nomura N, Yamamoto T, Toyoshima K, et al: DNA amplification of the c-myc and c-erbB-1 genes in a human stomach cancer. Jpn J Cancer Res 77:1188–1192, 1986.
243. Taira M, Yoshida T, Miyagawa K, et al: cDNA sequence of human transforming gene hst and identification of the coding sequence required for transforming activity. Proc Natl Acad Sci 84:2980–2984, 1987.
244. Czerniak B, Herz F, Gorczyca W, Koss LG: Expression of ras

244. [continued] oncogene p21 protein in early gastric carcinoma and adjacent gastric epithelia. Cancer 64:1467–1473, 1989.
245. Inoue H, Hirohashi S, Shimosato Y, et al: Establishment of an anti-A human monoclonal antibody from a blood group A lung cancer patient: Evidence for the occurrence of autoimmune response to difucosylated type-2 chain A. Eur J Immunol 19:2197–2203, 1989.
246. Yoshida K, Tsuda T, Matsumura T, et al: Amplification of epidermal growth factor receptor (EGFR) gene and oncogenes in human gastric carcinomas. Virchows Arch [B] 57:285–290, 1989.
247. Lundell L, Rosengren E: Polyamine levels in human gastric carcinoma. Scand J Gastroenterol 21:829–832, 1986.
248. Yonemura Y, Ooyama S, Sugiyama K, et al: Growth fraction in gastric carcinomas determined with monoclonal antibody Ki-67. Cancer 65:1130–1134, 1990.
249. Ohuchi N, Thor A, Nose M, et al: Tumor associated glycoprotein (TAG-72) detected in adenocarcinomas and benign lesions of the stomach. Int J Cancer 38:643–650, 1986.
250. Danova M, Riccardi A, Mazzini G, et al: Flow cytometric analysis of paraffin-embedded material in human gastric cancer. Anal Quant Cytol Histol 10:200–206, 1988.
251. Sasaki K, Takahashi M, Hashimoto T, Kawachnino K: Flow cytometric DNA measurement of gastric cancers: Clinico-pathological implication of DNA ploidy. Pathol Res Pract 184:561–566, 1989.
252. Okamura T, Korenaga D, Haraguchi M, et al: Growth mode and DNA ploidy in mucosal carcinomas of the stomach. Cancer 59:1154–1160, 1987.
253. Danova M, Mazzini G, Wilson G, et al: Ploidy and proliferative activity of human gastric carcinoma: A cytofluorometric study on fresh and on paraffin embedded material. Basic Appl Histochem 31:73–82, 1987.
254. Czerniak B, Herz F, Koss LG: DNA distribution patterns in early gastric carcinomas: A Feulgen cytometric study of gastric brush smears. Cancer 59:113–117, 1987.
255. Oda N, Tahara E, Taniyama K: Cytophotometric analysis on nuclear DNA contents of human scirrhous gastric carcinoma. Pathol Res Pract 184:390–401, 1989.
256. Sugihara H, Hattori T, Fugita S, et al: Regional ploidy variations in signet ring cell carcinomas of the stomach. Cancer 65:122–129, 1990.
257. Yonemura Y, Sugiyama K, Fugimura T, et al: Correlation of DNA ploidy and proliferative activity in human gastric cancer. Cancer 62:1497–1502, 1988.
258. Haraguchi M, Okamura T, Korenaga D, et al: Heterogeneity of DNA ploidy in patients with undifferentiated carcinomas of the stomach. Cancer 59:922–924, 1987.
259. Nanus DM, Kelsen DP, Niedzwiecki D, et al: Flow cytometry as a predictive indicator in patients with operable gastric cancer. J Clin Oncol 7:1105–1112, 1989.
260. Schneeberger AL, Finley RJ, Troster M, et al: The prognostic significance of tumor ploidy and pathology in adenocarcinoma of the esophagogastric junction. Cancer 65:1206–1210, 1990.
261. Wyatt JI, Quirke P, Ward DC, et al: Comparison of histopathological and flow cytometric parameters in prediction of prognosis in gastric cancer. J Pathol 158:195–201, 1989.
262. Korenaga D, Haraguchi M, Okamura T, et al: Consistency of DNA ploidy between primary and recurrent gastric carcinomas. Cancer Res 46:1544–1546, 1986.
263. Wurster K, Rapp W: Histological and immunohistological studies on gastric mucosa. 1. The presence of CEA in dysplastic surface epithelium. Pathol Res Pract 164:270–281, 1979.
264. Watanabe H, Jass JR, Sabin LH: Histological typing of oesophageal and gastric tumours. In World Health Organization International Histological Classification of Tumours. Berlin, Springer-Verlag, 1989, pp 20–26.
265. Brander WL, Needham PRG, Morgan AD: Indolent mucoid carcinoma of stomach. J Clin Pathol 27:536–541, 1974.
266. Arslan Pagnini C, Rugge M: Gastric cancer: Problems in histological diagnosis. Histopathology 6:391–398, 1982.
267. Lauren P: The two histological main types of gastric carcinoma. Diffuse and so-called intestinal type carcinoma: An attempt at histoclinical classification. Acta Pathol Microbiol Scand 64:31–49, 1965.
268. Stemmermann GN, Brown CA: Survival study of intestinal and diffuse types of gastric cancer. Cancer 33:1190–1195, 1974.
269. Ming SC: Tumors of the esophagus and stomach. Supplement. In Atlas of Tumor Pathology, 2nd series, fascicle 7. Washington, DC, Armed Forces Institute of Pathology, 1985, pp 533–554.
270. Ribeiro MM, Sarmento JA, Simoes S, Bastos J: Prognostic significance of Lauren and Ming classifications and other pathologic parameters in gastric carcinoma. Cancer 47:780–784, 1981.
271. Daves K Sr, Hale J, Kessimian N, Jauregui HO: Histological classification of gastric adenocarcinoma. Lab Invest 58:22A, 1988.
272. Nakamura K: Histogenesis of the gastric cancer and its clinical application. Tsukura International Center, Ibaraki, Japan, 1983.
273. Jass JR: Role of intestinal metaphasia in the histogenesis of gastric carcinoma. J Clin Pathol 33:801–810, 1980.
274. Mulligan RM: Histogenesis and biological behavior of gastric carcinoma. Pathol Annu 7:349–415, 1972.
275. Beahrs OH, Henson DE, Hutter RVP, Myers MH: Manual for Staging of Cancer, 3rd ed. Philadelphia, Lippincott, 1988, pp 69–74.
276. Tso PL, Bringaze WL 3rd, Dauterive AH, et al: Gastric carcinoma in the young. Cancer 59:1362–1365, 1987.
277. Grabiec J, Owen DA: Carcinoma of the stomach in young persons. Cancer 56:388–396, 1985.
278. Bloss RS, Miller TA, Copeland EM III: Carcinoma of the stomach in the young adult. Surg Gynecol Obstet 150:883–886, 1986.
279. Allum WH, Brearley S, Wheatley KE, et al: Acute haemorrhage from gastric malignancy. Br J Surg 77:19–20, 1990.
280. Wilson TS: Free perforation in malignancies of the stomach. Canad J Surg 9:357–364, 1966.
281. Macdougall IC, Fleming S, Frier BM: Hypoglycaemic coma associated with gastric carcinoma. Postgrad Med J 62:761–764, 1986.
282. Obara T, Ito Y, Kodama T, et al: A case of gastric carcinoma associated with excessive granulocytosis: Production of a colony-stimulating factor by the tumor. Cancer 56:782–788, 1985.
283. Bhathal PS, Brown RW, Doyle TC, Gray SJ: Pneumatosis cystoides gastrica associated with adenocarcinoma of the stomach. Acta Cytol 29:147–150, 1985.
284. Zimmerman SE, Smith FP, Phillips TM, et al: Gastric carcinoma and thrombotic thrombocytopenic purpura: Association with plasma immune complex concentrations. Br Med J [Clin Res] 284:1432–1434, 1982.
285. Hugli A, Beris P: Eleven cases of neoplastic microangiopathy. Nouv Rev Fr Hematol 31:223–230, 1989.
286. Sawabe M, Ohashi I, Kitagawa T: Diffuse intrasinusoidal metastasis of gastric carcinoma to the liver leading to fulminating hepatic failure: A case report. Cancer 65:169–173, 1990.
287. Barentsz JO, Rosenbusch GR, Strijk SP, Yap SH: Radiologic examination in gastric cancer: A retrospective study of 188 patients. Acta Radiol 27:547–552, 1986.
288. Vyberg M, Hougen HP, Tnnesen K: Diagnostic accuracy of endoscopic gastrobiopsy in carcinoma of the stomach: A histopathological review of 101 cases. Acta Pathol Microbiol Immunol Scand [A] 91:483–487, 1983.
289. Isaacson P: Biopsy appearances easily mistaken for malignancy in gastrointestinal endoscopy. Histopathology 6:377–389, 1982.
290. Au FC, Koprowska I, Berger A, et al: The role of cytology in the diagnosis of carcinoma of the stomach. Surg Gynecol Obstet 151:601–603, 1980.
291. Yap P, Pantangco E, Yap A, Yap R: Surgical management of gastric carcinoma: Follow-up results in 465 consecutive cases. Am J Surg 143:284–287, 1982.
292. Bizer LS: Adenocarcinoma of the stomach: Current results of treatment. Cancer 51:743–745, 1983.
293. Dupont BJ Jr, Cohn I Jr: Gastric adenocarcinoma. Curr Prob Cancer 4:1–46, 1980.
294. Boddie AW Jr, McBride CM, Balch CM: Gastric cancer. Am J Surg 157:595–606, 1989.
295. Bedikian AY, Chen TT, Khankhanian N, et al: The natural history of gastric cancer and prognostic factors influencing survival. J Clin Oncol 2:305–310, 1984.
296. Wilke H, Preusser P, Fink U, et al: New developments in the treatment of gastric carcinoma. Semin Oncol 17(Suppl 2):61–70, 1990.

297. Kremer B, Henne-Bruns D, Weh HJ, Effenberger T: Advanced gastric cancer: A new combined surgical and oncological approach. Hepatogastroenterology 36:23–26, 1989.
298. Habu H, Takeshita K, Sunagawa M, Endo M: Prognostic factors of early gastric cancer—results of long-term follow-up and analysis of recurrent cases. Jpn J Surg 17:248–255, 1987.
299. Kampschoer GH, Fujii A, Masuda Y: Gastric cancer detected by mass survey: Comparison between mass survey and outpatient detection. Scand J Gastroenterol 24:813–817, 1989.
300. Noguchi Y, Imada T, Matsumoto A, et al: Radical surgery for gastric cancer. Cancer 64:2053–2062, 1989.
301. Newbold KM, Thompson H, Dykes PW: The effect of routine endoscopy on the detection rate of T1 gastric cancer (early gastric cancer) in Birmingham. Endoscopy 21(2):56–59, 1989.
302. Okada M, Kojima S, Murakami M, et al: Human gastric carcinoma: Prognosis in relation to macroscopic and microscopic features of the primary tumor. J Natl Cancer Inst 71:275–279, 1983.
303. Haraguchi M, Okamura T, Sugimachi K: Accurate prognostic value of morphovolumetric analysis of advanced carcinoma of the stomach. Surg Gynecol Obstet 164:335–339, 1987.
304. Arslan Pagnini C, Rugge M: Advanced gastric carcinoma and prognosis. Virchows Arch [A] 406:213–222, 1985.
305. Shennib H, Lough J, Klein HW, Hampson LG: Gastric carcinoma: Intestinal metaplasia and tumor growth patterns as indicators of prognosis. Surgery 100:774–780, 1986.
306. Kaibara N, Iitsuka Y, Kimura A, et al: Relationship between area of serosal invasion and prognosis in patients with gastric carcinoma. Cancer 60:136–139, 1987.
307. Baba H, Korenaga D, Haraguchi M, et al: Width of serosal invasion and prognosis in advanced human gastric cancer with special reference to the mode of tumor invasion. Cancer 64:2482–2486, 1989.
308. Santini D, Bazzocchi F, Mazzoleni G, et al: Signet-ring cells in advanced gastric cancer: A clinical, pathological and histochemical study. Acta Pathol Microbiol Immunol Scand [A] 95:225–231, 1987.
309. Schachenmayr W, Haferkamp O: Prognostic significance of stromal reaction in gastric carcinoma. In Herfarth CH, Schlag P (eds): Gastric Cancer. Berlin, Springer-Verlag, 1979, pp 182–183.
310. Tsujitani S, Furukawa T, Tamada R, et al: Langerhans cells and prognosis in patients with gastric carcinoma. Cancer 59:501–505, 1987.
311. Gaffney EF: Favourable prognosis in gastric carcinoma with parietal cell differentiation. Histopathology 11:217–218, 1987.
312. Yamamoto T, Yasui W, Ochiai A, et al: Immunohistochemical detection of c-myc oncogene product in human gastric carcinomas: Expression in tumor cells and stromal cells. Jpn J Cancer Res 78:1169–1174, 1987.
313. Kojima O, Ikeda E, Uehara Y, et al: Correlation between carcinoembryonic antigen in gastric cancer tissue and survival of patients with gastric cancer. Gann 75:230–236, 1984.
314. Ito H, Tahara E: Human chorionic gonadotropin in human gastric carcinoma: A retrospective immunohistochemical study. Acta Pathol Jpn 33:287–296, 1983.
315. Sjostedt S, Pieper R: Gastric cancer: Factors influencing long term survival and postoperative mortality. Acta Chir Scand [Suppl]: 530:25–29, 1986.
316. Ohman U, Wetterfors J, Moberg A: Histologic grading of gastric cancer. Acta Chir Scand 138:384–390, 1972.
317. Hermanek P: Prognostic factors in stomach cancer surgery. Eur J Surg Oncol 12:241–246, 1986.
318. Kalish RL, Clancy PE, Orringer MB, Appelman HD: Clinical, epidemiologic and morphologic comparison between adenocarcinomas arising in Barrett's esophageal mucosa and in the gastric cardia. Gastroenterology 86:461–467, 1984.
319. Wang HH, Antonioli DA, Goldman H: Comparative features of esophageal and gastric adenocarcinomas: Recent changes in type and frequency. Hum Pathol 17:482–487, 1986.
320. MacDonald WC: Clinical and pathologic features of adenocarcinoma of the gastric cardia. Cancer 29:724–732, 1972.
321. Bruni HC, Nelson RS: Carcinoma of the esophagus and cardia. Diagnostic evaluation in 113 cases. J Thorac Cardiovasc Surg 70:367–370, 1975.
322. Kampschoer GH, Nakajima T, van de Velde CJ: Changing patterns in gastric adenocarcinoma. Br J Surg 76:914–916, 1989.
323. Allum WH, Powell DJ, McConkey CC, Fielding JW: Gastric cancer: A 25-year review. Br J Surg 76:535–540, 1989.
324. Mori M, Kitagawa S, Iida M, et al: Early carcinoma of the gastric cardia: A clinicopathologic study of 21 cases. Cancer 59:1758–1766, 1987.
325. Li L, Pan GL: Pathology of the gastric cardia. In Huang GJ, Wu YK (eds): Carcinoma of the Esophagus and Gastric Cardia. Berlin, Springer-Verlag, 1984, pp 117–155.
326. Okamura T, Tsujitani S, Marin P, et al: Adenocarcinoma in the upper third part of the stomach. Surg Gynecol Obstet 165:247–250, 1987.
327. Mori M, Iwashita A, Enjoji M: Squamous cell carcinoma of the stomach: Report of three cases. Am J Gastroenterol 81:339–342, 1986.
328. Straus R, Heschel S, Fortmann DJ: Primary adenosquamous carcinoma of the stomach: A case report and review. Cancer 24:985–995, 1969.
329. Urban A, Oszacki J, Szczygiel K: Squamous cell metaplasia in carcinoma of the stomach. Acta Med Pol 7:227–243, 1966.
330. Callery CD, Sanders MM, Pratt S, Turnbull AD: Squamous cell carcinoma of the stomach: A study of four patients with comments on histogenesis. J Surg Oncol 29:166–172, 1985.
331. Sato N, Wada K, Kobayashi K, et al: A case of primary adenosquamous carcinoma of the stomach associated with gastric polyposis. [In Japanese.] Gan No Rinsho 30:292–295, 1984.
332. Boswell JT, Helwig EB: Squamous cell carcinoma and adenoacanthoma of the stomach: A clinicopathologic study. Cancer 18:181–192, 1965.
333. Ruck P, Wehrmann M, Campbell M, et al: Squamous cell carcinoma of the gastric stump: A case report and review of the literature. Am J Surg Pathol 13:317–324, 1989.
334. Mingazzini PL, Barsotti P, Malchiodi-Albedi F: Adenosquamous carcinoma of the stomach: Histological, histochemical and ultrastructural observations. Histopathology 7:433–443, 1983.
335. Mori M, Iwashita A, Enjoji M: Adenosquamous carcinoma of the stomach: A clinicopathologic analysis of 28 cases. Cancer 57:333–339, 1986.
336. Saito T, Iizuka T, Kato H, Watanabe H: Esophageal carcinoma metastatic to the stomach: A clinicopathologic study of 35 cases. Cancer 56:2235–2241, 1985.
337. Talerman A, Woo-Ming MO: The origin of squamous cell carcinoma of the gastric cardia. Cancer 22:1226–1232, 1968.
338. Vaughan WP, Straus FH II, Paloyan D: Squamous carcinoma of the stomach after luetic linitis plastica. Gastroenterology 72:945–948, 1977.
339. Won OH, Farman J, Krishnan MN, et al: Squamous cell carcinoma of the stomach. Am J Gastroenterol 69:594–598, 1978.
340. Mori M, Fukuda T, Enjoji M: Adenosquamous carcinoma of the stomach: Histogenetic and ultrastructural studies. Gastroenterology 92:1078–1082, 1987.
341. Shibuya H, Azumi N, Abe F: Gastric small-cell undifferentiated carcinoma with adeno and squamous cell components. Acta Pathol Jpn 35:473–480, 1985.
342. Szogi S: Muco-epidermoid carcinoma of the stomach. Acta Pathol Microbiol Scand 46:37–42, 1959.
343. Hayashi I, Muto Y, Fujii Y, Morimatsu M: Mucoepidermoid carcinoma of the stomach. J Surg Oncol 34:94–99, 1987.
344. Eusterman GB, Senty EG: Benign tumors of the stomach: Report of 27 cases. Surg Gynecol Obstet 34:5–15, 1922.
345. Cairo MS, Grosfeld JL, Weetman RM: Gastric teratoma: Unusual cause for bleeding of the upper gastrointestinal tract in the newborn. Pediatrics 67:721–724, 1981.
346. Moriuchi A, Nakayama I, Muta H, et al: Gastric teratoma of children: A case report with review of the literature. Acta Pathol Jpn 27:749–758, 1977.
347. Haley T, Dimler M, Hollier P: Gastric teratoma with gastrointestinal bleeding. J Pediatr Surg 21:949–950, 1986.
348. Regan JF, Kremin JH: Chorioepithelioma of the stomach. Am J Surg 100:224–233, 1960.
349. Mori H, Soeda O, Kamano T, et al: Choriocarcinomatous change with immunocytochemically HCG-positive cells in the gastric carcinoma of the males. Virchows Arch [A] 396:141–153, 1982.

350. Ramponi A, Angeli G, Arceci F, Pozzuoli R: T1 Gastric choriocarcinoma: An immunohistochemical study. Pathol Res Pract 181:390–396, 1986.
351. Saigo PE, Brigati DJ, Sternberg SS, et al: Primary gastric choriocarcinoma: An immunohistological study. Am J Surg Pathol 5:333–342, 1981.
352. Fukayama M, Hayashi Y, Koike M: Human chorionic gonadotropin in gastric carcinoma: An immunohistochemical study suggesting independent regulation of subunits. Virchows Arch [A] 411:205–212, 1987.
353. Garcia RL, Ghali VS: Gastric choriocarcinoma and yolk sac tumor in a man: Observations about its possible origin. Hum Pathol 16:955–958, 1985.
354. Tanimura H, Furuta M: Carcinosarcoma of the stomach. Am J Surg 113:702–709, 1967.
355. Robey-Cafferty SS, Grignon DJ, Ro JY, et al: Sarcomatoid carcinoma of the stomach: A report of three cases with immunohistochemical and ultrastructural observations. Cancer 65:1601–1606, 1990.
356. Kumagai K, Kawai K, Kusano H, et al: A case of so-called carcinosarcoma of the stomach. [In Japanese.] Gan No Rinsho 30:1931–1936, 1984.
357. Minamoto T, Okada Y, Nakanishi I, Sawasaki K: So-called gastric carcinosarcoma: A case of chondrosarcomatous undifferentiated in the metastatic foci. [In Japanese.] Gan No Rinsho 30:1321–1326, 1984.
358. Dundas SA, Slater DN, Wagner BE, Mills PA: Gastric adenocarcinoleiomyosarcoma: A light, electron microscopic and immunohistological study. Histopathology 13:347–350, 1988.
359. Hussein AM, Otrakji CL, Hussein BT: Small cell carcinoma of the stomach: Case report and review of the literature. Dig Dis Sci 35:513–518, 1990.
360. Fukuda T, Ohnishi Y, Nishimaki T, et al: Early gastric cancer of the small cell type. Am J Gastroenterol 83:1176–1179, 1988.
361. Honmyo U, Misumi A, Murakami A, et al: Clinicopathological analysis of synchronous multiple gastric carcinoma. Eur J Surg Oncol 15:316–321, 1989.
362. Esaki Y, Hirokawa K, Yamashiro M: Multiple gastric cancers in the aged with special reference to intramucosal cancers. Cancer 59:560–565, 1987.
363. Iishi H, Tatsuta M, Okuda S: Diagnosis of simultaneous multiple gastric cancers by the endoscopic Congo red–methylene blue test. Endoscopy 20:78–82, 1988.
364. Yoshino K, Asanuma F, Hanatani Y, et al: Multiple primary cancers in the stomach and another organ: Frequency and the effects on prognosis. Jpn J Clin Oncol 15(Suppl 1):183–190, 1985.
365. Hoar SK, Wilson J, Blot WJ, et al: Second cancer following cancer of the digestive system in Connecticut, 1935–82. Natl Cancer Inst Monogr 68:49–82, 1985.
366. Sasaki M, Matsuda T, Hohara T: Multiple primary cancers subsequent to gastric cancer in Hokkaido Cancer Center. Jpn J Clin Oncol 15(Suppl 1):235–241, 1985.
367. Lynge E, Jensen OM, Carstensen B: Second cancer following cancer of the digestive system in Denmark, 1943–80. Natl Cancer Inst Monogr 68:277–308, 1985.
368. Ming SC: Tumors of the esophagus and stomach. In Atlas of Tumor Pathology, 2nd series, fascicle 7. Washington, DC, Armed Forces of Pathology. 1973, pp 253–255.
369. Green LK: Hematogenous metastases to the stomach: A review of 67 cases. Cancer 65:1596–1600, 1990.
370. Maeta M, Koga S, Shimizu N, et al: Clinicopathologic study of esophageal cancer associated with simultaneous metastatic lesions in the stomach. J Surg Oncol 38:143–146, 1988.
371. Choi SH, Sheehan FR, Pickren JW: Metastatic involvement of the stomach by breast cancer. Cancer 17:791–797, 1964.
372. Walker Q, Bilous M, Tiver KW, Langlands AO: Breast cancer metastases masquerading as primary gastric carcinoma. Aust N Z J Surg 56:395–398, 1986.
373. Gutman M, Klausner JM, Inbar M, et al: Surgical approach to malignant melanoma in the gastrointestinal tract. J Surg Oncol 36:17–20, 1987.
374. Klausner JM, Skornick Y, Lelcuk S, et al: Acute complications of metastatic melanoma to the gastrointestinal tract. Br J Surg 69:195–196, 1982.

PART 5

SMALL INTESTINE, COLON, AND RECTUM

CHAPTER 26

Infectious Disorders of the Intestines

GERALD D. ABRAMS, M.D.

THE GASTROINTESTINAL TRACT
  AS AN ECOSYSTEM
The Normal Microbial Flora
**Stabilizing Factors in the
  Gastrointestinal Ecosystem**
Gastric Acidity
Intestinal Motility
Mucosal Immune System
Colonization Resistance of Normal
  Flora
**Perturbations of the Gastrointestinal
  Ecosystem**
Contaminated Small-Bowel Syndrome
Clostridium Difficile Infection and
  Pseudomembranous Colitis
Neutropenic Enterocolitis

EXOGENOUS INFECTION
Virulence Factors
Mucosal Adhesion
Tissue Invasion
Microbial Toxins
Patterns of Host-Microbe Interaction
Mucosal Adhesion of Organisms with
  Enterotoxin Production
Mucosal Adhesion of Organisms with
  Microvillous Damage
Mucosal Invasion of Organisms with
  Intracellular Proliferation
Mucosal Translocation of Organisms
  with Proliferation in Lamina Propria
  and Regional Lymph Nodes
Mucosal Translocation of Organisms
  with Systemic Spread
Hemorrhagic Colitis

PATHOLOGY OF INTESTINAL
  INFECTIONS
General Considerations
Acute Self-Limited Enterocolitis
Exclusion of Noninfectious Causes
Viral Infections
Nonspecific Enteritis
Specific Viral Enteritis
Herpesvirus Infection
Cytomegalovirus Infection
Chlamydial Infections
Bacterial Infections
Salmonellosis and Shigellosis
Campylobacter Enterocolitis
Yersinia Enterocolitis
Tuberculosis
Actinomycosis
Intestinal Spirochetosis
Gonorrhea and Syphilis
Fungal Infections
Candidiasis and Mucormycosis
Histoplasmosis
Protozoan Infection
Amebiasis
Giardiasis
Coccidiosis
Helminthic Infection

THE GASTROINTESTINAL TRACT AS AN ECOSYSTEM

The Normal Microbial Flora

The gastrointestinal tract, in addition to being a complex apparatus for the digestion and absorption of nutrients, is actually a vast interface between the host and the environment. In approaching the infectious disorders of the intestine, it is therefore essential to view the subject with an ecologic perspective, recognizing the true relationship between the gastrointestinal mucosa and its surroundings.

Beginning at the moment of birth and throughout the life of the individual, the gastrointestinal tract is exposed to a continual stream of living microbial agents and is quite literally "infected." From early infancy the tract comes to be inhabited by a huge microbial population, from one end to the other. The microbial strains that associate in this fashion with the healthy host constitute the normal flora.

This complex microbial population, which reaches concentrations of 10^{12} cells per milliliter of intestinal content, is of reasonably predictable composition, given the fact that only a fraction of the microbial species encountered in the environment can survive and

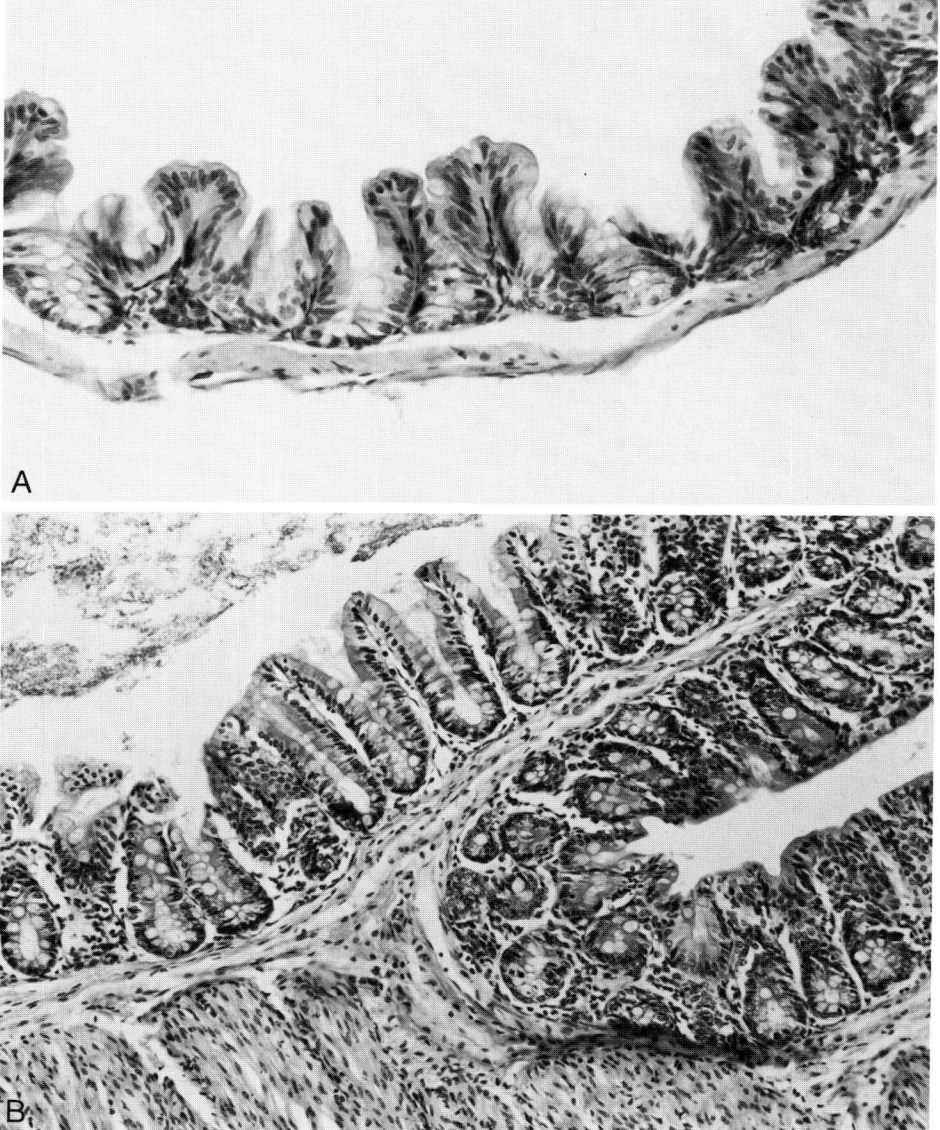

FIGURE 26–1. Large intestine of the germ-free (A), as compared with the conventional (B), mouse. The impact of the indigenous, normal flora in the latter animal is evident from the differences in mucosal architecture and the expansion of the lamina propria to its "normal" state as a response to the flora.

establish themselves in the particular conditions afforded by the gut.[1] Moreover, within the gastrointestinal tract, the distribution of various species is predictable. This is true because the physiochemical microenvironment of one level of the tract differs from that of the others (with respect to pH, oxidation-reduction potential, nutrient concentrations, and the like), and a different set of microbial strains is adapted to each set of conditions. Finally, even at a given level of the gastrointestinal tract, there may be a predictable ordering of the flora, with some strains associating closely with or even adhering to the mucosal surface and others living within the luminal contents.[2] In the normal host, all available "niches" are thus occupied; and the various microbial strains of the flora in each location interact with one another and with the host.

The inevitable infection of the gastrointestinal tract with this normal flora obviously does not produce disease and in fact even contributes to the physiologic well-being of the individual. The flora is a large, metabolically active mass, normally responsible for the biotransformation of many substances both exogenous and endogenous within the lumen.[3] The normal luminal environment itself is actually the reflection of this metabolic activity, and even certain enzymes normally active within the lumen are known to be of microbial origin.[4] The normal transit time of intestinal contents through the tract reflects a significant influence of the flora on peristaltic activity.[5] In the same fashion, even the normal histologic features of the gastrointestinal mucosa are shaped by the flora (Figure 26–1). Comparison of germ-free animal hosts with those harboring a conventional flora has shown that the customarily observed cellularity of the lamina propria is largely a reaction to the flora, and that the normal histology of the gut-associated lymphoid tissues in general is likewise a response to the flora.[6] The rate of epithelial cell renewal in the mucosa of normal or conventional animals is significantly faster than that of animals without the usual microbial load, and the mucosal content of certain enzymes is also influenced by the normal microbial presence.[6,7] Thus, the gastrointestinal tract normally "infected" by its resident flora is, in a general biologic sense, an ecosystem in which many complex interlocking equilibria are established and maintained within fairly narrow limits under ordinary conditions. The conditions that we view as infectious disorders of the intestines can be comprehended in this perspective as significant perturbations of the ecosystem due either to invasion of exogenous agents capable of gaining a foothold among the normal residents or to a change in the balance of endogenous strains and their relationship to one another and to the host.

Stabilizing Factors in the Gastrointestinal Ecosystem

A number of features of the normal gastrointestinal ecosystem, including both host and microbial factors, act in concert to maintain equilibrium and the status quo, and to make it difficult for exogenous microbial strains to invade and successfully colonize the host. These stabilizing influences can be viewed as mucosal defense mechanisms.

Gastric Acidity

One factor that acts as an important initial defense mechanism, by diminishing the microbial load impinging on the small and large intestine, is the strongly acid pH of the normal stomach. Many microbial strains that might be ingested from the environment are promptly killed upon exposure to a pH of less than 4.0.[8] This microbicidal effect of acid has been clearly shown not only in vitro by direct test, but also in vivo by a number of observations. The variety of microbial strains that can be cultured from samples of gastric juice has been found to be much greater in patients with achlorhydria (pH ranging between 6.8 and 8.4) than in patients with acid gastric juice (pH between 1.3 and 3.4).[9] Furthermore, in a controlled experimental setting, the size of the dose of certain pathogens required to establish infection is significantly reduced if challenge occurs simultaneously with neutralization of gastric acidity.[10] Finally, certain infections of the gastrointestinal tract have been found with greater frequency in postgastrectomy patients and in those achlorhydric for other reasons.[11]

Intestinal Motility

Those organisms that remain viable as they pass through the stomach are generally prevented from colonizing the small intestine by a set of defenses of a very different sort. The major factor at this second level is the speedy propulsion of contents to the colon. Even in the absence of any significant microbicidal activity of the sort encountered in the stomach, simple mechanical flushing of the entering organisms prevents buildup of the intraluminal microbial population.[12] It is primarily for this reason that microbial counts characteristically remain low in the small intestine. This mechanical defense of the small intestine is undoubtedly assisted by the constant production of mucus, which coats the mucosal surface and tends to minimize the chance that organisms can contact and perhaps adhere to the mucosa. The importance of intestinal motility in mucosal defense is highlighted by certain observations in situations of impaired motility. It has been shown, for instance, that an efficient means of ensuring the establishment of active infection following experimental challenge is the pharmacologic inhibition of peristalsis with opiates.[13] Similarly, it has been observed that the clinical manifestations of shigellosis may actually be prolonged by antimotility drugs.[14] Observations such as these argue strongly against the widespread use of antimotility preparations in the treatment of infectious diarrheal disease.

Mucosal Immune System

An important additional factor, working in concert with rapid peristaltic propulsion of microbial agents through the small intestine, is the mucosal immune system, discussed in Chapter 5. One major immunologic protection mechanism is mediated by secretory IgA, which inhibits microbial adherence to the epithelial lining of the gut, thus assuring rapid expulsion of microbes by mechanical means.[15] The importance of antibody and cell-mediated defenses in the intestine has been vividly underscored in recent years by the patterns of illness seen in immunocompromised patients, particularly those with acquired immunodeficiency syndrome (AIDS) as outlined in Chapter 14. These patients are frequently overwhelmed by environmental microbes that are so unlikely to colonize normal subjects that we are generally unaware of their presence in our surroundings.

Colonization Resistance of Normal Flora

In the lower gastrointestinal tract a very different set of conditions exists. At the colonic level there is neither a strongly acid intraluminal pH nor a rapid defensive expulsion of contents. Rather, the major defensive mechanism is one of microbial ecology. This effect has been variously designated as "colonization resistance," "bacterial interference," or "bacterial antagonism," and is the direct result of a massive normal flora. The potential invaders that retain their viability on their way through the stomach and small intestine enter the colon in relatively small numbers and immediately confront a dense, established, resident flora.

The ability of this flora to inhibit the growth of invaders appears to be a reflection of competition for limited nutrients and/or the effects of metabolic inhibitors produced by the flora.[16] Suppression of the resident flora is a well-recognized means of manipulating this ecologic defense experimentally. Furthermore, recent studies of the epidemiology of certain *Salmonella* infections in the community have implicated the use of antibiotics as a risk factor in the development of infection, possibly reflecting a lowered colonization resistance, resulting from a disturbance in the normal flora.[17,18]

Perturbations of the Gastrointestinal Ecosystem

The importance of viewing the gastrointestinal tract from an ecologic perspective lies in the recognition of the fact that much of the infectious disease encountered in the gut is in reality not simply the result of an unlucky encounter with a passing pathogen. Actually, it is a reflection of some perturbation of the mucosal ecosystem, broadly defined. A microbial strain that functions as a colonizing pathogen in one situation may be handled as a transient visitor or even trivial symbiont in another situation with different conditions prevailing in the ecosystem. In fact, given sufficient disturbance of the gastrointestinal ecosystem, even components of the normal flora assume the role of pathogens.

Contaminated Small-Bowel Syndrome

An excellent example of the normal flora becoming pathogenic is the so-called contaminated small bowel syndrome, in which a large microbial population, especially the anaerobes normally inhabiting the colon, come to colonize the upper intestine.[19] This can occur when the continuous unidirectional peristaltic cleansing of the small intestine is hampered, as it might be with various strictures and obstructions, or after surgical construction of loops and bypasses. Such colonization may also accompany continuous microbial seeding of the small intestine, as in the presence of hypochlorhydria, enterocolic fistulas, or multiple, stagnant, small-intestinal diverticula. Since the normal characteristics of the tract reflect certain host-microbe equilibria, it stands to reason that such a dramatic change in the habitat of the flora will alter these equilibria. In the contaminated small bowel syndrome, the results include steatorrhea due to altered bile salt metabolism, macrocytic anemia reflecting microbial interaction with vitamin B^{12}, malabsorption of various nutrients, and even morphologic evidence of mucosal damage (Figure 26–2). Somewhat analogous conditions may be obtained in another sort of ecologic aberration, when subjects are exposed chronically to a grossly polluted environment that affords essentially continuous exposure to exogenous fecal contamination.[19]

Clostridium Difficile Infection and Pseudomembranous Colitis

Another far more important example of an ecologic perturbation is seen in the recent emergence of *Clostridium difficile* in the role of intestinal pathogen. This organism is harbored by some healthy asymptomatic subjects, presumably in small numbers held in check by ecologic defenses. Many other individuals are ordinarily resistant to the organism even though it is frequently present in the environment. When, however, the normal intestinal flora is sufficiently altered, usually by antibiotic therapy, colonization resistance decreases and *C. difficile* is able to flourish, colonize the gut lumen, and produce an array of toxins.[20] Two of these have been well characterized: toxin A, which is both cytotoxic and enterotoxic, and toxin B, a potent cytotoxin that is largely responsible for the changes seen in diagnostic toxin assays.[21] Proliferation of *C. difficile* can be associated with a variety of conditions, including pseudomembranous colitis and antibiotic-associated diarrhea. Although the histologic lesions of pseudomembranous colitis have been reproduced by exposure of the mucosa to cell-free, toxin-containing filtrates,[22] the range of variation in the clinical expres-

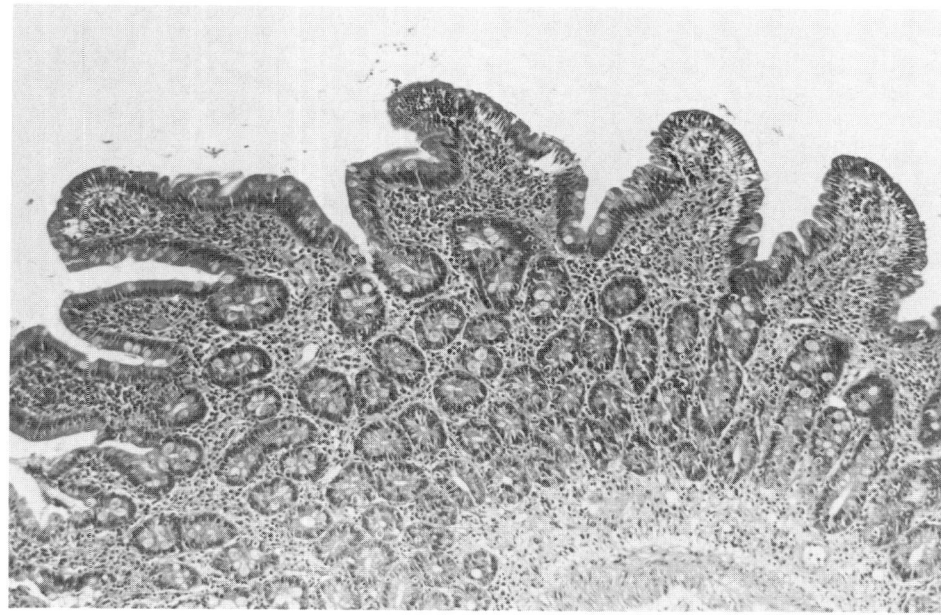

FIGURE 26–2. Mucosa of contaminated small bowel showing that even the normal (colonic) flora in an abnormal setting is capable of altering host tissues, as evidenced by expansion of the lamina propria and architectural distortion.

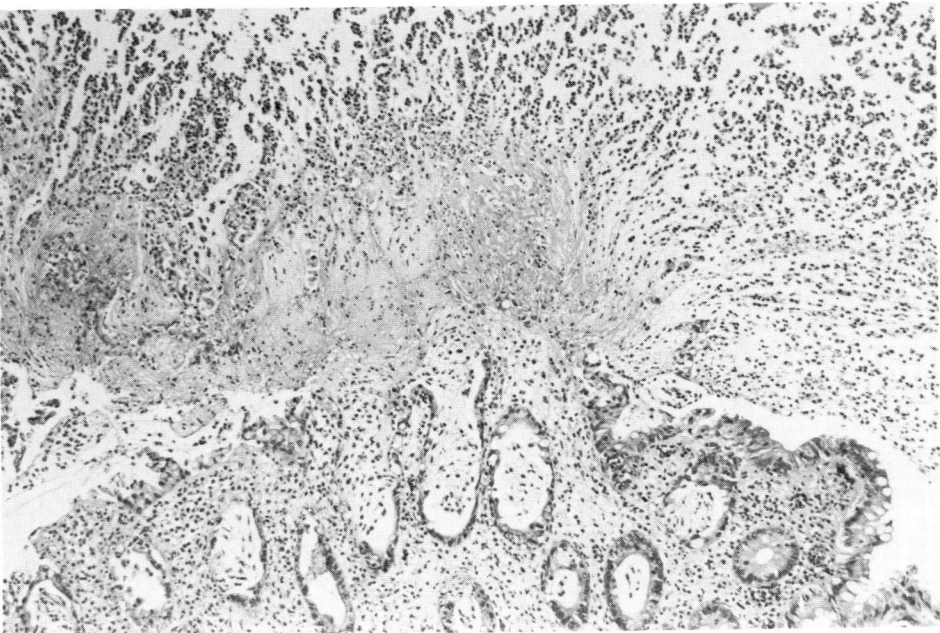

FIGURE 26–3. Antibiotic-associated pseudomembranous colitis, type II lesion. A "mushroom" of exudate is adherent to the superficially damaged mucosal surface. Deeper portions of the mucosa survive.

sion of *C. difficile* infection has not been completely explained. Presumably, it is related to quantitative variations in bacillary proliferation and/or toxin production.

The morphologic lesion characteristically associated with *C. difficile* is pseudomembranous colitis, typified in type II lesions by groups of superficially damaged crypts covered by a mushrooming cloud of fibrinopurulent exudate, epithelial debris, and admixed mucus (Figure 26–3). Price and Davies have shown that the diagnosis of pseudomembranous colitis can also be made on finding a more limited lesion, which they designated as a type I lesion, type II being the classic pseudomembranous lesion.[23] The type I lesion consists of a focus of epithelial damage on the intercryptal surface or "summit," associated with a small cluster of leukocytes (Figure 26–4). At the other extreme, *C. difficile* infection may produce a full-thickness mucosal necrosis, designated as a type III lesion by these authors.

It should be recognized that a wide range of mucosal appearances can be produced by infection with *C. difficile*. In one published study of biopsy material from patients with proven *C. difficile* infection, 8% were found to have no lesion, 8% had congestion and edema, 31% had a nonspecific colitis, and 53% had the classic pseudomembranous lesion.[24]

Our experience has been similar and has emphasized the importance of recognizing subtle variants of the

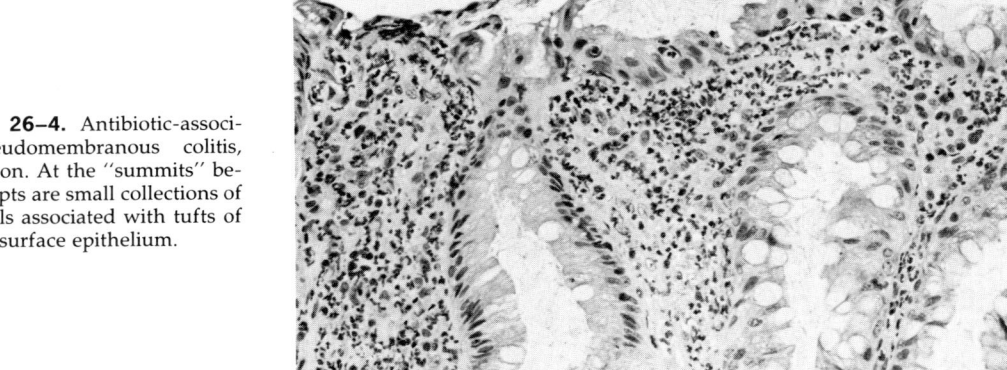

FIGURE 26–4. Antibiotic-associated pseudomembranous colitis, type I lesion. At the "summits" between crypts are small collections of neutrophils associated with tufts of damaged surface epithelium.

early type I lesion. Conversely, we have seen transmural colonic inflammation in C. difficile infection, and there have been published reports of massive mural edema and toxic megacolon necessitating colonic resection.[25,26]

While antibiotic therapy is the usual factor behind the ecologic perturbation allowing C. difficile infection, this organism has occasionally been found colonizing patients without prior antibiotic exposure, has been associated with antineoplastic chemotherapy, and has been found in association with symptomatic flares of chronic inflammatory bowel disease.[20,27,28]

Neutropenic Enterocolitis

A third example of ecologic perturbation of the gastrointestinal tract leading to the disease is the syndrome of necrotizing enterocolitis encountered in patients with malignancies, especially leukemia. This condition has been variously termed agranulocytic or neutropenic colitis, typhlitis, and ileocecal syndrome; and is generally seen in patients receiving aggressive chemotherapy.[29] In this instance the ecologic disturbance is complex, involving the host as well as possibly the flora. The lesions of neutropenic enterocolitis center about the terminal ileum and right colon and consist of patchy areas of transmural edema, necrosis, and microbial (bacterial and fungal) invasion, with minimal cellular response (Figure 26–5). These gastrointestinal lesions are frequently associated with positive blood cultures, most often with recovery of intestinal organisms. On the host side of the ecosystem, the critical pathogenetic factors are thought to include neutropenia and damage to the integrity of the mucosa, both related to chemotherapy. Given these alterations, microbial invasion could be a secondary phenomenon. However, the patients generally have also been exposed to antibiotics; and it has been suggested that under these conditions, *Clostridium septicum* may be favored in a manner analogous to C. difficile in antibiotic-associated colitis. In neutropenic enterocolitis, however, there appears to be actual invasion in the wall by the *Clostridium*.[30]

A final related example of microecologic disturbance associated with significant disease is the observation that the combination of neutropenia and C. difficile infection may lead to polymicrobial bacteremia. This phenomenon may reflect entry of organisms from the bowel lumen through areas of clostridial mucosal damage.[31]

EXOGENOUS INFECTION

Virulence Factors

In the examples thus far discussed, infections have been secondary to a significant derangement of one or more elements of the digestive ecosystem. Under ordinary circumstances, this ecosystem has an impressive degree of stability and resistance to exogenous agents

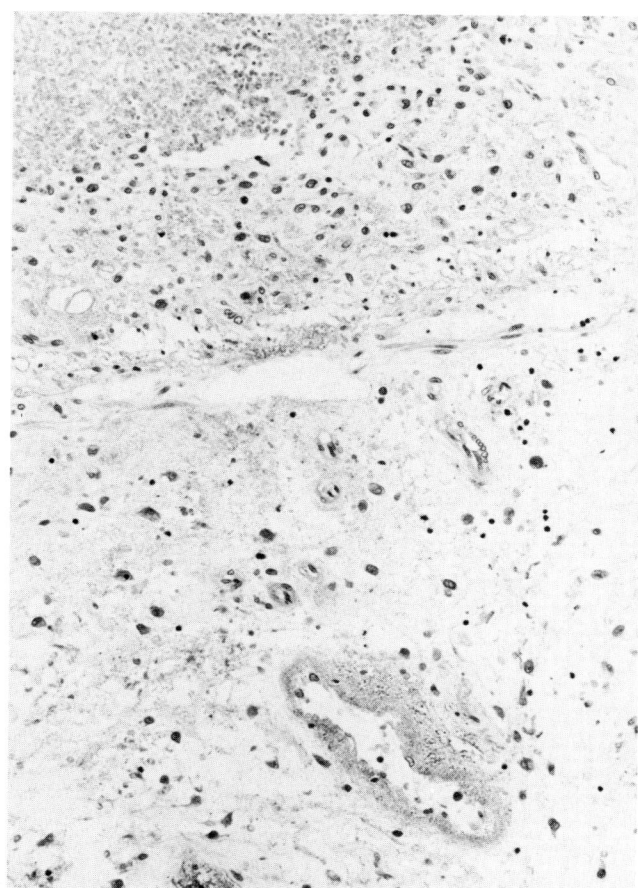

FIGURE 26–5. Neutropenic enterocolitis, showing *Candida* overgrowth in the mucosa (upper left) and diffuse bacterial spread into the submucosa, lending a fuzzy character to the edematous tissue, evident especially around the blood vessel near the lower margin of the field. Note the paucity of cellular response.

because of the defensive mechanisms intrinsic to it. Even so, there is a significant worldwide incidence of infection with enteric pathogens, reflecting not only unfavorable environmental conditions but also the development in some microbial species (i.e., the "pathogens") of mechanisms enabling them to overcome gastrointestinal defenses. The microbial attributes responsible for this are viewed as virulence factors, and many of these have been mapped to microbial plasmids and chromosomes. These virulence factors are of several sorts.

Mucosal Adhesion

One set of virulence factors endows certain microbes with the ability to resist being swept rapidly through the gut. If peristaltic elimination can be avoided, colonization may then occur. This is accomplished by actual microbial adhesion to the surface of the intestine effected by ligand-receptor interaction between microbial surface structures and the host epithelial cell membrane. Such microbial factors, termed adhesins, are known to reside on fimbriae or pili projecting from the microbial surface as in the case of certain *Escherichia coli*, or to be associated with surface structures other than fimbrial proteins, as in the case of *Vibrio cholerae*.[32,33] Antibody directed against these adhesins effectively prevents colonization and, thereby, production of disease. Certain organisms such as the cholera *Vibrio* are also equipped to supplement their adhesive properties with additional virulence factors conferring the ability to penetrate quickly through the layer of mucus protecting the mucosa and reach the epithelial surface. These ancillary factors include motility, chemotactic responsiveness, and mucinase production.[34,35]

Tissue Invasion

A second set of virulence factors endows certain agents (e.g., *Shigella, Salmonella, Yersinia, Campylobacter*) with the ability to invade the mucosa after initial colonization. The first step in invasion involves entry into epithelial cells, apparently accomplished by a microbially stimulated endocytosis on the part of the host cell.[36] Some organisms such as *Salmonella* are transported within phagosomes in the enterocyte to be discharged into the lamina propria. Others, e.g., *Shigella*, apparently spread laterally into other epithelial cells. In order to establish disease, the entering organisms must also be capable of intracellular multiplication, an attribute mediated by yet another set of virulence factors. The attributes of some organisms permit survival only in the lamina propria, whereas other agents are able to spread to regional lymph nodes or even systemically.

Microbial Toxins

Toxins, i.e., damaging substances produced by microbial agents, constitute yet another class of virulence factors. The toxins of enteropathogens fall into two major groups, enterotoxins and cytotoxins. Enterotoxins, without killing the epithelial cells or producing a significant histologic lesion, sharply alter cellular transport of electrolytes and water, producing a net secretion of water that may overwhelm the absorptive capacities of the colon, producing diarrhea.[37] Cytotoxins injure and kill cells and are therefore associated with histologic lesions of the mucosa.

Whereas the pathogenic role of toxins is precisely defined in some of the enterotoxigenic secretory diarrheas such as cholera, the details of pathogenesis have not been as clearly elaborated in the case of most invasive pathogens. For these agents, toxic production alone is insufficient and must be accompanied by invasion of the mucosa. Furthermore, diarrhea in these latter cases cannot be explained simply as a result of anatomic mucosal disruption. There is some evidence of a role for activated inflammatory mediators in some invasive infections.[38,39] Toxins may also act as virulence factors by altering the intestinal environment in a way that directly favors the microbial agent (e.g., release of some essential nutrient from the affected mucosa).[40] Less directly, it can be argued, they augment microbial spread in the environment through the provocation of diarrhea.

Patterns of Host-Microbe Interaction

Because various microbial strains are endowed with different sets of virulence factors, it follows that these agents should manifest a variety of patterns of interaction with the host. Levine has proposed a classification of enteric pathogens based on their relative degrees of invasiveness.[33] The classification is as follows:

Mucosal Adhesion of Organisms with Enterotoxin Production

In the infections of this class, the mucosa is not invaded and there is no discernible histopathologic lesion. Organisms attach to and colonize the mucosal surface of the small intestine, then elaborate and release enterotoxin, which leads to secretory diarrhea. Cholera, the classic example of this class of disease, involves enterotoxic activation of the adenylate cyclase system of the epithelium and secretion of large quantities of water with a histologically intact mucosa.[33,40,41] Simultaneously, there is suppression of water absorption in the colon.[42] Enterotoxogenic *E. coli* organisms also exemplify this class of infection, producing infant diarrhea and traveler's diarrhea, especially in developing countries.

Mucosal Adhesion of Organisms with Microvillous Damage

The best example of this type of infection is infant diarrhea associated with enteropathogenic *E. coli*. In this condition, microbial adherence is followed not by true cellular invasion, but by significant injury to microvilli. This ultrastructural cellular damage, together with the effects of the toxin, may produce the diarrhea.[43]

Mucosal Invasion of Organisms with Intracellular Proliferation

Shigella infections with invasion of the epithelial cells of distal small intestine and colon typify this class. Bacteria tend to remain localized in epithelial cells, with some spread into the lamina propria. Cell damage leads to the inflammation, hemorrhage, and ulceration associated with signs and symptoms of dysentery. Varying degrees of watery diarrhea may also be seen in *Shigellosis*. The pathogenic role of *Shigella*-associated toxin, which is cytotoxic, neurotoxic, and enterotoxic, is not entirely clear.[44] Fluid secretion may be related in part to increased concentration of prostaglandins associated with inflammation.[38] A similar pattern of disease is also seen in the dysenteric syndrome produced by enteroinvasive *E. coli*.

Mucosal Invasion of Organisms with Proliferation in Lamina Propria and Regional Lymph Nodes

This class of infection includes diseases related to nontyphoid *Salmonella* species, *Yersinia*, and *Campy-

lobacter. Although toxins have been associated with these organisms, details of pathogenesis are incompletely understood.

Mucosal Translocation of Organisms with Systemic Spread

Infections with *Salmonella typhi* and *Salmonella paratyphi* are of this class. These agents, through their virulence factors, are able to survive the inflammatory response in the lamina propria, spread into the regional lymph nodes, and ultimately spread to the bloodstream. Survival within macrophages of the nonimmune host appears to be a key factor.[33]

Hemorrhagic Colitis

Recently, yet another pattern of host-microbe interaction, not conforming precisely to those listed above, has been recognized. This is exemplified by the hemorrhagic colitis caused by strains of *E. coli* that produce toxins cytopathic for HeLa and Vero cells. These toxins are similar or identical to Shiga toxins. *E. coli* 0157:H7 is the most prominent of several verotoxin-producing strains. These "enterohemorrhagic" *E. coli* organisms cause an illness, generally nonfebrile, characterized by abdominal cramps and diarrhea, which is initially watery but eventually bloody. The organisms are noninvasive, but the mucosa can nonetheless be significantly damaged, either by direct contact or through the effect of the cytoxins. Lesions are nonspecific and can resemble those of acute self-limited (infectious) colitis described below but can also have the pattern of ischemic injury or even pseudomembranous colitis.[109,110] Although the colitis is most often self-limited, the hemolytic uremic syndrome or thrombotic thrombocytopenic purpura may be a complication.

PATHOLOGY OF INTESTINAL INFECTIONS

General Considerations

Given the multiple types of microbial agents that are capable of infecting the digestive tract, their differing degrees of invasiveness, and the variety of their virulence factors, it is difficult to characterize the pathology of intestinal infections succinctly.

At one extreme, some infectious agents may be associated with dramatic or even lethal physiologic derangements but produce no significant pathologic lesion. In cholera, the classic example of this sort of disease, enterotoxin production by the *Vibrio* organisms colonizing the gut triggers a massive secretion of water, but without an accompanying enteritis. The recognition of this important principle is a relatively recent event historically, correcting a misconception that originated in the time of Virchow. Observations at *autopsy*, confounded by inevitable autolytic changes in the intestinal mucosa, had led to the concept that the diarrhea of cholera was the result of mucosal denudement; and it remained for a relatively recent *biopsy* study to show that the mucosa was actually intact during the active disease.[45] A corollary to this principle is that even in those diseases associated with a significant histopathologic lesion, all of the clinically observed derangements are not necessarily correlated with that particular lesion.

At the opposite extreme, some enteric infections are associated with a characteristic or even pathognomonic histopathologic appearance. This is true, for instance, of certain viral infections (e.g., cytomegalovirus) wherein cytopathologic changes are virtually diagnostic. It is obviously the case for those infectious agents (e.g., protozoans, helminths, certain fungi) that can be readily recognized in tissue sections.

For most enteric infections encountered by the pathologist, however, the recognition of a particular histopathologic lesion does not in itself allow a specific etiologic diagnosis. Many diverse infections are associated with the same spectrum of mucosal changes, including damage to the surface and/or crypt epithelium, regenerative alterations in epithelial cell renewal patterns, altered mucin secretion, hyperemia and edema of the lamina propria, and leukocytic infiltration of varying degree. Only when these changes are correlated with microbial, immunologic, and clinical information can a specific diagnosis be made.

Acute Self-Limited Enterocolitis

An issue of crucial practical importance for the pathologist is distinguishing between mucosal lesions of the sort produced by various microbial agents and those of idiopathic bowel disease such as chronic ulcerative colitis or Crohn's disease. Patients presenting with bloody diarrhea of sudden onset may have an acute infectious enterocolitis or may be suffering the first clinical manifestations of idiopathic inflammatory bowel disease. In the former instance, the disease is usually short-lived and even self-limited, whereas in the latter, a protracted chronic course can be expected. Although stool cultures would appear to be the obvious way to make the distinction, most estimates suggest that enteric pathogens will be recovered in only half of the instances of self-limited colitis. Therefore, biopsy of such patients assumes great importance.

Kumar and her colleagues have delineated the histopathologic features that are helpful in making this distinction.[46] They studied a group of patients with "acute self-limited colitis" (ASLC), defined as a first episode of bloody diarrhea, accompanied by a sigmoidoscopic appearance consistent with inflammatory bowel disease, a rapid clinical resolution (usually within 2 weeks), and normal clinical follow-up examinations. Their study group included patients from whom *Campylobacter*, *Salmonella*, *Shigella*, and *Yersinia* were recovered; but in 57.5% no "pathogen" was recovered. The most important characteristic changes in sigmoidoscopic biopsies were seen within the first 4 days after the onset of clinical disease. These changes

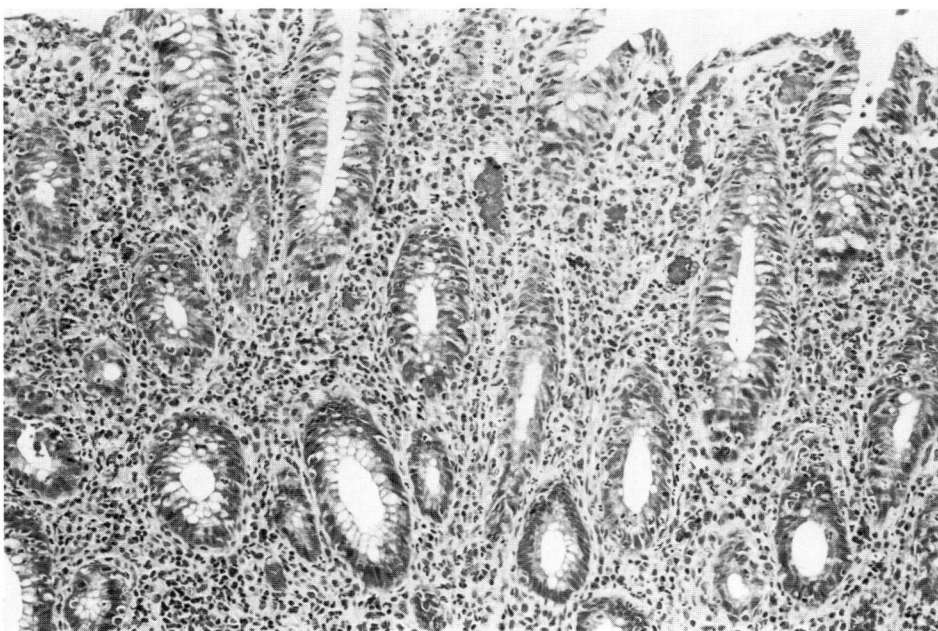

FIGURE 26–6. Acute self-limited colitis. Goblet cells are partly depleted of mucin, and the mucosa is diffusely inflamed, with a neutrophilic infiltrate in the epithelium. The appearance differs from that of ulcerative colitis in the lack of basal plasmacytosis and of significant crypt distortion.

included mucosal edema; superficial ulcers with a neutrophilic surface exudate; cryptitis, crypt ulcers, and crypt abscesses; diminution in intracellular mucin; and increased cellularity of the lamina propria, with neutrophils and lesser numbers of lymphocytes, plasma cells, and eosinophils (Figure 26–6). During the next several days the edema was variable; regenerative epithelial changes appeared; active crypt lesions became more focal; and neutrophils were less prominent in the lamina propria. In the later stages of resolution, at the latter part of the second week, mucosal edema had disappeared; active crypt lesions had resolved, leaving some persistent features of regeneration; increase in lamina propria cellularity was slight; and some biopsies were essentially normal. At none of these stages was there evidence of significant crypt distortion (abnormal shapes, branching, loss of parallelism) or plasmacytosis in the lower fifth of the mucosa. The absence of these two features, crypt distortion and basal plasmacytosis, was the most useful criterion in separating a self-limited colitis from a chronic colitis. In a follow-up study, patients with ASLC were compared with ulcerative colitis patients, and the differential diagnostic validity of these features was confirmed.[47] However, the resolving phase of ASLC with its residual *focal* cryptitis may be confused with Crohn's disease, and appropriate clinical follow-up is required. The utility of biopsy and distinguishing between ASLC and idiopathic inflammatory bowel disease has been independently confirmed by other workers.[48]

Exclusion of Noninfectious Causes

One additional factor that must be taken into account in the interpretation of biopsy material is the effect of agents used to prepare the bowel for endoscopic examination, because occasionally these effects may include mild "colitic" changes. (See Chapters 3 and 9 for additional information.) Hypertonic phosphate enemas can produce damage and/or detachment of surface epithelium, partial depletion of cellular mucin, and edema of the lamina propria.[49] Bisacodyl has been associated with similar changes as well as with deeper crypt damage and occasional neutrophilic accumulation.[50] Finally, it should be noted that a mild colitis (with crypt abscesses, epithelial cell degeneration, regenerative changes, and inflammatory infiltrates) has been seen in excluded segments of colon after diversion of the fecal stream (see Chapter 28). This colitic lesion does not appear to be related to known intestinal "pathogens" and is reversible with correction of the diversion.[51]

Viral Infections

Nonspecific Enteritis

Acute viral gastroenteritis is an exceedingly common ailment in many parts of the world; it is responsible for abundant, generally self-limited morbidity, and occasional mortality. Although multiple viral agents may be responsible for these frequent infections, the rotavirus and Norwalk virus are the two agents currently recognized as etiologically most important in nonbacterial acute gastroenteritis.[52] These infections are characterized by invasion of mature epithelial cells of the small intestine.[53] Mucosal injury leads to shortening of villi and lengthening of crypts, with heightened mitotic activity and cellular infiltration of the lamina propria.[54] The diarrhea associated with these infections represents a net secretion of water by the intestine. There is evidence in rotavirus enteritis that the functional ab-

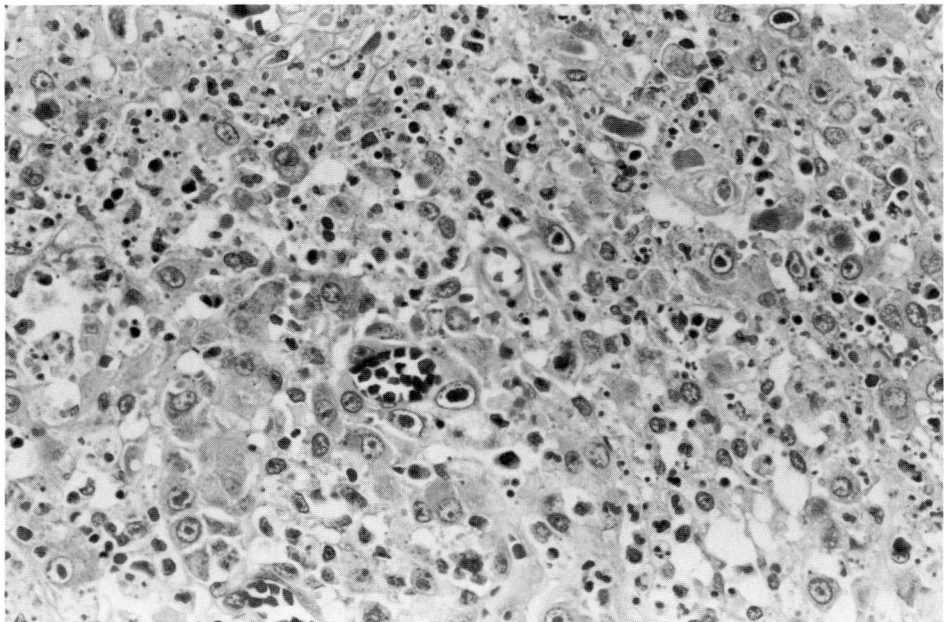

FIGURE 26–7. Granulation tissue in a colon with ulcerative colitis. The cytopathologic features of cytomegalovirus infection, centered especially around small vessels, are evident.

normalities are related not to direct damage of enterocytes, but to altered differentiation of epithelial cells as cell renewal patterns change.[53] Although the histopathologic lesions of these infections have been characterized in limited biopsy studies, diagnosis is most often circumstantial or immunologic.

Specific Viral Enteritis

Although much less common than the above conditions, infections with two members of the herpes group, herpes simplex virus and cytomegalovirus, are more likely to be encountered by the pathologist. Both of these viruses have been recognized recently in the gastrointestinal tract of immunoincompetent individuals and in homosexual males. Lesions associated with these viruses can be identified by demonstration of characteristic giant cells and intranuclear inclusions in the case of herpes simplex, and the presence of cytomegaly with intranuclear and/or cytoplasmic inclusions in the case of cytomegalovirus. Immunoperoxidase techniques can be utilized to show specific antigen in these lesions.

Herpesvirus Infection

Herpes simplex virus is recognized as an important cause of proctitis in homosexual males having anal receptive intercourse.[55] Signs and symptoms include anorectal pain, tenesmus, constipation, difficult in urinating, sacral paresthesias, and inguinal adenopathy. Physical examination may reveal perianal vesicular lesions, and sigmoidoscopic findings include mucosal friability and distal rectal ulcers or vesicles. Histopathologic findings in herpetic proctitis may be largely nonspecific, with crypt abscesses and increased numbers of neutrophils in the lamina propria. Some patients manifest more characteristic findings in addition, including perivascular lymphocytic cuffing in the submucosa, intranuclear inclusions, and multinucleated giant cells with "ground-glass" nuclei in the submucosa.

Cytomegalovirus Infection

Cytomegalovirus infection of the digestive tract is being seen with increasing frequency because of its common occurrence in patients with AIDS and in iatrogenically immunosuppressed transplant patients.[56,57] The infection has also been noted as a complicating feature of ulcerative colitis.[58,59] In the colon, cytomegalovirus has been associated with hemorrhage, ulceration, and perforation; but the role of the virus in *initiating* the mucosal damage is not clear. Some evidence suggests that the virus is simply an opportunist that colonizes established lesions, whereas other data point to a primary role. There is some indication that cytomegalovirus preferentially infects rapidly proliferating granulation tissue, perhaps aggravating various primary injuries.[60] Some authors have claimed that such cytomegalovirus infection may lead to worsening or intractability of underlying ulcerative colitis, whereas others have considered the infection without effect on the course of the colitis.[59,61] In most instances, the cytomegalovirus associated with ulcerative lesions seems to have a special affinity for cells in and around small vessels (Figure 26–7) but is rarely found in epithelial cells. Infected cells are significantly enlarged, with an increase in both nuclear and cytoplasmic volume. The typical virocyte has a large, basophilic to amphophilic intranuclear inclusion surrounded by a zone of nuclear clearing. Somewhat granular inclusion material of similar tinctorial character may be seen in the cytoplasm as well.

Chlamydial Infections

Chlamydiae, well recognized as etiologic agents of ocular, respiratory, and genital infections, are increasingly being documented as a cause of disease in the distal large intestine. Certain subtypes of the species *Chlamydia trachomatis* are known to produce a spectrum of infection, ranging from trachoma and inclusion conjunctivitis to salpingitis and nongonococcal urethritis; others are associated with lymphogranuloma venereum (LGV). Both LGV and non-LGV immunotypes have been found infecting the large bowel.[62] Anorectal LGV is a recognized secondary complication of genital LGV, especially in women.[63] Primary chlamydial bowel infection, however, is recognized most often in homosexual males and can involve non-LGV as well as LGV immunotypes of *C. trachomatis*. Definitive diagnosis of chlamydial proctitis is based on isolation of the agent from the rectum or serologic evidence of its presence.

LGV strains appear to be associated with more severe disease than non-LGV strains.[62] Some patients with proven infection are essentially asymptomatic; at the opposite extreme, others present with significant pain, bleeding, and discharge of exudate. Endoscopically, findings also range from mild erythema and friability to severe mucosal disruption with ulceration and formation of fistulas. The histologic appearance of chlamydial infection is similarly variable. Some cases show only nonspecific changes of mild ASLC; others can easily be confused with chronic inflammatory bowel disease. In proctocolitis produced by LGV strains of *C. trachomatis*, biopsy specimens with chronic focally granulomatous mucosal lesions can be indistinguishable from those of Crohn's disease; and this differential diagnosis must be kept in mind. A detailed autopsy study of the bowel in patients with clinically recognized genital LGV suggests that the lesions of LGV, as contrasted with those of Crohn's colitis, are almost never seen proximal to the midportion of the descending colon.[63]

Bacterial Infections

Bacteria of many different types infect the human digestive tract and produce various combinations of gastroenteritis and/or enterocolitis. As outlined above, the pathogenesis and pathophysiology of these infections are complex and involve colonization of the small and large intestines in varying combination. Clinical manifestations of these diseases may involve simple diarrhea related to enterotoxin-induced alterations in mucosal water absorption and secretion, dysentery due to the invasive and destructive action of the bacteria, or a combination of the two. Specific diagnosis of bacterial infections generally involves cultural or serologic identification of the etiologic agent, because clinical syndromes tend to overlap and pathologic features are most often nonspecific.

Salmonellosis and Shigellosis

The "classic" bacterial pathogens of the intestinal tract are *Salmonella* organisms, typically agents of "food poisoning," and *Shigella* organisms of various species, often associated with epidemics of bacillary dysentery. These organisms can actually produce a range of signs and symptoms from watery diarrhea to full-blown dysentery, with fever, abdominal pain, and bloody diarrhea. These agents are thought to colonize both the small intestine and the large intestine, but the detailed pathologic features of the small intestine have not been as well studied as has the appearance of the large intestine, especially the rectum. Findings of a recent colonoscopic study on shigellosis indicate that the rectosigmoid is the most frequently and most severely infected level of the colon, and that there are lesser degrees of proximal extension during the course of the disease.[64] The endoscopic appearance of *Salmonella* and *Shigella* colitis can vary from relatively mild mucosal inflammation with hyperemia and contact bleeding to a raggedly eroded surface. Biopsy studies in both salmonellosis and shigellosis have shown the proctocolitis to be characterized by nondistortive, relatively superficial changes detailed above as those of ASLC[65,66] (Figure 26-8). These histopathologic characteristics do not permit the designation of a specific etiologic agent without collateral microbiologic or serologic data, but do generally allow the distinction between "acute infectious colitis" and chronic inflammatory bowel disease, such as ulcerative colitis. A study from West Bengal reports, to the contrary, that lesions of shigellosis may mimic the crypt distortion of ulcerative colitis.[67] This may be a reflection of the particular characteristics and environment of that study population.

Campylobacter Enterocolitis

Since 1977, when effective and practical means of culture became available, members of the genus *Campylobacter*, especially *C. jejuni*, have emerged as important intestinal pathogens.[68,69] These organisms are widespread in mammals and birds and can survive well in the environment. Thus, sources of human infection include food, milk, water, and animal contact. The infection tends to involve young patients with no particular predisposing factors. The clinical features of *Campylobacter* infection do not allow it to be distinguished from other enteric infections without culture. Like many other enteric infections, the disease is usually self-limited. At one extreme, some patients have a mild diarrheal disease suggestive of viral gastroenteritis; at the other, signs and symptoms of a severe colitic illness with grossly bloody stools may closely mimic ulcerative colitis. The colonoscopic appearance may like-

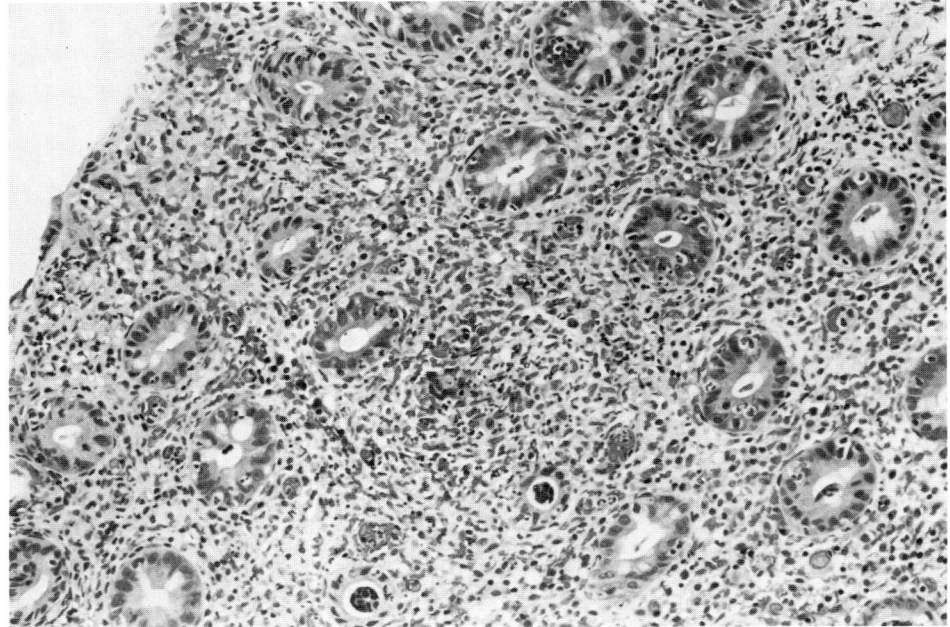

FIGURE 26–8. *Salmonella* colitis. The neutrophilic infiltrate, acute cryptitis, and the lack of significant crypt distortion are characteristic of acute infectious colitis or so-called acute self-limited colitis. Compare with Figure 26–6.

wise easily be confused with that of ulcerative colitis, with mucosal congestion and edema, friability, and granularity.

Campylobacter infection apparently involves the small intestine as well as the colon, but the disease in the small intestine has not been as well characterized by biopsy study. There is evidence that *C. jejuni* may produce an enterotoxin leading to a secretory diarrhea of the sort seen in cholera.[68] Other evidence demonstrates that the organisms are invasive in the manner of *Shigella* and *Salmonella*, usually within the bowel wall but occasionally extending parenterally.

The biopsy appearance of *Campylobacter* colitis has been well characterized, and it does not differ from that associated with other enteric agents, such as *Salmonella* or *Shigella*, i.e., with a range of appearances from mild mucosal edema and increased cellularity of the lamina propria to a full-blown picture of acute ASLC[70,71] (Figure 26–9). Because of the clinical mimicry of ulcerative colitis by *Campylobacter* infection, it is of obvious importance to distinguish between the two. Because a significant fraction of truly infected patients may appear "negative" on culture, biopsy assumes great practical significance and has been shown to be an effective means of making this important distinction.[47]

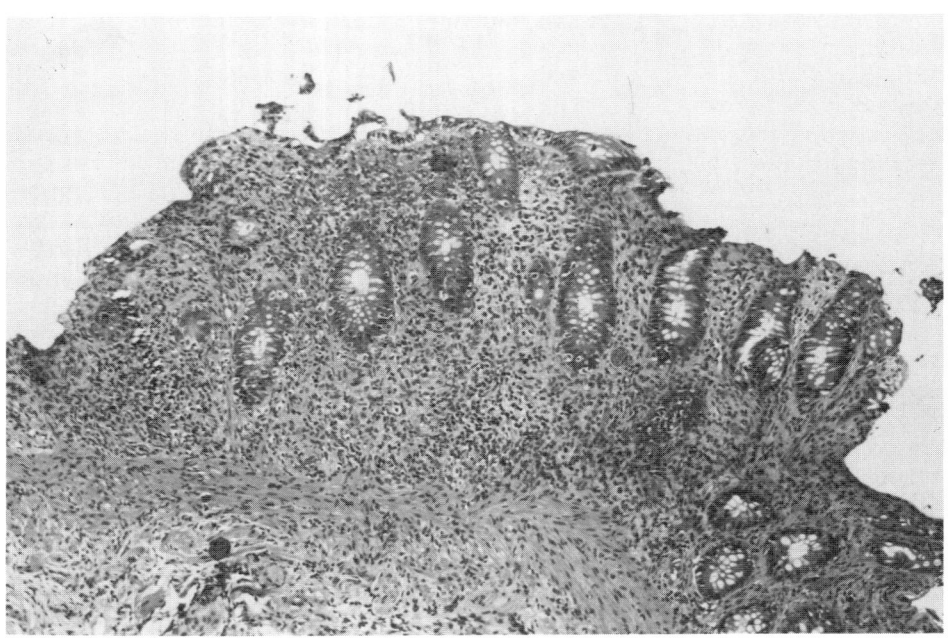

FIGURE 26–9. *Campylobacter* colitis. This infection is also characterized by the pattern of acute self-limited colits.

Yersinia Enterocolitis

Another group of enteric bacterial infections being recognized with increased frequency are those involving members of the genus *Yersinia*, aerobic, gram-negative organisms formerly classified in the genus *Pasteurella*.[72,73] Infection with these organisms has been traced to contaminated food, animal contact, and even person-to-person transmission. Infants, children, and young adults are most often affected. The commonest manifestations of *Yersinia* infection are those of a self-limited enterocolitis with abdominal pain, diarrhea, fever, and bloody stools. In a significant fraction of patients, particularly older children and adults, signs and symptoms point to right lower quadrant disease closely mimicking appendicitis. In a small number of patients, yersinial septicemia may ensue.

Yersinial lesions are most often recognized in material obtained at laparotomy for presumed appendicitis. The usual gross features in such cases are those of a striking mesenteric lymphadenopathy, often a normal-appearing appendix, and evidence of inflammation of terminal ileum and proximal colon, with thickening and edema of the bowel wall, prominence of Peyer's patches, and scattered mucosal ulcers. The findings may be suggestive of Crohn's disease or even tuberculosis. In *Y. enterocolitica* infections, the characteristic microscopic feature is lymphofollicular hyperplasia with microabscesses in the mesenteric lymph nodes and bowel wall. In the ileum, colon, and appendix, mucosal ulcers of various sizes are seen surfaced by fibrinopurulent exudate and sometimes associated with clusters of gram-negative bacteria. Characteristically, the small aphthous ulcers are situated over hyperplastic lymphoid follicles (Figure 26–10).[74] Similar changes have been described in association with *Y. pseudotuberculosis* but with a distinct granulomatous component surrounding the microabscesses in lymphoid tissue.[75] In addition to the lesions recognized in the ileocecal area, colorectal endoscopy has revealed more widespread colitic lesions, including aphthous ulcers.[72]

Tuberculosis

Mycobacteria of various types are also encountered occasionally as a cause of intestinal disease. *Mycobacterium tuberculosis*, long recognized as an etiologic agent of enteric disease, remains an important pathogen in developing countries but a less common one in the western world. *Mycobacterium avium*, on the other hand, has emerged as a "new" infectious agent in immunocompromised hosts. Infection of AIDS patients with this later agent is discussed in Chapter 14.

Tubercle bacilli are apparently capable of penetrating the intestinal mucosa after being swallowed. At one time, bovine strains of *M. tuberculosis* were important in this regard, but bovine tuberculosis has been virtually eliminated in economically developed countries. It appears that most gastrointestinal tuberculosis in much of the world now represents infection with human strains, presumably with a pulmonary route of initial entry. Older studies[76] showing the greater incidence of intestinal tuberculosis in patients with more advanced pulmonary tuberculosis with cavitation suggest swallowing of infected sputum as an initiating event. However, it has become increasingly apparent that at the time of clinical presentation of the enteric tuberculous lesion, there may be no radiographic evidence of pulmonary infection.

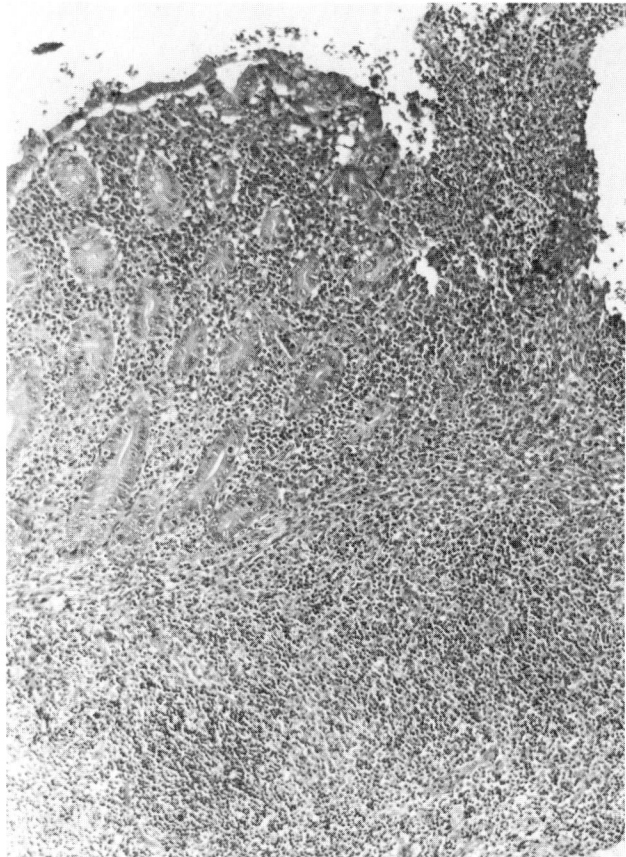

FIGURE 26–10. *Yersinia* appendicitis. This infection is characterized by aphthous ulcers (top) overlying hyperplastic lymphoid follicles, and microabscesses in regional nodes.

The signs and symptoms associated with enteric tuberculosis are highly variable, given the fact that various levels of the small and large bowel may be involved and that perforation, hemorrhage, obstruction, and fistula formation may all occur. Some cases have presented as mechanical small-bowel obstruction, apparent appendicitis, and even segmental colonic stricture.[77] Abdominal pain is a universal finding, as is the demonstration of abnormality on contrast radiography. Reflecting the fact that the ileocecal region is by far the commonest site of intestinal tuberculosis, the presence of a right lower quadrant mass is a common sign.[78]

Intestinal tuberculosis is grossly characterized by an inflammatory mass in the affected segment of gut, usually with secondary mesenteric lymphadenopathy. Lesions exhibit various combinations of mucosal ulceration, classically transverse, and inflammatory thickening of the wall. Grossly, as well as radiographically, the features of enteric tuberculosis and Crohn's disease may be virtually identical. Microscopically, intestinal lesions of tuberculosis are similar to tuberculous lesions

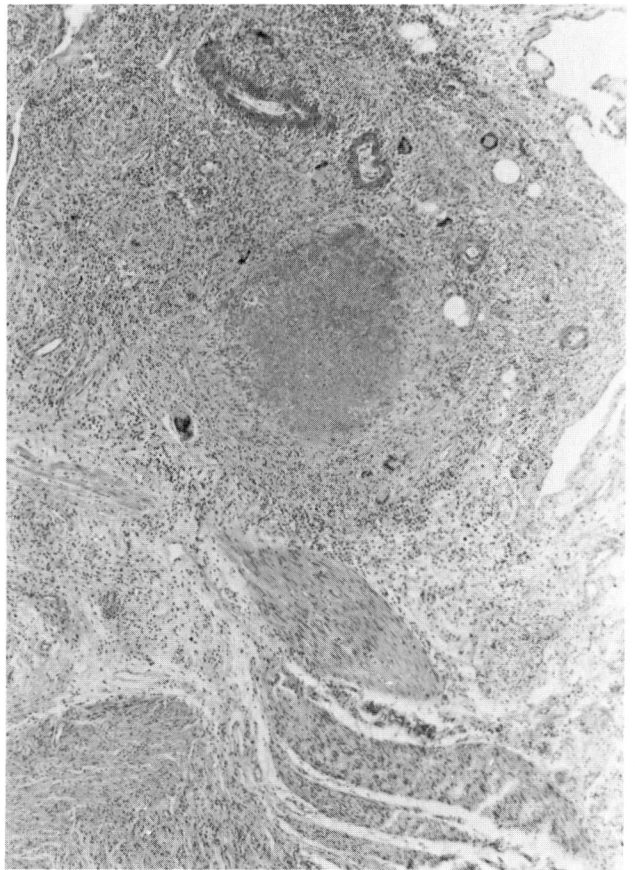

FIGURE 26–11. Ileocecal tuberculosis. This large granuloma in the submucosa, unlike those of Crohn's disease, shows central caseation.

elsewhere in the body, with necrotizing granulomata as their hallmark. The granulomata tend to be more florid than those of Crohn's disease, and caseation is found in the larger granulomata (Figure 26–11). Even when necrosis is not especially prominent in the intramural lesions, the associated lymph nodes usually show caseation.[76] As in any tuberculous lesions, acid-fast bacilli are variably demonstrable histologically with appropriate stains.

Actinomycosis

Actinomycosis is another infection with one of the "higher bacteria" (i.e., organisms related to *Streptomyces, Mycobacterium,* and *Nocardia*) that may be encountered in the bowel. *Actinomyces israelii* is the usual etiologic agent of human actinomycosis, other species of the genus being found only occasionally.[79] The organism is a normal commensal inhabitant of the digestive tract, especially in the oropharyngeal region. Actinomycosis apparently results from the introduction of the organism from the lumen into the tissues in the course of some other disease or after accidental or surgical trauma. Some have claimed a synergistic role for other microbes, occasionally demonstrated in actinomycotic lesions; but the evidence is not conclusive. Abdominal actinomycosis accounts for one fifth to one third of cases, the majority being cervicofacial and thoracic.[80] Many abdominal cases have been reported to follow appendectomy, cholecystectomy, or operation for diverticular disease, trauma, or neoplasm. The clinical manifestations are extremely variable but are generally those of local inflammation with draining abscesses.

The typical gross lesions of actinomycosis associated with the gut, as elsewhere in the body, are abscesses with tough, fibrous walls enclosing loculi filled with yellow to white pus, often associated with sinus tracts. Although classically "sulfur granules" are described in the exudate, these may not be evident grossly in many cases. Microscopically, the typical actinomycotic lesion is an abscess, often multiloculated, with a surrounding zone of vascular granulation tissue and scar. Large, foamy macrophages typically surround the suppura-

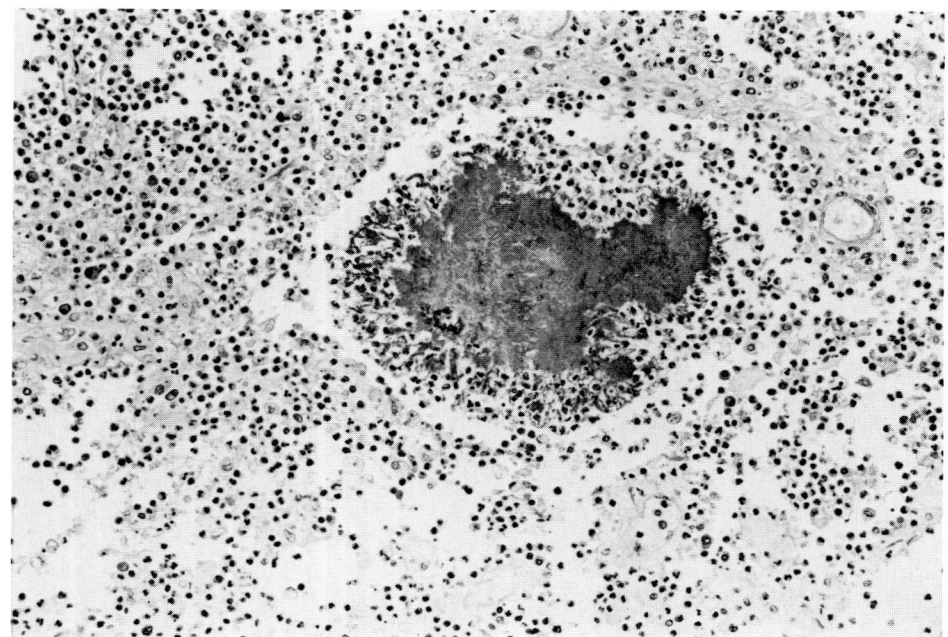

FIGURE 26–12. Actinomycosis. This infection is characterized by the presence of "granules" within areas of suppuration, such as the one shown.

tive centers of the lesions, with scattered lymphocytes and plasma cells in the granulation tissue.[80] The feature that is histologically diagnostic of the infection (cultural verification is often difficult) is the grain or granule found floating in the pus. In preparations stained with hematoxylin and eosin, the granules are spherical to ovoid masses averaging approximately 300 µm in diameter with lightly basophilic to amphophilic central regions and a peripheral fringe of radiating eosinophilic clubs (Figure 26–12). Organisms *per se* cannot be resolved well in routine preparations. In Brown-Brenn–stained sections, gram-positive, slender, branching, beaded bacilli can be demonstrated, tangled in the center of the granules, more parallel in their arrangement at the periphery in relation to the clubs. Differential diagnosis includes nocardiosis, staphylococcal botryomycosis, and fungal infections, all of which may involve granular clusters of organisms. *Nocardia* tends to form loose masses without clubs and, unlike actinomyces, is acid-fast. Staphylococci and fungi can be distinguished by their morphologic characteristics.

Intestinal Spirochetosis

Mention should be made of so-called intestinal spirochetosis, although its inclusion with the intestinal infections is somewhat debatable. The morphologic features of spirochetal colonization of the colon were first specifically delineated in 1967, although the presence of spirochetes in the gut flora had long been known.[81] This study revealed a 9% incidence of spirochetosis in consecutive biopsy specimens. The dense population of spirochetes is readily recognized by light microscopy (Figure 26–13) and can be seen by electron microscopy

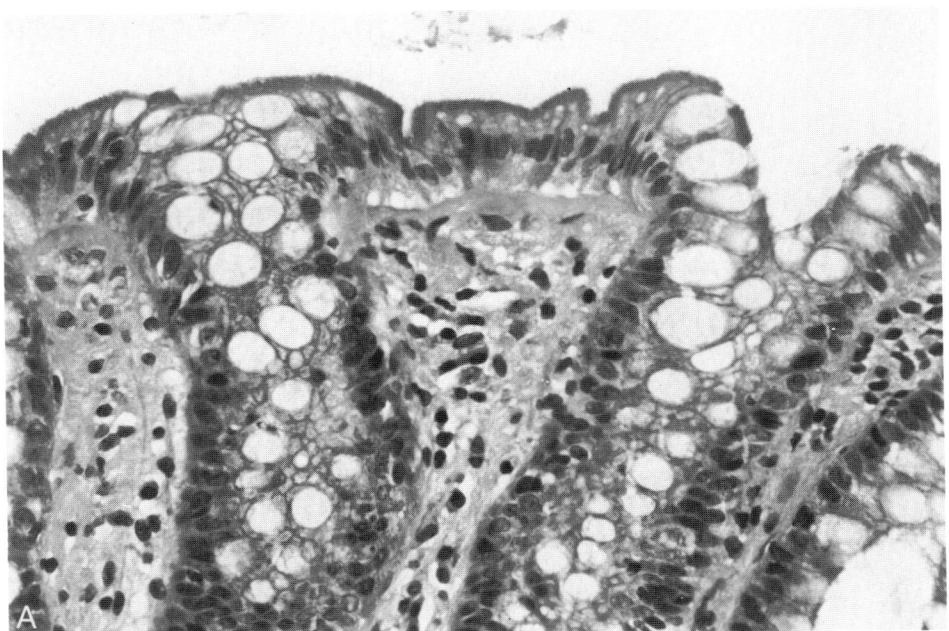
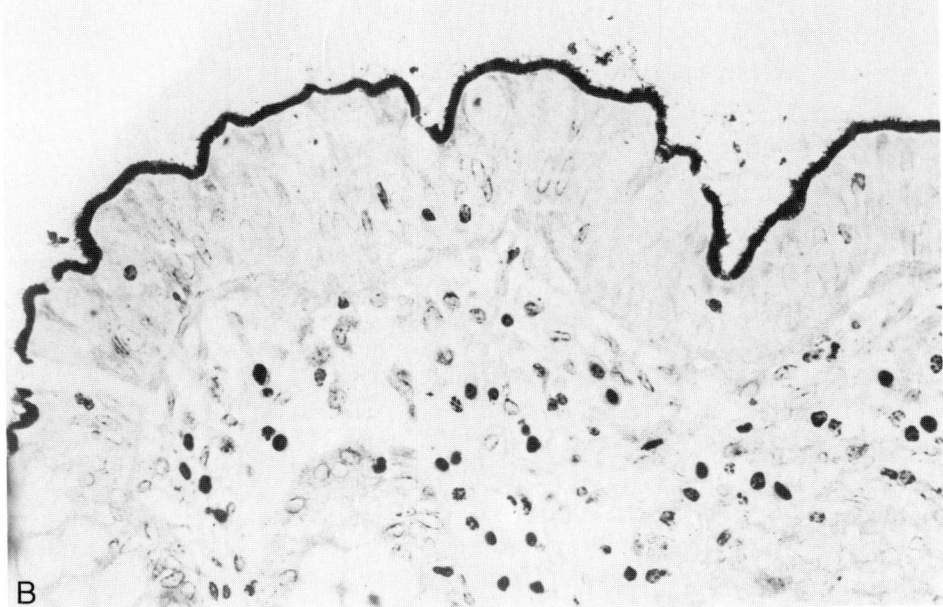

FIGURE 26–13. Colonic spirochetosis. In routine preparations (A) there is "accentuation" of the luminal border of epithelial cells, which is seen with the Warthin-Starry (or Churukian-Schenk) silver stain (B) to be an oriented layer of bacteria.

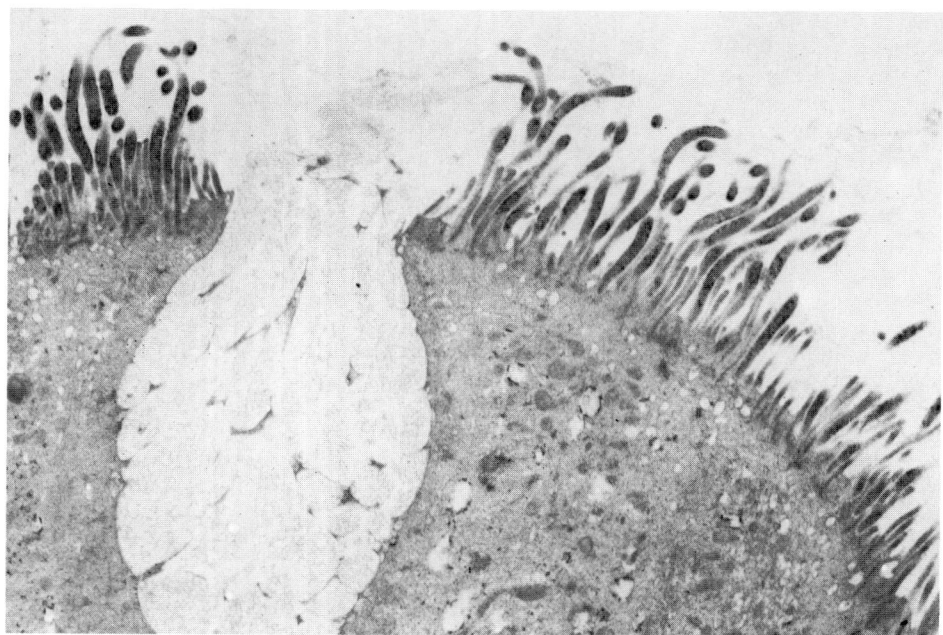

FIGURE 26–14. Colonic spirochetosis. The electron micrograph reveals spirochetes oriented longitudinally among microvilli.

to be regularly oriented among the microvilli of epithelial cells (Figure 26–14). In many published studies, the incidence of colorectal or appendiceal spirochetosis ranges between 1% and 10%, and the evidence suggests that the organisms are nonpathogenic.[82,83] In some instances, however, spirochetosis has been associated with symptoms, with resolution of the symptoms and disappearance of the spirochetes after antimicrobial therapy.[84,85] Spirochetosis has also been found to have a higher incidence in "pseudoappendicitis" (i.e., cases in which the appendix was removed because of symptoms of appendicitis and found to be not inflamed) than in appendices removed incidentally through other procedures.[86] Spirochetosis has also been found with significantly greater frequency in male subjects with a history of anal intercourse, although the significance of this is as yet obscure.[87]

Gonorrhea and Syphilis

In addition to the various bacteria listed above, others not ordinarily thought of as intestinal pathogens can be found infecting the gut. Because most of these do not have unique symptoms or produce pathognomonic morphologic changes, diagnosis generally depends on demonstration of the specific organisms or serologic evidence of their presence. In particular, sexually transmitted agents of many sorts, including *Neisseria gonorrhoeae* and *Treponema pallidum* have been found frequently in homosexual males with symptomatic anorectal disease.[88]

In a series of men with culture-proven rectal gonorrhea but without concomitant gastrointestinal infections, many had no anorectal symptoms, and in 84% the rectal mucosa appeared normal by proctoscopic examination. A small number had signs of distal proctitis. Histologically, only 42% showed any abnormality—most often an increase in lymphocytes and plasma cells in the lamina propria. Only a few subjects had an acute inflammatory infiltrate in the mucosa.[89] In another study of 89 homosexual men with intestinal symptoms, less than half had histologic abnormalities on biopsy.[90] No sigmoidoscopic appearance or histologic pattern was specific for any infection. Acute inflammatory changes were the most common histologic abnormalities. Chronic inflammatory changes (including increased chronic inflammatory cells in the submucosa, granulomas, and lymphoid follicles) were uncommon but were significantly associated syphilis, herpes simplex virus, and *C. trachomatis*. The authors concluded that when histologic features of idiopathic inflammatory bowel disease are found in a homosexual man, syphilis and chlamydial infection in particular need to be ruled out carefully before a diagnosis of idiopathic inflammatory bowel disease is entertained.[90]

Fungal Infections

Candidiasis and Mucormycosis

Mycotic infections of the gut are usually encountered as secondary phenomena in debilitated patients, especially those with leukemia or lymphoma; those with other diseases associated with immunologic impairment; and those who have been treated with cytotoxic agents, steroids, and antibiotics. Candidiasis and mucormycosis (Figure 26–15) appear to be the most important of the opportunistic infections. Although any level of the tract may be involved, infections with *Candida* species are more likely to be found in the mouth, esophagus, and stomach; lesions of mucormycosis show a predilection for the stomach and colon.[91,92] The organisms are ordinarily recognized in profusion in the lesions, which vary from areas of superficial erosion to foci of transmural hemorrhage and necrosis.

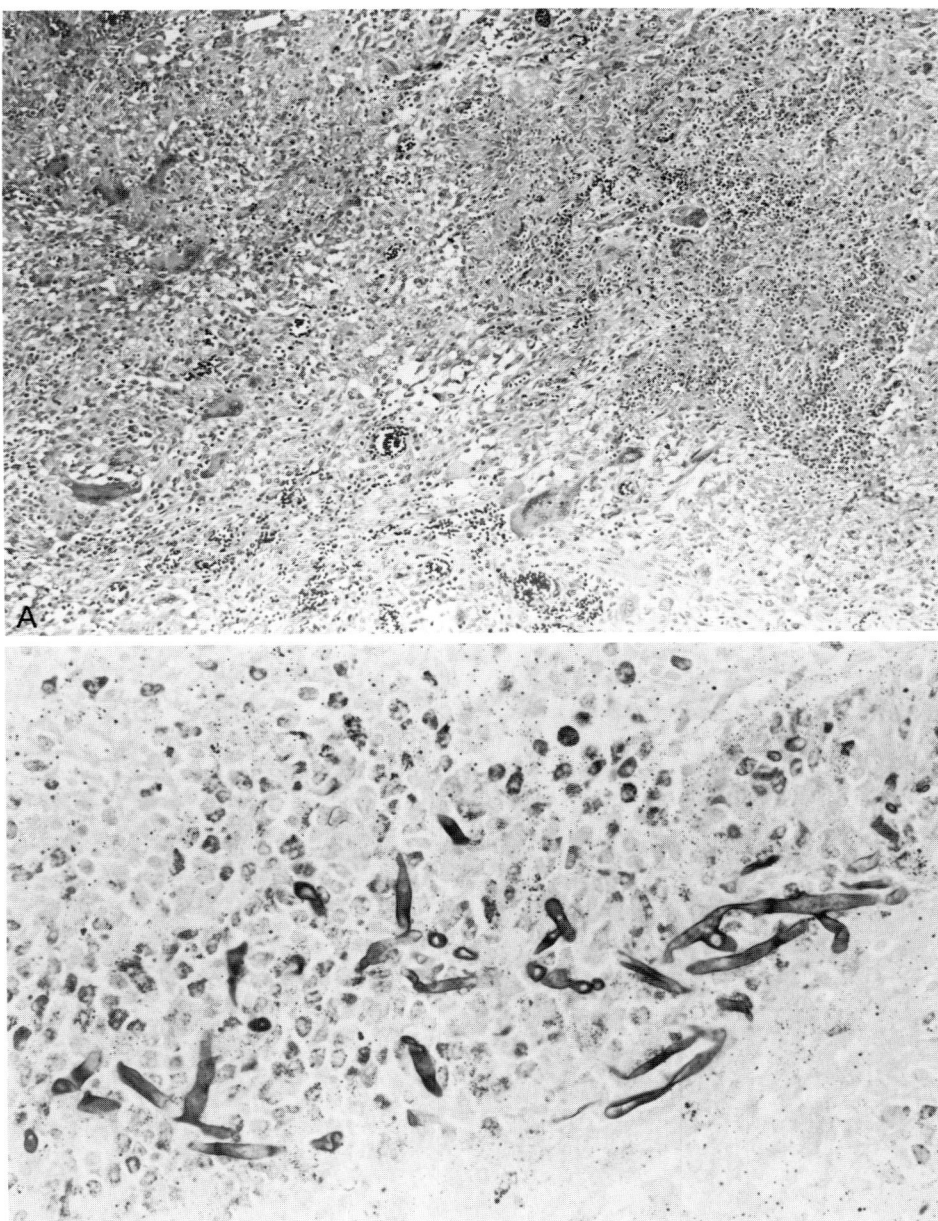

FIGURE 26–15. Colonic mucormycosis. An area of necrotizing, suppurative, and granulomatous inflammation in the wall (A) is seen with the methenamine silver stain (B) to be mycotic.

Histoplasmosis

The digestive tract is occasionally involved as part of a primary mycotic infection, i.e., in individuals who are not first overtly debilitated by some other disease. Infection with *Histoplasma capsulatum*, found in many parts of the world, but endemic in the eastern central United States, is usually acquired by inhalation of spores from organisms residing in the soil. Although histoplasmosis is most often a benign, asymptomatic pulmonary infection, in a small fraction of affected individuals disseminated infection develops.[93] Autopsy studies indicate that approximately 75% of patients with disseminated histoplasmosis have lesions in the small intestine, colon, or liver. The ileum is most frequently involved, closely followed by the colon, with occasional lesions in the appendix or at various other levels of the digestive tract. These gastrointestinal lesions are evident clinically in only a small minority of cases. In these few patients, the fungal lesions may mimic carcinoma, lymphoma, tuberculosis, or idiopathic inflammatory bowel disease, pain and diarrhea being the most frequent complaints. Although it seems probable that intestinal lesions reflect spread of organisms from the lung, the possibility of an enteric portal of primary entry cannot be excluded in all cases. The intestinal lesions are ulcerative and granulomatous, with presumptive diagnosis resting on demonstration of budding yeast forms in the lesions and definitive diagnosis, on culture of the organism.[94]

Protozoan Infection

Amebiasis

Infection with *Entamoeba histolytica* is prevalent in much of the world and is sometimes endemic in developing countries. Amebiasis has also been recognized recently as a particular problem in homosexual males.[88] The possibility of confusion clinically and endoscopically with ulcerative colitis and with Crohn's disease makes recognition of this infection important.

The amebae are ingested as cysts from the environment; after excystation, the trophozoites colonize the large intestine. This process is facilitated by an association between the amebae and bacteria resident in the gut. As is true for many other enteric organisms, specific adherence of the *E. histolytica* to mucosal lining cells is a critical step in pathogenesis. The organisms are then capable of invading the bowel wall and destroying host tissue, a process apparently mediated by proteolytic enzymes, cell-free cytotoxins, and a process of contact-dependent cytolysis.[95]

On the basis of autopsy study, the primary target of amebic attack appears to be the cecum and ascending colon, with subsequent spread to other locations. The usual lesions in the gut are ulcerative, but occasionally exuberant inflammation and formation of granulation tissue produce an ameboma, which may simulate a neoplasm. Complications of amebiasis include direct extension to perineal skin, intestinal perforation, and parenteral dissemination via blood vessels and lymphatics.[96]

In a detailed rectal biopsy study, Prathap and Gilman[97] recognized several types of amebic lesions:

1. A nonspecific lesion characterized by mucosal hyperemia, edema, patchy mucin depletion, and focal neutrophilic infiltration. At best, few amebae are seen in surface exudate.
2. A mucopenic depression in the mucosa, produced by depletion of epithelial mucin, with focal surface erosion. Amebae are present immediately adjacent to the area of superficial lysis of epithelium.
3. An early invasive lesion with superficial ulceration and amebae present in the tissue.
4. A late invasive lesion with deep ulceration, the classic flask-shaped ulcer. Amebae are present in the exudate, which is not especially cellular.
5. A granulating ulcer with a nonspecific appearance and no amebae.

In general, the diagnosis is suggested only when the amebae happen to be visualized in the biopsy (Figure 26–16), and strands of mucus associated with the mucosa therefore deserve careful scrutiny. In a sigmoidoscopic biopsy study in patients with documented amebic colitis, Pittman and Hennigar[98] stressed that a diffuse *nonspecific* inflammatory response was characteristic and that amebae might be absent from a significant fraction of biopsies. Conversely, many accounts suggest that amebae may often evoke little or no inflammatory response. Conceivably, amebae may differ in this regard, or possibly a brisk inflammatory response reflects secondary infection. Chances for making the diagnosis of amebiasis are best in any event, if the organisms are sought in fresh stool or exudate obtained at the time of endoscopy.

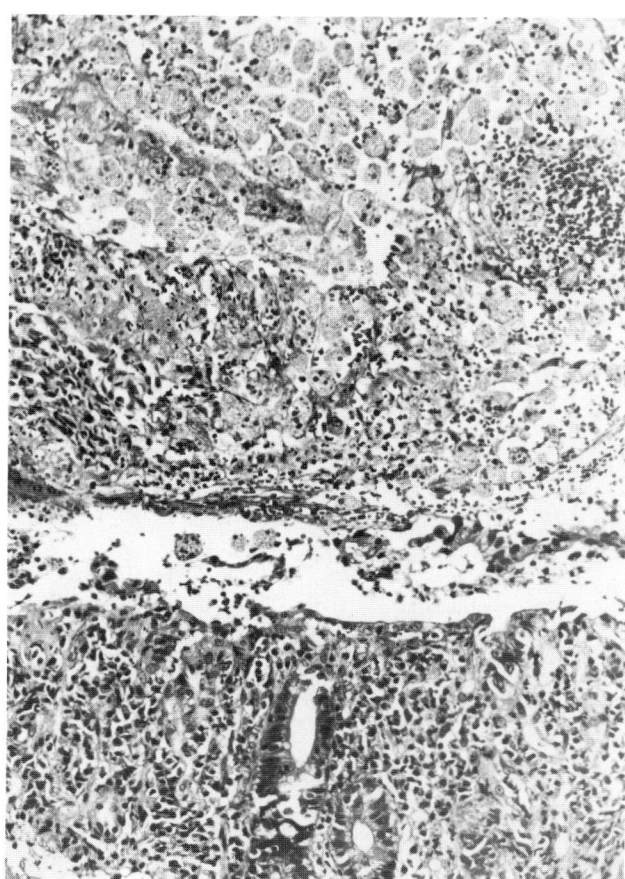

FIGURE 26–16. Amebiasis. The features of the mucosal inflammatory process (lower part of field) are nonspecific. Diagnosis rests on recognition of amebae in the surface exudate, in profusion at the top of this field.

Giardiasis

Giardia lamblia is another protozoan found worldwide that is often a cause of infectious diarrhea.[99] Water, containing the cyst forms of the organism, appears to be the major source of infection. After ingestion, excystation is begun in the stomach, and the small intestine is then colonized by the trophozoites. The organisms attach to the microvillous border of enterocytes by means of adhesive disks, and they can often be seen in biopsy specimens as arched or sickle-shaped forms attached to the microvillous border (Figure 26–17).

Clinically, giardiasis varies from an asymptomatic infection to a severe diarrheal disease that may become chronic, with malabsorption and weight loss.[100] There is a particular association with various hypogammaglobulinemic disorders. Biopsy of the upper small intestine yields a spectrum of appearances, many infected patients having a normal histologic appearance. Varying degrees of enterocyte damage can be seen, with shortening of the villi, expansion of lamina pro-

INFECTIOUS DISORDERS OF THE INTESTINES 639

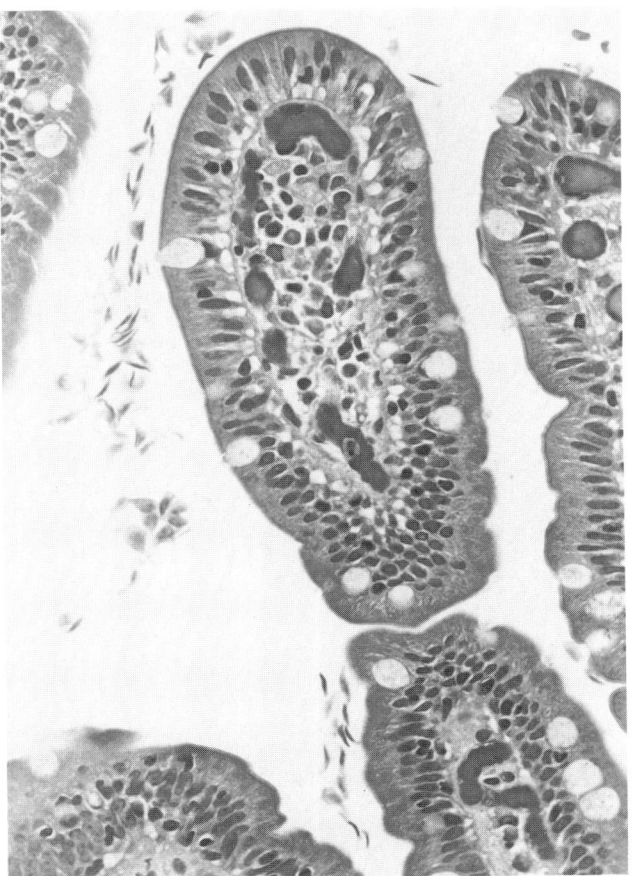

FIGURE 26–17. Giardiasis. Numerous organisms are seen along the villous surface (separation is an artefect), in profile, as crescent or sickle shapes, or occasionally *en face*, as at the lower left.

pria, and an increase in epithelial mitotic activity. In the extreme, the histologic picture may resemble that of sprue. More severe structural abnormalities tend to be found in immunodeficient patients. The pathogenesis of the disease is not completely understood but may involve enzymatic alterations associated with direct damage to enterocytes, loss of surface area associated with atrophy of the villi, altered turnover of epithelial cells, and release of prostaglandin from macrophages.[99] Diagnosis is based on demonstration of the organisms in duodenal jejunal biopsy specimens, aspirates of duodenal fluid, or stool specimens.

Coccidiosis

Protozoans of the subclass Coccidia have also been implicated recently in human infection, having long been recognized in infection of other animal species. These infections may be zoonotic or person-to-person and are associated with variable syndromes of diarrhea and malabsorption.[101,102] Organisms of the genus *Isospora* and the genus *Cryptosporidium* have been identified in human hosts, the former as intracytoplasmic parasites within enterocytes of the small intestine and the latter closely associated with the microvillous border of enterocytes, possibly within host-cell membrane.[103] *Isospora* infection has been identified as a rare cause of intractable diarrhea and malabsorption.[104]

Cryptosporidiosis, first identified as a human problem just over a decade ago, is seen as an opportunistic infection in immunocompromised patients, especially those with AIDS, but also infects immunocompetent subjects. The diarrheal disease in the latter group tends to be of short duration, whereas in the former it may often be intractable, persistent to the death of the subject. The small bowel seems to be the main site of colonization; but in immunocompromised subjects, organisms may be seen from pharynx to rectum. Infection of the small intestine may be accompanied by abnormalities in crypt architecture and variable inflammation in the lamina propria. The organisms are seen as tiny basophilic spheres seemingly attached to the microvillous border (Figure 26–18). Diagnosis can be

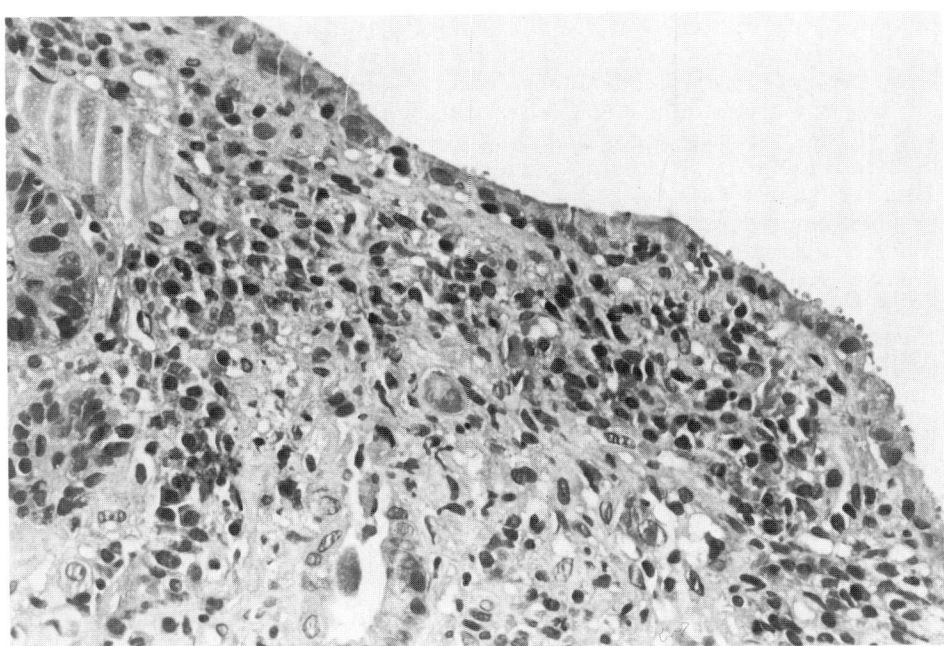

FIGURE 26–18. Cryptosporidiosis. The organisms have the appearance of tiny spheres along the microvillus border.

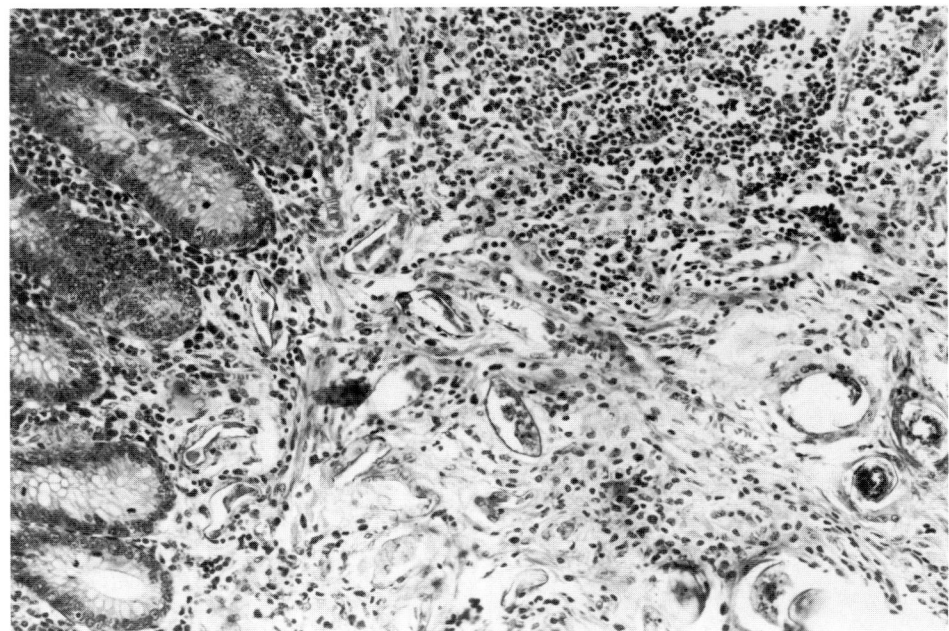

FIGURE 26–19. Schistosomiasis. Diagnosis rests on recognition of ova, surrounded by an inflammatory reaction, which is often granulomatous (right), and fibrosis.

confirmed not only by biopsy but also by examination of fecal concentrates.[105]

Helminthic Infection

The human gut can be infected by a wide variety of helminthic parasites; descriptions of them are beyond the scope of this discussion but are detailed in standard references.[106] Specific mention, however, should be made of schistosomiasis, a serious disease in many parts of the world that may be associated with significant lesions of the bowel. Adult *Schistosoma japonicum* and *Schistosoma mansoni* live in the mesenteric circulation, and the large numbers of ova produced by the parasites pass through the bowel wall. The granulomatous inflammatory reaction elicited by the ova may lead to polypoid and ulcerative gross lesions of the distal large bowel reminiscent of Crohn's disease or even a neoplasm.[107] It has been reported that the continuing mucosal proliferative changes in chronic schistosomiasis may be associated with the development of colonic carcinoma in a manner analogous to that in ulcerative colitis.[108] Accurate diagnosis of colonic schistosomiasis rests on recognition of the ova. The inflammatory reaction to the ova varies with time, ranging from diffuse cellular to granulomatous to fibrotic (Figure 26–19).

References

1. Simon G, Gorbach SL: Intestinal flora in health and disease. Gastroenterology 86:174–193, 1984.
2. Savage DC: Overview of the association of microbes with epithelial surfaces. Microecol Ther 14:169–182, 1984.
3. Drasar BS, Hill MS: The metabolic activities of gut bacteria. In Drasar BS, Hill MS: Human Intestinal Flora. Academic Press, New York, 1974, pp 51–168.
4. Prizont R, Konigsberg N: Identification of bacterial glycosidases in rat cecal contents. Dig Dis Sci 26:773–777, 1981.
5. Abrams GD, Bishop JE: Effect of the normal microbial flora on gastrointestinal motility. Proc Soc Exp Biol Med 126:301–304, 1967.
6. Abrams GD, Bauer H, Sprinz H: Influence of the normal flora on mucosal morphology and cellular renewal in the ileum: A comparison of germfree and conventional mice. Lab Invest 12:355–364, 1963.
7. Yolton DP, Stanley C, Savage DC: Influence of the indigenous gastrointestinal microbial flora on duodenal alkaline phosphatase activity in mice. Infect Immun 3:768–773, 1971.
8. Gianella RA, Broitman SA, Zamcheck N: The gastric barrier to microorganisms in man: In vivo and in vitro studies. Gut 13:251–256, 1972.
9. Borriello SP, Reed PJ, Dolby JM, et al: Microbial and metabolic profile of achlorhydric stomach: Comparison of pernicious anemia and hypogammaglobulinaemia. J Clin Pathol 38:946–953, 1985.
10. Hornick RB, Music SI, Wenzel R, et al: The Broad Street pump revisited: Response of volunteers to ingested cholera vibrios. Bull NY Acad Med 47:1181–1191, 1971.
11. Gianella RA, Broitman SA, Zamcheck N: Influence of gastric acidity on bacterial and parasitic enteric infections. Ann Intern Med 78:271–276, 1973.
12. Dixon JMS: The fate of bacteria in the small intestine. J Pathol Bacteriol 79:131–140, 1960.
13. Formal SB, Abrams GD, Schneider H, Sprinz H: Experimental Shigella infections. VI. Role of the small intestine in an experimental infection in guinea pigs. J Bacteriol 85:119–125, 1963.
14. Dupont HL, Hornick RB: Adverse effect of lomotil therapy in Shigellosis. JAMA 226:1525–1528, 1973.
15. Abraham SN, Beachey EH: Host defenses against adhesion of bacteria to mucosal surfaces. In Gallin JI, Fauci AS (eds): Advances in Host Defense Mechanisms 4. New York, Raven Press, 1985, pp 63–88.
16. Freter R: Interdependence of mechanisms that control bacterial colonization of the large intestine. Microecol Ther 14:89–96, 1984.
17. Holmberg SD, Osterholm MT, Senger KA, Cohen ML: Drug resistant *Salmonella* from animals fed antimicrobials. N Engl J Med 311:617–622, 1984.
18. Spika JS, Waterman SH, Soo Hoo GW, et al: Chloramphenicol resistant *Salmonella newport* traced through hamburger to dairy farms. N Engl J Med 316:565–570, 1987.

19. Gracey M: The contaminated small bowel syndrome: Pathogenesis, diagnosis and treatment. Am J Clin Nutr 32:234–243, 1979.
20. Trnka YM, LaMont JT: Clostridium difficile colitis. Adv Intern Med 29:85–107, 1984.
21. Bartlett JG, Laughon B: *Clostridium difficile* toxins. Microecol Ther 14:35–42, 1984.
22. Abrams GD, Allo M, Rifkin GD, et al: Mucosal damage mediated by clostridial toxin in experimental clindamycin-associated colitis. Gut 21:493–499, 1980.
23. Price AB, Davies DR: Pseudomembranous colitis. J Clin Pathol 30:1–12, 1977.
24. Rocca JM, Pieterse AS, Rowland R, et al: *Clostridium difficile* colitis. Aust NZ J Med 14:606–610, 1984.
25. Cone JB, Wetzel W: Toxic megacolon secondary to pseudomembranous colitis. Dis Colon Rectum 25:478–482, 1982.
26. Schnett S, Antonioli A, Goldman H: Massive mural edema in severe pseudomembranous colitis. Arch Pathol Lab Med 107:211–213, 1983.
27. Cudmore M, Silva J, Fekety R: Clostridial enterocolitis produced by antineoplastic agents in hamsters and humans. Curr Chem Infect Dis 2:1460–1461, 1980.
28. Trnka YM, LaMont JT: Association of Clostridium difficile toxin with symptomatic relapse of chronic inflammatory bowel disease. Gastroenterology 80:693–696, 1981.
29. Steinberg D, Gold J, Brodin A: Necrotizing enterocolitis in leukemia. Arch Intern Med 131:538–544, 1973.
30. King A, Rampling A, Wight DGD, Warren RE: Neutropenic entero-colitis due to *Clostridium septicum* infection. J Clin Pathol 37:335–343, 1984.
31. Rampling A, Warren RE, Bevan PC, et al: *Clostridium difficile* in hematological malignancy. J Clin Pathol 38:445–451, 1985.
32. Klemm P: Fimbrial adhesins of *Escherichia coli*. Rev Infect Dis 7:321–340, 1985.
33. Levine MM, Kaper JB, Black RE, CLements ML: New knowledge on pathogenesis of bacterial infections as applied to vaccine development. Microbiol Rev 47:510–550, 1983.
34. Freter R, O'Brien PCM: Role of chemotaxis in the association of motile bacteria with intestinal mucosa: In vivo studies. Infect Immun 34:234–240, 1981.
35. Burnet FM: The mucinase of *Vibrio cholerae*. Aust J Exp Med Sci 26:71–80, 1948.
36. Formal SB, Hale TL, Sansonetti PJ: Invasive enteric pathogens. Rev Infect Dis 5(Suppl 4):S702–S707, 1983.
37. Gianella RA: Pathogenesis of acute diarrheal disorders. Ann Rev Med 32:341–357, 1981.
38. Gots RE, Formal SB, Gianella RA: Indomethacin inhibition of *Salmonella typhimurium, Shigella flexneri* and *cholerae* mediated rabbit ileal secretion. J Infect Dis 130:280–284, 1974.
39. Rask-Madsen J: Eicosanoids and their role in the pathogenesis of diarrheal diseases. Clin Gastroenterol 15:546–566, 1986.
40. Mekalanos JJ: Cholera toxin: Genetic analysis, regulation, and role in pathogenesis. Cur Top Microbiol Immunol 118:97–118, 1985.
41. Rabbani GH: Cholera. Clin Gastroenterol 3:507–528, 1986.
42. Speelman P, Butler T, Kabir I, et al: Colonic dysfunction during cholera infection. Gastroenterology 91:164–170, 1986.
43. Ulshen MH, Rollo JL: Pathogenesis of *Escherichia coli* gastroenteritis in man: Another mechanism. N Engl J Med 302:99–101, 1980.
44. O'Brien AD, Marques LRM, Newland JW, et al: Shiga and Shiga-like toxins. Microecol Ther 14:25–30, 1984.
44a. Griffin PM, Olmstead LC, Petras RE, *Escherichia coli* 0157:H7-associated colitis. A clinical and histological study of 11 cases. Gastroenterology 99:142–149, 1990.
44b. Kelly J, Oryshak A, Wenetsek M, Grabiec J, Handy S: The colonic pathology of *Escherichia coli* 0157:H7 infection. Am J Surg Pathol 14:87–93,1990.
45. Gangarosa EG, Beisel WR, Benyajati C, et al: The nature of the gastrointestinal lesion in Asiatic cholera and its relation to pathogenesis: A biopsy study. Am J Trop Med Hyg 9:125–135, 1960.
46. Kumar NB, Nostrant TT, Appelman HD: The histopathologic spectrum of acute self-limited colitis (acute infectious-type colitis). Am J Surg Pathol 523–529, 1982.
47. Nostrant TT, Kumar NB, Appelman HD: Histopathology differentiates acute self-limited colitis from ulcerative colitis. Gastroenterology 92:318–328, 1987.
48. Surawicz CM, Belic L: Rectal biopsy helps to distinguish acute self-limited colitis from idiopathic inflammatory bowel disease. Gastroenterology 86:104–113, 1984.
49. Leriche M, Devroede G, Sanchez G, Rossano J: Changes in the rectal mucosa induced by hypertonic enemas. Dis Colon Rectum 21:227–236, 1978.
50. Meisel JL, Bergman D, Graney D, et al: Human rectal mucosa: Proctoscopic and morphological changes caused by laxatives. Gastroenterology 72:1274–1279, 1977.
51. Glotzer DJ, Glick ME, Goldman H: Proctitis and colitis following diversion of the fecal stream. Gastroenterology 80:438–441, 1981.
52. Cukor G, Blacklow NR: Human viral gastroenteritis. Microbiol Rev 48:157–179, 1984.
53. Davidson GP: Viral diarrhoea. Clin Gastroenterol 15:39–53, 1986.
54. Schreiber DS, Blacklow NR, Trier JS: The mucosal lesion of the proximal small intestine in acute infectious nonbacterial gastroenteritis. N Engl J Med 288:1318–1323, 1973.
55. Goodell SE, Quinn TC, Mkrtichian E, et al: Herpes simplex proctitis in homosexual men. N Engl J Med 308:868–871, 1983.
56. Bodey GP, Fainstein V: Infections of the gastrointestinal tract in the immunocompromised patient. Ann Rev Med 37:271–281, 1986.
57. Foucar E, Mukai K, Foucar K, et al: Colon ulceration in lethal cytomegalovirus infection. Am J Clin Pathol 76:788–801, 1981.
58. Keren DF, Milligan FD, Strandberg JD, Yardley JH: Intercurrent cytomegalovirus colitis in a patient with ulcerative colitis. Johns Hopkins Med J 136:178–182, 1975.
59. Cooper HS, Raffansperger EC, Jonas L, Fitts WT: Cytomegalovirus inclusions in patients with ulcerative colitis requiring colonic resection. *Gastroenterology* 72:1253–1256, 1977.
60. Goodman ZD, Boitnott JK, Yardley JH: Perforation of the colon associated with cytomegalovirus infection. Dig Dis Sci 24:376–380, 1979.
61. Eyre-Brook IA, Dundas S: Incidence and clinical significance of colonic cytomegalovirus infection in idiopathic inflammatory bowel disease requiring colectomy. Gut 27:1419–1425, 1986.
62. Quinn TC, Goodell SE, Mkrtichian E, et al: *Chlamydia trachomatis proctitis*. N Engl J Med 305:195–200, 1981.
63. dela Monte SM, Hutchins GM: Follicular proctocolitis and neuromatous hyperplasia with lymphogranuloma venereum. Hum Pathol 16:1025–1032, 1985.
64. Speelman P, Kabir I, Islam M: Distribution and spread of colonic lesions in shigellosis: A colonoscopic study. J Inf Dis 150:899–903, 1984.
65. Day DW, Mandal BK, Morson BC: The rectal biopsy appearances in Salmonella colitis. Histopathology 2:117–131, 1978.
66. McGovern VJ, Slavutin LJ: Pathology of Salmonella colitis. Am J Surg Pathol 3:483–490, 1979.
67. Anand BS, Malhotra V, Bhattacharya SK, et al: Rectal histology in acute bacillary dysentery. Gastroenterology 90:654–660, 1986.
68. Walker RI, Caldwell MB, Lee EC, et al: Pathophysiology of Campylobacter enteritis. Microbiol Rev 50:81–94, 1986.
69. Blaser MJ, Reller LB: Campylobacter enteritis. N Engl J Med 305:1444–1452, 1981.
70. Price AB, Jewkes J, Sanderson PJ: Acute diarrhea: Campylobacter colitis and the role of rectal biopsy. J Clin Pathol 32:990–997, 1979.
71. Colgan T, Lambert JR, Newman A, Luk SC: *Campylobacter jeduni* enterocolitis. Arch Pathol Lab Med 104:571–574, 1980.
72. Vantrappen G, Agg HO, Panette E, et al: Yersinia enteritis and enterocolitis: Gastroenterological aspects. Gastroenterology 72:220–227, 1977.
73. Simmonds SD, Noble MA, Freeman JH: Gastrointestinal features of culture-positive *Yersinia enterocolitica* infection. Gastroenterology 92:112–117, 1987.
74. Gleason TH, Patterson SD: The pathology of *Yersinia enterocolitica* ileocolitis. Am J Surg Pathol 6:347–355, 1982.
75. El-Maraghi NRH, Mair NS: The histopathology of enteric infection with *Yersinia pseudotuberculosis*. Am J Clin Pathol 71:631–639, 1979.

76. Abrams JS, Holden WD: Tuberculosis of the gastrointestinal tract. *Arch Surg* 84:282–293, 1964.
77. Breiter JR, Hajjar JJ: Segmental tuberculosis of the colon diagnosed by colonoscopy. Am J Gastroenterol 76:369–373, 1981.
78. Palmer KR, Patil DH, Basran GS, et al: Abdominal tuberculosis in urban Britain— a common disease. Gut 26:1296–1305, 1985.
79. Bennhoff DF: Actinomycosis: Diagnostic and therapeutic considerations and a review of 32 cases. Laryngoscope 94:1198–1217, 1981.
80. Brown JR: Human actinomycosis: A study of 181 subjects. Hum Pathol 4:319–330, 1973.
81. Harland WA, Lee FD: Intestinal spirochetosis. Br Med J 3:718–719, 1967.
82. Henrik-Nielsen R, Orholm M, Pederson JO, et al: Colorectal spirochetosis: Clinical significance of the infestation. Gastroenterology 85:62–67, 1983.
83. Lee FD, Kraszewski A, Gordon J, et al. Intestinal spirochaetosis. Gut 12:126–133, 1971.
84. Burns DG, Hayes MM: Rectal spirochetosis: Symptomatic response to metronidazole and mebendazole. S Afr Med J 68:335–336, 1985.
85. Gebbers JO, Ferguson DJP, Mason C, et al: Spirochaetosis of the human rectum associated with an intraepithelial mast cell and IgE plasma cell response. Gut 81:588–593, 1987.
86. Henrik-Nielson R, Lundbeck FA, Stubbe-Teglbjaerg P, et al: Intestinal spirochetosis of the vermiform appendix. Gastroenterology 88:971–977, 1985.
87. McMillan A, Lee FD: Sigmoidoscopic and microscopic appearances of the rectal mucosa in homosexual men. Gut 22:1035–1041, 1981.
88. Quinn TC, Corey L, Chaffee RG, et al: The etiology of anorectal infections in homosexual men. Am J Med 71:395–406, 1981.
89. McMillan A, McNeillage G, Gilmour HM, Lee FD: Histology of rectal gonorrhoea in men, with a note on anorectal infection with *Neisseria meningitidis*. J Clin Pathol 36:511–514, 1983.
90. Surawicz CM, Goodell SE, Quinn TC, et al: Spectrum of rectal biopsy abnormalities in homosexual men with intestinal symptoms. Gastroenterology 91:651–659, 1986.
91. Smith JMB: Mycoses of the alimentary tract. Gut 10:1035–1040, 1969.
92. Eras P, Goldstein MJ, Sherlock P: Candida infection of the gastrointestinal tract. Medicine 51:367–379, 1972.
93. Goodwin RA, Loyd JE, DesPrez RM: Histoplasmosis in normal hosts. *Medicine* 60:231–266, 1981.
94. Miller DP, Everett ED: Gastrointestinal histoplasmosis. J Clin Gastroenterol 1:233–236, 1979.
95. Ravdin J: Pathogenesis of disease caused by *Entamoeba histolytica*: Studies of adherence, secreted toxins, and contact-dependent cytolysis. Rev Infect Dis 8:247–260, 1986.
96. Brandt H, Perez Tamayo R: Pathology of human amebiasis. Hum Pathol 1:351–385, 1970.
97. Prathap K, Gilman R: The histopathology of acute intestinal amebiasis. Am J Pathol 60:229–245, 1970.
98. Pittman FE, Hennigar GR: Sigmoidoscopic and colonic mucosal biopsy findings in amebic colitis. Arch Pathol 97:155–158, 1974.
99. Smith PD: Pathophysiology and immunology of giardiasis. Ann Rev Med 36:295–307, 1985.
100. Hartong WA, Gourley WK, Arvanitakis C: Giardiasis: Clinical spectrum and functional-structural abnormalities of the small intestinal mucosa. Gastroenterology 77:61–69, 1979.
101. Navin TR, Juranek DD: Cryptosporidosis: Clinical, epidemiologic, and parasitologic review. Rev Infect Dis 6:313–327, 1984.
102. Casemore DP, Sands RL, Curry A: Cryptosporidum species a "new" human pathogen. J Clin Pathol 38:1321–1336, 1985.
103. Bird RG, Smith MD: Cryptosporidiosis in man: Parasite life cycle and fine structural pathology. J Pathol 132:217–233, 1980.
104. Liebman WM, Thaler MM, DeLorimer A, et al: Intractable diarrhea of infancy due to intestinal coccidiosis. Gastroenterology 78:579–584, 1980.
105. Casemore DP, Armstrong M, Sands RL: Laboratory diagnosis of cryptosporidiosis. J Clin Pathol 38:1337–1341, 1985.
106. Marcial-Rojas RA (ed): Pathology of Protozoal and Helminthic infections. Baltimore, Williams & Wilkins, 1971.
107. Dimmette RM, Sproat HF: Rectosigmoid polyps in schistosomiasis. Am J Trop Med Hyg 4:1057–1067, 1955.
108. Chen MC, Chuang CY, Chang FY, Hu JC: Evolution of colorectal cancer in schistosomiasis. Cancer 46:1661–1675, 1980.

CHAPTER 27

Ulcerative Colitis and Crohn's Disease

HARVEY GOLDMAN, M.D.

ULCERATIVE COLITIS
General Aspects
Etiology and Pathogenesis
Clinical Features
Pathology
Differential Diagnosis
Complications
Toxic Megacolon
Secondary Infections
Colitis Cystica
Postsurgical Ileal Abnormalities
Extraintestinal Manifestations
Dysplasia and Carcinoma

CROHN'S DISEASE
General Aspects
Etiology and Pathogenesis

Clinical Features
Pathology
Differential Diagnosis of Intestinal Disease
Small Intestine
Colon
Disease of Other Parts of the Alimentary Tract
Oral Cavity
Esophagus
Stomach and Proximal Duodenum
Appendix
Anal Region
Complications
Toxic Megacolon
Secondary Infections
Colitis and Enteritis Cystica

Postsurgical Ileal and Colonic Abnormalities
Extraintestinal Manifestations
Dysplasia and Carcinoma

COMPARATIVE FEATURES
Pathologic and Diagnostic Features
Discriminating Features in Colonic Disease
Shared Features in Colonic Disease
Indeterminate Colitis
Clinical Course

MUCOSAL BIOPSY
Rectal and Colonic Biopsy
Ileal Biopsy

Two common disorders affecting the intestinal tract, particularly in persons from the more developed countries, are ulcerative colitis and Crohn's disease.[1-3] They are often referred to by the common term *inflammatory bowel disease*, or IBD. Because many other intestinal diseases with known etiologies also have an inflammatory basis, it has been suggested that ulcerative colitis and Crohn's disease should more appropriately be linked under *idiopathic inflammatory bowel disease*, but this latter term has not as yet been widely accepted.

The precise cause and pathogenesis of ulcerative colitis and Crohn's disease are unknown, but the conditions share many common features.[4,5] Accordingly, the diagnostic separation of these two disorders depends at all times on a consideration of the combined clinical, distributional, macroscopic, and histologic characteristics.[5-9] In this regard, the results obtained from radiographic and gross endoscopic examinations are vital for accurate determination of the location of the disease and other gross features prior to pathologic study of the resected intestinal specimen. In the following sections of this chapter, the two conditions are presented separately; there follows a discussion of comparative features. A final section deals with the uses and interpretations of endoscopic biopsies in these disorders.

ULCERATIVE COLITIS

General Aspects

Definition. Ulcerative colitis is a chronic inflammatory disorder of unknown etiology that involves exclu-

Table 27–1 DIAGNOSTIC FEATURES OF ULCERATIVE COLITIS

Absence of known cause
Rectum always involved
Colonic disease in the majority of cases; when present, it is always diffuse and there are no skip areas
Appendix may be affected, but there is no involvement of other parts of the gut
Inflammation and ulceration are usually limited to the mucosa and submucosa; involvement of deeper parts of bowel wall is seen in one third of surgical resections and in toxic megacolon
Absence of discrete inflammatory sinus tracts, fissures, and fistulas; must distinguish from multiple "cracks" in the wall that may be seen in cases with toxic megacolon
Absence of well-formed, sarcoid-type granulomas; must distinguish from granulomas due to ruptured crypts or foreign bodies

sively the large intestine, and it is the most common cause of chronic colitis in the United States. Because the rectum is invariably affected, the disease has also been termed *ulcerative proctocolitis*. It was originally suspected that it may have an infectious cause, because of similarities in the inflammatory reaction; but a constant agent has never been established. The study by Warren and Summers in 1949 provided a detailed account of the pathologic features[10]; although these investigators initially thought that ulcerative colitis might be caused by a vasculitis, this has not been confirmed.

Diagnostic Criteria. Before the diagnosis of ulcerative colitis can be considered, all other possible causes of inflammatory colitis must be excluded, including infections, ischemic disease, known immune and toxic disorders, and mechanical effects. Because there is no pathognomonic feature, the diagnosis of ulcerative colitis depends on a combination of clinical, distributional, and structural characteristics (Table 27–1). There is constant involvement of the rectum, variable extension of the disease to the more proximal portions of the colon in a diffuse fashion without the appearance of skip areas of normal colon, and limitation of the disorder to the large intestine and appendix.[1–3,5,10] The dominant inflammatory effect, at least in the initial stages, is in the mucosa, and the inflammatory reaction is essentially nonspecific. Compared with Crohn's disease and some infections of the colon, there is usually less inflammation in the deeper portions of the bowel wall, and there are no skip areas, discrete inflammatory sinus tracts, or granulomas.

Epidemiology. The disease may affect persons of all ages, including children and older adults, with a major peak in the third decade.[11–14] A second, smaller peak has been suggested for the sixth and seventh decades, but it is uncertain whether the diagnosis in this group is not confounded by the presence of other disorders in elderly persons such as ischemic disease.[15] There is a slight preponderance of females, and ulcerative colitis is decidedly more common in persons from the Western developed countries, in the white population, and in Jewish people. The overall incidence in areas where the disease is more common is approximately 5 to 6 per 100,000 persons. About 1% to 2% of the cases are familial.

Etiology and Pathogenesis

The cause and pathogenesis of ulcerative colitis are not known.[4] An infectious cause was once considered because of the similarity of the inflammatory reaction to that seen in some human intestinal infections and animal models. Furthermore, some of the relapses may be associated with or actually precipitated by secondary infections, such as those due to *Salmonella* and *Clostridium difficile*. However, the inflammatory reaction has proven to be completely nonspecific, there is no response to antimicrobial drugs except in the special case of secondary infections, and a constant infectious agent has not been identified as the primary cause of the colitis. There is also no evidence of a vasculitis or a reaction to known toxins. Although stressful situations may induce diarrhea in general and may be a precipitating factor in a relapse in a patient with ulcerative colitis, there is as yet no solid evidence to support stress as being a primary etiologic factor.

It is currently believed that immune mechanisms are the probable cause of ulcerative colitis. Some patients have other disorders with a probable immunologic basis, such as rheumatoid arthritis; serum autoantibodies are commonly found, including those directed to elements of the colonic mucosa; and the disease usually responds to corticosteroids and other immunosuppressive therapy. However, most of these features could be of a secondary or nonspecific nature, and the actual immunologic event responsible for the colitis has not been established. A subset of cases, mainly involving the rectum, has been identified in which there is a high concentration of IgE-bearing plasma cells in the lamina propria and a beneficial response to antihistamine medications.[16–18] It has been suggested that these cases might be caused by an immediate hypersensitivity type of allergic reaction, but it is unclear how they relate to the overall condition of ulcerative colitis.

The primary lesion in ulcerative colitis appears to be in the mucosa and is characterized by a pronounced acute inflammation and degeneration of the surface and crypt epithelia. With sloughing of the necrotic mucosa, secondary ulcers develop that are usually superficial. The disease exhibits multiple episodes of healing and recurrences, and the reparative phase is frequently associated with the appearance of inflammatory or regenerative polyps (pseudopolyps). Very severe cases lead to marked dilatation of the lumen and thinning of the bowel wall (toxic megacolon), with the threat of perforation, and in long-standing cases fibrosis and neoplasia may develop.

Clinical Features

There is usually an abrupt onset, and major symptoms include crampy abdominal pain, tenesmus, mucous discharge in milder cases, diarrhea, and bleeding.[19,20] Laboratory tests reveal, in the severe cases, leukocytosis, anemia, hypokalemia, and hypoproteinemia. The presence of proctitis or proctocolitis is established by radiographic and/or sigmoidoscopic exami-

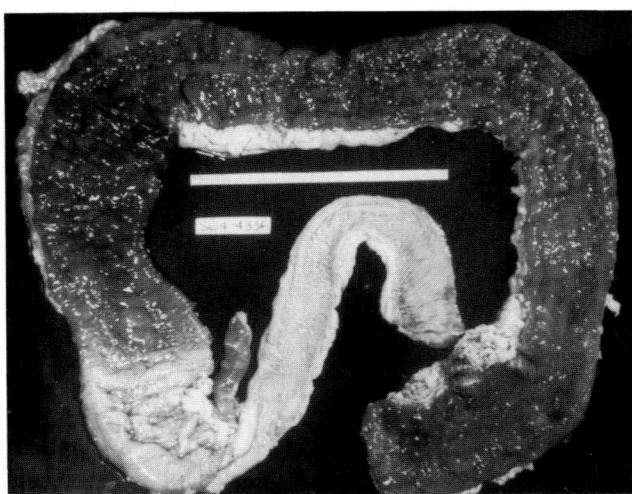

FIGURE 27-1. Ulcerative colitis. Subtotal colectomy specimen, showing diffuse involvement with hemorrhagic mucosa from the distal resection margin (bottom right) to the mid ascending colon. The more proximal part of the colon and cecum, the appendix, and the ileal segment are normal.

nations. As noted above, other known causes of colonic inflammation must be excluded before the diagnosis of ulcerative colitis can be made. It may be difficult to distinguish an initial episode of ulcerative colitis from a case of acute self-limited colitis. Mucosal biopsy may be especially helpful at this time in the detection or confirmation of the colitis and in the determination of whether it is in the acute stage or the chronic stage.[21-24]

About 90% of the patients present with disease that appears to be confined to the rectum and sigmoid colon, but over half will eventually progress to develop more extensive colitis. The disease is characterized by periods of remission (inactive or quiescent colitis) and relapses (active colitis), and the recurrences are often associated with proximal extension of the colitis. The presence of proctitis appears to accentuate the development of perianal complications, including fissures and abscesses, which occur in about 15% of the patients (see Chapter 34). Medical therapy includes mainly sulfasalazine and corticosteroids, and antibiotics are used for secondary infections. Surgery is reserved for intractable disease and complications and requires a complete proctocolectomy, which is performed in one or two stages. The surgery is associated with the creation of a permanent ileostomy of the standard or continent type or with the formation of an ileal reservoir and ileoanal anastomosis. It is essential that the complete rectal mucosa be removed because of the concern for the late development of carcinoma in this area.[25-27] The overall mortality for ulcerative colitis is very low, with deaths mainly related to perforated megacolon, to septic complications of surgery or immunosuppressive therapy, and to carcinoma.

Pathology

The pathologic features of ulcerative colitis are similar in all age groups, including young children and elderly patients.[28,29]

Distribution of Disease. There is always involvement of the rectum and a variable extension of the disease upward in a diffuse fashion into the colon.[1-3,30] The disease remains limited to the rectum (ulcerative proctitis) in approximately 5% to 10% of the cases, proceeds at time of recurrence to involve the sigmoid and descending colon (left-sided colitis) in about a third of the cases, and extends to the proximal transverse colon or beyond (extensive colitis) in over half of the patients (Figures 27-1 and 27-2). When the colitis involves the entire colon, it is also referred to as universal colitis or pancolitis. There is a disproportionate number of cases with extensive involvement in surgical specimens, because they tend to be derived from patients with more severe and complicated disease.

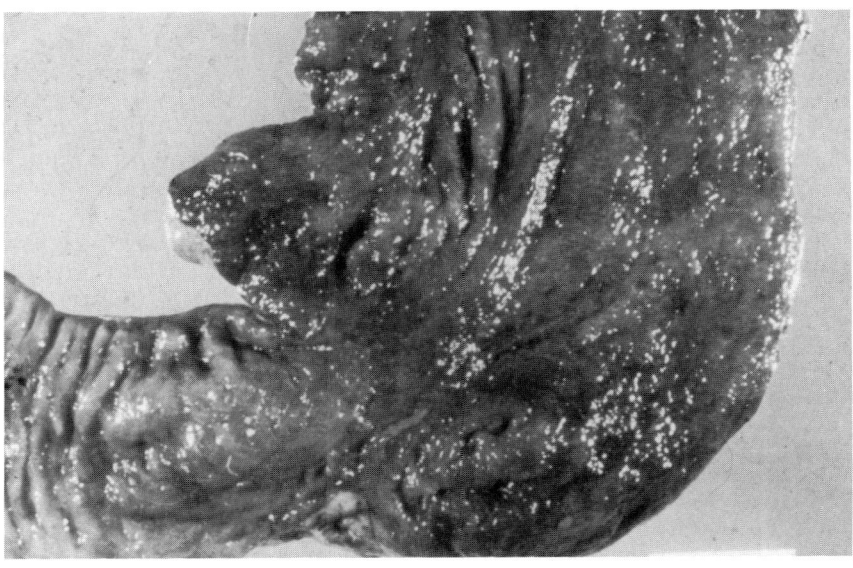

FIGURE 27-2. Ulcerative colitis. There is diffuse inflammation of the mucosa in the right colon, including the cecum, that stops abruptly at the ileocecal valve. The ileum (left) is slightly dilated but not ulcerated.

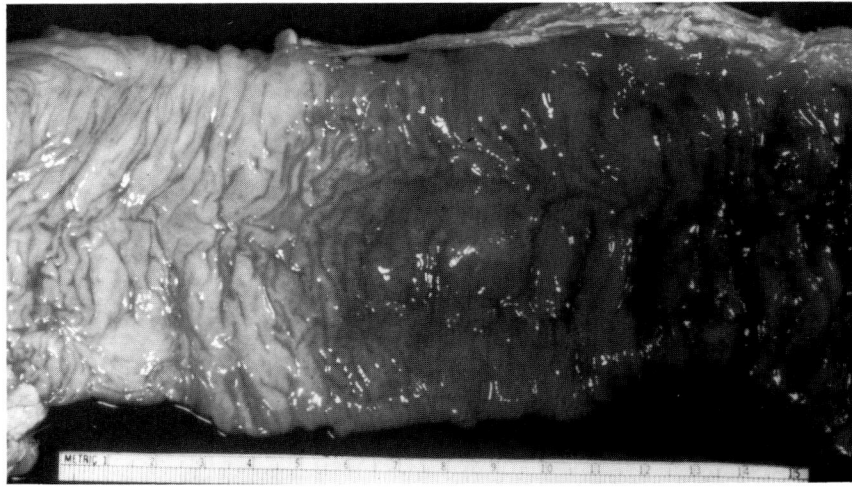

FIGURE 27–3. Segment of colon in ulcerative colitis, revealing a sharp demarcation between the inflamed, hemorrhagic mucosa at the right and the normal mucosa at the left.

There are no skip areas of normal colon amidst the inflamed segment of colon. Occasionally, there is an uneven degree of inflammation and repair resulting in areas that grossly simulate a skip region, but histologic examination of such areas confirms the presence of diffuse colitis.[31] Also, patients with severe colitis associated with colonic dilation who have a normal right colon may develop a localized area of colitis in the cecum, probably due to the effect of higher pressure in this region. Appendiceal involvement is usually associated with universal colitis but may occur in the face of relative sparing of the right side of the colon. The lesion in the appendix is typically diffuse and limited to the superficial layers, in contrast to the transmural acute inflammation noted in an ordinary case of acute suppurative appendicitis (see Chapter 33).

The terminal portion of the ileum, usually limited to the distalmost 10 cm, may be dilated, particularly in cases with universal colitis. It is thought that this results from regurgitation of colonic secretions through a dilated, relatively incompetent ileocecal valve; and this has been termed "backwash ileitis." It should be stressed, however, that there is no ulceration of the ileal mucosa; at most, there may be a patchy increase in inflammatory cells within the lamina propria together with the dilation. Accordingly, there is no evidence to support that the ileum is involved with the same process that is damaging the colonic mucosa. There are also no ulcerative lesions of any other portion of the small intestine or upper gastrointestinal tract in cases of ulcerative colitis—i.e., the disease, true to its name, is limited to the colon and rectum. When a destructive lesion is found in some other portion of the gut, an alternative explanation must be sought.

In cases limited to the rectum, referred to as ulcerative proctitis, the symptoms are characteristically less severe, there are fewer complications, and surgical excision is rarely needed.[20] The pathologic features of ulcerative proctitis, as determined by study of mucosal biopsies, are otherwise similar to those of ulcerative colitis.

Gross Features. Many of the early changes are best appreciated *in vivo* at the gross endoscopic examination.[32–35] The lesion begins with a diffuse erythema and patchy hemorrhage of the mucosa and proceeds to a stage of friability and overt ulceration. The disease involves the rectum and colon in a continuous fashion, and there is usually a relatively sharp demarcation between the inflamed mucosa at the proximal end of the lesion and the adjacent normal colon (Figure 27–3). More advanced lesions show extensive undermining of the intact but inflamed mucosa by the ulcerations, resulting in the formation of mucosal bridges (Figure 27–4). The ulcers tend to be superficial, usually limited to the mucosa or upper submucosa, and there are typically no gross abnormalities of the underlying muscularis propria or serosa. In about one third of surgically resected specimens, which presumably represent the more severe cases, ulcers are found to extend into the muscularis. This is associated with focal inflammation of the serosa, but the change is usually not grossly conspicuous. There are no discrete inflammatory sinus tracts or fistulas in uncomplicated cases of ulcerative colitis.

With time and intermittent repair of the colitis, there is the variable formation of inflammatory polyps, which are also commonly termed pseudopolyps.[36–38] These inflammatory polyps result in part from a persistence of intact mucosa that is relatively raised next to an ulcerated area but also from the intense inflammation and repair that is present in that mucosa (Figure 27–5). The presence of such polyps is a good indicator of chronic colitis, but it is not specific for ulcerative colitis, because they may be seen in other causes of chronic inflammation such as in Crohn's disease of the colon and in ischemic colitis.[39] The polyps vary considerably in their amount, size, and distribution. One may encounter a few scattered inflammatory polyps or a veritable sea of such lesions over a large portion of the colon (Figure 27–6). Most inflammatory pseudopolyps are sessile or have a short stalk, and they exhibit a relatively smooth surface, in contrast to the more convoluted or frankly papillary surface contour of adenomas. Occasionally, an inflammatory polyp may be very large and localized (giant pseudopolyp) and mimic the appearance of a polypoid neoplasm.[40–42] Close inspec-

FIGURE 27–4. Ulcerative colitis. There is extensive ulceration and the presence of mucosal bridges. The bowel wall is not thickened.

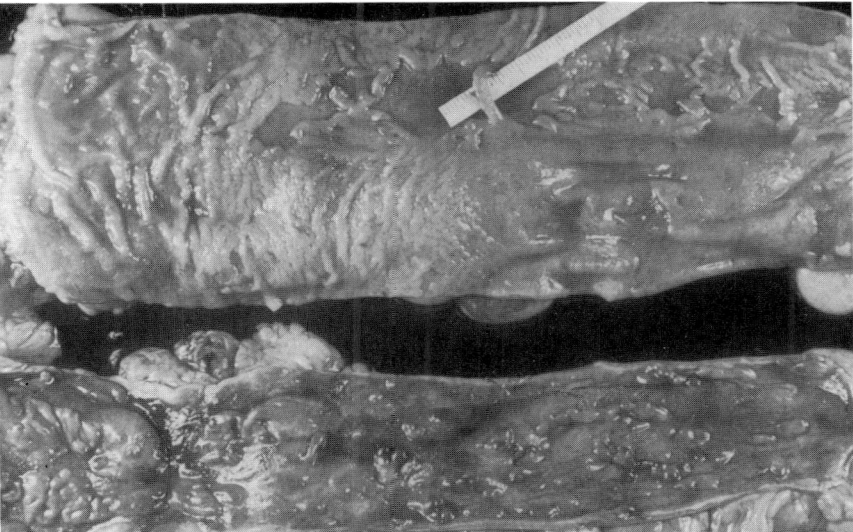

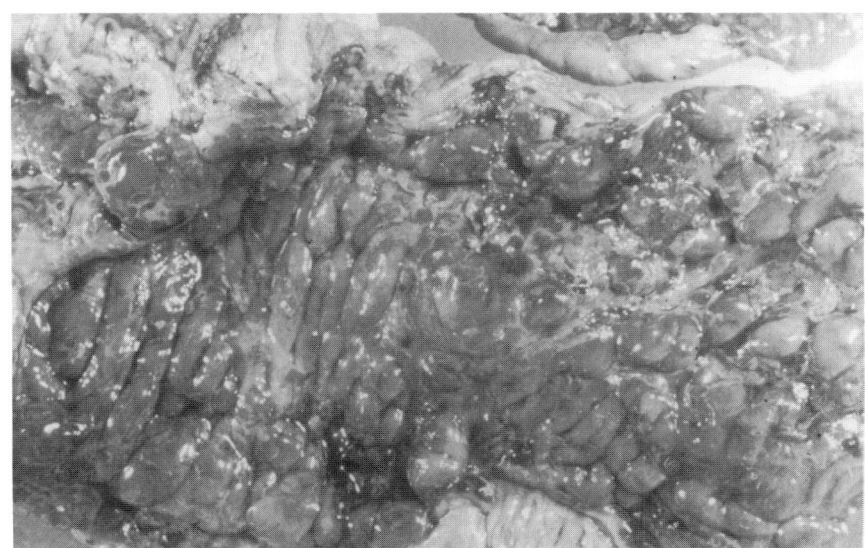

FIGURE 27–5. Ulcerative colitis, showing an admixture of ulceration and inflammatory pseudopolyps.

FIGURE 27–6. Ulcerative colitis. The mucosal surface is altered by the presence of a massive number of small inflammatory pseudopolyps.

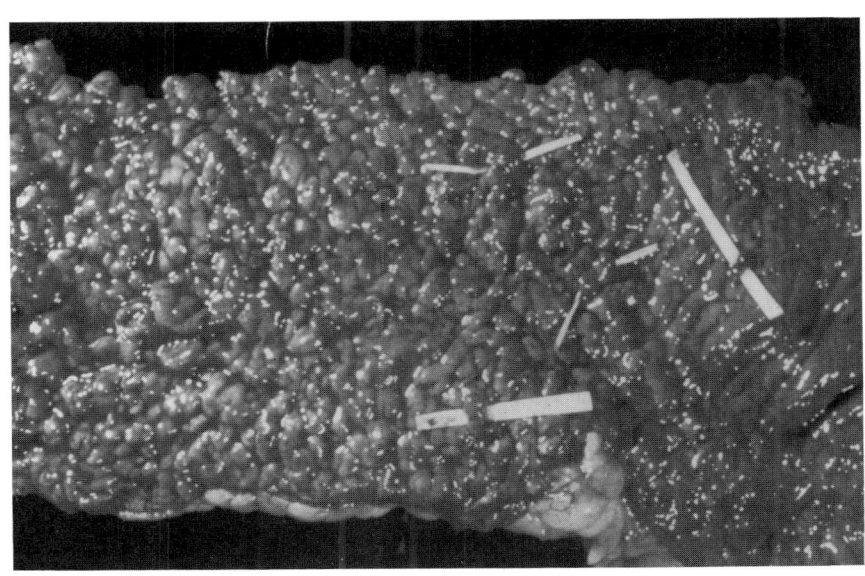

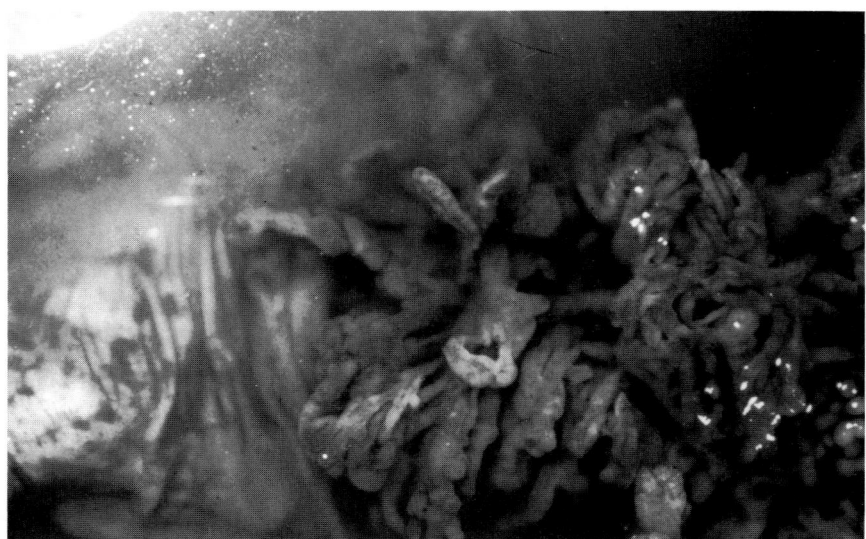

FIGURE 27-7. Single large inflammatory pseudopolyp in a case of chronic ulcerative colitis. The polyp is composed of numerous, fine mucosal bridges.

tion of such polyps reveals that they are composed of anastomosing strands of mucosa, which can be readily demonstrated by passing a probe through the various channels and arches of the lesion (Figure 27-7); a neoplasm, in contrast, is composed of a more solid mass and has a continuous attachment at its base with the mucosa. The polyps may also persist after the cessation of the ulcerating and inflammatory phase of active colitis. This appears to be due to the formation of a fibromuscular core in the polyp, analogous to the development of fibroepithelial polyps in other tissues. The overlying mucosa in such polyps may lose all signs of active inflammation, and superficial mucosal biopsies may fail to show their nature. These persistent polyps frequently have a villous or fingerlike configuration and have also been called filliform polyps.[43] Lesions in the rectum may develop a covering of squamous metaplasia and have an opaque surface.

The inactive or quiescent phase of ulcerative colitis is characterized grossly by the absence of ulcers and the occasional persistence of inflammatory pseudopolyps. There is usually a simplification of the haustral markings, and severe cases show a relatively flat mucosa. By endoscopic examination, there may be enhanced vascular markings due to the greater visualization of the submucosal vessels through an atrophic mucosa. Upon recurrence and progression of the disease, there may be an uneven degree of inflammation. In most cases, the worst disease remains in the distal colon and rectum; but some cases show more prominent disease in the proximal front of the colitis. More severe cases of active ulcerative colitis may be associated with pronounced dilation of the lumen and thinning of the bowel wall, and late lesions include a shortening of the colon and fibrous stricture formation. These are discussed below in the section on complications.

Histologic Features. The microscopic features noted in ulcerative colitis are essentially nonspecific.[1-3,5-10,31,44-47] Indeed, it is often impossible to distinguish the initial stage of ulcerative colitis from other causes of acute colitis, particularly in the examination of small mucosal biopsy specimens. With progression of the disease, however, the mucosa undergoes a series of architectural and inflammatory changes that serve to identify the lesion as a chronic disorder.[21-23] In the initial acute phase, there is marked infiltration of the mucosa, with neutrophils, together with signs of degeneration of the surface and crypt epithelia (Figure 27-8). The neutrophils are present both in the lamina propria and in the damaged epithelial layer. The injury to the crypt ranges from the simple presence of neutrophils in the epithelium to focal denudation of the epithelial cells and finally to complete destruction of the crypt surrounding a pool of luminal neutrophils (crypt abscess). The term *cryptitis* may be applied to the full variety of inflammatory changes affecting the crypts.[46-48] Also present are features of prominent regeneration of the epithelial cells, including elongation and pallisading of the nuclei, with central enlarged nucleoli, and numerous mitoses.

Mucosal erosions and superficial ulcerations, usually limited to the upper submucosa, develop in the more severe cases and are typically associated with inflammatory pseudopolyps in the adjacent mucosa (Figures 27-9 and 27-10). In nonulcerated areas, the normal architecture of relatively straight and parallel crypts with minimal branching may remain in an acute case of ulcerative colitis.[22] Giant cells, representing multinucleated macrophages, may be present in the mucosa that is actively inflamed and eroded, and these are thought to result from a nonspecific reaction to luminal contents. Occasionally seen are poorly formed granulomas surrounding a ruptured crypt (Figure 27-11), and multiple sections may be required for identification of the crypt injury as the source of the lesion.[49] Well-formed granulomas of the sarcoid type that are unassociated with necrosis or foreign material are not seen in ulcerative colitis.

Complete regeneration and restoration of the mucosa to normal are observed after most cases of acute self-limited colitis such as those due to various acute

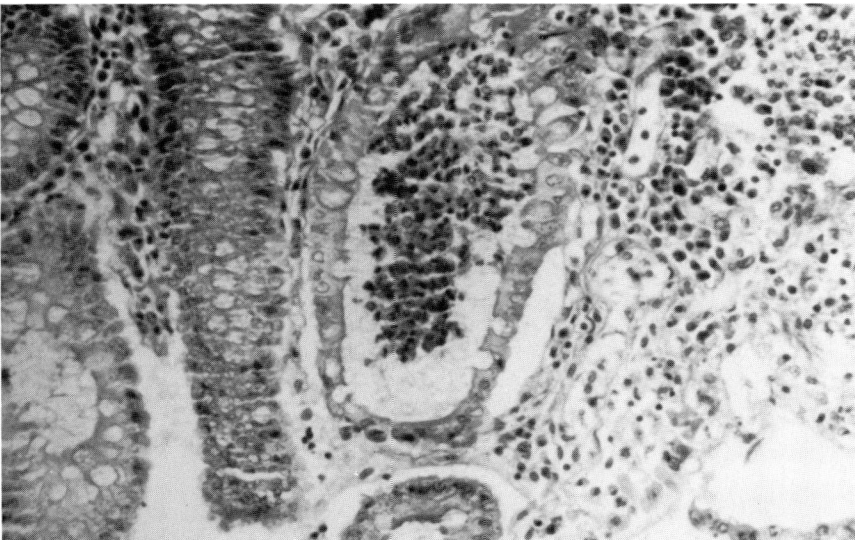

FIGURE 27-8. Colonic mucosa in an active case of ulcerative colitis, showing acute cryptitis with a crypt abscess. (H&E, × 100)

infections. In contrast, when a patient with ulcerative colitis attains a remission, there usually are present persistent and characteristic alterations in the mucosa that serve to identify the disorder as a chronic colitis (Table 27-2). Some of these features have been observed as early as three weeks after the onset of ulcerative colitis. The major mucosal changes are an abnormal architecture characterized by extensive budding and branching of the crypts (Figure 27-12); an atrophy of the crypts, as evidenced by their shortening and diffuse separation from the muscularis mucosae (Figure 27-13); and a villous-like transformation of the mucosal surface.[22] Also commonly present are an overall increase in mononuclear inflammatory cells and eosinophils in the lamina propria,[50-52] the presence of small lymphoid nodules and increased plasma cells at the base of the mucosa separating the crypts and the muscularis mucosae[21] (Figure 27-14), and the appearance of Paneth cell metaplasia in the crypt epithelium[23,53] (Figure 27-15). It should be remembered that Paneth cells are normally indigenous to the cecum and proximal ascending colon and that their presence, therefore, can only be considered abnormal if seen in the mid and distal portions of the colon. It has been estimated that at least one of these features of chronic colitis can be found in almost 80% of mucosal biopsies in cases of ulcerative colitis.[22] In contrast, they are never present in a case of acute self-limited colitis. By immunocytochemical staining, the increase in plasma cells is seen to affect all classes, including IgG, IgM, and IgA types.[54] Some cases of ulcerative proctitis show a preferential increase in IgE-type plasma cells and are thought to have an allergic component[16-18] (see Chapter 10).

Also noted in chronic colitis to a variable degree are a hyperplasia of the crypt endocrine cells[55]; small

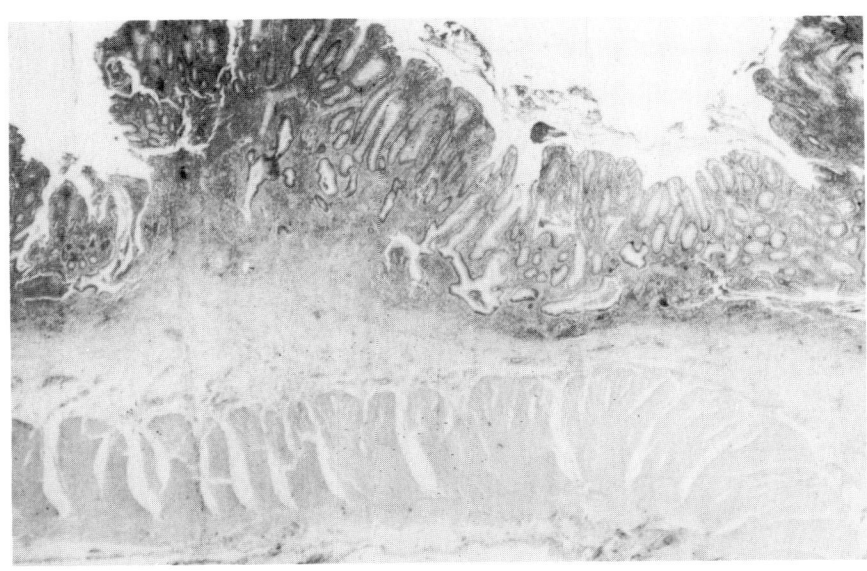

FIGURE 27-9. Ulcerative colitis, active. There is diffuse damage to the mucosa consisting of alternating ulcers and inflamed mucosa. The inflammation extends into the upper submucosa; but the deeper parts of the wall, including the mucularis propria and serosa, are usually normal. (H&E, × 20)

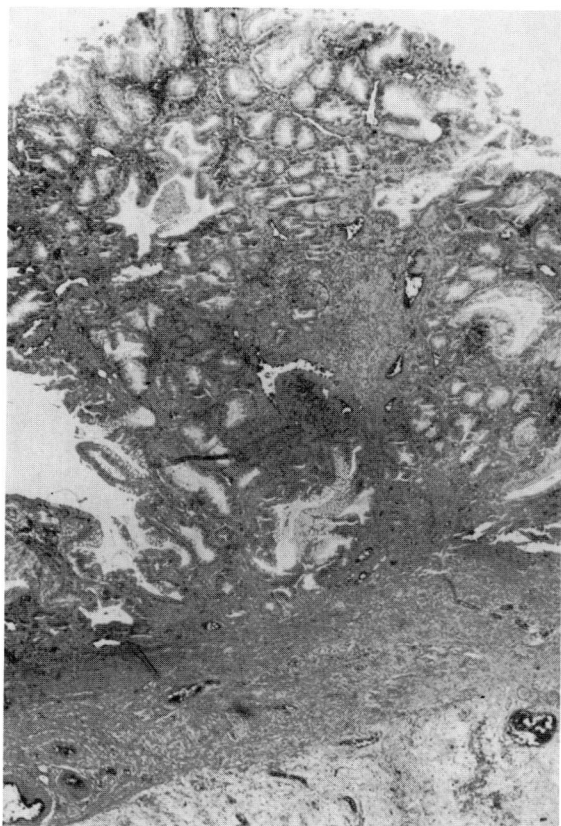

FIGURE 27-10. Ulcerative colitis, showing an inflammatory pseudopolyp. The polyp is composed of regenerating glands and inflamed mucosa. (H&E, × 60)

Table 27-2 HISTOLOGIC FEATURES OF CHRONIC COLITIS

Common Features
Abnormal mucosal architecture characterized by prominent branching of crypts
Atrophy of crypts
Villiform surface
Increase of mononuclear inflammatory cells and eosinophils in lamina propria
Presence of lymphoid nodules and increased plasma cells at base of lamina propria
Paneth cell metaplasia

More Variable Features
Endocrine cell hyperplasia
Pyloric gland metaplasia
Squamous metaplasia
Adipose tissue in lamina propria
Fibrosis of lamina propria

---

patches of pyloric glandular metaplasia; foci of squamous metaplasia in distal lesions; the incorporation of adipose tissue in the mucosa, probably resulting from prior ulceration; and fibrosis of the base of the lamina propria in long-standing cases. It is important to distinguish artifactual spaces in the lamina propria, referred to as pseudolipomatosis and commonly present in distorted biopsy specimens, from true adipose tissue in the mucosa[56]; the latter is usually associated with disruption of the muscularis mucosae. Although these various features of chronic colitis are commonly seen, they may not be appreciated in small biopsy samples in all cases. Furthermore, it appears that the mucosa more often appears normal during a remission if the patient has been treated with steroid enemas.

During a relapse, one encounters a mixture of the features described in acute colitis and in the remission phase. Thus, there are both the changes of chronic colitis and the inflammatory and degenerative effects of the active disease. Considering the duration of the disease and the histologic features in the mucosa, cases of ulcerative colitis can be categorized into three groups: acute colitis in the initial episode, chronic inactive colitis at the time of remission, and chronic active colitis during relapses.

The primary and dominant injury in ulcerative colitis is at the level of the mucosa, and the disease has also been called mucosal colitis for distinguishing it from the transmural colitis seen in most cases of Crohn's dis-

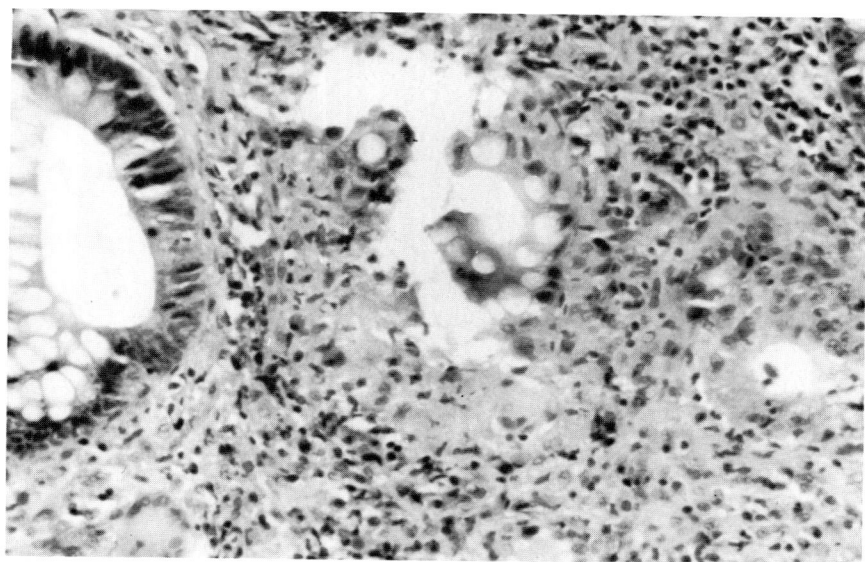

FIGURE 27-11. Colonic mucosa in active ulcerative colitis, revealing a poorly formed granulomatous reaction to a ruptured crypt. (H&E, × 400)

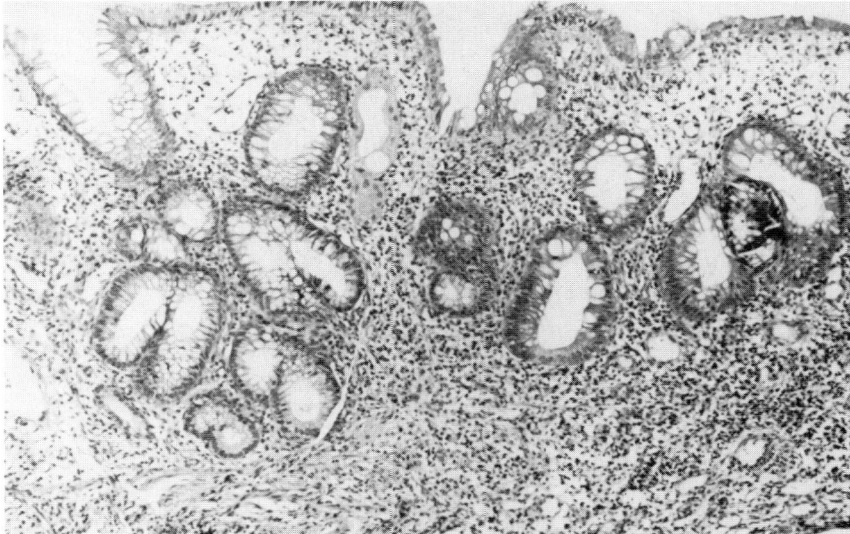

FIGURE 27–12. Colonic mucosa in chronic ulcerative colitis. There is a prominent architectural alteration due to multiple branching and slight shortening of the crypts. (H&E, × 60) (From Goldman H, Antonioli DA: Mucosal biopsy of the rectum, colon, and distal ileum. Hum Pathol 13:981–1012, 1982.)

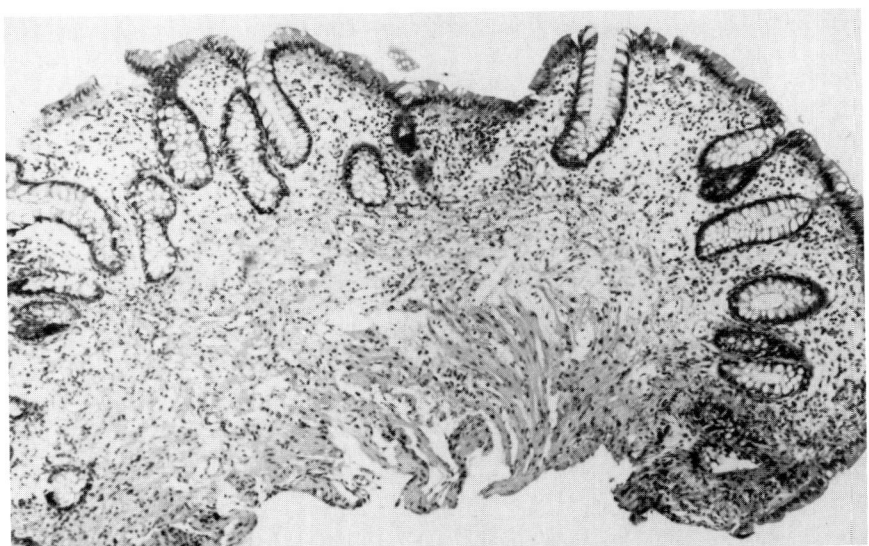

FIGURE 27–13. Colonic mucosa in chronic ulcerative colitis. An example of the inactive phase, showing crypt atrophy. The crypts are fewer in number and markedly shortened, as evidenced by the increased space between their bases and the muscularis mucosae (at bottom). (H&E, × 60) (From Goldman H, Antonioli DA: Mucosal biopsy of the rectum, colon, and distal ileum. Hum Pathol 13:981–1012, 1982.)

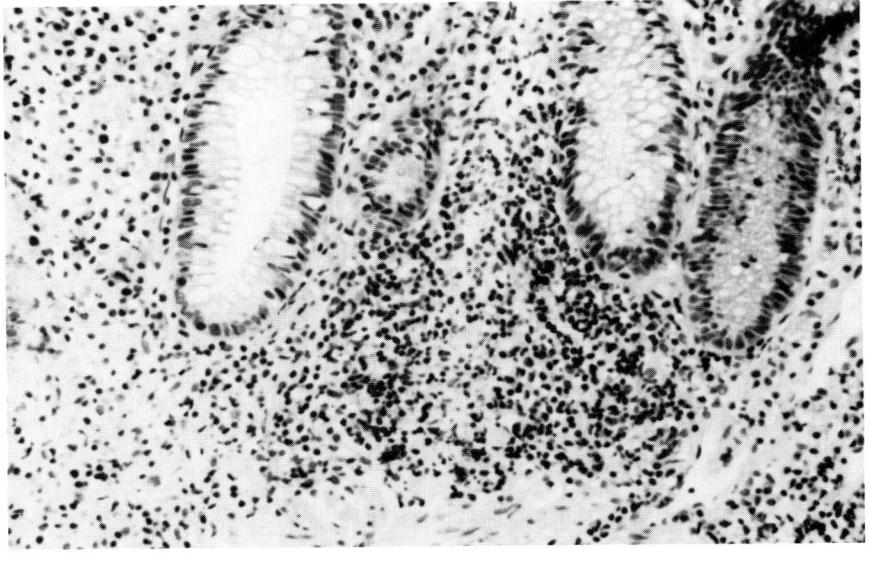

FIGURE 27–14. Colonic mucosa in chronic ulcerative colitis, showing a small lymphocytic nodule at the base of the mucosa between the crypts and the muscularis mucosae. (H&E, × 250)

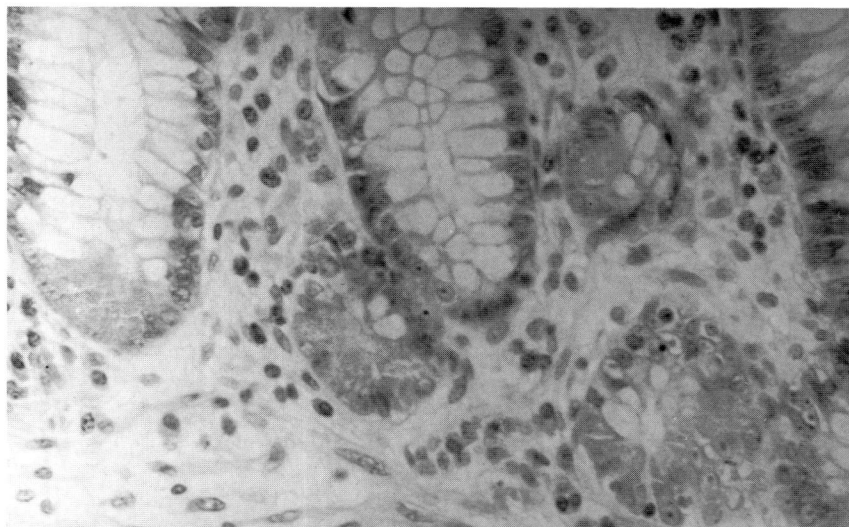

FIGURE 27-15. Colonic mucosa in chronic ulcerative colitis, revealing Paneth cell metaplasia in the bottom of the crypts. (H&E, × 250)

ease. When the mucosa is completely destroyed, there is sloughing of the necrotic tissue and formation of ulcers. The ulcers are usually superficial and limited to the upper submucosa (see Figure 27-9), but they may in severe cases extend to the muscularis propria, as noted in about one third of surgical resections. A nonspecific acute inflammatory response, consisting of edema and neutrophils, surrounds the ulcers. This inflammation is usually confined to the submucosa but may extend through the wall when there is deeper ulceration. Other alterations in the submucosa are nonspecific and include congestion, the presence of mononuclear inflammatory cells (plasma cells, lymphocytes, and macrophages) and occasional lymphoid nodules, and slight lymphatic dilatation. Underlying areas of prior ulceration, the muscularis mucosae may be either thinned out and disrupted or show focal areas of hypertrophy. In long-standing cases, there may be focal areas of fibrosis and neural proliferation in the submucosa, but this change is rarely as prominent as that seen in Crohn's disease. The muscularis propria and serosa are usually normal or show, at most, a patchy acute and chronic inflammation in cases with deep ulcers. There are no discrete inflammatory fissures extending into the muscularis. In some patients requiring surgery, an initial subtotal colectomy is performed, and the rectum is temporarily left *in situ* as a mucous fistula. The rectal mucosa continues to show the effects of chronic colitis and intermittent changes of active disease. Occasional cases reveal marked hyperplasia of lymphoid nodules within the mucosa and submucosa, and this has been referred to as follicular proctitis[45]; it is possible that this change reflects a reaction to substances in the static segment of rectum. This alteration may also be seen, but usually to a lesser degree, in cases with an intact colon.

Pathologic Diagnosis. Lacking any specific markers, the diagnosis of ulcerative colitis is essentially one of exclusion. Other types of acute and chronic colitis of known cause must be ruled out by appropriate clinical and laboratory studies. The diagnosis of ulcerative colitis (see Table 27-1) is established by the demonstration of *all* of the following features: (1) absence of a known or presumed cause; (2) rectal involvement and a variable degree of colonic and appendiceal disease, which is always diffuse (i.e., it has no skip areas); (3) no involvement of other portions of the gut; (4) absence of discrete inflammatory sinus tracts extending into the wall; and (5) a relatively nonspecific inflammatory reaction, largely confined to the mucosa and submucosa, without the presence of well-formed granulomas of sarcoid type. After the first few weeks, most cases also reveal characteristic changes in the mucosa that signify a chronic colitis.

Differential Diagnosis

Acute infections of the colon can usually be distinguished from ulcerative colitis in the very early stages because they more often exhibit focal lesions.[47,57,58] In some infections, such as those due to *Campylobacter* and *Chlamydia*, granulomas may also be present.[22,49,59] The later stage of infections is commonly associated with a more diffuse colitis, and only the demonstration of the microorganism, typically by culture of the stool or its examination for ova, serves to distinguish it from an acute case of ulcerative colitis.[60-65] Furthermore, some infections, including those due to *Shigella* and *Chlamydia* organisms, may persist and develop features of a chronic colitis, but this event is uncommon, and the histologic alterations are usually not as prominent as those seen in ulcerative colitis. Pseudomembranous colitis, typically due to *Clostridium difficile*, reveals characteristic small, sharply demarcated, yellow to white patches on the mucosa, and histology shows a relatively normal mucosa next to the inflamed areas.[66-69] Amebic colitis due to *Entamoeba histolytica* can cause an acute and chronic colitis with diffuse lesions that is identical to ulcerative colitis.[70] There may be extensive ulcerations, and the diagnosis is established by the identification of the characteristic ova in the stool or in smears obtained by direct imprints of the lesion. See Chapter 26 for further details.

Cases of ischemic colitis are more common in older patients, and there is a tendency for segmental involvement with frequent sparing of the rectum; microscopy reveals extensive necrosis, which is more often concentrated in the superficial half of the mucosa.[71–74] There also may be prominent hemorrhage and hemosiderin deposits in cases of ischemic colitis, but this is not a distinguishing feature, since it may be seen in any case of colitis with prominent bleeding. In the differential diagnosis of ulcerative colitis, particularly in the chronic phase, the major possibility is Crohn's disease.[1,2,5–9,47,75] Most cases can be readily distinguished either by the histologic features or by the gross and distributional characteristics. Thus, the diagnosis of Crohn's disease is manifested by the presence of some combination of focal lesions in the colon and other parts of the gut, the development of mural sinus tracts, and the appearance of granulomas.

Complications

Clinical problems resulting from severe episodes of ulcerative colitis include anemia from repeated hemorrhages, hypovolemia and hypokalemia due in part to the inflammation but mostly to reduced absorption, and hypoproteinemia resulting from oozing of protein from the mucosal ulcerations.

Toxic Megacolon

A severe episode of active colitis, either in the acute phase or at the time of a recurrence, can result in extreme outpouring of fluid and hemorrhage into the colonic lumen. This leads to progressive dilatation of the lumen, pressure-induced extension of the necrosis and thinning of the bowel wall, and ultimately perforation if this complication is not checked. The patient is very sick and exhibits a high fever and prominent leukocytosis; the lesion is best monitored by serial abdominal films, and surgery becomes indicated if there is progression of the bowel dilation over a period of 3 to 5 days. Inspection of the bowel wall reveals thinning due to ischemic necrosis with prominent vascular congestion and focal cracks or fissures in the most inflamed areas (Figure 27–16). These fissures must be distinguished from the discrete sinus tracts that occur in an otherwise normal or thickened bowel wall in Crohn's disease.[31] Perforation of the colon in a case of toxic megacolon results in a generalized peritonitis and an overall poor prognosis.

Secondary Infections

Some of the relapses seen in ulcerative colitis are due to the development of secondary infections, rather than to recrudescence of the primary disease. This may be caused by any of the ordinary pathogens,[76–77] but more commonly noted are infections due to *Salmonella* and *C. difficile*.[78–80] It is important to recognize this possibility at the time of relapse and to perform the appropriate stool culture and toxin assays, because these cases respond preferentially to specific antimicrobial therapy. The pathologic features of these infections are identical to those seen in ordinary recurrent ulcerative colitis; specifically, the pseudomembranes associated with *C. difficile* disease in noncolitis patients are not present in cases complicating ulcerative colitis. Occasionally, in patients receiving high doses of corticosteroids or other immunosuppressive therapy, opportunistic infections due mainly to herpes simplex virus and cytomegalovirus occur.[81–83] These tend to be associated with very severe cases and may promote increased necrosis and perforation. Occasionally there is spread of the opportunistic infection to internal organs, and death may result from generalized sepsis or mas-

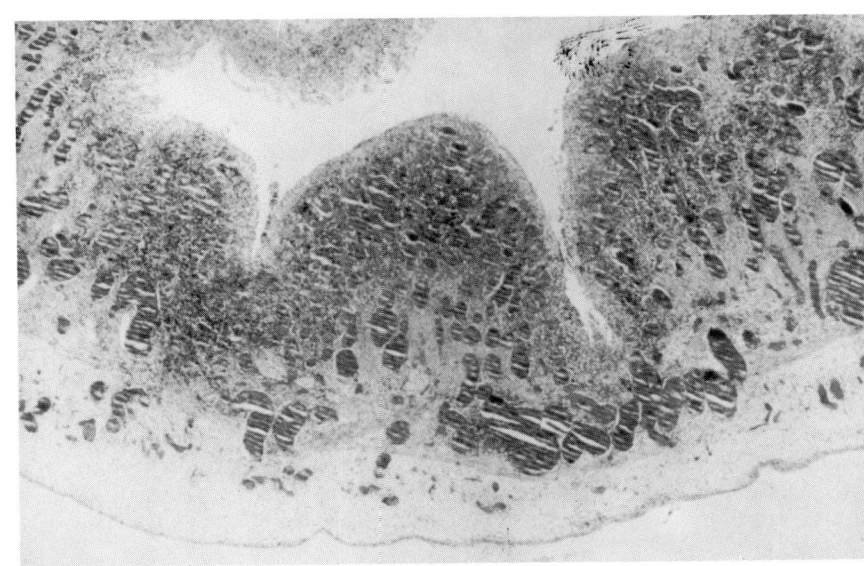

FIGURE 27–16. Colonic wall in a case of severe ulcerative colitis. There is deep ulceration, and the underlying muscularis propria shows marked congestion, granulation tissue, and superficial cracks in the tissue. (H&E, × 20)

sive hepatic necrosis. In such cases, one should look for the characteristic inclusions of the viruses, and this search can be abetted by specific immunocytochemical stains.

Colitis Cystica

In cases with extensive ulceration, there may be the downgrowth and persistence of dilated colonic glands into the submucosa and occasionally the muscularis propria, which has been called colitis cystica profunda.[84] The lesions may also be associated with inflammatory pseudopolyps, and the overall mass may be confused with an adenocarcinoma. The distinction is made by noting that the misplaced glands are either normal or show at most the effects of inflammation, and there is no dysplasia of the epithelium. Although there have been many descriptions of colitis cystica, it appears that the prominent and polypoid form is very uncommon. Other benign conditions in ulcerative colitis that reveal spaces or nodules in the submucosa include pneumatosis intestinalis, which is due to the growth of gas-forming bacteria in areas of acute or active colitis, and clusters of macrophages containing barium, the so-called barium granuloma (see Chapter 28).

Postsurgical Ileal Abnormalities

Because ulcerative colitis is a disease that is limited to the rectum and colon, it is expected that total proctocolectomy will be curative. Nevertheless, a small proportion of the patients later have problems with the ileum, associated either with an ileostomy or an ileal reservoir following an ileoanal anastomosis.[9,85-89] Up to 5% of patients who have had a regular ileostomy require one or more revisions of this structure, due mainly to a tight stoma, mucosal prolapse, or local sepsis. The resected ileum is frequently normal or shows just mucosal atrophy characterized by an increase in mononuclear inflammatory cells in the lamina propria, together with a variable degree of villous shortening.[90-94] Occasionally noted is a complete loss of villi and transformation to a colonic type of mucosa with sulfomucins in the goblet mucous cells.[92,93] Other abnormalities that may be present include hemorrhagic necrosis in cases of prolapse, focal ulceration, and sinus tracts. These changes are usually confined to the stoma and distal 5 cm of the ileostomy segment. Also, some patients develop what has been termed prestomal ileitis, characterized by the presence of focal and shallow ulcers in a longer segment of ileum proximal to the stoma.[95] The involved ileal segment is either of normal caliber or dilated, in contrast to the stenosis that is commonly seen in cases of recurrent Crohn's disease of the ileum. It is thought that prestomal ileitis might be due to a relative obstruction and formation of stasis ulcers. Histologic study of the ulcers shows nonspecific inflammation, and there are no mural fissures or granulomas. Occasionally one may encounter prominent granulomas at an ileostomy stoma and in the adjacent skin, due to suture reaction or to the insertion of foreign objects in the opening.

The incidence of abnormalities affecting continent ileostomies is much higher, with some estimates of 40% to 50%, and they are due largely to vascular compromise and obstruction.[96] This is ordinarily corrected by conversion to a standard ileostomy. In an effort to retain the anal sphincter in patients with ulcerative colitis who require a colectomy, there has been a recent increase in operations involving an ileoanal anastomosis with creation of an ileal reservoir. Some of these patients develop superficial ulcerations of the ileal mucosa, termed "pouchitis," which appear to be due mainly to stasis or to secondary infection by various microbial agents, including fungi such as *Candida*. There have been few detailed studies of the pathology of the ileal reservoir lesions, and most of the information has been based on the examination of superficial mucosal biopsies. The ileum in the reservoir usually shows a mild to moderate degree of mucosal atrophy, and there may be focal erosion or ulcers with a relatively nonspecific acute inflammatory reaction.[87,90,91,97] Occasional lesions are covered with a prominent inflammatory membrane. Later lesions may show signs of chronicity in the form of atrophy and prominent branching of the crypts, together with an increase in mononuclear inflammatory cells.[88,89]

In situations in which disease appears in an ileostomy area or an ileal reservoir, particularly in cases with ulceration, concern may arise that the original diagnosis of ulcerative colitis was an error and that the patient has, instead, Crohn's disease. It may prove useful, in such instances, to review the clinical findings and the pathologic features of the prior colectomy specimen. One must require stringent criteria in assessing the ileal lesions. Features sought to support the diagnosis of Crohn's disease in the ileum would include transmural inflammation, with fibrosis and stricture formation, and the presence of inflammatory sinus tracts or granulomas away from the area of the stoma or anastomosis[94] (see the section on Crohn's disease for further details).

Extraintestinal Manifestations

A variety of inflammatory conditions affecting other organ systems may occur at some time during the course of about one-third of the patients with ulcerative colitis.[98] These include uveitis, joint abnormalities in the form of polyarthritis or ankylosing spondylitis, and the skin diseases of erythema nodosum and pyoderma gangrenosum. The conditions are much more common in patients with extensive colitis than in those with left-sided colitis or proctitis.[99] It is thought that these manifestations are due to effects of circulating immune complexes, induced by antigens that are derived from the gut lumen or the damaged colonic mucosa. In support of this notion, all of these conditions disappear when the patient undergoes a total colectomy. Alterations are also commonly seen in the liver, consisting of fatty changes due to poor nutrition or high-dose corticosteroid therapy and the appearance of focal infiltration of mononuclear inflammatory cells in the portal triads (chronic pericholangitis), probably representing a nonspecific reaction to toxic substances that are absorbed from the inflamed colon.

A rarer effect noted in the liver and biliary tract in cases of ulcerative colitis is sclerosing cholangitis, characterized by the development of progressive fibrosis that encircles the large extra- and intrahepatic bile ducts as well as the ductules in the portal tracts. This results in a characteristic beaded appearance of the large bile ducts that is best visualized by radiographic study and in obstruction of the ductal system. The liver may show the added features of obstructive injury in the form of prominent bile stasis and acute cholangiolitis. The etiology of sclerosing cholangitis is unknown and, unlike the other extraintestinal manifestations seen in ulcerative colitis, this lesion does not regress after the performance of a total colectomy.[100] In cases of sclerosing cholangitis, there is a further problem, an increased incidence of bile duct adenocarcinoma.[101] The tumors may affect any part of the intra- and extrahepatic ducts, typically present as advanced lesions with progression of the stenosis and obstruction, and are rarely amenable to surgical resection. Primary sclerosing cholangitis is a rare disorder. Because most cases are associated instead with chronic inflammatory bowel disease, either ulcerative colitis or Crohn's disease, these latter conditions should be considered in any patient with the appearance of sclerosing cholangitis or stenotic bile duct carcinoma.

Dysplasia and Carcinoma

Incidence and Risk Factors. Patients with ulcerative colitis have an increased incidence of colonic adenocarcinoma.[102-104] The two major risk factors are the extent and the duration of the colitis.[105,106] It has been estimated that cases of extensive colitis (i.e., disease extending to at least the hepatic flexure) have an overall incidence of tumor development in 15%, whereas the rate in those with left-sided colitis is about 5% (Table 27-3). The incidence clearly increases with respect to time with a 1% to 2% rise in tumors after 10 years of extensive disease. Although the risk of tumor occurrence is least in the first decade, this is the period when most patients have not yet had a colectomy for other indications, and it appears that about one fifth of the tumors arise at this time, particularly after 5 years of disease.[107] The degree of cancer risk is variable, however, and probably depends on the geographic location and the particular group of patients studied.[108-110] There is no independent relation of tumor development to the age of onset of the colitis; to the activity or severity of the disease; to the type of medical therapy; or to the sex, race, or ethnic background of the patients.

It has been claimed that the incidence of leukemia and colonic lymphomas is increased in patients with ulcerative colitis,[111-113] but this does not appear to be a major problem. Also recorded have been increases of bile duct carcinoma,[101] colonic carcinoid tumors,[114,115] and possibly uterine and vaginal cancers.[113,116] It has been noted recently that there may be an increased chance of primary adenocarcinoma occurring in ileostomy sites, typically 20 or more years after colectomy for ulcerative colitis.[117,118] A carcinoma has also been detected in an ileoanal reservoir, but this may be related to inadvertently retained rectal mucosa.[119] There is no enhanced frequency of other tumors of the colon or other portions of the gastrointestinal tract.

Carcinoma. There are approximately 1000 new cases of carcinoma complicating chronic inflammatory bowel disease in the United States every year, accounting for about 1% of all new colonic adenocarcinomas.[120] When compared with persons without colitis, younger patients with ulcerative colitis develop tumors with an average age that is about 10 years less, and the tumors are frequently multiple.[104,121-123] They are also distributed more diffusely throughout the colon and do not show the strong predilection for the rectosigmoid area; indeed, recent studies suggest that there are an increasing number of cases in the right portion of the colon.[124,125] The tumors tend to be restricted to areas of prior inflammation, and they may also develop in rectal stumps after a subtotal colectomy.[25-27]

The majority of symptomatic cases present with stenotic lesions, and one does not see the usual adenoma-carcinoma sequence that is noted in patients without colitis. A comparison of tumors with and without colitis at equivalent stages of growth reveals similar behavior.[122,126,127] Nevertheless, because it may be exceedingly difficult to distinguish stenosing tumors from the effects of the underlying colitis, most cases of carcinoma complicating ulcerative colitis in symptomatic patients appear at an advanced stage, and the prognosis is generally poor. The advanced tumors vary in size, with lesions extending over several centimeters, and they frequently are circumferential (Figure 27-17). The adjacent mucosa is often raised, which may represent areas of residual dysplasia. The overall spread of the carcinomas is similar to that seen in patients without colitis, and there is invasion into and through the bowel wall to the peritoneum and metastases to regional lymph nodes and liver. The earlier carcinomas, which are presently being detected with greater frequency because of the use of surveillance programs,

Table 27-3 CARCINOMA IN ULCERATIVE COLITIS

Type	Incidence	
Extensive colitis*		15%
10 years	1%	
15 years	4.5%	
20 years	13%	
30 years	34%	
Left-sided colitis		5%

*Colitis extending to at least the hepatic flexure.
Modified from Greenstein AJ, Sachar DB, Smith H, et al: Cancer in universal and left-sided ulcerative colitis: Factors determining risk. Gastroenterology 99:290-294, 1979.

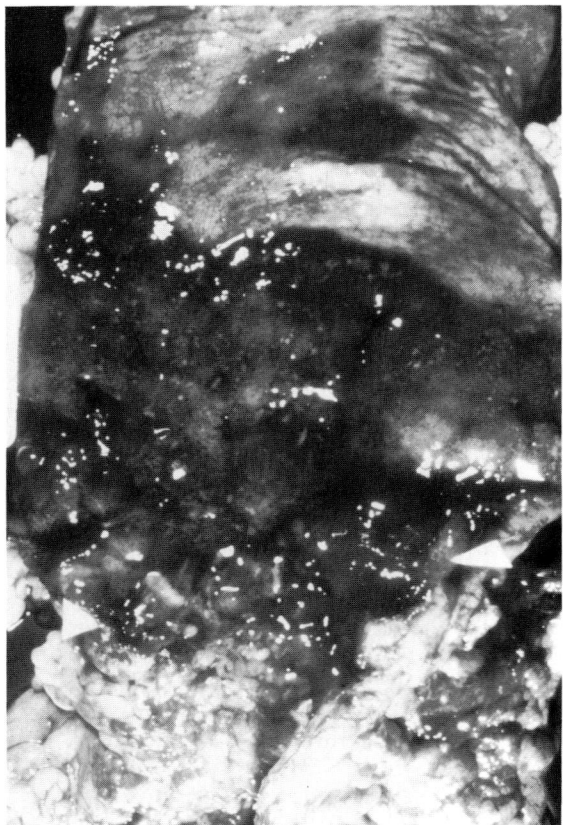

FIGURE 27–17. Adenocarcinoma of the colon in a case of chronic ulcerative colitis. The carcinoma is located in the stenotic portion (at bottom), and the adjacent mucosa is slightly raised as a result of associated dysplasia.

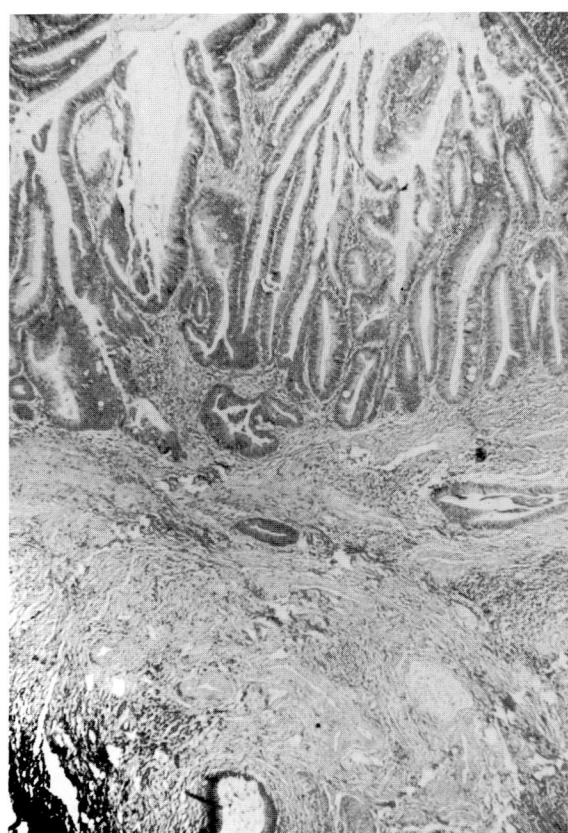

FIGURE 27–18. Well-differentiated adenocarcinoma of the colon, complicating chronic ulcerative colitis. The carcinomatous glands are well formed, and their nature is revealed only by invasion into the submucosa and muscularis propria. The overlying mucosa (top) shows the dysplastic glands. (H&E, × 20)

tend to be smaller and appear as more discrete, slightly raised or polypoid lesions.[128] These early tumors are associated with prominent dysplasia in the mucosa and usually show less invasion by the carcinoma. The remaining colonic mucosa shows signs of chronic colitis, which is usually in the inactive stage and may reveal other foci of gross or microscopic dysplasia alone or together with other carcinomas.

Histologic examination of the adenocarcinomas in ulcerative colitis reveals variable gland formation, and a high proportion, about 35% to 40%, are very well differentiated or the mucinous type[129,130] (Figure 27–18). Indeed, it may be difficult to appreciate the carcinoma in mucosal biopsies because the samples may be too superficial for detection of the invasion. All other histologic forms are encountered, including poorly differentiated carcinoma, signet-ring cell type, and tumors mixed with neuroendocrine cells (adenocarcinoid tumors).[48,115,131–133] There is no relation between the degree of differentiation of the carcinomas and their behavior.

A clinical suspicion of carcinoma complicating ulcerative colitis is raised if obstructive signs, bleeding, or weight loss develop that cannot be explained by the underlying inflammatory disease. The tumors are localized by radiographic and endoscopic studies, and a specific diagnosis is obtained by directed mucosal biopsy. The level of serum carcinoembryonic antigen has not proved to be of value, because it may vary considerably as a result of active colitis and its repair. Because of the common presence and occasional large size of inflammatory pseudopolyps, it was once thought that these lesions might be a precursor of the carcinoma, but this view is no longer accepted. Indeed, it is rare for an inflammatory polyp to be the site for even the presence of dysplasia.

Dysplasia. Dysplasia represents a neoplastic transformation of the colonic epithelium and serves as a marker that a patient with ulcerative colitis either already has or is particularly prone to the development of carcinoma.[48] Synonyms for colonic dysplasia include precancer, precarcinoma, and adenomatous epithelium. Early studies of carcinoma in ulcerative colitis noted the presence of such dysplasia at the edge of many tumors,[134] and Morson and Pang in 1967 demonstrated that this could be detected in mucosal biopsies that were obtained from sites away from the overt tumor.[135] Subsequent investigations have shown that about 90% of cases of ulcerative colitis with carcinoma contain foci of dysplasia, either adjacent to or remote from the gross cancer.[107,122,136–149] The dysplasia, like the carcinoma, may be present in any portion of the

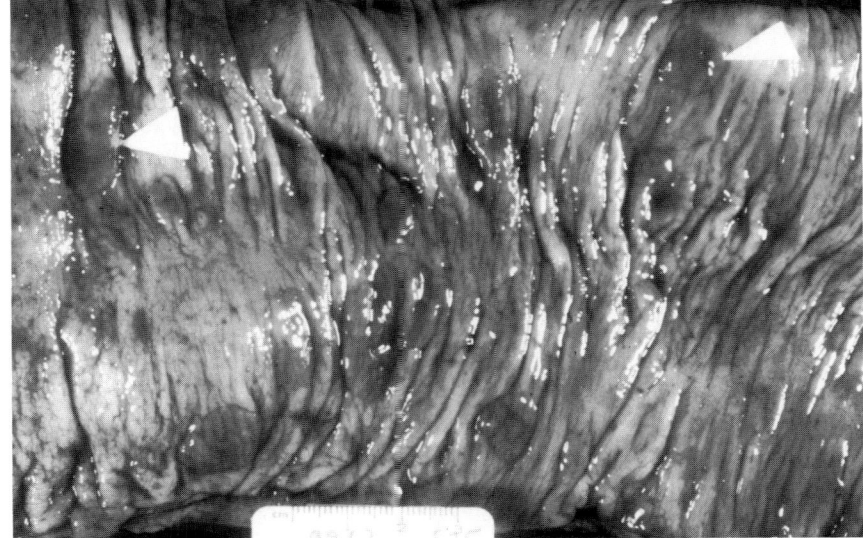

FIGURE 27–19. Colon segment in a case of inactive ulcerative colitis. There are several small plaques (arrows) in the mucosa, which revealed epithelial dysplasia on histologic examination (see Figure 27–32).

colon, and only two thirds of the lesions will be detected if the inspection is limited to the left side of the colon.[125,150,151] It may be observed as a microscopic alteration in the flat atrophic mucosa or, when severe, associated with a gross lesion (referred to as dysplasia-associated lesion or mass, or DALM.[152] The gross areas of dysplasia vary from a few millimeters to several centimeters in diameter, and they are typically sessile and slightly raised lesions with a prominent velvety or villous surface[137] (Figures 27–19 and 27–20). Ordinary inflammatory polyps (pseudopolyps), in contrast, tend to have a smoother or rounded surface contour. Signs of carcinoma within a gross dysplastic lesion include the presence of ulceration, induration, or stenosis. However, many of the carcinomas lack these surface changes and are revealed only by detection of invasion into the colonic wall, particularly in early and well-differentiated tumors (see Figure 27–18). It has been estimated that the appearance of dysplasia, particularly in the flat mucosa, may precede the development of overt carcinoma by as much as 7 years.[143] On the other hand, in grossly evident lesions, the dysplasia may be the first sign of an underlying invasive tumor.

The histologic diagnosis of dysplasia in cases of ulcerative colitis is often difficult because of the persistent inflammatory and reparative effects of the underlying disease. The latter features cause complex branching of the crypts and other architectural changes that may be confused with a neoplastic proliferation, especially in cases that also show regenerative effects in the epithelium. It is essential, therefore, that one is aware of the full range of inflammatory changes that may affect the mucosa in cases of chronic ulcerative colitis before one makes the diagnosis of dysplasia.[46,47] To assist in this distinction, a standardized classification of colonic dysplasia with uniform nomenclature and criteria has been provided (Table 27–4).[48] This was primarily designed for the interpretation of mucosal biopsy samples but can be applied to the general examination of the mucosa. Tissues are rated in this classification as "negative," "indefinite," or "positive" for dysplasia on the basis of a combination of histo-

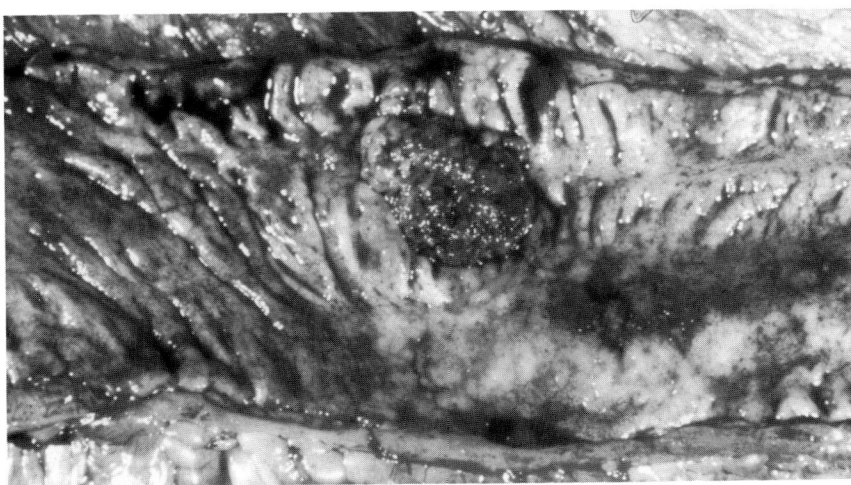

FIGURE 27–20. Polypoid lesion of dysplasia in ulcerative colitis.

Table 27-4 CLASSIFICATION OF DYSPLASIA IN CHRONIC COLITIS

Negative for dysplasia
    Normal mucosa
    Inactive (quiescent) colitis
    Active colitis
Indefinite for dysplasia
    Probably negative (inflammatory)
    Unknown
    Probably positive (dysplastic)
Positive for dysplasia
    Low-grade dysplasia
    High-grade dysplasia

Modified from Riddell RH, Goldman HG, Ransohoff DF, et al: Dysplasia in inflammatory bowel disease: Standardized classification with provisional clinical applications. Hum Pathol 14:931-968, 1983.

logic and cytologic characteristics. The negative category includes tissues that are normal or show the expected effects of inactive or active colitis (see Histologic Features, under Pathology). There is rarely any difficulty in evaluating tissues with inactive colitis; these may show irregular branching and shortening of the crypts, but the epithelial cells have a normal or slightly regenerative appearance without prominence of the nuclei (Figure 27-21).

As noted above, the greatest caution must be applied in the examination of specimens in cases of active colitis to avoid the overdiagnosis of dysplasia (Figure 27-22). The features should not be compared with those of the normal mucosa; rather, the changes of chronic colitis should serve as the baseline. Because of the severe confounding effects of active inflammation, one should try to avoid the examination of ulcerated areas or ordinary pseudopolyps; rather, samples should be taken from the regions that appear flat and more atrophic or from villous lesions. Active colitis is associated with greater regeneration, and some crypts may show prominent elongation and pallisading of the nuclei (Figure 27-23). Also present are numerous mitoses and occasional "dystrophic" goblet cells with mucin displaced to the basal portion of the cell (Figure 27-24). There is, however, no hyperchromatism (or a minimal amount) or pleomorphism. Although the nuclear changes may be similar to those seen in low-grade dysplasia, the inflammatory nature is usually evident because of the associated neutrophilic infiltration of the crypts and lamina propria.

The category "indefinite" for dysplasia is employed when the mucosal changes appear to exceed those usually seen in active colitis, but the features are insufficient for an unequivocal diagnosis of dysplasia. It is often used when signs of active disease are less conspicuous in the mucosa sampled (Figure 27-25) or when there are unusual forms of inflammation or growth. The latter include the degenerative effects in the surface cells overlying lymphoid nodules in cases of follicular proctitis or colitis (Figure 27-26), a hyperplastic type of growth with prominent papillary infoldings similar to those seen in hyperplastic polyps, and the appearance of incomplete maturation of the crypts, with uniformly enlarged nuclei (Figure 27-27). In all of these instances, the assessment is based primarily on the quality of the nuclei. Nevertheless, tissues showing a prominent villous surface or a hyperplastic type of growth are more likely to be dysplastic. Uncertainties in diagnosis may also be due to technical factors, including mainly the effects of fixatives, and to reactions to toxic enema solutions. Whenever possible, the rating of indefinite should be further qualified as probably negative (inflammatory) or probably positive (dysplastic) because of the implications for further management, as described below.

A two-tier system is used for the rating of colonic dysplasia, consisting of low-grade and high-grade degrees, to match the potential clinical options of further biopsy or colectomy. Low-grade dysplasia reveals no architectural changes in excess of those seen in chronic colitis and a mild to moderate degree of cytologic atypism of the epithelial cells in the absence of any signif-

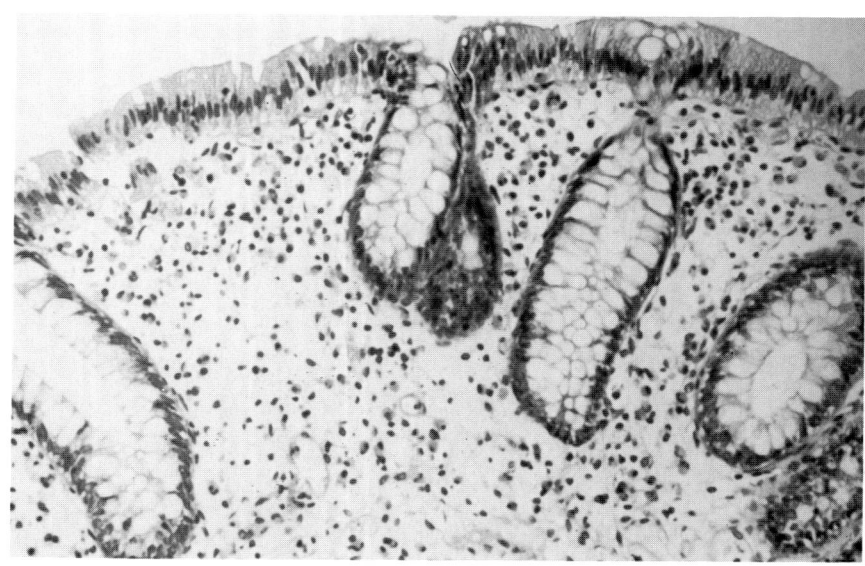

FIGURE 27-21. Colonic mucosa in ulcerative colitis, rated as negative for dysplasia. There is crypt atrophy but no cytologic atypism. (H&E, × 100)

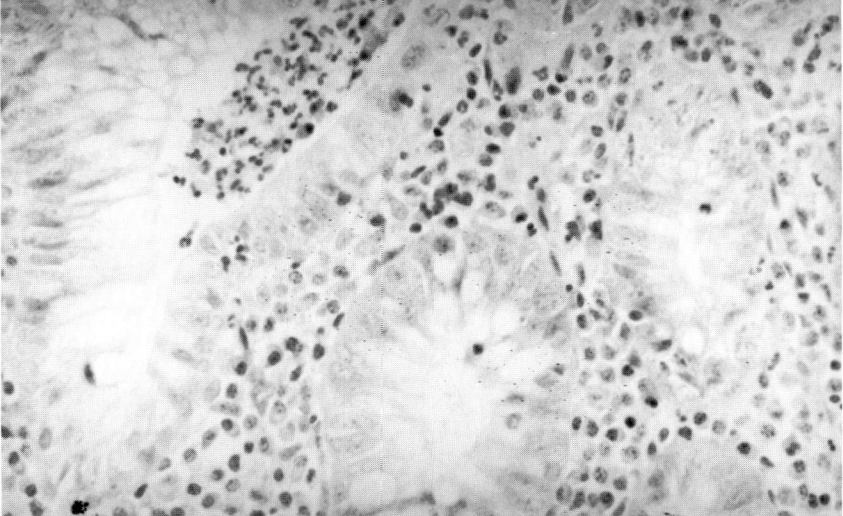

FIGURE 27–22. Colonic mucosa in ulcerative colitis, rated as negative for dysplasia. There is active colitis with crypt abscesses and increased inflammation in the lamina propria. Some of the epithelial cells contain elongated nuclei without hyperchromasia. (H&E, × 250) (From Goldman H, Antonioli DA: Mucosal biopsy of the rectum, colon, and distal ileum. Hum Pathol 13:981–1012, 1982.)

icant active inflammation (Figure 27–28). There is elongation and stratification of the nuclei, which tend to occupy about half of the cell height. The cells are otherwise fairly regular and show only focal and modest hyperchromatism. High-grade dysplasia, in contrast, shows some combination of stratified nuclei that extend beyond the midpoint of the cells (Figure 27–29); glandular proliferation that is more than expected in chronic colitis; a greater number of dystrophic goblet cells; and more prominent hyperchromatism and pleo-

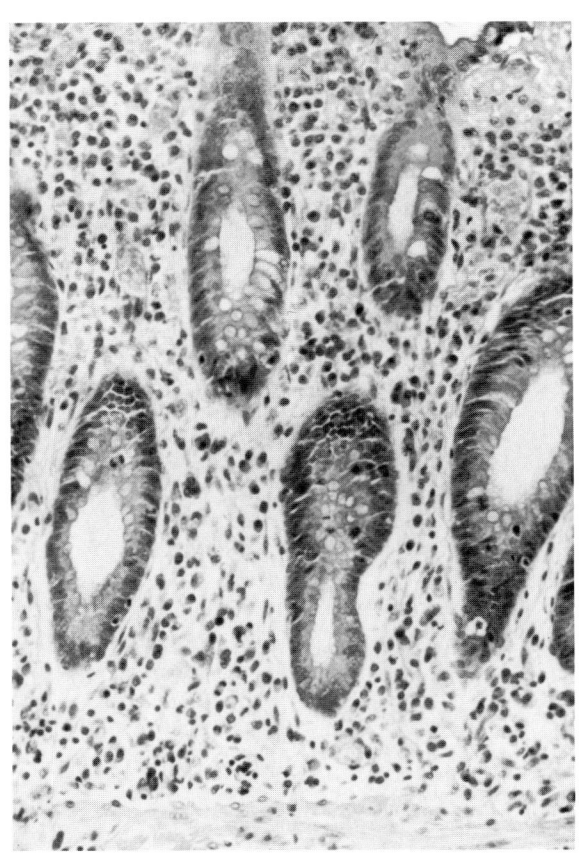

FIGURE 27–23. Colonic mucosa in ulcerative colitis, rated as negative for dysplasia. There is prominent regeneration of the crypts with reduction in the cytoplasmic mucin. The epithelial cell nuclei are slightly enlarged but uniform and not hyperchromatic. (H&E, × 100)

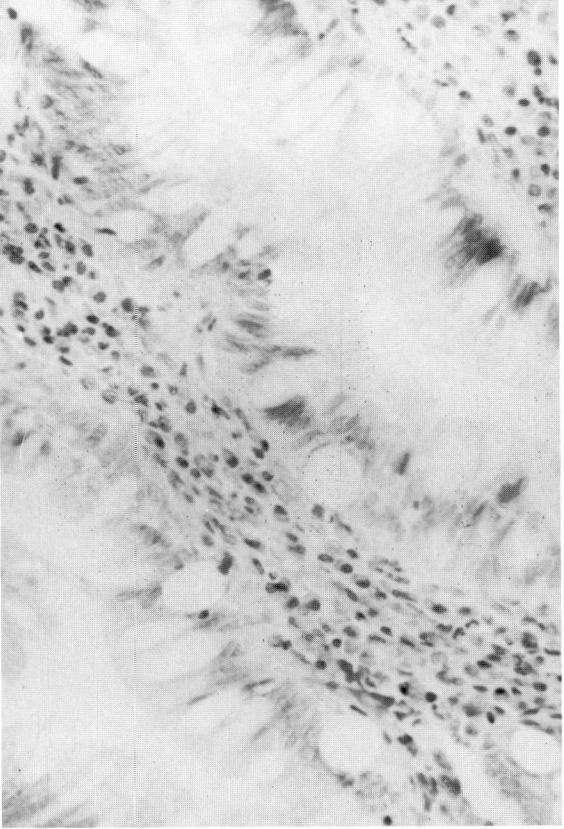

FIGURE 27–24. Colonic mucosa containing dystrophic goblet mucous cells, rated as negative for dysplasia. The dystrophic goblet cells are characterized by the presence of cytoplasmic mucin in the basal rather than the normal luminal position of the cell. Although dystrophic goblet cells are more often seen in dysplasia, there is no nuclear atypism in this example. (H&E, × 250)

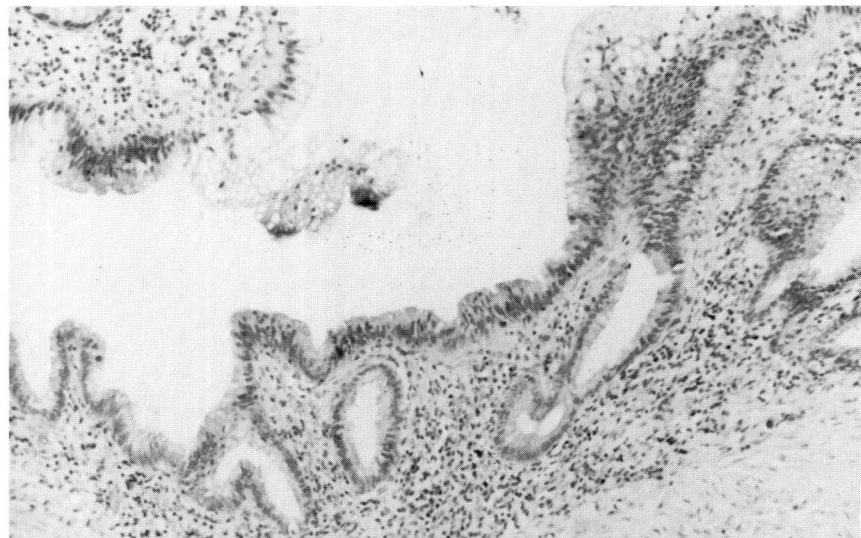

FIGURE 27-25. Colonic mucosa in ulcerative colitis, rated as indefinite for dysplasia. The surface epithelium (center) shows loss of mucin and enlarged pallisading nuclei suspicious of dysplasia. However, the affected region is depressed, and it is more likely that this represents active regeneration of a previously ulcerated area. (H&E, × 100)

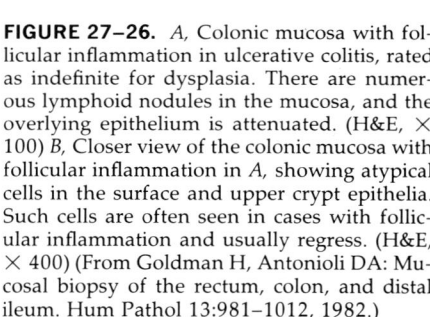

FIGURE 27-26. *A,* Colonic mucosa with follicular inflammation in ulcerative colitis, rated as indefinite for dysplasia. There are numerous lymphoid nodules in the mucosa, and the overlying epithelium is attenuated. (H&E, × 100) *B,* Closer view of the colonic mucosa with follicular inflammation in *A,* showing atypical cells in the surface and upper crypt epithelia. Such cells are often seen in cases with follicular inflammation and usually regress. (H&E, × 400) (From Goldman H, Antonioli DA: Mucosal biopsy of the rectum, colon, and distal ileum. Hum Pathol 13:981–1012, 1982.)

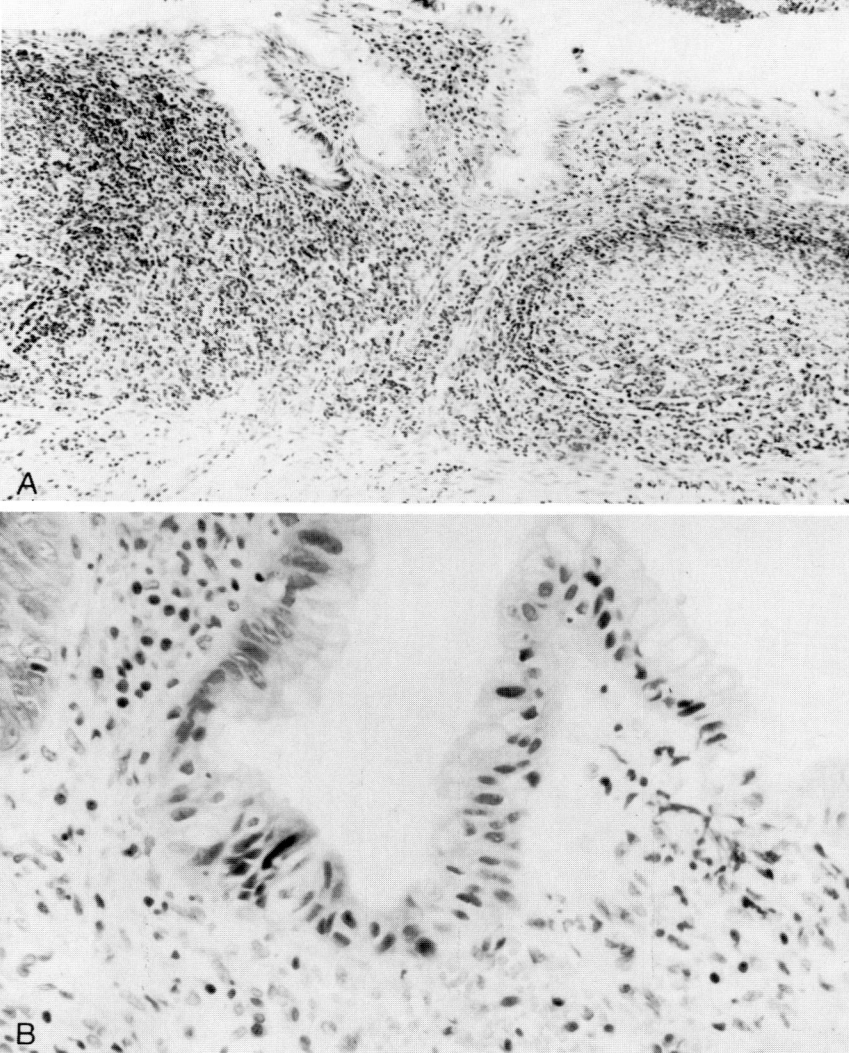

FIGURE 27-27. Colonic mucosa with incomplete maturation of the crypts, rated as indefinite for dysplasia. The mucin is reduced and limited to the luminal portion of the cells, and the nuclei are generally enlarged. Such changes can occur in regeneration but have also been noted next to overt dysplastic lesions. (H&E, × 400)

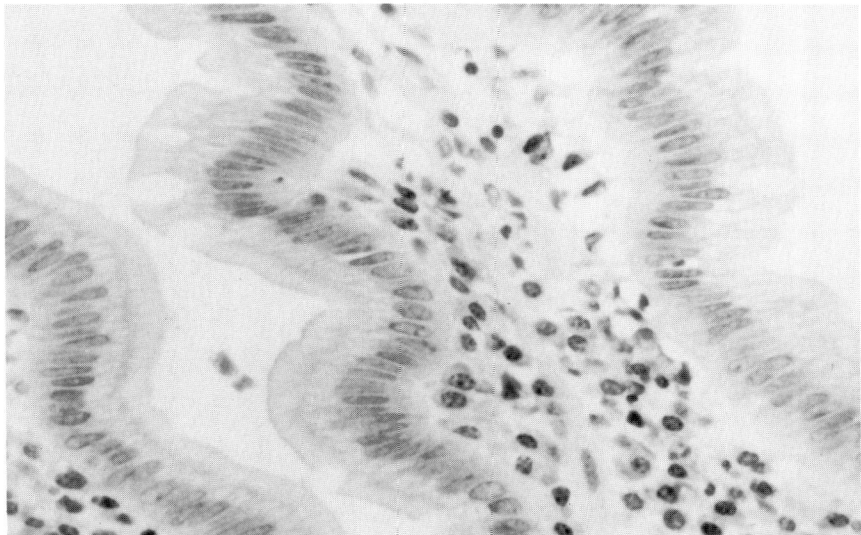

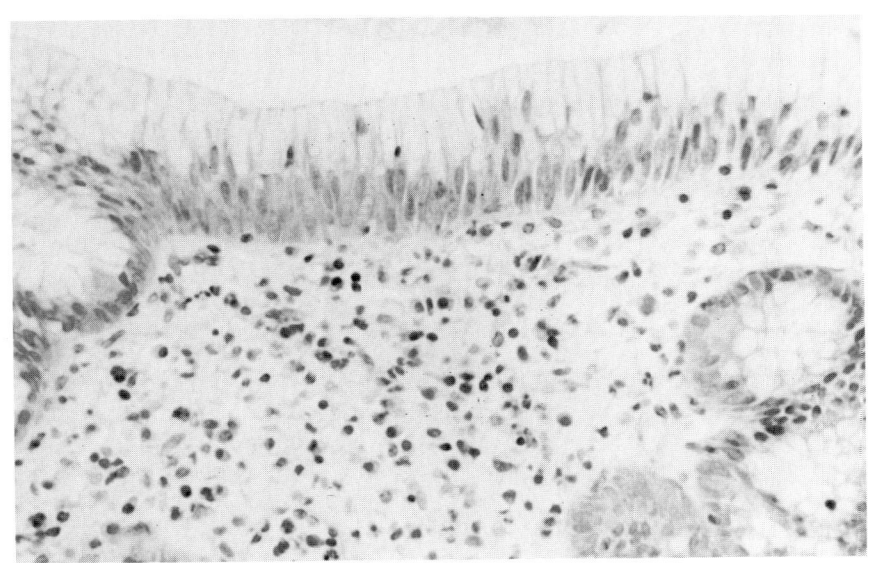

FIGURE 27-28. Colonic mucosal biopsy in ulcerative colitis, rated as positive for low-grade (or slight) dysplasia. There is a prominent elongation and stratification of the nuclei in the surface epithelial cells in the absence of acute inflammation. The nuclei occupy the basal half of the epithelial cells, and there is no hyperchromasia. (H&E, × 400) (From Goldman H: Dysplasia and carcinoma in inflammatory bowel disease. In Rachmilewitz D (ed): Inflammatory Bowel Diseases. The Hague, Martinus Nijhoff, 1982, pp 27–40. With permission from Kluwer Academic Publishers.)

FIGURE 27-29. Colonic mucosal biopsy of a raised mucosal lesion in ulcerative colitis, rated as positive for high-grade (or moderate) dysplasia. In contrast to Figure 27–28, this figure shows the glands to be more irregular, the nuclear stratification more prominent, and the nuclei extending into the luminal half of the cells. (H&E, × 400) (From Goldman H: Dysplasia and carcinoma in inflammatory bowel disease. In Rachmilewitz D (ed): Inflammatory Bowel Diseases. The Hague, Martinus Nijhoff, 1982, pp 27–40. With permission from Kluwer Academic Publishers.)

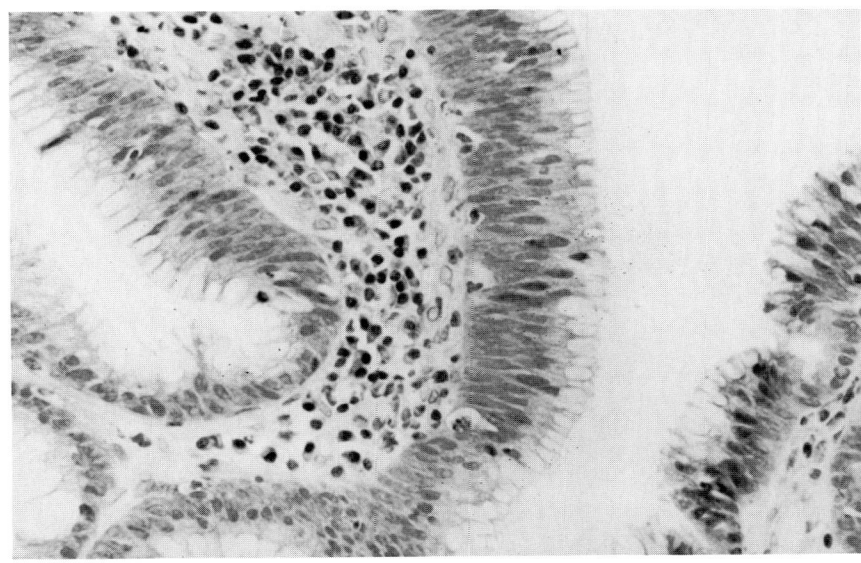

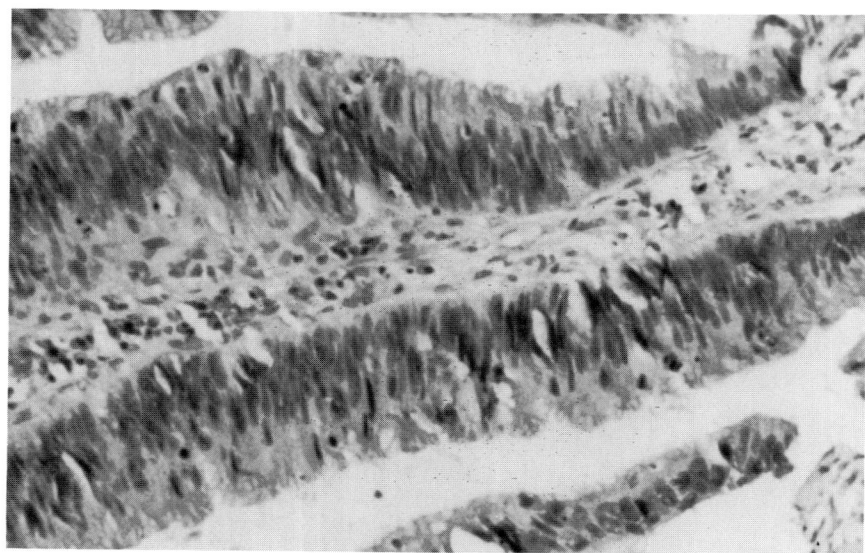

FIGURE 27–30. Colonic mucosal biopsy of a raised mucosal lesion in ulcerative colitis (same case as in Figure 27–17), rated as positive for high-grade (or severe) dysplasia. There was a villiform surface, and the epithelial cell nuclei show considerable pleomorphism and hyperchromatism. (H&E, × 400)

morphism (Figure 27–30). There may also be many mitoses, but these are also seen in ordinary regeneration. Carcinoma in situ, characterized by severe epithelial changes and a cribriform glandular arrangement, is not considered a separate entity but, rather, is included in the diagnostic term of high-grade dysplasia because the clinical implication is the same (Figure 27–31). In any case of dysplasia, one should also look for infiltrating carcinoma, either limited to the lamina propria and muscularis mucosae (intramucosal carcinoma) or extending into the submucosa or beyond (invasive carcinoma). In this regard, many of the carcinomas are well differentiated and only identified by the feature of invasion.

The dysplasia is usually most prominent in the crypt bases when associated with a gross mass (Figure 27–32), whereas it tends to be concentrated on the surface of flat atrophic mucosa (see Figure 27–28); in all instances, the degree of dysplasia, whether of low or high grade, is rated by the worst area. Inflammatory polyps (pseudopolyps) may show considerable glandular proliferation, but it is rare for dysplasia to develop in such lesions. One problem that is seen in older patients is how to distinguish a polypoid area of dysplasia from the incidental development of an adenoma. The neoplastic growth tends to be limited to the head of an adenoma and spares the stalk mucosa, whereas a dysplastic lesion often extends to involve parts of the stalk and adjacent colonic mucosa.

Other methods that have been tested for diagnosing dysplasia without success have included immunocytochemical stains for carcinoembryonic antigen and secretory component.[153] A reduction in sulfomucins and an increase in sialomucins have been noted in many cases of dysplasia,[154] but this alteration is also seen in most of the negative cases and may be a nonspecific

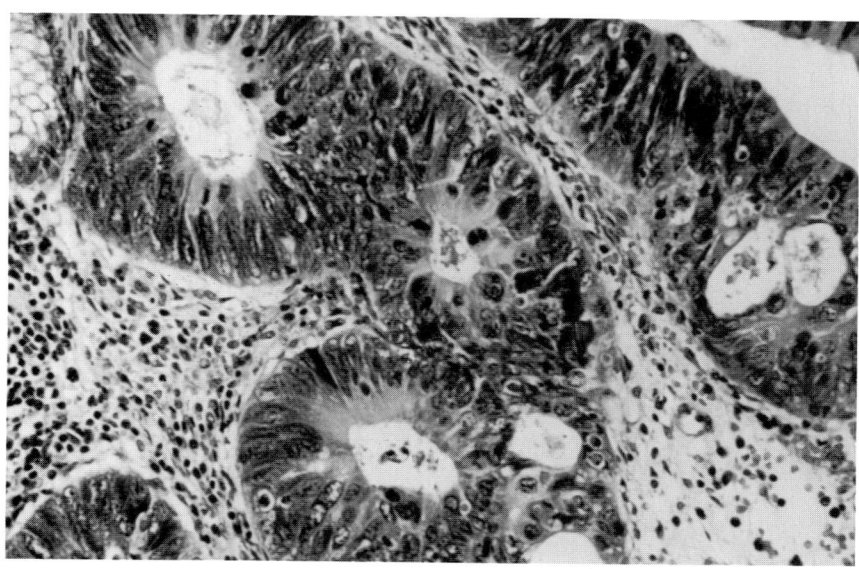

FIGURE 27–31. Colonic mucosa in ulcerative colitis, rated as positive for high-grade dysplasia. There is marked nuclear atypicality and cribriform glands without invasion into the lamina propria. Such features have also been called adenocarcinoma in situ but fit within the category of high-grade dysplasia. (H&E, × 250) (From Goldman H: Dysplasia and carcinoma in inflammatory bowel disease. In Rachmilewitz D (ed): Inflammatory Bowel Diseases. The Hague, Martinus Nijhoff, 1982, pp 27–40. With permission from Kluwer Academic Publishers.)

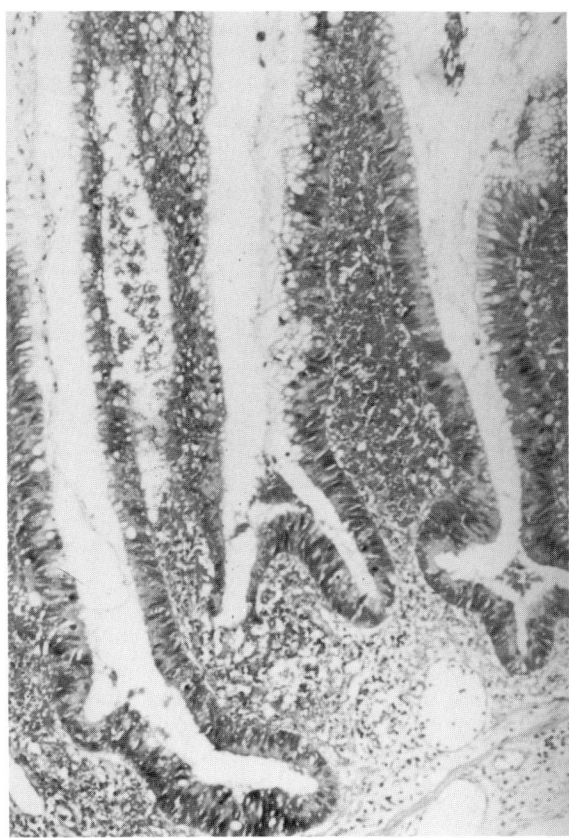

FIGURE 27-32. Colonic mucosa of a raised lesion in ulcerative colitis (same case as in Figure 27-19), showing a villiform surface. The dysplastic cells are concentrated in the basal portion of the crypts, whereas the cells at the surface appear mature. (H&E, × 100)

reaction of the colonic mucosa in inflammatory states. Similarly, the colonic mucosa in cancer cases reveals a reduction in the number of the large-intestinal type of mucous antigens and the appearance of the small-intestinal type of antigens. An increase in abnormal glycoconjugates, identified by lectin-binding studies, has been observed in patients who subsequently develop dysplasia, and it is possible that the appearance of such mucin abnormalities may serve to identify patients in special need of a surveillance program.[156]

The application of scanning electron microscopy with quantitative analyses has revealed reductions in the density and size of the surface cells and their microvilli in dysplastic lesions.[157-159] The changes in microvilli, particularly a reduction in their density and thickness, appear to be fairly specific and may help to distinguish dysplasia from inflammatory effects in cases that require repeat biopsy because of uncertainties in the diagnosis. The identification of aneuploid cells by DNA flow cytometry has been noted in about one half of cases of dysplasia, and this method may also prove useful in problem cases.[160-165]

Clinical Applications. Considering the statistical data, it has been recommended that patients with extensive ulcerative colitis lasting more than 10 years should have a prophylactic colectomy, but this has not been accepted by most patients. An effort to detect early carcinoma by periodic radiographic and endoscopic studies has proved difficult because of the flat and stenosing character of most tumors, which are similar to the inflammatory effects of the underlying colitis. Furthermore, many of the carcinomas are well differentiated and not easily appreciated in mucosal biopsy. It is currently recommended that patients with extensive ulcerative colitis lasting more than 8 to 10 years should have periodic colonoscopic examinations for the purpose of looking for dysplasia and determining which patients should undergo a colectomy.[48,107,143] From past cumulative studies of all patients with ulcerative colitis, including those seen for the first time and those with symptoms, it appeared that if high-grade dysplasia was identified in an endoscopic biopsy, there was about one chance in three that the patient had an occult carcinoma of the colon and some of these were deeply invasive.[150] More recent investigations have revealed that this chance of carcinoma is much less, even if the dysplasia is derived from a gross lesion, in patients who are asymptomatic and seen as part of a surveillance program. Accordingly, the primary aim of the surveillance program is to detect significant dysplasia and to prevent the appearance of carcinoma. The increased incidence of carcinoma is not as great in patients with left-sided ulcerative colitis,[106] and it is not certain whether they should be part of a surveillance program. Because the lag period appears to be longer in these patients, the starting points for surveillance could be later, perhaps after 15 years.

Raised velvety lesions should be sought for biopsy at endoscopy, and overtly inflamed areas and ordinary pseudopolyps should be avoided.[48] In the absence of a gross lesion, which is the usual case, multiple (8 to 12) random biopsies should be obtained from the flat mucosa in all parts of the colon. The biopsies are rated by light microscopy as negative, indefinite, or positive for dysplasia, and all positive cases should be confirmed by additional examiners or repeat study. If the biopsy specimens are taken from the flat mucosa, regular surveillance can be continued if they are rated as negative or indefinite-probably negative; earlier repeat biopsy should be done if they are rated as other indefinite or as low-grade dysplasia; and colectomy is considered if the confirmed diagnosis is high-grade dysplasia. These actions are slightly modified if the biopsies are taken from a gross lesion, with repeat biopsy for any indefinite lesion and consideration of colectomy for both low- and high-grade dysplasia. Further accumulation of data from prospective studies is needed to determine whether these recommendations will prove valid in the prevention of carcinoma in patients with ulcerative colitis.[166-169]

CROHN'S DISEASE

General Aspects

Definition and Terminology. Crohn's disease is a chronic inflammatory disorder of unknown etiology that may affect any portion of the alimentary tract. The disease is characterized by the frequent presence of transmural inflammation, strictures, fistulas, and granulomas.[1-3] It most commonly involves the small intestine, particularly the distal ileum, and the colon. Because of the tendency for there to be a segmental distribution, the disease has also been termed regional enteritis (or ileitis), regional enterocolitis, and segmental or regional colitis. Since predominant involvement of the colon was at one time considered to be uncertain, another old term for the disease in that area was *granulomatous colitis*.[5-7] The entity was firmly established and separated from other known inflammatory disorders such as infections in 1932 by Crohn, who described involvement of the terminal ileum.[170] Several reports over the ensuing 5 years illustrated disease in other portions of the small intestine, colon, and upper gastrointestinal tract. However, there remained a tendency to ascribe idiopathic inflammatory disease that affected mainly the colon to ulcerative colitis until 1960s, when studies by Lockhart-Mummery and others reestablished that Crohn's disease could affect the colon.[171,172] The spelling of the eponym has been a persistent challenge, as aptly documented in a published letter.[173]

Diagnostic Criteria. Before the diagnosis of Crohn's disease can be considered, other known causes of inflammation of the gut must be excluded by relevant laboratory tests and by radiographic and endoscopic procedures. The principal disorders to be distinguished include infections, ischemic disease, and diverticulitis. Furthermore, when the disease is confined to or predominantly affects the colon, the differential diagnosis includes ulcerative colitis.[5-8] The diagnosis of Crohn's disease is best accomplished by using a combination of distributional, gross, and microscopic features, including the presence of skip or segmental disease, sinus tracts and fistulas, and granulomatous inflammation (Table 27-5). Further details are provided below in the section on pathologic diagnosis.

Epidemiology. Crohn's disease has many epidemiologic features in common with ulcerative colitis.[12,174] Thus, it is more common in the Western developed countries, and it is about two to five times more frequent in the white population and two to three times more frequent in Jewish persons. The annual incidence in countries where the disease is more often seen is about 1 to 3 per 100,000, and there is a familial history in 3% to 11% of reported series. The disease has a peak incidence in the third decade but may affect all age groups, including children and elderly persons; and there is no definite gender predilection. It was formerly thought that Crohn's disease was much less common than ulcerative colitis, by a factor of one-fifth to one-seventh, but this was due to the misplacement of many cases of colonic Crohn's disease into the ulcerative colitis category. Overall, ulcerative colitis is slightly more frequent, whereas studies of surgical specimens reveal more cases of Crohn's disease because they more often require surgery.

Etiology and Pathogenesis

The cause and evolution of Crohn's disease are not known. Because of the character of the inflammatory reaction, with the presence of prominent lymphoid nodules and occasional granulomas, a chronic infection has long been suspected. Transfer studies in animals, employing ultrafiltrates of disease tissue, have implicated viruses and cell wall–defective bacteria, but a consistent agent has not been identified.[175,176] More recent investigations have noted the appearance of bacteria with an antigenic profile resembling *Mycobacterium paratuberculosis*.[177] An immunologic mechanism has also been considered because of the frequent presence of allergic and other immune disorders in the patients and by the beneficial response to immunosuppressive therapy.[4,178] There have been extensive investigations of the immune cells, and it has been suggested that Crohn's disease is due to an altered T-cell response to various antigens, including infectious agents. Other theories have included vascular disease,[179] lymphatic obstruction, and emotional stress; but there are no firm data to support their roles in the primary etiology of the disease.

The earliest lesion, well seen by scanning electron microscopy, appears to be a tiny erosion of the surface overlying normal mucosal lymphoid tissue.[180] These coalesce to form small aphthous ulcers and eventually more diffuse ulceration of the mucosa. With progression of the disease, there is marked hyperplasia of the lymphoid tissue, which extends through the wall; fibrosis and muscular hypertrophy, leading to strictures; and discrete inflammatory sinus tracts that pierce the wall. Granulomas are also present in about one half of the cases. The mechanisms responsible for this advancement of the disease are not known.

Clinical Features

The clinical findings are variable and depend on the particular distribution of the disease.[181] Most patients have involvement of the ileum and present with fever, crampy abdominal pain from obstruction, and watery

Table 27-5 DIAGNOSTIC FEATURES OF CROHN'S DISEASE

Absence of known etiology

Common involvement of the distal small intestine and/or colon; disease tends to have a focal or segmental distribution, and the rectum is often spared

May affect all other parts of the gut, including the oral cavity, esophagus, stomach, proximal small intestine, appendix, and anal region

Characterized by ulceration and inflammation extending deep into the bowel wall and by early fibrous stricture formation

Presence of discrete inflammatory sinus tracks, fissures, or fistulas in two thirds of cases; must distinguish from multiple "cracks" in wall that may be seen in cases with toxic megacolon

Presence of well-formed, sarcoid-type granulomas in one half of cases; must distinguish from granulomas due to ruptured crypts or foreign bodies

NOTE: All of the features may not be present in an individual case

diarrhea due mainly to the toxic effects of unabsorbed bile salts on the colonic mucosa. An acute attack, seen in about 20% of the cases, may simulate a case of acute appendicitis. More marked small-intestinal disease is characterized by the appearance of abdominal masses and sepsis due to localized perforations; sinus tracts and fistulas that may extend to other viscera and the skin; and malabsorption due to various factors, including reduced bile salt reabsorption from the diseased or bypassed ileum, bacterial proliferation states, and, least often, extensive mucosal loss in the jejunum. The nutritional deficit can be a special problem in preadolescents, since it may interfere with the normal maturation and cause a stunting of growth.[182] When there is prominent colonic disease, the clinical features are similar to those seen in cases of ulcerative colitis and include the acute onset of purulent diarrhea and rectal bleeding. Perianal disease in the form of fistulas and abscesses is seen in about 20% to 25% of all cases and is the presenting feature in about 5% of the patients. Exceptionally, the disease may affect the upper gastrointestinal tract and reveals focal ulceration of the oral cavity or lesions that mimic reflux esophagitis and chronic peptic ulcer disease.

Medical therapy consists of nutritional support, various anti-inflammatory and immunosuppressive agents, including corticosteroids, and antibiotics for secondary infections and perforations. The disease is characterized by frequent periods of relapses and remissions, and there is often extension and worsening of the lesions at the time of recurrence. Surgery is commonly required for the various complications and intractable disease in the intestines, and an attempt is made to limit this to conservative resections of the bowel[183,184]; there is a strong likelihood of postoperative recurrence, which is independent of the amount of normal tissue removed.[185,186] The distribution of the disease permits in most cases a segmental resection and anastomosis of the bowel, with an expected recurrence rate of about 5% per year. The recurrent disease tends to appear at the site, either the small intestine or the colon, of the original lesion, usually next to the anastomosis.[186,187] When surgery is needed for severe colonic disease with rectal involvement, a total colectomy is required. Despite the tendency for repeated relapses and for the need of multiple resections, it is rare for the patients to become nutritional cripples,[9,188] and the overall mortality from Crohn's disease and its complications is only about twice that of the general population.[189]

Pathology

There have been several detailed studies of the pathology of Crohn's disease affecting the small intestine and the colon.[1,2,190-192] The pathologic features are generally similar in cases of all age groups, including children and elderly patients.[28,193]

Distribution of Disease. Any part of the alimentary tract may be affected in Crohn's disease. At the microscopic and ultrastructural level there is often evidence, in the form of patchy inflammation, axonal degeneration or granulomas, of widespread lesions in the mucosa and submucosa throughout the gut.[180,194-200] These features may serve as a marker of Crohn's disease but do not predict that a clinically significant gross lesion will develop in that particular region. At the onset of the disease, there is gross involvement of the small intestine alone in about 45%, the small bowel and colon in 35%, and the colon alone in 15% of the cases. When there is involvement of both the small and large intestines, it is frequently dominant in one or the other area. As the disease progresses, the lesions tend to remain in their original tissues, and only a small proportion of the cases later extend between the small and large bowel. Most of the cases with small-intestinal disease affect the terminal portion of the ileum, and this frequently but not invariably extends to the ileocecal valve region (Figure 27-33). In about 5% to 10% of the

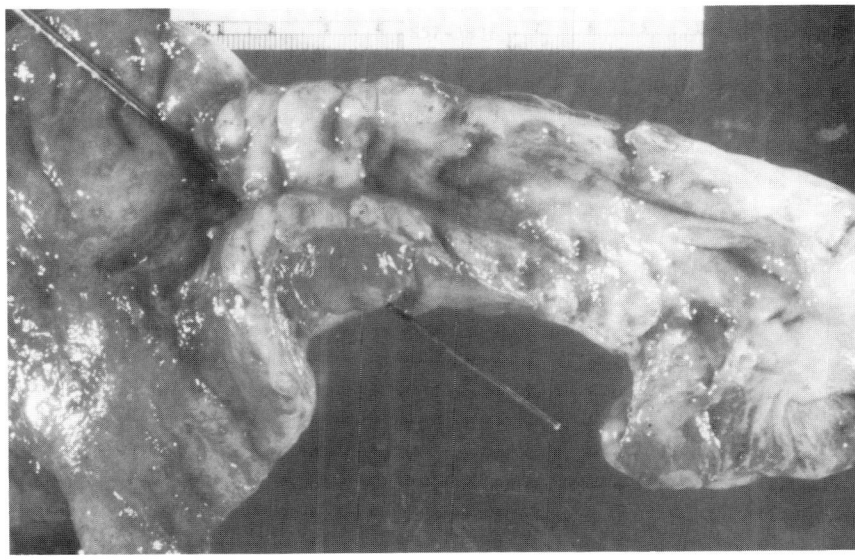

FIGURE 27-33. Crohn's disease of the terminal ileum, characterized by stenosis, mucosal ulceration, marked mural thickening, and a transmural sinus tract (identified by probe). The lesion appears to stop at the ileocecal valve, and the contiguous cecum (left) is not overtly involved.

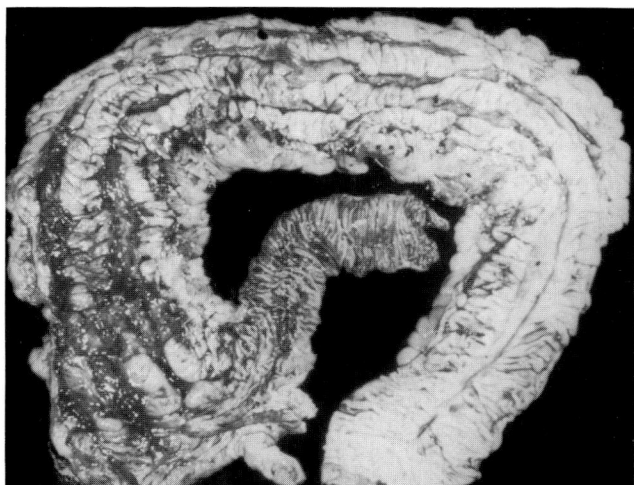

FIGURE 27-34. Crohn's disease, involving mainly the colon. There are prominent longitudinal ulcers extending from the cecum (lower left) to the descending colon, but the more distal part of the colon and the rectum were normal. In this figure, in contrast to Figure 27-33, there is no stenosis, and the wall is not thickened. The disease also crosses the ileocecal valve and extends into the terminal ileum for a short distance.

small-intestinal cases there is eventually involvement, either by direct extension or over skip areas, to the proximal ileum and jejunum.

The pattern of colonic disease is highly variable.[1-3,173,201] More commonly noted are a predominantly right-sided colitis or segmental disease of the colon with a normal rectum (Figure 27-34). About one quarter of the colonic cases reveal proctitis; this may be associated with continuous disease of the left colon, simulating ulcerative colitis. Intrinsic involvement of the appendix is frequent in patients with the small-intestinal disease and less often noted in those with mainly colonic lesions. Perianal disease is noted in about one quarter of patients with either small-intestinal or colonic disease.

Patients with Crohn's disease have a propensity for the development of sinus tracts and fistulas that frequently extend to other parts of the intestinal tract. It is important to distinguish these secondary openings from intrinsic disease in that region, because this information may be needed in the planning of surgical resections. A small number of cases reveal gross lesions in the upper part of the gut, including the oral cavity, esophagus, stomach, and proximal duodenum. These lesions are usually seen in conjunction with gross disease of the small or large intestine, but occasionally they may be the presenting feature of Crohn's disease. There have been several reports that purport to show the presence of primary Crohn's disease in tissues outside the alimentary tract, including the skin, musculoskeletal system, lung, gallbladder, and genital region.[202-212] In the absence of a histologic marker for Crohn's disease, however, there remains the possibility that these nonintestinal lesions are of a nonspecific or secondary nature.

Gross Features of Intestinal Disease. The earliest grossly evident lesion in Crohn's disease is a small, sharply demarcated ulcer of the mucosa (Figure 27-35), referred to as an aphthous ulcer. It is well visualized at endoscopic examination.[32,33,213,214] They may also be seen away from the major site of the disease, and this offers evidence that the lesions of Crohn's disease are often segmental and widespread. The aphthous ulcers are often multiple and vary from 1 to 2 mm up to a centimeter in greatest diameter. The intervening mucosa is either edematous or normal in appearance. Radiographic studies reveal in some cases a nodule, or "hump," of edema and inflammatory tissue around the ulcers.[215] These small lesions may eventually coalesce to form more diffuse ulceration of the intestinal mucosa.

The larger ulcers extend over a variable length of intestine, and they may be separated by patches or segments of normal mucosa, causing a cobblestone-like appearance in the affected areas. There is a tendency for the ulcers to occupy the deep part of the submucosa, and about two thirds of the cases are further associated with the presence of fine inflammatory fissures or sinus tracts that extend well into the muscularis propria[216] (Figure 27-36). These tracts are best seen by making multiple longitudinal cuts into the specimen and inspecting the bowel wall in profile. They must be distinguished from the multiple short cracks in the tissue that accompany the severe dilata-

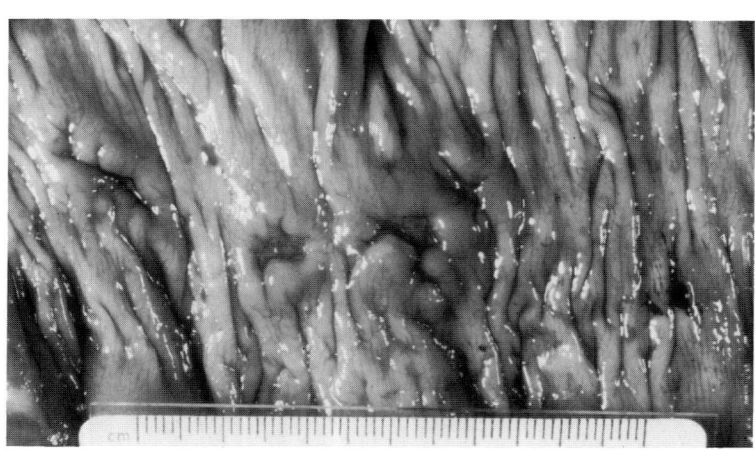

FIGURE 27-35. Crohn's disease of the colon, showing an early lesion with multiple small aphthous ulcers. The mucosa next to the ulcers is slightly raised as a result of inflammation, but the rest of the mucosa appears normal.

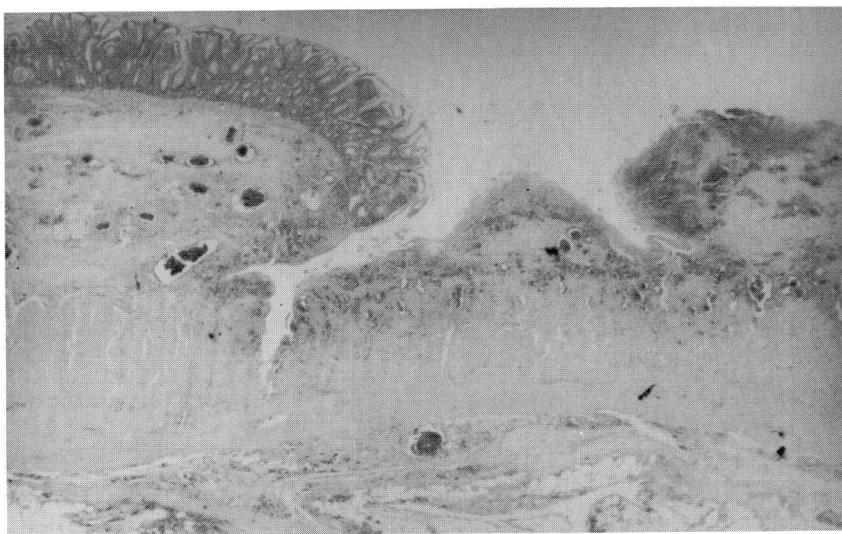

FIGURE 27-36. Crohn's disease of the colon, revealing superficial fissure into the muscularis propria. (H&E, × 20)

tion and secondary ischemic necrosis of the bowel wall in any case of severe colitis[31] (see Figure 27-16). Further extension of the sinus tracts through the bowel wall leads to localized perforation and external abscess formation (see Figure 27-33). The containment of the inflammatory process and the abscesses in a limited region is a characteristic feature of Crohn's disease. Free perforation of the gut with the development of generalized peritonitis can occur but is much less common than in cases of ulcerative colitis.[217,218]

The sinus tracts and external inflammatory reaction may further adhere to other tissues and promote the development of fistulous communications. The gross fistulas are observed at some time during the course of the disease in about one third of the cases and may connect the previously diseased area with other parts of the bowel and anal canal, the urinary bladder, the vagina, and the skin of the abdomen and perineal regions. Concomitant with the burrowing ulcers and deep inflammation, there is commonly a marked submucosal fibrosis that leads to early and progressive stricture formation.[219] The muscularis propria may undergo considerable hypertrophy, and the adjacent fat tends to wrap itself around the external surface and to obscure most of the serosal surface (Figure 27-37); this has been referred to as "creeping fat." There are also prominent peritoneal adhesions that often bind together and distort adjacent segments of bowel, particularly of the small intestine.

The gross features of Crohn's disease vary to some degree in the different regions. Disease of the small intestine, especially the terminal ileum, is much more commonly characterized by marked stenosis, muscular hypertrophy, encircling adipose tissue, and fistula formation (see Figure 27-33). Abscesses may surround nearby structures such as the appendix and uterine adnexa, and the sinus tracts frequently undermine the adjacent cecal mucosa. Colonic disease usually has less

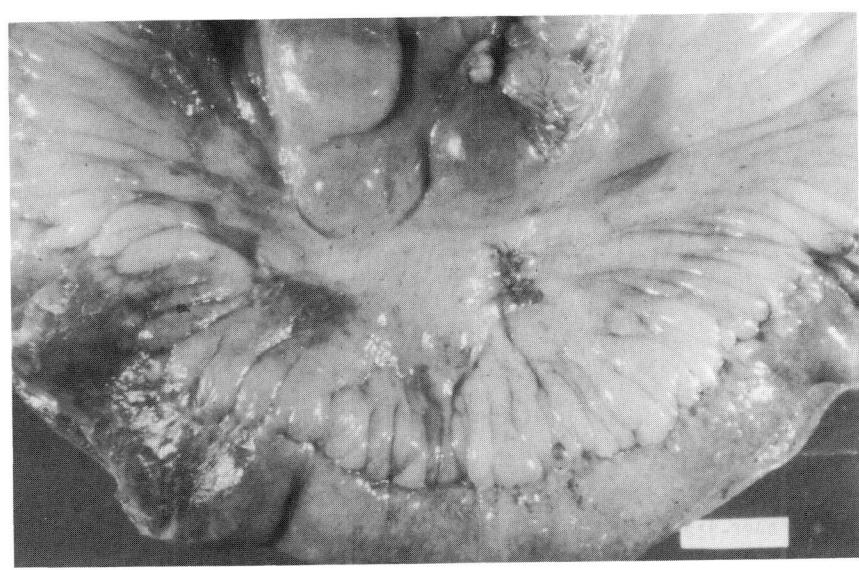

FIGURE 27-37. Crohn's disease of the small intestine, demonstrating serosal inflammation, creeping fat (left), and enlargement of the mesenteric lymph nodes (top).

prominent thickening of the bowel wall, and frequently noted are longitudinal ulcers that overlie the region of the teniae coli (see Figure 27–34). About 20% of the colonic cases are characterized by more superficial ulceration[220] and the presence of numerous inflammatory pseudopolyps,[221] similar to those seen in ulcerative colitis; the diagnosis of Crohn's disease in these cases depends on the demonstration of definite skip areas or coexisting ileal disease.[5] The absence of prominent muscular thickening and of serosal inflammation in many cases probably contributed to the underdiagnosis of Crohn's disease of the colon in the past. Longitudinal sinus tracts may result from multiple fissures piercing the colon wall, and these tracts may extend for a considerable distance. Similar lesions are seen in diverticular disease, and the distinction from Crohn's disease often requires histologic examination (see Differential Diagnosis). Indeed, the colon may be affected concurrently by both disorders.

In the examination of a surgically resected specimen, it is important to determine the exact location and extent of the disease and to decide whether the resection margins are affected or not. Only the presence of gross ulceration, usually in the form of the small aphthous lesions, at a margin is a strong indicator that the disease will progress and clinically recur.[184,186] The appearance of various histologic abnormalities such as increased inflammatory cells or granulomas in the absence of mucosal necrosis at the margin does not affect the clinical course. Accordingly, at the time of operating room consultation, one should rely on the gross extent of the disease and use frozen sections only for doubtful cases to confirm the presence of an ulcer at a margin. Indeed, considerable errors are noted if one depends on the finding of other features in the frozen sections.[222]

Histologic Features of Intestinal Disease. The early lesion of the aphthous ulcer reveals relatively superficial necrosis that is usually limited to the mucosa and upper submucosa, and the inflammatory reaction at the edge of the ulcer is nonspecific.[180,223] There is prominent edema and neutrophilic infiltration in the initial stage, followed by the appearance of granulation tissue and mononuclear inflammatory cells. There are often no granulomas or proliferation of lymphoid nodules in these early lesions. The mucosa between the ulcers is intact and lacks any features of active or chronic colitis.

The histologic features of the larger and advanced lesions in Crohn's disease are more striking and characteristic (Table 27–6). These include a relatively sharp demarcation between the edge of the ulcer and the adjacent normal mucosa (Figure 27–38); a marked proliferation of small lymphoid nodules, which is often most pronounced in the submucosa but may involve any layer from the mucosa to the serosa (Figure 27–39); prominent dilatation of the lymphatics, which is best seen in the submucosa (Figure 27–40); considerable expansion of the submucosa by fibrosis, which is often associated with marked proliferation of neural elements (see Figure 27–39; Figure 27–41); variable hypertrophy of the muscularis propria; and foci of inflammation in the muscle and serosa (see Figure 27–38). The larger ulcers have a variable depth but frequently extend into the lower submucosa or reach the muscularis propria. The lining of the sinus tracts and

Table 27–6 HISTOLOGIC FEATURES OF CROHN'S DISEASE

Focal (segmental) ulceration
Proliferation of lymphoid nodules
Dilatation of submucosal lymphatics
Submucosal fibrosis
Neuronal hyperplasia
Hypertrophy of muscularis propria
Serosal inflammation
Inflammatory sinus tracts that extend into or through the muscularis propria
Sarcoid-type granulomas

NOTE: The frequency of the features varies with the location of the disease (see text)

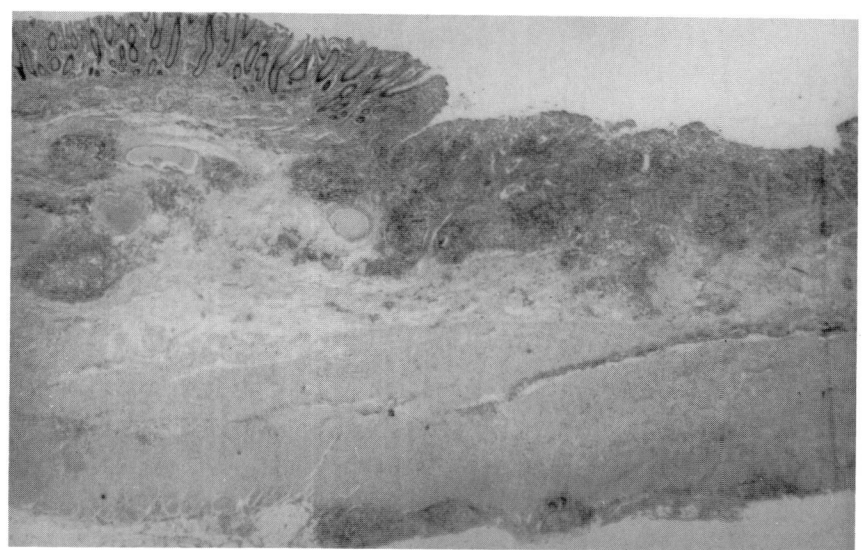

FIGURE 27–38. Crohn's disease of the colon, revealing a relatively sharp demarcation between the ulcerated area and the adjacent intact mucosa (top left) and prominent serosal inflammation in the absence of deep ulceration. (H&E, × 20)

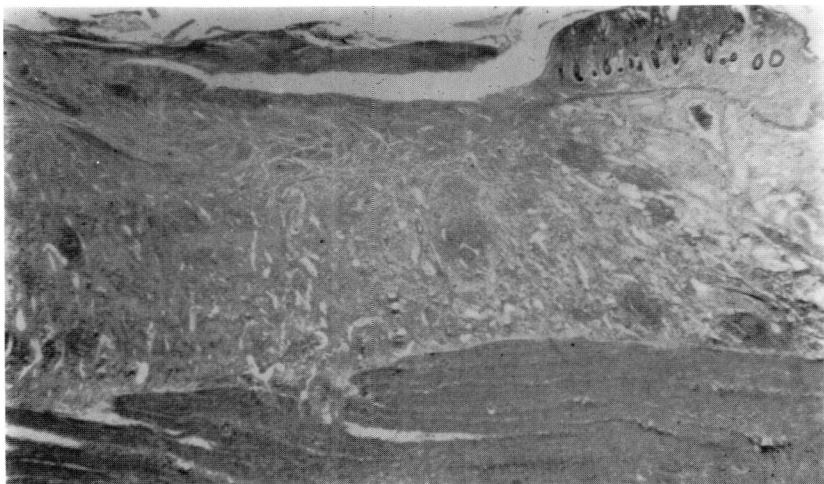

FIGURE 27–39. Crohn's disease of the ileum. There is marked thickening of the submucosa due to fibrosis and the presence of numerous small lymphoid nodules. The overlying mucosa is ulcerated (top). (H&E, × 20)

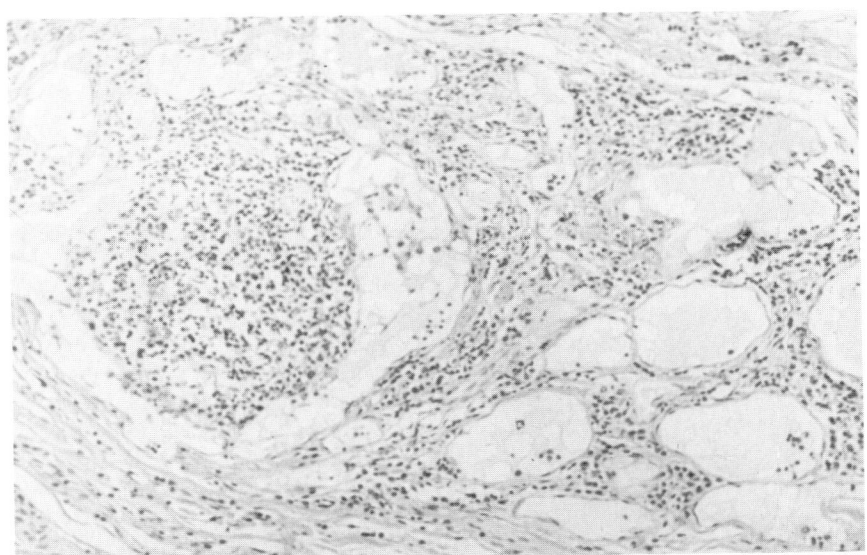

FIGURE 27–40. Crohn's disease of the small intestine, showing marked lymphatic dilatation and lymphoid nodules in the submucosa. (H&E, × 100)

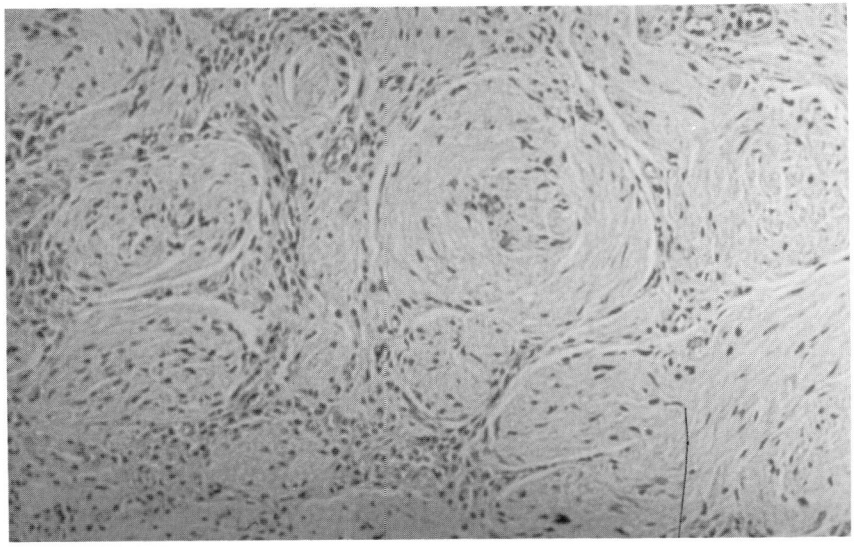

FIGURE 27–41. Crohn's disease of the small intestine, revealing prominent neural proliferation in the submucosa. (H&E, × 100)

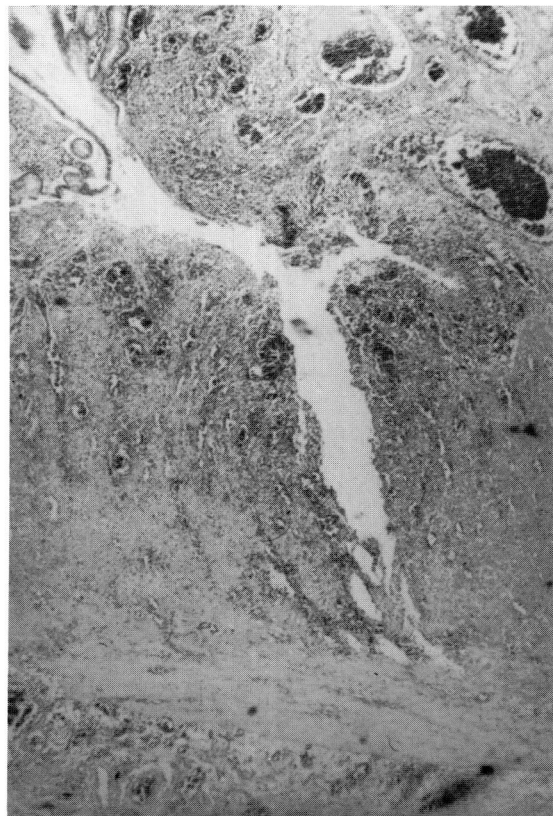

FIGURE 27-42. Crohn's disease of the colon, with an inflammatory sinus tract extending through the muscularis propria to the serosa. The tract is lined with nonspecific inflammatory cells and granulation tissue. (H&E, × 60)

fistulas is composed of acute and chronic inflammatory cells with varying degrees of granulation tissue and fibrosis (Figure 27-42); they may contain scattered foreign body giant cells, but well-formed granulomas are not typically found in these tracts. Vascular alterations are also commonly seen in the chronic cases and consist of intimal fibrous thickening, thrombosis, and old occlusions affecting the medium-sized arteries and veins.[224] Occasionally noted is a focal inflammation of the media, but this is not associated with prominent necrosis of the vessel wall. The vascular changes are typically located in the outer part of the wall and in the mesentery and are most often observed in cases with deep ulcerations. They are thought to represent a secondary phenomenon, and there is no conclusive evidence to support vasculitis as an etiologic factor in Crohn's disease.

Variations in the histologic features are noted in the different regions, especially during the reparative phase. Crohn's disease of the small intestine reveals a more constant and greater degree of submucosal fibrosis, neural proliferation, and muscular hypertrophy. In the regenerated mucosa there is a reduction or absence of villi, and frequently noted are a hyperplasia of Paneth cells, causing the cells to be higher in the crypts, and a pyloric glandular metaplasia, which is typically concentrated at the base of the glands (Figure 27-43). The intact mucosa often shows numerous slightly raised nodules, and these are usually due to lymphoid tissue or to florid pyloric gland metaplasia.[225]

In Crohn's disease of the colon, the submucosal and muscular features are often less pronounced, with a normal muscle thickness noted in over half of the cases. Indeed, when prominent muscular hypertrophy is seen in a case of Crohn's disease of the colon but is not associated with deep ulcers or fissures, the possible presence of concomitant diverticular disease of the colon must be considered. In about 20% of the colonic cases, the ulcers are relatively shallow and limited to the mucosa or upper submucosa. In Crohn's disease, in contrast to ulcerative colitis, however, there is usually present some inflammation in the muscle and serosa even in areas of superficial ulceration (see Figure 27-38). This observation supports the notion that the presence of marked and often transmural inflammation

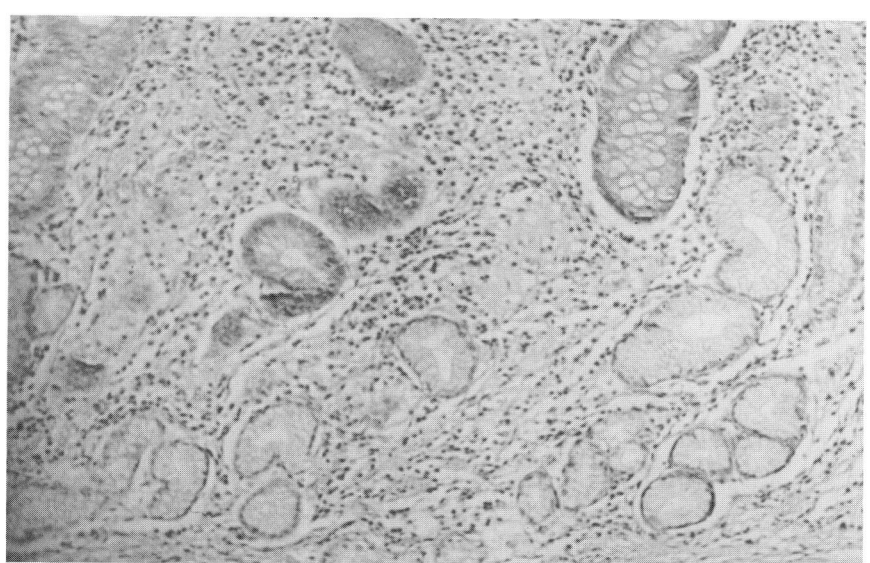

FIGURE 27-43. Crohn's disease of the small intestine. Section of granular mucosa revealing prominent pyloric gland metaplasia in the basal portion. The cells of the pyloric glands are mature, are distended with mucus of the neutral type, and have flattened basal nuclei. (H&E, × 100)

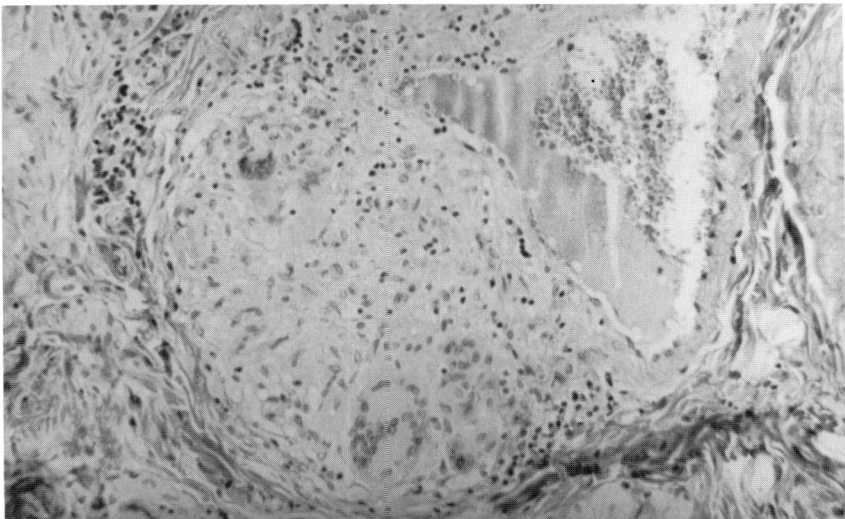

FIGURE 27–44. Well-formed granuloma, located in the intestinal submucosa, in a case of Crohn's disease. The granuloma is composed primarily of enlarged macrophages and giant cells. Other inflammatory cells, especially plasma cells and eosinophils, are often admixed at the edge, but there is no necrosis. (H&E, × 100)

with strong predominance of lymphoid nodules in Crohn's disease is an independent phenomena and not directly related to the depth of ulceration. The histologic characteristics of chronic colitis that are so prominent in the mucosa in cases of ulcerative colitis may also be seen in Crohn's disease, but they tend to exhibit a patchy distribution and to be separated by areas of completely normal mucosa. The mucosal features of chronic colitis include complex branching or atrophy of the crypts, a marked increase of mononuclear inflammatory cells and eosinophils in the lamina propria, a villiform surface, and the presence of Paneth cell metaplasia (see the section on the Pathology of ulcerative colitis for further details). Many of the colonic cases of Crohn's disease also contain inflammatory pseudopolyps, which are identical in size, configuration, and other characteristics to those seen in ulcerative colitis.[221]

One of the histologic hallmarks of Crohn's disease is the presence of granulomas.[226–229] However, these are noted in only one half of the cases, and there are no clinical or morphologic differences between the cases with granulomas and the cases without them. It has been suggested that granulomas are more commonly noted in younger patients, that they are seen earlier in the course of the disease, and that their presence might have prognostic significance; but none of these proposals has been substantiated.[230,231] The mechanism responsible for the development of granulomas is not known, and there is no explanation for the fact that many of the cases of Crohn's disease do not form granulomas. The granulomas may be observed in any portion of the bowel wall, from the mucosa to the serosa, and are also noted in the regional lymph nodes in about 5% to 10% of the cases. They typically appear as discrete nodules of compact macrophages with giant cells, and there is a variable admixture with other inflammatory cells such as lymphocytes and eosinophils (Figure 27–44). Necrosis is usually not present, and the granulomas resemble most those seen in sarcoidosis.[49] Occasionally, granulomas in the serosa may exhibit extensive necrosis; it is probable that this is a consequence of adjacent sinus tracts and abscesses or represents a reaction to foreign material, including suture material, vegetable matter, talc, and starch. Some of the granulomas are less well formed and consist of just a small aggregate of macrophages; these are usually observed in the mucosa and referred to as microgranulomas.[232] Before considering a granuloma as a supportive feature for the diagnosis of Crohn's disease, it is important to exclude lesions due to a reaction to ruptured crypts (see Figure 27–11) or to foreign material, especially in the perianal region.

The granulomas may appear in the inflamed and ulcerated areas but are more frequently noted in the otherwise normal mucosa. Overall, the presence of granulomas is not considered a sign of active disease, but, rather, may serve as a marker that the patient has Crohn's disease. Thus, granulomas may be seen in the mucosa of both the upper and lower gastrointestinal tract that is far removed from the grossly evident disease, and biopsies of such accessible areas can be helpful in making the diagnosis in uncertain cases.[194–197] In this regard, it may be difficult to distinguish by radiographic study some cases of Crohn's disease of the small intestine from other disorders such as malignant lymphoma, and endoscopic examination and random biopsies of the colon can be employed in looking for microscopic evidence of colitis or granulomas.[233] In the colon, the incidence of granulomas appears to relate to the presence and extent of grossly evident areas of disease. Thus, granulomas are seen in random biopsies of the rectum in about 5% of cases with gross lesions limited to the small intestine, 10% to 15% of those with right-sided colonic lesions, and 25% of patients with left-sided involvement. It has also been demonstrated that granulomas can be detected with increased frequency by the examination of *en face* sections of the intestinal mucosa.[234]

Pathologic Diagnosis of Intestinal Disease. Before considering the diagnosis of Crohn's disease, all other known inflammatory disorders of the gut must be excluded. Furthermore, when Crohn's disease affects the colon, it must be distinguished from chronic ulcerative colitis. The diagnosis of Crohn's disease, and its separation from ulcerative colitis, depends on the demonstration of any one or more of the following features (see Table 27–5): (1) involvement of the small intestine or the upper part of the alimentary tract; (2) segmental disease of the colon, including a normal rectum or the presence of other skip areas; (3) the appearance of fissures or sinus tracts, or fistulas that are not a secondary result of severe acute colitis; and (4) the presence of well formed, granulomas of the sarcoid type. More than one of these features is usually present, but it should be emphasized that the diagnosis of Crohn's disease does not require the finding of all of them in an individual case. Overall, the appearance of focal or segmental disease is the most frequent feature and seen in about 90%, microscopic fissures in two thirds, gross sinus tracts in one third, and granulomas in one half of the cases. Other common findings in Crohn's disease include stricture formation due to submucosal fibrosis, transmural inflammation, and prominent perianal disease; but none of these is specific.

Differential Diagnosis of Intestinal Disease

Small Intestine

About 20% of the cases of Crohn's disease affecting the terminal ileum have an abrupt onset and may mimic primary inflammation of the appendix or uterine adnexal structures. If an operation is performed for a case of suspected acute appendicitis, it is usually recommended that the appendix be removed so that future confusion with Crohn's disease is avoided, provided the appendix is not in direct contiguity with the intestinal lesion. The principal disorders that must be distinguished from Crohn's disease of the small intestine are lymphoma, ischemic disease, and chronic granulomatous infections with a predilection for the ileocecal area, including those due to tuberculosis, *Yersinia*, *Histoplasma*, and *Anisakis*. The similarity with lymphoma is largely at a clinical or radiographic level, and the tumor usually forms a mass that extends into the lumen and is readily identified by its characteristic histologic features. Rarely, ischemic disease may be localized to the terminal ileum and mimic Crohn's disease.[235]

Cases of intestinal tuberculosis are rare in the United States but may totally resemble Crohn's disease at a gross level.[236] They tend to display stenosing lesions of the terminal ileum and the contiguous cecum, transmural inflammation, and occasional sinus tracts. The granulomas, however, including those in the bowel wall as well as in the mesentery, show prominent caseous necrosis; the specific diagnosis is provided by special stains and cultures. Because of the large number and coalescence of the granulomas, tuberculosis may be suspected grossly by the presence of numerous tiny nodules on the serosal and free peritoneal surfaces. Histoplasmosis may show disease in the ileocecal area or patchy involvement of the colon, and the diagnosis depends on the finding of caseous necrosis and specific stains and cultures.[237–239] Anisakiasis is a helminthic infection due to the ingestion of raw fish containing the nematode eggs and is more prevalent in countries where this is a common practice.[240,241] It results in a destructive lesion of the small intestine with prominent sinus tracts; there is an intense eosinophilic reaction, and the worm is identified in the inflamed areas. Yersinial infections, due to *Y. pseudotuberculosis* and *Y. enterocolitica*, cause acute and chronic inflammatory lesions of the terminal ileum.[242–244] They may be associated with pronounced lymphoid hyperplasia and contain characteristic microabscesses and granulomas that may have spotty necrosis. Although the organism may be identified in the tissues by immunocytochemical stains, the diagnosis is usually obtained by specific culture. See Chapter 26 for further details.

Colon

The differential diagnosis of Crohn's disease of the colon is dependent on the particular distribution of the cases. Examples of right-sided colitis must be distinguished from certain infections, including tuberculosis and amebiasis. Infection due to *E. histolyticum* may reveal more widespread colonic lesions, resembling ulcerative colitis, or be concentrated in the cecal region.[70] There are characteristic discrete ulcers, which often penetrate deeply into the wall and show undermining of the adjacent heaped-up mucosa. Abundant organisms are present in the submucosa of the ulcerated areas, and these can be readily identified with conventional stains or the periodic acid–Schiff (PAS) reaction. When Crohn's disease of the colon presents with segmental disease, the differential diagnosis includes consideration of ischemic colitis, diverticular disease, and neoplasms. Chronic ischemic disease may be associated with patchy ulceration, stricture formation from submucosal fibrosis, and inflammatory pseudopolyps.[71–74] Distinguishing features include a tendency for the ulcers to be relatively shallow, the appearance of much less chronic inflammation without prominent lymphoid nodules, and the absence of discrete inflammatory sinus tracts and fistulas in the cases of ischemic colitis (see Chapter 12).

Diverticular disease of the colon, particularly when complicated by rupture and peridiverticulitis, may share clinical and radiographic features with Crohn's disease.[245–246] The lesions may be segmental and associated with complex transmural and pericolic tracts and abscesses, and hypertrophy of the muscularis propria is often present.[247–249] The discriminating features of diverticular disease (Table 27–7) include the lack of intrinsic colitis that can be assessed by endoscopic examination, the frequent presence of colonic mucosa in the inner lining of the diverticula, the occurrence of muscular hypertrophy that is not associated with inflammatory fissures, and the appearance of loosely formed granulomas or simply a collection of giant cells containing foreign material that are limited to the per-

ULCERATIVE COLITIS AND CROHN'S DISEASE 673

Table 27-7 CROHN'S DISEASE VERSUS DIVERTICULAR DISEASE OF THE COLON

	CDC	DDC
Intrinsic colitis	Present	Absent
Lining of mural sinus tracts	By inflammatory tissue only	In part by colonic mucosa
Granulomas	Well-formed, sarcoid type in all parts of bowel wall	Loose, foreign body type only in pericolic tissue

CDC, Crohn's disease of colon; DDC, diverticular disease of colon.

icolic tissue (see Chapter 30). Since Crohn's disease and colonic diverticulosis are each fairly common disorders, there are cases in which both disorders are present. A neoplasm must be considered in some cases of Crohn's disease with a large pseudopolyp, a progressive stricture, and sinus or fistulous tracts that are unassociated with prominent mucosal disease. In cases of Crohn's disease with mainly left-sided or diffuse colitis, the differential diagnosis includes consideration of other common colonic infections and ulcerative colitis; this was discussed previously in the section on differential diagnosis of ulcerative colitis.

Disease of Other Parts of the Alimentary Tract

Crohn's disease may also affect all other portions of the gut, including the oral cavity, esophagus, stomach and proximal duodenum, appendix, and anal region. The presence in these other locations is usually seen in conjunction with disease of the small or large intestine, but it may rarely be the initial or dominant site. The diagnosis is based on the finding of the characteristic pathologic features and is abetted by the demonstration of the disease in the more common regions.

Oral Cavity

Lesions of the mucosa of the oral cavity develop in about 5% to 10% of patients with Crohn's disease.[250-254] They are usually in the form of multiple, small, nonhealing aphthous ulcers, which must be distinguished from those due to more common viral and other infections. Biopsies reveal granulomatous inflammation, and the ulcers are typically superficial and uncommonly associated with nodular inflammation and sinus tracts. Less often noted is inflammation of the gingiva and lips. Granulomatous lesions have also been observed rarely in the salivary glands, where they may cause rupture of the ducts and localized mucocele formation.[255]

Esophagus

This is the least commonly affected area, and primary Crohn's disease in this site is extremely rare.[256-258] The lesions may be in the form of multiple superficial aphthous ulcers, or there may develop a more diffuse lesion with stenosis and sinus tracts (see Chapter 17 for further details).

Stomach and Proximal Duodenum

In cases of Crohn's disease affecting the intestines, random biopsies of the gastric and proximal duodenal mucosa reveal patchy inflammation or granulomas in about one quarter of the cases[195,196] (Figure 27-45). This does not signify, however, the presence or subsequent development of clinically significant gross lesions in this area. Ulcerated lesions of the stomach and contiguous duodenum are observed in about 5% of patients with Crohn's disease (Figure 27-46), and they are almost always seen together with involvement of the distal small intestine.[259-264] The lesions usually cause a diffuse erosion of the gastric antral and/or duodenal mucosa and resemble peptic inflammation; biopsy examination may reveal extensive necrosis over a large area and occasional granulomas to support the diagnosis of Crohn's disease. In some cases there is a more localized, deeper ulcer; and the distinction from chronic peptic ulcer usually depends on the radiographic demonstration of an odd location, multiple lesions, or sinus tracts.[265] Furthermore, the stomach and

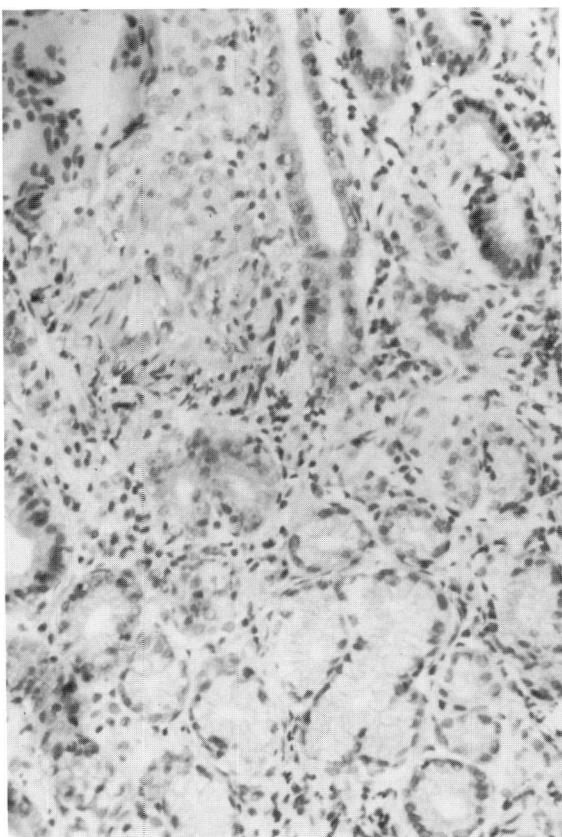

FIGURE 27-45. Crohn's disease of the stomach. The gastric mucosa reveals slight inflammation and irregularity of the glands and a granuloma (upper left). (H&E, × 100)

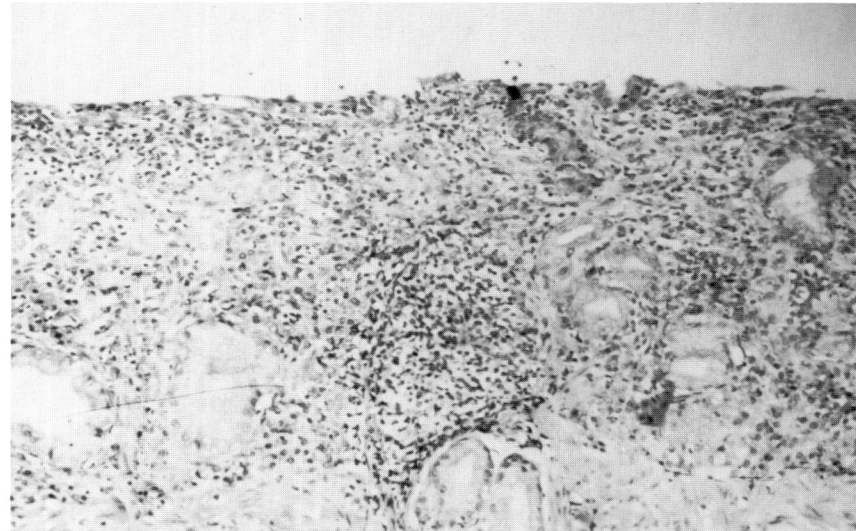

FIGURE 27-46. Crohn's disease of the duodenum, showing ulceration and inflammation of the mucosa (top). (H&E, × 40)

duodenum may be secondarily involved by fistulas that extend from active disease of the small intestine or colon. In these instances, the mucosa and wall immediately adjacent to the fistulas show inflammation, but there is no evidence of intrinsic disease in the stomach or duodenum (see Chapters 20 and 29 for further details).

Appendix

The appendix is commonly involved in cases of Crohn's disease affecting the intestines, and it may be the initial specimen examined because of the performance of an appendectomy in an unsuspected case of Crohn's disease.[266-269] Intrinsic disease is characterized by the presence of patchy or diffuse mucosal ulceration, marked mural thickening with numerous lymphoid nodules in all layers, occasional sinus tracts, and scattered granulomas. The major disorders to be distinguished are persistent inflammation following a previous appendiceal rupture and helminthic infections. In addition, the appendix may be secondarily involved and simply encased by an abscess or adhesions resulting from the rupture of an adjacent area of diseased intestine. The inflammation in such cases, typically of a nonspecific nature, is limited to the periappendiceal and serosal regions, and the mucosa and wall of the appendix are of normal caliber and show no intrinsic signs of inflammation (see Chapter 33 for further details).

Anal Region

Lesions in the anal and perianal region are seen in about 20% to 25% of patients with Crohn's disease of the small or large intestine.[270,271] It starts in this location in up to 5% of the cases and may precede the development of overt intestinal disease by 2 to 3 years. The lesions are characterized by the appearance of multiple and complex fissures and perianal abscesses. Fistulas frequently extend to the perineal skin and to other adjacent organs. The contiguous rectum may show signs of proctitis or be completely normal. Biopsy samples of the anal area show marked but nonspecific acute and chronic inflammation with granulation tissue and fibrosis and frequent multinucleated giant cells. Granulomas are also often present, particularly in the anal skin, but most of these are loosely formed and appear to be of the foreign body type. Since granulomas of this nature are also frequently seen in patients with perianal disease that is not associated with Crohn's disease, it is unsafe to use this feature for the diagnosis. Rather, it is recommended that additional biopsy specimens be obtained from the rectal mucosa, even if it appears grossly normal, in a search for evidence of proctitis or granulomas (see Chapter 34 for further details).

Complications

Clinical problems may result from fluid and electrolyte losses, anemia from repeated hemorrhages, which is more prevalent with disease of the colon, and malabsorption in cases involving the small intestine. Most of the cases of malabsorption are due to decreased bile salts from a reduction in their reabsorption in the distal ileum. This occurs after about 100 cm of terminal ileum is lost because of mucosal disease, bypass from fistulas or by surgical resections. Disease of the more proximal small intestine and bacterial proliferation states due to stenoses and fistulas also contribute to the malabsorption. Additional complications of Crohn's disease include intestinal obstruction, most common in the terminal ileum and at sites of anastomosis, due to stenosis from fibrotic strictures and to extensive peritoneal adhesions; secondary sepsis that results from the localized bowel perforations and peri-intestinal abscesses; and fistulous communication with adjacent tissues and organs. The fistulas may connect with and cause secondary inflammation in the abdominal and perineal skin; other segments of the gut; the urinary bladder; and the genital region, particularly the vagina. Secondary amyloidosis may also uncommonly develop, as a consequence of the long-standing inflammatory condition. Most of the other complications, including those principally affecting the colon and the extraintestinal manifestations, are similar to those seen in ulcerative colitis. Detailed descriptions are given in the previous section on complications of ulcerative colitis, and they are briefly summarized here.

Toxic Megacolon

Toxic megacolon is less common in Crohn's disease than in ulcerative colitis, presumably because of the tendency for the development of considerable fibrosis, which walls off the inflammatory lesions. It occurs in cases in which there is extensive colitis and is due to a great production of fluid and blood in the lumen, which leads by increased pressure to a dilation of the lumen and thinning of the bowel wall. Further complications include an ischemic type of necrosis of the wall and perforation into the free peritoneal cavity.

Secondary Infections

Aside from the septic complication of the fistulas and abscess, secondary infections may also occur at the level of the mucosal lesions. Some of the relapses may be due to infectious agents such as *C. difficile* and respond best to specific antimicrobial therapy.[76–80] In addition, opportunistic infections such as herpesvirus and cytomegalovirus infections may develop in patients who are receiving high doses of anti-inflammatory and immunosuppressive drugs, and these may lead to greater necrosis and the threat of systemic spread of the infection.[81–83]

Colitis and Enteritis Cystica

In areas of mucosal regeneration, some of the glandular tissue may extend through breaks in the muscularis mucosae and be misplaced in the submucosa.[272–274] The submucosal glands are often dilated, and there may be an overlying inflammatory polyp. The lesions are usually small and only an incidental finding. Larger lesions may be confused grossly with carcinoma but readily distinguished by the mature nature of the epithelium. See Chapter 28 for further details.

Postsurgical Ileal and Colonic Abnormalities

After surgery, the ileum just proximal to an anastomosis or an ileostomy stoma frequently shows some degree of mucosal atrophy. This is possibly due to stasis or to the exposure of the mucosa to an increased number of bacteria.[90–94] The features noted include some shortening of villus height and associated crypt hyperplasia, an increase in the number of goblet mucous cells in the villi, a hyperplasia of the Paneth cells, with extension of the cells to upper part of the crypts, and greater lymphoid nodules and patchy infiltrates of mononuclear inflammatory cells in the lamina propria. There is, however, no evidence of active ileitis in the form of erosion or neutrophilic infiltration in this atrophic mucosa, and the changes have no clinical significance.

Whenever an ulcerated lesion is noted in the ileum following surgery, the immediate concern is whether it represents recurrent Crohn's disease.[86,275] It should be remembered, however, that other ileal abnormalities may occur, as evidenced by their presence in patients who have undergone a colectomy for ulcerative colitis or for familial polyposis.[9,85] Thus, less specific alterations are seen in about 5% of patients who have an ileostomy and include hemorrhagic necrosis from mucosal prolapse, suture abscesses, and ulcers and occasional sinus tracts in the distal few centimeters and stoma that are due to mechanical effects or localized sepsis. Uncommonly, a longer segment of ileum may reveal focal ulcerations, called prestomal ileitis, which is thought to be due to a tight stoma.[95] In all of these situations, the problem is ordinarily corrected by a revision of the ileostomy. Similar changes are less frequently noted in the ileum just proximal to an anastomosis; these tend to be milder and usually do not require corrective surgery.

More prominent inflammation and erosions can develop in ileal reservoirs, called pouch ileitis,[88,97] in patients with ulcerative colitis who have undergone total colectomy and ileoanal anastomosis. The presence of this ileitis can lead to questions concerning the original diagnosis of the colitis, and this subject is discussed above in the section on complications of ulcerative colitis. Because of the propensity of Crohn's disease to involve the small intestine, a Kocks type of continent ileostomy and ileoanal reservoir procedures are not performed in these patients.

Recurrent Crohn's disease of the ileum proximal to a stoma or an anastomosis has a variable appearance.[94] Milder cases may show only focal ulcerations, and it may be impossible to distinguish them from the nonspecific ileal alterations unless there is granulomatous inflammation in the ulcerated areas. The finding of random granulomas in the intact mucosa cannot by itself be considered conclusive evidence that the patient has recurrent Crohn's disease, since such isolated granulomas may be seen in cases without active disease. Furthermore, granulomas are seen in only one half of cases of Crohn's disease; and, interestingly, they are found in recurrences only if granulomas were evident in the primarily resected disease. Advanced lesions show more certain features, in the form of sinus tracts away from the stoma or anastomosis and prominent stenosis that may extend over a long segment of the ileum. About one third of the ilea resected for recurrent disease lack characteristic features, and the diagnosis is determined by the subsequent clinical course.

The lesions of recurrent Crohn's disease following surgery tend to appear in the region, whether the small intestine or the colon, where the primary disease occurred.[186] Thus, if the previous intestinal resection contained Crohn's disease in the colon, the recurrent disease is also apt to be in the colon just distal to the anastomosis. Indeed, a patient with recurrent Crohn's disease of the colon is more likely to require a total colectomy eventually than one with primarily small-bowel disease. There is usually no diagnostic difficulty in assessing the colonic lesions, because nonspecific mechanical changes such as those described previously in the ileum do not apparently affect the colon that is immediately distal to the anastomosis. In patients who have undergone ileocolic resection and temporary ileostomy, however, mild nonspecific inflammatory changes in the mucosa can develop in the bypassed segment of distal colon and rectum. This condition has been called diversion-related colitis and is thought to be due to stasis in the excluded segment[276,277]; the lesion completely regresses after continuity of the bowel is restored by anastomosis (see Chapter 28 for further details).

Extraintestinal Manifestations

Several inflammatory conditions, possibly due to the effects of circulating immune complexes, are seen in 25% to 30% of patients with Crohn's disease.[98,270] These are similar to those seen in ulcerative colitis and include uveitis, polyarthritis and ankylosing spondylitis, and the skin lesions of erythema nodosum and pyoderma gangrenosum. The lesions tend to regress after surgical extirpation of the intestinal disease but may reappear with recurrent disease. Hepatic and biliary abnormalities include fatty change of the liver, due to nutritional deficiency; chronic pericholangitis; sclerosing cholangitis, which further promotes the development of bile duct carcinoma; and an increased incidence of gallstones. Granulomas may also be found in the portal tracts in a small percentage of the cases. In addition, renal calculi are commonly noted in patients with active small-bowel disease, and hydronephrosis may occur because of extrinsic compression of a ureter due to an adjacent abscess.

Dysplasia and Carcinoma

The major description of these conditions is provided above in the section on dysplasia and carcinoma under Ulcerative Colitis, and only the salient points relating to Crohn's disease are presented here.

Incidence and Risk Factors. An increased incidence of adenocarcinoma of both the small intestine and the colon is seen in patients with long-standing Crohn's disease, although it is not as great as that observed in cases of ulcerative colitis.[278-281] It has been estimated that patients with chronic disease of the small intestine have a 20-fold increase in carcinoma in that area, and that the overall incidence for tumor development in the colon is about 3%. The tumor formation is directly related to the duration of disease, with the major rise noted after 15 to 20 years. In Crohn's disease, compared with ulcerative colitis, there is a lower incidence of and longer interval before the appearance of carcinoma of the colon. This may be because there is less colonic tissue at risk, since the lesions tend to be more focal and earlier surgery is done for other indications in Crohn's disease.[282] Aside from the occurrence of bile duct carcinomas complicating sclerosing cholangitis and a possible slight increase in intestinal lymphomas, there is no evidence of an enhanced frequency of other tumors affecting the intestines and upper part of the gut.[101,113]

Carcinoma. In patients with Crohn's disease, compared with the normal population, the carcinomas occur in younger patients by an average of 10 years, are more often multiple, and tend to be more evenly distributed in the intestines, at sites of inflammatory disease.[283-290] At an earlier time, bypass of a diseased segment of small intestine was favored over primary resection, and it was later noted that almost 40% of the carcinomas developed in these excluded segments. Most of the cases present at an advanced stage with stenosis and evidence of deep invasion. Tumors may also arise in fistulous tracts. Since stricture and fistula formations are common characteristics of Crohn's disease, it is extremely difficult to detect the development of a superimposed carcinoma at an early stage. Occasionally, an early carcinoma is detected, more often in the colon; and these are usually associated with dysplasia; they appear as smaller, more circumscribed and flat lesions.

The histologic characteristics of the adenocarcinomas are the same as those seen in ulcerative colitis, with over one third of the cases of the well-differentiated and mucinous types. This factor adds to the difficulty of the preoperative diagnosis of carcinoma, even if the tumors are in the colon and accessible to endoscopic biopsy.

Dysplasia. As in cases of ulcerative colitis, epithelial dysplasia can often be identified in the marginal mucosa of carcinomas of both the small intestine and colon in Crohn's disease.[287-292] This dysplasia can also be found occasionally in the mucosa away from the carcinoma, but its utility in early diagnosis is limited to the colon, where the mucosa can be surveyed by colonoscopic examination.[293] The histologic features of dysplasia are identical to those seen in ulcerative colitis, and the same classification can be employed, with the following categories: negative for dysplasia, including normal and inactive and active inflammatory disease; indefinite for dysplasia, which is further rated, if possible, as probably negative or probably positive; and positive for dysplasia, including low-grade and high-grade types.[48] A full description is provided in the section on ulcerative colitis.

Clinical Applications. There have been insufficient data collected for a decision as to whether a surveillance program to detect dysplasia in Crohn's disease is warranted.[282] Part of the reason is that there are relatively few cases of chronic disease of the colon in which most or all of the colon has not been surgically removed for other reasons.[280] Nevertheless, in cases of long-standing Crohn's disease of the intact colon with relatively diffuse lesions (i.e., those resembling ulcerative colitis), surveillance might be considered. Considering the longer lag period before the carcinoma formation, such a program might be started later, perhaps after 15 years of disease. It has also been suggested that regions with persistent strictures and fistulas should be excised, because these may be preferred sites for tumor formation.

COMPARATIVE FEATURES

Because the precise etiology of ulcerative colitis and Crohn's disease is unknown and the two share several clinical and morphologic features, it has been long suspected that the two conditions might be variants of the same common disorder. Both are chronic inflammatory conditions that appear to have an immunologic basis, are often precipitated by stressful situations, and respond to equivalent anti-inflammatory and immunosuppressive drugs. There is a common set of extraintestinal manifestations, and the incidence of dysplasia and carcinoma is increased in both conditions. Major differences in the distributional and structural characteristics and in the overall behavior are noted, however, that justify the current separation of the two diseases. There are also dissimilarities in the immunologic studies, T-cell alterations being more typical of Crohn's disease. Until the exact cause is established, the issue of whether cases of idiopathic inflammatory bowel disease represent one or two diseases, or even more, will remain in doubt. For the present, we tentatively accept the division into the two disorders. There are rare cases in which both patterns appear to be present, the colon showing features of ulcerative colitis and the ileum showing those of Crohn's disease.[294] Again, without any truly specific markers, it is impossible to ascertain whether these patients have both conditions or only Crohn's disease with a variable pattern in different regions of the intestine.

Pathologic and Diagnostic Features

It should be stressed at the outset that before the diagnosis of either ulcerative colitis or Crohn's disease can be made, other known causes of inflammatory conditions must be excluded. This is not always possible at the start of the disease, and the definitive diagnosis may depend on the response to therapy and the subsequent clinical course. The diagnosis of Crohn's disease becomes evident when the disease dominantly affects the small intestine or the upper part of the gut. In contrast, considerable difficulty may be encountered in separating the two diseases in the colon.

Discriminating Features in Colonic Disease

The information obtained from all modalities, including the results of radiographic and endoscopic examinations, are usually needed to distinguish ulcerative colitis and Crohn's disease of the colon, particularly in patients who have not yet undergone surgical resection. Mucosal biopsy study may be especially

Table 27–8 ULCERATIVE COLITIS VERSUS CROHN'S DISEASE OF THE COLON: DISCRIMINATING FEATURES

	UC	CDC
Rectal involvement	100% (diffuse)	50% (usually focal)
Colonic disease	Always diffuse	Focal in 90%
Level of inflammation	Limited to mucosa and submucosa in 67%	Extends to muscularis propria and serosa in 80%
Mural sinus tracts	Absent	About 67%
Fistulas	Absent	About 33%
Granulomas	Absent	About 50%

UC, ulcerative colitis; CDC, Crohn's disease of colon.

helpful in determining the presence or absence of a grossly suspected skip area and in the detection of granulomas.[45,47,75,227,295–303] The separation is best made by considering the combined distributional, gross, and histologic features (Table 27–8). Ulcerative colitis is characterized by constant involvement of the rectum; a variable extent of disease of the colon, which is always diffuse; the absence of ulcerating lesions of the ileum; *and* the lack of discrete inflammatory sinus tracts or granulomas of the sarcoid type. Crohn's disease, in contrast, is distinguished by the identification of an atypical distribution (in the form of a normal rectum, other skip areas of disease in the colon, or ulcerating lesions of the ileum); the presence of discrete inflammatory sinus tracts or fistulas; *or* the appearance of well-formed granulomas. Difficulty may arise in a case of severe active ulcerative colitis, when multiple cracks or superficial fissures can appear in the bowel wall as a result of the increased intraluminal pressure (see Figure 27–16); and these must be distinguished from the more isolated and longer sinus tracts (see Figures 27–36 and 27–42) of Crohn's disease.[31] During the reparative phase, some cases of ulcerative colitis may reveal an uneven degree of residual inflammation resulting in the gross appearance of a skip area, but histologic examination confirms the presence of diffuse disease. Also, nonspecific granulomas reacting to ruptured crypts or foreign material are occasionally seen in ulcerative colitis (see Figure 27–11) and must be discounted.[49]

Shared Features in Colonic Disease

There are many other morphologic features that may be present in both ulcerative colitis and Crohn's disease of the colon, although they may be more frequent or prominent in one or the other disorder.[5,8,303,304] Thus, inflammatory pseudopolyps tend to be more extensive in ulcerative colitis, whereas stenosis is more frequent and appears earlier in Crohn's disease. Crypt abscesses, mononuclear inflammatory cells, eosinophils, and microscopic features of chronic colitis are common in both disorders. Cases of Crohn's disease show a greater frequency and degree of lymphoid nodular hyperplasia, fibrosis, neural and muscular proliferation, and serosal inflammation (see Figures 27–38 to 27–41). The notion that ulcerative colitis takes the form of a mucosal colitis and Crohn's disease, a transmural colitis is at best an idealization; the reverse may be seen in both conditions.[9,220]

Indeterminate Colitis

In about 10% to 15% of cases of idiopathic inflammatory bowel disease, there are either insufficient data or the presence of prominent overlapping features that interfere with the clear distinction between ulcerative colitis and Crohn's disease of the colon; these cases have been called indeterminate colitis.[31,305] Most of the difficulties arise in patients who have not had an intestinal resection and in whom the exact distribution of the disease has not yet been adequately defined by complete radiographic and endoscopic studies. In some instances, the term appears to be misused because of the failure to consider the combined information provided by the various diagnostic procedures. For example, a rectal mucosal biopsy may reveal a chronic active inflammation without granulomas, suggesting ulcerative colitis; whereas the roentgenographic examination may show segmental disease and/or sinus tracts in the colon; in such instances, it should be recognized that the results of the radiographic study are more specific and that the patient has Crohn's disease despite the limited findings of the rectal biopsy.

In the examination of surgical specimens, the diagnosis of indeterminate colitis is often applied to cases that grossly resemble ulcerative colitis, with diffuse involvement of the rectum and colon, but have one or more of the following added features: (1) cracks or superficial fissures in the bowel wall in regions of severe disease that may be difficult to distinguish from discrete inflammatory sinus tracts; (2) one or a few small, isolated ulcers with the appearance of aphthous lesions, that are proximal to the main site of the colonic disease; and (3) poorly formed granulomas that are usually related to ruptured crypts or reactions to foreign material. It is probable that most of these cases are ulcerative colitis; in these instances, the diagnosis of Crohn's disease would depend on the finding of characteristic lesions in the proximal colon or ileum. Some cases of idiopathic inflammatory bowel disease have been called indeterminate because of the unwillingness of the observer to completely accept segmental disease in the colon as a proven and solitary criterion of Crohn's disease. Thus, one may encounter descriptions of ulcerative colitis with a normal rectum and segmental ulcerative colitis; or, as a compromise, they may be called indeterminate colitis. If the spared areas of mucosa are confirmed to be completely normal by histologic examination, these cases should more appropriately be diagnosed as Crohn's disease, because ileal recurrences have been documented in such patients.

It is the author's impression that the category of indeterminate colitis has been overused. It may be employed as a tentative or provisional term in cases in which one does not have complete information about the distribution of the lesions, with the understanding that the more specific diagnosis of either ulcerative colitis or Crohn's disease will eventually be forthcoming.[31] Even in these instances, however, it might be sufficient to classify the disease as chronic idiopathic colitis and thus avoid the addition of a new term, and simply to await further data before making the particular diagnosis. If one considers the combined information provided by the radiographic and endoscopic procedures as well as the results of biopsy and specimen examinations, the great majority of cases can be classified readily as ulcerative colitis or Crohn's disease. *Indeterminate colitis* is best regarded as a descriptive term, and it should not be used to indicate a separate and distinct disease entity.

Clinical Course

The major reason for attempting to distinguish ulcerative colitis and Crohn's disease is that there are differences in their clinical behavior.[5,86,172] Recurrences are essentially limited to the colon and rectum in ulcerative colitis, and the disease can be ultimately controlled, if necessary, by a total colectomy. In contrast, most cases of Crohn's disease affect mainly the small intestine, which cannot be completely eliminated. Thus, there is a high incidence of recurrent disease in the residual intestine after surgical resections, which results in greater functional problems.[185,186]

Some cases of Crohn's disease are characterized by dominant or exclusive involvement of the colon, and their clinical course may be initially similar to that of ulcerative colitis. Compared with patients with ulcerative colitis, patients with Crohn's disease of the colon less often develop toxic megacolon but more frequently require earlier surgery for complications such as strictures and fistulas, and they are at risk for the occurrence and progression of disease in the small intestine. Because Crohn's disease frequently spares the rectum and the distal colon, segmental resections of the colon or of the ileum and colon with preservation of intestinal continuity is often possible. In patients who have an ileostomy, revisions for various mechanical, vascular, and septic problems may be required in both conditions; overall, the revision rate is greater in cases of Crohn's disease because of the added complication of recurrent disease.

The types and frequency of extraintestinal manifestations involving the eyes, joints, skin, liver, and biliary tract are similar in the two disorders, whereas renal calculi are mainly seen in Crohn's disease.[98] Dysplasia and carcinoma can occur in both conditions but are decidedly more common in cases of extensive ulcerative colitis.

MUCOSAL BIOPSY

The general information pertaining to endoscopic procedures and biopsies is provided in Chapter 3. We are concerned here with the particular uses and interpretations of mucosal biopsies as they relate to cases of ulcerative colitis and Crohn's disease, with special reference to biopsies of the rectum, colon, and ileum. Consonant with the development of flexible colonoscopes and with the overall increase in endoscopic procedures, the examination of the colon is being performed more often in cases of inflammatory bowel disease, and there is now greater reliance on the microscopic findings than in previous years.[21,22,32–35,45–47,213,227,295–304]

Rectal and Colonic Biopsy

There are several reasons for performing endoscopy and obtaining mucosal biopsies of the rectum and colon in inflammatory bowel disease (Table 27–9), and it is important that the particular indication be conveyed by the clinician and that there be a relevant response by the pathologist to the questions posed.[46,47,303,304]

Other Causes. In some instances, a biopsy is performed to detect or to exclude other inflammatory conditions that may have a fairly distinctive or specific histology. Thus, the biopsy may reveal the characteristic pseudomembrane in antibiotic-associated colitis, the bland hemorrhagic necrosis in early ischemic disease, and the particular microorganisms or their typical effects in fungal, protozoal, and some viral infections. Endoscopy may also assist in the distinction of diverticular disease of the colon from Crohn's colitis by showing the absence of intrinsic mucosal disease.

Identification of Colitis. There are times when the results of the radiographic and gross endoscopic examinations are equivocal and it is uncertain whether the patient has colitis. Some of the endoscopic features observed, such as edema and erythema, may be a consequence of the preparatory enemas or of the mechanical effects of the procedure itself.[303,306,307] A biopsy is often performed, in these situations, to establish, confirm, or exclude the presence of an inflammatory disease. Even if the gross appearance is normal, it is probably good practice to secure a biopsy specimen, because there may still be evidence of colitis at a microscopic level. Conversely, one might also consider biopsy in cases with flagrant signs of colitis to obtain an objective confirmation and permanent record, in the form of the histologic slide, of the existence of colitis.

Table 27–9 RECTOCOLONIC MUCOSAL BIOPSY IN INFLAMMATORY BOWEL DISEASE: USES

Detection or exclusion of other colonic diseases
Identification or confirmation of colitis
Separation of acute and chronic colitis
Distinction between ulcerative and Crohn's colitis
Determination of extent and severity of disease
Detection of dysplasia and carcinoma

In this regard, provided one avoids taking biopsies from deeply ulcerated areas, which may have an underlying thin wall, the chance of complications appears to be very low.[308]

Acute versus Chronic Colitis. Once a definite diagnosis of proctitis or colitis is made in a case with a relatively abrupt onset, the question usually arises as to whether it is an example of an acute self-limited colitis or of the early phase of a chronic colitis. Stool cultures will identify the common pathogens, but there remain cases of acute colitis without a clear cause. Biopsy can assist in this distinction and often provides definite evidence that the patient has a chronic disorder.[21–24] Major and common signs of chronic colitis that are noted in the mucosa include prominent branching or atrophy of the crypts, Paneth cell metaplasia, a villiform surface, and a marked increase of mononuclear inflammatory cells in the lamina propria with the appearance of lymphoid nodules and increased plasma cells just above the muscularis mucosae (see Figures 27–12 to 27–15). One or more of these features is seen in almost 80% of the cases of chronic colitis, as early as 3 weeks after the onset of the disease, whereas they are never seen in patients with acute self-limited colitis. Furthermore, if the results of the initial biopsy are not discriminatory, a repeat biopsy should be considered at the time that the patient is well. The mucosa will revert to normal if the case was one of acute self-limited colitis, whereas the mucosal alterations will usually progress and become evident in the chronic cases.

Ulcerative versus Crohn's Colitis. Having established that the patient has a chronic colitis and that it is of the idiopathic type, biopsy examination is often of assistance in deciding whether the case is ulcerative colitis or Crohn's disease of the colon.[45–47,295,299,303,304] Certain features that are characteristic of Crohn's disease, such as deep fissures and transmural inflammation, cannot be detected in the superficial biopsies. The possible appearances that can be observed in the mucosal biopsies include a normal mucosa, a diffuse colitis (Figure 27–47), a focal colitis (i.e., that part of the biopsy is completely normal or shows only a slight lengthening of the crypts) (Figure 27–48), and the presence of granulomas of the sarcoid type that may occur in the otherwise normal mucosa or in the inflamed mucosa (Figure 27–49). The finding in the biopsy specimens of normal mucosa to confirm rectal sparing or other skip areas, of focal colitis, or of granulomas offers evidence for the diagnosis of Crohn's disease, since these features are not seen in ulcerative colitis. Only the demonstration of diffuse colitis in the biopsy would be consistent with ulcerative colitis; because this pattern may also be identified in an area of Crohn's disease, however, the specific diagnosis in such cases must depend on further data. At the time of initial biopsy in a patient with colitis, the differential diagnosis is usually broader, and the finding of a biopsy pattern other than diffuse colitis serves simply to exclude ulcerative colitis. In these cases, showing a focal colitis and/or granulomas in the biopsy, the major differential diagnosis includes consideration of certain infections as well as Crohn's disease.

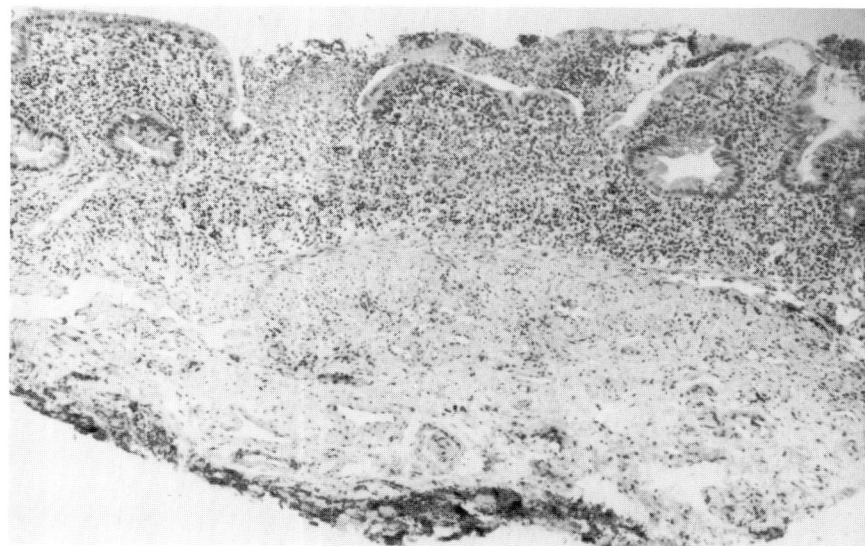

FIGURE 27–47. Colonic mucosal biopsy, revealing the pattern of diffuse active colitis. The mucosa (top) of the entire sample is inflamed. (H&E, × 40) (From Goldman H, Antonioli DA: Mucosal biopsy of the rectum, colon, and distal ileum. Hum Pathol 13:981–1012, 1982.)

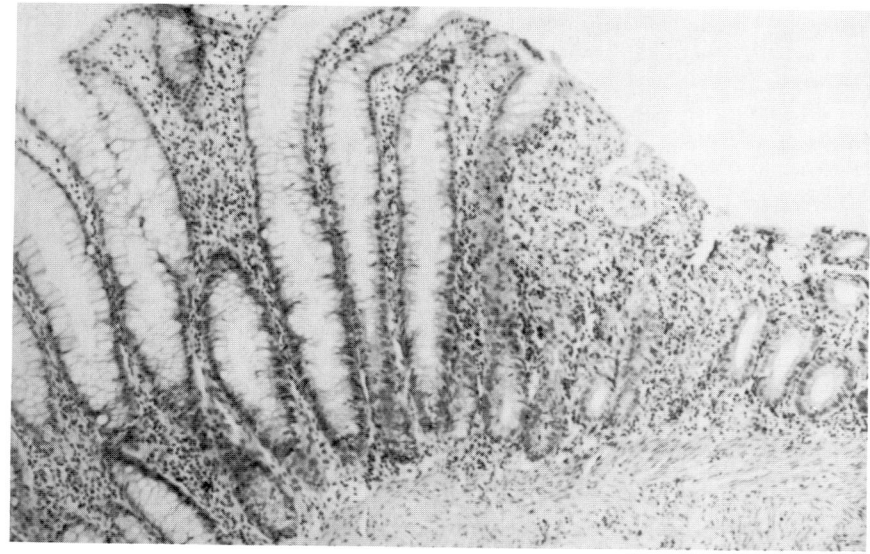

FIGURE 27–48. Colonic mucosal biopsy, demonstrating the pattern of a focal active colitis. Ulceration is noted on the right, whereas the crypts on the left are intact, are not inflamed, and show only slight elongation. (H&E, × 100) (From Goldman H, Antonioli DA: Mucosal biopsy of the rectum, colon, and distal ileum. Hum Pathol 13:981–1012, 1982.)

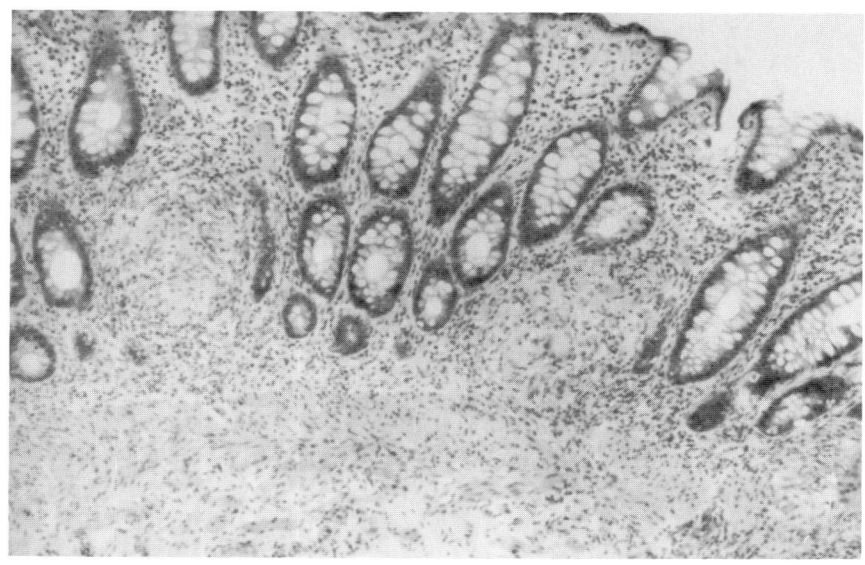

FIGURE 27–49. Colonic mucosal biopsy, showing two well-formed granulomas in the basal portion. The rest of the mucosa, including the crypts, appears normal. (H&E, × 100)

Extent and Severity of Disease. Whatever the particular type of idiopathic colitis present, endoscopy and mucosal biopsy offer the most sensitive tools for determining the extent and severity of the lesions, monitoring the response of the disease to therapy, and detecting recurrences.[44,309] Before surgery for Crohn's disease of the distal ileum, colonoscopy is often performed for accurate determination of the presence and extent of any colonic involvement; this information is needed for deciding on the amount of colon that should be resected. The determination is based primarily on the degree of gross disease found, because microscopic lesions alone do not necessarily presage the early development of clinically significant colitis. In particular, isolated granulomas in an otherwise normal mucosa are simply a marker for Crohn's disease; they are not an indicator of impending colitis in the region where they are noted. At the preoperative colonoscopy, biopsies are usually obtained of suspected lesions to confirm the appearance of an ulceration. Another important indication for the performance of colonoscopic examination is long-standing ulcerative colitis in patients in whom radiographic studies have identified only left-sided disease. Because the incidence of carcinoma is much greater in cases with extensive ulcerative colitis than in those with only distal disease, one performs the procedure to determine the true extent of the disease and to decide whether a surveillance program for the detection of dysplasia should be started. In this regard, although the radiographic and even the gross endoscopic appearances of the colonic mucosa may be normal, evidence of chronic colitis can be more sensitively detected by histologic examination. In all of these situations, it should be emphasized that the information sought is not the particular diagnosis, whether ulcerative or Crohn's colitis, which is already known, but the extent or severity of the disease. Accordingly, the pathologic report should attempt to address these specific issues.

Neoplasia. Mucosal biopsies are also obtained from large or other unusual polypoid lesions, from strictures, and from the flat atrophic mucosa, as part of a surveillance program, to look for dysplasia and carcinoma. This subject is presented above in detail in the sections on dysplasia and carcinoma under Ulcerative Colitis and Crohn's Disease.

Ileal Biopsy

Examination of the intact terminal ileum is limited, usually by the inability of the endoscopist to pass the colonoscope through the ileocecal valve.[310,311] Even when biopsies are taken from the valve region, they are almost always from the colonic side. There have been a few studies in which a more concerted and successful effort has been made to obtain samples from the terminal ileum, and useful information has been obtained in about 29% of the cases.[312] Features observed include those of typical Crohn's disease or of other causes of ileitis such as infections and ischemic disease; in many instances, the identification of normal mucosa helps to exclude Crohn's disease from consideration. In the assessment of the distal ileum, the histologic features of the normal mucosa of this region must be appreciated. Compared with the mucosa of the jejunum, there is usually an increased number of goblet mucous cells in the villi and a greater prominence of lymphoid tissue with mature lymphoid follicles (Peyer's patches) in the mucosa and submucosa of the ileum.

After surgical resections, mucosal biopsy specimens may be obtained from the ileum proximal to a stoma or an anastomosis with the colon or anal region. As a consequence of the surgical procedure itself, the ileal mucosa often reveals some degree of atrophy in the form of variable shortening of the villi and reactive crypt hyperplasia, more goblet mucous cells in the villous region, the appearance of Paneth cells higher in the crypts, and increased mononuclear inflammatory cells (macrophages, lymphocytes, and plasma cells) in the lamina propria[47,90–93] (Figure 27–50). These histo-

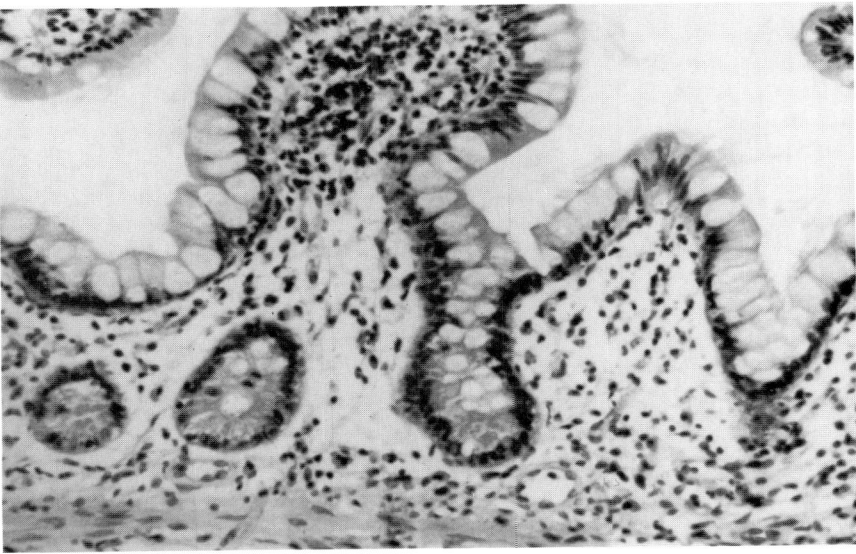

FIGURE 27–50. Ileal mucosal biopsy. There is a mild atrophy, characterized by a slight shortening of the villi and an increased number of goblet mucous cells over the surface of the villi. More marked cases show greater shortening of the villi, hyperplasia of the crypts, and proliferation of Paneth cells. (H&E, × 100)

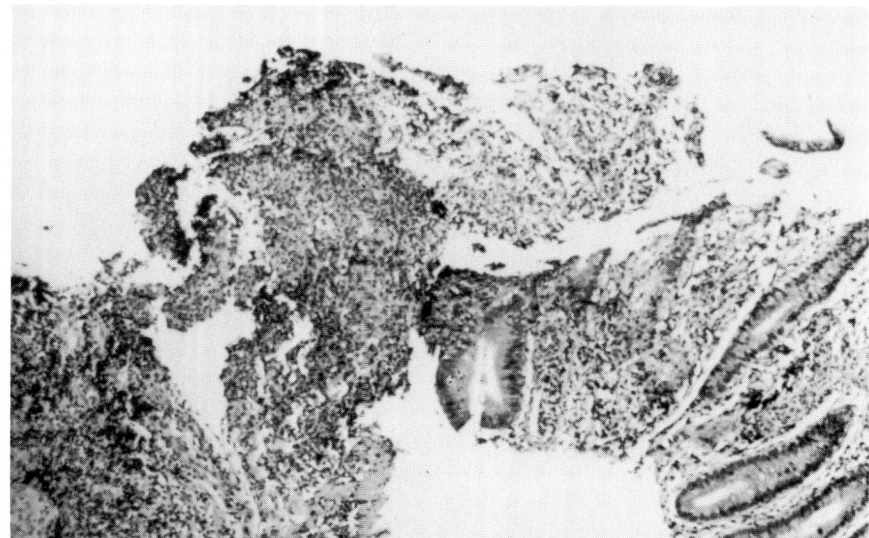

FIGURE 27–51. Ileal mucosal biopsy, revealing active ileitis. There is prominent erosion of the surface (top) and acute inflammation. (H&E, × 100)

logic features are usually unassociated with any gross changes, and they have no functional or clinical significance. Accordingly, they must be discounted before the diagnosis of ileitis can be considered. The major features sought to define a case of active ileitis[87,88,97] are (1) destructive lesions, ranging from erosion of the surface epithelium to overt ulceration (Figure 27–51); (2) the presence of neutrophils in the surface or crypt epithelium (cryptitis and crypt abscesses) and in the lamina propria; and (3) the appearance of granulomas in cases of Crohn's disease. It is important to remember that in patients with ulcerative colitis who have had a total colectomy, the mucosa proximal to an ileostomy stoma may reveal ileitis due to various mechanical, vascular, and septic causes.[85,95] Similar alterations can occur in the ilea proximal to a stoma or an anastomosis in cases of Crohn's disease, and these must be distinguished from recurrent disease in such patients.[94,313] The details of this subject are presented in the sections on postsurgical ileal abnormalities under Ulcerative Colitis and Crohn's Disease.

References

1. Mottet NK: Histopathologic Spectrum of Regional Enteritis and Ulcerative Colitis. Philadelphia, WB Saunders, 1971.
2. Price AB, Morson BC: Inflammatory bowel disease: The surgical pathology of Crohn's disease and ulcerative colitis. Hum Pathol 6:7–29, 1975.
3. Hamilton SR: Diagnosis and comparison of ulcerative colitis and Crohn's disease involving the colon. In Norris HT (ed): Pathology of the Colon, Small Intestine, and Anus. New York, Churchill Livingstone, 1983, pp 1–19.
4. Sachar DB, Auslander MD, Walfish JS: Aetiological theories of inflammatory bowel disease. Clin Gastroenterol 9:231–257, 1980.
5. Glotzer DJ, Gardner RC, Goldman H, et al: Comparative features and course of ulcerative and granulomatous colitis. N Engl J Med 282:582–589, 1970.
6. Lewin KJ, Swales JD: Granulomatous colitis and atypical ulcerative colitis: Histologic features, behavior and prognosis. Gastroenterology 50:211–223, 1966.
7. Schachter H, Goldstein MJ, Rappaport H, et al: Ulcerative and "granulomatous" colitis: Validity of differential diagnosis criteria: A study of 100 patients treated by total colectomy. Ann Intern Med 72:841–851, 1970.
8. Cook MG, Dixon MF: An analysis of the reliability of detection and diagnostic value of various pathological features in Crohn's disease and ulcerative colitis. Gut 14:255–262, 1973.
9. Fawaz KA, Glotzer DJ, Goldman H, et al: Ulcerative colitis and Crohn's disease of the colon: A comparison of the long-term postoperative courses. Gastroenterology 71:372–378, 1976.
10. Warren S, Sommers SC: Pathogenesis of ulcerative colitis. Am J Pathol 25:657–679, 1949.
11. Mendeloff A: The epidemiology of inflammatory bowel disease. In Kirsner J, Shorter R (eds): Inflammatory Bowel Disease. Philadelphia, Lea & Febiger, 1975, p 1.
12. Garland CF, Lilienfeld AM, Medeloff AI, et al: Incidence rates of ulcerative colitis and Crohn's disease in fifteen areas of the United States. Gastroenterology 81:1115–1124, 1981.
13. Monsen U, Brostrum O, Nordenvall B, et al: Prevalence of inflammatory bowel disease among relatives of patients with ulcerative colitis. Scand J Gastroenterol 22:214–218, 1987.
14. Mayberry JF: Some aspects of the epidemiology of ulcerative colitis. Gut 26:968–974, 1985.
15. Brandt L, Boley S, Goldberg L, et al: Colitis in the elderly: A reappraisal. Am J Gastroenterol 76:239–245, 1981.
16. Heatley RV, Calcroft BJ, Fifield R, et al: Immunoglobulin E in rectal mucosa of patients with proctitis. Lancet 2:1010–1012, 1975.
17. Rosekrans PCM, Meijer CJLM, VanDerWal AM, et al: Allergic proctitis, a clinical and immunopathological entity. Gut 21:1017–1023, 1980.
18. Murdock DL, Piris J: Immunoglobulin E in non-specific proctitis and ulcerative colitis: Studies with a monoclonal antibody. Digestion 25:201–204, 1983.
19. Edwards FC, Truelove SC: The course and prognosis of ulcerative colitis. Gut 4:299–315, 1963.
20. Sparberg M, Fennessey J, Kirsner JB: Ulcerative proctitis and mild ulcerative colitis: A study of 220 patients. Medicine 45:391–412, 1966.
21. Kumar NB, Nostrant TT, Appelman HD: The histopathologic spectrum of acute self-limited colitis (acute infectious colitis). Am J Surg Pathol 6:523–529, 1982.
22. Surawicz CM, Belic L: Rectal biopsy helps to distinguish acute self-limited colitis from idiopathic inflammatory bowel disease. Gastroenterology 86:104–113, 1984.
23. Goldman H: Acute versus chronic colitis: How and when to distinguish by biopsy. (Editorial) Gastroenterology 86:199–210, 1984.
24. Nostrant TT, Kumar NB, Appelman HD: Histopathology dif-

ferentiates acute self-limited colitis from ulcerative colitis. Gastroenterology 92:313–328, 1987.
25. Lavery FC, Jagelman DG: Cancer in the excluded rectum following surgery for inflammatory bowel disease. Dis Colon Rectum 25:523–524, 1982.
26. Johnson WR, McDermott FT, Hughes ESR, et al: The risk of rectal carcinoma following colectomy in ulcerative colitis. Dis Colon Rectum 26:44–46, 1983.
27. Filipe MI, Edwards MR, Ehsanullah M: A prospective study of dysplasia and carcinoma in the rectal biopsies and rectal stump of eight patients following anastomosis in ulcerative colitis. Histopathology 9:1139–1153, 1985.
28. Chong SKF, Blackshaw AJ, Boyle S, et al: Histologic diagnosis of chronic inflammatory bowel disease in childhood. Gut 26:55–59, 1985.
29. Zimmerman J, Gavish D, Rachmilewitz D: Early and late onset ulcerative colitis: Distinct clinical features. J Clin Gastroenterol 7:492–498, 1985.
30. Lumb G: Pathology of ulcerative colitis. Gastroenterology 40:290–298, 1961.
31. Price AB: Overlap in the spectrum of nonspecific inflammatory bowel disease: "Colitis indeterminate". J Clin Pathol 31:567–577, 1978.
32. Spencer JR: Endoscopy in chronic ulcerative colitis and Crohn's colitis. In Kirsner JB, Shortes RG (eds): Inflammatory Bowel Disease. Philadelphia, Lea & Febiger, 1975.
33. Waye JD: The role of colonoscopy in the differential diagnosis of inflammatory bowel disease. Gastrointest Endosc 23:150–154, 1977.
34. Powell-Tuch J, Day DW, Buchell NA, et al: Correlations between defined sigmoidoscopic appearances and other measures of disease activity in ulcerative colitis. Dig Dis Sci 27:533–537, 1982.
35. Holdstock G, DuBoulay CE, Smith CL: Survey of the use of colonoscopy in inflammatory bowel disease. Dig Dis Sci 29:731–734, 1984.
36. Teague RH, Read AE: Polyposis in ulcerative colitis. Gut 16:792–795, 1975.
37. Price AB: Benign lymphoid polyps and inflammatory polyps. In Morson BC (ed): Pathogenesis of Colorectal Cancer. Philadelphia, WB Saunders, 1978, p 33.
38. Jalan KN, Walker RJ, Sircus W, et al: Pseudopolyposis in ulcerative colitis. Lancet 2:555–559, 1969.
39. Levine DS, Surawicz CM, Spencer GD, et al: Inflammatory polyposis two years after ischemic colon injury. Dig Dis Sci 31:1159–1167, 1986.
40. Hinrichs HR, Goldman H: Localized giant pseudopolyposis of the colon. JAMA 205:248–249, 1968.
41. Goldenberg B, Mori K, Friedman IH, et al: Fused inflammatory polyps simulating carcinoma in ulcerative colitis. Am J Gastroenterol 73:441–447, 1980.
42. Kelly JK, Langevin JM, Price IM, et al: Giant and symptomatic inflammatory polyps of the colon in idiopathic inflammatory bowel disease. Am J Surg Pathol 10:420–428, 1986.
43. Brozna JP, Fisher RL, Barwick KW: Filiform polyposis: An unusual complication of inflammatory bowel disease. J Clin Gastroenterol 7:451–458, 1985.
44. Dick AP, Grayson MJ: Ulcerative colitis: A follow-up investigation with mucosal biopsy studies. Br Med J 1:160–165, 1961.
45. Morson BC: Rectal biopsy in inflammatory bowel disease. N Engl J Med 287:1337–1339, 1972.
46. Yardley JH, Donowitz M: Colo-rectal biopsy in inflammatory bowel disease. In Yardley JH, Morson BC, Abell MR (eds): The Gastrointestinal Tract. Baltimore, Williams & Wilkins, 1977, pp 50–94.
47. Goldman H, Antonioli DA: Mucosal biopsy of the rectum, colon, and distal ileum. Hum Pathol 13:981–1012, 1982.
48. Riddell RH, Goldman HG, Ransohoff DF, et al: Dysplasia in inflammatory bowel disease: Standardized classification with provisional clinical applications. Hum Pathol 14:931–968, 1983.
49. Haggitt RC: Granulomatous diseases of the gastrointestinal tract. In Ioachim HL (ed): Pathology of Granulomas. New York, Raven Press, 1983, pp 257–305.
50. Sommers SC, Korelitz BI: Mucosal cell counts in ulcerative and granulomatous colitis. Am J Clin Pathol 63:359–365, 1975.
51. Heatley RJ, James PD: Eosinophils in rectal mucosa. Gut 20:787–791, 1978.
52. Sarin SK, Malkotra V, Gupta SS, et al: Significance of eosinophil and mast cell counts in rectal mucosa in ulcerative colitis: A prospective controlled study. Dig Dis Sci 32:363–367, 1987.
53. Symonds DA: Paneth cell metaplasia in diseases of the colon and rectum. Arch Pathol 97:343–347, 1974.
54. Scott BB, Goodall A, Stephenson P, Jenkins D: Rectal mucosal plasma cells in inflammatory bowel disease. Gut 24:519–524, 1983.
55. Skinner JM, Whitehead R, Piris J: Argentaffin cells in ulcerative colitis. Gut 12:636–638, 1971.
56. Snover DC, Sandstad J, Hutton S: Mucosal pseudolipomatosis of the colon. Am J Clin Pathol 84:575–580, 1985.
57. Dickinson RJ, Gilmour HM, McClelland DBL: Rectal biopsy in patients presenting to an infectious disease unit with diarrhoeal disease. Gut 20:141–148, 1979.
58. Jewkes J, Larson HE, Price AB, et al: Aetiology of acute diarrhoea in adults. Gut 22:388–392, 1981.
59. Quinn TC, Goodell SE, Mhrtichian PAC, et al: Chlamydia trachomatis proctitis. N Engl J Med 305:195–200, 1981.
60. Day DW, Mandal BK, Morson BC: The rectal biopsy appearances in salmonella colitis. Histopathology 2:117–131, 1978.
61. McGovern VJ, Slarutin LJ: Pathology of salmonella colitis. Am J Surg Pathol 3:483–490, 1979.
62. Lambert ME, Shofield PF, Ironside AG, et al: Campylobacter colitis. Br Med J 1:857–859, 1979.
63. Willoughby CP, Piris J, Truelove SC: Campylobacter colitis. J Clin Pathol 32:986–989, 1979.
64. Price AB, Jewkes J, Sanderson PJ: Acute diarrhea: Campylobacter colitis and the role of rectal biopsy. J Clin Pathol 32:990–997, 1979.
65. Van Spreeuwel JP, Duursma GC, Meijer CJLM, et al: Campylobacter colitis: Histological, immunohistochemical and ultrastructural findings. Gut 26:945–951, 1985.
66. Medline A, Shin DH, Medline NM: Pseudomembranous colitis associated with antibiotics. Hum Pathol 7:693–703, 1976.
67. Cammerer RC, Anderson DL, Boyce HW Jr, et al: Clinical spectrum of pseudomembranous colitis. JAMA 235:2502–2505, 1976.
68. Bartlett JG: Antibiotic-associated colitis. Clin Gastroenterol 8:783–801, 1979.
69. Price AB, Davies DR: Pseudomembranous colitis. J Clin Pathol 30:1–12, 1977.
70. Pittman FE, Hennigar GR: Sigmoidoscopic and colonic mucosal biopsy findings in amebic colitis. Arch Pathol 97:145–158, 1974.
71. Whitehead R: The pathology of ischemia of the intestines. Pathol Annu 11:1–52, 1976.
72. Alschibaja T, Morson BC: Ischemic bowel disease. J Clin Pathol 11:68, 1977.
73. Ming SC, Bonakdarpour A: The evolution of lesions in intestinal ischemia. Arch Pathol Lab Med 101:40, 1977.
74. Norris HT: Reexamination of the spectrum of ischemic bowel disease. In Norris HT (ed): Pathology of the Colon, Small Intestine, and Anus. New York, Churchill Livingstone, 1983, pp 109–120.
75. Hellstrom HR, Fisher ER: Estimation of mucosal mucin as an aid in the differentiation of Crohn's disease of the colon and chronic ulcerative colitis. Am J Clin Pathol 48:259–268, 1967.
76. Lambert JR, Karmali MA, Newman A: Campylobacter enterocolitis. Ann Intern Med 91:929–930, 1979.
77. Gebhard RL, Greenberg HB, Singh N, et al: Acute viral enteritis and exacerbation of inflammatory bowel disease. Gastroenterology 83:1207–1209, 1982.
78. Lindemann RJ, Weinstein L, Levitan R, Patterson JF: Ulcerative colitis and intestinal salmonellosis. Am J Med Sci 254:855–861, 1967.
79. LaMont JT, Trnka YM: Therapeutic implications of *Clostridium difficile* toxin during relapse of chronic inflammatory bowel disease. Lancet 1:381–384, 1980.
80. Trnka YM, LaMont JT: Association of *Clostridium difficile* toxin with symptomatic relapse of chronic inflammatory bowel disease. Gastroenterology 80:393–396, 1981.
81. Tamura H: Acute ulcerative colitis associated with cytomegalic inclusion virus. Arch Pathol 96:164–167, 1973.

82. Cooper HS, Roffensperger EC, Jonal L: Cytomegalovirus inclusions in patients with ulcerative colitis and toxic dilatation requiring colonic resection. Gastroenterology 72:1253–1256, 1977.
83. Sidi S, Gragam JH, Razvi SA, Banks PA: Cytomegalovirus infection of the colon associated with ulcerative colitis. Arch Surg 114:857–859, 1979.
84. Magidson JG, Lewin KC: Diffuse colitis cystica profunda: Report of a case. Am J Surg Pathol 5:393–399, 1981.
85. Turnbull RB Jr, Weakley FL, Farmer RG: Ileitis after colectomy and ileostomy for non-specific ulcerative colitis. Dis Colon Rectum 7:427–435, 1964.
86. Steinberg DM, Allan RN, Brooke BN, et al: Sequelae of colectomy and ileostomy: Comparison between Crohn's colitis and ulcerative colitis. Gastroenterology 68:33–39, 1975.
87. Klein K, Stenzel P, Katon RM: Pouch ileitis: Report of a case with severe systemic manifestations. J Clin Gastroenterol 5:149–153, 1983.
88. Knober H, Ligumchy M, Ohon E, et al: Pouch ileitis: Recurrence of the inflammatory bowel disease in the ileal reservoir. Am J Gastroenterol 81:199–220, 1986.
89. Shepherd NA, Jass JR, Moskowitz RL, et al: Restorative proctocolectomy with ileal reservoir: Histopathology of mucosal biopsies. (Abstract) J Pathol 149:211A, 1986.
90. Philipson BM, Kock NG, Jagenburg R, et al: Functional and structural studies of ileal reservoirs used for continent urostomy and ileostomy. Gut 24:392–398, 1983.
91. Bechi P, Romagnoli P, Cortesini C: Ileal mucosal morphology after total colectomy in man. Histopathology 5:667–678, 1981.
92. Go PM, Lens J, Bosmon FT: Mucosal alterations in the reservoir of patients with Kock's continent ileostomy. Scand J Gastroenterol 22:1076–1080, 1987.
93. Berman JJ, Ullah A: Colonic metaplasia of ileostomies: Biological significance for ulcerative colitis patients following total colectomy. Am J Surg Pathol 13:955–960, 1989.
94. Bull DM, Peppercorn MA, Glotzer DJ, et al: Crohn's disease of the colon. (Clinical conference) Gastroenterology 76:607–621, 1979.
95. Knill-Jones RP, Morson BC, Williams R: Prestomal ileitis: Clinical and pathological findings in five cases. Q J Med 63:287–297, 1970.
96. Cranley B: The Kock reservoir ileostomy: A review of its development, problems, and role in modern surgical practise. Br J Surg 70:94–99, 1983.
97. Madden MV, Farthing MJG, Nicholls RJ: Inflammation in ileal reservoirs: "pouchitis." Gut 31:247–249, 1990.
98. Greenstein AJ, Janowitz HD, Sachar DB: The extra-intestinal complications of Crohn's disease and ulcerative colitis: A study of 700 patients. Medicine 55:401–412, 1976.
99. Monsen V, Sorstad J, Hellers G, Johansson C: Extracolonic diagnoses in ulcerative colitis: An epidemiological study. Am J Gastroenterol 85:711–716, 1990.
100. Cangemi JR, Wisner RH, Beaver SJ, et al: Effect of proctocolectomy for chronic ulcerative colitis on the natural history of primary sclerosing cholangitis. Gastroenterology 96:790–794, 1989.
101. Wee A, Ludwig J, Coffey RJ, et al: Hepatobiliary carcinoma associated with primary sclerosing cholangitis and chronic ulcerative colitis. Hum Pathol 16:719–726, 1985.
102. Goldgraber MC, Humphreys EM, Kirsner JB, Palmer WL: Carcinoma and ulcerative colitis: A clinical-pathologic study. II. Statistical analysis. Gastroenterology 34:840–846, 1958.
103. Devroede GJ, Taylor WF, Sauer WG, et al: Cancer risk and life expectancy of children with ulcerative colitis. N Engl J Med 285:17–21, 1971.
104. Lennard-Jones JE, Morson BC, Ritchie JK, et al: Cancer in colitis: Assessment of the individual risk by clinical and histological criteria. Gastroenterology 73:1280–1289, 1977.
105. Kewenter J, Ahlman H, Hulten L: Cancer risk in extensive ulcerative colitis. Ann Surg 188:824–828, 1978.
106. Greenstein AJ, Sachar DB, Smith H, et al: Cancer in universal and left-sided ulcerative colitis: Factors determining risk. Gastroenterology 99:290–294, 1979.
107. Nugent FW, Haggitt RC, Colcher H, et al: Malignant potential of chronic ulcerative colitis. Preliminary report. Gastroenterology 76:1–5, 1979.
108. Gilat T, Fireman Z, Grossman A, et al: Colorectal cancer in patients with ulcerative colitis: A population study in central Israel. Gastroenterology 94:870–877, 1988.
109. Gyde SN, Prior P, Allan RN, et al: Colorectal cancer in ulcerative colitis: A cohort study of primary referrals from three centers. Gut 29:206–217, 1988.
110. Brostrom O, Lofberg R, Nordenvall B, et al: The risk of colorectal cancer in ulcerative colitis: An epidemiologic study. Scand J Gastroenterol 22:1193–1199, 1987.
111. Hanauer SB, Wong KK, Frank PH, et al: Acute leukemia following inflammatory bowel disease. Dig Dis Sci 27:545–548, 1982.
112. Baker D, Chirput RO, Rimer D, et al: Colonic lymphoma in ulcerative colitis. J Clin Gastroenterol 7:379–386, 1985.
113. Greenstein AJ, Gennuso R, Sachar DB, et al: Extraintestinal cancers in inflammatory bowel disease. Cancer 56:2914–2921, 1985.
114. Owen DA, Hwang WS, Thorlakson RH, Walli E: Malignant carcinoid tumor complicating chronic ulcerative colitis. Am J Clin Pathol 76:333–338, 1981.
115. Miller RR, Sumner HW: Argyrophilic cell hyperplasia and an atypical carcinoid tumor in chronic ulcerative colitis. Cancer 50:2920–2925, 1982.
116. Mir-Madjlessi SH, Farmer RG, Easley KA, Beck GJ: Colorectal and extracolonic malignancy in ulcerative colitis. Cancer 58:1569–1574, 1986.
117. Carter D, Choi H, Otterson M, Telford GL: Primary adenocarcinoma of the ileostomy after colectomy for ulcerative colitis. Dig Dis Sci 33:509–512, 1988.
118. Suarez V, Alexander-Williams J, O'Connor HJ, et al: Carcinoma developing in ileostomies after 25 or more years. Gastroenterology 95:205–208, 1988.
119. Stern H, Wolfisch S, Mullen B: Cancer in an ileoanal reservoir: A new late complication? Gut 31:473–475, 1990.
120. Riddell RH: Dysplasia in inflammatory bowel disease. Clin Gastroenterol 9:439–458, 1980.
121. Edwards FC, Truelove SC: The course and prognosis of ulcerative colitis. IV. Carcinoma of the colon. Gut 5:1–22, 1964.
122. Cook MG, Goligher JD: Carcinoma and epithelial dysplasia complicating ulcerative colitis. Gastroenterology 68:1127–1136, 1975.
123. Greenstein AJ, Sachar DB, Smith H, et al: Patterns of neoplasia in Crohn's disease and ulcerative colitis. Cancer 46:403–407, 1980.
124. Yardley JH, Ransohoff DF, Riddell RH, Goldman H: Cancer in inflammatory bowel disease: How serious is the problem and what should be done about it? (Editorial) Gastroenterology 85:197–200, 1983.
125. Vatn MH, Elgjo K, Bergan A: Distribution of dysplasia in ulcerative colitis. Scand J Gastroenterol 19:893–895, 1984.
126. Lavery IC, Chiulli RA, Jagelman DG, et al: Survival with carcinoma arising in mucosa ulcerative colitis. Ann Surg 195:508–512, 1982.
127. Gyde SN, Prior P, Thompson H, et al: Survival of patients with colorectal cancer complicating ulcerative colitis. Gut 25:228–231, 1984.
128. Butt JH, Konishi F, Morson BC, et al: Macroscopic lesions in dysplasia and carcinoma complicating ulcerative colitis. Dig Dis Sci 28:18–26, 1983.
129. Symonds DA, Vickery AL: Mucinous carcinoma of the colon and rectum. Cancer 37:1891–1900, 1976.
130. Goldman H: Dysplasia and carcinoma in inflammatory bowel disease. In Rachmilewitz D (ed): Inflammatory Bowel Diseases. The Hague, Martinus Nijhoff, 1982, pp 27–40.
131. Riddell RH: The precarcinomatous lesion of ulcerative colitis. In Yardley JH, Morson BC, Abell MR (eds): The Gastrointestinal Tract. Baltimore, Williams & Wilkins, 1977, pp 109–123.
132. Gledhill A, Enticott ME, Howe S: Variation in the argyrophil cell population of the rectum in ulcerative colitis and adenocarcinoma. J Pathol 149:287–291, 1986.
133. Lyss AP, Thompson JJ, Glick JH: Adenocarcinoid tumor of the colon arising in pre-existing ulcerative colitis. Cancer 48:833–839, 1981.
134. Dawson IMP, Pryse-Davies J: The development of carcinoma of the large intestine in ulcerative colitis. Br J Surg 47:113–128, 1959.
135. Morson BC, Pang LSC: Rectal biopsy as an aid to cancer control in ulcerative colitis. Gut 8:423–434, 1967.
136. Fenoglio CM, Pascal RR: Adenomatous epithelium, intraepi-

thelial anaplasia, and invasive carcinoma in ulcerative colitis. Am J Dig Dis 18:556–562, 1973.
137. Yardley JH, Keren DF: "Precancer" lesions in ulcerative colitis: A retrospective study of rectal biopsy and colectomy specimens. Cancer 34:835–844, 1974.
138. Myrvold HE, Koch NG, Ahren CHR: Rectal biopsy and precancer in ulcerative colitis. Gut 15:301–304, 1974.
139. Gewertz BL, Dent TL, Appelman HD: Implications of precancerous rectal biopsy in patients with inflammatory bowel disease. Arch Surg 111:326–329, 1976.
140. Dickinson RJ, Dixon MF, Axon ATR: Colonoscopy and the detection of dysplasia in patients with long-standing ulcerative colitis. Lancet 2:620–622, 1980.
141. Butt JH, Morson BC: Dysplasia and cancer in inflammatory bowel disease. Gastroenterology 80:865–868, 1981.
142. Kewenter J, Hulten L, Ahren C: The occurrence of severe epithelial dysplasia and its bearing on the treatment of long-standing ulcerative colitis. Ann Surg 195:209–212, 1982.
143. Lennard-Jones JE, Ritchie JK, Morson BC, Williams CB: Cancer surveillance in ulcerative colitis. Experience over 15 years. Lancet 2:149–152, 1983.
144. Nugent FW, Haggett RC: Results of a long-term prospective surveillance program for dysplasia in ulcerative colitis. (Abstract) Gastroenterology 86:1197, 1984.
145. Rosenstock E, Farmer RG, Petras R, et al: Surveillance for colonic carcinoma in ulcerative colitis. Gastroenterology 89:1342–1346, 1985.
146. Ransohoff DF, Riddell RH, Lewin B: Ulcerative colitis and colonic cancer: problems in assessing the diagnostic usefulness of mucosal dysplasia. Dis Colon Rectum 28:383–388, 1985.
147. Fochios SE, Sommers SC, Korelitz BI: Sigmoidoscopy and biopsy in surveillance for cancer in ulcerative colitis. J Clin Gastroenterol 8:249–254, 1986.
148. Brostrom O, Lofberg R, Ost A, Reichard H: Cancer surveillance of patients with longstanding ulcerative colitis: A clinical, endoscopical, and histological study. Gut 27:1408–1413, 1987.
149. Manning AP, Bulgin OR, Dixon MF, Axon ATR: Screening by colonoscopy for colonic epithelial dysplasia in inflammatory bowel disease. Gut 28:1489–1494, 1987.
150. Dobbins WO, Stock M, Ginsberg AL: Early detection and prevention of carcinoma of the colon in patients with ulcerative colitis. Cancer 40:2542–2548, 1977.
151. Riddell RH, Morson BC: Value of sigmoidoscopy and biopsy in detection of carcinoma and premalignant change in ulcerative colitis. Gut 20:575–580, 1979.
152. Blackstone MO, Riddell RH, Rogers RHG, et al: Dysplasia-associated lesion or mass (DALM) detected by colonoscopy in long-standing ulcerative colitis: An indication for colectomy. Gastroenterology 80:366–374, 1981.
153. Isaacson P: Tissue demonstration of carcinoembryonic antigen (CEA) in ulcerative colitis. Gut 17:561–567, 1976.
154. Ehsanullah M, Morgan MN, Filipe MI, Gazzard B: Sialomucins in the assessment of dysplasia and cancer risk patients with ulcerative colitis treated with colectomy and ileo-rectal anastomosis. Histopathology 9:223–235, 1985.
155. Filipe MI, Sandey A, Ma J: Intestinal mucis antigens in ulcerative colitis and their relationship to malignancy. Hum Pathol 19:671–681, 1988.
156. Boland CR, Lance P, Levin B, Riddell RH, Kim YS: Abnormal goblet cell glycoconjugates in rectal biopsies associated with an increased risk of neoplasia in patients with ulcerative colitis: Early results of a perspective study. Gut 25:1364–1371, 1984.
157. Shields HM, Bates ML, Goldman H, et al: Scanning electron microscopic appearance of chronic ulcerative colitis with and without dysplasia. Gastroenterology 89:62–72, 1985.
158. Shields HM, Best CJ, Goldman H: Use of scanning electron microscopy with morphometric analyses in the distinction of dysplasia from inflammatory changes in ulcerative colitis. Surg Pathol 1:183–192, 1988.
159. Goldman H, Shields HM: Diagnosis of dysplasia in ulcerative colitis by combined light microscopy and scanning electron microscopy. In Rachmilewitz D (ed): Inflammatory Bowel Diseases 1986, Developments in Gastroenterology. The Hague, Martinus Nijhoff, 1986, pp 125–136.
160. Hammarberg C, Rubio C, Slezak P, et al: Flow-cytometric DNA analysis as a means for detection of malignancy in patients with ulcerative colitis. Gut 25:905–908, 1984.
161. Fozard JBJ, Quirke P, Dixon MF, et al: DNA aneuploidy in ulcerative colitis. Gut 27:1414–1418, 1987.
162. Cuvelier CA, Morson BC, Roels HJ: The DNA content in cancer and dysplasia in chronic ulcerative colitis. Histopathology 11:927–929, 1987.
163. Borkje B, Hostmark J, Shagen DW, et al: Flow cytometry of biopsy specimens from ulcerative colitis, colorectal adenomas, and carcinomas. Scand J Gastroenterol 22:1231–1237, 1987.
164. Melville DM, Jass JR, Shepherd NA, et al: Dysplasia and deoxyribonucleic acid aneuploidy in the assessment of precancerous changes in chronic ulcerative colitis: Observer variation and correlations. Gastroenterology 95:668–675, 1988.
165. Lofberg R, Caspersson T, Tribukait B, Ost A: Comparative DNA analyses in longstanding ulcerative colitis with aneuploidy. Gut 30:1731–1736, 1989.
166. Collins RH Jr, Feldman M, Fordtram JS: Colon cancer, dysplasia, and surveillance in patients with ulcerative colitis: A critical review. N Engl J Med 316:1654–1658, 1987.
167. Jones HW, Grogono J, Hoare AM: Surveillance in ulcerative colitis: Burdens and benefit. Gut 29:325–331, 1988.
168. Fozard JBJ, Dixon MF: Colonoscopic surveillance in ulcerative colitis: Dysplasia through the looking glass. Gut 30:285–292, 1989.
169. Melville DM, Jass JR, Morson BC, et al: Observer study of the grading of dysplasia in ulcerative colitis: Comparison with clinical outcome. Hum Pathol 20:1008–1014, 1989.
170. Crohn BB, Ginzburg L, Oppenheimer GD: Regional ileitis: A pathologic and clinical entity. JAMA 99:1323–1329, 1932.
171. Lockhart-Mummery HE, Morson BC: Crohn's disease (regional enteritis) of the large intestine and its distinction from ulcerative colitis. Gut 1:87–105, 1960.
172. Lennard-Jones JE, Lockhart-Mummery HE, Morson BC: Clinical and pathological differentiation of Crohn's disease and proctocolitis. Gastroenterology 54:1162–1170, 1968.
173. Yardley JH: Crohnology (letter). Gastroenterology 87:744, 1984.
174. Mayberry JF, Rhodes J: Epidemiologic aspects of Crohn's disease: A review of the literature. Gut 25:886–899, 1984.
175. Gitnick GL, Arthus MH, Shibata I: Cultivation of viral agents from Crohn's disease: A new sensitive system. Lancet 2:215–221, 1976.
176. Parent K, Mitchell P: Cell wall-defective variants of pseudomonas-like (group Va) bacteria in Crohn's disease. Gastroenterology 75:368–372, 1978.
177. Chiodini RJ, Van Kruiningen HJ, Thayer WR, et al: Possible role of Mycobacteria in inflammatory bowel disease. I. An unclassified *Mycobacterium* species isolated from patients with Crohn's disease. Dig Dis Sci 29:1073–1079, 1984.
178. Keren DF: Immunopathogenesis of inflammatory bowel disease. In Norris HT (ed): Pathology of the Colon, Small Intestine, and Anus. New York, Churchill Livingstone, 1983, pp 61–76.
179. Wakefield GJ, Sawyerr AM, Dohillon AP, et al: Pathogenesis of Crohn's disease: Multifocal gastrointestinal infarction. Lancet 2:1057–1062, 1989.
180. Rickert RR, Carter HW: The "early" ulcerative lesion of Crohn's disease: Correlative light and scanning electron microscopic studies. J Clin Gastroenterol 2:11–19, 1980.
181. Farmer RJ, Hawk WA, Turnbull RB Jr: Clinical patterns in Crohn's disease: A statistical study of 615 cases. Gastroenterology 68:627–635, 1975.
182. Homer DR, Grand RJ, Colodny AH: Growth, course, and prognosis after surgery for Crohn's disease in children and adolescents. Pediatrics 59:717–725, 1977.
183. Farmer RG, Hawk WA, Turnbull RB Jr: Indications for surgery in Crohn's disease: Analysis of 500 cases. Gastroenterology 71:245–250, 1976.
184. Pennington L, Hamilton SR, Bayless TR, et al: Surgical management of Crohn's disease: Influence of disease at margin of resection. Ann Surg 192:311–318, 1980.
185. Greenstein AJ, Sachar DB, Pasternack BS, Janowitz HD: Reoperation and recurrence in Crohn's colitis and ileocolitis: Crude and cumulative rates. N Engl J Med 293:685–690, 1975.
186. Trnka YM, Glotzer DJ, Kasdon EJ, et al: The long-term outcome of restorative operation in Crohn's disease: Influence of location, prognostic factors, and surgical guidelines. Ann Surg 196:345–355, 1982.

187. Rutgeerts P, Geboes K, Vantrappen G, et al: Natural history of Crohn's disease at the ileocolonic anastomosis after curative surgery. Gut 25:665–672, 1984.
188. Nugent FW, Veidenheimer MC, Meissner WA, Haggitt RC: Prognosis after colonic resection for Crohn's disease of the colon. Gastroenterology 65:398–402, 1973.
189. Prior P, Gyde S, Cooke WT, et al: Mortality in Crohn's disease. Gastroenterology 80:307–312, 1981.
190. Warren S, Sommers SC: Cicatrizing enteritis (regional ileitis) as a pathologic entity: Analysis of 120 cases. Am J Pathol 24:475–501, 1948.
191. Rappaport H, Burgoyne FH, Smetana HP: Pathology of regional enteritis. Milit Surg 109:463–502, 1951.
192. Geboes K: Morphological Aspects of Crohn's Disease. Maldegem, Druk Van Hoetenberghe, 1984.
193. Shapiro PA, Peppercorn MA, Antonioli DA, et al: Crohn's disease in the elderly. Am J Gastroenterol 76:132–137, 1981.
194. Goodman MJ, Skinner JM, Truelove SC: Abnormalities in the apparently normal bowel mucosa in Crohn's disease. Lancet 1:275–278, 1976.
195. Rutgeerts P, Onette E, Vantrappen G, et al: Crohn's disease of the stomach and duodenum: A clinical study with emphasis on the value of endoscopy and endoscopic biopsies. Endoscopy 12:288–294, 1980.
196. Korelitz BI, Waye JD, Kreuning J, et al: Crohn's disease in endoscopic biopsies of the gastric antrum and duodenum. Am J Gastroenterol 76:103–109, 1981.
197. Dunne WT, Cooke WT, Allan RN: Enzymatic and morphometric evidence for Crohn's disease as a diffuse lesion of the gastrointestinal tract. Gut 18:290–294, 1977.
198. Dvorak AM, Osage JE, Monahan RA, et al: Crohn's disease: Transmission electron microscopic studies. III. Target tissues: Proliferation and injury to smooth muscle and the autonomic nervous system. Hum Pathol 11:620–635, 1980.
199. Steinhoff MM, Kodner JJ, De Schryver-Kecskemeti K: Axonal degeneration/necrosis: A possible ultrastructural marker for Crohn's disease. Modern Pathol 1:182–187, 1988.
200. Nyhlin H, Stenling R: The small intestinal mucosa in patients with Crohn's disease assessed by scanning electron and light microscopy. Scand J Gastroenterol 19:433–440, 1984.
201. Whitehead R: Pathology of Crohn's disease of the colon. In Kirsner JB, Shorter RG (eds): Inflammatory Bowel Disease. Philadelphia, Lea & Febiger, 1975, pp 182–198.
202. Sutphen JL, Cooper PH, Mackel SE, Nelson DL: Metastatic cutaneous Crohn's disease. Gastroenterology 86:941–944, 1984.
203. Tweedie JH, McCann BG: Metastatic Crohn's disease of thigh and forearm. Gut 25:213–214, 1984.
204. Boerr LA, Bai JC, Olivares L, et al: Cutaneous metastatic Crohn's disease: Treatment with metronidazole. Am J Gastroenterol 82:1326–1327, 1987.
205. Nugent FW, Glaser D, Fernandez-Herlihy L: Crohn's disease associated with granulomatous bone disease. N Engl J Med 294:262–263, 1976.
206. Bayless TM, Stevens MB: Granulomatous synovitis and Crohn's disease. N Engl J Med 294:903, 1976.
207. Menard DB, Haddad H, Blain JG, et al: Granulomatous myositis and myopathy associated with Crohn's colitis. N Engl J Med 295:818–819, 1976.
208. Lemann M, Messing B, D'Agay F, Modigliani R: Crohn's disease with respiratory tract involvement. Gut 28:1669–1672, 1987.
209. McClure J, Banerjee SS, Schofield PS: Crohn's disease of the gallbladder. J Clin Pathol 37:516–518, 1984.
210. Kremer M, Nussenson E, Steinfeld M, Zuckerman P: Crohn's disease of the vulva. Am J Gastroenterol 79:376–378, 1984.
211. Schulman D, Beck LS, Roberts IM, Schwartz AM: Crohn's disease of the vulva. Am J Gastroenterol 82:1328–1330, 1987.
212. Slaney G, Muller S, Clay J, et al: Crohn's disease involving the penis. Gut 27:329–333, 1986.
213. Geboes K, Vantrappen G: The value of colonoscopy in the diagnosis of Crohn's disease. Gastrointest Endosc 22:18–23, 1975.
214. Watier A, Devroede G, Perey B, et al: Small erythematous mucosal plaques: an endoscopic sign of Crohn's disease. Gut 21:835–839, 1980.
215. Joffe N, Antonioli DA, Bettman M, Goldman H: Focal granulomatous (Crohn's) colitis: Radiological-pathological correlation. Gastrointest Radiol 3:73–80, 1978.
216. Kelly JK, Siu TO: The strictures, sinus, and fissures of Crohn's disease. J Clin Gastroenterol 8:594–598, 1986.
217. Steinberg DM, Cooke WT, Alexander-Williams J: Free perforation in Crohn's disease. Gut 14:187–190, 1973.
218. Greenstein AJ, Mann DA, Sachar DB, Aufses AH Jr: Free perforation in Crohn's disease. I. A survey of 99 cases. Am J Gastroenterol 80:682–689, 1985.
219. Kelly JK, Sutherland LR: The chronological sequence in the pathology of Crohn's disease. J Clin Gastroenterol 10:28–33, 1988.
220. McQuillon AC, Appelman HD: Superficial Crohn's disease: A study of 10 patients. Surg Pathol 2:231–239, 1989.
221. Kahn E, Daum F: Pseudopolyps of the small intestine in Crohn's disease. Hum Pathol 15:84–86, 1984.
222. Reese J, Hamilton SR: An evaluation of the role of resection margin frozen sections in the surgical management of Crohn's disease. (Abstract) Lab Invest 44:54A, 1981.
223. Dourmashkin RR, Davies H, Wells C, et al: Epithelial patchy necrosis in Crohn's disease. Hum Pathol 14:643–648, 1983.
224. Geller SA, Cohen A: Arterial inflammatory-cell infiltrates in Crohn's disease. Arch Pathol Lab Med 107:473–475, 1983.
225. Ming SC, Simon M, Tandar BN: Gross gastric metaplasia of ileum after regional enteritis. Gastroenterology 44:63–68, 1963.
226. Chambers TJ, Morson BC: The granuloma in Crohn's disease. Gut 20:269–274, 1979.
227. Surawicz CM, Meisel JL, Ylvisaker T, et al: Rectal biopsy in the diagnosis of Crohn's disease: Value of multiple biopsies and serial sectioning. Gastroenterology 80:66–71, 1981.
228. Petri M, Poulson SS, Christensen K, Jarnum S: The incidence of granulomas in serial sections of rectal biopsies from patients with Crohn's disease. Acta Path Microbiol Immunol Scand 90:145–147, 1982.
229. Kuramoto S, Oohara T, Ihara O, et al: Granulomas of the gut in Crohn's disease. A step sectioning study. Dis Colon Rectum 30:6–11, 1987.
230. Glass RE, Baker WNW: Role of the granuloma in recurrent Crohn's disease. Gut 17:75–77, 1976.
231. Wolfson DM, Sachar DB, Cohen A, et al: Granulomas do not affect postoperative recurrence rates in Crohn's disease. Gastroenterology 83:405–409, 1982.
232. Rotterdam H, Korelitz BI, Sommers SC: Microgranulomas in grossly normal rectal mucosa in Crohn's disease. Am J Clin Pathol 67:550–554, 1977.
233. Hyams JS, Goldman H, Katz AJ: Differentiating small bowel Crohn's disease from lymphoma: Role of rectal biopsy. Gastroenterology 79:340–343, 1980.
234. Hamilton SR, Bussey HJR, Morson BC: En face histopathologic technique for examining colonic mucosa of resection specimens. Am J Clin Pathol 78:514–517, 1982.
235. Brophy CM, Frederick WG, Schlessel R, Barwick KW: Focal segmental ischemia of the terminal ileum mimicking Crohn's disease. J Clin Gastroenterol 10:343–347, 1988.
236. Tandon HD, Prakash A: Pathology of intestinal tuberculosis and its distinction from Crohn's disease. Gut 13:260–269, 1972.
237. Miller DP, Everett ED: Gastrointestinal histoplasmosis. J Clin Gastroenterol 1:233–236, 1979.
238. Orchard JL, Luparello F, Brushill D: Malabsorption syndrome occurring in the course of disseminated histoplasmosis. Am J Med 66:331–335, 1979.
239. Lee SH, Barnes WG, Hodges GR, Dixon A: Perforated granulomatous colitis caused by *Histoplasma capsulatum*. Dis Colon Rectum 28:171–176, 1985.
240. Pinkus GS, Coolidge C, Little MD: Intestinal anisakiasis: First case report from North America. Am J Med 59:114–120, 1975.
241. Valdiserri RO: Intestinal anisakiasis: Report of a case and recovery of larvae from market fish. Am J Clin Pathol 76:329–333, 1981.
242. El-Maraghi NRH, Mair NS: The histopathology of enteric infection with *Yersinia pseudotuberculosis*. Am J Clin Pathol 71:631–639, 1979.
243. Bradford WD, Norce PS, Gutman LT, et al: Pathologic features of enteric infection with *Yersinia enterocolitica*. Arch Pathol 98:17–22, 1974.

244. Gleason TH, Patterson SD: The pathology of *Yersinia enterocolitica* ileocolitis. Am J Surg Pathol 6:347–355, 1982.
245. Ming SC, Fleischner FG: Diverticulitis of the sigmoid colon: Reappraisal of the pathology and pathogenesis. Surgery 58:627–633, 1965.
246. Morson BC: Pathology of the diverticular disease of the colon. Clin Gastroenterol 4:37–52, 1975.
247. Marshak RH, Janovitz HD, Present DH: Granulomatous colitis in association with diverticula. N Engl J Med 283:1080–1084, 1970.
248. Meyers MA, Alonso DR, Morson BC, et al: Pathogenesis of diverticulitis complicating granulomatous colitis. Gastroenterology 74:24–31, 1978.
249. Mershak RH, Lindner AE, Maklansky D: Paracolic fistulous tracts in diverticulitis and granulomatous colitis. JAMA 243:1943–1946, 1980.
250. Bishop RP, Brewster AC, Antonioli DA: Crohn's disease of the mouth. Gastroenterology 62:302–306, 1972.
251. Basu MK, Asquith P, Thompson RA, et al: Oral manifestations of Crohn's disease. Gut 16:249–254, 1975.
252. Wilder WM, Slagle GW, Hand AM, Watkins WJ: Crohn's disease of the epiglottis, aryepiglottic folds, anus and rectum. J Clin Gastroenterol 2:87–91, 1980.
253. Scully C, Cochran KM, Russell RI, et al: Crohn's disease of the mouth: an indicator of intestinal involvement. Gut 23:198–201, 1982.
254. Ward CS, Dunphy EP, Jagoe WS, Sheahan DG: Crohn's disease limited to the mouth and anus. J Clin Gastroenterol 7:516–521, 1985.
255. Schnitt SJ, Antonioli DA, Jaffe B, Peppercorn MA: Granulomatous inflammation of minor salivary gland ducts: A new oral manifestation of Crohn's disease. Hum Pathol 18:405–407, 1987.
256. Li Volsi VA, Jaretzki A: Granulomatous esophagitis: A case of Crohn's disease limited to the esophagus. Gastroenterology 64:313–319, 1973.
257. Freedman PG, Dietrich DT, Balthazar EJ: Crohn's disease of the esophagus: Case report and review of the literature. Am J Gastroenterol 79:835–838, 1984.
258. Geboes K, Janssen J, Rugeerts P, Van Trappen G: Crohn's disease of the esophagus. J Clin Gastroenterol 8:31–37, 1986.
259. Fielding JF, Toye DKM, Beton DC, et al: Crohn's disease of the stomach and duodenum. Gut 11:1001–1006, 1970.
260. Hermos JA, Cooper HL, Kramer P, Trier JS: Histologic diagnosis by peroral biopsy of Crohn's disease of the proximal intestine. Gastroenterology 59:868–873, 1970.
261. Wise L, Kyreakos M, McCown A, et al: Crohn's disease of the duodenum. Am J Surg 121:184–194, 1971.
262. Nugent FW, Richmond M, Park SK: Crohn's disease of the duodenum. Gut 18:115–120, 1977.
263. Schuffler MD, Chaffee RE: Small intestinal biopsy in a patient with Crohn's disease of the duodenum (The spectrum of abnormal findings in the absence of granulomas). Gastroenterology 76:1009–1014, 1979.
264. Frandsen PJ, Jarnum S, Malmstrom J: Crohn's disease of the duodenum. Scand J Gastroenterol 15:683–688, 1980.
265. Marshak RH, Maklansky D, Kurzban JD, Lindner AE: Crohn's disease of the stomach and duodenum. Am J Gastroenterol 77:340–341, 1982.
266. Ewen SWB, Anderson J, Galloway JMD, et al: Crohn's disease initially confined to the appendix. Gastroenterology 60:853–857, 1971.
267. Yang SS, Gibson P, McCaughey RS, et al: Primary Crohn's disease of the appendix: Report of 14 cases and review of the literature. Ann Surg 189:334–339, 1979.
268. Ariel I, Vinograd I, Hershlag A, et al: Crohn's disease isolated to the appendix: Truths and fallacies. Hum Pathol 17:1116–1121, 1986.
269. Timmcke AE: Granulomatous appendicitis: Is it Crohn's disease? Report of a case and review of the literature. Am J Gastroenterol 81:283–287, 1986.
270. Rankin GB, Watts HD, Melnyk CS, Kelley MI Jr: National Cooperative Crohn's Disease Study: Extraintestinal manifestations and perianal Crohn's. Gastroenterology 77:914–920, 1979.
271. Alexander-Williams J, Bachman P: Perianal Crohn's. World J Surg 4:203, 1980.
272. Aftalion B, Lipper S: Enteritis cystica profunda associated with Crohn's disease. Arch Pathol Lab Med 108:532–533, 1984.
273. Saul SH, Wong LK, Zinsser KR: Enteritis cystica profunda: Association with Crohn's disease. Hum Pathol 17:600–603, 1986.
274. Alexis J, Lubin J, Wallach M: Enteritis cystica profunda in a patient with Crohn's disease. Arch Pathol Lab Med 113:947–949, 1989.
275. Sachar DB, Wolfson DM, Greenstein AJ, et al: Risk factors for postoperative recurrence of Crohn's disease. Gastroenterology 85:917–921, 1983.
276. Glotzer DJ, Glick ME, Goldman H: Proctitis and colitis following diversion of the fecal stream. Gastroenterology 80:438–441, 1981.
277. Korelitz BI, Cheskin LJ, Sohn N, Sommers SC: Proctitis after fecal diversion in Crohn's disease and its elimination with reanastomosis: Implications for surgical management: Report of four cases. Gastroenterology 87:710–713, 1984.
278. Weedon DD, Shorter RG, Ilstrup DM, et al: Crohn's disease and cancer. N Engl J Med 289:1099–1103, 1973.
279. Lightdale CJ, Sternberg SS, Posner G, et al: Carcinoma complicating Crohn's disease. Am J Med 59:262–268, 1975.
280. Gyde SN, Prior P, Macartney JC, et al: Malignancy in Crohn's disease. Gut 21:1024–1029, 1980.
281. Shorter RG: Risks of intestinal cancer in Crohn's disease. Dis Colon Rectum 26:686–689, 1983.
282. Glotzer DJ: The risk of cancer in Crohn's disease. Gastroenterology 89:438–441, 1985.
283. Fresko D, Lazarus SS, Daton J, Reingold M: Early representation of carcinoma of the small bowel in Crohn's disease ("Crohn's carcinoma"): Case report and review of the literature. Gastroenterology 82:783–789, 1982.
284. Hawkes PC, Gyde SN, Thompson H, Allan RN: Adenocarcinoma of the small intestine complicating Crohn's disease. Gut 23:188–193, 1982.
285. Thompson EM, Clayden G, Price AB: Cancer in Crohn's disease: An "occult" malignancy. Histopathology 7:365–376, 1983.
286. Collier PE, Turowski P, Diamond DL: Small intestinal adenocarcinoma complicating regional enteritis. Cancer 55:516–521, 1985.
287. Hamilton SR: Colorectal carcinoma in patients with Crohn's disease. Gastroenterology 89:398–407, 1985.
288. Petras RE: Mir-Madjlessi SH, Farmer RG: Crohn's disease and intestinal carcinoma: A report of 11 cases with emphasis on associated epithelial dysplasia. Gastroenterology 93:1307–1314, 1987.
289. Cuvelier C, Bekaert E, DePother C, et al: Crohn's disease with adenocarcinoma and dysplasia: Macroscopical, histological, and immunohistochemical aspects of two cases. Am J Surg Pathol 13:187–196, 1989.
290. Senay E, Sachar DB, Keohane M, Greenstein AJ: Small bowel carcinoma in Crohn's disease: Distinguishing features and risk factors. Cancer 63:360–363, 1989.
291. Craft CF, Mendelsohn G, Cooper HS, et al: Colonic "precancer" in Crohn's disease. Gastroenterology 80:578–584, 1981.
292. Simpson S, Traube J, Riddell RH: The histologic appearance of dysplasia (precarcinomatous change) in Crohn's disease of the small and large intestine. Gastroenterology 81:492–501, 1981.
293. Warren R, Barwick KW: Crohn's colitis with carcinoma and dysplasia: Report of a case and review of 100 small and large bowel resections for Crohn's disease to detect incidence of dysplasia. Am J Surg Pathol 7:151–159, 1983.
294. White CL, Hamilton SR, Diamond MP, Cameron JL: Crohn's disease and ulcerative colitis in the same patient. Gut 24:857–862, 1983.
295. Goodman MJ, Kirsner JB, Riddell RH: Usefulness of rectal biopsy in inflammatory bowel disease. Gastroenterology 72:952–956, 1977.
296. Malatjalian DA: Pathology of inflammatory bowel disease in colorectal mucosal biopsies. Dig Dis Sci 32:5S–15S, 1987.
297. Dyer NH, Stansfeld AG, Dawson AM: The value of rectal biopsy in the diagnosis of Crohn's disease. Scand J Gastroenterol 5:491–496, 1970.
298. Hill RB, Kent TH, Hansen RN: Clinical usefulness of rectal biopsy in Crohn's disease. Gastroenterology 77:938–944, 1979.

299. Iliffe GD, Owen DA: Rectal biopsy in Crohn's disease. Dig Dis Sci 26:321–324, 1981.
300. Surawicz CM: Serial sectioning of a portion of a rectal biopsy detects more focal abnormalities: A prospective study of patients with inflammatory bowel disease. Dig Dis Sci 27:434–436, 1982.
301. Rotterdam H, Sommers SC: Biopsy Diagnosis of the Digestive Tract. New York, Raven Press, 1981.
302. Whitehead R: Mucosal Biopsy of the Gastrointestinal Tract, 3rd ed. Philadelphia, WB Saunders, 1985.
303. Goldman H: Colonic mucosal biopsy in inflammatory bowel disease. Surg Pathol (In press).
304. Haggitt RC: Differential diagnosis of colitis. In Goldman H, Appelman HD, Kaufman N (eds): Gastrointestinal Pathology. Baltimore, Williams & Wilkins, 1990, pp 325–355.
305. Lee KS, Medline A, Shockey S: Indeterminate colitis in the spectrum of inflammatory bowel disease. Arch Pathol Lab Med 103:173–176, 1979.
306. Meisel JL, Bergman D, Graney D, et al: Human rectal mucosa: Proctoscopic and morphological changes caused by laxatives. Gastroenterology 72:1274–1279, 1977.
307. Levine DS, Haggitt RC: Normal histology of the colon. Am J Surg Pathol 13:966–984, 1989.
308. Shahmis M, Schuman BM: Complications of fiberoptic endoscopy. Gastrointest Endosc 26:86–91, 1960.
309. Korelitz BI, Sommers SC: Responses to drug therapy in ulcerative colitis. Am J Dig Dis 21:441–447, 1976.
310. Goldin E, Rachmilewitz D: Ileoscopic diagnosis of terminal ileitis. Gastrointest Endosc 30:11–14, 1984.
311. Coremans G, Rutgeerts P, Geboes K, et al: The value of ileoscopy with biopsy in the diagnosis of intestinal Crohn's disease. Gastrointest Endosc 30:167–172, 1984.
312. Borsch G, Schmidt G: Endoscopy of the terminal ileum: Diagnostic yield in 400 consecutive specimens. Dis Colon Rectum 28:499–501, 1985.
313. Goldblatt MS, Corman ML, Haggitt RC, et al: Ileostomy complications requiring revision: Lahey Clinic experience, 1964–1973. Dis Colon Rectum 20:209–214, 1977.

CHAPTER 28

Other Inflammatory Disorders of the Intestines

HARVEY GOLDMAN, M.D.

DUODENITIS
Peptic Duodenitis
Other Types of Duodenitis
Infections
Physical and Chemical Injuries
Vascular Disease
Crohn's Disease
Celiac Disease
Allergic Disease
Other Immune Disorders
Stress Ulcers of the Duodenum

MISCELLANEOUS INFLAMMATORY DISORDERS OF THE SMALL INTESTINE
Ulcerative Jejunoileitis
Bypass Enteritis
Enteritis Cystica Profunda

Other Ulcers of the Small Intestine
Nonspecific Ulcers of the Small Intestine

MISCELLANEOUS INFLAMMATORY DISORDERS OF THE COLON
Microscopic (Lymphocytic) Colitis
Collagenous Colitis
Diversion-Related Colitis
Acute Self-Limited Colitis
Colitis Cystica Profunda
Solitary Rectal Ulcer Syndrome
Effects of Laxatives and Enemas
Melanosis Coli
Cathartic Colon
Laxative Abuse Syndrome
Effects of Enemas

Other Ulcers of the Colon
Behçet's Disease
Stercoraceous Ulcers
Nonspecific Ulcers of the Colon
Secondary Ulcers of the Colon
Irritable Bowel Syndrome

OTHER TUMOR-LIKE LESIONS OF THE INTESTINES
Pneumatosis Intestinalis
Endometriosis
Gastric Heterotopia
Foreign Body Reactions
Foreign Objects
Localized Granulomatous Reactions
Barium Granuloma
Oil Granuloma

There are numerous conditions that are characterized by the presence of inflammatory lesions in the small and large intestines (Table 28–1). The inflammation may be the primary pathologic event, or it may develop as a consequence or complication of some other disease process. The most common inflammatory disorders are those due to infections and the idiopathic diseases of ulcerative colitis and Crohn's disease. Inflammatory lesions may occur and become the dominant finding during the course of many other diseases, including allergic and other immune disorders, radiation and chemical injuries, motor and mechanical disturbances, ischemic disease, and various metabolic conditions. Since all of these inflammatory lesions affect the mucosa, considerable information has been acquired by the increasing study of mucosal biopsies of the various segments of the intestinal tract.[1–9]

This chapter deals with those inflammatory diseases and tumor-like lesions of the small and large intestines that are not completely covered in other parts of the book. Lesions primarily involving the jejunum are detailed in Chapter 29, on malabsorptive disorders; and other inflammatory conditions that can affect multiple organs of the alimentary tract are included in Chapter 16, on systemic and miscellaneous disorders. Necrotizing enterocolitis is presented in Chapter 12 on vascular diseases.

DUODENITIS

Peptic Duodenitis

Definition. Peptic duodenitis is an acute and chronic inflammatory disorder of the duodenal mucosa that is

Table 28-1 INFLAMMATORY DISEASES OF THE INTESTINES

Idiopathic inflammatory bowel disease
    Ulcerative colitis
    Crohn's disease
Infections
Ischemic bowel disease and vasculitis
Motor and mechanical diseases
Radiation and chemical injuries
Allergic and other immune disorders
Miscellaneous conditions
    Peptic duodenitis and ulcer
    Bypass enteritis and diversion colitis
    Collagenous colitis and microscopic colitis
    Enteritis and colitis cystica profunda
    Stercoraceous and nonspecific ulcers

---

largely due to the toxic effect of excess gastric acid and possibly abetted by activated gastric proteolytic enzymes.[10,11] It is a highly prevalent condition, which, in the acute form, probably affects all persons at some time; and it is estimated that 5% to 10% of the population in Western developed countries have prolonged or chronic disease. The condition is thought to be a part of the spectrum of peptic ulcer disease, in which the patients have the characteristic symptoms and mucosal inflammation but lack overt ulceration.[12–14] Furthermore, there are many cases in which the inflammation is minimal and difficult to identify, and yet the patients respond to specific antacid therapy.

Etiology and Pathogenesis. The cause of peptic duodenitis is believed to be the same as that of peptic ulcer disease of the duodenum. Most patients have increased gastric acid secretion, either at the basal level or, more commonly, after stimulation by a test meal, histamine, or pentagastrin. The acid acts on the mucosa of the proximal duodenum, which is not protected by the neutralizing effect of the biliary secretions, and causes damage of the surface epithelium.[15] Whether the injury is directly due to the erosive action of the acid and enzymes or is mediated by vasoconstrictive effects on the small vessels in the lamina propria is not established. In either event, the inflammation that follows is of a secondary or reactive nature. Some cases of peptic duodenitis progress to the development of discrete ulcers, or the duodenitis may appear and persist after the healing of an ulcer. This supports the notion that peptic duodenitis is a variant and milder form of peptic ulcer disease. It has been recently noted that about two thirds to three quarters of patients with peptic ulcer disease of the duodenum have *Helicobacter pylori* in the gastric antral mucosa, but the role of these organisms in the evolution of the ulcer disease or of the associated duodenitis is not known.[16,17] Interestingly, they are not seen in the mucosa of the normal or acutely inflamed duodenum, but are frequently present when there is gastric mucous cell metaplasia in cases of chronic duodenitis.[18] The organisms are located on the surface adjacent to the gastric mucous cells, and they are best visualized with silver and Giemsa stains. See Chapter 20 on gastritis, and Chapter 21 on peptic ulcer disorders, for further details.

Clinical Features. The clinical aspects of peptic duodenitis are essentially the same as those of duodenal peptic ulcer disease, and the condition often follows a chronic course with repeated recurrences.[10] The most common symptom is a burning midepigastric pain that appears when the stomach is relatively empty, at about 1 to 2 hours after eating or during the night. Severe cases may reveal more persistent pain, episodes of nausea and vomiting, and evidence of bleeding. Medical therapy is mainly intended to buffer the gastric acid by the use of frequent small meals, antacids, and H_2-blockers. There is also the avoidance of stressful situations and of the ingestion of any substances that may precipitate or promote acid-peptic injury, such as ethanol, aspirin, and other medications. Surgical procedures to reduce gastric acid secretion are infrequent but may be needed in severe cases with erosions and bleeding.

Gross Pathology. The lesion of peptic duodenitis primarily affects the mucosa, and the inflammation extends at most into the upper part of the submucosa, sparing the deeper portions of the bowel wall. Because surgical resections of the inflamed duodenum are not performed, the information on the pathology of duodenitis is mainly derived from endoscopic examination and the histologic study of mucosal biopsy specimens. The lesion is typically limited to the first portion of the duodenum, except in cases with extreme acid production such as is seen in the Zollinger-Ellison syndrome, where the inflammation may extend throughout the organ. Early gross features of duodenitis include edema, erythema, and patchy hemorrhages of the mucosa, and severe cases reveal friability and superficial erosions.[12,19–21] On the basis of the dominant appearance of the lesions, some cases have been categorized as hemorrhagic or erosive duodenitis, but these terms simply denote a more severe form of the disease and do not imply any differences in development.[22,23]

Microscopic Pathology. There have been a large number of histologic studies of the mucosa in peptic duodenitis.[13,14,24–29] The examination is made difficult because of the relatively distorted appearance of the normal duodenal mucosa when compared with that of the jejunum.[1,3,11,26,30,31] The villi of the normal duodenum are not as straight and frequently show slight shortening, which is due in part to the presence of variable numbers of Brunner glands in the mucosa (Figure 28–1). In addition, the first part of the duodenum is normally exposed to large quantities of unbuffered gastric acid and is, therefore, the site of what might be called physiologic peptic injury. These features are often seen in biopsies of patients who are shown to have other disorders and in the rim of the duodenum attached to the gastrectomy specimen. Accordingly, these changes must be discounted before one can consider the diagnosis of clinically significant acid-peptic injury.

More certain histologic features of acute or active duodenitis include evidence of degeneration of the surface epithelium and the presence of neutrophils and a variable increase of mononuclear inflammatory cells in

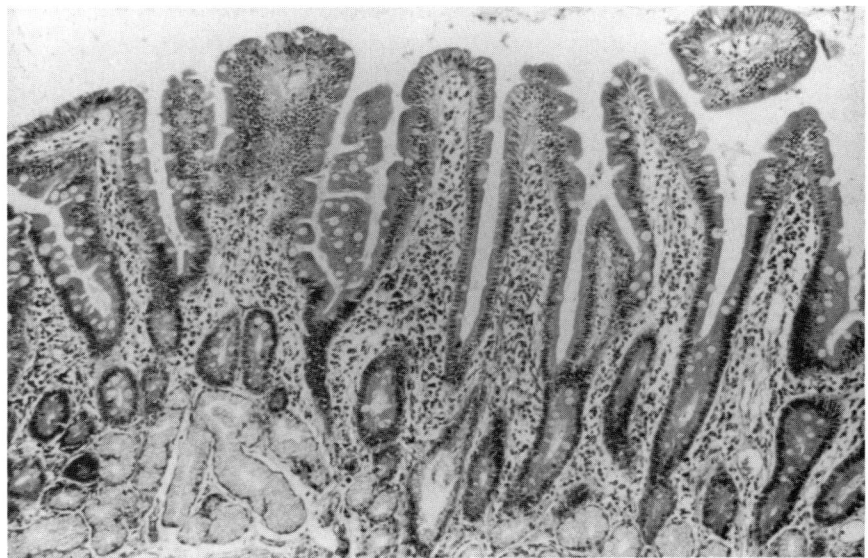

FIGURE 28–1. Normal duodenal mucosa. Compared with the normal jejunum, the duodenal villi are slightly shortened and irregular, in part because of the nests of Brunner glands at the base of the mucosa (bottom). There is a moderate amount of inflammatory cells, mainly of the mononuclear types, in the lamina propria; and the epithelial cells are intact. (H&E, × 120)

the lamina propria and epithelial layer (Figure 28–2). Milder cases show further shortening of the villi, with the inflammation limited to this region. The more severe cases are associated with greater blunting and occasional loss of the villi, extension of the epithelial damage and inflammation to the crypts, focal hemorrhages in the lamina propria, and superficial erosions. The lesions may be diffuse, which is more common, or show a patchy distribution. There may also be acute inflammation in the upper submucosa in the marked cases, but the muscularis propria is normal. The healing phase of duodenitis is characterized by the transient persistence of shortened villi; crypt hyperplasia, which is best visualized in areas with few Brunner's glands; remaining foci of increased mononuclear inflammatory cells in the lamina propria, an increased number of intraepithelial lymphocytes; and a reduction or absence of neutrophils.

As a result of repeated episodes of peptic injury, features of chronic duodenitis appear in the mucosa, and these include a retention of the changes noted in the healing phase, a hyperplasia of the Brunner glands,[32,33] and a gastric mucous cell metaplasia over the surface of the villi.[29,34,35] The proliferation of the Brunner glands is often diffuse, which results in the greater distortion of the villi and crypts, or it may produce a localized nodule (Figure 28–3). Such nodules may become grossly evident and have been called in the past Brunner's gland "adenomas"; there is, however, no cytologic atypism to indicate a neoplasm, and it is more appropriate to refer to them as hyperplastic nodules to signify their reparative nature. The gastric mucous cells in the metaplastic areas are of the surface-foveolar type, and they typically appear as a continuous layer of cells that is concentrated at the top or over the upper third of the villous surface (Figure 28–4). The character

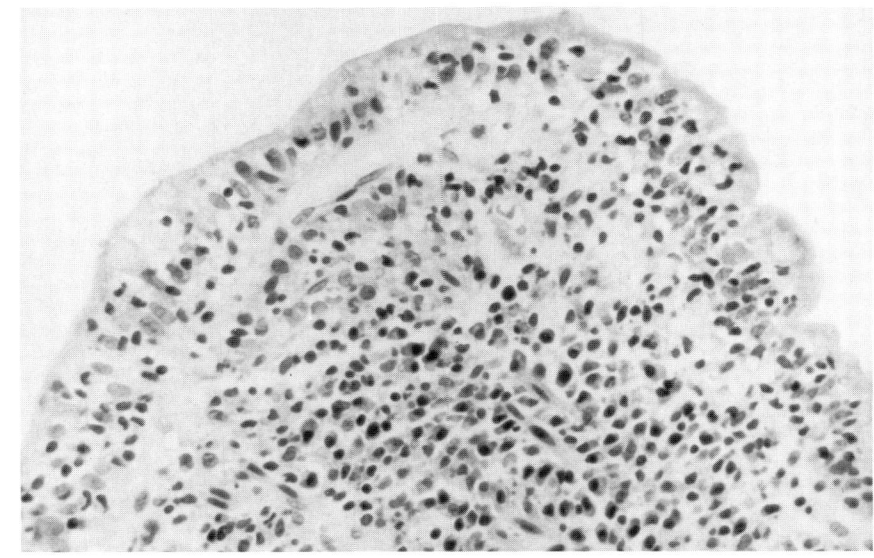

FIGURE 28–2. Duodenal mucosa in a case of active peptic duodenitis. The villus is blunted and widened, and the surface epithelial cells are markedly shortened and infiltrated with inflammatory cells. There is also an increase of inflammatory cells, including neutrophils as well as mononuclear cells, in the lamina propria. (H&E, × 400)

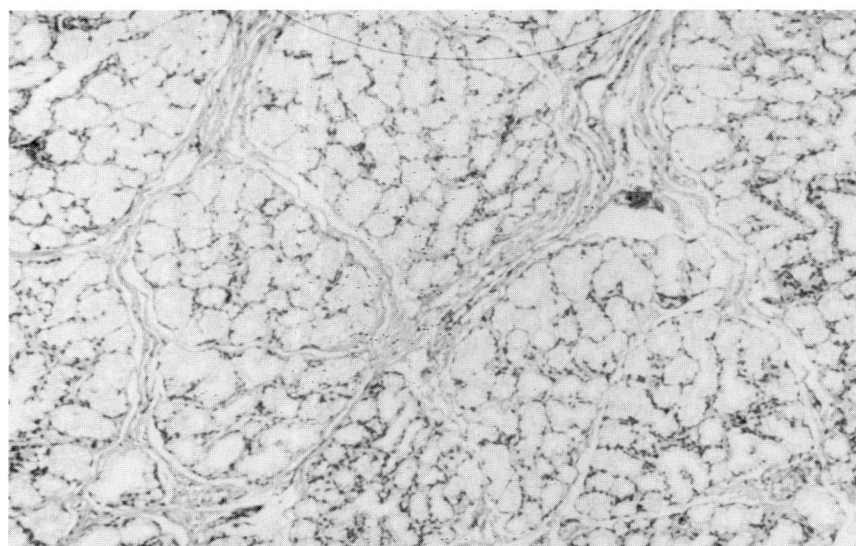

FIGURE 28-3. Nodule of Brunner gland hyperplasia in a case of chronic peptic duodenitis. There are a marked number of mature Brunner glands without any nuclear atypicality. (H&E, × 100)

of the gastric mucous cells is easily recognized in standard hematoxylin and eosin (H&E) preparations and can be accentuated by the use of differential mucin stains.[18] Whereas the intestinal goblet mucous cells have a distended shape and contain acid mucins that stain with alcian blue, the mucous cells of the gastric surface type are relatively thin and have mucous granules that are restricted to the luminal end of the cytoplasm and that stain intensely with the periodic acid–Schiff (PAS) reaction for neutral glycoproteins. As noted above, *Helicobacter pylori* may be seen in the areas of gastric mucous cell metaplasia. The mere presence of mononuclear inflammatory cells in the lamina propria, even if they appear slightly increased in number, in the absence of other features does not constitute evidence of chronic duodenitis, since they may be seen in the intestinal mucosa of normal persons.

Complications. In long-standing cases of duodenitis, the mucosal surface may be irregularly raised; this condition has been termed nodular duodenitis.[36] Some of these cases are caused by hyperplasia of the Brunner glands, but most appear to be the result of marked proliferation of lymphoid tissue in the mucosa and upper submucosa. Because the lesion of a peptic duodenitis is largely confined to the mucosa, one does not encounter complications of the sort that are seen in diseases with deeper lesions, such as fibrous stricture, sinus tracts, and perforation. Despite the persistence of the inflammation over many years, there is apparently no increase in the incidence of carcinoma, lymphoma, or other tumors in this condition. Patients with peptic duodenitis are more prone to the development of acid-peptic disease of other organs, mainly the stomach and the esophagus, presumably because excess gastric acid production may also be a contributing factor in the pathogenesis of the lesions in the other areas.

Diagnosis. The diagnosis of peptic duodenitis is based mainly on the clinical features, including the

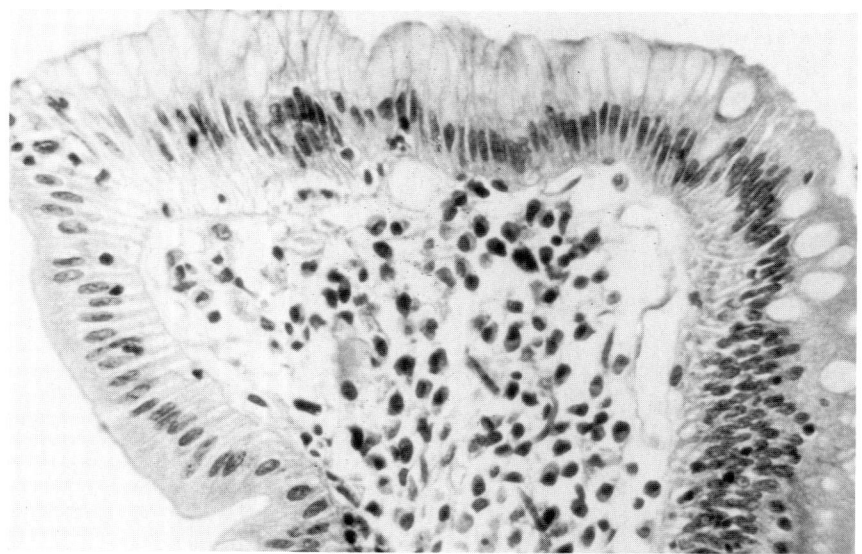

FIGURE 28-4. Duodenal mucosa in a case of chronic peptic duodenitis, showing gastric mucous cell metaplasia on the top of the villus. The gastric mucous cells are columnar, and the cytoplasmic mucin is concentrated in the luminal portion of the cells. (H&E, × 400)

characteristic pain and response to antacid therapy in a patient who does not have a demonstrable ulcer.[10] Radiographic study is commonly performed to exclude the presence of a peptic ulcer; the findings are usually normal, or they may reveal edema and, in late cases, a nodular appearance of the mucosa due to hyperplasia of the Brunner glands or lymphoid nodules. Endoscopic examination with mucosal biopsy is added in many cases for identifying or documenting the presence of inflammation, determining the exact site of the injury (whether the esophagus, stomach, or duodenum), excluding other causes, and monitoring the disease after therapy. Overall, there is a relatively poor correlation between the gross and microscopic features in the milder cases of duodenitis.[19,20] The gross features of early or mild disease, such as edema and erythema of the mucosa, may be difficult to distinguish from the traumatic effects of the endoscopic procedure. Conversely, there may be microscopic evidence of active duodenitis in cases with a normal gross appearance. The histologic interpretation of duodenitis must be conservative, since it is usually impossible to separate the various architectural and traumatic effects from the changes of early disease. Accordingly, the clinical diagnosis of active duodenitis is usually dependent on the characteristic symptomatology and on the presence of a compatible gross or microscopic appearance.

Differential Diagnosis. The pathologic features noted in peptic duodenitis are entirely nonspecific, and the diagnosis depends on the finding of disease restricted to the proximal duodenum and on the exclusion of other causes. Equivalent inflammation may be seen in many other disorders, including radiation, chemical and drug reactions, and ischemic disease; and the separation requires the relevant clinical information. Infections may be associated with prominent mucosal inflammation and are distinguished by the identification of the organism or viral inclusions in the tissue or by appropriate cultures. In allergic disease affecting the duodenum, the lesions are usually patchy; occasionally noted are large clusters of eosinophils in the lamina propria. The duodenum is ordinarily involved in celiac disease, with active lesions showing marked or complete villous atrophy, together with prominent crypt hyperplasia; but neutrophilic infiltration is usually minimal or absent. Crohn's disease may occasionally involve the duodenum, and severe lesions reveal greater destruction with a tendency for deep ulceration; the disease may be present in any portion of the duodenum, and granulomas are noted in many of the cases. The gross appearance of nodular duodenitis can raise the suspicion of a tumor, and biopsy examination is usually required to make the distinction.

Other Types of Duodenitis

Many other inflammatory conditions can affect the duodenum (Table 28–2). The detailed information about these disorders is provided in other chapters, and only some of the salient points that relate to disease in the duodenum are presented here.

Table 28–2 INFLAMMATORY DISEASES OF THE DUODENUM

Peptic duodenitis and chronic peptic ulcer
Acute stress ulcer
Infections
    Post–gastric surgery
    Opportunistic
Radiation, drug, and toxic injuries
Vasculitis
Crohn's disease
Celiac disease
Allergic disease

Infections

The common viral and bacterial infections of the intestines do not usually involve the duodenum, possibly because of the antagonistic effects of acid and other toxic substances in this area.[37] It has been noted, however, that some peptic ulcers reveal a localized overgrowth of bacteria and fungi; these are associated with greater severity and with delay in healing.[38–40] After a Billroth II operation, the afferent loop leading to the gastrojejunostomy may become stagnant and favor the development of bacterial proliferation in the lumen.[3,41] The functional problems that ensue are largely due to the effects of bacteria on the bile salts and to the utilization of vitamins, and the mucosa may be normal or show a variable degree of usually mild and patchy inflammation. Numerous opportunistic infections may involve the duodenal mucosa and that of the rest of the small intestine, including those due to cytomegalovirus,[42–44] fungi,[45] *Giardia*,[46–48] *Isospora*,[49–52] and *Cryptosporidium*[53–63]; and their distinctive structures can be readily visualized in the tissues. The amount of mucosal destruction and inflammatory reaction is highly variable in these infections, which are usually associated with marked immunosuppression, and ranges from minimal alterations to overt ulceration. The lesions are typically confined to the mucosa and submucosa.

Infection with *Mycobacterium avium-intracellulare* is most commonly seen in patients with the acquired immunodeficiency syndrome (AIDS).[64–66] The mucosa typically shows clusters of foamy macrophages or poorly formed granulomas but occasionally may be completely normal in appearance on H&E sections; the specific diagnosis is provided by the acid-fast stain, which reveals abundant organisms both in the macrophages and in the intervening lamina propria (Figure 28–5). The organisms also react with other stains, including PAS, which has caused confusion with Whipple's disease in the past. A variety of helminthic infections,[67–70] identified by the specific ova, and foci of Whipple's disease[71] have also been observed in the duodenum. It appears that the overall identification of duodenal infections, particularly of the opportunistic types, has increased in recent years, and this is mainly attributable to the greater performance of endoscopy and mucosal biopsy. See Chapter 26 for further details.

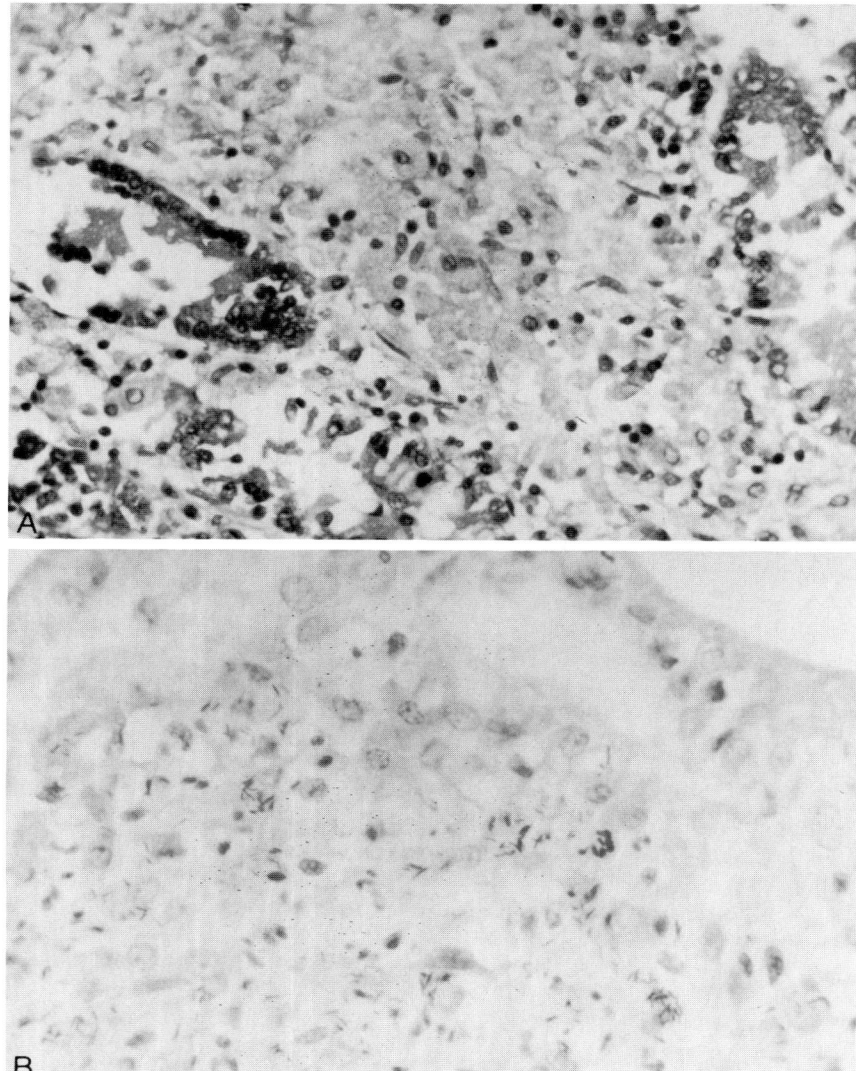

FIGURE 28–5. *A*, Duodenal mucosa in a case of acquired immunodeficiency syndrome. There is a sheet of vacuolated macrophages in the lamina propria (center). (H&E, × 400) *B*, Same duodenal mucosa as in *A*, showing numerous acid-fast bacilli in the lamina propria. (Ziehl-Neelsen, × 400)

Physical and Chemical Injuries

The duodenum may be damaged by radiation, which is usually applied for tumors in adjacent tissues.[72–74] The acute changes include prominent edema and hemorrhage of the mucosa and submucosa, followed by ulceration and marked inflammatory reaction. Obstruction may result from the inflammatory edema or fibrous stricture formation. Chronic effects include persistence of the ulcers, which may penetrate the deeper parts of the bowel wall; fibrosis and sinus tract formation; and progressive thickening of the small vessels leading to secondary ischemic effects. Histologic examination may reveal enlarged and atypical mesenchymal cells in the inflamed and fibrotic areas, and the diagnosis is based on the clinical history and the finding of compatible pathologic features. Muscosal biopsy of ulcerated areas is often obtained to exclude the presence of tumor or opportunistic infections. Various chemicals, such as ethanol,[75] and medications,[76–82] acting as direct toxins or mediated by immunologic injury, can also damage the duodenum. The lesions are typically in the mucosa and consist of patchy inflammation or ulceration. In addition, the duodenal epithelium may reveal marked atypism, following infusion chemotherapy for hepatic tumors.[83,84] After the toxic substances are discontinued, there is usually prompt healing; but in some cases, possibly because of secondary infections, persistence and progression of the lesions are seen. See Chapter 9 for further details.

Vascular Disease

Because of the extensive vascular collaterals encircling the duodenum, ischemic disease due to thrombotic occlusion of vessels or to low blood flow is rarely observed. In an effort to stop or reduce a massive hemorrhage from a peptic ulcer, vasoconstrictive agents and preformed clots or gelfoam are inserted into the mesenteric vessels at time of angiography, and this sometimes results in extensive ischemic damage of the duodenal mucosa and wall.[85] Vasculitis[86–88] and atheromatous emboli[89] may affect any part of the intestine, including the duodenum, and may lead to focal infarction and ulceration of the overlying tissues. See Chapter 12 for further details.

Crohn's Disease

In cases of Crohn's disease affecting the ileum and colon, microscopic abnormalities are commonly noted in the duodenal mucosa, consisting of focal cryptitis and/or granulomas.[90,91] Such changes are seen in random sections of the mucosa in one quarter to one half of the cases and in about 80% if serial sections are obtained, but their presence is not associated with any functional problems. Gross lesions, indicating clinically significant disease, are much less commonly observed and reveal prominent mucosal necrosis and ulceration that may affect any part of the duodenum (see Chapter 27, Figure 27–46).[92–95] The pathologic features are similar to those seen in the distal intestine and include the tendency for deep ulceration, fibrous stricture and sinus tract formation, muscular hypertrophy, and transmural inflammation. The distinction from peptic duodenitis and duodenal peptic ulcer is readily accomplished by noting the more diffuse distribution of the lesions in the duodenum and by the presence of sinus tracts and granulomas. Separation of Crohn's disease from other necrotizing lesions of the duodenum such as severe infections is often dependent on finding associated lesions in the more characteristic sites of the distal ileum and colon. See Chapter 27 for further details.

Celiac Disease

The duodenum is invariably involved in cases of celiac disease, which is also termed nontropical sprue and gluten-sensitive enteropathy.[96–98] The lesion is identical to that described in the jejunum and consists of a diffuse and uniform injury in the mucosa; the deeper parts of the bowel wall are uninvolved.[3,98–102] Major histologic features include a marked shortening ("atrophy") or absence of the villi; reactive crypt hyperplasia, which is proportional to the degree of villous damage; evidence of degeneration of the surface epithelial cells, with increased intraepithelial lymphocytes; and a prominent infiltrate of mononuclear inflammatory cells (mostly plasma cells and lymphocytes) in the lamina propria. Neutrophils may be present but are usually not conspicuous. The healing phase is characterized by the reappearance of the normal tall surface epithelial cells with well-formed brush borders, a decline in the inflammation, a slow reformation of the villi, and persistence of the crypt hyperplasia until the villi are completely normal.[103] Because the histologic features are nonspecific in nature and can be seen in many other conditions, including peptic disease, infections, and allergic conditions, the diagnosis of celiac disease depends on the response to a gluten-free diet; in children, a gluten challenge is also often required after the patient is well to effectively exclude the other causes of enteritis.[104] It has recently been demonstrated that the effects of gluten can be seen in the rectal mucosa, and after dietary challenge this area may prove to be more readily accessible for biopsy.[105]

With the greater use of endoscopy, mucosal biopsy of the duodenum is being increasingly used as a screening test for celiac disease.[1,4] If the duodenal biopsy is normal or shows only minimal changes in a patient with suspected celiac disease, that disorder is effectively excluded because of the expected involvement of the duodenum in all active cases. Conversely, the finding of duodenal disease on biopsy, particularly if there is not complete villous loss, could be the result of the much more common disorder of peptic duodenitis; in such cases, a jejunal microsal biopsy is needed. See Chapter 29 for further details.

Allergic Disease

The proximal small intestine, including the duodenum, is one of the preferential sites for involvement by allergic disease.[106] The lesions may be isolated to the small intestine but are more often associated with disease affecting other parts of the upper tract, including the esophagus and the stomach.[107–109] A specific causative food substance such as milk[110,111] or soy[112,113] protein is identified in many of the patients with small-bowel disease, whereas other cases (called allergic or eosinophilic gastroenteritis) are related to multiple allergens.[109,114,115] Severe cases may be associated with prominent mucosal edema, which can be appreciated by radiographic and endoscopic examinations.[116] In most cases, however, the lesions are detected by microscopic study of the duodenum or jejunum, which reveals a variable shortening of the villi, together with a patchy infiltrate of eosinophils in the lamina propria and adjacent epithelium.[3,102–113,117] The inflammation may extend into the upper submucosa, but the deeper parts of the bowel wall are unaffected. Because the lesions are so focal, multiple biopsy samples of the duodenum and jejunum may be required for establishing the diagnosis.[118] In this regard, it has been observed that the gastric antrum is more constantly and severely involved, and biopsy samples of this region should also be obtained in cases of suspected allergic disease.[108] See Chapter 10 for further details.

Other Immune Disorders

The proximal small intestine is often involved in the various primary and acquired immunodeficiency diseases, leading to alterations of the mucosa.[46,66,119] Abnormalities that are identified in duodenal and jejunal mucosal biopsies include the appearance of a focal or diffuse enteritis, a variable reduction of plasma cells in the lamina propria, and the presence of opportunistic microorganisms. In transient hypogammaglobulinemia of infants, the mucosa is usually normal, but about one quarter of the cases show signs of an active or healing enteritis in mucosal biopsies.[120] The small-intestinal mucosa is one of the target tissues in graft-versus-host reactions, and the lesions observed range from a patchy enteritis[121] to extensive ulceration.[122] See Chapters 5, 14, and 29 for further details on the immune-mediated disorders.

Stress Ulcers of the Duodenum

This subject is covered in Chapter 21.

MISCELLANEOUS INFLAMMATORY DISORDERS OF THE SMALL INTESTINE

Ulcerative Jejunoileitis

Definition and Etiology. This is a rare condition of uncertain etiology, characterized by the appearance of multiple and persistent ulcers of the jejunum and ileum.[123-125] The disorder was originally delineated and separated from Crohn's disease by noting the absence of mural thickening and granulomas and that lesions did not develop in the colon. The existence of ulcerative jejunoileitis as a distinct entity has been subsequently questioned, however; it has been suggested that it may represent an uncommon complication of long-standing celiac disease and of cases of refractory sprue in which ulcers may develop.[126,127]

Clinical Features. The patients typically present with abdominal pain and fever, together with signs of malabsorption and hypoproteinemia, and the ulcers are often not fully appreciated until the time of surgical exploration. Medical therapy consists of corticosteroids and supportive measures, and the ulcerated lesions do not respond to a gluten-free diet. Furthermore, there is a tendency for the ulcers to extend deep into the wall, leading to intestinal perforations, requiring surgical resection, and high morbidity and mortality.

Pathology. The ulcers vary in size, are usually sharply demarcated, and are concentrated in the jejunum and proximal ileum. The intervening mucosa appears grossly intact, and there are no diffuse alterations of the bowel wall. The inflammatory reaction surrounding the ulcers is entirely nonspecific, and there are no granulomas or sinus tracts. In support of the notion that ulcerative jejunoileitis may simply be a complication of celiac disease, the mucosa of the nonulcerated areas frequently reveals some degree of villous shortening, crypt hyperplasia, and increased mononuclear inflammatory cells in the lamina propria.[126-128]

Differential Diagnosis. The disorder must be distinguished from other conditions that are associated with multiple small-intestinal ulcerations, mainly infections, by cultures, and Crohn's disease, by the presence of mural thickening, sinus tracts, granulomas, and colonic lesions. As noted previously, the separation of ulcerative jejunoileitis from the ulcerated phase of celiac disease[129] or of refractory sprue[97] is probably a moot point. In addition, the appearance of ulcers in a case of celiac disease may signal the development of the further complication of malignant lymphoma.[126-128] It may be exceedingly difficult to appreciate the tumor grossly because of the absence of a discrete mass, and mucosal biopsies may be too superficial to detect the tumor, which is usually concentrated in the intestinal wall and the mesentery. The diagnosis of lymphoma, which is often of the T-cell type,[130] may be accomplished occasionally by multiple mucosal biopsies but usually requires a full-thickness sample at operation. See Chapter 29 for further details.

Bypass Enteritis

Definition, Etiology, and Clinical Features. Bypass of long segments of the jejunum and of the ileum was formerly performed in patients with extreme obesity, and subsequent examinations of these excluded segments often revealed inflammatory changes in the mucosa.[131] Although the mucosal alterations have usually been mild and not associated with prominent clinical problems in the intestine, it is possible that drainage of toxic substances from the inflamed areas may have contributed to the portal tract lesions of the liver that were frequently noted in these patients.[132] Occasionally, a more pronounced degree of enteritis has been observed.[133] The mucosal inflammation seen in the excluded tissues is probably a consequence of stasis, but a specific microbiologic agent or other toxic substance has not been established. The intestinal lesions typically disappear when the bypass is eliminated and normal luminal flow is restored in the gut segment. A temporary bypass or diverting ileostomy may be performed for other inflammatory conditions of the small intestine to allow time for some healing and localization to occur prior to resection, and it is important to recognize, in all of these situations, that newly developed inflammatory charges may simply be the effect of stasis, rather than extension of the primary disease. Such information might prove important in determining the extent of any planned surgical resections or in decisions to restore intestinal continuity.

Pathology. The changes noted in the excluded intestinal segments are mainly limited to the mucosa and are of a nonspecific nature.[131,132] There often are an increased number of hypertrophied lymphoid nodules and an overall increase of mononuclear inflammatory cells in the lamina propria, which may result in a slight granularity of the mucosal surface. Changes of active enteritis are less frequent and range from focal areas of cryptitis and villous atrophy to overt erosions and ulcers.[133] Neutrophils predominate in the active lesions, and the presence of granulomas has only rarely been noted.[134] In some cases, particularly in those who have had a long-standing bypass for a chronic enteritis such as Crohn's disease, there may develop a marked contraction of the bowel, with the lumen narrowed to 1 to 2 cm in diameter; there is often an associated hypertrophy of the muscularis propria,[135] but this may reflect the underlying condition of chronic enteritis.

Enteritis Cystica Profunda

Definition, Etiology, and Clinical Features. This is an uncommon condition of the small intestine, characterized by the extension of mature or regenerative epithelium through the muscularis mucosae into the submucosa and occasionally the deeper parts of the bowel wall.[136,137] The lesion is seen most commonly in chronic inflammatory disorders such as Crohn's disease[138,139] and in association with the hamartomatous polyps of the Peutz-Jeghers syndrome.[140,141] It is thought to result from disruptions of the muscularis mucosae that permit the proliferating mucosal tissue to extend past the natural barrier into the underlying tissues. The clinical features are usually dominated by the underlying disease, and the enteritis cystica lesion is typically an incidental finding. Rarely, when the lesion is large, the features of an expanded or polypoid mucosa, together with presence of glands in the wall, may simulate a neoplasm; this can be an important consideration because the primary diseases are prone to the development of carcinomas. Similar lesions are observed in other parts of the gut and are named according to their specific location as gastritis cystica profunda and colitis cystica profunda.

Pathology. The lesions may rarely be isolated but are more often multiple and observed as a complication of a chronic inflammatory or polypoid condition. They vary in size and location, the majority detected in the ileum; and most are grossly obscured by the underlying disease. Larger lesions may reveal cystic spaces or a mucinous appearance of the wall and mimic a neoplastic mass but are readily distinguished by microscopic examination. There is an irregular proliferation of glands, many of which are cystic; and the lesion is usually limited to the submucosa. More pronounced cases show further extension of the glands into the muscularis propria and, rarely, to the serosa. The epithelium lining the glands and cystic spaces is usually completely mature, with small basal-oriented nuclei and abundant mucus-filled cytoplasm, or it may show the features of inflamed or regenerating cells. There is typically no inflammatory reaction around the misplaced glands, unless there is rupture of the cysts and extravasation of mucus, which may evoke a mild proliferation of macrophages. Mucinous carcinomas, in contrast, show some degree of atypism of the epithelial nuclei (in the form of elongated and pallisading nuclei, hyperchromasia, and pleomorphism) and often the presence of a loose connective tissue stroma (so-called tumor stroma) between the glands and the indigenous tissues. The appearance of the overlying mucosa reflects the primary disease, revealing inflammation and pseudopolyps in Crohn's disease and other chronic forms of enteritis or the characteristic features of the hamartomatous polyps.

Other Ulcers of Small Intestine

Multiple ulcers are seen in the major diffuse inflammatory conditions of the small intestine (see Table 28–1), including infections (see Chapter 26) and Crohn's disease (Chapter 27), and as a complication of some cases of celiac disease (Chapter 29). In addition, ulcers can occur as a result of radiation and chemical injuries (Chapter 9), stasis and mechanical obstruction (Chapter 11), vasculitis and ischemic disease (Chapter 12), graft-versus-host disease and other immunologic conditions (Chapter 14), and various systemic disorders (Chapter 16). In the Zollinger-Ellison syndrome, multiple ulcers are occasionally noted in the distal duodenum and proximal jejunum and are due to the sustained, marked elevations in gastric acid secretion (see Chapter 21). Ulcerated lesions of the ileum are also noted in many patients with the Behçet's syndrome, described below in the section on miscellaneous disorders of the colon.

Nonspecific Ulcers of the Small Intestine

Nonspecific ulcers of the small intestine include ulcers of unknown or uncertain cause that involve the jejunum and/or the ileum.[142-145] It is clearly a mixed group and includes cases with single or multiple lesions that may be acute or associated with fibrous stricture formation. The ulcers may affect either sex and all age groups, but there is a tendency for lesions of the jejunum to be more common in children and those of the ileum to occur in adult patients.[143] Overall, about three quarters of the cases involve the ileum, but deep ulcers and perforation are more frequent in the jejunum. The major presenting symptoms are those of intestinal obstruction, bleeding, and perforation; and surgery is often required for these complications and to establish the diagnosis. The pathologic features are nonspecific, revealing ulcers of variable size and depth, acute and chronic inflammatory cells, and the formation of prominent granulation tissue and fibrosis, which can extend deep into the wall and cause marked stenosis. There are no sinus tracts or granulomas, and the mucosa and bowel wall adjacent to or between the ulcers is typically normal. The diagnosis of a case of nonspecific ulcer(s) of the small intestine depends on the identification by radiographic study or operative findings of ulcerated or stenotic lesions and on the exclusion of all other possible causes. In particular, ulcers due to less common infections such as the Yersinia agents,[146,147] to drug effects (from enteric-coated potassium,[148-150] gold,[151,152] nonsteroid anti-inflammatory agents,[153] digitalis, and oral contraceptive pills),[77,154] and to ischemic lesions resulting from constricting fibrous bands in the serosa and adjacent mesentery[155] may often present without a clear history, and these conditions should be considered in the differential diagnosis.

MISCELLANEOUS INFLAMMATORY DISORDERS OF THE COLON

Microscopic (Lymphocytic) Colitis

Definition and Etiology. The term *microscopic colitis* was applied by Bo-Linn et al. in 1985 to a group of patients with recurrent secretory diarrhea of unknown etiology, in whom morphologic investigations revealed only histologic alterations that were limited to the colonic mucosa.[156] The condition was initially identified in patients with suspected Crohn's disease who lacked and did not develop the characteristic features of that disease after a long follow-up period.[157] Considering the disparity between the functional problem and the microscopic features, it is highly unlikely that the structural change is a cause of the diarrhea; rather, the histologic findings serve as a potential marker of the disease and also to exclude other causes of chronic inflammatory bowel disease. It is possible as well that the microscopic changes are a simple consequence of the diarrhea and potential colonic stagnation or that they represent a nonspecific response to a primary etiologic agent. The use of the term *microscopic colitis* is not ideal, because it is often employed as a descriptive phrase in other inflammatory conditions. Furthermore, it is not as yet established that microscopic colitis is a distinct entity, and it has been suggested that it may be a variant of collagenous colitis,[158] another condition characterized by secretory diarrhea and minimal histologic changes that are limited to the colonic mucosa (see the section on collagenous colitis for further details). A recent study of a larger series of cases noted the constant presence of an increased number of lymphocytes in the surface epithelial layer, and the term *lymphocytic colitis* was proposed as a preferred name for this condition.[159] The appearance of the increased intraepithelial lymphocytes is similar to that observed in chronic erosive (lymphocytic) gastritis (see Chapter 20) and in celiac disease (Chapter 29), but there is no established connection between these three disorders.

Clinical Features. This is a rare condition, and the described cases have been mainly in middle-aged and older women.[156,157] Unlike collagenous colitis, however, cases have been noted in men and in younger patients as well. All patients present with persistent, watery diarrhea, and functional studies have revealed reduced colonic absorption of water due to a decrease in the active and passive absorption of sodium and chloride.[157] Interestingly, a decrease in water absorption in the small intestine has also been noted in some cases, but this has been unassociated with any structural abnormalities in the jejunal mucosa. There are no radiographic or gross endoscopic alterations, and stool cultures are normal. Other investigators have noted the appearance of anemia, hypokalemia, and hypoproteinemia in cases referred to as microscopic colitis, but it is not at all clear whether these represent the same condition as that with watery diarrhea alone.[160] The diarrhea tends to persist, and some cases respond to antiinflammatory drugs with improvement of the symptoms and the colonic biopsy features.

Pathology. There are no gross alterations, and histologic examination of the small-intestinal mucosa is normal. Studies of mucosal biopsy specimens have shown a focal colitis characterized by the presence of neutrophils and increased mononuclear cells in the lamina propria in the absence of cryptitis.[156] The overlying surface epithelium may show signs of degeneration and increased intraepithelial lymphocytes, but there are no overt erosions or ulcers.[159] The inflammatory reaction is entirely nonspecific, and granulomas or a prominence of lymphoid nodules is not observed. The histologic features, even in patients with recurrent or chronic disease, resemble most a mild acute colitis, except for the presence of the increased mononuclear inflammatory cells in the surface layer. The more characteristic findings of chronic colitis,[161] such as complex branching or atrophy of the crypts, a villiform surface, and Paneth cell metaplasia, have not been described (see section on ulcerative colitis in Chapter 27 for further details).

Differential Diagnosis. The diagnosis of microscopic (lymphocytic) colitis depends on the exclusion of other causes of recurrent or chronic colitis and secretory diarrhea and on the finding of patchy inflammation that is restricted to the colonic mucosa. Mild cases of acute colitis due to infections, known toxic substances, vascular diseases, and immunologic disorders are separated by stool cultures, relevant clinical information, and the limited duration of the disease. A diffuse colitis and gross alterations are seen in ulcerative colitis; and Crohn's disease of the colon ultimately reveals ulceration, mural inflammation, and often granulomas. In cases in which the secretory diarrhea is the dominant or sole feature, other diagnostic considerations would include celiac disease, which is identified by the typical alterations in the small bowel mucosa and by the absence of colitis, and functional endocrine tumors, which lack structural alterations. Fully developed cases of collagenous colitis show a characteristic thickening of the basement membrane in the colonic mucosa and typically lack signs of acute inflammation and rectal bleeding.

Collagenous Colitis

Definition and Etiology. First described by Lindström in 1976,[162] collagenous colitis is an uncommon condition characterized by prolonged episodes of watery diarrhea and the presence of marked thickening of the basement membrane region beneath the surface epithelial cells of the colonic mucosa.[158,163–191] The cause of this disorder is not known, but it has been suggested that the collagenous band may interfere with the normal reabsorption of water by the colonic mucosa, resulting in the diarrhea.[162,172] Alternatively, both the diarrhea and the structural change may be the consequences of a common etiologic event. In studies of serial mucosal biopsies, there is a general correlation between the degree of the diarrhea and that of the thickened membrane but also the observation that the diarrhea may be the initial feature.[178] It is currently thought that one or more toxic substances, as yet not identified, can cause this condition and that the colonic mucosa reveals a patchy inflammation, together with the gradual development of the collagenous band.[158,190] As noted previously, it is also possible that some cases of the condition referred to as microscopic colitis[156] may be variants of collagenous colitis. There are rare cases of collagenous colitis in which there are abnormalities of other tissues, including atrophy of the small-intestinal mucosa[192,193] and pulmonary fibrosis,[194] but it is not clear whether this association is real or simply coincidental.

Clinical Features. The exact incidence of collagenous colitis is not known, but it has been noted recently with increasing frequency.[172] The disorder ap-

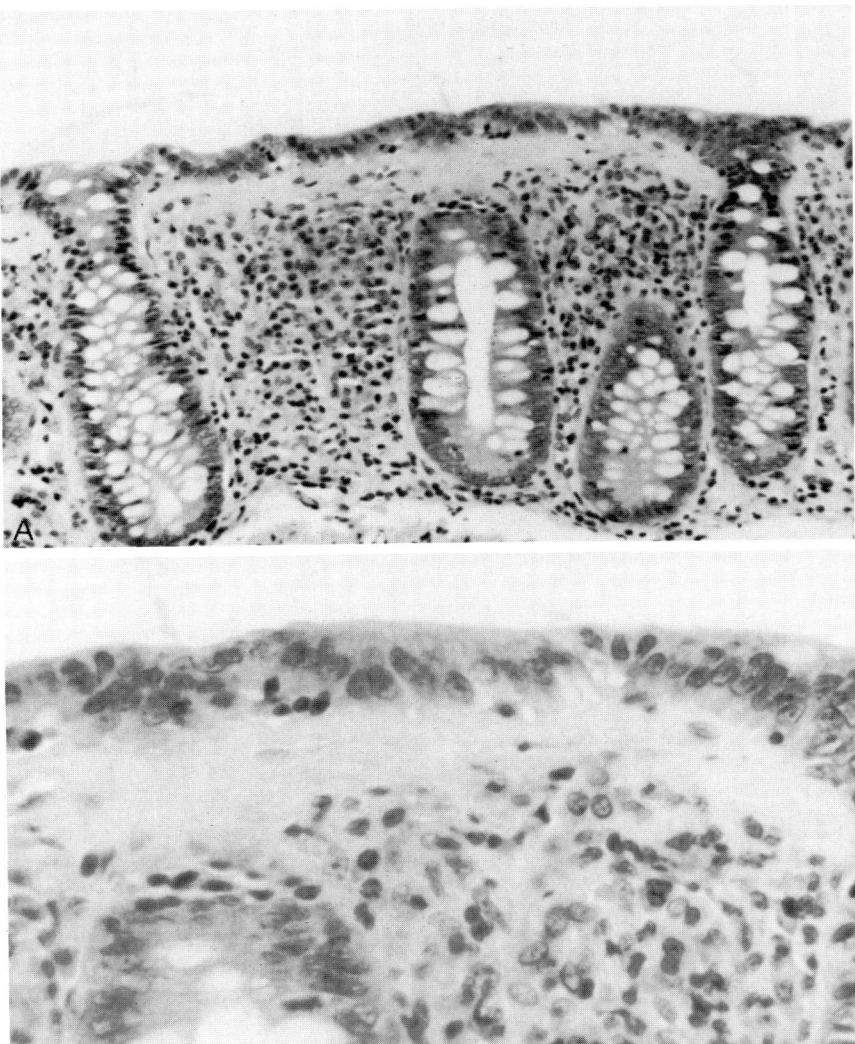

FIGURE 28-6. *A,* Colonic mucosa in collagenous colitis. There is a marked thickening of the collagen layer that is limited to the region just beneath the surface epithelium. The crypts are normal. (H&E, × 100) *B,* Colonic mucosa in collagenous colitis. Closer view of tissue seen in *A,* showing a thickened collagen layer and increased mononuclear inflammatory cells in the surface epithelial layer. (H&E, × 400)

pears to occur exclusively in middle-aged and older women, and patients usually are first seen with the gradual onset of watery diarrhea and abdominal crampy pain. The diarrhea often progresses or remits and recurs[181,186] and has a variable duration of up to several years, but it eventually subsides in most cases.[168,175] Radiographic and stool culture examinations are normal, and the diagnosis has been often overlooked in the past because the colonic mucosa appears normal at endoscopic study and biopsy has not been obtained. The patients have frequently been given a diagnosis of irritable bowel syndrome or psychosomatic illness and are often relieved once the diagnosis of collagenous colitis has been established by colonic mucosal biopsy.

Pathology. There are no gross abnormalities, and the histologic lesion is limited to the mucosa of the large intestine; the abnormality is more commonly noted and usually more severe in the colon than in the rectum.[187,190,191] In the fully developed lesion, there is marked thickening of the basement membrane region by collagen deposition, ranging from 15 to 65 μm in width, immediately beneath the surface epithelial cells (Figure 28-6). In contrast, the thickness of the basement membrane in the colonic mucosa of normal persons is typically less than 5 to 6 μm.[195] The lesion at this stage is usually diffuse within the biopsy and easily appreciated by H&E staining, and it can be accentuated by the use of trichrome stains for connective tissues. Ultrastructural studies have demonstrated that the basement lamina of the epithelial cells is of normal dimension and appearance and that the thickening is due solely to the deposition of mature type I and type III collagens in the subjacent tissue.[169,176] Amyloid stains are negative, and no other proteins including immune complexes have been identified by immunocytochemical stains in the abnormal area. The thickened band is limited to the surface area and does not extend down to involve the basement membrane region of the underlying crypts. Other histologic features in cases of collagenous colitis include a patchy increase of mononuclear inflammatory cells in the superficial part of the lamina propria and in the surface epithelial layer[185,190]; less commonly observed are tiny foci of epithelial de-

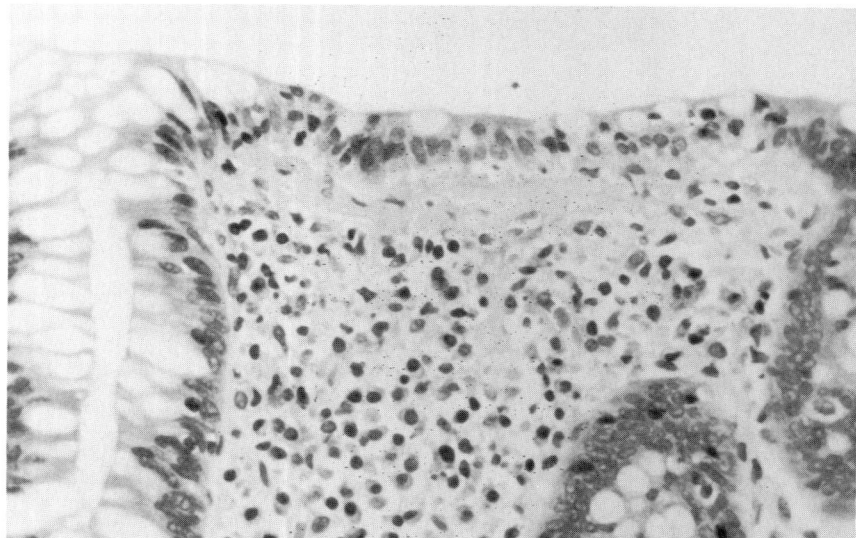

FIGURE 28–7. Colonic mucosa in an earlier case of collagenous colitis. The thickened collagen band beneath the surface epithelium is less prominent and more patchy in distribution. (H&E, × 250)

generation and small numbers of neutrophils. There are no granulomas or other signs of chronic colitis, such as complex branching and atrophy of the crypts, a villiform surface, or Paneth cell metaplasia.[161]

Serial biopsy examinations have been performed in some patients in whom the classic lesion of collagenous colitis eventually developed, and these have permitted a delineation of the earlier phases of the lesion.[178] The earliest biopsies, obtained only days or a few weeks after the onset of the symptoms, are often nonspecific, revealing only patchy areas of increased inflammation and occasional surface erosion but no collagen deposition. Samples taken even after several weeks of disease may show variable persistence of the inflammation and a definite but focal and usually slight collagen increase in the superficial basement membrane area (Figure 28–7). At this stage, the diagnosis of collagenous colitis can be suspected but not made with certainty, because equivalent degrees of collagen deposition can be seen in other forms of colitis, notably in radiation damage, ischemic disease, ulcerative colitis, and Crohn's disease.[191,195–197] The final and diagnostic biopsies contain the fully developed and diffuse lesions. Recovery from the condition is associated with elimination of the collagenous band and return of the mucosa to a completely normal appearance, but the condition may recur.[190]

Differential Diagnosis. The diagnosis of collagenous colitis is established by finding the characteristic lesion in the mucosa of a patient with a purely secretory form of diarrhea. It should be remembered that the lesion may be less obvious or absent in the rectum, and therefore, biopsies should be obtained from the colon if the disease is suspected. Patients with acute and chronic colitis, including infections and the idiopathic forms of ulcerative colitis and Crohn's disease of the colon, are typically first seen with purulent and bloody diarrhea and reveal ulcerations or other gross abnormalities of the colon. A patchy thickening of the basement membrane by collagen beneath the surface epithelial cells is occasionally seen in cases of ischemic, radiation-induced, and ulcerative colitis, but the collagen band is usually less than 10 μm in thickness, and the distinction from collagenous colitis is apparent from the presence of other features.[191,195] It is of interest that the identical collagenous thickening of the surface basement membrane is noted in many cases of hyperplastic (or metaplastic) polyps of the colon.[176] This should cause no confusion with the diagnosis of collagenous colitis, because the clinical setting is entirely different, but the presence of the fibrous band may help in identifying the particular type of polyp when the lesion is small and tangentially sectioned.

Other disorders that may be manifested by a secretory diarrhea include celiac disease and Crohn's disease of the small intestine, which are readily distinguished by lesions in that area of the gut, and functional endocrine tumors, which show no structural changes. Cases of so-called microscopic (lymphocytic) colitis may present with prominent watery diarrhea, but they often have other signs of an active colitis such as bleeding and foci of acute inflammation in the mucosa and lack the collagenous band.[156] As noted above, however, there is still the possibility that microscopic colitis and collagenous colitis might be variants of the same disorder or syndrome.[190] Probably the biggest problem in the diagnosis of collagenous colitis has been the failure to consider the possibility in an otherwise healthy patient who complains simply of watery diarrhea. Since there are no gross abnormalities evident upon radiographic and endoscopic examinations, the diagnosis can be secured only by biopsy of the colon, preferably above the rectal area.

Diversion-Related Colitis

Definition and Etiology. After a diverting ileostomy or colostomy, inflammatory changes of a nonspecific nature occasionally appear in the mucosa of the ex-

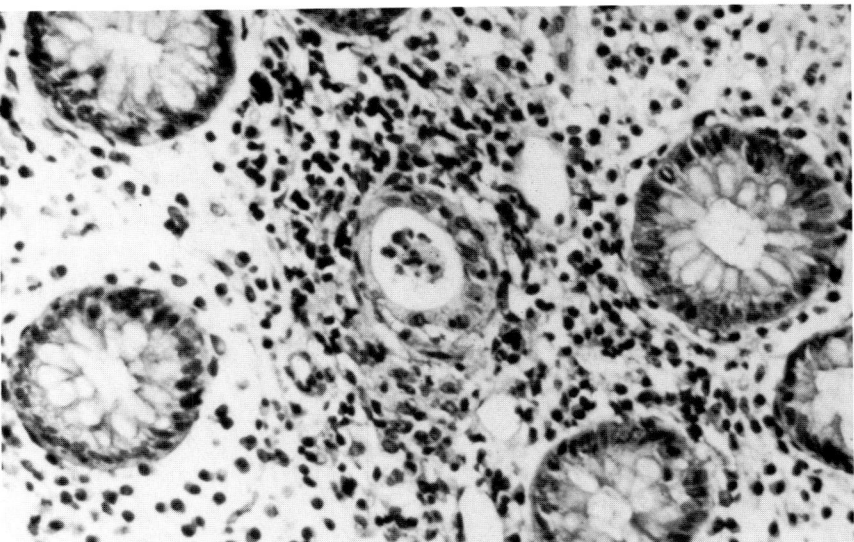

FIGURE 28-8. Rectal mucosa in a case of diversion-related colitis. There is a focal crypt abscess (center) in otherwise normal mucosa. (H&E, × 400)

cluded colonic segment that is distal to the stoma.[198-207] The gross features observed at endoscopy may mimic a mild case of ulcerative colitis, but the condition also occurs in patients without an antecedent history of inflammatory bowel disease, and lesions are not observed in the gut proximal to the stoma. Furthermore, the inflammatory changes completely resolve after intestinal continuity is restored. It is thought that the disorder results from the effects of stagnation in the excluded segment, but a specific microbiologic agent or another toxic substance has not been identified.

Clinical Features. There have been no detailed prospective studies of this disorder, and its frequency and time of onset after the diverting procedure are not known. It has been observed following ileostomy or, more often, colostomy at all sites for various conditions, including diverticular disease, motor disturbances, drug reactions, antibiotic-associated colitis, and Crohn's disease.[198,199,207] Most patients are asymptomatic, and the lesion is only detected at time of endoscopy that might be performed in advance of a planned reanastomosis of the intestine. In some patients, particularly in cases with a long duration, a mucous discharge, diarrhea, and rectal bleeding develop.[199-207] Amelioration of symptoms and histologic improvement have been observed after rectal irrigation with short-chain fatty acids.[205] The condition can persist for many months to years and does not appear to resolve completely until the intestine is reconnected, permitting normal fecal flow. In the past, finding of such inflammatory changes has resulted in delays in reanastomosis or even in resection of involved areas because of uncertainty in the diagnosis or significance of the lesion.[198,204] This is of particular importance in patients with known Crohn's disease who have had a temporary diverting procedure, and the dilemma arises as to whether the mucosal changes in the excluded segment are related to the surgery or represent evidence of persistent or recurrent Crohn's disease.[199] Since the lesions due to diversion are typically most prominent in the rectum, at stake is the decision to connect the bowel to the inflamed area or to resect the rectum and leave the patient with a permanent enterostomy. In the absence of certain signs of Crohn's disease such as granulomatous inflammation and sinus tracts in the rectum of such cases, it is probably worthwhile to explain the situation to the patient and to perform an anastomotic procedure. Ultimately, the determination of whether a patient had diversion-related colitis rests on its complete resolution following elimination of the stoma and reconnection of the intestine.

Pathology. The lesions are limited to the mucosal layer and are often confined to or most severe in the distal colon and rectum.[198] The gross appearance, as observed at endoscopic examination, typically reveals some combination of erythema, granularity, and mild friability, and discrete ulcers of the aphthous type have been noted in the more prolonged cases.[200,206,207] The changes may be very similar to those seen in idiopathic inflammatory bowel disease, but the distinction can be readily made by microscopic study of mucosal biopsy specimens. Since the lesions are often patchy, the mucosa may be completely normal or show only a prominence of lymphoid nodules. Signs of active colitis or proctitis are observed in most cases and include the focal presence of acute cryptitis and degeneration of surface epithelial cells with neutrophils in the adjacent lamina propria (Figures 28-8 and 28-9). The ulcers that sometimes develop have a nonspecific inflammatory reaction. There may also be regenerative signs in the crypts and foci of mononuclear inflammatory cells, and rarely observed are features of chronic colitis such as branching or atrophy of the crypts.[206,207] Loose granulomas of the foreign body type may uncommonly be found in the anorectal region in long-standing cases. The inflammatory changes appear to be restricted to the mucosa, and the deeper parts of the bowel wall are uninvolved. In particular, submucosal fibrosis and mural sinus tracts have not been observed. After reanastomosis and recovery from the condition, the mucosa

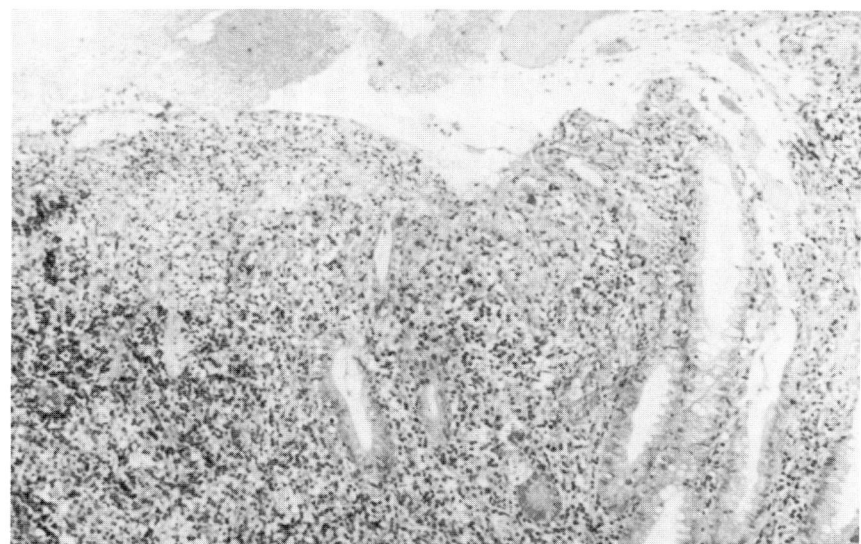

FIGURE 28–9. Rectal mucosa in diversion-related colitis, showing a more advanced lesion, characterized by superficial ulceration and greater inflammation. (H&E, × 100)

reverts to normal, and there are no sequelae seen in biopsy samples.

Differential Diagnosis. The diagnosis of diversion-related colitis is tentatively suspected by the finding of nonspecific, mild inflammatory changes in the mucosa of an excluded colonic and rectal segment and secured by reversion of the mucosa to normal after intestinal continuity is restored. The differential diagnosis includes consideration of any of the several conditions that may complicate a surgical procedure. Ordinary infections are excluded by stool cultures and ischemic disease by the absence of the typical features of hemorrhagic necrosis and extensive ulceration; furthermore, ischemic lesions are much less common in the rectum and tend not to persist at such a mild level of injury. Antibiotic-associated colitis is characterized by the frequent presence of small pseudomembranes on the mucosal surface and by the positive assay for *Clostridium difficile* in the stool.[208] In ulcerative colitis, there is usually a prior history of the disease, and the lesions are invariably diffuse and frequently associated with histologic features of chronic colitis. As noted previously in the section on the clinical course, the distinction between diversion colitis and extension of Crohn's disease in a patient with overt gross lesions in the ileum or proximal colon may be a particular challenge, since both conditions may reveal microscopic patches of inflammation and aphthous ulcers. In such cases, the definite diagnosis of Crohn's disease affecting the distal colon and rectum would require the finding of characteristic features such as prominent submucosal fibrosis, sinus tracts, transmural inflammation, or granulomas, except those of the foreign body type.

Acute Self-Limited Colitis

Acute self-limited colitis is not a specific disease entity, but, rather, a descriptive term that is applied to cases of acute colitis and proctitis that ultimately recover and leave no traces of injury in the mucosa.[161,209–211] Although an infectious agent or toxic substance is often identified, the particular course is not established in about one quarter to one third of the cases. The major importance of this category, particularly of those without an apparent etiology, is in the distinction from early or acute cases of idiopathic inflammatory bowel disease. Both groups may have an abrupt onset of colitis and identical radiographic and gross endoscopic appearances. Mucosal biopsy can be of considerable assistance in sorting out these disorders. Changes of chronic colitis are frequently seen in cases of ulcerative colitis and Crohn's disease, and include an altered architecture by complex branching and atrophy of the crypts, a villiform surface, Paneth cell metaplasia, a marked increase of mononuclear inflammatory cells in the lamina propria, and the interposition of numerous plasma cells and small lymphoid nodules between the crypt bases and the muscularis mucosae. In contrast, none of these histologic features is observed in cases of acute self-limited colitis. In the acute stage, there is evidence of cryptitis and a marked infiltrate of neutrophils, which are concentrated in the superficial half of the mucosa; but the crypts remain relatively straight, and there is no prominence of mononuclear inflammatory cells. Upon recovery, there is complete restoration of the mucosa to normal in cases of acute self-limited colitis, whereas the changes of chronic colitis persist in the great majority of cases of ulcerative colitis.

Colitis Cystica Profunda

Definition and Etiology. Colitis cystica profunda is a condition in which mature colonic epithelium extends through the muscularis mucosae into the submucosa or deeper parts of the intestinal wall.[212–215] It is most commonly observed as an isolated lesion in the late stages of the solitary rectal ulcer syndrome, which is described subsequently in a separate section. Multiple small lesions are less often seen as a consequence of a chronic inflammatory condition of the colon such as ulcerative colitis,[216] Crohn's disease,[217] radiation colitis,[218] and colonic schistosomiasis; rare cases have been observed in an apparently normal colon.[219,220] In these inflammatory disorders, it is believed that the colitis cystica forms as a result of an ulceration with destruction of the muscularis mucosae and subsequent regeneration of the mucosal glands that extend through the gap into the underlying tissues of the bowel wall. When one considers the high frequency of ulceration in such disorders, however, it is not clear why colitis cystica is not more commonly seen, which suggests that additional factors may be involved in its genesis. Equivalent lesions are seen in the stomach and small intestine and referred to respectively as gastritis cystica profunda and enteritis cystica profunda.

Clinical Features. Colitis cystica is usually a small and incidental histologic finding, and the clinical course is determined by the underlying inflammatory disease. Occasionally, there may be a larger lesion associated with a polypoid mucosa or deep extension into the wall, and the appearance may grossly resemble a tumor.[220] This circumstance takes on special significance because the underlying inflammatory conditions are particularly prone to the development of adenocarcinomas.

Pathology. Gross alterations may be observed in the larger lesions and include a raised or polypoid mucosa and a mucinous appearance of the wall. The histologic features are distinctive and reveal the presence of cystically dilated colonic glands within the submucosa and occasionally into the deeper parts of the intestinal wall. The epithelial cells lining the glands are usually normal or hyperplastic, containing basal nuclei and abundant cytoplasm, or they may show signs of regeneration. There is no dysplasia of the epithelium, and inflammatory reaction around the misplaced glands is usually minimal or absent.

Differential Diagnosis. The diagnosis of colitis cystica profunda is based on the finding of colonic glands with mature or regenerative epithelium beneath the mucosal layer. In the normal colonic mucosa, there are numerous lymphoid follicles, which frequently extend into the uppermost portion of the submucosa. The muscularis mucosae is interrupted at these points, and small portions of the crypt bases are often present in the superficial submucosa in such areas. This appearance may cause some difficulty, particularly in tangential or peripheral microscopic sections that do not reveal the complete lymphoid follicle; but it can be readily separated from colitis cystica by knowing of its existence and by noting that the glands are collapsed, rather than cystic, and that they are invariably associated with lymphoid tissue. It is most important that one make the distinction between colitis cystica and adenocarcinoma, which can also develop as a complication of chronic colitis. In this regard, well-differentiated or mucinous carcinomas are often encountered in these inflammatory diseases. The diagnosis of carcinoma is dependent on finding some degree of dysplasia of the epithelial cells and on the frequent presence of inflammation and a loose stroma between the neoplastic glands and the normal tissues. Some cases of hyperplastic polyps[221] and adenomas[222] of the colon reveal misplacement of the glands into the submucosa, but these lesions can be easily recognized by noting the characteristic features of the mucosal component and the epithelium.

Solitary Rectal Ulcer Syndrome

Definition and Etiology. Solitary rectal ulcer syndrome is characterized by the presence of ulcers or polypoid inflammatory lesions in the rectum and is often associated with mucosal prolapse.[223-237] It is thought to be due to a malfunction of the internal anal sphincter or of the overall rectal musculature, resulting in chronic straining upon defecation and the development of rectal prolapse and mucosal erosions.[229,230,237-239] After repeated episodes, there is often exuberant repair, leading to the formation of a polyp and to the extension of glands into the submucosa. The term *syndrome* has been applied to this condition, because the initial ulcerative phase may be either not identified or associated with multiple lesions. If one considers the variability of the early features and of the manometric studies as well as the frequent dominance of the polypoid stage, it has also been suggested that the condition might be due to a hamartomatous process.[225] Other names that have been proffered to describe the various features include *localized colitis* (or *proctitis*) *cystica profunda* in cases with submucosal involvement,[223,235] *inflammatory cloacogenic polyp* in those with a prominent mass,[238,240] and *mucosal prolapse syndrome*[234] to depict the full range of changes associated with rectal prolapse.

Clinical Features. Although the solitary rectal ulcer syndrome was once considered to be rare, it is now being encountered with increased frequency, and it is probable that the condition was greatly overlooked in the past.[236] In this regard, the clinical diagnosis is often delayed and is suspected in only about one third of the cases; its initial recognition is usually provided by morphologic study. The lesion is more common in women, and the peak incidence is in the third and fourth decades. Major symptoms include straining on defecation, constipation, anorectal or abdominal pain, rectal bleeding, and a mucous discharge.[233,239,241] Rectal prolapse is identified in about 80% of the cases, and recognition of the mucosal lesions often requires that the patient strain down at time of proctoscopic examination.[230,234] There is no definitive medical therapy, and attempts of local surgical resection are usually not successful.[233] The disorder typically persists or recurs, and only a minority of cases completely resolve. Treatment is typically limited to the use of laxatives and the assurance to the patient that a more serious condition is not present.

Pathology. About 85% of the lesions are noted on the anterior wall of the rectum, and they are located up to 18 cm above the anal verge, most occurring in the distal 3 to 5 cm.[229,233,236] The early lesion is typically a single small and shallow ulcer, up to a centimeter in

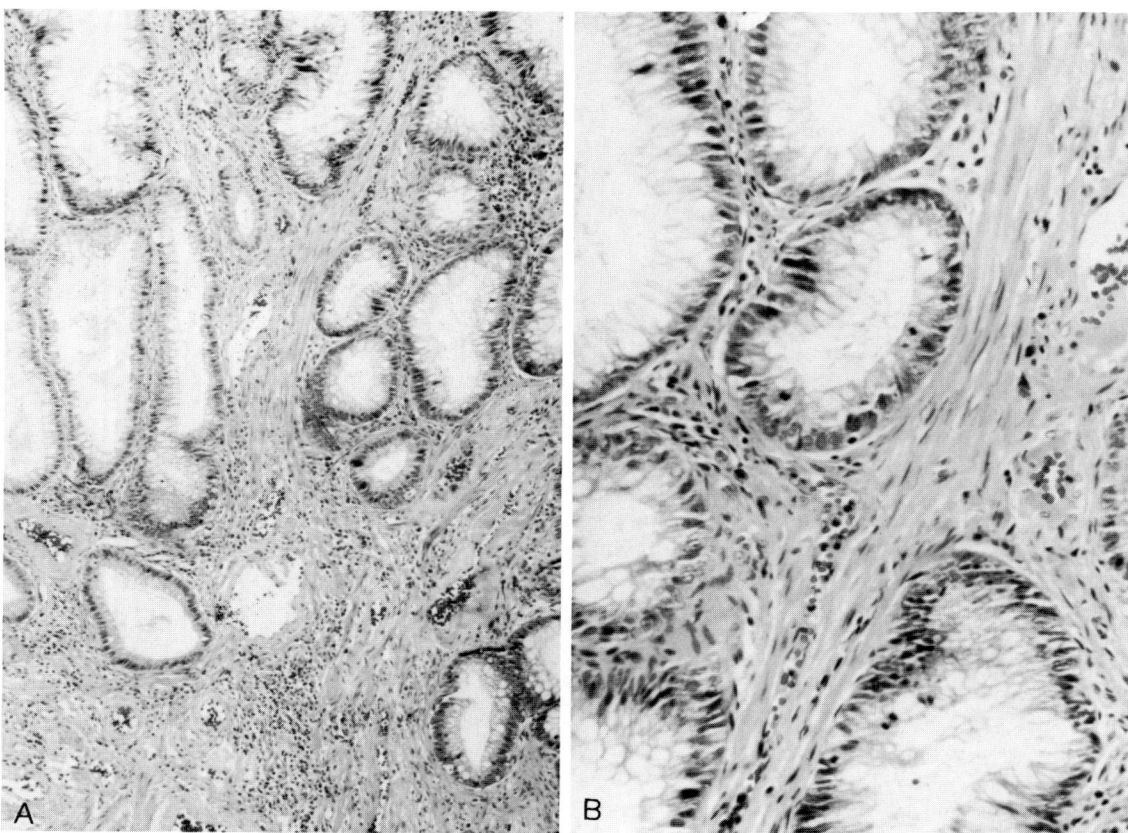

FIGURE 28-10. *A*, Rectal mucosa in solitary ulcer syndrome. Section of mucosa next to an ulcer, showing the prominent fibromuscular stroma and the serrated appearance of the glands. (H&E, × 100) *B*, Rectal mucosa in solitary ulcer syndrome. Closer view of the mucosa in *A*, revealing fibromuscular hyperplasia in the lamina propria. (H&E, × 400)

diameter, that is relatively well demarcated and often associated with erythema and slight elevation of the adjacent mucosa. Larger ulcers of up to 6 cm have been uncommonly observed. Multiple ulcers are infrequently seen, whereas the initial ulcerated lesion may be absent in about one third of the cases,[241] possibly because the patient is not evaluated during the early stage of the disease. Histologic examination reveals necrosis that is often limited to the superficial half of the mucosa, together with acute inflammation and often prominent hemorrhage in the adjacent mucosa. In addition, there is a characteristic fibromuscular hyperplasia in the lamina propria, which is best visualized by examination of the adjacent nonulcerated mucosa. Accordingly, biopsy samples should be selected from the edges of the ulcer to permit its detection.

The older lesions are associated with the development of a polypoid mass in the majority of the cases. The polyps vary in size, ranging up to 3 or 4 cm in diameter, are typically sessile, and have either a smooth surface or a papillary contour resembling an adenoma. There may be patches of superficial necrosis, but there is usually no discrete ulceration at this stage. The polyps are composed of regenerating glands with variable reduction of mucus and a faint serrated appearance, similar to that seen in hyperplastic polyps, and they are distinguished by the presence of a marked fibromuscular proliferation in the lamina propria[242] (Figure 28-10). The larger polyps are often associated with a villiform surface (Figure 28-11) and occasionally reveal focal loss of the muscularis mucosae and extension of cystic colonic glands into the submucosa (Figure 28-12), representing a localized form of colitis cystica profunda.[223,226] There is no dysplasia of the epithelium, and the misplaced glands are not associated with any inflammation or newly formed stroma (Figure 28-13). Other features of mucosal prolapse may be observed in the adjacent mucosa, including foci of hemorrhagic necrosis and patchy inflammation.[234] The submucosal ganglia and nerves appear to be normal, and there are no abnormalities of the muscularis propria.

Differential Diagnosis. The diagnosis of the solitary rectal ulcer syndrome depends on the findings of the characteristic fibromuscular hyperplasia in the lamina propria at the edge of an ulcer or in a polyp and of the absence of any epithelial dysplasia. Rectal ulcers may be seen in many other common inflammatory conditions, including infections, ischemic injury, ulcerative colitis, and Crohn's disease. However, the lesions in these disorders are more often multiple or diffuse, and diarrhea is a prominent feature. Localized ulcers can also occur as a result of stasis, pressure necrosis from a stercoraceous lesion and various generalized diseases, and they are separated by the nonspecific nature of the

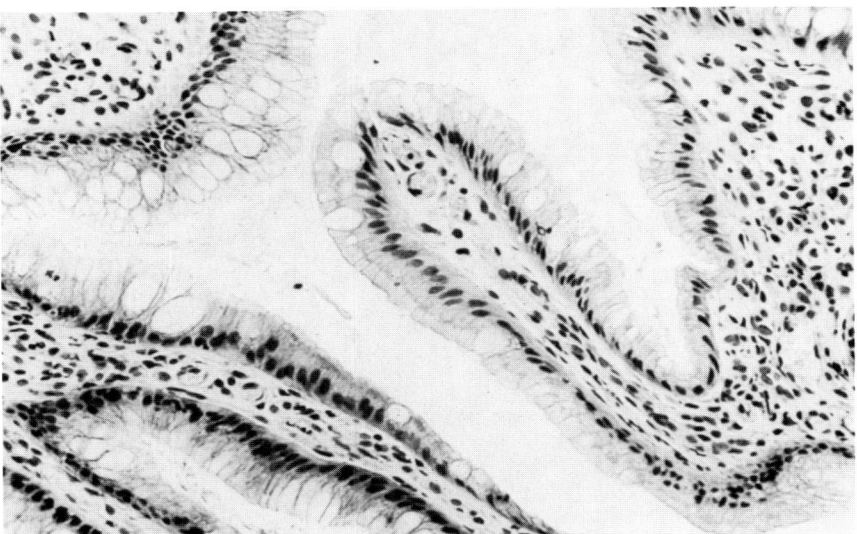

FIGURE 28–11. Rectal polyp in an advanced case of solitary ulcer syndrome. The surface has a prominent villous configuration, but there is no nuclear atypicality. (H&E, × 400)

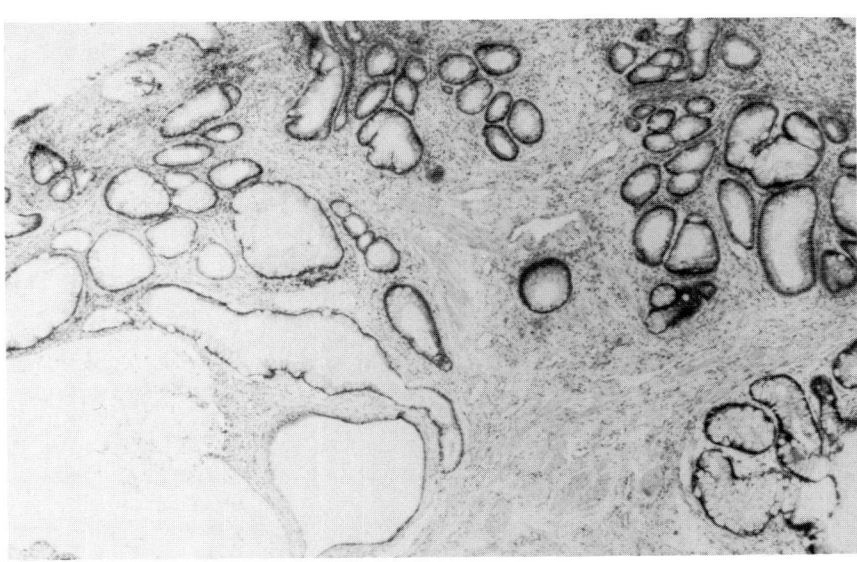

FIGURE 28–12. Rectal polyp in solitary ulcer syndrome. The glands are irregular and extend into the submucosa (lower left), representing a localized form of colitis cystica profunda. (H&E, × 60)

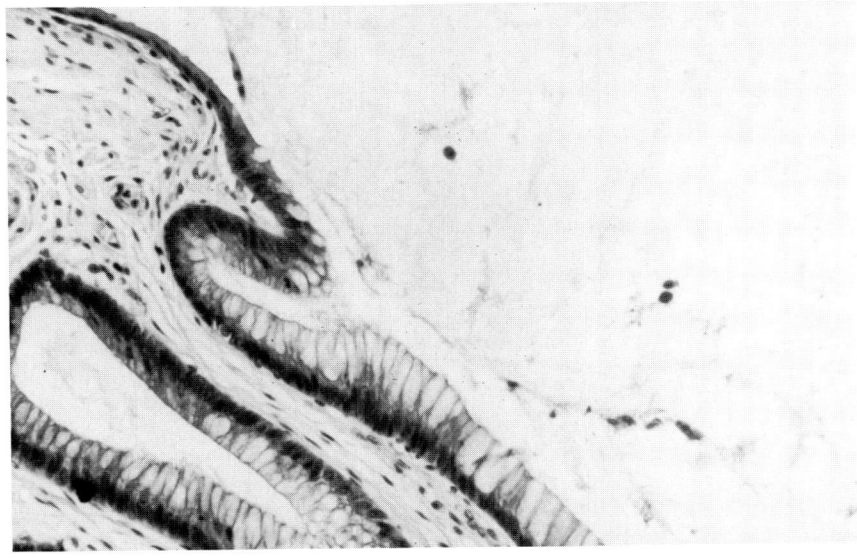

FIGURE 28–13. Rectal polyp in solitary ulcer syndrome. Section of submucosa, revealing the misplaced glands with mature cells. There is no cellular atypicality. (H&E, × 400)

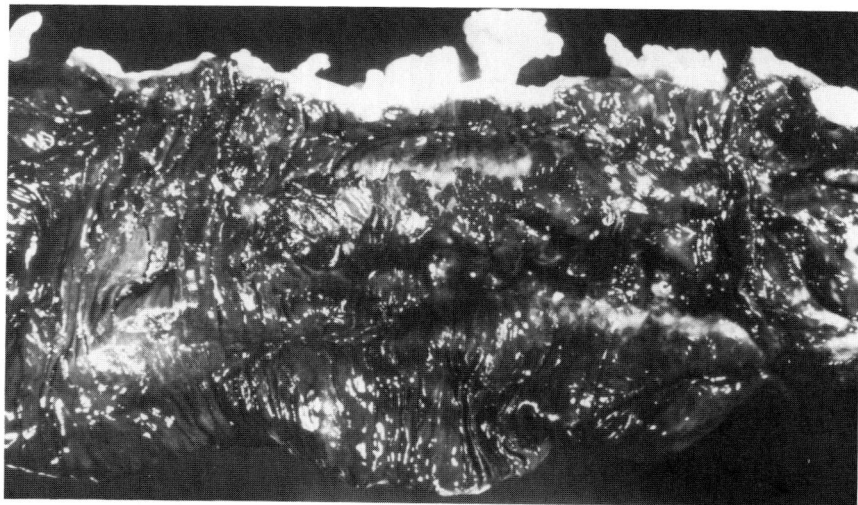

FIGURE 28–14. Melanosis coli. Mucosal surface of colon, showing the dark brown color. The haustral folds are intact, and the mucosa is otherwise normal.

histologic features or by the clinical information. It is most important that distinction be made between the lesions in the later stages and other polyps and adenocarcinoma of the rectum. It may be very difficult to separate the polyps of the solitary ulcer syndrome from inflammatory polyps and the juvenile type of polyps on the basis of the histologic features alone, and one must rely on the clinical findings in such cases. Hyperplastic polyps are typically small and barely raised; and they lack necrosis, inflammation, and the fibromuscular proliferation in the lamina propria. Adenomas, with or without misplaced epithelium, and carcinomas are readily distinguished by the presence of dysplasia of the epithelium; furthermore, there is often prominent inflammation and a loose connective tissue stroma around the submucosal glands in cases of invasive carcinoma.

Effects of Laxatives and Enemas

Melanosis Coli

Melanosis coli is a common asymptomatic condition that is characterized by the prominent presence of a pigment of the lipofuscin type in the macrophages of the lamina propria of the large bowel.[243–247] Because the pigment is not melanin, it has been suggested that the condition might be termed instead *pseudomelanosis coli*. It is thought to be due mainly to the continued use of anthracene-containing laxatives, which include cascara sagrada, senna, aloe, rhubarb, and frangula. The condition is more commonly noted in adult females, which may simply reflect the rate of laxative usage. Estimates of its frequency range from 5% in endoscopic studies to 10% in autopsy surveys, and it has been determined that it takes from 4 to 12 months for the lesion to appear on gross examination and an equivalent time for its regression after the cessation of laxative use. There are no clinical problems that are directly related to the pigment deposition. The lesion involves all parts of the rectum, colon, and appendix but tends to spare the regions of the mucosa occupied by lymphoid nodules, polyps, and carcinomas. When the deposition is very marked, the mucosa may be dark brown on gross examination (Figure 28–14); this appearance must be distinguished from that of old hemorrhages and necrosis, which would show a loss of the normal mucosal luster. Histologic study reveals that the brown, finely granular pigment is within the macrophages (Figure 28–15) and that it has the tinctorial characteristics of a lipofuscin, based on positive staining with fat stains and the PAS reaction. Similar pigment deposition may be seen in various storage diseases and in chronic granulomatous disease (see Chapter 16), but the macrophages in these disorders tend to be larger and arranged in clusters or nodules. The storage diseases also show pigment in other mesenchymal cells and in nerves. Scattered macrophages containing lesser amounts of lipofuscin are occasionally seen in the mucosa of normal persons, and the distinction from melanosis coli is a matter of degree.[248]

Patches of pseudomelanin deposition have also been noted in the duodenal mucosa at endoscopic examination,[249–253] particularly in patients with chronic renal failure.[254] The pigment appears to be an iron derivative and may be due to episodes of mucosal hemorrhage in these patients.[255] There does not appear to be any relationship to laxative use or to the colonic condition.

Cathartic Colon

Cathartic colon is an uncommon disorder that can result from the extensive and long-term use of laxatives, leading to the development of a dilated and hypotonic colon.[256,257] It is more common in women and usually requires over 15 years of laxative use before its formation. The laxatives employed have been of all sorts, including anthracene compounds, resins, and irritant oils. The patients typically present with chronic constipation and abdominal pain, and there are no signs of fever, diarrhea, or bleeding. It is thought that the cause is a toxic effect on the nerves and plexuses leading to secondary muscle damage in the bowel

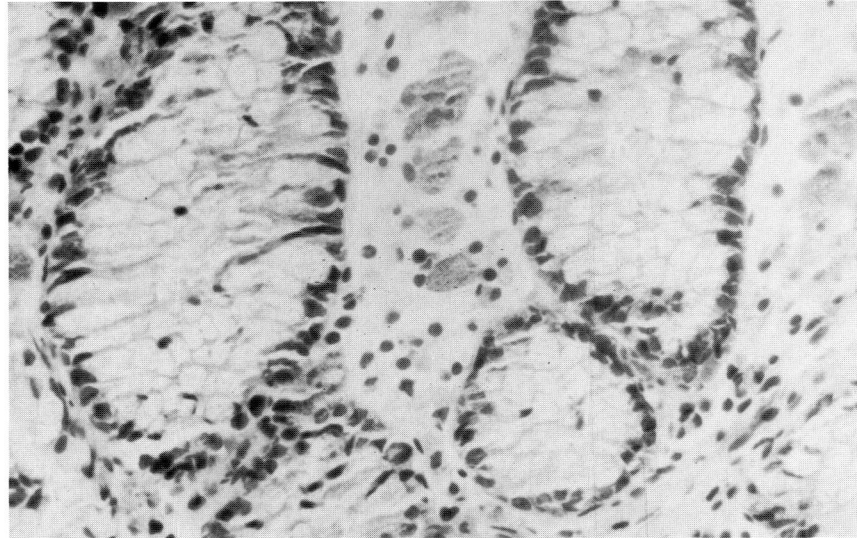

FIGURE 28-15. Colonic mucosa in melanosis coli. There are clumps of macrophages in the lamina propria, containing the finely granular and refractile lipofuscin material. The crypts are normal, and there is no increase of other inflammatory cells. (H&E, × 400)

wall.[258] The effects typically begin in the region of the ileocecal valve and right colon and progress with time to the distal portion, showing a dilated and tubular bowel with loss of the haustral markings and a dried-out mucosal surface.[259,260] Histologic features include the variable presence of mucosal and crypt atrophy, a thickening of the muscularis mucosae, and a vacuolization of the ganglion cells. Melanosis coli may also be present but is an independent effect of some of the laxatives. The cathartic colon must be distinguished from other causes of colonic dilatation such as pseudo-obstruction disorders,[261] and this distinction is accomplished by the history and the lack of lesions in other parts of the gut (see Chapter 11).

Laxative Abuse Syndrome

The laxative abuse syndrome is due to the excessive and surreptitious use of laxatives, leading to the appearance of unexplained chronic diarrhea and loss of protein and potassium.[262,263] It must be suspected when thorough gross and microscopic evaluation of the intestines fails to reveal any pathologic lesions.

Effects of Enemas

Saline enemas and other mild solutions used in the preparation of patients for colonoscopy often cause an edema of the lamina propria but no damage to the epithelium.[5,264-266] More prominent alterations are commonly noted with enemas containing Fleet Phospho-Soda solution, biscadyl, hydrogen peroxide, and other hypertonic solutions[266-269]; the changes noted include a flattening and sloughing of the surface epithelium, a decrease in the staining of the upper crypt epithelial cells, a depletion of the goblet cell mucus, and the occasional presence of neutrophils in the lamina propria (Figure 28-16). There are usually no symptoms from

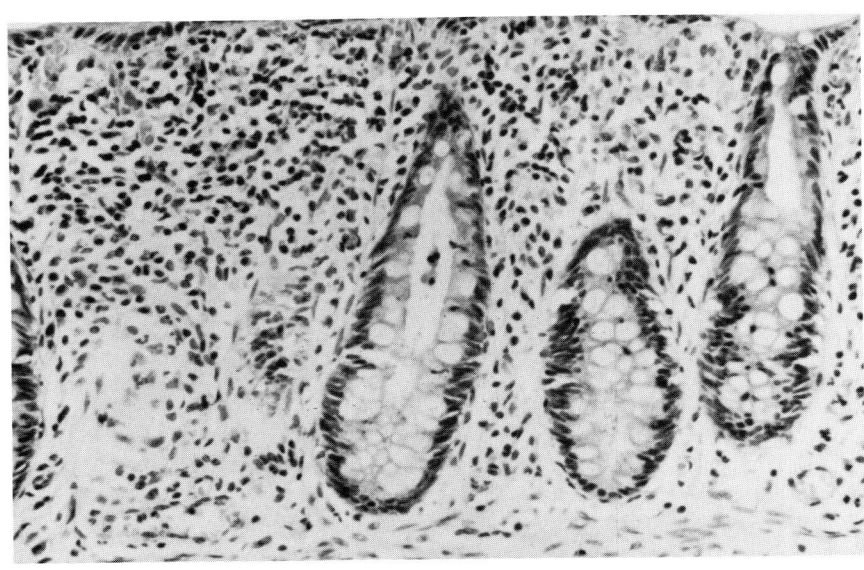

FIGURE 28-16. Rectal mucosa in a mild case of enema-induced colitis. There is a flattening of the surface epithelium, a slight pallor of the superficial mucosa, and the presence of rare neutrophils. (H&E, × 100) (From Goldman H, Antonioli DA: Mucosal biopsy of the rectum, colon, and distal ileum. Hum Pathol 13:981-1012, 1982.)

these enemas, but the histologic features may resemble those seen in a mild case of acute colitis or proctitis and must be discounted in the assessment of a mucosal biopsy. The enema changes typically resolve within a week. A much more severe form of colitis has been observed with enemas using a soap solution, characterized by mucosal necrosis and greater inflammation, leading to diarrhea and rectal bleeding.[270,271] The lesion is usually confined to the mucosa but may occasionally extend deeper into the bowel wall.[272,273] Because of the frequency of these effects as well as the uncertain need for such irritating solutions, soap enemas are no longer recommended.

Other Ulcers of the Colon

Ulceration of the mucosa is a feature of many intrinsic colonic diseases, and the lesions tend to be multiple or diffuse and are associated with inflammatory changes in the intervening mucosa (see Table 28–1). This section deals with those ulcers that are localized and have a relatively nonspecific histologic appearance.

Behçet's Disease

Behçet's disease is an uncommon disorder characterized by the presence of small aphthous ulcers of the oral cavity and the external genital region together with uveitis or iriditis.[274,275] It is thought to be an immune disorder, possibly mediated by a vasculitis, and lesions have also been noted in the skin, joints, and neuromuscular system. The gastrointestinal tract is involved in about one half of the cases, and the ulcers tend to be concentrated in the distal ileum and proximal colon.[276–279] The lesions are small and cause slight undermining of the adjacent mucosa; although most are superficial, they can occasionally extend into the wall and cause perforation. The inflammatory reaction around the ulcers is nonspecific, and a vasculitis has not been well documented in the intestinal lesions. Based on the distribution of the disease in the intestine and the appearance of the aphthous ulcers, the syndrome may resemble Crohn's disease in its early stage but is readily separated by the lack of progression to larger ulcerated and strictured lesions, of sinus tracts and of granulomas. Multiple, small shallow ulcers have also been noted in the esophagus[280–282] and in the stomach and duodenum[283–284] in some cases of Behçet's disease.

Stercoraceous Ulcers

Stercoraceous ulcers are most common in the distal colon and rectum and are due mainly to fecal impactions resulting in pressure-induced necrosis of the mucosal surface.[285] They are analogous to the decubitus ulcers that occur on other surfaces, such as the skin. The patients typically present with severe constipation, abdominal or rectal pain, and bleeding; and the clinical diagnosis is usually apparent. The ulcers may be single or multiple, vary from a few millimeters to several centimeters in diameter, and usually display sharply defined edges with congestion of the adjacent mucosa. They are most often confined to the submucosa, but deeper lesions and perforation may occur.[286–288] The histologic features are fairly distinctive in the early lesions, revealing an ischemic type of injury characterized by extensive necrosis, marked congestion, patchy hemorrhage, entrapped fecal material, and little inflammation. Chronic ulcers show the effects of repair and secondary infection, including neutrophilic reaction, variable fibrosis, and the appearance of giant cells and poorly formed granulomas in response to the fecal matter. Mucosal biopsy may be obtained in large lesions to exclude other inflammatory causes of ulceration and neoplasms.

Nonspecific Ulcers of the Colon

Isolated ulcers of unknown or uncertain cause spontaneously appear in all parts of the colon.[289–299] Before one considers this category, it is essential that ulcers due to the various intrinsic and secondary colonic diseases be excluded. In particular, localized ulcers of the rectum are usually part of the solitary rectal ulcer syndrome and are distinguished by their characteristic clinical and histologic features,[223–236] as described in the previous section. Localized ulcers of the colon and rectum have also been noted in patients with radiation injury,[72–74] with reactions to ergotamine suppositories,[300,301] contraceptive pills,[302,303] and other drugs,[76–78,304] and with atheromatous emboli and vasculitis.[88,306,307] A predilection for cecal lesions occurs in cases of renal failure,[308–310] agranulocytosis,[311–313] and colonic obstruction.[314] Rare cases have been recorded as a result of cocaine ingestion[315] and retained cleansing solutions on endoscopes.[316] The nonspecific ulcers of the colon have been noted most commonly in the cecum and proximal ascending portion, followed by the sigmoid colon, and appear to be least frequent in the transverse and descending parts. They may be seen in all age groups and typically present with bleeding from right-sided lesions and hemorrhage or obstruction from sigmoid cases. The lesions are identified by radiographic and endoscopic examination, and the diagnosis is obtained by noting the nonspecific nature on biopsy study and by the exclusion of other known causes of colonic ulceration.

Detailed pathologic studies have concentrated on the cecal ulcers, revealing that they are typically located on the antimesenteric border and that they vary in size and depth.[295,298] The ulcers may be up to several centimeters in diameter, and deep penetration of the intestinal wall and perforation have been described. The histologic features are essentially nonspecific: acute and chronic inflammation, prominent granulation tissue, variable fibrosis, and fibrin thrombi in small vessels. It has been considered that the ulcer might be a consequence of inflammation and effacement of a localized diverticulum of the cecum,[317] and this might apply in the younger patients in whom such limited diverticula away from the mesenteric border are more commonly observed. In older patients, an ischemic process has been postulated, based in part on its greater probability in this age group but also on the histologic character of the lesion.[296] In this regard, the lesion of vascular ectasia (or angiodysplasia) is known to occur in the cecum of older patients and is thought to be the result of chronic constipation leading to increased transmural pressure in this area.[318] Although these vascular cases usually present with massive hemorrhage and inconspicuous mucosal lesions, it is possible that they might be a nidus for secondary injury and the development of some of the cecal ulcers.

Secondary Ulcers of the Colon

Colonic ulcers can occur in other conditions that may affect the entire alimentary tract, and these are mentioned above and presented in detail in other parts of the book: radiation and chemical injury in Chapter 9; motor and mechanical disorders in Chapter 11; vasculitis and other vascular diseases in Chapter 12; graft-versus-host reaction[319,320] and other immunologic injuries in Chapter 14; and uremia,[308–310] chronic granulomatous disease,[321,322] and other systemic disorders in Chapter 16.

Irritable Bowel Syndrome

The irritable bowel syndrome is a common condition in which the patients are first seen with intermittent crampy abdominal pain and watery or mucus-filled diarrhea, and the symptoms are often precipitated by stressful situations.[323] It has long been suspected that this is a functional disorder, but recent manometric studies have suggested the possibility of a motor disturbance. There are no gross or microscopic alterations. Endoscopy and mucosal biopsy are often obtained to exclude some form of enteritis or colitis. As noted previously, some of these patients are found to have collagenous colitis.

OTHER TUMOR-LIKE LESIONS OF THE INTESTINES

Pneumatosis Intestinalis

Definition and Etiology. Pneumatosis intestinalis is a relatively uncommon disorder characterized by the presence of air or other gas-filled cysts in the intestinal wall.[324–327] Other names for this condition are *pneumatosis cystoides intestinalis* to honor the prominent cysts that may be present and *pneumatosis coli* when the lesion is limited to the colon. It may involve the small or the large intestine, and there appear to be two major forms of the disease. The more common type often appears as an asymptomatic radiographic abnormality of the small intestine, and it is seen in patients with pulmonary emphysema or an obstructing peptic ulcer of the gastric pylorus.[328] In these situations, it is believed that air under high pressure escapes from a ruptured pulmonary bleb or through a penetrating posterior ulcer and passes through the retroperitoneum and along the adventitia of the mesenteric vessels to reach the bowel wall, where it is deposited. The other type, which is seen more often in the colon, is thought to be the consequence of mucosal disease causing the penetration of luminal gases or gas-forming bacteria into the mucosa and underlying tissues.[326,327,329,330] Pneumatosis has been observed in a wide variety of inflammatory conditions affecting the small intestine and colon, including infections, necrotizing enterocolitis, ischemic disease, ulcerative colitis, Crohn's disease, and mechanical obstruction. It may also be seen following trauma to the mucosa as a result of an endoscopic procedure.[327,331] Other theories of the genesis of pneumatosis suggest that there is a primary chemical injury to the mucosal and submucosal tissues[332] or that the gas is mainly contained within the mural lymphatics.[333]

Clinical Features. The disease may affect all age groups, including infants and children, and is more common in males, possibly reflecting their higher incidence of pulmonary disease and peptic ulcers. Most of the cases related to pulmonary disease or to pyloric obstruction are asymptomatic, and the lesion is typically an incidental radiographic finding.[328] Symptoms are more often present in the cases of pneumatosis that are associated with intestinal disease and reflect the underlying enteritis or colitis. Uncommonly, the lesion may be localized and large, resembling a polypoid mass on radiographic and endoscopic examination, or there may be signs of intestinal obstruction.[329] The finding of pneumatosis in a patient with a clinically evident inflammatory or ischemic condition is often an ominous sign because it tends to correlate with cases that have greater necrosis. The pneumatosis may persist after the initiating event has subsided, or it may regress after a variable period of time.[330] Therapy is mainly directed at the underlying disease, and treatment is not required for the pneumatosis lesion.

Pathology. The lesions are more common in the small intestine than in the colon and may involve any part of the bowel wall but are particularly prominent in the looser submucosal and subserosal layers.[326,327] There is a marked expansion of the submucosa by the gas-filled cystic spaces, which range from a few millimeters to several centimeters in diameter, imparting a honeycomb or spongelike appearance. The mucosa is usually elevated over the cysts, and localized lesions may look like a broad-based polyp (Figure 28-17). Less pronounced changes are noted in the subserosal area, and the muscularis propria is often spared except for the region around the piercing vessels in its superficial portion. The histologic features differ somewhat in the two major types of pneumatosis, particularly in the character of the inflammatory reaction. Both reveal cystic spaces of variable size that are lined mainly by

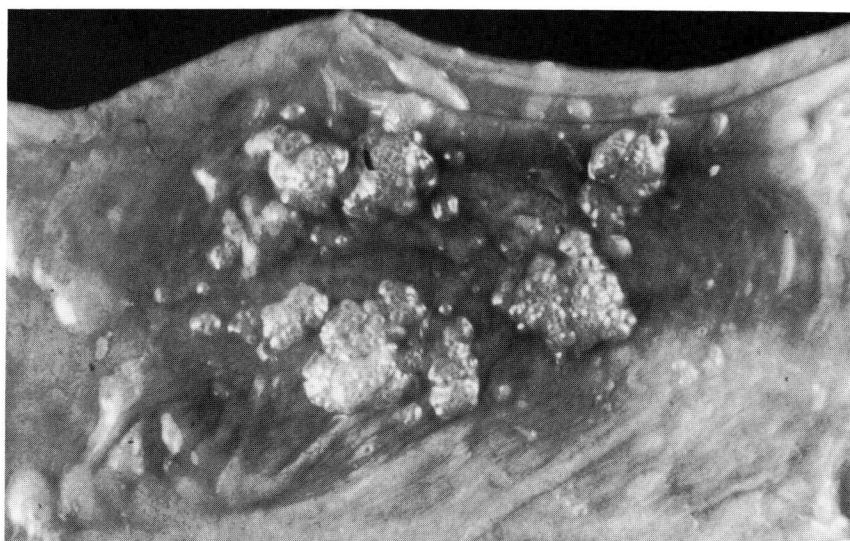

FIGURE 28-17. Pneumatosis coli. Mucosal surface showing an irregularly polypoid lesion composed of numerous gas-filled cysts.

flattened cells. It has long been debated whether these might be endothelial cells, in support of the theory that the gas is contained within dilated lymphatics,[333] but most believe that the lining is composed of indigenous mesenchymal cells that are compressed by the gas. There may be small foci of inflammation in the adjacent tissues in both types of pneumatosis, and cases related to mucosal disease often show more prominent proliferation of macrophages and giant cells at the edges of the cystic spaces[326] (Figure 28-18). It is thought that this might represent a reaction to luminal products, although bacteria and fecal matter are not ordinarily found in the spaces. The mucosa frequently reveals inflammation, dilatation, and rupture of crypts as well as microcysts with giant cells in the lamina propria[332,334]; and these features, together with the cysts in the upper submucosa, can be readily detected in biopsy samples[5,335] (Figure 28-19).

Differential Diagnosis. The diagnosis of pneumatosis intestinalis is easily accomplished by the demonstration of gas-filled spaces in the bowel wall. This is ordinarily done by radiographic and gross examinations and may be abetted by mucosal biopsy of lesions that protrude into the lumen. It is important that the intestine, particularly the mucosa, be carefully inspected for evidence of inflammatory or ischemic lesions, since the clinical course is largely dependent on the presence and extent of any primary intestinal disease. The postmortem formation of gas gangrene, due to invasion and proliferation of gas-forming bacteria such as *Clostridium welchii*, can also produce the appearance of large gaseous cysts in the intestinal wall. This can be readily distinguished from pneumatosis by histologic examination, which reveals extensive autolysis of the tissues in the absence of an inflammatory reaction, together with the finding of many large bacterial rods. In patients with severe neutropenia, a necrotizing colitis that is mainly due to virulent streptococci can occur, and irregular spaces are often seen in the intestinal wall upon microscopic examination.[311-313]

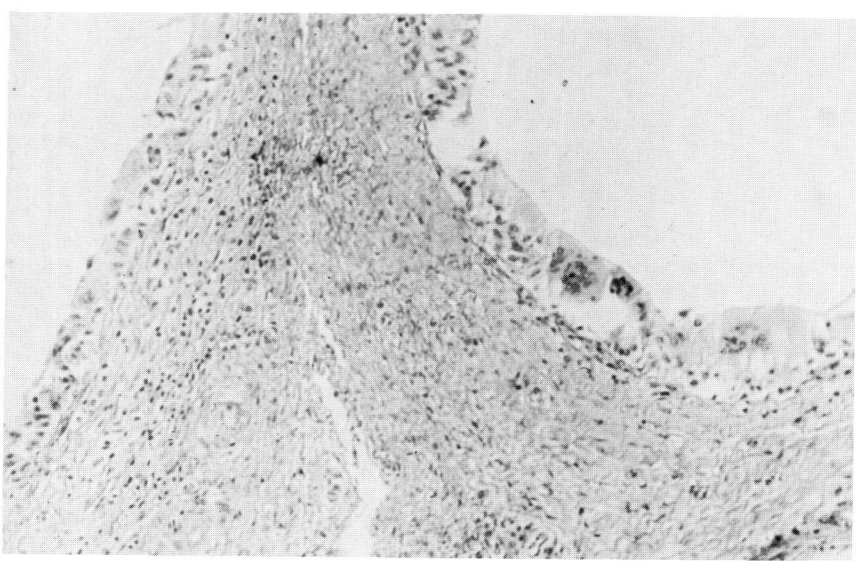

FIGURE 28-18. Colonic wall in a case of pneumatosis coli. There is a large gas-filled cyst (upper right), lined by inflammatory tissue and a few multinucleated giant cells. (H&E, × 100)

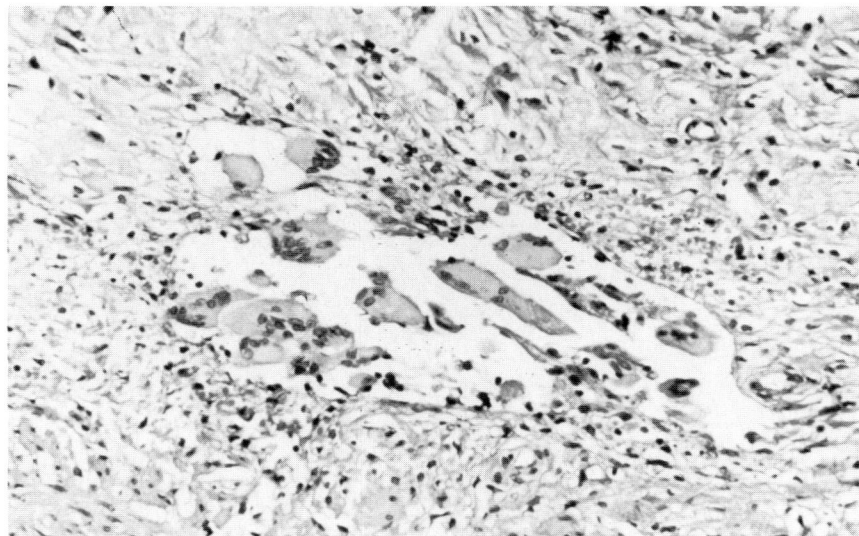

FIGURE 28–19. Colonic biopsy in a case of pneumatosis coli, revealing slitlike spaces lined by inflammatory giant cells in the submucosa. (H&E, × 400) (From Goldman H, Antonioli DA: Mucosal biopsy of the rectum, colon, and ileum. Hum Pathol 13:981–1012, 1982.)

There are typically no gross cystic lesions, however; and the specific diagnosis is provided by the finding of many bacteria in the wall and by cultures of the stool and tissues.

Other conditions that may need to be distinguished from pneumatosis intestinalis because of the presence of irregular or cystic spaces include areas of fat necrosis; foreign body reactions to other fatty substances that are dissolved during the tissue preparation, such as an oleogranuloma; enteritis or colitis cystic profunda; and lymphangioma. Areas of fat necrosis, which can be seen in any inflammatory disorder affecting the submucosa, are characterized by the appearance of small spaces and a marked inflammatory reaction with many foamy lipid-filled macrophages and fibrosis. A similar inflammatory reaction is noted in oleogranulomas, and these lesions are typically solitary and confined to the rectal area. In enteritis and colitis cystica profunda, the cysts are filled with mucus and lined by tall columnar epithelial cells. Lymphangiomas are usually solitary and more often circumscribed, and they may reveal lymph fluid within the cystic spaces and an attenuated, incomplete muscular wall.

Endometriosis

Definition and Etiology. Endometriosis is a common condition characterized by the presence of ectopic endometrial tissue. It is most often encountered in the uterine wall, the pelvic adnexa and soft tissues, and the peritoneum; and it may rarely be found in regional lymph nodes and in distant sites such as the lungs and pleura. Gastrointestinal involvement is noted in about one third of the cases, and the most common location is in the distal colon and rectum.[336–341] There are two major theories regarding the development of endometriosis. It has been suggested that endometrial tissue may extrude through the fallopian tubes at the time of normal menstruation, and this would explain the concentration of the lesions in the pelvic tissues and on the peritoneal surface. Alternatively, it is known that the coelomic epithelium is capable of pluripotential differentiation and is the probable source of tumors of müllerian origin affecting the uterine adnexa, and this hypothesis would allow for the finding of endometriosis in all regions, including areas that are remote from the uterus. In either situation, the ectopic endometrial tissue can respond to the cyclic hormonal stimulation, resulting in hemorrhage, fibrosis, and pressure effects in the affected tissues.

Clinical Features. The disorder is typically seen in women during their reproductive years, with a peak incidence of severe symptoms in the fourth decade; and it declines or abates during pregnancy and after menopause. In most cases affecting the intestinal tract, the lesions are at a microscopic level and not productive of clinical problems in this area. Symptoms referable to involvement of the distal colon and rectum include constipation, abdominal or rectal pain, and occasional diarrhea, which may be cyclic. Rectal bleeding is only rarely observed, presumably because the lesions do not often extend into the mucosal layer.[342,343] Obstruction is less common and is usually seen with larger lesions in the sigmoid colon and ileum; this condition is the result of an intraluminal mass or stricture,[336,343] an intussusception,[344] or serosal fibrosis and peritoneal adhesions. Such masses, which are composed mainly of fibrosis and hypertrophied smooth muscle, may persist in older patients and simulate a neoplasm. Patients with intestinal endometriosis may present with prominent symptoms but lack any findings on radiographic and endoscopic examination, and they are often initially thought to have the irritable bowel syndrome or a functional complaint. Furthermore, even when gross lesions of intestinal endometriosis are detected by such studies, their exact nature is not revealed and the clinical diagnosis is typically dependent on the finding of compatible features of the disease in other, more common locations. Treatment is identical to that for endometriosis in general and in-

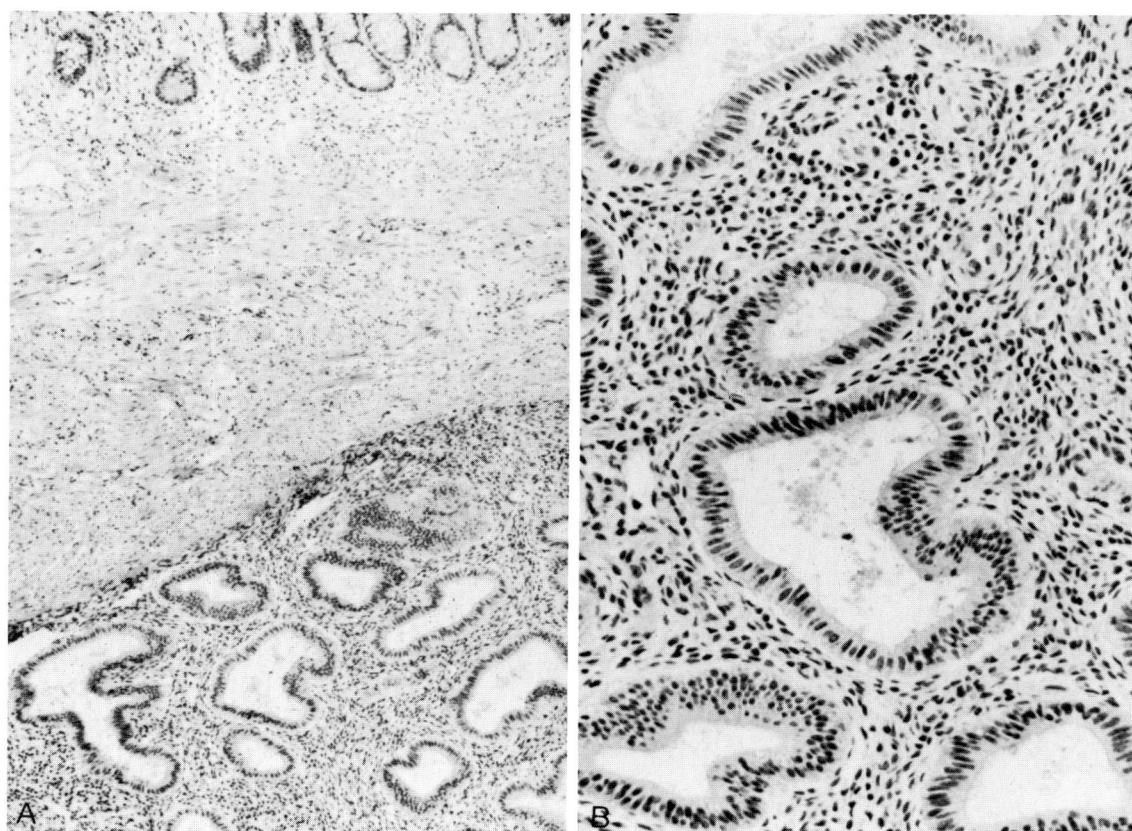

FIGURE 28–20. *A,* Endometriosis of the ileum, with the mucosal surface at the top. There is a large nodule of endometriotic tissue in the intestinal wall (bottom). (H&E, × 60) *B,* Endometriosis of the ileum. Closer view of the endometriotic tissue *A*, showing the characteristic glands and stroma. (H&E, × 250)

cludes hormones and analgesics; surgery may be required for the cases with obstruction, a mass of undetermined nature, or a rare perforation.[345]

Pathology. Estimates of involvement of the gastrointestinal tract by endometriosis have ranged up to 34%.[336–340,344] Of these cases, lesions have been noted in the sigmoid colon and rectum in over 80%; the appendix, in 5% to 10%; the cecum, in 4%; and the small intestine, usually the distal ileum, in about 7%. Rare examples have also been noted in the proximal small intestine and in a Meckel's diverticulum. The endometriosis is most commonly present in the serosal surface and in the muscularis propria, and it may extend into the submucosa but only rarely into the mucosa. Lesions range in size from microscopic foci to several centimeters in diameter, and the smaller implants are soft and red because of the dominant presence of the endometrial tissue and hemorrhage. In contrast, most of the mass of the large lesions is composed of fibrous and muscle tissue, which imparts a pale and hard appearance. The gross features of endometriosis are also somewhat dependent on its location in the bowel wall. Lesions concentrated in the serosa are often associated with prominent fibrosis, which may extend into the mesentery or mesocolon, whereas those embedded in the muscularis propria typically evoke a hypertrophy of the smooth muscle that may simulate a tumor of the intestinal wall. Least frequent is the appearance of a polypoid mass in the submucosa and mucosa.[342,343] Histologic examination reveals the characteristic endometrial tissue with glands and stroma, foci of fresh and old hemorrhage with inflammation and hemosiderin deposits, and variable fibrosis and smooth muscle hypertrophy (Figure 28–20). In the larger lesions that are usually dominated by the presence of fibrous and muscular tissues, multiple histologic sections may be required for identification of the endometriotic foci (Figure 28–21). The major complication is intestinal obstruction, which is most often at the level of the sigmoid colon[336] or the terminal ileum,[338] and this usually results from a constricting lesion of the bowel wall or peritoneal fibrous adhesions. Obstruction due to a polypoid mass or its intussusception, major hemorrhage into the gut lumen, and perforation of the bowel wall are rarely seen.[344,345] Endoscopic examination and mucosal biopsy are mainly used for exclusion of other diseases and occasionally may detect the endometriosis when it involves the mucosa or upper submucosa[343] (Figure 28–22). Rare cases of adenocarcinoma arising in endometriotic tissue within the colon have been reported,[346] and these must be distinguished from the spread of a primary uterine tumor.

Differential Diagnosis. The diagnosis of endometriosis is dependent on the histologic finding of the typical glands and stroma of the ectopic tissue in the wall of the intestine. As noted previously, the residual foci

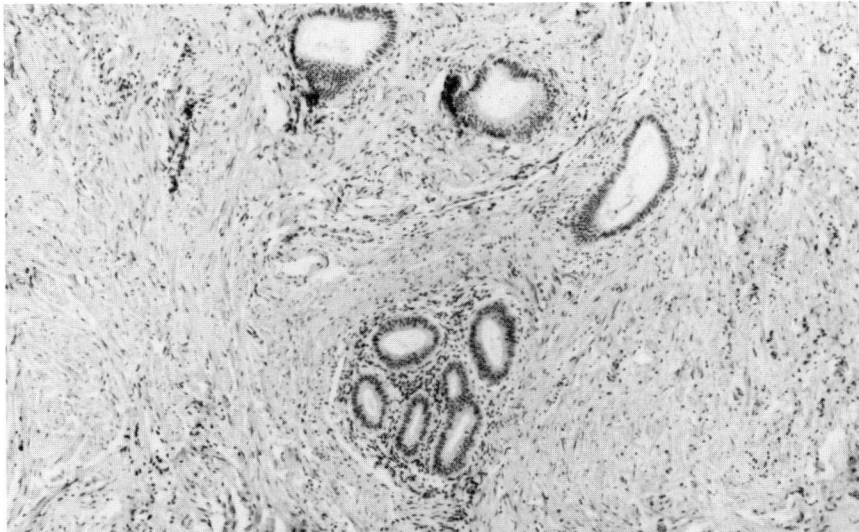

FIGURE 28–21. Endometriosis of rectosigmoid colon. There is a small focus of endometriotic tissue in the muscle layer, together with a proliferation of the smooth muscle tissue. (H&E, × 60)

of the endometriotic tissue may be sparse in the larger lesions, particularly in those affecting the muscularis propria; and it may be necessary to examine multiple tissue sections. Furthermore, repeated hemorrhages may result in considerable distortion and even loss of the stromal component, but the finding of the glands together with a surrounding fibromuscular proliferation should alert one to the possibility of endometriosis. The disease must be distinguished from other conditions that may be associated with an intestinal stricture, including mainly ischemic disease, which usually affects older persons and causes prominent bleeding; Crohn's disease, distinguished by the presence of greater diarrhea and the characteristic lesions of sinus tracts and granulomas; and adenocarcinoma of the colon, distinguished by the finding of dysplastic features of the glandular epithelium. Difficulties may arise in the assessment of mucosal biopsies containing endometriosis if there has been distortion or loss of the stroma component, but there should still be no atypism of the glands. In cases of endometriosis that are mainly in the muscularis propria, the associated muscular hypertrophy can mimic the appearance of a leiomyoma. The smooth muscle tumors tend to be well circumscribed, whereas endometriosis is more often circumferential or has ill-defined margins; the separation is provided by histologic examination of multiple sections in search of foci of ectopic tissue. The appearance of mural lesions, particularly in the distal ileum and appendix, with surrounding fibrosis that may extend into the contiguous mesentery, can also be caused by carcinoid tumors; the distinction from endometriosis is readily made by the histologic findings of the typical neuroendocrine cells.

Gastric Heterotopia

Definition and Etiology. Gastric heterotopia is an uncommon condition characterized by the presence of mature mucosa of gastric corpus-fundic type in ectopic locations throughout the alimentary tract.[347,348] The lesions are usually observed in the upper esophagus,[349–352] proximal duodenum,[353–358] and rectum,[359–363] possibly because these are sites that are commonly inspected by endoscopic examination. Nodules have also

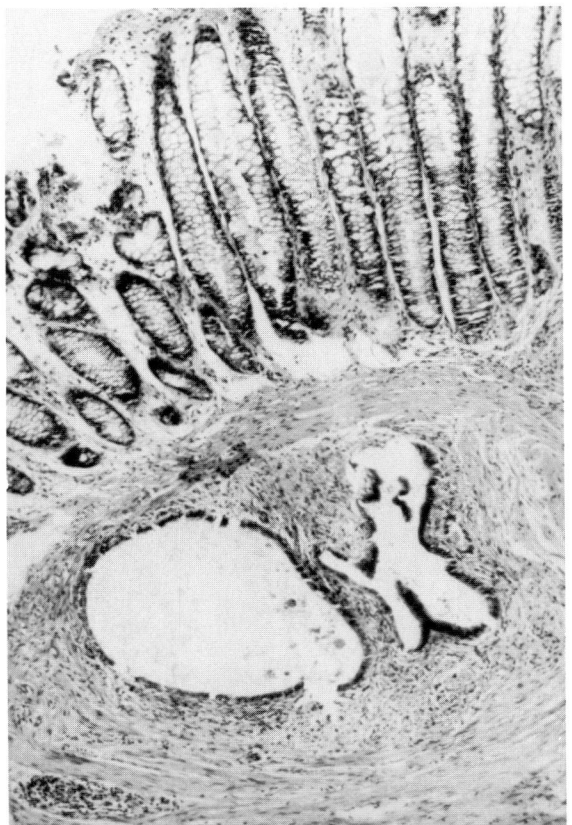

FIGURE 28–22. Colonic biopsy in a case of endometriosis, showing a small focus of endometrial glands in the submucosa. There is no cytologic atypicality. (H&E, × 60)

been noted in the jejunum,[364] in Meckel's diverticulum,[365-367] and in enteric and colonic duplication cysts[366,368,369] whereas they are rarely seen in the normal distal ileum and proximal colon. The lesions are thought to arise from congenital rests, and this concept is supported by the appearance of fully developed gastric corpus mucosa, by the more common occurrence in children and young adults, by the frequent association with other anomalies of the intestinal tract, and by the absence of an underlying inflammatory condition in the affected tissues.

Such heterotopias in the intestines must be distinguished from the more common process of gastric metaplasia, which typically consists of the appearance of gastric pyloric glands[1,3,5] or mucous cells of the surface-foveolar type[34,35] and which develops as a consequence of chronic inflammatory disorders such as peptic duodenitis, celiac disease, Crohn's disease, and ulcerative colitis. Similarly, gastric heterotopia of the esophagus must be separated from Barrett's esophagus, which occurs in patients with chronic esophagitis. The ectopic gastric tissue is typically confined to the upper esophagus and is composed of mature corpus tissue, whereas the Barrett lesion is located in the distal portion and shows a mixture of gastric and intestinal mucous cells.[1]

Clinical Features. Gastric heterotopia of the intestines may be seen in either sex and in all age groups, but the symptomatic cases appear to be more common in children. Most cases are asymptomatic and are observed as incidental findings during endoscopic examination of the duodenum[354] or as part of the pathologic study of excised diverticula and cysts.[366,368,369] The specialized glandular cells are functional and secrete acid and proteolytic enzymes,[350,359] but the occurrence of peptic injury is mainly related to the location of the lesions. Thus, ulceration of the adjacent unprotected mucosa is often observed when gastric heterotopia involves relatively stagnant areas such as the rectum[360-363] and congenital diverticula[366,367] and duplication cysts,[366] whereas peptic injury is rarely seen in cases affecting the duodenum, possibly because of the prompt dilution of the acid by biliary secretions in this area. Lesions of the duodenum typically present with a small solitary nodule at endoscopy, and the diagnosis is readily established by biopsy study. It is important to separate gastric heterotopia, which may be seen in any part of the duodenum, from the changes of peptic duodenitis, which are concentrated in the first portion, because there is no relation between these two conditions. Occasionally, there may be larger heterotopic nodules in the duodenum or jejunum, and these can bleed or be the source for an intussusception.[364] The esophogeal cases are usually asymptomatic but may occasionally develop ulceration and stricture.[352]

Patients with lesions of the rectum and of developmental diverticula and cysts more often present with painless rectal bleeding, and the diagnosis is commonly made by a technetium scan. In the rectal cases, the luminal pH is typically less than 4, and vital stains such as Congo red can be applied for detection of the parietal cells.[359] Patients with ulceration are prone to deep penetration of the wall and perforation, and fistulas may develop in the rectal lesions.[362] Surgical excision is ordinarily required for these symptomatic cases.

Pathology. The primary lesion of gastric heterotopia is essentially the same in whatever part of the intestinal tract it is located. It consists of a fairly well circumscribed nodule of variable size—most less than 1 cm in diameter—that is typically sessile and slightly raised and has a smooth surface contour. The lesions are usually single, but multiple nodules and simultaneous involvement of different parts of the tract (e.g., both the esophagus and the duodenum) are occasionally noted. The histologic features are distinctive, revealing completely normal gastric corpus-fundic mucosa in most cases (Figure 28–23). The flat surface and short foveolae (or pits) are lined by a continuous layer of tall columnar cells with mucous granules, which stain strongly with the PAS reaction, concentrated in the luminal portions of the cytoplasm. Interestingly, *H. pylori* organisms have been noted next to the gastric mucous cells in a case involving the rectum.[370] Most of the mucosa is occupied by the specialized glands, which are closely packed and contain abundant parietal and chief cells, and the margins of the lesions are sharply separated from the adjacent intestinal mucosa. As noted above, the duodenal cases are rarely associated with ulceration, and the finding of inflammation should alert one to the possible presence of a coexisting but unrelated duodenitis. Larger lesions of the small intestine are rare, and these can become inflamed or cause obstruction by an intussusception.[364] In addition, a case of adenocarcinoma of the jejunum thought to arise in an area of gastric heterotopia has been described.[371]

In the cases of gastric heterotopia involving the rectum and developmental cysts and diverticula, the ulcerations that may occur are typically located in the intestinal mucosa that is immediately adjacent to the ectopic tissue,[360,365,366] since this area is unprotected and would receive the highest concentration of gastric acid. This is analogous to the selective appearance of peptic injury in the first part of the duodenum or on the jejunal side of a gastrojejunostomy stoma. The ulcers vary in size and are often deep, which leads to free perforation or to the development of localized fistulas, the latter more commonly observed in the rectal cases.[362] It is also likely that the chance of perforation is enhanced in the cases involving diverticula and cysts by the pressure effects of inflammation and secondary ischemic damage in these relatively contained structures. The inflammation around the ulcerated areas may extend into the heterotopic nodules and cause damage and loss of some or all of the ectopic tissue. In this regard, gastric heterotopic tissue is noted in only about half of the cases of ruptured Meckel's diverticulum,[367] and it is possible that some of these cases may have lost the identifiable ectopic tissue, rather than representing examples of simple mechanical perforation.

Differential Diagnosis. The diagnosis of gastric heterotopia depends simply on the histologic identification of normal gastric corpus-fundic mucosa in any

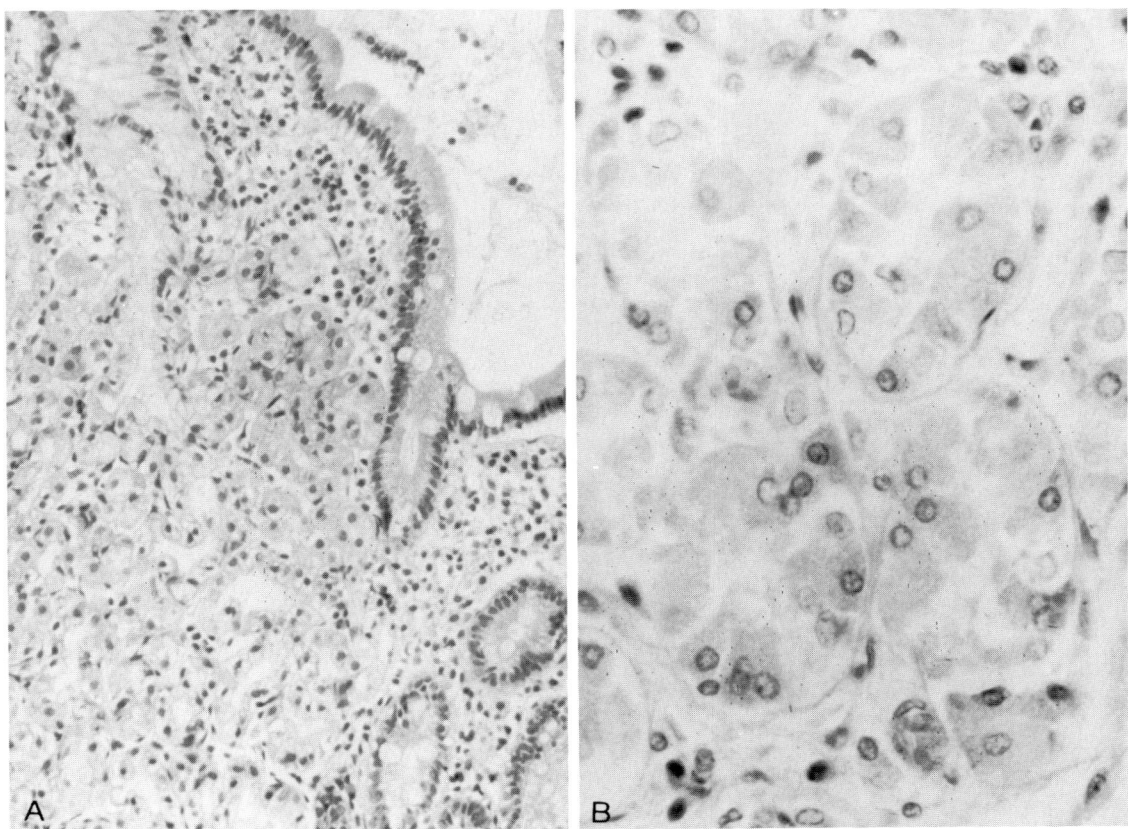

FIGURE 28–23. *A*, Heterotopic gastric mucosa in the duodenal mucosa. There is a sharply demarcated nodule of normal gastric corpus-fundic type mucosa in the left portion, consisting of surface-foveolar mucous cells at the top and the specialized glands at the bottom. A small area of normal duodenal mucosa is at the right, and there is no inflammatory reaction. (H&E, × 60) *B*, Heterotopic gastric mucosa in the duodenal mucosa. Closer view of the specialized corpus glands in *A*, showing both normal parietal cells and normal chief cells. There is no inflammation. (H&E, × 400)

other part of the alimentary tract. At a microscopic level, it must be distinguished from gastric metaplasia, which is a frequent finding in many chronic inflammatory conditions of the esophagus and intestinal tract. The metaplasia typically consists of a proliferation of pyloric glands[1,3,5] and a more variable presence of the surface-foveolar type of mucous cells. Scattered parietal and chief cells or small clusters of these cells may uncommonly be present, particularly in cases affecting the esophagus; but the appearance of a completely normal gastric corpus is not seen in the metaplastic process. In cases of Barrett's esophagus, the gastric metaplasia is admixed with the intestinal type of mucous cells, and distal samples may show some parietal and chief cells. The presence of a normal gastric fundus in this area is typically indicative of a hiatal hernia. Furthermore, gastric heterotopia is usually in the cervical part of the esophagus,[349] whereas the changes of Barrett's esophagus start in and are concentrated in the distal portion. Chronic peptic duodenitis often reveals a partial transformation of the epithelial cells overlying the villi into those of the gastric surface type[34,35]; and similar changes, together with patches of pyloric glands, have been noted in long-standing cases of celiac disease. Pyloric gland metaplasia is also a common finding in Crohn's disease, particularly of the small intestine, where it appears as patches of mature glands at the base of the inflamed mucosa. Gastric heterotopia of the duodenum frequently presents with small nodules, and the gross differential diagnosis includes consideration mainly of Brunner's gland hyperplasia and lymphoid hyperplasia in this area.

Foreign Body Reactions

Foreign Body Reactions are presented in part in the section on foreign bodies in Chapter 11 and in the section on granulomatous disorders in Chapter 16, and this section concentrates on those conditions that have their major or exclusive effects in the intestinal tract.

Foreign Objects

Foreign objects that are ingested or that are introduced through the rectum or a stoma can cause clinical problems by laceration of the mucosal surface and by obstruction of the lumen. The inflammatory reaction in such cases is often nonspecific but may reveal focal granulomas, and the intensity is largely determined by

Table 28-3 FOREIGN BODY GRANULOMAS IN THE INTESTINES

Mucin from ruptured crypts
Fecal matter from perforation
Suture, talc, and starch
Barium and other minerals
Oils

the degree of trauma to the intestinal wall. The foreign body may lodge in an area of pre-existing intestinal disease, and the combination may be responsible for the onset of symptoms. Perforation and fibrous stricture can develop, and surgery is often required for these complications and for the removal of objects that are not spontaneously passed in the feces.

Localized Granulomatous Reactions

Localized granulomatous reactions in the intestinal mucosa and wall can occur in response to a wide assortment of foreign substances (Table 28-3). These include mucin that has escaped from ruptured crypts in cases of enteritis or colitis or from tissues that have been traumatized by prior biopsy or a surgical procedure; fecal matter at the sites of bowel perforations and, less commonly, in the wall of sinus tracts; and suture material that is part of a healing process or in a stitch abscess[372] (Figure 28-24). The nature of the foreign substance can be readily identified in standard histologic sections in all of these situations, and there are usually no clinical problems that can be attributed to the granulomas alone. Reactions to talc[373-375] or to starch[376-378] that was introduced during prior surgery have been most often noted on the peritoneal surface, where they may be the cause of an exudative peritonitis; the character of the substance is defined by its birefringent appearance. In any of these circumstances, if the foreign body nature of the granuloma is not evident, it may be necessary to consider other causes of granulomatous inflammation of the intestines, principally infections and Crohn's disease.

Barium Granuloma

A barium granuloma is a nodule of barium sulfate and reactive macrophages that is most commonly seen in the submucosa of the rectum.[379,380] It results from the passage of barium through the mucosal layer at the time of radiographic study, and its occurrence is facilitated by prior endoscopic or biopsy examination and by the presence of pre-existing mucosal disease.[381] Most lesions are small incidental findings, whereas patients with larger nodules typically present with rectal pain and constipation. The granulomas vary in size, ranging up to 10 cm in diameter, are usually concentrated in the submucosa as a fairly well circumscribed mass, and may contain pale green crystals of barium upon gross inspection. The larger lesions may also show a central umbilication or a small ulcer on a mucosal aspect, and the barium may extrude into the perirectal tissues.[382] The histologic appearance is fairly distinctive, revealing a mass of macrophages that contain the barium granules, which have a faint brownish color on H&E-stained slides and are refractile but not birefringent[383] (Figure 28-25). There may be an occasional giant cell, but well-formed, discrete granulomas of the sarcoid type are not seen. Since the barium is an inert substance, there are no other signs of inflammation unless the nodule has occurred in an area of prior disease. Most of the lesions eventually regress, and surgical excision is usually not required. Barium granulomas are less commonly seen in other parts of the intestine and are typically revealed as incidental findings on histologic examination.[381]

Oil Granuloma

An oil granuloma is an uncommon condition that represents an inflammatory reaction to exogenous oily

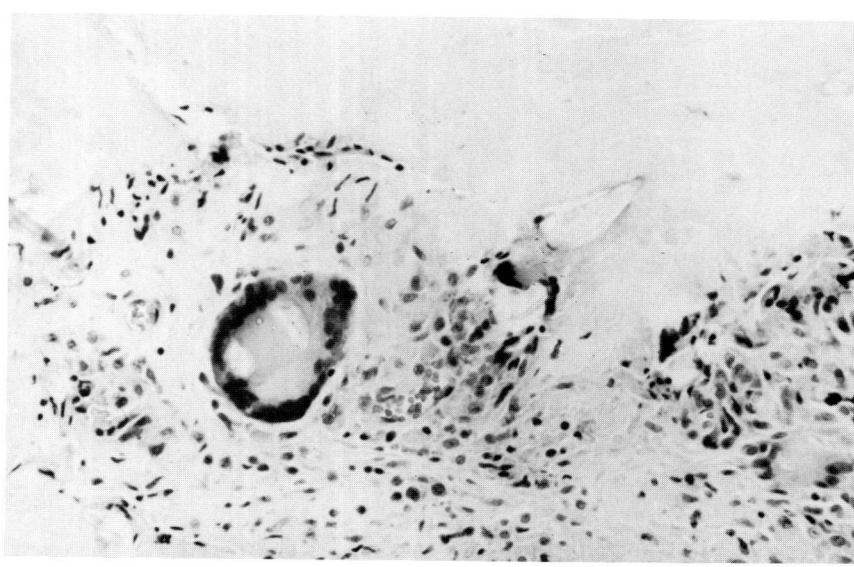

FIGURE 28-24. Suture reaction in colonic wall. There are many multinucleated inflammatory giant cells that contain and surround the suture material. (H&E, × 250)

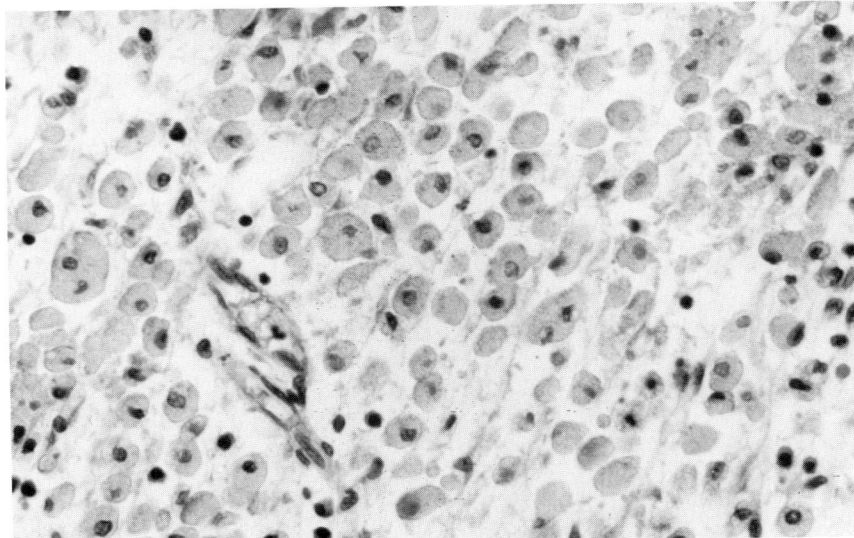

FIGURE 28-25. Barium granuloma in colonic submucosa. There is a mass of macrophages containing the fine brown, refractile barium material. Otherwise, there is very little inflammatory reaction. (H&E, × 400)

substances, and it has also been called an oleogranuloma.[372,384–387] The lesions are located in the rectum and are due to the introduction of a lubricant in this area or of an oil-based medium at time of local sclerosis of hemorrhoidal varices.[384,387] As noted in other tissues in the body, the strongest inflammatory reactions are caused by mineral oil. Most cases are observed as a small incidental finding during a rectal examination, or the patient may present with pain, constipation, and occasional bleeding. It is usually a single well-circumscribed nodule, ranging up to a few centimeters in diameter, and it is concentrated in the submucosa but may show focal extension into the mucosa and muscularis propria. The histologic features are characteristic: irregular spaces that are surrounded by macrophages and prominent fibrosis (Figure 28-26). Giant cells containing lipid are sparse, and well-formed granulomas of the sarcoid type are not observed. Some cases, possibly representing an earlier stage or a reaction to more toxic oils, show a greater amount of acute and chronic inflammatory cells, including eosinophils.[372] The spaces result from the extraction of the lipid during the slide preparation, and their nature can be confirmed by fat stains performed on frozen sections, but this is usually not needed for the diagnosis. The lesions appear as a solitary mass or, uncommonly, as a stricture in the rectum resembling a neoplasm[385]; and biopsy and surgery may be required to establish the diagnosis and to relieve any obstruction.

Oil granulomas must be distinguished from other rectal lesions that reveal cystic changes in the submucosa. Areas of fat necrosis are usually associated with less fibrosis and reveal a greater prominence of foamy macrophages due to the deposition of the triglycerides

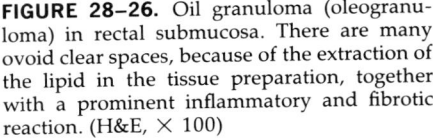
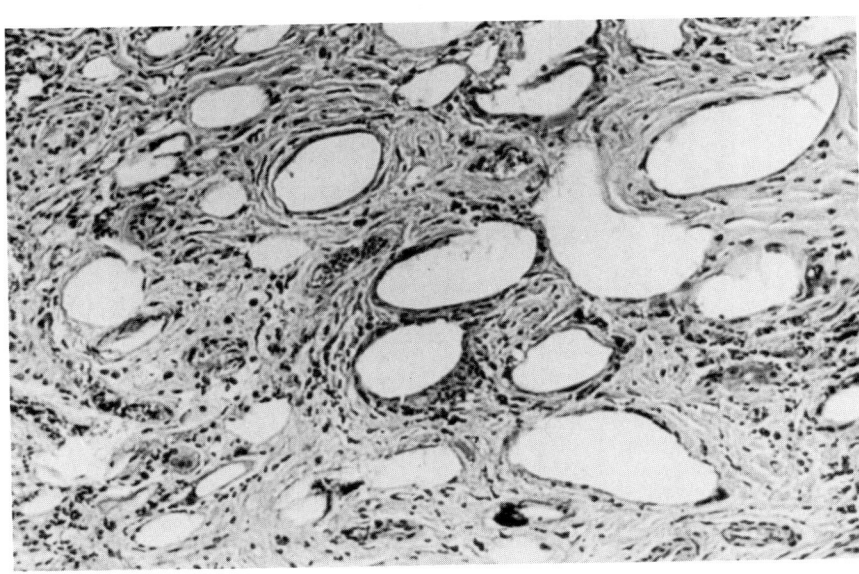

FIGURE 28-26. Oil granuloma (oleogranuloma) in rectal submucosa. There are many ovoid clear spaces, because of the extraction of the lipid in the tissue preparation, together with a prominent inflammatory and fibrotic reaction. (H&E, × 100)

within the cells in the form of fine droplets, and there is often other evidence of proctitis. The lesions of pneumatosis intestinalis typically show very little inflammation and fibrosis and are more diffuse. In the solitary rectal ulcer syndrome involving the submucosa, the cystic spaces are filled with mucus and lined by tall, columnar epithelial cells.

References

1. Goldman H, Antonioli DA: Mucosal biopsy of the esophagus, stomach and proximal duodenum. Hum Pathol 13:423–448, 1982.
2. Chang MH, Wang TH, Hsu JY, et al: Endoscopic examination of the upper gastrointestinal tract in infancy. Gastrointest Endosc 29:15–17, 1983.
3. Perera DR, Weinstein WM, Rubin CE: Small intestinal biopsy. Hum Pathol 6:157–217, 1975.
4. Scott BB, Jenkins D: Endoscopic small intestinal biopsy. Gastrointest Endosc 27:162–167, 1981.
5. Goldman H, Antonioli DA: Mucosal biopsy of the rectum, colon and distal ileum. Hum Pathol 13:981–1012, 1982.
6. Yardley JH, Donovitz M: Colo-rectal biopsy in inflammatory bowel disease. In Yardley JH, Morson BC, Abell MR (eds): The Gastrointestinal Tract. Baltimore, Williams & Wilkins, 1977, pp 50–94.
7. Whitehead R: Mucosal Biopsy of the Gastrointestinal Tract, 3rd ed. Philadelphia, WB Saunders, 1985.
8. Rotterdam H, Sommers SC: Biopsy Diagnosis of the Digestive Tract. New York, Raven Press, 1981.
9. Haggitt RC: Differential diagnosis of colitis. In Goldman H, Appelman HD, Kaufman N (eds): Gastrointestinal Pathology. Baltimore, Williams & Wilkins, 1990, pp 325–355.
10. Jaffe SN, Lee FD, Blumgart LH: Duodenitis. Clin Gastroenterol 7:635, 1978.
11. Owen DA: Gastritis and duodenitis. In Appelman HD (ed): Pathology of the Esophagus, Stomach, and Duodenum. New York, Churchill Livingstone, 1984, pp 37–77.
12. McCallum RW, Singh D, Wollman J: Endoscopic and histologic correlations of the duodenal bulb: The spectrum of duodenitis. Arch Pathol Lab Med 103:169–172, 1979.
13. Greenlaw R, Sheahan DG, DeLuca V, et al: Gastroduodenitis: A broader concept of peptic ulcer disease. Dig Dis Sci 25:660, 1980.
14. Hasan M, Sirius W, Ferguson A: Duodenal mucosal architecture in non-specific and ulcer-associated duodenitis. Gut 22:637–641, 1981.
15. Steer HW: Surface morphology of the gastroduodenal mucosa in duodenal ulceration. Gut 25:1203–1210, 1984.
16. Rathbone BJ, Wyatt JI, Heatley RV: *Campylobacter pyloridis*—a new factor in peptic ulcer disease. Gut 27:635–641, 1986.
17. Hazell SL, Hennessy WB, Brody TJ, et al: Campylobacter pyloridis gastritis. II. Distribution of bacteria and associated inflammation in the gastroduodenal environment. Am J Gastroenterol 82:297–301, 1987.
18. Frierson HF, Caldwell SH, Marshall BJ: Duodenal biopsy findings for patients with non-ulcer dyspepsia with or without Campylobacter pylori gastritis. Modern Pathol 3:271–276, 1990.
19. Paoluzi P, Pallone F, Palazzesi P, et al: Frequency and extent of bulbar duodenitis in duodenal ulcer: Endoscopic and histological study. Endoscopy 14:193–195, 1982.
20. Odeida G, Forni M, Farina L, et al: Duodenitis in children: Clinical, endoscopic and pathological aspects. Gastrointest Endosc 33:366–369, 1987.
21. Shousha S, Spiller RC, Parkins RA: The endoscopically abnormal duodenum in patients with dyspepsia: Biopsy findings in 60 cases. Histopathology 7:23–34, 1983.
22. Lance P, Filipe I, Wastell C: A new classification for duodenitis. Br J Surg 66:360–361, 1979.
23. Weinstein WM: The diagnosis and classification of gastritis and duodenitis. J Clin Gastroenterol 3(Suppl 2):7–16, 1981.
24. Cotton PB, Price AB, Tighe JR, et al: Preliminary evaluation of duodenitis by endoscopy and biopsy. Br Med J 3:430–433, 1973.
25. Whitehead R, Roca M, Meikle DD, et al: The histological classification of duodenitis in fiberoptic biopsy specimens. Digestion 13:129–136, 1975.
26. Jenkins D, Goodall A, Gille FR, Scott BB: Defining duodenitis: Quantitative histological study of mucosal responses and their correlations. J Clin Pathol 38:1119–1126, 1985.
27. Earlam RJ, Amerigo J, Kakavoulis T, Pollock DJ: Histological appearances of oesophagus, antrum and duodenum and their correlation with symptoms in patients with duodenal ulcer. Gut 26:95–100, 1985.
28. Scott BB, Goodall A, Stephenson P, Jenkins D: Duodenal bulb plasma cells in duodenitis and duodenal ulceration. Gut 26:1032–1037, 1985.
29. Yardley JH: Pathology of chronic gastritis and duodenitis. In Goldman H, Appelman HD, Kaufman N (eds): Gastrointestinal Pathology. Baltimore, Williams & Wilkins, 1990, pp 69–143.
30. Korn ER, Foroozan P: Endoscopic biopsies of normal duodenal mucosa. Gastrointest Endosc 21:51, 1974.
31. Kreunig R, Bosman FT, Kuiper G, et al: Gastric and duodenal mucosa in healthy individuals. J Clin Pathol 31:69–77, 1978.
32. Franzin G, Musola R, Ghidini O, et al: Nodular hyperplasia of Brunner's glands. Gastrointest Endosc 31:374–378, 1985.
33. Maratka Z, Kocianova J, Kudrmann J, et al: Hyperplasia of Brunner's glands: Radiology, endoscopy and biopsy. Acta Hepato-Gastroenterol 26:64–69, 1979.
34. James AH: Gastric epithelium in the duodenum. Gut 5:285–294, 1964.
35. Shousha S, Parkins RA, Bille TB: Chronic duodenitis with gastric metaplasia: Electron microscopic study, including comparison with normal. Histopathology 7:873–885, 1983.
36. Zukerman GR, Mills BA, Koehler RE, et al: Nodular duodenitis: Pathologic and clinical characteristics in patients with end-stage renal disease. Dig Dis Sci 28:1018–1024, 1983.
37. Giannella RA, Brastman SA, Zamcheck N: Influence of gastric acidity on bacterial and parasitic enteric infections. Ann Intern Med 78:271–276, 1973.
38. Peters M, Weiner J, Whelan G: Fungal infection associated with gastroduodenal ulceration: Endoscopic and pathologic appearances. Gastroenterology 78:350–354, 1980.
39. Reference deleted.
40. Steer HW: The gastro-duodenal epithelium in peptic ulceration. J Pathol 146:355–362, 1985.
41. King CE, Toskes PP: Small intestine bacterial overgrowth. Gastroenterology 76:1035–1055, 1979.
42. Freeman HJ, Shnitka TK, Piercey JRA, et al: Cytomegalovirus infection of the gastrointestinal tract in a patient with late onset immunodeficiency syndrome. Gastroenterology 73:1397–1403, 1977.
43. Knapp AB, Horst DA, Eliopoulos G, et al: Widespread cytomegalovirus gastroenterocolitis in a patient with acquired immunodeficiency syndrome. Gastroenterol 85:1399–1402, 1983.
44. Hinnant KL, Rotterdam HZ, Bell ET, Tapper ML: Cytomegalovirus infection of the alimentary tract: a clinicopathological correlation. Am J Gastroenterol 81:944–950, 1986.
45. Eras P, Goldstein MJ, Sherlock P: Candida infection of the gastrointestinal tract. Medicine 51:367–379, 1972.
46. Ament ME, Rubin CE: Relation of giardiasis to abnormal intestinal structure and function in gastrointestinal immunodeficiency syndromes. Gastroenterology 62:216–226, 1972.
47. Sun T: The diagnosis of giardiasis. Am J Surg Pathol 4:265–271, 1980.
48. Marshall JB, Kelley DH, Vogele K: Giardiasis: Diagnosis by endoscopic brush cytology of the duodenum. Am J Gastroenterol 79:517–519, 1984.
49. Trier JS, Moxey PC, Schimmel EM: Chronic intestinal coccidiosis in man: intestinal morphology and response to treatment. Gastroenterology 66:923–935, 1974.
50. Liebman WM, Thaler MM, DeLorimier A, et al: Intractable diarrhea of infancy due to intestinal coccidiosis. Gastroenterology 78:579–584, 1980.
51. Shein R, Gelb A: Isospora belli in a patient with acquired immunodeficiency syndrome. J Clin Gastroenterol 6:525–528, 1984.
52. DeHovitz JA, Pape JN, Boncy M, Johnson WD Jr: Clinical man-

ifestations and therapy of Isospora belli infection in patients with the acquired immunodeficiency syndrome. N Engl J Med 315:87–90, 1986.
53. Nime FA, Burek JD, Page DL, et al: Acute enterocolitis in a human being infected with the protozoon Cryptosporidium. Gastroenterology 70:592–598, 1976.
54. Meisel JL, Perera DR, Meligro C, et al: Overwhelming watery diarrhea associated with cryptosporidium in an immunosuppressed patient. Gastroenterology 70:1156–1160, 1976.
55. Lasser KH, Lewin KJ, Ryning FW: Cryptosporidial enteritis in a patient with congenital hypogammaglobulinemia. Hum Pathol 10:234–240, 1979.
56. Weisburger WR, Hutcheon DF, Yardley JH, et al: Cryptosporidiosis in an immunosuppressed renal-transplant recipient with IgA deficiency. Am J Clin Pathol 72:473–478, 1979.
57. Current WL, Reese NC, Ernst JV, et al: Human cryptosporidiosis in immunocompetent and immunodeficient persons: Studies of an outbreak and experimental transmission. N Engl J Med 308:1252–1257, 1983.
58. Chiampi NP, Sundberg RD, Klompus JP, Wilson AJ: Cryptosporidial enteritis and pneumocystic pneumonia in a homosexual man. Hum Pathol 14:734–737, 1983.
59. Guarda LA, Stein SA, Cleary KA, Ordonez NG: Human cryptosporidiosis in the acquired immune deficiency syndrome. Arch Pathol Lab Med 107:562–566, 1983.
60. Lefkowitch JH, Krumholz S, Feng Chen KC, et al: Cryptosporidiosis of the human small intestine: a light and electron microscopic study. Hum Pathol 15:746–752, 1984.
61. Casemore DP, Sands RL, Curry A: Cryptosporidium species—a "new" human pathogen. J Clin Pathol 38:1321–1336, 1985.
62. Isaacs D, Hunt GH, Phillips AD, et al: Cryptosporidiosis in immunocompetent children. J Clin Pathol 38:76–81, 1985.
63. Wolfson JS, Richter JM, Waldron MA, et al: Cryptosporidiosis in immunocompetent patients. N Engl J Med 312:1278–1282, 1985.
64. Gillin JS, Urmacher C, West R, Shuke M: Disseminated Mycobacterium avium-intracellulare infection in acquired immunodeficiency syndrome mimicking Whipple's disease. Gastroenterology 85:1187–1191, 1983.
65. Roth RI, Owen RZ, Keren DF, Volberding PA: Intestinal infection with Mycobacterium avium in acquired immune deficiency syndrome (AIDS): Histological and clinical comparison with Whipple's disease. Dig Dis Sci 30:497–504, 1985.
66. Dworkin B, Wormser GP, Rosenthal WS, et al: Gastrointestinal manifestations of the acquired immunodeficiency syndrome: A review of 22 cases. Am J Gastroenterol 80:774–778, 1985.
67. Witham RR, Mosser RS: An unusual presentation of schistosomiasis duodenitis. Gastroenterology 77:1316–1318, 1979.
68. Thatcher BS, Fleischer D, Rankin GB, Petras R: Duodenal schistosomiasis diagnosed by endoscopic biopsy of an isolated polyp. Am J Gastroenterol 79:927–929, 1984.
69. Bone MF, Chesner LM, Oliver R, Asquith P: Endoscopic appearances of duodenitis due to strongyloidiasis. Gastrointest Endosc 28:190–191, 1982.
70. Ainley CC, Clarke DG, Timothy AR, Thompson RPH: Strongyloides stercoralis hyperinfection associated with cimetidine in an immunosuppressed patient: Diagnosis by endoscopic biopsy. Gut 27:337–338, 1986.
71. Volpicelli NA, Salyer WR, Milligan FD, et al: The endoscopic appearance of the duodenum in Whipple's disease. Johns Hopkins Med J 138:19–23, 1976.
72. Novak JM, Collins JT, Donowitz M, et al: Effects of radiation on the human gastrointestinal tract. J Clin Gastroenterol 1:9, 1979.
73. Berthrong M, Fajardo LF: Radiation injury in surgical pathology. Part II. Alimentary Tract. Am J Surg Pathol 5:153–178, 1981.
74. Galland RB, Spencer J: The natural history of clinically established radiation enteritis. Lancet 1:1257–1258, 1985.
75. Millan MS, Morris GP, Beck IT, et al: Villous damage induced by suction biopsy and by acute ethanol intake in normal human small intestine. Dig Dis Sci 25:513–525, 1980.
76. Cooke AR: Drug damage to the gastroduodenum. In Sleisenger MH, Fordtran JS (eds): Gastrointestinal Disease, 2nd ed. Philadelphia, WB Saunders, 1978, pp 807–826.
77. Riddell RH: The gastrointestinal tract. In Riddell RH (ed): Pathology of Drug-Induced and Toxic Diseases. New York, Churchill Livingstone, 1982, pp 515–606.
78. Lewis JH: Gastrointestinal injury due to medicinal agents. Am J Gastroenterol 81:819–834, 1986.
79. Pemberton RE, Strand JL: A review of upper gastrointestinal effects of the newer nonsteroidal anti-inflammatory agents. Dig Dis Sci 24:53–64, 1979.
80. Eliakim R, Ophir M, Rachmilewitz D: Duodenal mucosal injury with nonsteroidal anti-inflammatory drugs. J Clin Gastroenterol 9:395–399, 1987.
81. Graham DY, Smith JL: Gastroduodenal complications of chronic NSAID therapy. Am J Gastroenterol 83:1081–1084, 1988.
82. Cunningham D, Morgan RJ, Mills PR, et al: Functional and structural changes of the human proximal small intestine after cytotoxic therapy. J Clin Pathol 38:265–270, 1985.
83. Jewell LD, Fields AL, Murray CJW, Thomson ABR: Erosive gastroduodenitis with marked epithelial atypia after hepatic infusion chemotherapy. Am J Gastroenterol 80:421–424, 1985.
84. Schuger L, Peretz T, Goldin E, et al: Duodenal epitheleal atypia: A specific complication of hepatic arterial infusion chemotherapy. Cancer 61:663–666, 1988.
85. Shapiro N, Brandt L, Sproyregan S, et al: Duodenal infarction after therapeutic gel-foam embolization of bleeding duodenal ulcer. Gastroenterology 80:176–180, 1981.
86. Shepherd HA, Patal C, Bamforth J, Isaacson P: Upper gastrointestinal endoscopy in systemic vasculitis presenting as an acute abdomen. Endoscopy 15:307–311, 1983.
87. Weiser MM, Adreas GA, Brentjens JR: Systemic lupus erythematosus and intestinal venulitis. Gastroenterology 81:570–579, 1981.
88. Camilleri M, Pusey CD, Chadwick VS, Rees AJ: Gastrointestinal manifestations of systemic vasculitis. Q J Med 206:141–149, 1983.
89. Socinski MA, Frankel JP, Morrow PL, Krawitt L: Painless diarrhea secondary to intestinal ischemia: Diagnosis of atheromatous emboli by jejunal biopsy. Dig Dis Sci 29:674–677, 1984.
90. Rutgeerts P, Onette E, Vantrappen G, et al: Crohn's disease of the stomach and duodenum: A clinical study with emphasis on the value of endoscopy and endoscopic biopsies. Endoscopy 12:288, 1980.
91. Korelitz BI, Waye JD, Kreuning J, et al: Crohn's disease in endoscopic biopsies of the gastric antrum and duodenum. Am J Gastroenterol 76:103–109, 1981.
92. Fielding JF, Toye DKM, Beton DC, et al: Crohn's disease of the stomach and duodenum. Gut 11:1001, 1970.
93. Wise L, Kyriakos M, McCown A, et al: Crohn's disease of the duodenum. Am J Surg 121:184–194, 1971.
94. Frandsen PJ, Jarnum S, Malmstrom J: Crohn's disease of the duodenum. Scand J Gastroenterol 15:683–688, 1980.
95. Tanaka M, Kimura K, Sakai H, et al: Long-term follow-up for minute gastroduodenal lesions in Crohn's disease. Gastrointest Endosc 32:206–209, 1986.
96. Rubin CE, Brandborg LL, Phelps PC, Taylor HC, Jr: Studies of celiac disease. I. Apparent identical and specific nature of duodenal and proximal jejunal lesion in celiac disease and idiopathic sprue. Gastroenterology 38:28–49, 1960.
97. Trier JS, Falchuck ZM, Carey MC, et al: Celiac sprue and refractory sprue. Gastroenterology 75:307–316, 1978.
98. Falchuk ZM: Update on gluten-sensitive enteropathy. Am J Med 67:50, 1979.
99. Yardley JH, Bayless TM, Norton JH, et al: Celiac disease: A study of the jejunal epithelium before and after a gluten-free diet. N Engl J Med 267:1173–1179, 1962.
100. Schenk EA, Samloff IM, Klipstein FA: Morphologic characteristics of jejunal biopsy in celiac disease and tropical sprue. Am J Pathol 47:765–781, 1965.
101. Variend S, Phillips AD, Walker-Smith JA: The small intestinal mucosal biopsy in childhood. Perspect Pediatr Pathol 1:57–78, 1984.
102. Dobbins WO III: Small bowel biopsy in malabsorptive states. In Norris HT (ed): Pathology of the Colon, Small Intestine, and Anus. New York, Churchill Livingstone, 1983, pp 121–165.
103. Kluge F, Koch HK, Grosse-Wilde H, et al: Follow-up of treated adult celiac disease: Clinical and morphological studies. Acta Hepato Gastroenterol 29:17–23, 1982.

104. Bramble MG, Zucolato S, Wright NA, Record CC: Acute gluten challenge in treated adult coeliac disease: A morphometric and enzymatic study. Gut 26:159–174, 1985.
105. Loft DE, Marsh MN, Crowe PT: Rectal gluten challenge and diagnosis of coeliac disease. Lancet 335:1293–1295, 1990.
106. Grybowski JD: Gastrointestinal milk allergy in infants. Pediatrics 40:354–360, 1967.
107. Dobbins JW, Sheahan DG, Behar J: Eosinophilic gastroenteritis with esophageal involvement. Gastroenterology 72:1312–1316, 1977.
108. Katz AJ, Goldman H, Grand RJ: Gastric mucosal biopsy in eosinophilic (allergic) gastroenteritis. Gastroenterology 73:705–709, 1977.
109. Goldman H, Proujansky R: Allergic proctitis and gastroenteritis in children. Clinical and mucosal biopsy features in 53 cases. Am J Surg Pathol 10:75–86, 1986.
110. Shiner M, Ballard J, Brook CGD, et al: Intestinal biopsy in the diagnosis of cow's milk protein intolerance without acute symptoms. Lancet 2:1060–1063, 1975.
111. Walker-Smith JA, Harrison M, Kilby A, et al: Cow's milk–sensitive enteropathy. Arch Dis Child 53:375–380, 1978.
112. Ament M, Rubin CE: Soy protein—another cause of the flat intestinal lesion. Gastroenterology 62:227–234, 1972.
113. Perkkio M, Savilahti E, Kuitunen P: Morphometric and immunohistochemical study of jejunal biopsies from children with intestinal soy allergy. Fin Eur J Pediatr 137:63–69, 1981.
114. Waldmann TA, Wochner RD, Laster L, et al: Allergic gastroenteropathy: A cause of excessive gastrointestinal protein loss. N Engl J Med 276:761–769, 1967.
115. Klein NC, Hargrove RL, Sleisenger MH, et al: Eosinophilic gastroenteritis. Medicine 40:299–319, 1970.
116. Teele RL, Katz AJ, Goldman H, et al: Radiographic features of eosinophilic gastroenteritis (allergic gastroenteropathy) of childhood. Am J Radiol 132:575–580, 1979.
117. Rosekrans PCM, Meijer CJLM, Cornelisse CJ, et al: Use of morphometry and immunohistochemistry of small intestinal biopsy specimens in the diagnosis of food allergy. J Clin Pathol 33:125–130, 1980.
118. Leinbach GE, Rubin CE: Eosinophilic gastroenteritis: A simple reaction to food allergies? Gastroenterology 59:874–889, 1970.
119. Ament ME, Ochs HD, Davis SD: Structure and function of the gastrointestinal tract in primary immunodeficiency syndromes: A study of 39 patients. Medicine 52:227–248, 1973.
120. Perlmutter PH, Leichtner AM, Goldman H, Winter HS: Chronic diarrhea associated with hypogammaglobulinemia and enteropathy in infants and children. Dig Dis Sci 30:1149–1155, 1985.
121. Snover DC, Weisdorf SA, Vercolotti GM, et al: A histopathologic study of gastric and small intestinal graft-versus-host disease following allogeneic bone marrow transplantation. Hum Pathol 16:387–392, 1985.
122. Spencer GD, Shulman HM, Mayerson D, et al: Diffuse intestinal ulceration after marrow transplantation: A clinicopathologic study of 13 patients. Hum Pathol 17:621–633, 1986.
123. Jeffries GH, Steinberg H, Sleisenger MH: Chronic ulcerative (nongranulomatous) jejunitis. Am J Med 44:47–59, 1968.
124. Corlin RF, Pops MA: Nongranulomatous ulcerative jejunoileitis with hypogammaglobulinemia. Gastroenterology 62:473–478, 1972.
125. Modigliani R, Poitras P, Galian A, et al: Chronic non-specific ulcerative duodenojejunoileitis: Report of four cases. Gut 20:318–328, 1979.
126. Isaacson P, Wright DH: Malignant histiocytosis of the intestine: Its relationship to malabsorption and ulcerative jejunitis. Hum Pathol 9:661–677, 1978.
127. Baer AN, Bayless TM, Yardley JH: Intestinal ulceration and malabsorption syndromes. Gastroenterology 79:754–765, 1980.
128. Robertson DAF, Dixon MF, Scott BB, et al: Small intestinal ulceration: Diagnostic difficulties in relation to coeliac disease. Gut 24:565–574, 1983.
129. Bayless TM, Kapelowitz RF, Shelley WM, et al: Intestinal ulceration—a complication of celiac disease. N Engl J Med 276:996–1002, 1967.
130. Isaacson PG, Spencer J, Connolly CE, et al: Malignant histiocytosis of the intestine: A T cell lymphoma. Lancet 2:688–691, 1985.
131. Passaro E Jr, Drenick E, Wilson SE: Bypass enteritis: A new complication of jejunoileal bypass for obesity. Am J Surg 131:169–174, 1976.
132. Drenick EJ, Ament ME, Finegold SM, et al: Bypass enteropathy: Intestinal and systemic manifestations following small bowel bypass. JAMA 236:269–272, 1976.
133. Francis WW, Iannuccilli E: Acute fulminating transmural ileocolitis after small bowel bypass for morbid obesity. Am J Surg 135:524–528, 1978.
134. Causey JQ: Granulomatous colitis and ileitis complicating jejunoileal bypass. Arch Intern Med 138:1727, 1978.
135. Morson BC, Dawson IMP: Gastrointestinal Pathology, 2nd ed. London, Blackwell Scientific Publishers, 1979, p 565.
136. Baillie EE, Abell MR: Enteritis cystica polyposa. Am J Clin Pathol 54:643–649, 1970.
137. Kyriakos M, Condon SC: Enteritis cystica profunda. Am J Clin Pathol 69:77–85, 1978.
138. Aftalion B, Lipper S: Enteritis cystica profunda associated with Crohn's disease. Arch Pathol Lab Med 108:532–533, 1984.
139. Saul SH, Wong LK, Zinsser KR: Enteritis cystica profunda: Association with Crohn's disease. Hum Pathol 17:600–603, 1986.
140. Bolwell JS, James PD: Peutz-Jeghers syndrome with pseudoinvasion of hamartomatous polyp and multiple epithelial neoplasms. Histopathology 3:39–50, 1979.
141. Shepherd NA, Bussey HJR, Jass JR: Epithelial misplacement in Peutz-Jeghers polyps: A diagnostic pitfall. Am J Surg Pathol 11:743–749, 1987.
142. Watson MR: Primary nonspecific ulceration of the small bowel. Arch Surg 87:600–603, 1963.
143. Boydstan JS Jr, Gaffey TA, Bartholomew LG: Clinicopathologic study of non-specific ulcers of the small intestine. Dig Dis Sci 26:911–916, 1981.
144. Wayte DM, Helwig EB: Small bowel ulceration: Iatrogenic or multifactorial origin? Am J Clin Pathol 49:26–40, 1968.
145. Wilson IH, Cooley NV, Luibel FJ: Non-specific stenosing small bowel ulcers. Am J Gastroenterol 50:449–455, 1968.
146. Bradford WD, Norce PS, Gutman LT, et al: Pathologic features of enteric infection with Yersinia enterocolitica. Arch Pathol 98:17–22, 1974.
147. El-Maraghi NRH, Mair NS: The histopathology of enteric infection with Yersinia pseudotuberculosis. Am J Clin Pathol 71:631–639, 1979.
148. Lawrason FD, Alpert E, Mohr FL, McMahon FG: Ulcerative-obstructive lesions of the small intestine. JAMA 191:641–644, 1965.
149. Weiss SM, Rutenberg HL, Paskin DL, Zoren HA: Gut lesions due to slow-release KCl tablets. N Engl J Med 296:111–112, 1977.
150. Barloon T, Moore SA, Mitros FA: A case of stenotic obstruction of the jejunum secondary to slow-release potassium. Am J Gastroenterol 81:192–194, 1986.
151. Jackson CW, Haboubi NY, Whorwell PJ, Schofield PF: Gold-induced enterocolitis. J Clin Gastroenterol 27:452–456, 1986.
152. Geltner D, Sternfeld M, Becker SA, Kori M: Gold-induced ileitis. J Clin Gastroenterol 8:184–186, 1986.
153. Bjarnson I, Price AB, Zanelli G, et al: Clinicopathological features of nonsteroidal anti-inflammatory drug-induced small intestinal strictures. Gastroenterology 94:1070–1074, 1988.
154. Davies DR, Brightmore T: Idiopathic and drug-induced ulceration of the small intestine. Br J Surg 57:134–139, 1970.
155. Kiser JL: Focal lesions of the small intestine. Am J Surg 112:48–51, 1966.
156. Bo-Linn GW, Vendrell DD, Lee E, Fordtran JS: An evaluation of the significance of microscopic colitis in patients with chronic diarrhea. J Clin Invest 75:1559–1569, 1985.
157. Read NW, Krejs GJ, Read MG, et al: Chronic diarrhea of unknown origin. Gastroenterology 78:264–271, 1980.
158. Giardiello FM, Bayles TM, Jesserun J, et al: Collagenous colitis: Physiologic and histopathologic studies in seven patients. Ann Intern Med 106:46–49, 1987.
159. Lazenby AJ, Yardley JH, Giardiello FM, et al: Lymphocytic ("microscopic") colitis: A comparative histopathologic study with particular reference to collagenous colitis. Hum Pathol 20:18–28, 1989.

160. Kingham JGC, Levinson DA, Ball JA, Dawson AM: Microscopic colitis—a cause of chronic watery diarrhea. Br Med J 285:1601–1604, 1982.
161. Surawicz CM, Belic L: Rectal biopsy helps to distinguish acute self-limited colitis from idiopathic inflammatory bowel disease. Gastroenterology 86:104–113, 1984.
162. Lindstrom CG: "Collagenous colitis" with watery diarrhea: A new entity? Pathol Eur 11:87–89, 1976.
163. Freeman HF, Weinstein WM, Shnitka TK, et al: Watery diarrhea syndrome associated with a lesion of the colonic basement membrane-lamina protein interface. Ann Roy Coll Phys Surg Canada 9:45, 1976.
164. Nielsen VT, Vetner M, Harslof E: Collagenous colitis. Histopathology 4:83–86, 1980.
165. Bogomoletz WV, Adnet JJ, Birembaut P, et al: Collagenous colitis: An unrecognized entity. Gut 21:164–168, 1980.
166. Colina F, Solis-Herruzo JA, et al: Collagenous colitis: The clinical and morphological features. Postgrad Med J 58:390–395, 1982.
167. Bamford M, Matz LR, et al: Collagenous colitis: A case report and review of the literature. Hum Pathol 14:481–484, 1982.
168. Pieterse AS, Hecker R, Rowland R: Collagenous colitis: a distinctive and potentially reversible disorder. J Clin Pathol 35:338–340, 1982.
169. Teglbjaerg PS, Tharpen EH: Collagenous colitis: An ultrastructural study of a case. Gastroenterology 82:561–563, 1982.
170. Van den Oord JJ, Geboes K, Desmet VJ: Collagenous colitis: An abnormal collagen table? Two new cases and review of the literature. Am J Gastroenterol 77:377–381, 1982.
171. Grouls V, Vogel J, Sorger M: Collagenous colitis. Endoscopy 14:31–33, 1982.
172. Bogomoletz WV: Collagenous colitis. Gastroenterology 83:727, 1982.
173. Guarda LA, Nelson R, Stroehlein JR, et al: Collagenous colitis. Am J Clin Pathol 80:503–507, 1983.
174. Eaves ER, Wallis PL, McIntyre RL, et al: Collagenous colitis: A recently recognized reversible clinicopathological entity. Aust NZ J Med 13:630–632, 1983.
175. Debongnie JC, DeGalocsy C, Caholessur O, Hoat J: et al: Collagenous colitis: A transient condition? Report of two cases. Dis Colon Rectum 27:672–676, 1984.
176. Flejou JF, Grimaud JA, Molas G: Collagenous colitis: Ultrastructural study and collagen immunotyping of four cases. Arch Pathol Lab Med 198:977–982, 1984.
177. Yeshaza C, Novis B, Bernheim J, et al: Collagenous colitis: Report of a case. Dis Colon Rectum 27:111–113, 1984.
178. Teglbjaerg PS, Tharpen EH, Jensen HH: Development of collagenous colitis in sequential biopsy specimens. Gastroenterology 87:703–709, 1984.
179. Weidner N, Smith J, Pattee B: Sulfasalazine in treatment of collagenous colitis. Am J Med 77:162–166, 1984.
180. Farar DA, Mills PR, Lee FD, et al: Collagenous colitis: Possible response to sulfasalazine and local steroid therapy. Gastroenterology 88:792–797, 1985.
181. Palmer KR, Berry H, Wheeler PJ, et al: Collagenous colitis: A relapsing and remitting disease. Gut 27:578–580, 1986.
182. Kingham JGC, Levison DA, Morson BC, Dawson AM: Collagenous colitis. Gut 27:550–557, 1986.
183. Hwang WS, Kelley JK, Shaffer EA, Hershfield NB: Collagenous colitis: A disease of pencryptal fibroblastic sheath. J Pathol 149:33–40, 1986.
184. Coverlizza S, Ferrari A, Scevola F, et al: Clinico-pathological features of collagenous colitis: Case report and literature review. Am J Gastroenterol 81:1098–1103, 1986.
185. Lazenby A, Jessurun J, Levine E, et al: Comparative study of microscopic and collagenous colitis. (Abstract) Lab Invest 56:42A, 1987.
186. Rask-Madsen J, Grove O, Hansen MGJ, et al: Colonic transport of water and electrolytes in a patient with secretory diarrhea due to collagenous colitis. Dig Dis Sci 28:1141–1146, 1983.
187. Mason CH, Jewell DP: Collagenous colitis: A report of five cases. (Abstract) Gut 26:A1152, 1985.
188. Rams H, Rogergs AI, Ghandus-Mnaymneh L: Collagenous colitis. Ann Intern Med 106:108–113, 1987.
189. Salt WB II, Llaneza PP: Collagenous colitis: A cause of chronic diarrhea diagnosed only by biopsy of normal appearing colonic mucosa. Gastrointest Endosc 32:421–423, 1986.
190. Jesserun J, Yardley JH, Giardiello FM, et al: Chronic colitis with thickening of the subepithelial collagen layer (collagenous colits): Histopathologic findings in 15 patients. Hum Pathol 18:839–848, 1987.
191. Wang HH, Owings DV, Antonioli DA, Goldman H: Increased subepithelial collagen deposition is not specific for collagenous colitis. Modern Pathol 1:329–335, 1988.
192. Hamilton I, Sander S, Hopwood D, Bouchier IAD: Collagenous colitis associated with small intestinal villous atrophy. Gut 27:1394–1398, 1986.
193. Eckstein RP, Dowsett JF, Riley JW: Collagenous enterocolitis: A case of collagenous colitis with involvement of the small intestine. Am J Gastroenterol 83:767–771, 1988.
194. Wiener MD: Collagenous colitis and pulmonary fibrosis: Manifestations of a single disease? J Clin Gastroenterol 8:677–680, 1986.
195. Gledhill A, Cole FM: Significance of basement membrane thickening in the human colon. Gut 25:1085–1088, 1984.
196. Guller R, Anabitarte M: "Collagenous colitis": New entity or simply a histologic anomaly? Schweiz Med Wochenschr 111:1076–1079, 1981.
197. Gardiner GW, Goldberg R, Currie D, Murray D: Colonic carcinoma associated with an abnormal collagen table. Cancer 54:2973–2977, 1984.
198. Glotzer DJ, Glick ME, Goldman H: Proctitis and colitis following diversion of the fecal stream. Gastroenterology 80:438–441, 1981.
199. Korelitz BI, Cheskin LJ, Sohn N, Sommers SC: Proctitis after fecal diversion in Crohn's disease and its elimination with reanastomosis: Implication for surgical management: Report of four cases. Gastroenterology 87:710–713, 1984.
200. Lush LB, Reichen J, Levine JS: Aphthous ulceration in diversion colitis: Clinical applications. Gastroenterology 87:1171–1173, 1984.
201. Bosshardt RT, Abel ME: Proctitis following fecal diversion. Dis Colon Rectum 27:605–607, 1984.
202. Ona FV, Bogar JN: Rectal bleeding due to diversion colitis. Am J Gastroenterol 80:40–41, 1985.
203. Bories C, Miazza B, Galian A, et al: Idiopathic chronic watery diarrhea from excluded rectosigmoid with goblet cell hyperplasia cured by restoration of large bowel continuity. Dig Dis Sci 31:769–772, 1986.
204. Murray FE, O'Brien MJ, Birkett DH, et al: Diversion colitis: Pathologic findings in a resected sigmoid colon and rectum. Gastroenterology 93:1404–1408, 1987.
205. Harig JM, Soergel KH, Komorowski RA, Wood CM: Treatment of diversion colitis with short-chain fatty acid irrigation. N Engl J Med 320:23–28, 1989.
206. Ma CK, Gottlieb C, Haas PA: Diversion colitis: A clinicopathologic study of 21 cases. Hum Pathol 21:429–436, 1990.
207. Komorowski RA: Histologic spectrum of diversion colitis. Am J Surg Pathol 14:548–554, 1990.
208. Price AB, Davies DR: Pseudomembranous colitis. J Clin Pathol 30:1–12, 1977.
209. Kumar NB, Nostrant TT, Appelman HD: The histopathologic spectrum of acute self-limited colitis (acute infectious colitis). Am J Surg Pathol 6:523–529, 1982.
210. Nostrant TT, Kumar NB, Appelman HD: Histopathology differentiates acute self-limited colitis from ulcerative colitis. Gastroenterology 92:318–328, 1987.
211. Goldman H: Acute versus chronic colitis: How and when to distinguish by biopsy. (Editorial) Gastroenterology 86:199–201, 1984.
212. Goodall HB, Sinclair ISR: Colitis cystica profunda. J Pathol Bacteriol 73:33–42, 1957.
213. Epstein SE, Ascari WQ, Ablow RC, et al: Colitis cystica profunda. Am J Clin Pathol 45:186–201, 1966.
214. Herman AH, Nabseth DC: Colitis cystica profunda: Localized, segmental, and diffuse. Arch Surg 106:337, 1973.
215. Martin JK Jr, Culp CE, Werland LH: Colitis cystica profunda. Dis Colon Rectum 23:488, 1980.
216. Dyson JD; Hernation of mucosal epithelium into the submucosa in chronic ulcerative colitis. J Clin Pathol 28:189, 1975.
217. Clark RM: Microdiverticula and submucosal epithelial elements

218. Gardiner GW, McAuliffe N, Murray D: Colitis cystica profunda occurring in a radiation-induced colonic stricture. Hum Pathol 15:295–298, 1984.
219. Magidson JG, Lewin KJ: Diffuse colitis cystica profunda: Report of a case. Am J Surg Pathol 5:393, 1981.
220. Bentley E, Chandrasoma P, Cohen H, et al: Colitis cystica profunda: Presenting with complete intestinal obstruction and recurrence. Gastroenterology 89:1157–1161, 1985.
221. Sobin LH: Inverted hyperplastic polyps of the colon. Am J Surg Pathol 9:265–272, 1985.
222. Muto T, Bussey HJR, Morson BC: Pseudo-carcinomatous invasion in adenomatous polyps of the colon and rectum. J Clin Pathol 26:25–31, 1973.
223. Wayte DM, Helwig EB: Colitis cystica profunda. Am J Clin Pathol 48:159–169, 1966.
224. Haskell B, Rovner H: Solitary ulcer of the rectum. Dis Colon Rectum 8:333, 1965.
225. Allen MS: Hamartomatous inverted polyps of the rectum. Cancer 19:257, 1966.
226. Fechner RE: Polyp of the colon possessing features of colitis cystica profunda. Dis Colon Rectum 10:359, 1967.
227. Madigan MR, Morson BC: Solitary ulcer of the rectum. Gut 10:871–881, 1969.
228. Tallerman A: Enterogenous cysts of the rectum (colitis cystica profunda). Br J Surg 58:643, 1971.
229. Rutter K, Riddell RH: The solitary ulcer syndrome of the rectum. Clin Gastroenterol 4:505–530, 1975.
230. Schweiger M, Williams JA: Solitary ulcer syndrome of the rectum: Its association with occult rectal prolapse. Lancet 2:170–171, 1977.
231. Bogomoletz W, Fenzy A: Histopathological features of the solitary ulcer syndrome of the rectum. Arch Anat Cytol Pathol 28:329, 1980.
232. Franzin G, Dina R, Scarpa A, Fratton A: The evolution of the solitary ulcer of the rectum: An endoscopic and histopathological study. Endoscopy 14:131–134, 1982.
233. Ford MJ, Anderson JR, Gilmour HM, et al: Clinical spectrum of "solitary ulcer" of the rectum. Gastroenterology 84:1533–1540, 1983.
234. DuBoulay CE, Fairbrother J, Isaacson PG: Mucosal prolapse syndrome: A unifying concept for solitary ulcer syndrome and related disorders. J Clin Pathol 36:1264–1268, 1983.
235. Stuart M: Proctitis cystica profunda: Incidence, etiology and treatment. Dis Colon Rectum 27:153–156, 1984.
236. Saul SH, Sollenberger LC: Solitary rectal ulcer syndrome: Its clinical and pathological underdiagnosis. Am J Surg Pathol 9:411–421, 1985.
237. Levine DS: Solitary rectal ulcer syndrome: Are "solitary" rectal ulcer syndrome and "localized" colitis cystica profunda analogous syndromes caused by rectal prolapse? Gastroenterology 92:243–253, 1987.
238. Saul SH: Inflammatory cloacogenic polyp: Relationship to solitary rectal ulcer syndrome/mucosal prolapse and other bowel disorders. Hum Pathol 18:1120–1125, 1987.
239. Keighley MR, Shouler P: Clinical and manometric features of the solitary rectal ulcer syndrome. Dis Colon Rectum 27:507–512, 1984.
240. Lobert PF, Appelman HP: Inflammatory cloacogenic polyp: A unique inflammatory lesion of the anal transitional zone. Am J Surg Pathol 5:761–766, 1981.
241. Niv Y, Bat L: Solitary rectal ulcer syndrome: Clinical, endoscopic, and histological spectrum. Am J Gastroenterol 81:486–491, 1986.
242. Levine DS, Surawicz CM, Ajer T, et al: Diffuse excess mucosal collagen in rectal biopsies facilitates differential diagnosis of solitary rectal ulcer syndrome from other inflammatory bowel diseases. Dig Dis Sci 33:1345–1352, 1988.
243. Bockus HL, Willard JH, Bank J: Melanosis coli: The etiologic significance of the anthracene laxatives: A report of 41 cases. JAMA 101:1–6, 1933.
244. Schrodt GR: Melanosis coli: A study with the electron microscope. Dis Colon Rectum 6:277–283, 1963.
245. Ghadially FN, Parry EW: An electronmicroscope and histochemical study of melanosis coli. J Pathol Bacteriol 92:313–317, 1966.
246. Wittoesch JH, Jackman RJ, MacDonald JR: Melanosis coli: General review and study of 887 cases. Dis Colon Rectum 1:172–180, 1958.
247. Steer HW, Colin-Jones DG: Melanosis coli: Studies of the toxic effects of irritant purgatives. J Pathol 115:199, 1975.
248. Levine DS, Haggitt RC: Normal histology of the colon. Am J Surg Pathol 13:966–984, 1989.
249. Breslaw L: Melanosis of the duodenal mucosa. Gastrointest Endosc 26:45–46, 1980.
250. Cowen ML, Humphries TJ: Pseudomelanosis of the duodenum. Gastrointest Endosc 26:107–108, 1980.
251. Ganju S, Adomavicius J, Salgia K, Steigmann F: The endoscopic picture of melanosis in the duodenum. Gastrointest Endosc 26:44–45, 1980.
252. Sharp JR, Insalaco SJ, Johnson LF: "Melanosis" of the duodenum associated with a gastric ulcer and folic acid deficiency. Gastroenterology 78:366–369, 1980.
253. Yamare H, Norris M, Gillier C: Pseudomelanosis duodeni: A clinicopathologic entity. Gastrointest Endosc 31:83–86, 1985.
254. Gupta TP, Weinstock JV: Duodenal pseudomelanosis associated with chronic renal failure. Gastrointest Endosc 32:358–360, 1986.
255. Kang JY, Wu AYT, Chia JLS, et al: Clinical and ultrastructural studies in duodenal pseudomelanosis. Gut 28:1673–1681, 1987.
256. Smith B: Pathology of cathartic colon. Proc Roy Soc Med 65:288, 1972.
257. Urso FP, Urso MJ, Lee CH: The cathartic colon: Pathological findings and radiological/pathological correlation. Radiology 116:557–559, 1975.
258. Smith B: Pathologic changes in the colon produced by antraquinone purgatives. Dis Colon Rectum 16:455–458, 1973.
259. Heilbrun N, Bernstein C: Roentgen abnormalities of the large and small intestine associated with prolonged cathartic ingestion. Radiology 65:549–556, 1955.
260. Ziter FMH Jr: Cathartic colon. NY State J Med 67:546–549, 1967.
261. Anuras S, Shirazi SS: Colonic pseudoobstruction. Am J Gastroenterol 79:525–532, 1984.
262. Heizer WD, Warshaw AL, Walkman TA: Protein-losing gastroenteropathy and malabsorption associated with factitious diarrhea. Ann Intern Med 68:839–852, 1968.
263. Oster JR, Materson BJ, Rogers AI: Laxative abuse syndrome. Am J Gastroenterol 74:451–458, 1980.
264. Sommers SC, Korelitz BI: Mucosal cell counts in ulcerative and granulomatous colitis. Am J Clin Pathol 63:359–365, 1975.
265. Pockros PJ, Foroozan P: Golytely lavage versus standard colonoscopy preparation: Effect on normal colonic mucosal histology. Gastroenterology 88:845–848, 1985.
266. Meisel JL, Bergman D, Graney D, et al: Human rectal mucosa: Proctoscopic and morphological changes caused by laxatives. Gastroenterology 72:1274–1279, 1977.
267. Leriche M, Devroede G, Sanchez G, et al: Changes in the rectal mucosa induced by hypertonic enemas. Dis Colon Rectum 21:227–236, 1978.
268. Meyer CT, Brand M, DeLuca VA, Spriro HM: Hydrogen peroxide colitis: A report of three patients. J Clin Gastroenterol 3:31–35, 1981.
269. Hardin RD, Tedesco FJ: Colitis after Hibiclens enema. J Clin Gastroenterol 8:572–575, 1986.
270. Barker CS: Acute colitis resulting from soapsuds enema. Can Med Assoc J 52:285–286, 1945.
271. Pike BF, Phillippi PJ, Lawson EH: Soap colitis. N Engl J Med 285:217–218, 1971.
272. Bendit M: Gangrene of the rectum as a complication of an enema. Br Med J 1:664, 1945.
273. Segal I, Tim LO, Hamilton DG et al: Ritual-enema-induced colitis. Dis Colon Rectum 22:195–199, 1979.
274. Chajek T, Fainaru M: Behçet's disease: Report of 41 cases and a review of the literature. Medicine 54:179–196, 1975.
275. Lakhanpal S, Tani K, Lie JT, et al: Pathologic features of Behçet's syndrome: A review of Japanese autopsy registry data. Hum Pathol 16:790–795, 1985.

276. Smith GE, Kime LR, Pitcher JL: The colitis of Behçet's disease: A separate entity? Colonoscopic findings and literature review. Dig Dis Sci 18:987–1000, 1973.
277. Baba S, Maruta M, Ando K, et al: Intestinal Behçet's disease: Report of five cases. Dis Colon Rectum 19:428–440, 1976.
278. Johnson DA, Everhart CW: Colitis in Behçet's syndrome. Gastrointest Endosc 32:58–59, 1986.
279. Lee RG: The colitis of Behçet's syndrome. Am J Surg Pathol 10:888–893, 1986.
280. Mori S, Yoshihira A, Kawamura H, et al: Esophageal involvement in Behçet's disease. Am J Gastroenterol 78:548–553, 1983.
281. Yashiro K, Nagasako K, Hasegawa K, et al: Esophageal lesions in intestinal Behçet's disease. Endoscopy 18:57–60, 1986.
282. Anti M, Marra G, Rapaccini GL, et al: Exophageal involvement in Behçet's syndrome. J Clin Gastroenterol 8:514–519, 1986.
283. Good AE, Mutchnick MG, Weatherbee L: Duodenal ulcer, hepatic abscess, and fatal hemobilia with Behçet's syndrome: A case report. Am J Gastroenterol 77:905–909, 1982.
284. Satake K, Yada K, Ikehara T, et al: Pyloric stenosis: An unusual complication of Behçet's disease. Am J Gastroenterol 81:816–818, 1986.
285. Grinvalsky HT, Bowerman CI: Stercoraceous ulcers of the colon: Relatively neglected medical and surgical problem. JAMA 171:1941–1946, 1959.
286. Milliser RV, Greenberg SR, Neiman BH: Exsanguinating stercoral ulceration. Am J Dig Dis 15:485–488, 1970.
287. Liedberg G: Stercoraceous perforations of the colon. Acta Clin Scand 135:552, 1969.
288. Gekas P, Schuster MM; Stercoral perforation of the colon: Case report and review of the literature. Gastroenterology 80:1054–1058, 1981.
289. Barlow D: Simple ulcer of the cecum, colon and rectum. Br J Surg 28:575–581, 1941.
290. Friedman MH, MacKenzie WC: Simple ulcer of the colon. Can J Surg 2:279, 1959.
291. Yates LN, Clausen EG: Simple nonspecific ulcers of the sigmoid colon. Arch Surg 81:535–541, 1960.
292. Miller SM, Juhl JH: Nonspecific ulcers of the colon. Minn Med 50:1327, 1967.
293. Smithwick W, Anderson RP, Ballinger WF: Nonspecific ulcer of the colon. Arch Surg 97:133–138, 1968.
294. Butsch JL, Dockerty MB, McGill DM, Judd ES: Solitary nonspecific ulcer of the colon. Arch Surg 98:171–174, 1969.
295. Benninger GW, Honig LJ, Fein HD: Non-specific ulceration of the cecum. Am J Gastroenterol 55:594–601, 1971.
296. Corry RJ, Bartlett NK, Cohen RB: Erosions of the cecum: A cause of massive hemorrhage. Am J Surg 119:106–110, 1970.
297. Mahoney TJ, Bubrick MP, Hitchcock CR: Nonspecific ulcers of the colon. Dis Colon Rectum 21:623–626, 1978.
298. Blundell CR, Earnest DL: Idiopathic cecal ulcer: Diagnosis by colonoscopy followed by nonoperative management. Dig Dis Sci 25:494–503, 1980.
299. Shah NC, Ostrov AH, Cavallero JB, Rodgers JB: Benign ulcers of the colon. Gastrointest Endosc 32:102–104, 1986.
300. Wormann B, Hochter W, Seib H-J, Ottenjann R: Ergotamine-induced colitis. Endoscopy 17:165–166, 1985.
301. Eckardt VF, Kanzler G, Remmele W: Anorectal ergotism: Another cause of solitary rectal ulcers. Gastroenterology 91:1123–1127, 1986.
302. Bernardino ME, Lawson TL: Discrete colonic ulcers associated with oral contraceptives. Dig Dis Sci 21:503–506, 1976.
303. Tedesco FJ, Volpicelli NA, Moore FS: Estrogen- and progesterone-associated colitis: A disorder with clinical and endoscopic features mimicking Crohn's colitis. Gastrointest Endosc 28:247–249, 1982.
304. Fortson WC, Tedesco FJ: Drug-induced colitis: A review. Am J Gastroenterol 79:878–883, 1984.
305. Korelitz BL: Atherosclerotic emboli. (Letter) Dig Dis Sci 30:506, 1985.
306. Tribe CR, Scott DGI, Bacon PA: Rectal biopsy in the diagnosis of systemic vasculitis. J Clin Pathol 34:843–850, 1981.
307. Geraghty J, Machay IR, Smith DC: Intestinal perforation in Wegener's granulomatosis. Gut 27:450–451, 1986.
308. Mason EE: Gastrointestinal lesions occurring in uremia. Ann Intern Med 37:96–105, 1952.
309. Sutherland DER, Chan FY, Foucar E, et al: The bleeding cecal ulcer in transplant patients. Surgery 86:386–398, 1979.
310. Huded F, Posner GL, Tick R: Non-specific ulcer of the colon in a chronic hemodialysis patient. Am J Gastroenterol 77:913–916, 1982.
311. Dosik GM, Luna M, Valdiviesv M, et al: Necrotizing colitis in patients with cancer. Am J Med 67:646–656, 1979.
312. Kies MS, Luedke DW, Boyd JF, McCue MJ: Neutropenic enterocolitis. Cancer 43:730–734, 1979.
313. Ryan ME, Morrissey JF: Typhlitis complicating methimazole-induced agranulocytosis. Gastrointest Endosc 29:299–302, 1983.
314. Saegesser F, Sandblom P: Ischemic lesions of the distended colon: A complication of obstructive colorectal cancer. Am J Surg 129:309–315, 1975.
315. Nalbundian H, Sketh N, Dietrich R, et al: Intestinal ischemia caused by cocaine ingestion: Report of two cases. Surgery 97:374–376, 1985.
316. Jonas G, Mahoney A, Murray J, Gertler S: Chemical colitis due to endoscopic cleansing solutions: A mimic of pseudomembranous colitis. Gastroenterology 95:1403–1408, 1988.
317. Williams KL: Acute solitary ulcers and acute diverticulitis of the cecum and ascending colon. Br J Surg 47:351–358, 1960.
318. Mitsudo SM, Boley SJ, Brandt LJ, et al: Vascular ectasias of the right colon in the elderly: A distinct pathologic entity. Hum Pathol 10:585–600, 1979.
319. Sale GE, Shulman HM, McDonald JB, et al: Gastrointestinal graft-versus-host disease in man: A clinicopathologic study of the rectal biopsy. Am J Surg Pathol 3:291, 1979.
320. Gallucci BB, Sale GE, McDonald GB, et al: The fine structure of human rectal epithelium in acute graft-versus-host disease. Am J Surg Pathol 6:293–305, 1982.
321. Ament ME, Ochs HD: Gastrointestinal manifestations of chronic granulomatous disease. N Engl J Med 288:382–387, 1973.
322. Werlin SL, Chusid MJ, Caya J, et al: Colitis in chronic granulomatous disease. Gastroenterology 82:328–331, 1982.
323. Lennard-Jones JE: Functional gastrointestinal disorders. N Engl J Med 308:431–435, 1983.
324. Hughes DTD, Gordon KCD, Swann JC, Bolt GL: Pneumatosis cystoides intestinalis. Gut 7:553–557, 1966.
325. Ecker JA, Williams RG, Clay KL: Pneumatosis cystoides intestinalis—bullous emphysema of the intestine: A review of the literature. Am J Gastroenterol 56:125–136, 1971.
326. Yale CE, Balish E: Pneumatosis cystoides intestinalis. Dis Colon Rectum 19:107–111, 1976.
327. Galondiuk S, Fazio VW: Pneumatosis cystoides intestinalis: A review of the literature. Dis Colon Rectum 29:358–363, 1986.
328. Keyting WS, McCarver RR, Kovarik JL, et al: Pneumatosis intestinalis: A new concept. Radiology 76:733, 1961.
329. Smith BH, Welter LH: Pneumatosis intestinalis. Am J Clin Pathol 48:455–465, 1967.
330. Nelson SW: Extraluminal gas collections due to diseases of the gastrointestinal tract. Am J Roentgenol 115:225–248, 1972.
331. Heer M, Altorfer J, Pirovino M, Schmid M: Pneumatosis cystoides coli: A rare complication of colonoscopy. Endoscopy 15:119–120, 1983.
332. Pieterse AS, Leong AS, Rowland R: The mucosal changes and pathogenesis of pneumatosis cystoides intestinalis. Hum Pathol 16:683–688, 1985.
333. Haboubi NY, Honan BP, Hasleton PS, et al: Pneumatosis coli: A case report with ultrastructural study. Histopathology 8:145–155, 1984.
334. Suarez V, Chesner IM, Price AB, Newman J: Pneumatosis cystoides intestinalis: Histological mucosal changes mimicking inflammatory bowel disease. Arch Pathol Lab Med 113:898–901, 1989.
335. Pemberton HW, Smith WG, Holman CB: Pneumatosis cystoides intestinalis diagnosed sigmoidoscopically. Am J Surg 94:472–477, 1957.
336. Jenkinson EL, Brown WH: Endometriosis: A study of 117 cases with special reference to constricting lesions of the rectum and sigmoid colon. JAMA 122:349–354, 1943.
337. Colcock BP, Lamphier TA: Endometriosis of the large and small intestine. Surgery 28:997–1004, 1950.

338. Boles RS, Hodes PJ: Endometriosis of the small and large intestine. Gastroenterology 34:367–380, 1958.
339. Tagart REB: Endometriosis of the large intestine. Br J Surg 47:27–34, 1959.
340. Spjut HJ, Perkins DE: Endometriosis of the sigmoid colon and rectum: A roentgenologic and pathologic study. AJR 82:1070–1075, 1959.
341. Parr NJ, Murphy C, Holt S, et al: Endometriosis and the gut. Gut 29:1112–1115, 1988.
342. Caccese WJ, McKinley MJ, Bronzo RL, Bronson R: Endoscopic confirmation of colonic endometriosis. Gastrointest Endosc 30:191–193, 1984.
343. Bashist B, Forde KA, McCaffrey RM: Polypoid endometrioma of the rectosigmoid. Gastrointest Radiol 8:85–88, 1983.
344. Aronchuck CA, Brooks FP, Dyson WL, et al: Ileocecal endometriosis presenting with abdominal pain and gastrointestinal bleeding. Dig Dis Sci 28:566–572, 1983.
345. Ledley GS, Shenk IM, Heit HA: Sigmoid colon perforation due to endometriosis not associated with pregnancy. Am J Gastroenterol 83:1424–1426, 1988.
346. Amano S, Yamada N: Endometrioid carcinoma arising from endometriosis of the sigmoid colon: A case report. Hum Pathol 12:845–849, 1981.
347. Wolff M: Heterotopic gastric epithelium in the rectum: A report of three new cases with a review of 87 cases of gastric heterotopia in the alimentary canal. Am J Clin Pathol 55:604–616, 1971.
348. Yokoyama I, Kozuka S, Ito K, et al: Gastric gland metaplasia in the small and large intestine. Gut 18:214–218, 1977.
349. Jabbori M, Goresky CA, Lough J, et al: The inlet patch: Heterotopic gastric mucosa in the upper esophagus. Gastroenterology 89:352–356, 1985.
350. Shah KK, DeRidder PH, Shah KK: Ectopic gastric mucosa in proximal esophagus: Its clinical significance and hormonal profile. J Clin Gastroenterol 8:509–513, 1986.
351. Truong LD, Stroebein JR, McKechnie JC: Gastric heterotopia of the proximal esophagus: A report of four cases detected by endoscopy and review of the literature. Am J Gastroenterol 81:1162–1166, 1986.
352. Steadman C, Kerlin P, Teague C, Stephenson P: High esophageal stricture: A complication of "inlet patch" mucosa. Gastroenterology 94:521–524, 1988.
353. Hoedemacher PJ: Heterotopic gastric mucosa in the duodenum. Digestion 3:165, 1970.
354. Franzin G, Musola R, Negri A, et al: Heterotopic gastric (fundic) mucosa in the duodenum. Endoscopy 14:166–167, 1982.
355. Spiller RC, Shousha S, Barrison IG: Heterotopic gastric tissue in the duodenum: A report of eight cases. Dig Dis Sci 27:880–883, 1982.
356. Lessells AM, Martin DF: Heterotopic gastric mucosa in the duodenum. J Clin Pathol 35:591–595, 1982.
357. Vizcarrondo FJ, Wang T-Y, Brady PG: Heterotopic gastric mucosa: Presentation as a rugose duodenal mass. Gastrointest Endosc 29:107–111, 1983.
358. Kundrotas LW, Camara DS, Meenaghan MA, et al: Heterotopic gastric mucosa: A case report. Am J Gastroenterol 80:253–256, 1985.
359. Debas HT, Chaun H, Thomson FB, et al: Functioning heterotopic oxyntic mucosa in the rectum. Gastroenterology 79:1300–1302, 1980.
360. Edouard J, Jouannelle A, Amor A, et al: Ulcerated heterotopic gastric mucosa located in the rectum. Gastroenterol Clin Biol 7:39–42, 1983.
361. Pistoia MA, Guadagni S, Tisiano D, et al: Ulcerated ectopic gastric mucosa of the rectum. Gastrointest Endosc 33:41–43, 1987.
362. Kaloni BP, Vaezzadeh K, Sieber WK: Gastric heterotopia in rectum complicated by rectovesical fistula. Dig Dis Sci 28:378–380, 1983.
363. Schwarzenberg SJ, Whitington PF: Rectal gastric mucosa heterotopia as a cause of hematochezia in an infant. Dig Dis Sci 28:470–472, 1983.
364. Galligan ML, Uhlich T, Lewin KJ: Heterotopic gastric mucosa in the jejunum causing intussusception. Arch Pathol Lab Med 107:335–336, 1983.
365. Seagram CG, Louch RE, Stephens CA, Wentworth P: Meckel's diverticulum: A 10-year review of 218 cases. Can J Surg 11:369–373, 1968.
366. Case Records of the Massachusetts General Hospital. N Engl J Med 302:958–962, 1980.
367. Meguid M, Erakis AJ: Complications of Meckel's diverticulum in infants. Surg Gynecol Obstet 139:541–544, 1974.
368. Gross RE, Holcomb GW Jr, Farber S: Duplications of the alimentary tract. Pediatrics 9:449–467, 1952.
369. Bower RJ, Sieber WK, Kiesewetter WB: Alimentary tract duplications in children. Ann Surg 188:669–674, 1978.
370. Dye KR, Marshall BJ, Frierson HF, et al: Campylobacter pylori colonizing heterotopic gastric tissue in the rectum. Am J Clin Pathol 93:144–147, 1990.
371. Caruso ML, Marzullo F: Jejunal adenocarcinoma in congenital heterotopic gastric mucosa. J Clin Gastroenterol 10:92–94, 1988.
372. Haggitt RC: Granulomatous diseases of the gastrointestinal tract. In Ioachim HL (ed): Pathology of Granulomas. New York, Raven Press, 1983, pp 257–305.
373. Lichtman AL, McDonald JR, Dixon CF, Mann FC: Talc granuloma. Surg Gynecol Obstet 83:531–546, 1946.
374. Eiseman B, Seelig MG, Wormach NA: Talcum powder granuloma: A frequent and serious postoperative complication. Ann Surg 126:820–832, 1947.
375. Anani PA, Ribaux C, Gardiol D: Unusual intestinal talcosis. Am J Surg Pathol 11:890–894, 1987.
376. Humphrey SR, Cameron AJ, Harrison EG Jr: Acute granulomatous peritonitis due to starch glove powder. Gastroenterology 63:1062–1065, 1972.
377. Case Records of the Massachusetts General Hospital. N Engl J Med 293:393–399, 1975.
378. Nissim F, Ashkenazy M, Borenstein R, Czernobilsky B: Tuberculoid corn starch granulomas with caseous necrosis: A diagnostic challenge. Arch Pathol Lab Med 105:86–88, 1981.
379. Carney JA, Stephens DH: Intramural barium (barium granuloma) of colon and rectum. Gastroenterology 65:316, 1973.
380. Lewis JW, Kerstein MD, Koss N: Barium granuloma of the rectum: An uncommon complication of barium enema. Ann Surg 81:418–423, 1980.
381. McKee PH, Cameron CHS: Barium granuloma of the transverse colon. Postgrad Med J 54:698–702, 1968.
382. Phelps JE, Sanowski RA, Kozarek RA: Intramural extravasation of barium simulating carcinoma of the rectum. Dis Colon Rectum 24:388, 1981.
383. Levison DA, Crocker PR, Smith A: Varied light and scanning electron microscopic appearance of barium sulphate in smears and histologic sections. J Clin Pathol 37:481–487, 1984.
384. Susnow DA: Oleogranulomas of the rectum: Following rectal installation of petrolatum or ointments containing petrolatum. Am J Surg 83:496–499, 1952.
385. Hernandez V, Hernandez IA, Berthrong M: Oleogranuloma simulating carcinoma of the rectum. Dis Colon Rectum 10:205–209, 1967.
386. Greaney MG, Jackson PR: Oleogranuloma of the rectum produced by Lasonil ointment. Br Med J 2:997–998, 1977.
387. Mazier WP, Sun KM, Robertson WG: Oil-induced granuloma (oleoma) of the rectum. Dis Colon Rectum 21:292–294, 1978.

CHAPTER 29

Malabsorptive Disorders

JOHN H. YARDLEY, M.D.

BIOPSY—SPECIAL
 CONSIDERATIONS

CLINICOPATHOLOGIC
 CONSIDERTIONS

PROTEIN-LOSING ENTEROPATHY

DISEASES ASSOCIATED WITH
 NORMAL MUCOSAL
 HISTOLOGY

DISEASES PRIMARILY SHOWING
 NONSPECIFIC INFLAMMATION
 AND MUCOSAL ALTERATIONS
Celiac Disease
Etiology and Pathogenesis
Pathology
Differential Diagnosis and Diagnostic
 Pitfalls
Complications
Celiac-Related Conditions
Refractory Celiac Disease and
 Refractory Sprue
Collagenous Sprue

Dermatitis Herpetiformis
Celiac-like and Celiac-Related
 Conditions Elsewhere in the
 Gastrointestinal Tract
**Tropical Sprue (Postinfective
 Tropical Malabsorption)**
Etiology and Pathogenesis
Pathology
Clinicopathologic Correlation
Differential Diagnosis
Stasis (Blind Loop) Syndrome
Pathogenesis
Pathology
Deficiency States
Protein Deficiency
Iron Deficiency
Zinc Deficiency and Acrodermatitis
 Enteropathica
**Unclassified Nonspecific
 Inflammatory Lesions**

INFECTION-ASSOCIATED
 MUSCOSAL LESIONS
Viral Infections
Bacterial Infections

Whipple's Disease
Fungal Infections
Moniliasis
Histoplasmosis
Protozoan Parasitosis
Microsporidiosis
Metazoan Parasitosis
Ascariasis
Strongyloidiasis
Capillariasis

MUCOSAL LESIONS ASSOCIATED
 WITH ALTERED IMMUNE
 RESPONSE
Idiopathic AIDS Enteropathy
Autoimmune Enteropathy

MISCELLANEOUS DISEASES
 ASSOCIATED WITH
 CHARACTERISTIC MUCOSAL
 LESIONS
Mastocytosis
Microvillus Inclusion Disease
Lymphangiectasia
Waldenström's Macroglobulinemia

This chapter deals with those chronic conditions that can lead to abnormal absorption of nutrient substances from the small intestine. The classification of these conditions is given in Table 29–1. Major attention is given to disorders such as celiac disease and Whipple's disease, for which malabsorption is a central feature of the clinical presentation. Clinicopathologic correlation is included to enhance general comprehension of pathologic changes and because it is often essential for full and correct pathologic interpretation. Diseases that can be associated with malabsorption, but which are discussed more fully elsewhere in the book (e.g., infections and Crohn's disease), are considered only briefly.

Useful reviews covering malabsorption and associated pathologic changes are included in the reference list.[1-5]

BIOPSY—SPECIAL CONSIDERATIONS

Pathologic study of malabsorptive disorders depends almost entirely on duodenal and small-intestinal biopsy. Prior to availability of fiberoptic endoscopy,

Table 29-1 CLASSIFICATION OF DISORDERS OF MALABSORPTION*

Diseases Associated with Normal Mucosal Histology
  Alcoholism
  Bile acid insufficiency
  Inborn disaccharidase deficiencies
    Adult lactase deficiency
    Other disaccharidase deficiencies
  Pancreatic insufficiency
  Postgastrectomy
  Short-bowel syndrome

Diseases Associated with Nonspecific Mucosal Inflammatory Lesions
  Peptic duodenitis and jejunitis (Chapter 28)
  Celiac disease (Gluten-induced enteropathy)
  Celiac-related conditions
    Refractory celiac disease
    Refractory sprue (some cases)
    Collagenous sprue
    Dermatitis herpetiformis
  Celiac-like reactions to agents other than gluten
    Soy milk, MER-29 (triparanol),
  Lymphocytic enterocolitis (Chapter 28)
  Tropical sprue
  Stasis (blind loop) syndrome
    Various motor and mechanical disturbances
  Deficiency states
    Protein deficiency
    Zinc deficiency and acrodermatitis enteropathica
    Iron deficiency
  Unclassified nonspecific imflammatory lesions

Infection-Associated Mucosal Lesions
  Viral infections (Chapters 14 and 26)
  Bacterial infections
    Mycobacterium avium intracellulare (Chapter 14)
    Whipple's disease
    Various other agents (Chapter 26)
  Fungus infections
    Moniliasis (Chapters 14 and 26)
    Histoplasmosis (Chapter 26)
  Protozoan parasitic infections
    Giardiasis (Chapter 26)
    Cryptosporidiosis (Chapter 14)
    Microsporidiosis
    Coccidiosis *(Isospora)* (Chapter 26)
  Metazoan parasitic infections
    Ascariasis (with protein deficiency)
    Hookworm
    Strongyloidiasis
    Capillariasis

Mucosal Lesions Associated with Altered Immune Response
  AIDS-associated diseases
    AIDS enteropathy (idiopathic)
    Opportunistic infections (Chapter 14)
  Autoimmune enteropathy
  Chronic granulomatous disease (Chapters 14 and 16)
  Graft-versus-host disease (Chapter 14)
  Immune deficiency states (Chapter 14)

Miscellaneous Diseases Associated with Characteristic Mucosal Lesions
  Abetalipoproteinemia (Chapter 16)
  Amyloidosis (Chapter 16)
  Crohn's disease (Chapter 27)
  Drug-associated lesions (Chapter 9)
  Eosinophilic gastroenteritis (Chapter 10)
  Histiocytosis X (Chapter 16)
  Lipid storage disease (Chapter 16)
  Lymphangiectasis
    Primary
    Secondary (Chapter 16)
  Lymphomas (Chapter 14)
  Mastocytosis
  Microvillus inclusion disease
  Radiation changes (Chapter 9)
  Waldenström's macroglobulinemia

*Chapter numbers in parentheses refer to the location where the disorder is discussed.

most biopsies of the small intestine were obtained by using a fluoroscopically guided capsule device. Capsule biopsy, which can be performed anywhere in the small intestine, is now largely supplanted by endoscopically guided biopsy of the duodenum. Although endoscopic biopsy is often adequate for diagnosis of such conditions as celiac disease,[6] the presence of peptic duodenitis (or just the possibility of its presence) frequently confounds interpretation of inflammatory and degenerative changes, especially if the specimen is taken from the duodenal bulb. (For additional discussion of this problem see Celiac Disease). Furthermore, the proximal and distal small intestine are not necessarily involved to comparable degrees in all conditions. Thus, "blind" biopsy from the jejunum and beyond by means of a capsule device is still needed at times for adequate study of the diseases and lesions described in this chapter.

The small-intestinal mucosa is often not uniformly involved in malabsorption-associated conditions, a fact that should always be kept in mind, especially in examining biopsies obtained blindly via a capsule instrument. For instance, celiac disease alters the mucosa diffusely, and all capsule biopsies taken from the same level of the small intestine can be expected to have a similar appearance, whereas biopsies from patients with segmental and focal disorders (e.g., Crohn's disease, dermatitis herpetiformis, and lymphoma) have an unpredictable degree of involvement. In addition, even with endoscopically guided biopsy, a specimen may not necessarily come from the intended biopsy site, since the operator does not always have full control over the location of the forceps at the moment when tissue is obtained.

Two special procedures that can be of value for studying small-intestinal biopsies in malabsorptive disorders are (1) macrosopic examination and photography of specimens, and (2) study of smears prepared from the biopsy specimen. Direct macroscopic study is most often done for indentification of changes in the configuration of villi. It is also helpful for correlating endoscopic and histologic findings and is immediately available for verifying that small-intestinal mucosa was obtained and for making preliminary assessment of mucosal architecture. An ordinary dissecting microscope, or even a strong hand lens, can provide useful observations. Correct lighting of the specimen with the light source set in the near horizontal plane is needed for good visualization and for photography of villi and other surface features.[7]

Stained smears obtained from a biopsy specimen by dabbing it against a clean glass slide are useful for examining luminal contents and for assessing cytologic characteristics. They can be especially helpful for detecting *Giardia lamblia* and other protozoan parasites.

CLINICOPATHOLOGIC CONSIDERATIONS

When used alone, the term *malabsorption* broadly describes dysfunction in the uptake of *any* substance by the small intestine. By this definition, malabsorption occurs in a wide range of disorders having varied clinical presentations. For instance, in pancreatic insufficiency the clinical picture is often dominated by abnormal lipid absorption, whereas the defect in adult lactase deficiency is malabsorption of lactose. The term *malabsorption syndrome* pertains more narrowly to a constellation of clinical findings that includes chronic diarrhea, steatorrhea, and variable secondary changes such as weight loss and evidence of vitamin deficiencies. The term *sprue* is an older generic term for diseases that are associated with steatorrhea, weight loss, deficiency states, etc., and thus is a synonym for *malabsorption syndrome*.

When considering biopsy findings in patients with malabsorption, it is often useful to consider whether the malabsorption has come about because of (1) abnormalities of intraluminal digestion, (2) abnormalities of uptake of nutrients by the mucosa, or (3) some combination of the two.

Abnormalities of digestion (maldigestion) chiefly result from derangements in intraluminal breakdown of foodstuffs and can occur with (1) inadequate mixing and time for interaction of enzymes and food, as in altered motility, with a short bowel, and after gastrectomy; (2) bile salt deficiency; (3) pancreatic insufficiency; and (4) deficiency of a specific digestive enzyme, lactase deficiency being the most common example. In general, the mucosa will show little or no abnormality when the principal cause of malabsorption is maldigestion.

Abnormalities of uptake occur when the ability of the mucosa to absorb foodstuff is reduced either because of mucosal injury, as in celiac disease, or functionally as in ileal bypass and in altered motility.

PROTEIN-LOSING ENTEROPATHY

Protein-losing enteropathy (PLE) occurs when serum proteins, especially albumin, leak across the mucosal barrier in excessive amounts and are lost in the fecal stream or are resorbed as breakdown products after digestion. Since patients with PLE can develop severe hypoalbuminemia, peripheral edema is often the presenting manifestation. PLE can be "primary," i.e., develop as a *de novo* condition in patients who demonstrate only widespread intestinal lymphangectasia (see below under Miscellaneous Diseases Associated with Characteristic Mucosal Lesions), or it can be "secondary" (see Chapter 16), resulting from mucosal injury, as in celiac disease, or because of lymphatic obstruction as in constrictive pericarditis or Whipple's disease. Thus, PLE is an important accompanying manifestation in some patients with malabsorption.

DISEASES ASSOCIATED WITH NORMAL MUCOSAL HISTOLOGY

Normal mucosal histology is most often seen in conditions where the malabsorption has resulted chiefly from intraluminal maldigestion (see Table 29–1). Examples are patients with *chronic pancreatic insufficiency* or intraluminal bile salt deficiency.[8,9] These patients characteristically show elevated stool fat because of resulting fat maldigestion,[10] whereas they have normal d-xylose uptake because their mucosa is unaffected. Normal histology can also be seen in patients with *rapid transit* of foodstuffs through the small intestine, with resulting reduction in total mucosal surface and inadequate mixing of foodstuffs and digestive enzymes. Examples are *postgastrectomy* patients and patients who have a *short bowel*. Again, the mucosa in these individuals will be normal or show insufficient alterations to account for the malabsorption. *Alcoholism* presents a special problem, particularly for the "binge drinker," who may, through a combination of incompletely understood factors, show malabsorption of a variety of substances even though by light microscopy the mucosa is normal when alcohol alone is administered.[11,12] On the other hand, chronic alcoholics often have dietary deficiencies that may be crucial to the resulting mucosal changes, as was shown in those patients with associated folate deficiency.[12] Pancreatic insufficiency secondary to alcoholism may also play a role.[13]

Patients with *primary disaccharidase deficiency* represent another class of patients in whom a normal intestinal mucosa accompanies a highly specific form of maldigestion-malabsorption. A large percentage of the world's adult population has lactase deficiency, especially among Oriental and black races. Lactase is concentrated on the surface of the microvilli of the small-intestinal absorptive cells.[14] Patients with lactase deficiency are unable to split adequate amounts of lactose into its constituent monosaccharides, glucose and galactose, an essential step before absorption can occur. When lactose remains in the intestinal lumen, the patient experiences symptoms of milk intolerance (abdominal cramps, bloating, diarrhea) as a result of osmotic retention of water in the lumen and bacterial action on the retained lactose in the colon, with resulting production of gas and irritant substances such as lactic acid.[15]

Mucosal biopsies obtained from patients with primary lactase deficiency are entirely normal by light microscopy (Figure 29–1) even though these same biopsies will demonstrate the enzyme abnormality by chemical analysis. Other types of disaccharidase defi-

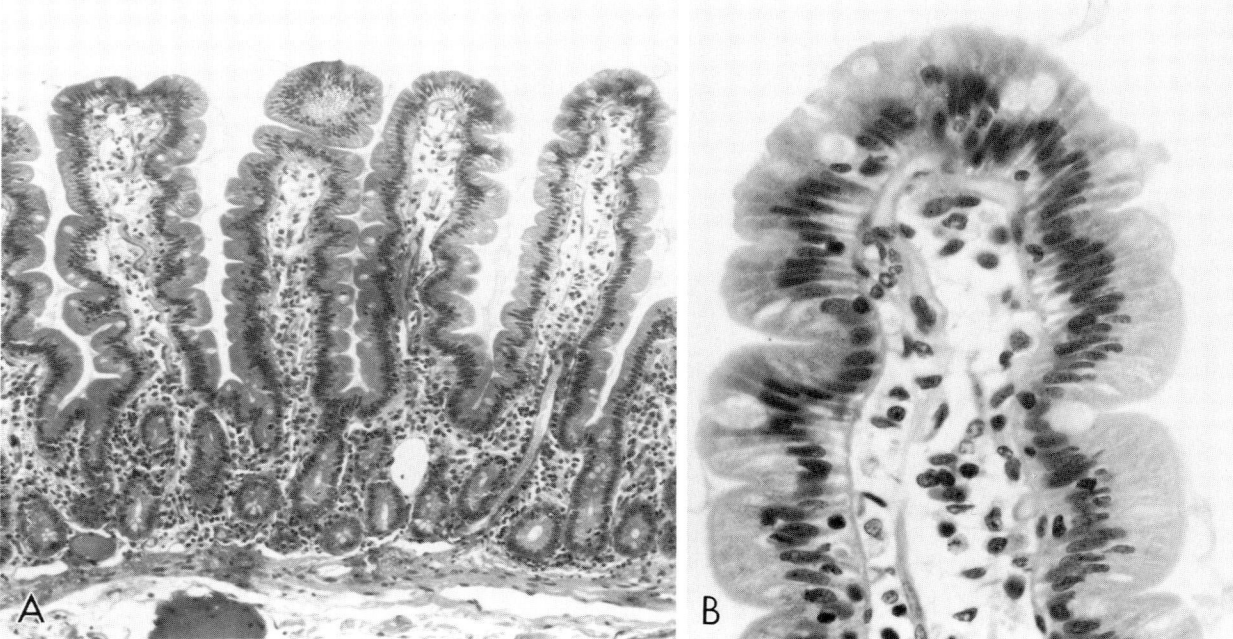

FIGURE 29–1. Primary lactase deficiency. *A,* Normal-appearing small intestinal mucosa in primary lactase deficiency. Villi are narrow; they have a ruffled outline and a villus-to-crypt ratio of almost 3:1. (× 125) *B,* Villus tip showing tall columnar epithelial cells with intact brush border. There are only scattered intraepithelial lymphocytes and lamina propria mononuclear cells. (× 450)

ciency are rare (e.g., sucrase and maltase deficiencies); the intestinal mucosa also appears normal in these patients even though the clinical consequences may be severe. There have been various attempts to demonstrate ultrastructural alterations in the microvilli related to the enzymic abnormalities, but these have not shown convincing changes.

From a practical standpoint, the important point is to recognize that clinically significant and demonstrable malabsorption can occur in the absence of mucosal alterations. On the other hand, it should also be stressed that a normal biopsy can be obtained because the biopsy instrument is fortuitously located away from any lesion.

DISEASES PRIMARILY SHOWING NONSPECIFIC INFLAMMATION AND MUCOSAL ALTERATIONS

Malabsorptive disorders in this group show variable assortments of mucosal inflammatory changes, none of which are by themselves diagnostic or even characteristic. Inflammatory changes can vary as to severity, predominant cell types, and location. Accompanying cellular injury and architecural alterations are frequent but also variable. Despite these limitations, important diagnostic insights and comprehension of underlying pathophysiology are possible from the histopathologic findings, especially when correlated with clinical observations.

Celiac disease is the major entity in this group of diseases among patients in developed Western countries.[16] Celiac disease is also an excellent reference point from which to consider other disorders in this group (see Table 29–1).

Celiac Disease

Synonyms for celiac disease, some no longer appropriate, are *nontropical sprue, idiopathic sprue, idiopathic steatorrhea, celiac sprue,* and *gluten-induced enteropathy*. Excellent reviews of this subject are available and should be consulted for detailed descriptions of clinical and pathophysiologic observations.[16–18] Revised criteria for the diagnosis of celiac disease were published recently.[16]

Etiology and Pathogenesis

Etiology. The central finding in celiac disease is an unusual sensitivity of the small intestinal mucosa to *gluten,* the major protein constituent of wheat flour and to a lesser degree of rye, oats, and barley.[19–22] The relevant protein in gluten has been further identified as the alcohol-soluble fraction *gliadin*; and a symptom-provoking subfraction of crude gliadin, α-gliadin (or A-gliadin), has also been identified. Most patients who adhere closely to a *gluten-free diet* show both clinical remission and eventual restoration of normal or near normal mucosal histology. Although by no means fully established, the underlying mechanism of mucosal injury in celiac patients is widely considered to be autoimmune.

Table 29–2 CELIAC DISEASE: CARDINAL FEATURES UNDER VARIED CONDITIONS OF GLUTEN EXPOSURE

Before Gluten-Free Diet (Full Exposure to Gluten)
Malabsorption syndrome
Flat jejunal biopsy (*absent* or severely blunted villi) with:
  Surface epithelium, thinned, injured
  Intraepithelial lymphocytes increased at surface
Chronic inflammation increased in lamina propria
Crypt mitoses increased; crypts elongated

Gluten-Free Diet—Short-Term (1 week to 3 months)
Marked clinical improvement
Diminished surface epithelial injury
Reduced number of intraepithelial lymphocytes
Villi return partially

Gluten-Free Diet—Long-Term (> 3 months)
Villi gradually become fully normal
Mitotic hyperactivity gradually subsides
Chronic inflammation much diminished

Gluten Restored to Diet
Rapid return of all lesions and malabsorption findings
Early increase in intraepithelial lymphocytes and injury to epithelium over villi

---

Findings in serial biopsies of the small intestine before and at various intervals after gluten withdrawal have shown a clear relation between the mucosal findings and exposure to dietary gluten.[23–26] The central feature is epithelial injury during gluten exposure that disappears on gluten withdrawal and reappears after reinstituting dietary gluten.[25,26] Parallel functional studies demonstrating impaired epithelial transport of lipid in active celiac disease, with recovery on a gluten-free diet, have also emphasized the central role of epithelial damage in celiac disease.[24]

It is useful to consider the typical response to a gluten-free diet in celiac disease in three stages (Table 29–2). At each stage the pathologist must anticipate a different set of findings, and definitive assessment without knowledge of the patient's dietary history should not be attempted.

Pathogenesis. The mechanisms by which gluten injures the absorptive epithelium in celiac disease are not fully established, but current knowledge fits well with a combined genetic, environmental, and autoimmune pathogenesis.

Genetic Factors. There is much evidence favoring genetic factors. There is often familial occurrence, including occult jejunal lesions in asymptomatic relatives.[27,28] Furthermore, monozygotic twins show a high frequency of concordance for celiac disease.[29] In one family study evidence of the disorder was found in 11% of first-degree relatives of patients examined[27] while other investigators noted that 22% were affected.[28] More recently, striking associations between celiac disease and class II major histocompatibility genes in the HLA-D region, especially DR3, DR7, DQw2, and a 4-kd restriction fragment in the DP subregion, were identified.[30–32] Marsh et al. have recently demonstrated increased intraepithelial lymphocytes in first-degree relatives of patients with celiac disease, especially in HLA-DR3 relatives.[33] A close association exists, too, between celiac disease and the class I HLA-B8 haplotype that is thought to reflect strong linkage disequilibrium with HLA-DR3.[32] Thus the available data strongly support a multigenic, HLA-associated susceptibility to celiac disease.[32] (See Chapter 6 for further details.)

The importance of genetic factors in celiac disease is further confirmed by the close connection between celiac disease and dermatitis herpetiformis (see below) and by the heightened association between celiac disease and other autoimmune diseases that demonstrate genetically determined susceptibility (e.g., type I diabetes mellitus, pernicious anemia).[34–36] (See Chapter 6 for further details.)

Immunologic Factors. The prominent lymphocytic and plasma cell infiltrates suggest the fundamental importance of immune response in celiac disease. But in addition, elegant *in vitro* (organ culture) techniques used by Falchuk and colleagues demonstrated that not only gluten but also an endogenous mediator present only in actively affected intestine is needed to cause injury (summarized in Walker-Smith et al.[16]). The local (intramucosal) immune system—humoral or cellular, or both—is the best candidate as "endogenous mediator." The favorable response by celiac patients to corticosteroids both *in vivo*[37] and *in vitro*[38] adds further weight to a role for immunity.

Elevated circulating antibodies to gluten and its fractions have long been noted, but celiac patients also often show parallel increases in antibodies to unrelated foodstuffs such as casein.[39,40] Increased IgA antibodies to gluten and its products are found, too, in persons with other forms of intestinal disease; and antigliadin antibodies (usually IgG) have sometimes been detected in normal individuals.[41–43] Thus, it is possible that there is only nonspecific immune response to gluten, as well as to other foodstuffs, which results when the damaged mucosa absorbs undigested peptides. Furthermore, since celiac patients can have selective IgA deficiency (perhaps with greater than expected frequency), it is hard to see how IgA antibodies could be an essential causative factor. Nonetheless, there is strong correlation between level of circulating IgA antigliadins and both the clinical status and the histologic status of the celiac disease[41–43]; and IgA antigliadin-producing mucosal lymphocytes are increased in active celiac disease.[45] In fact, these findings can be the basis of a screening test for celiac disease.

Along with the antibodies against gluten and its fractions, celiac patients with active disease often show circulating IgA antibodies against reticulin,[46] a feature that it shares with dermatitis herpetiformis. Furthermore, a 90-kd gliadin-binding glycoprotein is found in the intestine and skin of normal individuals. It is noteworthy that both observations are consistent with autoantibody production. The incidence of other autoantibodies (antinuclear, antiparietal cell, antithyroid, etc.) has been described as high in adults, although celiac children seldom show them.[36]

There are also observations which suggest a role for cellular immunity in celiac disease: A striking correlation has been noted between exposure to gluten and the number of intraepithelial lymphocytes. These lym-

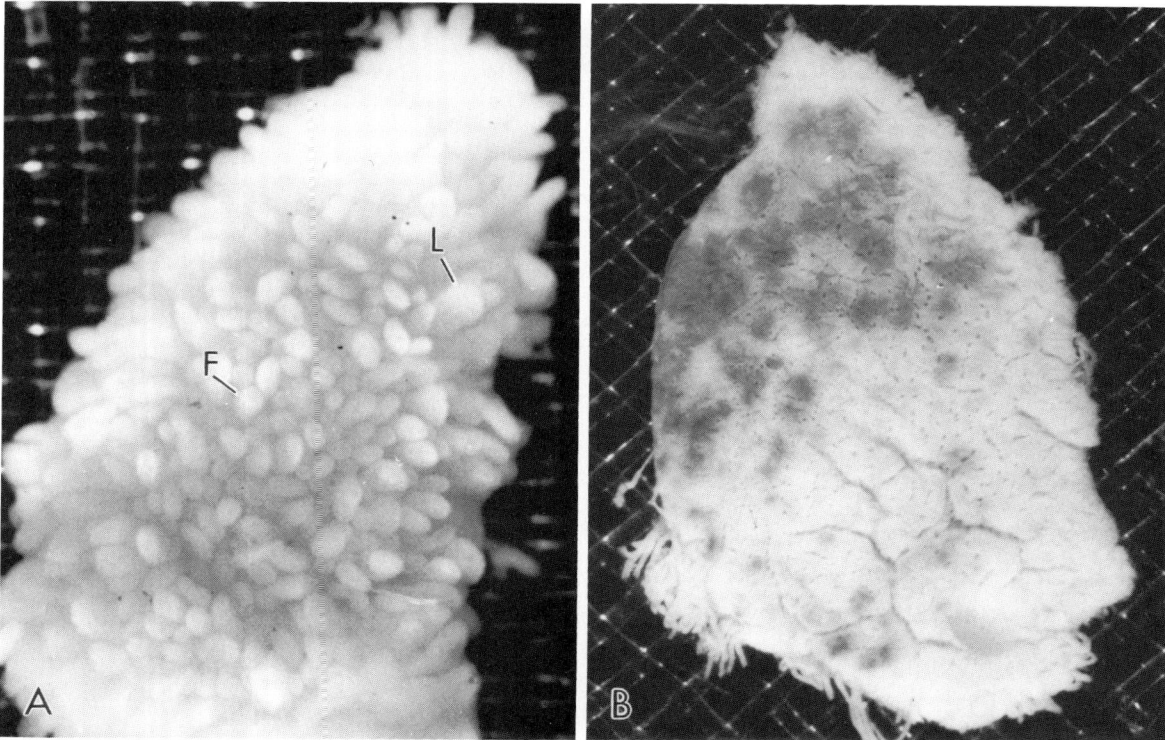

FIGURE 29–2. Macroscopic appearance of jejunal mucosa. *A,* Specimen from a healthy individual showing a typical normal pattern of predominantly fingerlike (F) and scattered leaf-shaped (L) villi. *B,* Active (untreated) celiac disease. No villi are detected. Numerous crypt openings are evident (small dots). Dark splotches are artifactual hemorrhage, probably induced during suction biopsy. (*A* and *B,* × 13)

phocytes, which are predominantly cytotoxic/suppressor T cells, diminished in number on gluten withdrawal and reappeared in as little as 2 hours when gluten was restored to the diet.[25,47,48] A similar response occurred in the rectum and was suggested as a diagnostic test for celiac disease.[49–51] It is reasonable to postulate that these intraepithelial lymphocytes, in concert with gluten, actually effect epithelial damage through release of injurious mediator substances. In other studies T cells from celiac patients demonstrated enhanced migration inhibition when exposed in vitro to α-gliadin.[52,53] Investigations using an α-gliadin peptide that was homologous to a peptide derived from type 12 adenovirus (see below) gave similar results.[54,55]

Kagnoff and colleagues have provided highly provocative evidence that individuals who develop celiac disease are first "primed" to become susceptible by initial exposure to a specific viral agent—type 12 adenovirus (Ad12).[56] The central observation is that the Ad12 virus contains a protein that shares homology with α-gliadin.[57] In addition, however, the authors demonstrated that celiac patients show a high frequency of circulating antibodies to the Ad12 virus.[56] It is their general hypothesis that the viral protein may play a role in the pathogenesis of celiac disease, "perhaps by virtue of immunologic cross-reactivity between determinants shared by the viral protein and α-gliadins."[17]

The concept of a preceding infectious component in the genesis of celiac disease is highly attractive from a clinicopathologic standpoint. It helps account for individual variations in findings, especially as demonstrated by celiac disease in identical twins. Although some identical twin pairs have shown similar clinical presentations,[27,29,58] in others the celiac-related findings were dissimilar, with absence of clinical and pathologic changes in the second twin,[59,60] with the second twin developing symptoms at a later time,[61] or with marked discrepancy in severity between twins.[62] In another report a second twin manifested dermatitis herpetiformis instead of celiac disease.[63]

Pathology

A jejunal biopsy specimen from a patient with untreated celiac disease is strikingly abnormal. Villi are completely absent, as shown both by examination using the dissecting microscope (Figure 29–2) and histologically (Figure 29–3). Indeed, the absence of villi can be so complete that the first impression is that one is examining a biopsy of colon rather than jejunum. The loss of villi is often referred to as *villus atrophy,* but the term, along with its various degrees—partial and subtotal—is a misnomer, because the villi are not atrophic in the literal sense. The mucosal flattening seems to result from remolding of the mucosa by a combination of increased inflammation, surface epithelial injury, and altered epithelial turnover. It has been noted that overall mucosal thickness is not significantly al-

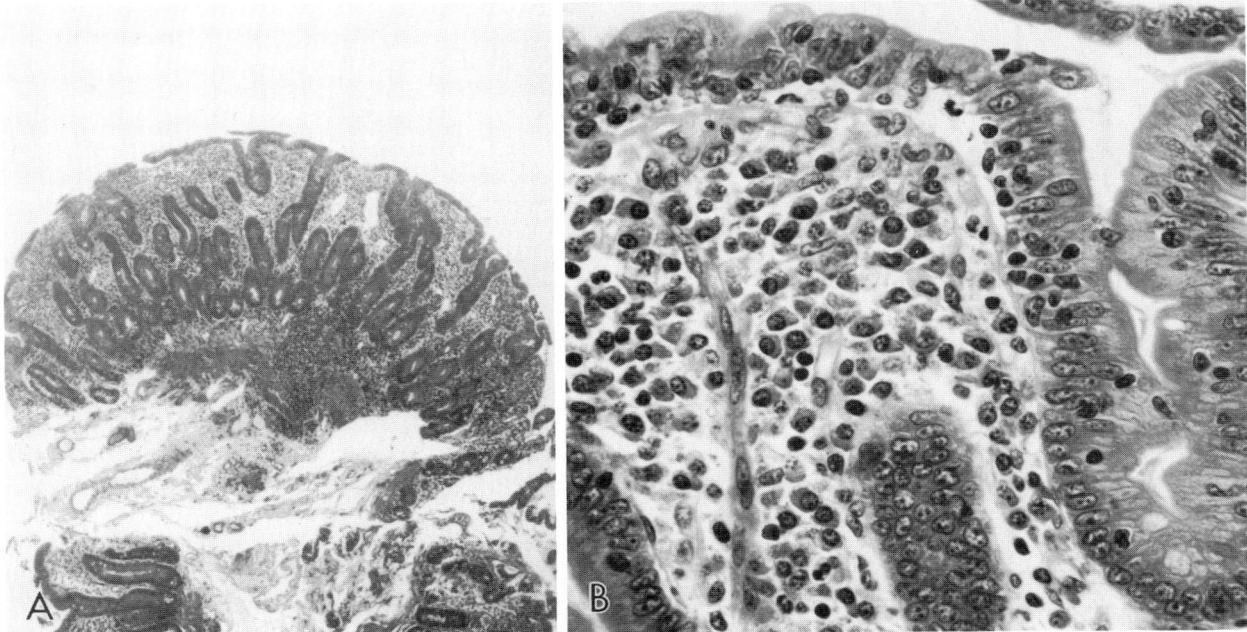

FIGURE 29-3. Active (untreated) celiac disease. Jejunal biopsy. *A*, The typical colonlike appearance at low power fits well with the macroscopic appearance seen in Figure 29-2B. (× 50) *B*, Same specimen, detail of surface and upper crypt epithelium. The surface epithelium appears thinned, damaged, and "pseudostratefied." It is also infiltrated by lymphocytes (small dark nuclei) and has detached from the basement membrane. The crypt epithelium is much less affected. Plasma cells and lymphocytes are increased in the lamina propria. (× 430)

tered in celiac disease,[64] and Padykula demonstrated that the epithelium lining the upper ends of the lengthened ("hyperplastic") crypts in celiac disease have the histochemical characteristics of villus epithelium.[65]

Comparison of the surface and crypt epithelia in active celiac disease demonstrates that the surface epithelium shows strikingly greater evidence of damage.[23] Its cells often appear cuboidal rather than columnar, the cytoplasm looks condensed and eosinophilic, the brush border is absent or thinned, the epithelial nuclei are scattered rather than basally placed ("pseudostratification"), and numerous lymphocytes are intercalated between the epithelial cells (see Figure 29-3B). Histochemical and electron-microscopic study of the surface epithelium have confirmed their damaged state.[24,65-68] The crypt epithelium shows little or no evidence of damage or inflammation, but there is usually moderate to marked increase in mitotic figures[23] (Figure 29-4). Goblet and Paneth cells are normal in appearance, although they may be reduced in number. The inflammatory response in the lamina propria is predominantly mononuclear, with numerous plasma cells (Figures 29-3 and 29-4), except in those rare individuals with immunodeficiency. Acute inflammation is usually absent, although it may be observed in occasional cases.

Response to a gluten-free diet is both clinically and morphologically dramatic in the patient with previously untreated celiac disease. Patients may report an improved sense of well-being within a few days; and in the ensuing days and weeks, there is rapid improvement, with diminution of malabsorption findings and rapid weight gain.[23] Re-biopsy of the jejunum soon

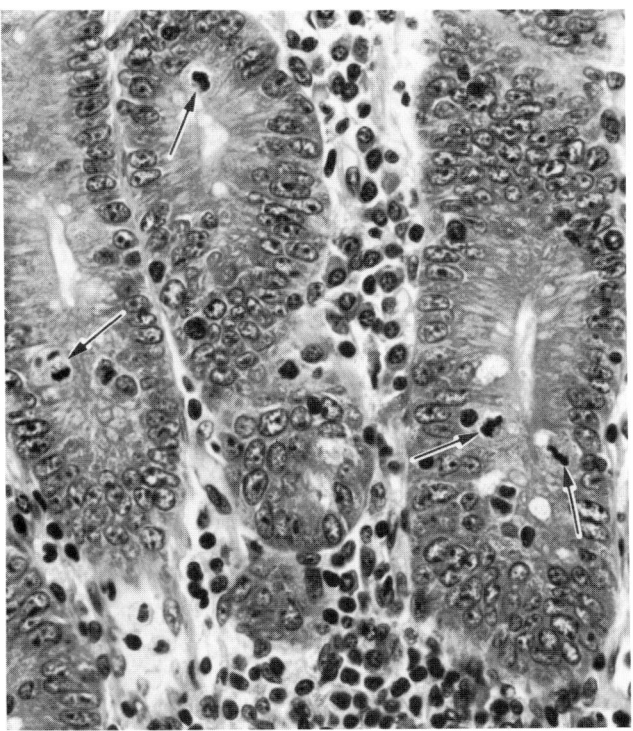

FIGURE 29-4. Crypts in active (untreated) celiac disease. Mitotic figures (arrows) are increased in number and some are located in the upper crypt (top of figure), findings that indicate heightened epithelial proliferation. (Conventionally prepared histologic material from the small intestine typically demonstrates about one mitotic figure per two to three crypts, and these are largely located near the crypt bases.) (× 430)

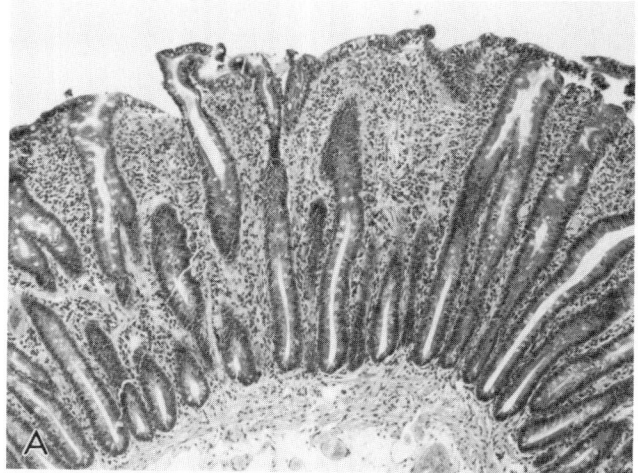
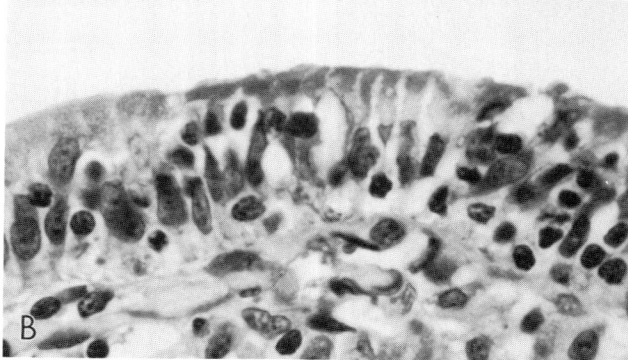
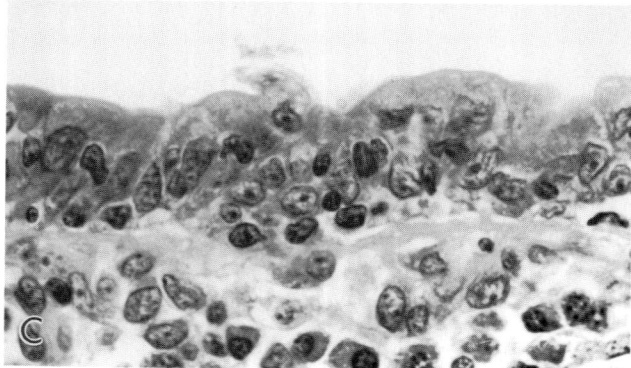

FIGURE 29–5. Celiac disease 3 weeks after instituting a gluten-free diet. *A*, The surface has a faintly wavy outline, suggesting incipient return of villi. (× 90) *B*, The surface epithelium is more columnar and probably taller, and its nuclei are more basally located as compared with the biopsy shown in C. (× 675) *C*, For comparison, surface epithelium from the untreated patient shown in Figure 29–3. (× 675)

after beginning the gluten-free diet (see Table 29–2) reveals little or no return of villi or reduction in chronic inflammation (Figure 29–5). There is, however, evidence of improvement in the surface epithelium, with partial restoration of healthy-looking columnar cells and reduction in intraepithelial lymphocytes (see Figure 29–5B) in as little as 1 week after initiating the gluten-free diet.[23] That this restoration of the surface epithelium accounts well for the patient's rapid improvement is evident from the return of intracellular enzymes by histochemical tests as well as the regained ability to transport lipid contained in a test meal.[66] There may be reduction in epithelial mitoses by actual count,[23] but the elevated mitotic levels typically persist long after gluten withdrawal. Since the heightened epithelial turnover is a response to injury, persistent elevation of epithelial mitoses may reflect the continued presence of small amounts of gluten in the diet; because wheat products are ubiquitous, total avoidance of all gluten is difficult even with rigorous compliance.

There is progressive morphologic improvement with continued adherence to the gluten-free diet. Although the time required for return of villi varies from patient to patient, all who respond clinically will show at least some return of villi after about 3 months. This is accompanied by a gradual reduction in chronic inflammation and diminution of epithelial mitoses. After 1 to 2 years on a strict diet, the villus-to-crypt ratio may be near normal (Figure 29–6), as will be the covering epithelium (see Figure 29–6C). On the other hand, even limited exposure to gluten seems to cause some continuing chronic inflammation, villus blunting, and epithelial injury.

Patients who have undergone long-term treatment with a gluten-free diet retain their sensitivity to gluten. This was confirmed for both the small intestine[25,69] and the rectum.[49,50] Furthermore, the histologic response of the mucosa in treated patients when they are re-exposed to gluten gives additional insight into the nature of the response. The time required for reappearance of histologic changes can vary from 2 hours to 6 days.[25,48] Initially, intraepithelial lymphocytes are increased and the epithelium over the upper part of the villus is damaged (Figure 29–6D); a rapid and specific intraepithelial lymphocytic response has also been seen in the rectum on exposure to gluten.[49,50] These observations fit well with the hypothesis that the surface epithelium in these patients is sensitive to gluten and that intraepithelial lymphocytes play a key role in the injurious response (see above). With continued exposure to gluten, there is further increase in chronic inflammation; and if gluten ingestion continues, the full-blown syndrome can return.

Differential Diagnosis and Diagnostic Pitfalls

Changes in the jejunal mucosa in celiac disease are so highly characteristic, especially in full-blown active disease with a flat small-intestinal biopsy, that one usually will not fail to consider the diagnosis. On the other hand, one should never make the diagnosis of celiac disease solely on the basis of histologic findings, because it is possible to have a flat small-intestinal biopsy in a variety of other entities (Table 29–3). Furthermore, the range of diagnostic possibilities becomes very large, encompassing most of the disorders described in this section, when intermediate degrees of villus shortening and blunting ("partial villus atrophy") and mucosal inflammation are considered.

It is curious and potentially important to our understanding of pathogenetic mechanisms in celiac disease

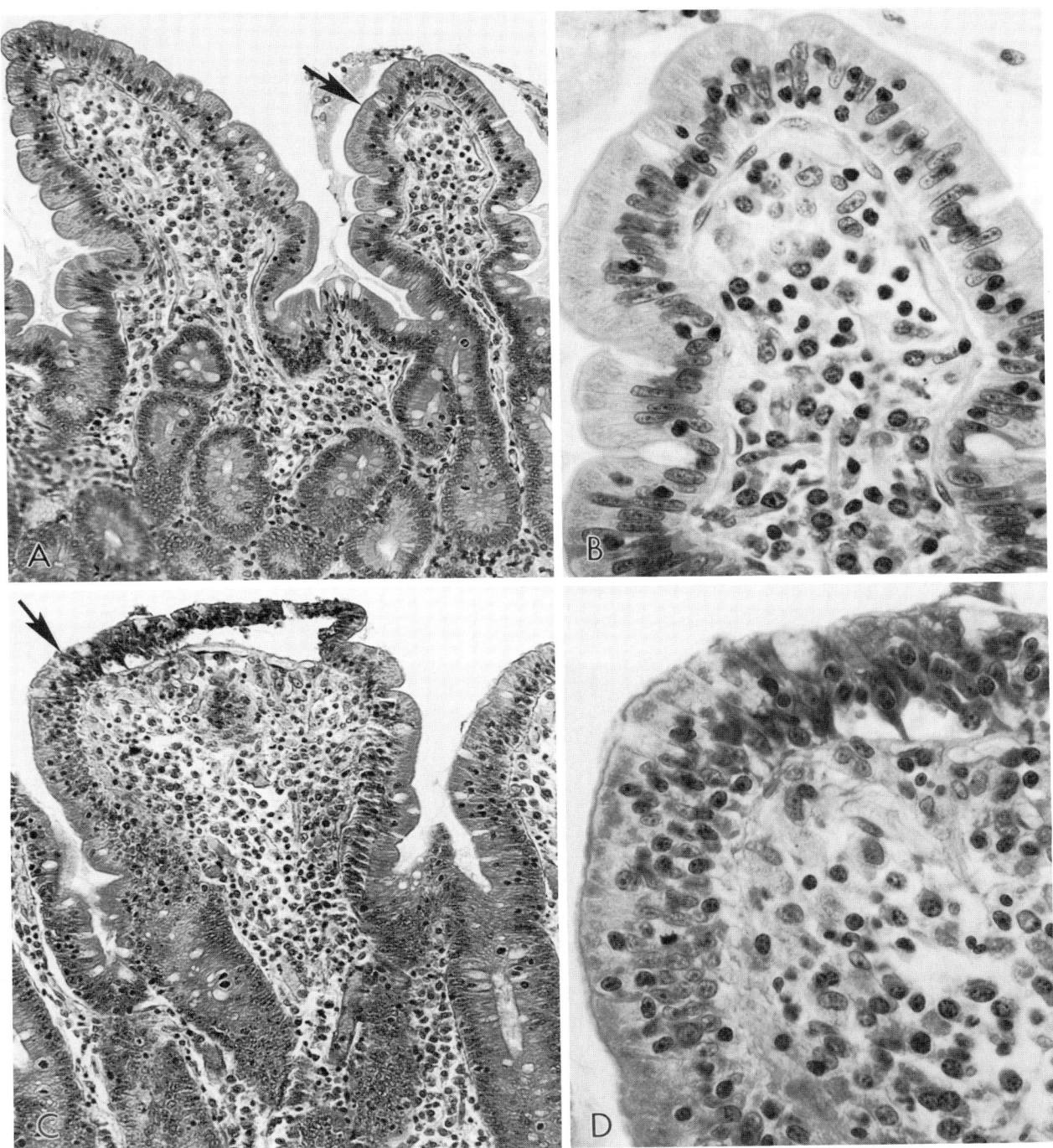

FIGURE 29–6. Celiac disease. Effects of a long-term gluten-free diet followed by restoration of dietary gluten. All frames are of biopsies from the same patient made 2 years after commencing a gluten-free diet. A and B, Before administering gluten, the villi were somewhat short but otherwise normal-looking. Lamina proprial and intraepithelial chronic inflammation were near normal. The surface epithelium was columnar and had a prominent brush border. The villus indicated by the arrow in A is seen in B. C and D, Intestinal mucosa 6 days after reinstituting dietary gluten. The villi appear bulbous and shortened, and chronic inflammation has increased. Numerous lymphocytes are now seen in the epithelium over the villus tips, and the surface epithelium is strikingly condensed and shows detachment from the basement membrane. The arrow in C indicates the area shown in D. (A and C, × 200; B and D, × 575) (B, C, and D from Bayless TM, Rubin S, Topping T, et al: Morphologic and functional effects of gluten feeding on jejunal mucosa and celiac disease. In Booth CC, Dowling RH (ed): Coeliac Disease. Edinburgh, Churchill Livingstone, 1970, pp 76–89.)

Table 29–3 MALABSORPTIVE DISORDERS FOR WHICH BIOPSIES CAN RESEMBLE UNTREATED CELIAC DISEASE*

Disorder/Agent	Comments
Dermatitis herpetiformis	Focal or patchy lesions
Autoimmune enteropathy[36,221]	Other autoimmune features
Lymphocytic enterocolitis[102]	See Chapter 14
Lymphoma	
Microvillus inclusion disease[246]	Infants; inborn abnormality
Peptic disease	Chiefly duodenal bulb (except Zollinger-Ellison syndrome)
Soy protein[70]	Probably soy allergy
Triparanol (MER-29)[71]	Historical interest only; drug removed from market
Tropical sprue	Unusual for mucosa to be completed flat

*Disorders that can demonstrate a flat or nearly flat mucosa. Other features of celiac disease (thinned surface epithelium, intraepithelial lymphocytes, chronic inflammation, increased mitoses, etc.) may not be present.

that, with minor exceptions, gluten remains the only noninfectious agent to have been established as a specific cause of severe chronic, mucosal injury and resulting malabsorption of the type seen in celiac disease. Isolated cases have been encountered in which soy protein, used as a milk substitute in infants, has caused a celiac-like lesions.[70] The mucosa shows chronic inflammation and flattening, and there is recovery after soy protein withdrawal. Only a few additional cases of this nature have been reported.

Patients given the drug triparanol (MER-29) on occasion developed a strikingly celiac-like mucosal lesion with loss of villi, chronic inflammation, and so forth. Withdrawal of the drug led to recovery from malabsorption and disappearance of the mucosal lesion.[71]

Neomycin is another drug that is associated with nonspecific inflammation and blunting of villi,[72] but it is less of a mimic of celiac disease than are the lesions associated with soy protein and triparanol. The neomycin lesion is said to be dose-related and to regress when the drug is discontinued.

Diagnostic Pitfalls. Depending on the patient's dietary status, plus individual variation, the pathologist must be alert to the wide spectrum of findings that can be seen in small-intestinal biopsy specimens from celiac patients. Difficulties for pathologists are compounded when they are asked to assess duodenal or jejunal mucosa for possible celiac disease in patients who have already been placed on a gluten-free diet without a pretreatment biopsy or in those who may not be fully compliant with their diet, or when the dietary history is incomplete.

The biopsy site along the small intestine can profoundly affect the pathologic findings. To a degree that varies widely among patients, the severity of the lesion diminishes distally in celiac disease, as does the total length of intestine involved. Thus, a typical flat biopsy can be obtained occasionally from an asymptomatic person if most of the small intestine is still functioning normally. The reduced severity distally is presumed to result from progressive proteolysis and hence dilution of intact gluten as it moves down the intestine.

Another pitfall for the pathologist is overreliance on biopsy specimens obtained from the duodenum. This can cause either over- or underdiagnosis of celiac disease, especially with specimens that have come from the duodenal bulb. On the one hand, severe peptic duodenitis, with or without associated peptic ulcer, occasionally causes a biopsy specimen to appear flat and heavily inflamed, thereby mimicking the changes of celiac disease. On the other hand, proximal duodenal biopsies from celiac patients who also have peptic duodenitis with marked replacement of absorptive cells by gastric mucous cells can show an intact villus architecture (Figure 29–7). Presumably the gastric metaplasia leads to localized protection against the effects of gluten.

Complications

Malignancy in Celiac Disease. There is no doubt that malignancy occurs with significantly higher than expected frequency in patients with celiac disease.[73–75] Primary non-Hodgkins lymphoma of the small intestine is the most commonly seen tumor (see Chapter 14), accounting for about 50% of all malignant conditions found in patients with celiac disease.[73,74] The lymphomas that arise in celiac disease are in all likelihood derived from mucosal T cells, probably those that migrate into the epithelial layer.[76,77] Furthermore, the T-cell subset characteristics of the lymphoma are similar to those that predominate in celiac disease (see Pathogenesis), thereby additionally supporting a direct relationship between the lymphoma and the celiac disease.[78]

Adenocarcinoma of the small intestine, carcinoma of the esophagus, and carcinoma of the mouth and pharynx are the principal other malignancies that arise with greater than expected frequency in celiac disease.[73–75] Swinson et al. found 19 instances of small-intestinal adenocarcinoma, compared with 0.23 case expected, among 119 non-lymphomatous malignancies in their registry.[74] Those tumors occur predominantly in the jejunum and duodenum. One patient with celiac disease demonstrated villous adenoma, a likely precursor of carcinoma, and others have been seen with multiple adenocarcinomas.[79–81] Conventional squamous esophageal and oropharyngeal tumors are also increased in celiac disease patients; Holmes et al. found the relative risk for those lesions to be 12.3 ($P < 0.01$) and 9.7 ($P < 0.01$) respectively.[75] There is no obvious explanation for the increased squamous lesions, but vitamin A deficiency associated with the malabsorption syndrome has been suggested.[74]

Holmes et al. observed a significantly reduced risk of malignancy among patients who adhered closely to a gluten-free diet for 5 or more years. While nonlymphomatous malignancy has been seen at numerous other sites in celiac patients (e.g., pancreas, stomach, colon, bladder, breast, brain), with the exception of the testes ($P < 0.001$) in one report,[74] it has not occurred in excess numbers in other locations.

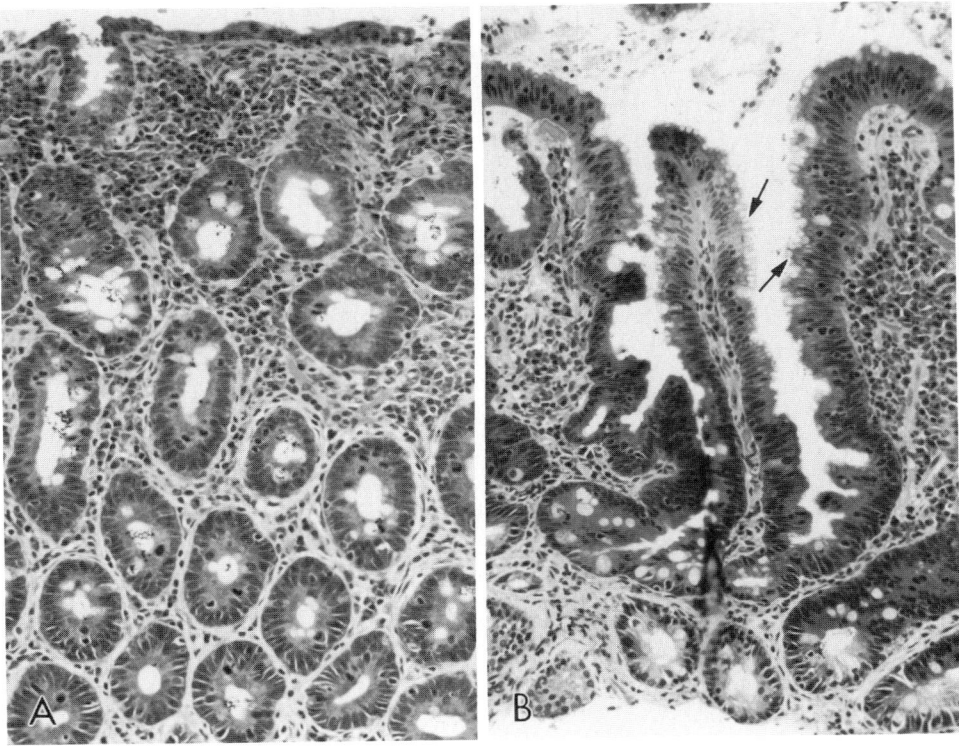

FIGURE 29-7. Celiac disease. Biopsies from two locations illustrating that the diagnosis may be overlooked if only the duodenal bulb is biopsied. *A*, Biopsy from second portion of duodenum demonstrating the typical flat appearance of celiac disease. *B*, Biopsy of the bulb obtained at the same time as *A*. Findings are consistent with peptic duodenitis, with inflammation and distorted villi demonstrating gastric mucous cell metaplasia (arrows). (*A* and *B*, × 180) (From Yardley JH: Pathology of chronic gastritis and duodentitis. In Goldman H, Appelman HD, Kaufmann N (eds): Gastrointestinal Pathology. USCAP Monograph in Pathology 31. Baltimore, Williams & Wilkins, 1990, pp 49-143.)

Celiac-Related Conditions

Refractory Celiac Disease and Refractory Sprue

Most persons with celiac disease remain well on a gluten-free diet for many years, but some patients later develop recurrent symptoms despite close adherence to the diet. Loss of responsiveness to the gluten-free diet is usually termed *refractory celiac disease* or (generically) *refractory sprue*[82] (Figure 29-8). There are also some patients with malabsorption and a typical flat biopsy who do not respond to gluten withdrawal even at the time their illness is first diagnosed (Figure 29-9). The condition afflicting these individuals is termed *refractory sprue* (synonyms: unclassified sprue, atypical sprue) because their intestinal lesion is of uncertain or unknown etiology, although some of these persons probably have underlying celiac disease.[83]

Refractory sprue, whether associated with gluten sensitivity (refractory celiac disease) or not, is often accompanied by ulcerations in the small intestine (Figure 29-10A). The ulcerations can cause bleeding, perforation, or stricture.[82-84] They can be small and superficial or large and extend to the muscularis propria. The ulcers may be accompanied by pyloric metaplasia or ec-

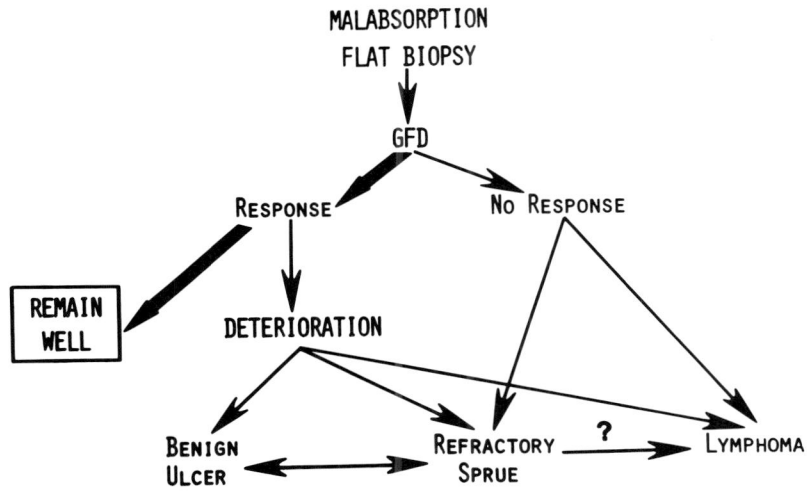

FIGURE 29-8. Celiac disease. Summary of possible clinical courses. Most patients who are found to have a flat biopsy and who subsequently adhere to a gluten-free diet (GFD) improve and remain well (thick arrows). A few, however, fail to respond to the diet at the outset or after an initial satisfactory response. The major unfavorable outcomes are indicated in the lower portion of the diagram.

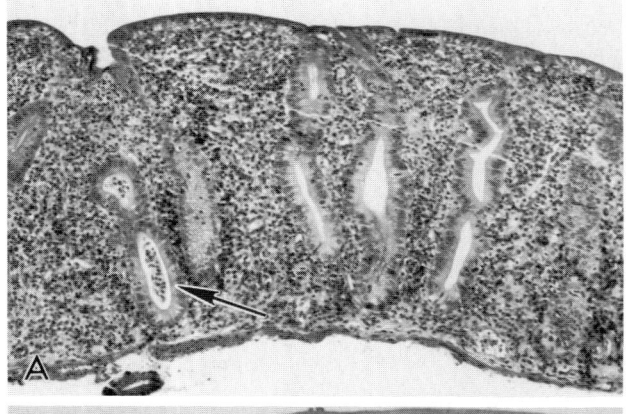
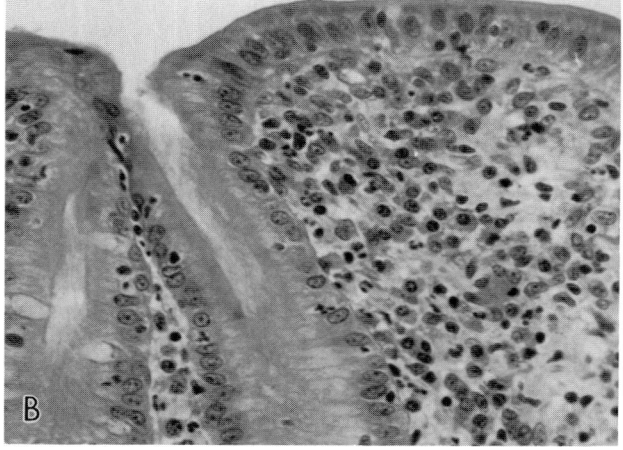
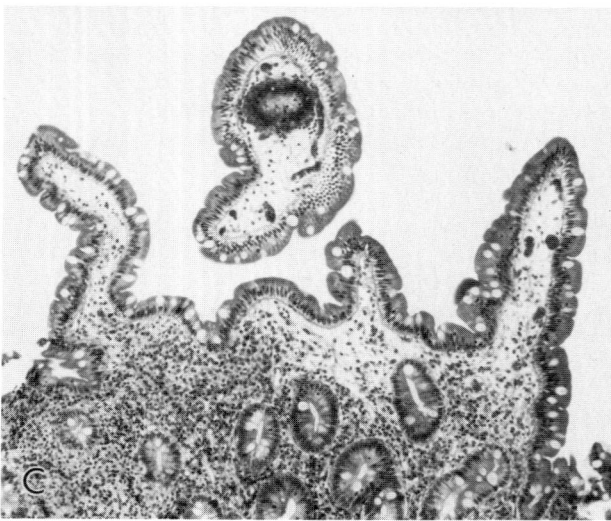

FIGURE 29-9. Refractory sprue in an adult. A gluten-free diet was ineffective, but malabsorption improved dramatically on corticosteroids. *A*, Initial flat biopsy with intense inflammation, including gland abscess (arrow). (× 90) *B*, Detail of specimen shown in *A*; the surface epithelium appears thinned and regenerating. Acute and chronic inflammation are present in the lamina propria, but the paucity of intraepithelial lymphocytes is in striking contrast to the typical findings in untreated celiac disease. (× 340) *C*, Restoration of villi seen shortly after initiating corticosteroid therapy. (× 90)

topic gastric mucosa,[85] but those features are typically lacking, and the pathogenesis of the ulcers is not known. Patients in full remission from their celiac disease as a result of treatment with either a gluten-free diet or corticosteroids can also develop ulcers (Figure 29-10B).[83,84] The presence of ulcers in refractory celiac disease or refractory sprue should always lead to a high index of suspicion of intestinal lymphoma, too.

Some ulcer-associated cases, especially those with refractory sprue, have been categorized in the past as "chronic ulcerative (nongranulomatous) jejunoileitis."[86] This is thought, however, to be a misleading term that should be avoided because it gives the impression that a distinct entity is described while failing to focus attention on the underlying malabsorptive disorder.

Acute inflammation is seen only rarely in celiac patients who respond well to gluten withdrawal. Thus, a biopsy specimen showing acute inflammation, with or without demonstrated ulceration (which could be nearby), should always cause suspicion that the individual may have ulcers and possibly refractory sprue or refractory celiac disease. The patient may also have an infection or other condition unrelated to celiac disease.

Lymphoma can present clinically as refractory celiac disease or refractory sprue and should be included in the differential diagnosis for unexplained or recrudescent malabsorption. Furthermore, in addition to the inherent sampling problem, early histologic changes in celiac disease–associated malignant lymphoma may be subtle and all but impossible to recognize, being noted only as scattered atypical lymphoid (often "histiocytic") cells that tend to infiltrate crypt epithelium. Lymphoma accompanying ulceration is also easily overlooked.[83,87]

In some patients with refractory celiac disease the poor response to a gluten-free diet may be related to associated hyperaciditiy that leads to additional mucosal injury.[88] Biopsies from the duodenum in these patients show peptic duodenitis combined with changes of celiac disease. The Brunner's gland enlargement associated with the peptic disease leads to a nodular appearance in the duodenum that at times is seen radiologically as a bubbly barium column ("bubbly bulb") (Figure 29-11).[88] The importance of hyperacidity in genesis of the lesion is supported by a favorable response in some patients to combined treatment with a gluten-free diet and H_2 blocking drugs.[88]

Cavitation of mesenteric lymph nodes and *hyposplenism* are two additional findings that are especially prone to occur in refractory celiac disease.[85,89] Cavitated mesenteric nodes are readily detected as an abdominal mass either by palpation or by computed tomography (Figure 29-12).[90] The nodes tend to concentrate in the jejunal mesentery; individual nodes can measure 5 cm or more. Lymphoma is frequently suspected in these individuals but is an infrequent associated lesion.[85] The cavitated nodes demonstrate a large central "pseudocystic" cavity from which fluid may gush on sectioning; histologically the cavitory space contains hyaline material and is surrounded by fibrosis and an outer rim of surviving lymphoid tissue. Patients with this condition also typically show hyposplenism clinically (presence of Howell-Jolly bodies and target cells in circulating erythrocytes) and have an atrophic spleen. The two findings are presumably associated in some

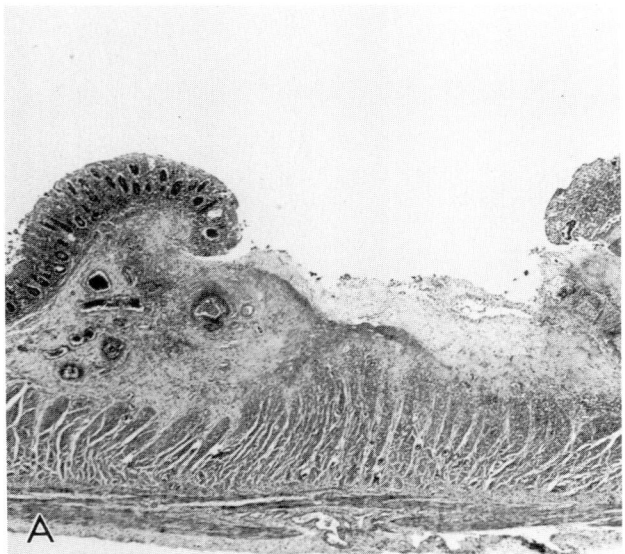
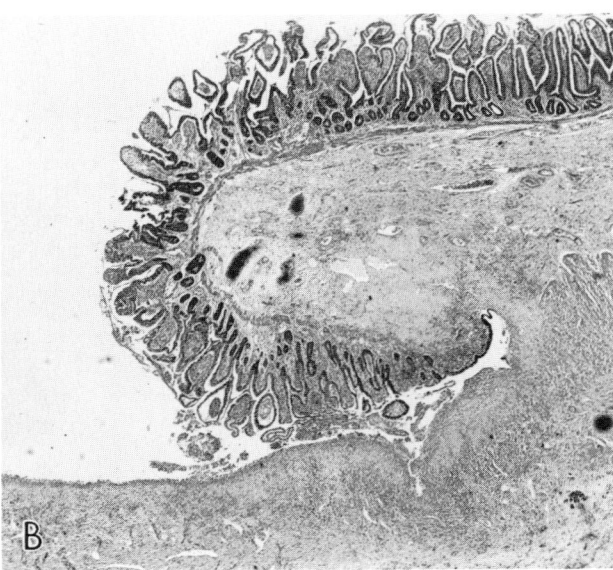

FIGURE 29–10. Ulceration in refractory sprue and in celiac disease. *A,* Ulcer in patient with malabsorption who never responded to a gluten-free diet (refractory or "unclassified" sprue). *B,* Ulcer in a patient with long-standing celiac disease responsive to a gluten-free diet who nonetheless developed multiple ulcers. Note absence of villi in *A* and their presence in *B.* (*A* and *B,* × 18) (From Baer AN, Bayless TM, Yardley JH: Intestinal ulceration and malabsorption syndromes. Gastroenterology 79:754–765, 1980, © copyright by The American Gastroenterological Association.)

way, although their pathogenesis is otherwise unknown. Some degree of hyposplenism is also common in celiac disease when cavitated mesenteric nodes are not detected.[90a] Studies of its possible relationship to malignant disease[91] and to autoimmune phenomena[90a] have been negative.

Collagenous Sprue

A curious and uncommon subset of patients with flat mucosal biopsies are those with so-called *collagenous sprue.*[92] In this condition the flattened mucosa shows intense scarring in the lamina propria. Bossart et al.

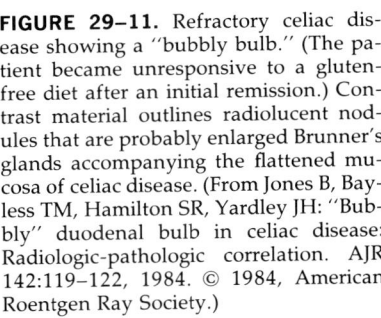

FIGURE 29–11. Refractory celiac disease showing a "bubbly bulb." (The patient became unresponsive to a gluten-free diet after an initial remission.) Contrast material outlines radiolucent nodules that are probably enlarged Brunner's glands accompanying the flattened mucosa of celiac disease. (From Jones B, Bayless TM, Hamilton SR, Yardley JH: "Bubbly" duodenal bulb in celiac disease: Radiologic-pathologic correlation. AJR 142:119–122, 1984. © 1984, American Roentgen Ray Society.)

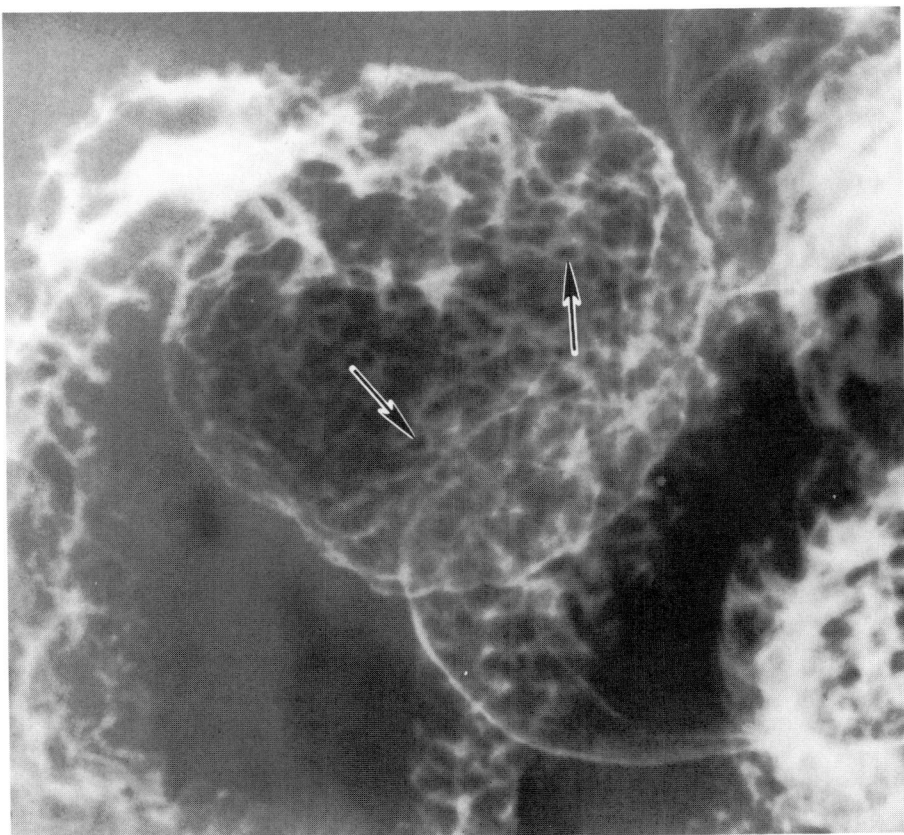

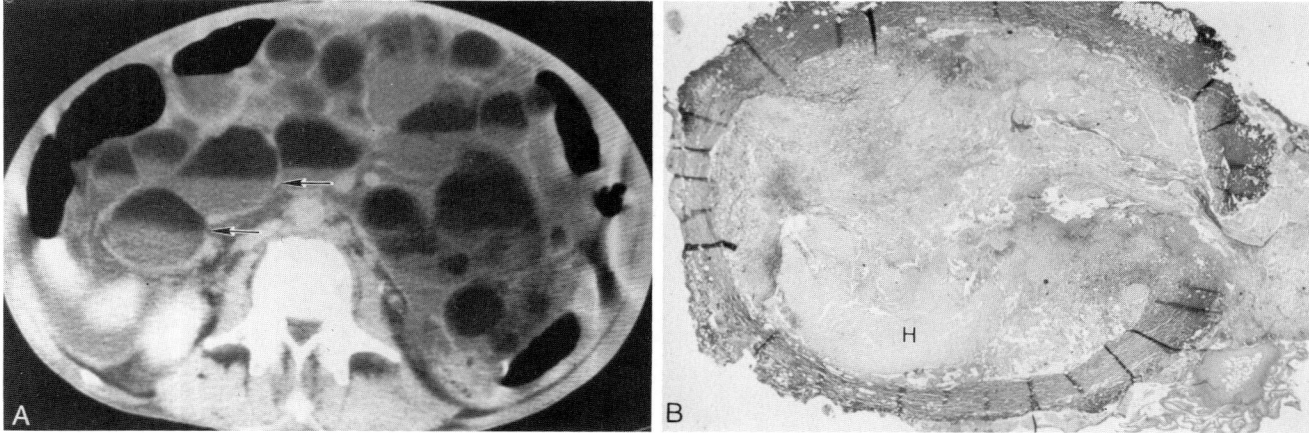

FIGURE 29–12. Cavitated mesenteric nodes in refractory Celiac disease. A, Computed tomographic scan showing greatly enlarged, cavitated node demonstrating fat-fluid levels (arrows). B, Histologic section of a largely destroyed cavitated node demonstrating hyaline material (H) and a separate upper region that contained abundant lipid. (From Rubesin SE, Herlinger H, Saul SH, et al: Adult celiac disease and its complications. Radiographics 9:1045–1066, 1989.)

found some degree of subepithelial collagen deposition in about a third of their patients with untreated celiac disease, and the collagen diminished on a gluten-free diet.[93] The clinical presentation in collagenous sprue is comparable to other instances of refractory celiac disease and refractory sprue, and the condition is now generally viewed as a variant form of celiac disease.[94,95]

Dermatitis Herpetiformis

Most patients with *dermatitis herpetiformis* have an associated derangement in the intestinal mucosa that closely resembles that seen in active celiac disease.[34,96–98] However, in dermatitis herpetiformis the mucosal lesion varies markedly in severity from patient to patient; also, its distribution in the intestine is less uniform than in celiac disease. Although up to 20% of patients with dermatitis herpetiformis have abnormal results in laboratory tests for malabsorption, only about 4% of the patients have intestinal symptoms.[34]

It was believed initially that dermatitis herpetiformis was not related to celiac disease or to gluten sensitivity. Subsequent experience, however, showed that individuals with dermatitis herpetiformis also have a high frequency of the same histocompatibility antigens (e.g., HLA-B8 and HLA-DR3) as celiac patients have, and that both the intestinal lesions and the skin lesions in dermatitis herpetiformis can be improved by adherence to a gluten-free diet. Reinstitution of dietary gluten in dermatitis herpetiformis leads to worsening of skin and gastrointestinal lesions with an increase in IgA- and IgM-containing plasma cells.[99]

Although the skin and intestinal lesions are histopathologically dissimilar, dermatitis herpetiformis patients almost always demonstrates deposition of IgA in the skin at the basement membrane, and this may be related to intestinal involvement.[34] The full pathogenesis of dermatitis herpetiformis and the nature of its relationship to celiac disease remain to be clarified. (See Chapter 16 for further details.)

Celiac-like and Celiac-Related Conditions Elsewhere in the Gastrointestinal Tract

Lymphocytic infiltration into the epithelium comparable to that seen in celiac disease is a prominent feature in lymphocytic gastritis (Chapter 20) and in lymphocytic ("microscopic") and collagenous colitis (Chapter 28). In fact, collagenous colitis resembles and took its name from collagenous sprue.[100]

Although these various forms of gastritis and colitis that share features with celiac disease most often occur as free-standing clinical entities in patients who give no historical or other evidence of celiac disease, lymphocytic gastritis and lymphocytic and collagenous colitis are sometimes seen in celiac patients. Among a group of patients with celiac-type disease from whom gastric biopsy specimens were available, lymphocytic gastritis was noted in 45%.[101] In one investigation lymphocytic colitis was found in 11% of celiac patients[102]; in another a much higher frequency (31%) was noted.[103] Celiac disease has also been reported in at least three patients with collagenous colitis.[104–106]

Small intestinal inflammatory changes that resemble celiac disease but that are refractory to gluten withdrawal can also be found in patients with lymphocytic ("microscopic") or collagenous colitis.[36,102,105,107] The accompanying small-intestinal lesion has consisted only of chronic inflammation and villus blunting in some patients, whereas in others there was collagenous change. Still other patients with small-intestinal changes resembling celiac disease who had never responded to a gluten-free diet (and hence had "refractory sprue") have also demonstrated lymphocytic infiltration of colonic epithelium. One such group of patients are said to have lymphocytic enterocolitis.[102]

Occurrence of celiac-like and celiac-related findings outside the small intestine has obvious significance from the standpoint of differential diagnosis. It is also of theoretic interest because autoimmune phenomena that are similar and/or related to celiac disease may be

Tropical Sprue (Postinfective Tropical Malabsorption)

Numerous definitions for tropical sprue have been proposed over the years, many with varying emphasis on particular findings. For all-encompassing conciseness, however, it is hard to improve upon the definition provided by Baker and Mathan[109]: "Intestinal malabsorption of unknown etiology, occurring among residents in, or visitors to, the tropics."

Noteworthy points about tropical sprue are as follows: (1) The malabsorption is *chronic* and is typically accompanied by various nutritional deficiencies with folate deficiency a usual hallmark. However, the deficiencies are secondary and do not, as was believed at one time, seem to be a primary etiologic factor. (2) Tropical sprue occurs only in certain areas, chiefly the West Indies (especially Puerto Rico, Haiti, and the Dominican Republic), portions of Central America and the northern countries of South America, the Indian subcontinent, south China, Southeast Asia, and central and southern Africa. (3) Adults are affected much more commonly than children. Expatriates such as military personnel who immigrate to endemic areas are often afflicted, but their illness tends to be more acute and they are less likely to present with severe folate and/or vitamin B_{12} deficiency and anemia. (4) The disorder is found in endemic and epidemic forms. Under both circumstances the patients' findings suggest an infectious etiology, including a frequent history of onset following an episode of an acute and presumably infectious diarrheal illness.

Etiology and Pathogenesis

The etiology of tropical sprue is unknown; indeed, there may be no single inciting agent. It is widely postulated, however, that tropical sprue begins with an episode of infectious diarrhea from a bacterial, parasitic, or viral organism. This is believed to be followed by residual and persistent damage to the mucosa, including absorptive cells. In addition, there is bacterial overgrowth by enterotoxigenic organisms (most commonly *Escherichia coli* and *Haemophilus*), which may be important in sustaining the disease.[110] Thus, broad-spectrum antibiotics are of major importance in treatment of tropical sprue.[111,112] The reason for the chronic bacterial overgrowth is poorly understood, but excess production of enteroglucagon with resulting reduced motility and stasis, thereby favoring heavy colonization, has been suggested.[113] At the same time, it should be stressed that the bacteria that colonize the intestine in tropical sprue are not predominantly of the anaerobic, bile salt–depleting variety found in the *stasis syndrome* (see further).[114–116]

Because it is a major site of folate and vitamin B_{12} absorption, damage to ileal mucosa leads to malabsorption of those vitamins with resulting deficiencies, especially of folate.[117] Individuals who are already malnourished are especially vulnerable. At the same time, there is evidence that folate and vitamin B_{12} deficiency can each *cause* derangements in intestinal mucosal structure and function.[12,118] Thus, the vitamin deficiencies, once in place in tropical sprue, are able to further enhance the intestinal mucosal damage and lead to megaloblastic anemia and other associated clinical findings.[117] Further support for the concept of direct damage by deficiency of the two vitamins is found in the favorable response to treatment with folic acid and/or vitamin B_{12} alone. Epithelial mitotic figures tend to reappear, nuclear size diminishes, and villi become more normal.[119] Ethyl alcohol, either ingested by the patient or produced locally by resident bacteria, may also be an important cofactor in mucosal damage.

Pathology

Histologically, the most common pattern in small intestinal biopsies is blunting and shortening of villi without total absence (Figure 29–13). This appearance matches well findings with the dissecting microscope of altered villus architecture with a shift toward leaves and ridges instead of tubular villi (Figure 29–14). There is chronic inflammation with increased lymphocytes, plasma cells, and eosinophils; and the surface epithelium is usually cuboidal, somewhat pseudostratified, and infiltrated by lymphocytes (see Figure 29–13B). The lymphocytic infiltration appears *after* onset of epithelial derangement and involves upper crypts and crypt-villus interzones, which suggests that cell-mediated immune response in the epithelium in tropical sprue is secondary.[120] This is in striking contrast to celiac disease, in which lymphocyte infiltration precedes or is concurrent with epithelial injury due to gluten and is focused almost entirely on surface epithelium.[120]

Total absence of villi comparable to that seen in celiac disease is only rarely noted in tropical sprue. Marsh et al.[120] stated: "Biopsies of proximal jejunum in over 1500 South Indian patients with tropical sprue have not revealed any with the "flat" mucosa characteristic of untreated celiac sprue." On the other hand, in tropical spruce unlike celiac disease, overall mucosal thinning occurs in more severely affected persons; and thus it can be said that a true mucosal and villous atrophy can be seen.[64,121] In the severest forms of untreated tropical sprue, the crypt epithelium shows reduced mitoses and nuclear enlargement (Figure 29–15).[122] Another noteworthy feature of the mucosal changes in tropical sprue is their *variability* both from patient to patient and from area to area in the small intestine of single individuals; this can be especially apparent with the dissecting microscope.[64,121] Despite the variability, the severity of the mucosal alterations tend to correlate with the severity of the clinical symptoms and laboratory findings.

Although epithelial changes are usually less prominent in tropical sprue than in celiac disease, there is good evidence that they contribute importantly to the malabsorption. Schenk et al. demonstrated diminished

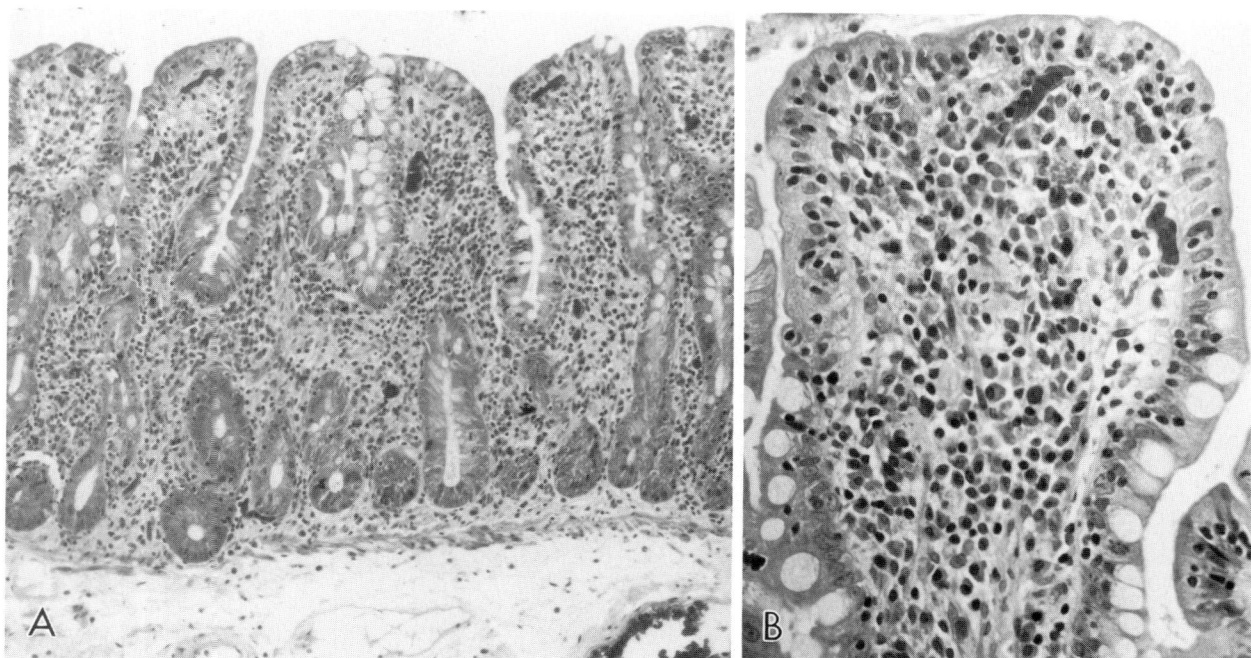

FIGURE 29-13. Moderately severe tropical sprue. *A*, The villi are blunted and shortened and the crypts elongated. On the other hand, there is not the *complete* absence of villi seen in celiac disease. There is overall increased chronic inflammation involving the lamina propria and epithelium. (× 120) *B*, The epithelium and lamina propria are infiltrated by lymphocytes and other mononuclears. The epithelium is cuboidal and somewhat stratified. (× 250)

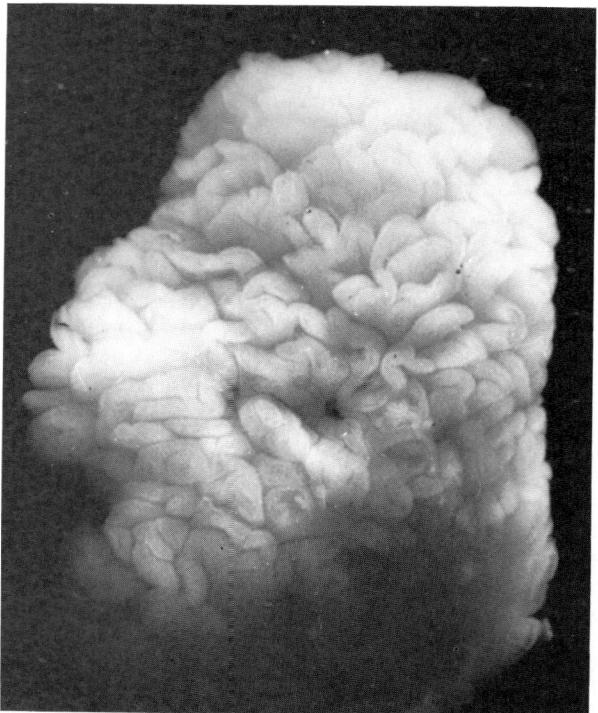

FIGURE 29-14. Alcoholic patient with malabsorption and folate deficiency comparable to that seen in tropical sprue. Ridges and large leaves have replaced the predominantly finger architecture of normal small intestine (compare with Figure 29-2A). Although an architectural shift of this type is characteristic of tropical sprue, it is in fact generally observed in conditions that demonstrate chronic blunting and shortening of villi.

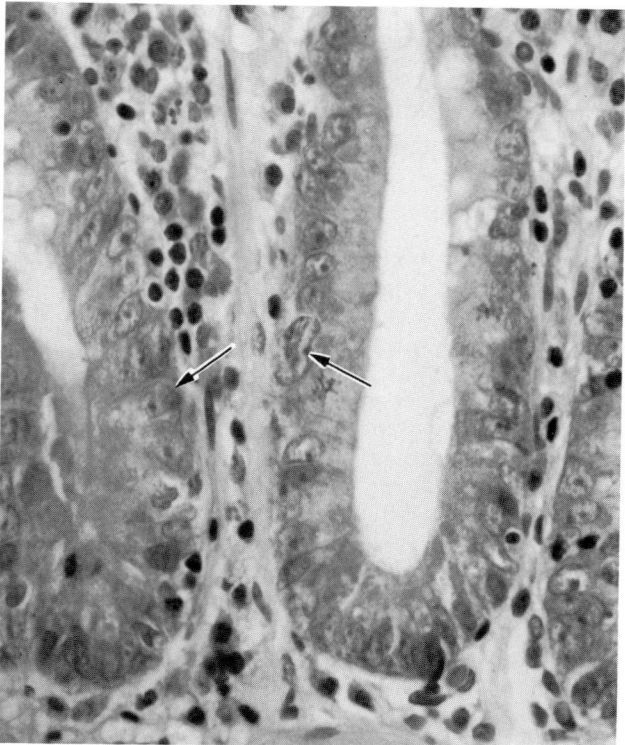

FIGURE 29-15. Tropical sprue. The lower portion of the crypts show enlarged, pale nuclei (arrows). Epithelial mitotic figures are generally sparse in this specimen. All are characteristic features of more severe degrees of tropical sprue. (× 550)

epithelial adenosine triphosphatase (ATPase) activity[64] and increased numbers of lipid droplets in the surface epithelium and just below the basement membrane.[64,123] The subepithelial region also often shows increased collagen and, by electron microscopy, finely granular and sometimes fibrillar material of unknown nature and significance. Similar material is occasionally seen in asymptomatic persons from the same part of the world and in other conditions affecting the small bowel, including celiac disease.[123]

The presence of mild to severe gastritis in about one half of a group of patients with tropical sprue led to the suggestion that the stomach is a possible additional site of disease.[124] However, there has been no confirmation of these findings. Furthermore, the available photomicrographs[124] show a nonspecific chronic gastritis comparable to that which is now recognized to be due to *Helicobacter pylori*. There is no evidence that deficiency of intrinsic factor plays a role in the B_{12} deficiency sometimes seen in tropical sprue. Instead, the deficiency is thought to result from consumption of the vitamin by intraluminal bacteria combined with ileal malabsorption.

Rare comments about histopathology of the colorectum suggest only that it appeared normal. Impaired absorption of water and electrolytes from the colorectum has, however, been described in tropical sprue,[125] and the mucosa showed low levels of sodium-potassium adenosine triphosphatase.[126] These abnormalities in the colorectum could contribute to the diarrhea. Findings in both the stomach and the colorectum in tropical sprue probably deserve further investigation.

Clinicopathologic Correlation

The occurrence of histologic changes of the type seen in tropical sprue does not always correlate well with the clinical and laboratory findings of malabsorption. Jejunal biopsies from symptom-free individuals living in areas where tropical sprue is endemic often show some blunting of villi and inflammatory changes that are qualitatively and at times quantitatively comparable to those seen in patients with demonstrated malabsorption. Although there are undoubtedly many variables, such as malnutrition, the patient's microflora, and the nature of inciting agents, that determine the final clinical picture, in all likelihood *distribution* of the lesion is a factor in the discrepancy between pathologic changes and clinical findings, too. In the earlier and milder stages of the disease, the mucosal changes diminish distally, but in chronic and advanced disease the ileum and jejunum typically are affected histologically to a similar degree.[127]

Differential Diagnosis

Because of the nonspecific character of the histopathologic changes, the importance of a maximal effort to exclude the many other possible causes of villus blunting and inflammation (see Table 29–1) before arriving at a diagnosis of tropical sprue cannot be overstressed. It is especially important to rule out malabsorption-associated syndromes due to known infectious causes (e.g., *Giardia lamblia*, *Stronglyloides stercoralis*, *Capillaria phillipinensis*). Obviously, demonstration of clinical features such as folate and/or B_{12} deficiency and a history of residence in the appropriate area of the world are also crucial.

Stasis (Blind Loop) Syndrome

The stasis syndrome is characterized by stagnation of intestinal contents and secondary proliferation of colonic-type bacteria occurring in a patient who has an underlying small-intestinal disorder that has led to delayed or altered movement of its contents. There is accompanying malabsorption of fat and, at times, of vitamin B_{12}, carbohydrates, and other substances. Synonyms are *blind loop syndrome*, *stagnant loop syndrome*, and *bacterial overgrowth syndrome*.

Conditions associated with the stasis syndrome include primary motor disturbance (see Chapter 11) and mechanical abnormalities resulting from a gastrointestinal disease or following surgical alterations (Table 29–4). It occurs in the small subset of *scleroderma* patients who develop saccular dilatations and diverticula of the small intestine secondary to degeneration of the muscularis propria. In patients with *pseudo-obstruction* there is dysmotility[128] and, at times, diverticulum formation due to nerve or muscle degeneration from an inherited defect. Bacterial overgrowth in even a single diverticulum in the duodenum can lead to malabsorption.[116] Patients with *diabetes mellitus* occasionally show motility disturbances as a result of peripheral neuropathy. Among various mechanical disturbances, stasis syndrome can be seen with spontaneous strictures and fistulas (as in Crohn's disease) or in a surgically isolated segment of intestine (blind loop). An enteroenterostomy can functionally become an isolated segment; in gastrojejunocolic fistulas, bacteria are constantly fed from the colon into the proximal small intestine. Stasis syndrome has also been described occasionally in elderly patients who lack demonstrable underlying disease.[129,130]

Table 29–4 DISEASES AND CONDITIONS ASSOCIATED WITH THE BLIND LOOP (STASIS) SYNDROME

Motor Disturbances
  Scleroderma
  Pseudo-obstruction
  Diabetes mellitus
  Amyloidosis
  Thyroid

Structural Abnormalities
  Diverticula of small intestine
  Strictures and narrowings
    Crohn's disease
    Tuberculosis
    Adhesions
  Surgically isolated segments
    Self-filling "pouches"
    Afferent limb in gastrojejunostomy
  Enteroenterostomy
  Gastrojejunocolic fistula

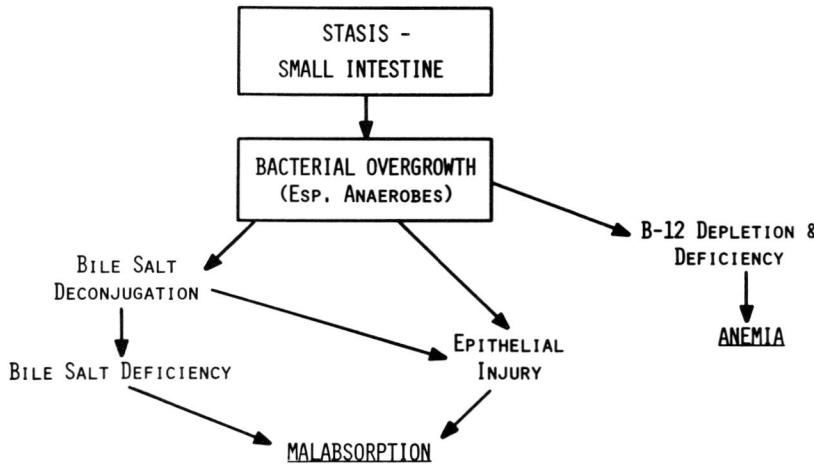

FIGURE 29-16. Blind loop (stasis) syndrome. Summary of pathogenetic factors leading to malabsorption and to anemia in some patients.

Pathogenesis

The roles of bacterial overgrowth in stasis syndrome have been studied extensively[116,131] and are summarized in Figure 29-16. At first the major focus was the effects of anaerobic bacteria on conjugated bile salts, compounds that are important to solubilization of fat into absorbable micelles. Anaerobic bacteria are not normally found in the small intestine, but typically occur in large numbers in patients with stasis syndrome. Certain of the anaerobic bacteria (Bacteroides and several others) can deconjugate bile salt to free bile acids. Free bile acids are ineffective as fat solubilizers, and fat malabsorption is felt to result from reduced availability of the conjugated bile salt. On the other hand, an association between fat solubilization and amounts of conjugated and free bile acids is not always demonstrated.[132]

The absorptive epithelium is also altered in stasis syndrome, and this could have as much or more importance than effects of changes in luminal bile salts and bile acids on micelle formation. Ultrastructural studies in patients[132] and in experimental animals[133] have shown epithelial damage and evidence of abnormal epithelial fat transport. Defective absorption and reduced brush border and other epithelial enzymes have been noted as well.[133-135] The cause of the epithelial injury is unclear, but unconjugated bile acids and bacterial metabolic products are suggested factors.

Depletion of nutrients by the luminal bacteria is an important factor in the vitamin B_{12} deficiency that these patients often show. Bacterial depletion may also cause other nutrient deficiencies, as suggested by the loss of administered d-xylose that occurs from bacterial action.

Definitive correction of mechanical conditions causing stasis syndrome such as blind loop is typically curative.[136] Furthermore, significant improvement in malabsorption is usually seen after reduction in intestinal flora from antibiotic treatment, thus confirming the importance of bacterial overgrowth.[131,137]

Pathology

Descriptions of the underlying disorders that can lead to stasis syndrome are covered in other chapters. Obviously, a mucosal biopsy will not serve to demonstrate changes in deep musculature or nerves or to identify gross mechanical disturbances that have led to to stasis syndrome.

The light-microscopic changes in small-intestinal biopsies from patients with stasis syndrome are easily summarized: They are nonspecific in character and variable in severity and do not necessarily correlate with clinical findings.[132] Although moderate and even severe changes may be noted, many biopsies show few if any abnormalities, and the changes are usually limited to chronic inflammation, with some villus blunting and reduction in the villus-to-crypt ratio (Figure 29–17).[132] Vesicles may be seen in the absorptive epithelium, especially over the villus tips; they probably reflect "hang-up" of absorbed lipid by damaged cells. The mucosal changes are often patchy in distribution

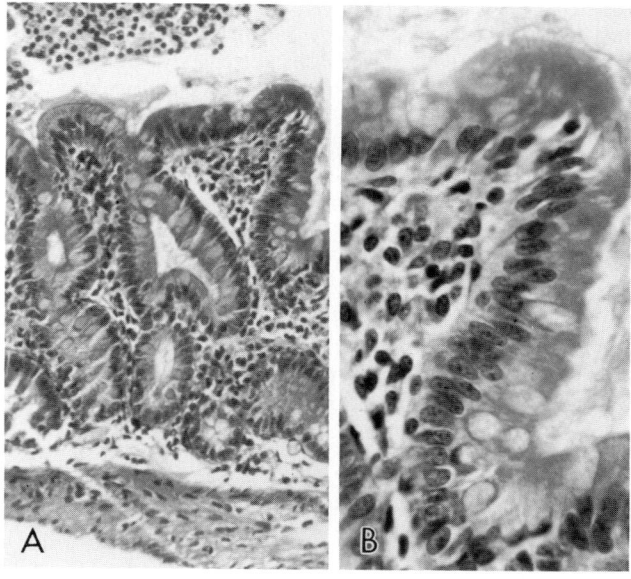

FIGURE 29-17. Jejunal biopsy from patient with gastrocolic fistula (post-Billroth II), leading to a "stasis syndrome." *A*, Villi are blunted and shortened, and there is increased chronic inflammation. *B*, The epithelium is not especially damaged or inflamed-looking. This is in keeping with the frequent poor correlation noted between pathologic changes and clinical findings in this condition. (× 675)

and severity, and multiple biopsy specimens may be needed to demonstrate them. On occasion, a smear prepared from the jejunal biopsy will show numerous bacteria in the mucus overlying the epithelium; but because of possible saliva-asociated organisms, their presence must be interpreted cautiously.

Experience with the markedly deranged mucosa of celiac disease during the early period after invention of the biopsy capsule was probably responsible for widespread initial failure to appreciate the potential importance in bacterial overgrowth conditions of relatively inconspicuous changes seen in villus epithelium by light microscopy.[138] The ultrastructural, enzymatic, and functional changes in absorptive epithelium described above in Pathogenesis do not always correlate closely with alterations seen by light microscopy, being typically more frequently observed and more prominent. This is a point to be kept in mind when one is evaluating biopsies from these patients.

Deficiency States

In addition to the numerous deficiency states that *result* from malabsorption, some deficiency states can *cause* malabsorption by damaging the small-intestinal mucosa. The direct effects of folate and vitamins B_{12} deficiency on the small intestine are discussed in the section on tropical sprue (see Etiology and Pathogenesis).

Protein deficiency (or protein-calorie malnutrition when total calorie intake is also inadequate), iron deficiency, and zinc deficiency have been shown to cause mucosal alterations *per se* and will be considered here. There are undoubtedly other deficiency states, too, whose relation to malabsorption has gone unrecognized or is less well defined.

Protein Deficiency

It is known from experimental studies that protein deficiency can lead to alterations in the small intestine with overall mucosal and muscle layer thinning, blunting of villi, epithelial thinning, and increased chronic inflammation (predominantly lymphocytes and plasma cells), especially when total calorie intake is also deficient (Figure 29–18).[139,140] There is frequently malabsorption, although not necessarily with steatorrhea or diarrhea; associated infection can lead to enhancement of histologic and clinical changes.[140] However, the effects of protein deficiency are variable. Rats placed on a low-protein diet for 22 weeks developed reduction in some epithelial enzymes such as acid phosphatase and succinic dehydrogenase, but epithelial ultrastructure remained normal.[141] On the other hand, only 3 weeks on a no-protein diet were required for rats to develop ultrastructural changes in absorptive epithelium.[139]

Although it is difficult to verify the impact on the human intestine of isolated protein deficiency, changes comparable to those produced experimentally have been reported in humans subjected to chronic protein malnutrition.[142–146] Klipstein et al. have summarized the difficulties of distinguishing among protein-calorie

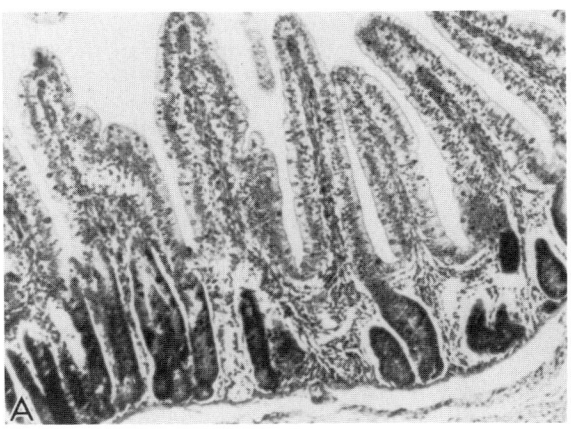
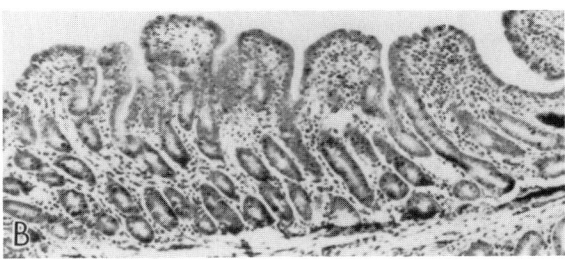
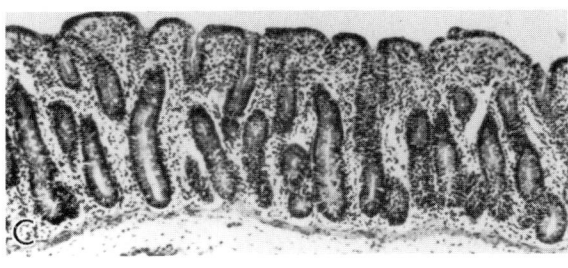

FIGURE 29–18. Effect of experimental protein-calorie deficiency on the jejunum in 3-week-old pigs. *A*, Normal-appearing jejunum after 52 days on a balanced commercial diet. *B*, Increased lymphocyte infiltration and blunting of villi after 53 days on reduced protein and calories. *C*, Severe changes produced after 205 days on slightly higher but still deficiency protein and calorie intake. Note the similarity of crypt depth in all three specimens. (From Platt BS, Heard CRC, Stewart RJC: The effects of protein-calorie deficiency on the gastrointestinal tract. In Munroe HN (ed): The Role of the Gastrointestinal Tract in Protein Metabolism. Philadelphia, FA Davis, 1964, 227–237.)

malnutrition, tropical sprue, superimposed infection, and other unknown factors in producing intestinal changes and malabsorption in Haitian patients.[147] Those authors considered patients who demonstrated both diarrhea and megaloblastic anemia to have tropical sprue, whereas those who showed reduced serum albumin without megaloblastic anemia, with or without diarrhea, were considered to have protein deficiency. Mucosal changes were more severe in those with tropical sprue, but lesser degrees of villus blunting, chronic inflammation, and so forth, were seen in both protein-deficient and asymptomatic patients.

In other studies, conducted in a tropical area where superimposed parasitic infection was common, it was found that treatment of protein-calorie malnutrition in children led to improvement in mucosal thickness, epithelial cell height, and brush border thickness.[148] However, when there was also chronic diarrhea (cause not specified), the epithelium showed greater inflammatory infiltrate. Control patients without past or present malnutrition showed minimal epithelial inflammatory infiltrate but nonetheless demonstrated macroscopic changes in villus architecture with blunting and ridge formation. Furthermore, inflammatory cells in the lamina propria were comparable in number and type for protein-calorie–malnourished children before and after recovery and for controls.[148] These studies emphasize that in the real world "pure" malnutrition rarely if ever exists and that multiple associated factors are the rule and usually always include undefined acute and chronic infections.

Iron Deficiency

Malabsorption associated with nonspecific mucosal abnormalities, including blunted villi and chronic inflammation, can occur in dietary iron deficiency anemia, and the abnormalities are corrected by adequate iron intake.[149] It is noteworthy that the malabsorption associated with iron-deficiency anemia in children may include impaired iron absorption, so that parenteral iron repletion may be needed for these patiens.[150] The mechanism by which iron deficiency causes gastrointestinal abnormalities is incompletely understood, but cellular enzymes are reduced in the mucosa of iron-deficient patients, including iron-dependent enzymes such as cytochrome oxidase.

Zinc Deficiency and Acrodermatitis Enteropathica

Zinc is an essential component of a number of metalloenzymes that participate in a variety of metabolic processes, including carbohydrate, lipid, protein, and nucleic acid synthesis.[151] Zinc deficiency can arise in a variety of clinical settings through diminished intake, competitive binding by certain foodstuffs, increased demand by the body, or increased excretion; and it can be accompanied by a wide range of clinical manifestations.[151]

Zinc deficiency is the underlying cause of acrodermatitis enteropathica, an inherited autosomal recessive disease in children. In addition to severe skin changes, the patient has diarrhea and malabsorption; if left untreated, the condition can lead to death. On the other hand, administration of zinc sulfate brings about rapid, complete remission. A similar syndrome can also occur at any age when zinc-free intravenous solutions are used for total parenteral alimentation over a prolonged (more than 1 month) period.[152–154]

The exact abnormality in zinc transport and/or metabolism in acrodermatitis enteropathica is not understood, but it has been suggested that the patient has a defective intestinal oligopeptidase that serves in normal persons to eliminate a zinc-chelating oligopeptide.[155] As a result, zinc remains bound to the oligopeptide and thus is unavailable for absorption. Symptoms of acrodermatitis enteropathica typically appear soon after weaning, perhaps because normal human milk provides the necessary enzyme. A smaller subset of patients with acrodermatitis enteropathica do not show reduced serum zinc, yet respond to zinc administration.[156]

Studies of the small intestine in acrodermatitis enteropathica have given variable results. Three untreated patients investigated by Kelly et al. showed "loss of villous architecture with flattening of villi, which in some areas was as severe as that seen in coeliac disease."[157] The surface epithelium was cuboidal, and increased chronic inflammation was seen in the lamina propria and epithelium. Some improvement occurred after treatment with human milk and diiodohydroxyquinoline (an older therapy for acrodermatitis enteropathica). Normal mucosal architecture was totally restored after 6 months of zinc administration. In another study, conducted before the importance of zinc was recognized, numerous proximal small-bowel biopsies showed *patchy* moderate to severe mucosal abnormalities with thinning, flattening, focal crypt necrosis, and reduction in crypts; rectal biopsies also showed abnormalities.[158]

Other investigators have described normal or minimally abnormal intestinal mucosa by light microscopy in acrodermititis enteropathica.[159,160] The discrepancies between these observations and the severe changes cited above are not readily explained, but possible differences in the degree and duration of zinc deficiency needed to produce skin versus intestinal lesions could be a factor. It is known that clinical manifestations can vary according to the severity of the zinc deficiency.[151] Another possible factor is the treatment other than zinc supplementation that was sometimes used.

Bohane et al. noted rodlike, spherical, and fibrillar inclusions in Paneth cells in small-intestinal biopsy specimens from patients with acrodermatitis enteropathica even though the specimens from patients with acrodermatitis enteropathica even though the specimens were normal by dissecting and light microscopy.[160] The Paneth cells became normal after zinc replacement. Similar changes in Paneth cells were described in experimental zinc deficiency in rats.[161] Ultrastructural abnormalities in Paneth cells were used to support a diagnosis of acrodermatitis enteropathica in a patient whose serum zinc levels were normal.[156] Other authors, however, believe that the Paneth cell findings are not specific for zinc deficiency, occurring also in malnutrition from a variety of other causes.[162]

Unclassified Nonspecific Inflammatory Lesions

It is important to recognize that in the last analysis a significant proportion of small-intestinal biopsies from patients with malabsorption show nonspecific chronic inflammation, villus blunting, and other changes that are not accounted for by any known or identifiable causative factor or aspect of the patient's clinical history. Absence of known causation is especially true for biopsies from patients who live in or have lived in tropical and developing countries, but can also occur elsewhere. Many such idiopathic cases could be infectious, but it is usually not possible to verify this in individual patients. Also, more than one factor may be operative, including multiple deficiency states and infections. It is preferable, therefore, for the pathologist to take a conservative stance and to consider such cases "unclassified."

INFECTION-ASSOCIATED MUCOSAL LESIONS

In this section some general points about infection-associated malabsorption will be mentioned, and the infections that bear a special relation to chronic malabsorption such as Whipple's disease will be covered in detail. Discussions of additional gastrointestinal infections are found in Chapters 14 and 26.

Viral Infections

Only nonspecific histopathologic changes (e.g., epithelial damage, villus blunting, and chronic inflammation) are found in most known viral infections of the small intestine. Pathologists are, therefore, usually unable to detect viral infection from conventional histologic material alone.[163] Nevertheless, it is important, if only from the standpoint of differential diagnosis, that they be aware that virally induced lesions in the small intestine can (1) be limited to that portion of the gastrointestinal tract and (2) be associated with significant clinical findings, including malabsorption.

It is also important to realize that many types of viruses have been implicated as causes or potential causes of gastroenteritis (Table 29-5) and that the list will undoubtedly grow. Furthermore, although viral infections of the gastrointestinal tract are largely associated with acute gastroenteritis from which the patient soon recovers, it is entirely possible that some viruses will be shown to be associated with chronic disease in the small intestine. Viruses may also play an indirect but essential role in chronic malabsorptive disease, as is being suggested for type 12 adenovirus and celiac disease.[55]

Bacterial Infections

The principal bacterial infection having a significant association with the malabsorption syndrome is Whipple's disease.

Whipple's Disease

This rare disorder was originally termed "intestinal lipodystrophy" by Dr. George Whipple because of the prominent accumulation of lipids in the intestinal mucosa and mesenteric lymph nodes.[164] Although Whipple himself saw bacteria in the tissues and remarked on their possible causative significance, for many years the disorder was viewed as a lipid storage abnormality.

Table 29-5 VIRUS INFECTIONS OF THE SMALL INTESTINE

Major Causes of Enteritis*
  Norwalk-like viruses
  Rotaviruses

Other Known or Possible Causes of Enteritis
  Enteric adenoviruses
  Astroviruses
  Caliciviruses
  Minirotaviruses
  Cytomegaloviruses*

*See Chapters 14 and 26 for additional information.

The bacterial causation of Whipple's disease was only (re)discovered with the advent of ultrastructural techniques.[165,166]

Patients with Whipple's disease typically present with the malabsorption syndrome, including steatorrhea and weight loss; protein-losing enteropathy is noted in some patients. Arthralgia and low-grade fever may also be prominent. Although it has long been recognized that Whipple's disease is a systemic, multiorgan disorder, awareness of nonintestinal forms of Whipple's disease has increased in recent years, especially after success with antibiotic treatment of the intestinal disease was followed by recognition of late-onset involvement of the nervous system and eyes.[167,168]

A jejunal biopsy in full-blown active Whipple's disease has a characteristic appearance and should be diagnosable from the hematoxylin and eosin (H&E)–stained preparations (Fig 29.). The villi often have a rounded and somewhat blunted appearance. Large extracellular lipid accumulations in the lamina propria that result from lymphatic blockage are frequently noted. Grossly, this can lead to a spectacular appearance with multiple white spots on the mucosa due to accumulations of chyle (Figure 29-19).[176] But the di-

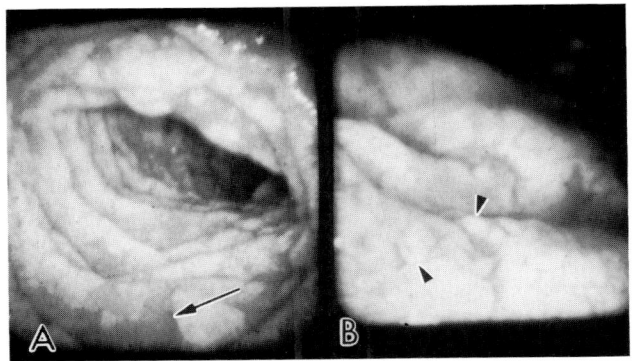

FIGURE 29-19. Whipple's disease. *A,* Low-power endoscopic view of the second portion of the duodenum. Thickened folds seem to be coated with granular, yellow-white material in a patchy distribution. Darker areas (arrow) represent more normal mucosa. *B,* Close-up view demonstrating prominent valvulae and enlargement of villi (arrowheads) because of chylous distention in paler areas. (From Volpicelli NA, Salyer WR, Milligan FD, et al: The endoscopic appearance of the duodenum in Whipple's disease. Johns Hopkins Med J 138:19–23, 1976.)

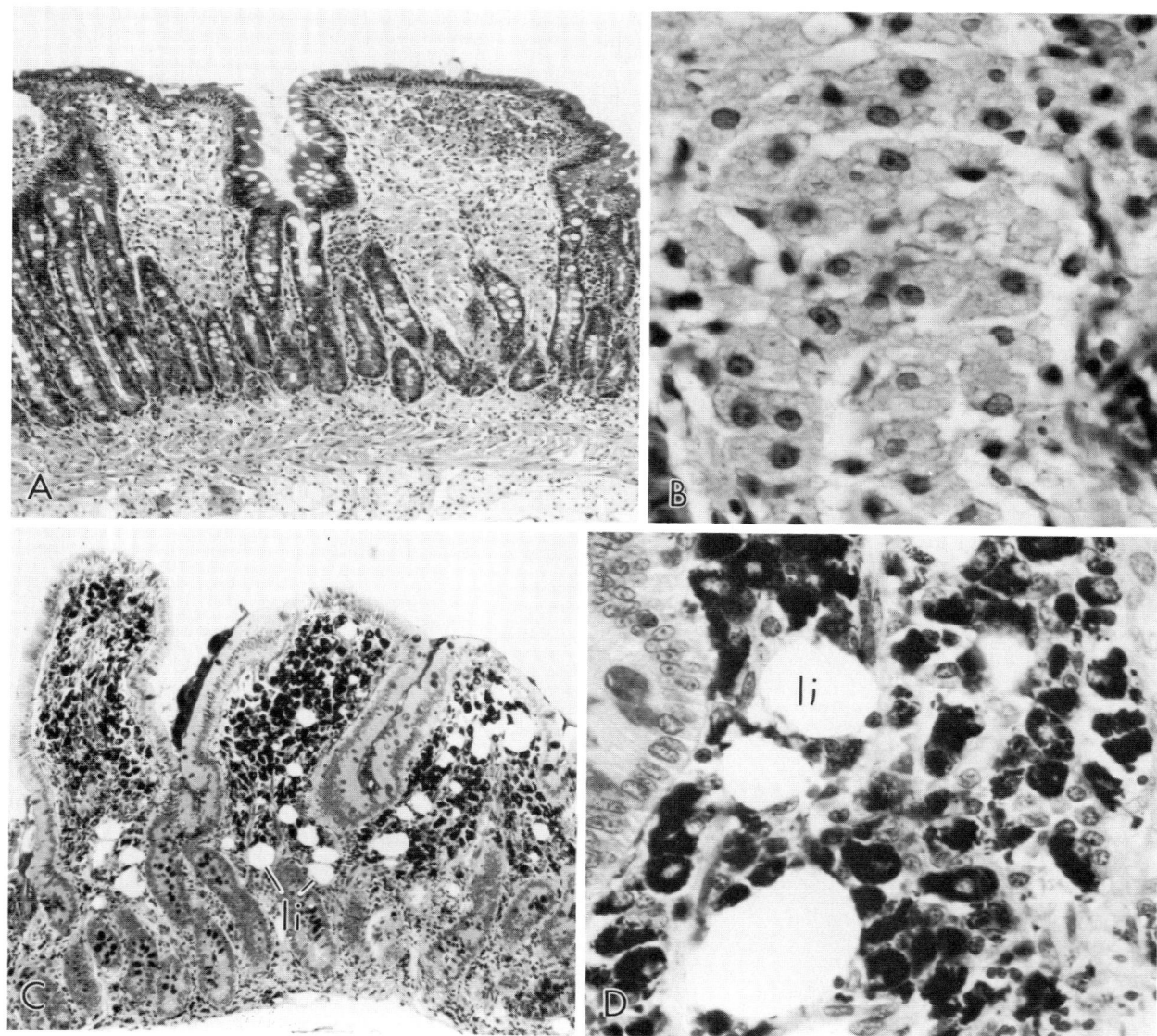

FIGURE 29-20. Whipple's disease—histopathology. A, Blunted and fused villi containing pale, foamy-looking macrophages. (× 90) B, Detail of foamy macrophages occupying lamina propria. (× 675) C, Periodic acid–Schiff (PAS) stain of another case demonstrating intensely PAS-positive (dark) macrophage contents. Extracellular lipid droplets (li) are also seen. (× 100) D, The macrophages are crammed with granular PAS-positive material. Lipid droplets are indicated (li). (× 510)

agnostic *sine qua non* is the presence there of numerous macrophages showing pink, foamy cytoplasm. Other inflammatory cell types are reduced in number, and on occasion polymorphonuclear leukocytes are observed (Figure 29–20A and B). A periodic acid–Schiff (PAS) stain demonstrates that the cytoplasm of the macrophage is packed with PAS-positive granules (Figure 29–20C and D). On occasion it is also possible to discern very small, rod-shaped PAS-positive, gram-positive objects in the extracellular space that are consistent with the causative organisms.

By electron microscopy, the small (1.0 to 1.5 μm) rod-shaped bacteria are seen both extracellularly and in the macrophages (Figure 29–21A). The macrophage granules are membrane-bound and show a variable content (Figure 29–21B–D). Some granules contain intact bacteria; in others the bacteria are degenerating; and still other granules contain no recognizable bacteria, showing only a membranous-looking material in irregularly patterned parallel array. These ultrastructural findings are consistent with the view that the bacteria are the causative agent in Whipple's disease and that they proliferate in the extracellular space, followed by phagocytosis by macrophages. The intracellular granules begin, therefore, as phagosomes containing the bacteria, which then undergo degeneration, becoming less and less recognizable in the granules until only the membranous structural elements remain.

It has been shown in detailed ultrastructural studies that the bacteria have an outer membrane of uncertain nature and an underlying cell wall with dimensions that are consistent with a gram-positive species. The

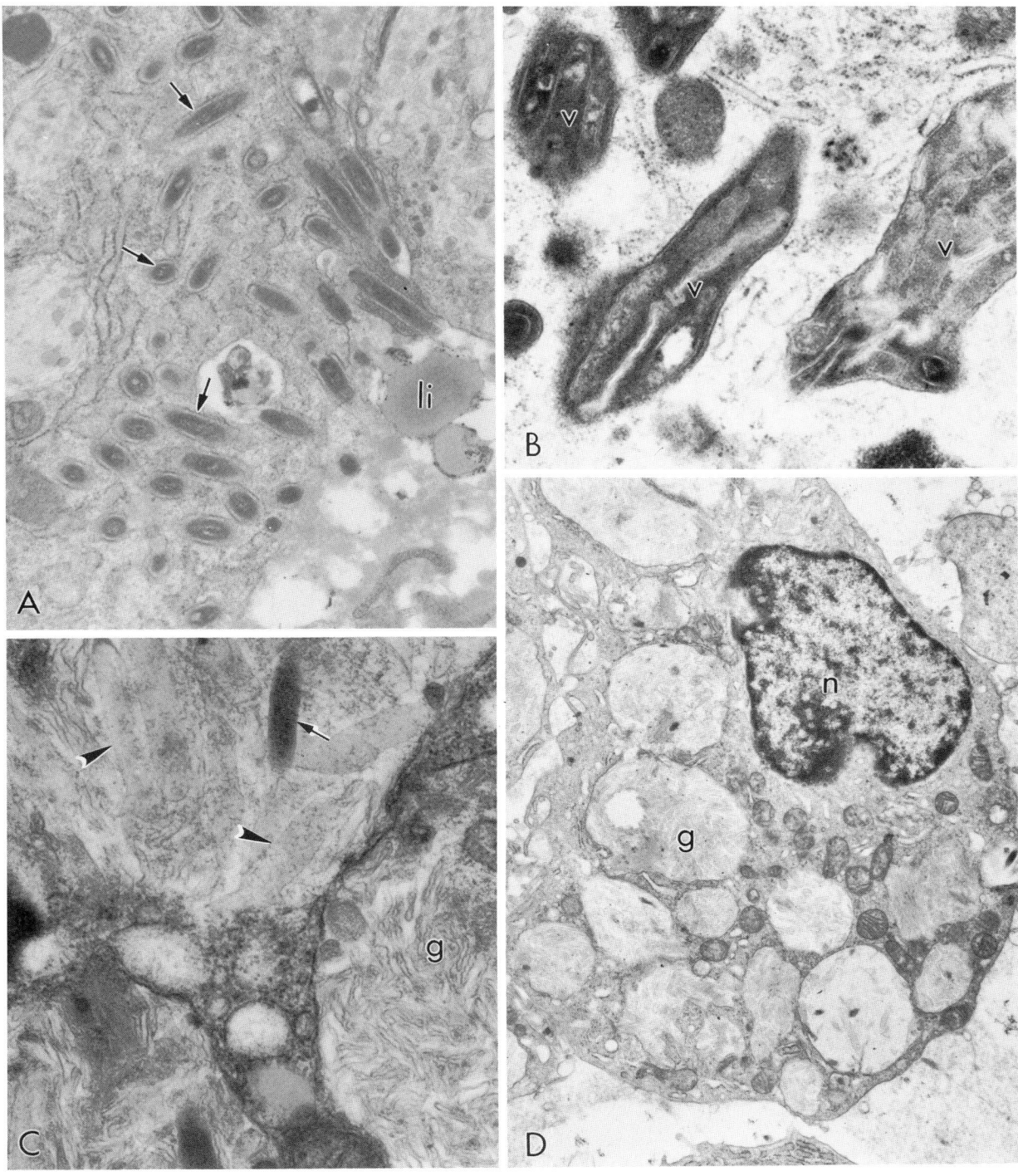

FIGURE 29-21. Whipple's disease—ultrastructural findings in lamina propria. *A*, Bacilli (arrows) are located in the cytoplasm of a macrophage, presumably soon after ingestion. Dark (osmiophilic) extracellular lipid droplets (li) are also evident. (× 15,400) *B*, Phagocytic vacuoles (v) in macrophages, each containing outlines of organisms undergoing digestion. (× 27,500) *C*, Transformation of phagocytic vacuoles into mature granules containing occasional residual bacilli (arrow) and ghostlike outlines of bacilli (arrowheads) (× 28,400) *D*, Overview of a "mature" Whipple macrophage; the nucleus (n) and a granule (g) are identified. (× 7300) (Courtesy of Dr. Jean Olson and Mr. Gerald Horne.)

cell wall also includes an inner membrane that is believed to be the origin of the residual PAS-positive membranous material in the macrophage granules after degradation of other bacterial components.[169] Rod-shaped intracellular bacteria are also found in other cell types in Whipple's disease. These include epithelium, fibroblasts, endothelium, leukocytes, lymphocytes, mast cells, and smooth muscle cells. This observation suggests that the causative agent is primarily an intracellular pathogen.[170]

There have been numerous attempts to isolate the causative agent of Whipple's disease and with extremely varied results that are largely unconvincing.[171] Immunohistochemical staining of the granules using a variety of antibacterial antisera has demonstrated strong cross-reactive affinity by the granules for antisera to certain classes of organisms.[172,173] Furthermore, macrophage granules in different patients from different geographic areas have shown affinity for antisera against comparable bacterial species. This finding supports the concept that Whipple's disease is caused by a single class of organism.[172] The most prominent affinity has been for antisera against streptococcal groups A, C, and G. This finding fits with previously published suggestions that Whipple's disease might be due to some form of streptococcus.[174,175]

Whipple's disease is a rare infectious disease, it being frequently noted that the number of patients ever seen is probably less than the number of articles ever published on the subject. This fact, combined with the unusual nature of the host response, suggests that host factors, such as abnormalities in macrophage function or immune response, are operative in addition to the causative bacterium. Studies so far have shown that macrophage function and the immune system is largely intact in patients with Whipple's disease.[171] However, while immunoglobulin production is normal, there may be some reduction in cell-mediated immune response.[171]

Whipple's disease is a systemic infection, and the characteristic PAS-positive macrophages have been noted in virtually all organ systems, including other regions of the gastrointestinal tract, the liver, lymphoid tissue, the heart, the central nervous system, and the eyes. Indeed, the major clinical manifestations may center on the heart, brain, or eye, either on first presentation of the patient or later on in those who are treated successfully for their gastrointestinal illness.

Whipple's disease is most reliably diagnosed from a small-intestinal biopsy. But there are pitfalls: (1) The diagnosis may be missed because of sampling difficulties. Small-intestinal biopsy specimens taken from adjacent areas of mucosa can show marked variation in numbers of PAS-positive macrophages.[176] Also, the diagnosis of Whipple's disease can be overlooked because PAS-positive cells may be located only in the submucosa, and this area is not always included in bi-

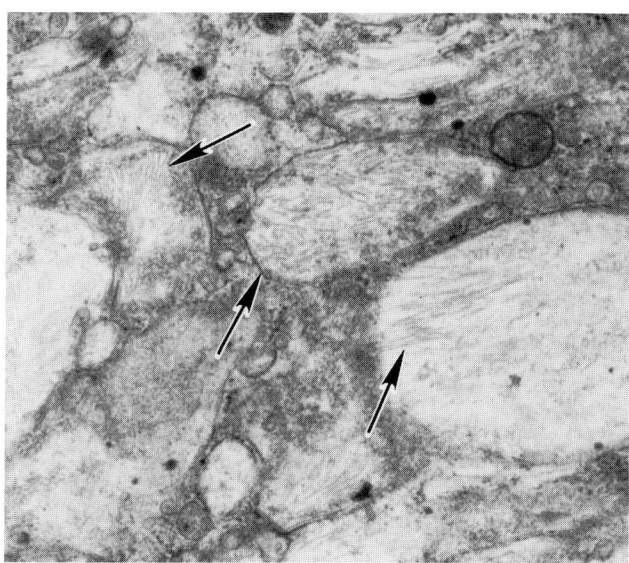

FIGURE 29-22. Posttreatment findings in Whipple's disease. By light microscopy a few macrophages with pale PAS-positive granularity were seen after antibiotic treatment. By electron microscopy these same macrophages are seen to demonstrate intracytoplasmic membrane-bound bundles of fibrillar material (arrows). Granules containing bacteria and residual membranous material (see Fig. 29-21C) were no longer detected. ($\times$ 37,800)

opsy specimens.[177] (2) Even partial treatment of Whipple's disease with antibiotics can reduce the number of PAS-positive macrophages. Furthermore, by electron microscopy, the residual macrophages may no longer show bacteria but may now contain characteristic posttreatment fibrillary material (Figure 29-22). (3) The pathologist must also be wary of a false-positive diagnosis: Normal intestinal mucosa will show occasional PAS-positive macrophages, although their appearance is usually atypical for Whipple's disease (Table 29-6). In questionable cases electron microscopy will help demonstrate the characteristic organisms and/or membranous intracellular granules. *Mycobacterium avium-intracellulare* infection in a patient with acquired immunodeficiency syndrome (AIDS) presenting with diarrhea and malabsorption is another potential source of error; a positive acid-fast stain will distinguish the lesion from Whipple's disease.[178] (See Chapter 14

Table 29-6 PAS-POSITIVE CELLS IN VARIOUS ORGANS THAT CAN MIMIC MACROPHAGES OF WHIPPLE'S DISEASE

Organ	Mimicking Cell(s)	Typical Staining		
		PAS	Alcian Blue*	AFB
Small intestine	Macrophages: Nongranular or granular (lipofucsin)	+	−	−
	Mycobacterium avium-intracellulare in AIDS	+	−	+
Lymph nodes and liver	Macrophages: nongranular or granular (lipofucsin?)	+	−	−
Stomach	Macrophage as above	+	−	−
	Carcinoma	+	+ (usual)	−
Colorectum	Muciphages	+	+	−

*Alcian blue at pH 2.5.
PAS, periodic acid-Schiff; AFB, acid-fast bacteria.

under AIDS for additional information about *Mycobacterium avium-intracellulare*.)

It is possible to diagnose Whipple's disease by demonstrating PAS-positive macrophages in an organ other than the small intestine. Indeed, this may be essential in those situations where PAS-stained macrophages are absent in the small intestine, especially in CNS Whipple's disease arising after treatment. However, diagnosis of the disorder from tissues other than small intestine must be approached with particular skepticism because PAS-positive cells of various types can be seen in multiple locations in persons without Whipple's disease (see Table 29–6). When the spurious cells are in fact macrophages, they often contain lipofuscin ("wear-and-tear pigment"). Such macrophages can frequently be recognized by their small size and because the PAS-positive granules are either absent or show more variation in size than those seen in Whipple's disease. In addition, the lipofuscin may impart a brownish or yellowish hue to the granules or cytoplasm in H&E sections. Mucin-positive cells in the lamina propria of the stomach should additionally be considered as possible isolated cancer cells.

Muciphages are foamy-looking macrophages that are commonly noted in colorectal biopsies; they contain PAS-positive granules that are believed to represent mucosubstances from the colon. Muciphages can lead to either over- or underdiagnosis of Whipple's disease. There are some differences between muciphages and Whipple macrophages that may be helpful in distinguishing between the two entities: muciphage granules are usually (but not universally) also alcian blue–positive at pH 2.5 and tend to have a broader size range than the strictly PAS-positive and smaller granules of Whipple's disease. Unfortunately, however, there is another limitation that renders colorectal biopsies essentially useless for definitive diagnosis of Whipple's disease by light microscopy: by electron microscopy Whipple's disease granules *and* muciphage granules can occur in the *same* colorectal mucosal macrophages.[179] Fortunately, similar cells do not occur elsewhere in the gastrointestinal tract.

Fungal Infections

Fungal infections of the alimentary tract are discussed in Chapters 14 and 26. They are not a significant cause of malabsorption. However, *Monilia* and *Histoplasma* are rarely mentioned as infectious agents in the small intestine and is briefly discussed here.

Moniliasis

Ten hospitalized patients with severe noncolitic, secretory diarrhea due to overwhelming infection caused by monilial (candidal) organisms have been described.[180] Most were elderly individuals being treated with multiple antibiotics or chemotherapeutic agents. We have seen severe moniliasis in an immunodeficient patient under treatment for leukemia. There was monilial esophagitis and marked destruction of villi over the entire length of the small bowel. The stomach was largely spared, presumably because of low pH. Histologically, the small intestine revealed a heavy superficial coating of yeast and pseudohyphae. The underlying villi had undergone necrosis and acute inflammation. The patient experienced cholera-like watery diarrhea, presumably because of diminished absorptive capacity combined with secretion from intact crypts.

Histoplasmosis

Although *Histoplasma capsulatum* is capable of infecting all parts of the gastrointestinal tract from the mouth to the anus, the ileum being most frequently involved, it is an extremely rare cause of malabsorption.[181] In the single case report of that association in the world's literature, there was disseminated histoplasmosis, and the patient presented with watery diarrhea of explosive onset along with laboratory evidence of malabsorption.[181] *H. capsulatum* was grown from a small-bowel biopsy specimen. Histologically, the specimen showed blunted villi and a heavy mononuclear infiltration. Organisms were seen in the mononuclear cells in the intestine as well as in liver, breast, and skin.

Protozoan Parasitosis

For a general discussion of parasitic disease and malabsorption, see Brasitus.[182]

The principal protozoan infections that can cause malabsorption are giardiasis, coccidiosis, cryptosporidiosis, and microsporidiosis. Pathologists should be able to recognize these protozoan organisms in small-intestinal biopsies and develop the habit of searching for them in all patients with diarrhea and/or malabsorption. There is also some evidence to suggest that malaria may be associated with malabsorption, perhaps because of effects on the microcirculation.[182] Giardiasis and coccidiosis are covered in Chapter 26, and cryptosporidiosis is considered in Chapter 14. Microsporidiosis is increasingly recognized as a common cause of diarrhea and malabsorption in immunocompromised patients, especially in those with AIDS,[183] and is discussed here.

Microsporidiosis

Although long known to occur in arthropods and fish, infections due to organisms of the phylum Microspora were only rarely described in warm-blooded animals, including man, until recently.[183] They are obligate intracellular parasites whose life cycle has both proliferative and spore-producing phases.[184] The defining feature is the presence in each spore of a coiled *polar filament* that is used to transmit the infection to a host cell by injecting it with the spore contents. Intestinal microsporidiosis in humans is largely due to a newly described agent—*Enterocytozoon bieneusi*.[185]

E. bieneusi is the apparent causative agent in a siza-

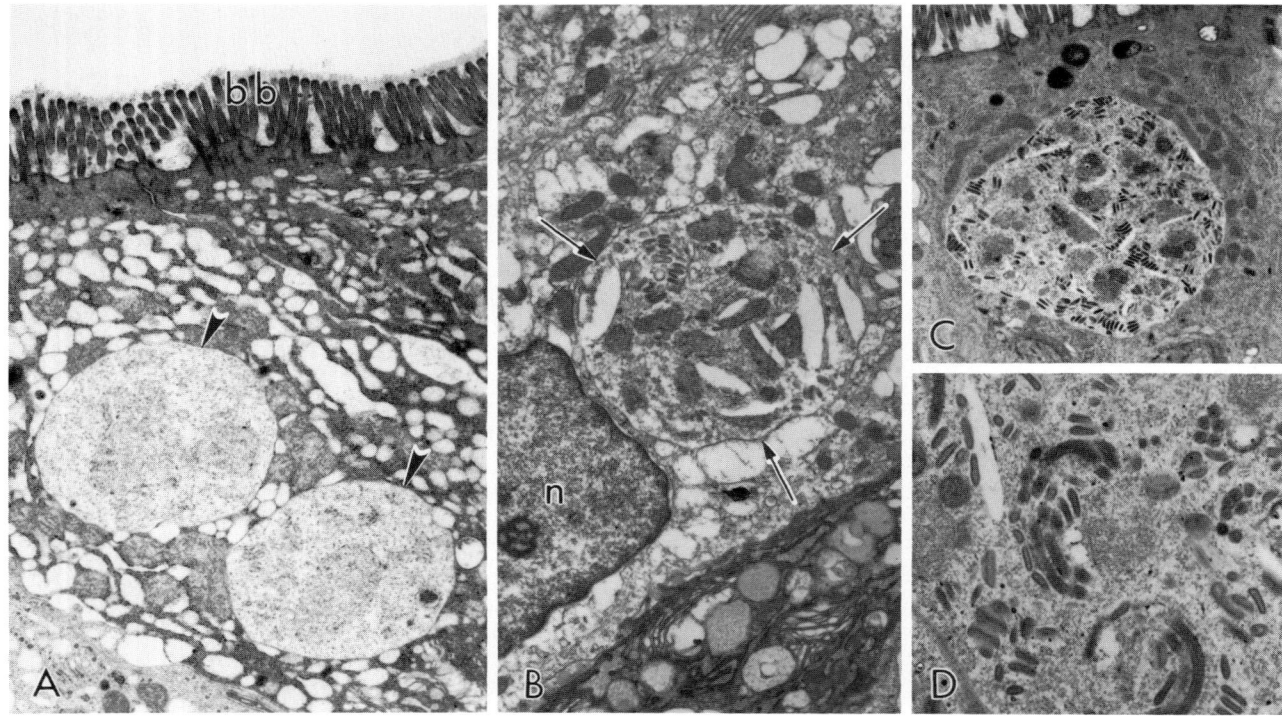

FIGURE 29–23. Microsporidiosis (*E. bieneusi* infection). Electron microscopy of infected villus tip enterocytes in a patient with AIDS. *A*, Two pale, early plasmodia (arrowheads) are seen just beneath the brush border (bb). The enterocyte epithelium is vacuolated—evidence of cellular injury. (× 8400) *B*, Plasmodium (outlined by arrows) undergoing sporogeny; nuclear material has divided into separate darker clumps. Note the characteristic open clefts in the organism and the typical concave deformity in the adjacent enterocyte nucleus (n). (× 7200) *C*, Multiple polar filaments have appeared in this organism during sporogeny. (× 6200) *D*, Detail of polar filaments during their formation. (× 18,200) (Courtesy of Drs. Joel Greenson and Audrey Lazenby.)

ble proportion of AIDS patients who have chronic diarrhea. Orenstein et al. found the organisms in small-intestinal epithelium from 20 of 67 AIDS patients who had chronic diarrhea and no other pathogen demonstrable by either light microscopy or by microbiologic techniques.[186] Similarly, other investigators demonstrated Microsporida in 5 of 11 AIDS patients with diarrhea and no additional pathogen.[187]

E. bieneusi organisms were demonstrated much more commonly in jejunal than in duodenal biopsies.[186] Electron microscopy is the most reliable method for detecting the infection and is required for species identification.[183,187,188] The plasmodial (meront) form of the organism occurs chiefly in the supranuclear cytoplasm of villus epithelium, especially those at the villus tips. The plasmodia have an average diameter of about 5 μm; a characteristic feature is the presence of one or more empty clefts or slits in the organism (Figure 29–23). The spores can be observed in various stages of development and when mature measure about 1.0 by 1.5 μm (Figures 29–23 and 29–24). Demonstration of the polar filaments either during spore development or in mature spores is crucial to positive identification of microsporidia.

Light-microscopic study of methylene blue–azure II–stained thick (~ 1 μm) sections from plastic-embedded tissue is almost as reliable as electron microscopy for demonstration of both plasmodia and spores (Figure 29–25).[186] In these preparations the plasmodia may be paler than the surrounding cytoplasm, whereas the spores are denser. Another approach that could prove to be both simple and reliable for detecting Microsporida is the use of Giemsa-stained dried smears prepared from small-intestinal biopsies or stool[188,189]; duodenal fluid can also be effective.[190]

Detection of microsporidan organisms in H&E-stained paraffin sections is possible and should be attempted, although it is more difficult and less dependable than electron microscopy or use of the methylene blue–azure II–stained thick sections. Optimal results with conventional histologic material require thin sections of well-preserved and uniformly stained tissue.[186] The plasmodial form, which is basophilic in H&E-stained sections, is especially difficult to demonstrate because not only is it small, but its staining is often only slightly darker than that of the surrounding epithelial cytoplasm. The organisms are typically most numerous in degenerating and sloughing epithelium at the villus tips (Figure 29–26A). Associated intraepithelial spores may also be seen in H&E-stained paraffin sections as very small refractile bodies.[186] The spores are, however, gram-positive and thus at times easily identified in paraffin sections with the use of bacterial stains (e.g., Brown and Brenn)[191] (Figure 29–26B). Unfortunately, the spores may be sparse or even absent.[188]

Histologically, the mucosa in patients with microsporidiosis shows some blunting and shortening of villi, chronic inflammation with numerous lympho-

MALABSORPTIVE DISORDERS 751

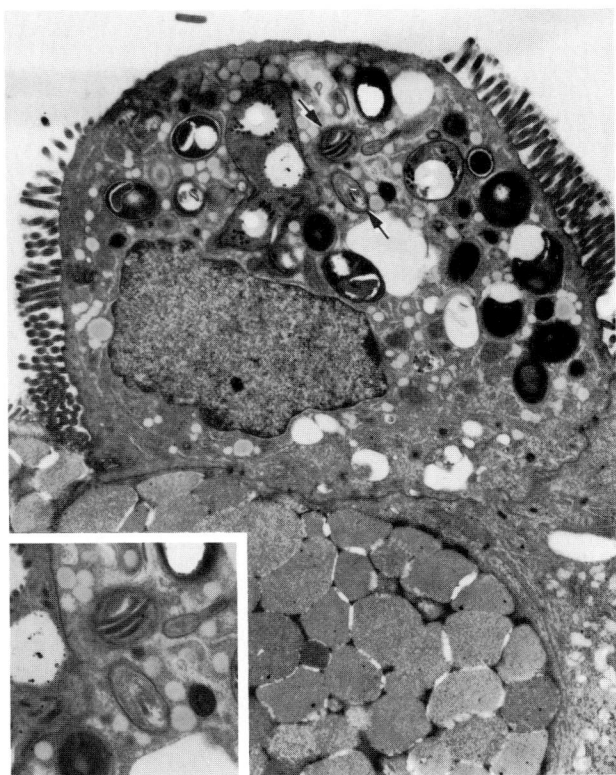

FIGURE 29–24. Microsporidiosis (*E. bieneusi* infection in AIDS). An enterocyte that contains multiple mature spores is about to be extruded from the villus tip. An adjacent goblet cell is present at the bottom of the picture. Coiled polar filaments are visible inside two of the spores (arrows). (× 6300) *Inset,* Closer view of spores, revealing the thin, tightly coiled polar filaments. (× 17,250) (Courtesy of Dr. Joel Greenson.)

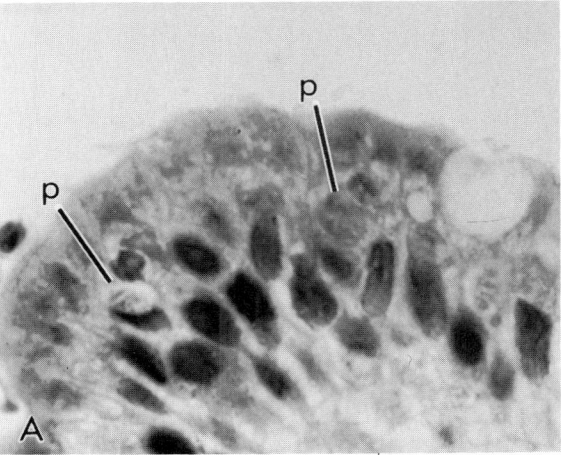

FIGURE 29–26. Microsporidiosis (*E. bieneusi* infection in AIDS) as seen in formalin-fixed, paraffin-embedded tissue. *A,* H&E staining. Plasmodia (p) are visible, one with indentation of the subjacent nucleus. (× 1225) *B,* Brown and Brenn bacterial staining demonstrating gram-positive staining of spores (arrow). (× 1850)

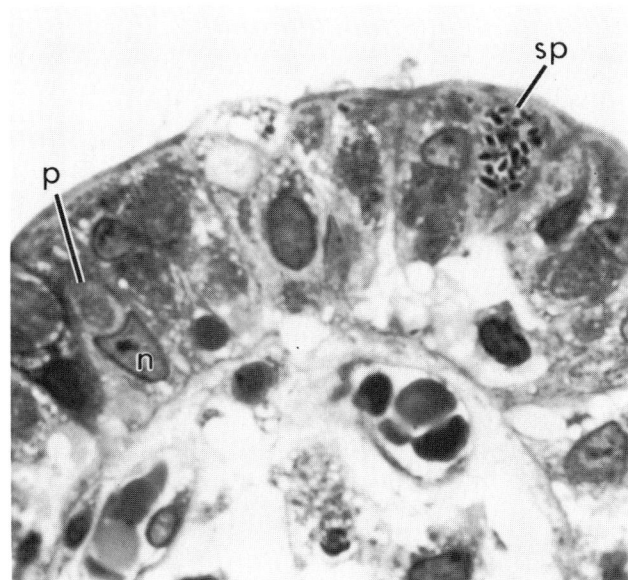

FIGURE 29–25. Microsporidiosis (*E. bieneusi* infection in AIDS). Plastic "thick" (1 μm.) section of a villus tip. A plasmodium (p) containing faintly visible open clefts is sharply outlined. The adjacent enterocyte nucleus (n) is indented. Dark-staining spores (sp) are seen elsewhere. Clumps of dark, amorphous material in other enterocytes are of uncertain significance. (Methylene blue–azure II stain, × 1225)

cytes and plasma cells in the lamina propria, and increased intraepithelial lymphocytes.[186,187] Small-intestinal microsporidiosis has so far been limited to patients with AIDS, and it should be noted that the mucosal changes are also consistent with that condition alone (see below on AIDS).

Metazoan Parasitosis

Nematodes (round worms) and cestodes (tapeworms) are the principal metazoan parasites that infect the small intestine. Most are largely asymptomatic or cause minimal discomfort. The larger nematodes and cestodes do rarely cause obstructive symptoms. Also, intestinal tapeworms (especially *Diphylobothrium latum*) can be associated with secondary vitamin B_{12} deficiency,[182] and hookworm infection can lead to iron-deficiency anemia and be accompanied by hypoproteinemia if the worm burden is large.[192] In general, however, visible changes in the mucosa and associated malabsorption are not found in metazoan parasite infections. The exceptions are possibly ascariasis, strongyloidiasis, capillariasis, and schistosomiasis (especially *Schistosoma japonicum*, since the egg-laying

Ascariasis

Infection with *Ascaris lumbricoides* is frequent in economically deprived individuals living under poor sanitary conditions in tropical and subtropical areas. Although *Ascaris* sometimes causes obstruction to hollow viscera, the large (up to 35 cm) organism lives free in the lumen and is not known to cause mucosal injury or inflammation or to lead to malabsorption by direct means. However, its potential importance in small-bowel function when malnutrition is also present was shown in one investigation in which malabsorption was noted in children having both a large *Ascaris* burden and poor protein intake.[193] Steatorrhea and d-xylose absorption improved after *Ascaris* organisms were eradicated, even though the children continued their low protein intake. Unfortunately, jejunal biopsies could not be done in that study, and the exact nature of the role played by the *Ascaris* in the malabsorption was not examined further.

Strongyloidiasis

The causative agent of strongyloidiasis is *Strongyloides stercoralis*. The infection, like capillariasis and schistosomiasis, differs from the other intestinal worm infections in that mucosal alterations may be present and the diagnosis can be made from an intestinal biopsy. *Strongyloides* occurs in tropical and temperate areas throughout the world but is most common in warm, moist climates, where in some instances (e.g., Brazil) up to 85% of the population may be infected.[194] It also is endemic in warmer areas of the United States, and can be found in individuals who have traveled to heavily infested regions such as Southeast Asia.

The mature adult female resides indefinitely (e.g., 30 years or longer) in mucosal crypts, typically in the duodenum, where eggs are probably produced by parthenogenesis. Eggs become larvae in the crypt epithelium. The larvae usually then escape into the bowel lumen and pass harmlessly out of the host with the stool. If, however, the host is subjected to generalized debilitation as from tumor, or becomes malnourished, or if there is supervening immunosuppression or other immunodeficiency state, including AIDS, the patient can develop an *internal autoinfection* or *hyperinfection* with *Strongyloides* larvae.[195] In this condition larvae reinvade the host instead of passing into the stool. This leads to widespread vascular dissemination and a resulting severe systemic illness. There may be malabsorption and hypoproteinemia and, rarely, associated urinary, cardiac, or central nervous system symptoms. Eosinophilia, which is common in the mild cases, will frequently disappear during hyperinfection. Early diagnosis of hyperinfection is critical because it is potentially lethal.

Unexplained bacteremia due to enteric organisms associated with hyperinfection in strongyloidiasis has been described.[195] It is believed that the larvae carry

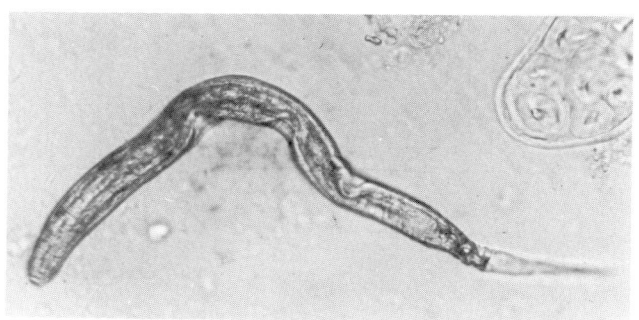

FIGURE 29–27. Strongyloidiasis. Rhabditiform larva in stool. The stool examination was crucial to this patient's diagnosis since a mucosal biopsy showed only nonspecific inflammation, prominent eosinophils, and villus blunting.

bacteria into the host either by surface adherence or in the larval intestine. Gram-negative bacillary meningitis can be a prominent aspect of the illness.

Diagnosis of strongyloidiasis is most frequently based on demonstration of larvae in duodenal drainage or stool (Figure 29–27).[196] A fresh specimen is needed, because if stool-containing hookworm eggs are allowed to stand around, they will hatch into larvae that closely resemble *Strongyloides*. Also, specimens containing *Strongyloides* larvae can, if stored, mature into different-looking free-living filariform larvae or adults. In a newer test, the larval forms of various species are distinguished by their characteristic tracks in soft agar.[197]

The appearance of *Strongyloides* in small-intestinal biopsies is characteristic. Organisms may be recognized as eggs or as embryonating larvae and, more rarely, adult worms. The adult female is recognized by its larger size and presence of reproductive tubes. All stages of the *Strongyloides* organism can be seen in the crypts, with eggs and hatching larvae being noted within the crypt epithelium (Figure 29–28).

Reactive changes in the mucosa are nonspecific. However, eosinophilia may be striking, and there is usually chronic inflammation and some blunting of villi. Thus, even when it is often not possible to demonstrate the organisms, heavy concentrations of eosinophils suggest the diagnosis, which is in turn verified by examining duodenal drainage or stool. Hyperinfection may be associated with large numbers of larvae in the mucosa, along with erosion, and larvae may be demonstrated in deeper structures (Figure 29–29). The colon may also be involved in hyperinfection,[194] so that it is also possible that the diagnosis will be made from a colonic or rectal biopsy.

Capillariasis

The causative agent is a nematode *Capillaria philippinensis*.[198,199] Capillariasis has been described only since 1964. Most patients reside in the Philippines, although cases have been noted more recently in Taiwan, Southeast Asia, and the Middle East.[200,201] Thus, although capillariasis is confined to a relatively small

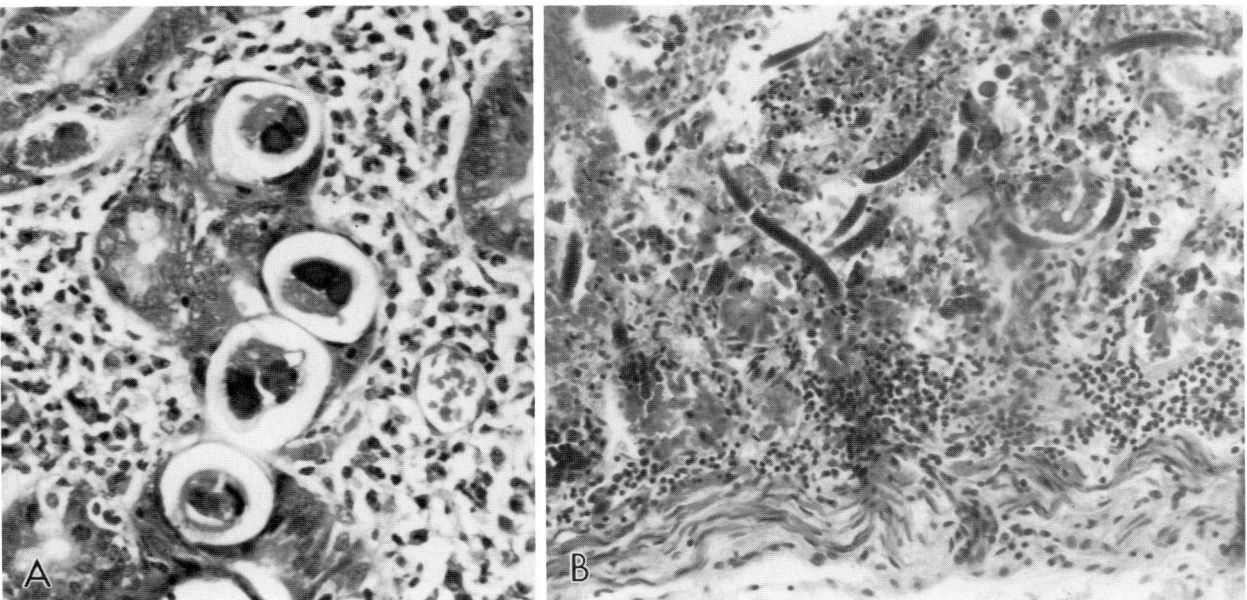

FIGURE 29-28. Strongyloidiasis. *A,* Jejunal biopsy specimen. Eggs undergoing embryonation in crypt epithelium. (× 340) *B,* Jejunum at autopsy showing heavy *S. stercoralis* infection. Numerous rhabditiform larvae are moving from the mucosa toward the lumen. (× 210)

region of the world, it may be spreading, and the high mobility of modern society could eventually lead to much wider dissemination.

Patients are believed to acquire the infection by eating fish whose flesh contains larvae; birds may also be an important vector.[202] It is uncertain whether ingestion of nematode eggs can infect human beings directly. Autoinfection is believed to occur in the human host, with resulting huge numbers of worms. Intestinal capillariasis can be epidemic. In its chronic form the symptoms resemble tropical sprue; emaciation can be severe and lead to death.[199]

The infection is centered primarily in the jejunum and ileum, although the duodenum is sometimes involved.[203] The nematodes are found burrowing into crypts of the small intestine, both adults and larvae being noted side by side.[198] The adult worms are small and slender, measuring about 2.5 to 4 mm in length by 20 to 50 μm in width.[198] Eggs and embryonating eggs are observed developing internally in adult female worms. The anterior ends of the infecting worms reach into the lamina propria, and the mucosa shows chronic inflammation with blunting and shortening of villi. Adult worms are occasionally found in the liver.[198,203]

A major differential point for the pathologist is to distinguish between capillariasis and strongyloidiasis. A key feature in making the distinction is to note the location of embryonating eggs; they occur only inside the female adults in capillariasis,[198] in contrast to their presence in crypt epithelium in stronglyloidiasis.

MUCOSAL LESIONS ASSOCIATED WITH ALTERED IMMUNE RESPONSE

The possibility that altered immunity may underlie a patient's intestinal dysfunction should be routinely considered when one is examining a small-bowel biopsy. Presence of a viral, bacterial, fungal, or parasitic agent should suggest that there may be an abnormal immune response, especially in those infections that are typical of AIDS. Common variable immune deficiency should be considered whenever giardiasis is noted. It should also be remembered that malnutrition, treatment with corticosteroids, cytotoxic agents, or other immunosuppressants, and the presence of protein-losing enteropathy can all lead to reduction in both humoral and cellular immune response.

Entities associated with alterations in immune response are largely covered elsewhere in this volume. Most primary and secondary immunodeficiency states

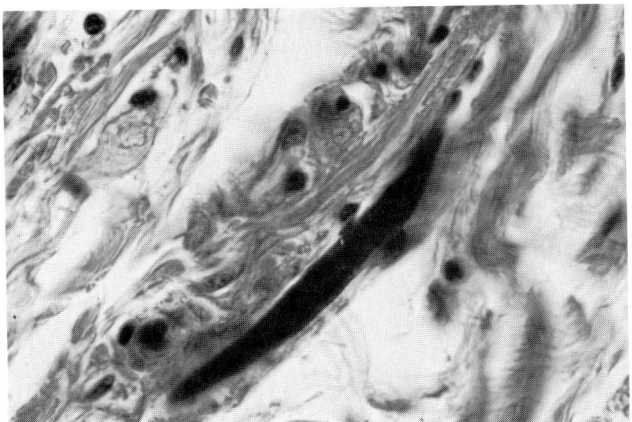

FIGURE 29-29. Internal autoinfection in strongyloidiasis. A larva is seen in the submucosa in the specimen shown in Figure 29-28B. (× 540)

are described in Chapter 14; graft-versus-host disease is considered there and additionally in Chapter 5. Eosinophilic gastroenteritis is reviewed in Chapter 10 along with other allergic conditions. In addition, see Kagnoff[204] for a thorough general discussion of altered immune states in gastrointestinal disease.

Two specialized aspects of altered immunity in the small intestine that are associated with malabsorption are considered here: idiopathic AIDS enteropathy and autoimmune enteropathy.

Idiopathic AIDS Enteropathy

Chronic diarrhea, often with malabsorption and weight loss, is an important finding in AIDS,[205,206] representing a major complaint in about half of all AIDS patients.[187,206] In approximately 50% of such cases the diarrheal malabsorption syndrome results from secondary infection in the small intestine and/or colorectum[207,208] (see Chapter 14 and see above for microsporidiosis). Altered gastrointestinal immunity with diminished mucosal CD4$^+$ (helper) cells and increased CD8$^+$ (cytotoxic/suppressor) cells correlate well with the AIDS patient's enhanced vulnerability to infection.[209] However, no secondary infectious agents can be demonstrated in the intestine of many AIDS patients with diarrhea even after all available methods have been used. This condition is here termed *idiopathic AIDS enteropathy*.

Mucosal biopsies from patients with idiopathic AIDS enteropathy have shown by morphometry decreased villus-to-crypt ratios because of villus atrophy and crypt elongation (Figure 29–30). In addition, however, the architectural changes were also found in AIDS patients without diarrhea as compared with normal controls ($P < 0.001$) (Figure 29–30).[187] Furthermore, AIDS patients witout diarrhea, and those with diarrhea, whether demonstrating an enteropathogen or not, all showed comparable frequencies of epithelial mitoses. Thus, the altered villus and crypt architecture and the patients' epithelial proliferative activity were independent of the presence of diarrhea or demonstrable enteric infection in advanced HIV infection.

Possible causes of idiopathic AIDS enteropathy include (1) undetected secondary infection, (2) the direct effect of the human immunodeficiency virus (HIV) or its products on the intestine, and (3) indirect effects of immunodeficiency or other immune dysregulation.

The role played by HIV in the mucosal morphometric changes is unclear. The virus has been described by some investigators in epithelial cells, leading them to postulate that the virus itself is responsible for idiopathic AIDS enteropathy,[210,211] but others failed to confirm those findings and noted HIV only in monocytes of the lamina propria.[212,213] The relatively sporadically seen HIV could in fact be a chance occurrence without direct bearing on the mucosal alterations.

The effects of HIV virus on T cells might also explain the villus atrophy and crypt hyperplasia seen in HIV-infected patients. Similar striking villus atrophy and

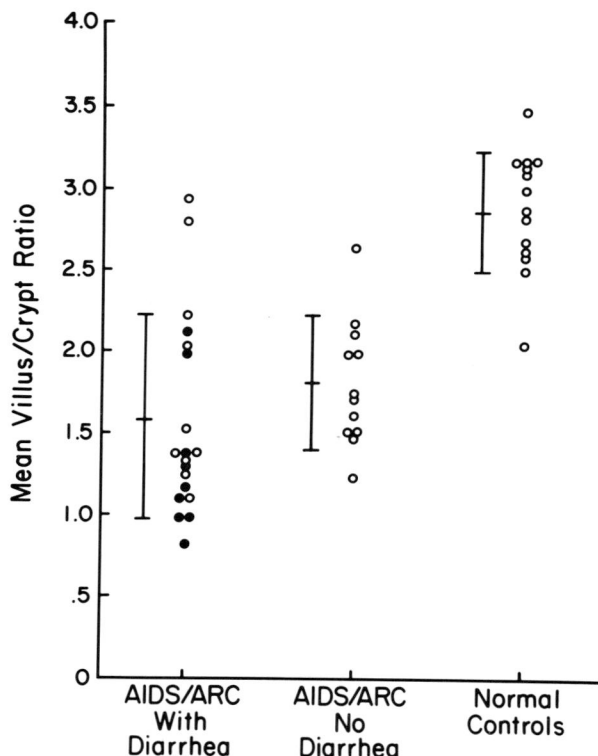

FIGURE 29–30. Morphometric data for duodenal mucosa in patients with AIDS or AIDS-related complex (ARC) and chronic diarrhea, in other patients with AIDS or ARC but without diarrhea, and for normal controls. Open circles, no pathogens identified. Closed circles, occult enteropathogens present (chiefly *Mycobacterium avium-intracellulare* and microsporidia). The mean villus to crypt ratios were reduced for patients with AIDS or ARC irrespective of whether or not diarrhea was present ($P > .001$). For patients with AIDS, diarrhea, and an enteropathogen, as compared with patients with AIDS and diarrhea without infections, $P = .06$; and as compared with patients with AIDS without diarrhea, $P < .03$. (Reproduced with permission from Greenson JK, Belitsos PC, Yardley JH, Bartlett JG: AIDS enteropathy—occult enteric infections and duodenal mucosal alterations in chronic diarrhea. Ann Intern Med 114:366–372, 1991.)

crypt hyperplasia were noted in fetal small-bowel explants when T cells were activated with pokeweed mitogens or anti-CD3 monoclonal antibody.[214,215] Comparable findings were also observed after rejection of mouse small intestine allografts and in graft-versus-host disease of the intestine following bone marrow transplantation.[216] Thus, it is conceivable that alterations in mucosal T cells in AIDS somehow lead to down-regulation of small-bowel epithelial proliferation and maturation with resulting alterations in mucosal architecture. Additional support for this hypothesis is suggested by the marked decrease in duodenal brush border lactase activity that was noted in HIV-infected patients.[217]

Autoimmune Enteropathy

The term *autoimmune enteropathy* is used for a condition seen in a group of pediatric patients, usually in-

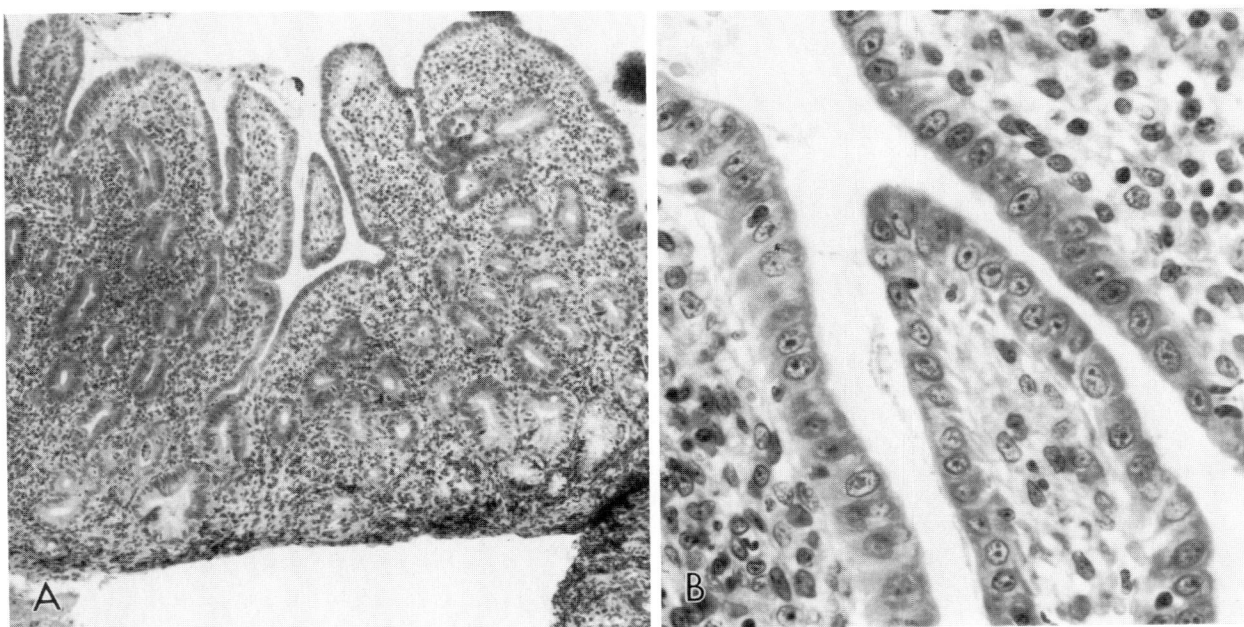

FIGURE 29-31. Autoimmune enteropathy in an infant who demonstrated autoimmune phenomena involving several systems and severe malabsorption. *A*, Villi are markedly rounded and shortened, and there is intense inflammation, which is chiefly chronic. ($\times$ 100) *B*, The villi are covered with regenerating epithelium that, however, shows a striking *absence* of lymphocytic infiltration. ($\times$ 510)

fants, who have watery diarrhea, derangement of the intestinal mucosa with inflammation and loss of villi, and evidence of circulating autoantibodies against intestinal epitehelium.[36,218,219] The patients characteristically have multiple other autoimmune reactions such as type I diabetes and hemolytic anemia and demonstrate other organ-specific or nonspecific autoantibodies. The disease is typically severe and intractable, requiring intravenous feeding; a favorable response to imunosuppressive agents may be noted.[220] These patients represent a distinctive subset among young patients, most of whom are infants, who have unexplained intractable diarrhea.[219,221]

A small-intestinal biopsy in autoimmune enteropathy typically appears flat, with markedly attenuated or absent villi (Figure 29-31). Chronic inflammation is increased in the lamina propria, whereas there is only limited if any increase in intraepithelial lymphocytes, an important feature distinguishing this conditon from celiac disease. Acute inflammation may also be seen. The severity of the lesion is proportional to the titer of circulating anti-enterocyte antibodies.[219] There is evidence of epithelial damage to both villus and crypt epithelium,[218] and the presence of crypt necrosis has been regarded as an especially poor prognostic sign.[221] It has recently been emphasized that these patients frequently also show colitis, which in some patients is severe and may resemble ulcerative colitis.[222]

The cause of autoimmune enteropathy is unknown. However, there is frequent mention of a similar disorder in siblings and of the presence of other autoimmune and allergic disorders in other relatives.[219,221]

Also, in some patients the illness has begun as an acute diarrheal episode that coincided with a similar acute illness in other family members in at least one instance.[218] Furthermore, it is noteworthy that the illness is *not* present at birth and that the anti-enterocyte antibodies appear *after* the illness has begun.[218] These findings suggest that a combination of one or more extrinsic agents and inherited factors are operative, and that although autoimmunity is unlikely to be the primary mechanism of epithelial injury, it probably does play an important secondary pathogenetic role. Cuenod et al. noted that activated T cells, as indicated by presence of interleukin-2 receptor-bearing cells, were markedly increased in number in their patients and have suggested that this might account for the villus atrophy.[221] They and others have also noted enhancement of epithelial HLA-DR antigens, with especially prominent involvement of crypts in those patients with high anti-epithelial antibody titers.[223] It is of special interest that treatment with cyclosporine has led to dramatic and prolonged clinical and histologic improvement with appearance of villi[220] (Fig 29-31*B*).

Miscellaneous Diseases Associated with Characteristic Mucosal Lesions

This section encompasses an otherwise diverse collection of disorders all of which have in common the presence of one or more characteristic features that allow them to be definitively recognized or strongly suspected solely from a mucosal biopsy. Most of the entities included under this heading are described in other chapters (see Table 29–1 for locations). Mastocytosis, microvillus inclusion disease, primary lymphangiectasia, and Waldenström's macroglobulinemia are discussed here.

Mastocytosis

This condition is characterized by abnormal accumulation of mast cells in various tissues, accompanied by symptoms that result from excessive release of vasoactive and possibly other substances by the mast cells, especially histamine. Mastocytosis presents most commonly during childhood as a localized disease manifested as a pigmented rash (*urticaria pigmentosa*), although the disorder can first appear during adulthood, too. Pruritis and dermatographia are the principal manifestations. About 10% of all patients with urticaria pigmentosa also have, or later develop, *systemic mastocytosis* with increased mast cells in other organs—most frequently bone marrow, lymph nodes, liver, and spleen.[224] Systemic mastocytosis in the absence of skin lesions is usually viewed as rare, although at least one group found no skin involvement in 44% of their patients.[224] Major clinical findings in systemic mastocytosis are episodic headache, flushing, weakness, abdominal pain, and diarrhea. Cherner et al. found that among 16 consecutive patients with systemic mastocytosis, 9 had either duodenal ulcer or duodenitis and 5 showed impaired absorption from the small intestine, although it was usually mild.[225] More severe malabsorption is an infrequent but well-recognized finding in systemic mastocytosis.[226–234]

For the pathologist to deal effectively with mastocytosis it is crucial that he know the techniques required to demonstrate mast cells, including aspects that are peculiar to the gastrointestinal tract: (1) Special stains such as Giemsa and toluidine blue are needed to reveal the characteristic mast cell granules and their metachromasia. Mast cells *cannot* be distinguished from other mononuclear cell types in hematoxylin and eosin stained sections. (2) After releasing their granule contents in response to immunologic or other stimulation, mast cells become undectable even by special stains, and electron microscopy is then required for their identification. (3) As was shown in rats and mice,[235,236] and more recently in human beings,[237,238] at least two types of mast cells are recognizable. The more widespread and common type occurs in dermis and connective tissue in many organs, including intestinal submucosa and muscularis. This type, termed a connective tissue mast cell (CTMC), is well shown by an appropriate stain such as toluidine blue after fixation in buffered or other ordinary formalin solutions. On the other hand, *the mast cells found in the lamina propria of the intestinal mucosa are predominantly of a different type and are termed mucosal mast cells (MMCs).* MMCs are poorly demonstrated after conventional

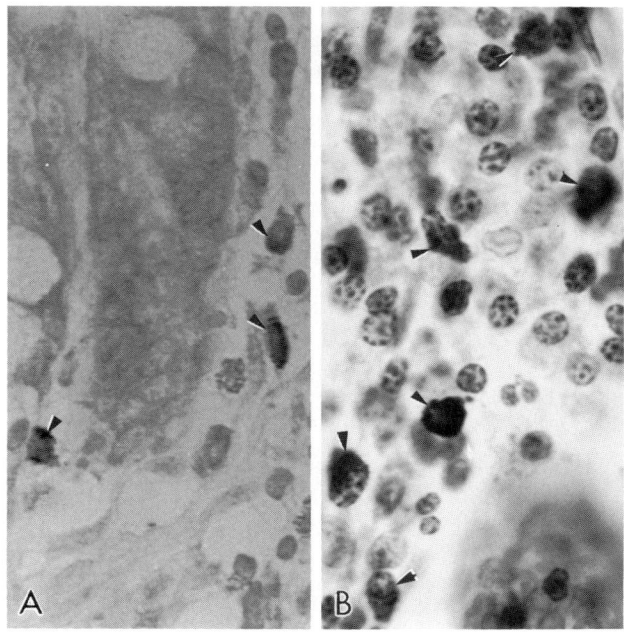

FIGURE 29–32. Relation of tissue fixation to demonstration of mucosal mast cells. Portions of small intestine from the same patient were used. *A*, Fixation in 10% buffered formalin. A typical field showing no more than three widely scattered, small-sized mast cells (arrowheads). In addition, they contain a limited number of metachromatic granules. *B*, Carnoy's fixation. A greater concentration of mast cells (arrowheads), each containing a large number of intracellular granules, is evident. Differences in background staining are an unrelated phenomenon. Toluidine blue stain. ($\times$ 875) (Preparations kindly provided by Dr. Audrey Lazenby.)

types of formalin fixation, requiring especially chosen fixatives such as Carnoy's fluid (Figure 29–32). Pulmonary mast cells have similar properties.

Strobel et al. found that whereas only a few mast cells could be seen in the lamina propria after buffered formalin, formol-sublimate, or saline-formol fixation, a four- to sixfold increase in visible mast cells was observed with Carnoy's fixative. Other fixatives tested, including basic lead acetate, formalin-acetic acid, Baker's (formalin-calcium chloride), and Bouin's, gave intermediate results (and in descending order).[237] Similarly, formalin-acetic acid was found by Ruitenberg et al. to be much more effective than standard 10% formalin for demonstrating MMC.[238] Later quantitative studies have shown that formaldehyde treatment can block cationic dye binding to granules in most MMCs, suggesting that this is a special property of the particular glycosoaminoglycan composition of the proteoglycan core in MMCs.[225] Submucosal mast cells, in keeping with the predominance of CTMC in that location, showed a less pronounced relationship to the type of fixation.

There are other features of human MMCs said to distinguish them from CTMCs: smaller size; fewer and smaller granules, which tend to be located in peripheral cytoplasm; differences in the content of the granules[237,238]; and different reactivities to monoclonal antibodies against tryptase and chymase.²³⁹ A possible additional mast cell type occurs under the crypt epithelium in humans.²³⁸ These findings are in keeping with the constantly expanding evidence of morphologic, cytochemical, and functional heterogeneity of mast cells generally.²⁴⁰

Gross and microscopic changes have often been described in the intestine in systemic mastocytosis with severe malabsorption. The wall may appear thickened,²²⁸,²⁴¹ and several authors have reported mucosal nodularity.²²⁹,²²⁴ One group of investigators saw "exudative duodenitis."²³³ Ammann et al. have suggested that the mucosal changes can result from exposure to extrinsic substances, observing by endoscopy that "papular edema" and hyperemia appeared after a provocation test using a peptone- or polymyxin-containing solution.²³⁰

Histologically, villus shortening ("atrophy"), edema, and increased mucosal lymphocytes and plasma cells are typically described; most authors also have stated that eosinophils are prominent.²²⁶,²²⁸⁻²³³ Braverman et al. saw short, clubbed villi and absence and destruction of some crypts,²³³ which led them to an initial diagnosis of celiac disease.

In contrast to the architectural and nonspecific inflammatory changes that are consistently described in the intestinal mucosa in systemic mastocytosis with malabsorption, there is inconsistency between authors with regard to the number of mucosal mast cells. Only normal or unimpressive numbers were described in the lamina propria in several reports,²²⁶,²²⁸,²³⁰,²³² e.g., three to four mast cells per high-power field (usually defined as with a 40× objective and 10× eyepiece).²³² On the other hand, other investigators found definite increases²²⁷,²²⁹,²³³,²³⁴,²⁴¹ with values for mast cells per high-power field ranging between 7 to 10²³⁴ and 50 to 100.²³³ In addition, degranulated mast cells and abnormal mast cells with irregular and double nuclei have been reported by electron microscopy.²³³

The variability in observed numbers of lamina propria mast cells in mastocytosis could occur in several ways. These include *true* variation in numbers between patients, or variable numbers at different times in the same patient, or only *apparent* lack of increase that results from granule depletion that in turn leads to reduced ability to detect their presence. However, before the nature of variation in number of lamina propria mast cells found in mastocytosis can be determined with certainty, it is obviously essential to consider the type of fixation used. In fact, of the authors mentioned above who describe malabsorption in mastocytosis by light microscopy, only two²²⁷,²³³ have provided information about fixation. And if it is assumed that ordinary formalin was the fixative used in the many of the reported cases, it is very possible, in view of the cited studies on the effects of fixation,²³⁷,²³⁸ that many if not all of the cases described as showing normal numbers of lamina propria mast cells in mastocytosis would have shown an increase if Carnoy's, formalin-acetic acid, or another more appropriate fixation had been used. This conclusion is supported by the observation of Braverman et al. that whereas mast cells were not increased in formalin-fixed intestine, an estimated 50 to 100 per high-power field were seen after fixation in Bouin's solution.²³³

Among authors who mention the status of *submucosal* mast cells in mastocytosis, several describe an increase,²²⁷⁻²²⁹ and this was seen in one case²²⁸ even when no increase was noted in lamina propria mast cells. Such an observation would fit with the fact that the submucosa largely contains CTMCs, which are not affected by ordinary formalin fixation.

It is not clear how the increase in mast cells comes about in systemic mastocytosis, or how it can sometimes lead to malabsorption and to altered mucosal architecture. It is generally agreed, however, that local increase in mast cells occurs in humans during a variety of acute and chronic inflammatory responses, during certain immune responses, and in fibrotic reactions. It is also known from experiments in rats that the intestinal mast cell population undergoes marked expansion following infection with a parasite, *Nippostrongylus brasiliensis*,²⁴² and that such expansion appears to be under T-cell control.²³⁶ Furthermore, a 30-fold increase in intestinal mast cells occurred in nude mice after interleukin-3 injections.²⁴³ Although *in vitro* studies did not confirm a similar relationship of mast cell proliferation to IL-3 in humans,²⁴⁴ observations of this type are consistent with the hypothesis that abnormal regulation of mast cell proliferation is of central importance in mastocytosis.

Microvillus Inclusion Disease

This is an autosomally inherited recessive condition in newborns, presenting as severe, intractable diarrhea with steatorrhea.²⁴⁵,²⁴⁶ The diarrhea does not abate on total parenteral alimentation. Absorptive tests and transepithelial electrolyte fluxes in microvillus inclusion disease have indicated sugar malabsorption and profound net secretion of fluid and electrolytes.²⁴⁵,²⁴⁷ Few if any of the infants live beyond the eighteenth month of life.

By endoscopy, atrophic folds may be seen in the duodenum. Small-intestinal biopsies show markedly blunted or absent villi and a thin surface epithelium resembling that seen in celiac disease except that intraepithelial lymphocytes are not increased (Figure 29–33).

Electron microscopy is definitive, consistently demonstrating striking and highly characteristic ultrastructural abnormalities in the surface enterocytes.²⁴⁶ The microvilli at the apical border are shortened, disorganized, and in places greatly reduced in number or even absent. At the same time, many enterocytes demonstrate large, pathognomonic microvillus inclusions just below the surface and in the apical cytoplasm. These inclusions consist of an apparently circularized fragment of complete microvillus border that are bounded externally by a terminal web (Figure 29–34). There is also evidence of autophagocytosis with various other

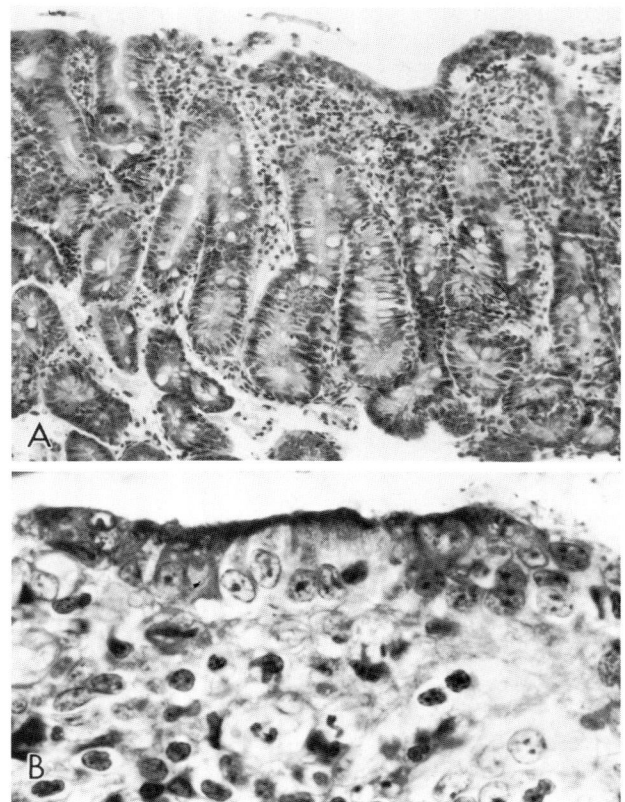

FIGURE 29-33. Microvillus inclusion disease. *A*, Flat mucosa. (H&E, × 120) *B*, Disorganized appearance of surface epithelium, which shows a prominent apical PAS-positive layer but lacks a clearly defined brush border. (PAS, × 675)

lysosome-like vesicular inclusions that sometimes contain microvilli.

It has been suggested that abnormalities in assembly of the microvilli at the apical surface of the enterocytes are responsbile for microvillus inclusion disease.[246] Goblet cells, Paneth cells, and endocrine cells are not affected. Similar changes have been noted in surface epithelium in the colon, rectum, and gallbladder.[246,247] The crypt enterocytes show well-preserved brush borders, although the cells are said to demonstrate increased numbers of vesicular bodies.[246]

While transmission electron microscopy is the diagnostic *sine qua non*, microvillus inclusion disease can also be strongly suspected from conventional histologic preparations. The brush border in places can be so thin as to be barely visible. In addition, the absorptive cells show prominent PAS-positive material in their apical cytoplasm (see Figure 29-33*B*). In addition, staining for alkaline phosphatase, which is normally found in the brush border, also stains the vesicles, thereby adding further specificity to light-microscopic study.[248]

Primary Intestinal Lymphangiectasia

Patients with this condition present with protein-losing enteropathy (PLE) (see introduction), hypoproteinemia, and peripheral edema.[249-251] Diarrhea and steatorrhea are often noted, and reductions in serum globulins and peripheral lymphocytes with associated immunologic disorders may be found.[252] The presence of dilated lymphatics in the mucosa of the small intestine is the cardinal finding in intestinal lymphangiectasia, and the only apparent cause is "disturbance of the lymphatic system."[249] The condition develops mainly as a sporadic disorder in children and young adults, although familial occurrence is described. The patient and other family members may also show evidence of abnormal lymphatic drainage in one or more extremities (primary or idiopathic lymphedema), and there may be chylous ascites.[249,253] In a study of 52 patients with primary lymphedema, 12 (22%) were found to have significant PLE.[254] Isolated instances of intestinal blood loss in patients with lymphangiectasia are described.[255]

Grossly (or endoscopically), the mucosa shows white spots, white villi, and an overlying chyle-like substance.[256] The lesions are focal and may require multiple biopsies or serial sections to demonstrate their presence.[251,257] The reader is reminded that similar gross findings are present in Whipple's disease (see Figure 29-19) and in macroglobulinemia with intestinal involvement.[176,258]

In some persons the subserosal intestinal and mesenteric lymphatics have shown evidence of chylous distention indicative of more distal obstruction (Figure 29-35). The cause of this condition is unclear. However, Waldman et al. demonstrated mesenteric lymphatic obstruction associated with thickening and fragmentation of the elastica interna and luminal fibrosis in four of five patients for whom specimens were available; mesenteric lymph nodes were also fibrotic.[249] It was not clear whether the changes were congenital or acquired.

Histologically, the dilated mucosal lymphatics are seen typically in the villi just under the epithelium (Figure 29-36) but can occur throughout the lamina propria and in the submucosa. The lymphatic endothelium is usually well outlined, and protein and scattered foamy macrophages may be present in the lumen and lamina propria. Mild to moderate blunting of villi and slight chronic inflammation are sometimes described[251]; and generalized edema of the lamina propria, presumably secondary to hypoproteinemia, may be seen. Intraepithelial lymphocytes were noted to be reduced, whereas plasma cells were present in normal numbers.[259] Ultrastructural studies have shown increases in collagen, basal lamina, and supporting cells around the dilated lymphatics along with prominent intracellular fibrils in the lymphatic endothelium.[260] Additionally, large lipid droplets were observed at the base of the absorptive cells, and chylomicrons were seen in the extracellular spaces and lymphatic lumina.[256,260]

The luminal protein loss probably occurs through a combination of leakage through the epithelium and rupture of the lymphangiectatic lesions with release of chyle. The steatorrhea seen in primary intestinal lymphangiectasia appears to result from enteric loss of fat rather than malabsorption.[261]

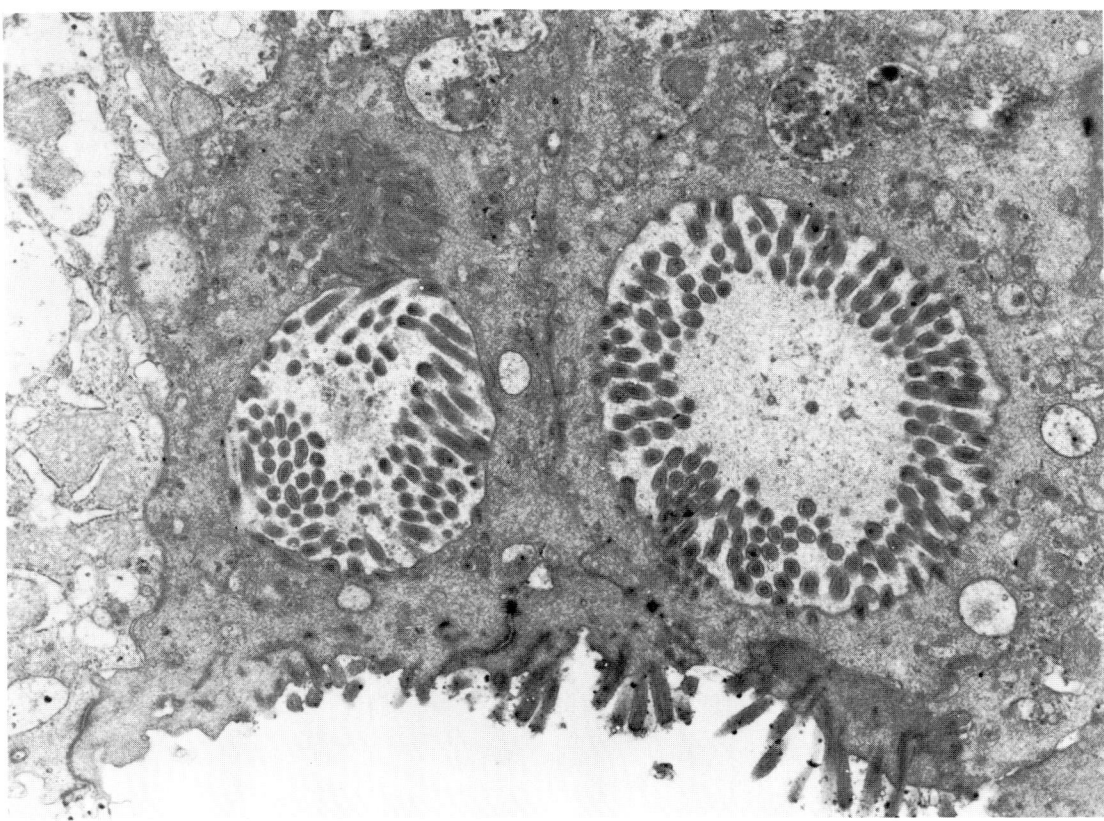

FIGURE 29–34. Microvillus inclusion disease. Electron micrograph of an abnormal surface enterocyte. Characteristic intracytoplasmic inclusions with apparent internalized microvilli are present beneath a markedly attenuated and abnormal brush border. ($\times$ 14,750) (Courtesy of Drs. Joy Young-Ramsaran and Jean Olson.)

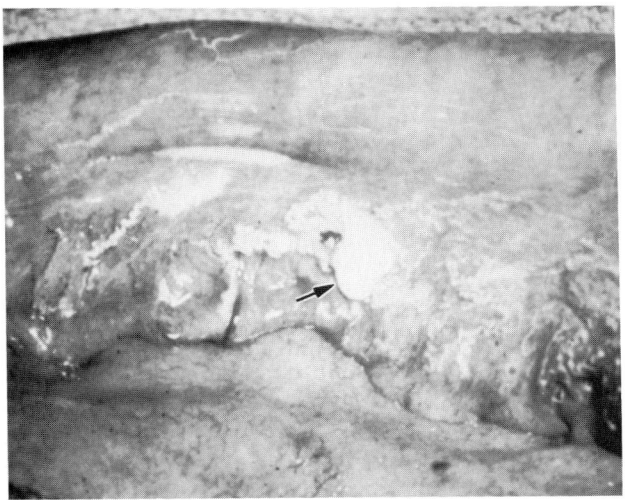

FIGURE 29–35. Primary lymphangiectasia. External appearance of the small intestine at laparotomy, showing tortuous, dilated lymphatic vessels filled with chyle. A large drop of chyle has formed where a vessel was nicked (arrow).

It should be stressed that lymphangiectasia may be found incidentally during endoscopy or in an isolated biopsy of the small intestine in the absence of any clinical evidence of PLE or hypoproteinemia. In addition, Patel and DeRidder described patients with "functional lymphangiectasia" in whom the changes were not associated with PLE, appeared to be transient, and required no follow-up.[262]

Waldenström's Macroglobulinemia

Intestinal involvement in Waldenström's macroglobulinemia is a rare complication of that disorder. These patients present with diarrhea, malabsorption, and PLE along with typical findings of a monoclonal IgM spike by serum immunoelectrophoresis and neoplastic plasmacytoid cells in the bone marrow.

Grossly, myriads of small, white nodules comparable to those seen in primary lymphangiectasia and in Whipple's disease carpet an edematous, thickened, small-intestinal mucosa (Figure 29–37).[258,263] The mesenteric nodes are enlarged and contain pale, cheesy material, as can the dilated lymphatics that may be seen draining into them.[263] Involvement of the stomach or colon has not been described.

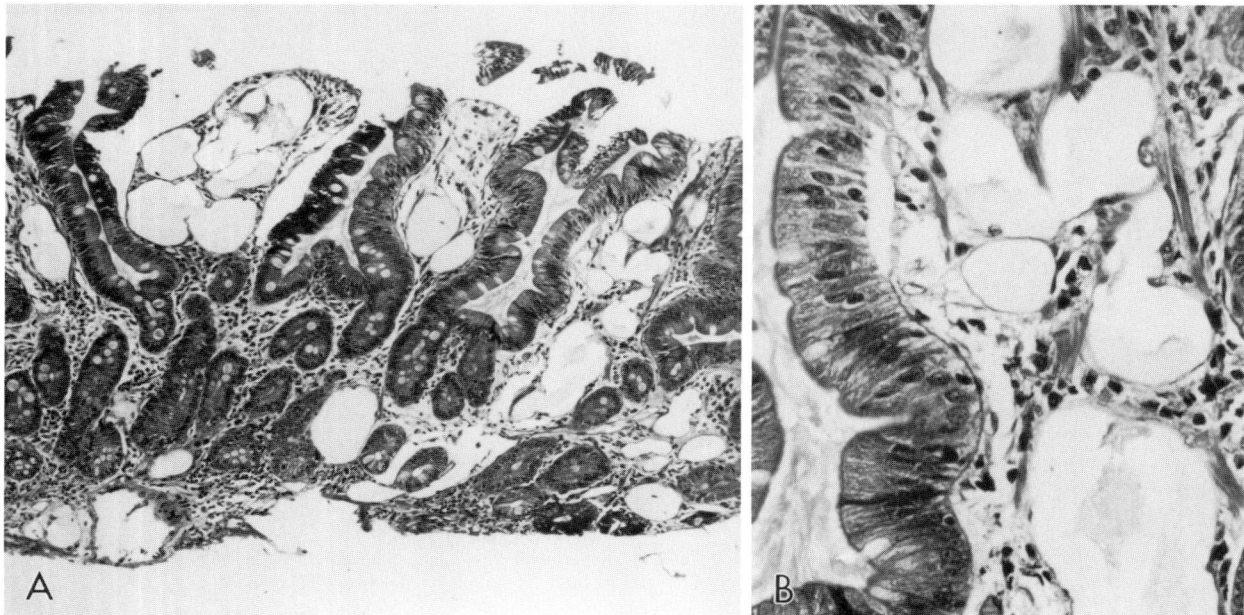

FIGURE 29–36. Primary lymphangiectasia in a patient with long-standing edema involving the extremities. A, Greatly dilated, tortuous central lacteals are present in villi and deeper parts of an otherwise unremarkable-looking mucosa. Detachment of surface epithelium is artifactual. (× 105) B, The multiple lymphatic channels are lined by an intact endothelial layer. (× 340)

Deposition of large amounts of eosinophilic, amorphous-looking proteinaceous material that is located in the mucosal lymphatics and lamina propria is the principal finding in the intestine histologically (Figure 29–38). By electron microscopy the material is also seen between epithelial cells. The proteinaceous material is PAS-positive and Congo red–negative[263-265]; it also stains immunohistochemically for monoclonal IgM, thereby demonstrating its identity with the circulating monoclonal macroglobulin.[258,266,267] Lipid droplets can be found extracellularly, sometimes admixed with the macroglobulin.[266] In addition, there are lipid-containing, largely PAS-negative foam cells (see Figure 29–38), but very little evidence of intracellular protein deposits is noted by either light or electron microscopy. The proteinaceous material involving the regional lymph nodes has the same characteristics as that in the intestine.

Neoplastic cellular infiltration is seen much less commonly than macroglobulin deposition as the cause of intestinal symptoms in patients with Waldenström's macroglobulinemia (summarized by Amrein and Compton[267]). Furthermore, the mononuclear cellular infiltrate that is associated with massive intestinal macroglobulin deposition is usually considered benign. Nevertheless, in some cases of macroglobulin deposition several authors have described accompanying plasmacytoid lymphoctyes, atypical plasma cells, and Dutcher bodies (intranuclear globulin deposits) (Figure 29–39).[263-265] Those observations suggest that neoplastic infiltration in the mucosa may at times be involved in local deposition of macroglobulin.[264] In all likelihood, however, deposition of circulating macroglobulins *per se*, with secondary lymphatic obstruction, is the underlying mechanism of the mucosal disease and malabsorption. This conclusion is supported by the demonstration of accompanying massive macroglobulin deposition in mesenteric lymph nodes in most if not

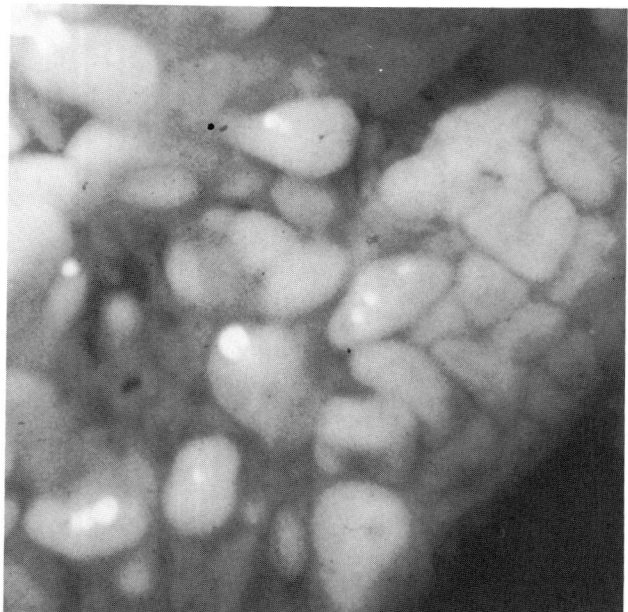

FIGURE 29–37. Intestinal involvement in Waldenström's macroglobulinemia. Macroscopic view of mucosa. Enlarged villi appear as multiple whitish nodules.

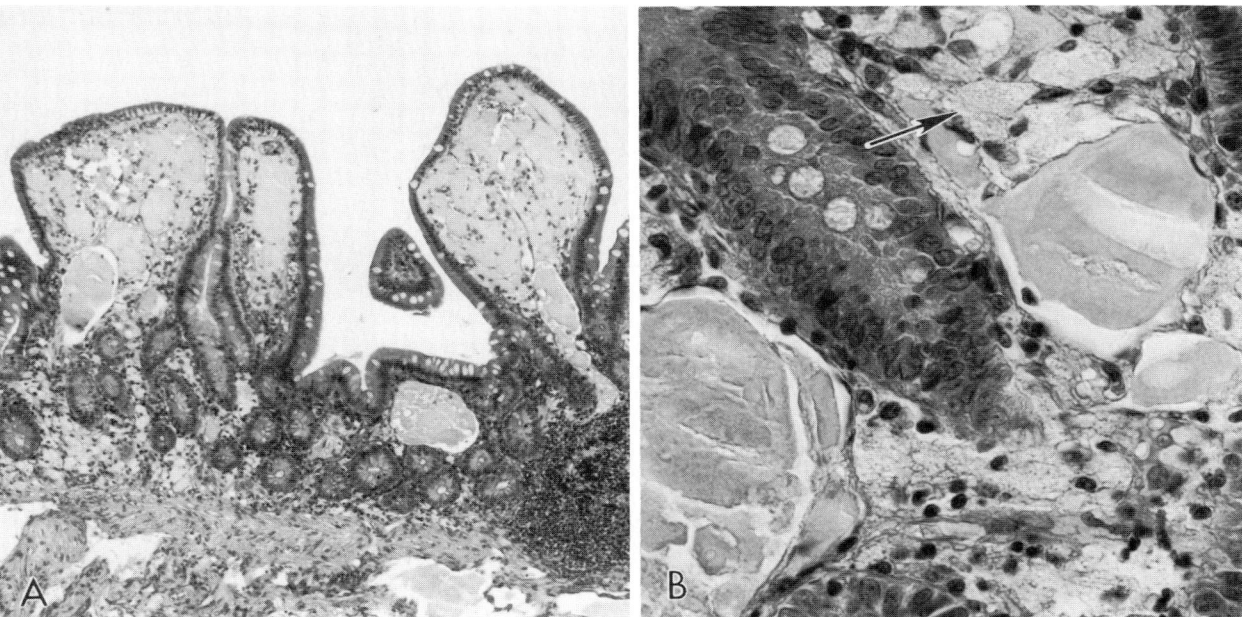

FIGURE 29-38. Intestinal involvement in Waldenström's macroglobulinemia. *A,* Macroglobulin has accumulated in the lymphatics and interstitium of the lamina propria, creating the nodules seen in Figure 29-37. (× 90) *B,* Macroglobulin accumulations in lymphatics. Numerous foamy macrophages are present in the interstitium (arrow). (× 400) (Courtesy of Dr. Geoffrey Mendelsohn.)

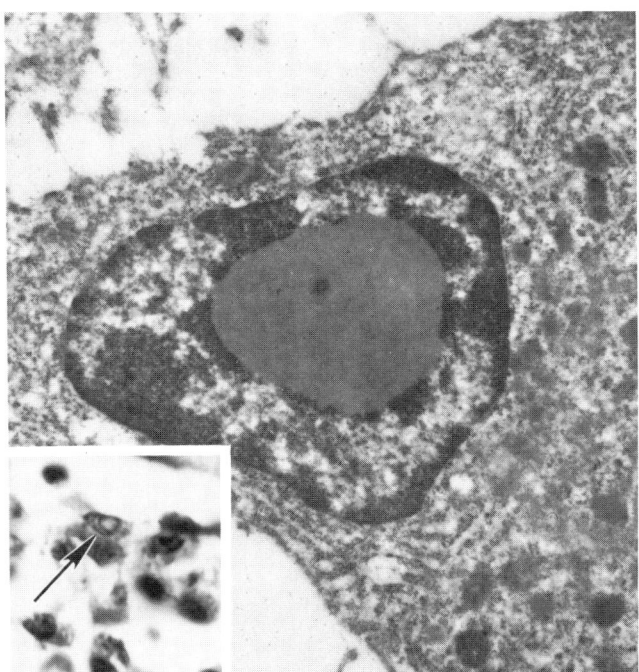

FIGURE 29-39. Possible mucosal Dutcher bodies in Waldenström's macroglobulinemia. Electron micrograph demonstrating an amorphous intranuclear inclusion consistent with accumulated macroglobulin in a lymphoplasmacytoid cell. (× 18,700) *Insert,* Light micrograph of a mucosal Dutcher body–like inclusion (arrow). (H&E, × 900) (From Bedine MS, Yardley JH, Elliott HL, et al: Intestinal involvement in Waldenström's macroglobulinemia. Gastroenterology 65:308–315, 1973, © copyright by The American Gastroenterological Association.)

all patients and by the dramatic regression of thickened mucosa and enlarged lymph nodes that can be seen after circulating macroglobulins are reduced therapeutically by means of plasmaphoresis.[258,268]

Acknowledgments. The collaboration and help of my many clinical colleagues in studies of malabsorption over the years are gratefully acknowledged. Special thanks go to Drs. Thomas R. Hendrix and Theodore M. Bayless, who first introduced me to the subject of malabsorption and contributed much to my understanding of it. Original photomicrographs are by Raymond E. Lund, RBP, FBPA.

References

1. Perera DR, Weinstein WM, Rubin CE: Small intestinal biopsy. Hum Pathol 6:157–217, 1975.
2. Dobbins WO III: Small bowel biopsy in malabsorptive states. In Norris HT (ed): Pathology of the colon, small intestine and anus. New York, Churchill Livingstone, 1983, pp 121–167.
3. Piris J: Malabsorption and protein intolerance. In Whitehead R (ed): Gastrointestinal and Oesophageal Pathology. Edinburgh, Churchill Livingstone, 1989, pp 468–496.
4. Sleisenger MH, Fordtran JS: Gastrointestinal Disease, 4th ed. Philadelphia, Saunders, 1989.
5. Shiner M: Ultrastructure of the small intestinal mucosa: Normal and disease related appearances. New York, Springer-Verlag, 1983.
6. Holdstock G, Eade DE, Isaacson P, Smith CL: Endoscopic duodenal biopsy in coeliac disease and duodenitis. Scand J Gastroenterol 14:717, 1979.
7. Brackenbury W, Stewart JS: Macroscopic appearances of mucosal biopsies from the small intestine. Med Biol Illus 13:220–227, 1963.
8. Atkinson M, Nordin BEC, Sheshock S: Malabsorption and bone

disease in prolonged obstructive jaundice. J Med 25:299–312, 1956.
9. Marin GA, Clark ML, Senior JR: Studies of malabsorption occurring in patients with Laennec's cirrhosis. Gastrenterology 56:727–736, 1969.
10. Bo-Linn GW, Fordtran JS: Fecal fat concentration in patients with steatorrhea. Gastroenterology 87:319–322, 1984.
11. Rubin E, Ryback BJ, Lindenbaum J, et al: Ultrastructural changes in the small intestine induced by ethanol. Gastroenterology 63:801–814, 1972.
12. Hermos JA, Adams WH, Liu Yong K, et al: Mucosa of the small intestine in folate-deficient alcoholics. Ann Intern Med 76:957–965, 1972.
13. Mezey E: Intestinal function in chronic alcoholism. Ann NY Acad Sci 252:215–227, 1975.
14. Crane RK: Hypothesis for mechanism of intestinal active transport of sugars. Fed Proc 21:891–895, 1962.
15. Bayless TM, Christopher NL. Disaccharidase deficiency. Am J Clin Nutr 22:181–190, 1969.
16. Walker-Smith JA, Guandalini S, Schmitz J, et al: Revised criteria for diagnosis of coeliac disease. Arch Dis Child 65:909–911, 1990.
17. Kagnoff MF: Immonopathogenesis of celiac disease. Immunol Invest 18:499–508, 1989.
18. Trier JS: Celiac sprue. In Sleisenger MH, Fordtran JS (eds): Gastrointestinal Disease, 4th ed. Philadelphia, WB Saunders, 1989, pp 1134–1141.
19. Dicke WK: Coeliac disease: Investigation of harmful effects of certain types of cereal on patients with coeliac disease (English summary). Doctoral thesis, University of Utrecht, Netherlands, 1950, pp 106–116.
20. Dicke WK, Weijers HA, v d Kamer JH: Coeliac disease. II. The presence in wheat of a factor having a deleterious effect in cases of coeliac disease. Acta Paediatr 42:34–42, 1953.
21. Rubin CE, Brandborg LL, Phelps PC, Taylor HC Jr: Studies of celiac disease. I. Apparent identical and specific nature of duodenal and proximal jejunal lesion in celiac disease and idiopathic sprue. Gastroenterology 38:28–49, 1960.
22. Sleisenger MH, Rynbergen HJ, Pert JH, Almy TP: Treatment of nontropical sprue: wheat-, rye-, and oat-free diet. J Am Dietet Assoc 33:1137–1140, 1957.
23. Yardley JH, Bayless TM, Norton JH, Hendrix TR: Celiac disease: A study of the jejunal epithelium before and after a gluten-free diet. N Engl J Med 267:1173–1179, 1962.
24. Samloff IM, Davis JS, Schenk EA: A clinical and histochemical study of gluten-free diet. Gastroenterology 48:155–172, 1965.
25. Bayless TM, Rubin S, Topping T, et al: Morphologic and functional effects of gluten feeding on jejunal mucosa and celiac disease. In Booth CC, Dowling RH (eds): Coeliac Disease. Edinburgh, Churchill-Livingstone, 1970, pp 76–89.
26. McNicholl B, Egan-Mitchell B, Stevens F, et al: Mucosal recovery in treated childhood celiac disease (gluten-sensitive enteropathy). J Pediatr 89:418–424, 1976.
27. MacDonald WC, Dobbins WO, Rubin CE: Studies on the familial nature of celiac sprue using biopsy of the small intestine. N Engl J Med 272:448–455, 1965.
28. Stokes PL, Ferguson R, Holmes, GK, Cooke WT: Familial aspects of coeliac disease. Q J Med 45:567–582, 1976.
29. Khuffash FA, Barakat MH, Majeed HA, et al: Coeliac disease in monozygotic twin girls. Synchronous presentation. Gut 25:1009–1012, 1984.
30. Mearin ML, Biemond I, Peña AS, et al: HLA-DR phenotypes in Spanish coeliac children: Their contribution to the understanding of the genetics of the disease. Gut 24:532–537, 1983.
31. Niven MJ, Caffrey C, Sachs JA, et al: Susceptibility to coeliac disease invovles genes in HLA-DP region. Lancet 2:805, 1987.
32. Kagnoff MF: Understanding the molecular basis of coeliac disease. Gut 31:497–499, 1990.
33. Marsh MN, Bjarnason I, Shaw J, et al: Studies of intestinal lymphoid tissue: XIV-HLA status, mucosal morphology, permeability, and epithelial lymphocyte populations in first degree relatives of patients with coeliac disease. Gut 31:32–36, 1991.
34. Katz SI, Hall RP III, Lawley TJ, Strober W: Dermatitis herpetiformis: The skin and the gut. Ann Intern Med 93:857–874, 1980.
35. Mulder CJJ, Tytgat GNJ: Coeliac disease and related disorders. Netherlands J Med 31:286–299, 1987.
36. Unsworth DJ, Walker-Smith JA: Autoimmunity in diarrhoeal disease. J Pediatr Gastroenterol Nutr 4:375–380, 1985.
37. Wall AJ, Douglas AP, Booth CC, Pearse AGE: Response of the jejunal mucosa in adult coeliac disease to oral prednisolone. Gut 11:7–14, 1970.
38. Katz AJ, Falchuk ZM, Strober W, Schwachman H: Gluten-sensitive enteropathy: Inhibition by cortisol of the effect of gluten protein in vitro. N Engl J Med 295:131–136, 1976.
39. Ferguson A, Carswell F: Precipitins to dietary proteins in serum and upper intestinal secretions of coeliac children. Br Med J 1:75–77, 1972.
40. Kendrick KG, Walker-Smith AJ: Immunoglobulins and dietary protein antibodies in childhood coeliac disease. Gut 11:635–640, 1970.
41. Lindberg T, Nilsson LA, Borulf S, et al: Serum IgA and IgG gliadin antibodies and small intestinal mucosal damage in children. J Pediatr Gastroenterol Nutr 4:917–22, 1985.
42. Juto P, Fredrikzon B, Hernell O: Gliadin-specific serum immunoglobulins A, E, G, and M in childhood: Relation to small intestine mucosal morphology. J Pediatr Gastroenterol Nutr 4:723–729, 1985.
43. Stahlberg MR, Savilahti E, Viander M: Antibodies to gliadin by ELISA as a screening test for childhood celiac disease. J Pediatr Gastroenterol Nutr 5:726–729, 1986.
44. Kilander AF, Nilsson L-A, Gillberg R: Serum antibodies to gliadin in coeliac disease after gluten withdrawal. Scand J Gastroenterol 22:29–34, 1987.
45. Lycke N, Kilander A, Nilsson L-A, et al: Production of antibodies to gliadin in intestinal mucosa of patients with coeliac disease: A study at the single cell level. Gut 30:72–77, 1989.
46. Unsworth DJ, Leonard NL, Fry L: Antireticulin and antigliadin antibodies in dermatitis herpetiformis and celiac disease. In Beutner EH, Chorzelski TC, Kumar V (eds): Immunopathology of the Skin, 3rd ed. New York, John Wiley & Sons, 1987, pp 455–470.
47. Ferguson A, Murray D: Quantitation of intraepithelial lymphocytes in human jejunum. Gut 12:988–994, 1971.
48. Freedman AR, Macartney JC, Nelufer JM, Ciclitira PJ: Timing of infiltration of T lymphocytes induced by gluten into the small intestine in coeliac disease. J Clin Pathol 40:741–745, 1987.
49. Austin LL, Dobbins WO: Studies of the rectal mucosa in coeliac sprue: The intraepithelial lymphocyte. Gut 29:200–205, 1988.
50. Loft DE, Marsh MN, Crowe PT: Rectal gluten challenge and diagnosis of coeliac disease. Lancet 335:1293–1295, 1990.
51. Loft DE, Marsh MN, Sandle GI, et al: Studies of intestinal lymphoid tissue. XII. Epithelial lymphocyte and mucosal responses to rectal gluten challenge in celiac sprue. Gastroenterology 97:29–37, 1989.
52. Corazza GR, Sarchielli P, Londei M, et al: Gluten specific suppressor T cell dysfunction in coeliac disease. Gut 27:392–398, 1986.
53. Guan R, Rawcliffe PM, Priddle JD, Jewell DP: Cellular hypersensitivity to gluten derived peptides in coeliac disease. Gut 28:426–434, 1987.
54. Karagiannis JA, Priddle JD, Jewell DP. Cell-mediated immunity to a synthetic gliadin peptide resembling a sequence from adenovirus 12. Lancet 1:884–886, 1987.
55. Mantzaris GJ, Karagiannis JA, Priddle JD, Jewell DP: Cellular hypersensitivity to a synthetic dodecapeptide derived from adenovirus 12 which resembles a sequence of A-gliadin in patients with coeliac disease. Gut 31:668–673, 1990.
56. Kagnoff MF, Paterson YJ, Kumar PJ, et al: Evidence for the role of a human intestinal adenovirus in the pathogenesis of coeliac disease. Gut 28:995–1001, 1987.
57. Kagnoff MF, Austin RK, Hubert JJ, Kasarda DD: Possible role for human adenovirus in the pathogenesis of celiac disease. J Exp Med 160:1544–1557, 1984.
58. Penna FJ, Mota JA, Roquete ML, et al: Coeliac disease in identical twins. Arch Dis Child 54:395–397, 1979.
59. Hoffman HN, Wollaeger EE, Greenberg E: Discordance for nontropical sprue (adult coeliac disease) in a monozygotic twin pair. Gastroenterology 51:36–42, 1966.

60. Walker-Smith JA: Discordance of childhood celiac disease in monozygotic twins. Gut 14:374–375, 1973.
61. Salazar-de-Sousa J, Ramos-de-Almeida JM, Monteiro MV, Magalhaes-Ramalho P: Late onset coeliac disease in the monozygotic twin of a coeliac child. Acta Paediatr Scand 76:172–174, 1987.
62. Lee FI, Prior J, Murray SM: Celiac disease in monozygous twin boys: Asynchronous presentation. Dig Dis Sci 27:1137–1140, 1982.
63. Jepsen LV, Ullman S: Dermatitis herpetiformis and gluten-sensitive enteropathy in monozygotic twins. Acta Dermatol Venereol (Stockh) 60:353–355, 1980.
64. Schenk EA, Samloff IM, Lipstein FA: Morphologic characteristics of jejunal biopsy in celiac disease and tropical sprue. Am J Pathol 47:765–781, 1965.
65. Padykula HA: Recent functional interpretations of intestinal morphology. Fed Proc 21:873–879, 1962.
66. Schenk EA, Samloff IM: Clinical and morphologic changes following gluten administration to patients with treated celiac disease. Am J Pathol 52:579–593, 1968.
67. Zetterqvist H, Hendrix TR: A preliminary note on an ultrastructural abnormality of intestinal epithelium in adult celiac disease (nontropical sprue) which is reversed by a gluten free diet. Bull Johns Hopkins Hosp 106:240–249, 1960.
68. Rubin W, Ross LL, Sleisenger MH, Wesser E: An electron microscopic study of adult celiac disease. Lab Invest 15:1720–1747, 1966.
69. Rubin CE, Brandborg LL, Flick AL, et al: Studies of celiac sprue. 3. The effect of repeated wheat instillation into the proximal ileum of patients on a gluten free diet. Gastroenterology 54:793, 1968.
70. Ament ME, Rubin CE: Soy protein—another cause of the flat intestinal lesion. Gastroenterology 62:227–234, 1972.
71. McPherson JR, Shorter RG: Intestinal lesions associated with triparanol: A clinical and experimental study. Am J Dig Dis 10:1024–1033, 1965.
72. Rogers AI, Vloedman DA, Bloom EC, Kalser MH: Neomycin-induced steatorrhea. JAMA 197:185–190, 1966.
73. Cooper BT, Holmes GK, Ferguson R, Cooke WT: Celiac disease and malignancy. Medicine 59:249–261, 1980.
74. Swinson CM, Slavin G, Coles EC, Booth CC: Coeliac disease and malignancy. Lancet 1:111–115, 1983.
75. Holmes GK, Prior P, Lane MR, et al: Malignancy in coeliac disease—effect of a gluten free diet. Gut 30:333–338, 1989.
76. Isaacson PG, O'Connor NTJ, Spencer J, et al: Malignant histiocytosis of the intestine: A T-cell lymphoma. Lancet 2:688–691, 1985.
77. Spencer J, Cerf-Bensussan N, Jarry A, et al: Enteropathy-associated T cell lymphoma (malignant histiocytosis of the intestine) is recognized by a monoclonal antibody (HML-1) that defines a membrane molecule on human mucosal lymphocytes. Am J Pathol 132:1–5, 1988.
78. Spencer J, MacDonald TT, Diss TC, et al: Changes in intraepithelial lymphocyte subpopulations in coeliac disease and enteropathy associated T cell lymphoma (malignant histiocytosis of the intestine). Gut 30:339–346, 1989.
79. Fishman MJ, Jeejeebhoy KN, Gopinath N, et al: Small intestinal villous adenoma and celiac disease. Am J Gastroenterol 85:748–751, 1990.
80. Dannenberg A, Godwin T, Rayburn J, et al: Multifocal adenocarcinoma of the proximal small intestine in a patient with celiac sprue. J Clin Gastroenterol 11:73–76, 1989.
81. Straker RJ, Gunasekaran S, Brady PG: Adenocarcinoma of the jejunum in association with celiac sprue. J Clin Gastroenterol 11:320–323, 1989.
82. Trier JS, Falchuk ZM, Carey MC, Schreiber DS: Celiac sprue and refractory sprue (clinical conference). Gastroenterology 75:307–316, 1978.
83. Baer AN, Bayless TM, Yardley JH: Intestinal ulceration and malabsorption syndromes. Gastroenterology 79:754–765, 1980.
84. Bayless TM, Kapelowitz RF, Shelley WM, et al: Intestinal ulceration—a complication of celiac disease. N Engl J Med 276:996–1002, 1967.
85. Freeman HJ, Chiu BK: Small bowel malignant lymphoma complicating celiac sprue and the mesenteric lymph node cavitation syndrome. Gastroenterology 90:2008–2012, 1986.
86. Jeffries GH, Steinberg H, Sleisenger MH: Chronic ulcerative (nongranulomatous) jejunitis. Am J Med 44:47–59, 1968.
87. Robertson DA, Dixon MF, Scott BB, et al: Small intestinal ulceration: Diagnostic difficulties in relation to coeliac disease. Gut 24:565–574, 1983.
88. Jones B, Bayless TM, Hamilton SR, Yardley JH: "Bubbly" duodenal bulb in celiac disease: Radiologic-pathologic correlation. Am J Roentgenol 142:119–122, 1984.
89. Matuchansky C, Colin R, Hemet J, et al: Cavitation of mesenteric lymph nodes, splenic atrophy, and a flat small intestinal mucosa. Gastroenterology 87:606–614, 1984.
90. Rubesin SE, Herlinger H, Saul SH, et al: Adult celiac disease and its complications. Radiographics 9:1045–1066, 1989.
90a. O'Grady JG, Stevens FM, Harding B, et al: Hyposplenism and gluten-sensitive enteropathy: Natural history, incidence, and relationship to diet and small bowel morphology. Gastroenterology 87:1326–1331, 1984.
91. O'Grady JG, Stevens FM, McCarthy CF: Celiac disease: Does hyposplenism predispose to the development of malignant disease? Am J Gastroenterol 80:27–29, 1985.
92. Weinstein WM, Saunders DR, Tytgat GN, Rubin CE: Collagenous sprue—an unrecognized type of malabsorption. N Engl J Med 283:1297–1301, 1970.
93. Bossart R, Henry K, Booth CC, Doe WF: Subepithelial collagen in intestinal malabsorption. Gut 16:18–22, 1975.
94. Holdstock DJ, Oleesky S: Successful treatment of collagenous sprue with combination of prednisolone and gluten-free diet. Postgrad Med J 49:664–667, 1973.
95. Guller R, Anabitarte M, Mayer M: Kollagensprue und ulzerierende Jejunoileitis bei einem Patienten mit gluteninduzierter Enteropathie. Schweiz Med Wochenschr 116:1343–1349, 1986.
96. Marks J, Shuster S, Watson AJ: Small bowel changes in dermatitis herpetiformis. Lancet 2:1280–1282, 1966.
97. Shuster S, Watson AJ, Marks J: Coeliac syndrome in dermatitis herpetiformis. Lancet 1:1101–1106, 1968.
98. Gebhard RL, Falchuk ZH, Katz SI, et al: Dermatitis herpetiformis: Immunologic concomitants of small intestinal disease and relationship to histocompatibility antigens HL-A8. J Clin Invest 54:98–103, 1974.
99. Kosnai I, Karpati S, Savilahti E, et al: Gluten challenge in children with dermatitis herpetiformis: A clinical, morphological and immunohistological study. Gut 27:1464–1470, 1986.
100. Lindstrom CG: "Collagenous colitis" with watery diarrhea: A new entity? Pathol Eur 11:87–89, 1976.
101. Wolber R, Owen D, DelBuono L, et al: Lymphocytic gastritis in patients with celiac sprue of spruelike intestinal disease. Gastroenterology 98:310–315, 1990.
102. Dubois RN, Lazenby AJ, Yardley JH, et al: Lymphocytic enterocolitis in patients with 'refractory' sprue. JAMA 262:935–937, 1989.
103. Wolber R, Owen D, Freeman H: Colonic lymphocytosis in patients with celiac sprue. Hum Pathol 21:1092–1096, 1990.
104. O'Mahony S, Nawroz IM, Ferguson A: Coeliac disease and collagenous colitis. Postgrad Med J 66:238–241, 1990.
105. Hamilton I, Sanders S, Hopwood D, Bouchier IA: Collagenous colitis associated with small intestinal villous atrophy. Gut 27:1394–1398, 1986.
106. Breen EG, Farren C, Connolly CE, McCarthy CF: Collagenous colitis and coeliac disease. Gut 28:364, 1987.
107. Eckstein RP, Dowsett JF, Rilet JW: Collagenous enterocolitis: A case of collagenous colitis with involvement of the small intestine. Am J Gastroenterol 83:767–771, 1988.
108. Yardley JH, Lazenby AJ, Giardiello FM, Bayless TM: Collagenous, "Microscopic," lymphocytic, and other gentler and more subtle forms of colitis. Hum Pathol 21:1089–1091, 1990.
109. Baker SJ, Mathan VI: Syndrome of tropical sprue in South India. Am J Clin Nutr 21:984–993, 1968.
110. Klipstien, FA, Holdeman LV, Corcino JJ, et al: Enterotoxigenic intestinal bacteria in tropical sprue. Ann Intern Med 79:632–641, 1973.
111. Guerra R, Wheby MS, Bayless TM: Long-term antibiotic therapy in tropical sprue. Ann Intern Med 63:619–634, 1965.
112. Rickles R, Klipstein FA, Tomasini J, et al: Long-term follow-up

113. Cook GC: Aetiology and pathogenesis of postinfective tropical malabsorption (tropical sprue). Lancet 1:721–723, 1984.
114. Gorbach SL, Banwell JG, Mitra R, et al: Bacterial contamination of the upper small bowel in tropical sprue. Lancet 74–77, 1969.
115. Cassells JS, Banwell JG, Gorbach SL, et al: Tropical sprue and malnutrition in West Bengal. IV. Bile salt deconjugation in tropical sprue. Am J Clin Nutr 23:1579–1581, 1970.
116. Simon GL, Gorbach SL: Intestinal microflora. Med Clin North Am 66:557–574, 1982.
117. Klipstein FA: Folate in tropical sprue. Br J Haematol 23 (Suppl):119–133, 1972.
118. Foroozan P, Trier JS: Mucosa of the small intestine in pernicious anemia. N Engl J Med 277:553–559, 1967.
119. Hendrix TR: Interpretation of intestinal biopsies. Gastroenterology 54:976–978, 1968.
120. Marsh MN, Mathan M, Mathan VI: Studies of intestinal lymphoid tissue. VII. The secondary nature of lymphoid cell "activation" in the jejunal lesion of tropical sprue. Am J Pathol 112:302–312, 1983.
121. Swanson VL, Thomassen RW: Pathology of the jejunal mucosa in tropical sprue. Am J Pathol 46:511–581, 1965.
122. Swanson VL, Wheby MS, Bayless TM: Morphologic effects of folic acid and vitamin B_{12} on the jejunal lesion of tropical sprue. Am J Pathol 49:167–191, 1966.
123. Brunser O, Eidelman S, Klipstein FA: Intestinal morphology of rural Haitians: A comparison between overt tropical sprue and asymptomatic subjects. Gastroenterology 58:655–668, 1970.
124. Vaish SK, Sampathkumar J, Jacob R, Baker SJ: The stomach in tropical sprue. Gut 6:458–465, 1965.
125. Ramakrishna BS, Mathan VI: Role of bacterial toxins, bile acids, and free fatty acids in colonic malabsorption in tropical sprue. Dig Dis Sci 32:500–505, 1987.
126. Ramakrishna BS, Mathan VI: Absorption of water and sodium and activity of adenosine triphosphatases in the rectal mucosa in tropical sprue. Gut 29:665–668, 1988.
127. Wheby MS, Swanson VL, Bayless TM: Comparison of ileal and jejunal biopsies in tropical sprue. Am J Clin Nutr 24:117–123, 1971.
128. Goyal RK, Compton CC, Ferrucci JT: Case records of the Massachusetts General Hospital: Weekly clinicopathological exercises. Case 25-1990: A 63-year-old man with recurrent diarrhea. N Engl J Med 322:1796–1806, 1990.
129. McEvoy A, Dutton J, James OFW: Bacterial contamination of the small intestine is an important cause of occult malabsorption in the elderly. Br Med J 287:789–793, 1983.
130. Roberts SH, James O, Jarvis EH: Bacterial overgrowth syndrome without "blind loop": A cause for malnutrition in the elderly. Lancet 2:1193–1195, 1977.
131. King CE, Toskes PP: Small intestine bacterial overgrowth. Gastroenterology 76:1035–1055, 1979.
132. Ament ME, Shimoda SS, Saunders DP, Rubin CE: Pathogenesis of steatorrhea in three cases of small intestinal stasis syndrome. Gastroenterology 63:728–747, 1972.
133. Toskes PP, Giannella RA, Jervis HR, et al: Small intestinal mucosal injury in the experimental blind loop syndrome: Light- and electron-microscopic and histochemical studies. Gastroenterology 68:193–203, 1975.
134. Giannella RA, Rout WR, Toskes PP: Jejunal brush border injury and impaired sugar and amino acid uptake in the blind-loop syndrome. Gastroenterology 67:965–974, 1974.
135. Riepe SP, Goldstein J, Alpers DH: Effect of secreted Bacteroides proteases on human intestinal brush border hydrolases. J Clin Invest 66:314–322, 1980.
136. Drenick EJ, Roslyn JJ: Cure of arthritis-dermatitis syndrome due to intestinal bypass by resection of nonfunctional segment of blind loop. Dig Dis Sci 35:656–660, 1990.
137. Kahn IJ, Jeffries GH, Sleisenger MH: Malabsorption in intestinal scleroderma: Correction by antibiotics. N Engl J Med 274:1339–1344, 1966.
138. Paulley JW: Gut damage in human blind-loop syndrome. Gastroenterology 81:195, 1981.
139. Takano J: Intestinal changes in protein-deficient rats. Exp Mol Pathol 3:224–231, 1964.
140. Platt BS, Heard CRC, Stewart RJC: The effects of protein-calorie deficiency on the gastrointestinal tract. In Munro HN (ed): The role of the gastrointestinal tract in protein metabolism. Philadelphia, FA Davis, 1964, pp 227–237.
141. Tandon BN, Newberne PM, Young VR: A histochemical study of enzyme changes and ultrastructure of the jejunal mucosa in protein-depleted rats. J Nutr 99:519–530, 1969.
142. Herskovic T: The effect of protein malnutrition on the small intestine. Am J Clin Nutr 22:300–304, 1969.
143. James WPT: Intestinal absorption in protein caloric malnutrition. Lancet 1:333–335, 1968.
144. Mayoral LG, Bolanos O, Lotero H, Duque E: Enteropathy in adult protein malnutrition: A review of the Cali experience. Am J Clin Nutr 28:894–900, 1975.
145. Duque E, Bolanos O, Lotero H, Mayoral LG: Enteropathy in adult protein malnutrition: Light microscopic findings. Am J Clin Nutr 28:901–913, 1975.
146. Duque E, Lotero H, Bolanos O, Mayoral LG: Enteropathy in adult protein malnutrition: Ultrastructural findings. Am J Clin Nutr 28:914–924, 1975.
147. Klipstein FA, Samloff IM, Smarth G, Schenk E: Malabsorption and malnutrition in rural Haiti. Am J Clin Nutr 21:1042–1052, 1968.
148. Schneider RE, Viteri FE: Morphological aspects of the duodenojejunal mucosa in protein-calorie malnourished children and during recovery. Am J Clin Nutr 25:1092–1102, 1972.
149. Naiman JL, Oski FA, Diamond LK, et al: The gastrointestinal effects of iron-deficiency anemia. Pediatrics 33:83–99, 1964.
150. Gross SJ, Stuart MJ, Swender PT, Oski FA: Malabsorption of iron in children with iron deficiency. J Pediatr 88:795–799, 1976.
151. Prasad AS: The role of zinc in gastrointestinal and liver disease. Clin Gastroentol 12:713–741, 1983.
152. Kay RG, Tasman-Jones C, Pybus J, et al: A syndrome of acute zinc deficiency during total parenteral alimentation in man. Ann Surg 183:331–340, 1976.
153. Brazin SA, Johnson WT, Abramson LJ: The acrodermatitis enteropathica-like syndrome. Arch Dermatol 115:597–599, 1979.
154. Strobel CT, Byrne WJ, Abramovits W, et al: A zinc-deficiency dermatitis in patients on total parenteral nutrition. Int J Dermatol 17:575–581, 1978.
155. Moynahan EJ: Acrodermatitis: A lethal inherited human zinc deficiency disorder. Lancet 2:399–400, 1974.
156. Mack D, Koletzko B, Cunnane S, et al: Acrodermatitis enteropathica with normal serum zinc levels: Diagnostic value of small bowel biopsy and essential fatty acid determination. Gut 30:1426–1429, 1989.
157. Kelly R, Davidson GP, Townley RRW, Campbell PE: Reversible intestinal mucosal abnormality in acrodermatitis enteropathica. Arch Dis Child 51:219–222, 1976.
158. Ament ME, Broviac J: Acrodermatitis enteropathica (AE). Demonstration of small and large intestinal mucosal lesions: Failure of hyperalimentation, Intralipid, and Diodoquin to reverse the intestinal lesions and generalized malabsorption syndromes. Gastroenterology 64:A-9/692, 1973.
159. Braun OH, Heilmann K, Pauli W, et al: Acrodermatitits enteropathica: Recent findings concerning clinical features, pathogenesis, diagnosis and therapy. Eur J Pediatr 121:247–261, 1976.
160. Bohane TD, Hamilton JR, Gall DG: Acrodermatitis enteropathica, zinc and the Paneth cell: A case report with family studies. Gastroenterology 73:587–592, 1977.
161. Elmes ME, Jones JG: Ultrastructural changes in the small intestine of zinc deficiency rats. J Pathol 130:37–43, 1980.
162. Kobayashi Y, Suzuki H, Konno T, et al: Ultrastructural alterations of Paneth cells in infants associated with gastrointestinal symptoms. Tohoku J Exp Med 139:225–230, 1983.
163. Blacklow NR, Cukor G: Viral gastroenteritis. N Engl J Med 304:397–406, 1981.
164. Whipple GH: A hitherto undescribed disease characterized anatomically by deposits of fat and fatty acids in the intestinal and mesenteric lymphatic tissue. Bull Johns Hopkins Hosp 18:382–391, 1907.
165. Chears WC, Ashworth CT: Electron microscopic study of intestinal mucosa in Whipple's disease: Demonstration of encapsulated bacilliform bodies in the lesion. Gastroenterology 41:129–138, 1961.
166. Yardley JH, Hendrix TR: Combined electron and light micros-

copy in Whipple's disease: Demonstration of "bacillary bodies" in the intestine. Bull Johns Hopkins Hosp 109:80–95, 1961.
167. Fleming JL, Wiesner RH, Shorter RG: Whipple's disease: clinical, biochemical, and histopathologic features and assessment of treatment in 29 patients. May Clin Proc 63:539–551, 1988.
168. Knox DL, Bayless TM, Pittman FE: Neurologic disease in patients with Whipple's disease. Medicine 55:467–476, 1976.
169. Silva MT, Macedo PM, Moura Nunes JF: Ultrastructure of bacilli and the bacillary origin of the macrophagic inclusions in Whipple's disease. J Gen Microbiol 131:1001–1013, 1985.
170. Dobbins WO 3d, Kawanishi H: Bacillary characteristics in Whipple's disease: An electron microscopic study. Gastroenterology 80:1468–1475, 1981.
171. Keren DF: Whipple's disease: A review emphasizing immunology and microbiology. Crit Rev Clin Lab Sci 14:75–108, 1981.
172. Keren DF, Weisburger WR, Yardley JH, et al: Whipple's disease: Demonstration by immunofluorescence of similar bacterial antigens in macrophages from three cases. Johns Hopkins Med J 139:51–59, 1976.
173. Kirkpatrick PM, Kent SP, Mihas A, Pritchette P: Whipple's disease: A case report with immunological studies. Gastroenterology 15:297–301, 1978.
174. Charache P, Bayless TM, Shelley WM, Hendrix TR: Atypical bacteria in Whipple's disease. Trans Assoc Am Physicians 79:399–408, 1966.
175. Clancy RL, Tompkins WAF, Muckle TH, et al: Isolation and characterization of an etiological agent in Whipple's disease. Br Med J 2:568–570, 1975.
176. Volpicelli NA, Salyer WR, Milligan FD, et al: The endoscopic appearance of the duodenum in Whipple's disease. Johns Hopkins Med J 138:19–23, 1976.
177. Kuhajda FP, Belitsos NJ, Keren DF, Hutchins GM: A submucosal variant of Whipple's disease. Gastroenterology 82:46–50, 1982.
178. Roth RI, Owen RL, Keren DF, Volbering PA. Intestinal infection with Mycobacterium avium in acquired immune deficiency syndrome (AIDS): Histological and clinical comparison with Whipple's disease. Dig Dis Sci 30:497–504, 1985.
179. Gonzalez-Licea AG, Yardley JH: Whipple's disease in the rectum. Light and electron microscopic findings. Am J Pathol 52:1191–1206, 1968.
180. Gupta TP, Ehrinpreis MN: Candida-associated diarrhea in hospitalized patients. Gastroenterology 98:780–785, 1990.
181. Orchard JL, Luparello F, Brunskill D: Malabsorption syndrome occurring in the course of disseminated histoplasmosis: Case report and review of gastrointestinal histoplasmosis. Am J Med 66:331–336, 1979.
182. Brasitus TA: Parasites and malabsorption. Clin Gastroenterol 12:495–510, 1983.
183. Cali A, Owen RL: Microsporidiosis. In Balows A (ed): Laboratory Diagnosis of Infectious Disease: Principles and Practices. Vol 1. New York, Springer-Verlag, 1988, pp 929–950.
184. Cali A, Owen RL: Intracellular development of Enterocytozoon, a unique microsporidian found in the intestine of AIDS patients. J Protozool 37:145–155, 1990.
185. Desportes I, LeCharpentier Y, Galian A, et al: Occurrence of a new microsporidian Enterocytozoon bieneusi n. g., n. sp., in the enterocytes of a human patient with AIDS. J Protozool 32:250–254, 1985.
186. Orenstein JM, Chiang J, Steinberg W, et al: Intestinal microsporidiosis as a cause of diarrhea in human immunodeficiency virus-infected patients. Hum Pathol 21:475–481, 1990.
187. Greenson JK, Belitsos PC, Yardley JH, Bartlett JG: AIDS enteropathy—occult enteric infections and duodenal mucosal alterations in chronic diarrhea. Ann Intern Med 114:366–372, 1991.
188. Rijpstra AC, Canning EU, Ketel RJV, et al: Use of light microscopy to diagnose small intestinal microsporidiosis in patients with AIDS. J Infect Dis 157:827–831, 1988.
189. van Gool T, Hollister WS, Schattenkerk JE, et al: Diagnosis of Enterocytozoon bieneusi microsporidiosis in AIDS patients by recovery of spores from faeces. Lancet 336:267–268, 1990.
190. Orenstein JM, Zierdt W, Zierdt C, Kotler DP: Identification of spores of enterocytozoon-bieneusi in stool and duodenal fluid from AIDS patients. Lancet 336:1127–1128, 1990.
191. Lucas SB, Papadaki L, Conlon C, et al: Diagnosis of intestinal microsporidiosis in patients with AIDS. J Clin Pathol 42:885–890, 1989.
192. Saraya AK, Tandon BN: Hookworm anaemia and intestinal malabsorption associated with hookworm infestation. Prog Drug Res 19:108–118, 1975.
193. Tripathy K, Gonzalez F, Lotero H, Bolanos O: Effects of Ascaris infection on human nutrition. Am J Trop Med Hyg 20:212–218, 1970.
194. Meyer WM, Connor DH, Neafie RC: Strongyloidiasis. In Binford CH, Connor DH (eds): Pathology of Tropical and extraordinary diseases. Washington, DC, Armed Forces Institute of Pathology, 1976, pp 428–432.
195. Scowden EB, Schaffner W, Stone WJ: Overwhelming strongyloidiasis: An unappreciated opportunistic infection. Medicine 57:527–544, 1978.
196. Milder JE, Walzer PD, Kilgore G, et al: Clinical features of Strongyloides stercoralis infection in an endemic area of the United States. Gastroenterology 80:1481–1488, 1981.
197. Arakaki T, Iwanaga M, Kinjo F, et al: Efficacy of agar-plate culture in detection of Strongyloides stercoralis infection. J Parasitol 76:425–428, 1990.
198. Neafie RC, Connor DH, Cross JH: Capillariasis (intestinal and hepatic). In Binford CH, Connor DH (eds): Pathology of tropical and extraordinary diseases. Washington, DC, Armed Forces Institute of Pathology, 1976, pp 402–408.
199. Intestinal capillariasis: A new disease of man. (Editorial) Lancet 1:587–588, 1973.
200. Chen CY, Hsieh WC, Lin JT, Liu MC: Intestinal capillariasis: Report of a case. Taiwan I Hsueh Hui Tsa Chih 88:617–620, 1989.
201. Youssef FG, Mikhail EM, Mansour NS: Intestinal capillariasis in Egypt: a case report. Am J Trop Med Hyg 40:195–196, 1989.
202. Cross JH, Basaca-Sevilla V: Experimental transmission of Capillaria philippinensis to birds. Trans R Soc Trop Med Hyg 77:511–514, 1983.
203. Fresh JW, Cross JH, Reyes V, et al: Necropsy findings in intestinal capillariasis. Am J Trop Med Hyg 21:169–173, 1972.
204. Kagnoff MF: Immunology and disease of the gastrointestinal tract. In Sleisenger MH, Fordtran JS (eds): Gastrointestinal Disease, 4th ed. Philadelphia, WB Saunders, 1989, pp 114–143.
205. HIV-associated enteropathy. (Editorial) Lancet 2:777–778, 1989.
206. Bartelsman JFWM, Sars PRA, Tytgat GNJ: Gastrointestinal complications in patients with acquired immunodeficiency syndrome. Scand J Gastroenterol 24 (Suppl 171):112–117, 1989.
207. Laughon BE, Druckman DA, Vernon A, et al: Prevalence of enteric pathogens in homosexual men with and without acquired immunodeficiency syndrome. Gastroenterology 94:984–993, 1988.
208. Rodgers VD, Fassett R, Kagnoff MF: Abnormalities in intestinal mucosal T cells in homosexual populations including those with the lymphadenopathy syndrome and acquired immunodeficiency syndrome. Gastroenterology 90:552–558, 1986.
209. Rodgers VD, Kagnoff MF: Abnormalities of the intestinal immune system in AIDS. Gastroenterol Clin North Am 17:487–494, 1988.
210. Nelson JA, Wiley CA, Reynolds-Kohler C, et al: Human immunodeficiency virus detected in bowel epithelium from patients with gastrointestinal symptoms. Lancet 1:259–262, 1988.
211. Mathijs JM, Hiug M, Grierson J, et al: HIV infection of rectal mucosa. (Letter) Lancet 1:1111, 1988.
212. Fox CH, Kotler D, Tierney A, et al: Detection of HIV-1 RNA in the lamina propria of patients with AIDS and gastrointestinal disease. J Infect Dis 159:467–471, 1989.
213. Jarry A, Cortez A, Rene E, et al: Infected cells and immune cells in the gastrointestinal tract of AIDS patients: An immunohistochemical study of 127 cases. Histopathology 16:133–40, 1990.
214. Ferreira RD, Forsyth LE, Richman PI, et al: Changes in the rate of crypt epithelial cell proliferation and mucosal morphology induced by a T-cell-mediated response in human small intestine. Gastroenterology 98:1255–1263, 1990.
215. MacDonald TT, Spencer J: Evidence that activated mucosal T cells play a role in the pathogenesis of enteropathy in human small intestine. J Exp Med 167:1341–1349, 1988.
216. MacDonald TT, Ferguson A: Hypersensitivity reactions in the

small intestine. 3. The effects of allograft rejection and of graft-versus-host reaction on epithelial cell kinetics. Cell Tissue Kinet 10:301-312, 1977.
217. Ullrich R, Zeitz M, Heise W, et al: Small intestinal structural and function in patients infected with human immunodeficiency virus (HIV): Evidence for HIV-induced enteropathy. Ann Intern Med 111:15-21, 1989.
218. Unsworth J, Hutchins P, Mitchell J, et al: Flat small intestinal mucosa and autoantibodies against the gut epithelium. J Pediatr Gastroenterol Nutr 1:503-513, 1982.
219. Mirakian R, Richardson A, Milla PJ, et al: Protracted diarrhoea of infancy: Evidence in support of an autoimmune variant. Br Med J 293:1132-1136, 1986.
220. Seldman EG, Localle F, Russo P, et al: Successful treatment of autoimmune enteropathy with cyclosporine. J Pediatr 117:929-932, 1990.
221. Cuenod B, Brousse N, Goulet O, et al: Classification of intractable diarrhea in infancy using clinical and immunohistological criteria. Gastroenterology 99:1037-1043, 1990.
222. Hill SM, Milla PJ, Bottazzo GF, Mirakian R: Autoimmune enteropathy and colitis: Is there a generalised autoimmune gut disorder? Gut 32:36-42, 1991.
223. Mirakian R, Hill S, Richardson A, et al: HLA product expression and lymphocyte subpopulations in jejunum biopsies of children with idiopathic protracted diarrhoea and enterocyte autoantibodies. J Autoimmun 1:263-277, 1988.
224. Webb TA, Li CY, Yam LT: Systemic mast cell disease: A clinical and hematopathologic study of 26 cases. Cancer 49:927-938, 1982.
225. Enerbäck L, Pipkorn U, Aldenborg F, Wingren U: Mast cell heterogeneity in man: Properties and function of human mucosal mast cells. In Galli SJ, Austen FK (eds): Mast Cell and Basophil Differentiation and Function in Health and Disease. New York, Raven Press, 1989, pp 27-37.
226. Bank S, Marks IN: Malabsorption in systemic mast cell disease. Gastroenterology 45:535-549, 1963.
227. Jarnum S, Zachariae H: Mastocytosis (urticaria pigmentosa) of skin, stomach, and gut with malabsorption. Gut 8:64-68, 1967.
228. Broitman SA, McCray RS, May JC, et al: Mastocytosis and intestinal malabsorption. Am J Med 48:382-389, 1970.
229. Dantzig PI: Tetany, malabsorption, and mastocytosis. Arch Intern Med 135:1514-1518, 1975.
230. Ammann RW, Vetter D, Deyhle P, et al: Gastrointestinal involvement in systemic mastocytosis. Gut 17:107-112, 1976.
231. Fishman RS, Fleming CR, Li CY: Systemic mastocytosis with review of gastrointestinal manifestations. Mayo Clin Proc 54:51-54, 1979.
232. Bredfeldt JE, O'Laughlin JC, Durham JB, Blessing LD: Malabsorption and gastric hyperacidity in systemic mastocytosis. Am J Gastroenterol 74:133-137, 1980.
233. Braverman DZ, Dollberg L, Shiner M: Clinical, histological, and electron microscopic study of mast cell disease of the small bowel. Am J Gastroenterol 80:30-37, 1985.
234. Reisberg IR, Oyakawa S: Mastocytosis with malabsorption, myelofibrosis, and massive ascites. Am J Gastroenterol 82:54-60, 1987.
235. Enerbäck L: Mast cells in rat gastrointestinal mucosa. I. Effects of fixation. Acta Pathol Microbiol Scand 66:289-302, 1966.
236. Befus AD, Pearce FL, Gauldie J, et al: Isolation and characteristics of mast cells from the lamina propria of the small bowel. In Pepys J, Edwards AM (eds): The Mast Cell: Its Role in Health and Disease. Baltimore, University Park Press, 1979, pp 702-709.
237. Strobel S, Miller HRP, Ferguson A: Human intestinal mucosal mast cells: Evaluation of fixation and staining techniques. J Clin Pathol 34:851-858, 1981.
238. Ruitenberg EJ, Gustowska L, Elgersma A, Ruitenberg HM: Effect of fixation on the light microscopical visualization of mast cells in the mucosa and connective tissue of the human duodenum. Int Arch Allergy Appl Immunol 67:233-238, 1982.
239. Irani AM, Bradford TR, Kepley CL, et al: Detection of MCT and MCTC types of human mast cells by immunohistochemistry using new monoclonal anti-tryptase and anti-chymase antibodies. J Histochem Cytochem 37:1509-1515, 1989.
240. Barrett KE, Metcalfe DD: Mast cell heterogeneity: Evidence and implications. J Clin Immunol 4:253-261, 1984.
241. Scott BB, Hardy GJ, Losowsky MS. Involvement of the small intestine in systemic mast cell disease. Gut 16:918-924, 1975.
242. Befus AD, Denburg J, Bienenstock J: Mechanisms of intestinal mastocytosis. In Pepys J, Edwards AM (eds): The Mast Cell: Its Role in Health and Disease. Baltimore, University Park Press, 1979, pp 115-122.
243. Abe T, Ochiai H, Minamishima Y, Nawa Y: Induction of intestinal mastocytosis in nude mice by repeated injection of interleukin-3. Int Arch Allergy Appl Immunol 86:356-358, 1988.
244. Saito H, Hatake K, Dvorak AM, et al: Selective differentiation and proliferation of hematopoietic cells induced by recombinant human interleukins. Proc Natl Acad Sci USA 85:2288-2292, 1988.
245. Davidson GP, Cutz E, Hamilton JR, Gall DG: Familial enteropathy: a syndrome of protracted diarrhea from birth, failure to thrive, and hypoplastic villus atrophy. Gastroenterology 75:783-790, 1978.
246. Cutz E, Rhoads JM, Drumm B, et al: Microvillus inclusion disease: An inherited defect of brush-border assembly and differentiation. N Engl J Med 320:646-651, 1989.
247. Rhoads JM, Vogler RC, Lacey SR, et al: Microvillus inclusion disease: In vitro jejunal electrolyte transport. Gastroenterology 100:811-817, 1991.
248. Lake BD: Microvillus inclusion disease: Specific diagnostic features shown by alkaline phosphatase histochemistry. J Clin Pathol 41:880-882, 1988.
249. Waldman TA, Steinfeld JL, Dutcher TF, et al: The role of gastrointestinal system in "idiopathic hypoproteinemia." Gastroenterology 41:197-207, 1961.
250. Waldmann TA: Protein-losing enteropathy. Gastroenterology 50:422-443, 1966.
251. Abramowsky C, Hupertz V, Kilbridge P, Czinn S: Intestinal lymphangiectasia in children: A study of upper gastrointestinal endoscopic biopsies. Pediatr Pathol 9:289-297, 1989.
252. Strober W, Wochner RD, Carbone PP, Waldman TA: Intestinal lymphangiectasia: A protein-losing enteropathy with hypogammaglobulinemia, lymphocytopenia and impaired homograft rejection. J Clin Invest 46:1643-1656, 1967.
253. Pomerantz M, Waldman TA: Systemic lymphatic abnormalities associated with gastrointestinal protein loss secondary to intestinal lymphangiectasia. Gastroenterology 45:703-711, 1963.
254. Eustace PW, Gaunt JI, Croft DN: Incidence of protein-losing enteropathy in primary lymphoedema using chromium-51 chloride technique. Br Med J 4:737, 1975.
255. Perisic VN, Kokai G: Bleeding from duodenal lymphangiectasia. Arch Dis Child 66:153-154, 1991.
256. Asakura H, Miur S, Morishita T, et al: Endoscopic and histopathological study on primary and secondary intestinal lymphangiectasia. Dig Dis Sci 26:312-320, 1981.
257. Hart MH, Vanderhoof JA, Antonson DL: Failure of blind small bowel biopsy in the diagnosis of intestinal lymphangiectasia. J Pediatr Gastroenterol Nutr 6:803-805, 1987.
258. Harris M, Burton IE, Scarffe JH: Macroglobulinemia and intestinal lymphangiectasia: a rare association. J Clin Pathol 36:30-36, 1983.
259. Myszor MF, Davidson A, Hodgson HJF: The local mucosal immune system in intestinal lymphangiectasia. J Clin Lab Immunol 26:1-3, 1988.
260. Dobbins WO III: Electron microscopic study of the intestinal mucosa in intestinal lymphangiectasia. Gastroenterology 51:1004-1017, 1966.
261. Mistilis SP, Skyring AP, Stephen DD: Intestinal lymphangiectasia. Mechanism of enteric loss of plasma protein and fat. Lancet 1:77-80, 1965.
262. Patel AS, DeRidder PH: Endoscopic appearance and significance of functional lymphangiectasia of the duodenal mucosa. Gastrointest Endosc 36:376-378, 1990.
263. Cabrera A, de la Pava S, Pickren JW: Intestinal localization of Waldenstrom's disease. Arch Intern Med 114:399-407, 1964.
264. Bedine MS, Yardley JH, Elliott HL, et al: Intestinal involvement in Waldenström's macroglobulinemia. Gastroenterology 65:308-315, 1973.
265. Brandt LJ, Davidoff A, Bernstein LH, et al: Small intestinal involvement in Waldenström's macroglobulinemia: Case report and review of the literature. Dig Dis Sci 26:174-180, 1981.
266. Pruzanski W, Warren RE, Goldie JH, Katz A: Malabsorption

syndrome with infiltration of the intestinal wall extracellular monoclonal macroglobulin. Am J Med 54:811–818, 1973.
267. Amrein PC, Compton CC: Case records of the Massachusetts General Hospital: Weekly clinicopathological exercises. Case 3-1990: A 66-year-old woman with Waldenstrom's macroglobulinemia, diarrhea, anemia, and persistent gastrointestinal bleeding. N Engl J Med 322:183–192, 1990.
268. Aspelin P, Adielsson G, Dimitrov N, et al: Abdominal computed tomography in macroglobulinemia (Waldenström's disease). Acta Radiol 30:197–200, 1989.

CHAPTER 30

Diverticular Disease of the Colon

SI-CHUN MING, M.D.

EPIDEMIOLOGY

ETIOLOGY AND PATHOGENESIS
Defects in the Colonic Wall
Abnormalities of the Muscular Layer
Intraluminal Pressure
Dietary Fiber
Other Factors

PATHOLOGY
Handling of Gross Specimens
Gross Features of Diverticulosis
Histologic Features of Diverticulosis

Classification
Prediverticular State
Simple Diverticulosis
Simple Massed Diverticulosis
Diverticulosis with Muscle
  Abnormality (Spastic Diverticulosis)
Giant Diverticula
Diverticulitis and Complications
Diverticula of the Right Colon

CLINICOPATHOLOGIC CORRELATION

Clinical Features
Complicated Diverticulitis with Perforation
Hemorrhage
Obstruction
Coexisting Colonic Conditions
Carcinoma
Inflammatory Bowel Diseases
Ischemic Colon Disease
Associated Extracolonic Conditions

A diverticulum of the gastrointestinal tract is a blind pouch leading off the gut. Its mucosa, including muscularis mucosae, is in continuance with that of the organ from which it arises, and it communicates with the main lumen of the gut. The diverticulum may partially or completely penetrate the muscularis propria so that the apex of diverticulum is covered only by the mesenteric tissue or the serosa. These features distinguish the diverticulum from a duplication of the alimentary tract, which is most commonly a noncommunicating cystic structure containing a full or partial layer of muscularis propria. The duplications are discussed in detail in Chapter 8.

The presence of diverticula is termed diverticulosis. In the majority of cases, the diverticulum is asymptomatic. Therefore, diverticulosis in a clinical sense may be considered an incidental phenomenon and not a disease. In many cases, however, the diverticulum may become inflamed, bleed, obstruct, and perforate, causing an extramural abscess, a fistula, or diffuse sepsis. The term *diverticular disease* encompasses the variable clinical spectrum of manifestations, particularly diverticulitis and its complications.

The diverticular disease of the colon is discussed in detail in this chapter. Those of the upper gastrointestinal tract are presented briefly. Additional information is presented in Chapter 8, on congenital diverticula; Chapter 17, on esophageal diverticula; Chapter 11, on small-intestinal diverticula; Chapter 33, on appendiceal diverticula; and, in brief passages, in various chapters on inflammatory and neoplastic disorders.

Classification of Diverticula. The diverticula have been classified in several ways. They can be divided into true and false types, the former with and the latter without a full muscularis propria. The congenital diverticulum is usually a true diverticulum, and the acquired diverticulum is usually a pseudodiverticulum.

The diverticula have also been classified into pulsion and traction types. The pulsion diverticulum is the result of increased intraluminal pressure pushing the mucosa through a weak point in the muscularis propria. It is therefore a pseudodiverticulum. The traction diverticulum is caused by scar tissue outside the gut pulling a portion of gut wall outward to form a sac. The traction diverticulum has a full-thickness muscular layer.

Diverticulosis of the Upper Gastrointestinal Tract.
Diverticula can occur in any segment of the gastrointestinal tract. The most common and most serious ones are found in the colon, in about 10% to 66% of barium enema examinations, increasing with the age of the patients.[1] Diverticula of the upper gastrointestinal tract are less frequent. Among 20,000 barium examinations, Wheeler found diverticula of the esophagus in 0.15%, of the stomach in 0.1%, and of the duodenum in 5.1%.[2]

In the esophagus, the diverticula are found at the pharyngoesophageal junction, just above the diaphragm and the midthorax, with a frequency ratio of approximately 7:1:2.[2] The diverticulum at midthoracic esophagus is usually a traction diverticulum caused by tuberculous lymphadenitis at the level of the bifurcation of the trachea. With marked decline of tuberculosis, the traction diverticula have virtually disappeared. The diverticula at either end of the esophagus are of the pulsion type. The pharyngoesophageal diverticulum, also known as Zenker's diverticulum, is invariably located at the posterior wall, between the oblique fibers of inferior constrictor and the crossing fibers of cricopharyngeus muscle.[3]

The epiphrenic diverticula occur just above the diaphragm and are often associated with conditons causing functional or structural obstruction of the distal esophagus, such as hiatus hernia,[4] diffuse esophageal spasm, and achalasia.[5,6] In one report, the diverticulum occurred in a boy with the Ehlers-Danlos syndrome.[7]

Clinically, the pulsion diverticula occur in the middle or later years of life and more frequently in males than in females. Many patients are asymptomatic. Symptoms are related to obstruction, inflammation, and hemorrhage.[8] Rarely, carcinoma develops in the diverticulum[9,10]; the incidence of malignancy in Zenker's diverticulum was reported to be 0.3%.[11]

The diverticula discussed above are usually single and large and project beyond the esophageal wall. In diffuse intramural esophageal diverticulosis[12,13] (also called pseudo-diverticulosis[14-16]), there are many small diverticula within the wall, more numerous in the upper esophagus. They were thought to be dilated ducts of the esophageal glands lined with metaplastic squamous cells.[14,15]

Diverticula of the stomach occur in the posterior wall near the cardia in three fourths of the cases and in the prepyloric region in 15%.[17-19] The former may be congenital or acquired.[18-21] They are often asymptomatic but may become ulcerated and bleed.[20-21] The prepyloric diverticula are usually acquired and probably related to peptic ulcer. Rarely, the diverticula are intramural.[22] Additional information on gastric diverticula is given in Chapter 20.

Diverticula of the small intestine occur most frequently in the duodenum. They are rare in the jejunum and ileum, found in about 0.1% of barium examinations.[23] They may be congenital or acquired. Meckel's diverticulum is the prototype of the congenital type. It is discussed in Chapter 8. It has been found in 0.3% to 2% of autopsies.[23,24] There is a slight male predominance in symptomatic patients. In the adult, it is located at the antimesenteric border of the ileum, 80 to 90 cm above the ileocecal valve. It measures up to 12 cm in length.[23] The mucosa is composed mostly of the small-intestinal type of tissue, but heterotopic mucosa of other parts of the gastrointestinal tract and pancreatic tissue may be present in up to 50% of examined specimens.[25,26] The oxyntic gastric mucosa is associated with peptic ulceration, often in the adjacent ileum. It may cause obstruction by kinking or volvulus. Rarely, neoplasms, epithelial or mesenchymal in origin, may arise in the diverticulum[27-29] (see Chapter 32).

Diverticula of the duodenum have been found in 1% to 6% of radiologic examinations, for an average of 1.7%, and in an average of 8.6% of autopsies.[23] They are mostly single, projecting at the medial aspect of the second portion of the duodenum. In about one third of the cases they are located in the third and fourth portions of duodenum.[30] Most patients are asymptomatic, but some diverticula may cause obstructive jaundice, hemorrhage, and perforation.[31,32] Congenital duodenal diverticula are rare. They may be extramural or intramural.[33] The intraluminal diverticulum is a pocket created by a membrane made of mucosa on both sides.[34] There is often a small opening on the membrane, allowing communication between the diverticulum and the duodenal lumen. The membrane may be excised endoscopically or surgically.[35]

Diverticula of the jejunum and ileum, other than Meckel's diverticulum, are mostly acquired, possibly because of defects in the muscular coat or nerve plexus (see Chapter 11). They are usually multiple and typically occur at the mesenteric border, where blood vessels enter the intestinal wall.[36] The diverticulum may be the seat of hemorrhage and inflammation.[37,38] The malabsorption syndrome, particularly vitamin B_{12} deficiency leading to macrocytic anemia, may occur, due to overgrowth of bacteria in the jejunal diverticula.[39,40]

EPIDEMIOLOGY

Accounts of historical events related to the description of colonic diverticula and their clinical consequences were given by Painter and Burkitt[1] and Localio and Stahl.[41] Cruveilhier[42] was credited for giving the first detailed description of diverticula of the colon in 1849. Four years earlier, in 1845, Gross[43] reported that obstruction caused the muscle fibers of the colon to separate, which permitted the mucous membrane to protrude through the colonic wall. In 1899, Graser[44] related the herniation of diverticulum to the point of vascular entrance to the colonic wall. In 1904, Beer[45] believed that fecal masses in the diverticula caused diverticulitis, which progressed to perforation and fistula. Thus the concept of diverticular disease of colon took shape around the turn of the twentieth century. However, the condition was uncommon, and its importance as a clinical problem was not generally appreciated until the advent of radiology, which demonstrated the prevalence of colonic diverticula in the general population.[1] Radiologic study and autopsy data showed that the incidence had increased dramatically in the United Kingdom, the United States, and Australia, from 5% in 1910[46] to 45% in 1969,[47] particularly in persons over 40 years of age. The increase in the incidence of colonic diverticula coincided with the change of lifestyle and eating habits in the Western countries, from a high-residue diet containing plenty of cereal fiber to a low-residue diet deficient in dietary fiber.[46]

The influence of westernization in dietary habit on the incidence of colonic diverticula is shown clearly by the geographic distribution of the disease. In native Africans and Asians the incidence is low. Kyle[48] noted in 1967 that whereas the incidence of diverticulitis per population of 1 million per year in Scotland was 12.88, the corresponding rate in Nigeria was only 0.17. A similar incidence was found among the Chinese and Indians in Singapore and Indians in Fiji, but Europeans in these places had incidences of 5.41 and 7.62, respectively. In recent reports the incidence has increased in urbanized Africans[49] and Indians[50] to over 2%. The incidence in Japan increased from 1% in 1975[51] to 7.8% in 1983.[52] In Hong Kong the rate was 5% in 1985.[53] There was a threefold increase in the Sephardic and Oriental Jews in Israel in 10 years to 16%, whereas the incidence among Ashkenazic Jews remained unchanged at 19%.[54] The rate among Arabs in Israel increased sevenfold to 9.5%. Although the sigmoid colon is affected in 90% of cases in the Western countries,[47] 75% of diverticula, mostly of congenital type, were found in the cecum and ascending colon in Asians.[52,53,55,56] Another difference is in the sex distribution, which is nearly equal between the sexes in Westerners and shows a 3:2 male predominance in Asians.[52]

ETIOLOGY AND PATHOGENESIS

Two factors determine the development of acquired colonic diverticula: (1) a higher intralumimal pressure in the gut than in the ambient peritoneal pressure and (2) a weak point in the intestinal wall, where herniation of the mucosa occurs. The effects of these factors on the diverticula of upper gastrointestinal tract are briefly mentioned above. The situation is more complicated in the colon. The muscularis propria, which generates the intraluminal pressure by contraction and maintains the integrity of the intestinal wall, has a unique anatomic arrangement, in that the longitudinal muscle is gathered into three equidistant bands: one mesenteric taenia at the attachment of mesocolon to colon and two antimesenteric taeniae on the opposing free wall. The blood vessels in the mesentery pass over the mesenteric taenia to enter the circular muscle coat between the mesenteric taenia and each antimesenteric taenia, corresponding to the usual location of diverticula (Figure 30–1).

Defects in the Colonic Wall

The occurrence of diverticula at the point of vascular penetration, which serves as a weak point in the co-

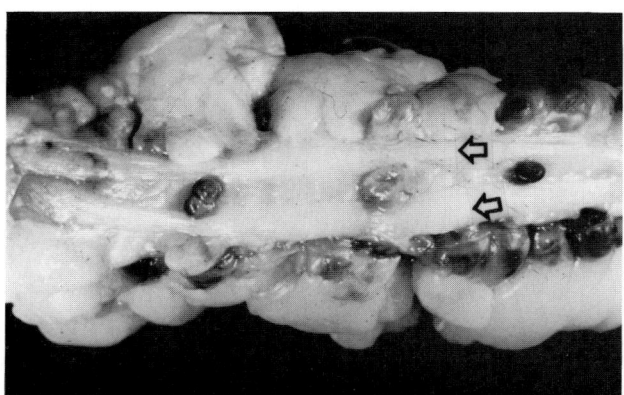

FIGURE 30–1. Gross photograph of a colon at postmortem examination. It shows many diverticula along the wall between the antimesenteric taeniae (arrows) and mesenteric taenia, which is not seen because it lies on the other side of the colon and is covered by adipose tissue. The diverticula are dark in color, more prominent in the lower row, because of feces within. Only three diverticula are between the antimesenteric taeniae. The taeniae are prominent in this specimen because of increased thickness. (From Fleischner FG, Ming SC, Henken EM: Revised concepts on diverticular disease of the colon. 1. Diverticulosis: Emphasis on tissue derangement and its relation to the irritable colon syndrome. Radiology 83:859–872, 1964.)

lonic wall, was recognized by Graser in 1899[44] and later by others.[57,58] The relationship was confirmed by Noer in specimens studied after injection of latex into the vessels.[59] He and others[60,61] recognized, however, that the relationship between vessels and diverticula was inconstant (Figure 30–2). The contribution of a weakened point in the colonic wall to the development of diverticulum is demonstrated in scleroderma. In this condition, diverticula occur at areas where the muscular layer is replaced by fibrous tissue[62] (see Figure 11–28). Since the fibrotic area is relatively broad, the opening of the diverticulum is wide. On the other hand, the opening of a usual diverticulum is small, and its neck is surrounded by circular muscle (Figure 30–3). The association of colonic diverticula with the Marfan[63] and Ehlers-Danlos syndromes,[64] diseases with a defect in collagen formation, suggests a possible defect in collagen tissue in diverticulosis. Electron microscopic examination of the submucosal collagen of the colon revealed that the fibrils become smaller and more compact with aging, and these features were more pronounced in colons with diverticula.[65] Elastic fibers in the muscular taeniae have also been shown to change with aging.[66,67] There is a 200% increase of elastin between normal-appearing muscle cells, causing shortening of the taeniae, which is a significant contributing factor in the development of colonic diverticula. There is also a decrease in the tensile strength and elasticity of the colon wall with age.[68]

Abnormalities of the Muscular Layer

The radiologic observation of a deformed colon, particularly the sigmoid, variously described as a saw-toothed pattern,[69] a serrated pattern,[70] a contracted

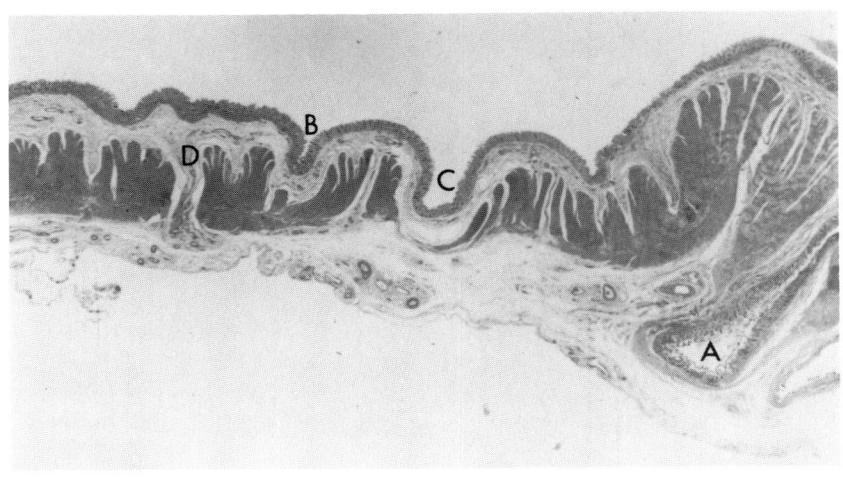

FIGURE 30–2. Photomicrograph of a colon sectioned longitudinally. It shows a well-developed diverticulum (A) in an area of thickened tunica muscularis. An artery runs alongside the diverticular wall. A beginning (B) and a partially developed diverticulum (C) burrow into the tunica muscularis between the fascicles of circular muscle. No large blood vessels are seen in these areas. At D, penetrating vessels are present, but without diverticulum. The relationship between the site of diverticulum and vascular distribution is inconstant, depending, in part, on the sampling of the tissue. ($\times$ 7)

haustral pattern,[71] and a prediverticular shape,[72] is commonly encountered in colonic diverticulosis. The last term was applied because the abnormality was also seen in colons without diverticula, presumably a precursor of diverticulosis. These terms describe the shortened and distorted appearance of the sigmoid colon, with prominent saccules separated by thick folds of colonic wall.[60] The cause of the deformity was thought to be inflammation and fibrosis.[69] Pathologic examination of the surgically resected as well as postmortem specimens by Morson[73,74] and us[60] revealed that inflammation and fibrosis were absent or mild in many cases. Instead, the deformity is caused by shortened longitudinal taeniae, which become thick and hard, with a cartilage-like consistency. Shortening of the taeniae causes the sigmoid colon to take on a concertina-like appearance, with bunched folds made of redundant mucosa and circular muscle layer (Figures 30–4 and 30–5). The folds narrow the lumen, causing obstruction in some cases and subsequent dilatation of colon proximal to it. Removal of the shortened taeniae restores the colon to the normal length and contour.[60] It was in these taeniae that Whitney and Morson found elastosis.[66,67] Elastosis is the probable cause of muscle shortening, not spasm, as suggested by the contracted appearance of the muscle, because the muscle changes are not related to the motility of the colon.[68]

The circular muscle is divided into small bands, the fasciculi,[60,74] between which the penetrating blood vessels reside (see Figure 30–1). It is not as markedly affected as the longitudinal taeniae. In the markedly contracted colon, the circular muscle is thickened, but the individual fiber does not appear hypertrophic.

The contracted state of the colon and the shortened taeniae suggest that the colon is in a state of spasm. The abdominal pain and constipation experienced by patients with spastic colon or irritable bowel syndrome are also major complaints of patients with colonic diverticular disease. It was therefore postulated that spastic colon was related to diverticulosis.[60,75] The development of colonic diverticulosis in two infants with total colonic aganglionosis has been explained on the basis of spasm.[76] Muscle relaxants may alleviate the symptoms in patients with diverticula.[77] Recent studies, however, indicate that the irritable bowel syndrome and diverticular disease may not be related,[78,79]

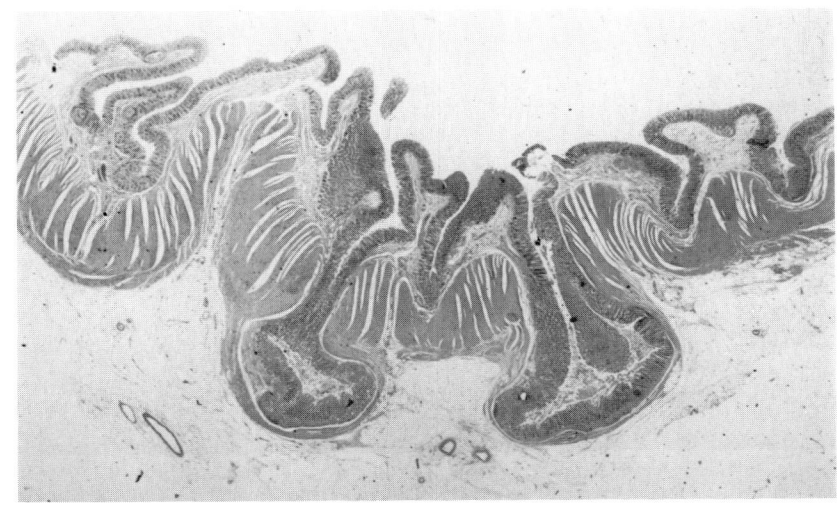

FIGURE 30–3. Photomicrograph of a longitudinal section of a resected colon, showing two well-developed diverticula and the beginning of one at the right margin. The patient had a documented episode of perforation of a diverticulum 6 months earlier. The section shows only mild peridiverticular fibrosis. The diverticula are flask-shaped. Their necks are narrow and surrounded by circular muscle. The colon was shortened, and the mucosa was thrown into many redundant folds. ($\times$ 7) (From Ming SC, Fleischner FG: Diverticulitis of the sigmoid colon: Reappraisal of the pathology and pathogenesis. Surgery 58:627–633, 1965.)

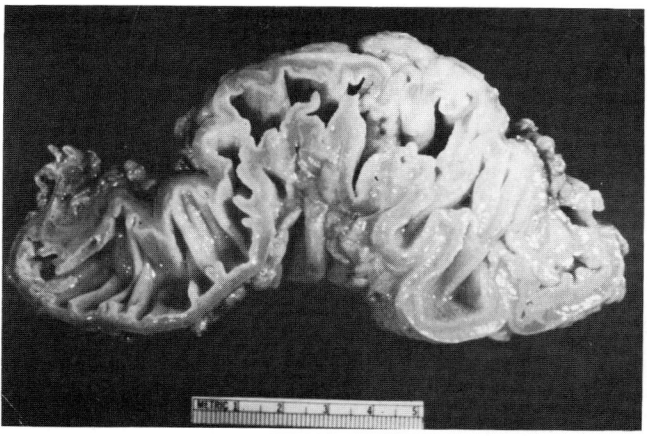

FIGURE 30–4. The longitudinal cut surface of a markedly contracted sigmoid colon, resected because of obstruction. The colon is markedly contracted, and the lumen is narrowed by folds of thick muscle and redundant mucosa. A few diverticula (not shown) were present. (From Ming SC, Fleischner FG: Diverticulitis of the sigmoid colon: Reappraisal of the pathology and pathogenesis. Surgery 58:627–633, 1965.)

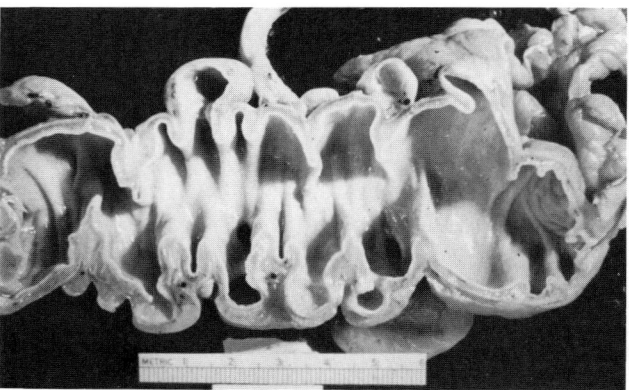

FIGURE 30–5. This longitudinally hemisectioned postmortem colon was fixed in a distended state by perfusing the lumen with formalin. Diverticula are present in the corrugated segment.

because they show different frequencies of myoelectric activity, predominantly 3 to 6 cycles per minute in the irritable bowel syndrome and 12 to 18 cycles per minute in diverticular disease. Clinically, patients with diverticular disease are usually old and have a short history of symptoms, whereas patients with the irritable bowel syndrome are young and usually have a long history of symptoms. The intraluminal pressure is increased in diverticular disease but not in irritable bowel syndrome.[80]

Intraluminal Pressure

The intraluminal pressure has been found to be increased in the sigmoid colon with diverticula.[81,82] The pressure recordings from adjacent areas of the colon show that the waves are independent of each other, implying that the pressure generated in one area is not always transmitted to the adjacent areas.[83] Painter showed that in diverticulosis there was increased segmentation of colonic activity.[84] The segmented colon was seen as a series of "little bladders" with obstruction at both ends by the contracting rings. The increased pressure generated by muscular contraction within the segment forced herniation of mucosa through the wall to form a diverticulum.[1] This sequence of events implies that muscle contraction is the cause of both segmentation and mucosal herniation. Subsequent studies by others, however, showed no relation between increased motility and diverticulosis, although the high pressure activity was related to the colicky pain experienced by patients with diverticular disease.[85] Furthermore, patients with asymptomatic diverticulosis have normal motility in the colon.[86]

Dietary Fiber

Epidemiologic data suggest that colonic diverticulosis is related to deficient fiber consumption.[1] Painter and Burkitt[87] postulated that a fiber-rich diet would increase the volume of feces and therefore the diameter of the colon. A wider colon would have lower pressure and less segmentation than a narrower colon, hence less diverticulosis. The low incidence of colonic diverticula in Africans was also related to the observation that the food residue stayed in the African's gut for a shorter period, allowing less time for absorption of water than the Westerner's. Therefore, the feces in the latter was drier and generated higher intraluminal pressure, thereby favoring the development of diverticula. This hypothesis was supported by the observation of Gear[88] that diverticulosis was three times more frequent in the nonvegetarians consuming an average of 21.4 gm of fiber per day than the vegetarians consuming an average of 41.5 gm of fiber per day. On the other hand, Eastwood et al.[89] found no difference in stool weight, transit time, or intraluminal pressure in individuals with and those without diverticulosis.

Supplementary bran fiber absorbs water and increases the volume and moisture of the stool, thus reducing the intraluminal pressure and spontaneous motility of the colon,[90] and has therefore been used to treat diverticular disease and has been found to reduce its symptoms.[91] Hyland and Taylor[92] treated 75 patients with acute complications of diverticular disease with a high-fiber diet. Ninety percent of them remained symptom-free for a period of 5 to 7 years.

Other Factors

Genetic influence has been implicated in a report of severe sigmoid diverticulitis in a pair of identical twins in their third decade[93] and in another report of colonic diverticula in three siblings in Nigeria,[94] where the incidence of the disease is low. These occurrences, however, are very rare.

Flynn and associates reported the possible effect of fecal bile acid.[95] Both fecal lithocholic and deoxycholic acids were lower in patients with colonic diverticula than in controls. Significant positive correlation was found between lithocholic acid concentration and myoelectric activity of 12 to 18 cycles per minute and between deoxycholic acid concentration and activity of 9 cycles per minute. It was suggested that in diverticulosis there was increased absorption of bile acids, causing alteration of myoelectric activity.

In summary, the formation of colonic diverticula follows the following sequence of events: biophysical alterations in the colonic wall of the aged person result in a reduction of tensile strength of the tissue and contraction and shortening of taeniae, particularly in the sigmoid. These changes in turn cause exaggerated haustration and redundant mucosal folds, narrowing the lumen. A low-fiber diet produces a small, dry fecal mass and generates an increase in intraluminal pressure. Elevated pressure in a narrowed segment of the colon forces herniation of mucosa through the weak point of the colonic wall to form a diverticulum.

PATHOLOGY

The etiologic factors discussed above contribute significantly to the morphologic appearance of diverticula of the colon as well as to the clinical presentation and the natural course of the disease.

Handling of Gross Specimens

The colon may be fixed in formalin before opening. In order to keep the diverticula distended, the colon should be filled with formalin under slight pressure and then immersed in a pail of formalin overnight. This treatment is suitable for a postmortem colon or a resected specimen that is not deformed by a muscle abnormality or an inflammatory process. Fixation will harden the tissue and make it difficult to identify all of the diverticula and to pinpoint the bleeding or perforated lesion. For such purposes it is better to examine the fresh specimen in detail, identify the diverticula by probing, fill them with cotton balls to maintain the shape, mark the diseased foci, and then fix the specimen in formalin for later sectioning for microscopic examination.

Gross Features of Diverticulosis

The diverticula appear as dark green or brown, round or oval nodules 0.5 to 1 cm in diameter, arranged in a longitudinal row along the lateral borders of the mesenteric taenia (see Figure 30-1). The color is that of the feces showing through the thin wall of the diverticulum. If the diverticulum is empty and collapsed, it will not be readily recognized on external examination of the bowel. Viewed from the mucosal aspect, the openings of diverticula are depressed dimples, 3 to 5 mm in diameter, from which fecal materials can be pressed out. The presence of diverticula can be confirmed by probing. Occasionally, the diverticulum inverts back into the lumen of the colon and appears as a wrinkled polyp. It can be pushed back into its seat. In cases of suspected bleeding from a diverticulum, it is important to probe each diverticulum for the presence of blood in order to identify the source of the bleeding. Angiography may be helpful in locating the bleeding vessel.

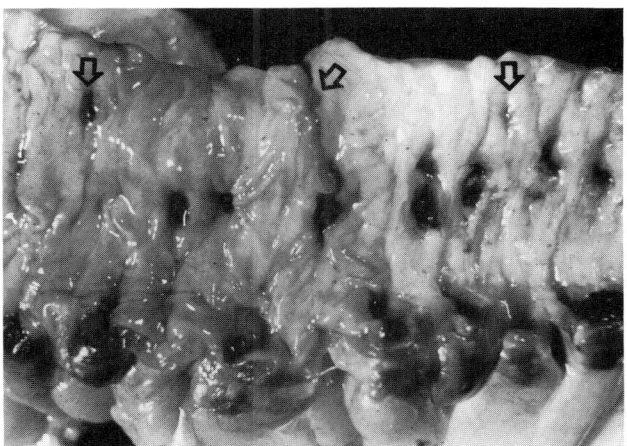

FIGURE 30-6. Luminal aspect of the colon shown in Figure 30-1. The colon was opened just above the lower row of diverticula shown in Figure 30-1. The upper row of diverticula is now in the middle of the colon, and the openings of three diverticula between the antimesenteric taeniae in the upper row (arrows). The redundant mucosa was stripped off. The openings of diverticula with fecal material within are clearly shown.

The gross features may be modified by the status of the tunica muscularis, the number of diverticula, and the amount of pericolic adipose tissue. Prominent mucosal folds in shortened, accordion-like colon, caused by either contraction of the taeniae or the presence of numerous diverticula, may obscure the openings of the diverticula. In this situation, removal of the mucosa will expose the openings and greatly facilitate the localization of diverticula (Figure 30-6). Externally, an excessive amount of mesocolic fat may cover up the diverticula. It is not unusual for the fat-covered diverticula to appear as appendices epiploicae.

Histologic Features of Diverticulosis

Basically, the diverticulum can be divided into two groups: true and false. A true diverticulum is a widemouthed pouch lined by a wall identical to that of the adjacent normal colon, including a full complement of muscular layer. It occurs most commonly as a single lesion in the cecum and ascending colon. The true diverticulum is a congenital anomaly, although the symptoms usually occur in late adult life.

Most diverticula of the colon are pseudodiverticula. They are shaped like a flask. The neck is surrounded by circular muscle. The wall consists of mucosa, muscularis mucosae, submucosa and, in some cases, a thin layer of longitudinal muscle (see Figure 30-3; Figure 30-7). The mucosa may appear normal or thinner than normal. At or near the apex, one or a few lymphoid nodules are often present. The lumen usually contains amorphous fecal material. The muscularis mucosae is thinner than that of the adjacent colon. When muscularis propria does not cover the apex, the submucosa of the diverticulum merges with the subserosal or meso-

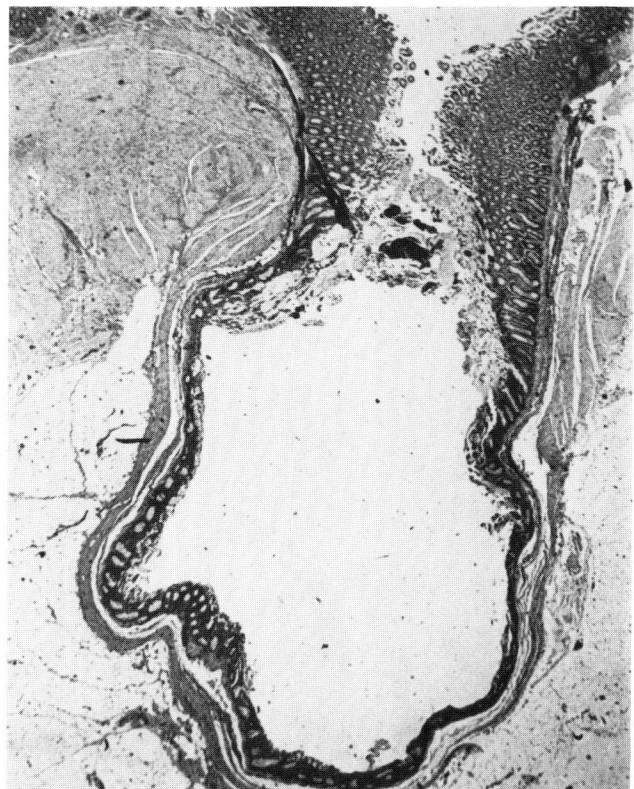

FIGURE 30–7. Photomicrograph of a simple diverticulum, showing a thin wall lined by atrophic mucosa, partial muscularis mucosae, and a thin layer of longitudinal muscle. (× 21)

colic adipose tissue, within which small and medium-sized blood vessels may be present. Occasionally, the diverticulum penetrates partially into the circular muscle layer, compressing the outer muscle fibers (see Figure 30–2). Such an early diverticulum probably corresponds to the transient diverticulum seen radiologically in 4.1% of patients with diverticula.[96]

Classification

On the basis of the gross and microscopic findings, diverticular disease of the colon can be classified as shown in Table 30–1. The specific pathologic characteristics of each category are described below.

Prediverticular State

The colon in prediverticular state is marked by the prominent muscle abnormalities described above, but without diverticula.[72,81] The disease affects principally the sigmoid colon. Externally the involved segment appears narrow, thickened, and shortened. The taeniae are thick and rigid. Between the taeniae the colon wall shows sacculation, with bulging segments alternating with circular depressions. On opening of the lumen, the depressions correspond to bunched-up muscle forming circular folds separating the contracted haustral sacs (see Figure 30–4). When the thick taeniae are trimmed off, the colon segment can be lengthened, and the sacculation disappears. This state is, therefore, created by the contraction of taeniae coli. The circular muscle is thickened only at a later stage. It is in this corrugated segment of colon that there is an increased intraluminal pressure resulting in the development of diverticula in the contracted haustral sacs. This sequence of events has been demonstrated by follow-up radiologic examinations for many years.[60,81] The chronology of these changes shows the contracted colon to be a prediverticular state.

Table 30–1 PATHOLOGIC CLASSIFICATIONS OF COLONIC DIVERTICULAR DISEASE

Prediverticular state
Simple diverticulosis
Simple massed diverticulosis
Diverticulosis with muscle abnormality (spastic diverticulosis)
Giant diverticulum
Diverticulitis
    Uncomplicated diverticulitis
    Complicated diverticulitis

Simple Diverticulosis

In simple diverticulosis, simple diverticula, described previously in the section on histologic features, are scattered along the colon of normal caliber and contour (Figure 30–8). The haustra are regularly spaced and have a smooth mucosal surface. The taeniae and circular muscle are normal.

Simple Massed Diverticulosis

The term *simple massed diverticulosis* is applied by Fleischner et al.[60] to the colon with numerous simple diverticula. The condition involves primarily the left colon. The colon is shortened because a large portion of the mucosa is consumed by diverticula. The colonic wall is wrinkled and shrunk. The resultant folds are close to each other and uniform in appearance. The taeniae and circular muscle are normal.

Diverticulosis with Muscle Abnormality (Spastic Diverticulosis)

The importance of the contracted state of the muscle layers of the colon in diverticulosis was recognized in 1910 by Keith,[97] who described contraction of taeniae causing the colon to assume the shape of a concertina and forcing the development of diverticula at the weak points of the muscular coat of the colon. His description fits well the pathology of spastic diverticulosis. The significance of muscle abnormality was emphasized also by Morson[73,74] and others.[60,98] We were so impressed by the contracted taeniae in sigmoid diverticulosis that the condition was given the name *spastic colon diverticulosis,* which implies a relationship with the spastic colon syndrome.[60] Although this relationship appears uncertain in view of their different clinical and myoelectric features, as discussed in the section on

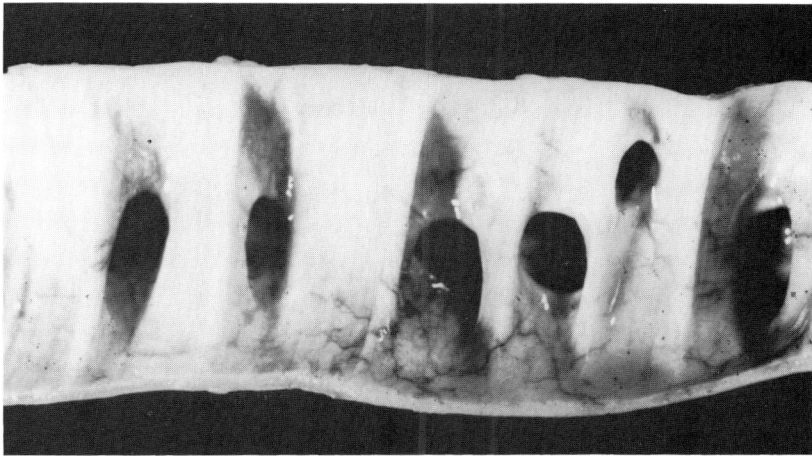

FIGURE 30–8. Hemisectioned strip of colon with simple diverticulosis, showing openings of diverticula in the haustral sacs. The wall of the colon is not thickened or deformed.

pathogenesis, spasm remains a significant factor in the development of this type of diverticulosis.

In spastic diverticulosis, the diverticula occur in the corrugated segment, usually close to the lateral borders of the thickened mesenteric taenia (Figures 30–9 to 30–11). The thickness of circular muscle is variable, shown best in the longitudinal section (Figure 30–12).

This type of diverticulosis is limited to the left colon, particularly the sigmoid, which is normally narrower and has thicker muscular tissue than the right colon. The effects of volume and consistency of the feces as related to dietary fiber intake are probably strongest in this region.

Giant Diverticula

Giant diverticula are large sacs measuring 6 to 27 cm in diameter.[99] Radiologically, they appear as persistent radiolucent "balloons."[100] They have also been described as air-filled cysts.[101,102] Fifty-two cases had been reported up to 1984.[103] They occur mostly in the sigmoid[101,104] and occasionally in the transverse colon.[104] McNutt and associates[105] described three types: (1) the gradually enlarged pseudodiverticulum, containing muscularis mucosae in the wall, but with the mucosal lining usually replaced by granulation tissue; (2) the diverticulum with focal perforation leading to abscess formation, with intermittent communication with the colon lumen, resulting in a large cavity filled with gas due to infection; and (3) the true diverticulum. Most reports described a granulation tissue–lined cavity possibly an infected diverticulum or a pseudocyst[101]; communication with the colonic lumen is present in 60% of cases.[105] The lesion may perforate the peritoneal cavity.[99,105] In one case, carcinoma was found in the diverticulum.[106]

Diverticulitis and Complications

Diverticulosis becomes a clinical entity when one or more diverticula are inflamed or the patient suffers abdominal pain, changes in bowel habits, or symptoms and signs of intra-abdominal infection. These symp-

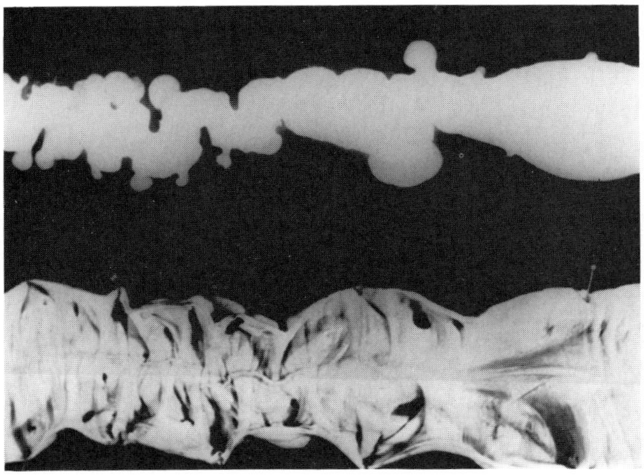

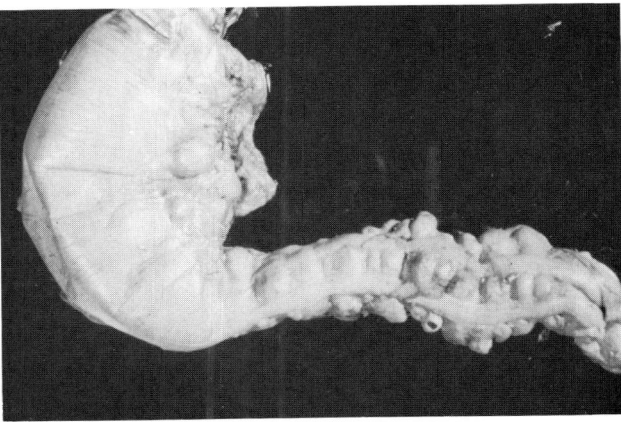

FIGURE 30–9. Radiograph (above) and the corresponding segment of a colon at postmortem examination (below), showing diverticula in the narrowed and corrugated area but not in the smooth area on the right.

FIGURE 30–10. Many diverticula in the narrowed portion on the right, where the taeniae are thickened and the intervening colonic wall is contracted and has many circular depressions corresponding to invaginating circular folds. The segment proximal to it is dilated, and the taeniae are inconspicuous. (From Fleischner FG, Ming SC, Henken EM: Revised concepts on diverticular disease of the colon. 1. Diverticulosis: Emphasis on tissue derangement and its relation to the irritable colon syndrome. Radiology 83:859–872, 1964.)

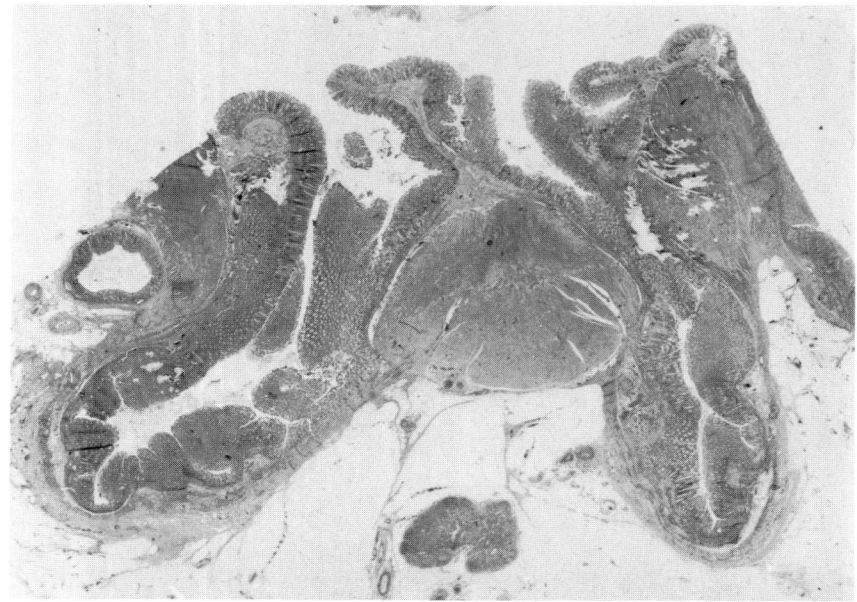

FIGURE 30–11. Photomicrograph of a cross section of a contracted segment of colon, showing two well-formed diverticula separated by the thickened mesenteric taenia. Redundant mucosal folds project into the lumen. ($\times$ 7)

toms occur in about 4% to 5% of all patients with diverticulosis or 20% of persons with diagnosed diverticulosis.[99] One quarter to one half of the patients are hospitalized, and 15% to 30% of the hospitalized patients are operated on.[107] Not all of the patients who undergo surgery are found to have pathologically confirmed diverticulitis, however.[73] In our own materials, 26% of surgical specimens resected for diverticulitis showed no inflammation but did show muscular distortion; 8% of specimens had localized inflammation limited to the diverticular wall; and 66% of specimens had severe peridiverticulitis, secondary to focal perforation of the diverticula.[108]

Pure acute diverticulitis, with inflammation limited to the diverticular wall (Figure 30–13), is uncommon in the resected specimens. It was found usually at or near the apex of a diverticulum.[73,108] The involved area is small, only a few millimeters in size. The mucosa is destroyed and replaced by acute inflammatory exudate. The muscularis mucosa is similarly affected. In some cases, the inflammation involves the submucosa and adjacent peridiverticular tissue. In three of seven such cases, there was erosion and rupture of small arteries in the involved submucosa, resulting in massive rectal bleeding requiring surgical resection of the colon.[108] The bleeding vessel was found only after every diverticulum in the specimen was examined microscopically.

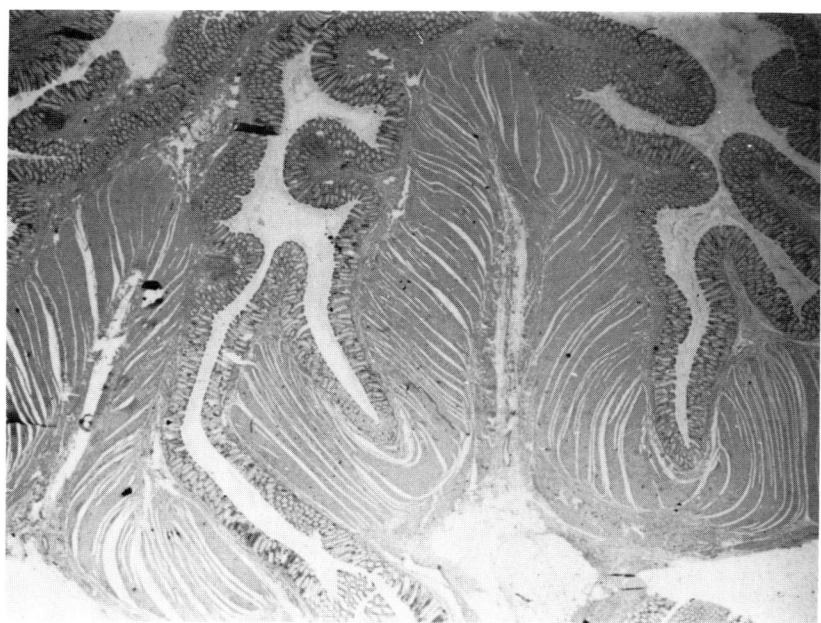

FIGURE 30–12. Photomicrograph of a longitudinal section of a markedly contracted sigmoid colon, showing thick, circular muscle, prominent mucosal folds, and three diverticula. ($\times$ 21)

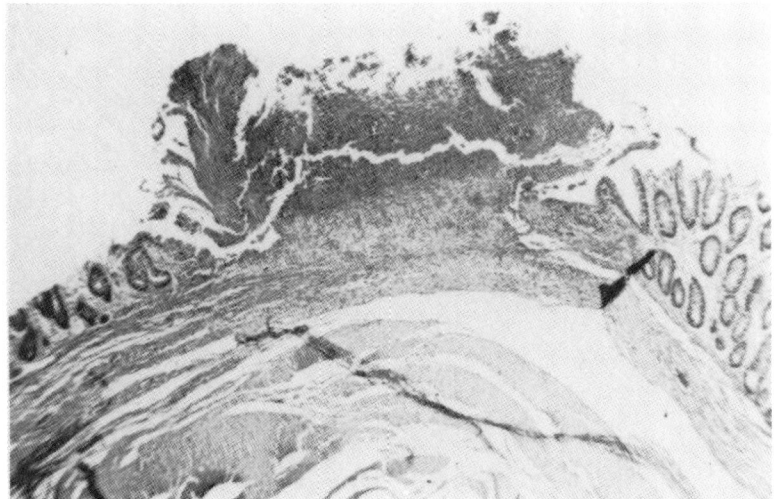

FIGURE 30–13. Acute diverticulitis with necrosis and inflammation involving the mucosa, muscularis mucosae, and adjacent submucosa. (× 35) (From Ming SC, Fleischner FG: Diverticulitis of the sigmoid colon: Reappraisal of the pathology and pathogenesis. Surgery 58:627–633, 1965.)

Minute foci of acute diverticulitis are probably quite common, but seldom documented, because they are not grossly visible and they may not cause symptoms. These small lesions may be readily healed, leaving no trace of inflammation or only slight fibrosis in the peridiverticular region, which is commonly seen in the surgical specimens.

Clinically manifest diverticulitis is in fact no longer pure diverticulitis, but complications of focal perforation (Figure 30–14) resulting in severe pericolitis (Figure 30–15), pericolic (Figure 30–16) or pelvic abscess, fistula formation involving pelvic organs, or free perforation to the peritoneum causing purulent or fecal peritonitis.[85,108,109] Histologic evidence of perforation of the diverticulum include foreign body granulomas containing food particles, fecal matter, or barium sulfate crystals (Figure 30–17). Such stigmas of perforation were present in 60% of resected specimens.[108] Radiologic evidence of perforation, such as extravasation of barium and free air in the peritoneal cavity, is readily demonstrated in the acute cases.[109] Occasionally, two or more diverticula are perforated, giving rise to the formation of intercommunicating or dissecting abscesses along the pericolic tissue[109] and double tracking of barium in radiologic examination.[110] A small perforation may heal, leaving a defect in the diverticular wall, accompanied by peridiverticular inflammation (Figure 30–18).

Marked pericolitis and abscess formation create an indurated mass (see Figures 30–14 and 30–15) that may compress and obstruct the bowel. Obstruction is encountered in 5% to 10% of complicated diverticula. The thickened wall may be erroneously interpreted as neoplastic. The accuracy of radiologic differentiation between a diverticular mass and carcinoma is only 50%, whereas the accuracy of diagnosing diverticula is 92%.[111]

The abscesses may rupture into other organs or the peritoneal cavity, producing fistulas, involving other organs in 2.4% to 20% of cases.[112,113] Among these cases, the colovesical fistula is most frequent, in 65% of patients, the colovaginal fistula in 25%, the coloenteric fistula in 6.5%, the colouterine fistula in 3%, and the colocutaneous fistula in 1%.[112] In one report, 35.6% of patients with diverticular disease had urinary tract symptoms, and 3.6% of patients had a colovesical fistula.[114] Uncommon sites of fistula formation include the hip joint,[115,116] the perineum, the scrotum, the buttock, the thigh, the lower extremity, the mediastinum,

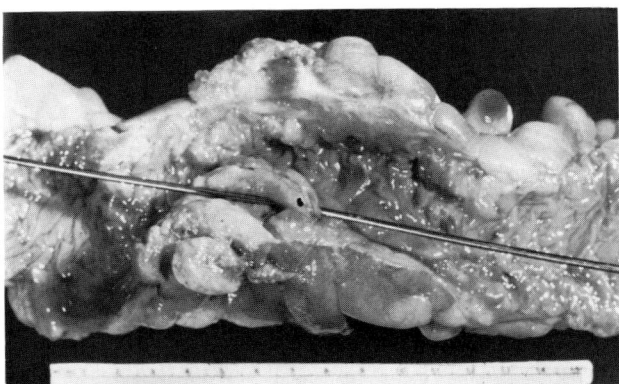

FIGURE 30–14. Opened colon, surgically resected for diverticulitis, showing a perforated diverticulum (with the probe through it) and a pericolic inflammatory mass compressing the lumen.

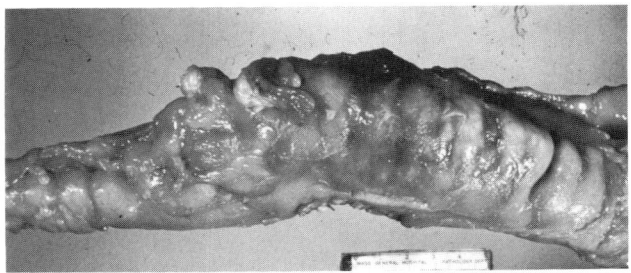

FIGURE 30–15. External view of a surgical specimen, showing markedly thickened pericolic tissue due to severe inflammation.

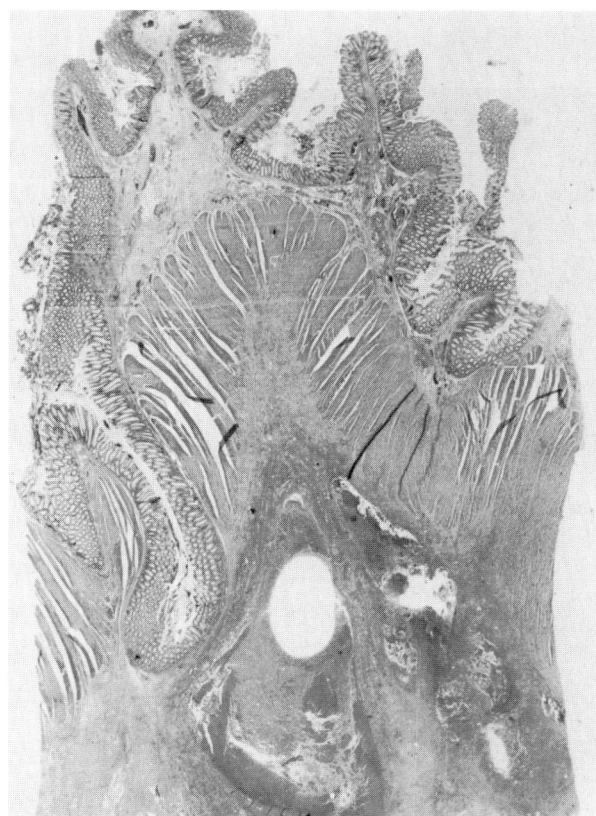

FIGURE 30–16. Photomicrograph of a colon with spastic diverticulosis, showing a pericolic abscess with gas bubbles (empty spaces) secondary to perforation of a diverticulum. (× 10)

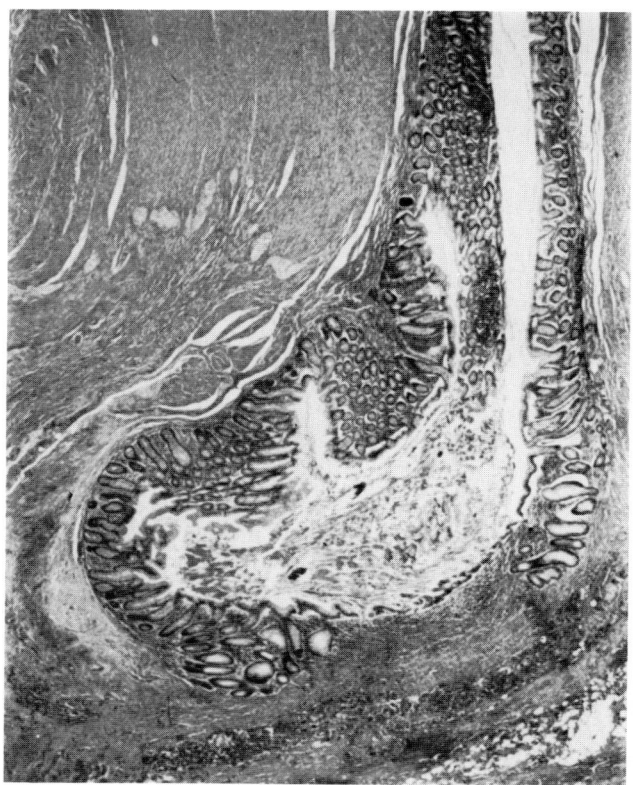

FIGURE 30–18. Photomicrograph of a perforated diverticulum, showing granulation tissue and regenerating surface epithelium at the site of perforation and severe chronic pericolitis. (× 30) (From Ming SC, Fleischner FG: Diverticulitis of the sigmoid colon: Reappraisal of the pathology and pathogenesis. Surgery 58:627–633, 1965.)

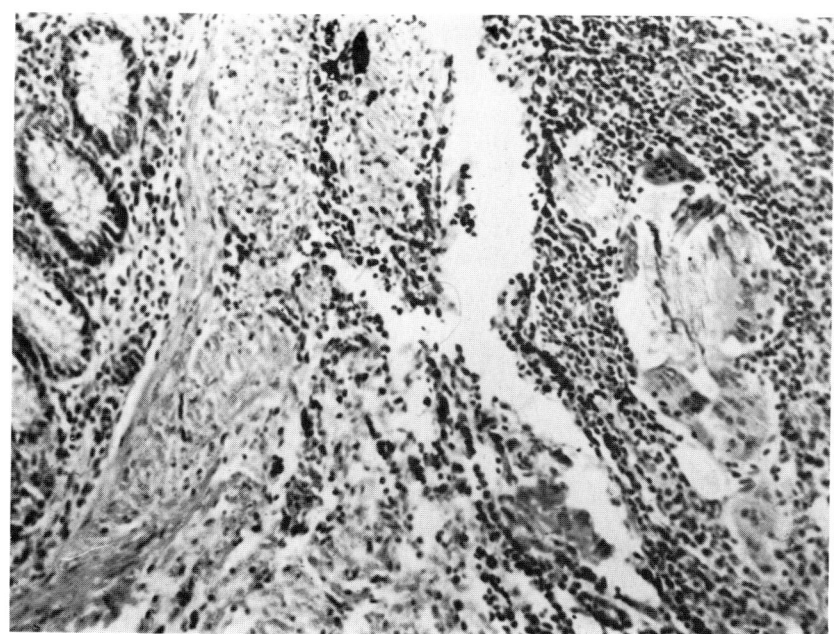

FIGURE 30–17. Photomicrograph of a colonic diverticulum, showing severe chronic inflammation and a foreign body granuloma containing vegetable fibers. (× 150)

Table 30–2 PATHOLOGIC STAGES OF COLONIC DIVERTICULITIS ACCORDING TO THE EXTENT OF INFLAMMATION

Stage 0: Diverticulitis confined to diverticular wall
Stage 1: Localized pericolitis and pericolic abscess, confined to peridiverticular tissue
Stage 2: Inflammation with abscess and fistula involving contiguous organs or tissue
Stage 3: Generalized peritonitis or sepsis involving distant organs
Stage 4: Fecal peritonitis

---

and the neck.[115] Sigmoid-appendiceal fistulas have also been reported.[117,118]

Free perforation is also common. Among 105 patients with diverticular sepsis operated on by Lambert et al.,[119] 73 had free peritonitis, 40 with communicating perforation and 33 with noncommunicating perforation. Intestinal obstruction was present in 9 patients, and a localized abscess or mass was present in 23 patients. In another report, 32 of 93 patients who underwent surgery had free perforation; obstruction was found in 14 and abscess in 11.[120] Mortality rate within 30 days was 10.8%. Rarely, the fistula perforates veins, causing pneumopylephlebitis and liver abscess.[121–124] Patients on steroid therapy for other diseases may develop perforation of colonic diverticula.[125] Hinchey et al.[126] classified the perforated cases into four stages. A modified staging system, including other inflammatory conditions, is shown in Table 30–2.

Diverticula of the Right Colon

The previous sections deal primarily with diverticula disease of the left colon, particularly the sigmoid. Diverticula of the right colon are different in several respects.

1. *Geographic distribution.* In Western countries colonic diverticula are found most frequently in the sigmoid colon[47,127–129]: the sigmoid only in 40% to 65%; the sigmoid and other areas in 20% to 35%; the entire colon in 7% to 16%; the right colon and cecum in 1% to 5%.[129–132] In Asians, including those living in Hawaii,[51–53,55,56] diverticula occur more frequently in the right colon. Of 979 cases of colonic diverticulosis reported by Kubo,[52] 76% were in the right colon.

2. *Type of diverticula.* Diverticula of the left colon are nearly all of the false type, whereas those in the right colon may be true or false. The false diverticula of the right colon resemble those of the left colon, being multiple and associated with high intraluminal pressure and abnormal motility.[133] They are accompanied by diverticula in the distal colon. The true diverticula are usually single or few and located mostly in the cecum. Wilkinson[134] reported a case of acute true diverticulitis in the transverse colon of a 13-year-old girl. The relative proportion of true diverticula varied in different reports. In one report, 70% of diverticula were of the true type.[135] In another report, only 2 of 16 diverticula were true.[136]

3. *Age of the patients.* Diverticula of the colon in general increase with age. The average age of patients was 63 years.[137] The average age of patients with diverticula of the right colon was 40 years,[41,138] with a range of 10 to 72 years.[135]

Cecal diverticulitis is rare. It was estimated that it constituted only 0.1% of all diverticular disease cases[139] and 1 in 40,000 laparotomies.[113] The congenital diverticulum is usually located on the anterior wall of the cecum, close to the ileocecal valve.[113,135] Acute cecal diverticulitis is misdiagnosed as acute appendicitis in 70% to 85% of cases.[135,138] The inflammatory mass may also be mistaken for a malignant tumor,[140–142] even at operation. Bleeding is the presenting symptom in some patients.[143] Free perforation occurs only rarely.[144] Computed tomography complements barium enema in the correct diagnosis of cecal diverticulosis.[145]

CLINICOPATHOLOGIC CORRELATION

Clinical Features

Diverticular disease of the colon is a disease of the aged. Its incidence increases progressively with age. According to Parks,[107] two thirds of patients at age 85 had diverticula by barium enema examination. Similar findings were noted by Rodkey and Welch.[137] Among patients with colonic diverticula, only 0.6% were under the age of 30 and 4.8% under the age of 40.[107] These observations coincide with the age-related decline in tensile strength and elasticity of colonic wall[68] and changes in the muscle of the colon.[66,73] There is an equal sex distribution. A slightly higher incidence of diverticular disease in females in some reports is unexplained.[107]

Symptoms of abdominal pain and the radiologic and sigmoidoscopic appearance of a narrowed and deformed colon segment could indicate either the prediverticular state with muscle abnormalities or pericolic inflammation. Pure diverticulitis with inflammation limited to the diverticular wall may be common, as suggested by the common observation of mild chronic inflammation and fibrosis in the peridiverticular region; but it is largely asymptomatic. Computed tomography gives better diagnostic results than contrast enema for the extent of inflammatory sequelae and extracolic abnormalities.[146–149] Sonography provides additional diagnostic accuracy for the recognition of inflamed pericolic tissue, which appears as a hypoechoic area.[150,151]

Diverticular disease of the colon may cause serious complications requiring surgical intervention. Orebaugh et al.[152] reported that recurrent diverticulitis was the most common indication for operation in 35% of cases; hemorrhage, in 25%; perforation, in 22%; suspicion of carcinoma, in 17%; obstruction, in 16%; fistula, in 10%; and more than one complication, in 25%. In a more recent report by Alexander et al.,[153] 14% of 673 patients with diverticular disease underwent surgery. Of 93 cases, the indication for operation was abscess in 36, bleeding in 18, perforation in 10, obstruction in 10, fistula in 5, recurrent symptoms in 7, and suspicion of cancer in 8. The problem is particularly grave in immunocompromised patients, who respond poorly to medical treatment and usually require operation.[154] Freischlag et al.[155] reported that patients younger than 40 years developed more severe complications. Eighty-eight percent of their patients required emergency surgery. A similar finding was reported by Ouriel and Schwartz.[156]

Some patients developed extraintestinal manifestations. Klein et al.[157] reported three patients with arthritis and pyoderma gangrenosum, which resolved after resection of the involved colon. In one patient, retroperitoneal fibrosis developed.[158]

Complicated Diverticulitis with Perforation

Limited diverticulitis is not significant until it is complicated by perforation. The abnormalities shown better by computed tomography and sonography than by contrast enema are extracolic manifestations of the perforated diverticulum. A small perforation causes pericolic abscess, from which a fistulous tract may form and extend into other organs. For proper management of patients suffering from these complications, the staging system according to the extent of extracolic infection by Hinchey et al.[126] (similar to that in Table 30-2) has been useful. Of 116 patients treated by Auguste et al.,[159] 21% were in stage 1, 35% in stage 2, 35% in stage 3, and 9% in stage 4. Primary resection with anastomosis is preferred for stages 1 and 2, but diseased-end colostomy with Hartmann's procedure (closure of the distal segment) is the treatment of choice for stages 3 and 4.[160] The primary resection has lower mortality (12% versus 20%), requires a shorter hospital stay (36 days versus 52 days), and causes a shorter duration of disability (81 days versus 148 days) than the staged resection.[159] A recurrence of diverticulitis had been reported in 30% to 40% of patients.[107] In a report by Larson,[161] three fourths of the patients required no further treatment after an average follow-up period of 9 years.

Hemorrhage

Rectal hemorrhage occurs in 10% to 30% of patients with diverticular disease, severely in 3% to 5%.[99] The bleeding stops spontaneously in 80% of cases but recurs in 20% to 25% of cases. It was said[99,162,163] that the source of bleeding was in the right colon in up to 70% of cases, "even if diverticula are seen only in the sigmoid colon."[163] This long-held view was clearly exaggerated, because this incidence equals or exceeds the incidence of right-sided colonic diverticula. The diverticula are found more often in the right than left colon in Japan. Bleeding occurred in only 3.9% of 1124 Japanese patients reported by Kubo et al.,[164] mostly in elderly patients with multiple diverticula in the left colon.

Another frequently stated belief, that most of the bleeding diverticulum is not inflamed, also requires qualification. Minor bleeding from granulation tissue is common in diverticulitis. Massive bleeding, on the other hand, is the result of erosion of an artery. Such a thick-walled vessel will not bleed without injury. In either situation, the precise location of the bleeding vessel is rarely demonstrated. The damaged artery is difficult to identify because it is usually not accompanied by overt, grossly evident inflammation to mark its location. It may be found only after a meticulous search in the pathologic specimen. When it is found, it is in an area of active inflammation (Figure 30-19). In our materials, the bleeding artery was identified in three resected colons only when every diverticulum was subjected to microscopic examination.[108] Rosenberg and Rosenberg[165] found the offending artery by serial sectioning of the tissue from the suspicious area.[165] Meyers et al.[166] noted the consistent finding of arterial changes in the diverticula, including eccentric intimal thickening, thinning of the media, and duplication of internal elastic lamina. These changes are commonly seen in an area of chronic inflammation, such as the base of a peptic ulcer. They are nonspecific but indicate past or continuing tissue injury. These arteries are not the source of bleeding in most instances.

Tedesco et al.[167] noted that 20% of distal intestinal bleeding occurred in patients with diverticular disease, but in 40% of these patients, the bleeding source was other than diverticulum. In the left colon, polyps, neoplasms, and other inflammatory conditions may coexist with diverticula and be the source of bleeding. In the right colon, angiodysplasia (also called arteriovenous malformation and vascular ectasia) is a recognized major source of colonic bleeding in older persons.[168-171] This condition is discussed in Chapter 12. The abnormal vessels are mostly dilated veins and capillaries located primarily in the submucosa and, in some cases, also in the mucosa. These vessels bleed easily because the walls are thin and their superficial location subject them to easy trauma. The bleeding can be successfully treated by endoscopic fulguration.[172,173] Compression by the tunica muscularis on the veins has been postulated as a possible cause of this condition in the colon.[169] They often coexist with diverticula.[172] Bleeding from angiodysplasia may have been mistaken for bleeding diverticular disease in the past.

The location of bleeding vessel in diverticular disease can be identified by angiography and radionuclide scintigraphy.[90,130,174,175] These techniques make surgical resection of only the involved segment of colon possi-

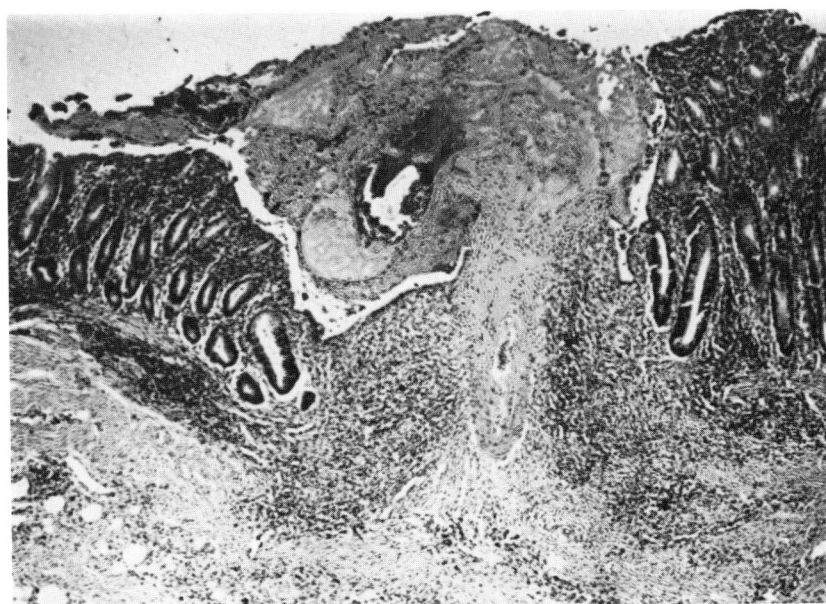

FIGURE 30-19. Photomicrograph of a bleeding diverticulum, showing a thrombus covering a partially necrotic artery in an area of severe inflammation. ($\times 70$)

ble, instead of total colectomy, as sometimes practiced in the past. They also help the pathologist to limit the search for the responsible vessel to a likely area.

Obstruction

Obstruction in diverticular disease of the colon can be due to muscle thickening and mucosal folds in the prediverticular state and uncomplicated diverticulosis. In diverticulitis, a large inflammatory mass, often with an abscess within it, may compress the lumen, sometimes circumferentially.[109] Obstruction is noted in about 10% of cases.[148,152,153] It is an important indication for surgical intervention, partly because an obstructive lesion may mimic carcinoma.

Coexisting Colonic Conditions

Carcinoma

There is no evidence that diverticular disease predisposes the colon to malignant transformation. However, the development of colonic carcinoma is related to dietary fiber deficiency (see Chapter 32 for details), as is the development of diverticular disease of the colon. It may be expected, therefore, that there may be an increased incidence of one condition when the other is present. In reality, the incidence of carcinoma in colons with diverticula and the incidence of diverticula in colons with carcinoma are the same as those in the control population: about 6% to 10% by colonoscopy in the former situation[176-179] and 39% by barium enema examination in the latter situation.[180] However, rare cases of carcinoma developing in a diverticulum have been reported.[180,181] In one case, a mucinous carcinoid was found in a rectosigmoid diverticulum.[182] The incidence of adenoma in the colon with diverticulosis was 27%, the same as that in the controls in one report[178] and twice that in the controls in another report.[177] The carcinoma may invade a coexisting diverticulum.[108] More importantly, it is often difficult to differentiate an inflammatory mass from a carcinoma, even during operation. In this situation, perioperative fine-needle aspiration biopsy has been found helpful.[183]

Inflammatory Bowel Diseases

Ulcerative colitis has bimodal development. Older persons may have coexisting diverticula. Such occurrences are uncommon. Jalan et al.[184] found 23 such cases in 399 ulcerative colitis patients. The typical mucosal lesions of ulcerative colitis are readily recognized. Crohn's disease of colon is more commonly associated with diverticular disease.[113] It is more difficult to differentiate these conditions radiologically because both are segmental, in both there may be a thickened colon wall and pericolic inflammation, and in both there may be fistulas. Marshak[185] outlined the major radiologic differences between them, which are applicable also to pathologic examination. Mainly, diverticular disease involves a shorter segment, a shorter fistulous tract, and a more localized lesion than Crohn's disease. Anal lesions, commonly seen in Crohn's disease, are absent in diverticular disease. Further discussions are provided in chapter 27.

Ischemic Colon Disease

The ischemic changes of the colon are characterized by coagulative necrosis of the mucosa and marked submucosal edema in the acute phase and cicatricial stricture in the chronic cases (see Chapter 12 for details). The splenic flexure of the colon is the favored site for ischemic changes. These lesions may be superimposed on the diverticular disease.

Associated Extracolonic Conditions

The patients with diverticular disease of the colon may have an increased incidence of other conditions. Saint's triad, with colonic diverticulosis, hiatal hernia, and gallstones, has been periodically reported since 1948.[186,187] Burkitt and Walker considered the triad to be manifestations of fiber deficiency.[186] Scaggion et al.[187] found 7 cases among 684 patients by barium examination. Eighty-six additional patients had two of the triad. In another report, cholelithiasis was present in 45% of patients with and in 22% of patients without colonic diverticula.[188] Other reported conditions, in addition to those mentioned in the section on etiology, included polycystic disease of the kidney,[189] ischemic heart disease,[190] and varicose veins.[191] There were reports of diverticulitis developing in patients in chronic renal failure[192] and following cardiac or other surgical procedures.[193,194] The reason for these associations is unknown.

References

1. Painter NS, Burkitt DP: Diverticular disease of the colon: A deficiency disease of Western civilization. Br Med J 2:450–454, 1971.
2. Wheeler D: Diverticula of foregut. Radiology 49:476–482, 1947.
3. Lahey FH: Pharyngoesophageal diverticulum: Its management and complications. Ann Surg 134:617–652, 1946.
4. Gage-Whote L: Incidence of Zenker's diverticulum with hiatus hernia. Larygnoscope 98:526–530, 1988.
5. Allen TH, Clagett OT: Changing concepts in the surgical treatment of pulsion diverticula of the lower esophagus. J Thorac Cardiovasc Surg 50:455–462, 1965.
6. Rasmussen PC, Jensen BS, Winther A: Oesophageal achalasia combined with epiphrenic diverticulum: A case report. Scand J Thorac Cardiovasc Surg 22:81–82, 1988.
7. Toyohara T, Kaneko T, Araki H, et al: Giant epiphrenic diverticulum in a boy with Ehlers-Danlos syndrome. Pediatr Radiol 19:437, 1989.
8. Hendren WG, Anderson T, Miller JI: Massive bleeding in a Zenker's diverticulum. South Med J 83:362, 1990.
9. Pierce WS, Johnson J: Squamous cell carcinoma in a pharyngoesophageal diverticulum. Cancer 24:1068–1070, 1969.
10. Wychulis AR, Gunnlaugsson GH, Claggett OT: Carcinoma occurring in pharyngoesophageal diverticulum: Report of three cases. Surgery 66:976–979, 1969.
11. Zitsch RP, O'Brien CJ, Maddox WA: Pharyngoesophageal diverticulum complicated by squamous cell carcinoma. Head Neck Surg 9:290–294, 1987.
12. Graham DY, Goyal RK, Sparkman J, et al: Diffuse intramural esophageal diverticulosis. Gastroenterology 68:781–785, 1975.
13. Watarai N, Kataoka M, Taniwaki S, Masaoka A: A rare type of intramural esophageal diverticulosis. Am J Gastroenterol 85:733–736, 1990.
14. Umlas J, Sakhuja R: The pathology of esophageal intramural pseudodiverticulosis. Am J Clin Pathol 65:314–320, 1976.
15. Medeiros LJ, Doos WG, Balogh K: Esophageal intramural pseudodiverticulosis: a report of two cases with analysis of similar, less extensive changes in "normal" autopsy esophagi. Hum Pathol 19:928–931, 1988.
16. Castillo S, Aburashed A, Kimmelman J, et al: Diffuse intramural esophageal pseudodiverticulosis: New cases and review. Gastroenterology 72:541–545, 1977.
17. Eells RW, Simril WA: Gastric diverticula: Report of thirty-one cases. AJR 68:8–14, 1952.
18. Eras P, Beranbaum SL: Gastric diverticula: Congenital and acquired. Am J Gastroenterol 57:120–132, 1972.
19. Palmer ED: Gastric diverticula. Int Abstr Surg 92:417–428, 1951.
20. Benhamou PH, Lenaerts C, Carnarelli JP, et al: Diverticulum of the stomach in children: Apropos of a case of congenital diverticulum. Ann Pediatr 36:467–478, 1989.
21. Gibbons CP, Harvey L: An ulcerated gastric diverticulum—a rare cause of haematemesis and melaena. Postgrad Med J 60:693–695, 1984.
22. Cockrell CH, Cho SR, Messmer JM, et al: Intramural gastric diverticula: A report of three cases. Br J Radiol 57:285–288, 1984.
23. Localio A, Stahl WM: Diverticular disease of the alimentary tract Part II: The esophagus, stomach, duodenum and small intestine. Curr Probl Surg 5:1–47, 1968.
24. Mackey WC, Dineen P: A fifty year experience with Meckel's diverticulum. Surg Gynecol Obstet 156:56–64, 1983.
25. Soderlund S: Meckel's diverticulum: A clinical and histologic study. Acta Chir Scand [Suppl] 248:1–233, 1959.
26. Artigas V, Calabuig R, Badia F, et al: Meckel's diverticulum: value of ectopic tissue. Am J Surg 151:631–634, 1986.
27. Moyana TN: Carcinoid tumors arising from Meckel's diverticulum: A clinical, morphologic, and immunohistochemical study. Am J Clin Pathol 91:52–56, 1989.
28. Niv Y, Abu-Avid S, Kopelman C, Oren M: Torsion of leiomyosarcoma of Meckel's diverticulum. Am J Gastroenterol 81:228–291, 1986.
29. Bloch T, Tejada E, Brodhecker C: Malignant melanoma in Meckel's diverticulum. Am J Clin Pathol 86:231–234, 1986.
30. Landor JH, Fulkerson CC: Duodenal diverticula. Arch Surg 93:182–188, 1966.
31. Juler JL, List JW, Stemmer EA, Connolly JE: Duodenal diverticulitis. Arch Surg 99:572–578, 1969.
32. Sheldon WC: Gastrointestinal hemorrhage from duodenal diverticulum. Am J Dig Dis 4:817–821, 1959.
33. Abdel-Hafiz AA, Birkett DH, Ahmed MS: Congenital duodenal diverticula: A report of three cases and a review of the literature. Surgery 104:74–78, 1988.
34. Soreide JA, Seime S, Soreide O: Intraluminal duodenal diverticulum: Case report and update of the literature 1975–1986. Am J Gastrotenterol 83:988–991, 1988.
35. Adams DB: Management of the intraluminal duodenal diverticulum: Endoscopy or duodenotomy? Am J Surg 151:524–526, 1986.
36. Nobles ER Jr: Jejunal diverticula. Arch Surg 102:172–174, 1971.
37. Hoover EL, Webb H, Walker C, Weaver WL: Perforated jejunal diverticulum with multiple hepatic abscesses. South Med J 83:54–56, 1990.
38. Wilcox RD, Shatney CH: Massive rectal bleeding from jejunal diverticula. Surg Gynecol Obstet 165:425–428, 1987.
39. Brinkman JH: Megaloblastic anemia associated with jejunal diverticula. J Iowa Med Soc 56:135–137, 1966.
40. Cooke WT, Cox EV, Fone DJ, et al: The clinical and metabolic significance of jejunal diverticula. Gut 4:115–131, 1963.
41. Localio A, Stahl WM: Diverticular disease of the alimentary tract. Part I: The colon. Curr Probl Surg 4:1–78, 1967.
42. Cruveilhier J: Traite d'Anatomie Pathologique Generale. Paris, 1849, p 592. Quoted in reference 41.
43. Gross S: Elements of pathological anatomy. Philadelphia, Blanchard and Lea, 1845, p 554. Quoted in reference 1.
44. Graser E: Das falsche darm divitkel. Arch Klin Chir 59:638, 1899. Quoted in reference 41.
45. Beer E: Some pathological and clinical aspects of acquired (false) diverticula of the intestine. Am J Med Sci 128:135, 1904. Quoted in reference 41.
46. Hartwell JA, Cecil RL: Intestinal diverticula: A pathological and clinical study. Am J Med Sci 140:174–203, 1910.
47. Hughes LE: Postmortem survey of diverticular disease of the colon. I. Diverticulosis and diverticulitis. II. The muscular abnormality in the sigmoid colon. Gut 10:336–351, 1969.

48. Kyle J, Adesola AD, Tinckler LF, de Beaux, J: Incidence of diverticulitis. Scand J Gastroenterol 2:77–80, 1967.
49. Segal I, Solomon A, Hunt JA: Emergence of diverticular disease in the urban South African black. Gastroenterology 72:215–219, 1977.
50. Kochhar R, Goenka MK, Nagi B, et al: The emergence of colonic diverticulosis in urbanised Indians: A report of 23 cases. Trop Geograph Med 41:254–256, 1989.
51. Narasaka T, Watanabe H, Yamagat S, et al: Statistical analysis of diverticulosis of the colon. Tohoku J Exp Med 115:271–275, 1975.
52. Kubo A, Ishiwata J, Maeda Y, et al: Clinical studies on diverticular disease of the colon. Jpn J Med 22:185–189, 1983.
53. Coode PE, Chan KW, Chan YT: Polyps and diverticula of the large intestine: A necropsy survey in Hong Kong. Gut 26:1045–1048, 1985.
54. Levy N, Stermer E, Simon J: The changing epidemiology of diverticular disease in Israel. Dis Colon Rectum 28:416–418, 1985.
55. Vajrabukka T, Saksornchai K, Jimakorn P: Diverticular disease of the colon in a far-eastern community. Dis Colon Rectum 23:151–154, 1980.
56. Sugihara K, Muto T, Morioka Y, et al: Diverticular disease of the colon in Japan: A review of 615 cases. Dis Colon Rectum 27:531–537, 1984.
57. Zollinger RW, Zollinger RM: Diverticular disease of the colon. Adv Surg 5:255–280, 1971.
58. Slack WW: The anatomy, pathology, and some clinical features of diverticulitis of the colon. Br J Surg 50:185–190, 1962.
59. Noer RJ: Hemorrhage as a complication of diverticulitis. Ann Surg 141:674–685, 1955.
60. Fleischner FG, Ming SC, Henken EM: Revised concepts on diverticular disease of the colon. 1. Diverticulosis: Emphasis on tissue derangement and its relation to the irritable colon syndrome. Radiology 83:859–872, 1964.
61. Watt J, Marcus R: The pathology of diverticulosis of the antimesenteric intertaenial area of the pelvic colon. J Pathol Bacteriol 88:97–105, 1964.
62. Heinz ER, Steinberg AJ, Sackner MA: Roentgenographic and pathologic aspects of intestinal scleroderma. Ann Intern Med 59:822–826, 1983.
63. Mielke JE, Becker KL, Gross JB: Diverticulitis of the colon in a young man with Marfan's syndrome. Gastroenterology 48:379–382, 1965.
64. Cook JM: Spontaneous perforation of the colon: Report of two cases in a family exhibiting Marfan stigmata. Ohio Med J 64:73, 1968.
65. Thomson HJ, Busuttil A, Eastwood MA, et al: Submucosal collagen changes in the normal colon and in diverticular disease. Int J Colorect Dis 2:208–213, 1987.
66. Whiteway J, Morson BC: Elastosis in diverticular disease of the sigmoid colon. Gut 26:258–266, 1985.
67. Whiteway J, Morson BC: Pathology of the ageing: Diverticular disease. Clin Gastroenterol 14:829–846, 1985.
68. Watters DA, Smith AN: Strength of the colon wall in diverticular disease. Br J Surg 77:257–259, 1990.
69. George AW, Leonard RD: Use of x-ray in study of multiple diverticulitis of the colon. Med Clin North Am 2:1503–1540, 1919.
70. Shanks SC, Kerley P: A textbook of X-ray diagnosis, 3rd ed. Vol 3. Philadelphia, WB Saunders, 1959, p 426.
71. Wolf BS, Khilnani M, Marshak RH: Diverticulosis and diverticulitis: Roentgen findings and their interpretation. AJR 77:726–743, 1957.
72. Spriggs EI, Marxer OA: Multiple diverticula of the colon. Lancet 1:1067–1074, 1927.
73. Morson BC: The muscle abnormality in diverticular disease of Sigmoid colon. Br J Radiol 36:385–392, 1963.
74. Morson BC: Pathology of diverticular disease of the colon. Clin Gastroenterol 4:37–52, 1975.
75. Ryle JA: Chronic sporadic affection of the colon and the disease which they simulate. Lancet 2:1115–1119, 1928.
76. Ivanoev K, Fork T, Hagerstrand J, et al: Diverticulosis in total colonic aganglionosis. Acta Radiol Diagn 26:447–451, 1985.
77. Srivastava GS, Smith AN, Painter NS: Steerculia, bulk-forming agent with smooth-muscle relaxant, versus bran in diverticular disease. Br Med J 1:315–318, 1976.
78. Almy TP, Howell, DA: Diverticular disease of the colon. N Engl J Med 302:324–331, 1980.
79. Snape WJ Jr, Carlson GM, Cohen S: Colonic myoelectric activity in the irritable bowel syndrome. Gastroenterology 70:326–330, 1976.
80. Trotman IF, Misiewicz JJ: Sigmoid motility in diverticular disease and the irritable bowel syndrome. Gut 29:218–222, 1988.
81. Arfwidsson S: Pathogenesis of mutliple diverticula of the sigmoid colon in diverticular disease. Acta Chir Scand [Suppl] 342:11–26, 1964.
82. Ritsema GH, Thijn CJ, Smout AJ: Motility of the sigmoid in irritable bowel syndrome and colonic diverticulosis. Ned Tijdschr Geneeskd 134:1398–1401, 1990.
83. Connell AM: Applied physiology of the colon: Factors relevant to diverticular disease. Clin Gastroenterol 4:23–36, 1975.
84. Painter NS, Truelove SC, Ardan GM, Tuckery M: Segmentation and the localization of intraluminal pressures in the human colon, with special reference to the pathogenesis of colonic diverticula. Gastroenterology 49:169–177, 1965.
85. Weinreich J, Andersen D: Intraluminal pressure in the sigmoid colon. II. Patients with sigmoid diverticula and related conditions. Scand J Gastroenterol 11:581–586, 1976.
86. Howell DA, Crow HC, Almy TP, Ramsey WH: A controlled double-blind study of sigmoid motility using psyllium mucilloid in diverticular disease (DD). Gastroenterology 74:1046, 1978.
87. Painter NS, Burkitt DP: Diverticular disease of the colon, a 20th century problem. Clin Gastroenterol 4:3–21, 1975.
88. Gear JSS, Ware A, Furdson P, et al: Symptomless diverticular disease and intake of dietary fibre. Lancet 1:511–514, 1979.
89. Eastwood MA, Smith AN, Brydon WG, Pritchard J: Colonic function in patients with diverticular disease. Lancet 1:1181–1182, 1978.
90. Findlay JM, Smith AN, Mitchell WD, et al: Effects of unprocessed bran on colon function in normal subjects in diverticular disease. Lancet 1:146–149, 1974.
91. Brodribb AJ, Humphreys DM: Diverticular disease: Three studies. Part II. Treatment with bran. Br Med J 1:425–428, 1976.
92. Hyland JM, Taylor I: Does a high fibre diet prevent the complications of diverticular disease? Br J Surg 67:77–79, 1980.
93. Frieden JH, Morgenstern L: Sigmoid diverticulitis in identical twins. Dig Dis Sci 30:182–183, 1985.
94. Omojala MF, Mangete E: Diverticulosis of the colon in three Nigerian siblings. Trop Geograph Med 40:54–57, 1988.
95. Flynn M, Hyland J, Hammond P, et al: Faecal bile acid excretion in diverticular disease. Br J Surg 67:629–632, 1980.
96. Rawlinson J, Brunton FJ: Transient diverticula of the colon. Br J Radiol 62:27–30, 1989.
97. Keith A: A demonstration on diverticula of the alimentary tract of complicated or of obscure origin. Br Med J 1:367–380, 1910.
98. Williams I: Changing emphasis in diverticular disease of the colon. Br J Radiol 36:393–406, 1963.
99. Noitove A, Almy TP: Diverticular disease of the colon. In Sleisenger MH, Fordtran JS (eds): Gastrointestinal Disease. Pathophysiology, Diagnosis, Management, 4th ed. Philadelphia, WB Saunders, 1989, pp 1419–1434.
100. Rosenberg RF, Naidich JB: Plain film recognition of giant colonic diverticulum. Am J Gastroenterol 76:59–69, 1981.
101. Harris RD, Anderson JE, Wolf EA: Giant air cyst of the sigmoid complicating diverticulitis: Report of a case. Dis Colon Rectum 18:418–424, 1975.
102. Van Niekerk AJ, Fourie PA: Giant colonic diverticulum—a radiological diagnostic problem: A case report. South Afr Med J 75:447–448, 1989.
103. Ellerbroek CJ, Lu CC: Unusual manifestations of giant colonic diverticulum. Dis Colon Rectum 27:545–547, 1984.
104. Lepeyrie H, Balmes P, Loizon P, Delhoume JY: Giant diverticulum of the transverse colon. J Chir 125:717–720, 1988.
105. McNutt R, Schmitt D, Schulte W: Giant colonic diverticula—three distinct entities: Report of a case. Dis Colon Rectum 31:624–628, 1988.
106. Kricun R, Stasik JJ, Reither RD, Dex WJ: Giant colonic diverticulum. AJR 135:507–512, 1980.

107. Parks, TG: Natural history of diverticular disease of the colon. Clin Gastroenterol 4:53–69, 1975.
108. Ming SC, Fleischner FG: Diverticulitis of the sigmoid colon: Reappraisal of the pathology and pathogenesis. Surgery 58:627–633, 1965.
109. Fleischner FG, Ming SC: Revised concept on diverticular disease of the colon. 2. So-called diverticulitis: Diverticular sigmoiditis and perisigmoiditis, diverticular abscess, fistula, frank peritonitis. Radiology 84:599–609, 1965.
110. Ferrucci JT, Ragsdale BD, Barrett PJ, et al: Double tracking in the sigmoid colon. Radiology 120:307–312, 1976.
111. Schnyder P, Moss AA, Thoeni RF, Margulis AR: A double-blind study of radiologic accuracy in diverticulosis, diverticulitis and carcinoma of the sigmoid colon. J Clin Gastroenterol 1:55–66, 1979.
112. Woods RJ, Lavery IC, Fazio VW, et al: Internal fistulas in diverticular disease. Dis Colon Rectum 31:591–596, 1988.
113. Small WP, Smith AN: Fistula and conditions associated with diverticular disease of the colon. Clin Gastroenterol 4:171–199, 1975.
114. Hafner CD, Ponka LJ, Brush BE: Genitourinary manifestations of diverticulosis of the colon: A study of 500 cases. JAMA 179:76–78, 1962.
115. Ravo B, Khan SA, Ger R, et al: Unusual extraperitoneal presentations of diverticulitis. Am J Gastroenterol 80:346–351, 1985.
116. McCrea ES, Wagner E: Femoral osteomyelitis secondary to diverticulitis. J Can Assoc Radiol 32:181–182, 1981.
117. Libson E, Bloom RA, Verstandig A, et al: Sigmoid-appendiceal fistula in diverticular disease. Diagn Imag Clin Med 53:262–264, 1984.
118. van Hillo M, Fazio VW, Lavery IC: Sigmoidoappendiceal fistula—an unusual complication of diverticulitis: Report of a case. Dis Colon Rectum 27:618–620, 1984.
119. Lambert ME, Knox RA, Schofield PF, Hancock BD: Management of the septic complications of diverticular disease. Br J Surg 73:567–579, 1986.
120. Berry AR, Turner WH, Mortensen NJ, Kettlewell MG: Emergency surgery for complicated diverticular disease: A five-year experience. Dis Colon Rectum 32:849–854, 1989.
121. Graham GA, Bernstein RB, Gronner AT: Gas in the portal and inferior mesenteric veins caused by diverticulitis of the sigmoid colon: Report of a case with survival. Radiology 114:601–602, 1975.
122. Jensen JA, Tsang D, Minnis JF, et al: Pneumopylephlebitis and intramesocolic diverticular perforation. Am J Surg 150:284–287, 1985.
123. Rodning CB, Williams L: Suppurative pylephlebitis due to pseudodiverticulosis coli. South Med J 77:1165–1167, 1984.
124. Sonnenshein MA, Cone LA, Alexander RM: Diverticulitis with colovenous fistula and portal venous gas: Report of two cases. J Clin Gastroenterol 8:195–198, 1986.
125. Arsura EL: Corticosteroid-association perforation of colonic diverticula. Arch Intern Med 150:1337–1338, 1990.
126. Hinchey EJ, Schaal PG, Richards GK: Treatment of perforated diverticular disease of the colon. Adv Surg 12:85–109, 1978.
127. Parks TG: Natural history of diverticular disease of the colon: A review of 521 cases. Br Med J 4:639–642, 1969.
128. Kocour EJ: Diverticulosis of colon. Am J Surg 37:433–436, 1937.
129. Ochsner HC, Barger JA: Diverticulosis of the large intestine: An evaluation of historical and personal observations. Ann Intern Med 9:283–296, 1935.
130. Haubrich WS: Diverticula and diverticular disease of the colon. In Berk JE, Haubrich WS, Kalser MH, et al (eds): Bockus Gastroenterology, 4th ed. Philadelphia, WB Saunders, 1985, pp 2445–2473.
131. Horner JL: Natural history of diverticulosis of the colon. Am J Dig Dis 3:343–350, 1958.
132. Case TC, Shea CE Jr: Acute diverticulitis of the caecum. Am J Surg 85:134–141, 1953.
133. Sugihara K, Muto T, Morioka Y: Motility study in the right sided diverticular disease of the colon. Gut 24:1130–1134, 1983.
134. Wilkinson S: Acute solitary diverticulitis of the transverse colon in a child: Report of a case. Dis Colon Rectum 31:574–576, 1988.
135. Lauridsen JR, Ross FP: Acute diverticulitis of cecum. Arch Surg 64:320–330, 1952.
136. Pieterse AS, Rowland R, Miliauskas JR, Hoffmann DC: Right-sided diverticular disease of the colon: A morphological analysis of 16 cases. Aust NZ J Surg 56:471–475, 1986.
137. Rodkey GV, Welch CE: Diverticulitis of the colon: Evolution in concept and therapy. Surg Clin North Am 45:1231–1243, 1965.
138. Sardi A, Gokli A, Singer JA: Diverticular disease of the cecum and ascending colon: A review of 881 cases. Am Surg 53:41–45, 1987.
139. Leichtling JJ: Acute cecal diverticulitis. Gastroenterology 29:453–460, 1955.
140. Magness LJ, Sanfelippo PM, Van Heerden JA, Judd ES: Diverticular disease of the right colon. Surg Gynecol Obstet 140:30–32, 1975.
141. Fischer MG, Farkas AM: Diverticulitis of the cecum and ascending colon. Dis Colon Rectum 27:454–458, 1984.
142. Luoma A, Nagy AG: Cecal diverticulitis. Can J Surg 32:283–286, 1989.
143. Mianglorra CJL: Diverticulitis of the right colon. Ann Surg 153:861–870, 1961.
144. Mittal VK, Cortez JA, Olson AM: Solitary perforated diverticulum of the ascending colon: Report of two cases. J Dis Colon Rectum 24:47–49, 1981.
145. Crist DW, Fishman EK, Scatarige JC, Cameron JL: Acute diverticulitis of the cecum and ascending colon diagnosed by computed tomography. Surg Gynecol Obstet 166:99–102, 1988.
146. Labs JD, Sarr MG, Fishman EK, et al: Complications of acute diverticulitis of the colon: Improved early diagnosis with computerized tomography. Am J Surg 155:331–336, 1988.
147. Feldberg MA, Hendriks MJ, van Waes PF: Role of CT in diagnosis and management of complications of diverticular disease. Gastrointest Radiol 10:370–377, 1985.
148. Hulnick DH, Megibow AJ, Balthazar EJ, et al: Computed tomography in the evaluation of diverticulitis. Radiology 152:491–495, 1984.
149. Cho KC, Morehouse HT, Alterman DD, Thornhill BA: Sigmoid diverticulitis: Diagnostic role of CT—comparison with barium enema studies. Radiology 176:111–115, 1990.
150. Verbanck J, Lambrecht S, Rutgeerts L, et al: Can sonography diagnose acute colonic diverticulitis in patients with acute intestinal inflammation? A prospective study. J Clin Ultrasound 17:661–666, 1989.
151. Wilson SR, Toi A: The value of sonography in the diagnosis of acute diverticulitis of the colon. AJR 154:1199–1202, 1990.
152. Orebaugh JE, Macris JA, Lee JF: Surgical treatment of diverticular disease of the colon. Am Surg 44:712–715, 1978.
153. Alexander J, Karl RC, Skinner DB: Results of changing trends in the surgical management of complications of diverticular disease. Surgery 94:683–690, 1983.
154. Perkins JD, Shield CF 3d, Chang FC, Farha GJ: Acute diverticulitis: Comparison of treatment in immunocompromised and nonimmunocompromised patients. Am J Surg 148:745–748, 1984.
155. Freischlag J, Bennion RS, Thompson JE Jr: Complications of diverticular disease of the colon in young people. Dis Colon Rectum 29:639–643, 1986.
156. Ouriel K, Schwartz SI: Diverticular disease in the young patient. Surg Gynecol Obstet 156:1–5, 1983.
157. Klein S, Mayer L, Present DH, et al: Extraintestinal manifestations in patients with diverticulitis. Ann Intern Med 108:700–702, 1988.
158. Harbrecht PJ, Ahmad W, Fry DE, Amin M: Occult diverticulitis, a cause of retroperitoneal fibrosis. Dis Colon Rectum 23:255–257, 1980.
159. Auguste L, Borrero E, Wise L: Surgical management of perforated colonic diverticulitis. Arch Surg 120:450–452, 1985.
160. Hackford AW, Veidenheimer MC: Diverticular disease of the colon: Current concepts and management. Surg Clin North Am 65:347–363, 1985.
161. Larson DM, Masters SS, Spiro HM: Medical and surgical therapy in diverticular disease: A comparative study. Gastroenterology 71:734–737, 1976.
162. Casarella WJ, Kanter IE, Seaman WB: Right-sided colonic diverticula as a cause of acute rectal hemorrhage. N Engl J Med 286:450–453, 1972.

163. Hughes LE: Complications of diverticular disease: inflammation, obstruction and hemorrhage. Clin Gastroenterol 4:147–170, 1975.
164. Kubo A, Kagaya T, Nakagawa H: Studies on complications of diverticular disease of the colon. Jpn J Med 24:39–43, 1985.
165. Rosenberg IK, Rosenberg BF: Massive haemorrhage from diverticula of the colon, with demonstration of the source of bleeding: A case report. Ann Surg 159:570–573, 1964.
166. Meyers MA, Alonso DR, Baer JW: Pathogenesis of massively bleeding colonic diverticulosis: New observations. AJR 127:901–908, 1976.
167. Tedesco FJ, Waye JD, Raskin JB, et al: Colonoscopic evaluation of rectal bleeding: A study of 304 patients. Ann Intern Med 89:907–909, 1978.
168. Boley SJ, Sammartano R, Adams WA, et al: On the nature and etiology of vascular ectasias of the colon. Gastroenterology 72:650–660, 1977.
169. Boley SJ, Brandt LJ: Vascular ectasias of the colon—1986. Dig Dis Sci 31(Suppl):26S–42S, 1986.
170. Welch CE, Athanasoulis CA, Galdabini JJ: Hemorrhage from the large bowel with special reference to angiodysplasia and diverticular disease. World J Surg 2:73–83, 1978.
171. Baum S, Athansoulis CA, Waltman AC, et al: Angiodysplasia of the right colon: a cause of gastrointestinal bleeding. AJR 129:789–794, 1977.
172. Santos JCM Jr, Aprilli F, Guimaraes AS, Rocha JJ: Angiodysplasia of the colon: Endoscopic diagnosis and treatment. Br J Surg 75:256–258, 1988.
173. Roberts PL, Schoetz DJ Jr, Coller JA: Vascular ectasia: Diagnosis and treatment by colonoscopy. Am Surg 54:56–59, 1988.
174. Talman EA, Dixon DS, Guiterrez FE: Role of arteriography in rectal hemorrhage due to arteriovenous malformation and diverticulosis. Ann Surg 190:203–213, 1979.
175. Athanasoulis CA, Baum S, Rosch J, et al: Mesenteric arterial infusions of vasopressin for hemorrhage from colonic diverticulosis. Am J Surg 129:212–216, 1975.
176. Stavorovsky M, Finkelstein T: Colonic cancer and associated diverticulitis. Int Surg 64:49–53, 1979.
177. Morini S, de Angelis P, Manurita L, Colavolpe V: Association of colonic diverticula with adenomas and carcinomas: A colonoscopic experience. Dis Colon Rectum 31:793–796, 1988.
178. Boulos PB, Cowin AP, Karamanolis DG, Clark CG: Diverticula, neoplasia, or both? Early detection of carcinoma in sigmoid diverticular disease. Ann Surg 202:607–609, 1985.
179. De Masi E, Bertolotti A, Fegiz GF: The importance of endoscopy in the diagnosis of neoplasms associated with diverticular disease of the colon, and its effect on surgical treatment. Ital J Surg Sci 14:195–199, 1984.
180. Hines JR, Gordon RT: Adenocarcinoma arising in a diverticular abscess of the colon: Report of a case. Dis Colon Rectum 18:49–51, 1975.
181. McCraw RC, Wilson SM, Brown FM, Gardner WA: Adenocarcinoma arising in a sigmoid diverticulum: Report of a case. Dis Colon Rectum 19:553–556, 1976.
182. Hernandez FJ, Fernandez BB: Mucus-secreting carcinoid tumor in a colonic diverticulum: Report of a case. Dis Colon Rectum 19:63–67, 1976.
183. Axelsson CK, Francis D: Peroperative fine-needle aspiration biopsy: An aid to differential diagnosis between diverticular disease and colonic cancer? A preliminary report. Dis Colon Rectum 21:319–321, 1978.
184. Jalan KN, Walker RJ, Prescot RJ, et al: Fecal stasis and diverticular disease in ulcerative colitis. Gut 11:688–696, 1970.
185. Marshak RH: Granulomatous colitis in association with diverticula. N Engl J Med 283:1080–1084, 1970.
186. Burkitt DP, Walker AR: Saint's triad: Confirmation and explanation. South Afr Med J 50:2136–2138, 1976.
187. Scaggion G, Poletti G, Riggo S: Saint's triad: Statistico-epidemiological research and case contribution. Minn Med 78:1183–1187, 1987.
188. Capron JP, Piperaud R, Dupas J-L, et al: Evidence for an association between cholelithiasis and diverticular disease of the colon. Dig Dis Sci 26:523–527, 1981.
189. Scheff RT, Zuckerman G, Harter H, et al: Diverticular disease in patients with chronic renal failure due to polycystic kidney disease. Ann Intern Med 92:202–204, 1980.
190. Foster KJ, Holdstock G, Whorwell PJ, et al: Prevalence of diverticular disease of the colon in patients with ischaemic heart disease. Gut 19:1054–1056, 1978.
191. Brodribb AJ, Humphreys DM: Diverticular disease: Three studies. Part I. Relation to other disorders and fibre intake. Br Med J 1:424–425, 1976.
192. Galbraith P, Bagg MN, Schabel SI, Rajagopalan PR: Diverticular complications of renal failure. Gastrointest Radiol 15:259–262, 1990.
193. Burton NA, Albus RA, Graeber GM, Lough FC: Acute diverticulitis following cardiac surgery. Chest 89:756–757, 1986.
194. Badia-Perez JM, Valverde-Sintas J, Franch-Arcas G, et al: Acute postoperative diverticulitis. Int J Colorect Dis 4:141–143, 1989.

CHAPTER 31

Benign Polyps of the Intestines

HARRY S. COOPER, M.D.

DEFINITION AND CLASSIFICATION

NONNEOPLASTIC POLYPS
Hyperplastic polyp
Peutz-Jeghers Polyps
Inflammatory Polyps
Inflammatory Fibroid Polyp
Inflammatory Pseudopolyp

Juvenile Polyp
Lymphoid Polyp

NEOPLASTIC POLYPS
Adenoma
Adenoma with Cancer
Adenoma with Pseudoinvasion

POLYPOSIS SYNDROMES

Familial (Adenomatosis) Polyposis Coli
Gardner's Syndrome
Turcot Syndrome
Juvenile Polyposis
Peutz-Jeghers Syndrome
Cronkhite-Canada Syndrome
Cowden's Disease
Intestinal Ganglioneuromatosis
Lymphoid Polyposis

DEFINITION AND CLASSIFICATION

Polyp is essentially a clinical term for or gross description of any circumscribed "tumor" that projects above the surrounding normal mucosa. *Polyp* should not be used as a histologic term. Polyps may be neoplastic, inflammatory, hyperplastic, or hamartomatous in nature (Table 31–1); only through histologic examination can one be certain of their nature and clinical significance. Solitary polyps (of whatever cause or whatever their histologic features) are much more common in the large intestine and rectum than in the small intestine; therefore, most of the chapter will cover lesions of the large intestine and rectum. However, in polyposis syndromes, involvement of the small intestine by these lesions is common.

NONNEOPLASTIC POLYPS

Hyperplastic Polyps

Hyperplastic (or metaplastic) polyps are small (most are less than 5 mm in size) convex elevations limited to the colon and rectum. They are most commonly seen in the rectums of patients 40 years of age or greater.[1] Morson was one of the early investigators to recognize that these lesions were nonneoplastic in nature.[2] However, our concepts regarding hyperplastic polyps are evolving and changing as a result of recent studies with mucin histochemistry, tumor-associated antigens, and simple light microscopy. These lesions may represent a more heterogeneous group than was previously thought.[3,4,4a]

Incidence and Epidemiology. In general, in the old literature, most investigators would agree that the vast majority of polyps of the colon and rectum less than 5 mm in size are hyperplastic polyps. In autopsy material Arthur[1] noted that 80% of polyps less than 5 mm in size were hyperplastic polyps. Similarly, Lane et al.,[3] in a study of 2136 colorectal polyps (1581 adenomas and 555 hyperplastic polyps) in symptomatic adults, noted that 90% of lesions less than 3 mm in size were hyperplastic polyps. However, recent data from biopsy material have challenged this. Estrada and Spjut[5] have found that 43.5% of lesions 5 mm or less were hyperplastic polyps, whereas 56.5% of such lesions were adenomas. Similarly, Waye et al.[5a] found that of polyps 6 mm or less in size, 61% were adenomas, while only 20% were hyperplastic polyps. In general, the inci-

Table 31-1 CLASSIFICATION OF INTESTINAL POLYPS

Solitary and multiple polyps
    Neoplastic polyps
        Tubular adenoma
        Tubulovillous adenoma
        Villous adenoma
    Nonneoplastic polyps
        Hyperplastic (metaplastic) polyp
        Juvenile polyp
        Peutz-Jeghers polyp
        Inflammatory polyp
            Inflammatory fibroid polyp
            Inflammatory pseudopolyp
        Lymphoid polyp
Polyposis syndromes
    Familial (adenomatosis) polyposis coli
    Gardner's syndrome
    Turcot syndrome
    Juvenile polyposis
    Peutz-Jeghers syndrome
    Cronkhite-Canada syndrome
    Lymphoid polyposis
    Cowden's disease
    Intestinal ganglioneuromatosis
    Hyperplastic polyposis

dence of hyperplastic polyps increases with the age of the population; these polyps are uncommon below the age of 40 years.[1,6] As for other types of polyps, the incidence of hyperplastic polyps varies depending upon the geographic area studied. In general, epidemiologic studies indicate that the incidence of hyperplastic polyps parallels that of large-bowel adenomas and cancers. Studies from Western countries, where there is a high incidence of adenomas and cancers, have reported the incidence of hyperplastic polyps to be as high as 85%; in underdeveloped countries, where the incidence of adenomas and cancers is low, the incidence of hyperplastic polyps may be as low as 2% to 3%.[6] Although it would appear that the incidence of hyperplastic polyps is proportional to the incidence of adenomas and cancers, these epidemiologic data are not meant to imply that hyperplastic polyps are markers for cancer or precancerous lesions. The incidence of hyperplastic polyps in the Japanese prefectures of Akita and Miyagi are almost identical; however, the Akita prefecture has an intermediate incidence of colorectal cancer, whereas the Miyagi has a low incidence of colorectal cancer.[7] Similarly the incidence of hyperplastic polyps is greater in São Paulo (a city with an intermediate incidence of cancer) than in New Orleans, which has a higher incidence of colorectal cancer. Most studies have shown that hyperplastic polyps are located mainly in the rectum and to a lesser extent in the sigmoid colon.[6-8] Depending on the study, the male-to-female ratio varies from unity to 4:1.[1,6-9]

Etiology and Pathogenesis. To date the etiology of hyperplastic polyps is unknown. Franzin et al.[10] believe that hyperplastic polyps may be of inflammatory or ischemic origin. They base this on the similar finding of a hyperplastic type of epithelium in cases of ischemic colitis, polypectomy scars, inflammatory polyps, juvenile polyps, and hyperplastic mucosa in the solitary rectal ulcer syndrome. Cell kinetic studies[11,11a] have shown that these hyperplastic polyps are non-neoplastic in nature. These studies have indicated also that the mode of cell renewal is the same as in the normal mucosa, but with a longer turnover time, a delayed migration from crypt to surface, and a slower exfoliation. In essence, these polyps represent "hypermature epithelial" changes. Morphologic findings to support this are the saw-toothed or serrated appearance of the epithelial cells. Also noted are increased length of the microvilli, accentuation of the lateral intercellular digitations, and increased breadth of the basal lamina attachment. Recent immunohistochemical studies of antigens related to cell differentiation indicate that hyperplastic polyps show hypermature epithelial changes.[11b]

Clinical Aspects. Hyperplastic polyps by themselves rarely produce symptoms referable to the gastrointestinal (GI) tract, probably because of their small size. However, there have been reports of patients with large or multiple hyperplastic polyps that were responsible for GI symptoms.[9,12-14] To date, most investigators believe that hyperplastic polyps are neither markers for colorectal cancer nor premalignant lesions themselves. In 1970 Goldman et al.[15] reported that 36% of villous adenomas less than 2 cm in size had hyperplastic polyp foci, whereas only 5% of villous adenomas greater than 2 cm in size had hyperplastic polyp foci. This led the authors to speculate that hyperplastic polyps may be a reservoir for villous adenomas. Over the past few years, several investigators have reported on hyperplastic polyps with foci of adenomatous change or rarely with adenocarcinoma.[9,10,12-14,16] Those patients with cancer also had foci of adenoma, and the cancer may have arisen in the adenoma. These hyperplastic polyps with adenomatous foci represent a very interesting entity. Many of the early studies regarding hyperplastic polyps have noted that adenomatous changes never occurred in hyperplastic polyps.[2,4] More recent studies have indicated that this is not true.[5,10,12-14,16] It would appear that the chance of adenomatous change in hyperplastic polyps probably is directly proportional to the size of the hyperplastic polyp. In a study of 173 hyperplastic polyps Franzin et al. found that five of seven hyperplastic polyps greater than 1 cm in size had adenomatous foci.[10] However, the finding of adenomatous foci in hyperplastic polyps is the exception, rather than the rule.

Although many patients with hyperplastic polyps may have multiple polyps, there have been occasional reports of patients who have so-called hyperplastic polyposis,[9,13] in which the number of polyps ranges from "numerous" to hundreds. In no case of hyperplastic polyposis was a familial incidence reported, as is known to occur in familial polyposis coli. In these reported cases there has been a marked male predominance. The author has personally examined one patient with hyperplastic polyposis, in whom 80 polyps were noted. In this case, two polyps had mixed hyperplastic and adenomatous foci.

Pathology. On gross examination, hyperplastic polyps appear as small sessile rounded excrescences that are the same color or paler than the surrounding mu-

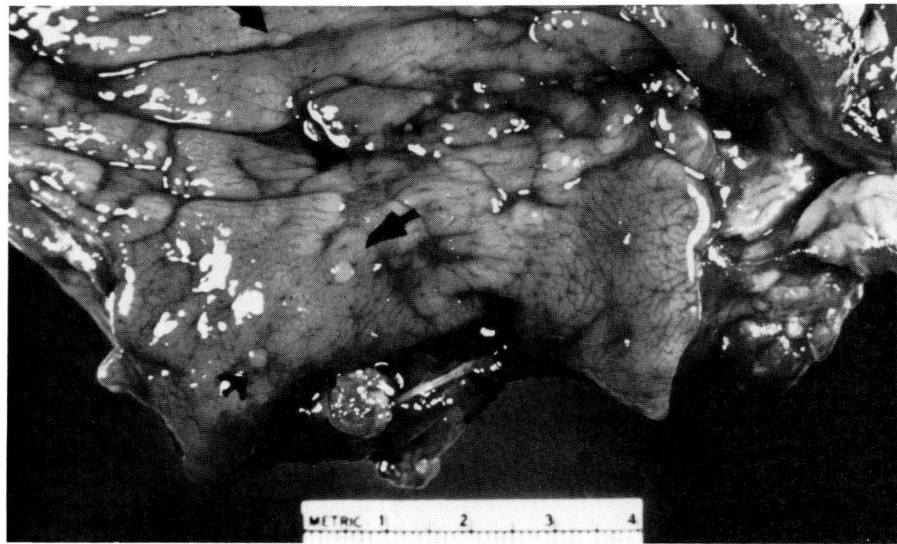

FIGURE 31-1. Gross appearance of hyperplastic polyps (arrows). The polyps are small and convex and appear to be of the same color as the surrounding mucosa.

cosa. They often sit on the mucosal folds and may be flattened or convex in nature (Figure 31–1). Occasionally, hyperplastic polyps may be pedunculated with a well-developed stalk. The vast majority of hyperplastic polyps range from 3 to 6 mm in size. However, in large series of hyperplastic polyps approximately 1% to 4% of polyps are greater than 1 cm in size.[9,10]

On microscopic examination, hyperplastic polyps have a serrated or saw-toothed appearance similar to that seen in a secretory endometrium. The serrated appearance is due to the extensive papillary infolding of epithelial cells. In most series columnar cells predominate over goblet cells;[1,2,10] however, it has been claimed that goblet cells predominate in earlier lesions.[1] The columnar cells take on a very bright eosinophilic appearance with a distinct brush border. The nuclei of both goblet cells and columnar cells are basally located and show no atypia. In well-oriented material the basal portion of the crypt shows an increased mitotic rate compared with the mitotic rate of the normal surrounding mucosa; however, mitoses are never located in the upper third of the crypt or surface epithelium (Figure 31–2). Arthur has claimed that in the earlier lesions, there is simply a dilatation of the superficial parts of the glands, whereas in "older" lesions, full-thickness involvement of the crypt is seen. Often the specimen is less well oriented and is cut tangentially, in which case the crypts take on a star-shaped appearance (Figure 31–3). Often one can appreciate a disordered muscularis mucosae, with muscle fibers radiating toward the surface. This disordered muscularis mucosa may account for pseudoinvasion of epithelium into the submucosa, or what has been recently described by Sobin[17] as inverted hyperplastic polyps. Occasionally Paneth cells may also be present. In hyperplastic polyps there is widening or exaggeration of the collagen table beneath the surface epithelium. This is in contrast to adenomas, in which there is thinning of this subepithelial basement membrane table.[3] The group from St. Mark's Hospital has noted that hyperplastic polyps greater than 1 cm in size may take on the low-power appearance of a villous or tubulovillous adenoma.[9]

In a review of a large number of adenomas, the St. Mark's group found hyperplastic foci in 0.6% of adenomas.[9] Franzin et al. found that 9.6% of adenomas had hyperplastic foci and five of seven hyperplastic polyps greater than 1 cm in size had adenomatous foci.[10] Similarly, Estrada and Spjut found 13% of hyperplastic polyps to have foci of adenomatous epithelium (Figure 31–4).[5] The significance of these "mixed polyps" is unknown, and more studies are needed for better definition of what these lesions actually represent. One must also be cautioned that on occasion small adenomas, when viewed at low power magnification, may take on the appearance of a hyperplastic polyp; however, on more careful inspection they are truly adenomas. Hyperplastic epithelium has also been noted in 20% to 85% of juvenile polyps, Peutz-Jeghers polyps, and inflammatory polyps.[10] Recently, Longacre et al. have described the entity of mixed hyperplastic adenomatous polyps, which they believe represent an adenoma, rather than a hyperplastic polyp.[4a]

Special Studies. In general, hyperplastic polyps have a distribution of sialomucins and sulfomucins similar to that of normal nonneoplastic colonic mucosa.[10,18] Occasionally, hyperplastic polyps with a predominance of goblet cells may show increased expression of sialomucins similar to that described in the transitional zone mucosa adjacent to colon cancers.[10] Jass et al. have studied hyperplastic polyps as they relate to expression of O-acylated sialomucins.[18] These authors found that hyperplastic polyps greater than 3.5 mm in size tended to have a reduction in the normal amount of O-acylated sialomucins, findings that have been noted in colorectal cancers and adenomas with severe dysplasia.[19] Jass and co-workers also noted that compared with hyperplastic polyps with normal O-acylated sialomucins, those with a reduced amount of mucins tended to have larger nuclei, more conspicuous mitoses in the lower half of the crypts, and a higher

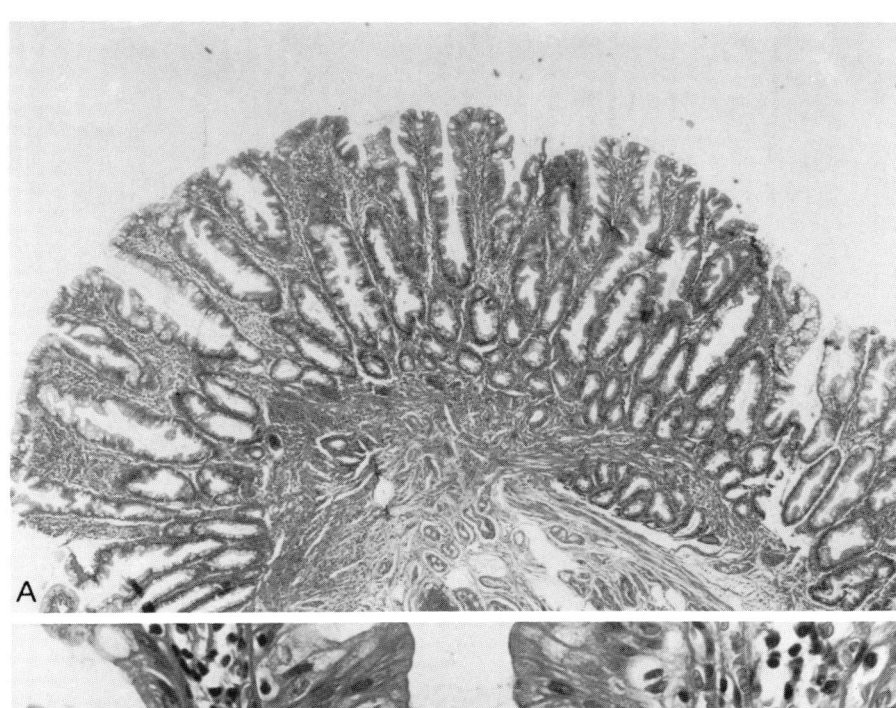
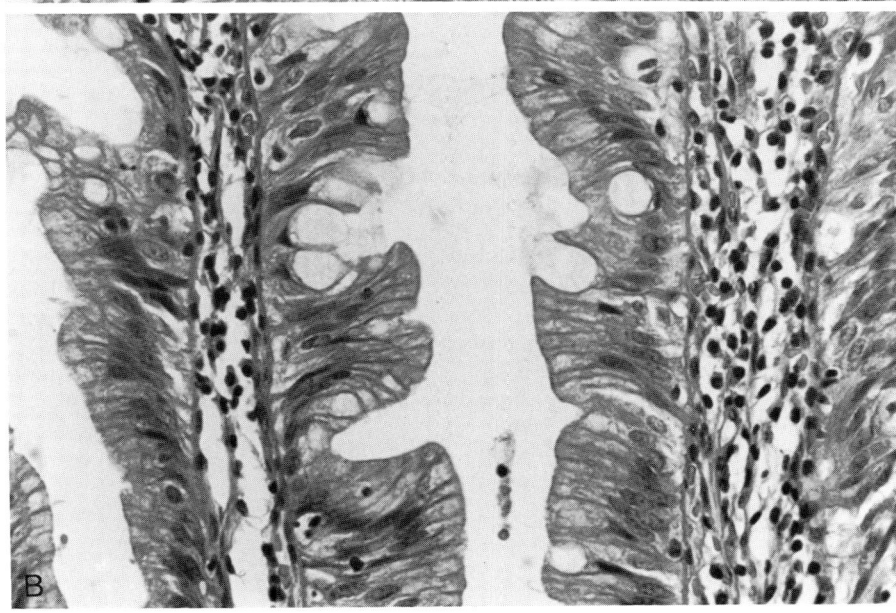

FIGURE 31–2. Hyperplastic polyp. *A,* Well-oriented specimen, showing the serrated, or papillary, infolding of epithelium. The muscularis mucosae is distorted and splayed. *B,* High-power view showing serrated epithelium with an admixture of columnar and goblet cells. No mitoses are noted, and the nuclei are bland in nature.

ratio of columnar cells to goblet cells. They further noted that such polyps tended to have marked papillary infolding and that their columnar cells had conspicuous brush borders with mucus in the apical cytoplasm; mature absorptive cells were not obvious. These hyperplastic polyps also showed a greater immunostaining for carcinoembryonic antigen (CEA). Based on these findings, Jass and colleagues postulated that smaller hyperplastic polyps may represent altered maturation of normal colonic epithelium, whereas larger hyperplastic polyps may be interpreted as showing maturation arrest and hyperplasia of intermediate cells normally found in the lower third of the colonic crypt, as shown by electron microscopy.[20]

Several investigators have studied hyperplastic polyps for tumor-associated antigens and have used lectins for studying changes in glycoconjugates. These studies have presented conflicting results, some reporting that hyperplastic polyps express antigenic changes noted in colonic neoplasms while others have noted just the opposite. Cooper and Reuter used peanut lectin (PNA) for studying glycoconjugate changes in hyperplastic polyps. PNA detects B-D-Gal (1→3)-D-GalNAc, which is the immediate precursor of the MN blood group antigens.[21] In hyperplastic polyps they noted that PNA localized to the supranuclear (Golgi) zone of both absorptive and columnar cells, findings that were noted also in the normal colonic epithelium. However, Boland et al. reported that PNA bound to the actual goblet cell theca, as they had noted for adenomas.[22] Jass et al.[18] and Skinner and Whitehead[23] have noted that the tumor-associated antigen CEA reacted with hyperplastic polyps; however, Skinner and Whitehead also noted that CEA reacted with normal colonic epithelium.[23] Other investigators studying the expression of ABH blood group antigens in the distal

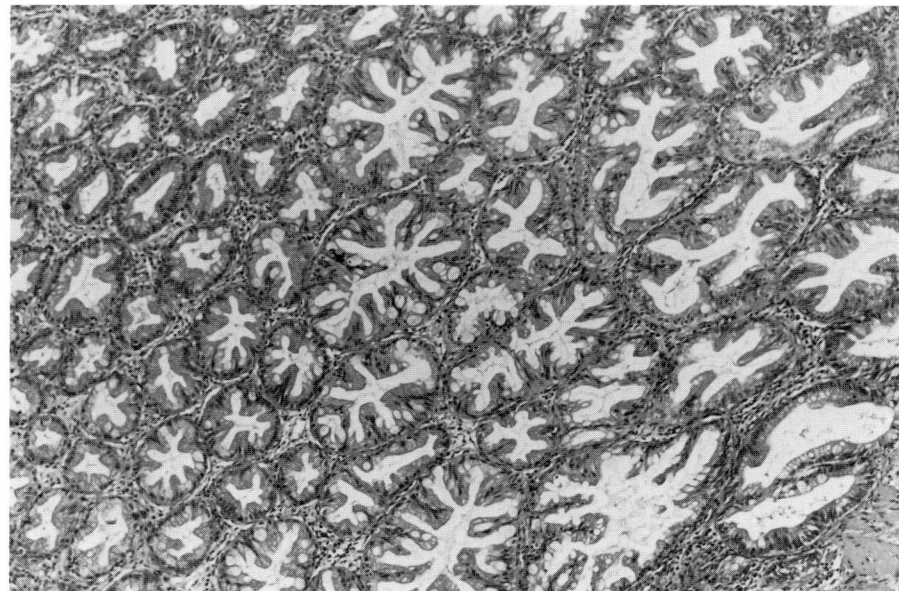

FIGURE 31-3. Low-power view of a poorly oriented hyperplastic polyp. One can identify the lesion as such by the star-shaped appearance of the glands.

colon have noted that hyperplastic polyps fail to express these antigens (which are normally absent in the normal distal colon), whereas adenomas express ABH blood group antigens.[24,11b] Bara et al. found that 100% of hyperplastic polyps expressed the M_1 antigen, which is an oncofetal antigen of the distal colon;[25] this antigen is normally absent in the distal colon but is found in cancers and adenomas.

Peutz-Jeghers Polyp

The Peutz-Jeghers polyp is a nonneoplastic hamartomatous polyp that occurs in the stomach, small intestine, and colon. One usually associates the Peutz-Jeghers polyp with the syndrome of intestinal polyposis and mucocutaneous pigmentation. However, it has been noted that these Peutz-Jeghers polyps may occur as solitary lesions in the stomach, small intestine, and colon in patients without the syndrome. In fact, it appears that those solitary polyps may be found as commonly as in patients with the syndrome.[26]

Etiology. Peutz-Jeghers polyps are true hamartomas. There is a genetic etiology in those people with the syndrome (see section on polyposis).

Clinical Aspects. These will be discussed under the section on polyposis.

Pathology. On gross examination these polyps may be sessile or pedunculated and may vary in size, some growing quite large (3.5 cm or more). The Peutz-Jeghers polyps are derived from intestinal glandular epithelium together with stroma that includes a branching muscular framework that comes from the muscularis mucosa. Both the epithelial and the smooth muscle

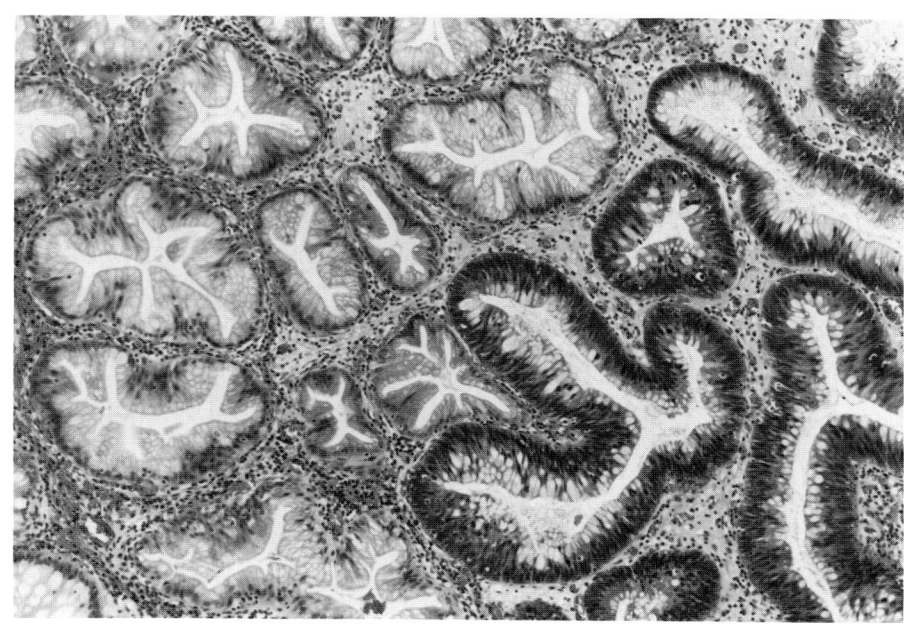

FIGURE 31-4. Hyperplastic polyp with focal adenomatous changes. The adenoma is on the right and the hyperplastic polyp on the left.

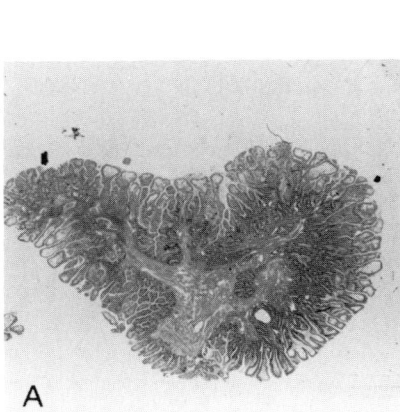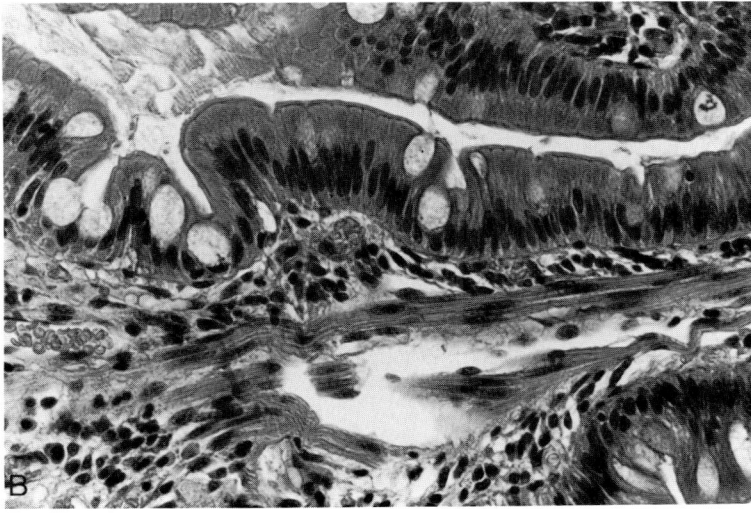

FIGURE 31–5. Peutz-Jeghers polyp of the small intestine. *A,* Whole mount view. *B,* Higher-power view, showing normal absorptive and goblet cells. Smooth muscle fibers are extending up through the core of the villus.

components give the Peutz-Jeghers polyp its characteristic appearance. Its arborescent arrangement should enable the pathologist to make the diagnosis at low-power magnification. The epithelium resembles the normal epithelium from the area of the gut from which it comes. In the small intestine the epithelium consists of both absorptive columnar cells and goblet cells (Figure 31–5). In the colon the glands often show extensive branching with predominantly hypertrophied goblet cells (Figure 31–6). A normal distribution of endocrine

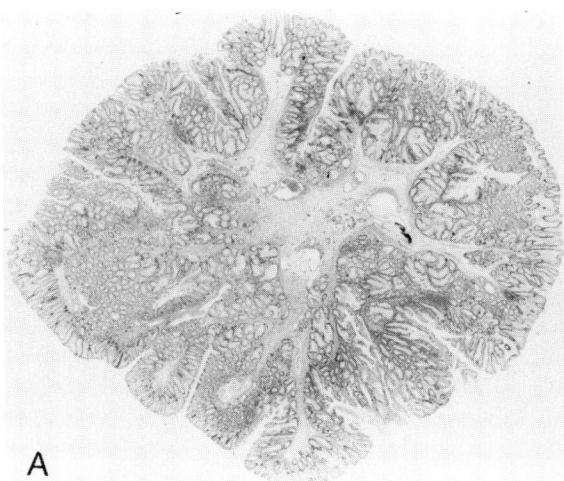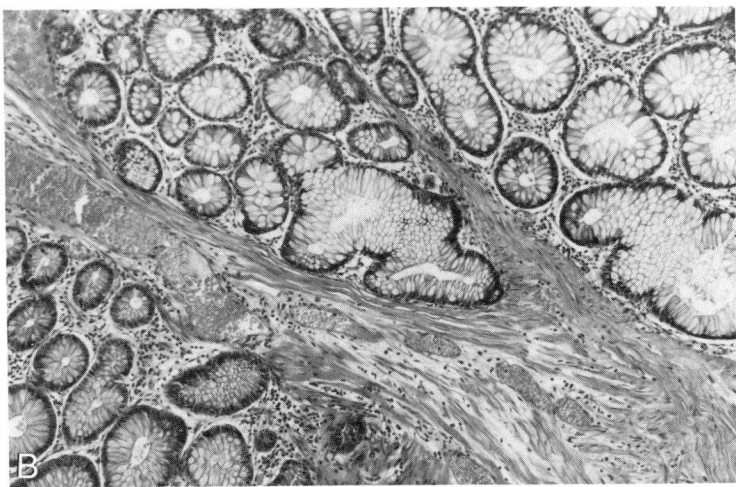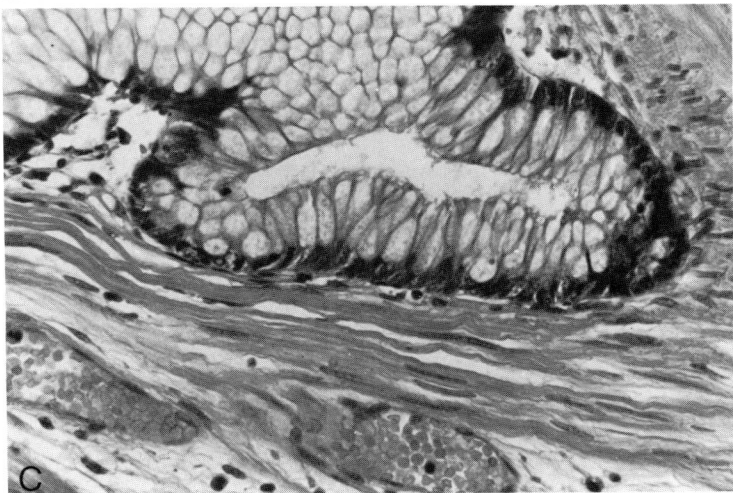

FIGURE 31–6. Peutz-Jeghers polyp of the colon. *A,* Whole-mount view showing the branching and tortuosity of glands. *B,* Medium-power view, showing branching smooth muscle fibers encircling and separating glands. *C,* High-power view, showing benign goblet cells with adjacent smooth muscle fibers.

cells is present. It is not uncommon to see areas of hyperplastic epithelium within these polyps. The epithelium in these polyps is nonneoplastic in nature; however, there have been occasional reports of dysplastic adenomatous changes and adenocarcinomas arising within Peutz-Jeghers polyps of the small intestine and those of the colon.[27-34] (The malignant potential of Peutz-Jeghers polyps will be discussed further under the section on polyposis. Occasionally one may see pseudoinvasion of the epithelium similar to that noted in adenomas, but this should not be taken as evidence of malignancy. Bolwell and James reported a case of ileal Peutz-Jeghers polyps that appeared grossly to form a tumor mass and infiltrate to the serosa.[35] On microscopic examination this proved to be herniation (pseudoinvasion of the mucosa with cystic formation that had extruded into the muscularis propria and serosa). Shepherd et al.[35a] have reported that pseudoinvasion or epithelial misplacement is present in 10% of small-intestinal Peutz-Jeghers polyps and is extremely uncommon in the large intestine. Recently there has been a report of an epithelioid leiomyosarcoma arising in a small-intestinal Peutz-Jeghers polyp that had metastasized to the liver.[36]

Inflammatory Polyps

Inflammatory Fibroid Polyp

General Aspects. Inflammatory fibroid polyps are benign tumor masses that occur in both the small and the large intestines. These uncommon lesions occur at all ages and have a worldwide distribution. Their cause is unknown, and they are not associated with any known medical conditions or syndromes. Other terms used to describe these lesions are eosinophilic granuloma, submucosal fibroma, hemangiopericytoma, inflammatory pseudotumor, and fibroma.[37-39]

Clinical Aspects. Inflammatory fibroid polyps can occur at any age (range, 3 to 80 years). The symptoms, in decreasing order of incidence, are episodic abdominal pain, vomiting, blood in the stool, diarrhea, constipation, abdominal distention, and weight loss; they may cause intussusception. The vast majority of the lesions are noted in the small intestine (mainly in the ileum); however, they can occur less commonly in the colon. Inflammatory polyps are benign, and surgical resection is curative.

Pathology. The pathology is similar whether the polyps arise in the small or the large intestine. They range in size from 1.5 to 13 cm (average, 3.0 to 4.0 cm). On gross examination most lesions are polypoid with a broad base. The bulk of the lesion resides in the submucosa; however, these polyps may infiltrate into the muscularis propria and serosa. On cut surface they tend to be tan, gray, or yellow, and the overlying mucosa is often ulcerated.

Microscopic examination reveals a fibrocytic lesion with variable blood vessels and an inflammatory infiltrate. Around muscular walled blood vessels one finds a characteristic rarefaction (myxoid change) to the stroma. In some areas the lesions are myxoid with sparse connective tissue fibers. Various cell types are randomly distributed throughout the lesion. There are stellate and spindle-shaped fibroblasts with indistinct basophilic cytoplasm. Eosinophils, lymphocytes, plasma cells, macrophages, and mast cells are noted. Eosinophils ranged from few to dense aggregates. Cellular fields may show cells with mitotic figures with some lesions showing two mitoses per high-power fields.

This lesion must be distinguished from malignant mesenchymal tumors. In addition to its characteristic histology, the inflammatory fibroid polyp may penetrate the bowel wall with a pattern of dissection between the muscle fibers, causing a splaying or splitting of the muscle wall layer. In contrast, mesenchymal neoplasms infiltrate by pushing aside the muscle wall layer.[38] To date, immunohistochemical studies with antibodies against S-100 protein have been negative,[37] suggesting that these lesions are not of neural nature.

Inflammatory Pseudopolyps

Incidence. Inflammatory pseudopolyps are noted in the colon and rectum. As their name suggests they are secondary to inflammatory disorders of the large intestine, such as ulcerative colitis and Crohn's disease. They may also be seen in amebiasis, schistosomiasis, ischemic colitis, at surgical anastomotic sites, and adjacent to ulcers (see Chapter 27). It has been noted that inflammatory polyps may be seen in 10% to 20% of patients with ulcerative colitis.[40] In Africa, inflammatory polyps account for 25% to 30% of all colonic polyps.[41,42]

Etiology and Pathogenesis. In ulcerative colitis and Crohn's disease, inflammatory pseudopolyps are primarily the result of ulceration and undermining of the adjacent intact mucosa. Because of this, the intact mucosa stands out and projects into the lumen. At times inflammatory pseudopolyps may become so extensive that they carpet a larger portion of the intestinal surface. In Africa there is a high incidence of bacterial proctocolitis, which may be etiologic, as is the incidence of schistosomal infestation.[41,42]

Pathology. In ulcerative colitis or Crohn's disease these polyps are nothing more than raised tags of mucosa or submucosa (Figure 31-7). In some polyps there is essentially no inflammation, and they consist simply of long fingers of normal mucosa. When inflammation is present they may consist of cystically dilated glands and an inflamed intervening stroma; there may also be changes of epithelial hyperplasia. Inflammatory polyps may closely resemble early juvenile polyps, which are believed by some to have an inflammatory etiology. In young children with no history of inflammatory bowel disease and only a few polyps, care should be taken not to misdiagnose a small inflamed juvenile polyp as an inflammatory polyp. The inflammatory polyps seen adjacent to ulcers, at surgical anastomotic sites, or in schistosomiasis tend to be small rounded nodules of granulation tissue with variable epithelial components

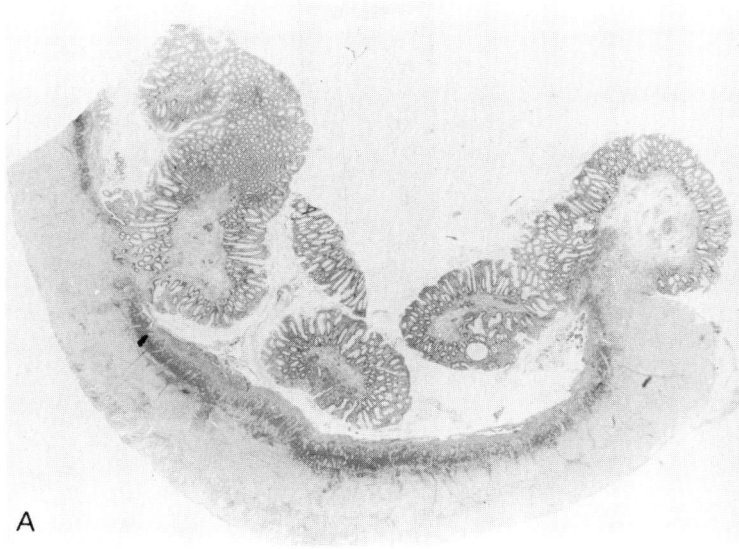
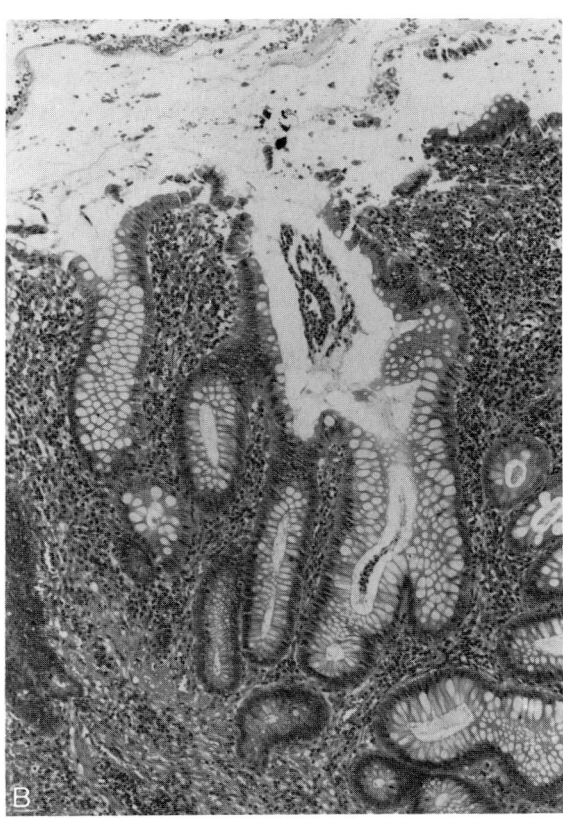

FIGURE 31–7. Inflammatory pseudopolyp in patient with ulcerative colitis. *A*, Whole-mount view. The polyps are due to residual mucosa adjacent to ulcerated epithelium. *B*, Medium-power view. The glands are distorted, and leucocytes are noted in the lumen. The lamina propria has a dense chronic inflammatory infiltrate.

(Figure 31–8). With schistosomal polyps ova can often be seen. Further details are presented in Chapter 27.

Juvenile Polyp

Incidence and Epidemiology. Juvenile polyps occur most commonly during the first two decades of life; however, they are not uncommonly seen in adults. They are essentially limited to the rectum, but the small intestine and stomach may be involved in cases of juvenile polyposis (see the section on polyposis). In a United States study of autopsied patients younger than 21 years of age, the incidence of juvenile polyps is 1%.[43] In Cali, Colombia, autopsy studies of children under 14 years of age reveal an incidence of 3.1%.[8] In Jordanians the calculated incidence is 1.6 per 100,000 of the total population and 2.8 per 100,000 in people under 10 years of age.[44] In general, the frequency of occurrence of juvenile polyps is not fully appreciated. However, on the African continent, they appear to be the most common type of polyp seen, representing from 53% to 60% of all polyps seen in surgically obtained material.[41,42] In these African studies the age distribution is similar to that seen in Western countries. Although the solitary juvenile polyp is not inherited, it will be discussed further in the section on juvenile polyposis, which does have a genetic etiology.

Etiology and Pathogenesis. Some authors believe that juvenile polyps are hamartomatous in nature,[2] and others have indicated an inflammatory etiology.[45] Recent studies of patients with juvenile polyposis suggest that the initiating event is mucosal hyperplasia and the formation of small hyperplastic polyps.[46–48] This is followed by inflammation and ulceration with sealing off of the surface, obstruction, and subsequent dilatation of crypts and the formation of a characteristic juvenile polyp.

Clinical Aspects. Juvenile polyps occur most commonly as solitary lesions (85% to 90% of the cases) localized mainly in the rectum. In the childhood and adult groups, rectal bleeding is the most common presenting symptom, occurring in approximately 80% of the patients. Abdominal cramps are an associated symptom. In the childhood group, approximately 20% present with prolapse or protrusion of the polyp; in about 10% of children the polyp is first discovered when it has been spontaneously passed in the stool (autoamputation).

Juvenile polyps are a benign proliferation and do not undergo neoplastic change. However, recently there have been two reports of adenomatous change in patients with solitary juvenile polyps[44,49] and three reported cases of adenocarcinoma arising in solitary juvenile polyps.[44,47,50] Another case involves a 17-year-old female patient with two juvenile polyps and a concomitant villous adenoma with carcinoma *in situ*.[51] The clinical manifestations and neoplastic changes associated with juvenile polyposis will be discussed under the section on polyposis.

Pathology. On gross examination, juvenile polyps have a smooth, glistening surface and are of a reddish-

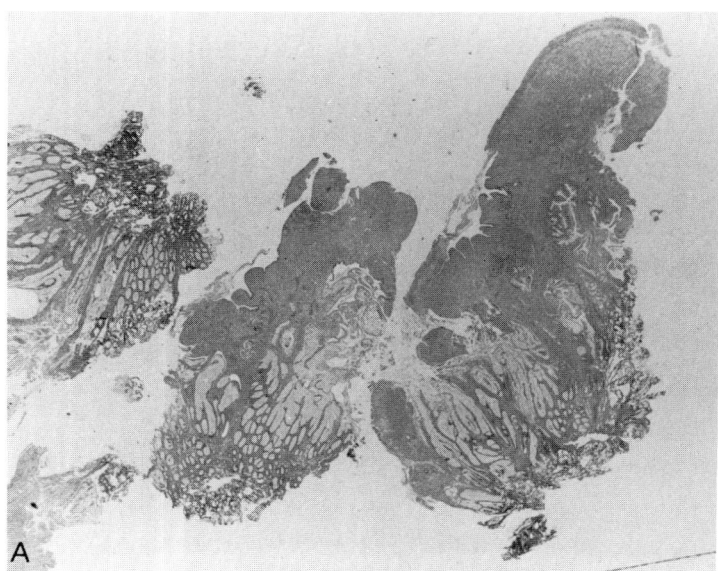
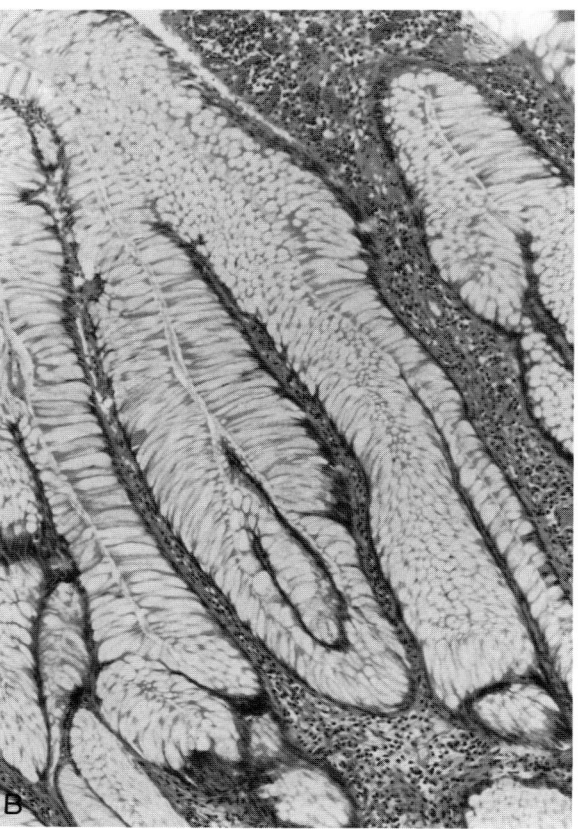
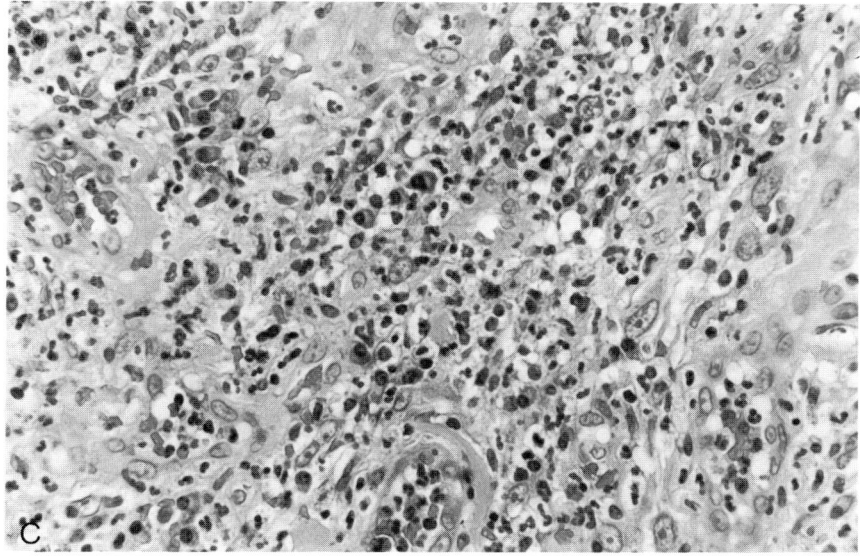

FIGURE 31–8. Colonic inflammatory pseudopolyp. *A*, The surface is capped with granulation tissue, and the basal glands are dilated and distorted. *B*, Medium-power view, showing distorted hypertrophic, benign goblet cells. *C*, High-power view of the cap of granulation tissue.

tan to red color (Figure 31–9). Cut section shows cystic spaces filled with grayish white or creamy yellow fluid. Most juvenile polyps are pedunculated, but occasionally they may be sessile.

In the "fully developed" juvenile polyp cystically dilated glands are seen in an inflamed stroma (Figure 31–10). The glands, which are often tortuous, may be made up of well-formed mucus-secreting cells. When the glands are filled with mucus the epithelial cells may be attenuated. Pink regenerative epithelium, similar to that in hyperplastic polyps, can be seen in 45% of the cases. When the cystically dilated glands mature they incite an inflammatory reaction in the stroma. Occasionally areas of osseous metaplasia are evident. The microscopic appearance of early juvenile polyps may be easily confused with that of inflammatory pseudopolyps, which appear as a cap of florid granulation tissue sitting on top of cystically dilated or hyperplastic crypts.

Although they are nonneoplastic, solitary juvenile polyps have been associated with adenomatous or carcinomatous change, but this is rare.[45,48,50,51] Neoplastic

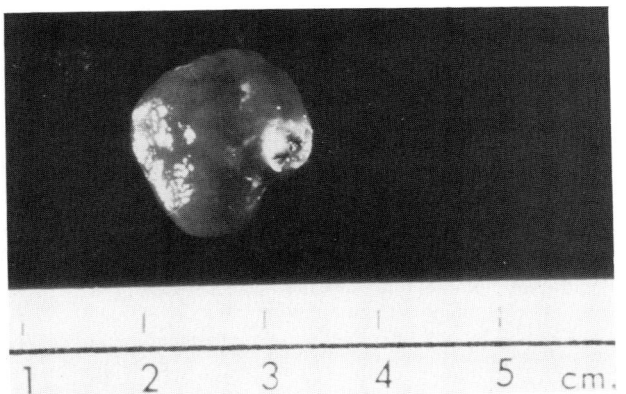

FIGURE 31–9. Juvenile polyp of the colon showing a smooth shiny surface. These polyps are of a tan, reddish color. In this instance the point of transection by fulguration can be appreciated.

Lymphoid Polyps

Lymphoid polyps occur mainly in the rectum and occasionally in the ileum. They occur in all age groups but most commonly in the second to fifth decades of life. They may be found incidentally or may occasionally cause symptoms such as rectal bleeding, discomfort, or prolapse. Lymphoid polyps vary in size from a few millimeters up to 3 cm. Approximately 80% of polyps are sessile and 20% are pedunculated. The polyps are solitary in 80% of the cases, but occur in groups of two to six in the remaining 20%. Microscopically they consist of prominent lymphoid follicles with active ger-

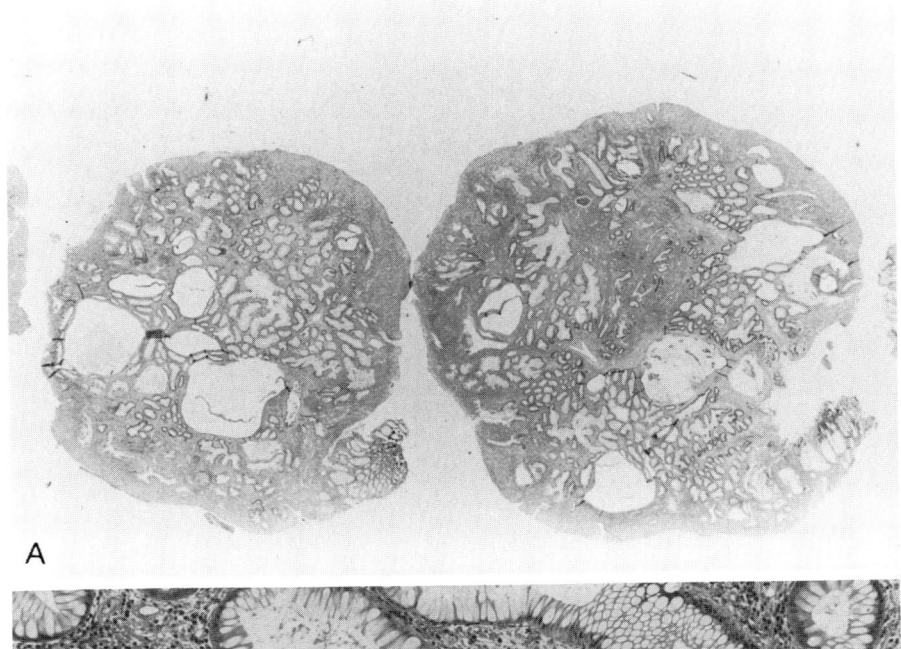

FIGURE 31–10. Juvenile polyp of the colon. *A*, Whole-mount section. There are cystically dilated glands interspersed with distorted branching glands. The intervening stroma is expanded. *B*, Branching glands. The epithelium is totally benign.
Illustration continued on following page

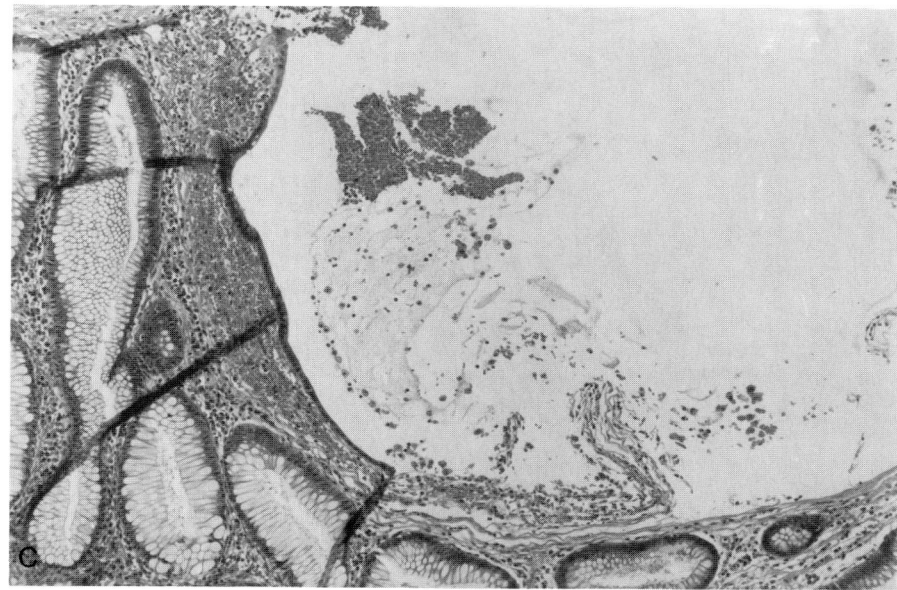
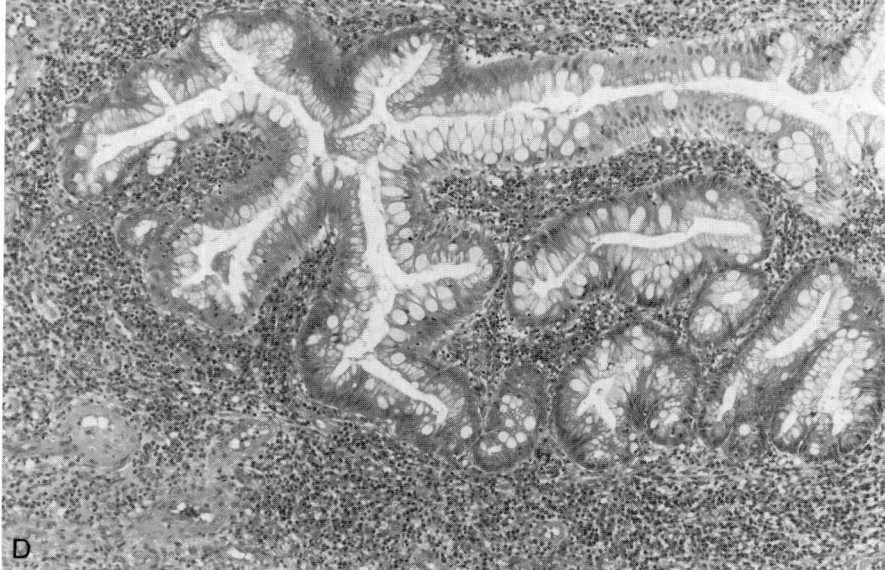

FIGURE 31–10 *Continued* C, Cystically dilated glands filled with mucin and polys. *D,* Focus of hyperplastic epithelium.

minal centers. These lymphoid aggregates are located mainly in the mucosa and the submucosa; however, they rarely may involve the muscularis propria. Local excision is curative, and recurrence is rare. Occasional spontaneous remission of these lesions has been noted.[52–53]

NEOPLASTIC POLYPS

Adenoma

Adenomas are benign neoplastic polyps of the small and the large intestines and are classified as either tubular, tubulovillous, or villous. Each of these lesions is not a different entity; rather, the classification serves to identify the characteristic growth pattern of adenomatous epithelium. Adenomas are important clinically because they are premalignant lesions that have the potential for developing into cancer. Although this chapter concerns polyps of both the small and the large intestines, the reader should be aware that adenomas are rare in the small intestine (except in hereditary polyposis syndrome) and quite common in the large intestine. Therefore, small-intestinal adenomas will be discussed briefly.

Incidence, Epidemiology, and Site Distribution. The incidence or prevalence of colonic adenomas varies in different parts of the world. Colonic adenomas tend to be fairly common in Western cultures (as high as 60% in one autopsy study[54]) and rare in underdeveloped countries (as low as 5.5% in another autopsy study[8]). All autopsy studies regardless of geographic location show an increased incidence of adenomas as the population ages, especially for the group 60 years of age and older.[8,54-56] In fact, in Cali, Colombia, the incidence of adenomas rises to 20% in the population over 65 years of age.[8] Although adenomas usually appear singly, it is important to be aware that they may occur in groups (synchronous and metachronous). Two large colonoscopic studies from New York[57] and London[58] report an incidence of multiple adenomas (two or more) as 36% and 50%, respectively. Autopsy studies have shown multiple lesions in 2% to 16% of the population,[8,54-56] the lower percentage reported from underdeveloped countries. This multiplicity is also related to age, because the older the population, the greater the chance for multiple lesions. As regards the incidence of histologic types of adenomas, most autopsy studies report that of all adenomas, 95% are tubular, 2% to 4% are tubulovillous, and the remaining lesions are villous.[8,54-56,59,60] For colonoscopic material, however, the incidence of tubular adenomas is 65% to 85%; of tubulovillous adenomas, 16% to 27%; and of villous adenomas, 3% to 9%.[57,58,61]

The incidence of adenomas generally parallels the incidence of cancer and the socioeconomic gradient, both of which are related to the Western lifestyle and diet. Race and country of origin, *per se,* do not have a role in the incidence of adenomas. Japanese and blacks who have migrated to Westernized societies take up the incidence of their new environment.[6]

Small-intestinal adenomas are found in the duodenum, particularly in the periampullary region. Distribution of colonic adenomas will vary depending on whether data were obtained from autopsy or colonoscopic material. Most colonoscopic studies report that 75% of adenomas occur in the left colon with the great preponderance in the sigmoid colon.[57,58,61] Autopsy studies report an even distribution of adenomas throughout the entire length of bowel.[54,56,59-60] This discrepancy may be explained on the basis of size of the polyp. Most adenomas less than 1.0 cm in size tend to show an even distribution throughout the entire large intestine, whereas those greater than 1.0 cm tend to be located in the distal colon. It is easier to identify smaller lesions in careful autopsy studies than in colonoscopic studies. In fact, 88% of adenomas in autopsy material tend to be under 1.0 cm in size whereas only 48% of adenomas in colonoscopic material are under 1.0 cm in size.

Etiology. Hypotheses regarding the etiology of adenomas have accounted for both genetic and environmental factors. Hill et al. have proposed that there is a recessive gene (p) that leads to the potential for development of adenomas.[62] Thus persons who carry two p genes (pp) would have a tendency for development of adenomas. However, the development of an adenoma would be predicated solely on some environmental factor working on the pp population. Furthermore, other environmental factors act on the already formed adenoma to transform it into a cancer. As mentioned previously, those Japanese and blacks who have left their native lands and moved to new environments in the West have a much greater incidence of adenomas than do those who remain in their native environment.[6] See Chapter 6 for a detailed discussion of the genetics of adenomas.

Clinical Aspects. In patients with adenomas, the predominant symptom is rectal bleeding, followed by varying symptoms of altered bowel habits, abdominal pain, flatulence, and mucus discharge. However, more and more patients today have no symptoms but are discovered with the multiple screening techniques (e.g., test for occult blood, barium enema, and colonoscopy) used in the population over 40 years of age.

Polyp Cancer Sequence. The major clinical significance of adenomas is that they are precancerous lesions, i.e., adenomas may undergo change into carcinomas. This is true for both large-bowel adenomas and small-intestinal adenomas. The polyp cancer sequence discussed relates to the large bowel only. Two major types of studies—epidemiologic and morphologic (size, histologic type, and atypia)—were used.

Many studies have shown that the incidence of adenomas parallels the incidence of large-bowel carcinoma[6,7,8]. In general, those countries with low rates of colon cancer have low rates of adenomas. In Cali, Colombia, where the incidence of colon cancer is low, the incidence of adenomas is 5.5%.[8] São Paulo, Brazil,[6] and Japan,[7] which have an intermediate incidence of colon cancer, have a 13% to 35% incidence of adenomas; countries with a high risk for colon cancer have a 50% to 65% incidence of adenomas.[6] The Akita prefecture of Japan has an intermediate incidence of colon cancer (30%), and the Miyagi prefecture has a low incidence (18%).[7] When these two groups were compared, the Akita prefecture was found to have a greater number of larger adenomas and adenomas with more atypia (dysplasia). While the parallel findings between adenomas and cancers tend to hold true, autopsy studies from Oslo[56] and northern Norway[59] showed an almost identical incidence of adenomas, although the incidence of colon cancer is 70% higher in Oslo than in northern Norway. Similarly, an autopsy study from Hong King[60] showed an incidence and distribution of adenomas similar to the data from Oslo; however, the cancer rate in Oslo is two times that in Hong Kong.

The relationship between sites and greatest number of adenomas and cancers is also important in the polyp cancer sequence. Most colon cancers arise in the distal colon; however, autopsy studies report an even distribution of polyps throughout the large intestine, whereas colonoscopic studies report a predominance of the left side. It must be remembered that such data must be considered in conjunction with other factors such as size and dysplasia as related to site. In conclusion, smaller adenomas tend to be distributed evenly throughout the large intestine, whereas larger adenomas with dysplasia tend to be located in the sigmoid colon.[54,55,57,58,61] In addition, size and dysplasia play important roles in the malignant transformation of adenomas.

The size of an adenoma is related to its malignant potential. A colonoscopic study from New York of 7000 endoscopically removed polyps revealed that carcinoma *in situ* was found in 5% of adenomas less than

1.0 cm, in 13% of adenomas from 1.0 to 1.9 cm, and in 18% of adenomas from 2.0 to 2.9 cm in size. It also noted that invasive cancer was present in 0.5% of adenomas under 1.0 cm, in 5% of adenomas from 1.0 to 1.9 cm, and in 10% of adenomas from 2.0 to 2.9 cm in size.[57] In another colonoscopic study from St. Mark's Hospital, of 49 adenomas with invasive cancer, 2.0% were less than 1.0 cm, 41% were from 1.0 to 1.9 cm, and 57% were 2.0 cm or larger.[58] An earlier study from the same institution found malignant changes in 1.3% of adenomas under 1.0 cm, in 9.5% of adenomas from 1 to 2 cm, and in 46% of adenomas over 2.0 cm in size.[63,64] Other studies have noted a relationship between size and site.[55,57,58,61] Lesions larger than 2.0 cm tend to be located in the sigmoid colon, the region of the large intestine with the greatest incidence of cancer.

The type of adenoma, or its growth pattern, has a role in its malignant potential. Large colonoscopic studies have shown that the incidence of carcinomatous change is higher in villous than in tubular adenomas, tubulovillous adenomas have an intermediate incidence.[57,58,61] In these studies the incidence of invasive cancer was 2% to 3% in tubular adenomas, 6% to 8% in tubulovillous adenomas, and 10% to 18% in villous adenomas. In a large study from St. Mark's Hospital, tumors that were partially malignant and partially benign were examined for the relative frequency with which the three different histologic types of adenomas occurred.[64] Investigators found that 33% of these lesions had a tubular adenoma component, 31% had a tubulovillous component, and 36% had a villous adenoma component. Considering that tubular adenomas are found more frequently than villous adenomas, one might determine that the villous growth pattern has a greater propensity for malignant change. When the size of the adenoma and its histologic type are considered, the incidence of invasive cancer in lesions smaller than 1.0 cm is 0.3% in tubular adenomas, 1.5% in tubulovillous adenomas, and 2.5% in villous adenomas; in lesions larger than 2.0 cm the incidence of invasive cancer is 6.5% in tubular adenomas, 11.4% in tubulovillous adenomas, and 17% in villous adenomas. These data show that although size is important in predicting malignant potential, villous adenomas of any size have a greater propensity for malignant changes than do tubular adenomas. Similar studies by Morson support this.[63] Another growth pattern that may be associated with a high malignant potential is the flat adenoma. Wolber and Owen[63a] noted that high-grade epithelial dysplasia was present in 41% of flat adenomas (<1.0 cm in diameter), compared with 4% of polypoid tubular adenomas of the same size. These flat adenomas may be precursors of small, flat, ulcerative carcinomas.

Atypia or dysplasia (defined in the section on pathology) is an important marker or determinant in the polyp cancer sequence. Colonoscopic studies have found that the sigmoid colon is the portion of the large intestine with the highest incidence of adenomas that show advanced dysplasia (*in situ* cancer or severe dysplasia).[57,58] This correlates with the major site for colon cancer. An autopsy study from Japan found that the Akita prefecture (with an intermediate incidence of colon cancer) had a statistically significant higher percentage of adenomas with dysplasia than did the Miyagi prefecture (with a low incidence of colon cancer).[7] Another autopsy study compared the incidence of dysplasia in adenomas among three different populations with different rates of cancer.[65] The respective incidences of dysplasia in Cali, Colombia, São Paulo, Brazil, and New Orleans were low, intermediate, and high, paralleling the rates of colon cancer in these regions. In the same study, among the different types of adenomas, the incidence of malignant change parallels the degree of dysplasia. The incidences of invasive cancer in tubular adenomas, tubulovillous adenomas, and villous adenoma with mild dysplasia were 2.0%, 13.9%, and 36.2%, respectively. In adenomas with severe dysplasia the incidence of invasive cancer rises to 27%, 34%, and 50% in tubular adenomas, tubulovillous adenomas, and villous adenomas, respectively. It would appear that severe dysplasia is a good marker for malignant change.

What is the time sequence for transformation from adenoma to cancer? A study of four patients with adenomas who were not treated for various reasons may lend insight.[64] Cancer developed in three of these patients at 5, 6, and 13 years of observation. The fourth patient was followed for 11 years, and when the adenoma was removed it was found to be benign. This observation suggests that the adenoma-to-cancer sequence, when it occurs, rarely takes less than 5 years but may average 10 to 15 years. Similarly, studies of patients with familial polyposis show a time interval of 12 years between detection of adenoma and the development of cancer.[64] It must be remembered, though, that these patients with polyposis have hundreds of adenomas and that their risk of cancer is much greater than that of the patient with only one or two adenomas. The relationship between adenoma and carcinoma is also discussed in Chapter 32.

Pathology. For adequate evaluation of the pathology of an adenoma in the polypectomy specimen, particularly when a malignancy is suspected, it is important that the specimen be grossly examined carefully so that the tissue is cut properly for optimal orientation. If this initial handling is done improperly, the information obtainable from the specimen may be inadequate. All polyps should be adequately fixed prior to sectioning. Larger lesions may require overnight fixation; however, most lesions smaller than 1.5 cm in diameter require less fixation. We have found that after 2 to 3 hours of fixation, most smaller lesions can be cut and allowed to fix for another 3 hours prior to processing. The gross lesion should be carefully examined for a stalk or pedicle. If a stalk or pedicle is short or absent, the transected site can be identified by the diathermy work, which is a white or tan color. The polyp should be transected longitudinally so that the slide shows all the landmarks in continuity (Figure 31–11).

When examining an adenoma, one must be familiar

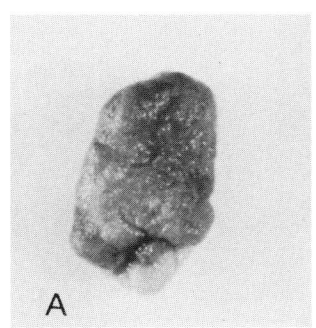 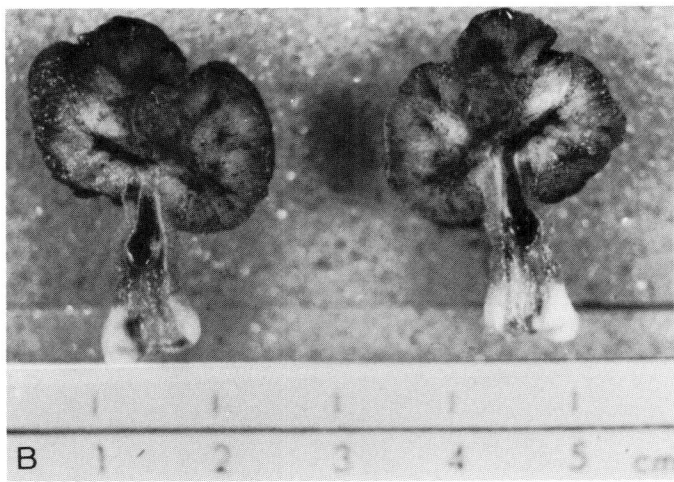

FIGURE 31–11. Adenoma of the colon. *A,* Surface view of an adenoma with a short stalk, *B,* Another adenoma with a long stalk, bisected after fixation. All important landmarks can be appreciated.

with its normal histologic landmarks, which become important for proper reporting of these lesions, especially those with cancer. The adenoma consists of three major regions: the head, the neck, and the stalk. The stalk consists of the nonneoplastic epithelium that makes up the pedicle of the adenoma. The point where the stalk meets the adenomatous epithelium is the neck, and the remainder of the polyp is the head (Figure 31–12). The muscularis mucosae, another important landmark, separates the mucosa from the submucosa. The margin of resection can be determined by the histologic appearance of the electrocautery diathermy mark.

Small-Intestinal Adenoma. Adenomas of the small intestine are uncommon but are of either the tubular or the villous type. They are usually flat or sessile. Microscopically they consist of papillary fronds with adenomatous epithelium, as in the colonic adenomas. All degrees of dysplasia, including *in situ* and invasive cancer, can occur (Figure 31–13).

Large-Intestinal Adenoma. In general, adenomas may be pedunculated (stalked) or sessile (flat). It has been generally taught that tubular adenomas were always pedunculated and that villous adenomas were characteristically sessile. In general this is probably true; however, tubular adenomas may be sessile and villous adenomas may be pedunculated. On gross examination, tubular adenomas tend to be spherical and have a relatively smooth surface that is often divided into what appears to be "lobules," as a result of intercommunicating clefts in the head of the adenoma. The adenoma is often darker or redder than the surrounding mucosa. A stalk may be present (Figure 31–14). Villous adenomas tend to have a "shaggy" surface with obvious papillary fronds (Figure 31–15). In autopsy material 88% of adenomas are smaller than 1.0 cm;[54,55] in colonoscopy material 48% of adenomas are smaller than 1.0 cm, 35% are 1 to 2 cm in size, and 17% are larger than 2.0 cm.[61] In general there is a correlation between the lesion's size and its histologic type. Regarding adenomas less than 1.0 cm in size, 91% are tubular adenomas, 7% are tubulovillous adenomas, and 2% are villous adenomas. However, of lesions greater than 2.0 cm in size, 48% are tubular adenomas, 38% are tubulovillous adenomas, 12% are villous adenomas, and 2% are polypoid carcinomas.[61]

Irrespective of type, all adenomas consist of neoplastic (adenomatous) epithelium. The overall growth pattern determines whether an adenoma qualifies as tubular, tubulovillous, or villous. In tubular adenomas there is a proliferation of adenomatous epithelium that forms tubules, which are usually separated from each other by normal lamina propria. In the usual tubular adenoma, the tubules are regular with little branching or tufting (changes that are seen with increasing dysplasia). The epithelial cells themselves show enlarged nuclei, which are hyperchromatic and elongated in shape; stratification of nuclei is common. Mucin may be absent or present, and can vary from well-formed

FIGURE 31–12. Diagram of normal landmarks of a pedunculated adenoma. M, mucosa; MM, muscularis; SM, submucosa; MR, margin of resection.

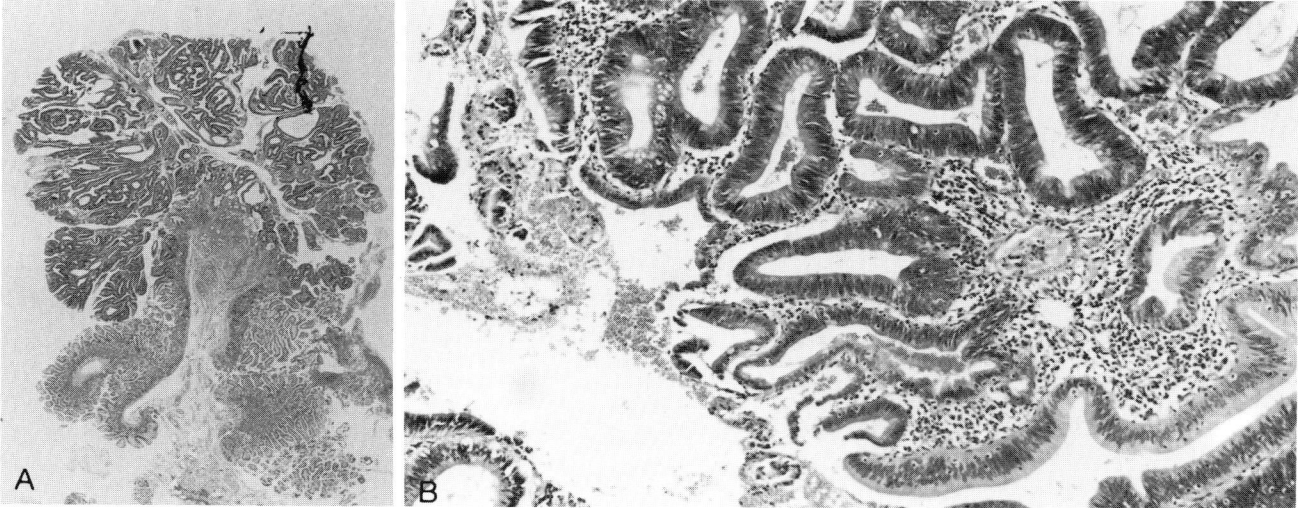

FIGURE 31–13. Small-intestinal adenoma. *A,* Whole-mount view. *B,* Microscopic view, showing classic changes of adenoma with hyperchromatic and stratifying nuclei.

goblets to small apical mucin vacuoles. In general the loss of mucin production correlates with degrees of dysplasia (Figure 31–16). In villous adenomas, one sees similar epithelial changes; however, the overall configuration is that of a growth of fine fingerlets or villi that project perpendicularly from the muscularis mucosae to the outer tip of the adenoma (Figure 31–17). Because many adenomas show mixed features of both tubules and villi, what determines the classification of a lesion as one or the other? Some authors say that if at least 80% of the lesion is either tubular or villous, then the lesion is classified as such, and all others as tubulovillous adenomas;[58] others use a standard of at least 75%.[57]

Adenomas can show degrees of dysplasia, the grading of which varies among observers. (British pathologists use the term *severe dysplasia* for what would be called *carcinoma in situ* by American pathologists.) In dysplasia one sees irregularity of the glands with infolding and buckling. The dysplastic epithelial cells tend to have hyperchromatic nuclei, and mucin production is often reduced (Figure 31–18). *In situ* cancer, or severe dysplasia, is diagnosed when a gland has a cribriform pattern. Mitoses are increased, and occasionally necrosis is present (Figure 31–19). In adenomas one may occasionally see foci of Paneth cell metaplasia, squamous metaplasia, and melanocytic metaplasia. In a study of 5778 adenomas or adenomas with cancer (3215 patients), squamous metaplasia, Paneth cell metaplasia, and melanocytic metaplasia were seen in 0.44%, 0.20%, and 0.017% of adenomas, re-

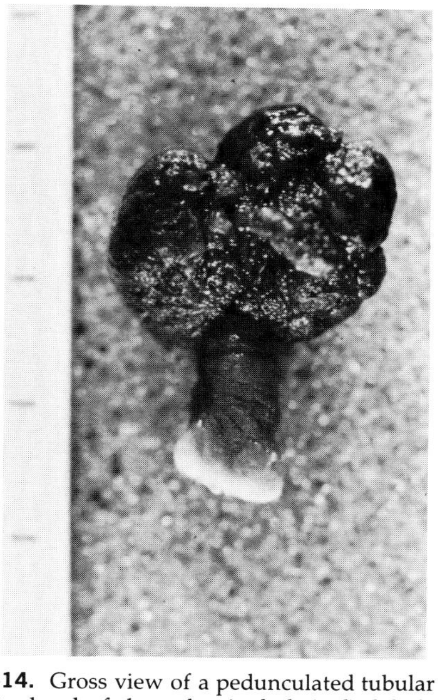

FIGURE 31–14. Gross view of a pedunculated tubular adenoma of the colon. The head of the polyp is dark (red), lobulated, and fissured. A long stalk (pedicle) is obvious.

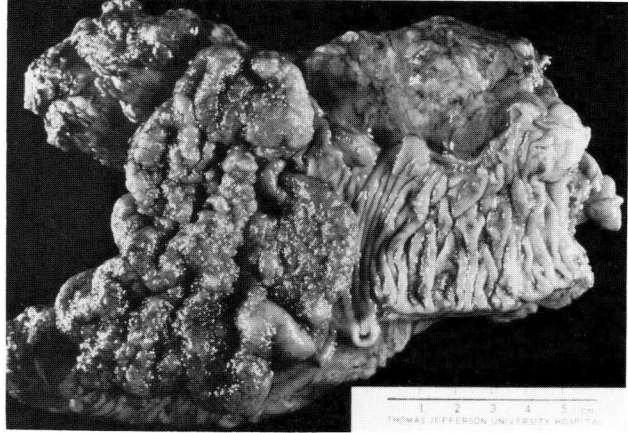

FIGURE 31–15. Gross photograph of a large villous adenoma. This lesion is spreading and sessile in nature.

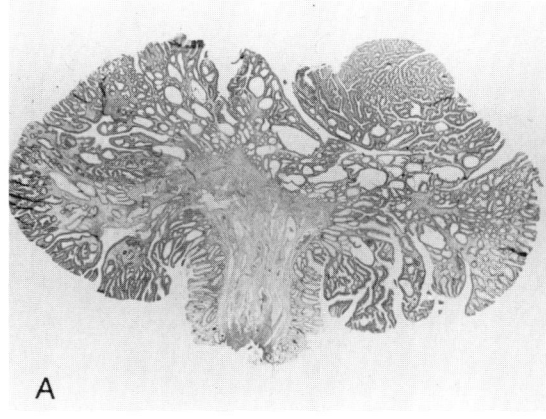
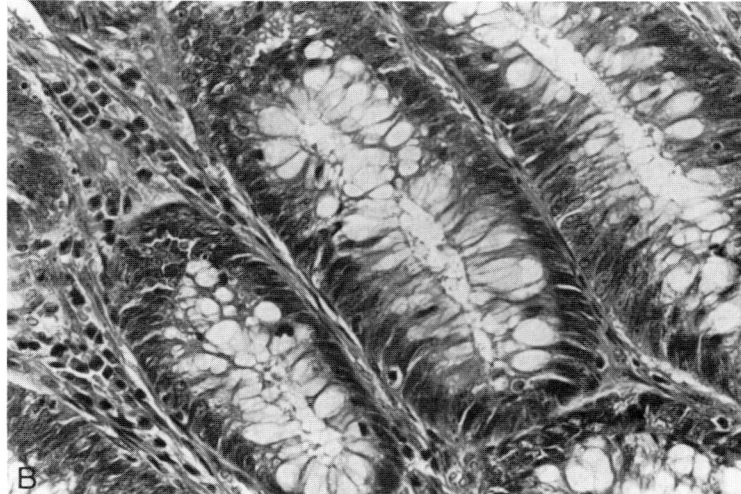
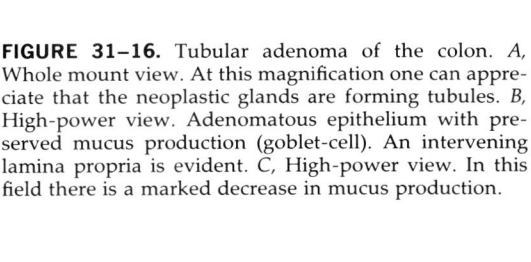
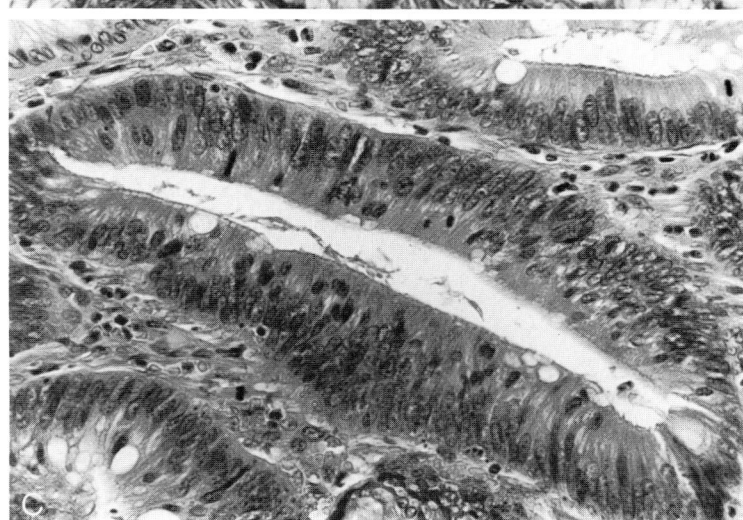

FIGURE 31-16. Tubular adenoma of the colon. *A,* Whole mount view. At this magnification one can appreciate that the neoplastic glands are forming tubules. *B,* High-power view. Adenomatous epithelium with preserved mucus production (goblet-cell). An intervening lamina propria is evident. *C,* High-power view. In this field there is a marked decrease in mucus production.

spectively.[66] The Grimelius stain was positive in 63% of all adenomas with metaplasia, and Paneth cells showed immunoreactivity with lysozyme. Occasionally squamous metaplasia may be so extensive that a diagnosis of adenoacanthoma is warranted.[67] There have been reports of adenomas with areas that could be called carcinoid,[68] and of adenomas with areas of small cell carcinoma.[68a]

Special Studies. Sulfomucins and sialomucins are the major carbohydrate-protein complex in goblet cell mucin. Both sulfomucins and sialomucins stain blue with the alcian blue stain at pH 2.5, whereas at pH 1.0 only sulfated mucins stain blue. The high iron diamine/Alcian blue stain will stain sulfated mucins brownish black and sialomucins blue. Neutral mucins (PAS-positive) are also present in goblet cells but are not a significant component.[69] Adenomas present a variety of mucus patterns, the quality and quantity of secretions differing from area to area. The majority of adenomas secrete a mixture of sialomucins and sulfomucins. Excess sialomucin may be seen in larger polyps, but polyps with severe dysplasia show no consistent pattern.[70] Using the PAT/KOH/PAS stain, Culling et al. found that normal colonic mucosa stains red and adenocarcinomas stain blue.[19] This is caused by the presence of O-acylated sialomucins in normal mucosa and reduced O-acylation of sialic acid in adenocarcinomas. Adenomas tend to stain both red and purple (owing to the mixture of normal O-acylation and reduced O-acylation); however, no benign lesions stained blue. Using the PAT/KOH/PAS stain, Greaves et al. noted that in the incidental adenomas, there essentially was no reduction in O-acylated sialomucins; however, loss of O-acylated sialomucins was observed in 14 of 47 patients with synchronous adenomas, mainly those with focal severe dysplasia.[70]

Lectins are glycoproteins that have the ability to bind to specific carbohydrate moieties. Various authors have used lectins to study changes in glycoconjugates in adenomas. PNA binding in adenomas has produced conflicting data. Cooper and Reuter have found that PNA binds to adenomas in a heterogeneous fashion.[21] Goblet cells bind PNA in the Golgi region, whereas columnar cells bind PNA in the glycocalyx/apical cytoplasm. (The Golgi pattern is seen in normal epithelium and hyperplastic polyp, and the glycocalyx/apical pattern

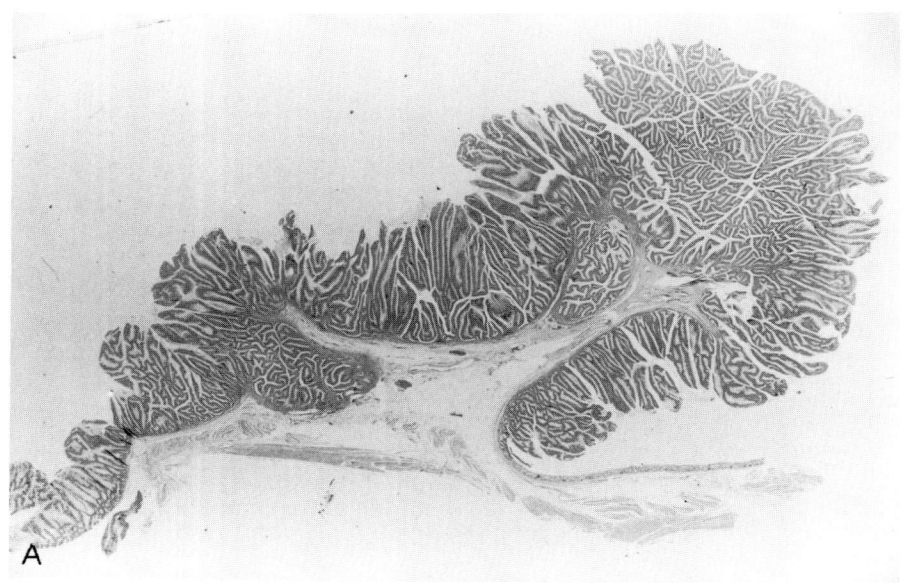
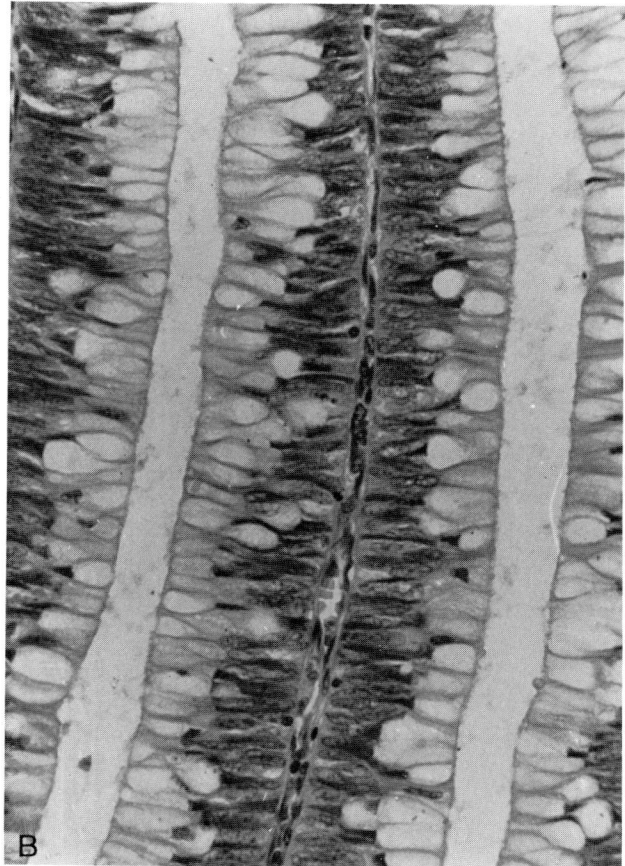

FIGURE 31–17. Villous adenoma of the colon. *A,* Whole-mount view. One can appreciate that the neoplastic epithelium is thrown up into villous projections. *B,* High-power view. The nuclei are stratified and atypical in nature. In this instance mucin production is preserved.

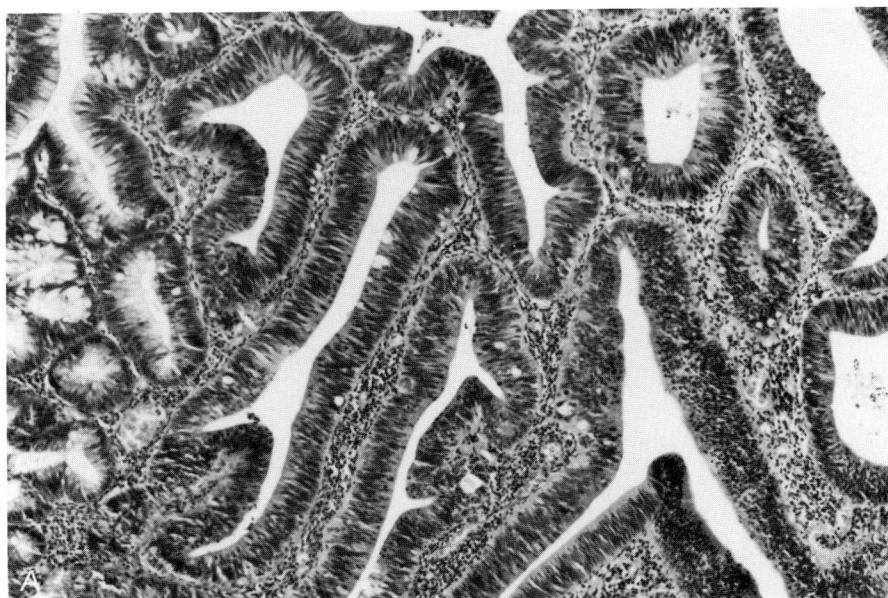
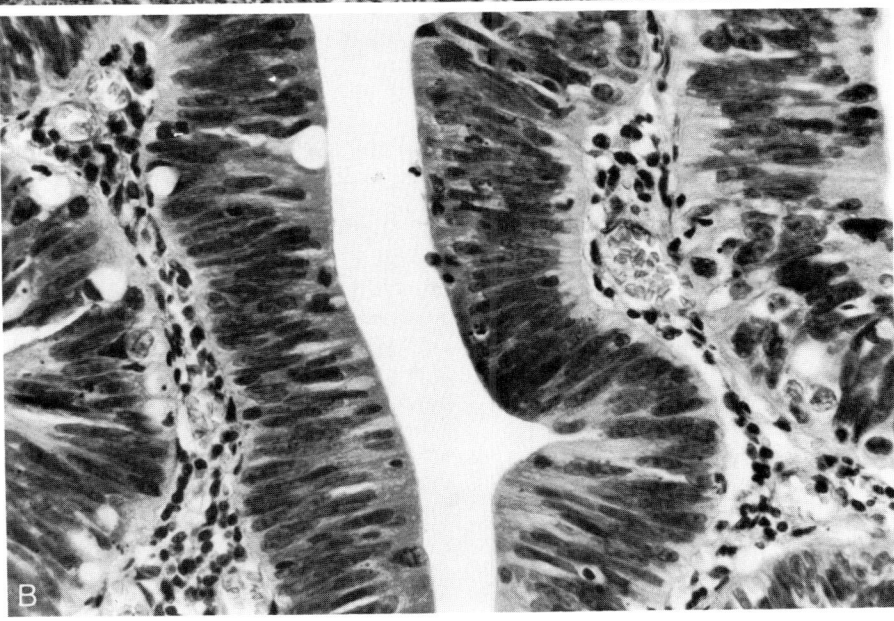

FIGURE 31–18. Colonic adenoma with dysplasia. *A,* Low-power view. The glands are tortuous and show buckling. *B,* High-power view, showing loss of mucin and presence of stratified hyperchromatic nuclei.

is noted in cancers.) Boland et al. have noted that in adenomas, PNA will bind to the actual goblet cells, findings they previously noted in cancers.[22] The lectin dolichos biflorus (DBA), which recognizes terminal GalNAc, binds to normal goblet cells; however, like cancers, adenomas show decreased binding of DBA.[22] Ulex Europaeus (UEA) reacts with α-fucose. The cells of the distal colon usually do not react with UEA. However, like cancers, adenomas of the distal colon express UEA–binding sites.[71]

Adenomatous lesions have been studied with antibodies against tumor-associated antigens (TAAs). Earlier studies used polyclonal antibodies, but more recent studies have used monoclonal antibodies (MAbs). Many of these studies have presented conflicting data.

Carcinoembryonic antigen (CEA) was one of the earlier TAAs studied. Isaacson and LeVann found immunoreactive CEA only in cancers.[72] CEA was not found in the vast majority of adenomas, but they did note focal staining in three adenomas with dysplasia. Burtin et al. found that CEA was in all adenomas.[73] Skinner and Whitehead noted that 16 of 22 adenomas had immunoreactive CEA.[23] O'Brien et al. noted that some CEA was found in virtually all 62 adenomas they studied.[74] Adenomas that showed severe dysplasia had the greatest amount of CEA. Within severely dysplastic adenomas, CEA reactivity was usually confined to areas of dysplasia and cancer. Both O'Brien et al.[74] and Skinner and Whitehead[23] reported that CEA reacted with normal colonic epithelium. It must be cautioned that

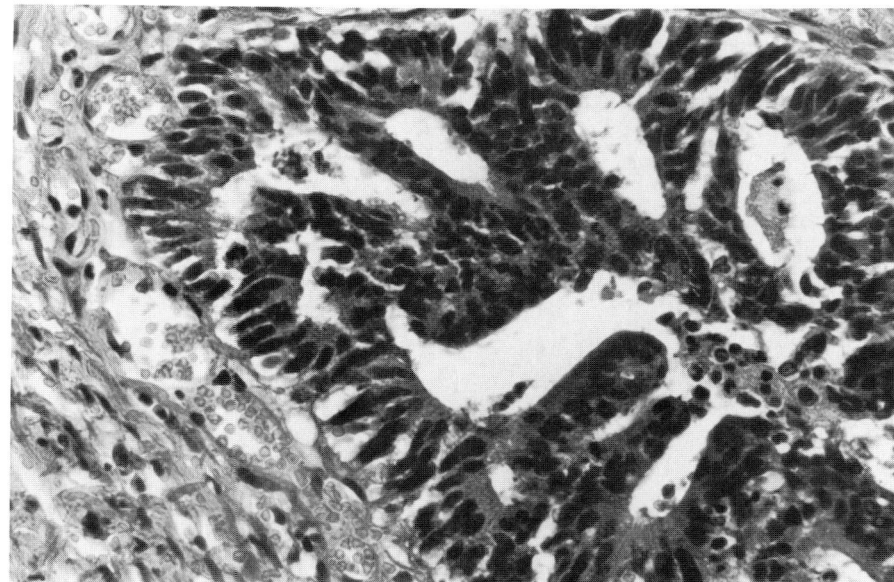

FIGURE 31–19. High-power view of *in situ* adenocarcinoma. There is a cribriform pattern and central necrosis.

antibodies to CEA raised in goat or rabbit may cross-react with related glycoproteins that are found in normal and neoplastic colorectal tissue. Stramignoni et al. using MAb against CEA (10 µg/ml) found that 83% of adenomas showed reactivity; however, when more dilute MAbs were used (1 µg/ml), the percentage of adenomas staining for CEA was somewhat lower.[75]

The ABH blood group isoantigens are normally absent in the adult distal colon but are present in the fetal distal colon. Cooper et al. found that 41% of adenomas and 57% of cancers of the distal colon express these blood group antigens and hence show oncofetal antigens.[24] Bara et al. have studied the M_1 (oncofetal fetal fucomucin) in adenomas of the colon.[25] M_1 is found in the fetal distal colon but is absent in the adult. They found M_1 in 66% of the adenomas studied; however, M_1 was found in 94% of adenomas that had a concomitant carcinoma. They also found a statistically significant difference between villous adenomas and tubular adenomas with regard to M_1 expression.

MAbs against the Lewis y hapten have been used to study adenomas. This antigen is usually present only in the deep crypt cells of the normal colon. Brown et al. found reactivity in 100% of colonic adenomas.[76] Studies with MAb against the gastrointestinal cancer antigen (a sialylated Lewis a antigen) have shown that adenomas do indeed express this antigen as do cancers.[77,77a]

To date, these TAAs have not been of any diagnostic use but serve as an aid to understanding the basic biology of colonic neoplasia.

Adenoma with Cancer

Both small-intestinal and large-intestinal adenomas are precancerous lesions. The incidence of *in situ* cancer arising in colonic adenomas is 12.3%, whereas the incidence of invasive cancer arising in colonic adenomas is about 5%.[57] The term *malignant polyp* should be restricted to those adenomas (or polypoid carcinoma) in which there is true invasive cancer. The term *invasive cancer* should be used to describe only those lesions in which cancer has invaded beyond the muscularis mucosae into the submucosa. The lymphatics of the colon are closely associated with the muscularis mucosae, and only after the cancer has invaded into the submucosa does it have the biologic potential for metastasis. Cancer that is limited to the mucosa has been termed carcinoma *in situ* or intramucosal cancer; and although both entities are morphologically cancer, they have no biologic potential for metastasis. Some researchers say that *carcinoma in situ* describes malignant changes within the crypt or the gland, whereas *intramucosal cancer* describes cancer that has "invaded" into the lamina propria and elicits a desmoplastic reaction.

Pathology. *In situ* cancer (severe dysplasia) is diagnosed when there is bridging or cribriform growth of epithelial cells with accompanying cytologic atypia. Intramucosal cancer shows the same epithelial changes; however, the cancer invades the mucosal stroma and elicits an inflammatory or desmoplastic reaction. In many adenomas the muscularis mucosae is quite irregular and appears splayed or splintered. This must be considered when a lesion with intramucosal or *in situ* cancer is examined, as this disordered muscularis mucosa may trap the uninitiated observer into making an incorrect diagnosis of invasive cancer. Invasive cancer should be diagnosed only when tumor cells have invaded beyond the muscularis mucosae into the submucosa.

In the case of an adenoma with invasive cancer, the following parameters should be reported: (*a*) extent of cancer (limited to head, neck, stalk invasion), (*b*) histologic grade of the cancer, (*c*) status of the resection

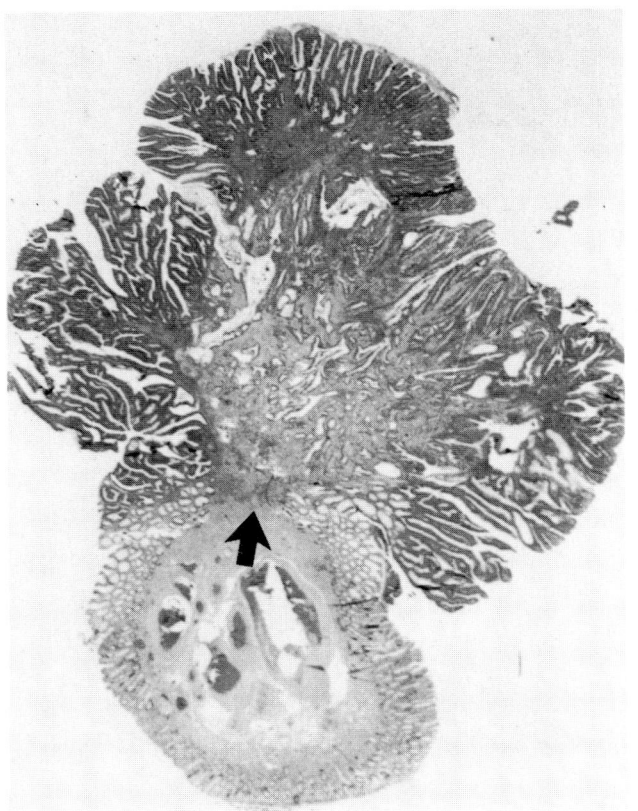

FIGURE 31-20. Pedunculated (long stalk) adenoma of colon with invasive cancer limited to the head of the polyp and up to the neck (arrow).

margin, and (d) the presence or absence of lymphatic invasion (Figures 31-20 to 31-24).

Patient Management in Large-Intestinal Malignant Polyps. The pathologist plays an important role in the management of the patient with the endoscopically removed malignant polyp.

In general, the pathologist attempts to predict which histologic features can signal the presence of lymph node metastases or local disease. Overall, the incidence of lymph node metastasis in endoscopically removed malignant polyps is approximately 10%.[78] However, in a large study from St. Mark's Hospital, Morson et al. reported that the incidence of lymph node metastases was 0%.[79] When cancer is limited to the head of the polyp, the incidence of lymph node metastases is essentially zero,[79-81] except when the cancer is grade III or when lymphatic invasion is present. These poorly differentiated cancers behave quite aggressively, the incidence of lymph node and distant metastasis being 66% for grade III cancers.[80] The significance of lymphatic invasion is currently a controversial issue. Cooper noted that one of six (17%) lesions with lymphatic invasion had lymph node metastases;[80] however, the sole lesion was a grade III cancer. Haggitt et al. found metastasis in one of two patients with lymphatic invasion.[81] More cases of lymphatic invasion must be studied in order to ascertain its significance, but its presence probably does denote some unfavorable factor, the magnitude of which remains to be determined. Regarding the status of the resection margin, Morson et al. reported that even with tumor at the resection margin, there were no lymph node metastases, but 2 of 11 (18%) cases did show residual cancer at the polypectomy site.[79] Cooper reported that the incidence of lymph node metastases in those lesions with tumor at or near the resection margin was 21%, whereas the incidence of recurrence or residual disease was 4.1%.[80] Haggitt et al. noted that the incidence of lymph node metastases was 25% in those lesions in which cancer invaded to what they defined as level 4.[81] Regarding the entity of polypoid carcinoma, most authors would

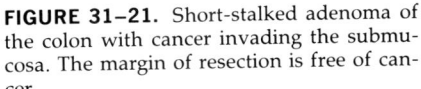

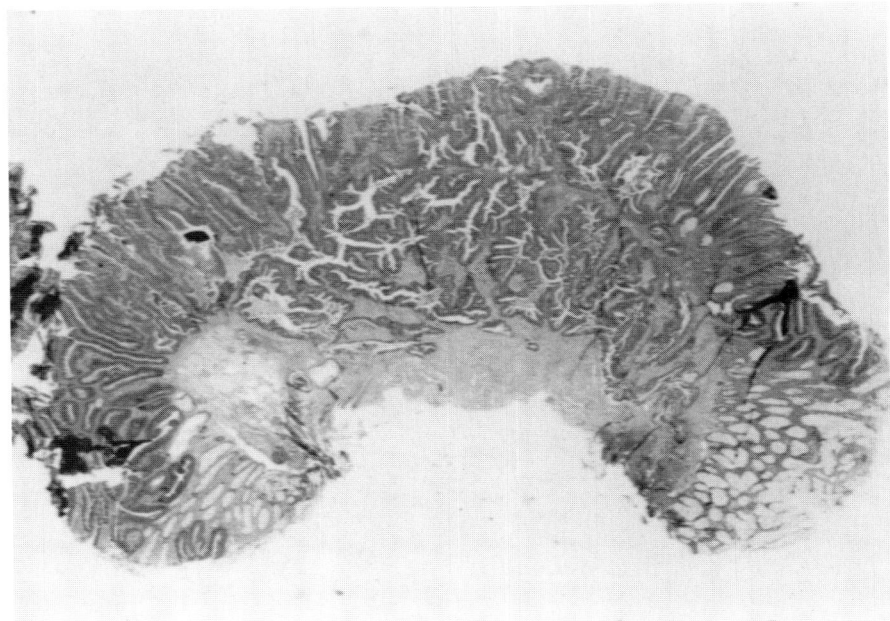

FIGURE 31-21. Short-stalked adenoma of the colon with cancer invading the submucosa. The margin of resection is free of cancer.

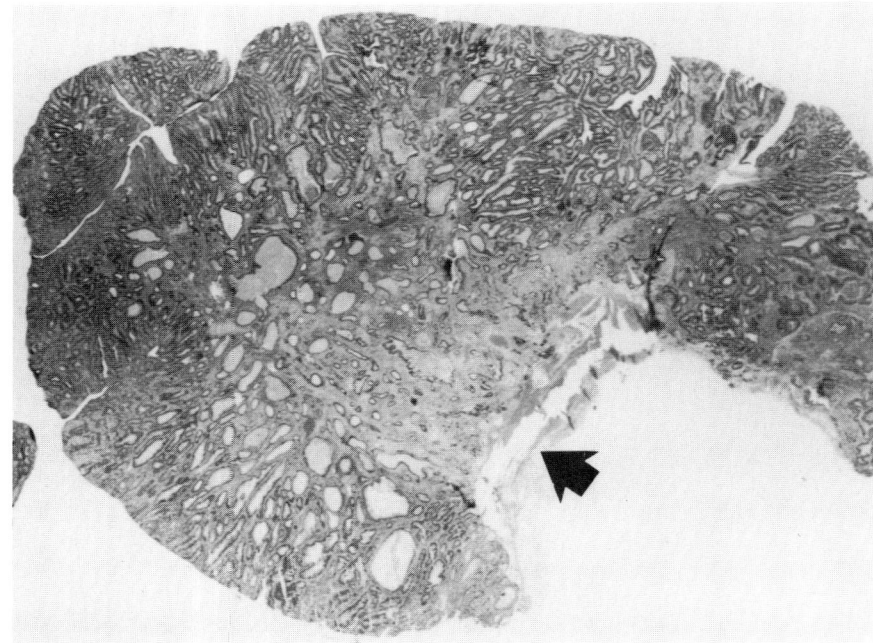

FIGURE 31-22. Sessile adenoma with invasive cancer extending to the transected margin of the resection (arrow).

agree that they are no more aggressive than malignant adenomas and should be treated under the same criteria.[80,81] Based on the studies cited,[79-81] the following guidelines are offered: Endoscopically removed malignant polyps should be treated with subsequent surgical resection if (*a*) the cancer involves the resection margin (or is close to it, less than 1.0 mm); (*b*) the cancer is grade III; or (*c*) lymphatic invasion is present (a controversial issue). For all other lesions, endoscopic polypectomy can be considered adequate. It is important to remember that if factors indicate that definite surgery is deemed necessary after polypectomy, no residual cancer or lymph node metastases will be found 70% to 80% of the time.[80]

Adenoma with Pseudoinvasion

Pseudoinvasion occurs when the mucosa of the polyp has been "misplaced" into the submucosa, and hence mimics invasive carcinoma. Other terms used to describe this entity are *epithelial misplacement* and *hamartomatous inverted polyps,* the latter term used also for colitis cystica. It is important to recognize pseudoin-

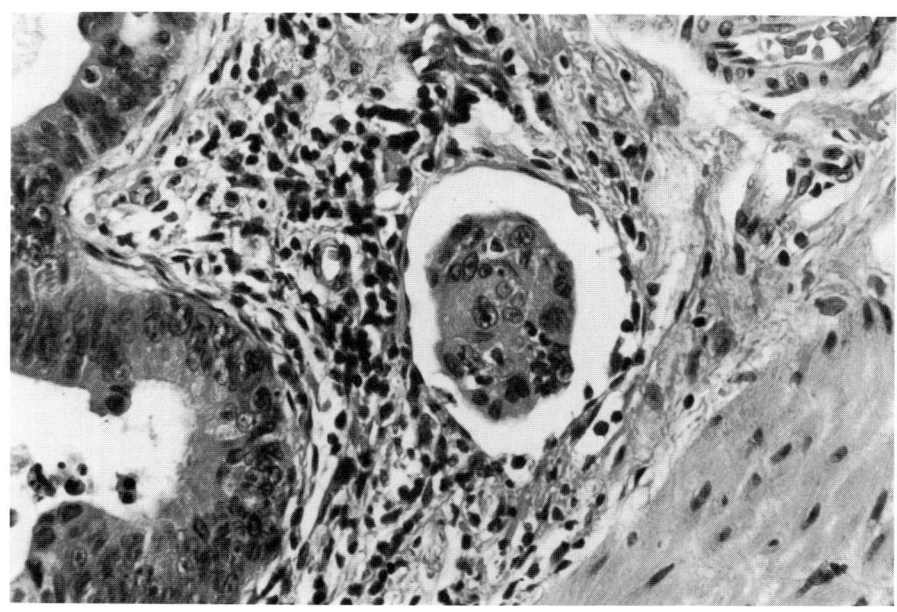

FIGURE 31-23. Malignant polyp with a tumor embolus in a lymphatic.

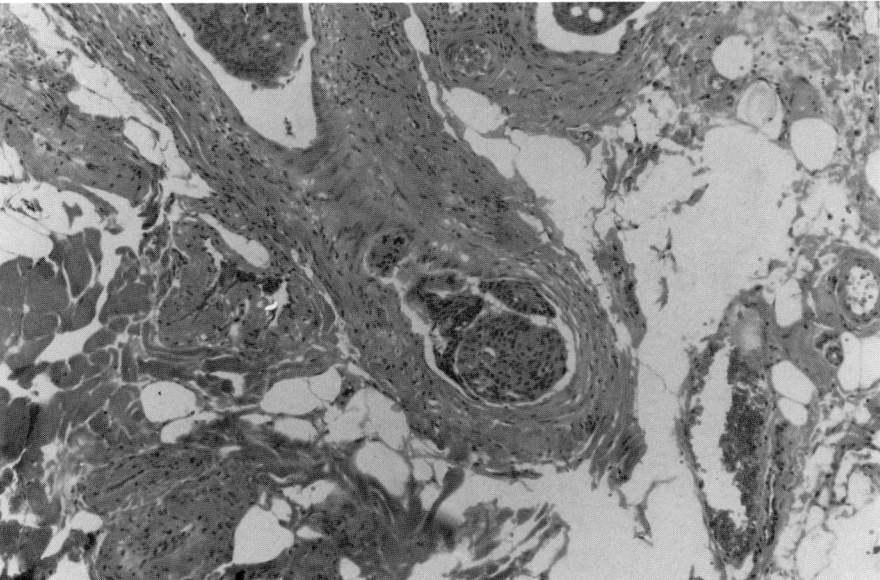

FIGURE 31–24. Malignant polyp with tumor emboli in muscular walled veins.

vasion so that a misdiagnosis of invasive carcinoma and unnecessary surgery are avoided. In one retrospective study it was reported that 18 of 21 cases of pseudoinvasion were originally diagnosed as some form of cancer.[82]

Incidence and Etiology. The incidence of pseudoinvasive adenomas in two large series of colonic lesions is 2.5% to 3.5%.[61,83] When one considers that 5% of adenomas will contain invasive cancer, the incidence of pseudoinvasion is not that uncommon. The male-to-female ratio is 3:1, and most of the polyps are located in the sigmoid colon and have long pedicles or stalks. The etiology probably has to do with rotation of the polyp's stalk and vascular compromise, which may act as a mechanical force that forces the mucosa to be misplaced and herniated into the submucosa through defects in the muscularis mucosae.[82,83]

Pathology. The basic pathology is that of misplaced benign epithelial structures in the submucosa, in contrast to truly invasive cancer, in which the malignant epithelial glands themselves infiltrate into the submucosa and elicit a desmoplastic reaction. In pseudoinvasion the misplaced structures consist of both epithelium and surrounding lamina propria (Figure 31–25). This may be somewhat analogous to adenomyosis in the uterus. These misplaced glands may be histologically normal epithelium or may show adenomatous changes, sometimes even with dysplasia. The submucosal glands often show cystic dilatation with rupture, causing leakage of mucin into the stroma and secondary inflammation. Often the submucosa shows extensive deposits of hemosiderin. Careful examination of the actual polyp will reveal whether the changes in the head of the lesion is cancerous or adenomatous. If the changes in the head are adenomatous, invasive cancer within an adenoma would be highly unlikely. Although many cases of pseudoinvasion are straightforward, there are some in which it is extremely difficult to differentiate pseudoinvasion from true invasive cancer.

POLYPOSIS SYNDROMES

Familial (Adenomatosis) Polyposis Coli

Familial polyposis coli (FPC) is an autosomal-dominant disorder in which the large intestine and rectum are carpeted with multiple adenomas.[84–86] (See Chapter 6 for a detailed discussion of the cytogenetics of FPC.) The number of adenomas ranges from hundreds to approximately 3000 (Figure 31–26). No true case of FPC has had fewer than 100 adenomas. The incidence of this disorder has been estimated to be 1 in 8000 births, 20% of which are the first instance in a family (a fresh mutation). The average age at detection in those patients who present with symptoms is 36.5 years. However, in those patients who are examined because of a family history of FPC, the average age at detection is 23.8 years. Adenomas usually do not appear before the age of 10; however, they have been reported rarely in younger children. Adenocarcinoma of the large intestine will develop in all patients who are left untreated. At the time of initial diagnosis, 67% of the probands will have colonic adenocarcinoma; however, only 7.5% of a screened group will have adenocarcinoma at initial examination.[86] The average age at diagnosis of adenocarcinoma in the FPC group is 39 years, which is at least 25 years younger than the average age of diagnosis of adenocarcinoma in the general population. The lesions in FPC are adenomas, and they are histologically similar to those seen in the non-

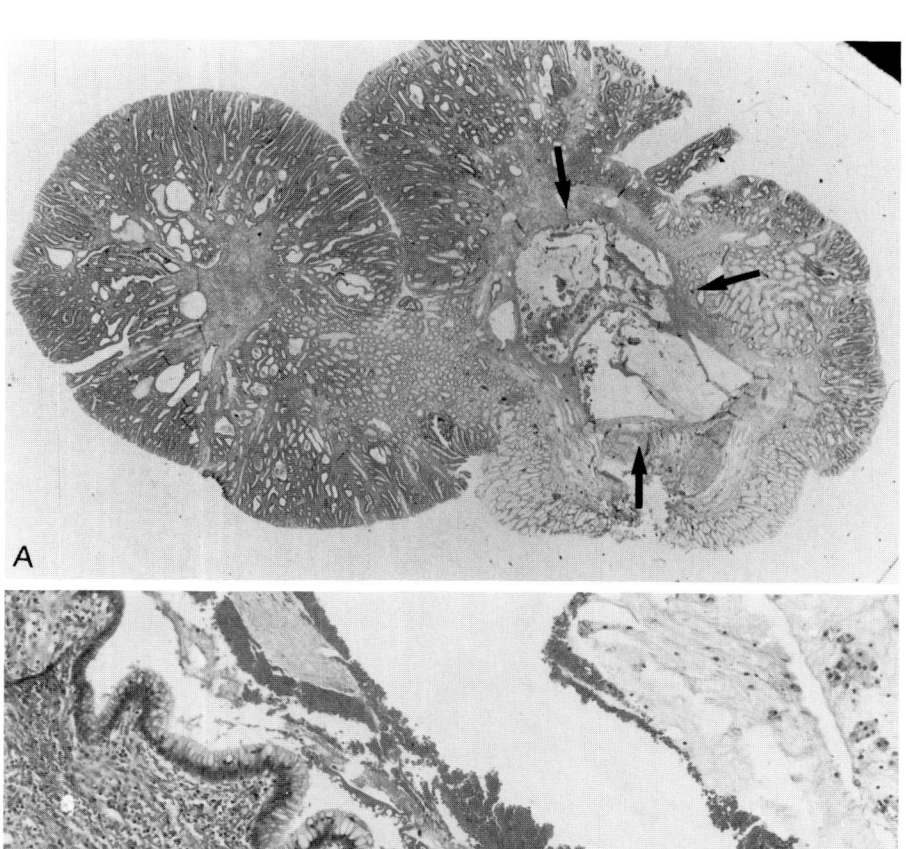

FIGURE 31-25. Colonic adenoma with pseudoinvasion. *A,* Cystically dilated epithelial structures are present in the submucosa of the stalk (arrows). *B,* Medium-power view of a pseudoinvasive submucosal gland. The gland is dilated and filled with blood and mucin. A lamina propria can be discerned surrounding this epithelial gland.

FPC patient. Samples of grossly normal mucosa can be examined, and microscopic adenomas consisting of only one or two glands may be found. Kinetic studies using tritiated thymidine have shown that histologically normal epithelial cells will show DNA synthesis at all levels of the crypt in contradistinction to the lower two-thirds seen in normal mucosa.[87] Additional information on kinetic studies is presented in Chapter 7. Mucin studies have shown that 82% of the flat mucosa (nonadenomatous) of patients with FPC will show decreased staining for O-acylated sialomucins,[88] findings noted also for colonic adenocarcinomas.[19] Studies with the lectin UEA, which detects an α-fucose, have shown that in FPC the histologically normal goblet cells of the distal colon will express UEA-binding sites, whereas the histologically normal goblet cells in the non-FPC population do not express UEA-binding sites.[89] Finally, one should be aware of the following reports: that patients with FPC may have benign lymphoid polyps of the terminal ileum,[90] and that a member of an FPC family had multiple benign lymphoid polyps of the colon and ileum and no adenomas.[91]

Gardner's Syndrome

Gardner's syndrome is an autosomal-dominant disorder that comprises the following triad: intestinal polyposis, soft tissue abnormalities, and abnormalities of bone.[84-86] The intestinal polyps are adenomas and occur mainly in the large intestine and rectum; adenomas may also occur in the stomach and small intestine. Also noted in the stomach are benign polyps that

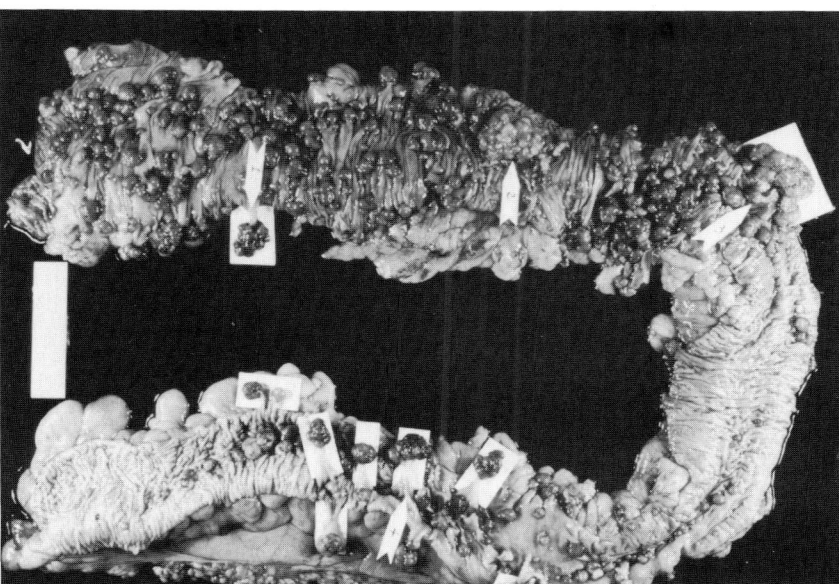

FIGURE 31–26. Gross specimen from patient with familial polyposis coli. Numerous adenomas of varying sizes can be appreciated.

have been called fundic gland polyps (see Chapter 23). Benign lymphoid polyposis of the ileum has been associated with this syndrome.[92,93] There is an increased incidence of adenocarcinoma of the pancreatic duodenal region. Cancers have also been reported in the thyroid gland and the adrenal gland. The soft tissue lesions are epidermal cysts, fibromas, lipomas, and desmoid tumors (occurring postoperatively or spontaneously). The bony lesions are osteomas and cortical thickening of the long bones and ribs. Dental abnormalities such as impacted teeth, supernumerary teeth, and dental cysts have been reported. At times, the soft tissue abnormalities may precede the intestinal manifestations by years. The colonic manifestations, numbers of adenomas, and the incidence of large-bowel cancer are as described for the FPC syndrome.

Turcot Syndrome

Turcot syndrome was originally described in two siblings with polyposis coli who developed malignant brain tumors.[85] This is probably an autosomal dominant disorder, but this is somewhat controversial. The lesions are adenomas, and the malignant potential may be the same as in FPC; however, patients may die of central nervous system lesions prior to the onset of intestinal carcinoma. The author has seen one 21-year-old male patient who had a glioblastoma multiforme and a rectal adenocarcinoma.

Juvenile Polyposis Syndrome

The subject of juvenile polyposis is quite complex and confusing. This disorder represents a heterogeneous group: (a) some patients have polyps limited to the colon, while others have polyps that involve the stomach and small bowel also; (b) some cases are familial, others are not; and (c) some patients have coexisting separate adenomas, whereas others have juvenile polyps with adenomatous changes.[46–48,94–99] First, one must differentiate those with polyps limited to the colon (juvenile polyposis coli)[47,94–96] from those with polyps in the large intestine, small intestine, and stomach (generalized juvenile polyposis).[46,96–97] In juvenile polyposis the number of polyps ranges from dozens to hundreds; however, they are not as numerous as in FPC. In general, one-third of the patients have a familial or genetic history that probably indicates autosomal dominance. Extraintestinal congenital anomalies have been reported in both familial and nonfamilial cases. The various anomalies reported are malrotation of the gut, mesenteric lymphangioma, hypertelorism, amyotonia congenita, hydrocephalus, tetralogy of Fallot, coarctation of the aorta, thyroglossal duct cyst, and idiopathic hypertrophic subaortic stenosis.[44,99] Patients with the polyposis syndrome present different clinical and pathologic findings than patients with solitary polyps. An increased but undetermined risk for development of large-bowel cancer in patients with the polyposis syndrome has been reported. These cancers have been reported to arise either in juvenile polyps or separately. There is one report of a kindred with associated gastric and colon cancer.[100] In this group the cancers occurred in relatives who had no juvenile polyps themselves. The pathology of the polyps is more variable than in the nonpolyposis patients. All patients have obvious classic polyps; however, others have polyps with features of both juvenile polyps and adenomas (mixed polyps). In some cases one can see concomitant separate adenomas and juvenile polyps.

Peutz-Jeghers Syndrome

The Peutz-Jeghers syndrome is an autosomal-dominant disorder of hamartomatous polyps associated with mucocutaneous pigmentation.[84-86,101] The polyps are located in the stomach and the small and large intestines. The number of polyps is usually counted in the dozens rather than in the hundreds, as it is in FPC. Most patients are diagnosed in their twenties, and the male-to-female ratio is one. The clinical symptoms vary depending upon the location of the polyps. Most patients present with GI complaints, such as obstruction, abdominal pain, bloody stools, and anal extrusion (in decreasing order of frequency). Obstruction and abdominal pain are associated with small-intestinal polyps, and bloody stools and anal extrusion with large-intestinal and rectal polyps. Approximately 23% of cases are initially diagnosed because of changes in pigmentation, consisting of melanin deposition forming spots or freckles that usually appear in infancy or early childhood. Pigmentation occurs on the lips, buccal mucosa, eyelids, digits, and rarely the intestinal mucosa. The pigmentation in the lips is the most consistent finding, but this tends to fade with age. Also associated with the syndrome is the presence of sex cord tumors with annular tubules of the ovary,[102] well-differentiated adenocarcinoma of the uterine cervix, and bilateral breast cancers.[102a]

A series of 222 Japanese patients with Peutz-Jeghers syndrome reported the following distribution of polyps: 49% had gastric polyps, 64% had small-intestinal polyps, 53% had colonic polyps, and 32% had rectal polyps.[32] In a series of 182 patients with Peutz-Jeghers at the Mayo Clinic, 24% of the patients had gastric polyps, 96% had small-intestinal polyps, 26% had colonic polyps, and 24% had rectal polyps.[103] In the Japanese study colonic polyps were twice as frequent as in the Mayo Clinic study, but the Mayo Clinic reported a much higher frequency of small-intestinal polyps.

The pathologic features of these polyps are described earlier in this chapter.

One major area of controversy has been whether there is a real association between this syndrome and malignancy. In the earlier literature it was claimed that malignant change in a Peutz-Jeghers polyp ran as high as 24%.[104] This claim is obviously false, but the interpretation of malignancy can be accounted for by the appearance of an unusual admixture of epithelial cells and smooth muscle bundles. Once the hamartomatous nature of these lesions was recognized, so was the fact that malignant change is uncommon. To date there have been eight documented cases of cancers arising in Peutz-Jeghers polyps of the small bowel.[27-32,34] Three of these have had lymph node metastases, two have been truly invasive adenocarcinomas, and three were *in situ* lesions. There have also been reports of three rectal adenocarcinomas arising in Peutz-Jeghers polyps (one invasive and two *in situ*).[31,33,105] Reid has estimated that 2% to 3% of patients with the Peutz-Jeghers syndrome will develop a GI malignancy, mainly in the duodenal region.[106] In a Japanese study of 222 histologically documented cases of Peutz-Jeghers syndrome, 15 (6.7%) had "early cancers" (three in the stomach, eight in the small intestine, and four in the intestine) and 11 (4.9%) had "advanced cancer" (three in the stomach, one in the small intestine, one in the small and the large intestines, and six in the large intestine).[32] However, the authors could document histologically malignant change in only two Peutz-Jeghers polyps. It is not known whether the cancers arose in Peutz-Jeghers polyps or in nonhamartomatous mucosa. Recent studies have shown an increased risk of both gastrointestinal and extraintestinal cancers in 48% of patients reported by Giardiello et al.[106a] and 22% of patients reported by Spigelman and associates.[106b] In the latter group, four of nine gastrointestinal cancers actually arose in Peutz-Jeghers polyps.

Cronkhite-Canada Syndrome

The Cronkhite-Canada syndrome (CCS) is a nonhereditary disorder of GI polyposis associated with alopecia, nail atrophy, and hyperpigmentation of the skin.[107,108] Since it was first described in 1955,[107] approximately 50 cases have been reported in the literature. CCS is noted worldwide, and unlike most cases of intestinal polyposis, the lesions first appear in late adult life, with approximately 80% of patients being 50 years or older at onset. The male-to-female ratio is close to one. The clinical symptoms (in decreasing order of frequency) are diarrhea, weight loss, abdominal pain, anorexia, weakness, and hematochezia. The physical findings are nail changes (dystrophy, thinning, and splitting), hair loss, and pigmentary changes. Hair loss usually occurs rapidly over a period of weeks and has been noted in all parts of the body. It is of interest that regrowth of hair has been noted after therapy or during spontaneous remission. Pigmentary changes include hyperpigmentation (lentigo-like area) and white patchy vitiligo. Approximately 50% of the cases are fatal, usually secondary to cachexia, anemia, and so forth. Supportive therapy may provide long-term remission; in fact it has been reported that polyps may decrease in size or number.[108] At present, surgery is recommended only for complications such as prolapse, bowel obstruction, or malignancy. Present data indicate that the potential risk for development of intestinal cancer is not great enough to indicate colectomy, although to date there have been seven reported cases of colorectal cancer arising in conjunction with CCS.[108-110]

The polyps of CCS are found in the stomach, small intestine, colon, and rectum and may be sessile or pedunculated. Histologically the polyps are identical to juvenile polyps. One sees tortuous glands that are cystically dilated and filled with inspissated mucus (Figure 31-27). The lamina propria is edematous and inflamed. However, in CCS, the intervening nonpolypoid mucosa shows cystic dilatation of crypts and inflammation and edema in the lamina propria (Figures 31-27 and 31-28). There have been a few reports of adenomatous changes in these polyps.[109,110]

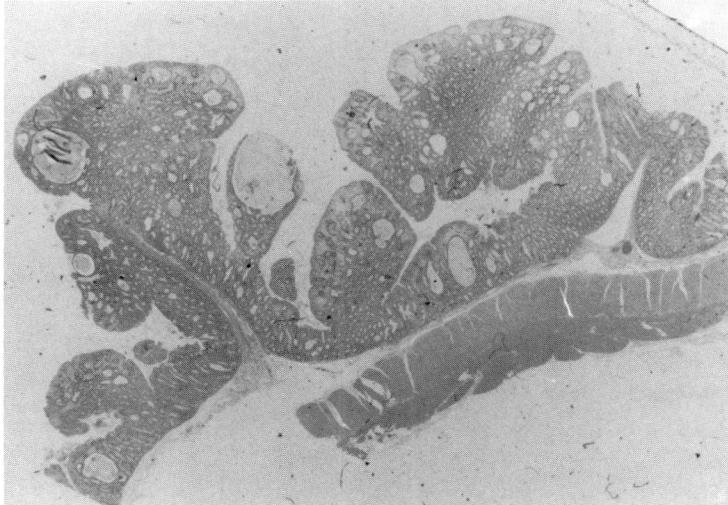

FIGURE 31-27. Whole-mount view of Cronkhite-Canada polyps. The polypoid mucosa shows cystically dilated glands. Also note that the intervening flat mucosa has cystically dilated glands. (Courtesy of Dr. Klaus Lewin, University of California, Los Angeles, Los Angeles, California.)

Cowden's Disease

Cowden's disease is an uncommon autosomal-dominant disorder. In Cowden's disease one sees facial trichilemmomas, acral keratosis, and oral mucosal papillomas. This disorder is also associated with breast and thyroid cancer. Cowden's disease is mentioned under the polyposis syndromes because one can see numerous colonic and small-intestinal polyps. Some have described these as hamartomatous lesions,[111] consisting of a mildly fibrotic, mildly disordered mucosa overlying a submucosa that displayed disorganization and splaying of smooth muscle fibers. These lesions show some similarities to the pathology seen in the solitary rectal ulcer syndrome. Other authors reported polyps that were described as inflammatory lesions, lipomas, and ganglioneuromas.[112]

Intestinal Ganglioneuromatosis

Intestinal ganglioneuromatosis is a familial disorder that has been associated with the multiple endocrine neoplasia syndrome, type 2b, and with Recklinghausen's disease.[113-116] There may be a diffuse proliferation of ganglioneuromatous elements, which at times may be polypoid. In some instances, the ganglioneuromatosis has been found in association with juvenile polyposis and adenomas.[115,116]

Lymphoid Polyposis

Multiple benign lymphoid polyposis of the large bowel has been reported. Most cases occurred in children.[91,117] Histologically similar to the solitary lymphoid polyps of the rectum, lymphoid polyposis consists of prominent active lymphoid nodules in the mucosa and submucosa (Figure 31-29). The lesions are entirely benign and in some cases have been reported to disappear spontaneously. In one series there was a family history of lymphoid polyposis.[117] In another report, a 12-year-old boy with a family history of familial adenomatosis coli was found to have multiple lymphoid polyps and no adenomas.[91] In patients with fam-

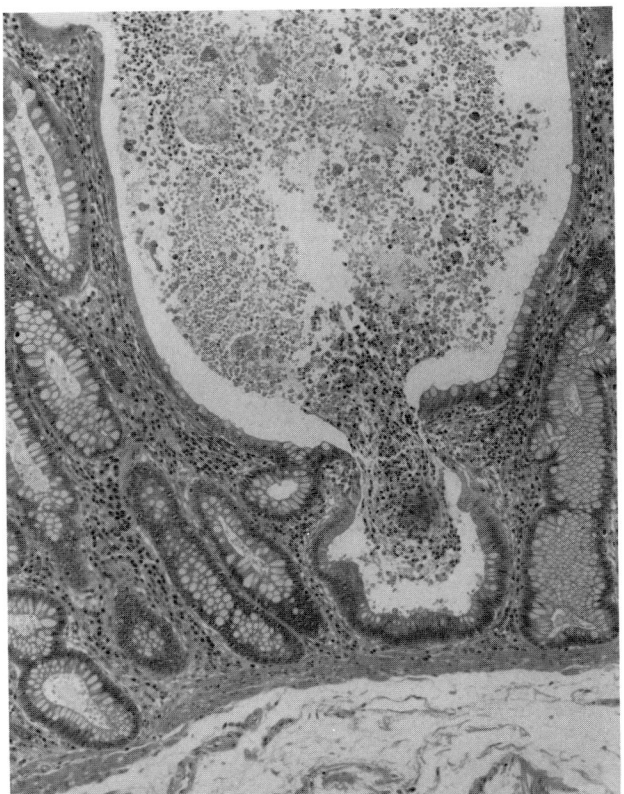

FIGURE 31-28. Flat, intervening mucosa in Cronkhite-Canada syndrome. There is a dilated gland filled with mucus and leucocytes. The epithelium is benign. (Courtesy of Dr. Klaus Lewis, University of California, Los Angeles, Los Angeles, California.)

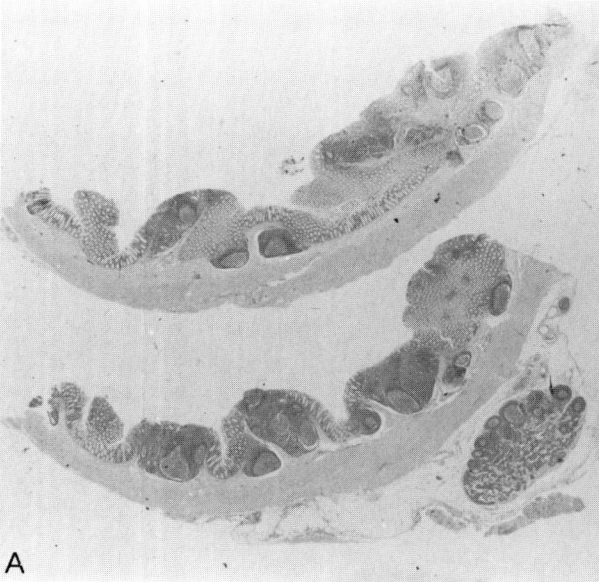
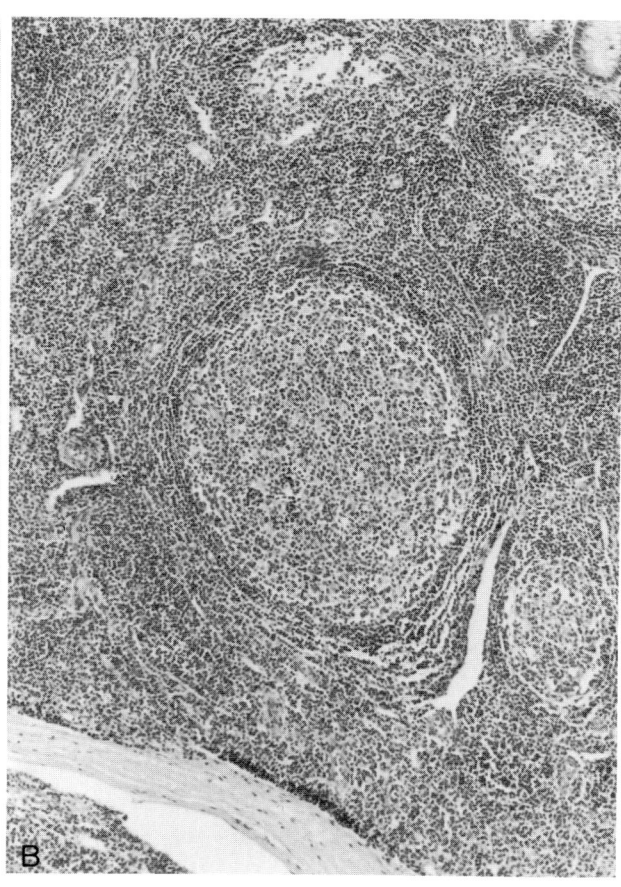

FIGURE 31-29. Lymphoid polyposis of the colon. *A*, Whole-mount view. One can appreciate that the polyps are due to prominent mucosal and submucosal lymphoid tissue. *B*, Microscopic view, showing lymphoid nodules with prominent germinal centers.

ily histories of polyps it is essential to determine the exact histologic nature of the lesions so that unnecessary surgery is not performed. Benign lymphoid polyposis of the terminal ileum has been reported in patients with Gardner's syndrome and familial polyposis coli.[90-93]

References

1. Arthur JF: Structure and significance of metaplastic nodules in the rectal mucosa. J Clin Pathol 21:735-743, 1968.
2. Morson BC: Some peculiarities in the histology of intestinal polyps. Dis Colon Rectum 5:337-344, 1962.
3. Lane N, Kaplan H, Pascal RR: Minute adenomatous and hyperplastic polyps of the colon: Divergent patterns of epithelial growth with specific associated mesenchymal changes; contrasting roles in the pathogenesis of carcinoma. Gastroenterology 60:537-551, 1971.
4. Lane N, Lev R: Observations on the origin of adenomatous epithelium of the colon: Serial section studies of minute polyps in familial polyposis. Cancer 16:751-764, 1963.
4a. Longacre TA, Fenoglio-Preiser CM: Mixed hyperplastic adenomatous polyps/serrated adenomas: A distinctive form of colorectal neoplasia. Am J Surg Pathol 14:524-537, 1990.
5. Estrada RG, Spjut HJ: Hyperplastic polyps of the large bowel. Am J Surg Pathol 4:127-133, 1980.
5a. Waye JD, Lewis BS, Frankel A, Geller SA: Small colon polyps. Am J Gastroenterol 83:899-906, 1988.
6. Correa P: Epidemiology of polyps in cancer. In Morson BC (ed): Pathogenesis of Colorectal Cancer. Philadelphia, WB Saunders, pp 126-152.
7. Sato E, Oughi A, Sussano N, Ishidate T: Polyps and diverticulosis of the large bowel in autopsy populations of Akita prefecture compared with Miyagi: High risk for colorectal cancer in Japan. Cancer 37:1316-1321, 1976.
8. Correa P, Duque E, Cuello C, Haenszel W: Polyps of the colon and rectum in Cali, Colombia. Int J Cancer 9:86-96, 1972.
9. Williams GT, Arthur JF, Busey HJR, Morson BC: Metaplastic polyps and polyposis of the colorectum. Histopathology 4:155-170, 1980.
10. Franzin G, Zamboni G, Scarpa A, et al: Hyperplastic (metaplastic) polyps of the colon: A histological and histochemical study. Am J Surg Pathol 8:687-698, 1984.
11. Hayoshi T, Yatani R, Apostal J, Stemmermann GN: Pathogenesis of hyperplastic polyps of the colon: A hypothesis based on ultrastructural and in vitro cell kinetics. Gastroenterology 66:347-356, 1974.
11a. Risio M, Coverlizza S, Ferrari A, et al: Immunohistochemical study of epithelial cell proliferation in hyperplastic polyps, adenomas, adenocarcinomas of the large bowel. Gastroenterology 94:899-906, 1988.
11b. Cooper HS, Marshall C, Ruggierio F, Steplewski Z: Hyperplastic polyps of the colon and rectum: An immunohistochemical study with monoclonal antibodies vs. blood group antigens (Sialosyl-Le^a, Le^a, Le^b, Le^x, Le^y, A, B, and H). Lab Invest 57:421-428, 1987.
12. Cooper HS, Patchefsky AP, Marks G: Adenomatous and carcinomatous changes within hyperplastic colonic epithelium. Dis Colon Rectum 22:152-156, 1979.
13. Sumner HW, Wasserman NF, McClain CJ: Giant hyperplastic polyposis of the colon. Dig Dis Sci 26:85-89, 1981.
14. Whittle TS, Varner W, Brown FM: Giant hyperplastic polyp of the colon simulating adenocarcinoma. Am J Gastroenterol 69:105-107, 1978.
15. Goldman H, Ming SC, Hickok DF: Nature and significance of

hyperplastic polyps of the human colon. Arch Pathol 89:349–354, 1970.
16. Urbanski SJ, Kossakowska AE, Marcou NN, Bruce WR: Mixed hyperplastic adenomatous polyps, an underdiagnosed entity: Report of a case of adenocarcinoma arising within a mixed hyperplastic adenomatous polyp. Am J Surg Pathol 8:551–556, 1984.
17. Sobin LH: Inverted hyperplastic polyps of the colon. Am J Surg Pathol 9:265–272, 1985.
18. Jass JR, Filipe MI, Abbas S, et al: A morphologic and histochemical study of metaplastic polyps of the colorectum. Cancer 53:510–515, 1984.
19. Culling CFA, Reid PE, Worth AJ, Dunn WL: A new histochemical technique of use in the interpretation and diagnosis of adenocarcinoma in villous lesions of the large intestine. J Clin Pathol 30:1056–1062, 1977.
20. Kaye GI, Fenoglio CM, Pascal RR, Lane N: Comparative electron microscopic features of normal, hyperplastic, and adenomatous human colonic epithelium: Variations and cellular structure relative to the process of epithelial differentiation. Gastroenterology 64:926–945, 1973.
21. Cooper HS, Reuter VE: Peanut lectin binding sites in polyps of the colon and rectum: Adenomas, hyperplastic polyps and adenomas with in situ carcinoma. Lab Invest 49:655–661, 1983.
22. Boland CR, Montgomery CK, Kim YS: A cancer associated mucin alteration in benign colonic polyps. Gastroenterology 82:664–672, 1982.
23. Skinner JM, Whitehead R: Tumor associated antigens in polyps and carcinoma of the human large bowel. Cancer 47:1241–1245, 1981.
24. Cooper HS, Cox J, Patchefsky AS: Immunohistochemical study of blood group substances in polyps of the distal colon: Expression of a fetal antigen. Am J Clin Pathol 73:345–350, 1980.
25. Bara J, Languille O, Gendron MC, et al: Immunohistochemical study of precancerous mucus modification in human distal colonic polyps. Cancer Res 43:3885–3891, 1983.
26. Gibbs NM: Juvenile and Peutz-Jegher polyps. In Morson BC (ed): Pathogenesis of Colorectal Cancer. Philadelphia, WB Saunders, 1978, pp 33–42.
27. Perzin KH, Bridge MF: Adenomatous and carcinomatous changes in hamartomatous polyps of the small intestine (Peutz-Jeghers syndrome): Report of a case and review of the literature. Cancer 49:971–983, 1982.
28. Williams JP, Knudsen A. Peutz-Jeghers syndrome with metastasizing duodenal carcinoma. Gut 6:179–184, 1965.
29. Matuchanuky C, Babin P, Costrot S, et al: Peutz-Jeghers syndrome with metastasizing carcinoma arising from a jejunal hamartoma. Gastroenterology 77:1311–1315, 1979.
30. Shibata HR, Phillips MJ: Peutz-Jeghers syndrome with jejunal and colonic adenocarcinoma. Can Med Assoc J 103:285–287, 1970.
31. Cochet B, Carrel J, Desbaillets L, Widgren S: Peutz-Jeghers syndrome associated with gastrointestinal cancer. Gut 20:169–175, 1979.
32. Utsunomiya J, Gocho H, Miyanga T, et al: Peutz-Jeghers syndrome: Its natural course in management. Johns Hopkins Med J 136:71–82, 1975.
33. Miller LJ, Bartholomew LG, Dozois RR, Dahlin DC: Adenocarcinoma of the rectum arising in a hamartomatous polyp in a patient with Peutz-Jeghers syndrome. Dig Dis Sci 28:1047–1051, 1983.
34. Horn RC Jr, Payne WA, Fine G: The Peutz-Jeghers syndrome. Arch Pathol 76:29–37, 1963.
35. Bolwell JS, James PD: Peutz-Jeghers syndrome with pseudoinvasion of hamartomatous polyps and multiple epithelial neoplasms. Histopathology 3:39–50, 1979.
35a. Shepherd NA, Bussey HJR, and Jass JR: Epithelial misplacement in Peutz-Jeghers polyps: A diagnostic pitfall. Am J Surg Pathol 11:743–749, 1987.
36. Patterson MJ, Kernen JA: Epithelioid leiomyosarcoma originating in a hamartomatous polyp from a patient with Peutz-Jeghers syndrome. Gastroenterology 88:1060–1064, 1985.
37. Shimer GR, Helwig EB: Inflammatory fibroid polyps of the intestine. Am J Clin Pathol 81:708–714, 1984.
38. Benjamin SP, Hawk WA, Turnbull RB: Fibrous inflammatory polyps of the ileum and cecum: Review of five cases with emphasis on differentiation from mesenchymal neoplasms. Cancer 39:1300–1305, 1977.
39. LiVolsi VA, Perzin KH: Inflammatory pseudotumor (inflammatory fibrous polyp) of the small intestine, colon: A clinicopathological study. Am J Dig Dis 20:325–336, 1975.
40. Price AB: Benign lymphoid polyps and inflammatory polyps. In Morson BC (ed): Pathogenesis of Colorectal Cancer. Philadelphia, WB Saunders, 1978, pp 33–42.
41. Williams AO, Prince DL: Intestinal polyps in the Nigerian African. J Clin Pathol 28:367–371, 1975.
42. Mabogunje OA, Subbuswamy SG, Lawrie JH: Rectal polyps in Zaria, Nigeria. Dis Colon Rectum 21:474–479, 1978.
43. Helwig EB: Adenomas of the large intestine in children. Am J Dis Child 72:289–295, 1946.
44. Dajani YV, Kamal MF: Colorectal juvenile polyps: An epidemiological and histopathological study of 144 cases in Jordanians. Histopathology 8:765–779, 1984.
45. Roth SI, Helwig EB: Juvenile polyps of the colon and rectum. Cancer 16:468–479, 1963.
46. Goodman ZD, Yardley JH, Milligan FD: Pathogenesis of colonic polyps in multiple juvenile polyposis: Report of a case associated with gastric polyps and carcinoma of the rectum. Cancer 43:1906–1913, 1979.
47. Lipper S, Kahn LB, Sandler RS, Varma V: Multiple juvenile polyposis: The study of the pathogenesis of juvenile polyps and their relationship to colonic adenomas. Hum Pathol 12:804–813, 1981.
48. Grigioni WF, Alampi G, Martinelli G, Piccaluga A: Atypical juvenile polyposis. Histopathology 5:361–376, 1981.
49. Freeman CJ, Fechner RE: A solitary juvenile polyp with hyperplastic and adenomatous glands. Dig Dis Sci 27:946–948, 1982.
50. Tung-Hua L, Min-Chang C, Hsien-Chiu LC, Chieh L: Malignant change of juvenile polyp of the colon: A case report. Chin Med J 4:434–439, 1978.
51. Baptist SJ, Sabatini MT: Co-existing juvenile polyps in tubulovillous adenoma of colon with carcinoma in situ. Hum Pathol 16:1061–1063, 1985.
52. Ranchod M, Lewin KJ, Dorfman RF: Lymphoid hyperplasia of the gastrointestinal tract: A study of 26 cases and review of the literature. Am J Surg Pathol 2:383–400, 1978.
53. Corres JS, Wallace MH, Morson BC: Benign lymphomas of the rectum and anal canal: A study of 100 cases. J Pathol Bacteriol 82:371–382, 1961.
54. Rickert RR, Auerbach O, Garfinkle L, et al: Adenomatous lesions of the large bowel and colon: An autopsy survey. Cancer 43:1847–1857, 1979.
55. Williams AR, Baisoorya BAW, Day DW: Polyps and cancer of the large bowel: A necropsy study in Liverpool. Gut 23:835–842, 1982.
56. Vatn MH, Stalsberg HH: The prevalence of polyps in the large intestine in Oslo: An autopsy study. Cancer 49:819–825, 1982.
57. Shinya H, Wolff WI: Morphology, anatomic distribution and cancer potential of polyps: An analysis of 7000 polyps endoscopically removed. Ann Surg 190:679–683, 1979.
58. Konishi F, Morson BC: Pathology of colorectal adenomas: A colonoscopic survey. J Clin Pathol 35:830–841, 1982.
59. Eide TJ, Stalsberg H: Polyps of the large intestine in Northern Norway. Cancer 42:2839–2848, 1978.
60. Coode PE, Chan KW, Chan YT: Polyps and diverticuli of large intestine: A necroscopy study in Hong Kong. Gut 26:1045–1048, 1985.
61. Gillespie PE, Chambers TJ, Chan KW, et al: Colonic adenomas: A colonoscopic survey. Gut 20:240–245, 1979.
62. Hill MJ, Morson BC, Bussey HJR: Etiology of adenoma carcinoma sequence in large bowel. Lancet 1:245–247, 1978.
63. Morson BC: A polyp sequence in the large bowel. Proc Soc Med 67:451–457, 1974.
63a. Wolber RA, Owen DA: Flat adenomas of the colon. Hum Pathol 22:70–74, 1991.
64. Day DW, Morson BC: The adenoma-cancer sequence. In Morson BC (ed): Pathogenesis of Colorectal Cancer. Philadelphia, WB Saunders, 1978, pp 58–71.
65. Cuello C, Marigo C, Correa P: Atypia in adenomas in three populations with different risks for large bowel cancer. Cali, Sao Paulo, and New Orleans. Natl Cancer Inst Mongr 53:171–173, 1979.

66. Bansal M, Fenoglio CM, Robboy SJ, King DW: Are metaplasias in colorectal adenomas truly metaplasias? Am J Pathol 115:253–265, 1984.
67. Comer TP, Beahrs OH, Dockerty MP: Primary squamous cell carcinoma and adenoacanthoma of the colon. Cancer 28:1111–1117, 1971.
68. Mori K, Shinya H, Kalisman M: A composite tumor in tubulo-villous adenoma. Dis Colon Rectum 21:506–509, 1978.
68a. Gaffey MJ, Mills SE, Lack EE: Neuroendocrine carcinoma of the colon and rectum: A clinicopathologic, ultra-structural, and immunohistochemical study of 24 cases. Am J Surg Pathol 14:1010–1023, 1990.
69. Filipe MI: Mucin histochemistry of the colon. Curr Top Pathol 65:143–178, 1978.
70. Greaves P, Filipe MI, Abbas S, Ormerod MG: Sialomucins and carcinoembryonic antigen in the evolution of colorectal cancer. Histopathology 8:825–834, 1984.
71. Yonezawa S, Nakamura T, Tanaka S, Sato E: Glycoconjugate with Ulex Europaeus agglutinin-I binding sites in normal mucosa, adenoma, and carcinoma of human large bowel. JNCI 69:777–785, 1982.
72. Isaacson P, LeVann HP: The demonstration of CEA in colorectal carcinoma in colonic polyps using an immunoperoxidase technique. Cancer 38:1348–1356, 1976.
73. Burtin P, Martin E, Sabine MC, VonKleist S: Immunological study of polyps of the colon. JNCI 48:25–29, 1972.
74. O'Brien MJ, Zamchek N, Burke B, et al: Immunocytochemical localization of carcinoembryonic antigen in benign and malignant colorectal lesions: Assessment of diagnostic value. Am J Clin Pathol 75:283–290, 1981.
75. Stramignoni D, Bowen R, Atkinson BF, Schlom J: Differential reactivity of monoclonal antibodies with human colon adenocarcinomas and adenomas. Int J Cancer 31:543–552, 1983.
76. Brown A, Ellis IO, Embleton MJ, et al: Immunohistochemical localization of Y hapten and structurally related H type 2 blood group antigen in large bowel tumors and normal adult tissues. Int J Cancer 33:727–736, 1984.
77. Gong EC, Hirohashi S, Shimosato Y, et al: Expression of carbohydrate antigen 19-9 and stage specific embryonic antigen 1 in non-tumorous and tumorous epithelium of the human colon and rectum. JNCI 75:447–454, 1985.
77a. Ruggerio F, Cooper HS, Steplewski Z: Immunohisto-chemical study of colorectal adenomas with monoclonal antibodies against blood group antigens (Sialosyl-Le^a, Le^a, Le^b, Le^x, Le^y, A, B, and H). Lab Invest 59:96–103, 1988.
78. Wilcox GM, Anderson PB, Colacchio TA: Early invasive cancer in colonic polyps: A review of the literature with emphasis of the assessment of the risk of metastasis. Cancer 57:160–171, 1986.
79. Morson BC, Whiteway JE, Jones EA, et al: Histopathology and prognosis of malignant colorectal polyps treated by endoscopic polypectomy. Gut 25:437–444, 1984.
80. Cooper HS: Surgical pathology of endoscopically removed malignant polyps of the colon and rectum. Am J Surg Pathol 7:613–623, 1983.
81. Haggitt RC, Glotczbach RE, Soffer EE, Wruble LD: Prognostic factors in colorectal carcinoma arising in adenomas: Implications for lesions removed by endoscopic polypectomy. Gastroenterology 89:329–336, 1985.
82. Greene FL: Epithelial misplacement in adenomatous polyps of the colon and rectum. Cancer 33:206–217, 1974.
83. Muto T, Bussey HJR, Morson BC: Pseudocarcinomatous invasion in adenomatous polyps of the colon and rectum. J Clin Pathol 26:25–31, 1973.
84. Erbe RW: Current concepts in genetics: Inherited gastrointestinal-polyposis syndrome. N Engl J Med 294:1101–1104, 1976.
85. Wennstrom J, Pierce ER, McKusick VA: Hereditary benign and malignant lesions of the large bowel. Cancer 34:850–857, 1974.
86. Bussey HJR, Veale AMO, Morson BC: Genetics of gastrointestinal polyposis. Gastroenterology 74:1325–1330, 1978.
87. Deschner EE, Lipkin M: Proliferative patterns in colonic mucosa in familial polyposis. Cancer 35:413–418, 1975.
88. Muto T, Kamiya J, Sawada T, et al: Mucin abnormality of colon mucosa in patients with familial polyposis coli. Dis Colon Rectum 28:147–148, 1985.
89. Yonezawa S, Nakamura T, Tanaka S, et al: Binding of Ulex europaeus agglutinin-I in polyposis coli: Comparative study with solitary adenoma in the sigmoid colon and rectum. JNCI 71:19–24, 1983.
90. Dorazio RA, Whelan TJ Jr: Lymphoid hyperplasia of the terminal ileum associated with familial polyposis coli. Ann Surg 171:300–302, 1970.
91. Venkitachalam PS, Hirsch E, Elguezabal A, Littman L: Multiple lymphoid polyposis and familial polyposis of the colon: A genetic relationship. Dis Colon Rectum 21:336–341, 1978.
92. Shaw EB Jr, Henningar GR: Intestinal lymphoid polyposis. Am J Clin Pathol 61:417–422, 1974.
93. Thomford NR, Greenberger NJ: Lymphoid polyps of the ileum associated with Gardner's syndrome. Arch Surg 96:289–291, 1968.
94. Veale AMO, McColl I, Bussey HJR, Morson BC: Juvenile polyposis coli. J Med Genet 3:5–16, 1966.
95. Rozen P, Baratz M: Familial juvenile polyposis with associated colon cancer. Cancer 49:1500–1503, 1982.
96. Jarvinen H, Franssila KO: Familial juvenile polyposis coli: Increased risk of colorectal cancer. Gut 25:792–800, 1984.
97. Sachatello CR, Pickren JW, Grace JT: Generalized juvenile gastrointestinal polyposis. Gastroenterology 58:699–708, 1970.
98. Velcek FT, Coopersmith IS, Chen CK, et al: Familial juvenile adenomatosis polyposis. J Pediatr Surg 11:781–787, 1976.
99. Restrepo C, Moreno J, Duque E, et al: Juvenile colonic polyposis in Colombia. Dis Colon Rectum 29:600–612, 1978.
100. Stemper EJ, Kents TA, Summers RW: Juvenile polyposis and gastrointestinal carcinoma: A study of a kindred. Ann Intern Med 183:639–646, 1975.
101. Jegher H, McKusick VA, Katz KH: General intestinal polyposis and melanin spots of the oral mucosa, lips and digits. N Engl J Med 241:993–1005, 1032–1036, 1949.
102. Scully RE: Sex cord tumor with annular tubules: A distinctive ovarian tumor of the Peutz-Jeghers syndrome. Cancer 25:1107–1121, 1970.
102a. Haggitt RC, Reid BJ: Hereditary gastrointestinal polyposis syndromes. Am J Surg Pathol 10:871–887, 1986.
103. Bartholomew LG, Dahlin DC, Waugh JM: Intestinal polyposis associated with mucocutaneous melanin pigmentation (Peutz-Jegher's syndrome). Gastroenterology 32:434–451, 1957.
104. Bailey D: Polyposis of the gastrointestinal tract: The Peutz-Jeghers syndrome. Br Med J 2:433–438, 1957.
105. Hsu SD, Zaharopoulus PA, May JT, Costanzi JJ: Peutz-Jeghers syndrome with intestinal carcinoma: Report of the association in one family. Cancer 44:1527–1532, 1979.
106. Reid JD: Intestinal cancer in the Peutz-Jeghers syndrome. JAMA 229:833–834, 1974.
106a. Giardiello FM, Welsh SB, Hamilton SR, et al: Increased risk of cancer in the Peutz-Jeghers syndrome. N Engl J Med 316:1511–1514, 1987.
106b. Spigelman AD, Murday V, Phillips RKS: Cancer and the Peutz-Jeghers syndrome. Gut 30:1588–1590, 1989.
107. Cronkhite LW, Canada WJ: Generalized gastrointestinal polyposis: An unusual syndrome of polyposis, pigmentation alopecia, and onychodystrophy. N Engl J Med 252:1011–1015, 1955.
108. Daniel ES, Ludwig SL, Lewin KJ, et al: The Cronkhite Canada syndrome: An analysis of clinical and pathological features and therapy in 55 patients. Medicine 61:293–309, 1982.
109. Katayama Y, Kimura M, Konn M: Cronkhite-Canada syndrome associated with rectal cancer and adenomatous changes in colonic polyps. Am J Surg Pathol 9:65–71, 1985.
110. Nomomura A, Ohta G, Ihata T, et al: Cronkhite-Canada syndrome associated with sigmoid cancer. Acta Pathol Jpn 30:825–845, 1980.
111. Carlson GJ, Nivatvongs S, Snover DC: Colorectal polyps in Cowden's disease (multiple hamartomatous syndrome). Am J Surg Pathol 8:763–770, 1984.
112. Weary PE, Gorlin RJ, Gentry WC Jr, et al: Multiple hamartoma syndrome: Cowden's disease. Arch Dermatol 106:682–690, 1972.
113. Carney JA, Hayles AB: Alimentary tract manifestations of multiple endocrine neoplasia, type II B. Mayo Clin Proc 52:543–548, 1977.

114. Snover DC, Weigent CE, Sumner HW: Diffuse mucosal ganglioneuromatosis of the colon associated with adenocarcinoma. Am J Clin Pathol 75:225–229, 1981.
115. Weidner N, Flanders DJ, Mitros FA: Mucosal ganglioneuromatosis associated with multiple colonic polyps. Am J Surg Pathol 8:779–786, 1984.
116. Mendelsohn G, Diamond MP: Familial ganglioneuromatosis polyposis of the large bowel: Report of a family with associated juvenile polyposis. Am J Surg Pathol 8:515–520, 1984.
117. Louw JH: Polypoid lesions of the large bowel in children with particular reference to benign lymphoid polyposis. J Pediatr Surg 3:195–209, 1968.

CHAPTER 32

Adenocarcinoma and Other Malignant Epithelial Tumors of the Intestines

SI-CHUN MING, M.D.

INCIDENCE AND TYPES OF INTESTINAL TUMORS

ADENOCARCINOMA OF THE INTESTINES
General Considerations
Epidemiology
Small-Intestinal Carcinoma
Colorectal Carcinoma
Etiology
Carcinogens
Modifying Agents
Systemic Risk Factors
Genetic Factors
Dietary Factors
Alcohol and Beer
Steroids and Hormones
Cancer History
Social Status and Physical Activity
Extraintestinal Conditions
Intestinal Risk Factors
Intestinal Contents
Tissue Susceptibility
Precancerous Conditions
Benign Epithelial Polyps
Inflammatory and Other Bowel Diseases

Experimental Carcinogenesis
Pathology
Histogenesis and Natural History
Histogenesis
Rate of Growth
Spread of Adenocarcinoma
Gross Morphology and Classification
Polypoid Type
Fungating Type
Ulcerative Type
Diffusely Infiltrative Type
Histologic Features and Cell Types
Histologic Features
Cell Types
Ultrastructural and Morphometric Studies
Variants of Adenocarcinoma
Mucinous Adenocarcinoma
Signet-Ring Cell Carcinoma
Staging of Adenocarcinoma
Small-Intestinal Adenocarcinoma
Pathology
Location
Pathologic Features and Pattern of Spread
Clinical Presentation

Colorectal Adenocarcinoma
Pathology
Location
Pathologic Features
Multiplicity
Patterns of Spread
Marker Substances
Clinical Presentation

SQUAMOUS CELL CARCINOMA AND ADENOSQUAMOUS CARCINOMA

ENDOCRINE (NEUROENDOCRINE) CARCINOMA
Composite Adenocarcinoma and Carcinoid and Adenocarcinoid
Small-Cell Carcinoma
Pleomorphic (Giant Cell) Carcinoma

OTHER RARE CARCINOMAS AND METASTATIC TUMORS

The small and the large intestines have similar structural organizations and histologic components. (Details are described in Chapter 2.) However, they exhibit a number of differences, primarily related to their different functions. The small intestine is principally an absorptive organ for nutrients and has abundant absorptive cells with well-developed microvilli that form a brush border recognizable under a light microscope. The large intestine contains few absorptive cells that do not have a distinct brush border. Goblet cells, on the other hand, are more abundant in the large than in the small intestine. The endocrine cells secrete more prod-

Table 32-1 ESTIMATED NEW CASES AND DEATHS FOR GASTROINTESTINAL CANCER IN 1990

Cancer Site	New Cases			Deaths		
	Male	Female	Total	Male	Female	Total
All Sites	520,000	520,000	1,400,000	510,000	270,000	240,000
Esophagus	7,400	3,200	10,600	7,000	2,500	9,500
Stomach	13,900	9,300	23,200	8,300	5,400	13,700
Small intestine	1,500	1,300	2,800	500	400	900
Colon	52,000	58,000	110,000	26,000	27,300	53,300
Rectum	24,000	21,000	45,000	4,000	3,600	7,600
TOTAL	98,800	92,800	191,600	45,800	39,200	85,000
Lung	102,000	55,000	157,000	92,000	50,000	142,000
Breast	900	150,000	150,900	300	44,000	44,300
Prostate Gland	106,000	—	106,000	30,000	—	30,000

Data from Silverberg E, Boring CC, Squires TS: Cancer statistics, 1990. CA 40:9-26, 1990.

ucts and lymphoid tissue is more abundant in the small than in the large intestine. Tumors of the endocrine and lymphoid cells are presented in Chapters 13 and 14, respectively, and the mesenchymal tumors in Chapter 15. This chapter deals primarily with malignant epithelial tumors. The benign epithelial tumors, namely adenomas and polyps, are presented in Chapter 31.

INCIDENCE AND TYPES OF INTESTINAL TUMORS

Incidence of Intestinal Tumors. A striking difference between the tumors of the small and large intestines is in the frequency of epithelial tumors. The average length of the small intestine is 7 m, and that of the large intestine 1.5 m.[1] Although the small intestine is much narrower than the large intestine, the presence of numerous circular mucosal folds (Kerckring's valves or plicae circulares) greatly increases the mucosal surface in the small intestine, so that it makes up about 90% of the total surface area of the gastrointestinal tract.[2-4] However, tumors of the small intestine are rare, constituting only 5% to 6% of all gastrointestinal tumors and 1% to 2% of all gastrointestinal cancers.[3,4] The estimated incidence of new cases and deaths of small-intestinal cancer in 1990 in the United States is 2800 and 900, respectively; this accounts for 1.5% of new cases and 1.1% of death from all gastrointestinal cancers.[5] On the other hand, cancers of the large intestine (colorectum) are much more common, accounting for 80.9% of new cases and 71.6% of death from all gastrointestinal cancers (Table 32-1). They are among the most common tumors in the United States and account for nearly 15% of all cancers diagnosed in 1990.

Small-intestinal tumors are rare in the hospital population, affecting less than 0.1% of all admissions.[6,7] At the Massachusetts General Hospital, from 1913 to 1957, among 17,070 autopsies, 93 patients (0.54%) had small-intestinal tumors, 24% of which were malignant.[8] Among the surgically treated symptomatic patients, 75% of small-intestinal tumors were malignant.[8]

The incidence of benign tumors in the small intestine is equally low.[9] The reported ratio between malignant and benign tumors ranged from nearly 1:1[8,10,11] to over 2:1.[12,13] In contrast, benign tumors, particularly adenomas and polyps, are common in the large intestine. In the data compiled by Berk and Haubrick, the incidence of polyps varied from 7.0% to 38.8% at autopsy and from 1.6% to 19.2% in clinic patients.[14]

Types of Intestinal Tumors and Their Frequency. The types of tumors and their distribution in the small intestine are listed in Table 32-2.[8,12,13,15-19] Among the benign tumors, only one third are epithelial lesions, and these are equally distributed among the segments of the small intestine. Although only 25 to 30 cm long, the duodenum has a disproportionately high number of adenomas and polyps per unit area. The mesenchymal tumors, both benign and malignant, occur more commonly in the jejunum and ileum. These tumors are discussed in Chapter 15. The angiomatous lesions are presented in Chapter 12.

Among the malignant tumors of the small intestine, adenocarcinoma is the most common. About 80% of the carcinomas occur in the duodenum and jejunum. Carcinoid and lymphoma, on the other hand, occur most commonly in the ileum. The carcinoids are presented in Chapter 13 and lymphomas in Chapter 14.

Epithelial tumors dominate in the large intestine. In contrast to the small intestine, adenomas and polyps of the large intestine are much more common than the carcinomas. The younger the patients, the more likely the tumors will be polyps. The constituent cells of these tumors, irrespective of their location in the intestine, are of the same lineage as the normal cells, mainly columnar absorptive type cells, mucous cells, endocrine cells, and occasionally Paneth cells.[20] Only rarely, cells of metaplastic or heterotopic origin play a role in the tumor development of the intestines. Two types of metaplasia or heterotopia may occur in the intestines: squamous metaplasia and gastric metaplasia or heterotopia (see Chapter 28). Squamous metaplasia is rare and has been seen mainly in the colon and rectum after tissue injury;[21,22] it may also occur in an adenoma.[23,24] Squamous cell carcinoma may develop from such

Table 32-2 FREQUENCY AND TYPES OF TUMORS OF THE SMALL INTESTINE IN NUMBER AND PERCENT

Tumor Type†	Duodenum	Jejunum	Ileum	Total
Benign	531 (22.6)	759 (32.4)	1057 (45.0)	2347 (100.0)
Adenoma, polyp	230 (30.5)	265 (35.1)	259 (34.4)	754 (100.0)
Leiomyoma	123 (19.0)	275 (42.4)	250 (38.6)	648 (100.0)
Lipoma	100 (19.1)	196 (37.4)	228 (43.5)	524 (100.0)
Fibroma	8 (3.0)	130 (48.9)	128 (48.1)	266 (100.0)
Angioma	21 (7.5)	136 (48.6)	123 (43.9)	280 (100.0)
Nerve tumor	16 (14.7)	48 (44.0)	45 (41.3)	109 (100.0)
Miscellaneous	33 (43.4)	19 (25.0)	24 (31.6)	76 (100.0)
Malignant	375 (20.0)	560 (29.8)	945 (50.2)	1880 (100.0)
Carcinoma	267 (38.5)	290 (41.8)	137 (19.7)	694 (100.0)
Carcinoid	57 (9.3)	41 (6.7)	512 (83.8)	610 (100.0)
Sarcoma	38 (17.3)	88 (40.0)	94 (42.7)	220 (100.0)
Lymphoma	12 (3.5)	137 (39.5)	198 (57.0)	347 (100.0)
Miscellaneous	1 (11.1)	4 (44.4)	4 (44.5)	9 (100.0)

†This table includes only reports that listed tumors in different parts of the small intestine. References: for benign cases, 12,13,15,16; for malignant cases, 8,12,13,16–19.

metaplastic cells. Pure squamous cell carcinomas of the colon are rare.[22,25] Adenosquamous cell carcinoma is slightly more common.[26] The squamous cells in the latter probably originate from the progenitor of the neoplastic cells rather than from a separate cell origin of metaplastic nature. Gastric metaplasia or heterotopia is common in the duodenum. The gastric cells are usually in association with duodenitis and consist primarily of surface and foveolar cells[27,28] and occasionally cells of fundic glands.[29] Pyloric glands are difficult to identify because of the presence of Brunner's glands in the normal duodenum. Polyp and adenoma in the gastric metaplastic tissue have been reported.[27,30,31] Gastric metaplasia with pyloric glands may be seen in the distal small intestine and colorectum, usually in association with chronic inflammatory bowel disease[32] and rarely as heterotopia.[33] There has been a case of jejunal adenocarcinoma in heterotopic gastric mucosa.[34] Neoplastic change in the gastric tissue in colorectum has not been reported.

ADENOCARCINOMA OF THE INTESTINES

General Considerations

Adenocarcinoma is the most important malignant tumor in the intestines. It is 50 times more frequent in the large intestine than in the small intestine (see Table 32-1). Colorectal carcinoma ranks as the second most common cause of cancer death in both men and women in the United States. The probability of dying of colorectal cancer in a lifetime is high. It is higher in the white than in the black population (Table 32-3).[35] The incidence, mortality rate, and survival rate for colorectal cancer are listed in Table 32-4.[36] Because of its high prevalence, colorectal carcinoma has attracted a great deal more attention and efforts than has the small-intestinal cancer. Consequently, much more information is available concerning colorectal carcinoma.

The small and large intestines are structurally similar and are exposed to a similar environment, namely, a mixture of ingested substances and bodily secretions that contain bile and metabolic products. Also present are a great many bacteria, many of which are anaerobic. If the carcinogenic agents are exogenous and environmental in sources as suspected, they are likely to be in this mixture, and the epithelium of both the small and the large intestines is exposed to them. It is, therefore, puzzling to see such a striking difference in the cancer incidence in the respective segments of the intestines. A number of possible factors have been postulated[3,17,37,38]:

1. Rapid transit time of bowel contents in the small intestine may have reduced the contact time with carcinogens, whereas the solid feces in the large intestine remains for a much longer time.

2. The liquid content of the small intestine may dilute the carcinogens, whereas absorption of water in the large intestine concentrates the carcinogens. Furthermore, liquid content may be less irritating and injurious to the small-intestinal mucosa than is the solid and particulate fecal matter in the large intestine.

3. The larger bacterial population with many anaerobes in the large intestine may be responsible for the conversion of bile salts and other procarcinogens into carcinogens.[39,40]

4. The small intestine may have a higher enzyme activity than the large intestine for detoxification of carcinogens. For instance, the benzpyrene hydroxylase in the small intestine may convert benzpyrene into less active metabolites.[41]

5. Rapid cell turnover in the small intestine may protect the mucosal cells by shedding. On the other hand, increased proliferation of mucosal cells may actually increase the malignant transformation,[42] and the neoplastic cells do not shed but accumulate at the site of origin.[43] Thus, the beneficial effect of rapid cell turnover may be limited to the initial stage of carcinogenesis.

Table 32-3 PROBABILITY AT BIRTH FOR PERSONS BORN IN 1985 OF EVENTUALLY DEVELOPING OR DYING OF GASTROINTESTINAL CANCER

Cancer Site	White Males (%)	Black Males (%)	White Females (%)	Black Females (%)
Developing Cancer				
Esophagus	0.5	1.5	0.3	0.7
Stomach	1.2	1.6	0.8	0.8
Colon-rectum	6.5	5.1	6.9	6.3
Dying of Cancer				
Esophagus	0.5	1.4	0.2	0.5
Stomach	0.7	0.9	0.6	0.8
Colon-rectum	2.9	2.2	3.1	2.7

Data from reference 35.

6. The effective immune system in the small intestine with immunologically active lymphocytes may protect the tissue against oncogenic viruses[41] and the T lymphocytes against the cancer cells.[44]

Epidemiology

Small-Intestinal Carcinoma

The low incidence of small-intestinal carcinoma seen in the United States (see Tables 32-1 and 32-4) is also found in other countries.[38] The incidence is higher in the developed western countries than in the underdeveloped countries[38,45] and parallels that of colon cancer.[41] Within the United States, the incidence in Hawaiian whites is higher than in Hawaiian Japanese; the incidence in Hawaiian Japanese is higher than that in Japan.[38] There is a slight male predominance,[46] and the incidence is higher in blacks than in whites.[36] The survival rate for small-intestinal cancer is lower than that for colorectal cancer, particularly in the male (see Table 32-4).

Colorectal Carcinoma

The annual incidence per 100,000 varies greatly in different countries (Figure 32-1) and ranges from a low of 2.8 for males and 2.9 for females in Peru to a high of 41.2 for males in Czechoslovakia and 26.9 for females in New Zealand.[5] In general, the incidence is high in the European and North American countries and low in Asian, South American, and African countries. There is a male predominance, particularly in the high-incidence regions.[46] The incidence of colon cancer is higher than that of rectal cancer in the high-incidence areas, but the difference is small in the low-incidence areas.[47] Furthermore, rectal cancer in the high-risk regions is located more frequently in the upper rectum, and in the low-risk regions more frequently in the lower rectum.[48] The ratio between the incidence and the mortality of colorectal cancer in the United States is about 2.5 (see Table 32-4). Between 1973 and 1987 there has been an increased incidence of colon cancer, only slightly among the white male, but prominently in both sexes of the black race (Table 32-5). The incidence of rectal cancer had increased only among the black male. The mortality for colonic cancer during these periods increased in blacks, while that for rectal cancer declined in blacks and whites.

Etiology

Migration studies show that the geographic, sex, and racial differences in the incidence of intestinal cancer appear to be caused by environmental rather than genetic factors. The incidence for migrants residing in a

Table 32-4 AGE-ADJUSTED INCIDENCE AND MORTALITY RATES PER 100,000 POPULATION AND 5-YEAR RELATIVE SURVIVAL RATE (%) OF GASTROINTESTINAL CANCER IN 1983-1987 SEER* PROGRAM

	Incidence Rate			Mortality Rate			Survival Rates		
Cancer Site	Male and Female	Male	Female	Male and Female	Male	Female	Male and Female	Male	Female
Esophagus	3.8	6.2	1.9	3.3	5.6	1.6	8.0	7.1	10.1
Stomach	8.2	12.1	5.4	5.5	8.2	3.6	17.0	15.8	19.1
Small intestine	1.0	1.3	0.8	0.3	0.4	0.3	40.5	37.1	44.3
Colon-rectum	50.9	61.2	43.4	19.9	24.1	17.0	55.5	55.2	55.6
Colon	36.5	42.2	32.1	17.0	20.3	14.8	56.4	56.8	55.9
Rectum	14.6	19.0	11.3	2.9	3.8	2.2	53.4	52.0	54.9

*SEER (Surveillance, Epidemiology and End Results) program is a project of the National Cancer Institute.
From Gloeckles-Ries LA, Hankey BF, Edwards BK: Cancer statistics review, 1973-1987. NIH publication 90-2789. Bethesda, Md, National Cancer Institute, 1990.

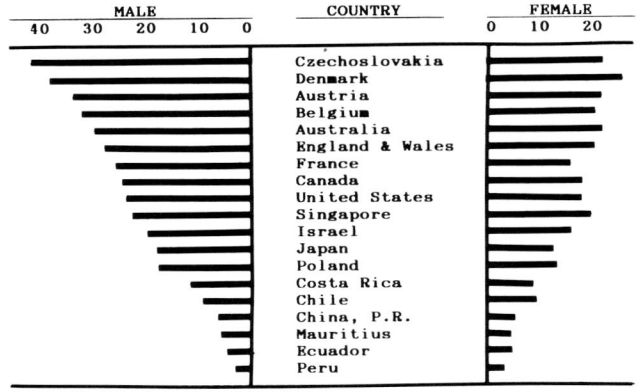

FIGURE 32–1. Geographic distribution of death rates per 100,000 for colorectal carcinoma 1984 to 1986. (Data from Silverberg E, Boring CC, Squires TS: Cancer Statistics, 1990. CA 40:9–26, 1990, except those for China, which are from Cancer Mortality Study in China, People's Health Publications, Beijing, China, 1979.)

new country for a long time, and for their next generations, usually shifts toward the prevailing rates for the local population.[48–52] Although racial genetics does not appear to be important, genetics does play a dominant role in the development of intestinal cancer in a number of hereditary diseases, such as familial adenomatous polyposis and Gardner's and Lynch syndromes. In addition, alterations in gene expression have been demonstrated in cancer cells. A detailed discussion of these findings is presented in Chapter 6.

Carcinogens

The carcinogenic agents for intestinal cancer in humans have not been identified. There are, however, reliable animal models for the induction of intestinal carcinoma with chemical carcinogens.[53] Two models in particular give information relevant to human intestinal carcinogenesis. One model involves the use of a strong direct-acting carcinogen, such as N-methyl-N'-nitro-N-nitrosoguanidine (MNNG) for induction of the carcinoma at points of contact with the tissue.[54,55] The other model uses chemicals that require metabolic activation before they exert their carcinogenic effect, such as analogs of cycasin and 1,2-dimethylhydrazine (DMH).[56,57] MNNG is not organ-specific. DMH and related chemicals, on the other hand, are strongly organotropic and cause intestinal tumors, mostly colonic, independent of the route of administration. It is unlikely that exposure to a direct carcinogen is a major cause of intestinal tumors in humans. The other indirect mechanism of carcinogenesis may be more applicable to the human situation. In addition to illustrating possible modes of carcinogenesis, the experimental models are used in evaluating suspected risk factors in the human through manipulation of dietary and other environmental conditions. Further discussion is found in the section on experimental carcinogenesis.

The sources of possible intestinal carcinogens may be environmental, occupational, diet-linked, or endogenous. The environmental agents include air pollutants such as sulfur dioxide in the acid haze,[58] hazardous chemical waste,[59] automobile emissions,[60] arsenics in well water,[61] and asbestos.[62] The importance of exposure to asbestos has been disputed, however.[63] Several occupations carry an increased risk for colon cancer,[64] including the petroleum product workers, printing machine operators, food manufacturing workers, and manufacturers of polypropylene.[65] Food may be contaminated by carcinogens or may serve as a substrate for an endogenous carcinogen.[66] Nitroso compounds have been found in the feces of persons on a diet that was high in protein and low in ascorbic acid and to-

Table 32–5 AGE-ADJUSTED INCIDENCE AND MORTALITY RATE (PER 100,000 POPULATION) AND SURVIVAL RATE (IN PERCENTAGE) OF COLORECTAL CANCER BETWEEN 1973 AND 1987, SEER PROGRAM

Cancer Site	Male and Female		Male		Female	
	White	Black	White	Black	White	Black
Incidence (1973/1987)						
Colon-rectum	46.8/48.8	41.6/51.4	54.2/60.5	42.4/58.5	41.6/40.5	40.6/46.7
Colon	31.9/34.5	30.0/39.6	34.7/41.6	31.3/44.7	30.2/29.7	29.2/36.1
Rectum	14.9/14.3	11.4/11.8	19.5/18.9	11.0/13.8	11.4/10.9	11.5/10.5
Mortality Rate (1973/1987)						
Colon-rectum	22.0/19.7	20.9/23.2	25.3/24.4	21.8/26.8	19.8/16.4	20.2/20.7
Colon	17.5/17.0	16.4/20.3	19.3/20.9	16.5/23.0	16.3/14.4	16.4/18.5
Rectum	4.5/2.6	4.4/2.9	6.0/3.5	5.3/3.8	3.5/2.0	3.8/2.2
Survival Rate (1974–6/1981–7)						
Colon-rectum	49.6/56.2	44.4/46.0	49.0/56.0	40.8/43.7	50.2/56.3	47.4/47.8
Colon	50.1/57.0	45.5/47.5	49.7/57.5	43.5/45.9	50.5/56.5	47.1/48.7
Rectum	48.5/54.3	41.3/41.3	47.7/53.1	34.2/37.8	49.5/55.6	48.2/44.9

*The improvement in the survival rate in white males is statistically significant.
From Gloeckles-Ries LA, Hankey BF, Edwards BK: Cancer statistics review, 1973–1987. NIH publication 90-2789. Bethesda, Md, National Cancer Institute, 1990.

copherol.[67] Nitroso compounds may be formed in the stomach with chronic gastritis.[68] Other endogenous substances that may be related to intestinal carcinogenesis include mutagenic agents such as the fecapentaenes, which are found in the human feces and thought to be produced by colonic microflora. They have been correlated with the incidences of colon cancer[69,70] and of polyp,[71] but no such relationship was found in a recent study.[72] Mutagenic compounds have also been found in cooked meat.[53,73-75] A study in New Zealand demonstrated DNA-damaging activity in fecal extract from persons on a mixed diet, but no such activity was reported in Seventh-Day Adventists on an ovolactovegetarian diet.[76]

Radiation as a possible carcinogenic agent is suspected when colonic carcinoma develops in patients who received radiation therapy to the pelvic region for various reasons, most often gynecologic malignancies.[77,78] Jao et al. reviewed 76 cases of colon or anorectal cancer after pelvic irradiation.[77] The mean interval between irradiation and cancer development was 15.2 years. About one third of the tumors were mucinous adenocarcinomas. The 5-year survival rate was 48%. Carcinomas of the colon or rectum had been reported also in patients who received a single massive dose of radiation[79] and in survivors of the atomic bomb.[80] The tissue surrounding the tumor may show the effects of radiation.

Tubulovillous adenoma was induced in the duodenum of guinea fowls by intravenous injection of virus strain pts-57.[81] The search for viral DNA for cytomegalovirus, Epstein-Barr virus, and human papillomavirus in biopsies of human colonic adenomas and adenocarcinomas has been negative.[82]

Modifying Agents

Chemical carcinogenesis appears to be the most important cause of intestinal carcinoma. Several substances have been found to have a modifying effect on the process. The promoters include bile acids[83,84] and 3-ketosteroids;[85] the inhibitors are generally antioxidants such as vitamins C and E and selenium. Vitamins C and E reduce the level of fecal mitogens in the stool and inhibit the formation of nitrosamines, cell proliferation, and carcinogenesis.[86] Vitamins C and E are associated with low risk for esophageal and gastric cancer,[87] but their effect on colonic carcinogenesis is not definitive.[88,89] Supplementary administration of these vitamins for 2 years to patients who underwent excision of colonic polyps showed a recurrence rate that was slightly lower than the rate for the control patients on placebo.[90] Selenium reduces tumor formation in the colon in experimental animals,[91,92] particularly in the right colon.[93] The reported increased incidence in western countries of cancer in the right colon has been attributed to a selenium deficiency.[94] Butylated hydroxytoluene, another antioxidant, reduces experimental colonic tumors in male mice but not in the female mice.[95] Indomethacin, a prostaglandin synthesis inhibitor, reduces the incidence of DMH-induced bowel tumor.[96] The mechanism appears to be the reduction of ornithine decarboxylase (ODC), a marker for tumor promotion, in the colonic mucosa.[97] Administration of prostaglandin to the animals restores ODC activity.

Table 32-6 RISK FACTORS FOR INTESTINAL CARCINOMA

Systemic risk factors
  Genetic factors
  Dietary factors
    Fat intake
    Protein intake
    Total calorie intake
    Cholesterol and its metabolites
    Fiber and vegetable intake
  Alcohol and beer
  Steroids and hormones
  Cancer history
  Social status and physical activity
  Extraintestinal conditions
    Cholecystectomy
    Gastrectomy and hypochlorhydria
Intestinal risk factors
  Intestinal contents
    Bile acids
    Intestinal flora
    Fecal contents
  Tissue susceptibility
Precancerous conditions
  Benign epithelial polyp and adenoma
    Adenoma and adenomatosis
    Nonneoplastic polyps and polyposis
      Hyperplastic polyp
      Hamartomatous polyposis
  Inflammatory and other bowel diseases
    Ulcerative colitis and Crohn's disease
    Schistosomiasis
    Mucosal hyperplasia

Systemic Risk Factors

Although precise etiologic agents for intestinal cancers are not known, many factors related to an increased risk for development of intestinal cancer, particularly colorectal cancer, have been identified. Some of these factors are systemic and affect the body as a whole. Others are regional changes that affect the site of tumor formation. Thus systemic factors are mainly metabolic in nature, and the regional factors are tissue alterations that precede carcinogenesis and thus are precancerous conditions. The risk factors are listed in Table 32-6.

The intestinal tract is exposed to many possible carcinogens, both exogenous and endogenous. Because the likely possibility involves one or more carcinogenic agents that require prior metabolic activation before the carcinogenic effect is manifested, the tumors are often the result of complex interplay among a number of risk factors rather than the product of a single factor. In some instances, conflicting observations were made.

Genetic Factors

The genetic aspects of intestinal cancers are discussed in Chapter 6; only information related to pathologic features are presented here. Genetic factors play a role in an estimated 20% of colorectal carcinomas.[98] They have a primary role in several rare syndromes in which intestinal polyposis is the main or prominent component: (1) familial adenomatous polyposis (FAP) and the related Gardner's syndrome, which manifests, in addition to polyposis, benign skin, soft tissue, and bone lesions;[99] (2) Peutz-Jeghers syndrome, in which, in addition to polyposis, there is mucocutaneous pigmentation;[100] and (3) juvenile polyposis.[101] Much more common are the hereditary nonpolyposis colorectal cancers (HNPCC), which account for about 5% of all colorectal cancers.[102,103] Although patients with HNPCC do not have polyposis, in about one third of the cases screened, adenomas occurred randomly, as in the general population.[98] In addition, heredity plays a role in patients with discrete familial clustering of colonic polyps,[104] the estimated gene frequency being 19%.[105]

Colorectal cancer can occur in all these conditions, usually at a young age. In FAP and Gardner's syndrome, all patients with polyposis will eventually develop colorectal cancer.[99] The carcinoma develops from the adenoma, and *de novo* carcinoma has not been seen in these cases.[99] Carcinoma and adenoma can occur also in the stomach and the small intestine, particularly the duodenum.[106] The polyps in Peutz-Jeghers syndrome and in familial juvenile polyposis are of the nonneoplastic hamartomatous type. Carcinoma develops from the hamartomatous polyp or the associated adenoma.[100,107–109]

The cases of HNPCC have been divided into two groups: Lynch syndromes I and II. The difference between these two syndromes is that familial aggregation of cancers in other organs—particularly the endometrial, ovarian, and pancreatic carcinomas—is present in Lynch syndrome I but not in Lynch syndrome II. Lynch syndrome II is also known as cancer family syndrome. The colorectal cancers in these syndromes have several characteristics:[98] They are located mostly in the right colon (72%), and the mean age at diagnosis is 45.6 years. Multiple colorectal carcinomas are common: synchronous in 18% and metachronous in 24% of cases. Histologically, mucinous and signet-ring cell carcinomas are more common than in the general population.[98,110] The associated adenomas may be of the flat type,[98] which has a high rate of malignant change.[111] Additional information on the polyposis syndromes is presented in Chapter 31, and the genetic aspects of these conditions are discussed in Chapter 6.

In addition to the genetics related to hereditary intestinal tumors, a change in the expression of one or more genes in the DNA is commonly involved in the carcinogenic process even though the tumor is not hereditary. A progressive series of steps in which tumor suppressor gene are deleted or mutated has been identified by biochemical and cytogenetic methods.[112,113] Additional information is provided in Chapter 6.

Dietary Factors

Epidemiologic studies implicate diet as the major risk factor for colonic cancer. The marked regional variations in the incidence rates for colorectal carcinoma can be correlated with dietary habits. Experimental studies on animals fed with various modified diets support these views.

Dietary Fat and Protein. It has been shown that the countries with high mortality from colorectal cancer have high fat and protein consumption.[50,114] Dietary fat constituted 41.8% of total calorie intake in the United States, a high-risk country, and only 12.2% in Japan, a low-risk country.[114] Similar positive correlation between the incidence of large-bowel cancer and animal fat, animal protein, and cholesterol, and an inverse correlation with intake of dietary fiber and vitamins C and A were found in other studies.[115] The mortality of colorectal cancer is low among the Seventh-Day Adventists, who consume less fat and cholesterol than their high-risk compatriots.[76,116] The type of fat or oil consumed is important.[117] For instance, saturated fat has a negative effect on carcinomas of right colon and a slightly positive effect on rectal cancer among the Japanese in Hawaii.[118] However, experiments comparing the effects of saturated fat with those of unsaturated fat gave conflicting results.[119,120] The combination of high-fat and low-fiber diet gives a high yield of colorectal tumors in rats.[121] The mechanism of these effects is an increase in endogenous bile acids and fatty acids, which promote colonic carcinogenesis.[83,84] The meat protein enhances carcinogenesis by serving as a substrate for possible carcinogenic substances and increasing bacterial growth.[122]

Total Calorie Intake. High total intake of calories increases the risk for colon cancer.[123] Calorie restriction reduces the yield of colon tumor in rats, even if the animals are on a high-fat diet.[124,125]

Cholesterol and Fecal Sterols. High-fat intake increases the fecal level of cholesterol and natural sterols and the serum levels of cholesterol and beta-lipoprotein, which are associated with increased risk of colon cancer in man[126] and experimental animals.[127] In some persons, however, high-cholesterol intake may be accompanied by a low serum cholesterol level but a high risk of colon cancer.[128] Reddy et al. found that the levels of fecal cholesterol and sterol excretion differed markedly in people with different dietary habits: at decreasing levels among Americans on a mixed diet, American vegetarians, Seventh-Day Adventists, Japanese, and Chinese,[129] in parallel with the incidence of colon cancer.

Dietary Fibers and Vegetables. People in countries at high risk for colorectal cancer consume less vegetables, fruits, and fibers than do those in countries at low risk.[115,130] The search for specific anticancer agents in vegetables has not been fruitful except for the finding of the tumor inhibitory action of diallyl sulfide in garlic[131] and the protective effects of vitamins and fibers they contain. The negative effect of dietary fiber has been extensively studied since it was recognized by Burkitt.[132] While most reports on the human show the protective effect of fiber against colon cancer, some reports show no effect.[133] In animal experiments conflicting data have also been obtained, apparently related to the types of fibers used.[130,134] Cellulose and wheat bran generally reduce cancer yield, whereas oat bran, peptin, and carrageenan enhance carcinogenesis.[133-136] The mechanisms of modulating effects of fiber on colon carcinogenesis are complex and involve interactions between fiber and many substances in the gut. Insoluble fibers increase the bulk of the feces, dilute the carcinogens and bile acids, and shorten the transit time. Carcinogens and bile acids can be bound to the fiber[137] and excreted with it. These effects reduce the exposure of colonic epithelium to the carcinogens and promoters.[130] Fiber such as peptin may modify microbial flora and may increase the production of enzymes such as β-glucuronidase,[136] which can activate procarcinogens in the gut lumen. Fibers are fermented by the anaerobic organisms to produce short-chain fatty acids and increase the fecal acidity, which can stimulate cell growth of colonic epithelium and facilitate carcinogenesis.[133,134] On the other hand, the acidic contents of the bowel may inhibit the metabolism of carcinogens and bile acids and reduce the carcinogenicity of these substances.[138]

Vitamins and Calcium. Vitamins C and E are antioxidants that may inhibit the formation of N-nitroso compounds, but their ability to reduce carcinogenesis is variable.[88,89,139] Vitamin A and related retinoid and beta-carotene are protective against esophageal carcinomas; their role in colon carcinogenesis is equivocal.[130,140] The intake of dietary vitamin D and calcium has been found to be inversely related to the incidence of colorectal cancer in a 19-year prospective study in man.[141] Insoluble calcium soap formed with fatty acid or bile acid prevents mucosal damage and hyperplasia caused by these agents.[130] Supplementary oral calcium has been shown to reduce the proliferative activity of colon epithelial cells in patients at high risk for familial colon cancer.[142,143] Finally, intestinal tumor fails to develop in vitamin B_{12}–deficient rat.[144]

Alcohol and Beer

Alcohol is an important etiolgic factor for esophageal cancer, but its relationship with colon cancer is unknown. Heavy beer drinking, on the other hand, has been associated with an increased incidence of rectal carcinoma.[50,140,145,146]

Steroids and Hormones

Among hormones of the digestive tract, gastrin[147] and vasoactive intestinal peptide[148] have been shown to promote the development of colon cancer because of their effect on increased cell proliferation.[148,149]

That sex hormones play a role in bowel cancer is suggested by the finding that males are more often affected than females.[50,150] Furthermore, protection was found in women who had previous pregnancies and never used estrogen.[151,152] The use of oral contraceptives increased the risk of rectal cancer in women, but not of colon cancer.[153] Estrogen receptors are present in the colon cancer and surrounding tissue, more frequently in tumors of women than men.[154] Androgen receptors are also present in colon tumors.[155] Injection of testosterone at birth increases the number of DMH-induced tumors in both male and female mice, but more so in the female; this has been attributed to the hyperestrogenization of the androgenized female.[156] However, data on the effect of testosterone on tumor growth are contradictory.[155,157] Patients with acromegaly have increased incidence of colon cancer and polyps,[158] probably because of the stimulation by insulin-like growth factors that are present in the tumor.[159] Colon cancer has been seen in patients with parathyroid adenoma;[160] the mechanism is not clear.

Cancer History

In genetic cancer syndromes, the patients' familial and personal history with regard to the occurrence of bowel tumors is a characteristic feature. The incidence of synchronous and metachronous colorectal cancers is about 20% in the nonpolyposis hereditary cases,[98] compared with 3% in the general population.[161] Enblad et al. found a high incidence of small-bowel cancer in patients with prior large-bowel cancer.[162] There was also a slight increase in the relative incidence of cancer in extraintestinal organs, including the bladder, in both sexes, and in the breast, endometrium, and ovary in the female.[162] In the relatives of patients with familial breast cancer, there is a high risk for colon cancer, mainly in the male.[163] There is no increased risk for the spouses of patients with colorectal cancer.[164]

Social Status and Physical Activity

The incidence of colorectal carcinoma is higher in urban than in rural regions and in the upper than in the lower socioeconomic class.[48,50] The incidence is lower in Mormons and Seventh-Day Adventists than in other groups.[75,165] Lifestyle and dietary habits are likely factors. Physical activity may also be a factor, as it reduces both the rate of mortality from colorectal cancer[166,167] and the incidence of DMH-induced colon tumors.[168]

Extraintestinal Conditions

Cholecystectomy. There have been many reports on the relationship between prior cholecystectomy and subsequent development of colon cancer. Most reports indicated a positive relationship for both cancer[169-171] and adenoma,[172,173] but some reports showed no relationship.[174,175] The increased risk affects the right colon but not the left colon or the rectum.[169,171] Women are affected more often than men.[170,171] The colon carcinoma generally develops several years after cholecystectomy.[169] The proposed mechanism is related to bile acid metabolism.[169] After cholecystectomy, the enterohepatic circulation of bile salts is increased. This leads to increased secondary bile acids in the bowel by action of intestinal bacteria and to enhanced tumor production. A recent study, however, did not reveal an increase in the bile acids.[176]

Gastrectomy and Hypochlorhydria. There is a twofold increase of colorectal cancer after remote gastrectomy for gastroduodenal disease.[177,178] Hypochlorhydria and bile reflux, which results in increased levels of carcinogens, and free secondary bile acids in the gastric remnant may be responsible factors for the increased risk for colorectal cancer as well as for gastric cancer.[178] The same mechanism may be applied to the finding of a slightly increased incidence of colorectal cancer in patients with pernicious anemia.[68]

Intestinal Risk Factors

Intestinal Contents

Bile Acids. Bile acids and their metabolites are involved in many ways in colorectal carcinogenesis. The bile acid conjugates can be hydrolyzed by the intestinal anaerobes, mainly clostridia,[179,180] to free bile acids, particularly deoxycholic and lithocholic acids. Their fecal concentration is higher in patients with colon cancer than in patients with adenoma.[129] The free bile acid concentration in patients with a small adenoma is the same as in normal persons, suggesting that the bile acids are involved in the growth but not the initiation of the adenomas.[115]

Deoxycholic acid causes inflammation and necrosis followed by proliferation of colonic epithelium. These changes can be prevented by calcium, which sequesters the bile acid.[181] Lithocholic acid has an even more important role in promoting tumor growth, as the ratio of lithocholic acid to deoxycholic acid in the feces is highest in patients with colon carcinoma, lowest in persons at low risk, and at middle level in patients with adenomas.[182] The free bile acids are potent inducers of chromosomal aneuploidy, whereas the conjugated bile acids are not.[183]

Intestinal Flora. Intestinal microorganisms, particularly the anaerobic clostridia, play a crucial role in carcinogenesis of the gut by producing or activating carcinogens.[184] Their enzymes, such as β-glucuronidase and hydroxylases, convert conjugated bile acids and carcinogens into free active forms that may initiate or promote tumorigenesis.[179,185] They influence the carcinogenic process[138] by fermenting plant fibers that produce short-chain fatty acids and lower the pH of bowel contents.[134] Germ-free animals produce fewer intestinal tumors than do conventional animals.[186] The treatment of animals with antibiotics during the induction period reduces the incidence of cancer.[187]

Fecal Contents. It is evident that fecal matter is a primary source of carcinogens, whether exogenous or endogenous, and of tumor-promoting and -inhibiting substances. In one experiment, in which a segment of distal colon was bypassed by the fecal stream as a result of a surgical operation, DMH induced tumors in the feces-filled segment and not in the empty bypassed segment.[188] However, fecal contact is not essential for tumor formation. In another experiment, the administration of DMH did produce tumors in the isolated, defunctionalized, and cleansed segment of colon, although in fewer animals and in smaller numbers than in the reanastomosed intact colon.[189] Because the isolated segment did not have contact with feces, the DMH probably reached the segment by circulation and was converted to active carcinogen by colonic cells.

Tissue Susceptibility

Colon is more susceptible to carcinogenic effects than is the small intestine. In rats with surgical transposition of the jejunum or cecum to the distal colon or vice versa, the administration of carcinogen produced tumors in the colorectum of all animals, but tumors were absent or few in the transposed jejunum or cecum.[190,191]

Precancerous Conditions

Precancerous conditions are diseases in which there is an increased risk for development of intestinal carcinoma. It is generally accepted that carcinomas do not develop from a totally normal cell but from an altered cell that may appear normal on routine histologic examination but has altered function so that it may contain abnormal markers such as carcinoembryonic antigen (CEA). On the other hand, many premalignant cells are already morphologically abnormal and show hyperchromatism, pleomorphism, abnormal size and shape, loss of polarity, and frequent mitoses. Such cells are dysplastic, and their propensity for malignancy is proportional to the degree of abnormality. The dysplastic cells are characteristic of adenomas, and premalignant lesions of ulcerative colitis.[192] It is the presence of such functionally or morphologically altered cells that marks the premalignant nature of the precancerous conditions.

Benign Epithelial Polyps

The pathologic features and malignant potential of intestinal polyps are presented in detail in Chapter 31.

Adenomas and Adenomatosis. The malignant potential of adenoma is proportional to the grades of dysplasia and the quantity of cell mass.[193,194] When the individual adenoma is small, the large number of adenomas increases the malignant potential, as in FAP. When the lesion is small but highly dysplastic, a high rate of malignant change is again evident, as in the flat adenomas.[111,195] The growth pattern is also a factor; e.g., the presence of villous configuration, a sign of heightened vertical expansion, is a marker of high malignant potential.[192,194] These features in concert determine the outcome of an adenoma or the adenomatosis syndrome. A comparable relationship between adenoma and carcinoma is also present in the small intestine.[196]

The process by which carcinoma develops into an adenoma is known as the adenoma-carcinoma sequence.[197] The evolution of carcinoma from adenoma is usually histologically evident, and the invasive carcinomas often contain a focus of remnant adenoma[198,199] (Figures 32–2 and 32–3). The reported incidence of residual adenoma in carcinoma ranged

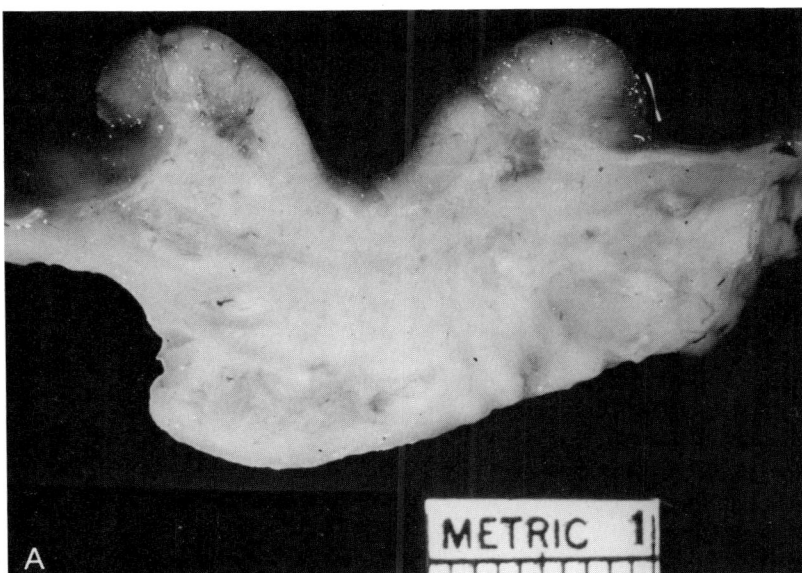
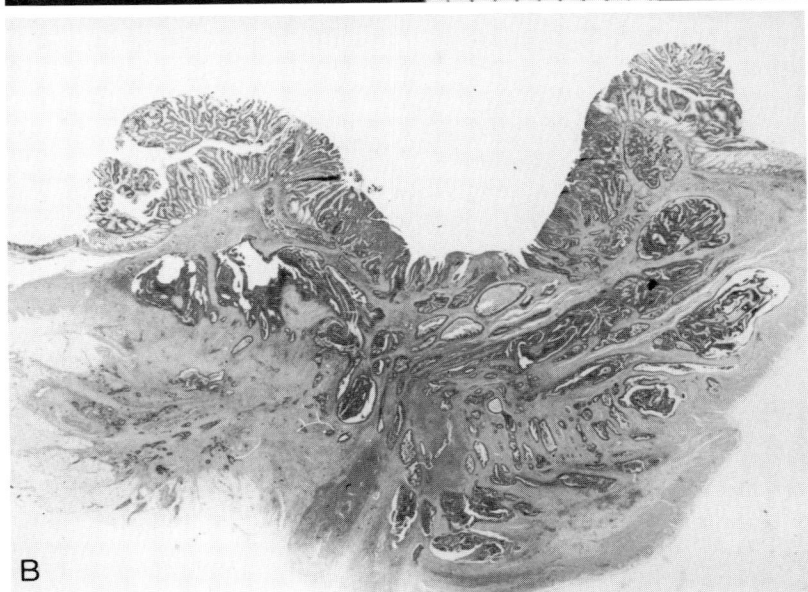

FIGURE 32–2. Small ulcerated adenocarcinoma of colon, showing adenomatous tissue at the border of the invasive lesion. A, Gross appearance of the cross-sectional surface of the lesion. B, Scanning view of the histologic section.

from 0%[200,201] to 56%,[202] for carcinomas with invasion of the submucosa only. When the carcinomas had invaded the pericolic fat, the incidence dropped to 7%. When the adenomas are serially sectioned, the incidence of malignant focus increased: even adenomas less than 1 cm in diameter showed a 27% rate of malignancy.[203]

Many adenomas have markers of malignancy, including blood group antigens, oncofetal antigens such as CEA and CA19-9,[204] T antigens,[205] and nuclear receptors for estrogen and progesterone.[206] Recent investigation using molecular biology techniques revealed multistep gene alteration in the colonic carcinogenesis sequence, with changes in the adenoma as the initial step (see Chapter 6). The question remains, however, whether all colorectal carcinomas, except those following long-standing inflammatory bowel disease, de-

velop from a pre-existing adenoma. Evidence against this was the finding of small nonpolypoid carcinomas without a trace of adenomatous tissue.[207,208] Furthermore, experimental studies show that colon carcinoma may develop without the adenoma stage.[309,310] The question of *de novo* carcinoma is further discussed in the section on the histogenesis of the carcinoma.

Nonneoplastic Polyps and Polypsis. *Hyperplastic Polyps.* Hyperplastic polyps are small and generally considered to be innocuous lesions. However, adenomas may contain areas showing features of a hyperplastic polyp,[198,211] and this suggests that hyperplastic polyps may become adenomatous and thus indirectly involved in malignant change.[212] Furthermore, features of malignant change such as CEA and O-acylated sialomucin have been found in hyperplastic polyps.[213] Recently, some adenomas have been found to contain

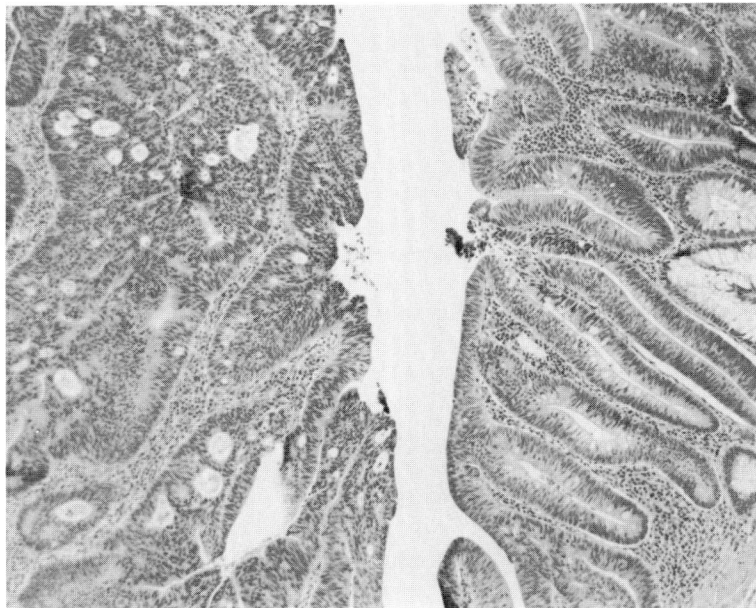

FIGURE 32–3. Area of adenocarcinoma (at left) in a tubular adenoma (at right). ($\times$ 55)

mixed hyperplastic and adenomatous features.[214] About one third of these lesions had significant dysplasia, and 11% had intramucosal carcinoma.

Hamartomatous Polyposis. There are two kinds of hamartomatous polyps: polyps in the Peutz-Jeghers syndrome and the juvenile polyposis. Both are composed of essentially normal epithelial cells and are not considered premalignant. However, intestinal cancers have been reported in both syndromes, mostly in the small intestine in the Peutz-Jeghers syndrome and in the colon in the juvenile polyposis syndrome. The carcinomas arise in the dysplastic or adenomatous lesions (Figure 32–4).[100,107–109,215]

Inflammatory and Other Bowel Diseases

Ulcerative Colitis and Crohn's Disease. Malignant and premalignant changes complicating ulcerative colitis and Crohn's disease are discussed in detail in Chapter 27.

The development of colon carcinoma in patients with ulcerative colitis is related to the extent and duration of colitis. The wide geographic variation in the incidence of malignancy in ulcerative colitis[216] raises the possibility of the role of environmental factors.[217] The colitis-carcinoma differs from colon carcinoma in the general population in its tendency to locate ran-

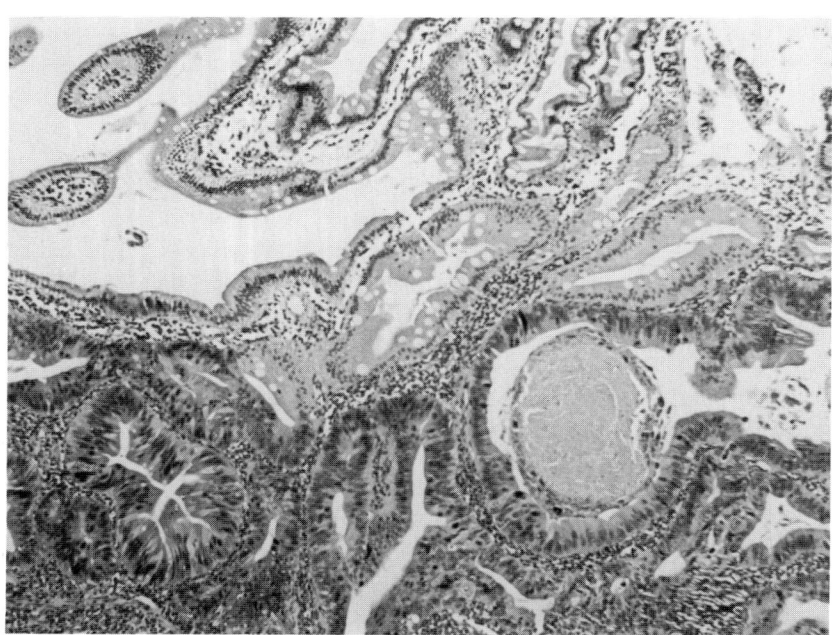

FIGURE 32–4. Focus of adenocarcinoma (bottom) in a Peutz-Jeghers polyp of the duodenum. ($\times$ 55) The adenomatous lesion was present in other areas.

domly in the colon, to be multiple, and to have an early age of onset.[216] It originates from dysplastic tissue rather than from adenoma.[217] Its survival rate is the same as for common carcinoma.

Carcinoma arises in the affected segments of the intestine in patients with Crohn's disease through the stage of dysplastic change, as in ulcerative colitis.[218–221] The incidence of colon carcinoma in Crohn's disease is lower than that in ulcerative colitis as a whole but is about the same as that in left-sided colitis.[219] The incidence is higher for the small intestine with a ratio of observed to estimated rates of 85.8,[219] perhaps because of the low rate of carcinoma at this site in the general population. The corresponding ratio for colorectal carcinoma is 6.9.

A natural model of intestinal carcinoma associated with inflammatory lesions has been found in a species of marmoset (*Saguinus oedipus oedipus*, the cotton-top tamarin).[222] In this case, the carcinomas occur multifocally, in the colon as well as the small intestine. However, this model differs from human colitis-carcinoma in a number of ways: Most of the carcinomas in the marmosets are undifferentiated,[223] the colitis is mild, and neither dysplasia nor adenoma is present.

Schistosomiasis. Among the infectious diseases of the bowel in man, only infestation with *Schistosoma japonicum* is known to be complicated by colorectal carcinoma.[224] The patients usually have a long history of diffuse involvement of the large intestine with pseudopolyps, disrupted muscularis mucosae, and ectopically regenerating glands. The carcinoma is often multicentric.[225]

Mucosal Hyperplasia. Proliferating cells may be at risk for altered DNA replication when exposed to carcinogen. Experimentally, adaptive hyperplasia of intestinal mucosa can be produced by jejunoileal resection, subtotal colectomy, enteric bypass, or pancreatobiliary diversion.[226] The administration of carcinogen to these animals postoperatively induces an increased number of intestinal tumors. A single dose of DMH induces more foci of atypia in the hyperplastic colon than in the normal colon.[227] In man, precancerous conditions usually have hyperplastic epithelium. Many of the risk factors in carcinogenesis may also be related to cell proliferation.[228] Tumor-promoting agents such as fat, bile acids, and short-chain fatty acids increase cell proliferation, whereas a vegetarian diet decreases it. Hyperplasia is probably responsible for the occurrence of dysplasia, adenoma, and carcinoma in the colon at or adjacent to the site of ureterosigmoidoscopy.[229,230]

Experimental Carcinogenesis

Experimental studies are useful for providing insight into the mechanisms of carcinogenesis by allowing evaluation of risk factors through manipulation of the experimental environments and sequential study of tissue changes in the target organ. Reliable animal models for intestinal carcinoma are available for these studies. The carcinomas have been produced by a variety of carcinogens in several species of rodents.[54–57] The most commonly used chemical is DMH, a procarcinogen that is not mutagenic. DMH produces tumors in the colon and, to a lesser degree, in the upper small intestine, whether it is given orally, subcutaneously, or intraperitoneally. It is oxidized primarily in the liver to form azoxymethane (AOM), then it is N-hydroxylated to methylazoxymethanol (MAM),[57,231,232] which is secreted in the bile in conjugated form. The bacterial β-glucuronidase frees MAM in the intestinal lumen, where it is metabolized to active carcinogen.[56] AOM and MAM have also been used to produce tumors. It is evident that this pathway to active carcinogen is subjected to modification by a variety of factors in the microenvironment of the intestinal tract. The DMH model is therefore commonly used to test the significance of risk factors. Another commonly used gastrointestinal carcinogen is MNNG, a direct-acting carcinogen that produces stomach and upper small-intestine tumors when given in the drinking water[233] and colorectal tumors by intrarectal instillation.[54,55]

In either model, the initial change is an increase in cell proliferation with expansion of the proliferative compartment in the crypt before tumorigenesis.[234] The DMH-induced tumors are adenomas and carcinomas. An adenoma-carcinoma sequence was noted in these tumors by some investigators.[235–237] Others found evidence for *de novo* origin of the carcinomas.[189,238,239] In our own experiments in mice,[190] DMH produced two types of adenomas: the polypoid adenoma with a single-crypt origin, and the flat adenoma with multiple-crypt origin. Carcinomas with superficial invasion arose in both of them (Figure 32–5). Crypt hyperplasia was common in the preneoplastic stage, but dysplasia was rare. In the MNNG-treated mice, dysplasia was common. In addition to polypoid adenoma, deeply infiltrative carcinoma without adenomatous elements were also frequent (Figure 32–6). Thus adenomas were produced in both models, but carcinomas differed in both origin and invasiveness. It appears that the origin of intestinal carcinoma is related to the type and perhaps also to the dose and the mode of action of the carcinogen.

Pathology

Although the gross and microscopic anatomies of the small and large intestines differ in many aspects, the pathologic features of adenocarcinoma are remarkably similar. All normally present cell types—including columnar cells, goblet cells, less-differentiated crypt cells, Paneth cells, and endocrine cells—have been identified in the adenocarcinomas of both the small and large intestines. Squamous cell differentiation has also been found in some tumors. Gross appearance of the carcinomas is also similar in the small and large intestines. On the other hand, the clinical presentations may vary regionally because of the relationship between the tumor and the neighboring organs. This relationship may affect the prognosis as well.

The common pathologic features are presented in this section, and the variable clinicopathologic features

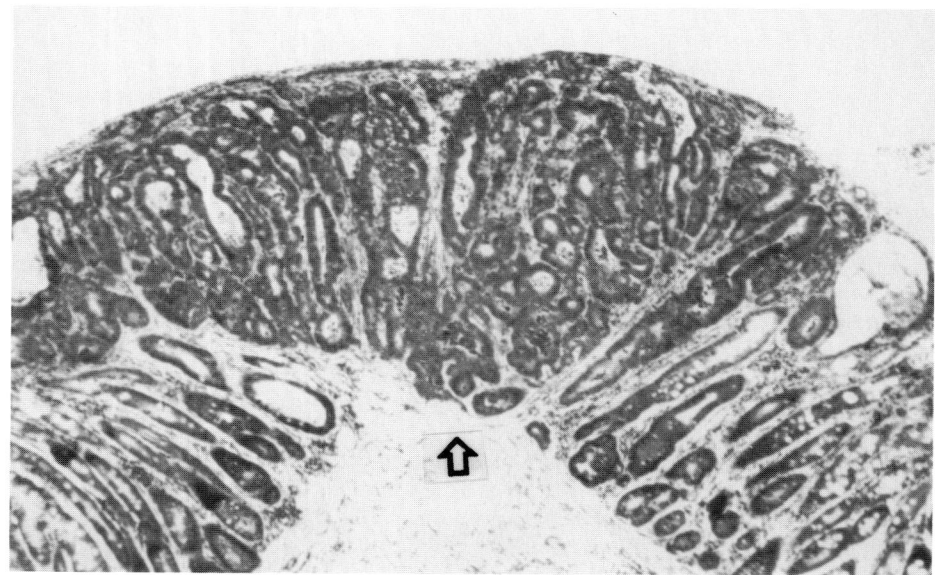

FIGURE 32–5. DMH-induced colonic adenoma in a mouse with a focus of adenocarcinoma at the center of the base invading the muscularis mucosae (arrow). ($\times$ 50)

are presented in the sections to follow on individual organs.

Histogenesis and Natural History

Histogenesis

Adenocarcinomas of the intestines develop along two major pathways. More commonly they occur in the highly dysplastic areas of an adenoma, and less commonly they arise in the dysplastic epithelium of the intestine, which is the site of chronic inflammatory disease of long duration. These events are discussed in this chapter in the section on precancerous conditions, as well as in Chapter 27 on ulcerative colitis and Crohn's disease and in Chapter 31 on benign intestinal polyps. The relatively recent recognition of small flat adenomas in the colon adds support to the adenoma-carcinoma pathway.[111]

The fact that residual adenoma might not be found by serial sectioning, even in the early carcinomas, raises the possibility of *de novo* development of intestinal carcinoma.[240] Evidence for this event must be searched for in the minute lesions. Kjeldsberg and Altshuler reported a case of colon carcinoma *in situ* without associated adenoma.[241] Crawford and Stromeyer[207] reported two minute colonic carcinomas: an intramucosal one measuring 0.3 by 0.3 by 0.1 cm and a submucosal one measuring 0.2 by 0.2 cm. Similar cases of early carcinoma without adenoma were reported by Ikegami.[242] Recently Shimoda et al. studied 178 early and 853 advanced carcinomas of the colorectum.[208] Of the early carcinomas 146 were polypoid and 32 nonpolypoid. The size of the polypoid lesions ranged from 7 to 45 mm. Adenomas were found in 96% of pedunculated polypoid carcinomas and 86% of sessile polypoid carcinomas. The size of the nonpolypoid early

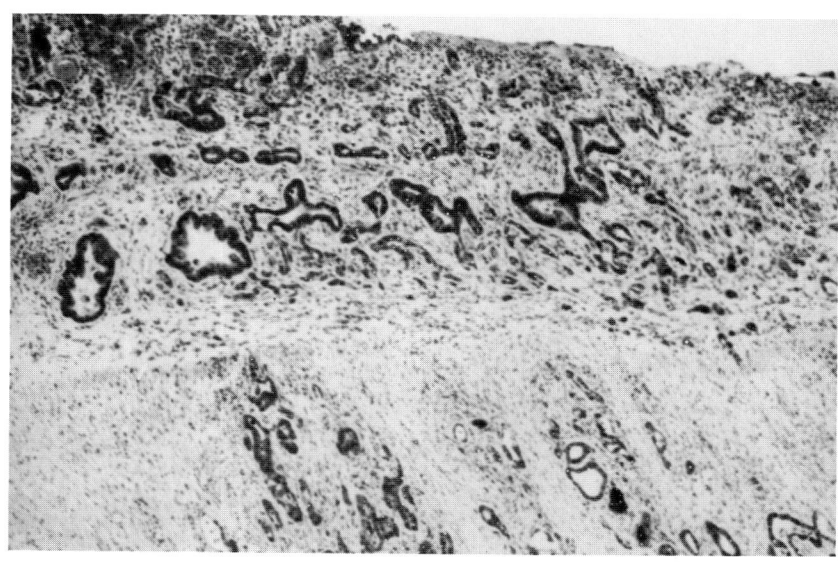

FIGURE 32–6. Infiltrative adenocarcinoma of the colon from a MNNG-treated mouse. There was no adenomatous tissue in the lesion. ($\times$ 50)

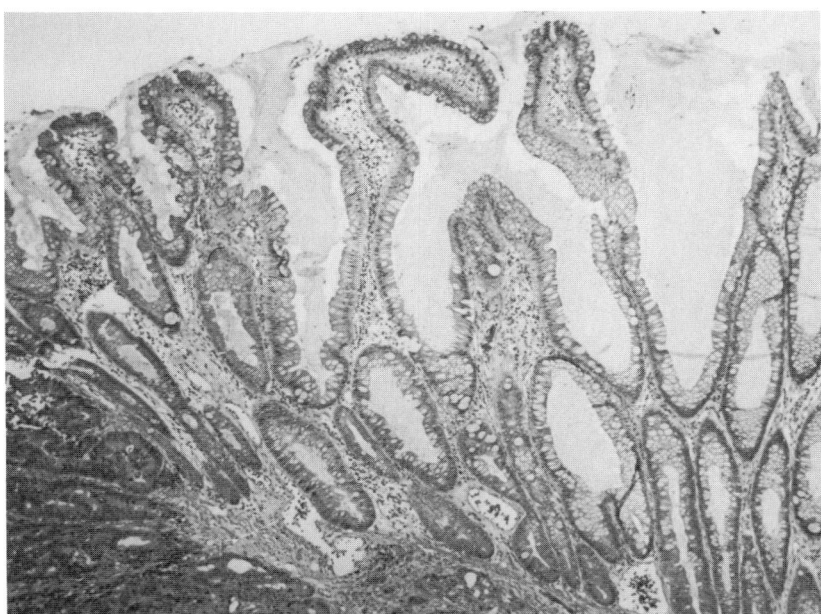

FIGURE 32-7. Transitional mucosa bordering an adenocarcinoma (left lower corner) of the colon, showing thickened mucosa containing dilated and hyperplastic glands. ($\times$ 32)

carcinomas ranged from 2 to 28 mm. Adenomatous tissue was absent in all. The advanced carcinomas had invaded muscularis propria or beyond. Polypoid lesions were seen in 186 cases, and adenoma in 40 of these lesions. The remaining advanced carcinomas were nonpolypoid. It was postulated that the carcinomas, which had not developed from adenoma, invaded early and grew rapidly to account for a higher percentage of nonpolypoid carcinomas among the advanced cases.

Hyperplasia is commonly observed in the colonic mucosa adjacent to carcinoma, so-called transitional mucosa, and occasionally in patchy areas remote from the carcinoma.[243] The transitional mucosa is hyperplastic and thickened, and the crypts are dilated and distorted[244,245] (Figure 32-7). Goblet cells are markedly increased. There is an increase of sialomucin,[243-245] which is more evident in the left colon, where sulfomucin normally predominates. Electron microscopy revealed an increased number of electron-dense bodies and an enlarged Golgi zone.[246] Immature and intermediate cells are retained in the upper level of the crypts. The absorptive cells are often vesiculated, and the microvilli are sparse. Similar changes can also be found in the mucosa adjacent to the adenoma.[245,247] The transitional mucosa shows an affinity for concanavalin A,[248] but there is no CEA.[247] It is not clear whether these changes are precancerous, incidental, or secondary to the neoplastic change.

Rate of Growth

Colonic carcinomas are slow-growing tumors. Cell kinetic studies (see Chapter 7) have shown variable doubling time of tumor cells grown *in vitro*. In general, their cell cycle time is longer than that of normal crypt cells, and the S phase is lengthened. The small carcinomas grow quickly, but the rate slows down as the tumor enlarges. Clinically the doubling time of the tumor, growing to twice its diameter as measured by radiologic examinations, is quite long.[249] The mean doubling time of the primary carcinomas was 620 days, with a range of 111 to 3430 days in 20 colorectal carcinomas.[250] This figure is undoubtedly influenced by the amount of necrosis, which may account for as much as 90% of the tumor mass. It was estimated that it might take 6 to 8 years for a colon carcinoma to reach the size of 6 cm.[251] The mean doubling time of pulmonary metastasis was 109 days,[252] and the doubling time of hepatic metastasis was 50 to 95 days.[253,254]

Spread of Adenocarcinoma

Depending on the location of the carcinoma, deep penetration of the tumor may cause direct involvement of the neighboring organs or tissues. Tumor cells may seed the peritoneum, surgical wound, or areas of inflammation. Venous permeation usually results in metastasis in the liver through the portal system. Cells of the lower rectal carcinoma may enter the systemic venous circulation directly and become lodged in the lung.

The lymphatic spread of carcinoma differs between the small and the large intestines. The small intestine has a rich lymphatic network in the mucosa. An intramucosal carcinoma, therefore, may be able to metastasize to the regional lymph node. However, the small-intestinal carcinoma is generally discovered at the advanced stage, and there are no data on lymph node status in early cancers. The lymphatics of the colon reach only to the level of muscularis mucosae,[255] so that only carcinomas with invasion into the submucosa or deeper layers may have lymphatic metastasis. Of 178 early colorectal carcinomas studied by Shimoda et al., 32 of 146 polypoid carcinomas and 22 of 32 nonpolypoid carcinomas had submucosal involvement. Lymph

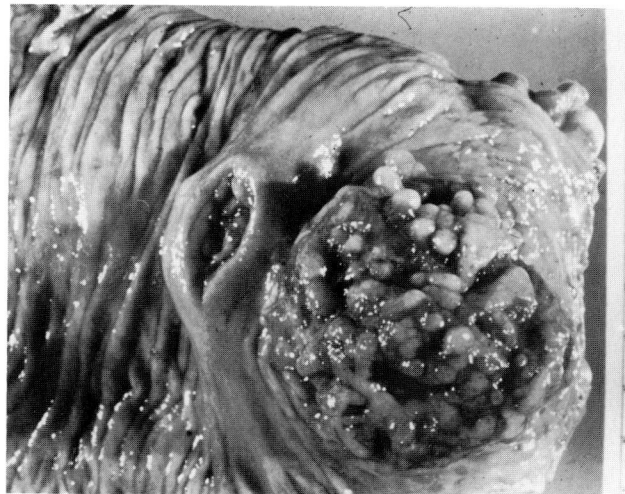

FIGURE 32–8. Polypoid carcinoma of cecum. The orifice of the ileum is shown on the left.

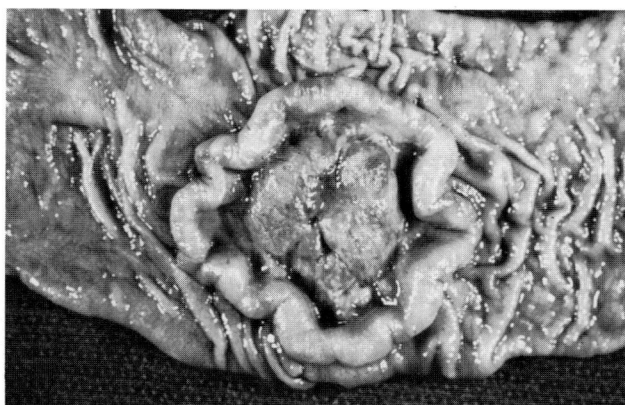

FIGURE 32–10. Fungating carcinoma of sigmoid colon, showing a raised rim of tumor tissue around a large ulceration.

node metastasis was present in only four cases, all nonpolypoid.[208]

Gross Morphology and Classification

Grossly the intestinal adenocarcinomas take one of four forms: polypoid, fungating, ulcerative, or diffusely infiltrative.

Polypoid Type

In this type, the carcinoma forms an exophytic intraluminal mass without significant ulcerative defects (Figure 32–8). It may have a nodular, lobulated or papillary surface. The small ones may closely resemble adenomas and may be, in fact, adenoma with carcinomatous focus. The large bulky ones are seen more commonly in the cecum and right colon than in the left colon or rectum. This type of carcinoma is likely to have arisen in an adenoma.

Fungating Type

This type of carcinoma is basically a polypoid carcinoma, superimposed by varying degrees of ulceration (Figure 32–9). In some tumors the ulceration destroys much of the tumor, and only a small portion of exophytic lesion at the border of the tumor remains. The tumor often has a raised and rolled border in which residual adenomatous tissue may be present (Figure 32–10). The carcinomatous tissue, including the marginal region, is firm, whereas the residual adenomatous tissue is relatively soft and pliable. Careful inspection and palpation of the nonulcerated tumor margin can usually identify the adenomatous areas.

Ulcerative Type

This type of carcinoma invades deep into the colonic wall, and the ulcerated surface is even with the normal mucosal surface or, more often, depressed (Figure 32–11). The tumor margin is flat or only slightly raised,

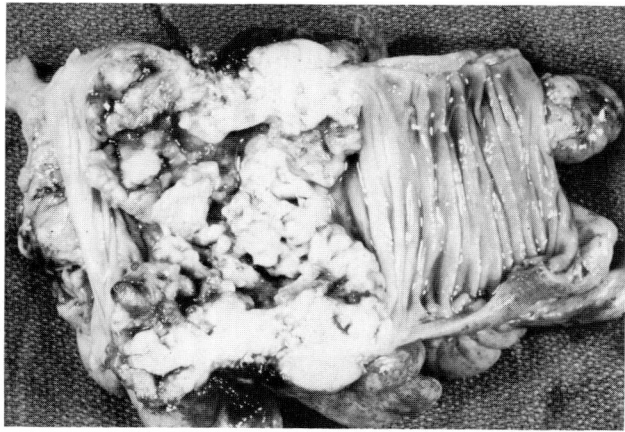

FIGURE 32–9. Fungating carcinoma of sigmoid colon, involving the entire circumference of the colon.

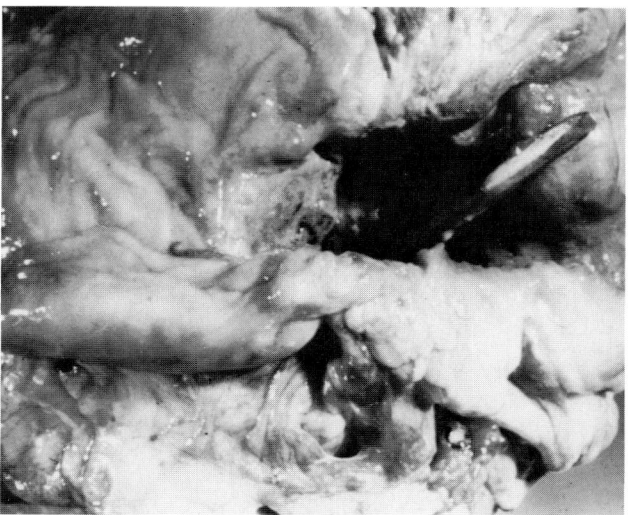

FIGURE 32–11. Ulcerative carcinoma of colon, with a probe through the perforated crater.

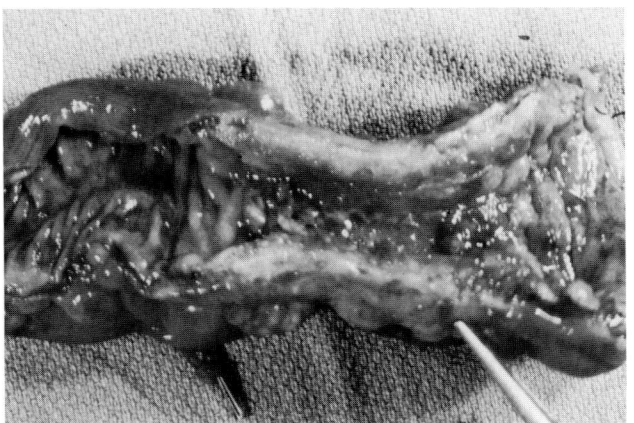

FIGURE 32-12. Diffusely infiltrative carcinoma of rectosigmoid, showing the uniformly thickened wall and shallow ulceration of the luminal surface. It was composed of signet-ring cells.

an appearance similar to that of the linitis plastica carcinoma of the stomach.[256,257] In this regard, it should be kept in mind that a metastatic lesion from the linitis plastica type of gastric carcinoma may have the same appearance. On the cut surface, the carcinoma is pale gray or white and has a firm and gritty consistency.

In the polypoid and fungating type, the periphery of the tumor tissue is sharply demarcated, at least focally. The periphery of infiltrative carcinoma, on the other hand, is indistinct. The border of an ulcerative carcinoma may have either appearance. The circumferential and obstructive lesions are also called stenosing or constrictive tumors.

The reported frequency of different types of carcinoma varied because of the variety of terms used. Shimoda et al. found that 20% of the carcinomas were polypoid and 80% nonpolypoid.[208] Jackman and Beahrs noted that 65% of the carcinomas were crater-like ulcerative lesions and 25% fungating tumors.[258] A similar frequency was found by Dionne.[259]

and there is no grossly discernible adenomatous tissue. The carcinoma infiltrates and thickens the intestinal wall, and this results in a discoid or saucerlike appearance of the lesion. The ulcerative carcinoma is more commonly seen in the left colon than in the right. Shimoda et al. considered that such nonpolypoid carcinomas arose *de novo*.[208] However, it remains possible that the pre-existing adenoma may have been destroyed by either the carcinoma or the ulceration, or both.

Diffusely Infiltrative Type

This type of carcinoma infiltrates a segment of the intestine diffusely and often circumferentially without forming a nodular mass (Figure 32-12). Diffuse thickening of a long segment of the bowel gives the lesion

Histologic Features and Cell Types

Histologic Features

Most intestinal adenocarcinomas are either well-differentiated (25%) or moderately differentiated (60%) glandular tumors[260] (Figures 32-13 and 32-14). Intraglandular papillary infoldings may be present in the well-differentiated carcinomas (Figure 32-15). Rarely groups of neoplastic cells with few fenestrations fill the glandular lumen.[261] About 15% of intestinal adenocarcinomas are either poorly differentiated or mostly undifferentiated. These tumors often grow expansively and form solid nodular masses (Figure 32-16). In spite of the lack of gland formation, the cells in some tumors are not particularly pleomorphic or bizarre, and the

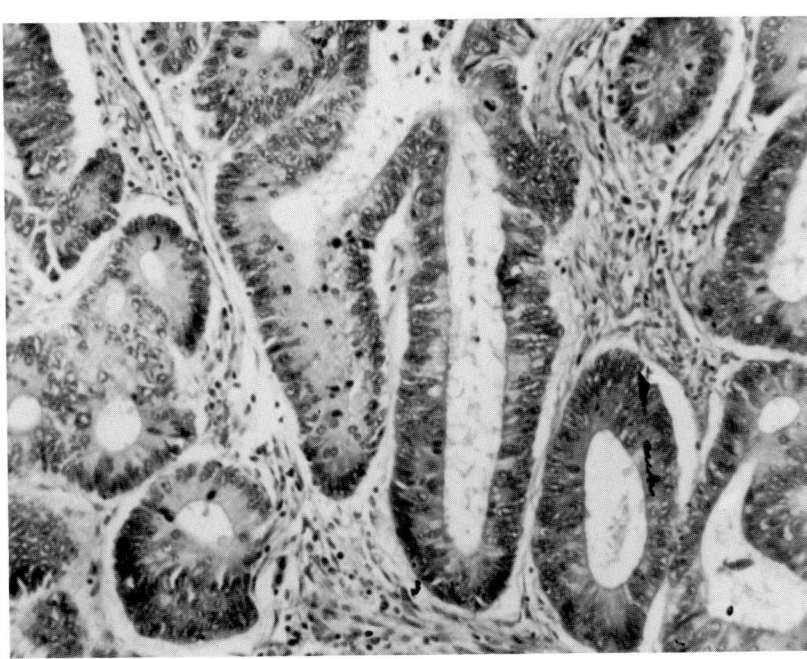

FIGURE 32-13. Well-differentiated adenocarcinoma of colon, showing glands composed mainly of columnar cell, some of which contain small globules of mucus in the apical cytoplasm. Many mitotic figures are present. (× 150)

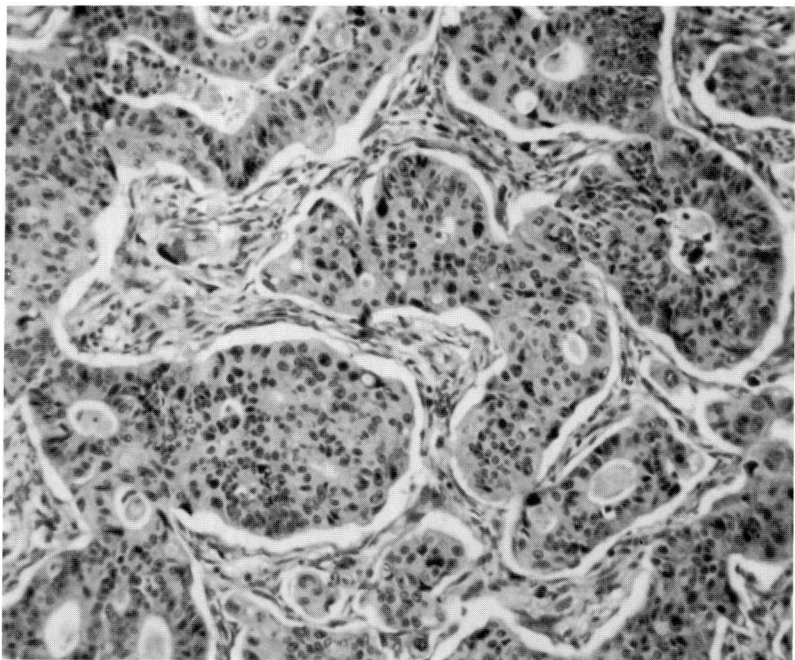

FIGURE 32–14. Moderately differentiated adenocarcinoma of the colon, with poor glandular formation in some areas. ($\times$ 180)

prognosis is relatively good.[262] The undifferentiated small cell carcinomas have been identified as endocrine tumors and carry a poor prognosis.

There are two main patterns of growth: expanding and infiltrative. The expanding growth pattern is characterized by nodular tumor aggregates of large interconnecting glands (Figure 32–17). In many tumors, the branching glands form a loosely intertwined network interposed by cellular fibrous tissue in which varying numbers of lymphocytic cells are present. The infiltrative growth pattern is characterized by narrow tubular glands with few bridging connections; the glands invade the gut wall individually or in small groups (Figure 32–18). The tubules are accompanied by varying amounts of relatively acellular collagenous tissue. Tumors with abundant fibrous stroma have been called scirrhous carcinomas, which can be recognized grossly as firm fibrous-appearing tissue without discrete nodules. Some carcinomas have a mixed pattern of growth (Figure 32–19) with the infiltrative tubules chiefly in the deeply invasive region, which suggests a change of biologic behavior as the carcinoma advances. Diffuse infiltration by individual carcinoma cells, as commonly seen with gastric carcinoma, is rare in the intestines. This pattern of invasion is characteristic of the signet-ring cell carcinoma. Diffuse infiltration by undifferentiated individual cells is extremely rare.

Expanding carcinomas are usually polypoid or fun-

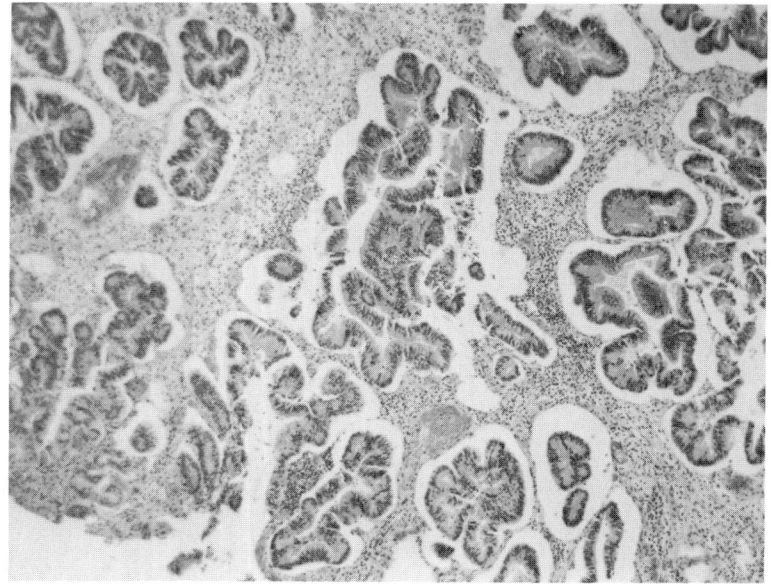

FIGURE 32–15. Papillary adenocarcinoma at the periampullary region of the duodenum. ($\times$ 50)

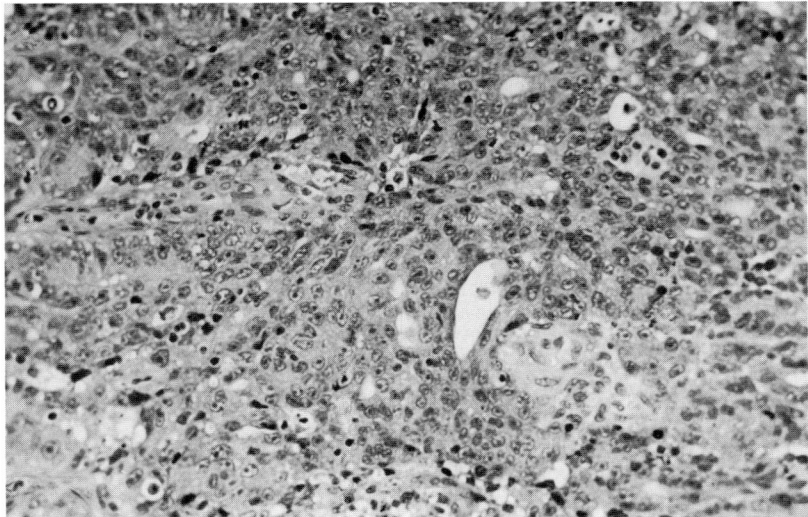

FIGURE 32-16. Poorly differentiated adenocarcinoma of colon, showing a compact sheet of tumor cells and a few small glandular spaces. (× 120)

gating on gross examination. Infiltrative carcinomas are ulcerative or diffusely infiltrative. The ulcerative carcinomas with a slightly raised border often show mixed patterns of growth.

Cell Types

The majority of carcinoma cells are columnar cells with no, or an ill-defined, striated border. Mucous cells are commonly present, and the intraluminal secretion usually contains mucus, predominantly sulfomucin mixed with lesser amounts of sialomucin. Neutral-type mucoprotein is rarely present. Many mucous cells have only small globules of secretion (see Figure 32–13). Goblet cells are infrequent.

Endocrine cells, mostly argyrophilic and less frequently argentaffin, are commonly present. Iwafuchi et al. found these cells in 18 of 24 small-intestinal carcinomas, secreting serotonin and a variety of peptides.[263] In the large intestine, endocrine cells have been found in 20%[264] to 75%[265] of the carcinomas. They were found in 4% of mucinous and 5% of undifferentiated carcinomas of the rectum and 52% of nonmucinous carcinomas of the colon.[264] Most often, the number of endocrine cells is small.[263-265] In some cases, however, they are prominent enough to justify the name *neuroendocrine carcinoma* or *adenocarcinoid*.[266,267] Additional information on endocrine cell tumors is presented in Chapter 13 and in the section on endocrine carcinomas.

Neoplastic Paneth cells have also been identified in the adenocarcinomas of both the small intestine[268,269] and the colon;[265,270-272] sometimes Paneth cells figure prominently.[269,272] The endocrine and Paneth cells are normally derived from stem cells in the intestinal crypt, as are the columnar and goblet cells. The clonal origin

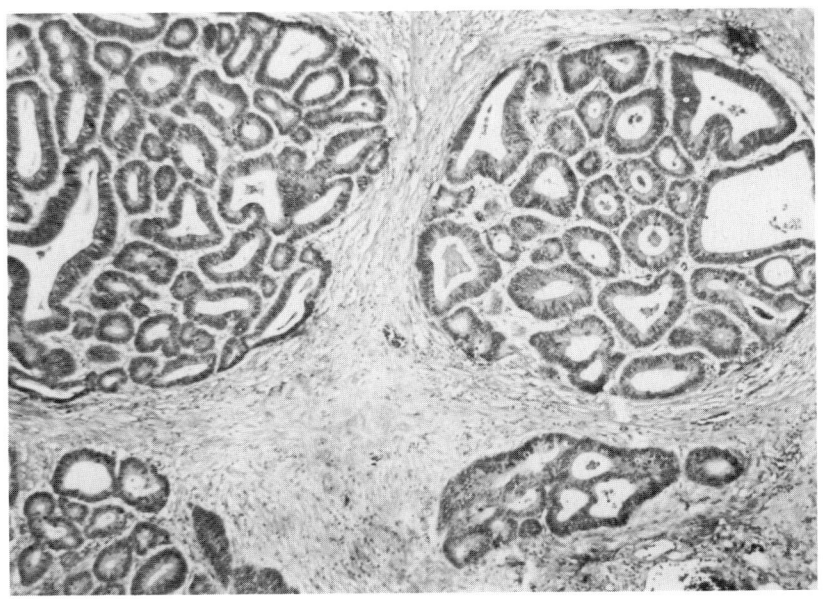

FIGURE 32-17. Well-differentiated adenocarcinoma of colon, showing an expanding type of growth. Groups of glands form circumscribed nodules separated by fibrous stroma. (× 50)

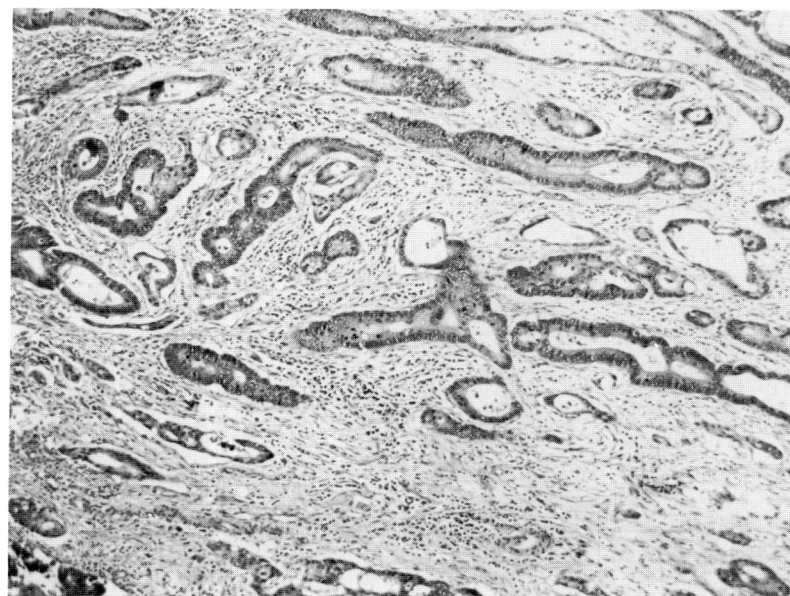

FIGURE 32–18. Well-differentiated adenocarcinoma, showing an infiltrative type of growth. Individual glands infiltrate the fibrous stroma, in which many lymphocytes are present. (× 50)

of these cells in the carcinoma is supported by the observation of differentiation into columnar, mucous, and endocrine cells in the culture of a single human rectal carcinoma cell.[273] In view of these findings, an intestinal adenocarcinoma with neoplastic endocrine and Paneth cells have been called crypt cell carcinoma[274] or stem cell carcinoma.[275,276] These tumors may also contain squamous cells. Tuft (caveolated) cells have been identified in two carcinoma cell lines.[277] Neoplastic M and cup cells have not been described.

Ultrastructural and Morphometric Studies

Colonic carcinomas have been studied with electron microscopy,[278–280] which shows various degrees of cell differentiation. The number of mucin granules decreases with lowering grade of differentiation. Conversely, the amount of apical dense bodies, glycocalyceal bodies, cytoplasmic vesiculation, and desmosomes increases. The microvilli are sparse and contain dense core microfilaments extending as long rootlets into a clear zone of apical cytoplasm. The long rootlets appear to be a marker for colonic adenocarcinoma.[280] The nucleus of the carcinoma cells shows thin, flat appendages that are connected with the main nucleus by lamellar bridges. These appendages were called nucleotesimals by Elias and Fong[281] and were thought possibly to be related to an unusual form of amitotic division. Electron microscopy is instrumental in the identification of special cell types in the carcinoma,

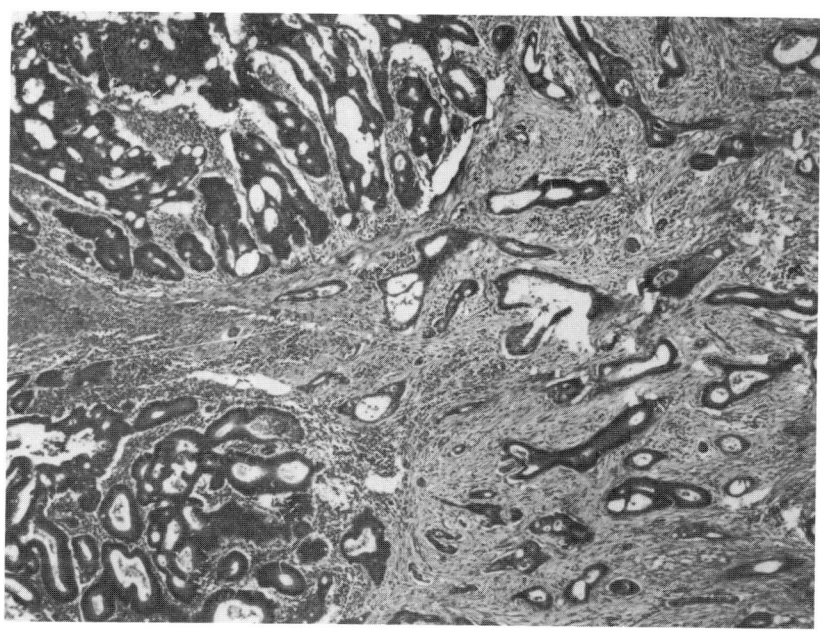

FIGURE 32–19. Well-differentiated adenocarcinoma of the colon, with mixed expanding and infiltrative types of growth. (× 32)

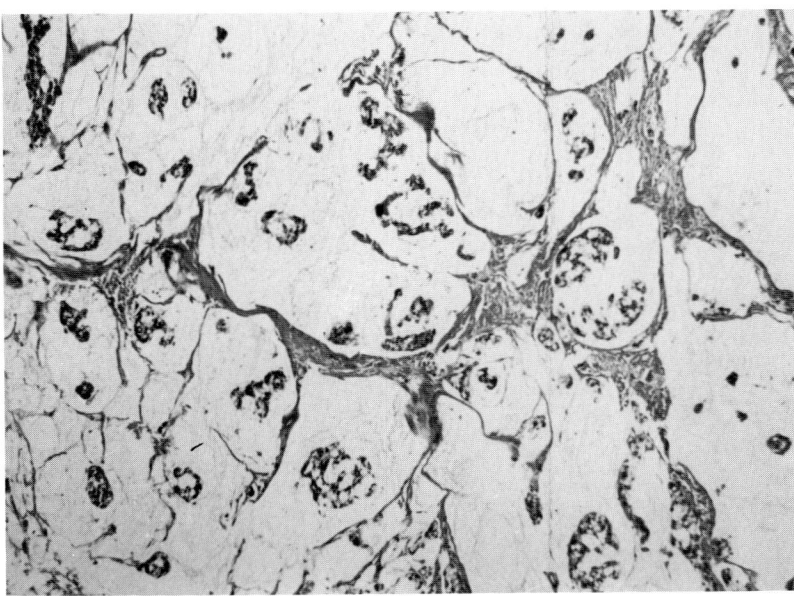

FIGURE 32-20. Mucinous adenocarcinoma of colon. More than 80% of the tumor mass is occupied by mucus. (× 50)

such as endocrine cells.[274,275] Morphometric studies of carcinoma show an expanded nuclear area, an increased nucleocytoplasmic ratio (from the normal mean of 20.4 to a mean of 39.7), displacement of nuclear position in the cells, and variable nuclear size and shape.[282,283] There is no significant difference in these parameters between a primary carcinoma and its metastatic lesion.[284]

Variants of Adenocarcinoma

Mucinous adenocarcinoma and signet-ring cell carcinomas are mucus-secreting variants of adenocarcinoma. The specific morphologic and biologic characteristics of each warrants a separate identity, as shown in the World Health Organization (WHO) Histological Typing of Intestinal Tumors.[285] In the mucinous adenocarcinoma the mucus is primarily extracellular (Figure 32-20), and in the signet-ring cell carcinoma the mucus is intracellular.

Mucinous Adenocarcinoma

In mucinous adenocarcinoma, abundant mucus forms a pool in the connective tissue, in or surrounding which the cancerous tissue resides. The amount of mucus required to qualify the tumor as mucinous is generally 50% or more of the tumor mass.[285-288] A minimum of 25% mucus is required for the tumor to be considered as having a mucinous component.[289] With these criteria, 5% to 15% of colonic carcinomas are mucinous[287,290,291] and an additional 5% to 6% of tumors have mucinous components.[286,289] The tumors with large amounts of mucus present a grossly gelatinous appearance and the term *colloid carcinoma* is applied. Most of the mucinous carcinomas appear to have originated from adenomas[290] and are composed of tubular structures. They occur more often in younger patients, and in the right colon and rectum than do the nonmucinous carcinomas.[287,291] These tumors are often in an advanced stage when diagnosed, are less resectable, and carry a poorer prognosis than other carcinomas.[286,290-292] They are seen frequently in the hereditary nonpolyposis colorectal cancers.[98,99] Purtilo et al. reported a familial occurrence of mucinous colonic carcinoma in 13 members of a black family.[293] The median age of the patients was 39 years. The transmission was by an autosomal-dominant trait.

Signet-Ring Cell Carcinoma

Signet-ring cell carcinoma occurs rarely in the intestines. In 1982 Ojeda et al. found only 52 reported cases in the English literature in a 50-year period.[294] The reported incidences were 0.2% to 1% for carcinomas[295,296] and 4% for mucinous carcinomas.[297] The tumor cells infiltrate diffusely to produce a linitis plastica type of gross appearance.[257] It is characterized by tumor cells shaped like a signet ring, with an eccentric crescent-shaped nucleus pushed by the intracytoplasmic mucus against the cell wall (Figure 32-21). These cells infiltrate the gut wall individually or in small groups. The prognosis is poor, and only a few patients live more than one year after diagnosis.[294,298]

Staging of Adenocarcinoma

With the same definition applied to gastric cancers,[208,209] intestinal adenocarcinomas have been divided into early and advanced cases. The early carcinomas are limited to mucosa or submucosa, and the advanced carcinomas have invaded muscularis propria or deeper layers. The status of lymph node metastasis is not taken into consideration. Hermanek and Gall had 130 early cases, 3% of which had lymph node metastasis.[300] The 10-year survival rate was 100%, and a limited resection of the lesion was adequate in some cases.

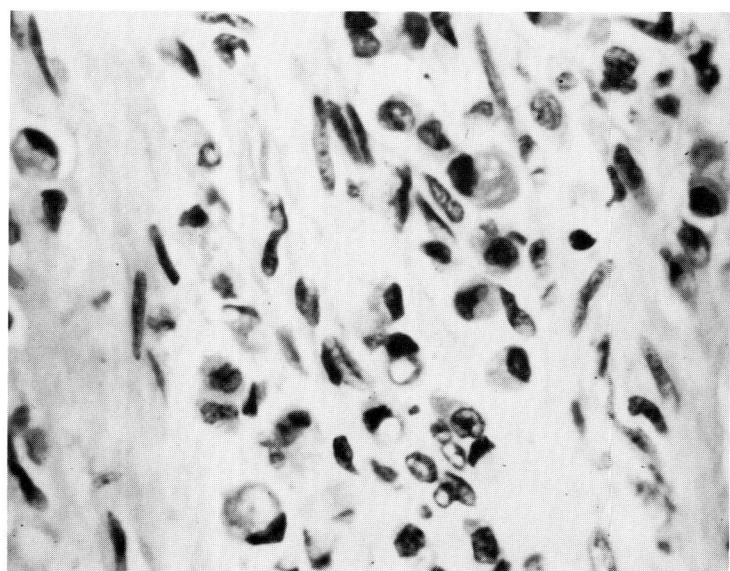

FIGURE 32–21. Signet-ring cell carcinoma of the colon. (× 480)

A comprehensive staging system, with specific reference to survival rate and prognosis, was introduced by Dukes in 1932.[301] It was designed originally for use with rectal cancers but now has been applied to all intestinal cancers. Dukes classified the tumors into three groups: group A—tumor is within the rectal wall, up to but not through the muscularis propria; group B—tumor penetrates through the rectal wall into the extramural tissue, but without lymph node metastasis; and group C—metastasis to the regional lymph nodes. The 5-year survival rates for the respective groups were 93%, 65%, and 23%.[302] With the recognition of additional factors, there have been several attempts to modify the grouping criteria. In 1949 Kirklin et al. divided group A cases into A with carcinoma limited to the mucosa and B1 with tumor extending into muscularis propria.[303] The original Dukes' group B became B2. There was no significant difference between the survival rates of these two subgroups. In 1954 this modification was adopted by Astler and Coller,[304] who introduced the subgroups C1 and C2 for cases with lymph node metastasis. C1 patients had B1 primary tumor, and C2 patients had B2 primary tumor. The 5-year survival rates were 100% for group A patients, 66.6% for group B1, 53.9% for group B2, 42.8% for group C1, and 22.4% for group C2 patients. The difference between survival rates for groups B1, B2, and C1 was not great. Dukes also introduced C1 and C2 categories in 1949 and 1958[305,306]: C1 for involvement of regional lymph nodes only, and C2 for positive nodes at the point of ligation of the blood vessel at the time of surgical resection of the tumor. (The positive nodes of the C2 category were called apical nodes, a term that refers to their location in the surgical specimen.) It was noted that the 5-year survival rate for C1 patients was 40.9% and for C2 patients, 13.6%.[306] Turnbull et al. introduced a D-category for patients with metastasis to distant organs.[307] In addition to the level of lymph node involvement, Dukes also recognized the importance of the number of involved nodes.[306] Recent analyses indicate that metastasis to more than four lymph nodes carries a poor prognosis.[308,309]

The American Joint Commission on Cancer (AJCC) has developed a staging system based on similar parameters: T—the extent of tumor invasion; N—the status of lymph node involvement; and M—distant metastasis. The TNM staging system has undergone several modifications. The recent version,[310] which takes into consideration the number of involved lymph nodes, is compared with the Dukes' classification[306] and the modified classifications of Astler and Coller[304] and Turnbull et al.[307] in Table 32–7.

The pathologic features of intestinal tumors are complex, and only a few of the features are used by the staging systems. Other significant prognostic factors include the pattern of tumor growth, grade of tumor cell differentiation, and the density of lymphocytic infiltration in the tumor.[311] Jass proposed a new classification of colorectal carcinomas for prognostic prediction based on the evaluation of all the features using numerical indicators.[311,312] In practice, Dukes' method remains popular because it is simple and easy to use.

Small-Intestinal Adenocarcinoma

Carcinomas of the small intestine share many pathologic features and precursor conditions with colorectal cancers. The etiologic factors are presumably similar also. The epidemiologic data, however, show less geographic variation than shown by carcinomas of other segments of the digestive tract.

Pathology

Location

Adenocarcinomas of the small intestine occur mostly in the upper segments, about 40% each in the duode-

Table 32–7 STAGING METHODS FOR COLORECTAL CARCINOMA

AJCC TNM System[310]	Dukes' Classification[306]	Astler and Coller[304] and Turnbull et al.[307] Modifications
0: Tis N0 M0	—	—
I: T1 N0 M0	A: intramural	A: mucosa
T2 N0 M0	A: intramural	B1: muscularis propria
II: T3,4 N0 M0	B: extramural	B2: extramural
III: T1-4 N1-3 M0	C1: regional nodes	C1: B1 and positive nodes
	C2: apical nodes	C2: B2 and positive nodes
IV: T1-4 N1-3 M1		D: distant metastases

Definition of TNM categories:[310]
T–Depth of primary tumor invasion:
  Tis: carcinoma *in situ*, T1: mucosa or submucosa
  T2: muscularis propria, T3: subserosa or periocolic tissue
  T4: through serosa or invading contiguous organs
N–Metastasis in regional lymph nodes:
  N0: no positive nodes
  N1: 1 to 3 positive nodes
  N2: 4 or more positive nodes
  N3: any positive node along a named vessel
M–Metastasis in distant organs:
  M0: absent
  M1: present

num and the jejunum (see Table 32–2). In one report, carcinoma of the duodenum was nearly twice as common as that of the jejunum and ileum combined.[196] Duodenal carcinomas account for 0.3% of all gastrointestinal malignancies.[313] They occur in the periampullary region in 65% of cases, the supra-ampullary region in 21%, and the infra-ampullary region in 14%.[10] Involvement of the duodenal bulb is rare.[314,315] In the jejunum the carcinomas are located primarily in the upper portion. In both the duodenum and the jejunum, adenocarcinoma is the most common malignant tumor. In the ileum, on the other hand, the most common tumor is the carcinoid, and the distal segment is the favored site for carcinoma.[17]

The location of adenocarcinoma is influenced by the precancerous conditions from which the tumors arise. Of carcinomas associated with Crohn's disease, for instance, 75% occur in the ileum,[316] the primary site for Crohn's disease. The jejunum is the site for carcinoma in Crohn's disease in 24% of cases. The duodenum is involved only rarely.[317] These carcinomas develop from the dysplastic epithelium.[219,318] In patients with familial adenomatous polyposis or Gardner's syndrome, carcinomas and adenomas often occur in the duodenum, particularly in the periampullary region.[319,320] In celiac disease and nontropical sprue, duodenal and jejunal carcinoma may occur.[321–323] Other sites of origin of small-intestinal carcinoma include Meckel's diverticulum,[324,325] aberrant pancreas,[326] ecoptic gastric mucosa,[34] the ileostomy,[327–329] and possibly Brunner's glands.[330]

Pathologic Features and Pattern of Spread

The adenocarcinomas of the proximal small intestine tend to be polypoid or fungating, possibly related to their origin in the adenoma (Figures 32–22 and 32–23), whereas those of the distal segment are often ulcerated and infiltrating. In about 80% of cases, the carcinoma

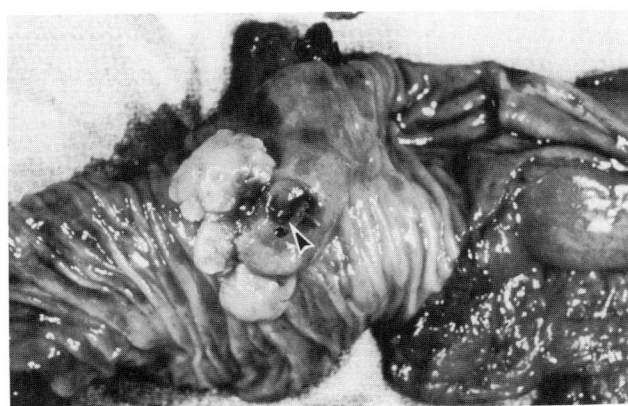

FIGURE 32–22. Carcinoma of the duodenum at the periampullary region. The orifice of ampulla of Vater is indicated by the arrowhead.

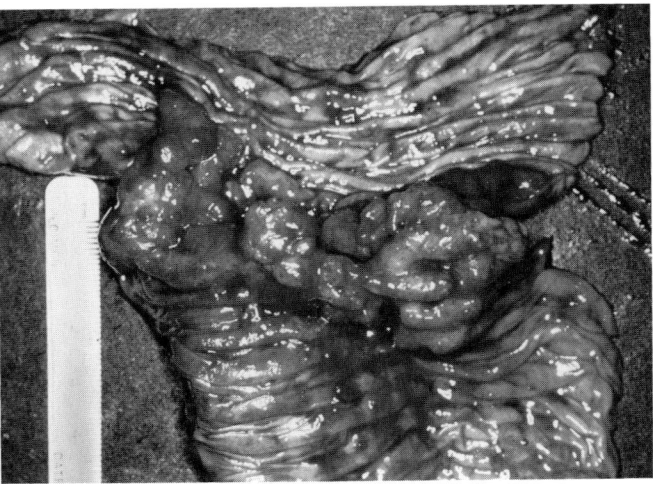

FIGURE 32–23. Circumferential polypoid carcinoma of jejunum. The lumen above the tumor is dilated.

is annular and constricting.[4] The carcinoma complicating Crohn's disease may not be grossly evident in one half of the cases.[316] Occasionally, they are multifocal.

Microscopically, most adenocarcinomas of the small intestine are well to moderately differentiated. Papillary and villous appearances are seen mainly in the polypoid tumors[315] (see Figure 32–15). About 20% of tumors are poorly differentiated.[331] Most cells are columnar, with varying degrees of microvillar development.[332] Mucous cells are commonly present and secrete both sialomucin and sulfomucin in most cases, although the adjacent normal mucosa secretes only sialomucin.[333] Argyrophilic cells are commonly found, particularly in carcinomas of the ileum.[263,333] Paneth cells may be present also, occasionally in large numbers.[269]

In most cases, the carcinoma is already deeply invasive at the time of diagnosis. Early carcinoma is rarely diagnosed, except as a focal lesion in an adenoma, mostly in the duodenum.[334] Carcinomas of the ampullary region can invade the head of the pancreas, pancreatic duct, or common bile duct. In such a situation, it may be difficult to decide the origin of the tumor. In an analysis of 233 periampullary tumors, Yamaguchi and Enjoji found 109 carcinomas of the ampulla of Vater, 19 of the duodenum, 38 of the distal bile duct, and 48 of the head of the pancreas.[334] In 12 cases the origin of the carcinoma was not determined. In other regions, penetration of the tumor through serosa may cause peritoneal dissemination or adherence between the tumor and loops of adjacent intestinal segments.

Because the small intestine is rich in lymphatics, lymphatic permeation is common in the primary lesion. Carcinomas of the duodenum metastasize to the posterior pancreaticoduodenal lymph nodes; those of the jejunum and ileum, to the mesenteric nodes; and those of the terminal ileum, to the ileocolic nodes and posterior cecal nodes. The carcinomas of the ampulla of Vater have lower rates of lymph node involvement in only 20% to 35% of cases.[315] Venous invasion of carcinoma in all parts of the small intestine leads to the portal venous system and eventually to the liver, from which further spread to the lung and other organs occurs.

Clinical Presentation

Adenocarcinomas of the small intestine occur mainly in elderly persons (mean age, around 60 years).[3,335] The annual incidence per 100,000 in the United States is 1.2 for white males, 0.8 for white females, 1.6 for black males, and 0.7 for black females.[336]

Because most carcinomas are annular, intestinal obstruction is common and pain is the most frequent complaint.[3] Tumors of the upper small intestine produce nausea and vomiting, whereas those in the distal small intestine cause abdominal distention and periumbilical pain. Weight loss is frequent.[337] Acute abdominal emergency due to perforation of the tumor is uncommon.[338] Bleeding commonly occurs, but usually it is occult and chronic. Acute massive bleeding is rare.

The periampullary carcinomas often cause obstruction of the common bile duct and jaundice. Of the cases reviewed by Yamaguchi et al., 111 were icteric and 31 nonicteric.[339] The carcinomas in the icteric group were more advanced and less papillary, and showed less intraluminal and more periductal growth than those in the nonicteric group. The 5- and 10-year survival rates were 57%, in both, for the nonicteric patients, and 32% and 23%, respectively, for the icteric patients.

The primary choice of treatment is surgical resection of the carcinoma. The reported resectability rate was, on average, 72% for carcinomas of the duodenum, 76% for those of the jejunum, and 82% for those of the ileum.[3] The 5-year survival rates of the resected cases were 20%, 17%, and 9% for the respective locations (duodenum, jejunum, and ileum). The reported 5-year survival rate for all carcinomas of the small intestine was 15%.[337] The poor survival rates are related to the advanced state of the tumor at the time of diagnosis.

Colorectal Adenocarcinoma

Colorectal cancer is the most common cancer and the second most common cause of death from cancer in the United States. The estimated number of new cases in 1990 is 191,600, and the estimated number of deaths is 85,000 (see Table 32–1).[5] The annual incidence rate per 100,000 in 1987 was 50.9, and the mortality rate was 19.9 (see Table 32–4).[36] Ninety-five percent of colorectal cancers are adenocarcinomas.

Pathology

Location

Most colorectal adenocarcinomas are located in the left colon, particularly the sigmoid and rectum. There have been reports of increasing incidence of carcinomas in the proximal colon and decreasing incidence of carcinoma in the distal colon.[340–343] The change is particularly evident within the same institution. Cady et al. reported that in the 40-year period from 1940 to 1979, the percentage of carcinoma in the right colon at The Lahey Clinic in Boston increased from 7% to 22%, whereas that of the sigmoid and rectal carcinoma decreased from 80% to 62%.[344] Slater et al. reported an increase from 18.7% to 27.5% for right colon cancer, and a decrease from 72.1% to 62.5% for left colon cancer.[343] A similar change is found by comparing the frequencies of tumors in different segments of the colorectum. In 1967 Wood[10] reported that the frequency of carcinoma in the cecum and ascending colon was only 10% and in sigmoid and rectum, 75%. In recent reports, the corresponding frequencies were about 25% and 60%, respectively.[260,344,345] The frequencies of carcinoma between these two segments showed minor variations, mostly in the range of 2% to 4% at the hepatic flexure, 5% to 7% in the transverse colon, 2% to 5% at the splenic flexure, and 5% to 11% in the descending colon. The shift of frequency to the right colon parallels a similar shift of the location of the adenomas and an increase in the age of the patients.[346]

The location of colorectal carcinoma is influenced by the location of the precancerous condition from which the cancer develops. In ulcerative colitis, the carcinoma is widely distributed. In Crohn's disease, carcinoma is located more often in the right colon than in the left colon.[347] Carcinoma has also been reported in the rectal stump after colectomy for colitis.[348,349] The location of colonic carcinoma is also affected by genetics. In Lynch syndromes, over 70% of the carcinomas occur in the right colon and only 25% in the sigmoid and rectum.[98]

Carcinomas of the right colon differ from those of the left colon in several respects. The carcinomas of the left colon tend to occur more frequently in males, have three times more concomitant adenomas, and are twice as likely to have adenomatous tissue in the tumor. Carcinoid and mucinous components are more prominent in the carcinomas of the right colon.

Pathologic Features

Grossly, carcinomas of the right colon, particularly the cecum, tend to be polypoid and fungating (see Figure 32–8), whereas those of the left colon tend to be ulcerative (see Figure 32–11) as well as fungating (see Figures 32–9 and 32–10). The diffusely infiltrative (linitis plastica) type of carcinoma occurs more often in the distal colon (see Figure 32–12). Circumferential involvement is more common in the left colon, which is normally narrower than the right colon. The carcinomas that complicate inflammatory bowel disease are often flat and may not be grossly evident.[350,351]

Histologically, the colorectal carcinomas are mostly well to moderately differentiated. Endocrine and mucinous elements are more common in the tumors of the right than the left colon.[351,352] The carcinomas associated with Crohn's disease may be less differentiated than others.[352]

Multiplicity

Adenocarcinomas of the colon and rectum are often multiple, occurring synchronously in 3% to 8% of patients and metachronously in 2% to 3% of patients surviving the first carcinoma.[161,353–355] The origin of synchronous carcinomas was investigated retrospectively by DNA ploidy of the tumors.[356] In four cases all tumors were diploid, and in three cases the tumors had identical aneuploid patterns, suggesting the possibility of a single origin of the tumors in these cases. Synchronous carcinomas are more common in patients with familial polyposis (21%),[357] Lynch syndromes (18%),[103] and ulcerative colitis (18%),[357] and after pelvic irradiation.[358] In one report each of a pair of monozygotic twins had three colonic carcinomas.[359] In a study in Japan, 35% of synchronous carcinomas were both advanced, 59% were mixed advanced and early, and 6% were both early.[360] In 62% of cases, both synchronous carcinomas were in the sigmoid and rectum.

In other cases, the tumors were randomly distributed. In another study, 88% of synchronous carcinomas were found in different segments of the colon.[361] Sixty percent of the colons that contain synchronous carcinoma have adenomas. Patients with synchronous carcinoma have a higher incidence of metachronous cancer than those with single cancer at first diagnosis.[362] The intervals between the first and the second carcinoma vary, between 2 and 5 years in 40% to 50% of cases,[355] but the interval may be longer than 20 years.[359]

The preoperative diagnosis of multiple carcinomas is achieved mainly by colonoscopy.[355,363] The early lesions can be easily missed, and correct preoperative diagnosis was made in only 42% of cases.[364] In 24% of cases the second carcinoma was discovered at operation; in 34% it was found incidentally in the resected specimen. Postoperative colonoscopy is mandatory for early diagnosis of metachronous carcinomas.[364]

Patterns of Spread

Local Spread. The mucosal origin of colorectal carcinoma causes the carcinomas to grow intraluminally, particularly in tumors arising in an adenoma. Intramural spread may be circumferential with production of a constrictive lesion, or longitudinal along the long axis of the bowel. The extent of intramural spread under an intact mucosa is an important concern at the time of surgical resection, in regard to the length of resection margin. Fortunately, in most cases, deep-seated lateral spread of the tumor is limited. A study by Lazorthes et al. on 119 rectal carcinomas[365] revealed that in 74% of cases, the extent of deep-seated carcinomatous tissue was the same as that seen grossly. In 21% of cases, the border of tumor spread was beyond the gross margin by less than 5 mm. In only 5% did the tumor extend for 5 to 15 mm beyond the gross margin. A similar observation was made by Madsen et al., who concluded that 1.5 cm was an adequate distal margin.[366] Kameda et al. noted that the intramural spread of the tumor was within 0.5 cm of the gross margin in a localized tumor and 2.1 cm in an infiltrative tumor and that lymph node with metastatic tumor was usually located within 1 cm of the margin of the primary lesion.[367] They, therefore, recommended a resection margin of 2 cm for localized carcinomas and 3 cm for infiltrative carcinomas. The highly infiltrative signet-ring cell carcinoma is an exception to this rule. Rarely, perineural invasion may extend beyond the gross tumor margin.[366]

The carcinomas may invade directly into the neighboring tissue. A cecal carcinoma may extend into the lateral abdominal gutter and the abdominal wall. Carcinoma of the transverse colon may involve the stomach, pancreas, liver, gallbladder, and spleen. Carcinomas of the ascending and descending colons may involve the retroperitoneal tissue. Carcinomas of the sigmoid and rectum may involve the pelvic organs, urinary bladder in males, and vagina in females. The anterior surface of the colon is covered by the peritoneum. The carcinoma may penetrate the serosa and seed the peritoneal surface. Fibrous adhesion forms when the carcinoma involves the adjacent loops of intestine, mesentery, or omentum.

Lymphatic Spread. In his study of rectal cancer Dukes noted that lymph node involvement rarely occurred when the primary carcinoma was still within the bowel wall.[301] When lymphatic permeation is present, the tumor emboli travel to regional nodes along the arteries: ileocolic artery for the cecum and ascending colon, middle colic artery for the transverse colon, inferior mesenteric artery for the descending colon and sigmoid, and hemorrhoidal vessels for the rectum. The first group of lymph nodes are in the pericolic or perirectal tissue. The ileocolic and middle colic lymphatic chains drain into the central nodes of the superior mesenteric artery. There may be aberrant lymphatics draining the lower rectum to nodes along the inferior mesenteric artery, skipping the nodes adjacent to the primary tumor.[368] Retrograde lymph node metastasis may occur when the normal lymphatic flow is blocked by metastatic tumor.[369] Lymph node metastasis is present in about 40% to 50% of colorectal carcinomas.[306,370]

Venous Spread. Venous invasion occurs in about one half of colorectal carcinomas,[371] and tumor cells have been found in both regional and peripheral venous blood.[372] Mesenteric venous flow lodges the tumor cells in the liver, and the liver is the most frequent site of visceral metastasis, in about 40% of autopsied patients.[373] From the liver, tumor cells advance to the lung and other organs. Metastasis may occur in the lung alone, however, from carcinomas of the lower rectum, which has a dual venous system: the superior hemorrhoidal veins to the portal system and liver, and the middle and inferior hemorrhoidal veins to the systemic circulation and lung. Occasionally, direct metastasis to the vertebrae occurs by way of Batson's venous plexus.[374] The frequency of venous spread is related to the extent of primary tumor invasion,[259,375] the stage of tumor, and the technique of tissue examination. The invaded vein may be too distorted to be readily recognized. Using elastic tissue stain to identify the venous wall, Grinnell found venous involvement in about one third of colorectal carcinomas.[376]

Metastasis. The frequency of metastasis in the visceral organs at autopsy was reported by Berge et al.[377] The liver was involved in 75.7% of colonic carcinomas and 61.9% of rectal carcinomas. The corresponding percentages for metastasis in the lung were 47.7% and 64.2%. Lymph node metastasis was present in 77% and 78.4%, respectively. The other organs, which were involved relatively frequently, included peritoneum (in 49.4% and 25.4% of cases, respectively), adrenal gland (13.8% and 18.7%), ovary (17.3% and 3.6%), bone (11.7% and 19.4%), pleura (11.3% and 12.7%), brain (6.3% and 8.2%), kidney (5.0% and 4.5%), skin (5.0% and 3%), and spleen (6.7% and 2.2%).

Metastasis to the ovary by signet-ring cell carcinoma produces Krukenberg tumors with bilateral enlargement of the ovaries.[378] In one report, metastasis of a cecal adenocarcinoma to the ovary caused excessive production of estrogen and postmenopausal uterine bleeding.[379] Other uncommon sites of metastasis include testis,[380] jaw,[381] nasopharynx,[382] pelvic bone,[383] and phalangeal bone.[384] The metastatic lesion may become ossified.[385]

Implantation. Peritoneal seeding of carcinoma cells is relatively common, particularly in patients with the infiltrative type of carcinoma. Occasionally the tumor implant grows in the rectouterine (pouch of Douglas) or rectovesical pouch and forms a palpable mass by rectal examination, known as Blumer's shelf. Implantation of tumor cells at the time of operation may be responsible for tumor growth in surgical wounds[386] and at the anastomotic suture line.[387,388] Intraluminal seeding of exfoliated cancer cells may cause implantation in anal fistulas.[389] The occurrence of some of the synchronous colonic carcinomas with identical DNA indices has been postulated to be on a similar basis.[356]

Marker Substances

Since the isolation of CEA in 1965,[390] many biochemical markers have been demonstrated in colorectal carcinomas.[391–394] The development of monoclonal antibody techniques and immunohistochemical methods further facilitated the investigation.

Carcinoembryonic antigen is the prototype of a group of oncofetal antigens. This glycoprotein is present in the fetal cells as well as some adult cells[395] and in an increased amount in many malignant tumors. In the colorectum it is associated with the striated border of the normal columnar cells and the apical cell wall of the carcinoma cells. Intracytoplasmic presence is seen mainly in the mucus-secreting cells.[396] CEA is demonstrable also in adenomas[391,397] and in inflammatory bowel disease.[397] CEA is drained from the tumor by the portal venous system.[398] The serum level of CEA is apparently related to the size of the tumor mass. Elevated serum levels of CEA were present in 18% of patients with early colonic carcinoma and 83% of patients with advanced carcinoma.[394] Although CEA is not specific enough for the diagnosis of colorectal carcinoma, its serum level has been used to monitor postoperative tumor recurrence.[345,399] In some reports, preoperative serum CEA level was found to be related to the stage of the carcinoma and the survival rate.[392,400,401]

CA19-9 is an example of newly synthesized antigen by cancer cells.[391,392] It is related to blood group antigen Le^a and is present in up to 80% of colonic carcinomas and other benign lesions such as polyps and dysplastic cells. CA19-9 is drained from the tumor by lymphatics.[398] Elevated serum levels of CA19-9 are present in up to 50% of cancer patients. It is less sensitive but more specific than CEA for cancer diagnosis.[402] Altered expressions of Lewis and ABH blood group antigens are often noted in colorectal adenomas and carcinomas.[391,403–405] T antigen, a precursor for blood group M and N antigens, is demonstrated by binding with peanut agglutinin in nearly all colonic carcinomas.[391] Other lectins have also been found to bind colonic carcinomas and polyps.[406–408] Colon-specific antigen p (CSAp) is another glycoprotein found in the serum of patients with advanced colonic carcinomas.[392,409] Several cancer-related antigens recognize mucin-type glycoproteins,[410-412] including M1 antigen and colon-ovarian tumor antigen (COTA).

DNA contents of carcinoma cells have been studied by many investigators. Aneuploidy was found in 53% of colonic carcinomas, 27% of tubular adenomas, and 19% of cases of ulcerative colitis.[413] However, 68% of hereditary nonpolypoid carcinomas were found to be diploid.[414] The polypoid carcinomas were aneuploid in 17%, whereas the crater-shaped carcinomas were aneuploid in 77%.[191] The ploidy of the carcinoma has been correlated with CEA serum level,[397] depth of tumor invasion,[415,416] stage of tumor,[416,417] and prognosis.[417,418] Some studies, however, did not find such relationship.[419,420] In any case, the ploidy of the tumor is not as significant a prognostic factor as the morphologic features of the carcinoma.[312] Using tritiated thymidine labeling or antibody Ki-67, more proliferating cells were found in carcinomas than in adenomas or normal mucosa.[421,422] However, the number of these cells in colonic carcinoma varied widely and there was no relation to any known parameter of prognostic significance.[423]

These and other biologic markers[424-442] of colorectal carcinoma are listed in Table 32-8.

Clinical Presentation

Age, Sex, and Race. Carcinomas of the colon and rectum are diseases of the elderly, with peak age in the seventh and eighth decades.[377] The mean age of the patients was 71.2 years for carcinoma of the right colon, 68.2 years for left colon cancer, and 65.6 years for rectal cancer.[443] Colorectal carcinoma occurs rarely in the young. Only 3% to 6% of patients were younger than 40 years.[444-446] The symptoms in these patients are not different from those in the older patients.[447] Some reports noted that the young patients had a high incidence of signet-ring cell and mucinous carcinomas,[444,448,449] a delay in diagnosis,[444] and poor prognosis.[444,445,448,449] Other reports found the survival rate to be no worse in the young patients than in older ones.[447,450]

There is no significant sex or racial difference in the incidence of colon carcinoma, but rectal carcinoma is more frequent in the white male (see Table 32-5).[36] Comparing the rates in 1973 and 1987, there was a 16% increase in the incidence for the white male and 31% increase in both black males and females (see Table 32-5). The rates of mortality from colon cancer increased in the black population, but that of rectal cancer decreased in both sexes and races.

Symptoms and Signs. The symptoms and signs of colorectal carcinoma are abdominal pain or cramp (78% of patients), change in bowel habits (67%), hematochezia (56%), weight loss (38%), palpable abdominal mass (37%), anemia (24%), intestinal obstruction (11%), and symptoms related to metastasis (7%).[451] There are regional variations in the frequency of these clinical manifestations because of differences in the caliber of bowel, the nature of feces, and the type of

Table 32-8 BIOLOGIC MARKERS OF COLORECTAL CARCINOMA

Glycoproteins
 Carcinoembryonic antigen (CEA)[390-402]
 CA19-9[391,392,398,402]
 Colon-specific antigen p (CSAp)[393,409]
 Colon-associated antigen[391]
Blood group antigens
 ABH antigens[391,403,405]
 Lewis antigens[391,404]
 T antigen[391,406]
Lectin-binding glycoconjugates[406-408]
Mucoproteins
 M1 antigen[411]
 Colonic mucoprotein antigen (CMA)[410]
 TAG-72[391]
 MAM-6[391]
 Colon-ovarian tumor antigen (COTA)[412]
Growth factors and receptors[424-427]
Enzymes
 Ornithine decarboxylase[391,392]
 Carcinoplacental alkaline phosphatase[428]
DNA ploidy and marker for cell proliferation[413-423]
Chromosomal aberrations and oncogenes (see Chapter 6)
Hormones[427,430]
 Human chorionic gonadotropin[429]
 Androgen receptors[155]
 Estrogen and progesterone receptors[154,431,436-439]
 Gastrin receptor[432]
 Glucocorticord receptor[433]
Polyamines[434]
Plasminogen activator[435]
Acute-phase reactive protein[394,400]
Other markers and monoclonal antibody–defined antigen[391,394]
HLA[440,441]
Immunocomplexes[442]

tumor. Fresh blood in the stool and a change of bowel habits are common in patients with carcinomas of the distal colon and rectum, whereas anemia, weight loss, and palpable mass are the main manifestations of carcinomas of the proximal colon.[452]

Unusual manifestations include symptoms of appendicitis in a case of cecal carcinoma,[453] rupture of iliac aneurysm into the fistula of a cecal carcinoma,[454] inappropriate secretion of antidiuretic hormone in a rectal carcinoma leading to a low serum sodium level,[455] dyspepsia,[456] glossodynia and xerostomia,[457] and an increased serum calcium level and hyperparathyroidism.[458,459]

Complications. Obstruction and perforation, the main complications, affect 29% of patients with colon carcinomas and 7% of those with rectal carcinomas.[460] Obstruction alone was present in 15% of cases, and perforation with or without obstruction in 4%. Compared with noncomplicated cases, these patients were older, the tumors were less resectable, the surgical mortality was four times higher, and the overall 5-year survival rate was only half that of uncomplicated cases.[460,461] The cases of perforation fared worse, with a 5-year survival rate of only 10%.[462]

Perforation of the carcinoma into the peritoneal cavity causes acute abdominal symptoms that require emergency operation. Small perforation results in pericolic abscess or fistula formation, which may involve adjacent organs or blood vessels. A case of aortoenteric fistula was reported, secondary to recurrent colon carcinoma.[463]

Acute obstruction due to intussusception is relatively common in association with benign tumors of the intestine but is only rarely reported in patients with carcinoma.[464] Chronic obstruction is due primarily to circumferential infiltration of the tumor with napkin-ring–shaped constriction.

The colorectal carcinomas are often ulcerated and bleed. The blood loss may be frank or occult. The ulcerated tumor may serve as a locus for infection, which induces further necrosis of the tumor and contributes to perforation and fistula formation. The infection may spread to other organs. There have been reports of *Streptococcus bovis* septicemia and endocarditis,[465–467] clostridial septicemia and soft tissue gangrene,[468,469] meningitis, and abscesses in various organs.[465]

The lower urinary tract is affected in 38% of patients, causing obstruction, gross hematuria, or neurogenic bladder,[470] associated more commonly with recurrent than with primary colorectal carcinoma. Other uncommon complications include coagulopathy in patients with metastasizing mucus-producing tumors,[471] microangiopathic hemolytic anemia,[472] dermatomyositis,[473] and extrahepatic obstructive jaundice.[474]

Associated Conditions. In addition to the common association of colorectal carcinoma with precancerous conditions listed in Table 32–6, colon carcinoma has been reported in patients with a variety of other conditions. Colonic diverticulosis is common in the western countries in which colorectal carcinoma prevails. Furthermore, diverticulosis affects mostly the distal colon, as does carcinoma. It is therefore not surprising to find that both conditions may coexist in a high percentage of cases in both men and women.[475,476] The carcinoma may fortuitously involve one or more diverticula.

Colorectal carcinoma was found to be associated with hyperplastic gastric polyps in 18.7% of cases and with gastric adenomas in 3.5%.[477] Appendicitis was present in 10 of 519 patients with cecal carcinoma.[478] Coexisting carcinomas are found in other parts of the digestive tract: ampulla of Vater,[479] gallbladder,[480] appendix,[412] and anus.[481] Other reported coexisting tumors were astrocytoma,[482] extragenital malignant mixed mesodermal tumor,[483] and mesenteric fibromatosis.[484] Colorectal carcinomas have been found in patients with acromegaly,[158,485] parathyroid adenoma,[160] acquired immune deficiency syndrome,[486] linear seborrheic keratosis,[487] malacoplakia of colon,[488] and ciliary dyskinesia.[489] They have also been found in patients with Hodgkin's disease after chemotherapy.[490]

Diagnosis, Screening, and Treatment. The diagnosis of colorectal carcinoma in symptomatic patients requires increasingly sophisticated imaging techniques, endoscopic examination with biopsy (see Chapter 3), and cytologic study (see Chapter 4). Local spread of carcinoma and lymph node metastasis can be detected by endoluminal ultrasonography, which has an accuracy rate of more than 80%, much better than computerized tomographic (CT) scan.[491] Endoscopy is indispensable in diagnosing colorectal tumors. Sigmoidoscopy up to 60-cm level may miss one third of the lesions.[492] Total colonoscopy is necessary to detect synchronous lesions preoperatively and metachronous lesions postoperatively.[355,363] Endoscopic biopsy is accurate for diagnosis in 90% of cases, and fine-needle aspiration cytology is particularly useful on the infiltrative type of growth. The accuracy rate of fine-needle aspiration cytology is 97%, and brush cytology is accurate in 83% of cases.[493] In terms of reliability of pathologic diagnosis on the resected specimens, routine histologic sections have been found to be quite adequate and representative.[494,495]

For the screening of asymptomatic persons in the general population, a variety of tests for occult blood in the feces have been used. A 6-day test resulted in the detection of adenoma in 8.77 and carcinoma in 2.54 per 1000 persons tested.[496] The detected carcinomas were in relatively early stages in most of the cases.[497,498] Screening with proctosigmoidoscopy has only limited benefit.[499] Colonoscopy is useful in screening the high-risk population, such as first-degree relatives of patients with familial traits. In one such study, adenoma was detected in 21% of 114 tested persons.[500]

The colorectal carcinomas are treated primarily by surgical resection. The resectability of the tumor depends on the stage of the tumor when first diagnosed and the surgical techniques used. In general, 85% of colorectal carcinomas are resectable for cure, 10% are unresectable or resectable for palliation only, and 5% are inoperable.[501] Endoscopic transrectal resection has been applied to patients who are poor operative risks or who have small tumors.[502,503] Adjuvant postoperative radiation has been used to control local recurrence and improve the survival rate.[504,505] Chemotherapy with 5-fluorouracil (5-FU) alone or in combination with interferon on patients with advanced cancer has elicited a partial response.[506,507] Recently, combined use of fluorouracil and levamisole, an immunostimulant, showed beneficial effects on postresection patients.[508] Liver metastasis has been treated surgically, with low operative mortality and a 5-year survival rate of 25%.[509,510] Arterial infusion of 5-FU to the liver results in partial remission and prolongs the survival interval.[511]

Survival Rates and Prognosis. The latest available 5-year survival rates of colorectal cancer in the SEER (surveillance, epidemiology, and end results) program of the National Cancer Institute are listed in Table 32–5.[36] The rates in the 1981-to-1987 period were about 6% higher than the corresponding rates in the 1974-to-1976 period in the white population, but not in the black population, as blacks had more advanced cases than whites.

The survival rates by stages of the tumors in SEER program are listed in Table 32–9.[36] The carcinomas were classified into three stages: localized tumors were limited to the bowel wall, regional tumors had extramural invasion or metastasis to local lymph nodes, and distant tumors had metastasis to the distant organs.

Table 32-9 STAGE DISTRIBUTION AND 5-YEAR RELATIVE SURVIVAL RATES OF INTESTINAL CANCER, SEER PROGRAM, 1974-1986 (IN PERCENTAGES)

Site	Stage				Survival Rate				
	L	R	D	U	L	R	D	U	T
Small intestine	20	39	35	6	58	48	21	28	39
Colon-rectum	34	38	21	7	85	55	6	30	53
Colon	32	40	22	6	88	58	6	28	54
Rectum	39	34	17	9	80	47	4	34	51

L, localized; R, regional; D, distant; U, stage unknown; T, all cases.
From Gloeckles-Ries LA, Hankey BF, Edwards BK: Cancer statistics review, 1973-1987. NIH publication 90-2789. Bethesda, Md, National Cancer Institute, 1990.

The survival rates were highest for the localized carcinomas and lowest for the distant tumors.

Survival rates are influenced by many factors (Table 32-10), but the stage of the tumor is the most important factor.

SQUAMOUS CELL CARCINOMA AND ADENOSQUAMOUS CARCINOMA

Occasional squamous cells are present in about 5% of colorectal adenocarcinomas. About one half of these tumors were found in the rectum and sigmoid and 20% in the cecum.[512] When the malignant squamous cells are prominent components of the tumor, the term *adenosquamous carcinoma* is applied. These tumors are rare (Figure 32-24), occurring in only 0.05% of carcinomas.[513] Squamous cell carcinoma of the colon was first reported in 1919.[514] By 1988 more than 60 cases had been reported.[515,516] The squamous cells have been identified by electron microscopy and immunohistochemistry.[517,518] The reported location of the tumor was

Table 32-10 PROGNOSIC FACTORS FOR COLORECTAL CARCINOMA

Pathologic factors
　Stage of carcinoma at time of diagnosis
　Extent of local invasion of carcinoma
　Lymph node metastasis
　Number of lymph nodes with metastasis
　Type of carcinoma
　Growth pattern of carcinoma
　Length of resection margin from tumor
　Grade of differentiation of carcinoma
　Vascular permeation by carcinoma
　Perineural invasion by carcinoma
　Serosal involvement by carcinoma
　Inflammatory reaction in carcinoma
　Lymph node reaction
　Fibrosis in carcinoma
　Location of carcinoma
　Size and shape of carcinoma
　DNA ploidy of carcinoma
Clinical factors
　Age of patient
　Sex of patient
　Symptoms and duration of symptoms
　Complications
　Carcinoembryonic antigen serum level
　Acute-phase reactive protein serum level

variable: more in the right colon in some reports[519,520] and more in the left colon in other reports.[521] The clinical presentation is similar to that of adenocarcinoma. In rare cases, hypercalcemia was present.[522,523] There is no sex difference. Grossly, the tumors form fungating masses.[515] They are aggressive tumors,[517,518] and 5-year survival rates were reported to be 50% for Dukes B, 33% for Dukes C, and 0% for Dukes D tumors.[516] In view of the occasional occurrence of squamous differentiation in adenocarcinomas, squamous cell and adenosquamous carcinoma probably originate from crypt cells. The presence of carcinoid cells in an adenosqua-

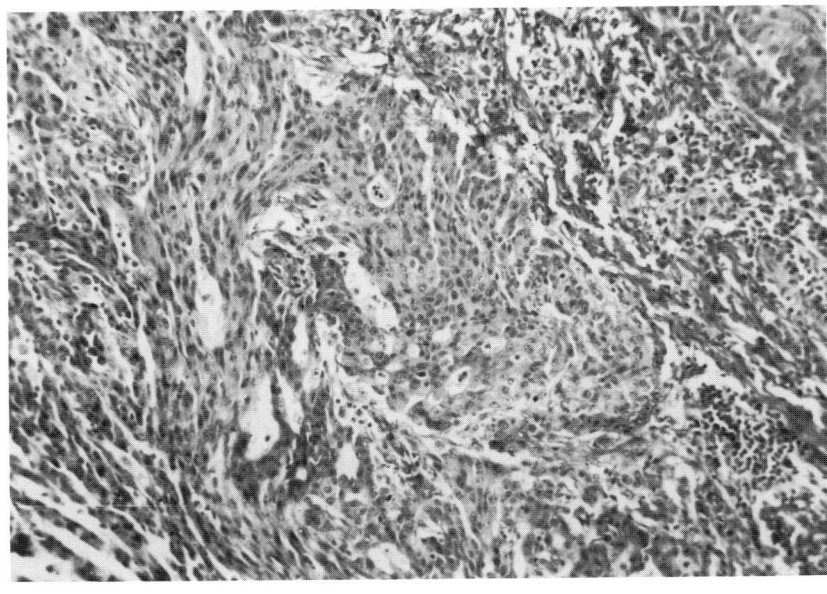

FIGURE 32-24. Adenosquamous carcinoma, showing squamous component of the tumor. (× 120)

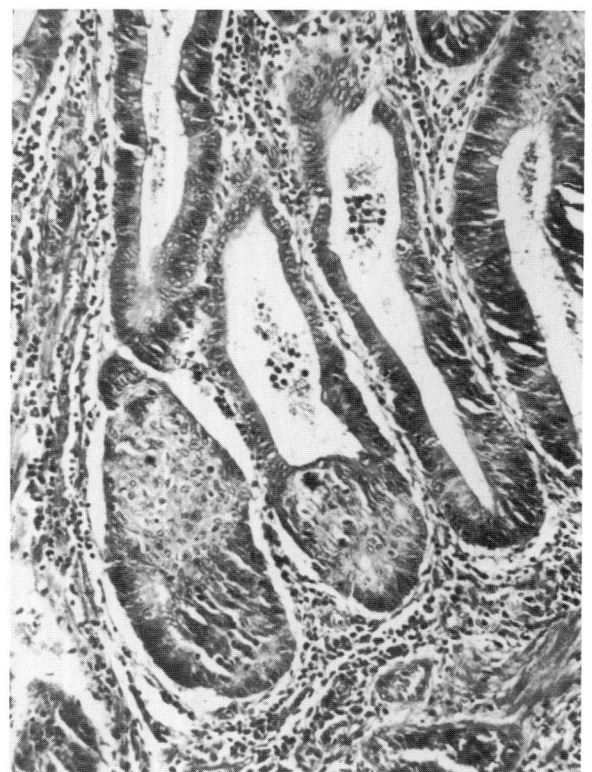

FIGURE 32–25. Focal squamous metaplasia in a tubular adenoma of the colon. (× 120)

mous carcinoma supports this view.[524] Colonic adenoma may have areas of squamous metaplasia (Figure 32–25), and squamous cell carcinoma may develop in such an adenoma.[519,525,526] These tumors have also been reported in patients with ulcerative colitis[516,527] and after radiation treatment for cervical carcinoma.[528] They may also arise from an area of squamous metaplasia in the flat mucosa.[529] In one case, the squamous cell carcinoma developed in a duplication of the colon.[530]

ENDOCRINE (NEUROENDOCRINE) CARCINOMA

Endocrine cells of the gut are of endodermal origin and are differentiated from stem cells in the crypt. The crypt origin of these cells explains their presence in a wide range of intestinal neoplasms,[263–265,274,531] occasionally in conjunction with Paneth[266] or squamous cells.[524,531] In addition, there are tumors that are composed of both carcinoid and carcinoma or of carcinomatous cells with endocrine functions. These tumors are discussed in detail in Chapter 13.

Composite Adenocarcinoma and Carcinoid and Adenocarcinoid

Carcinoid may coexist with either adenoma or adenocarcinoma (Figure 32–26) as composite tumors.[532–534] In other cases the carcinoma and carcinoid cells intimately intermingle to form adenocarcinoid.[535,536] The latter, particularly the variant known as goblet cell carcinoid, occurs most frequently in the appendix (see Chapter 33).

Small-Cell Carcinoma

Small-cell carcinomas of the intestines have been identified as an unusual form of endocrine carcinoma. They are histologically identical to the pulmonary tumor of the same name. The cells are uniformly small and have a dense chromatin pattern and scanty cytoplasm (Figures 32–27 and 32–28). Occasional glandu-

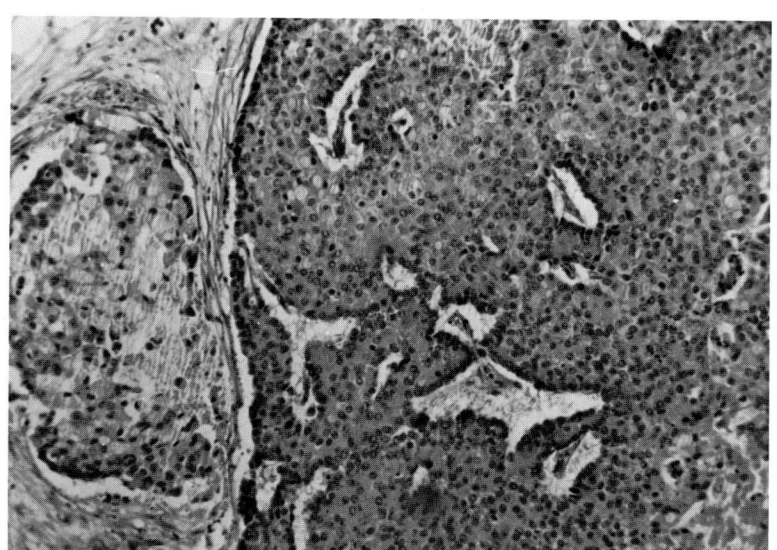

FIGURE 32–26. Composite adenocarcinoma and carcinoid of the colon, showing a small group of mucous carcinoma cells to the left of a patch of carcinoid cells. (× 120) In other areas, the carcinoma is mostly tubular and infiltrative.

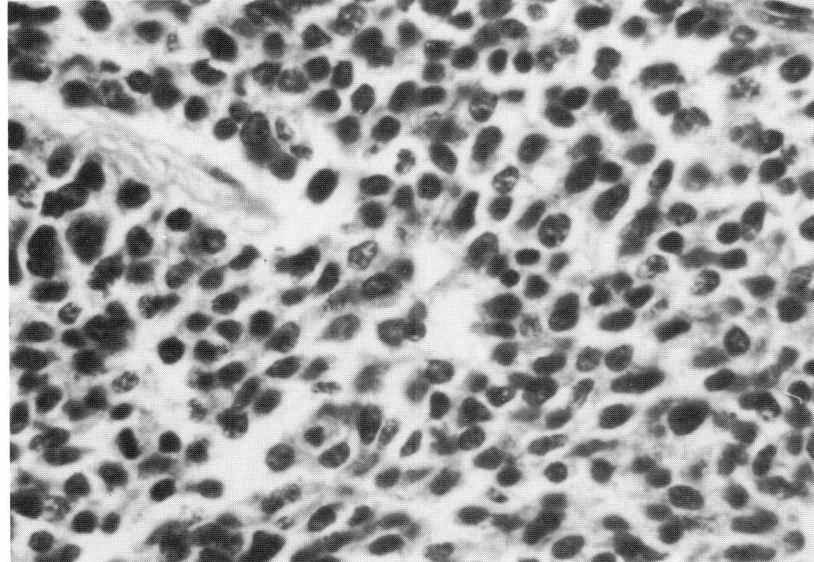

FIGURE 32-27. Small-cell carcinoma of colon. (× 480)

lar structures may be present.[267] Some tumors appear to have developed in an adenoma. Of five cases reported by Mills et al., four were associated with villous or tubulovillous adenoma.[537] Occasional cases have coexisting adenocarcinoma[538] (Figure 32-29). Grossly, small-cell carcinomas may be polypoid, fungating, or constrictive.[537,539]

Electron-microscopic examination of the tumor reveals neurosecretory dense-core granules of variable sizes, tonofilaments, and desmosomes.[267,539,540] Immunohistochemical studies show positive reaction for medium- and low-molecular-weight cytokeratin, epithelial membrane antigen, neuron-specific enolase, and neurofilaments.[541]

Small-cell carcinomas are quite aggressive; even a small superficial tumor may have already metastasized to the lymph node.[537] Of 20 colonic tumors reviewed by Redman et al., widespread metastasis was present in 85%.[538] Nearly all patients died, mostly within a year.[537] Radiation and chemotherapy may provide temporary remission.[538,539]

Pleomorphic (Giant Cell) Carcinoma

Bak reported four cases of pleomorphic (giant cell) carcinoma, two in the small intestine and two in the colon.[542] The tumors are composed of a mixture of giant cells, small polygonal cells, and spindle cells. Dense-core granules, keratin, vimentin, and neuron-specific enolase were present in the cells. There was early spread of the tumor, and the prognosis was poor.

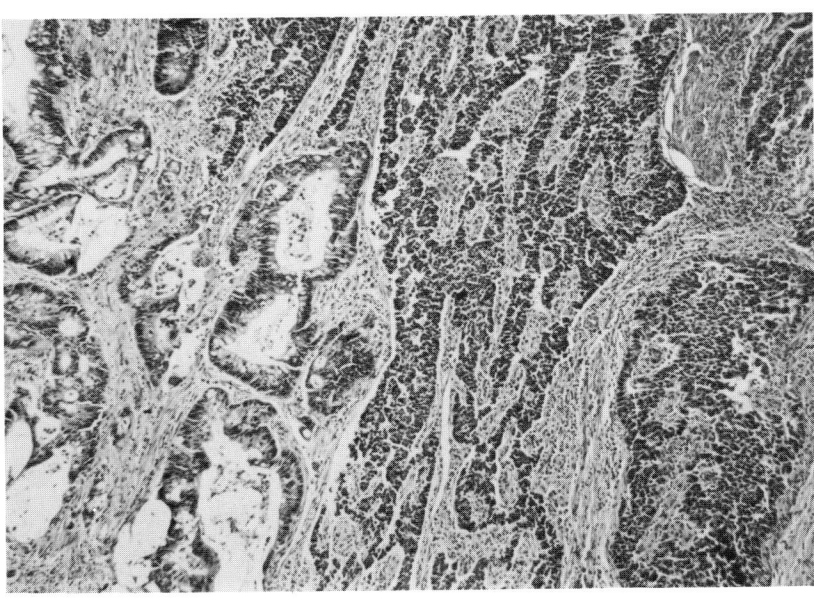

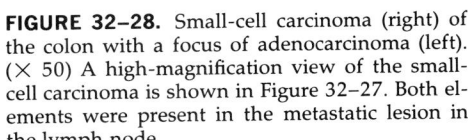

FIGURE 32-28. Small-cell carcinoma (right) of the colon with a focus of adenocarcinoma (left). (× 50) A high-magnification view of the small-cell carcinoma is shown in Figure 32-27. Both elements were present in the metastatic lesion in the lymph node.

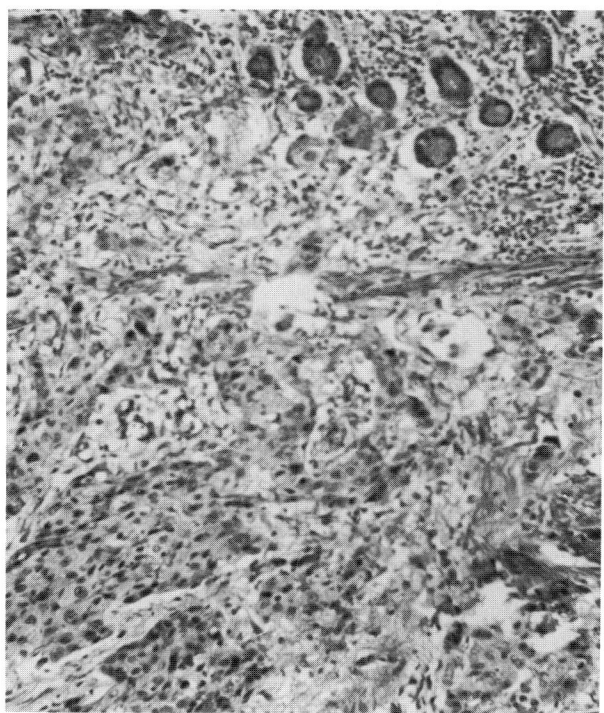

FIGURE 32–29. Metastatic squamous cell carcinoma of lung in the submucosa and adjacent mucosa of the jejunum. (× 120)

OTHER RARE CARCINOMAS AND METASTATIC TUMORS

Jewell et al. reported four cases of colonic adenoma and carcinoma composed of uniform clear cells with abundant glycogen instead of mucin in the cytoplasm.[543] Kubosawa et al. reported a case of choriocarcinoma, together with papillary adenocarcinoma, in the sigmoid colon of a 50-year-old woman with a high serum level of human chorionic gonadotropin.[544] The metastatic lesions contained only choriocarcinoma. Robey-Cafferty et al. reported six cases of anaplastic sarcomatoid carcinoma in the jejunum and ileum.[545] The tumors were large endophytic masses composed of large cells with prominent nucleoli and spindle cells, which by electron microscopy were shown to be epithelial cells. An aggressive course was followed, and five patients died within 40 months. Amano and Yamada reported an endometrioid carcinoma arising from endometriosis in the sigmoid.[546] Rare carcinomas in the duplication of the gastrointestinal tract have been reported.[547]

Primary melanomas of the anus and anal canal may extend into the lower rectum.[548] Primary melanoma of the rectum is rarely reported.[549] The diagnosis of primary melanoma of the small bowel is usually based on the lack of a known primary lesion elsewhere. Such cases are rare.[550,551] On the other hand, melanoma of the skin often metastasizes to the gut, particularly the small intestine.[552–554]

Carcinomas of other parts of the digestive tract may metastasize to the intestines. The linitis plastica type of gastric carcinoma may metastasize to the colon and cause segmental stricture, which can be mistaken for a primary colonic lesion.[555,556] Metastatic colon carcinoma may cause annular narrowing of the small intestine.[557] Other tumors that mestastasize relatively commonly to the intestines are carcinomas of the breast[558–560] and lung.[561,562] The metastatic lesions in the intestine are usually submucosally located (Figure 32–29) and small, and the covering mucosa is intact. Occasionally, a polypoid lesion may lead to intussusception.[563] The infiltrative lesions may cause obstruction, and ulcerated lesions may bleed or perforate.[561,562]

References

1. Goss CM: Gray's Anatomy, 29th ed. Philadelphia, Lea & Febiger, 1973, pp 1225–1244.
2. Garvin PJ, Herrmann V, Kaminski DL, Willman VL: Benign and malignant tumors of the small intestines. Curr Probl Cancer 3:1–46, 1979.
3. Sindelar WF: Cancer of the small intestine. In De Vita VT, Hellman S, Rosenberg SA (eds): Cancer: Principle and Practice of Oncology, 2nd ed. Philadelphia, JB Lippincott, 1985, pp 771–794.
4. Jaffe BM, McFadden D: Tumors of the small intestine. In Moossa AR, Robson MC, Schimpff SC (eds): Comprehensive Textbook of Oncology. Baltimore, Williams & Wilkins, 1986, pp 1052–1062.
5. Silverberg E, Boring CC, Squires TS: Cancer statistics, 1990. CA 40:9–26, 1990.
6. McPeak CJ: Malignant tumors of the small intestine. Am J Surg 114:402–411, 1967.
7. Eckel JH: Primary tumors of the jejunum and ileum. Surgery 23: 467–475, 1948.
8. Darling RC, Welch CE: Tumors of the small intestine. N Engl J Med 260:397–408, 1959.
9. River L, Silverstein J, Tope JW: Benign neoplasms of the small intestine. Int Abst Surg 102:1–38, 1956.
10. Wood DA: Tumors of the intestines. In Atlas of Tumor Pathology, fascicle 22. Washington DC, Armed Forces Institute of Pathology, 1967.
11. Moertel CG, Sauer WG, Dockerty MB, Baggenstoss AH: Life history of the carcinoid tumor of the small intestine. Cancer 14:901–912, 1961.
12. del Regato JA, Spjut HJ, Cox JD: Ackerman and del Regato's Cancer: Diagnosis, Treatment and Prognosis, 6th ed. St. Louis, CV Mosby, 1985, pp 512–530.
13. Herbsman H, Wetstein L, Rosen V: Tumors of the small intestine. Curr Probl Surg 17:121–184, 1980.
14. Berk JE, Haubrich WS: Benign tumors of the colon and rectum. In Bockus HL (ed): Gastroenterology, 2nd ed. Philadelphia, WB Saunders, 1964, pp 954–988.
15. Wilson JM, Melvin DB, Gray GF, et al: Benign small bowel tumor. Ann Surg 181:247–250, 1975.
16. Mason GR: Tumors of the duodenum and small intestine. In Sabiston DC Jr (ed): Textbook of Surgery, 13th ed. Philadelphia, WB Saunders, 1986, pp 868–873.
17. Kelsey JR Jr: Small bowel tumors. In Bockus HL (ed): Gastroenterology, 3rd ed. Philadelphia, WB Saunders, 1976, pp 459–472.
18. Barclay THC, Shapira DV: Malignant tumors of the small intestine. Cancer 51:878–881, 1983.
19. Wilson JM, Melvin DB, Gray GF, Thorbjarnarson B: Primary malignancies of the small bowel: A report of 96 cases and reviews of the literature. Ann Surg 180:175–179, 1974.
20. Ho SB, Itzkowitz SH, Friera AM, et al: Cell lineage markers in premalignant and malignant colonic mucosa. Gastroenterology 97:392–404, 1989.
21. Irnbaum W: Squamous cell carcinoma and adenoacanthoma of the colon. JAMA 212:1511–1513, 1970.

22. Lafreniere R, Ketcham AS: Primary squamous carcinoma of the rectum: Report of a case and review of the literature. Dis Colon Rectum 28:967–972, 1985.
23. Almagro UA, Pintar K, Zellmer RB: Squamous metaplasia in colorectal polyps. Cancer 53:2679–2682, 1984.
24. Williams GT, Blackshaw AJ, Morson BC: Squamous carcinoma of the colorectum and its genesis. J Pathol 129:139–147, 1979.
25. Pigott JP, Williams GB: Primary squamous cell carcinoma of the colorectum: Case report and literature review of a rare entity. J Surg Oncol 35:117–119, 1987.
26. Griesser GH, Schumacher U, Elfeldt R, Horny HP: Adenosquamous carcinoma of the ileum: Report of a case and review of the literature. Virchows Arch [A] 406:483–487, 1985.
27. Shousha S, Spiller RC, Parkins RA: The endoscopically abnormal duodena in patients with dyspepsia: Biopsy findings in 60 cases. Histopathology 7:23–34, 1983.
28. Franzin G, Musola R, Negri A, et al: Heterotopic gastric (fundic) mucosa in the duodenum. Endoscopy 14:166–167, 1982.
29. Tsadilas T: Duodenal polyp composed of ectopic gastric mucosa. Dig Dis Sci 29:475–477, 1984.
30. Johansen AA, Hansen OH: Macroscopically demonstrable heterotopic gastric mucosa in the duodenum. Scand J Gastroenterol 8:58–63, 1973.
31. Russin R, Krevsky B, Caroline DF, et al: Mixed hyperplastic and adenomatous polyp arising from ectopic gastric mucosa of the duodenum. Arch Pathol Lab Med 110:556–558, 1986.
32. Ming SC, Simon M, Tandar BN: Gross gastric metaplasia of ileum after regional enteritis. Gastroenterology 44:63–68, 1963.
33. Taylor AL: The epithelial heterotopias of the alimentary tract. J Pathol 30:415–449, 1930.
34. Caruso ML, Marzullo F: Jejunal adenocarcinoma in congenital heterotopic gastric mucosa. J Clin Gastroenterol 10:92–96, 1988.
35. Seidman H, Mushinski MH, Gelb SK, Silverberg E: Probabilities of eventually developing or dying of cancer—United States, 1985. CA 35:37–56, 1985.
36. Gloeckles-Ries LA, Hankey BF, Edwards BK: Cancer statistics review, 1973–1987. NIH publication 90-2789. Bethesda, Md, National Cancer Institute, 1990.
37. Lightdale CJ, Sherlock P: Small intestinal tumors. In Berk JE (ed): Bockus' Gastroenterology, 4th ed. Philadelphia, WB Saunders, 1985, pp 1887–1899.
38. Lightdale CJ, Koepsell TD, Sherlock P: Small intestine. In Schottenfeld D, Fraumeni JF (eds): Cancer Epidemiology and Prevention. Philadelphia, WB Saunders, 1982, pp 692–702.
39. Reddy BS, Martin CW, Wynder EL: Fecal bile acids and cholesterol metabolites of patients with ulcerative colitis, a high-risk group for development of colon cancer. Cancer Res 37:1697–1701, 1977.
40. Hill MJ, Aries BC: Faecal steroid composition and its relationship to cancer of the large bowel. J Pathol 104:129–139, 1971.
41. Lowenfels AB: Why are small bowel tumors so rare? Lancet 1:24–26, 1973.
42. Williamson RCN, Rainey JB: The relationship between intestinal hyperplasia and carcinogenesis. Scand J Gastroenterol [Suppl] 104:57–76, 1985.
43. Lipkin M: Phase 1 and phase 2 proliferative lesions of colonic epithelial cells in diseases leading to colonic cancer. Cancer 34:878–888, 1974.
44. Calman KC: Why are small bowel tumors rare? An experimental model. Gut 15:552–554, 1974.
45. WHO (World Health Organization): Cancer Incidence in Five Continents. Vol III. Lyon, France, International Agency for Research on Cancer, 1976.
46. Cutler SJ, Young JR Jr: Demographic patterns of cancer incidence in the United States. In Fraumeni J Jr (ed): Persons at High Risk of Cancer: An Approach to Cancer Etiology and Control. New York, Academic Press, 1975, pp 307–342.
47. Schottenfeld D, Winawer SJ: Large intestine. In Schottenfeld D, Fraumeni J (eds): Cancer Epidemiology and Prevention. Philadelphia, WB Saunders, 1982, pp 703–727.
48. Correa P: Comments on the epidemiology of large bowel cancer. Cancer Res 35:3395–3397, 1975.
49. Bert JW, Howell MA: The geographic pathology of bowel cancer. Cancer 34:807–814, 1974.
50. Correa P, Haenszel W: The epidemiology of large bowel cancer. Adv Cancer Res 26:1–141, 1978.
51. King H, Locke FB: Cancer mortality among Chinese in the United States. JNCI 65:1141–1148, 1980.
52. Locke FB, King H: Cancer mortality risk among Japanese in the United States. JNCI 65:1149:1156, 1980.
53. Weisburger JH, Reddy BS, Spinger NE, Wynder EL: Current views on the mechanisms involved in the etiology of colorectal cancer. In Winawer SJ, Schonttenfeld P, Sherlock P (eds): Colorectal Cancer: Prevention, Epidemiology and Screening. New York, Raven Press, 1980, pp 19–41.
54. Bralow SP, Grenstein M, Meranze DR, et al: Adenocarcinoma of glandular stomach and duodenum in Wistar rats ingesting N-methyl-N'-nitro-N-nitrosoguanidine: Histopathology and associated secretory changes. Cancer Res 30:1215–1222, 1970.
55. So BT, Magadia NE, Wynder EL; Induction of carcinomas of the colon and rectum in rats by intrarectal instillation of N-methyl-N'-nitro-N-nitrosoguanidine. JNCI 50:927–932, 1973.
56. LaMont JT, O'Gorman TA: Experimental colon cancer. Gastroenterology 75:1157–1169, 1978.
57. Pozharisski KM, Likhachev AJ, Klimashevski VF, Shaposhinikov JD: Experimental intestinal cancer research with special reference to human pathology. Adv Cancer Res 30:165–237, 1979.
58. Gorham ED, Garland CF, Garland FC: Acid haze air pollution and breast and colon cancer mortality in 20 Canadian cities. Can J Public Health 80:96–100, 1989.
59. Griffith J, Duncan RC, Riggan WB, et al: Cancer mortality in the U.S. countries with hazardous waste sites and ground water pollution. Arch Environ Health 44:69–74, 1989.
60. Ippen M, Fehr R, Krasemann EO: Cancer in residents of heavy traffic areas. Versicherungsmedizin. 41:39–42, 1989.
61. Chen CJ, Chuang YC, Lin TM, et al: Malignant neoplasms among residents of a blackfoot disease–endemic area in Taiwan: High-arsenic artesian well water and cancers. Cancer Res 45:5895–5899, 1985.
62. Frumkin H, Berlin J: Asbestos exposure and gastrointestinal malignancy review and meta-analysis. Am J Ind Med 14:79–95, 1988.
63. Edelman DA: Exposure to asbestos and the risk of gastrointestinal cancer: A reassessment. Br J Ind Med 45:75–82, 1988.
64. Brownson RC, Zahm SH, Chang JC, et al: Occupational risk of colon cancer: An analysis by anatomic subsite. Am J Epidemiol 130:675–678, 1989.
65. Acquavella JF, Douglass TS, Phillips SC: Evaluation of excess colorectal cancer incidence among workers involved in the manufacture of polypropylene. J Occup Med 30:438–442, 1988.
66. Habs M, Schmahl D: Carcinogenic substances in food. Inn Med 6:237–249, 1979.
67. Bruce WR, Varghese AJ, Wang S, Dion, P: The endogenous production of nitroso compounds in the colon and cancer at that site. Int Symp Princess Takamatsu Cancer Res Fund, 9:221–228, 1979.
68. Talley NJ, Chute CG, Larson DE, et al: Risk for colorectal adenocarcinoma in pernicious anemia: A population-based cohort study. Ann Intern Med 111:738–742, 1989.
69. Ehrich M, Aswell JE, Van Tassell RL, et al: Mutagens in the feces of three South African populations at different levels of risk for colon cancer. Mutat Res 64:231–240, 1979.
70. Bruch WR: Recent hypotheses for the origin of colon cancer. Cancer Res 47:4237–4242, 1987.
71. Correa P, Paschal J, Pizzolato P, et al: Fecal mutagens and colorectal polyps: Preliminary report of an autopsy study. In Bruce WR, Correa P, Lipkin M, et al (eds): Gastrointestinal Cancer: Endogenous Factors. Cold Spring Harbor, NY, Cold Spring Harbor Laboratory, 1981, pp 119–123.
72. Schiffman MH, Van Tassell RL, Robinson A, et al: Case-control study of colorectal cancer and fecapentaene excretion. Cancer Res 49:1322–1326, 1989.
73. Hatch FT, Felton JS, Stuermer DH, et al: Identification of mutagens from the cooking of food. Chem Mutagens 9:111–164, 1984.
74. Felton JS, Knize MG, Wood C, et al: Isolation and characterization of new mutagens from fried ground beef. Carcinogenesis 5:95–102, 1984.

75. Sugimura T: Carcinogenicity of mutagenic heterocyclic amines formed during the cooking process. Mutat Res 150:33–42, 1985.
76. Ferguson LR, Alley PG, Gribben BM: DNA-damaging activity in ethanol-soluble fractions from feces from New Zealand groups at varying risks of colorectal cancer. Nutr Cancer 7:93–103, 1985.
77. Jao SW, Beart RW Jr, Reiman HM, et al: Colon and anorectal cancer after pelvic irradiation. Dis Colon Rectum 30:953–958, 1987.
78. Gajraj H, Davies DR, Jackson BT: Synchronous small and large bowel cancer developing after pelvic irradiation. Gut 29:126–128, 1988.
79. Rotmensch S, Avigad I, Soffer EE, et al: Carcinoma of the large bowel after a single massive dose of radiation in healthy teenagers. Cancer 57:728–731, 1986.
80. Kato H: Radiation-induced cancer and its modifying factor among A-bomb survivors. Int Symp Princess Takamatsu Cancer Res Fund 18:117–124, 1987.
81. Kirev TT, Toshkov IA, Mladenov ZM: Virus-induced duodenal adenomas in guinea fowls. JNCI 79:1117–1121, 1987.
82. Boguszakova L, Hirsch I, Brichacek B, et al: Absence of cytomegalovirus, Epstein-Barr virus, and papillomavirus DNA from adenoma and adenocarcinoma of the colon. Acta Virol 32:303–308, 1988.
83. Suzuki K, Bruce WR: Increase by deoxycholic acid of the colonic nuclear damage induced by known carcinogens in C57B1/6J mice. JNCI 76:1129–1132, 1986.
84. Hill MJ, Draser BS, Williams RED, et al: Faecal bile-acid and clostridia in patients with cancer of the large bowel. Lancet 1:535–539, 1975.
85. Smith LL: Carcinogenic cholesterol products. In Smith LL (ed): Cholesterol Autoxidation. New York, Plenum Press, 1981, pp 432–446.
86. Mirvish SS: Blocking the formation of N-nitroso compounds with ascorbic acid in vitro and in vivo, Ann NY Acad Sci 258:175–180, 1975.
87. Raineri R, Weisburger JH: Reduction of gastric carcinogens with ascorbic acid. Ann NY Acad Sci 258:181–189, 1975.
88. Chen LH, Boissonneault GA, Glauert HP: Vitamin C, vitamin E and cancer. Anticancer Res 8:739–748, 1988.
89. Willett WC: Selenium, vitamin E, fiber, and the incidence of human cancer: An epidemiologic perspective. Adv Exp Med Biol 206:27–34, 1986.
90. Mckeown-Eyssen G, Holloway C, Jazmaji V, et al: A randomized trial of vitamins C and E in the prevention of recurrence of colorectal polyps. Cancer Res 48:4701–4705, 1988.
91. Jacobs MM: Effects of selenium on chemical carcinogens. Prev Med 9:362–367, 1980.
92. Temple NJ, Basu TK: Selenium and cabbage and colon carcinogenesis in mice. JNCI 79:1131–1134, 1987.
93. Soullier BK, Wilson PS, Nigro ND: Effect of selenium on azoxymethane-induced intestinal cancer in rats fed high fat diet. Cancer Lett 12:343–348, 1981.
94. Nelson RL: Is the changing pattern of colorectal cancer caused by selenium deficiency? Dis Colon Rectum 27:459–461, 1984.
95. Clapp NK, Bowels ND, Satterfield LC, et al: Selective protective effect of butylated hydroxytoulene against 1,2-dimethylhydrazine carcinogenesis in balb/c mice. JNCI 63:1081–1087, 1979.
96. Metzger U, Meier J, Uhlschmid G, et al: Influence of various prostaglandin synthesis inhibitors on DMH-induced rat colon cancer. Dis Colon Rectum 37:366–369, 1984.
97. Narisawa T, Takahashi M, Niwa M, et al: Involvement of prostaglandin E2 in bile acid–caused promotion of colon carcinogenesis and anti-promotion by the cyclooxygenase inhibitor indomethacin. Jpn J Cancer Res 78:791–798, 1987.
98. Lynch HT, Lanspa J, Bowman BM, et al: Hereditary nonpolypsis colorectal cancer–Lynch syndrome I and II. Gastroenterol Clin North Am 17:679–712, 1988.
99. Burt RW, Samowitz WS: The adenomatous polyp and the hereditary polyposis syndromes. Gastroenterol Clin North Am 17:657–678, 1988.
100. Perzin KH, Bridge MF: Adenomatous and carcinomatous changes in hamartomatous polyps of the small intestine (Peutz-Jeghers syndrome). Cancer 49:971–983, 1982.
101. Haggitt RC, Reid BJ: Hereditary gastrointestinal polypous syndromes. Am J Surg Pathol 10:871–877, 1986.
102. Mecklin JP. Frequency of hereditary colorectal cancer. Gastroenterology 93:1021–1025, 1987.
103. Lynch HT, Watson P, Lanspa SJ, et al: Natural history of colorectal cancer in hereditary nonpolyposis colorectal cancer (Lynch syndromes I and II). Dis Colon Rectum 31:439–444 1988.
104. Burt RW, Bishop OT, Cannon ML, et al: Dominant inheritance of adenomatous colonic polyps and colorectal cancer. N Engl J Med 312:1540–1544, 1985.
105. Cannon-Albright LA, Skolnick MH, Bishop T, et al: Common inheritance of susceptibility to colonic adenomatous polyps and associated colorectal cancers. N Engl J Med 319:533–537, 1988.
106. Jarvinen H, Nyberg M, Peltokallio P: Upper gastrointestinal tract polyps in familial adenomatosis coli. Gut 24:333–339, 1983.
107. Giardiello FM, Welsh SB, Hamilton SR, et al: Increased risk of cancer in the Peutz-Jeghers syndrome. N Engl J Med 316:1511–1514, 1987.
108. Jarvinen H, Franssila KO: Familial juvenile polyposis coli increased risk of colorectal cancer. Gut 25:792–800, 1984.
109. Jass JR, Williams CB, Bussey HJ, Morson BC: Juvenile polyposis: A precancerous condition. Histopathology 13:619–630, 1988.
110. Mecklin JP, Sipponen P, Järvinen HJ: Histopathology of colorectal carcinoma in cancer family syndrome kindreds. Dis Colon Rectum 29:849–853, 1986.
111. Muto T, Kamiya J, Sawada T, et al: Small "flat adenomas" of the large bowel with special reference to its clinicopathologic features. Dis Colon Rectum 28:847–851, 1985.
112. Faron ER, Vogelstein B: A genetic model for colorectal tumorigenesis. Cell 61:759–767, 1990.
113. Wildrick DM: Molecular genetic studies of colon cancer. Hematol Oncol Clin North Am 3:1–18, 1989.
114. Wynder EL: The epidemiology of large bowel cancer. Cancer Res 35:3388–3394, 1975.
115. Hill MJ: Environmental and genetic factors in gastrointestinal cancer. In Sherlock P, Morson BC, Barbara L, Veronesi U (eds): Precancerous Lesions of the Gastrointestinal Tract. New York, Raven Press, 1983, pp 1–22.
116. Phillips RL, Garfinkel L, Kuzma JW, et al: Mortality among California Seventh-Day Adventists for selected cancer sites. JNCI 65:1097–1107, 1980.
117. Reddy BS: Dietary fat and colon cancer: Animal models. Prev Med 16:460–467, 1987.
118. Stemmermann GN, Nomura AM, Heilburn LK: Dietary fat and the risk of colorectal cancer. Cancer Res 44:4633–4637, 1984.
119. Sakaguchi M, Minoura T, Hiramatsu Y, et al: Effects of dietary saturated and unsaturated fatty acids on fecal bile acids and colon carcinogenesis induced by azoxymethane in rats. Cancer Res 46:61–65, 1986.
120. Minoura T, Takata T, Sakaguchi M, et al: Effect of dietary eicosapentaenoic acid on azoxymethane-induced colon carcinogenesis in rats. Cancer Res 48:4790–4794, 1988.
121. Galloway DJ, Jarrett F, Boyle P, et al: Morphological and cell kinetic effects of dietary manipulation during colorectal carcinogenesis. Gut 28:754–763, 1987.
122. Cummings JH, Hill MJ, Bone ES, et al: The effect of meat protein and dietary fiber on colonic function and metabolism. II. Bacterial metabolites in feces and urine. Am J Clin Nutr 32:2094–2101, 1979.
123. Lyon JL, Mahone AW, West DW, et al: Energy intake: Its relationship to colon cancer risk. JNCI 78:853–861, 1987.
124. Kritchevsky D, Weber MM, Buck CL, et al: Calories, fat and cancer. Lipids 21:272–274, 1986.
125. Reddy BS, Wang CX, Maruyama H: Effect of restricted caloric intake on azoxymethane-induced colon tumor incidence in male f344 rats. Cancer Res 46:1226–1228, 1987.
126. Tornberg SA, Holm LE, Carstensen JM, et al: Risks of cancer of the colon and rectum in relation to serum cholesterol and beta-lipoprotein. N Engl J Med 315:1629–1633, 1986.
127. Hiramatsu Y, Takada H, Yamamura M, et al: Effect of dietary

128. Broitman SA: Dietary cholesterol, serum cholesterol, and colon cancer: A review. Adv Exp Med Biol 206:137–152, 1986.
129. Reddy BS, Cohen IA, McCoy GO, et al: Nutrition and its relationship to cancer. Adv Cancer Res 32:237–245, 1980.
130. Wargovich MJ, Baer AR, Hu PJ, et al: Dietary factors and colorectal cancer. Gastroenterol Clin North Am 17:727–745, 1988.
131. Wargovich MJ: Diallyl sulfide, a flavor component of garlic (Allium sativum), inhibits dimethylhydrazine-induced colon cancer. Carcinogenesis 8:487–489, 1987.
132. Burkitt DP: Epidemiology of cancer of the colon and rectum. Cancer 28:3–13, 1971.
133. Jacobs LR: Fiber and colon cancer. Gastroenterol Clin North Am 17:747–760, 1988.
134. Jacobs JR: Modification of experimental colon carcinogenesis by dietary fibers. Adv Exp Med Biol 266:105–118, 1986.
135. Prizont R: Absence of large bowel tumors in rats injected with 1,2-dimethylhydrazine and fed high dietary cellulose. Dig Dis Sci 32:1418–1421, 1987.
136. Freeman HJ: Effects of differing purified cellulose, pectin, and hemicellulose fiber diets on fecal enzymes in 1,2-dimethylhydrazine-induced rat colon carcinogenesis. Cancer Res 45:5529–5532, 1986.
137. Smith-Barbaro P, Hanson D, Reddy BS: Carcinogen binding to various types of dietary fiber. JNCI 67:495–497, 1981.
138. Thornton JR: High colonic pH promotes colorectal cancer. Lancet 1:1081–1083, 1981.
139. Reddy BS, Hirota N, Katayama S: Effect of dietary sodium ascorbate on 1,2-dimethylhydrazine- or methylnitrosourea-induced colon carcinogenesis in rats. Carcinogenesis 3:1097–1099, 1982.
140. Vogel VG, McPherson RS: Dietary epidemiology of colon cancer. Hematol Oncol Clin North Am 3:35–63, 1989.
141. Garland C, Skekelle RB, Barrett-Connor E, et al: Dietary vitamin D and calcium and risk of colorectal cancer: A 19-year prospective study in men. Lancet 1:307–309, 1985.
142. Lipkin M, Friedman E, Winawer SJ, et al: Colonic epithelial cell proliferation in responders and nonresponders to supplemental dietary calcium. Cancer Res 49:248–254, 1989.
143. Rozen P, Fireman Z, Fine N, et al: Oral calcium suppresses increased rectal epithelial proliferation of persons at risk of colorectal cancer. Gut 30:650–655, 1989.
144. Yamamoto RS: Effect of vitamin B12-deficiency in colon carcinogenesis. Proc Soc Exp Biol Med 163:350–353, 1980.
145. Kune S, Kune GG, Watson LF: Case-control study of alcoholic beverages as etiological factors: The Melbourne colorectal cancer study. Nutr Cancer 9:43–56, 1987.
146. Pollack E, Nomura AM, Heilburn LK, et al: Prospective study of alcohol consumption and cancer. N Engl J Med 310:617–621, 1984.
147. Karlin DA, McBath M, Jones RD, et al: Hypergastrinemia and colorectal carcinogenesis in the rat. Cancer Lett 29:73–80, 1985.
148. Iishi H, Tatsuta M, Baba M, et al: Enhancement by vasoactive intestinal peptide of experimental carcinogenesis induced by azoxymethane in rat colon. Cancer Res 46:4890–4893, 1987.
149. Hoosein NM, Kiener PA, Curry RC, et al: Antiproliferative effects of gastrin receptor antagonists and antibodies to gastrin of human colon carcinoma cell lines. Cancer Res 48:7179–7183, 1988.
150. Hahn DL: Sex and race are risk factors for colorectal cancer within reach of the sigmoidoscope. J Fam Pract 30:409–416, 1990.
151. Davis FG, Furner SE, Persky V, Koch M: The influence of parity and exogenous female hormones on the risk of colorectal cancer. Int J Cancer 43:587–590, 1989.
152. Weiss NS, Darling JR, Chow WH: Incidence of cancer of the large bowel in women in relation to reproductive and hormonal factors. JNCI 57:57–60, 1981.
153. Kune GA, Kune S, Watson LF: Oral contraceptive use does not protect against large bowel cancer. Contraception 41:19–25, 1990.
154. Francavilla A, DiLeo A, Polimeno L, et al: Nuclear and cytosolic estrogen receptors in human colon carcinoma and in surrounding noncancerous colonic tissue. Gastroenterology 93:1301–1306, 1987.
155. Smironova IO, Turusov VS: 1,2-dimethylhydrazine carcinogenesis in neonatally androgenized CBA mice. Carcinogenesis 9:1927–1929, 1988.
156. Izbicki JR, Wambach G, Hamilton SR, et al: Androgen receptors in experimentally induced colon carcinogenesis. J Cancer Res Clin Oncol 112:39–46, 1986.
157. Tutton PJ, Barkla DH: The influence of androgens, antiandrogens, and castration on cell proliferation in the jejunal and colonic crypt epithelia and in dimethylhydrazine-induced adenocarcinoma of rat colon. Virchows Arch [B] 38:351–355, 1982.
158. Ituarte EM, Petrini J, Hershman JM, et al: Acromegaly and colon cancer. Ann Intern Med 5:627–628, 1984.
159. Conteas CN, Desai TK, Arlow FA: Relationship of hormones and growth factors to colon cancer. Gastroenterol Clin North Am 17:761–772, 1988.
160. Feig DS, Gottesman IS: Familial hyperparathyroidism in association with colonic carcinoma. Cancer 60:429–432, 1987.
161. Franchini A, Giardino R, Cola B: Multiple tumors of the large bowel. Ann Gastroenterol Hepatol 18:309–311, 1982.
162. Enblad P, Adami HO, Glimelius B, et al: The risk of subsequent primary malignant diseases after cancers of the colon and rectum: A nationwide cohort study. Cancer 65:2091–2100, 1990.
163. Phipps RF, Perry PM: Familial breast cancer and the association with colonic carcinoma. Eur J Surg Oncol 15:109–111, 1989.
164. Mellemgaard A, Jensen OM, Lynge E: Cancer incidence among spouses of patients with colorectal cancer. Int J Cancer 44:225–228, 1989.
165. Lyon JL, Gardner JW, West DW: Cancer risk and life-style cancer among Mormons from 1967–1975. Banbury Rep Ser 4:3–30, 1980.
166. Gerhardsson M, Floderus B, Norell SE: Physical activity and colon cancer risk. Int J Epidemiol 17:743–746, 1988.
167. Garfinkel L, Stellman SD: Mortality by relative weight and exercise. Cancer 62:1844–1850, 1988.
168. Andrianopoulos G, Nelson RL, Bombeck CT, et al: The influence of physical activity in 1,2-dimethylhydrazine–induced colon carcinogenesis in the rat. Anticancer Res 7:849–852, 1987.
169. Vernick LJ, Kuller LH: A case-control study of cholecystectomy and right-side colon cancer: The influence of alternative data sources and differential interview participation proportions on odds ratio estimates. Am J Epidemiol 116:86–101, 1982.
170. Mamianetti A, Cinto RO, Altolaguirre D, et al: Relative risk of colorectal cancer after cholecystectomy: A multicentre case-control study. Int J Colorect Dis 3:215–218, 1988.
171. Alley PG, Lee SP: The increased risk of proximal colonic cancer after cholecystectomy. Dis Colon Rectum 26:522–524, 1983.
172. Moorehead RJ, Mills JO, Wilson HK, et al: Cholecystectomy and the development of colorectal neoplasia: A prospective study. Ann R Coll Surg Engl 71:37–39, 1989.
173. Sandler RS, Martin ZZ, Carlton NM, et al: Adenomas of the large bowel after cholecystectomy: A case-control study. Dig Dis Sci 33:1178–1184, 1988.
174. Adami HO, Krusemo UB, Meirik O: Unaltered risk of colorectal cancer within 14–17 years of cholecystectomy: Updating of a population-based cohort study. Br J Surg 74:675–678, 1987.
175. Kune GA, Kune S, Watson LF: Large bowel cancer after cholecystectomy. Am J Surg 156:359–362, 1988.
176. Castleden WM, Detchon P, Misso NL: Biliary bile acids in cholelithiasis and colon cancer. Gut 30:860–865, 1989.
177. Mizusawa K, Kaibara N, Yonekawa M, et al: A prospective cohort study on the development of colorectal cancer after gastrectomy. Dis Colon Rectum 33:298–301, 1990.
178. Offerhaus GJ, Tersmette AC, Tersmette KW, et al: Gastric, pancreatic, and colorectal carcinogenesis following remote peptic ulcer surgery: Review of the literature with the emphasis on risk assessment and underlying mechanism. Mod Pathol 1:352–356, 1988.

179. Thompson M: Aetiological factors in gastrointestinal carcinogenesis. Scand J Gastroenterol 104:77–89, 1985.
180. Owen RW: Biotransformation of bile acids by clostridia. J Med Microbiol 20:233–238, 1985.
181. Wargovich MJ, Eng VW, Newmark HL, et al: Calcium ameliorates the toxic effect of deoxycholic acid on colonic epithelium. Carcinogenesis 4:1205–1207, 1983.
182. Owen RW, Henly PJ, Day DW, et al: Fecal steroids and colorectal cancer: Bile acid profiles in low and high risk groups. Int Congr Ser 685:165–170, 1985.
183. Ferguson LR, Parry JM: Mitotic aneuploidy as a possible mechanism for tumor promoting activity in bile acids. Carcinogenesis 5:447–451, 1984.
184. Hill MJ: Bacterial metabolism and human carcinogenesis. Br Med Bull 37:89–94, 1980.
185. Rogers AE, Nauss KM: Rodent models for carcinoma of the colon. Dig Dis Sci 12:87S–102S, 1985.
186. Reddy BS, Narisawa T, Wright P, et al: Colon carcinogenesis with azoxymethane and dimethylhydrazine in germ-free rats. Cancer Res 35:287–290, 1975.
187. Goldin BR, Gorbach SL: Effect of antibiotics on incidence of rat intestinal tumors induced by 1,2-dimethylhydrazine dihydrochloride. JNCI 67:877–880, 1981.
188. Filipe MI, Scurr JH, Ellis H: Effects of fecal stream on experimental colorectal carcinogenesis morphologic and histochemical changes. Cancer 50:2859–2865, 1982.
189. Oravec CT, Jones CA, Huberman E: Activation of the colon carcinogen 1,2-dimethylhydrazine in a rat colon cell-mediated mutagenesis assay. Cancer Res 46:5068–5071, 1986.
190. Celik C, Mittleman A, Paolini NS, et al: Effects of 1,2-symmetrical dimethylhydrazine of jejunocolic transposition in Sprague-Dawley rats. Cancer Res 41:2908–2911, 1981.
191. Rainey JB, Maeda M, Williamson RC: Distal transposition of rat caecum does not render it susceptible to carcinogenesis. Gut 26:718–723, 1985.
192. Morson BC: Markers for increased risk of colorectal cancer. In Sherlock P, Morson BC, Barbara L, Veronesi U (eds): Precancerous Lesions of the Gastrointestinal Tract. New York, Raven Press, 1983, pp 253–259.
193. Potet F, Brousse N, Soullard J: Precancerous lesions of colonic mucosa: Epidemiological study and histological analysis of polyps. Eur J Cancer (Suppl) 1:59–68, 1978.
194. Ninto T, Bussey HJR, Morson BC: The evolution of cancer of the colon and rectum. Cancer 36:2251–2270, 1975.
195. Adachi M, Muto T, Moioka Y, et al: Flat adenoma and flat mucosal carcinoma (IIb type): A new precursor of colorectal carcinoma? Report of two cases. Dis Colon Rectum 31:236–243, 1988.
196. Perzin KH, Bridge MF: Adenomas of the small intestine: A clinicopathologic review of 51 cases and a study of their relationship to carcinoma. Cancer 48:799–819, 1981.
197. Day DW. The adenoma-carcinoma sequence. Scand J Gastroenterol [Suppl] 104:99–107, 1985.
198. Fenoglio CM, Pascal RR: Colorectal adenomas and cancer: Pathologic relationships. Cancer 50:2601–2608, 1982.
199. Eide TJ: Remnants of adenomas in colorectal carcinomas. Cancer 51:1866–1872, 1983.
200. Spratt JS, Ackerman LV, Moyer CA: Relationship of polyps of the colon to colonic cancer. Ann Surg 148:682–698, 1958.
201. Castleman B, Krickstein HI: Do adenomatous polyps of the colon become malignant? N Engl J Med 267:469–475, 1962.
202. Morson BC: Factors influencing the prognosis of early cancer of the rectum. Proc R Soc Med 59:607–608, 1966.
203. Muto T: Serial section study of colonic adenomas with special reference to minute carcinoma. Jpn J Cancer Res 80:356–359, 1989.
204. Enblad P, Busch C, Carlsson U, et al: The adenoma-carcinoma sequence in rectal adenomas: Support by the expression of blood group substances and carcinoma antigens. Am J Clin Pathol 90:121–130, 1988.
205. Boland CR: Lectin histochemistry in colorectal polyps. Prog Clin Biol Res 279:277–287, 1988.
206. Concolino G, Arrabito G, Buonomo O, et al: Nuclear steroid receptors and dysplasia in adenomas polyps of the colon as markers of high risk for malignant transformation. Cancer Detect Prev 9:466–484, 1986.
207. Crawford BE, Stromeyer FW: Small nonpolypoid carcinomas of the large intestine. Cancer 51:1760–1763, 1983.
208. Shimoda T, Ikegami M, Fujisaki J, et al: Early colorectal carcinoma with special reference to its development de novo. Cancer 64:1138–1146, 1989.
209. Maskens AP, Dujardin-Loits RM: Experimental adenomas and carcinomas of the large intestine behave as distinct entities. Cancer 47:81–89, 1981.
210. Ming SC, Yu PC: Histogenesis of experimental colonic carcinoma. Front Gastrointest Res 18:200–224, 1991.
211. Goldman H, Ming SC, Hickok DF: Nature and significance of hyperplastic polyps of the human colon. Arch Pathol 89:349–354, 1970.
212. Teoh HH, Delahunt B, Isbister WH: Dysplastic and malignant areas in hyperplastic polyps of the large intestine. Pathology 21:138–142, 1989.
213. Jass JR, Filipe MI, Abbas S, et al: A morphologic and histochemical study of metaplastic polyps of the colorectum. Cancer 53:510–515, 1984.
214. Longacre TA, Fenoglio-Preiser CM: Mixed hyperplastic adenomatous polyps/serrated adenomas: A distinct form of colorectal neoplasia. Am J Surg Pathol 14:524–537, 1990.
215. Bentley E, Chandrasoma P, Radin R, Cohen H: Generalized juvenile polyposis with carcinoma. Am J Gastroenterol 84:1456–1459, 1989.
216. MacDermott RP: Review of clinical aspects of cancer of the colon in patients with ulcerative colitis. Dig Dis Sci 30:1145–1185, 1985.
217. Gilat T, Rozen P: Risk of colon cancer in ulcerative colitis in low incidence areas: A review. In Winawer SJ, Schottenfeld D, Sherlock P (eds): Colorectal Cancer: Prevention, Epidemiology and Screening. New York, Raven Press, 1980, pp 335–339.
218. Riddell RH, Goldman H, Ransohoff DF, et al: Dysplasia in inflammatory bowel disease: Standardized classification with provisional clinical applications. Hum Pathol 14:931–968, 1983.
219. Greenstein AJ, Sachar DB, Smith H, et al: A comparison of cancer risk in Crohn's disease and ulcerative colitis. Cancer 48:2742–2745, 1981.
220. Korelitz BI: Carcinoma of the intestinal tract in Crohn's disease: Results of a survey conducted by the national foundation of ileitis and colitis. Am J Gastroenterol 78:44–46, 1983.
221. Hamilton SR: Colorectal carcinoma in patients with Crohn's disease. Gastroenterology 89:398–407, 1985.
222. Yardley JH: Comments on comparative pathology of colonic neoplasia in cotton-top marmoset (Saguinus oedipus oedipus). Dig Dis Sci 30:126S–133S, 1985.
223. Lushbaugh C, Humason G, Clapp N: Histology of colon cancer in Saguinus oedipus oedipus. Dig Dis Sci 30:119S–125S, 1985.
224. Xu Z, Su Dl: Schistosoma japonicum and colorectal cancer: An epidemiological study in the People's Republic of China. Int J Cancer 34:315–318, 1984.
225. Chen MC, Chuang CY, Chang PY, et al: Evolution of colorectal cancer in schistosomiasis: Transitional mucosal changes adjacent to large intestinal carcinoma in colectomy specimens. Cancer 46:1661–1675, 1980.
226. Williamson RCN, Rainey JB: The relationship between intestinal hyperplasia and carcinogenesis. Scand J Gastroenterol [Suppl] 104:57–76, 1985.
227. Barthold SW, Beck D: Modification or early dimethylhydrazine carcinogenesis by colonic mucosal hyperplasia. Cancer Res 40:4451–4455, 1980.
228. Jacobs R: Role of dietary factors in cell replication and colon cancer. Am J Clin Nutr 48:775–779, 1988.
229. Cendron J: Tumor of the colon following ureterosigmoidostomy for bladder exstrophy. Ann Urol 16:275–279, 1982.
230. Macrae FA, Stewart M, Williams CB: Colonic tumours and ureterosigmoidostomy: An endoscopic study. Gut 23:A453, 1982.
231. Duckrey H. Production of colonic carcinomas by 1,2-dialkylhydrazines and azoyalkanes. In Burdette WJ (ed): Carcinoma of Colon and Antecedent Epithelium. Springfield, Ill, Charles C Thomas, 1970, pp 267–279.
232. Fiala ES, Kulakis C, Bobotas G, Weisburger JH: Brief communication: Detection and estimation of azomethane in expired

air of 1,2-dimethylhydrazine-treated rats. JNCI 56:1271–1273, 1976.
233. Sumi Y, Miyakawa M: Gastrointestinal carcinogenesis in germ-free rats given N-methyl-N'-nitro-N-nitrosoguanidine in drinking water. Cancer Res 39:2733–2736, 1979.
234. Sunter JP: Cell proliferation in gastrointestinal carcinogenesis. Scand J Gastroenterol 104:45–55, 1985.
235. Rubio CA, Nylander G, Wahlin B, et al: Monitoring the histogenesis of colonic tumors in the Sprague-Dawley rat. J Surg Oncol 31:225–228, 1986.
236. Chang WWL: Histogenesis of symmetrical 1,2-dimethylhydrazine-induced neoplasms of the colon in the mouse. JNCI 60:1405–1418, 1978.
237. Madara JL, Harte P, Deasy J, et al: Evidence for an adenoma-carcinoma sequence in dimethylhydrazine-induced neoplasms of rat intestinal epithelium. Am J Pathol 110:230–235, 1983.
238. Maskens AP: Mechanisms of histogenesis and carcinogenesis in dimethylhydrazine-induced rat colon cancer. Eur J Cancer (Suppl) 1:95–104, 1978.
239. Inamori Y, Misumi A, Murakami A, Akagi M: The histogenesis of DMH-induced colonic carcinoma in rats. Gastroenterol Jpn 22:7–17, 1987.
240. Spratt JS, Ackerman LV: Small primary adenocarcinomas of the colon and rectum. JAMA 179:337–346, 1962.
241. Kjeldsberg CR, Altshuler JH: Carcinoma in situ of the colon. Dis Colon Rectum 13:376–381, 1970.
242. Ikegami M: A pathological study on colorectal cancer from de novo carcinoma to advanced carcinoma. Acta Pathol Jpn 37:21–37, 1987.
243. Dawson PM, Habib NA, Rees HC, Wood CB: Mucosal field change in colorectal cancer. Am J Surg 153:281–284, 1987.
244. Roby-Cafferty SS, Ro JY, Ordonez NG, Cleary KR: Transitional mucosa of colon: A morphological histochemical, and immunohistochemical study. Arch Pathol Lab Med 114:72–75, 1990.
245. Schmidbauer G, Heilmann KL: Morphology and histochemistry of the mucosa surrounding small oligotubular adenomas of the large bowel. Pathol Res Pract 180:45–48, 1985.
246. Dawson PA, Filipe MI: An ultrastructural and histochemical study of the mucous membrane adjacent to and remote from carcinoma of the colon. Cancer 37:2388–2398, 1976.
247. Mori M, Shimono R, Adachi Y, et al: Transitional mucosa in human colorectal lesions. Dis Colon Rectum 33:498–501, 1990.
248. Caccamo D, Telenta M, Celener D: Concanavalin A binding sites in fetal, adult, transitional, and malignant rectosigmoid mucosa. Hum Pathol 20:1186–1192, 1989.
249. Spratt JS Jr: Gross rates of growth of colonic neoplasms and other variables affecting medical decisions and prognosis. In Burdette WJ (ed): Carcinoma of the Colon and Antecedent Epithelium. Springfield, Ill, Charles C Thomas, 1970, pp 66–77.
250. Welin S, Youkers J, Spratt JS Jr: The rates and patterns of growth of 375 tumors of the large intestine and rectum observed serially by double contrast enema (Malmo technique). AJR 90:673–687, 1965.
251. Bolin S, Nilsson E, Sjodahl R: Carcinoma of the colon and rectum-growth rate. Ann Surg 198:151–158, 1983.
252. Spratt JS Jr: Rates of growth of pulmonary metastases and host survival. Ann Surg 159:161–171, 1964.
253. Havelaar I, Sugarbaker PH: Rate of growth of intraabdominal metastases from colon and rectal cancer followed by serial EOE CT. Cancer 54:163–171, 1984.
254. Finlay IG, Brunton GF, Meed K, et al: Rate of growth of hepatic metastasis in colorectal carcinoma. (Abstract) Br J Surg 69:689, 1982.
255. Fenoglio CM, Kaye GI, Lane N: Distribution of human colonic lymphatics in normal, hyperplastic and adenomatous tissue. Gastroenterology 64:51–66, 1973.
256. Sizer JS, Frederick PL, Osborne MP: Primary linitis plastica of the colon: Report of a case and review of the literature. Dis Colon Rectum 10:339–343, 1967.
257. Mathews JL, Cyle D Jr, Little WP: Primary linitis plastica of the rectum: Report of a case. Dis Colon Rectum 25:488–490, 1982.
258. Jackman RJ, Beahrs OH: Tumors of the Large Bowel. Philadelphia, WB Saunders, 1969.
259. Dionne L: The pattern of blood-borne metastasis from carcinoma of rectum. Cancer 18:775–781, 1965.
260. Qizilbash AH: Pathologic studies in colorectal cancer: A guide to the surgical pathology examination of colorectal specimens and review of features of prognostic significance. Pathol Annu 17 (Part 1):1–46, 1982.
261. Sarlin JG, Mori K: Morules in epithelial tumors of the colon and rectum. Am J Surg Pathol 8:281–285, 1984.
262. Gibbs NM: Undifferentiated carcinoma of the large intestine. Histopathology 1:77–84, 1977.
263. Iwafuchi M, Watanabe H, Ishihara N, Ito S: Neoplastic endocrine cells in carcinomas of the small intestine: Histochemical and immunohistochemical studies of 24 tumors. Hum Pathol 18:185–194, 1987.
264. Smith DM Jr, Haggitt RC: The prevalence and prognostic significance of argyrophil cells in colorectal carcinomas. Am J Surg Pathol 8:123–128, 1984.
265. Jansson D, Gould VE, Gooch DT, et al: Immunohistochemical analysis of colon carcinomas applying exocrine and neuroendocrine markers. Acta Pathol Microbiol Immunol Scand 96:1129–1139, 1988.
266. Staren ED, Gould VE, Warren WH, et al: Neuroendocrine carcinomas of the colon and rectum: A clinicopathologic evaluation. Surgery 104:1080–1089, 1988.
267. Gould VE, Jao W, Chejfec G, et al: Neuroendocrine carcinomas of the gastrointestinal tract. Semin Diagn Pathol 1:13–18, 1984.
268. Lundqvist M, Wilander E: Exocrine and endocrine cell differentiation in small intestinal adenocarcinomas. Acta Pathol Microbiol Immunol Scand [A] 91:469–474, 1983.
269. Stern JB, Sobel HJ: Jejunal carcinoma with cells resembling Paneth cells. Arch Pathol 72:47–50, 1961.
270. Scharfenberg JC, DeCamp PT: Neoplastic Paneth cells: Occurrence in an adenocarcinoma of a Meckel's diverticulum. Am J Clin Pathol 64:204–208, 1975.
271. Gibbs NM: Incidence and significance of argentaffin and Paneth cells in some tumours of the large intestine. J Clin Pathol 20:826–831, 1967.
272. Shousha S: Paneth cell-rich papillary adenocarcinoma and a mucoid adenocarcinoma occurring synchronously in colon: A light and electron microscopic study. Histopathology 3:489–501, 1979.
273. Kirkland SC: Clonal origin of columnar, mucous, and endocrine cell lineages in human colorectal epithelium. Cancer 61:1359–1363, 1988.
274. Watson PH, Alguacil-Garcia A: Mixed crypt cell carcinoma: A clinicopathological study of the so-called goblet cell carcinoid. Virchows Arch [A] 412:175–182, 1987.
275. Damjanov I, Amenta PS, Bosman FT: Undifferentiated carcinoma of the colon containing exocrine, neuroendocrine and squamous cells. Virchows Arch [A] 401:57–66, 1983.
276. Palvio DH, Sørensen FB, Kløve-Mogensen M: Stem cell carcinoma of the colon and rectum: Report of two cases and review of the literature. Dis Colon Rectum 28:440–455, 1985.
277. Barkla DH, Whitehead RH, Foster H, Tutton PJ: Tuft (caveolated) cells in two human colon carcinoma cell lines. Am J Pathol 132:521–525, 1988.
278. Balazs M, Dovacs A: Electron microscopic study of carcinoma of the colon. Exp Pathol 20:210–214, 1981.
279. Seiler MW, Reilova-Velez J, Hickey W, et al: Ultrastructural markers of large bowel cancer. Prog Cancer Res Therapy 29:51–65, 1984.
280. Hickey WF, Seiler MW: Ultrastructural markers of colonic adenocarcinoma. Cancer 47:140–145, 1981.
281. Elias H, Fong BB: Nuclear fragmentation in colon carcinoma cells. Hum Pathol 9:679–684, 1978.
282. Hamilton PW, Allen DC, Watt PC, et al: Classification of normal colorectal mucosa and adenocarcinoma by morphometry. Histopathology 11:901–911, 1987.
283. Graham AR, Paplanus SH, Bartels PH: Micromorphometry of colonic lesions. Lab Invest 59:397–402, 1988.
284. Watson PH, Carr I: A morphometric study of invasion and metastasis in human colorectal carcinoma. Clin Exp Metastasis 5:311–319, 1987.
285. Jass JR, Sobin LH: World Health Organization Histological

286. Minsky BD, Mies C, Recht A, Chaffey JT: Colloid carcinoma of the colon and rectum. Cancer 60:3103–3112, 1987.
287. Umpleby HC, Ranson DL, Williamson RCN: Peculiarities of mucinous colorectal carcinoma. Br J Surg 72:715–718, 1985.
288. Symonds DA, Vickery AL: Mucinous carcinoma of the colon and rectum. Cancer 37:1891–1900, 1976.
289. Spratt JS, Spjut HJ: Prevalence and prognosis of individual clinical and pathologic variables associated with colorectal carcinoma. Cancer 20:1976–1985, 1967.
290. Sundblad AS, Paz RA: Mucinous carcinomas of the colon and rectum and their relationship to polyps. Cancer 50:2504–2509, 1982.
291. Okuno M, Ikehara T, Nagayama M, et al: Mucinous colorectal carcinoma: Clinical pathology and prognosis. Am Surg 54:681–685, 1988.
292. Phil E, Nairn RC, Hughes ESR, et al: Mucinous colorectal carcinoma: Immunopathology and prognosis. Pathology 12:439–447, 1980.
293. Purtilo DT, Geelhoed GW, Li FP, et al: Mucinous colon carcinoma in a black family. Cancer Genet Cytogenet 24:11–15, 1987.
294. Ojeda VJ, Mitchell KM, Walters MN, Gibson MJ: Primary colo-rectal linitis plastica type of carcinoma: Report of two cases and review of the literature. Pathology 14:181–189, 1982.
295. Giacchero A, Aste H, Baracchini P, et al: Primary signet-ring carcinoma of the large bowel: Report of nine cases. Cancer 56:2723–2726, 1985.
296. Lui IOL, Kung ITM, Lee JMH, Boey JH: Primary colorectal signet-ring cell carcinoma in young patients: Report of 3 cases. Pathology 17:31–35, 1985.
297. Bonello JC, Sternberg SS, Quan SHQ: The significance of the signet-cell variety of adenocarcinoma of the rectum. Dis Colon Rectum 23:180–183, 1980.
298. Almagro UA: Primary signet-ring carcinoma of the colon. Cancer 52:1453–1457, 1983.
299. Muto T, Kamiya J: Histological features of early cancer of the large intestine. Gan No Rinsho 25:461–467, 1979.
300. Hermanek P, Gall FP: Early (microinvasive) colorectal carcinoma: Pathology, diagnosis, surgical treatment. Int J Colorectal Dis 1:79–84, 1986.
301. Dukes CE: The classification of cancer of the rectum. J Pathol Bacteriol 35:323–332, 1932.
302. Dukes CE: Cancer of the rectum: An analysis of 1000 cases. J Pathol Bacteriol 50:527–539, 1940.
303. Kirklin JW, Dockerty MD, Waugh JM: The role of the peritoneal reflection in the prognosis of carcinoma of the rectum and sigmoid colon. Surg Gynecol Obstet 88:326–331, 1949.
304. Astler VB, Coller FA: The prognostic significance of direct extension of the carcinoma of the colon and rectum. Ann Surg 139:846–851, 1954.
305. Dukes CE: The surgical pathology of rectal cancer. J Clin Pathol 2:95–98, 1949.
306. Dukes CE, Bussey HJR: The spread of rectal cancer and its effect on prognosis. Br J Cancer 12:309–320, 1958.
307. Turnbull RB, Kyle K, Watson FR, et al: Cancer of the rectum: The influence of the no-touch isolation technic on survival rates. Ann Surg 166:420–427, 1967.
308. Phillips RHS, Hittingger R, Blesovsky L, et al: Large bowel cancer: Surgical pathology and its relationship to survival. Br J Surg 71:604–610, 1984.
309. Gastrointestinal Tumor Study Group: Prolongation of the disease-free interval in surgically treated rectal carcinomas. N Engl J Med 312:1465–1472, 1985.
310. Beahrs OH, Henson DE, Hutter RVP, Myers MH: Manual for staging of cancer, 3rd ed. Philadelphia, JB Lippincott, 1988, pp 75–80.
311. Jass JR, Love SB, Northover JM: A new prognostic classification of rectal cancer. Lancet 1:1303–1306, 1987.
312. Jass JR, Morson BC: Reporting colorectal cancer. J Clin Pathol 40:1016–1023, 1987.
313. Zenklusen HR, Landmann J, Feess A, et al: Primary duodenal carcinoma arising in a non-vaterian tubulo-villous adenoma: A case report with immunocytochemical analysis and review of the literature. Virchows Arch [A] 414:529–533, 1989.
314. Barloon TJ, Lu CH, Honda H, et al: Primary adenocarcinoma of the duodenal bulb: Radiographic and pathologic findings in two cases. Gastrointest Radiol 14:223–225, 1989.
315. Qizilbash AH: Epithelial neoplasms of the duodenum and periampullary region. In Appelman HD (ed). Pathology of the Esophagus, Stomach and Duodenum. New York, Churchill Livingstone, 1984, pp 145–173.
316. Perzin KH, Perterson M, Castiglione CL, et al: Intramucosal carcinoma of the small intestine arising in regional enteritis (Crohn's disease): Report of a case studied for carcinoembryonic antigen and review of the literature. Cancer 54:151–162, 1984.
317. Meiselman MS, Ghahremani GG, Kaufman MW: Crohn's disease of the duodenum complicated by adenocarcinoma. Gastrointest Radiol 12:333–336, 1987.
318. Cuvelier C, Bekaert E, De Potter C, et al: Crohn's disease with adenocarcinoma and dysplasia: Macroscopical, histological, and immunohistochemical aspects of two cases. Am J Surg Pathol 13:187–196, 1989.
319. Spigelman AD, Williams CB, Talbot IC, et al: Upper gastrointestinal cancer in patients with familial adenomatous polyposis. Lancet 2:783–785, 1989.
320. Jagelman DG, DeCosse JJ, Bussey HJ: Upper gastrointestinal cancer in familial adenomatous polyposis. Lancet 1:1149–1151, 1988.
321. Dannenberg A, Godwin I, Rayburn J, et al: Multifocal adenocarcinoma of the proximal small intestine in a patient with celiac sprue. J Clin Gastroenterol 11:73–76, 1989.
322. Levine ML, Dorf BS, Bank S: Adenocarcinoma of the duodenum in a patient with nontropical sprue. Am J Gastroenterol 81:800–802, 1986.
323. Nielsen SN, Wold LE: Adenocarcinoma of jejunum in association with nontropical sprue. Archives Pathol Lab Med 110:822–824, 1986.
324. Yamaguchi K, Maeda S, Kitamura K: Adenocarcinoma in Meckel's diverticulum: case report and literature review. Aust NZ J Surg 59:811–813, 1989.
325. Chen KTK, Workman RD, Kierkegaard DD: Adenocarcinoma of Meckel's diverticulum. J Surg Oncol 23:41–42, 1983.
326. Persson GE, Biosen PT: Cancer of aberrant pancreas in jejunum: Case report. Acta Chir Scand 154:599–601, 1988.
327. Smart PJ, Sastry S, Wells S: Primary mucinous adenocarcinoma developing in an ileostomy stoma. Gut 29:1607–1612, 1988.
328. Suarez V, Alexander-Williams J, O'Connor HJ, et al: Carcinoma developing in ileostomies after 25 or more years. Gastroenterology 95:205–208, 1988.
329. Gadacz TR, McFadden DW, Gabrielson EW, et al: Adenocarcinoma of the ileostomy: The latent risk of cancer after colectomy for ulcerative olitis and familial polyposis. Surgery 107:698–703, 1990.
330. Christie AC: Duodenal carcinoma with neoplastic transformation of the underlying Brunner's gland. Br J Cancer 7:65–67, 1953.
331. Bridge MF, Perzin KH: Primary adenocarcinoma of the jejunum and ileum: A clinicopathologic study. Cancer 36:1876–1887, 1975.
332. Yamashina M: Primary adenocarcinoma of the small intestine with emphasis on microvillous differentiation. Acta Pathol Jpn 37:1061–1070, 1987.
333. Lien GS, Mori M, Enjoji M: Primary carcinoma of the small intestine: A clinicopathologic and immunohistochemical study. Cancer 61:316–323, 1988.
334. Yamaguchi K, Enjoji M: Carcinoma of the ampulla of Vater: A clinicopathologic study and pathologic staging of 109 cases of carcinoma and 5 cases of adenoma. Cancer 59:506–515, 1987.
335. Lioe TF, Biggart JD: Primary adenocarcinoma of the jejunum and ileum: Clinicopathological review of 25 cases. J Clin Pathol 43:533–536, 1990.
336. Cutler SJ, Young JL: Third National Cancer Survey: Incidence data. Natl Cancer Inst Monogr 41:1–454, 1975.
337. Williamson RCN, Welch CE, Malt RA: Adenocarcinoma and

lymphoma of the small intestine: Distribution and etiologic associations. Am Surg 197:172–178, 1983.
338. Brophy C, Cahow CE: Primary small bowel malignant tumors: Unrecognized until emergent laparotomy. Am Surg 55:408–412, 1989.
339. Yamaguchi K, Enjoji M, Kitamura K: Non-icteric ampullary carcinoma with a favorable prognosis. Am J Gastroenterol 85:994–999, 1990.
340. Del Regato JA, Spjut HJ, Cox JD: Ackerman and del Regato's Cancer: Diagnosis, Treatment and Prognosis, 6th ed. St Louis, CV Mosby, 1985, pp 530–567.
341. Netscher DT, Larson GM: Colon cancer: the left to right shift and its implications. Surg Gastroenterol 2:13–18, 1983.
342. Ghahremani GG, Dowlatshahi K: Colorectal carcinomas: Diagnostic implications of their changing frequency and anatomic distribution. World J Surg 13:321–324, 1989.
343. Slater GI, Haber RH, Aufses AH: Changing distribution of carcinoma of the colon and rectum. Surg Gynecol Obstet 158:216–218, 1984.
344. Cady B, Persson AV, Monson DO, Manuz DL: Changing patterns of colorectal carcinoma. Cancer 33:422–426, 1974.
345. Minton JP, Hoehn JL, Gerber DM, et al: Results of a 400-patient carcinoembryonic antigen second-look colorectal cancer study. Cancer 55:1284–1290, 1985.
346. Greene FL: Distribution of colorectal neoplasms: A left to right shift of polyps and cancer. Am Surg 49:62–65, 1983.
347. Lockhart-Mummery HE, Morson BC: Crohn's disease of the large intestine. Gut 5:493–509, 1964.
348. Filipe MI, Edwards MR, Ehsannulah M: A prospective study of dysplasia and carcinoma in the rectal biopsies and rectal stump of eight patients following ileorectal anastomosis in ulcerative colitis. Histopathology 9:1139–1153, 1985.
349. Thomas DM, Filipe MI, Smedley FH: Dysplasia and carcinoma in the rectal stump of total colitics who have undergone colectomy and ileo-rectal anastomosis. Histopathology 14:289–298, 1989.
350. Goldbrager MB, Humphreys EM, Kirshner JB, Palmer WL: Carcinoma and ulcerative colitis. Gastroenterology 34:809–839, 1958.
351. Hamilton SR: Colorectal carcinoma in patients with Crohn's disease. Gastroenterology 89:398–407, 1985.
352. Ponz de Leon M, Sacchetti C, Sassatelli R, et al: Evidence for the existence of different types of large bowel tumor: Suggestions from the clinical data of a population-based registry. J Surg Oncol 44:35–43, 1990.
353. Ekelund GR: Multiple carcinomas of the colon and rectum. Cancer 33:1630–1634, 1974.
354. Cuncliffe WJ, Hasleton PS, Tweedle DE, Schofield PF: Incidence of synchronous and metachronous colorectal carcinoma. Br J Sur 71:941–943, 1984.
355. Kiefer PJ, Thorson AG, Christensen MA: Metachronous colorectal cancer: Time interval to presentation of a metachronous cancer. Dis Colon Rectum 29:378–382, 1986.
356. Schwartz D, Banner BF, Roseman DL, et al: Origin of multiple "primary" colon carcinomas: A retrospective flow cytometric study. Cancer 58:2082–2088, 1986.
357. Greenstein AJ, Slater G, Heimann TM, et al: A comparison of multiple synchronous colorectal cancer in ulcerative colitis, familial polyposis coli, and de novo cancer. Ann Surg 203:123–128, 1986.
358. Gajraj H, Davies DR, Jackson BT: Synchronous small and large bowel cancer developing after pelvic irradiation. Gut 29:126–128, 1988.
359. Johnson CD, Thomson H: Six synchronous colonic cancers in a pair of monozygotic twins. Dis Colon Rectum 29:745–746, 1986.
360. Kaibara N, Koga S, Jinnai D: Synchronous and metachronous malignancies of the colon and rectum in Japan with special reference to a coexisting early cancer. Cancer 54:1870–1874, 1984.
361. Langevin JM, Nivatvongs S: The true incidence of synchronous cancer of the large bowel: A prospective study. Am J Surg 147:330–333, 1984.
362. Dasmahapatra KS, Lopyan K: Rationale for aggressive colonoscopy in patients with colorectal neoplasia. Arch Surg 124:63–66, 1989.
363. Evers BM, Mullins RJ, Matthews TH, et al: Multiple adenocarcinomas of the colon and rectum: An analysis of incidence and current trends. Dis Colon Rectum 31:518–522, 1988.
364. Finan PJ, Ritchie JK, Hawley PR: Synchronous and "early" metachronous carcinomas of the colon and rectum. Br J Surg 74:945–947, 1987.
365. Lazorthes F, Voigt JJ, Roques J, et al: Distal intramural spread of carcinoma of the rectum correlated with lymph nodal involvement. Surg Gynecol Obstet 170:45–48, 1990.
366. Madsen PM, Christiansen J: Distal intramural spread of rectal carcinomas. Dis Colon Rectum 29:279–282, 1986.
367. Kameda K, Furusawa M, Mori M, Sugimachi K: Proposed distal margin for resection of rectal cancer. Jpn J Cancer Res 81:100–104, 1990.
368. Wood WQ, Wilkie DPD: Carcinoma of the rectum: An anatomicropathologic study. Edinburgh Med J 40:321–331, 1933.
369. Grinnell RS: Lymphatic block with atypical and retrograde lymphatic metastasis and spread in carcinoma of the colon and rectum. Ann Surg 163:272–280, 1986.
370. Jass JR, Atkin WS, Cuzick J, et al: The grading of rectal cancer: Historical perspectives and a multivariate analysis of 447 cases. Histopathology 10:437–459, 1986.
371. Burns FJ, Pfaff J Jr: Vascular invasion in carcinoma of the colon and rectum. Am J Surg 92:704–709, 1956.
372. Watne AL, Moore GE, Burke E, et al: Cancer of the colon and rectum: A study of routes and metastases. Am J Surg 101:7–10, 1961.
373. Weiss L, Grundmann E, Torhorst J, et al: Hematogenous metastatic patterns in colonic carcinoma: An analysis of 1541 necropsies. J Pathol 150:195–203, 1986.
374. Vider M, Maruyama Y, Narvaez R: Significance of the vertebral venous (Batson's) plexus in metastatic spread in colorectal carcinoma. Cancer 40:67–71, 1977.
375. Brown CE, Warren S: Visceral metastasis from rectal carcinoma. Surg Gynecol Obstet 66:611–621, 1938.
376. Grinnell RS: The spread of carcinoma of the colon and rectum. Cancer 3:641–652, 1950.
377. Berge T, Ekelund G, Mellner C, et al: Carcinoma of the colon and rectum in a defined population: An epidemiological, clinical and postmortem investigation of colorectal carcinoma and coexisting benign polyps in Malmo, Sweden. Acta Chir Scand [Suppl] 438:1–86, 1973.
378. Holtz F, Hart WR: Krukenberg tumors of the ovary: A clinicopathologic analysis of 27 cases. Cancer 50:2438–2447, 1982.
379. Brennecke SP, McEvoy MI, Seymour AE, et al: Caecal adenocarcinoma metastatic to ovary inducing increased oestrogen production and postmenopausal bleeding. Aust NZJ Obstet Gynaecol 26:158–161, 1986.
380. Blefari F, Risi O: Rare secondary carcinoma from colon to testis: Review of literature and report of a new case. Arch Ital Urol 61:275–278, 1989.
381. Mast HL, Nissenblatt MJ: Metastatic colon carcinoma to the jaw: A case report and review of the literature. J Surg Oncol 34:202–207, 1987.
382. McKay MJ, Carr PJ, Jawarski R, Kalnins I: Cancer of distant primary site relapsing in the nasopharynx: A report of two cases and review of the literature. Head Neck 11:534–537, 1989.
383. Paling MR, Pope TL: Computed tomography of isolated osteoblastic colon metastases in the bony pelvis. J Comput Tomogr 12:203–207, 1988.
384. Hindley CJ, Metcalfe JW: A colonic metastatic tumor in the hand. J Hand Surg 12:803–805, 1987.
385. Morris DC, Tomita T, Anderson HC: Heterotopic ossification: A case report and immunohistochemical observation. Hum Pathol 20:86–88, 1989.
386. Boreham P: Implantation metastases from cancer of the large bowel. Br J Surg 46:103–108, 1958.
387. Slanetz CA, Herter FP, Grinnell RS: Anterior resection versus abdominoperineal resection for cancer of the rectum and rectosigmoid. Am J Surg 123:110–117, 1972.
388. Mason AY: Cancer of the colon and rectum: Carcinoma of the

389. Guiss RL: The implantation of cancer cells with a fistula in ano: Case report. Surgery 36:136–139, 1954.
390. Gold P, Freeman SO: Specific carcinoembryonic antigens of the human digestive system. J Exp Med 122:467–481, 1965.
391. Ho SB, Toribara NW, Bresalier RS, Kim YS: Biochemical and other markers of colon cancer. Gastroenterol Clin North Am 17:811–836, 1988.
392. Luk GD, Desai TK, Conteas CN, et al: Biochemical markers in colorectal cancer: Diagnostic and therapeutic implications. Gastroenterol Clin North Am 17:931–940, 1988.
393. Klavins JV: Gastrointestinal tumor markers, other than carcinoembryonic antigen, and alpha fetal protein. Cancer Detect Prev 6:131–136, 1983.
394. Mercer DW, Talamo TS: Multiple markers of malignancy in sera of patients with colorectal carcinoma: Preliminary clinical studies. Clin Chem 31:1824–1828, 1985.
395. Nap M, Mollgard K, Burtin P, et al: Immunohistochemistry of carcinoembryonic antigen in the embryo, fetus and adult. Tumour Biol 9:145–153, 1988.
396. Huitric E, Laumonier R, Burtin P, et al: An optical and ultrastructural study of the localization of carcinoembryonic antigen (CEA) in normal and cancerous human rectocolonic mucosa. Lab Invest 34:97–108, 1976.
397. Fischbach W, Mossner J, Seyschab H, Hohn H: Tissue carcinoembryonic antigen and DNA aneuploidy in precancerous and cancerous colorectal lesions. Cancer 65:1820–1824, 1990.
398. Tabuchi Y, Deguchi H, Saitoh Y: Carcinoembryonic antigen and carbohydrate antigen 19-9 levels of peripheral and draining venous blood in colorectal cancer patients: Correlation with histopathologic and immunohistochemical variables. Cancer 62:1605–1613, 1988.
399. Fletcher RE: Carcinoembryonic antigen. Ann Intern Med 104:66–73, 1986.
400. Stamatiadis AP, St Toumanidou M, Vyssoulis GP, et al: Value of serum acute-phase reactant proteins and carcinoembryonic antigen in the preoperative staging of colorectal cancer: A multivariate analysis. Cancer 65:2055–2057, 1990.
401. Sener SF, Imperato JP, Chmiel J, et al: The use of cancer registry data to study preoperative carcinoembryonic antigen level as an indicator of survival in colorectal cancer. CA 39:50–57, 1989.
402. Kuuselu P, Jalanko H, Roberts P, et al: Comparison of CA 19-9 and carcinoembryonic antigens (CEA) levels in the serum of patients with colorectal disease. Br J Cancer 49:135–139, 1984.
403. Dahiya R, Itzkowitz SH, Byrd JC, et al: ABH blood group antigen expression, synthesis, and degradation in human colonic adenocarcinoma cell lines. Cancer Res 49:4550–4556, 1989.
404. Kim YS, Yuan M, Itzkowitz SH, et al: Expression of ley and extended ley blood group-related antigens in human malignant, premalignant, and nonmalignant colonic tissues. Cancer Res 46:5985–5992, 1986.
405. Schoentag R, Williams V, Kuhns W: The distribution of blood group substance H and CEA in colorectal carcinoma. Cancer 53:503–509, 1984.
406. Boland CR, Kim YS: Lectin markers of differentiation and malignancy. Prog Cancer Res Ther 29:252–266, 1984.
407. Fischer J, Klein PJ, Vierbuchen M, et al: Characterization of glycoconjugates of human gastrointestinal mucosa by lectins. I. Histochemical distribution of lectin binding sites in normal alimentary tract as well as benign and malignant gastric neoplasms. J Histochem Cytochem 32:681–689, 1984.
408. Ota H, Nakayama J, Katsuyama T, Kanai M: Histochemical comparison of specificity of three bowel carcinoma-reactive lectins, Griffonia simplicifolia agglutinin-II, peanut agglutinin, and Ulex europaeus agglutinin-I. Acta Pathol Jpn 38:1547–1559, 1988.
409. Pant KD, Shochat D, Nelson MO, Goldenberg DM: Colon-specific antigen-p (CSAp). I. Initial clinical evaluation as a marker for colorectal cancer. Cancer 50:919–926, 1982.
410. Gold DV: Immunoperoxidase localization of colonic mucoprotein antigen in neoplastic tissues. Cancer Res 41:767–772, 1981.
411. Bara J, Gautier R, Daher N, et al: Monoclonal antibodies against oncofetal mucin M1 antigens associated with precancerous colonic mucosae. Cancer Res 46:3983–3989, 1986.
412. Pant KD, Fenoglio-Preiser CM, Berry CO, et al: COTA (colon-ovarian tumor antigen): An immunohistochemical study. Am J Clin Pathol 86:1–9, 1986.
413. Birkje B, Histmark J, Skagen DW, et al: Flow cytometry of biopsy specimens from ulcerative colitis, colorectal adenomas, and carcinomas. Scand J Gastroenterol 22:1231–1237, 1987.
414. Kouri M, Laasonen A, Mecklin JP, et al: Diploid predominance in hereditary nonpolyposis colorectal carcinoma evaluated by flow cytometry. Cancer 65:1825–1829, 1990.
415. Hamadas R, Itoh R, Nakanishik, Fujita S: DNA distribution pattern of early adenocarcinomas of the colon and rectum and its possible meaning in the tumor progression. Cancer 61:1555–1562, 1988.
416. Banner BF, Tomas De La Vega JE, Roseman DL, Coon JS: Should flow cytometric DNA analysis precede definitive surgery for colon carcinoma? Ann Surg 202:740–744, 1985.
417. Crissman JD, Zarbo RJ, Ma CK, Visscher DW: Histopathologic parameters and DNA analysis in colorectal adenocarcinomas. Pathol Annu 24:103–147, 1989.
418. Visscher DW, Zarbo RJ, Ma CK, Crissman JD: Flow cytometric DNA and clinicopathologic analysis of Dukes' A&B colonic adenocarcinomas: A retrospective study. Mod Pathol 3:709–712, 1990.
419. Melamed MR, Enker WE, Banner P, et al: Flow cytometry of colorectal carcinoma with three-year follow-up. Dis Colon Rectum 29:184–186, 1986.
420. Hood DL, Petras RE, Edinger M, et al. Deoxyribonucleic acid ploidy and cell cycle analysis of colorectal carcinoma by flow cytometry: A prospective study of 137 cases using fresh whole cell suspensions. Am J Clin Pathol 93:615–620, 1990.
421. Hoang C, Polivka M, Valleur P, et al: Immunohistochemical detection of proliferating cells in colorectal carcinomas and adenomas with the monoclonal antibody Ki-67: Preliminary data. Virchows Arch [A] 414:423–428, 1989.
422. Lipkin M, Higgins P: Biological markers of cell proliferation and differentiation in human gastrointestinal diseases. Adv Cancer Res 50:1–23, 1988.
423. Shepherd NA, Richman PI, England J: Ki-67 derived proliferative activity in colorectal adenocarcinoma with prognostic correlations. J Pathol 155:213–219, 1988.
424. Bradley SJ, Garfinkle G, Walker E, et al: Increased expression of the epidermal growth factor receptor of human colon carcinoma cells. Arch Surg 121:1242–1247, 1986.
425. Flanders KC, Thompson NL, Cissel DS, et al: Transforming growth factor-beta 1: Histochemical localization with antibodies to different epitopes. J Cell Biol 108:653–660, 1989.
426. Tahara E: Growth factors and oncogenes in human gastrointestinal carcinomas. J Cancer Res Clin Oncol 116:121–131, 1990.
427. Conteas CN, Desai TK, Arlow FA: Relationship of hormones and growth factors to colon cancer. Gastroenterol Clin North Am 17:761–772, 1988.
428. Skinner JM, Whitehead R: Carcinoplacental alkaline phosphatase in malignant and premalignant conditions of the human digestive tract. Virchows Arch [A] 394:109–118, 1981.
429. Campo E, Palacin A, Benasco C, et al: Human chorionic gonadotropin in colorectal carcinoma. Cancer 49:1611–1616, 1987.
430. Stebbings WS, Farthing MJ, Vinson GP, et al: Androgen receptors in rectal and colonic cancer. Dis Colon Rectum 29:95–98, 1986.
431. Alford TC, Do HM, Geelhoed GW, et al: Steroid hormone receptors in human colon cancers. Cancer 43:980–984, 1979.
432. Beauchamp RD, Townsend CM Jr, Singh P, et al: Prolimide, a gastrin receptor antagonist, inhibits growth of colon cancer and enhances survival in mice. Ann Surg 202:303–309, 1985.
433. Geelhoed GW, Crandall A, Lippman ME: Biologic implications of steroid hormone receptors in cancers of the colon. South Med J 78:252–254, 1985.
434. Loser C, Folsch UR, Paprotny C, Creutzfeldt V: Polyamines in colorectal cancer: Evaluation of polyamine concentrations in the colon tissues, serum and urine of 50 patients with colorectal cancer. Cancer 65:958–966, 1990.

435. de Bruin PA, Griffioen G, Verspaget HW, et al: Plasminogen activator profiles in neoplastic tissues of the human colon. Cancer Res 48:4520–4544, 1988.
436. Gong E, Hirohashi S, Shimosato Y, et al: Expression of carbohydrate antigen 19-9 and stage-specific embryonic antigen 1 in nontumorous and tumorous epithelia of the human colon and rectum. JNCI 75:446–454, 1985.
437. Drewinko B, Yang LY, Chang J, et al: New monoclonal antibodies against colon cancer-associated antigens. Cancer Res 46:5137–5143, 1986.
438. Decaens C, Gautier R, Bara J, et al: A new mucin-associated oncofetal antigen, a marker of early carcinogenesis in rat colon. Cancer Res 48:1571–1577, 1988.
439. Ernst CS, Shen JW, Litwin S, et al: Multiparameter evaluation of the expression in situ of normal and tumor-associated antigens in human colorectal carcinoma. JNCI 77:387–395, 1986.
440. Degener T, Momburg F, Moller P: Differential expression of HLA-DR, HLA-DP, HLA-DQ and associated invariant chain (II) in normal colorectal mucosa, adenoma and carcinoma. Virchows Arch [A] 412:315–322, 1988.
441. Momburg F, Ziegler A, Happrecht J, et al: Selective loss of HLA-A or HLA-B antigen expression in colon carcinoma. J Immunol 142:352–358, 1989.
442. Chester SJ, Maimonis P, Meitner PA, et al: An analysis of immunocomplexes for the detection of the early stages of colon cancer. Cancer 65:1338–1344, 1990.
443. Fleshner P, Slater G, Aufses AH Jr: Age and sex distribution of patients with colorectal cancer. Dis Colon Rectum 32:107–111, 1989.
444. Pitluk H, Poticha SM: Carcinoma of the colon and rectum in patients less than 40 years of age. Surg Gynecol Obstet 157:335–337, 1983.
445. Adkins RB Jr, DeLozier JB, McKnight WG, Waterhouse B: Carcinoma of the colon in patients 35 years of age and younger. Am Surg 53:141–145, 1987.
446. Haubrich WS, Berk JE: Malignant tumors of the colon and rectum. In Bockus HL (ed): Gastroenterology, 3rd ed. Philadelphia, WB Saunders 1976, pp 1009–1044.
447. Beckman EN, Gathright JB, Ray JE: A potentially brighter prognosis for colon carcinoma in the third and fourth decades. Cancer 54:1478–1481, 1984.
448. VanVoorhis B, Cruikshank DP: Colon carcinoma complicating pregnancy: A report of two cases. J Reprod Med 34:923–927, 1989.
449. Heydenrych JJ, Warren B: An unusual presentation of carcinoma of the colon in a child: A case report. S Afr Med J 65:617–618, 1984.
450. Sarma DP: Colorectal carcinoma in young adults: An autopsy study. J Surg Oncol 35:52–54, 1987.
451. Bockus HL, Kalser MH, Mouhran Y, et al: Early clinical manifestations of cancer of the colon and rectum. Dis Colon Rectum 2:58–68, 1959.
452. Bloem RM, Zwaveling A, Stijnene T: Adenocarcinoma of the colon and rectum: A report on 624 cases. Neth J Surg 40:121–126, 1988.
453. Becking WB, Quylaert JB, Feldberg MA, van Leeuwen MS: Appendiceal involvement in cecal carcinoma: Demonstration by ultrasound. Gastrointest Radiol 14:170–172, 1989.
454. Aladgem D, Mazor A, Kashtan H, et al: Colonic bleeding due to rupture of an isolated iliac artery aneurysm into a caecal carcinoma. Postgrad Med J 64:636–637, 1988.
455. Murakami S, Togo S, Yasuda S, et al: The syndrome of inappropriate secretion of antidiuretic hormone by rectal cancer: A case report. Jpn J Surg 17:293–296, 1987.
456. O'Reilly D, Long RG: Carcinoma of the colon presenting with dyspepsia. Postgrad Med J 63:215–216, 1987.
457. Gallager FJ, Baxter DL, Denobile J, Taybos GM: Glossodynia, iron deficiency anemia, and gastrointestinal malignancy: Report of a case. Oral Surg Oral Med Oral Pathol 65:130–133, 1988.
458. Berkelhammer CH, Baker AL, Block GE, et al: Humoral hypercalcemia complicating adenosquamous carcinoma of the proximal colon. Dig Dis Sci 34:142–147, 1989.
459. Strodel WE, Thompson NW, Eckhauser FE, Knol JA: Malignancy and concomitant primary hyperparathyroidism. J Surg Oncol 37:10–12, 1988.
460. Kyllonen LE: Obstruction and perforation complicating colorectal carcinoma: An epidemiologic and clinical study with special reference to incidence and survival. Acta Chir Scand 153:607–614, 1987.
461. Kaufman Z, Eiltch E, Dinbar A: Completely obstructive colorectal cancer. J Surg Oncol 41:230–235, 1989.
462. Bear HD, MacIntyre J, Burns HJ, et al: Colon and rectal carcinoma in the west of Scotland: Symptoms, histologic characteristics, and outcome. Am J Surg 147:441–446, 1984.
463. Armitage NC, Ballantyne KC: Primary aortoenteric fistula due to recurrent colorectal cancer: Report of a case. Dis Colon Rectum 33:148–149, 1990.
464. Nesbakken A, Haffner J: Colo-recto-anal intussusception: Case report. Acta Chir Scand 155:201–204, 1989.
465. Panwalker AP: Unusual infections associated with colorectal cancer. Rev Infect Dis 10:347–364, 1988.
466. Tabibian N, Clarridge JE: Streptococcus bovis septicemia and large bowel neoplasia. Am Fam Physician 39:227–229, 1989.
467. Emiliani VJ, Chodos JE, Comer GM, et al: Streptococcus bovis brain abscess associated with an occult colonic villous adenoma. Am J Gastroenterol 85:78–80, 1990.
468. Kornbluth AA, Danzig JB, Bernstein LH: Clostridium septicum infection and associated malignancy: Report of 2 cases and review of the literature. Medicine 68:30–37, 1989.
469. Buckley D, Kudsk K: Occult gastrointestinal carcinoma causing metastatic clostridial soft-tissue infection: Report of two cases. Dis Colon Rectum 31:306–310, 1988.
470. Lee PH, Khauli RB, Baker S, Menon M: Prognostic and therapeutic observations of manifestations in the genitourinary tract of adenocarcinoma of the colon and rectum. Surg Gynecol Obstet 169:511–518, 1989.
471. Amico L, Caplan LR, Thomas C: Cerebrovascular complications of mucinous cancers. Neurology 39:522–526, 1989.
472. Liel Y, Ariad S: Microangiopathic hemolytic anemia associated with metastatic carcinoma of the colon. South Med J 81:1320–1321, 1988.
473. Macpherson A, Berth-Jones J, Graham-Brown RA: Carcinoma-associated dermatomyositis responding to plasmapheresis. Clin Exp Dermatol 14:304–305, 1989.
474. Sung MW, Bruckner HW, Szabo S, Mitty HA: Extrahepatic obstructive jaundice due to colorectal cancer. Am J Gastroenterol 83:267–270, 1988.
475. McCallum A, Eastwood MA, Smith AN, Fulton PM: Colonic diverticulosis in patients with colorectal cancer and in controls. Scand J Gastroenterol 23:284–286, 1988.
476. Morini S, de Angelis P, Manurita L, Colavolpe V: Association of colonic diverticula with adenomas and carcinomas. A colonoscopic experience. Dis Colon Rectum 31:793–796, 1988.
477. Shemesh E, Czerniak A, Pines A, Bat L: Is there an association between gastric polyps and colonic neoplasms? Digestion 42:212–216, 1989.
478. Armstrong CP, Ahsan Z, Hinchley G, et al: Appendectomy and carcinoma of the caecum. Br J Surg 76:1049–1053, 1989.
479. Yoshida J, Morisaki T, Yamaguchi K, et al: Carcinoma in adenoma of the ampulla of Vater synchronous with cancer of the sigmoid colon. Dig Dis Sci 35:271–275, 1990.
480. Schmid KW, Galser K, Wykypiel H, Feichtinger H: Synchronous adenocarcinoma of the transverse colon, the gallbladder and the vermiform appendix. Klin Wochenschr 66:1093–1096, 1988.
481. Klompje J, Petrelli NJ, Herrera L, Mittelman A: Synchronous and metachronous colon lesions in squamous cell carcinoma of the anal canal. J Surg Oncol 35:86–88, 1987.
482. Takayama H, Nakagawa K, Onozuka S, et al: Nonfamilial Turcot syndrome presenting with astrocytoma: Case report. Neurol Med Chir 29:606–609, 1989.
483. el-Jabbour JN, Helm CW, McLaren KM, et al: Synchronous colonic adenocarcinoma and extragenital malignant mixed mesodermal tumour. Scott Med J 34:567–568, 1989.
484. Kinn AC, Haggmark T, Willems JS: Aggressive mesenteric fibromatosis: Case report. Acta Chir Scand 155:293–296, 1989.
485. Brunner JE, Johnson CC, Zafar S, et al: Colon cancer and pol-

yps in acromegaly: Increased risk associated with family history of colon cancer. Clin Endocrinol 32:65–71, 1990.
486. Cappell MS, Yao F, Cho KC: Colonic adenocarcinoma associated with the acquired immune deficiency syndrome. Cancer 62:616–619, 1988.
487. Heng MC, Soo-Hoo K, Levine S, Petresek D: Linear seborrheic keratoses associated with underlying malignancy. J Am Acad Dermatol 18:1316–1321, 1988.
488. Moran CA, West B, Schwartz IS: Malacoplakia of the colon in association with colonic adenocarcinoma. Am J Gastroenterol 84:1580–1582, 1989.
489. Yoshida J, Tsuneyoshi M, Nakamura KAU, et al: Primary ciliary dyskinesia with transverse colon carcinoma. Am J Clin Pathol 85:101–104, 1986.
490. Aggarwal P, Sharma SK, Wali JP, Sahani P: Colonic carcinoma after chemotherapy of Hodgkin's disease. J Clin Gastroenterol 11:340–342, 1989.
491. Hinder JM, Chu J, Bokey EL, et al: Use of transrectal ultrasound to evaluate direct tumour spread and lymph node status in patients with rectal cancer. Aust NZ J Surg 60:19–23, 1990.
492. Dasmahapatra KS, Lopyan K: Rationale for aggressive colonoscopy in patients with colorectal neoplasia. Arch Surg 124:63–66, 1989.
493. Kochhar R, Rajwanshi A, Wig JD: Fine needle aspiration cytology of rectal masses. Gut 32:334–336, 1990.
494. Vobecky J, Leduc CP, Devroede G, Madarnas P: The reliability of routine pathologic diagnosis of colorectal adenocarcinoma. Cancer 64:1261–1265, 1989.
495. Halvorsen TB: Tissue sampling and histological grading in colorectal cancer: Are routine sections representative? Acta Pathol Microbiol Immunol Scand 97:261–266, 1989.
496. Thomas WM, Pye G, Hardcastle JD, Mangham CM: Faecal occult blood screening for colorectal neoplasia: A randomized trial of three days or six days of tests. Br J Surg 77:277–279, 1990.
497. McGarrity TJ, Long PA, Peiffer LP: Results of a repeat television-advertised mass screening program for colorectal cancer using fecal occult blood tests. Am J Gastroenterol 85:266–270, 1990.
498. Hardcastle JD, Thomas WM, Chamberlain J, et al: Randomised, controlled trial of faecal occult blood screening for colorectal cancer: Results for first 107,349 subjects, Lancet 1:1160–1164, 1989.
499. Ow CL, Lemar HJ, Weaver MJ: Does screening proctosigmoidoscopy result in reduced mortality from colorectal cancer? A critical review of the literature. J Gen Intern Med 4:209–215, 1989.
500. Orrom WJ, Brzezinski WS, Wiens EW: Heredity and colorectal cancer: A prospective, community-based, endoscopic study. Dis Colon Rectum 33:490–493, 1990.
501. Beart RW: Colon, rectum, and anus. Cancer 33:684–688, 1990.
502. Ottery FD, Bruskewitz RC, Weese JL: Endoscopic transrectal resection of rectal tumors. Cancer 576:563–566, 1986.
503. Stearns MW Jr, Sternberg SS, DeCosse JJ: Treatment alternatives: Localized rectal cancer. Cancer 54:2691–2694, 1984.
504. Shehata WM, Meyer RL, Jazy FK, et al: Regional adjuvant irradiation for adenocarcinoma of the cecum. Int J Radiat Oncol Biol Phys 13:843–846, 1987.
505. Kopelson G: Adjuvant postoperative radiation therapy for colorectal carcinoma above the peritoneal reflection. I. Sigmoid colon. Cancer 51:1593–1598, 1983.
506. Wadler S, Wiernik PH: Clinical update on the role of fluorouracil and recombinant interferon alpha-2a in the treatment of colorectal carcinoma. Semin Oncol 17:16–21, 1990.
507. Farley PC, McFaden KH: Colorectal cancer: Are adjuvant therapies beneficial? Postgrad Med 84:175–178, 181–183, 1988.
508. Moertel CG, Gleming TR, MacDonald JS, et al: Levasimole and fluorouracil for adjuvant therapy of reseated colon carcinoma. N Engl J Med 322:352–358, 1990.
509. Coppa GF, Eng K, Ranson JH, et al: Hepatic resection for metastatic colon and rectal cancer: An evaluation of preoperative and postoperative factors. Ann Surg 202:203–208, 1985.
510. Bismuth H, Castaing D, Traynor O: Surgery for synchronous hepatic metastases of colorectal cancer. Scand J Gastroenterol [Suppl] 149:144–149, 1988.
511. Schlag P, Hohenberger P, Holting T, et al: Hepatic arterial infusion (HAL) chemotherapy for liver metastasis of colorectal cancer using 5-FU. Eur J Surg Oncol 16:99–104, 1990.
512. Yamagiwa H, Yoshimura H, Tomiyama H, et al: Squamous change of adenocarcinoma of the large intestine. Gan No Rinsho 30:233–238, 1984.
513. Comer TP, Beahrs OH, Docheertz MB: Primary squamous cell carcinoma and adenoacanthoma. Cancer 28:1111–1117, 1971.
514. Schmidtmaun M: Zur Kenntnis seltener Krebsformen. Arch Pathol Anat 226:100–118, 1919.
515. Latreniere R, Ketcham AS: Primary squamous carcinoma of the rectum: Report of a case and review of literature. Dis Colon Rectum 28:967–972, 1985.
516. Michelassi F, Mishlove LA, Stipa F, Block GE: Squamous-cell carcinoma of the colon: Experience at the University of Chicago—review of the literature, report of two cases. Dis Colon Rectum 31:228–235, 1988.
517. Cerezo L, Alvarez M, Edwards O, Price G: Adenosquamous carcinoma of the colon. Dis Colon Rectum 28:597–603, 1985.
518. Kontozoglou TE, Moyana TN: Adenosquamous carcinoma of the colon—an immunocytochemical and ultrastructural study: Report of two cases and review of the literature. Dis Colon Rectum 32:719–721, 1989.
519. Lundquest DE, Marcus JN, Thorson AG, Massop D: Primary squamous cell carcinoma of the colon arising in a villous adenoma. Hum Pathol 19:362–364, 1988.
520. Burgers PA, Lupton EW, Talbot IC: Squamous-cell carcinoma of the proximal colon: Report of a case and review of the literature. Dis Colon Rectum 22:241–247, 1979.
521. Pigott JP, Williams GB: Primary squamous cell carcinoma of the colorectum: Case report and literature reviews of a rare entity. J Surg Oncol 35:117–119, 1987.
522. Chevinsky AH, Berelowitz M, Hoover HC Jr: Adenosquamous carcinoma of the colon presenting with hypercalcemia. Cancer 60:1111–1116, 1987.
523. Berkelhammer CH, Baker AL, Block GE, et al: Humoral hypercalcemia complicating adenosquamous carcinoma of the proximal colon. Dig Dis Sci 34:142–147, 1989.
524. Peonim V, Thakerngpol K, Pacharee P, Stitnimankarn T: Adenosquamous carcinoma and carcinoidal differentiation of the colon: Report of a case. Cancer 52:1122–1125, 1983.
525. Almargo UA, Pintar K, Zellmer RB: Squamous metaplasia in colorectal polyps. Cancer 53:2679–2682, 1984.
526. Williams GT, Blackshaw AJ, Morson BC: Squamous carcinoma of the colorectum and its genesis. J Pathol 129:139–147, 1979.
527. Michelassi F, Montag AG, Block GE: Adenosquamous-cell carcinoma in ulcerative colitis: Report of a case. Dis Colon Rectum 31:323–326, 1988.
528. Pemberton M, Lendrum J: Squamous cell carcinoma of the caecum following ovarian adenocarcinoma. Br J Surg 55:273–276, 1969.
529. Vezeridis MP, Herrera LO, Lopez GE, et al: Squamous-cell carcinoma of the colon and rectum. Dis Colon Rectum 26:188–191, 1983.
530. Hickey WF, Corson JM: Squamous cell carcinoma arising in a duplication of the colon: Case report and literature review of squamous cell carcinoma of the colon and of malignancy complicating colonic duplication. Cancer 47:602–609, 1981.
531. Petrelli M, Tetangco E, Reid JD: Carcinoma of the colon with undifferentiated carcinoid and squamous cell features. Am J Clin Pathol 75:581–584, 1981.
532. Knight BK, Hayes MM: Mixed adenocarcinoma and carcinoid tumour of the colon: A report of 4 cases with postulates on histogenesis. S African Med J 72:708–710, 1987.
533. Klappenbach RS, Kurman RJ, Sinclair CF, James LP: Composite carcinoma-carcinoid tumors of the gastrointestinal tract: A morphologic, histochemical, and immunocytochemical study. Am J Clin Pathol 84:137–143, 1985.
534. Moyana TN, Qizilbash AH, Murphy F: Composite glandular-carcinoid tumors of the colon and rectum: Report of two cases. Am J Surg Pathol 12:607–611, 1988.
535. Jones MA, Griffith LM, West AB. Adenocarcinoid tumor of the periampullary region: A novel duodenal neoplasm presenting as biliary tract obstruction. Hum Pathol 20:198–200, 1989.

536. Levendoglu H, Cox CA, Nadimpalli V: Composite (adenocarcinoid) tumors of the gastrointestinal tract. Dig Dis Sci 35:519–525, 1990.
537. Mills SE, Allen MS, Cohen AR: Small-cell undifferentiated carcinoma of the colon: A clinicopathological study of five cases and their association with colonic adenomas. Am J Surg Pathol 7:643–651, 1987.
538. Redman BG, Pazdur R: Colonic small cell undifferentiated carcinoma: A distinct pathological diagnosis with therapeutic implications. Am J Gastroenterol 83:382–385, 1987.
539. Robidoux A, Monte M, Heppell J: Small-cell carcinoma of the rectum. Dis Colon Rectum 28:594–596, 1984.
540. Schwartz AM, Orenstein JM: Small cell undifferentiated carcinoma of the rectosigmoid colon. Arch Pathol Lab Med 109:629–632, 1985.
541. Wick MR, Weatherby RP, Weiland LH: Small cell neuroendocrine carcinoma of the colon and rectum: Clinical, histologic, and ultrastructural study and immunohistochemical comparison with cloacogenic carcinoma. Hum Pathol 18:9–21, 1987.
542. Bak M, Teglbjaerg PS: Pleomorphic (giant cell) carcinoma of the intestine: An immunohistochemical and electron microscopic study. Cancer 64:2557–2564, 1989.
543. Jewell LD, Barr JR, McCaughey WT, et al: Clear-cell epithelial neoplasms of the large intestine. Arch Pathol Lab Med 112:197–199, 1988.
544. Kubosawa H, Nagao K, Kondo Y, et al: Coexistence of adenocarcinoma and choriocarcinoma in the sigmoid colon. Cancer 54:866–868, 1984.
545. Robey-Cafferty SS, Silva EG, Cleary KR. Anaplastic and sarcomatoid carcinoma of the small intestine: A clinicopathologic study. Hum Pathol 20:858–863, 1989.
546. Amano S, Yamada N: Endometrioid carcinoma arising from encometriosis of the sigmoid colon: A case report. Hum Pathol 12:845–848, 1981.
547. Orr MM, Edwards AJ. Neoplastic change in duplication of the alimentary tract. Br J Surg 62:269–274, 1975.
548. Wanebo HJ, Woodruff JM, Farr GH, Quan SH. Anorectal melanoma. Cancer 47:1891–1900, 1981.
549. Hambrick E, Abacarian M, Smith D, Keller F: Malignant melanoma of the rectum in a negro man: Report of a case and review of the literature. Dis Colon Rectum 17:360–364, 1974.
550. Sroujieh AS: Spontaneous regression of intestinal malignant melanoma from an occult primary site. Cancer 62:1247–1250, 1988.
551. Raymond AR, Rorat E, Goldstein D, et al: An unusual case of malignant melanoma of the small intestine. Am J Gastroenterol 79:689–692, 1984.
552. Beardmoir GL, Davies NC, McLeod R, et al: Malignant melanoma in Queensland: A study of 219 deaths. Aust J Dermatol 10:158–168, 1969.
553. Wilson BG, Anderson JR: Malignant melanoma involving the small bowel. Postgrad Med J 62:355–357, 1986.
554. Das Gupta TK, Brasfield RD: Metastatic melanoma of the gastrointestinal tract. Arch Surg 88:969–973, 1964.
555. Katon RM, Brendler SJ, Ireland K: Gastric linitis plastica with metastases to the colon: A mimic of Crohn's disease. J Clin Gastroenterol 11:555–560, 1989.
556. Kanter MA, Isaacson NH, Knoll SM, Nochomovitz LE: The diagnostic challenge of metastatic linitis plastica: Two cases and a consideration of the problem. Am Surg 52:510–513, 1986.
557. Levine MS, Drooz AT, Herlinger H: Annular malignancies of the small bowel. Gastrointest Radiol 12:53–58, 1987.
558. Nyberg B, Sonnenfeld T: Metastatic breast carcinoma causing intestinal obstruction. Acta Chir Scand 530:95–96, 1986.
559. Graham WP III, Goldman L: Gastrointestinal metastases from carcinoma of the breast. Ann Surg 159:477–480, 1964.
560. Rabau MY, Alon RJ, Werbin N, Yossipov Y: Colonic metastases from lobular carcinoma of the breast: Report of a case. Dis Colon Rectum 31:401–402, 1988.
561. Wegener M, Borsch G, Reitemeyer E, Schafer K: Metastasis to the colon from primary bronchogenic carcinoma presenting as occult gastrointestinal bleeding: Report of a case. Z Gastroenterol 26:358–362, 1988.
562. Pang JA, King WK: Bowel haemorrhage and perforation from metastatic lung cancer: Report of three cases and a review of the literature. Aust NZ J Surg 57:779–783, 1987.
563. Fawaz F, Hill GJ 2d: Adult intussusception due to metastatic tumors. South Med J 76:522–523, 1983.

PART 6

APPENDIX AND ANAL REGION

CHAPTER 33

Disorders of the Vermiform Appendix

CHIK-KWUN TANG, M.D.

ANATOMY AND EMBRYOLOGY

DEVELOPMENTAL ABNORMALITIES
Congenital Absence (Agenesis)
Duplication
Diverticula
Malposition
Miscellaneous Conditions

INFLAMMATORY DISORDERS
Acute Appendicitis
Etiology and Pathogenesis
Pathology
Correlation of Clinical Diagnosis and Pathologic Observation
Chronic Appendicitis
Ulcerative Colitis and Crohn's Disease
Acquired Diverticulum and Diverticulitis
Infections

Bacterial Infections
Campylobacter-Associated Appendicitis
Tuberculosis
Yersiniosis
Spirochetosis
Actinomycosis
Viral Infections
Measles
Adenovirus
Mononucleosis
Cytomegalovirus
Parasitic Infections
Fungal Infections

EPITHELIAL HYPERPLASIA

NEOPLASIA
Adenoma and Cystadenoma
Adenocarcinoma and Cystadenocarcinoma
Mucocele and Pseudomyxoma Peritonei

Carcinoid Tumor
Adenocarcinoid Tumor
Other Tumors
Lymphoma
Leiomyoma and Leiomyosarcoma
Granular Cell Tumor
Neuroma
Ganglioneuroma
Metastatic Tumors

MISCELLANEOUS LESIONS
Fibrous Obliteration
Sarcoidosis
Periappendicitis
Intussusception
Endometriosis
Arteritis
Cystic Fibrosis
Septa
Other Lesions

The human vermiform appendix can be affected by a wide range of diseases, and its inflammatory condition, acute appendicitis, remains the most common acute abdominal condition.[1] Other diseases—including congenital anomalies, various infectious conditions, hyperplastic, and neoplastic diseases—have also been observed in the appendix. Diseases other than acute appendicitis may produce symptoms and signs indistinguishable from those of appendicitis. Conversely, a complicated acute appendicitis may resemble other diseases, such as tumor. The accuracy of diagnosing acute appendicitis is high but far from perfect. The decision when to operate thus continues to be one of the most common challenges to surgeons.

ANATOMY AND EMBRYOLOGY

Developmentally the human vermiform appendix can be regarded as a part of the cecum. In the sixth week of gestational age, a blind-ended pouch, the cecal diverticulum, is formed on the antimesenteric border of the primitive midgut.[2] The distal end of this pouch, which does not grow as rapidly as the proximal portion, becomes the appendix. The length of the appendix, however, increases during fetal development. Beginning at birth, the lateral wall of the cecum grows faster than the medial. This different growth rate results in the shift of the appendix from its end position to the side near the ileocecal valve.

In normal adults, approximately 65% of the appendices are located behind the cecum and descending colon, with its orifice opening into the cecum near the ileocecal valve. The appendix may also be found on the side of the ascending colon, in front of or behind the terminal ileum, lying on the psoas muscle or hanging over the pelvic brim.[3] The appendiceal orifice varies in shape, from round to slitlike. The length of the appendix ranges from 2 to 20 cm,[3,4] the average being 7 cm in normal adults; the appendix is usually shorter in children. The external diameter measures 0.5 to 0.6 cm[4] and that of its lumen, 0.1 to 0.2 cm.[3] The base of the appendix is anchored onto the posterior abdominal wall by the mesoappendix, which is an extension of the mesentery of the adjacent terminal ileum. The tip of the appendix is free. Although the three taeniae coli meet at the base of the appendix, none is present in the appendix proper.

The appendicular artery, a branch of the ileocecal artery, provides the arterial blood supply. Its venous blood drains into the portal system by means of the superior mesenteric vein. The lymphatics of the appendix drain into the lymph nodes in the mesoappendix and then into the right para-aortic lymph nodes and those in the ileocecal angle.[3] Externally the serosa is pink, smooth, and glistening, and small blood vessels are observed through it. On cross section, the appendiceal wall is a circular structure that displays a pink to white color. The mucosa is soft, smooth, and pink, and slightly protrudes into the lumen.

The cells of the appendiceal mucosa are cytologically identical to those of the colon: tall columnar epithelial cells, many of which contain mucus; and a basal zone of mitotically active primitive cells. They appear to differentiate toward columnar cells, including the goblet cells, early in fetal life (Figure 33–1). The mucosa of the appendix does not form villi[5] (Figure 33–2). Most columnar cells lining the surface of the mucosa function as absorptive elements. Nonbranching crypts (crypts of Lieberkühn) are also lined with columnar cells. Here the goblet cells are more prominent than those in the surface (see Figure 33–2). At the bases of the crypts

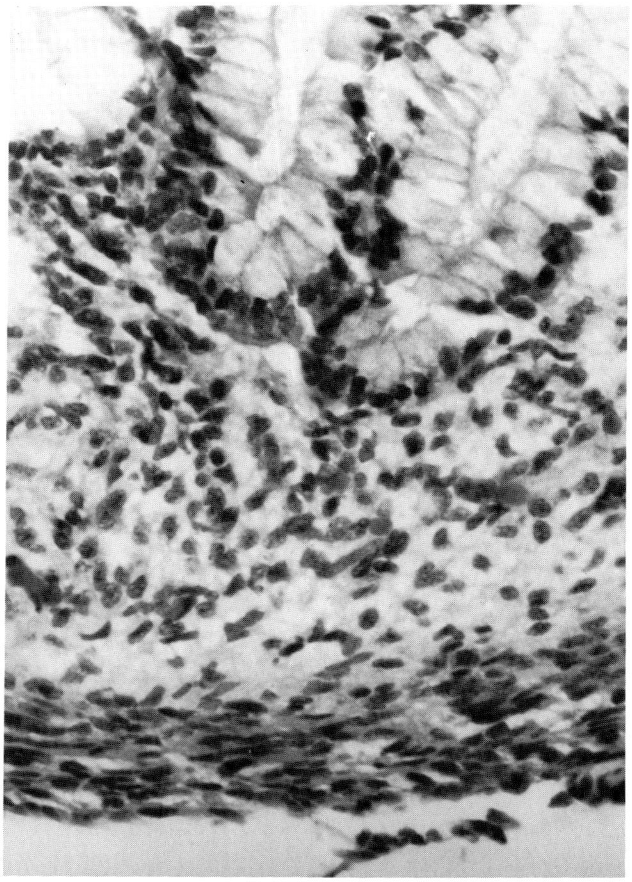

FIGURE 33–1. Normal vermiform appendix of a 13-week-old fetus (gestational age), showing well-developed goblet cells and a thin muscular coat. Lymphoid follicles are absent. (× 500) (Courtesy of Dr. Elizabeth Dellers, Temple University Hospital, Philadelphia, Pa.)

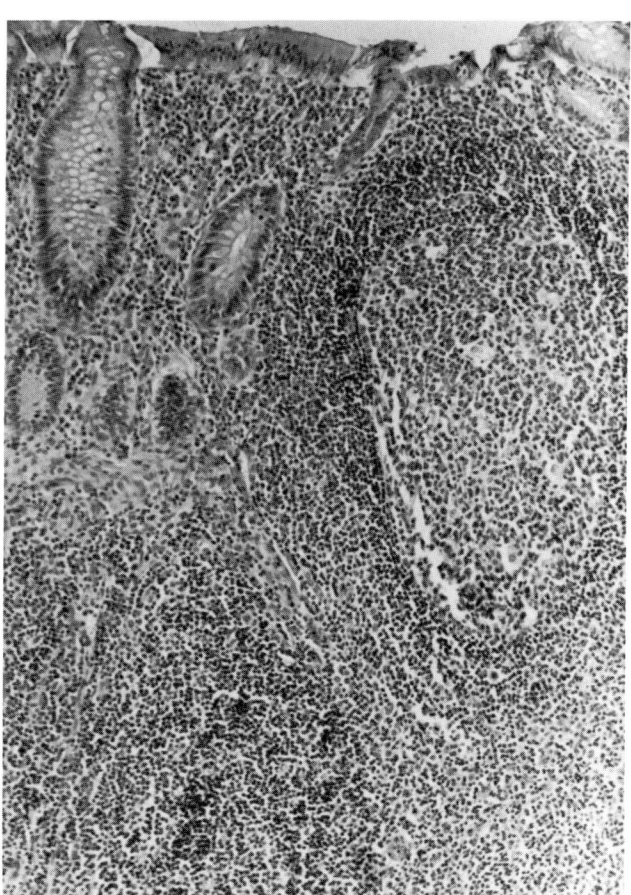

FIGURE 33–2. Normal vermiform appendix of an adult at the site of a lymphoid follicle. The epithelium lining the crypts of Lieberkühn has prominent goblet cells. Lymphocytes and plasma cells are abundant in the lamina propria, with follicle and germinal center formation. (× 125)

and mixed with the mucus-secreting cells are scattered enterochromaffin (Kulchitsky type) and Paneth cells.[5,6] Fewer of these cells are also found in the upper parts of the glands.[5]

Some of the endocrine cells are argentaffin cells and secrete 5-hydroxytryptamine (5-HT), whereas others are argyrophils.[3] These cells can further be demonstrated by immunohistochemical techniques for neuron-specific enolase (NSE) and serotonin and by electron microscopy.[6] Enterochromaffin cells can be found in the lamina propria as well; some of these appear to be associated with the large cells that resemble neurons in the submucosal Meissner's plexus, confirming Masson's original findings. These complexes, termed enterochromaffin–nerve fiber complexes, may play a modulatory role between the epithelium and the deeper enteric nervous system mediated by serotonin neurotransmission under physiologic conditions. Abnormal release of serotonin may cause acute inflammation, or pain, or both. This raises the question of whether the pain in the clinically inflamed but histologically normal appendix is secondary to the abnormally secreted serotonin.

Like the intestine, the appendix is composed of lamina propria, which comprises loosely arranged fibrous connective tissue where histiocytes and lymphocytes are easily seen. The lymphocytes begin to appear as lymphoid nodules during fetal life. The percentage of the lymphoid tissue in the appendix is the highest during the first decade of life and steadily decreases thereafter.[7] The lymphoid follicles in a normal appendix typically show germinal centers, each of which is surrounded by a mantle of small lymphocytes (see Figure 33–2). Both the germinal center and the mantle are composed of B cells and some admixed T cells, almost exclusively T-helper cells. Immediately above the follicle is a zone of mixed cells (small and large lymphocytes), most of which are B cells. The overlying epithelium shows intraepithelial B- and T-suppressor lymphocytes. On either side of the follicle are diffuse small lymphocytes, macrophages, and plasma cells, the latter being the most prominent component. Beneath the follicle is the T-cell area, where the ratio of helper to suppressor T cells is approximately 8:1.[8]

The muscularis mucosae is poorly developed. The submucosa is composed of fibrous connective tissue in which blood vessels, nerves, and varying amounts of adipose tissue are present.[5] The submucosa is surrounded by a circular coat and a longitudinal coat of smooth muscle, which is in turn covered by a serosa. Few ganglion cells are found in the submucosa. Other ganglion cells are haphazardly distributed in the muscle.[9]

DEVELOPMENTAL ABNORMALITIES

Congenital Absence (Agenesis)

Agenesis of the appendix is rare, the frequency being 0.006%.[10] It has been reported to be associated with other congenital anomalies caused by thalidomide.[11] Hypoplasia of the appendix is more common than agenesis.[12]

Duplication

Duplication of the appendix is rare and is commonly associated with duplication of the cecum,[3] but may also occur with a normal cecum.[13] Three different types of duplication may occur with a normal cecum: (1) "double-barreled" appendix, characterized by two separate lumens each lined by mucosa and separated by submucosa but confined by one muscular wall; (2) completely separate but symmetric appendices, one on either side of the ileocecal valve; this type occurs only in infants with multiple congenital abnormalities; and (3) one normal appendix and one rudimentary appendix.

Diverticula

Diverticula of the appendix are found in 0.004% to 2.8% of surgical and autopsy material[14] and are more often acquired than congenital. The congenital diverticula are distinguished from their acquired counterparts by the presence of muscular coats and the absence of inflammation. Multiple congenital diverticula have also been described.[15]

Malposition

Malposition of the appendix occurs occasionally with a maldescent of the cecum, resulting in a subhepatic cecum and appendix. Malpositions of appendix may also occur as consequences of different types of congenital malrotation of the intestine.[2] Malpositions may create diagnostic difficulty should acute appendicitis develop.

Miscellaneous Conditions

A unique case of appendix helicus was described in a 13-month-old child born with a lumbosacral meningomyelocele and a neurogenic bladder.[16] The appendix helicus was found incidentally during cystectomy. Hirschsprung's disease (aganglionosis) may rarely involve the appendix with dilatation and even perforation.[17] In neurofibromatosis (von Recklinghausen's disease), the appendix may rarely be involved, with associated inflammation.[18] Ectopic gastric and esophageal mucosa[19,20] and aberrant pancreas[10] have also been reported.

INFLAMMATORY DISORDERS

Acute Appendicitis

Acute appendicitis, the acute inflammation of the vermiform appendix, is the most common acute surgical condition of the abdomen.[1] It has been generally accepted that Fitz was the first investigator to recognize acute appendicitis as a distinct clinicopathologic entity in 1886.[21,22]

Acute appendicitis is far more common in western than eastern countries.[3,23] The annual incidence is approximately 1.5 in the male and 1.9 in the female per 1000 persons between the ages of 17 and 64.[24] The rate, however, has been noted to be declining after World War II.[4] It occurs in all ages but is rare before 2 years of age. The peak incidence is in the second and third decades, teenagers being the most frequently affected. The incidence begins to decline after the age of 40.[24] The male-to-female ratio is 1:1 before puberty, 2:1 between 15 and 25 years of age, and 1:1 after 25 years of age.[1]

Etiology and Pathogenesis

The etiology and pathogenesis of acute appendicitis are not entirely clear. However, observations and studies of the surgically removed appendix and experimental approaches have revealed contributory factors, among which obstruction, infection, and mucosal damage are the most important.

In their elegant study in dogs, Wangensteen and Bowers demonstrated that complete obstruction of the cecal appendage (an equivalent to the appendix in humans) without prewashing the content resulted in acute appendicitis in six of eight dogs 6 to 24 hours after the ligation; the remaining two dogs were normal.[25] Complete obstruction of washed cecal appendage failed to produce appendicitis. If feces were introduced into the prewashed cecal appendage, which had been ligated for 5 days, two of three animals developed appendicitis. For correlation with their experimental results, they also carefully observed 91 human appendices surgically removed for acute appendicitis. Evidence of obstruction, usually by fecaliths, was found in more than 70% of the specimens. The role of obstruction in the development of appendicitis was further confirmed in other experimental studies in rabbits,[26] apes, and humans.[27]

In a study of patients who had colonic cancer, the appendices were exteriorized and obstruction was created by ligating the base of the appendix. The intraluminal pressure increased up to 126 cm of water in the majority of appendices 7 to 49 hours after the initial obstruction. Histologic examination revealed a spectrum of changes, including mucosal appendicitis, diffuse appendicitis, and healing appendicitis. However, the unobstructed appendix that served as a control also demonstrated acute appendicitis.

Other factors may also be relevant and important in the development of appendicitis. Luminal pressure was increased after complete obstruction of the appendix was created.[25–27] The increased pressure would then interfere with circulation, resulting in accumulation of fluid in the lumen and a greater increase in pressure, creating a vicious circle. The deprivation of oxygen from the reduced blood flow would result in tissue damage, thus favoring the invasion of bacteria.[26]

Examination of the surgically removed appendix does not always reveal a fecalith or other evidence of obstruction. The incidence of fecaliths or other demonstrable obstruction in the surgically removed appendix ranges from 7% to 34%.[28,29] In a number of cases that appear to be due to a nonobstructive condition, lymphoid hyperplasia may play a role, especially in young patients in whom the lymphoid tissue is prominent and appendicitis is common.[4] Lymphoid hyperplasia of the appendix may be seen with measles,[4] Coxsackie B virus infection,[30,31] and mononucleosis. However, the incidence of appendicitis is not known to be increased in these conditions. Further complicating the interpretation is the fact that lymphoid hyperplasia may be secondary to inflammation of the appendix. The role of lymphoid hyperplasia in causing obstruction is therefore debatable or at best may only be a factor in a small number of cases of appendicitis. Butler found neither total obstruction of the appendiceal lumen by lymphoid hyperplasia nor distal dilatation in the specimens of acute appendicitis.[29]

Mucosal ulceration is definitely an important pathogenic factor, as it is found in 48 of 64 surgical specimens of acute appendicitis.[32] Butler[29] and Sisson et al.[32] postulated that appendicitis begins as mucosal ulceration, followed by invasion by bacteria. Because obstruction in their specimens was infrequent, these authors further suggested that obstruction was not fundamental in the development of appendicitis. However, in a significant number of specimens of acute appendicitis, fecaliths are found to occupy the lumens. Acute appendicitis does result from obstruction both in experimental animals and in man.[26,27] Perhaps it is time to investigate the possible role of obstruction in the development of mucosal ulcerations. The obstruction by a fecalith in man may be similar to that created by ligature of the base of appendix in that it might result in ischemia, which in turn would cause ischemic damage of the appendiceal mucosa. In some specimens, the changes in ulcerated and inflamed mucosa appear to be similar to the ischemic changes of, for instance, the large intestine. The fecaliths, which are hard and not entirely smooth,[25] may damage the mucosa mechanically.

Based on the circumstantial evidence of lymphoid hyperplasia and inflammatory involvement of the lymphoid follicles in acute appendicitis, Butler raised another intriguing speculation that immune complex injury or delayed hypersensitivity might play a role in pathogenesis.[29] There is conflicting evidence that diet may play a role in the pathogenesis of acute appendicitis. Studies have shown that Europeans who live in Africa and consume a low-fiber diet have a higher incidence of appendicitis than do native Africans who eat a high-fiber diet.[23] In contrast, a decreased incidence of appendicitis in Sweden occurred during a period in which fiber content of the average diet was reduced.[33]

From these studies, it is clear that the etiology and pathogenesis of appendicitis are mutlifactorial. Because the bacterial flora in the lumen of normal appendix is essentially the same as that in inflamed appendix, bacterial invasion into the appendiceal lymphoid tissue and other structures must be accomplished through the

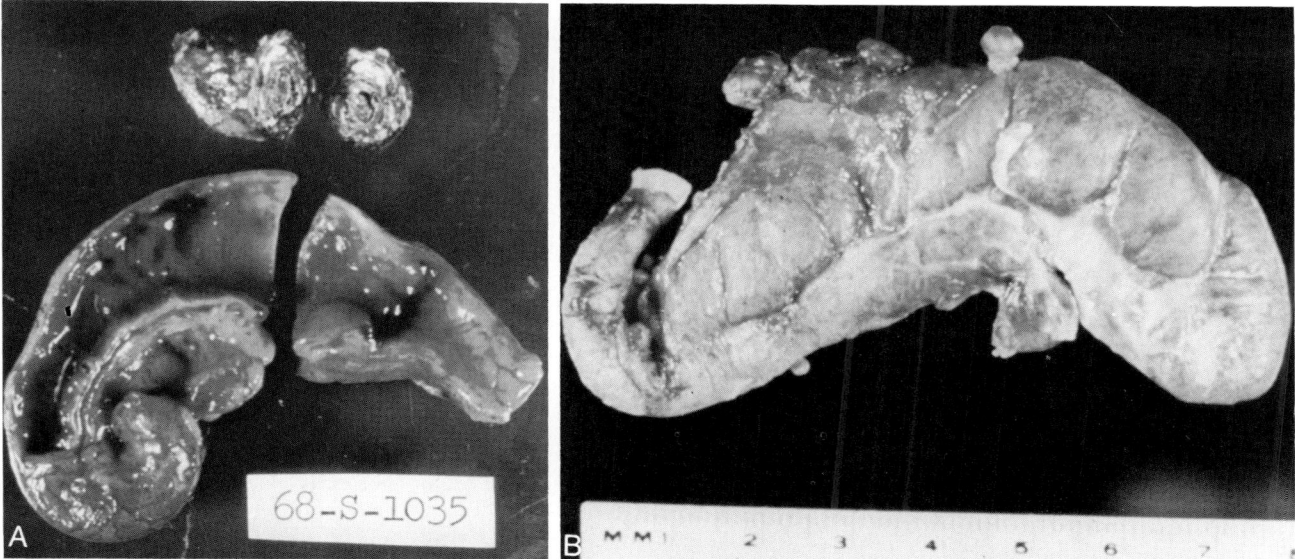

FIGURE 33–3. Acute purulent appendicitis. *A*, Bisected appendix, showing hemorrhage and pus in the dilated lumen. A laminated fecalith (top) is present in the appendiceal lumen. *B*, The serosa of an appendix with acute appendicitis is covered by purulent exudate. (Courtesy of Dr. Theodore Krouse, Episcopal Hospital, Philadelphia, Pa.)

damaged mucosa, as advocated by Sisson et al.[32] and Butler,[29] lest appendicitis be more common than it is. The mucosal damage may be the result of viral infection,[32] immune complex injury or delayed hypersensitivity,[29] mechanical injury by a fecalith, or ischemia due to obstruction. There remains a minority of cases in which the causative organism may itself be invasive without the assistance of pre-existent mucosal damage.

Pathology

The morphologic appearance of acute appendicitis is basically that of acute inflammation with variations that depend on the severity and duration of the inflammatory process.

The appendix is grossly congested and swollen and has an increased diameter. The lumen is dilated in many specimens and may contain pus, or a fecalith, or both (Figure 33–3A). The serosa is covered by fibrin, fibrinopurulent exudate, or pus (Figure 33–3B). The presence of pus does not necessarily indicate perforation because suppuration may dissect the entire appendiceal wall into the periappendiceal tissue without a perforation.[4] The mucosa is hyperemic (see Figure 33–3A) and may show necrosis or ulceration. In other instances, the lymphoid tissue may be so prominent that it forms soft, pink to tan, nodular protrusions into the appendiceal lumens. Microscopic examination shows characteristic features of acute appendicitis, including mucosal ulceration (Figure 33–4) and infiltration by polymorphonuclear leukocytes (PMNs), eosinophils, plasma cells, and histiocytes throughout all appendiceal layers and frequently into the serosa. PMNs are seen also in the prominent lymphoid follicles. The epithelial cells are likewise infiltrated by PMNs, many of which may be found spilling out into the lumen. The appendiceal wall is edematous.

In less severe cases, the gross appearance may reveal congestion on the serosa and may even be normal. The inflammatory infiltrate of PMNs is seen only in the

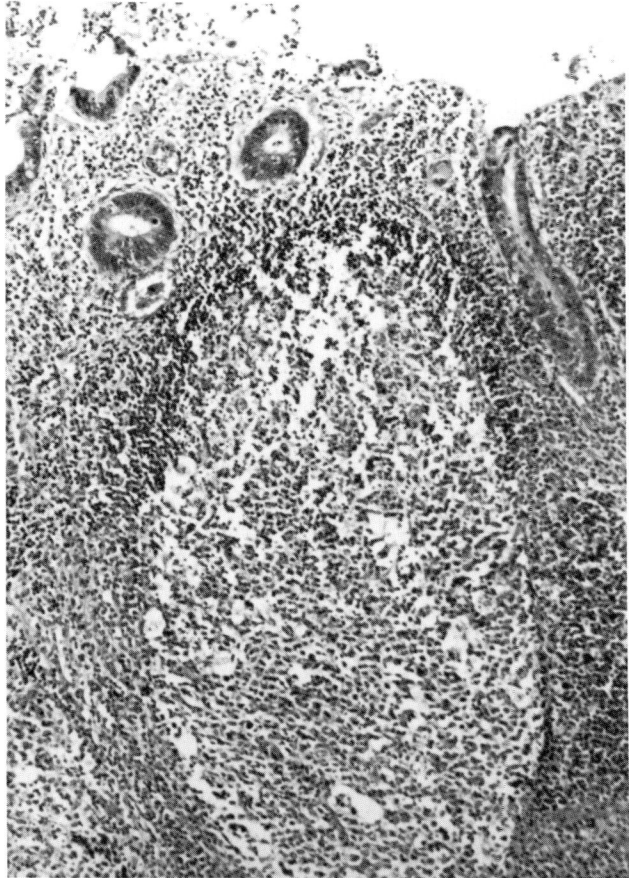

FIGURE 33–4. The mucosa is denuded in this case of acute appendicitis. The germinal center is enlarged. ($\times$ 125)

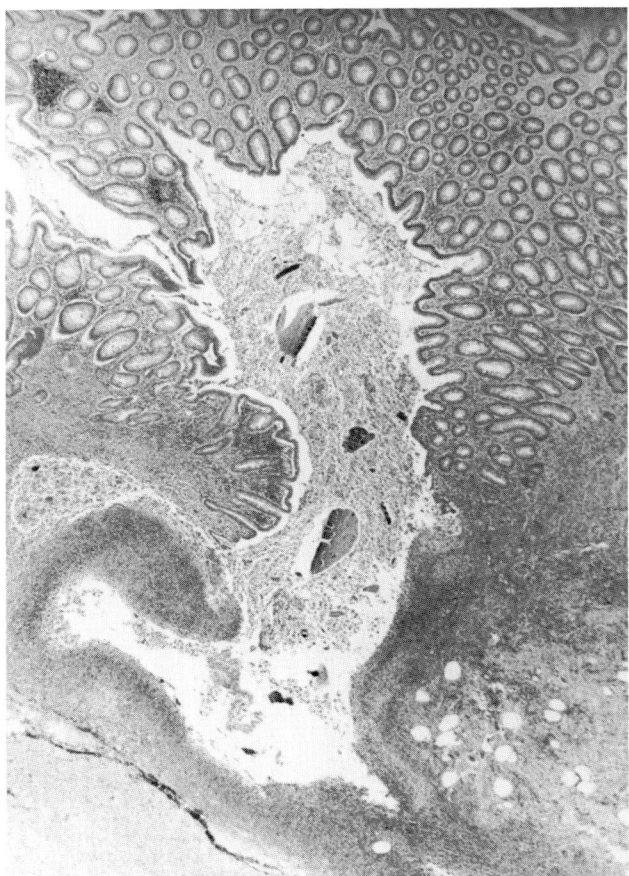

FIGURE 33–5. Acute gangrenous appendicitis, displaying complete destruction of part of the appendiceal wall at bottom, where only a layer of necrotic tissue is present. (× 25)

mucosa, lamina propria, and submucosa. When this feature is associated with mucosal ulcerations, it is diagnostic of acute appendicitis. The absence of ulceration would lead to a controversial interpretation between an early acute appendicitis and the result of surgical manipulation, especially in patients with a clinical presentation of acute appendicitis.

In the more advanced stage, the inflammatory process involves the full thickness of the appendiceal wall with partial necrosis or infarction of the wall where perforation may take place (Figure 33–5). The tissue adjacent to the perforation is dull gray and covered by pus. An abscess may be formed in the periappendiceal tissue with some degree of organization characterized by granulation and fibrous tissue, resulting in a periappendiceal mass with adhesion to the adjacent structures. This must be distinguished from a tumor or conditions other than appendicitis, such as endometriosis or walled-off, perforated diverticulitis of the adjacent bowel. Rarely the pus may extend along the paracolic gutter or may spread to cause generalized peritonitis, subhepatic abscess, or pyelophlebitis.[4] A fistulae rarely may be formed between the inflamed appendix and the adjacent organs.[4,10]

Occasionally, acute appendicitis occurs in the appendix with fibrosis of the lumen. Fibrous obliteration may have a protective mechanism.[29]

Correlation of Clinical Diagnosis and Pathologic Observation

Although the acceptable frequency of errors varies from institution to institution, it is well established that a certain percentage of appendices removed from patients with the clinical presentation of acute appendicitis would show no inflammation on microscopic examination. This is probably best illustrated by the scenario created by King Edward VII's acute appendicitis.[34]

In 1902, King Edward VII of England developed violent abdominal pain, nausea, vomiting, fast pulse, fever, and restlessness, which lasted for almost 2 weeks. That was 3 days before his coronation, when his doctors decided that they should not wait any longer. They successfully removed a well-encapsulated abscess by which the appendix was totally destroyed. King Edward VII's illness made appendicitis (perityphlitis) a fashionable disease and triggered arguments about when to operate. This decision remains a difficult one even today because an early and accurate diagnosis of an appendicitis is still a challenge to the surgeons. The highest rate of perforation (29%) had the best diagnostic accuracy (89%), and the lowest rate of perforation rate (14%) the worst accuracy (67%).[22] Three percent of patients with perforated appendicitis died of peritonitis, intra-abdominal abscesses, or gram-negative septicemia. The mortality rate in nonperforated appendicitis is about 0.1%.[1] Morbidity in perforated appendicitis is also more common than in nonperforated appendicitis. To minimize the mortality and morbidity, it is inevitable that some of the appendices removed from patients with clinical symptoms and signs are histologically normal. What is a standard rate of error is not agreed upon. Malt considers that a 23% error rate might be reasonable.[22]

Chronic Appendicitis

The existence of chronic appendicitis still is a subject of controversy.[4] Conceptually, an acute stage of appendicitis may subside and become a chronic stage, among other possible consequences. The histologic criteria should include the infiltration of both lymphocytes and plasma cells in the muscular coat and serosa.[3] Simple fibrosis obliterating the lumen may not necessarily result from an inflammatory process and may be a physiologic process and therefore not an acceptable diagnostic criterion for chronic appendicitis. Strictly following these morphologic criteria, one must find that true cases of chronic appendicitis are rare. Granulation tissue and fibrosis associated with a chronic inflammatory infiltrate are regarded as manifestations of organizing acute appendicitis.[4]

Ulcerative Colitis and Crohn's Disease

Approximately one half of the appendix removed from patients with ulcerative colitis involving the right colon also have involvement of the appendix.[35] The in-

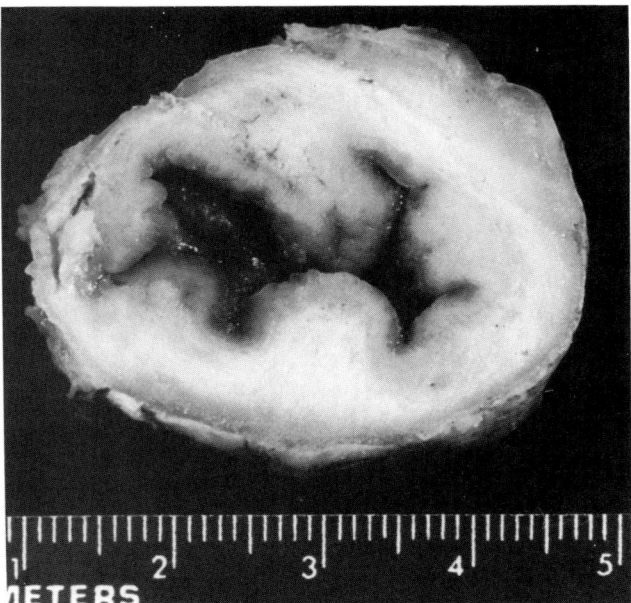

FIGURE 33–6. Cross section of an appendix involved by Crohn's disease. The entire organ is enlarged, and the appendiceal wall is markedly thickened. The patient, a 35-year-old woman, presented with symptoms of acute appendicitis. (Courtesy of Dr. Susan Yaron, Metropolitan Hospital, Springfield, Pa.)

volvement of the appendix is almost always part of a generalized colitis. The mucosa shows goblet cell depletion, crypt abscesses and, in some cases, mucosal ulceration associated with an inflammatory infiltrate, mostly of PMNs. The submucosa may also be infiltrated by inflammatory cells. The number of lymphocytes and plasma cells is increased in the lamina propria. These features are essentially similar to those of ulcerative colitis but may be difficult to distinguish from those of acute appendicitis.[36] The histologic features may change depending on the phase of the disease.[35]

Crohn's disease (transmural enteritis) can involve the appendix in approximately 25% of patients with Crohn's disease of the terminal ileum and in more than 50% of patients with colonic Crohn's disease.[37] Crohn's disease that is limited to the appendix is rare; over 60 cases have been reported since 1953.[37] Patients with Crohn's disease limited to the appendix present with pain in the right lower quadrant, frequently associated with a mass.[37] It can be cured by appendectomy and only rarely recurs.[38]

Grossly, the appendix is enlarged with a diameter of 1.5 cm or greater (Figure 33–6). The microscopic features are basically similar to those of Crohn's disease elsewhere, including mucosal ulceration with PMN infiltration, transmural thickening by fibrosis, transmural chronic inflammation, noncaseating granulomas and giant cells, and superficial mucosal and submucosal fissures (Figure 33–7). When granulomas are present and Crohn's disease is suspected, a differential diagnosis of yersiniosis, sarcoidosis, tuberculosis, and other granulomatous diseases should be considered.[38] See Chapter 27 for further details.

Acquired Diverticulum and Diverticulitis

Acquired diverticula of the appendix are more common than congenital ones. Careful examination of the surgically removed appendix reveals an incidence of approximately 1%.[39] They are usually small (0.2 to 0.5 mm) and found along both the mesenteric and the antimesenteric borders, as single or multiple beaded lesions.[40,41] The diverticula may be the site of inflammation, which may perforate or spread to cause appendicitis.[4] Most diverticula are incidental findings, but they commonly show inflammation without involving the adjacent appendix. Their walls are composed of appendiceal mucosa and submucosa, including muscularis mucosae but not muscularis propria (which the congenital diverticula do include), probably because of the protrusion of these structures through the appendiceal wall, which results from increased luminal pressure.[42] Gray and Wackym have identified diverticula in association with appendicitis, carcinoids, and retention mucoceles.[4] When symptomatic, diverticular disease may be similar clinically to acute appendicitis.[39]

Infections

Bacterial Infections

When cultured, most of the surgically removed, acutely inflamed appendices demonstrated a variety of bacteria,[43] without any responsible species in particular. There remain a few inflammatory conditions for which a specific agent may be solely responsible.

Campylobacter-Associated Appendicitis

Recently, *Campylobacter* has been found to be responsible for a spectrum of disorders of the digestive system, including the appendix.[44] The patients are young, usually children, who often present with an appendicitis-like clinical picture. The appendices are grossly normal, but the mesenteric lymph nodes are sometimes found to be swollen at operation.

The histologic abnormalities are similar to those of *Campylobacter* colitis. The mucosa is infiltrated by PMNs or eosinophils, or both, with degenerative changes or ulceration. Crypt abscesses may be present, and there is subepithelial edema. Sometimes the infiltration of histiocytes and lymphocytes in the mucosa gives rise to a granulomatous appearance. The submucosa, muscular layers, and serosa are not involved. *Campylobacter fetus* subspecies *jejuni* can be found in the appendiceal lumen with the use of the Warthin-Starry stain, indirect immunofluorescence, immunoperoxidase stains, and transmission electron microscopy.[44] *Campylobacter* organisms are curved rods.

Tuberculosis

Tuberculosis of the appendix more often presents as part of a gastrointestinal or pulmonary infection than an isolated lesion.[45] The rarity of an isolated lesion is reflected by the finding of only four cases in 4784 appendectomies.[46] The patients usually present with

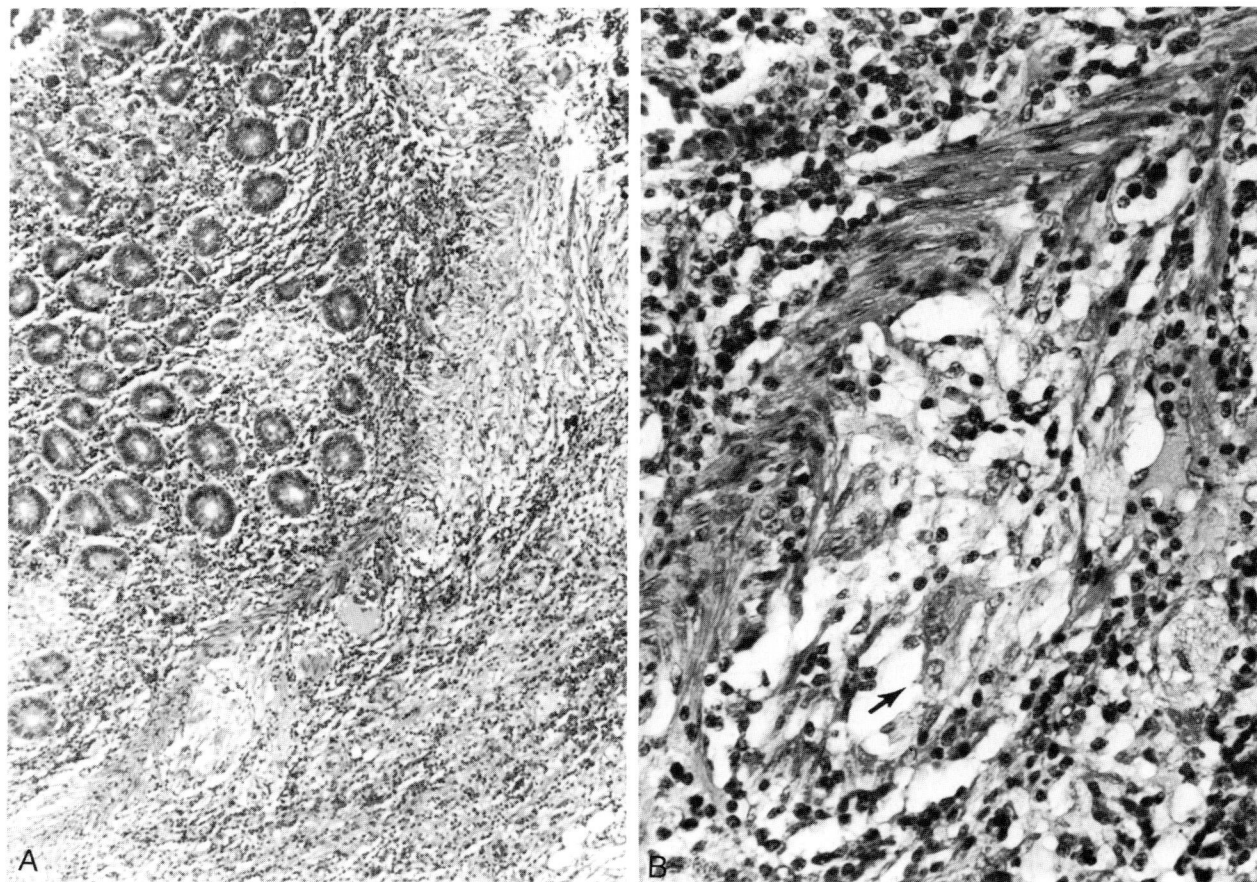

FIGURE 33-7. A, Microphotograph of Figure 33-6, demonstrating a mucosal and submucosal inflammation, where a noncaseous granuloma is observed. B, Scattered giant cells (arrow) are present in the granuloma. (× 125) (Courtesy of Dr. Susan Yaron, Metropolitan Hospital, Springfield, Pa.)

symptoms of acute appendicitis. The tuberculous appendix is grossly thickened. Its microscopic appearance is characterized by granulomas, which usually contain a necrotic center surrounded by epithelioid cells, lymphocytes, and histocytes. Despite characteristic features, the diagnosis of tuberculosis must be confirmed by either acid-fast stain, or culture, or both.[47] In the isolated tuberculosis of the appendix, as in that of the gastrointestinal tract, the causative organism is likely *Mycobaterium bovis*.

Yersiniosis

Yersinia infection (yersiniosis) is caused by *Yersinia pseudotuberculosis* or *Yersinia enterocolitica* in man. There have been reports of outbreaks of yersiniosis in the United States and other countries.[48] The patients are most commonly children and young adults who present with abdominal pain and fever. The organisms may be identified in culture and yield positive titers, both of which are important for confirming the diagnosis. Although systemic yersiniosis is usually fatal, enteric yersiniosis is a self-limited illness.[49] Because its clinical picture is often indistinguishable from that of acute appendicitis, many patients undergo an appendectomy.

Y. pseudotuberculosis and *Y. enterocolitica* are different but closely related, pleomorphic, gram-negative coccobacilli. The morphologic features produced by both organisms are similar.[49] The mesenteric lymph nodes are almost always enlarged and frequently matted, are fleshy and reddish gray, and have yellowish microabscesses. The appendices are either normal or congested. Microscopically, the appendiceal lymphoid follicles are enlarged with prominent reactive germinal centers in which granulomas may be present. The mucosa is infiltrated by eosinophils. The submucosal granulomas may be associated with ulceration of the overlying epithelium. Some of the granulomas have central necrosis, sometimes in the form of microabscess. Periappendiceal inflammation and fibrosis may be marked. Similar granulomas and lymphoid hyperplasia are found in the lymph nodes and other involved parts of the intestine. The differential diagnosis includes Crohn's disease, tuberculosis, sarcoidosis, tularemia, actinomycosis, ambiasis, and schistosomiasis.[49]

Spirochetosis

Spirochetes have been found in up to 12.3% of histologically normal appendices and in 2.6% to 4.4% of appendices showing inflammation.[50] These microorganisms are morphologically similar to *Brachyspira aalborgi*, a spirochete isolated from colorectal biopsy specimens of patients with intestinal symptoms. They measure 2.0 to 4.8 μm long and 0.2 μm wide and are one of the normal flora in the intestine and appendix. Why they flourish and colonize the epithelium is still unknown. Their colonization could account for the appendicitis symptoms in patients with histologically normal appendices.[50]

Actinomycosis

Actinomyces israelii can be found in the oral cavity and may survive the acidic content of the stomach to reach the lower gastrointestinal tract, including the appendix.[3] Infrequently these organisms may invade the appendiceal mucosa, causing mixed inflammation with symptoms indistinguishable from those of acute appendicitis. Colonies are formed by gram-negative filamentous forms, which can be observed grossly as yellow, friable "sulfur granules."[4] Polymorphonuclear leukocytes are found surrounding these granules and in the adjacent tissue, where granulation tissue and other types of inflammatory infiltrate are also present. Actinomycosis of the appendix may potentially cause either a fistulous tract with the adjacent organs or skin or a "metastatic abscess" to the liver.[3]

Viral Infections

Viral infection of the appendix is a difficult diagnosis to establish and may be reflected by lymphoid hyperplasia.

Measles

Measles is a viral infection in which lymphoid hyperplasia as well as multinucleated, Warthin-Finkeldey giant cells may be observed in the appendix. These changes are similar to those of the tonsils and adenoids and may precede the clinical presentation of measles.[51] The involvement of the appendix may produce a clinical picture indistinguishable from that of acute appendicitis.

Adenovirus

Adenovirus inclusions have been found in the appendices of young children presenting with ileal or ileocecal intussusception.[52,53] Grossly the appendix is normal. With light microscopy, the epithelial cells display budlike proliferation and the adjacent surface epithelium is destroyed.[53] Eosinophilic inclusions are found in the surface epithelial cells, usually intranuclearly and surrounded by a halo;[53] they may also be intracytoplasmic, as demonstrated by electron microscopy.[52] The submucosal lymphoid follicles show hyperplastic changes.

Mononucleosis

Mononucleosis is caused by the Epstein-Barr virus. All lymphoid tissues may be affected. When involved, the appendix shows lymphoid hyperplasia and marked infiltration of large immunoblasts (some of which resemble Reed-Sternberg cells) in the interfollicular zones, expanding the lamina propria.[54]

Cytomegalovirus

Cytomegalovirus inclusions have been reported in the appendix of a homosexual man who was not immunosuppressed.[55] The acutely inflamed and ruptured appendix was associated with a periappendiceal abscess. The inclusions were found in the histiocytes and endothelial cells but not in the epithelial cells.

Parasitic Infections

Parasites are occasionally found in the appendices with or without accompanying inflammation. It is not entirely clear why some parasites become invasive and cause tissue damage that is often complicated by bacterial infection. Many types of parasites have been observed in the appendix (Table 33-1).[10]

Oxyuris vermicularis (pinworm) is the parasite most commonly found in the appendix, usually without associated tissue changes. Ashburn reported an incidence of 3% in the United States.[62] Gray and Wackym observed a declining incidence.[4] At their hospital, several instances were found per year in the 1950s, but not a single case in the past 4 years. A survey of the surgical specimens at the Temple University Hospital fails to reveal any oxyuriasis in the 12-year period from 1974 through 1986.

Both the worm and the eggs may be found in the appendiceal lumen (Figure 33-8). The appendix itself usually shows no tissue reaction. Less frequently, the parasite may be associated with an inflammatory picture indistinguishable from that of acute appendicitis or may be seen in the mucosa, surrounded by numerous eosinophils.[63]

Table 33-1 PARASITIC INFECTIONS OF THE VERMIFORM APPENDIX AND ASSOCIATED PATHOLOGIC CHANGES

Type of Parasite	Associated Appendiceal Changes
Oxyuris (Enterobius) vermicularis	No significant changes (majority); appendicitis, abscess
Ascaris lumbricoides[56]	No significant changes; acute appendicitis with or without perforation
Entamoeba histolytica[57]	Changes similar to those of intestine, mimicking those of appendicitis
Balantidium coli[58]	No significant changes; mucosal ulceration, appendicitis
Schistosoma mansoni[4]	Granulomatous inflammation
Trichuris trichiura[59]	Not mentioned
Trichuris vulpis[59]	Eosinophilic appendicitis
Strongyloides stercoralis[60]	Eosinophilic appendicitis with eosinophilic granuloma
Rictularia[61]	No significant changes

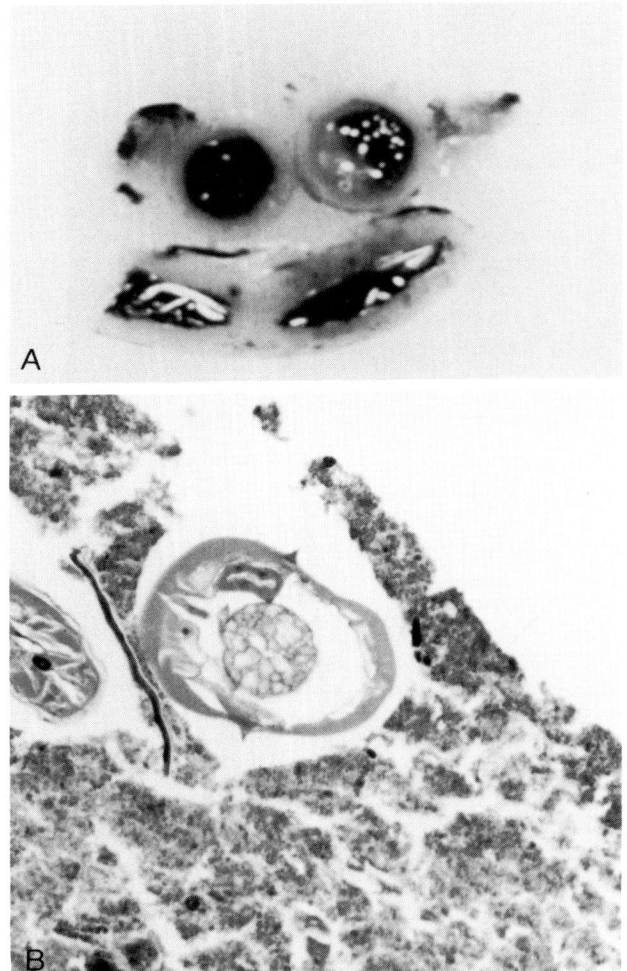

FIGURE 33–8. *A,* Adult pin worms in the lumen of the cross and longitudinal sections of an appendix that was embedded in paraffin. (Courtesy of Dr. Theodore Krouse, Episcopal Hospital, Philadelphia, Pa.) *B,* Sections of the adult female worms sowing ala on the sides, intestine, and uterus. ($\times 500$)

Fungal Infections

Histoplasma encapsulatum was found in 8.8% of 71,000 appendices.[10] Rare fungal infections such as coccidioidomycosis, South American blastomycosis, sporotrichosis, cryptococcosis, and geotrichosis have also been reported.[10]

EPITHELIAL HYPERPLASIA

Epithelial (or mucosal) hyperplasia is a benign proliferation of the appendiceal mucosa histologically and cytologically indistinguishable from hyperplastic polyps of the large intestine.[64,65] It is almost always found in appendices that are removed incidentally. Appelman was able to collect 59 published cases since 1956.[66] Patients range from adolescents to the elderly, but most are over 40 years of age. Women are more often affected than men, which is obviously related to the high frequency of "incidental appendectomy" in women.

The gross appearance is often not described or is described as normal. In a few cases, the appendices show a slightly dilated lumen with focal or diffuse thickening of the mucosa. Small papillary excrescences could be observed.[64] On microscopic examination, the luminal surface of hyperplastic focus is serrated or finely papillary. Cross sections of the glands show folded epithelium, which creates a stellate pattern. The columnar cells and goblet cells are interspersed in an orderly fashion. Paneth cells are found in more than 50% of cases, and argentaffin cells are found in all cases.[65] These changes are to be distinguished from those of villous adenomas of the appendix.[66]

Epithelial hyperplasia of the appendix may be found alone or associated with acute inflammation, mucocele, villous papilloma of the appendix, adenomatous and hyperplastic polyps and adenocarcinoma of the colon, and mucinous cystadenoma of the ovary.[64,65] This lesion is regarded as nonneoplastic by Qizilbash and probably represents a response to mucosal injury.[65]

NEOPLASIA

Though similar to the colonic epithelium, the appendiceal epithelium differs in that it rarely gives rise to neoplasms, both benign and malignant. Comparison between the two would inevitably raise a speculation that this difference is probably attributed to the smaller amount of appendiceal epithelium and the manner in which they are exposed to the environmental factors within their lumens. The small lumen of the appendix may account for the rare polypoid adenomas and the relatively common cystadenomas and cystadenocarcinomas. The etiology and tumorigenesis are unknown.

Adenoma and Cystadenoma

Adenomas of the appendix are benign epithelial tumors, which may rarely present as polyps or more frequently as diffuse lesions that involve the entire circumference of the organ. They are less common than their malignant counterparts. When the appendix is cystic due to large production of mucus by the neoplastic cells, the adenomas are regarded as cystadenomas.

Adenomas occur in patients in the second through ninth decades, with the peak in the seventh.[66] Clinically adenomas either are asymptomatic, especially when the adenomas are small polypoid lesions measuring less than 1 cm,[64] or present with symptoms and signs indistinguishable from those of acute appendicitis, or with a palpable abdominal mass. Plain abdominal roentgenography may demonstrate partial calcification of the wall of the cystadenoma.[64]

The appendix appears either normal or diffusely to cystically enlarged.[64,67,68] The polypoid lesions are small. The diffuse adenomas display thickened mucosa, which is soft and pink and protrudes into the

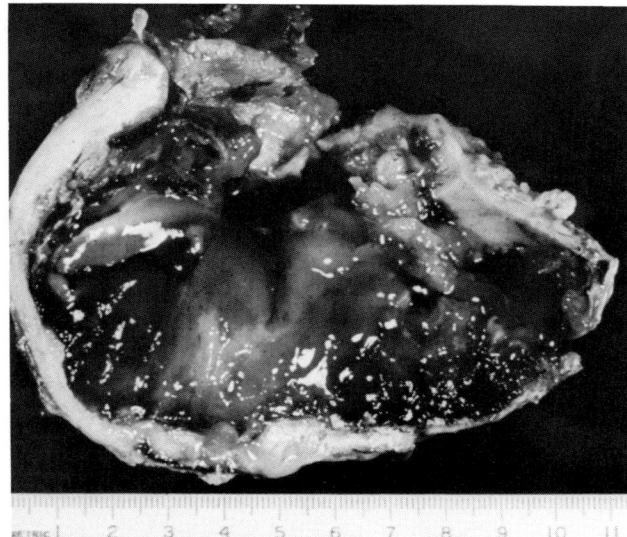

FIGURE 33–9. Cystadenoma of the appendix, characterized by glistening, nodular tumor tissue and gelantinous mucus admixed with blood in the cystic cavity. The wall is composed partly of the appendiceal muscular coat and partly of fibrous tissue. (Courtesy of Dr. Theodore Krouse, Episcopal Hospital, Philadelphia, Pa.)

lumen with many folds. The cystadenomas show a large amount of gelatinous and glistening mucus upon sectioning (Figure 33–9). The inner surface may show solid areas. There may be areas of fibrosis that disrupt the integrity of the wall, suggesting rupture. The mucus escapes from the ruptured site and into the adjacent tissue, creating the mass phenomenon pseudomyxoma peritonei.

Microscopically some appendiceal adenomas are composed of irregular glandular elements similar to those of tubular adenoma and characterized by increased immature columnar cells with reduction of goblet cells (or goblet cell depletion), hyperchromatism, and increased mitotic activity. Both the polypoid and the diffuse types, however, are often villous and display long, slender, branching papillary projections composed of tall columnar cells and fibrovascular cores (Figure 33–10). The columnar cells have basally located nuclei and often show eosinophilic or vacuolated cytoplasm. On cross section of the diffuse villous adenoma, the entire circumference is lined by these villous structures. In cystadenomas, the neoplastic epithelium shows similar changes; but these projections may be pushed toward the wall or even flattened to a thickness of one cell. Mucosal ulceration is commonly present. Argentaffin cells are found in 11 of 18 cystadenomas.[67] Fragments of the neoplastic mucosa may or may not be observed in the pools of mucus in ruptured cystadenomas with fibrosis and acute and chronic inflammation. When this is the case, the adenomas may be difficult or even impossible to be distinguished from an invasive carcinoma. Occasionally, small foci of well-differentiated adenocarcinoma may appear to arise from an otherwise benign adenoma.[69] It has been observed that some of the cystadenomas are associated with ovarian cystadenomas or colonic adenocarcinoma.

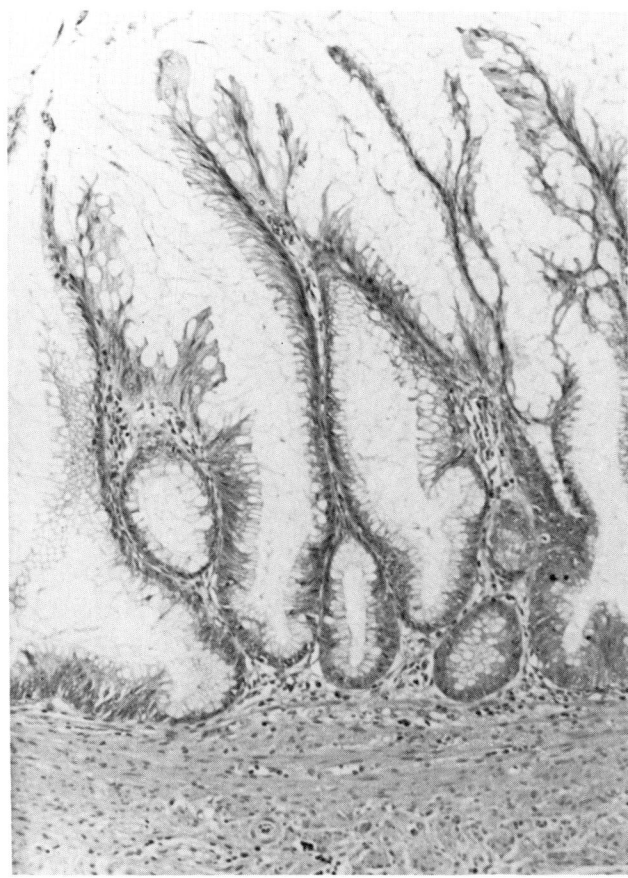

FIGURE 33–10. Tall villi lined by tall columnar and goblet cells with fibrovascular cores, characteristic of villous adenoma. (H&E, × 250)

Appendiceal cystadenomas have been treated either by simple appendectomy or right hemicolectomy. Follow-up study has shown good outcome even in the patients who had extension of mucus into the extra-appendiceal spaces.[64]

Adenocarcinoma and Cystadenocarcinoma

Adenocarcinoma and cystadenocarcinoma are two different forms of the same disease, namely, malignant epithelial tumor. The ratio of noncystic to cystic adenocarcinoma is approximately 3:1.[66] The age incidence is similar to that of appendiceal adenomas.[66] Males have a slight predominance. The rarity of appendiceal adenocarcinoma is reflected by the finding of only 57 cases out of 71,000 appendices (0.08%).[10]

Clinically patients may present with symptoms of acute appendicitis, palpable masses, or intestinal obstruction. At operation, it is not unusual for the surgeon to find an inflammatory mass. A suspicious surgeon might request an examination by a pathologist, who in turn diagnoses carcinoma on a frozen section. Occasionally, primary appendiceal adenocarcinoma

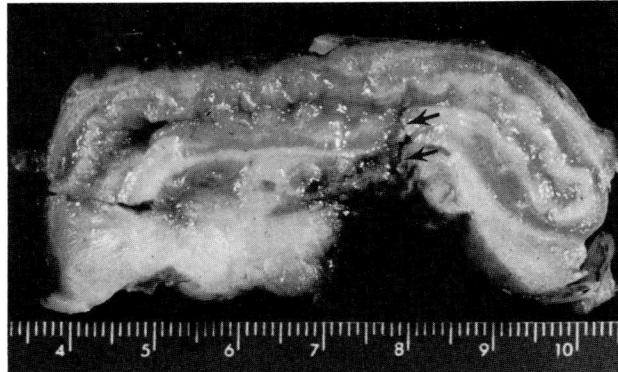

FIGURE 33–11. Noncystic adenocarcinoma of the appendix. The appendiceal mucosa and wall are markedly thickened by firm tumor and fibrous tissue, which is extending into the periappendiceal fat. A fistula tract is identified (arrows).

presents as a uterine tumor[70] or bilateral Krukenberg tumors.[64]

The gross appearance of a carcinomatous appendix may be indistinguishable from that of acute appendicitis with walled-off perforation. The appendix is usually irregularly enlarged in the portion that is involved by the carcinoma and the accompanying fibrosis (Figure 33–11). The latter may cause adhesion with the serosal surface of the adjacent cecum or other organs. The tumor is composed of creamy white or yellowish-tan hard tissue. In the cystic variant, the tumor is largely cystic with accumulation of varying amounts of mucus. The cystadenocarcinoma is grossly indistinguishable from its benign counterpart.[64] When the mucus has accumulated in the tissue outside the cystic tumor, either through rupture or produced by infiltrating tumor cells, it is invariably accompanied by fibrosis and inflammation, resulting in pseudomyxoma peritonei. Fibrous adhesion with the neighboring organs may be extensive. A fistulous tract may be formed (Figure 33–12).

Microscopically, the tumor cells form irregular glandular structures with focal clustering of tumor cells (see Figure 33–12). The tumor cells themselves are more atypical than those of appendiceal adenoma in that their nuclei are more pleomorphic and hyperchromatic. However, the cytologic difference is so subtle that the only reliable criterion for diagnosing adenocarcinoma is invasion of the appendiceal wall or tissue outside the appendix.[64,66,71,72] Metastasis to lymph nodes can occur but may not be apparent at operation. Other metastatic sites include liver, peritoneum, and lung.[73] Occasionally the neoplastic epithelium displays irregular microglandular glands and markedly atypical columnar cells, which are indistinguishable from those of colonic adenocarcinoma, thus allowing a diagnosis of carcinoma even in the absence of invasion.

It is common to find adenomatous epithelium in continuity with the malignant component. This association would naturally raise the possibility that there is an adenoma-carcinoma sequence. It is well accepted that this probably is the case in colonic neoplasms as it is supported by the remarkably common findings of car-

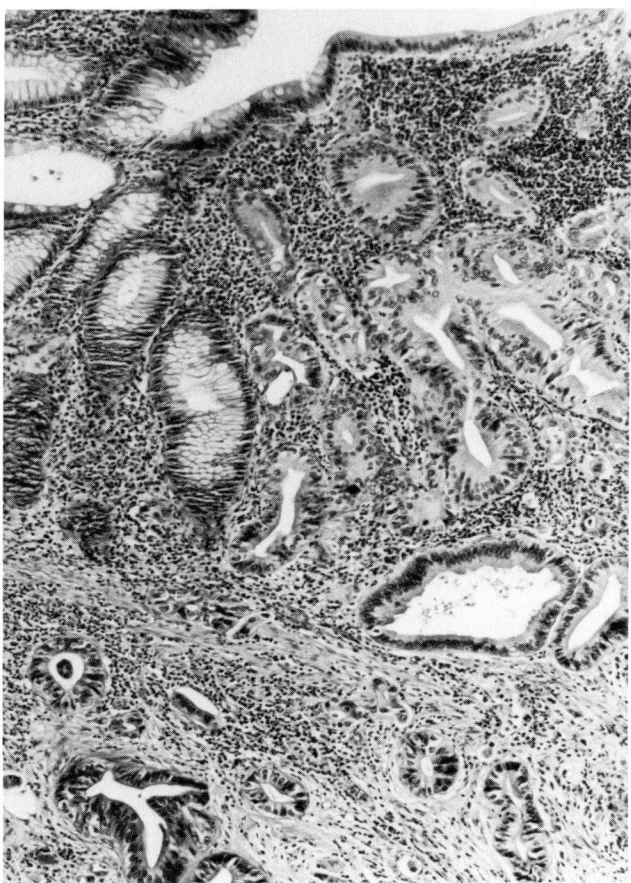

FIGURE 33–12. Noncystic adenocarcinoma of the appendix. The irregular, neoplastic glands invade the muscular wall. The tumor cells are pleomorphic and hyperchromatic. ($\times$ 250) (Courtesy of Dr. Telesforo Reyes, North Arundel Hospital, Glen Burnie, Md.)

cinoma in colonic polyps, especially the villous type, and by the follow-up study.[74] Though follow-up study of this type is impossible in appendiceal neoplasms, an endorsement of this concept is entirely reasonable because of the close similarity between the two epithelia. In some other instances, the malignant epithelium may be seen in connection with normal-appearing appendiceal epithelium. One must question then whether the phenotypically normal epithelium has undergone a subtle, preneoplastic change.

Rarely observed in the appendix is signet-ring cell carcinoma, which is histologically and cytologically identical to the signet-ring cell carcincoma arising elsewhere. The prognosis is poor.

Adenocarcinoma of the appendix may be present synchronously with tubular or villous adenomas or carcinoma of the colon. Some of the carcinomas that involve the proximal portion of the appendix may represent carcinoma of the cecum with an extension into the appendix.[66] Appendiceal adenocarcinoma has been associated with malignant tumors of the colon, uterine cervix, breast, prostate, esophagus, stomach, ovary, bladder, and lymph nodes.[75]

Appelman collected published cases and added his own for the statistical analysis.[66] Types of surgical approach are more contributory to survival than are the morphologic features of the tumor. Hemicolectomy results in 5-year and 10-year survival rates of 66%, and appendectomy results in a 5-year survival rate of 54% and a 10-year survival rate of 41.5%. The number of cases of *in situ* adenocarcinoma arising in adenomas is too small to obtain a significant prognostic figure.

Mucocele and Pseudomyxoma Peritonei

Mucocele of the appendix is defined as a distention of the appendix by accumulation of mucus within the lumen.[3] The accumulation of mucus may be due to obstruction of the proximal lumen with resulting cystic distention of the distal lumen, which is regarded as simple or retention mucocele.[4] Retention mucoceles are usually small and rarely exceed 5 cm at their greatest diameter (Figure 33–13). In addition to the content of mucus, retention mucoceles are lined by normal appendiceal epithelium (Figure 33–14), which may be flattened, or are without epithelial lining. Chronically inflamed granulation tissue is observed around the mucus. In rabbits, the intraperitoneal injection of chloroform-treated contents of mucocele resulted in a foreign-body peritonitis.[76] Obstruction of the appendix has resulted in mucoceles in rabbits.[77]

Myxoglobulosis is a variant of mucocele of the appendix, characterized by the contents of pearl-like globules of mucin, which are occasionally calcified.[78] At least 67 cases have been reported in the literature. The globules are composed of amorphous, granular, either mucinous or nonmucinous material in the center and laminated mucin at the periphery with scattered inflammatory cells. The mechanism of the formation of the mucinous globules is still unsettled.

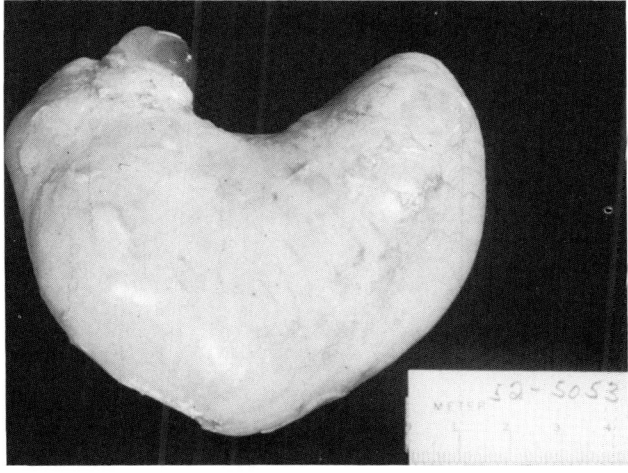

FIGURE 33–13. Mucocele of the appendix showing marked expansion of the organ, apparently as a result of accumulation of mucus. (Courtesy of Dr. Si-Chun Ming, Temple University School of Medicine, Philadelphia, Pa.)

Because of the large production of mucus, cystadenomas and cystadenocarcinomas are mucus-containing cysts. Although many authors have used the term *mucocele* to designate them, others[64] have recommended eliminating this term for all mucus-producing cystic appendiceal lesions that result from hyperplasia or neoplastic proliferation of the appendiceal epithelium. The author shares this view because the term *mucocele* does not indicate the nature of the proliferative lesion. If the lining epithelium is neither hyperplastic nor neoplastic, the cystic lesion then should be designated "retention mucocele."

Pseudomyxoma peritonei is characterized by implantation of mucus-producing epithelium on the peritoneal surface and accumulation of mucus in the

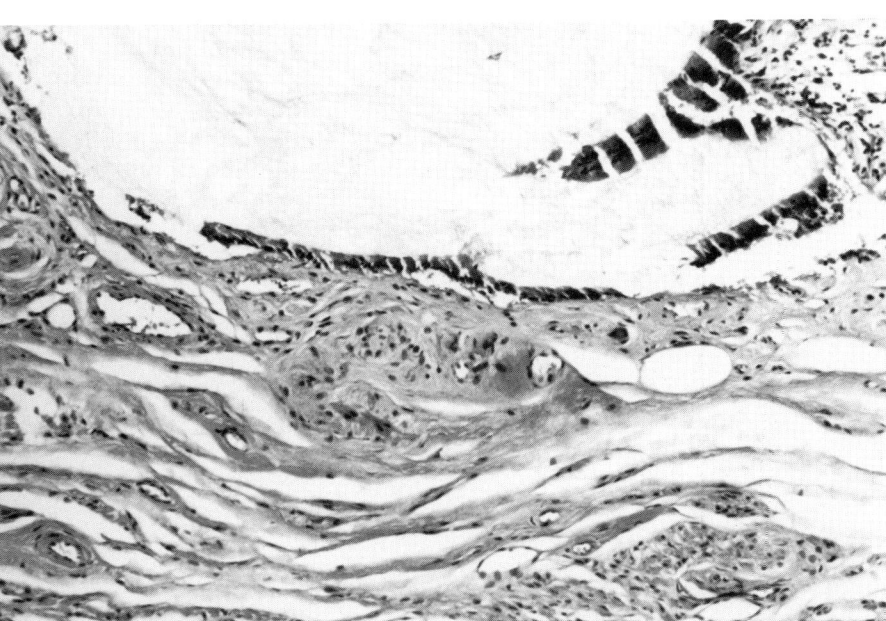

FIGURE 33–14. The retention mucocele is lined by a single layer of appendiceal epithelium. ($\times$ 250)

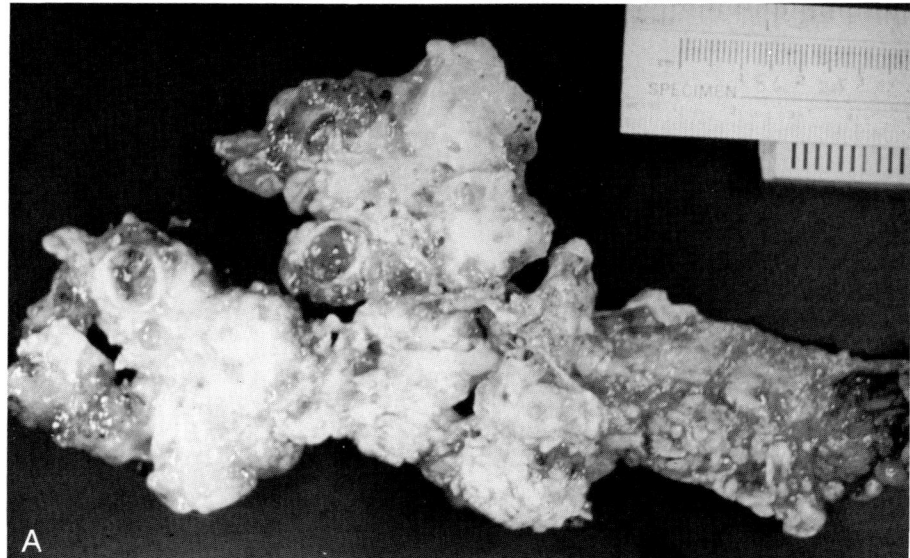
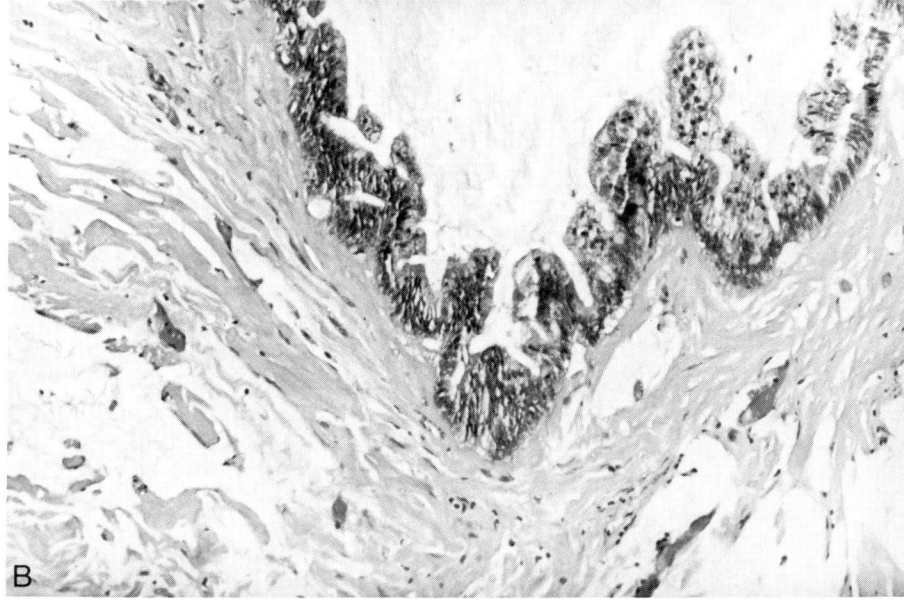

FIGURE 33-15. *A,* Gross appearance of pseudomyxoma peritonei. Lakes of mucus are surrounded by firm, white tissue. *B,* Microscopically, the firm areas are mostly fibrous connective tissue in which irregular, neoplastic glands are observed. Distinguishing between benign and malignant tumors may be impossible. (× 250)

peritoneal cavity[4] (Figure 33–15). Rupture of a cystadenoma or a cystadenocarcinoma of either appendiceal or ovarian origin or invasion by a cystadenocarcinoma may result in pseudomyxoma peritonei. The accumulation of mucus in the peritoneum is invariably associated with PMN infiltration and granulation tissue in the adjacent areas with fibrosis. The pseudomyxoma peritonei due to benign lesions may be self-limited, whereas those that result from a malignant lesion have a poor prognosis.[64] Adhesions and intestinal obstruction are frequent complications.[4]

Carcinoid Tumor

Carcinoid tumor is an endocrine tumor composed of intestinal enterochromaffin cells. The incidence of carcinoids is 0.32% (range, 0.06% to 0.69%) in surgically removed appendices; the incidence in autopsy series is 0.054% (range, 0.009% to 0.17%).[79] They are the most common tumors of the appendix. Adults between 20 and 39 years of age are most often affected. Females outnumber males, owing to the fact that women undergo appendectomy more often than men.

The majority of appendiceal carcinoids are smaller than 2 cm when discovered, and approximately 70% of carcinoids are located in the tip of the organ. The body of appendix is involved in 22% and the base in 7%. Both the small size and the location probably explain why the majority of patients are asymptomatic. The symptomatic patients most often present with symptoms and signs of appendicitis, and only occasionally their symptoms are related to the obstruction of the lumen. Patients may rarely present with carcinoid syndrome[4] and Cushing's syndrome.[80]

Appendiceal carcinoid tumors are oval or round, es-

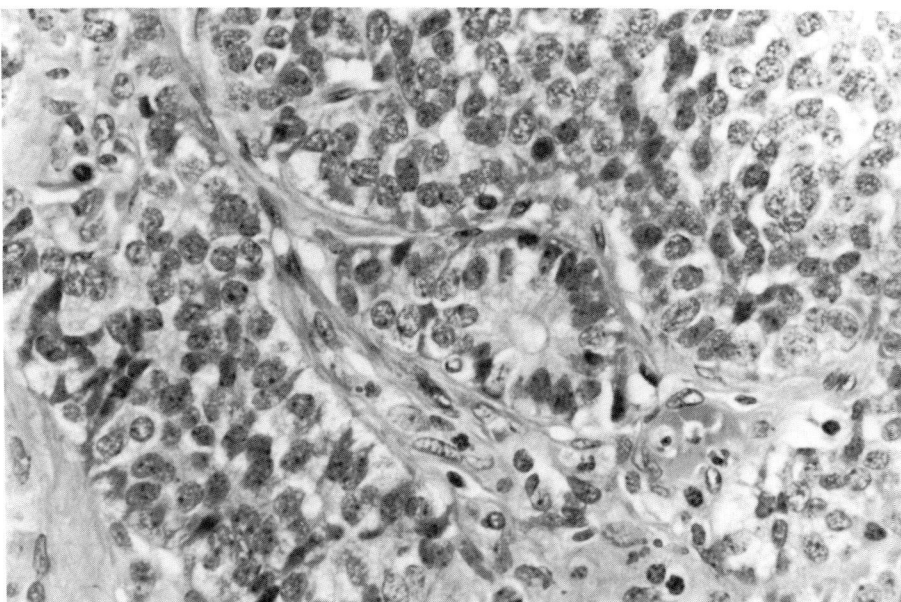

FIGURE 33–16. Carcinoid tumor of the appendix, characterized by sheets of relatively uniform tumor cells with round to oval nuclei and scanty cytoplasm. A small gland can also be seen. (× 500) (Courtesy of Dr. Telesforo Reyes, North Arundel Hospital, Glen Burnie, Md.)

pecially those arising in the tip, or appear to be a thickening of the wall. The tumors are usually firm, homogeneous, and gray to yellow. Because of their small size, they are often overlooked and only become evident microscopically. The appendiceal carcinoids are composed of uniform tumor cells with round to oval nuclei and relatively scanty amounts of cytoplasm. The tumor cells form sheets, nests of microglandular structures, or cords (Figure 33–16). The periphery of the sheets shows a palisading pattern characterized by parallel arrangement of their nuclei; inside, the tumor cells may form small, round structures, the so-called microglandular pattern. The cytoplasm may show vacuolation. Mitoses are virturally absent. Masson-Fontana (argentaffin) and Grimelius (argyrophil) stains are positive in tumor cells.[81] Immunohistochemical stain is positive for neuron-specific enolase (NSE).[4] Electron microscopy demonstrates neurosecretory granules similar to those of carcinoid tumor cells arising elsewhere. The muscular wall of the appendix is always invaded by tumor, and lymphatic invasion is common. Both of these features are somewhat paradoxical to the excellent prognosis for patients with appendiceal carcinoids. None of the patients who had tumors smaller than 2 cm developed either recurrence or metastasis or died of tumor 5 to 25 years after simple appendectomy.[79,82] Likewise, patients with localized carcinoids larger than 2 cm also had an excellent prognosis. However, those who had carcinoids larger than 2 cm as well as unresectable metastasis at the time of operation may have a fatal outcome. The appendiceal carcinoids invade the mesoappendix and metastasize to the regional lymph nodes in 1.4% to 8.8% of the cases.[4] The metastasizing tumors are usually larger than 2 cm, and the smaller tumors rarely metastasize.[4]

Additional information on carcinoid and adenocarcinoid tumors is given in Chapter 13.

Adenocarcinoid (Goblet Cell Carcinoid Tumor, Mucinous Carcinoid Tumor, Crypt Cell Carcinoma)

Adenocarcinoid of the appendix is composed of both mucus-producing and endocrine cells. It was first described in the late 1960s and has been labeled with several different names.[66] Some pathologists have regarded this entity as a variant of carcinoid.[3,4] Isaacson suggests that the so-called adenocarcinoid is derived from lysozyme-producing cells of the type normally present in small-intestinal crypts.[81] The histogenesis of this unusual tumor is controversial at best. The patients are usually in their sixties and present with symptoms of appendicitis. Adenocarcinoids may be an incidental finding, or rarely they present as bilateral ovarian tumors.[83]

Similar to the conventional appendiceal carcinoid, adenocarcinoid usually is less than 1 cm in diameter and is found at the tip. The tumor sometimes may be grossly inapparent, diffusely infiltrating the appendix, or may be associated with features of acute appendicitis.[66] The microscopic appearance is characterized by microglandular formation and small nests composed of signet-ring cells (Figure 33–17), identical to those of signet-ring cell carcinoma. Focally, the tumor cells appear to arise from the crypt of Lieberkühn (Figure 33–18). Mitotic figures are infrequent. The submucosa, muscular wall, and serosa are often infiltrated by tumor. Supporting both the glandular and the endocrine components are the findings of mucin content and neurosecretory granules in the tumor cells.[84] In Isaacson's study, however, the immunohistochemical stains have demonstrated lysozyme, secretory component, and IgA, all of which are also present in the small-intestinal crypt cells but are absent in the con-

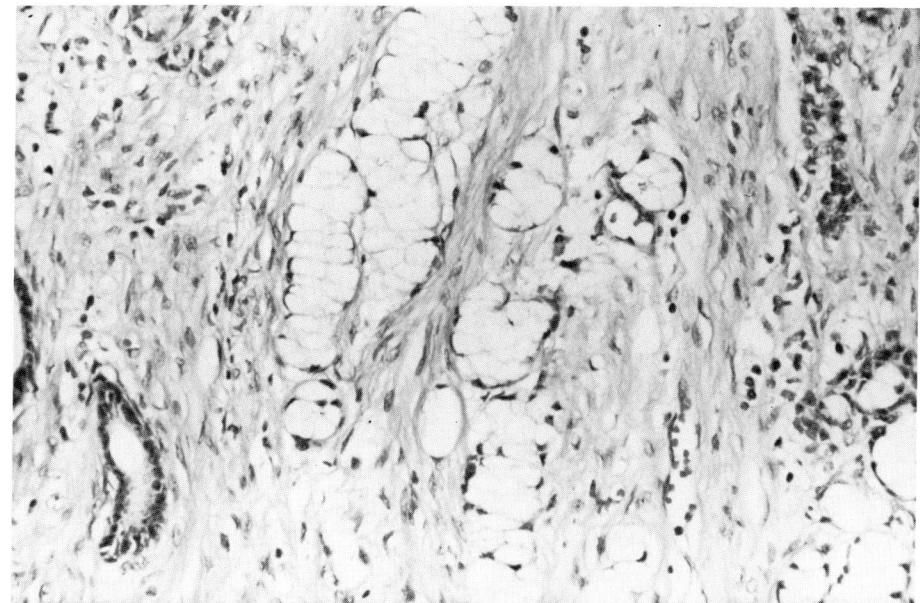

FIGURE 33–17. Adenocarcinoid of an appendix displaying prominent signet-ring cells. The tumor cells form small clusters or glandular structures infiltrating the lamina propria and appendiceal wall. (× 250) (Courtesy of Dr. Si-Chun Ming, Temple University School of Medicine, Philadelphia, Pa.)

ventional carcinoids. Further, only few endocrine cells and scattered Paneth cells are mixed with the mucin-containing cells, prompting Isaacson to conclude the aforementioned histogenesis. When both serotonin and mucosubstance are found in the same tumor cells, adenocarcinoid represents an amphicrine carcinoma.[85] With the concept that intestinal endocrine cells are of endodermal, rather than neural crest, origin, adenocarcinoids may well be neoplasms derived from intestinal stem cells that have the capability for differentiation along different cell lines.[84]

The behavior of adenocarcinoids is intermediate between that of conventional carcinoids and that of adenocarcinomas of the appendix, as reflected by their 5-year survival rate of 80%.[84]

Adenocarcinoid may be admixed with noncarcinoid adenocarcinoma; the latter is characterized by a glandular pattern or poorly differentiated pattern with signet-ring cells and a high mitotic rate with an average of 10 (range, 0 to 25) mitotic cells per 10 high-power fields.[85a] When the carcinomatous component in such a mixed lesion exceeds 50% of tumor volume, the tumor behaves aggressively. Of 14 patients reported by Burke et al., 8 died of metastatic disease after an average follow-up period of 16 months.[85a]

Table 33–2 compares the conventional carcinoids,

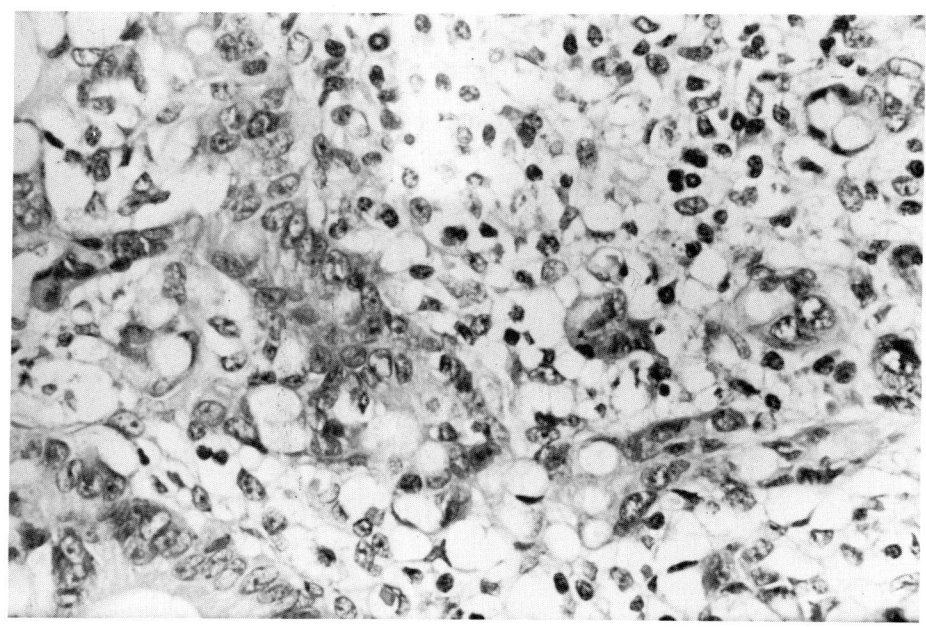

FIGURE 33–18. Same type of signet-ring cells as shown in Figure 33–17, found in one of the crypts in an adenocarcinoid. (× 500) (Courtesy of Dr. Si-Chung Ming, Temple University Hospital, Philadelphia, Pa.)

Table 33-2 COMPARISON BETWEEN CONVENTIONAL CARCINOIDS, ADENOCARCINOIDS, AND ADENOCARCINOMAS OF THE APPENDIX

	Conventional Carcinoids	Adenocarcinoids	Adenocarcinomas
Incidence	85% of all appendiceal tumors	Fewer than 100 cases reported in the literature	Infrequent but more common than adenocarcinoids
Age	Third and fourth decades	Sixth decade	Fifth to seventh decades
Size	Majority less than 2 cm	Usually less than 1 cm, rarely exceed 2 cm	Larger; may reach 15 cm
Gross appearance	Homogeneously firm, yellow	Thickening of appendiceal wall	Solid, or cystic with large amount of mucus
Microscopic Appearance	Uniform, round and polygonal tumor cells; sheets and trabeculae	Goblet and signet-ring cells, few endocrine and Paneth cells, microglandular structures	Irregular glands composed of atypical columnar cells; mucinous pools common
Clinical presentation	Majority are incidental findings	70% present as acute appendicitis	Symptoms of appendicitis or intestinal obstruction; palpable mass
Carcinoid syndrome	Rarely present	None reported	None reported
Cushing's syndrome	Rarely present	None reported	None reported
Survival 5 years	99%	80%	54-66%
10 years	99%	73%	41-66%

adenocarcinoids, and adenocarcinomas of the appendix.

Other Tumors

Lymphoma

Though the gastrointestinal tract is the most common extranodal site of primary lymphoma,[86] the appendix is rarely affected. Lymphoma of the appendix is more often an extension of the intestinal tumor than a solitary lesion. The overall incidence of primary appendiceal lymphoma is approximately 0.064% in 71,000 appendices.[10] It may occur both in adults and children. The pathologic features of the appendiceal lymphoma are those of non-Hodgkin's lymphomas, including the Burkitt type.[86,87] The prognosis largely depends on the extent of the tumor. Lymphomas limited to the appendix have an excellent prognosis.

Leiomyoma and Leiomyosarcoma

Both benign and malignant smooth muscle tumors are rare. In a series of 8699 appendices, 2 of the 101 appendiceal tumors were leiomyomas.[88] Collins found an incidence of 1.7% in 71,000 appendices.[10] In his series, leiomyomas were the most common benign tumors of the appendix. The leiomyomas are small and are usually incidental findings. The largest appendiceal leiomyoma recorded measured 15 by 11 by 12 cm and weighed 480 gm.[89]

The two reported appendiceal leiomyosarcomas were highly cellular and displayed marked cellular pleomorphism and a high mitotic rate. Both patients died of advanced tumor within 6 months.[90]

Granular Cell Tumor

Granular cell tumors of the appendix are rare. In a review of 74 granular cell tumors of the gastrointestinal tract, Johnston and Helwig found four cases of appendiceal origin.[91] Granular cells should be distinguished from the degenerated smooth muscle cells.[92]

Neuroma

Neuromas were first described by Masson and since then have been a subject of controversy.[93] Using immunoperoxidase and electron-microscopic techniques, Stanley et al. demonstrated the neural nature not only of the nodular forms but also of so-called fibrous obliteration.[93] Endocrine cells were also found in many neuromas.

Ganglioneuroma

Ganglioneuromas of the appendix have been described in the literature. They range from a few millimeters to a pedunculated mass, causing obstruction of the lumen and appendicitis.[94]

Metastatic Tumors

Carcinomas of the breast, stomach, bronchus, and prostate can metastasize infrequently to the appendix.[95-97] Metastatic breast carcinoma and prostatic carcinoma may be difficult to distinguish from carcinoid tumors. Metastatic gastric signet-ring cell carcinoma may resemble adenocarcinoid.[4] Kaposi's sarcoma was found in the appendix as one of multiple foci in a patient afflicted with the acquired immunodeficiency syndrome (AIDS).[98]

A variety of rare benign and malignant tumors were recorded in Collins' collection, including different types of mesenchymal tumors and melanomas.[10]

MISCELLANEOUS LESIONS

Fibrous Obliteration

Fibrous obliteration is characterized by occlusion of a portion of or the entire appendiceal lumen by bland spindle cells to replace the normal mucosal and lymphoid components. It is found in 35% of 71,000 appendices (91% were surgical and the remaining were autopsy specimens).[10] Most of these demonstrated obliteration of segments of the appendiceal lumens. In Butler's series, 14% of 276 surgically removed appendices showed fibrous obliteration.[29] The lack of preexisting appendicitis led to the belief that fibrous obliteration is a developmental event rather than the end-stage of inflammation.[99] Kazzaz demonstrated argentaffin and argyrophil cells in the neuroma-like structures and suggested that the argentaffin and argyrophil cells migrate and cause hyperplasia of the nerve plexus, leading to the obstruction of the lumen.[100] Recently, Stanley et al. further confirmed the neural nature of fibrous obliteration and concluded that most cases of fibrous obliteration actually represent appendiceal neuromas.[93] Although the pathogenesis is still uncertain, these morphologic findings support the notion that fibrous obliteration is a proliferative lesion.

Sarcoidosis

The appendix rarely may be involved in sarcoidosis.[101] The appendix shows noncaseating granulomas, with or without concomitant acute appendicitis. Because the granulomas are not diagnostic for sarcoidosis, the differential diagnosis should include infectious granulomas, Crohn's disease, and other conditions that may cause granulomas.

Periappendicitis

Periappendicitis is a condition in which the inflammatory infiltrate is seen in the serosa and periappendiceal adipose tissue, usually secondary to an inflammatory process in the adjacent organs. The appendix proper is devoid of inflammation, although a severe case of periappendicitis may spread into the appendiceal wall. The common origins of periappendicitis are salpingitis, ileal Crohn's disease, Meckel's diverticulitis, and others.[4]

Intussusception

Intussusception of the appendix occurs rarely; fewer than 200 cases have been reported in the medical literature.[102] They occur more often in males than in females and in patients ranging from 10 months to 75 years of age (average, 16 years). Clinically, intussusceptions may be asymptomatic or may present with symptoms and signs of intussusception or those mimicking acute appendicitis. There are four types of intussusception of the appendix: (1) the tip of the appendix is the intussusceptum, and its proximal portion is the intussuscipiens; (2) the base of the appendix is the intussusceptum, and the cecum is the intussuscipiens; (3) the proximal portion of the appendix is the intussusceptum, and its distal part is the intussuscipiens; and (4) complete inversion of the appendix (inside-out appendix), with accompanying ileocecal intussusception. All four types are well illustrated diagramatically by Langsam et al.[102] Intussusception develops when the peristalsis of the appendix is increased or becomes irregular due to foreign bodies, endometriosis, muco-celes, neoplasms, and others.[102]

Endometriosis

The appendix is an unusual site of endometriosis. However, when the intestinal tract is involved, the appendix is one of the affected sites in approximately one third of the patients.[103] Endometriosis either is an incidental finding or clinically presents as symptoms mimicking those of appendicitis. Foci of endometrial gland and stroma are found in the serosa or the appendiceal wall, which may or may not be associated with inflammation. There may be associated muscular hyperplasia, forming a mass.[104]

Arteritis

Arteritis may be found in up to 1% of appendices.[4] Almost all of these cases are local and asymptomatic, although the histologic features are indistinguishable from those of systemic arteritis nodosa. A case of polyarteritis nodosa, which presented as acute appendicitis, was reported recently.[105] Necrotizing vasculitis was found in this surgically removed appendix without evidence of appendicitis.

Cystic Fibrosis

Cystic fibrosis may clinically mimic "chronic appendicitis," resulting in appendectomy.[106] The appendix showed increased activity of the mucus-secreting cells with mucus filling the distended crypts. Rarely, the appendiceal lumen may be markedly distended by the viscid mucus, resulting in the appearance of a mucocele.

Septa

Septa in the appendix have recently been described.[107] By sectioning the appendix longitudinally, the septa are found to be complete and incomplete. All cases were found to be associated with acute appendicitis. Therefore, the question of whether it is a congenital lesion or an acquired lesion cannot be answered.

Other Lesions

Melanosis,[4] malakoplakia,[108] Whipple's disease,[109] and numerous other conditions[10] have been observed in the appendix.

References

1. Storer EH: Appendix. In Schwartz SI, Shires GT, Spencer FC, Storer EH (eds): Principles of Surgery, 3rd ed. New York, McGraw-Hill, 1979, pp 1257–1261.
2. Moore KL: The Developing Human: Clinically Oriented Embryology, 3rd ed. Philadelphia, WB Saunders, 1982, pp 242–244.
3. Morson BC, Dawson IMP: Gastrointestinal Pathology, 2nd ed. London, Blackwell, 1979, pp 449–451.
4. Gray GF Jr, Wackym PA: Surgical Pathology of the Vermiform Appendix. Pathol Annu 21(Part 2):111–144, 1986.
5. Bloom W, Fawcett DW: A Textbook of Histology, 11th edition. Philadelphia, WB Saunders, 1986, p 660.
6. Rode J, Dhillon AP, Papadaki L: Serotonin-immuoreactive cells in the lamina propria plexus of the appendix. Hum Pathol 14:464–469, 1983.
7. Huang JMS, Krumbhaar EB: The amount of lymphoid tissue of the human appendix and its weight at different age periods. Am J Med Sci 199:75–83, 1940.
8. Spencer J, Finn T, Isaacson PG: Gut-associated lymphoid tissue: A morphological and immunocytochemical study of the human appendix. Gut 26:672–679, 1985.
9. Emery JL, Underwood J: The neurological junction between the appendix and ascending colon. Gut 11:118–120, 1970.
10. Collins DC: 71,000 human appendix specimens: A final report summarizing 40 years' study. Am J Proctol 14:365–381, 1963.
11. Bremner DN, Mooney G: Agenesis of appendix: A further thalidomide anomaly. (Letter) Lancet 1:826, 1978.
12. Juca W: Intussusception of the vermiform appendix. Am J Surg 99:106–107, 1960.
13. Waugh TR: Appendix vermiformis duplex. Arch Surg 42:311–320, 1941.
14. George DH: Diverticulosis of the vermiform appendix in patients with cystic fibrosis. Hum Pathol 18:75–79, 1987.
15. Favara BE: Multiple congenital diverticula of the vermiform appendix. Am J Clin Pathol 49:60–64, 1968.
16. Mikat DM, Mikat KW: Appendix helicus: A unique anomaly of the vermiform appendix. Gastroenterology 71:304–305, 1976.
17. Stone WD, Hendrix TR, Schuster MM: Aganglionosis of the entire colon in an adolescent. Gastroenterology 48:636–641, 1965.
18. Merck C, Kindblom L-G: Neurofibromatosis of the appendix in von Recklinghausen's disease: A report of a case. Acta Pathol Microbiol Scand [A] 83:623–627, 1975.
19. Aubrey DA: Gastric mucosa in the vermiform appendix. Arch Surg 101:628–629, 1970.
20. Droga BW, Levine S, Baber JJ: Heterotopic gastric and esophageal tissue in the vermiform appendix. Am J Clin Pathol 40:190–193, 1963.
21. Fitz RH: Perforating inflammation of the vermiform appendix: With special references to its early diagnosis and treatment. Am J Med Sci 92:321–346, 1886.
22. Malt RA: The perforated appendix (Editorial). N Engl J Med 315:1546–1547, 1986.
23. Burkitt DP: The aetiology of appendicitis. Br J Surg 58:695–699, 1971.
24. Sleisinger MH: Acute appendicitis (including the acute abdomen). In Wyngaarden JB, Smith LH Jr (eds): Cecil's Textbook of Medicine, 18th ed. Philadelphia, WB Saunders, 1988, pp 800–804.
25. Wangansteen OH, Bowers WF: Significance of the obstructive factor in the genesis of acute appendicitis: An experimental study. Arch Surg 34:496–526, 1937.
26. Pieper R, Kager L, Tidefeldt U: Obstruction of appendix vermiformis causing acute appendicitis: An experimental study in the rabbit. Acta Chir Scand 148:63–72, 1982.
27. Buirge RE, Dennis C, Vardo RL, Wangensteen OH: Histology of experimental appendiceal obstruction (rabbit, ape and man). Arch Pathol 30:481–503, 1940.
28. Chang AR: An analysis of 3,003 appendices. Aust NZ J Surg 51:169–178, 1981.
29. Butler C: Surgical pathology of acute appendicitis. Hum Pathol 12:870–878, 1981.
30. Tobe T, Horikoshi Y, Hamada C, Hamashima Y: Virus infection as a trigger of appendicitis. Experimental investigation of Coxsackie B5 virus infection in monkey intestine. Surgery 62:927–934, 1967.
31. Tobe T: Inapparent virus infection as a trigger of appendicitis. Lancet 1:1343–1346, 1965.
32. Sisson RG, Ahlvin RC, Hartlow MC: Superficial mucosal ulceration and the pathogenesis of acute appendicitis in childhood. Am J Surg 122:378–380, 1971.
33. Arnbjornsson E, Asp N-G, Westin SI: Decreasing incidence of acute appendicitis with special reference to the consumption of dietary fiber. Acta Chir Scand 148:461–464, 1982.
34. Brooks SM: McBurney's Point: The Story of Appendicitis. London, AS Barnes, 1969, p 102.
35. Jahidi MR, Shaw ML: The pathology of the appendix in ulcerative colitis. Dis Colon Rectum 19:345–349, 1976.
36. Larsen E, Axelsson C, Johansen A: The pathology of the appendix in morbus Crohn and ulcerative colitis. Acta Pathol Micro Scand [Suppl] 212:161–165, 1970.
37. Timmicke AE: Granulomatous appendicitis: Is it Crohn's disease? Report of a case and review of the literature. Am J Gastroenterol 81:283–287, 1986.
38. Allen DC, Biggart JD: Granulomatous disease in the vermiform appendix. J Clin Pathol 36:632–638, 1983.
39. Payan HM: Diverticular disease of the appendix. Dis Colon Rectum 20:473–476, 1977.
40. Esparza AR, Pan CM: Diverticulosis of the appendix. Surgery 67:922–928, 1970.
41. Rabinovitch J, Arden M, Barrett T, et al: Diverticulosis and diverticulitis of the vermiform appendix. Ann Surg 155:434–440, 1962.
42. Deschenes L, Couture J, Garneau R: Diverticulitis of the appendix. Am J Surg 121:706–709, 1971.
43. Leigh DA, Simmons K, Norman E: Bacterial flora of the appendix fossa in appendicitis and postoperative wound infection. J Clin Pathol 27:997–1000, 1974.
44. van Spreeuwel JP, Lindeman J, Bax R, et al: Campylobacter-associated appendicitis: Prevalence and clinicopathologic features. Pathol Annu 22:55–65, 1987.
45. Mittal VK, Khanna SK, Gupta NM, Aikat M: Isolated tuberculosis of appendix. Am Surg 41:172–174, 1975.
46. Morrison H, Mixter CG, Schlesinger MJ, Ober WB: Tuberculosis localized to the appendix. N Engl J Med 246:329–331, 1952.
47. Parkin M, Robinson BL: Tuberculosis of the appendix. Br J Clin Pract 18:741–742, 1964.
48. Black RE, Jackson RJ, Tsai T, et al: Epidemic Yersinia enterocolitica infection due to contaminated chocolate milk. N Engl J Med 298:76–79, 1978.
49. El-Maraghi NRH, Mair NS: The histopathology of enteric infection with yersinia pseudotuberculosis. Am J Clin Pathol 71:631–639, 1979.

50. Henrik-Nielson R, Lundbeck FA, Teglbjaerg PS, et al: Intestinal spirochetosis of the vermiform appendix. Gastroenterology 88:971–977, 1985.
51. Herzberg M: Giant cells in the lymphoid tissue of the appendix in the prodromal stage of measles. JAMA 98:139–140, 1932.
52. Yunis EJ, Hashida Y: Electron microscopic demonstration of adenovirus in appendix vermiformis in a case of ileocecal intussuception. Pediatrics 51:566–569, 1973.
53. Reif RM: Viral appendicitis. Hum Pathol 12:193–196, 1981.
54. O'Brien A, O'Brien DS: Infectious mononucleosis: Appendiceal lymphoid tissue involvement parallels characteristic lymph node changes. Arch Pathol Lab Med 109:680–682, 1985.
55. Blackman E, Vimadalal S, Nash G: Significance of gastrointestinal cytomegalovirus infection in homosexual males. Am J Gastroenterol 79:935–940, 1984.
56. Arean VM, Crandall CA: Ascariasis. In Marcial-Rojas PA (ed): Pathology of Protozoal and Helminthic Diseases with Clinical Correlation. Baltimore, Williams & Wilkins, 1971, p 784.
57. Perez-Tamayo R, Brandt H: Amebiasis. In Marcial-Rojas PA (ed): Pathology of Protozoal and Helminthic Diseases with Clinical Correlation. Baltimore, Williams & Wilkins, 1971, p 159.
58. Arean VM, Echevarria R: Balantidiasia. In Marcial-Rojas PA (ed): Pathology of Protozoal and Helminthic Diseases with Clinical Correlation. Baltimore, Williams & Wilkins, 1971, p 238.
59. Kenney M, Yermakov V: Infection of man with Trichuris vulpis, the whipworm of dogs. Am J Trop Med Hyg 29:1205–1208, 1980.
60. Noodleman JS: Eosinophilic appendicitis demonstration of Strongyloides stercoralis as a causative agent. Arch Pathol Lab Med 105:148–149, 1981.
61. Kenney M, Eveland LK, Yermakov V, Kassouny DY: A case of rictularia infection of man in New York. Am J Trop Med Hyg 24:596–599, 1975.
62. Ashburn LL: Appendiceal oxyuris. Am J Pathol 17:841–856, 1941.
63. Mogensen K, Pahle E, Kowalski K: Enterobius vermicularis and acute appendicitis. Acta Chir Scand 151:705–707, 1985.
64. Higa E, Rosai J, Pizzimbono CA, Wise L: Mucosal hyperplasia, mucinous cystadenoma, and mucinous cystadenocarcinoma of the appendix: A re-evaluation of the appendiceal "mucocele." Cancer 32:1525–1541, 1973.
65. Qizilbash AH: Hyperplastic (metaplastic) polyps of the appendix: Report of 19 cases. Arch Pathol 97:385–388, 1974.
66. Appelman HD: Epithelial neoplasia of the appendix. In Norris HT (ed): Pathology of the Colon, Small Intestine and Anus. Churchill Livingstone, New York, 1983, pp 233–265.
67. Qizilbash AH: Mucoceles of the appendix: Their relationship to hyperplastic polyps, mucinous cystadenomas, and cystadenocarcinomas. Arch Pathol 99:548–555, 1975.
68. Wolfe M, Ahmed N: Epithelial neoplasms of the vermiform appendix (exclusive of carcinoid). II. Cystadenomas, papillary adenomas, and adenomatous polyps of the appendix. Cancer 37:2511–2522, 1976.
69. Mibu R, Itsh H, Iwashita A, et al: Carcinoma in situ of the vermiform appendix associated with adenomatosis of the colon. Dis Colon Rectum 24:482–484, 1981.
70. Alenghat E, Talerman A: Adenocarcinoma of the vermiform appendix presenting as a uterine tumor. Gynecol Oncol 13:265–268, 1982.
71. Qizilbash AH: Primary adenocarcinoma of the appendix: A clinicopathologic study of 11 cases. Arch Pathol 99:556–562, 1975.
72. Wolfe M, Ahmed N: Epithelial neoplasms of the vermiform appendix (exclusive of carcinoid). I. Adenocarcinomas of the appendix. Cancer 37:2493–2510, 1976.
73. Cohen SE, Wolfman EF Jr: Primary adenocarcinoma of the vermiform appendix. Am J Surg 127:704–707, 1974.
74. Lotfi AM, Spencer RJ, Ilstrup DM, Melton LJ III: Colorectal polyps and the risk of subsequent carcinoma. Mayo Clin Proc 61:337–343, 1986.
75. Ferro M, Anthony PP: Adenocarcinoma of the appendix. Dis Colon Rectum 28:457–459, 1985.
76. Cheng K-K: An experimental study of mucocele of the appendix and pseudomyxoma peritonei. J Pathol Bacteriol 61:217–225, 1949.
77. Dachman AH, Nicholas JB, Patrick DA, Lichtenstein JE: Natural history of the obstructed rabbit appendix: Observations with radiography, sonography and CT. AJR 148:281–284, 1987.
78. Gonzalez JEG, Haan SE, Trujillo YP: Myxoglobulosis of the appendix. Am J Surg Pathol 12:962–968, 1988.
79. Moertel CG, Dockerty MB, Judd ES: Carcinoid tumors of the vermiform appendix. Cancer 21:270–278, 1968.
80. Johnston WH, Waisman J: Carcinoid tumor of the vermiform appendix with Cushing's syndrome. Cancer 27:681–686, 1971.
81. Isaacson P: Crypt cell carcinoma of the appendix (so-called adenocarcinoid tumor). Am J Surg Pathol 5:213–224, 1981.
82. Moertel CG, Weiland LH, Nagorney DM, Dockerty MB: Carcinoid tumor of the appendix: Treatment and prognosis. N Engl J Med 317:1699–1701, 1987.
83. Hood IC, Jones BA, Watts JC: Mucinous tumor of the appendix presenting as bilateral ovarian tumors. Arch Pathol Lab Med 110:336–340, 1986.
84. Lewin KJ, Ulich T, Yang K, Layfield L: The endocrine cells of the gastrointestinal tract tumors. Pathol Annu 21(Part II):181–215, 1986.
85. Chejfec G, Capella C, Solicia E, et al: Amphicrine cells, dysplasias, and neoplasias. Cancer 56:2683–2690, 1985.
85a. Burke AP, Sobin LH, Federspiel BH, et al: Goblet cell carcinoids and related tumors of the vermiform appendix. Am J Clin Pathol 94: 27–35, 1990.
86. Lewin KJ, Ranchod M, Dorfman RF: Lymphomas of the gastrointestinal tract: A study of 117 cases presenting with gastrointestinal disease. Cancer 42:693–707, 1978.
87. Sin IC, Ling E-T, Prentice RSA: Burkitt's lymphoma of the appendix: Report of two cases. Hum Pathol 11:465–470, 1980.
88. Schmutzer KJ, Bayer M, Zaki AE, et al: Tumors of the appendix. Dis Colon Rectum 18:324–331, 1975.
89. Powell JL, Fuerst JF, Tapia RA: Leiomyoma of the appendix. South Med J 73:1298–1299, 1980.
90. Jones PA: Leiomyosarcoma of the appendix: Report of two cases. Dis Colon Rectum 22:175–178, 1979.
91. Johnston J, Helwig EB: Granular cell tumors of the gastrointestinal tract and perianal region: A study of 74 cases. Dig Dis Sci 26:807–816, 1981.
92. Sobel JH, Marquet E, Schwarz R: Granular degeneration of appendiceal smooth muscle. Arch Pathol 92:427–432, 1971.
93. Stanley MW, Cerwitz D, Hagen K, Snover DC. Neuromas of the appendix: A light-microscopic, immunohistochemical and electron-microscopic study of 20 cases. Am J Surg Pathol 10:801–815, 1986.
94. Zarabi M, LaBach JP: Ganglioneuroma causing acute appendicitis. Hum Pathol 13:1143–1146, 1982.
95. Latchis KS, Canter JW: Acute appendicitis secondary to metastatic carcinoma. Am J Surg 111:220–223, 1966.
96. Dieter RA Jr: Carcinoma metastatic to the vermiform appendix: Report of three cases. Dis Colon Rectum 13:336–340, 1970.
97. Ansari MA, Pintozzi RL, Choi YS, Ladove RF: Diagnosis of carcinoid-like metastatic prostatic carcinoma by an immunoperoxidase method. Am J Clin Pathol 76:94–98, 1976.
98. Baker MS, Goldman H, Wille M, Kim H-K: Metastatic Kaposi's sarcoma presenting as acute appendicitis. Milit Med 151:45–47, 1986.
99. Howie JGR: The Prussian-blue reaction in the diagnosis of previous appendicitis. J Pathol Bacteriol 91:85–92, 1966.
100. Kazzaz BA: Argentaffin and argyrophil cells in the appendix. J Pathol 104:206–209, 1971.
101. Clarke H, Pollett W, Chittal S, Ra M: Sarcoidosis with involvement of the appendix. Arch Intern Med 143:1603–1604, 1983.
102. Langsam LB, Raj PK, Galang CF: Intussusception of the appendix. Dis Colon Rectum 27:387–392, 1984.
103. Mittal VK, Chondhury SP, Cortez JA: Endometriosis of the appendix presenting as acute appendicitis. Am J Surg 142:519–521, 1981.
104. Panganiban W, Cornog JL: Endometriosis of the intestines and vermiform appendix. Dis Colon Rectum 15:253–260, 1972.
105. Fayemi AO, Ali M, Braun EV: Necrotizing vasculitis of the gallbladder and the appendix: Similarity in the morphology of rheumatoid arthritis and polyarteritis nodesa. Am J Gastroenterol 67:608–612, 1977.

106. Shwachman H, Holsclaw D: Examination of the appendix at laparotomy as a diagnostic clue in cystic fibrosis. N Engl J Med 286:1300–1301, 1972.
107. DeLaFuente AA: Septa in the appendix: A previously undescribed condition. Histopathology 9:1329–1337, 1985.
108. Blackshear W Jr: Malakoplakia of the appendix: A case report. Am J Clin Pathol 53:284–287, 1970.
109. Misra PS, Lebwohl P, Laufer H: Hepatic and appendiceal Wipple's disease with negative jejunal biopsies. Am J Gastroenterol 75:302–306, 1981.

CHAPTER 34

Disorders of the Anal Region

ROBERT R. RICKERT, M.D.

ANATOMY

DEVELOPMENTAL ABNORMALITIES

HEMORRHOIDS

PROLAPSE

INFLAMMATORY AND INFECTIOUS DISORDERS
Fissure
Fistula and Abscess
Hidradenitis Suppurativa
Anal Lesions in Inflammatory Bowel Disease
Ulcerative Colitis
Crohn's Disease
Sexually Transmitted Diseases

Syphilis
Gonorrhea
Herpes Simplex
Chlamydia
Molluscum Contagiosum
Lymphogranuloma Venereum, Chancroid, and Granuloma Inguinale
Tuberculosis
Other Conditions

BENIGN TUMORS AND TUMOR-LIKE LESIONS
Condyloma Acuminatum
Bowenoid Papulosis
Adnexal Tumors
Keratoacanthoma
Granular Cell Tumor and Neurilemoma

Leiomyoma
Oleogranuloma

MALIGNANT TUMORS
General Considerations
Anal Canal Carcinoma
Anal Margin Carcinoma
Carcinoma *in Situ*
Bowen's Disease
Cloacogenic Carcinoma
Squamous Cell Carcinoma
Verrucous Carcinoma
Giant Condyloma Acuminatum
Adenocarcinoma
Malignant Melanoma
Extramammary Paget's Disease
Basal Cell Carcinoma
Other Malignant Tumors

ANATOMY

Despite the frequency of many disorders of the anal region, their pathogenesis often is poorly understood. The confusion surrounding anal disorders relates largely to the rather complex gross and microscopic anatomy of the anal region, knowledge of which is essential to an understanding of its disease processes.[1] Although uncommon, neoplasms arising in this area are also attended by considerable confusion with respect to classification and histogenesis.

The anal canal is 3 to 4 cm long and extends from the upper to the lower borders of the internal sphincter muscle (Figure 34–1). It connects with the rectum superiorly and the true anal skin inferiorly. The most important macroscopic landmark noted on inspection of the mucosal surface is the dentate or pectinate line located at about the midlevel of the canal. This line corresponds to the location of the anal valves, which are separated from each other by small papillae that represent the lower ends of six to ten vertical mucosal folds known as the anal columns of Morgagni. Above each of the crescentic anal valves lies a small recess or anal crypt. The dentate line marks the site of the fetal anal membrane corresponding to the junction of the endodermal part of the anal canal developed from the cloaca and the ectodermal portion derived from the anal pit (proctodeum).

Microscopically the mucosal lining below the dentate line is of stratified squamous type. Because its bor-

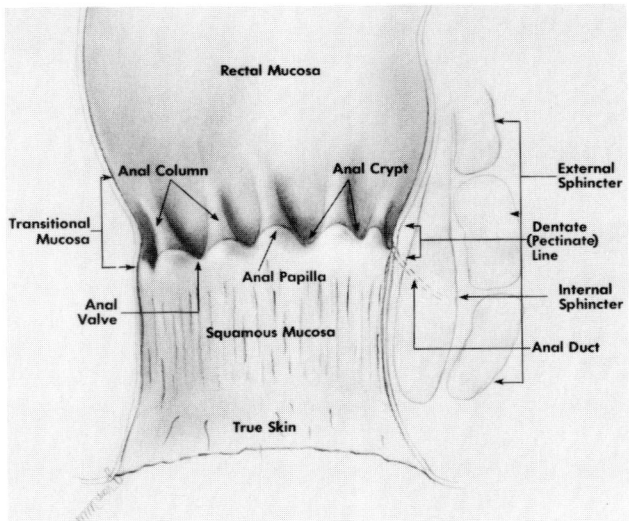

FIGURE 34–1. Diagram of the normal anatomy of anal region.

der with the dentate line grossly resembles a comb, it is also known as the pecten. The squamous mucous membrane of the anal canal is devoid of hair and other cutaneous appendages. The lower portion of the anal canal ends at the anal verge, where the squamous mucous membrane merges with true skin containing hair follicles, sweat, and apocrine glands.

The dentate line corresponds generally to the squamocolumnar junction. However, this is not an abrupt line of demarcation. Instead, there is an intervening or anal transitional zone (ATZ) that measures several millimeters to just over 1 cm in length. This narrow ring of transitional epithelium is of great interest and of presumed significance in the histogenesis of certain anal neoplasms (Figure 34–2). Its microscopic appearance varies from an epithelium resembling lower urinary tract to one of stratified squamous, columnar, or cuboidal type.[1,2] The most characteristic pattern is an epithelium containing cells of columnar to cuboidal shape arranged in four to nine rows.[3] Small islands of colorectal type or of squamous epithelium, or both, may also be seen in this transitional zone. The upper border of the transitional zone merges with the normal mucosa of the rectum.

The anal ducts or glands open into the anal crypts. These long tubular structures usually extend distally for a short distance before penetrating into and occasionally through the internal sphincter muscle (Figure 34–3). They may also extend proximally beneath the rectal mucosa. The ducts are lined by transitional or stratified columnar epithelium, and mucus-producing cells are commonly seen, especially in the terminal portion. Nodules of lymphoid tissue may surround the gland ducts.

Recent studies of the ATZ by scanning and transmission electron microscopy have suggested that the mucosa might be metaplastic squamous epithelium rather than urothelium, with which it is often compared.[4] The anal canal epithelium has also been shown to contain endocrine cells and melanin-containing cells.[5]

The hemorrhoidal plexus of veins surrounding the anal canal consists of an internal and an external portion. Above the dentate line the internal hemorrhoidal plexus drains into the portal venous system by means of the superior rectal and inferior mesenteric veins. The external hemorrhoidal plexus below the dentate line drains into the internal iliac veins of the systemic circulation by means of the internal pudendal veins, which receive blood from the inferior rectal veins.

The muscular wall of the anal canal consists of two portions. The internal sphincter is composed of smooth muscle and represents the expanded continuation of the circular layer of the muscularis propria of the rectum. The external sphincter is composed of skeletal (voluntary) muscle and is divided into a deep, superficial part and a subcutaneous part representing a downward extension of the puborectalis muscle.

The mucosa of the anal canal above the dentate line is supplied by autonomic nerves and is insensitive to pain. The squamous mucosa of the pecten, however, is supplied by inferior rectal nerves of somatic type, which render the lower canal sensitive to pain, touch, and temperature.

The lymphatic drainage of the anal canal, like the vascular supply, is in two directions. The drainage of the upper canal is into inferior mesenteric and internal iliac nodes, and that of the canal below the dentate line is into the inguinal nodes.

In this chapter the pathologic features of disorders of the anal region will be discussed. Several recent reviews elaborate more completely on the anatomic, clinical, and therapeutic aspects of diseases in this area.[6,7]

DEVELOPMENTAL ABNORMALITIES

Congenital abnormalities of the rectum and anus occur in about 1 in every 5000 live births. Most have been somewhat loosely classified as examples of imperforate anus. After a period of extensive worldwide collaboration, a proposed "International Classification of Anorectal Anomalies" was presented in 1970.[8] This scheme is based on the relationships of the abnormality to the puborectalis muscle or levator sling and classifies lesions as low (translevator), intermediate, or high (supralevator).

The *low anomalies* comprise about 40% and may include anal stenosis, covered anus, anocutaneous fistula, anovulvar fistula, anovestibular fistula, anterior perineal anus, and vestibular anus. These tend to be the least severe types of defects. Pelvic innervation is normal. *Intermediate anomalies* are uncommon and account for about 15% of the total. They consist of anal agenesis or anorectal stenosis with or without the formation of fistula. The most significant lesions are the *high anomalies*, which make up 40% and are frequently associated with other sacral, neurologic, or urinary tract abnormalities. These are lesions of anorectal agenesis, and fistulas between the intestinal and urinary tracts occur only in this group.[9] Rare additional

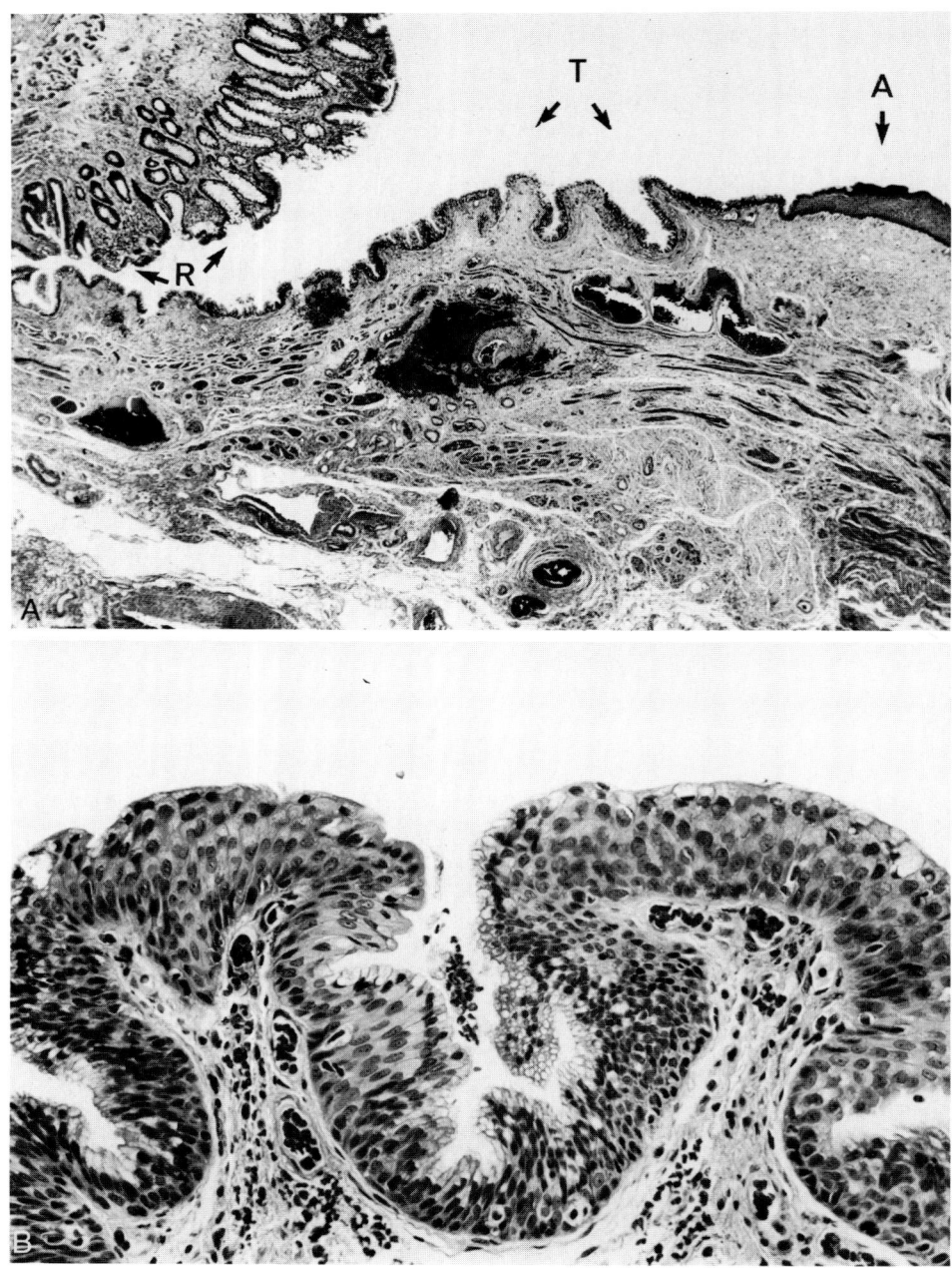

FIGURE 34–2. A, Scanning photomicrograph of normal anal transitional zone. Rectal mucosa is on left (R), transitional mucosa is in the broad central region (T), and anal stratified squamous mucosa is on the right (A). (H&E, × 35). B, Higher-power view of transitional mucosa, showing rows of cuboidal to columnar cells. Some mucus secreting cells are seen on the surface. (H&E, × 330)

anomalies that do not fit this classification include imperforate anal membrane. Further details on these anomalies are discussed in Chapter 8.

A recent report has suggested an increased risk of sacrococcygeal teratoma in patients with congenital anorectal malformations.[10] Because the frequency of malignant change in sacrococcygeal teratomas increases proportionately with age, recognition of this apparent association and early treatment are important.

HEMORRHOIDS

Recognized since the time of Hippocrates, hemorrhoids have traditionally been regarded as varicosities of the submucosal plexus of the superior hemorrhoidal veins. Recent evidence suggests, however, that hemorrhoids are "cushions" of tissue normally present in the anal submucosa and are composed of blood vessels, smooth muscle, and connective tissue.[11] They are located above the dentate line on the left lateral, right anterior, and right posterior aspects of the canal and are covered by transitional or rectal mucosa. They are normally present at birth. It is suggested that their engorgement during defecation serves a protective role for the anal canal.

Additional evidence that hemorrhoids are not simply varicosities is their lack of relationship with portal hypertension. Surgeons also recognize that they are more than distended veins because much of the bleeding during surgery is arterial.[12] Microscopically, hemor-

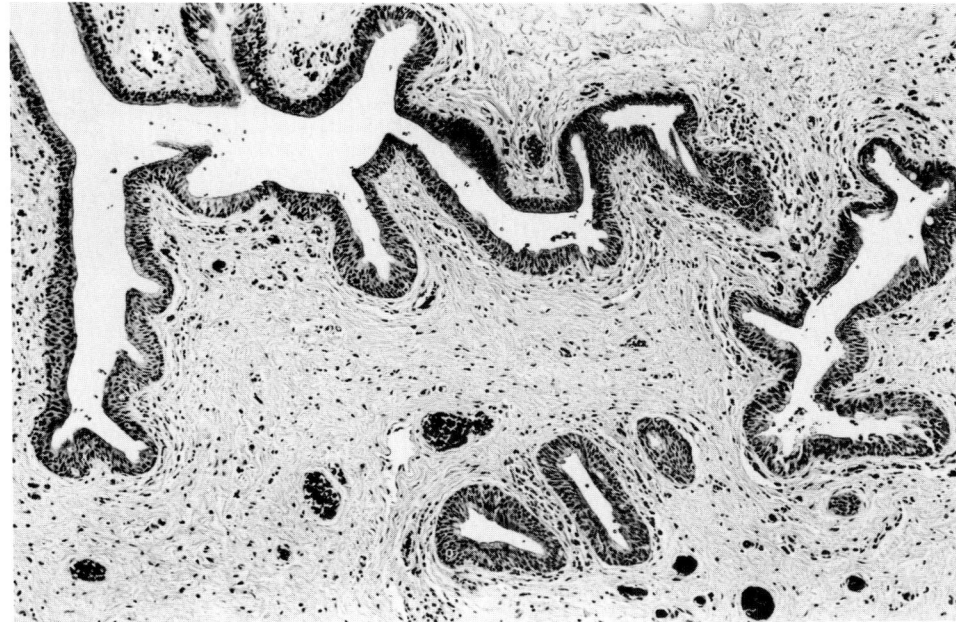

FIGURE 34–3. Anal ducts (glands) in the submucosal stroma, showing prominent branching. Ducts are lined by transitional epithelium. (H&E, × 125)

rhoids also contain more smooth muscle in their walls than do ordinary veins of similar size or in varicosities.

It has been suggested that with age these cushions bulge and then descend into the lumen of the anal canal.[12] As they lose their support, the lining becomes more susceptible to the effects of straining, resulting in the common symptoms of bleeding and protrusion. Hereditary and environmental factors as well as individual habits may be responsible for the variations in size of hemorrhoids, presentation, or symptoms in different individuals.

Hemorrhoids are commonly defined by their anatomic location.[6,7] Those above the dentate line are internal hemorrhoids and are covered mostly by rectal mucosa. Those below the dentate line are external hemorrhoids and are covered by the squamous mucosa of the pecten or by perianal skin. If the communications between the internal and external venus plexuses enlarge, combined internal and external hemorrhoids result.

Clinical classification of internal hemorrhoids is based on the degree of prolapse.[6,7] First-degree hemorrhoids bleed but do not protrude. Second-degree hemorrhoids protrude during defecation but reduce spontaneously. Third-degree hemorrhoids protrude and must be reduced manually. Fourth-degree hemorrhoids cannot be reduced. Complications such as thrombosis, necrosis, and inflammation may occur. Organization of thrombosed hemorrhoids may result in the formation of fibrous polyps or tags. Since internal hemorrhoids are innervated by the autonomic system, they generally present without pain.

External hemorrhoids present usually because of thrombosis, which is often painful, or because of the appearance of tags or polyps, which may result from organization of previously thrombosed hemorrhoids. In my opinion, tissues submitted following hemorrhoid surgery should be routinely examined microscopically. Although rare, microscopic evidence of infections, Crohn's disease, or early neoplasms that were unsuspected clinically may be identified.

PROLAPSE

Rectal prolapse (procidentia) is defined as the circumferential descent of rectum through the anal sphincter.[7] It is a condition seen most often in the very young or in the elderly. Prolapse of hemorrhoidal tissue also commonly occurs.

The reddened, protruding rectal mucosa in cases of procidentia and the surface of prolapsing hemorrhoids have a similar and very characteristic appearance (Figure 34–4). The features include fibromuscular obliteration of the lamina propria, thickening and often fragmentation of the muscularis mucosae, hyperplasia of mucosal glands often with a villous configuration, and telangiectasia of the surface vessels. Surface erosion may also occur.

These histologic features are entirely similar to the mucosal changes seen in the *solitary rectal ulcer syndrome*.[13–15] It has been suggested that the solitary rectal ulcer syndrome results from ischemia due to internal prolapse of the rectal mucosa.[13] In an effort to conceptually unify the similar nature of these processes the term *mucosal prolapse syndrome* has been proposed.[14] Recently added to this family of disorders has been *inflammatory cloacogenic polyp*, an unusual inflammatory polyp arising from the transitional zone of the anus (Figure 34–5).[16] This lesion has many histologic features similar to prolapsed mucosa, suggesting that prolapse of transitional zone mucosa may be important in its pathogenesis. Further details on these disorders are discussed in Chapter 28.

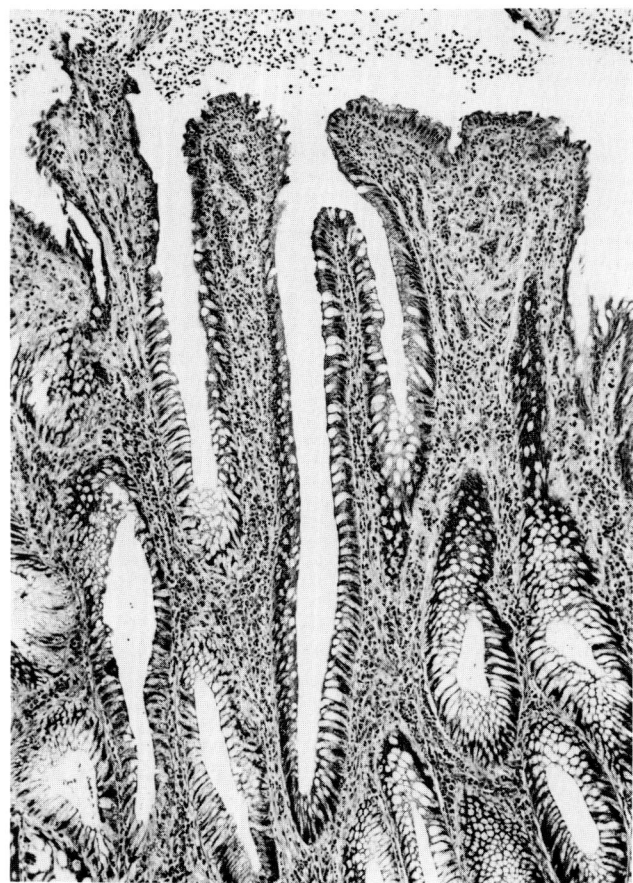

FIGURE 34–4. Prolapsed rectal mucosa. Note villous elongation and distortion of gland tubules, partial fibrous obliteration of lamina propria, and focal superficial erosion (upper left). (H&E, × 125)

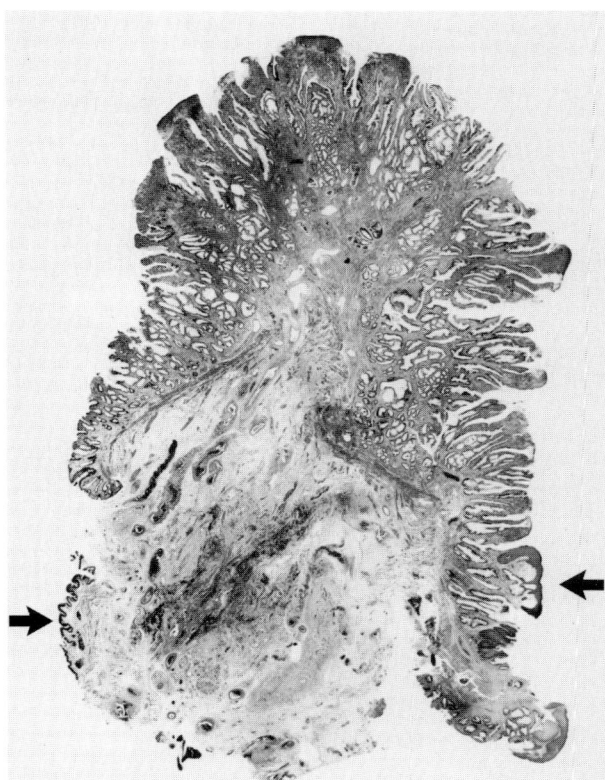

FIGURE 34–5. Scanning photomicrograph of inflammatory cloacogenic polyp. The mucosal surface has a microscopic appearance similar to that of the prolapsed mucosa in Figure 34–4. Remnants of transitional epithelium are present on the lower left (arrow) and of squamous epithelium on the lower right (arrow). (H&E, × 7)

INFLAMMATORY AND INFECTIOUS DISORDERS

Fissure

An anal fissure is an elongated, triangular ulcer of the anal canal.[6,7] Fissures typically extend from the dentate line to the anal verge. The great majority are located in the posterior midline of the canal overlying the lower portion of the internal sphincter. Most of the rest are in the anterior midline.

The precise pathogenesis is not clear, but most believe the lesion is the result of traumatic tearing, especially during defecation with the passage of large, firm stools. Most fissures are superficial and may heal rapidly. They may, however, become chronic. Dysfunction of the internal sphincter may contribute to the chronicity of the lesion. Histologically, fissures are characterized by nonspecific inflammation. Large, deep chronic fissures are known as *anal ulcers*. Frequently, chronic fissures are associated with hypertrophy of the anal papilla at the proximal end of the lesion to form a so-called *sentinel tag* or *pile*. Histologically, these are similar to other types of fibroepithelial papillomas and are covered by squamous mucosa. Occasionally, the stroma of large hypertrophied papillae may show cytologic atypia, which is regarded as a reactive phenomenon.[17]

When fissures are located in atypical positions or when they fail to heal following appropriate treatment, other diagnostic possibilities should be considered. These include inflammatory bowel disease, especially Crohn's disease, specific infections such as tuberculosis or syphilis, and carcinoma.

Fistula and Abscess

An anal fistula (fistula in ano) is a passage one end of which opens into an anal crypt at the dentate line. The fistula may extend to the skin or may terminate in the perineal soft tissue. Because most do not have openings at both ends of the track, these lesions are more accurately regarded as sinuses rather than fistulae.

Knowledge of the normal muscular anatomy of the region is important to an understanding of anorectal suppurative disease. Structurally, the muscles are arranged as two funnels, one located within the other.[18] The inner consists of the muscular wall of the rectum and anus including the terminal portion or internal sphincter. The outer funnel consists of the external sphincter and puborectalis muscles. Between the two is the intersphincteric space.

It is believed that the majority of suppurative processes in the area are the result of an initial infection of an anal duct, the anatomy of which provides a pathway between the anal canal and perianal soft tissues. The acute process in most cases is an abscess in the intersphincteric space. The formation of a fistula represents the chronic phase of this process. Anorectal abscess and fistula in ano are, therefore, different stages of the same basic condition.[18,19]

A detailed anatomic study has demonstrated that fistula in ano can be classified into four major groups based on the relationship of the track to the sphincteric muscles.[18]

1. *Intersphincteric,* the most common type, in which the fistula extends only into the intersphincteric space.

2. *Transsphincteric,* the next most common, in which the fistula passes from the intersphincteric space through the external sphincter to the ischiorectal fossa.

3. *Suprasphincteric,* in which the fistula extends in the intersphincteric space over the top of the puborectalis muscle, then downward through the levator to the ischiorectal fossa.

4. *Extrasphincteric,* the least common type, in which the fistula passes from rectum to perianal skin completely external to the external sphincteric complex.

Histologically the fistula is lined by granulation tissue and surrounded by a nonspecific acute and chronic inflammatory reaction. Giant cells of the foreign body type are frequently present and should not be confused with the granulomatous reaction seen in Crohn's disease. Fistulas do, however, occur in the course of inflammatory bowel disease, especially Crohn's disease, as well as in specific infections in the area. Carcinomas may also be associated with the formation of fistulas.

Hidradenitis Suppurativa

Hidradenitis suppurativa is a chronic and acute inflammatory process involving the skin and subcutaneous tissues, especially where aprocrine glands are found. The axilla is the most common site, but the anogenital area may also be affected. The term is actually a misnomer because involvement of the apocrine glands and adjacent deep structures is a secondary phenomenon. The primary event is probably related to follicular occlusion followed by a deep folliculitis, after which subcutaneous sinus tracts, abscesses, ulceration and scarring may develop.

It is important to distinguish this inflammatory process from other disorders in the area that are associated with fistula formation. Several differential diagnostic observations have been offered using the internal sphincter as a point of reference.[20] The sinus tract of hidradenitis is superficial to the sphincter muscle and involves the lower part of the canal distal to the dentate line. The fistula in ano penetrates and progresses deep to the sphincter muscle and originates in the crypt area of the dentate line. Finally, the fistula of Crohn's disease is often deep to all sphincter muscles and may involve rectal mucosa proximal to the dentate line.

Anal Lesions in Inflammatory Bowel Disease

The pathologic features of idiopathic inflammatory bowel disease are covered in detail in Chapter 27. Involvement of the anal region, however, is sufficiently common and important to merit additional comment here.

Ulcerative Colitis

In ulcerative colitis, anal involvement is usually nonspecific and not qualitatively different from that seen in patients without colitis. Superficial nonspecific inflammation is common, and acute lesions such as fissure, cryptitis, anorectal abscess, and fistula in ano may also occur.

Crohn's Disease

Anal involvement in Crohn's disease is more frequent and important than in ulcerative colitis. Reports of the frequency of anal manifestations vary rather widely based mainly on what types of lesions are included as anal involvement.[21-23] Generally, however, it is observed that 20% to 30% of patients with small-bowel involvement and 50% to 80% of patients with large-bowel involvement will develop anal lesions during the course of their disease. In some patients the anal manifestations may antedate by several years other clinical or radiographic evidence of disease in the more proximal intestinal tract.[24]

The typical clinical features of anal Crohn's disease have been well described.[21] Anal skin tags are common and tend to be larger, thicker, and firmer than tags in patients without Crohn's disease. Fissures are also common and are often large and deep with undermined edges. They also are more likely to occur in atypical positions than the non–Crohn's-associated fissure. Fistula in ano may be similar to that in patients without Crohn's disease but is more frequently complex with multiple openings often at a considerable distance from the anus. The features most characteristic of Crohn's disease in anal inflammatory processes are absence of pain and presence of chronicity, induration, multiplicity, and cyanotic coloration.

The diagnosis of anal Crohn's disease may be confirmed by the histologic demonstration of a sarcoid-like granulomatous reaction in the tissue lesions described above (Figure 34–6).[24] It is important to exclude anal tuberculosis with appropriate special stains. Care must also be taken not to confuse the giant-cell response to fecal debris commonly seen in fistula with the sarcoid-like reaction of Crohn's disease.

Recent attention has been given to a possible association between anal Crohn's disease and carcinoma of the anus. Several cases of anal squamous cell carcinoma and cloacogenic carcinoma in patients with anal

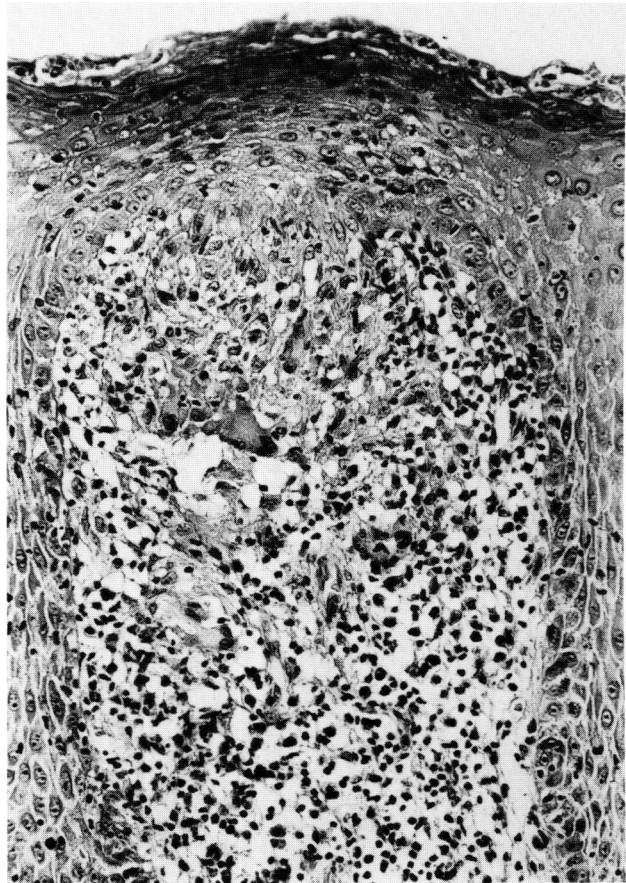

FIGURE 34-6. Sarcoid-like granulomatous reaction in an edematous anal tag from patient with advanced intestinal and anal Crohn's disease. Note the giant cell in the upper center of the field. (H&E, × 330)

Crohn's disease have been reported.[25-27] Although a definite relationship between the two has yet to be established conclusively, careful clinical observation of patients with anal Crohn's disease with special attention to any new or unusual lesions is important.

Sexually Transmitted Diseases

There has been a steady increase in the frequency of sexually transmitted diseases during the past several decades.[28] The increase has included not only such traditional venereal infections as syphilis, gonorrhea, lymphogranuloma venereum, chancroid, and granuloma inguinale but also, more dramatically, a host of other conditions including herpes, nonlymphogranulomatous chlamydial infections, candidiasis, condyloma acuminatum, and molluscum contagiosum. Anorectal venereal lesions are most commonly seen in male homosexuals who practice anorectal intercourse.[29,30] Patients may present with concurrent sexually transmitted infections of different types. In addition to the increased incidence of anorectal lesions in this population there is a risk of sexual transmission of enteric infections such as viral hepatitis, amebiasis, giardiasis, shigellosis, and *Campylobacter* enteritis.

During recent years there has been a dramatic increase in interest in sexually transmitted diseases. This is due to the noted increased frequency of these disorders as well as the enormous concern of both medical profession and general public with the acquired immunodeficiency syndrome (AIDS). Not only is AIDS most commonly transmitted sexually, but it is also often associated with other venereal disorders in the same patient. This section will review the common sexually transmitted diseases involving the anal region. Condyloma acuminatum will be considered later in a discussion of benign tumors.

Syphilis

Primary lesions of anogenital syphilis are frequently overlooked clinically. This is due both to the apparent trivial nature of the lesion as well as to its frequent similarity to other nonvenereal anal inflammatory disease, especially the common fissure. The typical lesion is an ulcer of the anal canal.[28,31] Unlike the primary ulcerated, indurated, and painless genital chancre, anal lesions of syphilis may be very painful.[7] Histologically the lesion is nonspecific. There is superficial ulceration with an underlying dense inflammatory infiltrate usually rich in plasma cells. Thick-walled blood vessels with prominent endothelial cells may be seen. Diagnosis may be accomplished by demonstration of spirochetes in fixed tissue by appropriate silver stains such as the Warthin-Starry stain, by darkfield microscopic examination of lesional scrapings, or by fluorescent treponemal antibody staining.

Secondary lesions of anogenital syphilis include the typical raised condylomata lata, which may be seen in association with a characteristic maculopapular rash.[28] Other anorectal lesions seen in syphilis include polyps and smooth lobulated masses that may simulate neoplasms.[32]

Gonorrhea

Anorectal gonorrhea is common in the male homosexual population.[28,30,33] In women anorectal involvement is the result either of anorectal intercourse or of secondary spread from the vagina. The usual lesion is an acute or subacute proctitis, but the upper anal canal including anal crypts and ducts may also be affected.

Herpes Simplex

Herpes of the anogenital region is usually due to infection by herpes simplex virus, type II (HSV-2).[7,28,32] It results in most cases from direct inoculation during anorectal intercourse. The patient first notes perianal itching and paresthesia several days to 2 weeks after exposure. This is followed by intense anal pain. Grossly the lesions are erythematous with small clustered vesicles that soon rupture and give rise to larger ulcers. The perianal skin and anal canal are most frequently involved, but the distal rectal mucosa may also be affected. Resolution usually occurs within 2 weeks, but recurrences are very common. Histologically, the lesions are similar to lesions of other cutaneous and mucosal surfaces caused by HSV-2. They are characterized by vesicle formation resulting from a reticular-type degeneration of the epithelium. Characteristic giant cells with prominent intranuclear inclusions are generally easily identified in early lesions.

Chlamydia

Nonlymphogranulomatous chlamydial infection of the genitals is the most common sexually transmitted inflammatory disease.[7,28] The usual presentation is as a nonspecific urethritis in men or a nonspecific infection of the lower genital tract in women, but anorectal infection may occur in patients practicing anorectal intercourse.

Molluscum Contagiosum

Molluscum contagiosum is a contagious disorder characterized clinically by the appearance of multiple small, waxy papules with umbilicated centers. Histologically the lesions consist of epidermal lobules that extend into the dermis. Prominent inclusion bodies are characteristic. The disease, caused by a member of the poxvirus family, is spread by close body contact and, therefore, may be sexually transmissible. The most common sites of involvement are skin of abdomen, thigh, perineum, penis, scrotum, and vulva. The buttocks and perianal area, however, may occasionally be affected.

Lymphogranuloma Venereum, Chancroid, and Granuloma Inguinale

These lesions are all rare venereal infections in industrialized countries.[28] Each may occasionally be associated with anorectal lesions. There is a suspected though not proven relationship between lymphogranuloma venereum and carcinoma of the anus.

Tuberculosis

Anorectal tuberculosis has steadily decreased in frequency in most parts of the world but remains quite common in those areas where pulmonary and intestinal tuberculosis are common. Involvement of the gastrointestinal tract results either exogenously from ingestion of contaminated milk or as endogenous spread from another site, especially the lung. Several types of anal and perianal tuberculosis have been described including ulcerative, hypertrophic, verrucous, lupoid, and miliary.[34,35] The ulcerative form is the most common. The verrucous form is the least common and presents as a warty mass in the anal canal (Figure 34–7).

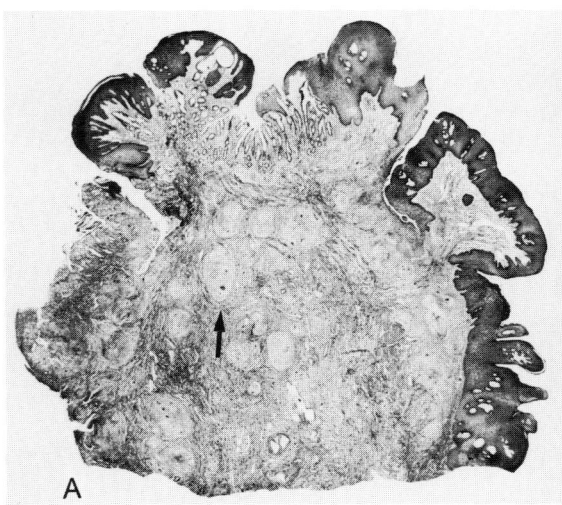
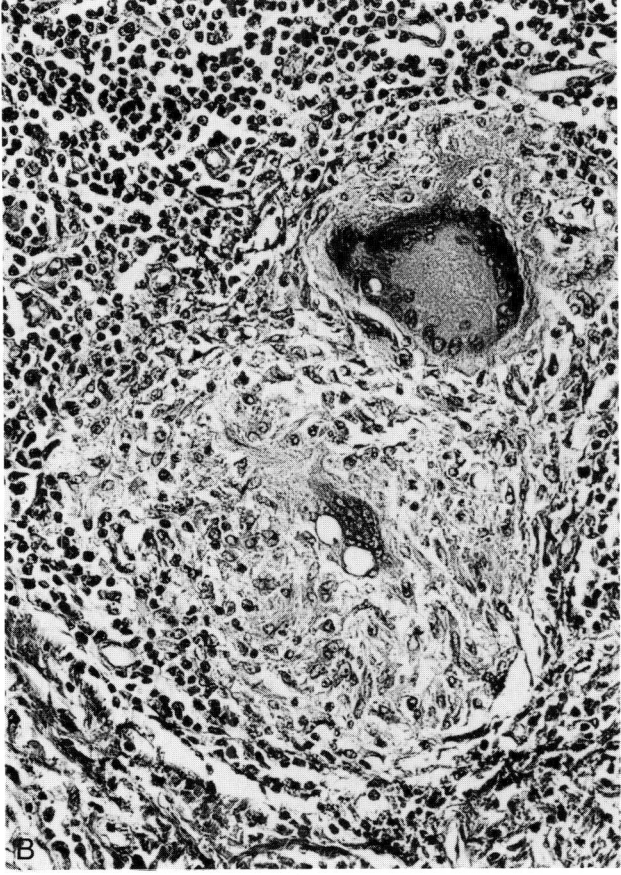

FIGURE 34–7 A, Scanning power of a polypoid lesion of verrucous tuberculosis of the anus. (H&E, × 7.5) B, Higher-power view of the area marked by the arrow in A, showing a granuloma with early caseation. Acid-fast bacilli were easily identified. (H&E, × 330)

All forms must be distinguished from other types of anal inflammatory disease, especially Crohn's disease. The verrucous variant must also be distinguished from carcinoma.

Other Conditions

A variety of other inflammatory, infectious, and nonneoplastic conditions are occasionally associated with anal involvement. Many dermatologic disorders may affect the anal region. Lichen sclerosus et atrophicus is rather common in the anogenital region of postmenopausal women but may also occur in children.[36] Rare examples of malakoplakia have been reported in the anus.[37] Eosinophilic colitis is usually seen in the proximal gastrointestinal tract, but anal involvement may occur.[38] A recent report presents a young patient with an anal abscess due to *Enterobious vermicularis*.[39] A wide spectrum of anal inflammatory lesions including ulcers and abscesses have also been described in patients with hematologic disorders.[40] A variety of microorganisms have been cultured from these lesions, the most frequent being *Escherichia coli* and *Pseudomonas aeruginosa*.

BENIGN TUMORS AND TUMOR-LIKE LESIONS

Condyloma Acuminatum

Condyloma acuminatum, or common genital wart, is a sexually transmitted disease caused by members of the human papillomavirus family (HPV). The typical condyloma is a soft, fleshy, gray-tan to pink papillomatous growth that frequently occurs in multiples. In men genital warts are usually located on the penis, anus, or uncommonly the scrotum. In women the lesions are most frequent on the vulva, vaginal introitus, perineum, anus, and cervix.

Condyloma acuminatum is the most common tumor of the anal and perianal region. In this area the perianal skin is most frequently involved, but many patients have anal canal lesions as well. Condylomata of the anal region may be seen in association with penile warts in men or with vulvar warts in women, but they may also occur as the sole manifestation of infection in male homosexuals who practice anorectal intercourse.[41] They frequently occur together with other sexually transmitted disorders.

Histologically the typical condyloma acuminatum is a papillomatous lesion characterized by pronounced acanthosis of the squamous epithelium (Figure 34–8). At the base of the lesion the proliferating epithelium shows no evidence of invasion. There is orderly and progressive maturation of the epithelium, and the surface usually shows parakeratosis. Commonly present near the surface of the lesion are squamous cells with vacuolated cytoplasm surrounding variably enlarged and hyperchromatic nuclei. This feature, known as "koilocytotic" change or atypia, is a histologic hallmark of HPV infection.

Within the past decade there has been increasing interest in the relationship between HPV infection and neoplasia of the lower female genital tract, especially cervix and vulva.[42-45] Of great significance in this area of active investigation is the observation that evidence of HPV infection of the cervix is usually in the subclinical form of a flat condyloma rather than the acuminate lesion described here. Several types of HPV have been implicated in anogenital lesions, including types 6, 11, 16, and 18. HPV-6 and HPV-11 are most likely to be associated with the grossly papillary benign condylomata acuminata, whereas HPV-16 and less commonly HPV-18 are associated with high-grade dysplastic lesions.[43-45] Anal warts have been found to contain virus in low concentration, usually HPV-6.[41]

An important and as yet incompletely resolved issue concerns the premalignant potential of the anal condyloma. Several examples of carcinoma *in situ* associated with anal condylomata have been described.[46,47] Of particular interest in one of these reports is the observation that five of the nine patients had developed AIDS.[47] Occasional cases of invasive squamous cell carcinoma arising in anal condylomata have also been described.[48,49] Care must be taken to distinguish malignant change in a condyloma from the bizarre atypia seen after topical treatment of these lesions with podophyllum resin.[50] These changes may persist for several weeks after application.

Bowenoid Papulosis

Bowenoid papulosis (dysplasia) was initially described as a lesion of the genitalia of young adults.[51,52] It is characterized clinically by multiple, small, pigmented papules. In addition to the common penile and vulvar involvement, anal lesions may also occur.[53] Although clinically benign in appearance, these lesions have histologic features that are very similar to those of *in situ* squamous cell carcinoma (Bowen's disease). In contrast to classic Bowen's disease, however, bowenoid papulosis (dysplasia) usually presents a more orderly maturation of keratinocytes, greater nuclear uniformity, and milder cellular anaplasia (Figure 34–9). Although clinical follow-up suggests that bowenoid papulosis (dysplasia) is a benign condition, it probably should be included within the spectrum of intraepithelial neoplasia.[45] HPV-16 has been demonstrated in these lesions.[54] In a study of vulvar lesions, many patients with these bowenoid lesions also had condylomata acuminata.[52]

Adnexal Tumors

Adnexal tumors of several varieties have been observed in the perianal skin. Most are of apocrine gland origin including such lesions as the apocrine gland adenoma and aprocrine fibroadenoma.[55,56] Hidradenoma

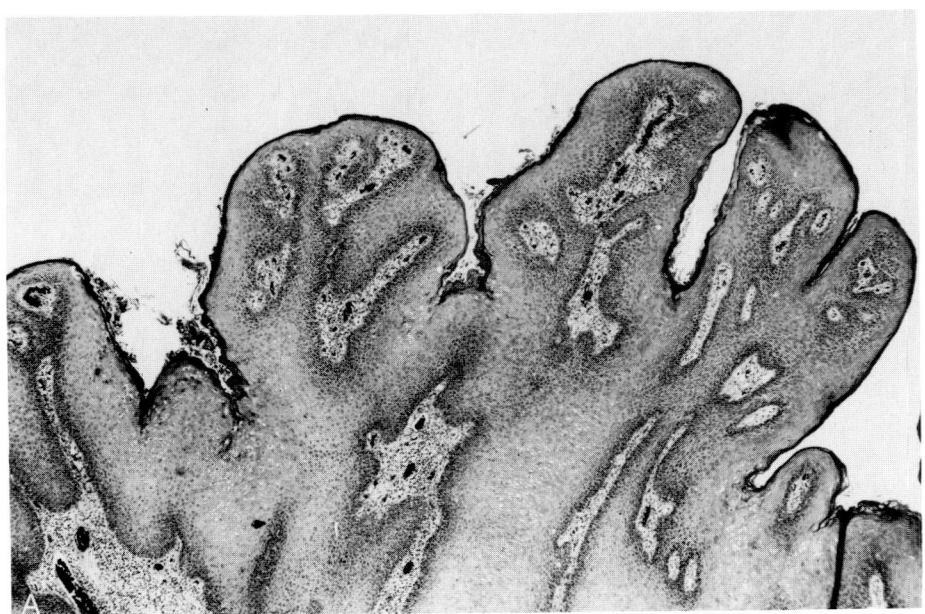
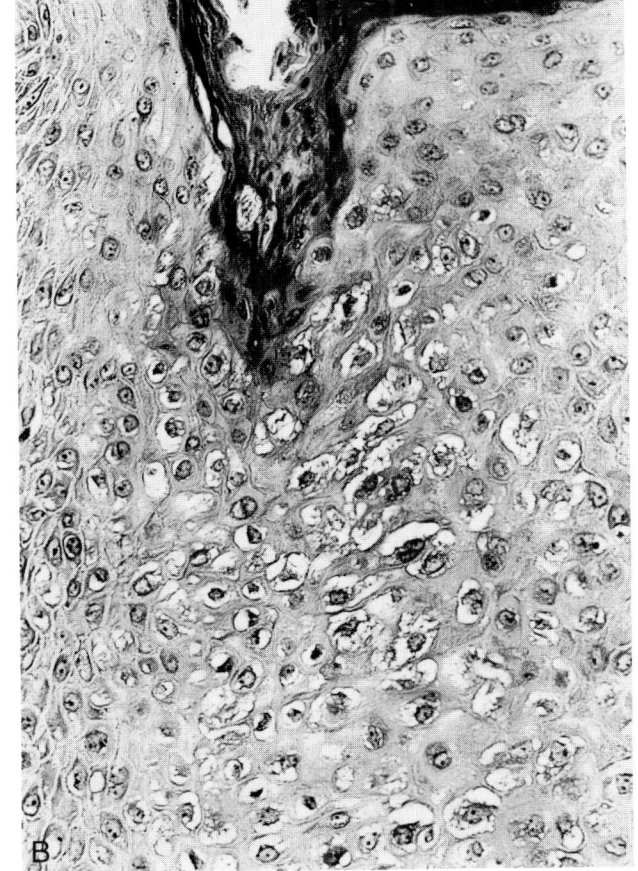

FIGURE 34–8. *A,* Scanning photomicrograph of condyloma acuminatum showing typical papillary architecture. (H&E, × 35) *B,* Higher-power view of condyloma acuminatum showing vacuolated cytoplasm of koilocytotic cells. (H&E, × 330)

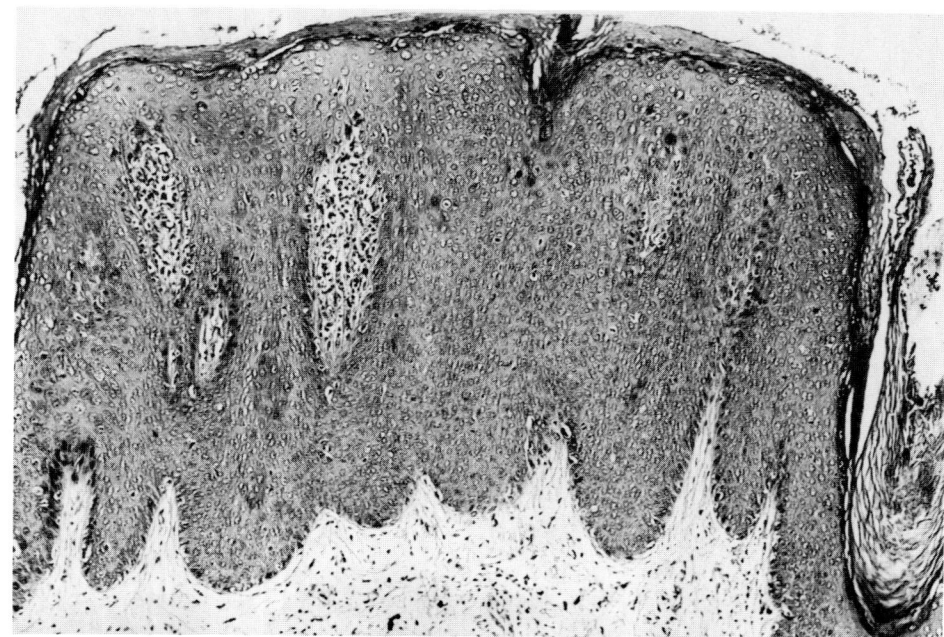

FIGURE 34–9. Perianal lesion of bowenoid papulosis (dysplasia) in a 31-year-old woman. Note the markedly atypical but orderly squamous epithelium with nuclear uniformity. (H&E, × 125)

papilliferum, a benign sweat gland tumor usually found in the vulva, may also occur in the anal region.

Keratoacanthoma

Keratoacanthoma is a benign exophytic tumor of skin usually found on sun-exposed surfaces such as the dorsum of the hands and the face. Rare examples from the anal region have been described.[57,58] Just as in lesions of sun-exposed skin, it is important to distinguish this rapidly growing, "infiltrative" but clinically benign tumor from squamous cell carcinoma.

Granular Cell Tumor and Neurilemoma

Granular cell tumors (myoblastomas) are common benign tumors that occur in a wide range of tissues and organs. The anal region is an infrequent site.[59,60] The lesions are composed of plump, granular cells that show diastase-resistant positivity with the periodic acid–Schiff (PAS) method. Although it was originally believed that the tumor was of muscle origin, it is now generally believed but not conclusively proved that the lesions are derived from Schwann's cells. A feature of special significance in granular cell tumors arising beneath mucosal surfaces is the frequent presence of pseudoepitheliomatous hyperplasia of the overlying epithelium (Figure 34–10). Other benign neural tumors such as neurilemomas have also been described in the anal area.[61]

Leiomyoma

Other benign lesions derived from mesenchymal tissue can also arise in this area. We have seen a single example of leiomyoma arising from the internal sphincter, and a few others have been reported.[62,63]

Oleogranuloma

Oleogranuloma is a benign reactive process that may grossly simulate a neoplasm. These lesions usually present as submucosal nodules in the lower rectum or anal canal, but ulcerated and annular lesions have also been described.[64] The lesion is a foreign body reaction to oily substances most commonly employed in the injection of hemorrhoids. Histologically there are lipid granulomas with associated inflammation and fibrosis.

MALIGNANT TUMORS

General Considerations

Before proceeding with a discussion of individual malignant neoplasms arising in the anal region, general considerations relating to the confusing subject of anal carcinoma will be addressed. The classification of malignant epithelial tumors of this region is complicated by an inadequate appreciation of the microscopic anatomy of the area as well as the related multiplicity of microscopic patterns expressed by these neoplasms.

The histologic junction between anus and rectum is not an abrupt interface between the squamous epithelium of the anal canal and the columnar, glandular mucosa of the lower rectum. Rather, there is an irregular, intervening "transitional" zone of presumed cloacogenic derivation. The existence of this special mucosa has been recognized for more than 100 years.[65] However, it was not until more than 75 years later that it was suggested that neoplasms of a characteristic but varied histologic type arose from this epithelium.[66] The

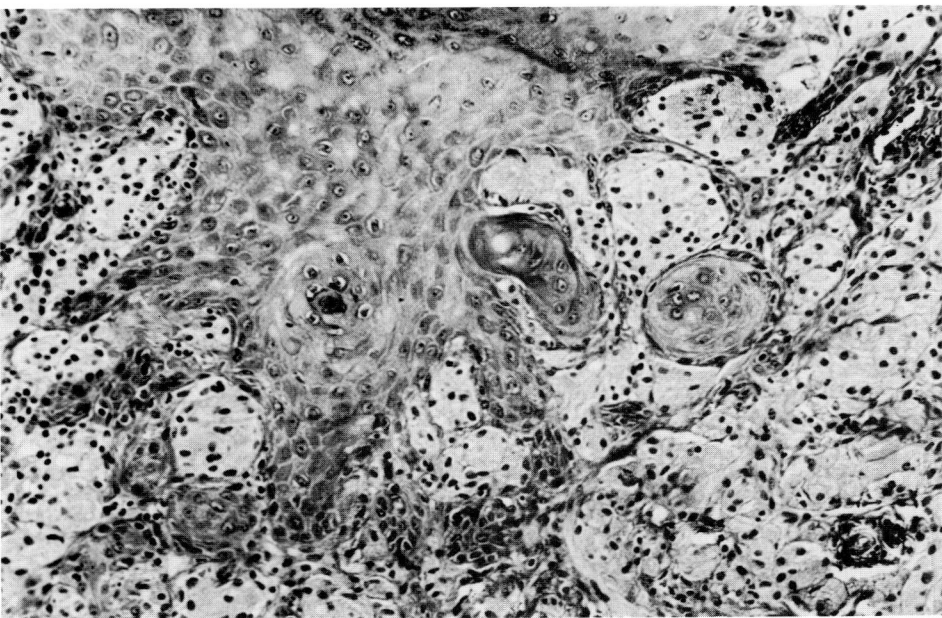

FIGURE 34-10. Granular cell tumor of the anal canal with pseudoepitheliomatous hyperplasia of the overlying squamous mucosa. The granular cells are noted between nests of proliferating squamous epithelium. (H&E, × 320)

term *transitional cloacogenic carcinoma* was proposed for these neoplasms. A host of descriptive terms have been used subsequently to designate members of this family of tumors including basaloid, transitional, nonkeratinizing squamous cell, cloacogenic, and mucoepidermoid carcinoma. It is appropriate to regard this multiplicity of microscopic patterns of anal carcinoma as a reflection of the histologic variability of the transitional zone.

It is likely that the subject of anal carcinoma has been made unnecessarily complicated by focusing too much attention on the diverse histologic characteristics of these tumors. It should be emphasized that the most important issue is the site of origin of these tumors, that is, the distinction between tumors arising in the anal canal from tumors arising at the anal margin.

Anal Canal Carcinoma

Anal canal carcinoma is nearly three times more common than anal margin carcinoma.[66] It is, however, an uncommon cancer, accounting for only 2% to 4% of all malignant tumors of the distal large bowel. These neoplasms arise grossly above or mainly above the dentate line. They arise from the mucous membrane of the upper anal canal and include those that have been designated as cloacogenic carcinoma. They may be grossly indistinguishable from adenocarcinoma of lower rectum.

Anal canal carcinoma is two to four times more common in women than men, and the average age in most series is from 55 to 60 years.[67-73] Common presenting symptoms are bleeding, anal pain, change in bowel habit, sensation of a mass, and pruritus ani. Treatment and survival data have been addressed in detail in several recent publications.[68,73] The most important prognostic indicators are depth of invasion and extent of spread of tumor. To date there has been no generally accepted and widely utilized staging system for anal canal carcinomas. Various centers presenting series have developed their own staging schemes usually based on depth of invasion and extent of tumor.[68,69,70] Specific histologic type has not yet been a significant predictor of survival, but differentiation has been useful and correlates with the frequency of lymph node metastases.[66,74] Anal canal carcinomas spread commonly into the lower one third of the rectum and most commonly involve the perirectal and later the inguinal lymph nodes. Generally, the 5-year survival rates for patients with carcinoma of the anal canal have been in the range of 45% to 50%. The American Joint Committee on Cancer (AJCC) has developed universal staging systems for all anatomic sites including the anal canal (Tables 34-1 and 34-2).[75] It is hoped that widespread use of a common staging system will permit easier comparison of data concerning therapy and prognosis.

Anal Margin Carcinoma

Carcinoma of the anal margin typically arises in the distal anal canal at the junction of anal squamous epithelium and true, hair-bearing perianal skin. These tumors are more common in men and occur in the same general age range as anal canal carcinoma. Most are well- to moderately well-differentiated squamous cell (epidermoid) carcinoma, usually of the keratinizing type.[66,76] Clinically, early lesions present as small, firm nodules, whereas more advanced tumors are often ulcerated. Verrucous forms of squamous cell carcinoma may also occur at this site. Coexisting conditions are much more common in association with cancer of the anal margin than of the anal canal.[76] These include condyloma, chronic fistulae, chronic pruritus, and a histology of previous radiation treatment. Coexisting Bowen's disease may also occur. Carcinoma of the anal

Table 34–1 TNM COMPONENTS IN THE AMERICAN JOINT COMMITTEE ON CANCER (AJCC) SYSTEM FOR STAGING CANCER OF THE ANAL CANAL

Category	Description
Tx	Primary tumor cannot be assessed
T0	No evidence of primary tumor
Tis	Carcinoma *in situ*
T1	Tumor 2 cm or less in greatest dimension
T2	Tumor more than 2 cm but not more than 5 cm in greatest dimension
T3	Tumor more than 5 cm in greatest dimension
T4	Tumor of any size invades adjacent organ(s), e.g., vagina, urethra, bladder (involvement of the sphincter muscle(s) *alone* is not classified as T4)
Nx	Regional lymph nodes cannot be assessed
N0	No regional lymph node metastasis
N1	Metastasis in perirectal lymph node(s)
N2	Metastasis in unilateral internal iliac and/or inguinal lymph node(s)
N3	Metastasis in perirectal and inguinal lymph nodes and/or bilateral internal iliac and/or inguinal lymph nodes
Mx	The presence of distant metastasis cannot be assessed
M0	No distant metastasis
M1	Distant metastasis present

From Beahrs OH, Henson DE, Hutter RVP, Myers MH: Manual for Staging of Cancer, 3rd ed. Philadelphia, JB Lippincott, 1988, pp 81–83.

Table 34–2 STAGE GROUPINGS IN THE AJCC SYSTEM FOR STAGING CANCER OF THE ANAL CANAL

Stage	Grouping		
0	Tis	N0	M0
I	T1	N0	M0
II	T2	N0	M0
	T3	N0	M0
IIIA	T4	N0	M0
	T1	N1	M0
	T2	N1	M0
	T3	N1	M0
IIIB	T4	N1	M0
	Any T	N2, N3	M0
IV	Any T	Any N	M1

From Beahrs OH, Henson DE, Hutter RVP, Myers MH: Manual for Staging of Cancer, 3rd ed. Philadelphia, JB Lippincott, 1988, pp 81–83.

margin grows more slowly than carcinoma of the anal canal, is more amenable to local treatment, and has a better prognosis. Metastasis to inguinal lymph nodes may occur, but visceral metastases are quite uncommon.

Studies investigating possible etiologic factors in anal carcinoma are somewhat confusing because of the failure of some reports to distinguish between anal canal and anal margin tumors. Nevertheless, several interesting observations have been made. It has been noted recently that homosexual males appear to be at increased risk for anal carcinoma, presumably related to the practice of anorectal intercourse.[77–80a] Both *in situ* and invasive squamous cell carcinomas have been described and, as noted earlier, malignant change has been observed in condylomata from this patient population.[47] A recent study that histologically examined all anal tissue submitted to a surgical pathology service identified 6.7% of 180 specimens from men with foci of mucosal atypia, whereas only 0.85% of 118 specimens from women had similar lesions.[81] Some of these lesions contained koilocytotic changes suggestive of infection by HPV. Of 14 men with these atypical lesions whose sexual orientation was known, 11 (79%) were homosexuals. Another study has demonstrated HPV antigens by immunohistochemistry in both condylomata and squamous cell carcinomas of the anus in homosexual men.[82] Only one of the eight homosexual men in this study had AIDS. A recent study applying a sensitive *in situ* hybridization technique detected HPV mesenger RNA in 12 of 18 anal carcinomas.[82a]

An additional observation in women with anal carcinoma is the increased frequency of other cancers of the lower genital tract.[83] The continuous epithelial surface of the area shares a closely related embryologic origin, a factor of possible etiologic and pathogenetic significance in multifocal anogenital cancer in women.

Carcinoma *in Situ*

Intramucosal carcinoma and varying degrees of dysplasia are frequently observed in mucosa adjacent to invasive carcinoma of both the anal canal and the anal margin (Figure 34–11). Anal canal carcinoma may also be associated with *in situ* involvement of the contiguous anal ducts. *In situ* squamous cell carcinoma has been demonstrated in condyloma acuminatum and in anal mucosa of homosexual males.[47] Extension of perineal *in situ* carcinoma to the contiguous anal mucosa in women has also been observed.[84]

An interesting but not entirely unexpected observation is the occurrence of atypical (dysplastic) mucosa in anal tissues removed for a variety of benign conditions.[81,85] In one study previously noted, a preponderance of the patients with atypical lesions were homosexual males.[81] Another study describing unsuspected dysplastic changes in 2.3% of 306 surgical specimens removed for benign diseases noted no difference in sex distribution and did not comment on homosexuality.[85]

Bowen's disease, a clinicopathologic variant of *in situ* squamous cell carcinoma, only rarely involves the anal area.[86,87] When anal involvement occurs, it is usually of the anal margin and adjacent perianal skin and may accompany more extensive perineal Bowen's disease. Clinically, Bowen's disease is manifested by discrete, red plaques with a scaly or fissured surface.[88] Symptoms of itching and burning may occur. Histologically the squamous epithelium exhibits striking disorganization with numerous large, atypical squamous cells and loss of normal polarity and orderly maturation (Figure 34–12). Mitotic figures, often of markedly atypical type, may be seen at all levels of epithelium. The process usually also involves the epithelium of the cutaneous appendages. Bowen's disease may be asso-

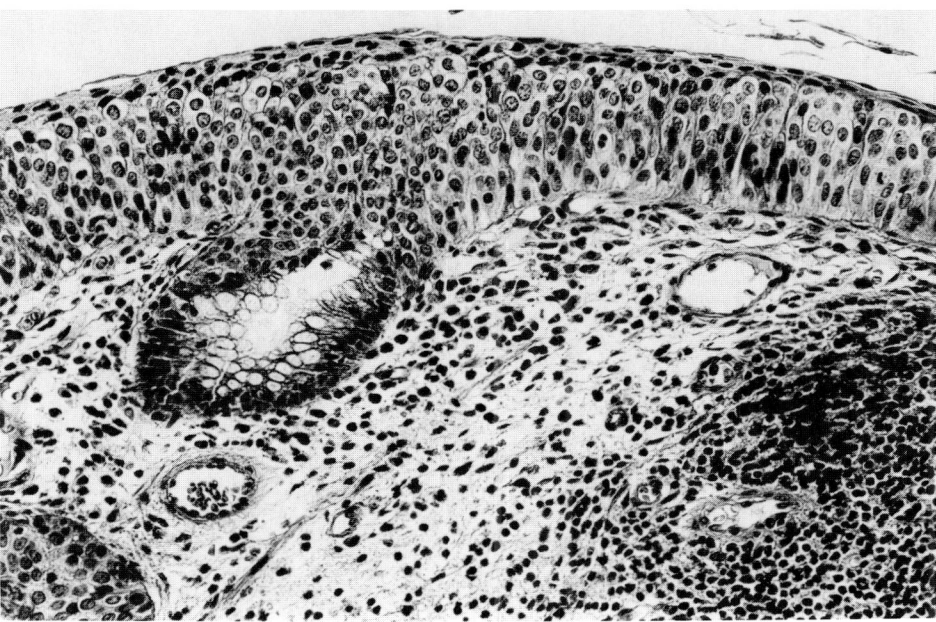

FIGURE 34–11. Carcinoma *in situ* extending into the lower rectum adjacent to invasive carcinoma of the anal canal. (H&E, × 330)

ciated with an increased risk of other cutaneous and internal cancers.[53]

"Cloacogenic" Carcinoma

So-called cloacogenic carcinoma is a tumor of the upper anal canal that is believed to arise from the transitional zone epithelium. Grinvalsky and Helwig were the first to suggest the potential of this special epithelium for giving rise to neoplasms morphologically distinct from usual squamous cell (epidermoid) carcinoma.[2] Others also have supported the contention that cloacogenic carcinoma is a distinct clinicopathologic entity.[67,89-90a] Electron microscopic observations have suggested that both anal transitional epithelium and cloacogenic carcinoma are morphologically different from urothelium and squamous epithelium.[90] A confusing profusion of descriptive terms has evolved, sometimes used as synonyms for cloacogenic carcinoma and sometimes to define histologic subtypes. These include basaloid, transitional, nonkeratinizing squamous cell (epidermoid), and mucoepidermoid carcinoma.

Regardless of the dominant histologic pattern, foci of more typical squamous differentiation are often ob-

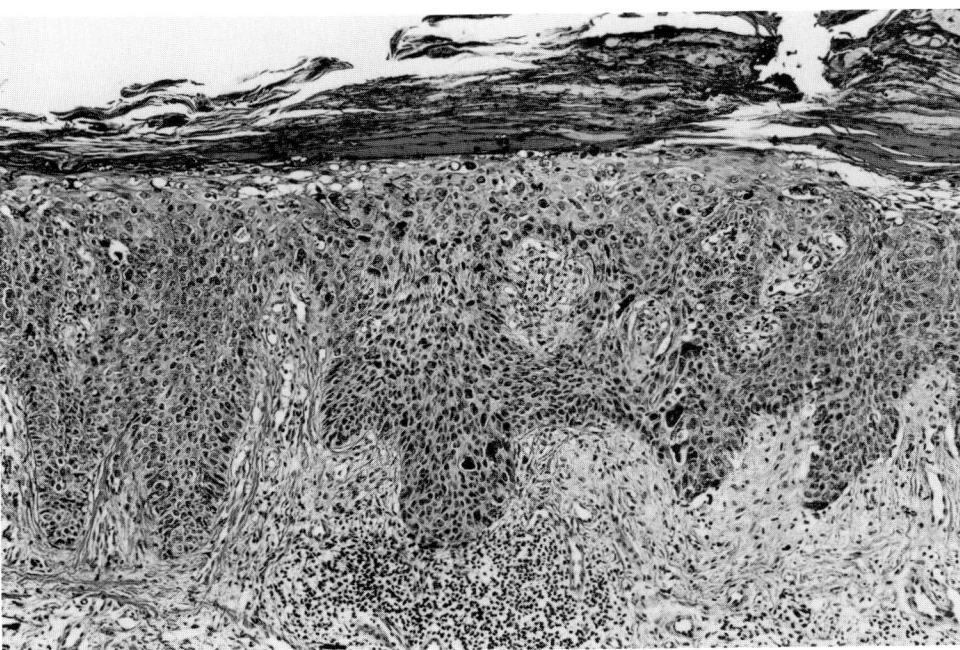

FIGURE 34–12. Bowen's disease (*in situ* squamous cell carcinoma). Note marked cellular anaplasia, disorderly maturation and overlying parakeratotic scale. (H & E, × 330)

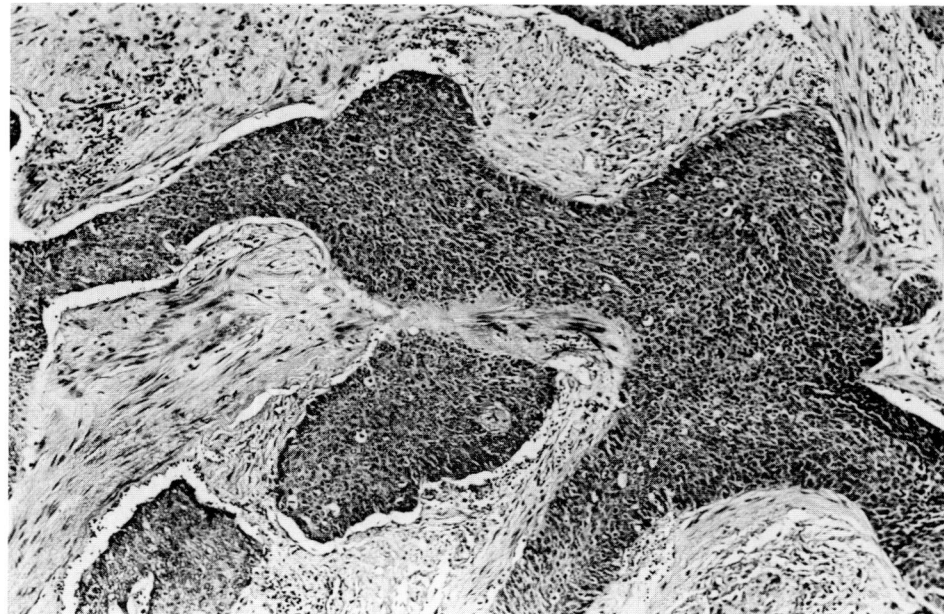

FIGURE 34–13. Low-power view of invasive "cloacogenic" carcinoma, showing a typical branching trabecular pattern. (H&E, × 125)

served. Low-power view frequently shows an irregular, angulated, and trabeculated pattern of infiltrating tumor (Figure 34–13). One or another histologic subtype may dominate the appearance at higher power (Figure 34–14). Basaloid or transitional type lesions are composed of nests and trabeculae of small cells without obvious intercellular bridges. Some observers reserve the term *basaloid* for those with palisading of cells at the periphery of the nests, a feature that is somewhat reminiscent of cutaneous basal cell carcinoma. Those without palisading have been morphologically compared with transitional cell tumors of urothelium. Many of these basaloid or transitional tumors contain small collections of squamoid cells or foci of indistinct pearl formation, often in the center of larger nests of tumor cells. Zones of central necrosis may also be a prominent feature. Other tumors are characterized by the presence of small cystic or acinar foci lined by mucus-producing cells, sometimes referred to as mucoepidermoid carcinomas. Even less common are tumors with features reminiscent of adenoid cystic carcinoma. Mitotic figures are not uncommon, but marked cellular pleomorphism is rare. It should be emphasized that any single tumor may show mixtures of all of these histologic patterns. The adjacent anal epithelium often shows *in situ* carcinoma (see Figure 34–11).

Neoplasms of this type may also occasionally arise from the anal duct epithelium, which shares a common embryologic origin with the transitional zone. With large, bulky tumors it may be difficult to identify the precise site of origin. Interestingly, some small lesions may rarely be associated with *in situ* carcinomatous changes in both anal duct and transitional zone epithelium.[53]

It has been suggested that despite this wide spectrum of histologic appearances, these neoplasms fundamentally are variants of squamous cell carcinoma.[66,69,71,72] In general, the higher the tumor arises in the anal canal, the more cloacogenic or basaloid are its features, and the more distal its origin, the more squamous is the appearance. Some have recognized a justification for retaining the descriptive terms for the various major histologic patterns such as basaloid (cloacogenic, transitional) or squamous cell carcinoma.[66,70,72] Others have asserted that because these terms have no prognostic or other biologic significance to justify a separation from squamous cell carcinomas of the anal canal, their use should be discontinued.[71] A recent study using rigid histologic criteria has suggested that anal cloacogenic and squamous cell carcinomas are distinct neoplasms.[90a] This conclusion was reinforced by the identification of HPV DNA by *in situ* hybridization in 14 of 21 squamous cell carcinomas (HPV types 16/18 in 12 and types 6/11 in 2), but in none of 14 cloacogenic carcinomas.

The significance of tumor grading and staging of anal canal carcinoma has been previously addressed. As noted, the degree of differentiation appears to be more significant than the specific histologic subtype. Within the basaloid or transitional group, the presence of distinct palisading of cells is a feature of better-differentiated tumors.[66,67] Extent of tumor remains the most reliable criterion for predicting survival, but comparison of published data has been hindered by the lack of a uniformly utilized staging system. Cloacogenic carcinoma, particularly that with a basaloid or transitional pattern, should be distinguished from small-cell (neuroendocrine) carcinoma, an uncommon tumor that may arise in the lower rectum or upper anal canal.

Squamous Cell Carcinoma

Many tumors that fit within the category of cloacogenic (basaloid, transitional) carcinoma of the anal

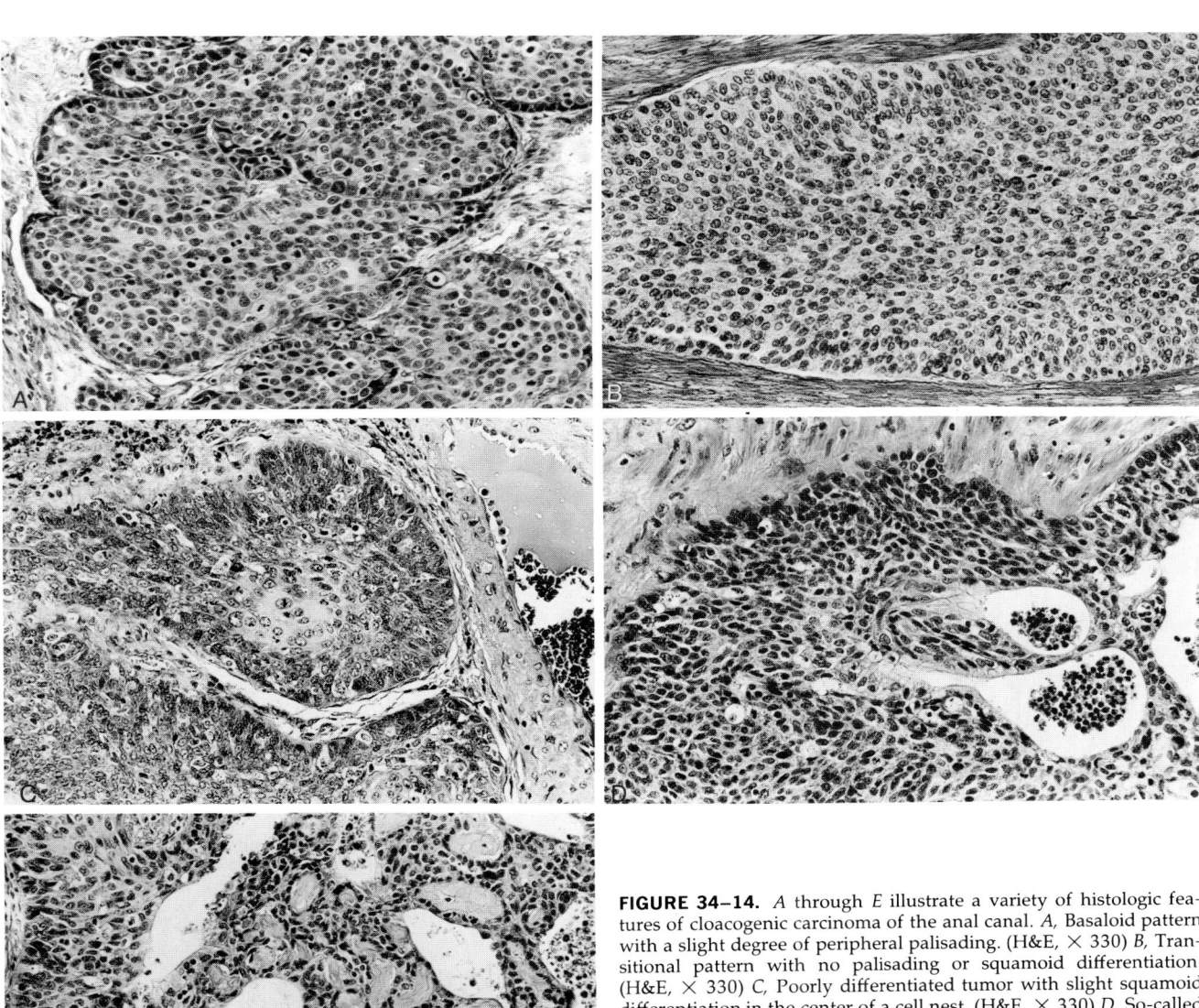

FIGURE 34–14. A through E illustrate a variety of histologic features of cloacogenic carcinoma of the anal canal. A, Basaloid pattern with a slight degree of peripheral palisading. (H&E, × 330) B, Transitional pattern with no palisading or squamoid differentiation. (H&E, × 330) C, Poorly differentiated tumor with slight squamoid differentiation in the center of a cell nest. (H&E, × 330) D, So-called mucoepidermoid pattern with mucus-secreting cells lining microcysts. (H&E, × 330) E, Pseudo-adenoid cystic pattern with microcysts and trabecular arrangement of hyalinized stroma. (H&E, × 330)

canal have variable degrees of squamous differentiation. The more distal lesions tend to have a greater degree of squamous differentiation. Carcinomas of the anal margin are typically pure squamous cell tumors, usually keratinizing, and of well- or moderately well-differentiated type (Figure 34–15).

Verrucous Carcinoma

Verrucous carcinoma is an exceedingly well-differentiated variant of squamous cell carcinoma that occurs most commonly in the oral cavity.[91] These tumors are characterized by a bulky, warty gross appearance and by a histologically benign appearance. They are locally invasive growths with pushing rather than infiltrating tumor margins. Only rare examples have been described involving the anal region.[92]

Giant Condyloma Acuminatum

Giant condyloma acuminatum (Buschke-Loewenstein's tumor) was initially described as a tumor of the penis. Rare examples arising from the anorectal area have now been reported.[93–96] These are large verrucous growths that tend to invade locally. It appears very likely that verrucous carcinoma and giant condyloma acuminatum are the same lesion.[96] Furthermore, it appears that the tumor does not result from malignant transformation of a condyloma acuminatum but is a low-grade squamous cell carcinoma from its inception.

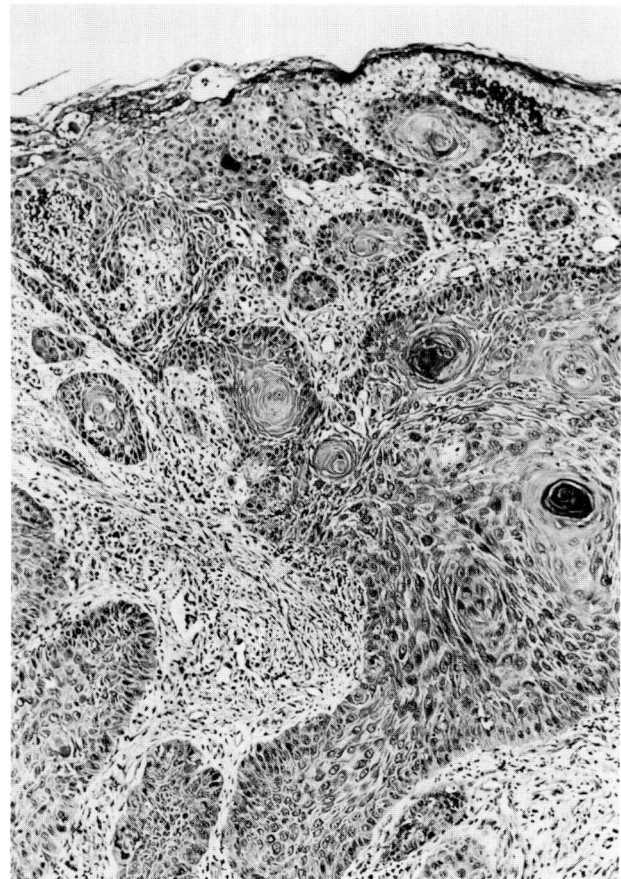

FIGURE 34-15. Moderately differentiated, focally keratinizing squamous cell carcinoma of the anal margin in a 64-year-old man. (H&E, × 125)

Adenocarcinoma

Adenocarcinomas of the anal region may arise from several available sources of glandular epithelium. These include the normal mucosa of the lower rectum, the mucus-secreting cells of the anal transitional epithelium, anal ducts (glands), and the apocrine glands of the perianal skin.

The most frequent type of adenocarcinoma to involve the anal region is simply a low-lying rectal cancer that extends downward into the upper anal canal. Differentiation from true anal adenocarcinoma is generally easy, as mucosal origin can usually be traced histologically to rectal glandular epithelium.

So-called cloacogenic carcinoma may show variable degrees of mucus secretion, a pattern sometimes referred to as mucoepidermoid carcinoma. These may arise from transitional epithelium of either the upper anal canal or the anal duct.

The most interesting type of primary adenocarcinoma of the anus is believed by most observers to arise from anal ducts (glands) and is known as perianal mucinous (colloid) adenocarcinoma.[97-100] These are very rare neoplasms that have several clinical and pathologic features in common. They are slow-growing tumors and are frequently associated with long-standing perianal fistulae and abscesses. They arise in the deep perianal tissues without evidence of surface mucosal involvement. Presentation may be due to a painful mass in the buttock, occasionally accompanied by a gelatinous discharge. Anorectal bleeding or obstruction is not usually seen. Histologically, these are generally well-differentiated adenocarcinomas with abundant mucus production. Diagnosis requires a high degree of clinical suspicion. Multiple deep biopsies may be necessary to establish a diagnosis because the abundant mucus may make identification of tumor cells difficult. The clinical course is often followed by frequent recurrences when excision has been inadequate. Late metastases to inguinal lymph nodes may occur.

The relationship of this tumor to the commonly associated fistulae and abscesses continues to be controversial. Some believe that the perianal fistulae and abscesses antedate the carcinoma, but others believe that these typically slow-growing neoplasms undergo secondary fistulization. Most observers believe that these tumors arise from the mucous cells of anal ducts (glands). However, an alternative explanation suggests that they may arise from duplications of the lower end of the hindgut.[101] Evidence offered in support of this theory is the occasional identification of normal rectal-type mucosa in anal fistulae, providing a possible epithelial source for this rare lesion. Recently, histochemical studies of mucinous adenocarcinoma associated with chronic anal fistulae have been performed.[102] In four of eight cases studied, the histochemical characteristics of the mucus were those of anal gland rather than rectal mucosa. Anal gland mucus has strong PAS reactivity, which is abolished by periodate borohydride saponification, indicating an absence or scarcity of O-acylated sialic acids.

Malignant Melanoma

Although rare, malignant melanoma of the anus is the third most common site after skin and eye and the most common primary site in the gastrointestinal tract. Several excellent reviews of this tumor have been published.[103-107] The median age (55 to 60 years) is similar to that of anal carcinoma. Reports of the largest numbers of cases suggest an approximately equal sex distribution. Bleeding is the most common presenting clinical symptom, followed by a mass, change in bowel habit, and pain.

Grossly, primary malignant melanoma of the anal canal usually appears as a polypoid mass that may be smooth or ulcerated. The average lesion measures 4 cm in diameter.[107] About two thirds are grossly pigmented. The most common site of origin is at the dentate line and contiguous transitional zone. Pigment-producing cells have been identified at these sites in normal anal mucosa.[5] Satellite nodules may be seen. Clinically the lesion may be confused with thrombosed hemorrhoids. Because extension of the growth into the lower rectum is common, a gross distinction between nonpigmented malignant melanoma and carcinoma of the anal canal or lower rectum is very difficult.

Histologically, malignant melanoma of the anal

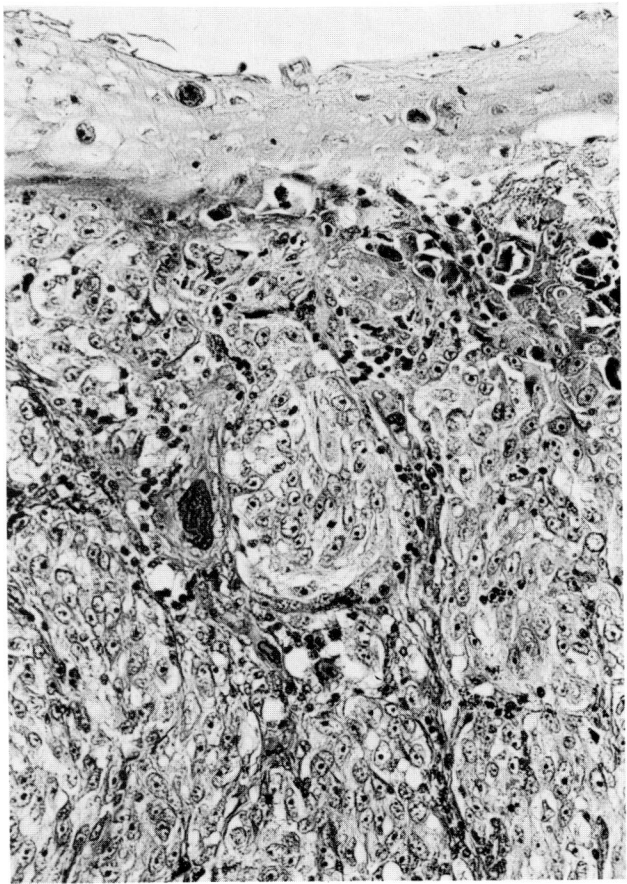

FIGURE 34–16. Malignant melanoma of the anal canal in an elderly women. The lesion presented clinically as a prolapsing, pigmented mass. (H&E, × 330)

canal resembles its cutaneous counterpart (Figure 34–16). Junctional change, either overlying or adjacent to the invasive mass, is common. The lateral junctional extension is often of the acral-lentiginous type similar to other primary mucosal melanomas.[106] In the absence of melanin pigment or identifiable junctional change, differentiation from a poorly differentiated anal carcinoma may be very difficult. A characteristic nesting pattern is helpful. Adjunctive techniques such as electron microscopy or the immunohistochemical demonstration of S-100 protein or cytoplasmic melanoma antigen (HMB45) may also aid in establishing a correct diagnosis.

Anal malignant melanoma is a highly aggressive and usually lethal tumor. More than one half of patients have evidence of metastasis at the time of diagnosis. The most common metastatic sites are the regional lymph nodes followed by liver and lung. The overall 5-year survival rate is 10% to 15% in most series.

Extramammary Paget's Disease

The most common site of involvement in extramammary Paget's disease is the vulva and contiguous perineal skin of postmenopausal white women. Much less commonly affected are sites such as the scrotum and axilla. Involvement of the contiguous perianal skin may also occur, but disease that is limited to perianal skin is rare. The clinical appearance of extramammary Paget's disease has been well described.[108,109] The typical lesions are erythematous patches or plaques, which may be scaly, crusted, eroded, or even ulcerated. Pruritus is common. The lesions vary greatly in size, and microscopic evidence of disease may extend beyond the grossly recognized limits of involvement.

Histologically the disorder is characterized by the presence of large, cytologically malignant cells with pale, granular, and vacuolated cytoplasm scattered within the epidermis and sometimes the underlying cutaneous appendages (Figure 34–17). The cells tend to be more numerous in the basal region, where they may form intraepidermal acinar structures. The involved epidermis may also show hyperkeratosis, parakeratosis, and acanthosis. The important differential diagnosis is distinction of extramammary Paget's disease from pagetoid malignant melanoma and Bowen's disease. An important feature of the Paget's cell is the presence of cytoplasmic acid mucopolysaccharide, which may be demonstrated by a variety of special stains. Recent studies have also reported the immunohistochemical detection of carcinoembryonic antigen (CEA) in Paget's cells.[110] The presence of melanin pigment within pagetoid cells does not establish a diagnosis of malignant melanoma, as melanin granules are occasionally seen both in Paget's cells and the neoplastic keratinocytes of Bowen's disease. Other differential diagnositic features of these disorders have been well described.[109] The histologic appearance of mammary and extramammary Paget's disease is the same.

The histogenesis and pathogenesis of extramammary Paget's disease remain controversial topics. The area of greatest agreement is that the Paget's cell is a secretory (glandular) epithelial cell. It is well known that mammary Paget's disease is virtually always associated with an underlying ductal carcinoma of the breast. This constant association with an underlying carcinoma does not obtain in extramammary disease.[108,109] In fact, there appear to be variations in this association depending on the site of extramammary involvement. For example, in one series, 86% of 14 cases with perianal disease had underlying adnexal or visceral carcinomas, whereas a similar association was noted in only 33% of patients with nonperianal extramammary Paget's disease.[108]

The most frequently espoused concepts of the nature of this disease suggest that (1) there is migration of Paget's cells into the epidermis from an underlying carcinoma or (2) the origin of the Paget's cells in the epidermis occurs independently or concomitantly with an underlying carcinoma.[53] Most observers now regard extramammary Paget's disease as a form of intraepithelial adenocarcinoma that may progress to invasion of adjacent stroma. Another area of incompletely resolved controversy is the histogenetic source of the Paget's cells. Some favor an eccrine sweat gland origin, and others believe they arise from apocrine gland epi-

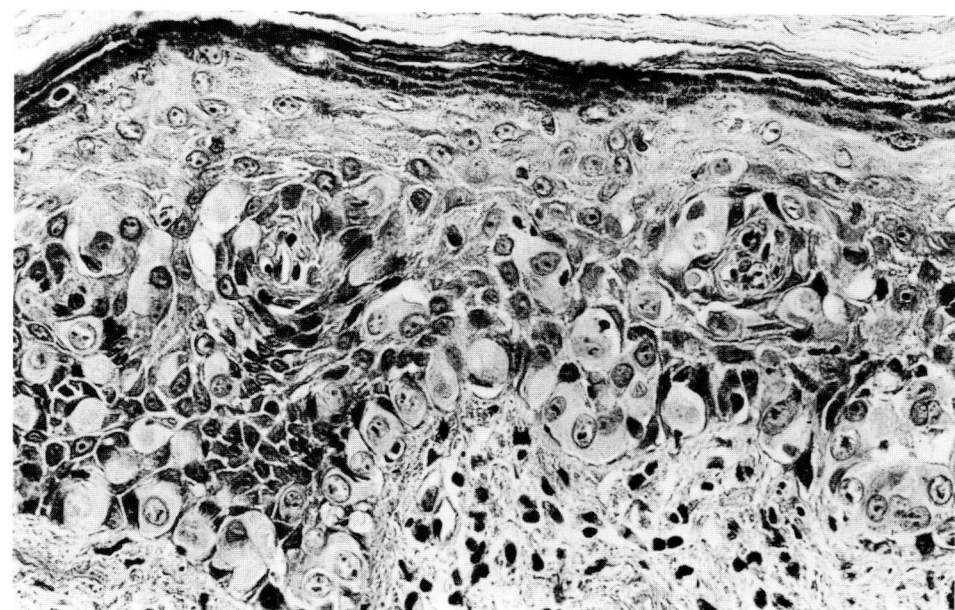

FIGURE 34–17. Perianal extramammary Paget's disease. Note the pale, granular cells singly and in nests in basal portion of the epidermis. (H&E, × 530)

thelium. Recent immunohistochemical demonstration of gross cystic disease fluid protein (GCDFP), a marker of apocrine epithelium, supports the most widely held view that extramammary Paget's disease is of apocrine cell derivation.[111,112]

Basal Cell Carcinoma

Basal cell carcinoma of the anus is a rare tumor that arises in the perianal skin. It is similar to cutaneous basal cell carcinoma arising in other sites and must be distinguished from the well-differentiated basaloid form of cloacogenic carcinoma of the anal canal (Figure 34–18).[113,114] The typical gross presentation is an ulcerated nodule with raised, pearly margins similar to that of other cutaneous basal cell carcinomas. The behavior is also similar to that of the usual basal cell carcinoma and distinctly different from that of carcinoma of the anal canal. Histologically, anal canal carcinoma of the basaloid type tends to have more cytologic atypia and greater numbers of mitoses than does basal cell carcinoma, but differential diagnosis may sometimes depend upon demonstration of the anal canal mucosal or perianal cutaneous origin of the particular neoplasm in question.

Other Malignant Tumors

Several other rare malignant tumors may arise in the anal region. Leiomyosarcoma of the anorectal area has been described.[63] Rare examples of embryonal rhabdomyosarcoma, usually of the botryoid type, have been seen in children.[115] An anal mass has been reported as the presenting sign in a case of chronic lymphocytic leukemia.[116]

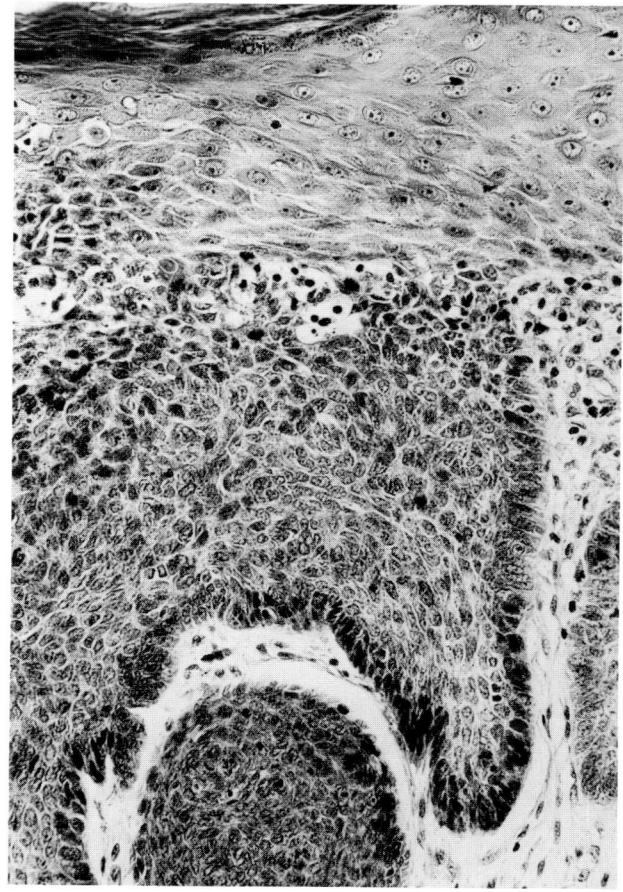

FIGURE 34–18. Basal-cell carcinoma of the perianal skin. Note the origin from the basal zone of the epidermis and the pronounced palisading of the cells at the periphery. (H&E, × 330)

Tumors from other sites may also secondarily involve the anus either as a result of metastasis or direct extension. The most common source of metastatic tumor of the anus is colorectal carcinoma. Extremely rare sources of metastatic disease such as the breast have also been reported.[117] Direct extension of cancer to the anal and perianal tissue may occur from any site in the region including the lower urinary and genital tracts and the lower bowel.

References

1. Fenger C: Histology of the anal canal. Am J Surg Pathol 12:41–55, 1988.
2. Grinvalsky HT, Helwig EB: Carcinoma of the anorectal junction: Histologic considerations. Cancer 9:480–488, 1956.
3. Fenger C: The anal transitional zone: Location and extent. Acta Pathol Microbiol Scand [A] 87:379–386, 1979.
4. Fenger C, Knoth M: The anal transitional zone: A scanning and transmission electron microscopic investigation of the mucosal surface. Ultrastruct Pathol 2:163–173, 1981.
5. Fenger C, Lyon H: Endocrine cells and melanin-containing cells in the anal canal epithelium. Histochem J 14:631–639, 1982.
6. Lieberman D: Common anorectal disorders. Ann Intern Med 101:837–846, 1984.
7. Fry RD, Kodner IJ: Anorectal disorders. Clin Symp 37:2–32, 1985.
8. Santulli TV, Kiesewetter WB, Bill AH Jr: Anorectal anomalies: A suggested international classification. J Pediatr Surg 5:281–287, 1970.
9. Parrott TS: Urologic implications of anorectal malformations. Urol Clin North Am 12:13–21, 1985.
10. Moazam F, Talbert JL: Congenital anorectal malformations: Harbingers of sacrococcygeal teratomas. Arch Surg 120:856–859, 1985.
11. Thomson WH: The nature of hemorrhoids. Br J Surg 62:542–552, 1975.
12. Haas PA, Fox TA Jr, Haas GP: The pathogenesis of hemorrhoids. Dis Colon Rectum 27:442–450, 1984.
13. Rutter KRP, Riddell RH: The solitary ulcer of the rectum syndrome. Clin Gastroenterol 4:505–530, 1975.
14. duBoulay CEH, Fairbrother J, Isaacson PG: Mucosal prolapse syndrome: A unifying concept for solitary ulcer syndrome and related disorders. J Clin Pathol 36:1264–1268, 1983.
15. Saul SH, Sollenberger LC: Solitary rectal ulcer syndrome: Its clinical and pathological underdiagnosis. Am J Surg Pathol 9:411–421, 1985.
16. Lobert PF, Appelman HD: Inflammatory cloacogenic polyp: A unique inflammatory lesion of the anal transitional zone. Am J Surg Pathol 5:761–766, 1981.
17. Schinella RA: Stromal atypia in anal papillae. Dis Colon Rectum 19:611–613, 1976.
18. Parks AG, Gordon PH, Hardcastle JD: A classification of fistula-in-ano. Br J Surg 63:1–12, 1976.
19. Hanley PH: Anorectal abscess fistula. Surg Clin North Am 58:487–503, 1978.
20. Culp CE: Chronic hidradenitis suppurativa of the anal canal: A surgical skin disease. Dis Colon Rectum 26:669–676, 1983.
21. Alexander-Williams J, Buchmann P: Perianal Crohn's disease. World J Surg 4:203–208, 1980.
22. Williams DR, Coller JA, Corman ML et al: Anal complications in Crohn's disease. Dis Colon Rectum 24:22–24, 1981.
23. Lockhart-Mummery HE: Anal lesions in Crohn's disease. Br J Surg 72:S95–S96, 1985.
24. Gray BK, Lockhart-Mummery HE, Morson BC: Crohn's disease of the anal region. Gut 6:515–524, 1965.
25. Daley JJ, Madrazo A: Anal Crohn's disease with carcinoma in situ. Dig Dis Sci 25:464–466, 1980.
26. Preston DM, Fiona EF, Lennard-Jones JE, Hawley PR: Carcinoma of the anus in Crohn's disease. Br J Surg 70:346–347, 1983.
27. Slater G, Greenstein A, Aufses AH Jr: Anal carcinoma in patients with Crohn's disease. Ann Surg 199:348–350, 1984.
28. Catterall RD: Sexually transmitted diseases of the anus and rectum. Clin Gastroenterol 4:659–669, 1975.
29. Quinn TC, Corey L, Chaffer RG, et al: The etiology of anorectal infections in homosexual men. Am J Med 71:395–406, 1981.
30. Rompalo AM, Stamm WE: Anorectal and enteric infections in homosexual men. West J Med 142:647–652, 1985.
31. Samenius B: Primary syphilis of the anorectal region. Dis Colon Rectum 11:462–466, 1968.
32. Quinn TC, Lukehart SA, Goodell S, et al: Rectal mass caused by Treponema pallidum: Confirmation by immunofluorescent staining. Gastroenterology 82:135–139, 1982.
33. Felman YM, Nikitas JA: Anorectal gonococcal infection. NY State J Med 80:231–233, 1980.
34. Nepomuceno OR, O'Grady JF, Eisenberg SW, et al: Tuberculosis of the anal canal: Report of a case. Dis Colon Rectum 14:313–316, 1971.
35. Alankar K, Rickert RR, Sen P, Lazaro EJ: Verrucous tuberculosis of the anal canal: Report of a case. Dis Colon Rectum 17:254–257, 1974.
36. Laude TA, Narayanaswamy G, Rajkumar S: Lichen sclerosus et atrophicus in an eleven year old girl: Report of a case. Cutis 26:78–80, 1980.
37. Colby TV: Malakoplakia: Two unusual cases which presented diagnostic problems. Am J Surg Pathol 2:377–382, 1978.
38. Lee FI, Costello FT, Cowley DJ, et al: Eosinophilic colitis with perianal disease. Am J Gastroenterol 78:164–166, 1983.
39. Mortensen NJ, Thomson JP: Perianal abscess due to Enterobius vermicularis: Report of a case. Dis Colon Rectum 27:677–678, 1984.
40. Vanheuverzwyn R, Delannoy A, Michaux JL, Dive C: Anal lesions in hematologic diseases. Dis Colon Rectum 23:310–312, 1980.
41. Oriel JD: Epidemiology of human papilloma viruses. In DePalo G, Rilke F, zur Hausen H (ed): Herpes and Papilloma Viruses. New York, Raven Press, 1986, pp 55–61.
42. Meisels A, Morin C, Casas-Cordero M: Human papilloma-virus infection of the uterine cervix. Int J Gynecol Pathol 1:75–94, 1982.
43. Crum CP, Ikenberg H, Richart RM, Gissman L: Human papillomavirus type 16 and early cervical neoplasia. N Engl J Med 310:880–883, 1984.
44. Kadish AS, Burk RD, Kress Y, et al: Human papillomaviruses of different types in precancerous lesions of the uterine cervix: Histologic, immunocytochemical and ultrastructural studies. Hum Pathol 17:384–392, 1986.
45. Gissman L, Schneider A: The role of human papilloma-viruses in genital cancer. In De Palo G, Rilke F, zur Hausen H (ed): Herpes and Papilloma Viruses. New York, Raven Press, 1986, pp 15–24.
46. Oriel JD, Whimster IW: Carcinoma-in-situ associated with virus-containing anal warts. Br J Dermatol 84:71–73, 1971.
47. Croxson T, Chabon AB, Rorat E, Barash IM: Intraepithelial carcinoma of the anus in homosexual men. Dis Colon Rectum 27:325–330, 1984.
48. Kovi J, Tillman L, Lee SM: Malignant transformation of condyloma acuminatum: A light microscopic and ultrastructural study. Am J Clin Pathol 61:702–710, 1974.
49. Ejeckman GC, Idikio HA, Nayak V, Gardiner JP: Malignant transformation in an anal condyloma acuminatum. Can J Surg 26:170–173, 1983.
50. Connors RC, Ackerman AB: Histologic pseudomalignancies of the skin. Arch Dermatol 112:1767–1780, 1976.
51. Wade TR, Kopf AW, Ackerman AB: Bowenoid papulosis of the penis. Cancer 42:1890–1903, 1978.
52. Ulbright TM, Stehman FB, Roth LM, et al: Bowenoid dysplasia of the vulva. Cancer 50:2910–2919, 1982.
53. Helwig EB: Neoplasms of the anus. In Norris HT (ed): Pathology of the Colon, Small Intestine and Anus. New York, Churchill Livingstone, 1983, pp 303–327.
54. Gross G, Hagedorn M, Ikenberg H, et al: Bowenoid papulosis: Presence of human papillomavirus (HPV) structural antigens

55. Weigand DA, Burgdorf WHC: Perianal apocrine gland adenoma. Arch Dermatol 116:1051–1053, 1980.
56. Assor D, Davis JB: Multiple apocrine fibroadenomas of the anal skin. Am J Clin Pathol 68:397–399, 1977.
57. Elliott GB, Fisher BK: Perianal keratoacanthoma. Arch Dermatol 95:81–83, 1967.
58. Jensen SL, Sjolin K-E: Keratoacanthoma of the anus: Report of three cases. Dis Colon Rectum 28:743–745, 1985.
59. Rickert RR, Larkey IG, Kantor EB: Granular-cell tumors (myoblastomas) of the anal region. Dis Colon Rectum 21:413–417, 1978.
60. Johnston J, Helwig EB: Granular cell tumors of the gastrointestinal tract and perianal region: A study of 74 cases. Dig Dis Sci 26:807–816, 1981.
61. Abel ME, Kingsley AEN, Abcarian H, et al: Anorectal neurilemomas. Dis Colon Rectum 28:960–961, 1985.
62. Kalima TV, Peltokallio P: Leiomyoma of the ischioanal region: Report of a case. Dis Colon Rectum 11:198–200, 1968.
63. Hishida Y, Ishida M: Smooth-muscle tumors of the rectum in Japanese. Dis Colon Rectum 17:226–234, 1974.
64. Hernandez V, Hernandez IA, Berthrong M: Oleogranuloma simulating carcinoma of the rectum. Dis Colon Rectum 10:205–210, 1967.
65. Herrmann G, Desfosses L: Sur la muqueuse de la region cloacale du rectum. Compt Rend Acad Sci 90:1301–1302, 1880.
66. Morson BC, Pang LSC: Pathology of anal cancer. Proc R Soc Med 61:623–624, 1968.
67. Klotz RG Jr, Pamukcoglu T, Souilliard DH: Transitional cloacogenic carcinoma of the anal canal: Clinicopathologic study of three hundred seventy-three cases. Cancer 20:1727–1745, 1967.
68. Singh R, Nime F, Mittelman A: Malignant epithelial tumors of the anal canal. Cancer 48:411–415, 1981.
69. Quan SHQ: Carcinoma of the anus. Int Adv Surg Oncol 6:323–335, 1983.
70. Boman BM, Moertel CG, O'Connell MJ, et al: Carcinoma of the anal canal: A clinical and pathologic study of 188 cases. Cancer 54:114–125, 1984.
71. Dougherty BG, Evans HL: Carcinoma of the anal canal: A study of 79 cases. Am J Clin Pathol 83:159–164, 1985.
72. Greenall MJ, Quan SHQ, Decosse JJ: Epidermoid cancer of the anus. Br J Surg [Suppl] 72:S97–S103, 1985.
73. Clark J, Petrelli N, Herrera L, Mittelman A: Epidermoid carcinoma of the anal canal. Cancer 57:400–406, 1986.
74. Hardcastle JD, Bussey HJR: Results of surgical treatment of squamous cell carcinoma of the anal canal and anal margin seen at St. Mark's Hospital, 1928–66. Proc R Soc Med 61:629–630, 1968.
75. Beahrs OH, Henson DE, Hutter RVP, Myers MH: Manual for Staging of Cancer, 3rd ed. Philadelphia, JB Lippincott, 1988, pp 81–83.
76. Greenall MJ, Quan SHQ, Stearns MW, et al: Epidermoid cancer of the anal margin: Pathologic features, treatment, and clinical results. Am J Surg 149:95–100, 1985.
77. Cooper HS, Patchefsky AS, Marks G: Cloacogenic carcinoma of the anorectum in homosexual men: An observation of four cases. Dis Colon Rectum 22:557–558, 1979.
78. Daling JR, Weiss NS, Klopfenstein LL, et al: Correlates of homosexual behavior and the incidence of anal cancer. JAMA 247:1988–1990, 1982.
79. Peters RK, Mack TM: Patterns of anal carcinoma by gender and marital status in Los Angeles County. Br J Cancer 48:629–636, 1983.
80. Daling JR, Weiss NS, Hislop TG, et al: Sexual practices, sexually transmitted diseases, and the incidence of anal cancer. N Engl J Med 317:973–977, 1987.
80a. Wexner SD, Milsom JW, Dailey TH: The demographics of anal cancer are changing: Identification of a high-risk population. Dis Colon Rectum 30:942–946, 1987.
81. Nash G, Allen W, Nash S: Atypical lesions of the anal mucosa in homosexual men. JAMA 256:873–876, 1986.
82. Gal AA, Meyer PR, Taylor CR: Papillomavirus antigens in anorectal condyloma and carcinoma in homosexual men. JAMA 257:337–340, 1987.
82a. Gal AA, Saul SH, Stoler MH: In situ hybridization analysis of human papillomavirus in anal squamous cell carcinoma. Mod Pathol 2:439–443, 1989.
83. Cabrera A, Tsukada Y, Pickren JW, et al: Development of lower genital carcinomas in patients with anal carcinoma: A more than casual relationship. Cancer 19:470–480, 1966.
84. Schlaerth JB, Morrow CP, Nalick RH, Otis G Jr: Anal involvement by carcinoma in situ of the perineum in women. Obstet Gynecol 64:406–411, 1984.
85. Fenger C, Nielsen VT: Dysplastic changes in the anal canal epithelium in minor surgical specimens. Acta Pathol Microbiol Scand 89:463–465, 1981.
86. Scoma JA, Levy EI: Bowen's disease of the anus: Report of two cases. Dis Colon Rectum 18:137–140, 1975.
87. Strauss RJ, Fazio VW: Bowen's disease of the anal and perianal area: A report and analysis of twelve cases. Am J Surg 137:231–234, 1979.
88. Rickert RR, Brodkin RH, Hutter RVP: Bowen's disease. CA 27:160–166, 1977.
89. Levin SE, Cooperman H, Freilich M, et al: Transitional cloacogenic carcinoma of the anus. Dis Colon Rectum 20:17–23, 1977.
90. Gillespie JJ, MacKay B: Histogenesis of cloacogenic carcinoma: Fine structure of anal transitional epithelium and cloacogenic carcinoma. Hum Pathol 9:579–587, 1978.
90a. Wolber R, Dupuis B, Thiyagaratnam P, Owen D: Anal cloacogenic and squamous carcinomas: Comparative histogenic anaylsis using in situ hybridization for human papillomavirus DNA. Am J Surg Pathol 14:176–182, 1990.
91. Kraus FT, Perez-Mesa C: Verrucous carcinoma: Clinical and pathological study of 105 cases involving oral cavity, larynx and genitalia. Cancer 19:26–38, 1966.
92. Gingrass PJ, Burbrick MP, Hitchcock CR, et al: Anorectal verrucose squamous carcinoma: Report of two cases. Dis Colon Rectum 21:120–122, 1978.
93. Knoblich R, Failing JF Jr: Giant condyloma acuminatum (Buschke-Löwenstein tumor) of the rectum. Am J Clin Pathol 48:389–395, 1967.
94. Elliot MS, Werner ID, Immelman EJ, Harrison AC: Giant condyloma (Bushke-Loewenstein tumor) of the anorectum. Dis Colon Rectum 22:497–500, 1979.
95. Alexander RM, Kaminsky DB: Giant condyloma acuminatum (Buschke-Loewenstein tumor) of the anus: Case report and review of the literature. Dis Colon Rectum 22:561–565, 1979.
96. Prioleau PG, Santa Cruz DJ, Meyer JS, Bauer WC: Verrucous carcinoma: A light and electron microscopic, autoradiographic and immunofluorescence study. Cancer 45:2849–2857, 1980.
97. Prioleau PG, Allen MS Jr, Roberts T: Perianal mucinous adenocarcinoma. Cancer 39:1295–1299, 1977.
98. Askin FB, Muhlendorf K, Walz BJ: Mucinous carcinoma of anal duct origin presenting clinically as a vaginal cyst. Cancer 42:566–569, 1978.
99. Honore LH: Anal gland adenocarcinoma presenting as painless scrotal swelling in a 73 year old man: A case report. J Surg Oncol 15:201–207, 1980.
100. Lee SH, Zucker M, Sato T: Primary adenocarcinoma of an anal gland with secondary perianal fistulas. Hum Pathol 12:1034–1036, 1981.
101. Dukes CE, Galvin C: Colloid carcinoma arising within fistulae in the anorectal region. Ann R Coll Surg Engl 18:246–261, 1956.
102. Fenger C, Filipe MI: Pathology of the anal glands with special reference to their mucinous histochemistry. Acta Path Microbiol Scand [A] 85:273–285, 1977.
103. Morson BC, Volkstadt H: Malignant melanoma of the anal canal. J Clin Pathol 16:126–132, 1963.
104. Mason JK, Helwig EB: Ano-rectal melanoma. Cancer 19:39–50, 1966.
105. Chiu YS, Unni KK, Beart RW Jr: Malignant melanoma of the anorectum. Dis Colon Rectum 23:122–124, 1980.
106. Wanebo HJ, Woodruff JM, Farr GH, Quan SH: Anorectal melanoma. Cancer 47:1891–1900, 1981.
107. Cooper PH, Mills SE, Allen MS Jr: Malignant melanoma of the anus: Report of 12 patients and analysis of 255 additional cases. Dis Colon Rectum 25:693–703, 1982.

108. Helwig EB, Graham JH: Anogenital (extramammary) Paget's disease. Cancer 16:387–403, 1963.
109. Jones RE Jr, Austin C, Ackerman AB: Extramammary Paget's disease: A critical reexamination. Am J Dermatopathol 1:101–132, 1979.
110. Nadji M, Morales AR, Girtanner RE, et al: Paget's disease of the skin: A unifying concept of histogenesis. Cancer 50:2203–2206, 1982.
111. Mazoujian G, Pinkus GS, Haagensen DE Jr: Extramammary Paget's disease: Evidence for an apocrine origin: An immunoperoxidase study of gross cystic disease fluid protein-15, carcinoembryonic antigen, and keratin proteins. Am J Surg Pathol 8:43–50, 1984.
112. Merot Y, Mazoujian G, Pinkus G, et al: Extramammary Paget's disease of the perianal and perineal regions: Evidence of apocrine derivation. Arch Dermatol 121:750–752, 1985.
113. Nielsen OV, Jensen SL: Basal cell carcinoma of the anus: A clinical study of 34 cases. Br J Surg 68:856–857, 1981.
114. White WB, Schneiderman H, Sayre JT: Basal cell carcinoma of the anus: Clinical and pathological distinction from cloacogenic carcinoma. J Clin Gastroenterol 6:441–446, 1984.
115. Srouji MN, Donaldson MH, Chatten J, Koblenzer CS: Perianal rhabdomyosarcoma in childhood. Cancer 38:1008–1012, 1976.
116. Cresson DH, Siegal GP: Chronic lymphocytic leukemia presenting as an anal mass. J Clin Gastroenterol 7:83–87, 1985.
117. Dawson PM, Hershman MJ, Wood CB: Metastatic carcinoma of the breast in the anal canal. Postgrad Med J 61:1081, 1985.

Index

Note: Page numbers in *italics* indicate illustrations; page numbers followed by (t) refer to tables.

Abdomen, embryology of, return of bowel in, 118
Abdominal distention, in aganglionic megacolon, 119
Abdominal pain, in allergic gastroenteritis, 175
Abetalipoproteinemia, small-intestinal effects of, 362, *363*
Abscess(es), anal, in adenocarcinoma, 898
  anorectal, fistula and, 886–887
  crypt, in ulcerative colitis, 648, *650*
  in Crohn's disease, 674
  pericolic, diverticulosis and, 777, *778*
  suture, 716, *716*
Absorptive cells, colonic, 34, *34–35*
  small-intestinal, 26(t), 26–28, *27–28*
    cytoplasm of, structural features of, *29*
    cytoskeleton of, 28–29, *29*
    intercellular tight junction of, functions of, 27–28, *27–28*
      structural features of, *29*
    microvilli of, structural features of, 28–29, *29*
    organelles of, *29*
    plasma membrane of, absorption and transport in, 27
      structural features of, *29*
      ultrastructural features of, 26–27, *27*
    polarity of, origin and maintenance of, 27–28
    undifferentiated crypt cells vs., 30, *30*
Acanthosis, glycogenic, of esophageal squamous epithelium, 385–386, *386*
Acanthosis nigricans, with ECL cell tumors, 248
Acetaminophen, toxic injury by, 143
Acetylcholinesterase, levels of, in Hirschsprung's disease, 208
Acetylcholinesterase stain, of aganglionic megacolon biopsy specimens, 121
Achalasia, esophageal, 423, *424*–425
  in carcinoma, 443
  squamous epithelial findings in, 425
Acids, esophageal injury from, *401*, 401–402
  gastrointestinal lesions from, 146
Acquired immunodeficiency syndrome (AIDS), candidiasis in, 268, 277–278
  condyloma acuminatum in, 890
  Cryptosporidium in, 268, *270*, 278
  cytomegalovirus infection in, 278, *279*
    gastric erosions with, 268, *269*
  duodenal mucosa in, 693, *694*
  Enterocytozoon bieneusi infection in, 749–751, *750–751*
  esophagitis in, 396
  gastric mucosa in, 361, *361*
  gastrointestinal infections in, 275(t)
    pathogenesis of, 279
  gastrointestinal manifestations of, 277–280, *277–281*
    opportunisitc infections in, 277–278, *277–279*
  idiopathic enteropathy in, 754, *754*

Acquired immunodeficiency syndrome (AIDS) (*Continued*)
  intestinal defense mechanisms in, impairment of, microbial infection from, 623
  intestinal spirochetes in, 279, *280*
  Kaposi's sarcoma in, gastrointestinal involvement in, 279–281, *280*
  Mycobacterium avium-intracellulare infection in, 277, *277–278*, *278*, 279
    esophagitis from, 400
    Whipple's disease vs., 748–749
  parasitic infestation in, 275(t)
  T cell alterations in, 274, 754
  villus atrophy and crypt hyperplasia in, 754
Acrodermatitis enteropathica, zinc deficiency and, 744
Actin, in intestinal absorptive cell cytoskeleten, 28–29, *29*
Actinomyces israelii infections. See *Actinomycosis*.
Actinomycin D, radiomimetic nature of, 144, 150
Actinomycosis, 634
  appendiceal, 869
  esophagitis from, 400
  gastric, 502
  intestinal, pathology of, 634, *634–635*
Ad12, exposure to, celiac disease from, 730
Addison's disease, gastrointestinal effects of, 355
Adenoacanthoma, esophageal, 469, *470*
Adenocarcinoid, appendiceal, carcinoids and adenocarcinomas vs., 877(t)
  microscopic appearance of, 875–876, *876*
  mixed with noncarcinoid adenocarcinoma, 876
  intestinal, 833
Adenocarcinoma, appendiceal, 871–873, *872*
  gross appearance of, 872, *872*
  microscopic appearance of, 872, *872–873*
  noncystic, 872, *872*
  colonic, colitis cystica profunda vs., 703
  composite, carcinoid with, 844, *844*
  cytogenetic changes in, 92
  cytology of, 62
    statistical evaluation of, 67, 67(t)
  MNNG-induced, 827, *828*
  moderately differentiated, 831, *832*
  mucinous, 835, *835*
  poorly differentiated, 831, *833*
  transitional mucosa in, 829, *829*
  ulcerated, 824, *825*
  well-differentiated, 831, *831*
    expanding growth patterns in, 831–832, *833*
    expanding-infiltrative mixed growth patterns in, 832, *834*
    in ulcerative colitis, 656, *656*
    infiltrative growth patterns in, 832, *834*

905

Adenocarcinoma (*Continued*)
    colorectal, 838
        age, sex, and race in, 841
        associated conditions in, 842
        clinical presentation of, 841–843, 843(t)
        complications of, 841–842
        diagnosis of, 842
        location of, 838–839
        marker substances for, 840–841, 841(t)
        multiplicity of, 839
        obstruction in, 841–842
        pathologic features of, 839
        patterns of spread of, implantation in, 840
            local, 839–840
            lymphatic, 840
            metastatic, 840
            venous, 840
        perforation in, 842
        prognosis of, 842–843, 843(t)
        screening for, 842
        survival rates of, 842–843, 843(t)
        symptoms and signs of, 841
        treatment of, 842
    duodenal, papillary, 831, *832*
        cytology of, 60, *60*
    esophageal, 460–470
        incidence of, 460, 461(t)
        location of, 460, 461(t)
        not associated with Barrett's epithelium, 469
    gastric, 586–606
        absorptive cells in, 599–600
        age distribution of, 605
        Borrmann's classification of, 596
        carcinogenesis of, experimental, 595, *596*
        cell types in, 599–601
        clinical presentation of, 605–606
        cytology of, 50, *51*
        diagnosis of, 605–606
        differentiated, 605
        diffuse, *603*, 603
        diffusely infiltrative, 597, *599*
        epidemiology of, 586, *586*
        etiology of, 586–587
        expanding, 604, *604*
            tubules and masses in, 598, *600*
        fungating, 597, *597*
        genetic basis of, 88–89
        gross morphology of, 596–597, *597–599*
        growth rates of, 596
        histologic classification of, Lauren's, *603*, 603–604
            Ming's, *604*, 604–605
            World Health Organization typing, 603
        histologic features of, epithelial elements in, 598–601, *599–601*
            stromal elements in, 601, *602*
        incidence of, blood type A in, 586
            pernicious anemia in, 586
        infiltrative, 604, *604*
            pyloric-type glands and signet-ring cells in, 599, *601*
            undifferentiated tumors cells in, 598, *600*
        intestinal, 603–604
        linitis plastica, 597, *599*
            mucosal thickening in, *544*, 545
        location of, 596
        marker substances in, 602(t), 602–603
        metastases in, 609–610
        mortality rate of, decline of, 586, *586*
            geographic variation in, 586, *586*
        mucinous, 579–580
        multiple primary, 609–610
        natural history of, 595–596
        papillary, histologic features of, 577, *579*
            projections in, 598, *599*
        pathology of, 596–603, *597–602*, 598(t), 602(t)

Adenocarcinoma (*Continued*)
    gastric, polypoid, 597, *597*
        poorly differentiated, histologic features of, 578–579, *580*
        precursors to, 587–595
            chronic gastric ulcer in, 590, *590*
            epithelial dysplasia in, 591–592, *592–595*, 594–595
            epithelial polyps in, 587
            gastric remnants in, 590–591
            hyperplastic gastropathy in, 591
            intestinal metaplasia in, *588–589*, 588–590, 589(t)
            precancerous conditions in, 587–591, *588–591*, 589(t)
        prognosis of, 606
        scirrhous, 597, *599*, 601
        sex distribution of, 605
        signet-ring cell type, 579, *580*
        size of, 596
        spread of, 601–602
        superficial (early or spreading), 596–597, *597*
            in intestinal metaplasia, 589, *589*
        TNM staging of, 605
        treatment of, 606
        tubular, histologic features of, 577–578, *579*
        tubular glands in, 598, *599*
        ulcerated, 597, *598*
            benign vs. malignant, 597, 598(t)
        undifferentiated, 605
        well-differentiated, absorptive cells in, 598, *601*
            goblet cells in, 598–599, *600*
            signet-ring cells in, 598, *601*
    in Barrett's esophagus, 411, 418, *418*, 460–469. See also under *Barrett's esophagus; Barrett's epithelium.*
    in Barrett's mucosa, 421, *422*
    in chronic gastritis, 498–499, *499*
    in Crohn's disease, 676
    in familial polyposis coli, 807
    in tubular adenoma, *826*
    in ulcerative colitis, histology of, 656, *656*
        incidence of, 655
        pathology of, 655–656, *656*
    intestinal, cell types of, 833–834
        classification of, 830–831, *830–831*
        diffusely infiltrative, 831, *831*
        epidemiology of, 819, *820*, 820(t)
        fungating, 830, *830*
        general considerations in, 818–819, 819(t)
        gross morphology of, 830–831, *830–831*
        growth rate of, 829
        histogenesis of, 828–829, *829*
        histologic features of, 831–833, *831–834*
        natural history of, 829–830
        pathology of, 827–836, *829–836*, 837(t)
        polypoid, 830, *830*
        spread of, 829–830
        staging of, 835–836, 837(t)
        ulcerative, *830*, 830–831
        ultrastructural and morphometric studies of, 834–835
        variants of, 835, *835–836*
        well-differentiated, endocrine cells in, 259
    intraepithelial, as extramammary Paget's disease, 899
    of anal region, 898
    of esophagogastric junction, 606–607
    of gastric cardia, 606–607
    perianal mucinous (colloid), 898
    poorly differentiated, lymphomas vs., 297
    small-intestinal, 836–838, *837*
        clinical presentation of, 838
        in celiac disease, 734
        location of, 836–837
        pathologic features of, *837*, 837–838
        pattern of spread of, 837–838
Adenocarcinoma *in situ*, colonic, 800, *804*
Adenocarcinoma-carcinoid tumors, endocrine components of, distinguishing of, 259
Adenoid cystic carcinoma, esophageal, 470

Adenoma, appendiceal, 870–871, *871*
  cecal, *338*
  colonic, classification of, 800
    clear cells in, 846
    cytogenetic changes in, 92
    DMH-induced, 827, *828*
    DNA synthesis abnormalities in, 105
    dysplasia in, 800–801, 803–804
    epidemiology of, 797
    epithelial cell proliferation in, 105–106
    genetic basis of, 91
    incidence of, 796–797
      carcinoma and, 797
    oncogene expression in, 92–93
    pathology of, 799–801, *800–804*
    pedunculated, invasive cancer in, *805*
      pathology of, 799, *800*
    polyp-cancer sequence in, 797–798
    sessile, invasive cancer in, *806*
      pathology of, 799
    short-stalked, submucosal cancer in, *805*
    site distribution of, 797
    size of, histologic type and, 799
      malignant potential and, 797–798
    squamous metaplasia in, 844, *844*
    tubular, cytology of, 62, *63*
      neoplastic (adenomatous) epithelium in, 799–800, *801*
      pathology of, 799
    type of, malignant potential and, 798
    villous, gross appearance of, 799, *800*
      hyperplastic polyps and, 787–788
      neoplastic epithelium in, 800, *801*
  dysplasia in, polyp-cancer sequence and, 798
  esophageal, 474
  gastric, as precancerous lesion, 582, *582*
    cell types in, 585
    dysplasia vs., 592
    flat, 551–552, *552–554*
      dysplasia vs., 552, *554*
      gross morphology of, 551, *552*
      histologic features of, 551–552, *553*
    histogenesis of, 550
    history of, 548
    incidence of, 550
    malignant change in, 554–555, 561(t)
    papillary (villous), 552, *554–556*
      histologic features of, 552, *555–556*
      nodular lesions in, 552, *554*
    pathology of, 550–552, *551–556*, 554–555
    subtypes of, 550–552, *551–556*, 554–555
      schematic presentation of, 551, *551*
  gastrointestinal, genetic basis of, 89
  hyperplastic polyp correlation with, 787
  in Barrett's epithelium, 464–465, *464–465*
  intestinal, 796–804
    cancer in, 804–806, *805–807*
      lymph node metastases in, 805–806
      parameters of, 804–805
      pathology of, 804–805, *805–807*
    clinical aspects of, 797
    epithelial misplacement in, 806
    etiology of, 797
    glycoconjugates in, 801, 803
    malignant potential of, 824–825, *825–826*
      genetics in, 822
    multiple, 807–808, *809*
    pathology of, 798–801, *799–804*
      landmarks in, 798–799, *799*
    pseudoinvasion in, 806–807
      etiology of, 807
      incidence of, 807
      pathology of, 807, *808*
    sialomucin and sulfomucin secretion by, 801
    special studies of, 801, 803–804

Adenoma (*Continued*)
  rectal, solitary ulcer syndrome vs., 706
  small-intestinal, pathology of, 799, *800*
    site distribution of, 797
  tubular, in adenocarcinoma, *826*
Adenoma-carcinoma sequence, 797–798, 824–825, *825–826*, 828
  in appendiceal adenocarcinoma, 872
Adenomatosis,
  gene alteration sequence of, 91–92
Adenomyoma, 566
Adenosine triphosphate (ATP), in mechanisms of cell injury, 142
Adenosquamous carcinoma, 843, *843*
  esophageal, 469
  gastric, 580, *607*, 607–608
Adenovirus, appendiceal, 869
  type 12, celiac disease from, 730
Adhesion(s), as virulence factors for exogenous infection, 626–627
  bowel infarcts from, 230, *231*
  mechanical obstruction from, 194
Adipose tissue, tumors of, 336–338, *337–338*
Adrenal disease, gastrointestinal involvement in, 355
Adrenaline, in small-intestinal epithelial cell proliferation, 103,103(t)
Adriamycin, radiomimetic nature of, 144, 150
Agammaglobulinemia, infantile X-linked, gastrointestinal manifestations of, 273
Aganglionosis, colitis with, allergic proctitis and colitis vs., 184
  diagnosis of, biopsy in, 121
Agar, liquid, for specimen orientation, 40
Agenesis, anorectal, 136
  appendiceal, 863
Agranulocytosis, drug treatment and, 144
Alcian blue, for biopsy specimen staining, 42–43, 43(t)
Alcohol, gastric injury from, *145*
  gastritis from, 482
  gastrointestinal lesions from, 146–147, 147(t), 153–154
  in etiology of carcinoma, 443, 823
Alcoholism, malabsorption in, folate deficiency with, *740*
  normal mucosal histology in, 727
Alimentary tract, duplications of, 133–135, *134*. See also *Duplication(s).*
Alkali, ingestion of, gastrointestinal lesions from, 146
Allergic disorders, 171–187. See also *Gastrointestinal food allergy.*
  aspects of, 171–172
  duodenal involvement in, 695
  food reactions in, causes of, 172(t)
  terminology in, 172
Amanita phalloides, effect on gastrointestinal motility of, 211
Amebiasis, 638, *638*
  vs. inflammatory bowel disease, 652, 672
American Joint Committee on Cancer, intestinal carcinoma classification of, 836, 837(t)
  TNM staging system of, for anal carcinoma, 894(t)
    for esophageal cancer, 451, 452(t)
    for gastric carcinoma, 605
Amphicrine cells, in adenocarcinomas, 259
Amyloid, histology of, 366–367, *366–367*
Amyloidosis, clinical features of, 366
  definition of, 365–366
  esophageal involvement in, 428, *429*
  gastrointestinal, pseudo-obstruction in, 208, *208*
  mucosal biopsy in, 367–368
  pathology of, 366–367, *366–367*
  pathophysiology of, 366
  secondary, in Crohn's disease, 675
    in rheumatoid arthritis, 357
  senile cardiovascular, 368
  systemic, 366
    histology of, *366–367*
  types of, 366
Anal agenesis, 136
Anal atresia, membranous, 136
Anal canal, carcinoma of, 893, 894(t)
  dentate (pectinate) line of, 882, *883*
    mucosal lining below, microscopic appearance of, 882

Anal canal (*Continued*)
  hemorrhoidal plexus of, 883
  lymphatic drainage of, 883
  malignant melanoma of, 898–899, *899*
  muscular wall of, 883
Anal duct(s), adenocarcinoma from, 898
  anatomy of, 883, *885*
  epithelium of, cloacogenic carcinoma of, 896
Anal fissure, 886
  in Crohn's disease, 887
Anal fistula, 886–887
  classification of, 887
  in anal adenocarcinoma, 898
  in Crohn's disease, 887
Anal margin, carcinoma of, 893–894, 894(t)
Anal mucosa, 883, *884*
Anal region. See also *Anus; Rectum.*
  abscesses of, in adenocarcinoma, 898
  adenocarcinoma of, 898
  adnexal tumors of, 890, 892
  anatomy of, 882–883, *883*
  basal cell carcinoma of, 900, *900*
  benign tumors and tumor-like lesions of, 890, *891–893*, 892
  bowenoid papulosis of, 890, *892*
  chancroid of, 889
  chlamydial infection of, 889
  cloacogenic carcinoma of, 895–896, *896–897*
  condyloma acuminatum of, 890, *891*
    giant, 897
  developmental abnormalities of, 883–884
  disorders of, 882–901
  gonorrhea of, 888
  granular cell tumors of, 892, *893*
  granuloma inguinale of, 889
  herpes simplex virus infection of, 888–889
  hidradenitis suppurativa of, 887
  inflammatory and infectious disorders of, 886–890, *888–889*
  keratoacanthoma of, 892
  leiomyoma of, 892
  lesions of, in inflammatory bowel disease, 887–888
  lymphogranuloma venereum of, 889
  malignant tumors of, 892–901, 894(t), *895–900*
  molluscum contagiosum of, 889
  neoplasms of, transitional epithelium in, 883, *884*
  neurilemoma of, 892, *893*
  oleogranuloma of, 892
  sentinel tag (pile) of, 886
  sexually transmitted diseases of, 888–889
  squamous cell carcinoma of, 896–899, *898–899*
  stenosis of, 136
  suppurative disease of, 886–887
  syphilis of, 888
  tuberculosis of, *889*, 889–890
  ulcers of, 886
  verrucous carcinoma of, 897
Anal transitional zone, anatomy of, 883, *884*
  neoplasms of, histology of, 892–893
Androgen receptors, in colon carcinoma, 823
Anemia, in gastric carcinoma, 585
  in stasis syndrome, 742, *742*
  iron deficiency, gastrointestinal absorption of iron in, 354
    in allergic gastroenteritis, 176
  megaloblastic, gastrointestinal epithelial changes in, 354
  pernicious, chronic atrophic gastritis with, *493–494*
    argyrophil cell hyperplasia with, 247
    in common variable hypogammaglobulinemia, 271
    in immunodeficiency, 271
  sickle cell, gastrointestinal ischemia in, 353–354
Aneurysm(s), gastrointestinal, 224, *224*
Angiitis, allergic granulomatous, gastrointestinal involvement in, 228
  hypersensitivity, gastrointestinal involvement in, 228

Angiodysplasia, colonic, 219–220, *220–221*
  etiology of, 220
  histology of, 220, *221*
  upper gastrointestinal bleeding from, 220
Angiography, in gastrointestinal bleeding diagnosis, 215
  in ischemic bowel disease diagnosis, 230
Angioma, gastrointestinal, 338–339
Angiosarcoma, primary, gastrointestinal, 225
Anisakiasis, Crohn's disease vs., 672
  gastric, 504
Anisocytosis, of gastric epithelial cells, 57, *57*
Anisokaryosis, of gastric epithelial cells, 57, *57–58*
Anorectal agenesis, 136
Anorectal anomalies, high, 883–884
  intermediate, 883
  international classification of, 883–884
  low, 883
Anorectal malformations, 136, 136(t)
Antacids, in prophylactic treatment of gastrointestinal hemorrhage, 518
  response to, in peptic duodenitis diagnosis, 693
Antibiotics, as risk factors in infection, 623–624
  esophagitis and inflammation from, 402(t)
  for familial visceral myopathy, 201
  gastrointestinal lesions from, 147(t), 151
  intolerance to, 151
  neutropenic enterocolitis from, 626
  pseudomembranous colitis from, 234–235, 624–626, *625*
Anticholinergic drugs, gastrointestinal lesions from, 147(t), 151
Anticoagulant drugs, gastrointestinal lesions from, 147(t), 151
Antidepressant drugs, gastrointestinal lesions from, 147(t), 151
Antigen(s), gastrointestinal processing of, 74–76, *75*
  oral exposure in, 75–76
  human leukocyte (HLA), 84
    relationship with celiac disease of, 84, 86
    relationship with duodenal ulcer of, 84, 86
  major histocompatibility, 84
  tumor-associated, in hyperplastic polyps, 789–790
Antimicrobial drugs, gastrointestinal lesions from, 147(t), 151
Antrum, gastric, allergic gastroenteritis of, 178–180, *179–180*
  biopsy of, in allergic disease, 185
  chronic inflammation of, 489–492, *490*
  muscle of, 191
  NSAID injury to, 148
  retained, after Billroth II operation, 531
  vascular ectasia of, 224
Anus. See also entries under *Anal; Anorectal.*
  carcinoma of, cytology of, 63
  Crohn's disease of, 674
  embryology of, 135–136
  imperforate, 136, 136(t)
  junction between rectum and, histologic, tumor classification and, 892–893
Appendiceal mucosa, cytology of, *862*, 862–863
Appendicitis, acute, adenocarcinoid vs., 875
  adenocarcinoma vs., 871–872, *872*
  clinical diagnosis of, correlation with pathology of, 866
  etiology of, 864–865
  gangrenous, 866, *866*
  history of, 863–864
  incidence of, 864
  lymphoid hyperplasia of terminal ileum and appendix in, 287, *287*
  mucosa in, 865, *865*
  pathogenesis of, 864–865
  pathology of, *865*, 865–866
  polymorphonuclear leukocytes in, 865
  purulent, 865, *865*
Campylobacter-associated, 867
chronic, 866
Crohn's disease vs., 665, 672
Yersinia, 633

Appendix, vermiform, actinomycosis of, 869
　　adenocarcinoid of, 875–876, *876*, 877(t)
　　　　carcinoids and adenocarcinomas vs., 877(t)
　　　　microscopic appearance of, 875–876, *876*
　　adenocarcinoma of, 871–873, *872*
　　　　carcinoid and adenocarcinoid vs., 877(t)
　　adenoma of, 870–871, *871*
　　adenovirus of, 869
　　anatomy of, 861–863, *862*
　　argentaffin (EC cell) carcinoids of, 253–254
　　arteritis of, 878
　　blood supply of, 862
　　carcinoid of, 874–875, *875*
　　　　adenocarcinoid and adenocarcinoma vs., 877(t)
　　congenital absence of, 863
　　Crohn's disease of, 674
　　cystadenocarcinoma of, 871–873
　　cystadenoma of, 870–871, *871*
　　cystic fibrosis of, 878
　　cytomegalovirus of, 869
　　developmental abnormalities of, 863
　　disorders of, 861–879
　　diverticula of, 863
　　duplication of, 863
　　embryology of, 861–863, *862*
　　endocrine cells of, classification of, 241(t)
　　endometriosis of, 878
　　epithelial hyperplasia of, 870
　　fibrous obliteration of, 878
　　fungal infections of, 870
　　ganglioneuroma of, 877
　　granular cell tumors of, 877
　　helicus of, 863
　　infections of, 867–870, 869(t), *870*
　　　　bacterial, 867–869
　　　　parasitic, 869, 869(t), *870*
　　　　viral, 869
　　inflammatory disorders of, 863–870, *865–868*, 869(t), *870*. See also *Appendicitis.*
　　intussusception of, 878
　　lamina propria of, 863
　　leiomyoma of, 877
　　leiomyosarcoma of, 877
　　lymphoid hyperplasia of, 287, *287–288*
　　lymphoma of, 877
　　malposition of, 863
　　measles of, 869
　　metastatic tumors of, 877–878
　　miscellaneous lesions of, 879
　　mononucleosis of, 869
　　mucocele of, 873, *873*
　　neoplasia of, 870–878, *871–876*, 877(t)
　　neuroma of, 877
　　neuromuscular structures of, 192
　　pseudomyxoma peritonei of, 873–874, *874*
　　role in mucosal immunity of, 71
　　sarcoidosis of, 878
　　septa of, 879
　　spirochetosis of, 868–869
　　tuberculosis of, 867–868
　　ulcerative colitis involving, 646, 866–867
　　yersiniosis of, 868
Arbuthnot Lane's disease, 203. See also *Constipation, idiopathic, severe.*
Areae gastricae, 19
Argentaffin (EC cell) tumors, 253–254, *254*
　　appendiceal, 253–254
　　sites of, 253
　　small-intestinal, 253, *254*
Argyrophil cell carcinoma, esophageal, 471–472
Argyrophil cells, hyperplasia of, 245, *245*
　　hypertrophy of, 245
Arterial occlusion, bowel infarcts from, 239
Arteriovenous malformation, colonic, angiodysplasia in, 219–220, *220–221*

Arteriovenous malformation (*Continued*)
　　gastrointestinal, 219–220, *220–223*
　　　　congenital, 223
　　　　submucosal, 220, *222–223*
Arteritis, appendiceal, 878
　　bowel infarcts from, 230
　　gastrointestinal, in rheumatoid disease, 229
　　necrotizing, biopsy in, 226, *227*
　　occurring in systemic lupus erythematosus, 228
Artery, ectatic small, in angiodysplasia, 220
Artery of Drummond, marginal, colonic, as anastomotic connection, 217
Arthritis, reactive, gastrointestinal effects of, 357–358
　　rheumatoid, 228, 357
Ascariasis, malabsorption in, 752
Ascorbic acid, effect on colonic epithelial cell proliferation of, 105
Aspergillus infection, esophagitis from, 391–392, *392–393*
Aspirin, alternatives to, 148–149
　　anti-inflammatory effect of, 148
　　gastric injury from, *145*
　　　　hemorrhage in, 148, *149*
　　gastrointestinal lesions from, 153–154
　　toxicity of, 148
　　injury from, 143–144
Astler and Coller's classification, of intestinal carcinoma, 836, 837(t)
Ataxia-telangiectasia, gastrointestinal manifestations of, 274
Atherosclerosis, bowel infarcts from, 230, *231*
　　in ischemic bowel disease, 231
Atony, gastric, 506
Atresia, anal membranous, 136
　　colonic, 122
　　duodenal, annular pancreas with, *122*
　　　　incidence of, 122
　　　　pathogenesis of, 123
　　esophageal, annular pancreas with, 124
　　　　with tracheoesophageal fistula, *114*, 114, 114(t)
　　　　without tracheoesophageal fistula, 114(t), 114–115
　　ileal, 123, *124*
　　ileojejunal, 122
　　intestinal, clinical manifestations of, 123–124, *124*
　　　　meconium ileus with, 132, *132*
　　　　pathogenesis of, *122*, 122–123
　　　　types of, *122*, 122–123
　　jejunal, multiple, 122
　　pyloric, congenital, 116
　　　　membranous, 116
　　rectal, 136
Atrophy, gastric, 487
　　villous, in celiac disease, 730–731
　　　　scleroderma and, 202
Atypia, colonic, in polyp-cancer sequence, 798
　　inflammatory, 8
　　usage of, 8
Auerbach's plexus. See *Myenteric plexus (Auerbach's plexus).*
Autonomic dysfunction, familial, intestinal pseudo-obstruction with, 210
Autonomic nervous system, stimulation of, gastrointestinal effects of, 352

B cells, circulating, in immunodeficiency disorders diagnosis, 267
　　dysfunction of, 274
　　　　gastrointestinal manifestations of, 273
　　　　immunodeficiency disorders from, 266
　　　　susceptibility to bacterial infection from, 267
　　IgA production of, in GALT, 76
　　precursor, in Peyer's patches, 71, *71*
Bacteremia, in strongyloidiasis, 752
Bacteria, esophageal location of, 387(t)
　　in chronic antral gastritis, 491
　　in Crohn's disease, 664
　　in esophagitis, 396, 398–400, *398–400*
　　in familial visceral myopathy, 200, *202*
　　in tropical sprue, 739

Bacterial infections, appendiceal, 867–869
  gastric, 500–503
  intestinal, clinical manifestations of, 631
    pathology of, 631–636, 632–636
Bacterial overgrowth syndrome. See also *Stasis syndrome*.
  in stasis syndrome, 742, 742
Balloon cells, in gastroesophageal reflux, 408
  of esophageal squamous epithelium, 386, 386
Barium, granuloma from, 716, 717
Barrett's epithelium, adenocarcinoma in, clinicopathologic correlation of, 468–469
    etiology of, 462–465, 462–465
    gastric cardia adenocarcinoma vs., 469
    gross morphology of, 465(t), 466
    incidence of, 461–462
    location of, 465
    microscopic features of, 465–466, 467–468, 468
    nodular, 466
    papillary, 466
    pathology of, 465(t), 465–466, 466–468
    prevalence of, 462
    prognosis of, 468–469
    risk factors for, 462–465, 462–465
    ulcerative, 466
  adenoma in, 464–465, 464–465
  cell proliferation in, 99
  columnar nature of, 460
  dysplasia of, 462–463, 462–464
    high-grade, 463, 463
    low-grade, 462, 462–463
    moderate-grade, 463, 463
  gastric epithelium vs., 460
  histologic patterns of, 461
  intestinal metaplasia in, 461, 461, 464
  origin and location of, 460
Barrett's esophagus, 411–423
  adenocarcinoma in, 418, 418. See also *Barrett's epithelium, adenocarcinoma in*.
    predisposition to, 411
  as premalignant condition, 418
  columnar-lined mucosa in, 412, 412, 416, 418
  complications of, 422
  definition of, 411
  diagnosis of, criteria for, 416
    histopathologic, 415–416
    mucosal biopsy specimens in, 416, 418
  diagrammatic representation of, 412
  differential diagnosis of, 416–418, 417
  etiology of, 411–412
  gastric heterotopia vs., 714, 715
  gastroesophageal reflux and, achalasia with, 424
  glandular epithelium in, congenital origin of, 16
  hiatal hernia in, 413
  histopathologic features of, 413(t), 413–415, 414–415
  pathogenesis of, 412
  prevalence of, 411
  reflux esophagitis in, 413
  stricture in, 412–413
  ulcer in, 412
Barrett's mucosa. See also *Barrett's epithelium*.
  biopsy of, for monitoring dysplasia and adenocarcinoma, 422–423
    for monitoring therapy, 422
  cardiac, 414–415, 415
  distinctive, 413–414, 414
    adenocarcinoma invasion in, 421, 422
    dysplasia in, high-grade epithelial, 420
      intermediate-grade epithelial, 419–420
      low-grade epithelial, 419
    dysplasia in, evolution to carcinoma of, 463–464
    histopathology of, 418–422, 419–421
      biopsy classification criteria in, 420–421
      nonneoplastic reactive changes in, 419, 421
    embryonic ciliated cell rests vs., 416
  fundic, 415

Barrett's mucosa (*Continued*)
  gastric heterotopia vs., 417–418
  histopathologic features of, 413(t), 413–415, 414–415
    classification of, 413(t)
  indeterminate, 415
  topographic appearance of, 412–413
  tracheobronchial remnants vs., 416–417, 417
  true gastric cardiac or fundic muscosa vs., 416
  ultrastructural studies of, 415
Barrett's syndrome, 412–413
Basal cell carcinoma, anal, 900, 900
Beckwith-Wiedemann syndrome, omphalocele in, 129
Beer, in etiology of rectal carcinoma, 823
Behçet's disease, colonic involvement in, 708
  esophageal involvement in, 426
Bezoars, gastric retention of, 506
Bicarbonate, gastric production of, by oxyntic cells, 23
Bile acid, binding to fiber of, colonic carcinoma risk reduction from, 823
  fecal, in pathogenesis of colonic diverticula, 772–773
  in colorectal carcinogenesis, 824
Bile duct, obstruction of, lipid maldigestion and steatorrhea in, 358
Bile salt, deficiency of, malabsorption with, normal mucosal histology in, 727
  reflux of, acute gastritis from, 482
  unabsorbed, in Crohn's disease, 665
Biliary secretions, in small-intestinal epithelial proliferation, 103
Biliary system, effect on colonic epithelial cell proliferation of, 104–105
Billroth I operation, gastritis after, 495, 495–496
  stomal ulcers after, 530–531, 531
Billroth II operation, gastritis after, 495, 495–496
  infections after, 693
  retained antrum after, 531
  stomal ulcers after, 530–531, 531
Biological markers, of colorectal carcinoma, 840–841, 841(t)
  of gastric adenocarcinoma, 602(t), 602–603
Biopsy, and autopsy, 11
  colonic, in antibiotic-associated pseudomembranous colitis, 155, 155–156
  in endometriosis, 712, 713
  duodenal, in celiac disease, disadvantages of, 734, 735
  endoscopic. See *Endoscopic biopsy*.
  for aganglionic megacolon, interpretation of, 121–122
  gross preparation and examination of, 11
  in malabsorptive disorders, special considerations in, 725–727
  in radiation esophagitis, 405, 405–406
  microscopic examination of, 11–12
  mucosal, examination of, fixation in, 11
    methods of, 10–11
      specimen orientation in, 10–11
    in gastrointestinal food allery, 185
    in pediatric allergic gastroenteritis, 185, 185(t)
    in vasculitis, 226, 227
  rectal, amebic lesions in, 638
  small-intestinal, altered immune response and, 753–754
    capsular, in malabsorptive disorders, 726
    in autoimmune enteropathy, 755, 755
    in stasis syndrome, 742, 742–743
    macroscopic study in, 726–727
    Strongyloides in, 752, 753
  surgical, 11
Bladder, urinary, increased collagen levels in, visceral myopathy and, 197, 197
Bleach, ingestion of, gastrointestinal lesions from, 146
Bleeding, endoscopic control of, 38
  gastrointestinal, diagnosis of, 215–216
    lower, 215
      colonic angiodysplasia and, 220
    upper, 215
  rectal, in allergic gastroenteritis, 175
Blind loop syndrome. See *Stasis syndrome*.
Blood flow, decreased, gastrointestinal effects of, 239
  hepatic, supply of, 217

Blood flow (*Continued*)
  increased viscosity of, necrotizing enterocolitis from, 233
  intestinal, during shock, 232
    experimental studies on, 231–232
  peripheral, macrophages of, characteristics of, 74, 74(t)
Blood group A, gastric carcinoma associated with, 84, 88
Blood group ABH, in study of intestinal adenomas, 804
Blood group O, duodenal ulcer associated with, 84
  reduced gastric carcinoma incidence in, 84
Blood vessels, colonic, relationship with diverticula of, 770, *771*
  gastrointestinal, injection studies of, 216
  tumors of, 338–339, *338–339*
Blue rubber bleb nevus syndrome, gastrointestinal involvement in, 225
Bombesin, role in gastrin cell hyperplasia of, 248
Bone marrow transplantation, gastrointestinal infection in, 275, 275(t)
  gastrointestinal injury in, causes of, 275
  graft-versus-host reaction in, gastrointestinal involvement in, 355
  parasitic infestation in, 275, 275(t)
Borrmann's classification, of gastric adenocarcinoma, 596
Bowel infarct. See *Infarction, gastrointestinal*.
Bowenoid papulosis, perianal, 890, *892*
Bowen's disease, anal, 894, *895*
Breast feeding, secretory IgA in, 75
Brown bowel syndrome, 206–207
  deposition in, 363(t)
  histology of, 206–207, *207*
  lipofuscin pigment deposition in, 364–365
  vitamin E deficiency and, 360
Brunner's glands, 25–26
  hyperplasia of, 566
    peptic duodenitis vs., 693
  in peptic duodenitis, 690–691, *691–692*
Burkitt's lymphoma, gastrointestinal, histology of, 296, *298*
Bypass, jejunoileal, enteritis from, 696
  megacolon from, 211

CA19-9, in colorectal carcinoma, 840
Calcinosis-Raynaud's-sclerodactyly-telangiectasia (CRST) syndrome, 222
Calcium, carcinogenesis reduction by, 823
  in mechanisms of cell injury, 142
  intracellular homeostasis of, changes in, ischemic bowel disease from, 233
Calcium channel blockers, in prevention of gastric stress ulcers, 233
Calories, total intake of, colonic carcinoma risk and, 822
Campylobacter infection, appendicitis from, 867
  colonic, ulcerative colitis vs., 652
  enterocolitis from, pathology of, 631–632, *632*
    ulcerative colitis vs., 632
  mucosal invasion in, with proliferation in lamina propria and lymph nodes, 627–628
Campylobacter jejuni, enterotoxin production by, diarrhea from, 632
Canaliculi, of oxyntic cells, 22
Cancer. See *Carcinoma; Tumors*.
Cancer family syndrome, genetic basis of, 90–91
Candidiasis, esophagitis from, 388–390, *390–391*
  gastric, 503, *503*
  in AIDS, 268, 277–278
  in chronic peptic ulcer, 524–525
  in immunocompromised patient, 268
  in neutropenic enterocolitis, *626*
  intestinal, pathology of, 636
  malabsorption from, 749
  mucocutaneous, chronic, clinical and histologic features of, 274
    esophagitis with, 389
    in immunodeficiency disorders, 268, *268*
Cantrell's pentalogy, 128
Capillariasis, geographic distribution of, 752–753
  strongyloidiasis vs., 753
  transmission of, 753
Carcinoembryonic antigen (CEA), in colorectal carcinoma, 840–841, 841(t)

Carcinoembryonic antigen (CEA) (*Continued*)
  in gastric adenocarcinoma, 602
  in hyperplastic polyps, 789
  in intestinal adenomas, 803–804
Carcinogenesis, chemical, in etiology of intestinal carcinoma, 821
  experimental, intestinal, 827, *828*
Carcinogens, for gastric carcinoma, 587
  for intestinal cancer, 820–821
Carcinoid, adenoma and adenocarcinoma with, 844, *844*
  appendiceal, 874–875, *875*
    incidence of, 874
    microscopic appearance of, 875, *875*
  argentaffin (EC cell), 253–254, *254*
    appendiceal, 253–254
    association with von Recklinghausen's multiple neurofibromatosis of, in duodenal neurocarcinoids, 252–253
    classification of, 244(t)
    sites of, 253
    small-intestinal, 253, *254*
  argyrophil, clinically nonfunctioning, 255–256
    gastric, cell type in, 245(t)
      chronic atrophic gastritis with, 244, 245(t)
      classification of, 244(t)
      site of, 245(t)
  argyrophil nonargentaffin, 256, *257*
  bronchial, diarrhea from, 352
  classification of, general, 243
  colonic, 255
  esophageal, 471, *472*
  gastric, 580
    chronic atrophic gastritis with, 247–248
      prognosis of, 248
    incidence of, 244
    mixed, 600–601
    Zollinger-Ellison syndrome with, 245
  goblet cell, appendiceal, 875–876
  hyperfunctional syndrome with, 243(t)
  in chronic gastritis, 498–499, *499*
  mucinous, appendiceal, 875–876
  rectal, 255
    histology of, 255, *256*
  trabecular (L cell), hindgut, 255, *256*
    classification of, 244(t)
Carcinoid syndrome, atypical, in argentaffin (EC cell) carcinoids, 253
  with gastric carcinoids, 248
Carcinoma. See also *Adenocarcinoma*.
  adenoid cystic, esophageal, 470
  adenoma-carcinoma sequence in, 824–825, *825–826*
  adenosquamous, 843, *843*
    esophageal, 469
    gastric, 580, *607*, 607–608
  anal, classification of, transitional zone mucosa in, 892–893
    relationship to Crohn's disease of, 887–888
    verrucous, 897
  anal canal, incidence of, 893
    rates of spread and survival in, 893
    staging of, 893, 894(t)
  anal margin, clinical presentation of, 893–894
    etiology of, 894
  argyrophil cell, esophageal, 471–472
  basal cell, anal, 900, *900*
  cloacogenic, of anal canal, basaloid lesions in, 896, *896*
    classification of, 896
    descriptive terms for, 895
    from transitional zone epithelium, 892–893
    histologic features of, 896, *896*
    trabeculated pattern of, 896, *896*
    transitional pattern in, 896, *896*
  colonic, cell cycle times in, 107
    cytology of, 62–63, *63*
    diverticular disease and, 781
    DNA synthesis abnormalities in, 105
    epithelial cell proliferation in, 106–107
    genetic basis of, 91

Carcinoma (*Continued*)
  colonic, hereditary site-specific, 91
    metastatic, 846
    polypoid, cytology of, 62, *63*
    relationship of adenomas to, 797–798
    risk of, after radiation, 165
    sigmoid, fungating, 830, *830*
    ulcerative, *830*, 830–831
  colorectal, cytogenetic changes in, 92
    death rates of, geographic distribution of, 819, *820*
    hereditary nonpolyposis, genetic basis of, 90–91
      Lynch syndromes in, 822
    incidence of, 819, 820(t)
      social status and physical activity in, 823
    nonpolyposis, manifestations of, 89, 89(t)
      tumor type in, 89, 89(t)
    oncogene expression in, 92–93
    polypoid lesions in, 828–829
    survival rates of, 818, 819(t)
  diagnosis of, biopsy artifacts vs., 44–45, *44–45*
  endocrine. See *Endocrine carcinoma.*
  esophageal, adenoid cystic, 470
    adenosquamous, 469
    argyrophil cell, 471–472
    cell proliferation in, 99–100
    cytology of, statistical evaluation of, 63(t), 63–64
    in celiac disease, 734
    mucoepidermoid, 469–470
    polypoid, 471
    risks factors for, 99
    small cell (oat cell), 471–472, *472*
    spindle cell, 451, *451*, 451, *451*
    verrucous, 450–451
  gastric. See *Gastric carcinoma.*
  gastrointestinal, probability of death from, 819(t)
    survival rate in, 819(t)
  genetic, cancer history in, 823
  in Crohn's disease, 676
    incidence of, 676
    risk factors for, 676
  in Peutz-Jeghers syndrome, 562–563
  in ulcerative colitis, incidence of, 655, 655(t)
    pathology of, 655–656, *656*
      dysplasia in, 656–657, *657*
    risk factors for, 655, 655(t)
  intestinal, etiology of, 819–820
      carcinogens in, 820–821
      modifying agents in, 821
    experimental carcinogenesis of, 827, *828*
    intramucosal, 804
    invasive, definition of, 804
      residual adenoma in, 824–825, *825*
    lymphatic spread of, 829–830
    pathology of, 827–836, *829–836*, 837(t)
    pleomorphic, 845
    precancerous conditions in, 824–827, *825–826*
    rare types of, 846
    risk factors for, 821, 821(t)
      alcohol in, 823
      cancer history in, 823
      dietary, 822–823
      extraintestinal conditions in, 823–824
      genetic, 821–822
      hormones in, 823
      intestinal, 824
      physical activity in, 823
      social status in, 823
      steroids in, 823
    signet-ring cell, 835, *836*
  neuroendocrine, classification of, 244(t)
    intestinal, 833, 844–845, *844–846*
  oat cell. See *Small cell carcinoma.*
  oral, in celiac disease, 734
  Paneth cell, gastric, 601
  parietal cell, gastric, 600
  poorly differentiated, lymphomas vs., 297

Carcinoma (*Continued*)
  rectal, cytology of, 63
    etiology of, beer in, 823
    risk of, after radiation, 165
    solitary ulcer syndrome vs., 706
  relation to Ménétrier's disease of, 543
  sarcomatoid, anaplastic, 846
  scirrhous, 601
  screening for, endoscopy in, 38
  small cell. See *Small cell carcinoma.*
  small-intestinal, colonic vs., 818–819
    incidence of, 819
  with lymphoid stroma, 601, *602*
Carcinoma cells, DNA contents of, 841
Carcinoma *in situ*, in colonic adenomas, 804
  in high-grade colonic dysplasia, 662, *662*
  of anal canal and margin, 894–895, *895*
Carcinosarcoma, esophageal, 470–471, *471*
  gastric, 608, *609*
Cardioesophageal junction, mucosal laceration of, in Mallory-Weiss syndrome, 504, *504*
Cardiopyloric glands, histology of, 22, *22*
Cardiopyloric mucous cells, histology of, 20(t)–21(t), 23
Cardiovascular drugs, esophagitis and inflammation from, 402(t)
  examples of, 151(t)
  gastrointestinal lesions from, 147(t), 151–152
  small-intestinal ischemia from, 154
Cardiovascular system, diseases of, gastrointestinal involvement in, 352
Carney's triad, gastric epithelioid sarcoma in, 323
  gastric epithelioid cell tumor in, 314, *315*
Cathartic colon, 204, 706–707
Caustic agents, gastrointestinal lesions from, 146, 147(t)
Caveolae, 33
Cecum, colitis of, 646
  congenital diverticula of, 131
  mobile, 125–126
  polypoid carcinoma of, relationship of vermiform appendix to, 862
Celiac artery, obstruction of, chronic intestinal ischemia from, 236
Celiac disease, allergic gastroenteritis vs., 182, *182*
  biopsy of, duodenal, missed diagnosis in, 734, *735*
    jejunal, absence of villi in, 730–731, *730–731*
    small-intestinal, resemblance to malabsorptive disorders of, 732, 734, 734(t)
    site of, 734
  clinical course of, possibilities in, 735, *735*
  collagenous colitis vs., 700
  complications of, 734
  dermatitis herpetiformis in, 356–357
  diagnostic pitfalls in, 734, *735*
  differential diagnosis of, 732, 734, 734(t)
  duodenal involvement in, 695
  epithelial cell proliferation in, 103–104
  etiology of, 728–729, 729(t)
  genetic basis of, 86
  gluten exposure in, epithelial injury during, 729
    features of, 729(t)
  HLA complex associated with, 84
  in diabetes mellitus, 355–356
  in esophageal carcinoma, 444
  malignancy in, 734
  pathogenesis of, genetic factors in, 729
    immunologic factors in, 729–730
    viral factors in, 730
  pathology of, 730–732, *730–733*
  refractory, 735–737, *735–737*
    "bubbly bulb" in, 736, *737*
    cavitated mesenteric lymph nodes in, 736–737, *738*
    definition of, 735, *735*
    ulcerations accompanying, 735–736, *737*
  somatostatin D cell growth in, 249
  surface and crypt epithelia in, 731, *731*
  synonyms for, 728
  tropical sprue vs., mucosal changes in, 739, *740*, 741
  ulcerative jejunoileitis vs., 696

Celiac-related conditions, *735–738, 735–739*
Cell cycle, in colonic carcinoma, 107
    in colonic mucosa, 103
    rectal, 104
Cell division, effect of radiation on, 158–159
    in gastrointestinal disease, 98–99
Cell injury, ATP in, 142
    calcium in, 142
    free radicals in, 142
    mechanisms of, in chemical gastrointestinal disorders, 142
    oxygen in, 142
    proteases in, 142
    radiation in, 158–159
Cell renewal, in health and disease, 98–110
Cells of Cajal, interstitial, histology of, 190, *193*
Central nervous system, gastrointestinal control by, 189
Central venous pressure, elevated, gastrointestinal effects of, 352
Ceroid pigment, deposition of, 364–365
Ceroidosis, gastrointestinal, histology of, 206–207, *207*
Chagas' disease, esophageal involvement in, 401
    intestinal pseudo-obstruction with, 209–210
Chancroid, anal, 889
Chemical disorders, classification of, 142–143
    clinical features of, 145–146
    definitions in, 142–143
    diagnosis of, 145–146
    duodenal, 694
    etiologic agents in, 146–152, 147(t)–148(t), *149*, 150(t)–151(t)
    pathogenesis of, 143, 143(t)
        foreign body deposition in, 144
        infection in, 144
        synergistic effects in, 144
        toxic injury in, 143–144
        vascular lesions in, 144
    pathologic features of, 144(t), 144–145, *145*
    specific organ involvement in, 152–156, 154(t)–155(t), *155–156*. See also specific organ.
Chemicals, effects of, 147(t)
    number of, 142–143
Chemotherapeutic drugs, colonic lesions from, 155–156
    esophageal epithelial effects of, 402, *404*
    esophagitis and inflammation from, 402(t)
    examples of, 150(t)
    gastric complications of, 145
    gastrointestinal lesions from, 147(t), 150–151
    synergistic effects of, in drug disorders, 144
Chicken, Chinese, incidence of esophageal cancer in, 442, *442*, 442(t)
Chief cells, gastric mucosal, proliferation of, 100–101
Children, chronic granulomatous disease in, 370
    colitis in, allergic, 183–184
    ileoileal intussusception in, 195, *195*
    lymphoma in, 298
    Ménétrier's disease in, 543
    polyps in. See *Polyp(s), juvenile.*
    proctitis in, allergic, 183–184, *183–184*
China, esophageal squamous cell carcinoma in, distribution of, 440–441, *440–441*
    incidence in fowl of, 442, *442*, 442(t)
    mass surveys of, *441*, 441–442
Chlamydia trachomatis, lymphogranuloma venereum–associated immunotypes of, 631
Chlamydial infections, anal, 889
    colonic, ulcerative colitis vs., 652
    intestinal, pathology of, 631
Cholangitis, sclerosing, in ulcerative colitis, 655
Cholecystectomy, colonic carcinoma after, 823
Cholecystokinin, in G cell tumor immunohistochemistry, 249
    in gastric epithelial renewal, 101, 101(t)
    in small-intestinal epithelial cell proliferation, 103, 103(t)
Cholelithiasis, in colonic diverticular disease, 782
Cholera, diarrhea in, undifferentiated crypt cells in, 30
    enterotoxin production in, water secretion from, 628
    immunization against, history of, 69–70
    mucosal adhesion by pathogen in, 627
    protection against, secretory IgA in, 71

Cholesterol, colonic carcinoma risk and, 822
    deposition of, in Wolman's disease, 365
Cholinergic fibers, colonic, in epithelial cell proliferation, 104
Choriocarcinoma, colonic, 846
    esophageal, 473
    gastric, 580–581, 608
Chorioepithelioma, malignant, gastric, 580–581
Chromosomal syndromes, gastrointestinal tract involvement in, 84–85, 85(t)
Chromosome(s), abnormalities of, correlation with pathologic examination of, 12
    in colorectal carcinoma, classification of, 92
    deletion of, in colorectal tumors, 91–92
Churg-Strauss syndrome, gastrointestinal involvement in, 228
    gastrointestinal vasculitis in, 226
    Wegener's granulomatosis vs., 228
Chyle, lymphatic, in primary intestinal lymphangiectasia, 758, *759*
Chylomicrons, formation of, in abetalipoproteinemia, 362
Cirrhosis, alcoholic, esophageal varices from, 218
    biliary, gastrointestinal effects of, 358–359
Cloaca, embryology of, 135–136
Cloacal exstrophy, 137
Cloacal membrane, embryology of, 136–137
Clofazimine, enteritis and colitis from, 145
Clostridium difficile, drug treatment and, 144
Clostridium difficile infection, colonic, ulcerative colitis vs., 652–653
    in Crohn's disease, 675
    pseudomembranous colitis from, 624–626, *625*
    toxins from, 624
Clostridium septicum, in neutropenic enterocolitis, 626
Clostridium welchii, intestinal wall invasion by, pneumatosis coli vs., 710
Coccidiosis, in immunocompromised patient, 271
    pathology of, *639*, 639–640
Coelom, extraembryonic, 118
Colectomy, for Crohn's disease, 676
    for severe idiopathic constipation, histologic analysis in, 204, *205*
    prophylactic, for extensive ulcerative colitis, 663
Colic cells, 61, *62*
Colitis, acute, chronic vs., rectocolonic mucosal biopsy in, 679
    enema-induced colitis vs., 707–708
    acute self-limited, 702
        idiopathic inflammatory bowel disease vs., histopathologic diagnosis of, 628–629, *629*
        mucosal regeneration in, 648–649
        pathology of, *632*
    allergic, 182–185, *183–184*, 185(t)
        adult cases of, 185
        childhood cases of, 183–184
        definition of, 182–183
        terminology for, 172
    amebic, ulcerative colitis vs., 652–653
    chronic, acute vs., rectocolonic mucosal biopsy in, 679
        allergic proctitis and colitis vs., 184
        histologic features of, 649, 650(t)
        microscopic (lymphocytic) colitis vs., 698
        radiation vs. ulcerative, 165
    collagenous, celiac disease–type features in, 738
        clinical features of, 698–699
        definition of, 698
    diversion-related, differential diagnosis of, 700
        etiology of, 698
        pathology of, 699–700, *699–700*
    cytomegalovirus-associated, in AIDS, 278, *279*
    diffuse active, mucosal biopsy of, 679, *680*
    diversion-related, 676
        clinical features of, 701
        definition of, 700–701
        differential diagnosis of, 702
        etiology of, 700–701
        pathology of, 701–702, *701–702*
    drug-induced, 157
    eosinophilic, anorectal, 890
    extensive, 645, *645*
    focal active, mucosal biopsy of, 679, *680*

Colitis (*Continued*)
  granulomatous, 664
  hemorrhagic, in exogenous infections, 628
  identification of, by rectocolonic mucosal biopsy, 679
  idiopathic, chronic, in Crohn's disease vs. ulcerative colitis differentiation, 678
    extent and severity of, endoscopic biopsy of, 681
  in Crohn's disease, 675
  indeterminate, 678
  ischemic. See *Ischemic colitis*.
  left-sided, 645
  localized, 703
  microscopic (lymphocytic), celiac disease–type features in, 738–739
    clinical features of, 698
    definition of, 697–698
    differential diagnosis of, 698
    etiology of, 697–698
    pathology of, 698
  mucosal, transmural colitis vs., 650, 652
  neutropenic, drug treatment and, 144
  obstructive, allergic proctitis and colitis vs., 184
  pseudomembranous, 234–235
    antibiotic-induced, 154–155, 155(t), 155–157
      Clostridium difficile growth in, 154–155
      drugs causing, 155(t)
      lesion characteristics in, 155, 155–156
      severe examples of, 155, 156–157
      Staphylococcus aureus growth in, 154
    drug-induced, 144
    ulcerative colitis vs., 652
  radiation, 164, 164–165
    mucosal changes in, 161
  Salmonella, pathology of, 632
  severe, sinus tracts vs., 667
  ulcerative. See *Ulcerative colitis*.
  universal, 645
Colitis cystica profunda, clinical features of, 703
  definition of, 702–703
  differential diagnosis of, 703
  etiology of, 702–703
  in ulcerative colitis, 654
  localized, 703
  pathology of, 703
Collagen formation, in radiation injury, 159, 160
Collagen tissue defects, relationship with diverticulosis of, 770
Collagen vascular–connective tissue disease, esophageal involvement in, 424–425
Colloidal carbon suspension, vascular lesion study with, 216
Colon, absorptive cells of, 34, 34–35
  aganglionic, in Hirschsprung's disease, parasympathetic nerve fibers in, 208, 209
  allergic disease of, clinical presentation of, 185
  allergic gastroenteritis of, 182
  atresia of, 122
  carcinoids of, 255
  carcinoma of. See *Carcinoma, colonic*.
  cathartic, 204, 706–707
  cavernous hemangioma of, 224
  cell types of, 104
  chemotherapeutic drug injury to, 150–151
  columnar cells of, 60
  Crohn's disease of, 665–666, 666. See also *Crohn's disease*.
    differential diagnosis of, 672–673, 673(t)
    gross features of, 667–668
    submucosal and mucosal features of, 670–671
    ulcerated vs. normal mucosa in, 668, 668
    ulcerative colitis vs., 677, 677(t)
  crypts of, hyperproliferative activity in, neoplastic transformation from, 105
  cytologic sampling of, 50
  diverticular disease of, 768–782
  drug injury to, 154–156, 155(t), 155–157, 157(t)
  duplications of, 135
  dysplasia of, in polyp-cancer sequence, 798

Colon (*Continued*)
  embryology of, 118–119
  endocrine cells of, classification of, 241(t)
  endoscopic biopsy of, techniques in, 39
  enema effects on, 707, 707–708
  epithelial cells of, number of, in ascending and descending colon, 104
    proliferation of, in disease states, 105–108, 106(t)
      in normal states, 104–105
  epithelium of, hyperplastic polyps as, 789
    injury to, in allergic colitis, 183, 183–184
  function of, 33
  ganglioneuromatosis of, 344, 347
  goblet mucous cells of, 35
  gross anatomy of, 33–34
  in ulcerative colitis, normal vs. pathologic mucosa of, 646, 646
  infections of, ulcerative colitis vs., 652–653
  inflammatory disorders of, 697–704, 699–702, 704–707, 706–709
  inflammatory pseudopolyps of, 792, 794
  ischemia of, 231
    estrogen usage and, 148
    progesterone usage and, 148
  juvenile polyps of, 795–796
  laxative effects on, 706–707, 706–707
  leiomyoma of, histology of, 329, 332
  leiomyosarcoma of, histology of, 329, 332
  lesions of, cytology of, 61–63, 62–63
    statistical evaluation of, 67, 67(t)
  lymphoid hyperplasia of, 286
  malacoplakia of, 371–372, 371–372
  mesenteric taeniae of, spastic diverticulosis and, 775, 775–776
  metaplasia of, 7(t), 8
  muscular layer of, abnormalities of, in diverticulosis, 770–772, 772
  neuromuscular structure of, 192, 194
  nodular lymphoid hyperplasia of, without hypogammaglobulinemia, 289–290
  periarteritis nodosa involvement of, 226, 227
  Peutz-Jeghers polyps of, 791, 792
  prediverticular state of, 774
  preneoplasia of, loss of DNA synthesis in, 105
  pseudo-obstruction of, drug-induced, 155, 157(t)
  radiation injury to, 164, 164–165
  rectosigmoid, diffusely infiltrative carcinoma of, 831
    endometriosis of, 712, 713
  scleroderma of, morphologic changes in, 205–206, 206
  sigmoid, deformities of, shortened taeniae in, 770–771, 772
    fungating carcinoma of, 830, 830
    incidence of adenomas in, 798
    intraluminal pressure of, in diverticulosis, 772
    leiomyoma of, 329, 333, 333
    volvulus of, 126
  sporadic visceral myopathy of, 200
  stromal tumors of, site specificity of, 312
  structure of, similarity to small intestine of, 816–817
  susceptibility to carcinoma of, 824
  undifferentiated columnar crypt cells of, 35
  varices of, 218, 218–219
Colonic mucosa, biopsy of, diffuse active colitis diagnosis by, 679, 680
    focal active colitis diagnosis by, 679, 680
    granuloma diagnosis by, 679, 680
    in inflammatory bowel disease, 679, 679(t), 680, 681
  cell turnover time in, 103
  colic cells of, 61, 62
  compartments of, 33
  crypts of, 34, 34
  DNA synthesis in, abnormal stages of, preneoplasia and, 105
  eosinophil levels in, in allergic proctitis and colitis, 184
  epithelial cells of, 26(t), 33–34
  epithelium of, 34
  hyperplasia of, as precancerous condition, 827
  in chronic ulcerative colitis, architectural alteration in, 649, 651
    crypt atrophy in, 649, 651
    lymphoid nodules in, 649, 651
    Paneth cell metaplasia in, 649, 652

Colonic mucosa (*Continued*)
  in collagenous colitis, 699–700, *699–700*
  in melanosis coli, 706, *706–707*
  in pneumatosis coli, 710, *710*
  in ulcerative colitis, follicular inflammation in, 658, *660*
    granulomatous reaction in, 648, *650*
    indefinite for dysplasia, 658, *660–661*
    negative for dysplasia in, 658, *658–659*
  lymphoid nodules of, 34
  mucin-filled macrophages in, 361–362, *362*
  neurofibroma of, in von Recklinghausen's disease, 344, *346*
  organization of, 33, *33*
  surface of, 34
  ulceration of, 708–709
    normal state vs., in Crohn's disease, 668, *669*
Colonic submucosa, barium granuloma in, 716, *717*
Colonic wall, defects in, effect on diverticular development of, 770, *771*
  suture reaction in, 716, *716*
Colonoscope, fiberoptic, history of, 38
Colonoscopy, cytologic sampling with, 50
    for ulcerative colitis, 663
    indications for, 38
    preoperative, for Crohn's disease severity and extent determination, 681
Colon-specific antigen, in colorectal carcinoma, 840–841
Colostomy, diverting, colitis after, 700–701
Columnar cells, colonic, 60
  gastric, 51, *51*, 55–56, *56*
  in papillary gastric adenoma, 552, *555*
Condyloma acuminatum, of anal region, 890, 897
  histology of, 890, *891*
Congenital anomalies, of gastrointestinal tract, 4, 4(t)
Connective tissue disorders, blood vessel involvement in, 222–223
Constipation, idiopathic, severe, as sporadic visceral neuropathy, 203–204
    histology of, 204, *205*
  in aganglionic megacolon, 119
  in intestinal pseudo-obstruction, 197
  trabecular rectal tumors and, 255
Contractile ring, in intestinal absorptive cells, 29
Contrasuppressor cells, in GALT, 76
Corticosteroid hormones, peptic ulcers from, 154
Corticosteroids, colonic injury from, 155
Cortisone, in gastric epithelial renewal, 101, 101(t)
Cowden's disease, intestinal polyps in, 811
Cow's milk protein allergy, definition of, 175
  in infants, 183
Crohn's disease, 663–677
  allergic gastroenteritis vs., 182
  anal, 674, 887–888
    diagnosis of, 887, *888*
    sarcoid-like granulomatous reaction in, *888*
  anorectal fistula in, 887
  aphthous ucler in, 666, *666*
    disease progression and, 668
  appendiceal, 674
    gross features in, 867, *867*
    microscopic features in, 867, *868*
  Behçet's disease vs., 708
  carcinoma in, 676
    colonic, 827
    incidence of, 676
  chronic peptic ulcer disease vs., 526
  clinical features of, 664–665
  colitis in, 675
  collagenous colitis vs., 700
  colonic, 666, *666*
    cytology of, 61, *62*
    differential diagnosis of, 672–673, 673(t)
    submucosal and mucosal features of, 670–671
    ulcerated vs. intact mucosa in, 668, *668*
    ulcerative colitis vs., clinical course in, 678
      discriminating features in, 677, 677(t)
      rectocolonic mucosal biopsy in, 679, *680*
      shared features in, 677–678

Crohn's disease (*Continued*)
  complications of, 674–676
  definition of, 663–664
  diagnosis of, features in, 664, 664(t)
    inflammatory conditions vs., 677
    pathologic, 671–672
  distribution of, 665–666, *665–666*
  diverticular disease in, 781
  diverting procedures for, temporary, colitis in, 701
  duodenal, 695
    cytology of, 60
    proximal, 673–674, *674*
  dysplasia in, 676
    surveillance of, 676–677
  enteritis cystica in, 675
  epidemiology of, 664
  esophageal, 425–426, 426(t), 673
  etiology of, 664
  extraintestinal manifestations of, 676
  fistulas in, 666
  gastric, 507–508, 673, *673–674*
  general aspects of, 663–664, 664(t)
  granulomas in, 369, 671, *671*
    in recurrent disease, 675
    mucosal biopsy of, 679, *680*
  gross features of, *666–667*, 666–668
    lesion distribution in, 666
  histologic features of, 668, 668(t), *668–671*, 670–671
    variation by region in, 670, *670–671*
  ileal, ileostomy complications vs., 654
    mucosal biopsy of, 681–682, *681–682*
    recurrent, lesions in, 675–676
    submucosal thickening in, 668, *669*
  inflammatory conditions in, 676
  intestinal obstruction in, 674
  malabsorption in, 674
  medical therapy for, 665
  mural eosinophilic gastroenteritis vs., 174
  myopathy vs., histologic features in, 200, *202*
  of oral cavity, 673
  pathogenesis of, 664
  pathology of, 665–668, *665–671*, 668(t), *670–672*
  recurrent disease in, 665
    in differentiation from ulcerative colitis, 678
  secondary infections in, 675
  severity and extent of, preoperative colonoscopy for, 681
  sinus tracts in, 666–667, *667*, 667(t)
    inflammatory, 669–670, *670*
  skip areas in, 677
  small-intestinal, creeping fat in, 667, *667*
    differential diagnosis of, 672
    lymphatic dilatation in, 668, *669*
    pyloric gland metaplasia in, 670, *670*
    submucosal neural proliferation in, 668, *669*
  stenosis in, 677
  stricture in, 196, *196*
  surgical resection for, 665
    ileal and colonic abnormalities after, 675–676
  terminology for, 663–664
  toxic megacolon in, 675
  ulcerative colitis vs., 653
    biopsy differentiation of, 46
    clinical course in, 678
    comparative features of, 677(t), 677–678
    indeterminate colitis in, 678
    mucosal features in, 670–671
    shared features of, 643
    surgical specimen examination in, 678
Cronkhite-Canada syndrome, clinical symptoms of, 810
  nonpolypoid mucosa in, 810, *811*
  polyposis in, 89
  polyps in, 810, *811*
    juvenile polyposis syndrome vs., 564
    retention, 565
CRST syndrome, 222

Crypt(s), colonic, atrophy of, in chronic ulcerative colitis, 649, *651*
  small-intestinal, effect of radiation on, *163*, 163–164
    hyperplasia of, in allergic gastroenteritis, 181, *181*
Crypt cell carcinoma, appendiceal, 875–876
Crypt cells, undifferentiated, absorptive cells vs., 30, *30*
  columnar, 35
  structure and function of, 26(t), 29–30, *30*
Cryptitis, in ulcerative colitis, 648, *649*
Cryptorchidism, congenital inguinal hernia with, 128
Cryptosporidiosis, in AIDS, 278
Cryptosporidium, in immunodeficiency disorders, 268, 270, 278
Culture techniques, in pathologic examination, 12
Cup cells, small-intestinal, 33
Curling's ulcer. See *Stress ulcer(s)*.
Cushing's ulcer. See *Stress ulcer(s)*.
Cyst(s), cloacal, in colonic duplications, 135
  esophageal, 474
    embryology of, 116
  glandular, 564
  intramucosal, in gastric carcinoma, 591, *591*
  mediastinal, of neurenteric origin, 115–116
    clinical manifestations of, 116
  mesenteric, 137–138, *137–138*
    clinical features of, 137
    pathologic features of, 137–138, *137–138*
  neurenteric, embryology of, 115
  omental, 138
  umbilical, 131
  unilocular, in duplications, 135
Cystadenocarcinoma, appendiceal, 871–873
Cystadenoma, appendiceal, 870–871, *871*
Cystic fibrosis, appendiceal, 878
  pancreatic, meconium ileus equivalent in, 132
    meconium ileus in, 131–132
  systemic effects of, 358
Cystinosis, deposition in, 363(t)
  histology of, 365
Cytodiagnosis, colonic, 60–63, *62–63*
  statistical evaluation of, 67, 67(t)
  duodenal, 60–61, *61*
  esophageal, 54–55, *55*
    assessment criteria in, 55(t)
    statistical evaluation of, 63(t), 63–64
  gastric, 55–60, *56–59*, 58(t)–59(t)
    statistical evaluation of, qualitative studies in, 64, 65(t)
    quantitative studies in, 64–66, 65–66, 66(t)
  rectal, 63
    statistical evaluation of, 67, 67(t)
Cytology, classification in, light microscropy vs. automated image analysis in, 54(t)
  collection of material in, 49–50
    abrasive balloon technique in, 49
    brush abrasion in, 49–50
    cell-swab method in, 49
    colorectal, 50
    duodenal, 50
    endoscopically guided, 49
    esophageal, 49
    gastric, 49
    needle aspiration in, 49
  microscopic examination methods in, 50–52, *50–54*, 54, 54(t)
    for fresh unfixed preparations, 50–52, *50–52*
      fluorescence microscopy in, 52
      Nomarski differential interference contrast microscopy in, 51, *51*
      phase contrast microscopy in, 50–51, *50–51*
      ultraviolet light microscopy in, 51–52, *52*
    mucosal biopsy and, 12
    quantitative, 53–54, *54*, 54(t)
      flow cytophotometry in, 53
      fluorescence cytophotometry in, 53
      high-resolution image analysis in, 53–54, *54*, 54(t)
      micromorphometry in, 53

Cytology (*Continued*)
  microscopic examination methods in, smear techniques vs. DNA flow cytometry in, 66(t)
  staining techniques in, 52–53
  role of, 48
Cytomegalovirus infection, appendiceal, 869
  esophagitis from, 396, *397*
  gastric, 500, *501*
  in AIDS, 278, *279*
    gastric erosions with, 268, *269*
  in Crohn's disease, 675
  intestinal, pathology of, 630, 630–631
Cytometry, flow DNA, of gastric cells, smear cytology vs., 66(t)
  statistical evaluation of, 65–66, *66*
Cytomorphology, colonic, 60–63, *62–63*
  duodenal, 60–61, *61*
  esophageal, 54–55, *55*, 55(t)
  gastric, 55–60, *56–59*, 58(t)–59(t)
  rectal, 63
Cytophotometry, flow, 53
  fluorescence, 53
  predictive potential of, in esophageal carcinoma, 100
Cytoskeleton, of intestinal absorptive cells, structural features of, 28–29, *29*
Cytotoxicity, cell-mediated, of interepithelial lymphocytes, 73
Cytotoxins, as virulence factors in exogenous infection, 627

Deficiency states, *743*, 743–744
Degeneration, epithelial, gastrointestinal injury and, 7
Deoxycholic acid, in colorectal carcinogenesis, 824
Depositions, 360–368. See also *Storage disease*.
  definition of, 360–361
Dermatitis, atopic, allergic basis of, 173
Dermatitis herpetiformis, celiac disease and, 356–357
  lesions in, 738
Dermatologic disease, esophageal involvement in, 427, 427(t)
Dermatomyositis, pseudo-obstruction in, 206
Dermatosis, linear-IgA bullous, 357
Detergents, esophageal injury from, *401*, 401–402
Developmental anomalies, of gastrointestinal tract, 4, 4(t)
Diabetes mellitus, gastrointestinal involvement in, 355–356
  motility disorders and, 210
  stasis syndrome in, 741
Diaphragm, embryology of, 126
  eventration of, 126
Diarrhea, bloody, chronic idiopathic inflammatory bowel disease vs., biopsy differentiation of, 46
  Campylobacter enterotoxin producing, 632
  chronic, in AIDS, morphometric data for duodenal mucosa in, *754*, 754
  enterotoxigenic *E. coli*, in newborns, breast milk and, 75
  enterotoxigenic secretory, role of toxins in, 627
  in aganglionic megacolon, 119
  in allergic gastroenteritis, 175
  in Crohn's disease, 665
  in diabetes mellitus, 355
  in intestinal pseudo-obstruction, 197
  in microscopic (lymphocytic) colitis, 698
  in microvillus inclusion disease, 757
  in shigellosis, 627
  infant, enterotoxin production in, 627
  infectious, in etiology of tropical sprue, 739
  secretory, bicarbonate loss in, mechanisms for, 35
    in collagenous colitis, 698–699
    undifferentiated crypt cells in, 30
  traveler's, enterotoxin production in, 627
Diet, as risk factor for colonic carcinoma, 822–823
  cholesterol and fecal sterols in, 822
  fiber and vegetables in, 822–823
  high fat and protein intake in, 822
  total calorie intake in, 822
  vitamins and calcium in, 823
  effect on colonic epithelial cell proliferation of, 105
  fiber, for diverticulosis, 772

Diet (*Continued*)
  gluten-free. See *Gluten-free diet.*
  in esophageal cancer etiology, 442–443
  in pathogenesis of acute appendicitis, 864
  westernization of, effect on incidence of colonic diverticula of, 770
Dieulafoy's disease, 223
DiGeorge's syndrome, 274
Digestion, abnormalities of, malabsorption from, 727
  occurrence in stomach of, 20
Dilatation, colonic, in intestinal pseudo-obstruction, 197, *197*
  in type I visceral myopathy, 198, *198*
  of muscularis propria, mechanical obstruction and, 196, *196*
Disaccharidase deficiency, malabsorption from, normal mucosal histology in, 727–728, *728*
Distention, in intestinal pseudo-obstruction, 197, *197*
  mechanical obstruction and, 194–195
Diversion procedures, colitis after, 700–702, *701–702*. See also *Colitis, diversion-related.*
Diverticula, acquired, appendiceal, 867
  classification of, 5, 768
  colonic, bleeding of, inflammation and, 780, *781*
    giant, 775
    gross features of, 773, *773*
    historical description of, 769
    location of, 770, *770*, 773, *773*
    pathogenesis of, colonic wall defects in, 770, *771*
      dietary fiber deficiency in, 772
      fecal bile acid in, 772–773
      genetic influence in, 772
      intraluminal pressure in, 772
      muscular layer abnormalities in, 770–772, *772*
    pathology of, 773–777, 774(t), *774–778*, 779, 779(t)
      handling of gross specimens in, 773
    perforation of, 777, *777*
      chronic inflammation in, 777, *778*
      foreign body granuloma in, 777, *778*
    pseudo-, 773–774, *774*
    right-sided, geographic distribution of, 779
      patient age in, 779
      types of, 779
    scleroderma and, 205–206, *206*
    sigmoidal, geographic distribution of, 779
  congenital, 768
    appendiceal, 863
    cecal, 131
    intestinal, 131
  duodenal, 769
  epiphrenic, 769
  esophageal, 424, 769
    in carcinoma, 444
  false, 768, 779
  formation of, in soft tissue diseases, 357
  gastric, 506, 769
  gastrointestinal, description of, 768
  ileal, 769
  jejunal, 769
  locations of, 769
  pulsion, 768
    clinical manifestations of, 769
  small-intestinal, location of, 769
  traction, 768
  true, 768, 773, 779
Diverticular disease, colonic, 768–782
  carcinoma in, 781
  clinical features of, 779–780
  clinicopathologic correlation of, 779–782, *781*
  coexisting colonic conditions in, 781–782
  Crohn's disease vs., 672–673, 673(t)
  epidemiology of, 769–770
  etiology of, *770–772*, 770–773
  extracolonic conditions associated with, 782
  hemorrhage in, 780–781, *781*
  history of, 769–770
  inflammation in, hemorrhage and, 780, *781*

Diverticular disease (*Continued*)
  colonic, inflammatory bowel diseases in, 781
    ischemic colon disease in, 781–782
    obstruction in, 781
    pathogenesis of, *770–772*, 770–773
    pathologic classification of, 774(t), 774–777, *775–778*, 779
Diverticulitis, appendiceal, 867
  cecal, 779
  colonic, perforation in, complications of, 780
  in Meckel's diverticulum, 130
Diverticulosis, colonic, acute, inflammation and necrosis in, 776, *777*
  complications of, 775–777, *777–778*, 779
  focal perforation in, complications of, 777, *777–778*, 779
  free perforation in, 779
  gross features of, 773, *773*
  histologic features of, 773–774, *774*
  muscle abnormality in, 774–775, *775–776*
  pathologic stages of, according to extent of inflammation, 779, 779(t)
  prediverticular state in, 774
  rectal bleeding in, 776
  relationship of muscle spasm to, 771–772
  simple, 774, *775*
  spastic, 774–775, *775–776*
  symptoms of, 775–776
  definition of, 768
  esophageal, diffuse intramural, 769
  jejunal, neuromuscular causes of, *207*, 207–208
  of upper gastrointestinal tract, 769
  small-intestinal, neuromuscular causes of, *207*, 207–208
DMH, in experimental carcinogenesis, 827, *828*
DNA synthesis, abnormalities of, in colonic adenoma, 105–106
  in colonic preneoplasia, 105
  effects of radiation on, 158
Double esophagus, 115
Down's syndrome. See *Trisomy 21.*
Drug(s), effects of, 147(t)
  esophageal ulceration from, 402, 402(t), *403*
  esophagitis from, 153(t)
  gastrointestinal lesions from, 147(t), 152
  malabsorption from, 154, 154(t)
  number of, 143
  pseudomembranous colitis from, 154–155, 155(t), *155–157*
  pseudo-obstruction from, 155, 157(t)
Drug disorders, classification of, 143
  clinical features of, 145–146
  colonic, 154–156, 155(t), *155–157*, 157(t)
  definitions in, 143
  diagnosis of, 145–146
  duodenal, 153–154
  esophageal, 153, 153(t)
  etiologic agents in, 146–152, 147(t)–148(t), *149*, 150(t)–151(t)
  gastric, 153–154
  ileal, 154, 154(t)
  jejunal, 154, 154(t)
  pathogenesis of, 143, 143(t)
    altered motility in, 144
    infection in, 144
    physical events in, 143
    synergistic effects in, 144
    toxic injury in, 143–144
    vascular lesions in, 144
  pathologic features of, 144(t), 144–145, *145*
    complications in, 145
    hemorrhage in, 144
    inflammation in, 145, *145*
    thrombosis in, 145
    ulceration in, 145
  specific organ involvement in, 152–156, 154(t)–155(t), *155–157*, 157(t). See also specific anatomic part.
Dukes' classification, of intestinal carcinoma, 836, 837(t)
Duodenal mucosa, in peptic duodenitis, microscopic features of, 690–692, *691–692*
  Mycobacterium avium-intracellulare infection of, in AIDS, 693, *694*
  opportunistic infection of, 693

Duodenitis, 689–696
    acute, drug-induced, 153–154
    chronic, drug and chemical usage and, 145
    cytology of, 60
    nodular, 692
    peptic, 689–693. See also *Peptic ulcer disease, chronic.*
        chronic peptic ulcer disease vs., 526–527
        clinical features of, 690
        complications of, 692
        definition of, 689–690
        diagnosis of, 692–693
        differential diagnosis of, 693
        etiology of, 690
        gastric heterotopia vs., 714, 715
        gross pathology of, 690
        malabsorptive disorders vs., 726
        microscopic pathology of, 690–692, *691–692*
        pathogenesis of, 690
        refractory celiac disease associated with, 736
        shortening of villi in, 690–691, *691*
    types of, 693, 693(t)
Duodenum, allergic disease of, 695
    annular pancreas involvement of, 124
    atresia of, 122, *123*
    biopsy of, in celiac disease, disadvantages of, 734, *735*
        in malabsorptive disorders, 725–727
    blood supply of, 24
    Brunner's glands of, 25–26
    celiac disease of, 695
    cell types in, 59
    chemical injury to, 153–154
    chronic peptic ulcer of. See also *Peptic ulcer disease, chronic.*
        gross features of, 523–524, *523–524*
    Crohn's disease of, 695
    cytologic sampling of, 50
    dilatation of, in type I visceral myopathy, 198, *198–199*
    diverticula of, 769
    drug injury to, 153–154
    duplications of, 135
    endocrine cells of, classification of, 241(t)
    gastric heterotopia of, peptic duodenitis vs., 714
    gross anatomy of, 24
    immune disorders of, 695
    infections of, 693, *694*
    inflammatory diseases of, types of, 693, 693(t)
    lesions of, cytology of, 60–61, *61*
        statistical evaluation of, 66
    metaplasia of, 7(t), 8
    obstruction of, mixed rotation and, 125
    papilla of, tumors of, cytology of, 60, *60*
    peptic ulcer of, 522
    periampullary region of, carcinoma of, *837*
    proximal, Crohn's disease of, 673–674, *674*
        NSAID injury to, 148
    stenosis of, 122, 123, 124
    tumors of, cytology of, 60
        somatostatin D cell, 249
            histology of, 250–251, *251*
            somatostatinoma with, *251*
    ulcers of. See *Ulcer(s), duodenal.*
    vacuolization of, 122
    vascular disease of, 694–695
Duplication(s), appendiceal, 863
    colonic, 135
    duodenal, 135
    esophageal, 135
    gastric, 135
    of alimentary tract, clinical features of, 134–135
        embryonic origin of, 133–134
        general features of, 133, *134*
        locations of, 135
        macroscopic appearance of, 135
        neuroenteric origin of, 134
        pathogenesis of, 133–134
        pathologic features of, 135
    small-intestinal, 135

Dutcher bodies, mucosal, in Waldenström's macroglobulinemia, 760, *761*
Dysentery, bacillary, 631
    immunization against, history of, 69–70
Dysplasia, as synonymous with premalignancy, 592
    colonic, classification of, 657–658, *658*, 658(t)
        diagnosis of, immunocytochemical stains in, 662–663
            scanning electron microscopy in, 663
        high-grade, 659, *661–662*, *662*
        in polyp-cancer sequence, 798
        low-grade, 658–659, *661*
        rating of, crypt base location and, 662, *663*
        synonyms for, 656
    definition of, general, 592
        in pathology and cytology, 592
    epithelial. See under *Barrett's epithelium; Barrett's mucosa.*
    esophageal, epithelial cell proliferation and, 99–100
        of squamous epithelium, cytologic classification of, 445
            follow-up study of, 445
            histology of, 444–445, *444–445*
    gastric, classification of, 592, *592–595*, 594–595
        epithelial, as precancerous lesion, 591–592, *592–595*, 594–595
        epithelial cell proliferation in, 102
        globoid, of foveolar cells, 595, *595*
        grading systems of, 592
        studies of, 592
    gastrointestinal, definition of, 8
    in chronic gastritis, 498–499, *499*
    in Crohn's disease, surveillance of, 676–677
    in ulcerative colitis, 656–659, *657–663*, 658(t), *662–663*
        carcinoma with, pathology of, 656–657, *657*
        chronic, histologic classification of, 657–658, *658*, 658(t)
        polypoid lesion of, 657, *657*
    intestinal, neuronal, 208–209, *210*
        giant ganglia in, 209, *210*
Dysplasia-associated lesion or mass (DALM), in ulcerative colitis, 657
Dystrophy, muscular, progressive, pseudo-obstruction in, 206

Ectasia, gastric antral vascular, 506–507
Eczema, allergic basis of, 173
Edema, inflammatory, duodenal, 694
Ehlers-Danlos syndrome, gastrointestinal bleeding in, 222–223
Elastosis, in sigmoid colon, muscle shortening from, 771
Electrolytes, uptake of, in colonic absorptive cells, 35
Electromagnetic waves, 157, 157(t)
Electron micrography, of esophageal squamous mucosa, 16, *17*
Electron microscopy, of colonic carcinoma, 834–835
    of microvillus inclusion disease, 757–758, *759*
    of stromal cell tumors, 311
    pathologic examination with, 12
    scanning, of colonic dysplasia, 663
Elements, trace, role in esophageal cancer of, 443
Emepronium bromide, pill-induced esophagitis from, 152
Emphysema, pulmonary, pneumatosis intestinalis in, 709
Endocrine carcinoma, intestinal, 844–845, *844–846*
    poorly differentiated, gastrointestinal, 256–258, *257*
        aggressive behavior of, 258
        histology of, *257*, 257–258
        small- to intermediate-cell, esophageal, 256–257
        gastric, 257, *257*
Endocrine cell tumors, gut, chronic atrophic gastritis with, 245(t)
    classification of, 243, 244(t)
        as "carcinoid," 255
        by cell type, 242–243, 245(t)
        functional, 242, 243(t)
    diagnosis of, 241–243, 243(t)
    histologic features of, 242
    hyperfunctional syndromes with, 242–243, 243(t)
    miscellaneous, 255–256, *257*
    prognosis of, 243–244
        invasiveness in, 243–244
        metastases in, 244
        site in, 243
    site of, 245(t)
    inappropriate, 255

Endocrine cells, gastroenteropancreatic, classification of, 241, 241(t)
　histochemical and ultrastructural features of, 241, 242(t)
　gut, origins of, 241
　　structure of, 241
　　study techniques for, 240–241
　histology of, 23
　hyperplasia of, in chronic atrophic gastritis, 246–248, 247
　in intestinal carcinoma, 833
Endocrine-exocrine tumors, combined, 258, 258–259
　composite, 259
　role of endocrine component in, 258
Endocrine neoplasia syndrome, multiple, neuronal intestinal dysplasia with, 209
　type 1, gastric carcinoids in, 245
Endocrine system, disorders of, 240–259
　categories of, 6
　gastrointestinal involvement in, 355–356
　secondary pseudo-obstruction in, 210–211
　normal structure and function of, 240–241, 241(t)–242(t)
Endometriosis, appendiceal, 878
　ileal, 712, 712
　intestinal, clinical features of, 711–712
　　definition of, 711
　　differential diagnosis of, 712–713
　　etiology of, 711
　　pathology of, 712, 712–713
　of rectosigmoid colon, 712, 713
Endoscope, design application of, 39
　fiberoptic, history of, 38
Endoscopic biopsy, accuracy of, factors affecting, 45–46
　bowel preparation in, colitic changes from, 629
　brush cytology with, 45–46
　channels in, 39
　colon sampling in, 39
　control of, 38
　false-positive results of, 46
　findings in, disease differentiation from, 46
　　interpretation of, 44–45, 44–46
　　　crush artifacts in, 44, 44–45
　　　edge artifacts in, 45, 45
　　　enema and laxative-induced changes in, 45
　　　hemorrhage in, 45
　　　value to patient of, 46
　　　villous architecture assessment in, 46
　forceps in, 39
　ileal mucosal, 681–682, 681–682
　in gastric lymphoid hyperplasia diagnosis, 285, 286
　in ulcer evaluation, 532–533
　in ulcerative colitis, 663
　of colonic mucosa, for epithelial dysplasia, in ureterosigmoidostomy patients, 353, 353
　of gastrointestinal lymphoproliferative disorders, 303, 303(t)
　rectocolonic mucosal, colitis identification by, 679
　　determination of extent and severity of colitis by, 681
　　in acute vs. chronic colitis, 679
　　in inflammatory bowel disease, 679, 679(t), 680, 681
　　uses of, 679, 679(t)
　　in ulcerative vs. Crohn's colitis, 679, 680
　　of neoplasia, 681
　specimens in, electron microscopy of, 43–44
　　embedding of, 41
　　fixation of, 40–41
　　　Hollande's solution for, 40, 40(t)
　　Giemsa staining of, 43
　　immunohistochemical preparation of, 43–44
　　number required, lesion type and, 45–46
　　orientation of, 39–40
　　processing of, 41, 41
　　sectioning of, 41–42, 42
　　size of, 39
　　special procedures for, 43–44
　　staining of, 42–43, 43(t)
　　technical factors and handling methods for, 39–44, 40(t), 41–42, 43(t)
　　touch preparations of, 43

Endoscopic biopsy (Continued)
　submucosal, 39
　suction, of small intestine, 39–40
　technique of, value to patient of, 46
Endoscopy, biopsy with. See Endoscopic biopsy.
　complications of, 39
　contraindications to, 38–39
　cytologic examination with, 12
　duodenal, anatomic features in, 24
　gastric, mucosal biopsy with, 509–510
　gastrointestinal bleeding diagnosis by, 215–216
　history of, 37–38
　in diagnosis of early gastric carcinoma, 571
　modern, 38–39
　mucosal biopsy with, specimen orientation in, 10–11
　therapeutic uses of, 38
Endothelial cells, effects of radiation on, 159
Enemas, colonic effects of, 707, 707–708
　effect on biopsy findings of, 45
　gastrointestinal lesions from, 147(t), 152
　proctitis from, 157
ENNG, gastrointestinal carcinoma induction with, 595, 596
Entamoeba histolytica infection, 638, 638
　Crohn's disease vs., 672
　ulcerative colitis vs., 652
Enteral feeding, necrotizing enterocolitis and, 234
Enteric nervous system, damage to, in diabetes mellitus, 355–356
Enteritis, bypass, clinical features of, 696
　　definition of, 696
　　etiology of, 696
　　pathology of, 696
　ischemic, 6
　lupus, 228
　nonspecific, pathology of, 629–630
　radiation, acute, 163
　　chronic, 163, 163–164
　　diagnosis of, 164
　small-intestinal viral infections and, 745, 745(t)
　specific viral, pathology of, 630
Enteritis cystica profunda, clinical features of, 696–697
　definition of, 696–697
　etiology of, 696–697
　in Crohn's disease, 675
　pathology of, 697
Enterochromaffin (EC) cells, hyperplasia of, in chronic atrophic gastritis, 246
　in ileal argentaffin carcinoids, 253, 254
Enterochromaffin-like (ECL) cell tumors, atypical carcinoid syndrome with, 248
　classification of, 242
　gastric argyrophil, 244–248, 245(t), 245–247
　　clinicopathologic aspects of, 248
　　in chronic atrophic gastritis, 245(t), 246–248, 247
　　in normal or hypertrophic mucosa, 244–246, 245(t), 245–247
　　histology of, 245–246, 245–256
Enterocolitis, acute, infantile, in aganglionic megacolon, 119, 121
　acute self-limited, idiopathic inflammatory bowel disease vs., histopathologic diagnosis of, 628–629, 629
　Campylobacter, pathology of, 631–632, 632
　necrotizing, in premature infants, 234, 235
　　increased blood viscosity and, 233
　　pathogenesis of, 234
　　polycythemia and, 233
　　stricture formation in, 234, 235
　neutropenic, as gastrointestinal ecologic perturbation, 626, 626
　Yersinia, pathology of, 633, 633
Enterocolitis lymphofollicularis, 289–290
Enterocyte(s), surface, in microvillus inclusion disease, 757–758, 759
Enterocytozoon bieneusi infections, electron microscopy of, 750, 750
　intestinal microsporidiosis from, in AIDS, 749–751, 750–751
　plasmodia identification in, 750, 751
　spore development in, 750, 750–751
Enteroglucagon, in small-intestinal epithelial cell proliferation, 103

Enteropathy, autoimmune, causes of, 755
  malabsorption in, 754–755, 755
  gluten-induced. See *Celiac disease.*
  hemorrhagic, 6
  idiopathic AIDS, malabsorption in, 754, 754
  protein-losing, in primary intestinal lymphangiectasia, 758–759
    in small-intestinal allergic gastroenteritis, 182
    primary vs. secondary, 727
Enterotoxin(s), as virulence factors in exogenous infection, 627
  production of, mucosal adhesion of organisms with, 627
Enzyme, proteolytic, peptic duodenitis from, 690
Eosinophils, in allergic reactions, 173. See also *Gastroenteritis, allergic; Gastroenteritis, eosinophilic.*
  increased levels of, in allergic colitis and proctitis, 183–184, 183–184
    in allergic gastroenteritis, 176, 177
      causes of, 177(t)
      in esophageal epithelium, 177, 178
      in small-intestinal mucosa, 181–182
Epigastric discomfort, in gastric carcinoma, 585
Epithelial cells, colonic, DNA synthesis abnormalities in, in preneoplasia, 105
  proliferation of, in disease states, 105–108, 106(t)
    in normal states, 104–105
  damage to, chemical and physical disorders and, 142
  disease states and, 98
  effect of radiation on, 159–160, 161
  esophageal, proliferation of, in disease states, 99–100
    in normal states, 99, 99(t)
  follicle-associated. See *Membranous (M) cells.*
  gastric, 20(t)
    mucin profiles of, 21(t)
    proliferation of, effects of humoral factors on, 101(t)
      in disease states, 101–102
      in normal states, 100(t)–101(t), 100–101
    ultrastructural characteristics of, 20(t)
  intestinal, proliferation of, defects in, atresia from, 122–123
      stenosis from, 122
    jejunal, phase contrast microscopy of, 50, 50
    normal vs. neoplastic, high-resolution image analysis of, 53, 53
    of gastric glands, 21–22, 21–22
    of gastric mucosa, maturational disturbances to, 56–58, 57–58
  proliferative characteristics of, analytic techniques for, 99
    in esophageal epithelium, 99(t)
    in gastric mucosa, 100, 100(t)
  rectal, radiation-induced changes in, 164
  small-intestinal. See also specific cell type.
    functions of, 26(t)
    mucin profiles of, 31(t)
    proliferation of, effect of humoral factors on, 103, 103(t)
      in disease states, 103–104
      in normal states, 102–103
    types of, 26–33, 27–32
    ultrastructural characteristics of, 26(t)
  structure and function of, metaplasia of, 6–7
Epithelial tumors, esophageal, type and origin of, 460(t)
Epithelioid cell tumors, gastric, gross characteristics of, 314, 315
Epithelium. See also under specific organ.
  mucosal, 14, 15
  pseudostratified columnar ciliated, in duplications, 135
Epstein-Barr virus, infection with, esophagitis in, 396
Ergot drugs, gastrointestinal lesions from, 151
Erosion, hemorrhagic, in chemical and drug disorders, 145, 145
Erythema multiforme, gastrointestinal effects of, 357
Erythema nodosum, in ulcerative colitis, 654
Erythromycin, intolerance to, 151
Escherichia coli, enterotoxigenic, diarrhea from, 627
  neonatal, breast milk and, 75
  esophagitis from, 398, 399
  hemorrhagic colitis from, 628
  mucosal adhesion by, 627
Esophageal atresia, with tracheoesophageal fistula, 114, 114, 114(t)
  without tracheoesophageal fistula, 114(t), 114–115

Esophageal disease, diagnosis of, esophagoscopy in, 38
Esophageal epithelium, bacterial colonization of, 396, 398
  columnar, as source of adenocarcinoma, 459–460
  embryology of, 113–114
  embryonic ciliated cell rests in, Barrett's mucosa vs., 416
  eosinophilic infiltration of, differential diagnosis of, 409, 409(t)
  eosinophils in, in allergic gastroenteritis, 177, 178
  intercellular spaces of, lymphocytes in, 409, 409
  squamous, alkaline reflux changes in, 410, 410
    balloon cells of, 386, 386
    basal zone of, 16, 17
      hyperplasia of, in allergic gastroenteritis, 177, 178
    dysplasia of, in carcinoma, cytologic classification of, 445
      follow-up study of, 445
      histology of, 444–445, 444–445
    glycogenic acanthosis of, 385–386, 386
    histology of, 16, 17–19, 18
    in achalasia, 425
    Langerhans cells in, 16, 18
    melanocytic proliferation of, 386
    papillae of, 17, 18
    reactive changes and vascular lakes in, 384, 384
    Z line junction of, 16
Esophageal hiatus, hernias at, 406–407
Esophageal mucosa, squamous, luminal surface of, 16, 17
  nuclear area of, 63(t)
Esophageal varices, causes of, 218
  location of, 217–218, 217–218
  sclerotherapy for, perforation after, 402, 403
Esophagitis, 383–401
  Actinomyces israelii, 400
  active, pathologic findings in, 384, 384
  Aspergillus, 391–392, 392–393
  bacterial, 396, 398–400, 398–400
    opportunistic, 398–399, 399
  blastomycotic, 393
  candidal, 387, 388–390, 389–392
    acute, 387
    biopsy in, 391–392
    causative organisms of, 387
    chronic, 389–390
    disseminated candidiasis from, 391
    histopathologic features of, 388–390, 390–391
    in AIDS, 278
    squamous epithelial changes in, 390–391
    subacute, 387, 389
  cell proliferation in, 99
  chronic, definition of, 385
    in esophageal carcinoma, 443
  cytomegalovirus, 396
    ulceration in, 396, 397
  definition of, 383–384
  drugs and, 402, 402(t), 403
  eosinophilic, differential diagnosis of, 409, 409(t)
  eosinophilic gastroenteritis and, 426
  Epstein-Barr virus infection and, 396
  Escherichia coli, 398, 399
  fungal, 387–393
    opportunistic, 387, 388–392, 389–393
    pathogenic, 393
  granulomatous, differential diagnosis of, 426, 426(t)
  herpes, 391, 393, 394–395, 395–396
    Candida infection with, 391, 393
    histopathologic diagnosis of, 395–396
    immunohistochemical studies of, 395, 395
    squamous epithelial inclusions in, 393, 394, 395
  histoplasmal, 393
  HIV infection and, 396
  infectious agents and, 386–401
    localization of, 387(t)
  mixed fungal, 390, 391
    viral esophagitis with, 390, 391
  mycobacterial, 399–400
  parasitic, 401
  pathologic findings in, 383–385, 384–385
  peptic, in sliding hiatal hernia, 406

Esophagitis (*Continued*)
　Phycomycetes and, 392–393
　pill-induced, 152
　　causes of, 153, 153(t)
　radiation, 162
　　acute, *405*, 405
　　chronic, 405–406
　reactive epithelial changes in, 384, *384*
　reflux, allergic gastroenteritis vs., 177
　　definitions of, 407
　　development of, 407
　　epithelial changes in, 408(t)
　　epithelial injury in, reactive changes vs., 410, *410*
　　gastroesophageal reflux vs., 407
　　in Barrett's esophagus, 413
　　pathophysiology of, histopathologic features in, 411
　　relationship between sliding hiatal hernia and, 406
　　ulcers with, 530
　rubella associated with, 396
　spirochetal (syphilitic), 400–401
　Streptococcus, 398, *399*
　varicella associated with, 396
　variola associated with, 396
　viral, 393, *394–395*, 395–396, *397*
Esophagogastric junction, adenocarcinoma of, 606–607
Esophagogastroduodenoscopy, upper gastrointestinal bleeding diagnosis by, 38
Esophagoscopy, in diagnosis of esophageal disease, 38
Esophagus, achalasia of, 423, *424–425*
　　squamous epithelial findings in, *425*
　adenoacanthoma of, 469, *470*
　adenocarcinoma of, 460–470. See also *Barrett's esophagus, adenocarcinoma in.*
　　not associated with Barrett's epithelium, 469
　adenoid cystic carcinoma of, 470
　adenoma of, 474
　adenosquamous carcinoma of, 469
　allergic gastroenteritis of, 177–178, *178*
　　mucosal biopsy of, 185
　amyloidosis of, 428, *429*
　arterial blood supply of, 15
　Behçet's disease involvement of, 426
　benign tumors of, 473–474
　carcinoid of, 471, *472*
　carcinosarcoma of, 470–471, *471*
　cardiac glands of, 18
　choriocarcinoma of, 473
　collagen vascular–connective tissue disease involvement of, 424–425
　Crohn's disease of, 425–426, 426(t), 673
　cysts of, 116, 474
　cytologic sampling of, 49
　dermatologic diseases affecting, 427, 427(t)
　diverticula of, 424, 769
　double, 115
　duplications of, 135
　ectopic sebaceous glands of, 386
　embryology of, 113–114
　epithelial cells of, proliferation of, in disease states, 99–100
　　in normal states, 99, 99(t)
　epithelial tumors of, type and origin of, 460(t)
　erosion of, 385
　giant fibrovascular polyps of, 342, *344*
　glands of, as source of adenocarcinoma, 459–460
　　deep (submucosal), 18, *19*
　　superficial (mucosal), 16, 18
　graft-versus-host disease of, 427–428, *427–428*
　granular cell tumors of, 346, *348*
　gross anatomy of, 15–16
　histologic features of, 16, *17–19*, 18
　　normal variants of, 385–386, *386*
　human papillomavirus infection of, 396
　immunodeficiency involvement of, 427
　infectious agents in, localization of, 386–387, 387(t)
　injury to, chemotherapy and, 150
　　drugs and, 153, 153(t)

Esophagus (*Continued*)
　injury to, exogenous chemicals and, 401–402, 402(t), *403–404*
　　physical agents and, *405*, 405–406
　　thermal, 406
　length of, 15
　lesions of, cytology of, 54–55, *55*, 55(t)
　　assessment criteria for, 55(t)
　　statistical evaluation of, 63(t), 63–64
　lymphatic drainage of, 15–16
　malignant melanoma of, 472–473
　metaplasia of, 7, 7(t)
　motor disorders of, 423–424, *424–426*
　mucoepidermoid carcinoma of, 469–470
　neuromuscular structure of, 190–191
　polypoid carcinoma of, 471
　polyps of, 474
　proliferative compartment of, 99
　propulsive functions of, 16
　radiation injury to, 162
　rings of, 423–424, *426*
　sarcoidosis of, 427
　scleroderma of, 205, *206*
　Sjögren's syndrome effects on, 358
　small cell (oat cell) carcinoma of, 471–472, *472*
　squamous cell carcinoma of, 439–456. See also *Squamous cell carcinoma, esophageal.*
　squamous cell papilloma of, 473
　squamous cells of, dysplastic, cytology of, 54, *55*
　stenosis of, congenital, 115
　　segmental, 115
　stricture of, in carcinoma, 443–444
　　tracheobronchial remnant as, 416–417, *417*
　stromal tumors of, 320–321, *321*
　　site specificity of, 312
　submucosa of, ganglion cells of, 18
　systemic diseases of, 424–428, 426(t), *427–429*
　trauma to, 404–405
　tumors of, 473–474
　　genetic basis of, 88
　ulcers of, active chronic, 385, *385*
　　acute, 385
　　bacterial colonization of, 396, *398*
　　drugs in, 402, 402(t), *403*
　　healing, 385
　webs of, 423–424
　Whipple's disease of, 400, *400*
Estrogen, colonic injury from, 155
　gastrointestinal lesions from, 147(t), 148
Estrogen receptors, in colon carcinoma, 823
Ethanol. See *Alcohol*.
Exogenous hormones, gastrointestinal effects of, 356
Exogenous infections, gastrointestinal, 626–628
　hemorrhagic colitis in, 628
　host-microbe interaction in, patterns of, 627–628
　microbial toxins in, 627
　mucosal adhesion of organisms in, with enterotoxin production, 627
　　with microvillous damage, 627
　mucosal invasion of organisms in, with intracellular proliferation, 627
　　with proliferation in lamina propria and lymph nodes, 627–628
　mucosal translocation of organisms in, with systemic spread, 628
　tissue invasion in, 627
　virulence factors in, 626–627
Exstrophy, cloacal, 137

Fabry's disease, deposition in, 363(t)
　gastrointestinal effects of, 364
　jejunal diverticulosis from, 208
Familial polyposis coli, 807–808, *809*
Fascicle, shunt, 190
Fat, and colonic epithelial cell proliferation, 105
　as risk factor for colonic carcinoma, 822

Fecal matter, as carcinogen, 824
Fecapentaenes, as intestinal carcinogen, 821
Fetal sulfoglycoprotein antigen (FSA), in gastric adenocarcinoma, 602
Fiber, dietary, deficiency of, colonic carcinoma risk and, 822–823
　relationship to colonic diverticulosis of, 772
Fibroblast, atypical, radiation and, 159
Fibrosis, colonic, collagen increase vs., 192, 194
　cystic. See *Cystic fibrosis.*
　in Crohn's disease, 668, 669
　muscular, myopathy vs., 200, 201
　peridiverticular, 770, 771
Fibrous tissue, tumors of, 339, 339(t), 340–344, 341–342
Fimbrin, in absorptive cells, 29, 29
Fissure(s), anal, 886
Fistula(s), colovesical, in colonic diverticulosis, 777
　H type, 115
　in Crohn's disease, 666, 667, 674–675, 677, 677(t), 887
　laryngotracheoesophageal, 115
　tracheoesophageal, with esophageal atresia, 114, 114, 114(t)
　　without esophageal atresia, 114(t), 115
　umbilical, 131
Fistula in ano, 886–887
　in adenocarcinoma, 898
Flow-cytometric analysis, in pathologic examination, 12
Fluorophotometry, single-cell, of gastric cytology, statistical evaluation of, 64–65, 65–66
5-Fluorouracil, gastrointestinal lesions from, 150–151
Folic acid deficiency, gastrointestinal effects of, 354, 360
　intestinal megaloblastic changes in, 354
　in tropical sprue, 739, 740
Follicle, lymphoid, of GALT, 71, 72
Food allergy, gastrointestinal. See also *Gastroenteritis, allergic.*
　aspects of, 171–172
　causes of, 172(t)
　diagnosis of, 171–172
　terminology for, 172
　in organ systems, 173
Food intake, in small-intestinal epithelial proliferation, 103
Foodstuffs, propulsion of, 16
　rapid transit of, through small intestine, malabsorption from, 727
Foramina of Morgagni, hernias through, 127–128
Foregut, endocrine tumors of, classification of, 243, 244(t)
　esophageal development from, 113
Foreign body deposits, chemical disorders from, 144
Foreign body granulomas, 369, 507
　in colonic diverticula, 777, 778
　intestinal, types of, 716(t)
Foreign body reactions, 715–718, 716(t), 716–717
　inflammatory, 715–716
　localized granulomatous, 716, 716, 716(t)
Foveolar mucous cells, hyperplasia of, in hypertrophic hypersecretory gastropathy, 543
　in Ménétrier's disease, 540–541, 541–542
Free radicals, in mechanisms of cell injury, 142
Fundic gland, polyps of, 564
Fungal infections, appendiceal, 870
　gastric, 503, 503
　in immunodeficiency disorders, 268
　intestinal, pathology of, 636–637, 637
　malabsorption from, 749
Fungi, esophageal location of, 387(t)

G_1 phase (presynthetic phase), of cell proliferation, 98–99
Ganglia, of myenteric plexus, interconnections of, 190, 190
　prevertebral, gastrointestinal control by, 189
Ganglion cells, gastrointestinal, 344
　giant, in neuronal intestinal dysplasia, 209, 210
　identification of, in aganglionic megacolon biopsy specimens, 121
　intestinal, congenital absence of, Hirschsprung's disease from, 119, 121
　of esophageal submucosa, 18
Ganglioneuroma, appendiceal, 877
　gastrointestinal, 344, 346, 347

Ganglioneuromatosis, colonic, 344, 346, 347
　intestinal, 811
　synonyms for, 346
　systemic syndromes associated with, 346
Ganglionic nerve cells, eosinophilic intranuclear inclusions in, in familial visceral neuropathy, 203, 203
Gangliosidosis, deposition in, 363(t), 363–364
Gangrene, gastrointestinal, 6
Gardner's syndrome, fundic gland polyps in, 564
　genetic basis of, 90
　intestinal polyps in, 808–809
Gastrectomy, antral, gastritis after, 495, 495–496
　colorectal carcinoma after, 823–824
　for gastric dysplasia, controversy over, 594–595
　malabsorption from, normal mucosal histology in, 727
　partial, gastric remnants following, carcinoma in, 590–591
Gastric acid, as defense mechanism, 623
　excess of, peptic duodenitis from, 690
　in etiology of chronic peptic ulcer disease, 521
　reduced levels of, in Ménétrier's disease, 540
Gastric Cancer Study Group (Japan), histologic classification of, 577
Gastric carcinoma. See also *Gastric tumors.*
　adenosquamous, 607, 607–608
　advanced, growth rates of, 596
　age distribution in, 605
　blood group A associated with, 84
　blood group O unassociated with, 84
　carcinogens for, 587
　cell proliferation in, 596
　cell types of, 584–585
　chronic ulcer in, 590, 590
　clinical presentation of, 585, 605–606
　combined, argyrophil endocrine cells in, 258, 258–259
　cytology of, 58–60, 59(t), 59–60
　　characteristic features in, 59(t)
　　statistical evaluation of, qualitative studies in, 64, 65(t)
　　quantitative studies in, 64–66, 65–66, 66(t)
　diagnosis of, 605–606
　dysplastic findings in, 594
　differential diagnosis of, 585
　differentiated type, 605
　early, 570–583
　　adenosquamous, 580
　　advanced cancer vs., 572, 572
　　age distribution in, 571–572, 572
　　carcinoid, 580
　　choriocarcinomatous, 580–581
　　clinical diagnosis of, endoscopy in, 571
　　combined, 573–574, 577–578
　　definitions of, 572, 572
　　frequency of, 573
　　geographic distribution of, 570
　　growth patterns of, 582
　　growth rates of, 582, 596
　　histogenesis of, 581–582
　　histologic classification of, 575, 577
　　histologic features of, 577–581, 579–580
　　histologic types of, 577–581, 578(t), 579–580. See also *Adenocarcinoma, gastric.*
　　　frequency of, 581
　　history of, 570–571, 571
　　incidence of, in precancerous lesions, 582, 582
　　location of, 572–573, 573
　　lymph node metastases in, 581
　　macroscopic classification of, 573, 573–574
　　　types in, 574(t)
　　　　distribution and prevalence of, 574–575
　　　　gross, 574
　　macroscopic features of, 573–575, 573–578, 574(t)
　　malignant chorioepitheliomatous, 580–581
　　morphology of, 573, 574–578
　　mucinous, 579–580
　　multiple occurrence of, 581
　　natural history of, 581–582
　　pathology of, 572–581

Gastric carcinoma (*Continued*)
  early, percentage of, chronologic trend in, 571, *571*
    precancerous lesions in, 582, *582*
    prognosis of, 582–583
    recurrence of, after surgery, 582
    sex distribution in, 571–572, *572*
    signet-ring cell type, 579, *580*
    size of, chronologic trend in, 575, *578*
    squamous cell, 580
    synonyms for, 570
    tubular, well-differentiated, 577, *579*
    type I, 573, *574*, 574(t)
    type IIa, 573, 574(t)
    type IIb, 573, 574(t)
    type IIc, 573, 574(t), *575–577*
      moderately differentiated tubular, 577–578, *579*
      poorly differentiated, 577–578, *579*
    type III, 573, 574(t)
    ulceration in, 581
    undifferentiated, 580
  endoscopy of, statistical evaluation of, 64, 65(t)
  epithelial cell proliferation in, 102
  etiology of, carcinogen exposure in, 595–596
  expanding, 604, *604*
  hepatoid, 600
  histogram of, 64, *65*
  in situ, diagnosis of, 594
  infiltrative, 604, *604*
  intestinal, dysplasia as precursor to, 595
  location of, 596
  lymphatic permeation in, 602
  metastases in, 609–610
  mixed, 600–601
  mucoepidermoid, 607, *607–608*
  peptic ulcer vs., 527, *527–528*
  ploidy patterns of, 603
  precancerous conditions and, 585
  prognosis of, 606
  proliferative activity of, 102
  relation with intestinal metaplasia of, intestinal cell type in, 585
  scirrhous, 601
  sex distribution of, 605
  size of, 596
  small cell, 609, *609*
  spread of, 601–602
  squamous cell, 607, *607–608*
  TNM staging of, 605
  treatment of, 606
  undifferentiated, 580, 605
  with lymphoid stroma, 601, *602*
Gastric cardia, adenocarcinoma of, 606–607
  Barrett's adenocarcinoma vs., 469
Gastric epithelium, abnormalities of, classification of, 592, *592–595*, 594–595
  dysplasia of, 592, *593*
    adenoma vs., 592
    carcinoma in, stromal invasion in, 594, *594*
    management of, conservative vs. surgical, 594–595
    mild, 592
    precancerous nature of, evidence of, 594
  esophageal, 417–418
  hyperplasia of, carcinoma in, 591
    classification of, 591
    severe, 592, *593*
    simple (regenerative), 592, *592*
    possible cancer of, 594–595, *594–595*
Gastric folds, enlarged, in Ménétrier's disease vs. allergic gastroenteritis, 180
Gastric foveolae, damage to, in allergic gastroenteritis, 179, *180*
  hyperplasia of, 558, *558*
Gastric freezing, 505–506
Gastric glands, corporal, in Zollinger-Ellison syndrome, 539, *540*
  dysplasia of, 592, *593*
  epithelial cells of, *21–22*, 21–22
  severe hyperplasia of, 592, *593*

Gastric glands (*Continued*)
  simple hyperplasia of, 592, *592*
  submucosal, carcinoma associated with, 591, *591*
Gastric mucosa, alcohol-induced damage to, 146–147, 147(t)
  allergic gastroenteritis of, 176, *177*
  antral, allergic gastroenteritis of, edema and erosion in, 179, *180*
    eosinophil infiltration in, 178–179, *179–180*
    biopsy of, in chronic active gastritis, 485–486, *487*
    in chronic gastritis, 485, *486*
    cell proliferative activity in, 100, 100(t)
    cellular structure of, 100
    destruction of, in atrophic gastritis, 493, *494*
    in isolated granulomatous gastritis, 508, *508*
  aspirin injury to, hemorrhage and necrosis from, *149*
  atrophic, intestinal metaplasia of, 587–588
  Barrett's mucosa vs., 416
  biopsy of, 509–510
    in acute gastritis, 483–484, *483–484*
    in disease diagnosis, 38
    in ulcer evaluation, 532–533
  cardiopyloric cells of, 20(t), 23, *23*
  columnar cells of, 51, *51*, 55–56, *56*
    in intestinal metaplasia, 588
  corporal, destruction of, in chronic gastritis, 493, *493*
    in gastritis cystica profunda, *509*
    in Ménétrier's disease, 540–541, *541*
    in postgastrectomy gastritis, 495, *495*
    in stress ulcer, 519, *519*
    in Zollinger-Ellison syndrome, 539, *539*
  corpus fundic type, in gastric heterotopia, 713–714
  eosinophilic infiltration of, differential diagnosis of, 179
  epithelial cells of, functions of, 20(t)
    mucin profiles of, 21(t)
    proliferation of, in disease states, 101–102
      in normal states, 100(t)–101(t), 100–101
    ultrastructural characteristics of, 20(t)
  epithelium of, 20
    dysplasia of, adenoma vs., 552, *554*
    regeneration of, cell types in, 58
      physiologic stimuli in, 101, 101(t)
  fundic, cell proliferation in, 100, 100(t)
    cellular structure of, 100
  glandular dysplasia of, 499, *499*
  goblet cells of, 56, *57*
  heterotopic, in duodenal mucosa, 714, *715*
  histology of, 20(t)–21(t), 20–23, *21–23*
  hypertrophy of, diffuse, 538–545
    causes of, 538–539, 539(t)
    hypertrophic hypersecretory gastropathy and, 543
    inflammatory disorders and, 543, *544*, 545
    tumors and, *544*, 545
    Zollinger-Ellison syndrome and, 539–540, *540*
    epithelial hyperplasia and, carcinoma in, 591
    focal, causes of, 537, 538(t)
      heterotopic pancreatic tissue and, 538, *538*
      inflammatory lesions and, 538
      polyps and, 537–538
    Ménétrier's disease and, 540–543, *541–543*
  in chronic erosive gastritis, 496, *496–497*
  in duplications, 135
  inflammation of, in congenital pyloric stenosis, 506
  intestinal type of, transformation to, 588
  intramucosal cysts in, carcinoma associated with, 591, *591*
  iron deposition in, in hemochromatosis, 359, *359*
  isolated granuloma in, 369, *370*
  lamina propria of, 20
  lesions of, cytology of, 55–60, *56–59*, 58(t)–59(t)
    statistical evaluation of, qualitative studies in, 64, 65(t)
      quantitative studies in, 64–66, 65–66, 66(t)
  mucous neck cells of, 20(t)–21(t), 21, 56, *57*
  muscularis mucosae of, 20
  oxyntic (parietal) cells of, 20(t), 22–23, 56, *57*
    ultrastructural features of, *23*
  resistance of, in etiology of chronic peptic ulcer disease, 521

Gastric mucosa (*Continued*)
    surface-foveolar mucous cells of, histology of, 20(t)–21(t), 20–21, *21*
    zymogenic (chief) cells of, 20(t), 23, *23*
Gastric tumors. See also *Gastric carcinoma*.
    frequency of, 584–585, 585(t)
    genetic basis of, 88–89
    mucosal thickening in, *544*, 545
    precursors of, 88
    radiation-induced, 162–163
Gastrin, gastric production of, 20
    in G cell tumor immunohistochemistry, 249
    in gastric epithelial renewal, 101, 101(t)
    in small-intestinal epithelial cell proliferation, 103, 103(t)
    serum levels of, in Zollinger-Ellison syndrome, 102
Gastrin (G) cell tumors, *248*, 248–249
    classification of, 244(t)
    duodenal, 249
    gastric, 248–249
        cell type in, 245(t)
        chronic atrophic gastritis with, 245(t)
        diagnostic immunohistochemistry for, 249, *250*
        histology of, 249, *250*
        site of, 245(t)
Gastrin (G) cells, hyperfunction of, 243(t)
    hyperplasia of, 248, *248*
        duodenal, 249
        pyloric, argyrophil ECL cell tumors in, 245, *245*
Gastrin (G) cell/somatostatin (D) cell tumors, gastric, 249
    classification of, 242
Gastrinoma, duodenal, gastrin cell hyperplasia with, *250*
    hyperfunctional syndrome with, 243, 243(t)
    pancreatic, malignancy rate of, 249
        Zollinger-Ellison syndrome from, argyrophil nonargentaffin tumor in, 256, *257*
    somatostatin (D) cell density in, 249
Gastritis, 481–510
    acute, clinical features of, 482–483
        definition of, 481–482
        differential diagnosis of, 484–485
        drug-induced, 153–154
        etiology of, 482
        healing phase of, histology of, 484, *484*
        histology of, 483–484, *483–484*
        mucosal biopsy of, 483–484, *483–484*
        pathogenesis of, 482
        pathology of, 483–484, *483–484*
    acute hemorrhagic, 482
    acute nonerosive, erosive gastritis vs., 482
    acute toxic, 482
    alcohol-induced, 146–147, 147(t)
    allergic gastroenteritis vs., inflammatory infiltrate in, 179–180
    antral, chronic, 489–492, *490*
        alcohol-induced, 147
        bacteria in, 491
        clinical features of, 491
        differential diagnosis of, 491–492
        drug and chemical usage and, 145
        etiology of, 489–490
        Helicobacter organisms in, *490*, 490–491
        pathogenesis of, 489–490
        pathology of, 491
    atrophic, chronic, 487
        argyrophil carcinoid with, 244, 245(t)
        argyrophil ECL cell hyperplasia with, 246–248, *247*
        as carcinoma precursor, 88, 587–588
        autoimmune, cancer development in, 587
        environmental, cancer development in, 587
        goblet cells in, 56, *57*
        histogram of, 64, *65*
        hypersecretory, 587
        metastases in, 248
        epithelial cell proliferation in, 101
        in Sjögren's syndrome, 358
        pernicious anemia with, pathology of, 493, *494*

Gastritis (*Continued*)
    chronic, 485(t)
        active, features of, 485–486, *487*
            in children, 509
        adenocarcinoma in, 498–499, *499*
        carcinoids in, 499
        complications of, 497–499, *499*
        definition of, 481–482
        dysplasia in, 498–499, *499*
        epithelial maturational disturbances in, 56–58, *57–58*
        epithelial polyps in, 498
        histologic features of, 485(t)
        in diabetes mellitus, 355
        intestinal metaplasia in, 487(t), 487–489, *488–489*
            as diagnostic finding, 489
            as precancerous lesion, 582
        Ménétrier's disease vs., 542
        pathologic features of, 485–489
            common, 485, *486*
        relationship to carcinoma of, 530
        special features and terms in, 486–487, 487(t)
        stages of, 487(t)
        types of, 485, 485(t)
        xanthoma in, 498
    classification of, 482, 482(t)
    corrosive, clinical features of, 499
        etiology of, 499
        pathology of, 499–500
    definitions of, 481–482
    diagnosis of, histologic, cytologic changes vs., 58, 58(t)
    emphysematous, acute, 501
    eosinophilic, 506
    erosive, chronic, 496, *497*
    fundic, chronic, 492–495, *493–494*
        clinical features of, 492
        differential diagnosis of, 493–495
        etiology of, 492
        pathogenesis of, 492
        pathology of, 492–493, *493–494*
    histogram of, 64, *65*
    hypertrophic, chronic, 497
    in tropical sprue, 741
    isolated granulomatous, 508, *508*
    location of, correlation with cause of, 482
    lymphocytic, 496–497
        celiac disease–type features in, 738
        mucosal hypertrophy in, 545
    metaplastic, columnar cells in, 56, *57*
    motor and mechanical disorders associated with, 506
    phlegmonous, acute, 501
    postgastrectomy, *495*, 495–496
        clinical features of, 495
        differential diagnosis of, 496
        etiology of, 495
        pathology of, *495*, 495–496
    superficial, chronic, 487
        epithelial cells in, 52
        progression of, cell kinetic studies of, 101
    vascular disease associated with, 506–507
    verrucous, as precancerous lesion, 582, *582*
Gastritis cystica polyposa, mucosal thickening in, *544*, 545
Gastritis cystica profunda, 508–509, *509*
Gastroduodenostomy, gastritis after, *495*, 495–496
    chronic, 530
Gastroenteritis, allergic, clinical and laboratory features of, 175–176
    colonic, 182
    definitions in, 175
    diagnosis of, 176–177, *177*, 177(t)
    differential diagnosis of, 177, 177(t)
    esophageal, 177–178, *178*
        diagnosis of, 177, *178*
        differential diagnosis of, 177–178, *178*
    gastric, 178–180, *179–180*
        gastritis vs., 179–180
        malabsorption in, 180
        mucosal changes in, 178–179, *179–180*

Gastroenteritis (Continued)
    allergic, increased eosinophils in, 176, 177
        causes of, 177(t)
        mucosal biopsy of, 185
        pathologic features of, 176–177, 177, 177(t)
        pediatric, mucosal biopsy of, 185(t)
        pulmonary symptoms in, 173
        rectal, 182
        small-intestinal, 180–182, 181–182
            diagnosis of, 181–182
            differential diagnosis of, 182
            mucosal changes in, 180–181, 181–182
        specific organ involvement in, 177–182, 178–182
        terminology for, 172
    eosinophilic, 173(t), 173–175, 174–175
        definitions in, 175
        esophagitis and, 426
        motility disorders in, 211
        mucosal, 173, 173(t)
        mural, 173, 173(t)
            diagnosis of, 174, 174
            differential diagnosis of, 174, 175
            pathologic features of, 174, 174
        serosal, 174–175
        terminology for, 172
        types of, 173(t)
Gastroenteropathy, allergic, terminology for, 172
Gastroenterostomy, gastritis cystica profunda after, 508
Gastroesophageal reflux, 407–423
    biopsy in, interpretation of, 411
        value of, 410, 410–411
    changes due to, alkaline reflux and, 410, 410
        high-grade, 409(t), 409–410, 409–411
            histopathologic classification of, 407–408
        low-grade, 408, 408–409, 409(t)
            histopathologic classification of, 407–408
    in etiology of Barrett's esophagus, 411–412. See also *Barrett's esophagus*.
    loss of antireflux mechanisms in, 407
    reflux esophagitis vs., 407
Gastrointestinal disorders, acute vs. chronic, determination of, 9–10
    categories of, 4(t)–5(t), 4–7
    cellular changes in, 81
    chemical, 141–170. See also *Chemical disorders*.
        mechanisms of cellular injury in, 142
    developmental, 4, 4(t)
    drug, 142–156. See also *Drug disorders*.
    endocrine and metabolic, 4(t), 6
    epithelial cell behavior in, 98–99
    examination of, general concepts and methods of, 3–13
    general concepts of, 4(t)–5(t), 4–10
    genetics of, 81
        in neoplastic conditions, 88–93, 89(t)
        in nonneoplastic conditions, 85–88
    HLA complex associated with, 84
    inflammatory, 4(t), 6
    inheritance of, autosomal dominant, 82(t)
        autosomal recessive, 83(t)
        multifactorial, 83–84
    injury response in, epithelial, 7(t), 7–8
        inflammatory, 8–9
    interepithelial lymphocytes in, 73
    kinetics of, 98–99
    malignant, 4(t), 6–7
    motor and mechanical, 4(t), 4–5. See also *Mechanical obstruction*.
    pathologic examination in, methods of, 10–13
    patterns and stages of, 9–10
    physical, 141–170
    subacute, definition of, 10
    vascular, 4(t)–5(t), 5–6, 214–239. See also *Vascular disorders*.
        cardiovascular drug usage and, 151–152
Gastrointestinal epithelium, injury to, degeneration from, 7
    dysplasia from, 8
    effects of, 7(t), 7–8
    metaplasia from, 7(t), 7–8

Gastrointestinal epithelium (Continued)
    injury to, neoplasia from, 8
    regeneration from, 7
Gastrointestinal food allergy, 171–172
    causes of, 172(t)
    histologic features of, 173
    immunologic mechanisms in, 172(t)
    pathogenetic mechanisms of, 172(t), 172–173
    terminology for, 172
Gastrointestinal hemorrhage, diagnosis of, 215–216
    in bleeding and coagulation disorders, 353
    in polycythemia, 354
    in vitamin K deficiency, 359–360
    liver disease and, 358
Gastrointestinal hormones, role in motility disorders of, 210
Gastrointestinal mucosa, eosinophilic infiltration of, differential diagnosis of, 177, 177(t)
    lymphoid cells of, 72(t)–74(t), 72–74, 73
    pathologic changes to, in ischemic bowel disease, 230, 231
Gastrointestinal stoma, varices from, 219
Gastrointestinal submucosa, pathologic changes to, in ischemic bowel disease, 230, 231
Gastrointestinal tract, adrenal diseases affecting, 355
    anastomotic network of, 217
    antigen processing in, 74–76, 75
    as ecosystem, 621–626, 622, 624–626
        perturbation(s) of, 624–626, 624–626
            contaminated small-bowel syndrome as, 624, 624
            neutropenic enterocolitis as, 626, 626
            pseudomembranous colitis as, 624–626, 625
        stabilizing factors in, 623–624
    celiac-like and celiac-related conditions in, 738–739
    chromosomal syndromes affecting, 84–85, 85(t)
    cytotoxic activity in, 74
    defense mechanisms of, 623–624
        colonization resistance of normal flora in, 623–624
        gastric acidity in, 623
        intestinal motility in, 623
        microbial ecology in, 623–624
        mucosal immune system in, 623
    dermatitis herpetiformis effects on, 356–357
    diabetes mellitus effects on, 355–356
    diverticula of, 769
    endocrine disorders affecting, 355–356. See also entries under *Endocrine*.
    epithelium of, necrosis of, in ischemic bowel disease, 230, 231
    erythema multiforme effects on, 357
    exogenous hormone effects on, 356
    food allergies of. See *Gastrointestinal food allergy*.
    function of, effect of temperature alteration on, 165
    functional anatomy of, 14–35. See also specific organ.
    granulomatous disorders of, 368–373, 369–372
        classification of, 368(t)
    hepatic disease effects on, 358–359
    histologic organization of, 14, 15
    host defense mechanisms of, 265
    hyperplastic polyps of, symptoms of, 787
    hyperthyroidism effects on, 355
    hypothyroidism effects on, 355
    immunodeficiency disorders of, 265–281. See also *Immunodeficiency disorders, gastrointestinal*.
    immunologic system of, anatomy of, 70(t), 70–72, 71–72
        concept of, 69–70
        role of appendix in, 71
        structure and function of, 69–77
    infarction of, in polycythemia, 354
    infections of, 621–640
        in radiation injury, 160
        secondary, renal disease and, 352–353
    intralumimal pressure of, ambient peritoneal pressure vs., effect on development of diverticula, 770
    intramural extramucosal lesions of, endoscopic diagnosis of, 38
    ischemia of, 352
        hypoxemia and, 352
        sickle cell anemia and, 353–354
    Köhlmeier-Degos disease effects on, 357

Gastrointestinal tract (*Continued*)
  leukemia effects on, 354–355
  lymphoma effects on, 354–355
  macrophages of, characteristics of, 74, 74(t)
  malignant lymphomas of. See *Lymphoma, malignant, gastrointestinal.*
  mechanical obstruction of, 194–196, *195–196*. See also *Mechanical obstruction.*
  megaloblastic cells of, anemia and, 354
  morphology of, 188–189
  motility of, altered, drug treatment and, 144
    as defense mechanism, 623
  muscular layer of, organization of, 188–189, *189*
  neural apparatus of, 189–190, *189–193*
    visceral neuropathy involvement of, 201–202
  neuromuscular apparatus of, 188–193, *189–194*
    study techniques for, 192–193
  nonspecificity symptoms referable to, 351–352
  normal anatomy of, 188–193, *189–194*
  normal flora of, 621–623, *622*
    colonization resistance of, 623–624
  organization of, 14–15, *15*
  pelvic lesion effects on, 356
  peristaltic activity of, flora in, 622
  pregnancy effects on, 356
  radiation injury to. See *Radiation injury.*
  radiation sensitivity of, 158
    whole-body irradiation and, 159
  reproductive disorders affecting, 356
  Sjögren's syndrome effects on, 358
  skin disease effects on, 356
  smooth muscle of, 310–311
  soft tissue disease effects on, 357
  storage diseases of, nature and localization of deposits in, 363(t)
  structural abnormalities of, stasis syndrome in, 741, 741(t)
  trauma to, 165
  tumors of, 4(t), 6–7
  varices of. See *Varices.*
  vascular abnormalities of, 219–224, *220–224*
    classification of, 219, 219(t)
  vascular anatomy of, 217
  vascular malformations of, acquired and congenital, *217–218*, 217–224, 219(t), *220–224*
  vasculitic lesions in, 226–229
  vitamin disorder effects on, 359–360
Gastrojejunostomy, gastric remnants after, carcinoma in, 591
  gastritis after, *495*, 495–496
    chronic, 530
Gastroparesis, in diabetes mellitus, 210
Gastropathy, hyperplastic, as precancerous lesion, 591
  hypersecretory, hypertophic, with and without protein loss, 543
Gastroschisis, 129
Gastroscope, fiberoptic, history of, 37–38
  flexirigid, history of, 37
Gastroscopy, in disease diagnosis, 38
G/D-cell tumors, classification of, 242
Gelatin-barium mixture, vascular lesion study with, 216
Gene(s), class II major histocompatibility, relationship with celiac disease of, 729
  tumor-suppressing, 91–92
Genetic markers, 84
Genetics, in celiac disease pathogenesis, 729
  in esophageal cancer, 443
  in gastrointestinal disorders, 81
  in intestinal carcinoma, 821–822
  in pathogenesis of diverticulosis, 772
  inheritance patterns in, 82(t)–83(t), *82–83*, 82–84
    Mendelian, autosomal dominant, 82, *82*, 82(t)
      autosomal recessive, 82–83, *83*, 83(t)
      X-linked, 83, *83*
    multifactorial, 83–84
  of gastrointestinal disorders, neoplastic, 88–93, 89(t). See also specific disease.
    nonneoplastic, 85–88. See also specific disease.
Genital wart, 890, *891*

Giant cell carcinoma, intestinal, 845
Giant cells, in ulcerative colitis, 648
Giardiasis, 638
  in immunocompromised patient, 268, *270*, 271
  malabsorption in, 749
  pathology of, 638–639, *639*
Giemsa stain, methods for, 52–53
Gliadin, sensitivity to, celiac disease from, 728
Glomus tumors, gastric, histology of, 338, *338–339*
Glucagonoma, hyperfunctional syndrome with, 243(t)
Glucocorticoids, gastrointestinal lesions from, 147(t), 148
Gluten, antibodies to, 729
  ingestion of, celiac disease from, genetic basis of, 86
  sensitivity to, association with refractory celiac disease or sprue, 735
    celiac disease from, 728–729, 729(t), 732
Gluten-free diet, for celiac disease, diagnosis with, 695
  hyperacidity associated with, 736, *737*
  inflammation in, 736
  responses to, 729, 729(t)
    mucosal, 731–732, *732–733*
  restoration of normal mucosa by, 728
  unresponsiveness to, 736, *737*
  for dermatitis herpetiformis, 738
Glycoconjugates, in intestinal adenoma, 801, 803
Glycogen storage disease, esophageal effects of, 365
Glycolipid disease, gastrointestinal involvement in, 362–364, 363(t)
Goblet cell carcinoid, appendiceal, 875–876
Goblet cell carcinoma, appendiceal, endocrine cells in, 259
Goblet cells, colonic, 35
  dystrophic, 658, *659*
  cytoplasm of, 30, *30*
  electron micrograph of, *31*
  gastric mucosal, 56, *57*
  in gastric carcinoma, 599
  in papillary gastric adenoma, 552, *556*
  mucin profile of, 31, 31(t)
  small-intestinal, *30–31*, 30–32, 31(t)
  theca of, 30
Gold salts, gastrointestinal lesions from, 152
Gonorrhea, anorectal, 636, 888
Graft-versus-host disease, esophageal involvement in, 427–428, *427–428*
  in bone marrow transplantation, pathogenesis of, 275
  pathology of, of acute form, 275, *276*, 277
    of chronic form, 277
Granular cell tumors, appendiceal, 877
  esophageal, 346, *348*
  gastrointestinal, 346
  of anal canal, 892, *893*
Granulation tissue, in radiation injury, 159, *160*
Granulocyte(s), mucosal, 74
Granuloma, barium, 716, *717*
  cellular features of, 368
  colonic, mucosal biopsy of, 679, *680*
  eosinophilic, 373
    in mural eosinophilic gastroenteritis, 173
  foreign body, 369
    gastric, 507
    in colonic diverticula, 777, *778*
    intestinal, types of, 716(t)
  in Crohn's disease, 369, 426, 426(t), 671, *671*, 677, 677(t)
  in infection, 368–369
  in ulcerative colitis, 648, *650*
  isolated, 369, *370*
  lymphoid nodule vs., 368, *369*
  miscellaneous presentation of, 373
  oil, 716–718, *717*
Granuloma inguinale, anal, 889
Granulomatosis, Wegener's, 226, 228–229
Granulomatous disease, chronic, clinical features of, 370
  definition of, 370
  differential diagnosis of, 370–371
  etiology of, 370

Granulomatous disease (*Continued*)
　chronic, gastrointestinal manifestations of, 274
　　melanosis coli vs., 706
　　pathology of, 274, 370
　gastric, 507–508, *508*
　gastrointestinal, 368–373, *369-372*
　　classification of, 368(t)
Granulomatous reactions, localized, 716, *716*, 716(t)
Guaiac test, in gastrointestinal bleeding diagnosis, 215
Gut-associated lymphoid tissue (GALT), antigen processing by, GALT to mucosa cycle of, 75
　M cells in, 74–75, *75*
　arrangement of, 264–265
　histology of, gastrointestinal flora in, 622
　lymphocytes of, 70(t)
　macrophages of, 74, 74(t)
　normal distribution of, 264–265, *265-266*
　structures of, 70

H_2-blockers, in prophylactic treatment of gastrointestinal hemorrhage, 518
Heartburn, pregnancy and, 356
Heavy metals, gastrointestinal lesions from, 147(t), 152
Helicobacter pylori infection, acute gastritis from, 482
　gastric, 500
　in chronic antral gastritis, *490*, 490–491
　in chronic peptic ulcer disease, 521–522, 524
　in duodenal peptic ulcer disease, 690
Helminthic infections, gastric, 504
　intestinal, pathology of, 640, *640*
Hemangiomas, gastrointestinal, classification of, 224
　location of, 224
　pathology of, 224
　syndromes involving, 224–225
Hemangiomatosis, diffuse intestinal, 224–225
　universal (miliary), 225
Hemangiopericytoma, gastrointestinal, 339
Hematemesis, in gastrointestinal bleeding diagnosis, 215
Hematologic disorders, gastrointestinal involvement in, 353–355
Hematoxylin and eosin (H&E), for biopsy specimen staining, 42–43, 43(t)
Hemochromatosis, gastrointestinal effects of, 359, *359*
Hemolytic-uremic syndrome, differential diagnosis of, 229
　gastrointestinal involvement in, 229
　gastrointestinal vasculitis in, 226
Hemoptysis, in mediastinal neurenteric cysts, 116
Hemorrhage, gastric, 223
　　aspirin injury and, *149*
　gastrointestinal, 353
　　anticoagulant usage and, 151
　　diagnosis of, 215–216
　　in chemotherapeutic drug injury, 150
　　in stress ulcer, 518
　　uremia and, 352
　in chemical and drug disorders, 144
　in colonic diverticular disease, 780–781, *781*
Hemorrhoids, as "cushions" of tissue vs. varicosities, 884–885
　external, 885
　internal, 885
　portal hypertension and, 219
Henoch-Schönlein purpura, gastrointestinal involvement in, 228
　gastrointestinal vasculitis in, 226
Heparin, deposition of, in mucopolysaccharidosis, 365
Hepatic disease, gastrointestinal effects of, 358–359
　gastrointestinal varices from, *217-218*, 217–219
Hepatoid carcinoma, gastric, 600
Hernia, congenital, affecting alimentary tract, 126(t), 126–128, *127*
　diaphragmatic, 126–128, *127*, 407
　　congenital posterolateral, clinical manifestations of, 126–127, *127*
　　　visceral displacement in, 127, *127*
　　epigastric, 128
　　femoral, 128

Hernia (*Continued*)
　hiatal, 19, 406–407
　　in Barrett's esophagus, 413
　　in esophageal carcinoma, 444
　　paraesophageal, 127
　　sliding, 127, 406
　inguinal, 128
　irreducible, bowel infarcts from, 230, *231*
　mechanical obstruction from, 194
　mesenteric, 126
　mesentericoparietal, 126
　omentomesenteric parietal, 126
　paraduodenal, 126
　paraesophageal, 406–407
　pericardiodiaphragmatic, 128
　　omphalocele with, *129*
　pleuroperitoneal, 126
　retrosternal, 127–128
　transmesenteric, 126
　transmesocolic, 126
　umbilical, 128
Herpes simplex virus, type 1, esophagitis from, 393
　type 2, esophagitis from, in neonates, 393
Herpesvirus infections, anal, 888–889
　gastric, 500
　in Crohn's disease, 675
　in immunocompromised patient, 268
　intestinal, pathology of, 630
Heterotopia, gastric, Barrett's mucosa vs., 417–418
　clinical features of, 714
　definition of, 713–714
　differential diagnosis of, 714–715
　etiology of, 713–714
　pathology of, 714, *715*
　ulceration in, 530
　metaplasia vs., 7
　of pancreatic tissue, 117
　　histology of, 117
Heterozygote, 82
Hidradenitis suppurativa, 887
Hindgut, endocrine tumors of, classification of, 243, 244(t)
Hirschsprung's disease, 119–122, *120*
　appendiceal involvement in, 863
　biopsy for, interpretation of, 121–122
　clinical features of, 119
　definition of, 119
　diagnosis of, 119–120, *120*
　genetic basis of, 87
　location of, 119
　neuromuscular features of, 208, *209*
　neuronal intestinal dysplasia vs., 208–209
　pathology of, *120*, 120–121
　sporadic visceral myopathy vs., *200*
Histamine, in gastric epithelial renewal, 101, 101(t)
　in small-intestinal epithelial cell proliferation, 103, 103(t)
Histiocytosis X, classification of, 372–373
　pathology of, 373
Histocompatibility complex, major, 84
Histogram, DNA flow, of gastric cells, statistical evaluation of, 64–66, *65-66*
Histoplasma capsulatum infection, 637
　appendiceal, 870
　gastric, 503
　intestinal, Crohn's disease vs., 672
　　pathology of, 637
　malabsorption from, 749
Hodgkin's disease, gastrointestinal, lymphomas vs., 296–297
Hollande's solution, fixation of biopsy specimens with, 40, 40(t)
Homosexuals, male, anal carcinoma in, 894
　anorectal gonorrhea in, 636, 888
　idiopathic inflammatory bowel disease in, syphilis and chlamydial infection vs., 636
　proctitis in, herpes simplex virus and, 630
Homozygote, 82

Honeycomb phenomenon, of gastric columnar cells, 56, *56*
Hormone(s), effects on epithelial cell proliferation of, colonic, 105
  gastric, 101, 101(t)
  small-intestinal, 103, 103(t)
  exogenous, gastrointestinal effects of, 356
  gastrointestinal, role in motility disorders of, 210
  inappropriate, endocrine tumor production of, 255
  sex, in colon carcinoma etiology, 823
  steroid, gastrointestinal lesions from, 147(t), 148
Household products, esophageal injury from, *401*, 401–402
Human immunodeficiency virus (HIV) infection. See *Acquired immunodeficiency syndrome (AIDS)*.
Human papillomavirus infection, esophageal, 396
  in anal carcinoma, 894
  of anal region, 890, *891*
Humoral factors, effects on epithelial cell proliferation of, gastric, 101(t)
  small-intestinal, 103(t)
Hydrocele, congenital inguinal hernia with, 128
Hydrochloric acid, gastric, physiologic roles of, 19–20
  production of, by oxyntic cells, 23
Hydrocortisone, effects on epithelial cell proliferation of, colonic, 105
  small-intestinal, 103, 103(t)
Hydroxyanisole, butylated, effects on colonic epithelial cell proliferation of, 105
Hydroxyl radicals, toxicity of, in cell injury, 142
Hydroxytoluene, butylated, tumor reduction by, 821
Hygroma, cystic, 137–138, *137–138*
Hyperacidity, in peptic duodenal ulcer, 522
Hypercalcemia, gastrointestinal effects of, in hyperparathyroidism, 355
Hyperchlorhydria, gastrin cell hyperplasia with, 248
  peptic ulcer disease with, pancreatic gastrinoma and, 256, *257*
  somatostatin (D) cell growth in, 249
Hypergastrinemia, chronic atrophic gastritis with, endocrine cell hyperplasia in, 246–247, *247*
  food-stimulated, gastrin cell hyperplasia with, 248, *248*
  hyperplastic argyrophil cells in, 245, *245*
Hyperparathyroidism, gastrointestinal effects of, 355
Hyperplasia, appendiceal, epithelial, 870
  atypical. See *Neoplasia*.
  esophageal, epithelial cell proliferation and, 99–100
  gastric, adenomatous, cancer from, 101–102
  intestinal, as precancerous condition, 827
  lymphoid. See *Lymphoid hyperplasia*.
  of Brunner's gland, 566
  polypoid foveolar, 559
Hypersensitivity, in food allergies, delayed, 172(t)
  immediate, 172, 172(t)
Hypertension, portal, hemorrhoids in, 219
  of extrahepatic origin, gastrointestinal varices with, 219
  of hepatic origin, gastrointestinal varices with, 217–219, *217–219*
Hyperthermia, gastrointestinal effects of, 165
Hyperthyroidism, gastrointestinal effects of, 355
Hypertrophy, of muscularis propria, mechanical obstruction and, 196, *196*
Hypervitaminosis D, gastrointestinal effects of, 360
Hypochlorhydria, in colorectal carcinogenesis, 824
Hypogammaglobulinemia, common variable, pathogenesis and clinical features of, 271
  pathology of, 271–273
  malabsorption with, *Giardia lamblia* in, 270
  nodular lymphoid hyperplasia with, 288
    giardiasis in, 289
    pathology of, 288–289, *289*
Hypoparathyroidism, intestinal pseudo-obstruction in, 210–211
Hyposplenism, in refractory celiac disease, 736–737
Hypothermia, gastrointestinal effects of, 165
Hypothyroidism, gastrointestinal effects of, 355
  intestinal pseudo-obstruction in, 210
Hypoxemia, intestinal ischemia from, 352
Hypoxia, gastrointestinal, causes and effects of, 5(t), 5–6

Ibuprofen, in reduction of bowel ischemia, 233
I-cell disease, deposition in, 363(t)
IgA, against gluten, 729
  against reticulin, 729
  circulating levels of, relationship to celiac disease of, 729
  deposition of, in dermatitis herpetiformis, 738
  secretory, as immunologic protection mechanism, 623
    characteristics of, 76–77, *77*
    in GALT, 75–76
    in gastrointestinal immune system, 265
    protective qualities of, 77
  subclasses of, 76
  synthesis of, 76–77, *77*
IgA deficiency, immune injury and, 271
  selective, clinical features of, 273
    pathogenesis of, 273
    pathology of, 273
IgE, in allergic gastroenteritis, 176
  in colonic allergic disease, 184–185
  in food allergies, 172
IgG, in food allergies, 172
  suppression of, in GALT, 76
IgM, in food allergies, 172
Ileal mucosa, aspirin injury to, 149
Ileal reservoir, for ulcerative colitis, complications of, 654
Ileitis, active, features of, mucosal biopsy of, 682, *682*
  backwash, 646
  pouch, in ulcerative colitis, 675
  prestomal, 654
Ileocecal valve, lipomatous hypertrophy of, 336–338, *338*
  muscular structure of, 192, *194*
Ileostomy, diverting, colitis after, 700–701
  for Crohn's disease, ileal abnormalities after, 675
    mucosal atrophy after, 675
  for ulcerative colitis, complications of, 654
Ileum, abnormalities of, postsurgical, after ulcerative colitis treatment, 654
  argentaffin (EC cell) carcinoids of, 253, *254*
  atrophy of, postresection, mucosal biopsy of, *681*, 681–682
  blood supply of, 24
  capillariasis of, 753
  chemical injury to, 154
  Crohn's disease of, differential diagnosis of, 672
    gross features of, 667
    mucosal biopsy of, 681–682, *681–682*
    recurrent lesions in, 675–676
    submucosal thickening in, 668, *669*
  diverticula of, 769
  drug injury to, 154
  endocrine cells of, classification of, 241(t)
  endometriosis of, 712, *712*
  gross anatomy of, 24
  malignant lymphoma of, 293, *294*
  mucosal biopsy of, 681–682, *681–682*
  nodular lymphoma of, 293, *294*
  terminal, Crohn's disease of, *665*, 665–666
    duplication of, 133, *134*
    lymphoid hyperplasia of, 287, *287–289*
  ulcerative colitis of, 646
Ileus, adynamic, pseudo-obstruction in, 196–197
  meconium, 131–132, 358
    atresia with, 123, 132, *132*
    histology of, 132, *133*
    volvulus with, 132, *132*
Image analysis, high-resolution, in cytology, 53–54, *54*, 54(t)
Immune complex disease, in food allergies, 172(t), 172–173
Immune disorders, duodenal involvement in, 695
  in etiology of Crohn's disease, 664
Immune response, in celiac disease, 729–730
  intestinal, afferent limb of, epithelial and lymphoid tissue in, 25
    altered, mucosal lesions associated with, 753–761, *754–756, 758–761*
  mucosal, summary of, 77
  secretory, maturation of, 75–76

Immune system, gastrointestinal, functions of, 265
  structure and function of, 69–77
  local (intramucosal), as mediator in celiac disease, 729–730
  mucosal, as gastrointestinal defense mechanism, 623
  concept of, 69–70
Immunity, cellular, in celiac disease, 729–730
  in food allergies, 172(t)
  humoral, in food allergies, 172(t), 172–173
  systemic, correlation with mucosal immunity of, 70
  suppression of, following oral immunization, 76
Immunocompromise, histologic changes in, 268
Immunocytochemistry, pathologic examination with, 12
Immunodeficiency disorders, chronic fundic gastritis with, 492
  duodenal, 695–696
  esophageal, 427
  gastrointestinal, 265–281
    acquired, 274–275, 275(t), 276–280, 277–281, 281(t)
      development of, 274–275
      infection in, 275
      neoplasia in, 275
    clinical aspects of, 266–267
    Cryptosporidium in, 268, 270
    cytomegalovirus infection in, 268, 269
    diagnosis of, immunologic tests in, 267
    general features of, 265–268, 267(t), 267–270, 271
    Giardia lamblia in, 268, 270
    histologic changes in, intrinsic and associated morphologic, 271
      minor, 267, 267–268
      mucosal, infection or bacterial overgrowth and, 268, 268–270, 271
      neoplastic, 271
    mucocutaneous candidiasis in, 268, 268
    pathologist's role in, 266
    pathology of, 267(t), 267–268, 267–270, 271
    primary, 271–274. See also specific disorder; e.g., *Hypogammaglobulinemia*.
      malignant lymphoma with, 291
      manifestations of, 272(t)
      nonimmunologic defects in, 272(t), 274
      pathology of, 267(t)
      phagocytic dysfunction in, 272(t), 274
      predominant antibody defects in, 271–273, 272(t)
      predominant cell-mediated, 272(t), 273–274
      types of, 266
    secondary, 266
    types of, 266
    workup of patient in, 281, 281(t)
  severe combined, abnormalities in, 273
    clinical manifestations of, 273–274
    pathology of, 274
    small-intestinal mucosa in, histology of, 267, 267
Immunoglobulin, in amyloidosis, 366
Immunohistochemical studies, of stromal cell tumors, 311
Immunologic mechanisms, in gastrointestinal food allergy, 172(t)
Immunologic reaction, humoral (type III), in food allergies, 172(t), 172–173
  immediate hypersensitivity (type I), in food allergies, 172, 172(t)
Immunoproliferative small-intestinal disease (IPSID), α-chain disease in, 299
  diagnosis of, 300–301
  etiology of, 299
  malignant lymphoma with, 291, 293, 299, 300, 301–302
  management of, 301–302
  pathology of, 299–300, 299–302
  prognosis of, 301–302
  stage 1 of, 300, 300–301
Immunosuppressive drugs, colonic lesions from, 155–156
  gastrointestinal lesions from, 147(t), 150–151
Imperforate anus, 136, 136(t)
Incisura angularis, 19
Indomethacin, bowel ischemia potentiation by, 233
  gastrointestinal lesions from, 153–154
  tumor reduction by, 821

Infants, autoimmune enteropathy in, 754–755, 755
  cow's milk protein allergy in, 183
  diarrhea in, 627
  herpes simplex virus infection in, esophageal involvement in, 393
  meconium ileus in, 131
  premature, necrotizing enterocolitis of, 234, 235
  spontaneous intestinal perforation in, 133
Infarct, hypoxia and, 6
  mucosal, 6
  mural, 6
  transmural, 6
Infarction, gastrointestinal, etiology of, 230, 232
  nonocclusive, 230
  transmural, classification of, 230
Infection(s), bacterial. See *Bacterial infections*.
  chemical-induced, 144
  chlamydial. See *Chlamydial infections*.
  colonic, allergic proctitis and colitis vs., 184
  drug-induced, 144
  duodenal, 693, 694
  exogenous. See *Exogenous infections*.
  fungal. See *Fungal infections*.
  gastric, 500(t), 500–504
  gastrointestinal, 621–640
    in AIDS, 275(t)
    in bone marrow transplantation, 275, 275(t)
    in chemotherapeutic drug injury, 150
    granulomas in, 368–369
    helminthic, 504, 640, 640
  in acquired immunodeficiency disorders, 275
  in etiology of Crohn's disease, 664
  intestinal. See *Intestinal infections*.
  mechanical obstruction and, 195
  opportunistic, in radiation injury, 160
  parasitic. See *Parasitic infections*.
  pyogenic, chronic granulomatous disease from, 370
  secondary, in Crohn's disease, 675
  in ulcerative colitis, 653–654
  viral. See *Viral infections*.
Inflammation, endothelial, 159, 161
  gastrointestinal, mechanical obstruction from, 194
    special features of, 9
    standard reaction in, 8–9
    subacute, 10
  in chemical and drug disorders, 145; 145
  radiation and, 159, 160
Inflammatory bowel disease, anal lesions in, 887–888
  anorectal fistula in, 887
  cancer incidence in, 106
  chronic idiopathic, bloody diarrhea vs., biopsy differentiation of, 46
  definition of, 643
  diverticular disease in, 781
  DNA synthesis defects in, 106
  genetic basis of, 86–87
  idiopathic, acute self-limited colitis vs., 702
    definition of, 643
    indeterminate, 678
    syphilis and chlamydial infection vs., in male homosexuals, 636
  malignant change in, 826–827
  malignant lymphoma with, 291
  rectocolonic mucosal biopsy in, uses of, 679, 679(t)
Inflammatory disorders, amyloidosis from, 366
  categories of, 4(t), 6
  colonic, 697–704, 699–702, 704–707, 706–709
  duodenal, types of, 693, 693(t)
  gastric mucosal thickening in, 543, 544, 545
  intestinal, 689–718. See also *Crohn's disease*; *Duodenitis*.
    types of, 689, 690(t)
  small-intestinal, 696–697
^{111}In-granulocyte scanning, in gastrointestinal vasculitis diagnosis, 226
Injection studies, of blood vessels, 216
Insulin, in gastric epithelial renewal, 101, 101(t)

Intestinal infections. See also specific type and *Bacterial infections; Fungal infections; Protozoan infections; Viral infections.*
  pathology of, 628–640
    acute self-limited vs. chronic progressive disease in, 628–629, *629*
    biopsy interpretation in, colitic bowel preparation changes and, 629
    exclusion of noninfectious causes in, 629
    general considerations in, 628–629, *629*
Intestinal wall, defects in, effect on diverticular development of, 770
  gas-filled spaces in, 710, *710*
Intestine(s). See also *Colon; Small intestine.*
  bacterial infections of, clinical manifestations of, 631
    pathology of, 631–636, *632–636*
  benign polyps of, 786–812
  chlamydial infections of, pathology of, 631
  congenital diverticula of, 131
  contents of, as carcinoma risk factors, 824
  embryology of, 118–119
  flora of, in carcinogenesis, 824
  inflammatory disorders of, 689–718. See also *Crohn's disease; Duodenitis.*
    types of, 689, 690(t)
  obstruction of. See *Obstruction, intestinal.*
  pseudo-obstruction of. See *Pseudo-obstruction, intestinal.*
  rotation of, anomalies of, 124(t), 124–126
    embryologic, 118
    mixed rotation in, 125
    nonrotation in, 124–125
    reversed rotation in, 125
  spontaneous perforation of, 133
  tumor-like lesions of, 709–718
  viral infections of, pathology of, 629–631, *630*
Intramural plexuses, gastrointestinal control by, 189
  myenteric. See *Myenteric plexus (Auerbach's plexus).*
  submucosal. See *Submucosal plexus (Meissner's plexus).*
Intrauterine accident, intestinal atresia and stenosis from, 123
Intrinsic factor, gastric, production of, by oxyntic cells, 23
Intussusception, appendiceal, 878
  ileal inflammatory fibroid polyps in, 341, *341*
  ileocecal, in lymphoid hyperplasia of terminal ileum and appendix, 287, *289*
  ileocolic, in meconium ileus equivalent, 132
  ileoileal, in children, 195, *195*
  small-intestinal, in adults, 195, *195*
Iron, deficiency of, mucosal abnormalities in, 744
  gastrointestinal ulceration from, 152
  parietal cell deposition of, in hemochromatosis, 359, *359*
Irradiation, whole-body, gastrointestinal effects of, 159
Irritable bowel syndrome, 709
  relationship of colonic diverticula to, 771–772
Ischemia, chronic, 6
  colonic, 231
    myopathy vs., histologic features in, 200, *201*
  drug-induced, small-intestinal, 154
  gastrointestinal, causes and effects of, 5(t), 5–6, 239
    mechanical obstruction and, 195
    pathophysiologic effects of, 239
  necrosis from, 142
  reversible, 6
  tissue injury from, 142
Ischemic bowel disease, clinical features of, 230–231
  diagnosis of, barium enema in, *233*
  entities of, 232(t), 233, *233–236, 235–236*
  experimental studies in, 231–232
  in elderly, differential diagnosis of, 234
  pathogenesis of, proposed mechanisms of, 232–233
  progression of, stages in, 230, *231*
  spectrum of, 230–231, 232(t)
  therapeutic considerations in, 233
Ischemic colitis, 6, *233*, 233–234
  hemolytic-uremic syndrome and, 229
  pseudopolyps in, *233*, 234
  syndromes of, *233*, 233–234
  ulcerative colitis vs., 653

Ischemic disease, colonic, Crohn's disease vs., 672
  diverticular disease in, 781–782
  duodenal, 694–695
  gastrointestinal, 229–236, *231–233*, 232(t), *235–236*, 352
    classification of, 230
    endometriosis vs., 713
    general considerations in, 229
    nomenclature of, 230
    pathology of, 230, *231*
Isospora infections, 271
Isotope(s), radioactive, epithelial cells analysis with, 99

Jejunal epithelium, in celiac disease, 731, *731*
  gluten-free diet response in, 731–732, *732*
Jejunal mucosa, hemochromatosis of, 359, *359*
  in celiac disease, macroscopic appearance of, 730–731, *730–731*
  injury to, aspirin usage and, 149
  response to gluten-free diet by, in celiac disease, 731–732, *732*
Jejunoileal bypass, megacolon from, 211
Jejunoileitis, chronic ulcerative, as misleading term, 736
  ulcerative, clinical features of, 696
    definition of, 696
    differential diagnosis of, 696
    etiology of, 696
    pathology of, 696
Jejunum, abetalipoproteinemia effects on, 362, *363*
  biopsy of, in stasis syndrome, 742, *742–743*
  blood supply of, 24
  capillariasis of, 753
  chemical injury to, 154
  circumferential polypoid carcinoma of, *837*
  diverticula of, 769
  diverticulosis of, neuromuscular causes of, 207, *207–208*
  drug injury to, 154, 154(t)
  endocrine cells of, classification of, 241(t)
  gross anatomy of, 24
  IPSID of, malignant lymphoma with, 300
  muscular layer of, 189
  type II visceral myopathy of, *199*

Kaposi's sarcoma, gastrointestinal involvement in, 225
  in AIDS, 279–281, *280*
Karyotype(s), in colorectal study, 92
Kayexalate, in sorbitol, esophagitis due to, 402, *403*
Keratoacanthoma, of anal region, 892
Kidneys, diseases of, gastrointestinal involvement in, 352–353, *353*
  enteroglucagon-producing tumor of, 255
Killer cells, in peripheral blood lymphocytes, 74
Kinetics, of gastrointestinal disorders, 98–99
Klippel-Trenaunay-Weber syndrome, gastrointestinal involvement in, 225
Köhlmeier-Degos disease, gastrointestinal effects of, 357

Labeling index, of epithelial cells, 99
  colonic, 104
    in adenoma and carcinoma, 106
  esophageal, 99, 99(t)
    in carcinoma, 100
  gastric, 100, 100(t)
  in ulcerative colitis, 106(t)
  small-intestinal, 103
Lactase deficiency, primary, malabsorption from, normal mucosal histology in, 727–728, *728*
Lamina propria, anatomy of, 14, *15*, 20
  appendiceal, 863
  diffuse lymphoid tissue in, distribution of, 265, *265*
  eosinophils in, in allergic colitis, 183, *184*
  inflammatory cells in, in alleric gastroenteritis, 176
  macrophages of, 74, 74(t)
  mast cells in, in intestinal mastocytosis, 756–757
  papillae of, in esophageal squamous epithelium, *17*, 18
  pathologic changes to, in ischemic bowel disease, 230, *231*
  plasma cells of, development of, 72, 72(t)
    IgA synthesis in, 76–77, *77*

Langerhans cells, in esophageal squamous epithelium, 16, *18*
Laparotomy, for gastrointestinal lymphomas, 303(t), 303–304
Large intestine. See *Colon.*
Laryngeal cleft, 114(t), 115
Laryngotracheal diverticulum, 113
Laryngotracheal groove, 113
Laryngotracheoesophageal fistula, 115
Lauren's classification, of gastric adenocarcinoma, *603*, 603–604
Laxative abuse syndrome, 707
Laxatives, cathartic colon from, 204, 706–707
　effects of, 706–707, *706–707*
　　on biopsy findings, 45
　gastrointestinal lesions from, 147(t), 152
　melanosis coli from, *706*, 706–707
Lectins, in study of intestinal adenomas, 801, 803
　in study of intestinal goblet cell mucin, 31
Leiomyoblastoma, gastric, definition of, 321
Leiomyoma, anal, 892
　appendiceal, 877
　colonic, histology of, 329, *332*
　duodenal, gross characteristics of, 313, *313*
　esophageal, 320–321
　　gross characteristics of, 314, *315*
　　"seedling," 320, *321*
　gastric, cellular, 321, *322–323*
　　epithelioid, glomus tumor vs., 338, *339*
　　　histology of, 321–323, *323–327*, 326
　　gross characteristics of, 313, *313–315*
　　microscopic features of, 315, *317–318*
　gastrointestinal, definition of, 312
　　differentiation of, 311
　jejunal, gross characteristics of, 313–314, *314*
　rectal, histology of, 333–335, *334*
　rectosigmoid, histology of, 329, *333*, 333
　small-intestinal, histology of, 326, 329, *329–331*
　　microscopic features of, 315, *316*, 318
Leiomyosarcoma, appendiceal, 877
　colonic, histology of, 329, *332*
　esophageal, 321
　gastric, epithelioid, histology of, 323, 326, *327*
　gastrointestinal, definition of, 312
　　differentiation of, 311
　rectal, deep intramural, 333–335, *334*
　　leiomyoma vs., 334, *334*
　small-intestinal, histology of, 326, 329, *331*
Lesion, low-flow, 6
Leukemia, gastrointestinal, 354–355
　complications of, 299
Leukocyte(s), polymorphonuclear, in acute appendicitis, 865–866
　intraepithelial, in gastroesophageal reflux, 409
Leukoencephalopathy, metachromatic, deposition in, 363(t)
Lichen sclerosus et atrophicus, anogenital, 890
Ligament of Treitz, gross anatomy of, 24
Linear energy transfer, of radiation, 158
Lipid(s), accumulation of, in abetalipoproteinemia, 362
　deposition of, in storage diseases, 362–364, 363(t)
　intracellular metabolism of, in intestinal absorptive cells, 26, 29
Lipid peroxidation, in cell injury, 142
Lipid pigment disorders, 364–365
　deposition in, 363(t)
Lipodystrophy, intestinal, 745
Lipofuscin pigment, deposition of, 364–365
Lipofuscinosis, neuronal ceroid, pigment deposition in, 364
Lipogranuloma, cellular features of, 368
Lipoma, esophageal, pedunculated, 474
　gastrointestinal, submucosal, gross features of, 336, *337*
　　microscopic features of, *336*, 337
Lipoprotein disorders, gastrointestinal effects of, 362
Liposarcoma, gastrointestinal, 336
Lithocholic acid, in colorectal carcinogenesis, 824
Liver, abnormalities of, in Crohn's disease, 676
Lupus erythematosus, systemic, gastrointestinal involvement in, 227–228
　differentiation of, 229
　gastrointestinal vasculitis in, 226

Lye, esophageal injury from, *401*, 401–402
Lymph nodes, mesenteric, cavitation of, in refractory celiac disease, 736–737, *738*
　of GALT, 71–72
　metastases to, in early gastric carcinoma, 581
Lymphangiectasia, gastrointestinal, 352
　intestinal, primary, clinical features of, 758
　　gross findings in, 758, *759*
　　histology of, 758, *760*
　　incidental discovery of, 759
Lymphangioma, gastrointestinal, 225
Lymphatics, dilatation of, in Crohn's disease, 668, *669*
　gastrointestinal, demonstration of, 216–217
　　lymphangiectasia involvement of, 352
　mesenteric, obstruction of, in primary intestinal lymphangiectasia, 758, *759*
Lymphocyte(s). See also *B cells* and *T cells.*
　in IPSID, 300, *300–301*
　in Peyer's patches, 71, *71*
　in vermiform appendix, 863
　intercellular, in esophageal epithelium, *409*, 409
　mucosal, interepithelial, 73, 73(t), 73–74
　　intraepithelial, 265, *265–266*
　　　gluten exposure and, 729–730
　　　in colitis, 698
　　lamina propria, 73(t), 73–74
　　phenotypes of, 73(t)
　peripheral blood, killer cells in, 74
Lymphogranuloma venereum, anal, 889
　intestinal, *Chlamydia trachomatis*–associated, 631
Lymphoid cells, mucosal, 72(t)–74(t), 72–74, *73*
Lymphoid hyperplasia, gastric, 282
　diagnosis of, endoscopic biopsy in, 285, *286*
　differential diagnosis of, 282, 284–285, *285*, 285(t)
　fibrosis in, 282, *283–284*
　histology of, 282, *282–284*
　infiltrate in, 282, *283–284*
　　monomorphous nature of, 282, *285*
　malignant lymphoma vs., 282, 284–285
　　histologic features in, 285(t)
　malignant predisposition of, 285
　mucosal ulceration in, 282, *283*
　pathology of, 282, *282–284*
　gastrointestinal, 281–282, *282–289*, 284–290, 285(t)
　　clinicopathology of, 281
　　secondary, 282
　lymphoma vs., 297
　malignant lymphoma with, 291
　nodular, *287–289*, 287–290
　　diffuse, without hypogammaglobulinemia, 289–290
　　　clinical implications of, 290
　　　pathology of, 290
　　hypogammaglobulinemia with, 288
　　　common variable, 272–273
　　giardiasis in, 289
　　pathology of, 288–289, *289*
　intestinal, 287–290, *289*
　of terminal ileum and appendix, 287, *287–289*
　　histology of, 287, *288–289*
　　intussusception in, 287, *289*
　rectal, 286
　　pathology of, *286*, 286–287
　　treatment of, 287
　small-intestinal, 285–286
Lymphoid nodules, granuloma vs., 368, *369*
　in chronic ulcerative colitis, 649, *651*
　in Crohn's disease, 668, *669*
Lymphoid polyps, rectal, *286*, 286–287
Lymphoid system, disorders of, 264–304
　functional anatomy of, 264–265, *265–266*
Lymphoid tissue, diffuse, distribution of, 265, *265–266*
　gut-associated. See *Gut-associated lymphoid tissue (GALT).*
　in ileoileal intussusception, 195, *195*
Lymphoma, appendiceal, 877
　as refractory celiac disease or sprue, 736
　Burkitt's, 296, *298*

Lymphoma (*Continued*)
  colonic, risk after radiation of, 165
  gastric, diffuse, mucosal thickening in, *544*, 545
    frequency of, 585, 585(t)
  gastrointestinal, workup of, endoscopic biopsy in, 303, 303(t)
    laparotomy in, 303(t), 303–304
  histiocytic, in celiac sprue, 290–291
    rarity of, 291
  malignant, gastric lymphoid hyperplasia vs., 282, 284–285
    histologic features in, 285(t)
    gastrointestinal, 290–293, *292–303*, 295(t), 295–304, 303(t), 355
      adult, clinical presentation of, 291
        course of, 298
        definition of, 291
        differential diagnosis of, 297
        etiology of, 291
        gross pathology of, 291–293, *292*
        histologic classification of, 295, 295(t)
        location of, 291–293, *292*
        microscopic features of, 293, *293–298*, 295–297
        pathogenesis of, 291
        prognosis of, 298
        treatment of, 298
      childhood, 298
      Crohn's disease vs., 672
        granulomas in, 671
      IPSID with. See *Immunoproliferative small-intestinal disease (IPSID)*.
      large-cell type, 295, *295–296*
      nodular, 293, *294*, 295
      peptic ulcer vs., 527–528
      risk of, conditions associated with, 290–291
      secondary, 299
      small cell type, 293, *293*, 295–296, *297*
      "Western type," 301
    ileal, 293, *294*
  non-Hodgkin's, gastrointestinal, cytology of, 59, *60*
    small-intestinal, in celiac disease, 734
  rectal, risk after radiation of, 165
Lymphoproliferative disorders, gastrointestinal, 281–282, *282–289*, 284–290, 285(t)
  workup of, by endoscopic biopsy, 303, 303(t)
Lynch syndromes, genetic basis of, 90–91
  types I and II, differentiation of, 822
Lysozyme, production of, in Paneth cells, 32

Macroglobulin, deposition of, in Waldenström's macroglobulinemia, 760, *761*
Macroglobulinemia, Waldenström's, intestinal involvement in. See *Waldenström's macroglobulinemia*.
Macromolecule, effect of radiation on, 158
Macrophage(s), enlarged, in chronic granulomatous disease, 370–371
  in glycolipid diseases, 363
  mucin-filled, in xanthomas, 361–362, *362*
  mucosal, characteristics of, 74, 74(t)
  PAS-positive, in diagnosis of Whipple's disease, 748, 748(t), 748–749
  vacuolated (foamy), in xanthomas, *360–361*, 361
Major histocompatibility complex, 84
Malabsorption, bacterial infections and, 745–748, 745–749, 748(t)
  causes of, intraluminal maldigestion in, 727
    nutrient uptake abnormalities in, 727
  ceroidosis with, 207
  clinicopathologic considerations in, 727
  deficiency states in, 743–744, *744*
  definition of, 727
  drug-induced, 154, 154(t)
  fungal infections and, 749
  histoplasmosis and, 749
  in allergic gastroenteritis, 180, 182
  in autoimmune enteropathy, 754–755, *755*
  in Crohn's disease, 674
  in idiopathic AIDS enteropathy, 754, *754*

Malabsorption (*Continued*)
  in rheumatoid disease, 229
  in stasis syndrome, 742, *742*
  in tropical sprue, 739
  in Waldenström's macroglobulinemia, 760–761
  inflammatory lesions in, unclassified nonspecific, 744–745
  mastocytosis and, 757
  metazoan parasitosis and, 751–753, *752–753*
  moniliasis and, 749
  mucosal lesions in, diseases associated with, 755–761, *756–761*
    infection-associated, 745(t), 745–748, 745–753, 748(t), 750–753
  postinfective tropical. See *Sprue, tropical*.
  protozoan parasitosis and, 749–751, *750–751*
  radiation injury and, 163–164
  viral infections and, 745, 745(t)
  Whipple's disease and, 745–748, 745–749, 748(t). See also *Whipple's disease*.
Malabsorption syndrome, definition of, 727
Malabsorptive disorders, 725–761
  biopsy in, resemblance to celiac disease of, 732, 734, 734(t)
    special considerations in, 725–727
  classification of, 725, 726(t)
  nonspecific inflammation and mucosal alterations in, 728–745. See also *Celiac disease*.
  normal mucosal histology in, 727–728, *728*
Malacoplakia, clinical features of, 371
  colonic, gross features of, 371, *371*
    histology of, 371–372, *372*
  definition of, 371
  differential diagnosis of, 372
  etiology of, 371
  pathology of, 371–372, *371–372*
Malaria, malabsorption in, 749
Maldigestion, malabsorption from, 727
Mallory-Weiss syndrome, gastric, clinical features of, 504
  etiology of, 504
  pathology of, *504*, 504–505
Malposition, appendiceal, 863
Malrotation, 124
  annular pancreas with, 124
Mannose, deposition of, in mannosidosis, 365
Mannosidosis, deposition in, 363(t)
  mannose deposition in, 365
Marker substances, in colorectal carcinoma, 840–841, 841(t)
  in gastric adenocarcinoma, 602(t), 602–603
Marmoset, colon carcinoma in, 827
Mast cells, connective tissue vs. mucosal, 756
  identification of, pathology stains for, 756, *756*
  mucosal, 74, 756
    CTMC vs., 756–757
  submucosal, in mastocytosis, 757
Mastocytosis, clinical presentation of, 756
  malabsorption in, 757
  pathology stains for, 756, *756*
  systemic, 756
    intestinal mucosal changes in, 757
Measles, appendiceal involvement in, 869
Mechanical disorders, 188–213. See also *Mechanical obstruction; Pseudo-obstruction*.
  categorization of, 4(t), 4–5
  gastritis associated with, 506
Mechanical obstruction, gastrointestinal, 194–196, *195–196*
  adhesions and, 194
  causes of, 194
  effects of, 194–195
  hernia and, 194
  inflammation and, 194
  intraluminal, 196
  intussusception in, 195, *195*
  neuromuscular features in, 196, *196*
  special forms of, 195–196, *195–196*
  symptoms of, 195
  volvulus in, 195–196

Meckel's diverticulum, 130
  aberrant pancreas in, *130*
  incidence of, 769
  pancreatic tissue in, 117
Meconium ileus, 123, 131–132, *132–133*, 358
Meconium ileus equivalent, 132
Meconium peritonitis, *132*, 132–133
Meconium plug syndrome, 133
Megacolon, congenital aganglionic. See *Hirschsprung's disease.*
  jejunoileal bypass and, 211
  toxic, in Crohn's disease, 675
    in ulcerative colitis, 653, *653*
Megaduodenum, in type I visceral myopathy, 198, *198*
Meissner's plexus. See *Submucosal plexus (Meissner's plexus).*
Melanocyte(s), proliferation of, in esophageal squamous epithelium, 386
Melanoma, malignant, anal, gross features of, 898
    histology of, 898–899, *899*
    metastases in, 899
  anorectal, 846
  esophageal, 472–473
Melanosis, deposition in, 363(t)
Melanosis coli, 365, 706, *706–707*
Membranous (M) cells, in Peyer's patches, 71
  small-intestinal, 25, 32, *32–33*
    electron micrograph of, *32*
    structure and function of, 74–75, *75*
Ménétrier's disease, childhood, 543
  clinical features of, 540
  definition of, 540
  diagnosis of, 541–542
  differential diagnosis of, 542
  endoscopic biopsy of, 542
  enlarged gastric folds in, 180
  epithelial cell proliferation in, 102
  etiology of, 540
  gastric carcinoma in, incidence of, 591
  pathogenesis of, 540
  pathology of, 540–541, *541–543*
  relation to carcinoma of, 543
Mesenchymal tumors. See also *Stromal tumors.*
  gastric, cytology of, 59
  gastrointestinal, 310–350
    general features of, 310–320, *313–319*
    inflammatory fibroid polyp vs., 792
Mesenteric artery, in intestinal embryology, 118
  inflammation of, in systemic lupus erythematosus, 228
  occlusion of, bowel infarcts from, 230, 239
    chronic intestinal ischemia from, 236
Mesenteric vein, thrombosis of, bowel infarcts from, 230
Metabolic disorders, categories of, 6
Metaplasia, gastric, heterotopia vs., 7, 714, 715
  gastrointestinal injury and, 7(t), 7–8
  intestinal, in Barrett's epithelium, 464
    in chronic gastritis, 487(t), 487–489, *488–489*
    of gastric mucosa, as precursor to adenocarcinoma, 588–589, 588–590, 589(t)
      carcinoma associated with, 102
        intestinal cell type in, 585
      classification of, 489, 588–589, 589(t)
      columnar cells in, 56, *57*
      complete (type I), 487–488, *488*, 588–589, *588–589*, 589(t)
      incomplete (type II), 488, *488*, 588–589, *588–589*, 589(t)
      mucin stains of, 488–489, *489*
      precancerous nature of, 589, 589–590
      superficial adenocarcinoma in, 589, *589*
      types of, 487(t)
        differences among, 588–589, 589(t)
    pseudopyloric, 19
    types of, in gut epithelium, 7(t), 7–8
Metastasis(es), in colorectal adenocarcinoma, 840
  in gastric carcinoma, 609–610
  lymph node, in early gastric carcinoma, 581
Michaelis-Guttman inclusions, in colonic malacoplakia, 372, *372*

Microcarcinoidosis, gastric, cellular features of, 242
Micromorphometry, 53
Microorganisms, immune protection against, secretory IgA in, 77
  in gastrointestinal flora, 621–623, *622*
Microscopy, electron. See *Electron microscopy.*
  fluorescence, 52
  Nomarski differential interference contrast, 51, *51*
  phase contrast, 50–51, *50–51*
  ultraviolet light, 51–52, *52*
Microsporidiosis, *Enterocytozoon bieneusi* infection and, 749–751, *750–751*
  malabsorption in, 749–751, *750–751*
Microvilli, damage to, mucosal adhesion of organisms with, 627
Microvillus inclusion disease, diarrhea in, 757
  electron microscopy of, 757–758, *759*
  small-intestinal biopsy of, 757, *758*
Midgut, endocrine tumors of, classification of, 243, 244(t)
  rotation of, 125
Milk, breast, secretory IgA in, 75
Mineral oil, granuloma from, 717
Ming's classification, of gastric carcinoma, *604*, 604–605
Mitosis, in gastrointestinal disease, 98–99
Mitotic index, of epithelial cells, 99
  in small intestine, 103
MNNG, gastrointestinal carcinoma induction with, 595, *596*
  in experimental carcinogenesis, 827, *828*
  intestinal carcinoma induction with, 820
Mobile cecum, 125–126
Molecular techniques, correlation with pathologic examination of, 12
Molecules, intercellular flow of, impedence of, 28
Molluscum contagiosum, anal, 889
Moniliasis. See *Candidiasis.*
Mononucleosis, appendiceal involvement in, 869
Morgagni's anal columns, 882
Motility disorders, neural causes of, 202–203
Motor disorders, 188–213. See also *Mechanical obstruction; Pseudo-obstruction.*
  categorization of, 4(t), 4–5
  gastritis associated with, 506
  stasis syndrome in, 741, 741(t)
Mucin, in gastric epithelial cells, 21(t)
  in intestinal function, 32
  in intestinal goblet cells, 31, 31(t)
Muciphage(s), colonic, 361–362, *362*
  in diagnosis of Whipple's disease, 749
Mucocele, appendiceal, 873, *873*
Mucoepidermoid carcinoma, esophageal, 469–470
  gastric, 607, *607–608*
Mucolipidosis, lipid deposition in, 364
Mucopolysaccharidosis, deposition in, 363(t), 365
Mucormycosis, gastric, 503
  intestinal, pathology of, 636, *637*
Mucosa, pathologic examination of, 11
  structure and function of, 14–15, *15*
Mucosal biopsy. See *Biopsy, mucosal; Endoscopic biopsy* and specific mucosal area.
Mucosal prolapse syndrome, 703, 885
Mucous cells, gastric, cardiopyloric, 20(t), 23, *23*
  division of, 100
  in peptic duodenitis, 692
  surface-foveolar, 20(t)–21(t), 20–21, *21*
Mucous neck cells, gastric, 20(t)–21(t), 21, 56, *57*
Muir-Torre syndrome, genetic basis of, 91
Muscle diseases, secondary pseudo-obstruction in, 205–208, *206–208*
Muscle fibers, degeneration of, in visceral myopathy, 200, *200–201*
Muscle spasm, colonic, relationship to diverticulosis of, 771–772
Muscularis mucosae, 14–15, *15*
  colonic, ulcerative colitis changes in, 652
  esophageal, 190–191
  interruption of, in ileal atresia, 123, *124*
  intestinal, in hyperplastic polyps, 788
  rectal, leiomyoma of, 329, 333, *333*
  sigmoid colonic, leiomyoma of, 329, 333, *333*

Muscularis mucosae (Continued)
    small-intestinal, structure of, 191–192
    visceral myopathic involvement of, 198
Muscularis propria, amyloid deposition in, 208, 208
    circular layer of, scleroderma involvement of, 205, 206
    colonic, 192, 194
        muscle fibers of, crisscrossing of, 190, 190
    dilatation of, mechanical obstruction and, 196, 196
    gastric, structure of, 191
    gastrointestinal, microscopic features of, in leiomyoma, 315, 316–318
    hypertrophy of, mechanical obstruction and, 196, 196
    myenteric plexus interface with, stromal tumors of, histology of, 335–336, 335–336
    neuromuscular apparatus of, study techniques for, 192–193
    scarring of, myopathy vs., 200, 201–202
    small-intestinal, creeping fat in, Crohn's disease and, 667, 667
    structure and function of, 14–15, 15
    visceral myopathic involvement of, 198, 199
myc gene, expression of, in colonic carcinoma, 93
Mycobacterium avium-intracellulare infection, 361, 361
    esophagitis from, 400
    gastric, 502
        granulomatous disease in, 507
    in AIDS, 277–278, 277–279
        Whipple's disease vs., 748–749
    in immunocompromised hosts, 633
Mycobacterium tuberculosis. See *Tuberculosis.*
Myenteric plexus (Auerbach's plexus), 15
    amyloid deposition in, 208, 208
    colonic, in severe idiopathic constipation, 204, 205
    degenerative inflammatory neuropathy of, morphologic changes in, 203, 204
    ganglion cells of, absence of, in Hirschsprung's disease, 208
    histology of, immunoperoxidase techniques in, 190, 192–193
        silver staining techniques in, 190, 190–191
    hyperplasia of, in neuronal intestinal dysplasia, 209
    in duplications, 135
    lesions of, jejunal diverticulosis from, 208
    muscularis propria interface with, stromal tumors of, histology of, 335–336, 335–336
Myocyte(s), gastrointestinal, organization of, 188–189, 189
    of muscularis propria, brown pigment in, 207, 207
Myopathy, visceral, characteristics of, 197, 197
    differential diagnosis of, 200, 201–202
    familial, pathologic features of, 198, 198–202, 200
        prognosis of, 200–201, 202
        treatment of, 200–201, 202
        type I, 198
            dilatation in, 198, 198
            histologic features of, 198, 199–200, 200
            prognosis of, 200–201
        type II, 198
            histologic features of, 199, 201
            prognosis of, 200–201, 202
            small-intestinal diverticulosis in, 208
        type III, 198
            prognosis of, 201
    sporadic, 198
        histologic features of, 198, 200, 200
Myxoglobulosis, appendiceal, 873

Naproxen, enteritis and colitis from, 145
Nausea, pregnancy and, 356
Necrosis, coagulative, in ischemic bowel disease, 230–231
    fat, oil granuloma vs., 717–718
        pneumatosis coli vs., 711
    gastric, aspirin injury and, 149
    hemorrhagic, 6
        gastrointestinal, 235, 235
            histology of, 236
        ischemia and, 142
        radiation and, 159, 160

Neomycin, lesions from, resemblance to celiac disease of, 734
Neoplasia, appendiceal, 870–878, 871–876, 877(t)
    gastrointestinal, definition of, 8
        in immunodeficiency disorders, 271
    in acquired immunodeficiency disorders, 275
    rectocolonic mucosal biopsy of, 681
Neoplasms. See *Carcinoma; Tumors.*
Nephrectomy, bilateral, ischemic colitis from, 236
Nerve fibers, histology of, staining in, 190, 192
    in aganglionic megacolon, 120, 120–121
    parasympathetic, in Hirschsprung's disease, 208, 209
Nervous tissue, tumors of, 342, 343–348, 344, 346
Neural diseases, secondary pseudo-obstruction in, 208–210, 209–210
Neurilemoma, anal, 892
Neurocarcinoid, 251–253, 252
    appendiceal, argentaffin microcarcinoid with, 254
    duodenal, histology of, 252, 252
Neurofibromatosis. See *von Recklinghausen's disease.*
Neuroma, appendiceal, 877
Neuron(s), argyrophilic, histology of, 190, 191
    argyrophobic, histology of, 190, 191
    decreased numbers of, in visceral neuropathy, 201–202
Neuronal intranuclear inclusion disease, 203, 203
Neuropathy, autonomic, visceral, in diabetes mellitus, 210
    inflammatory, degenerative, patterns of neural damage in, 203, 204
    noninflammatory, degenerative, patterns of neural damage in, 203, 204
    visceral, 201–204, 203–205
        familial, 202–203, 203
            inheritance patterns of, 203
        neuronal loss in, 201–202
        sporadic, 203–204, 204–205
Neutrophils, in colonic mucosa, in ulcerative colitis, 648, 650
Nevus syndrome, blue rubber bleb, gastrointestinal involvement in, 225
Nezelof syndrome, 273. See also *Immunodeficiency disorders, severe combined.*
Niacin deficiency, gastrointestinal effects of, 360
Niemann-Pick disease, deposition in, 363(t), 364
Nippostrongylus brasiliensis infection, mast cell proliferation in, 757
Nitrates, in gastric carcinoma risk, 587
Nitrosamines, in esophageal cancer, 443
Nitroso compounds, as intestinal carcinogen, 820–821
    in gastric carcinoma risk, 587
N-methyl-N'-nitro-N-nitrosoguanidine (MNNG), gastrointestinal carcinoma induction with, 595
    ethyl (ENNG) derivative in, 596
    propyl (PNNG) derivative in, 595
    in experimental carcinogenesis, 827, 828
    intestinal carcinoma induction with, 820
Nodule(s), in gastric heterotopia, 714–715, 715
Nomarski contrast microscopy, 51, 51
Nonrotation, of midgut, 124–125
Nonsteroidal anti-inflammatory drugs, acute gastritis from, 482
    colonic injury from, 155
    esophagitis and inflammation from, 402(t)
    examples of, 148(t)
    gastric injury from, 145
    gastric toxicity from, 143–144
    gastrointestinal lesions from, 147(t), 148–150, 149, 153–154
Noradrenaline, in intestinal epithelial cell proliferation, 103(t), 103–104
Nutrients, abnormal mucosal uptake of, malabsorption from, 727
Nutritional supplements, esophagitis and inflammation from, 402(t)

Oat cell carcinoma. See *Small cell carcinoma.*
Obstipation, in mechanical obstruction, 195
Obstruction, colonic, in diverticular disease, 781
    duodenal, mixed rotation and, 125

Obstruction (*Continued*)
  intestinal, in aganglionic megacolon, 119
    in argentaffin (EC cell) carcinoids, 253
    in Crohn's disease, 674
    in endometriosis, 711, 712
    in Meckel's diverticulum, 130
    meconium ileus and, 131
    meconium plug syndrome and, 133
  mechanical. See *Mechanical obstruction.*
  pseudo-. See *Pseudo-obstruction.*
Occult blood, in gastrointestinal bleeding diagnosis, 215
Ogilvie's syndrome, intestinal pseudo-obstruction in, 197
Oil granuloma, 716–718, *717*
  of anal region, 892
  pneumatosis coli vs., 711
Oligomucous cells, 30
Omphalocele, 128–129
  associated anomalies in, 129
  formation of, 129
  incidence of, 128
  mixed rotation of midgut with, 125
  pericardiodiaphragmatic hernia with, *129*
Omphalomesenteric artery, remnants of, in Meckel's diverticulum, 130
Omphalomesenteric duct, embryology of, 129–130
  remnants of, 129(t), 129–131, *130–131*
Oncogene(s), amplification of, in gastric carcinoma, 89
  expression of, in colorectal carcinoma, 92–93
Oral cavity, Crohn's disease of, 673
Osler-Weber-Rendu disease, gastrointestinal hemorrhagic telangiectasia in, 221–222, *223*
Oxygen, in mechanisms of cell injury, 142
Oxyuris vermicularis infection, appendiceal, 869, *870*

Paget's disease, extramammary, of perianal region, 899
  histology of, 899, *900*
  pathogenesis of, 899–900
Pancolitis, 645
Pancreas, aberrant, in Meckel's diverticulum, 130, *130*
  annular, clinical manifestations of, 124
    duodenal atresia with, *122*
  cystic fibrosis of, meconium ileus equivalent in, 132
    meconium ileus in, 131–132
  endocrine cells of, classification of, 241(t)
  heterotopic, 565–566
  secretions of, in small-intestinal epithelial proliferation, 103
Pancreatic insufficiency, chronic, malabsorption with, normal mucosal histology in, 727
Pancreatic tissue, heterotopic, 117
  gastric, 538, *538*
Pancreatitis, chronic, lipid maldigestion and steatorrhea in, 358
Paneth cell carcinoma, gastric, 601
Paneth cells, in intestinal carcinoma, 833–834
  metaplasia of, in chronic ulcerative colitis, 649, *652*
  small-intestinal, 32
  role in antigen processing of, 75
Papanicolaou stain, methods for, 52
Papilla of Vater, cytologic sampling of, 50
Papilloma, squamous, esophageal, 444, 473
Papulosis, bowenoid, perianal, 890, *892*
  malignant atrophic, in Köhlmeier-Degos disease, 357
Paraffin, embedding of biopsy specimens in, 41
Paraganglioma, gangliocytic, classification of, 244(t)
  ganglioneuromatous, 251–253, *252*
    association with von Recklinghausen's disease of, 252–253
    cellular components of, 251
    pancreatic vs. intestinal origin of, 251–252, *252*
Parasite(s), esophageal location of, 387(t)
Parasitic infections, appendiceal, 869, 869(t), *870*
  esophageal, 401
  gastric, 503–504
  in AIDS, 275(t)

Parasitic infections (*Continued*)
  in bone marrow transplantation, 275(t)
  in immunocompromised patient, 268, *270*, 271
  metazoan, intestinal obstruction from, 751–753, *752–753*
  protozoan, malabsorption from, 749–751, *750–751*
Parasympathetic nerve fibers, increased number of, in Hirschsprung's disease, 208, *209*
Parathyroid disease, gastrointestinal involvement in, 355
Paratyphoid, immune responses to, history of, 69–70
Parietal cell carcinoma, gastric, 600
Parietal cells, hyperplasia of, in hypertrophic hypersecretory gastropathy, 543
  of gastric mucosa, 20(t), 22–23, 56, *57*
  proliferation of, 100
  ultrastructural features of, *23*
Parkinson's disease, intestinal pseudo-obstruction with, 210
Particulate matter, 157, 157(t)
Pathogens, enteric, classification of, 627–628
  hemorrhagic colitis from, 628
  mucosal adhesion of, with enterotoxin production, 627
    with microvillous damage, 627
  mucosal invasion of, with intracellular proliferation, 627
    with proliferation in lamina propria and lymph nodes, 627–628
Pathologic examination, cytologic exam in, 12
  electron microscopy in, 12
  gross preparation and inspection in, 11
  immunocytochemistry in, 12
  methods of, 10–13
  microscopic examination in, 11–12
  nature of specimen in, 10–11
    mucosal, 10–11
    surgical and autopsy, 11
  report contents in, 12–13
  special techniques in, 12
  vascular injection in, 11
Pellagra, gastrointestinal effects of, 360
Pelvic lesions, gastrointestinal effects of, 356
Penetrance, 82
Pentalogy of Cantrell, 128
Pepsinogen, production by zymogenic cells of, 23
Peptic ulcer(s), acute, 520
  duodenal, 522
    duodenitis vs., 526–527
  gastric, 522
    carcinoma vs., *527*, 527–528
    in heterotopia, 530, 714
    pneumatosis intestinalis in, 709
Peptic ulcer disease, chronic, 519–530
  aspirin usage and, 148–149
  clinical features of, 522–523
  complications of, 528(t), 528–530, *528–530*
  conditions associated with, 521, 521(t)
  definition of, 520
  differential diagnosis of, 526–528, *527*
  dumping syndrome after, 529–530
  endoscopy of, 523
  epidemiology of, 520–521
  etiology of, 521–522
  gastric lymphoid hyperplasia in, 284–285
  gastric outlet obstruction in, 528, *530*
  gastric perforation in, 528, *529*
  genetic basis of, 521
  Helicobacter pylori in, 521–522
  hemorrhage in, 528, *528*
  hyperacidity in, 522
  location of, 523, 523(t)
  normal gastric secretion and, 521
  pathogenesis of, 521–522
  pathology of, 523(t), 523–526, *523–526*
    gross features in, 523–524, *523–525*
    histologic features in, 524–525, *525–527*
    surgical specimen examination in, 525–526
  precipitating factors in, 521, 521(t)

Peptic ulcer disease (*Continued*)
  chronic, psychologic factors in, 521
    recurrence of, 529, *531*
    relation of gastric carcinoma to, 530
    sex predilection of, 521
    surgery for, 528–529
    treatment of, 523
      stomal ulcers after, 530–531, *531*
  drug usage and, 154
  gastric, eosinophilic reaction in, mural eosinophilic gastroenteritis vs., 174, *174*
  gastrin cell hyperplasia with, 248
  genetic basis of, 85–86
  in alcoholics, 147
  in duplications, 135
  in Meckel's diverticulum, 130
  in rheumatoid disease, 229
  Zollinger-Ellison syndrome and, 531–532, *532–533*
Perforation, gastric, in peptic ulcer disease, 528, *529*
    traumatic, spontaneous rupture and 117–118
  intestinal, in aganglionic megacolon, 119
    in chemotherapeutic drug injury, 150
    in meconium ileus, 132
      meconium peritonitis from, 132
    spontaneous, 133
Perfusion, splanchnic, decreased, 5
Perianal region, basal cell carcinoma of, 900, *900*
  extramammary Paget's disease of, 899–900, *900*
Periappendicitis, 878
Periarteritis nodosa, colonic biopsy in, 226, *227*
Pericolitis, diverticulosis and, 777, *777–778*
Periodic acid–Schiff (PAS) stain, in Whipple's disease screening, 43
Peripheral blood, macrophages of, characteristics of, 74, 74(t)
Peritonitis, in aganglionic megacolon, 119
  meconium, 132, *132–133*
Peroxidation, lipid, in cell injury, 142
Peutz-Jeghers syndrome, carcinoma in, 562–563
  genetic basis of, 90
  hemangiomas in, 225
  polyps in, 561–563, *562*, 791–792, *792*
    association with malignancy of, 810
    etiology of, 790
    hamartomatous, adenocarcinoma in, 826, *826*
    malignant potential of, 562–563, 792
    microscopic features of, 562, *562*
    pathology of, 790–792, *791*
Peyer's patches, 24
  anatomy of, 70
  areas of, 71, *71*
  number of, 70, 70(t)
  size of, 70–71
  T-lymphocyte–dependent areas of, 71
pH, gastric, as defense mechanism, 623
  at birth, 116
Phagolysosomes, in colonic malacoplakia, 371, *372*
Pharmacologic agents, secondary pseudo-obstruction from, 211
Pheochromocytoma, gastrointestinal effects of, 355
  intestinal pseudo-obstruction in, 210–211
Photography, of small-intestinal biopsies, 726–727
Phycomycete(s), esophagitis from, 392–393
Phycomycosis, gastric, 503
Pinworm infections, appendiceal, 869, *870*
Plasma cells, gastrointestinal, development of, 72, 72(t)
  in chronic ulcerative colitis, 649
  in IPSID, 300, *300–301*
  in lamina propria, 71, *71*, 72, 72(t)
    IgA synthesis in, 76–77, *77*
  in solitary plasmacytoma, 302, *302–303*
Plasmacytoma, solitary, gastrointestinal, pathology of, 302, *302–303*
Platelet activating factor, in pathogenesis of ischemic bowel disease, 233
Plicae circulares, 24
Plummer-Vinson syndrome, in esophageal carcinoma, 444
  iron deficiency anemia in, 354

Pneumatosis coli, 709
  colonic mucosa in, 710, *710*
Pneumatosis cystoides intestinalis, clinical features of, 709
  definition of, 709
  differential diagnosis of, 710–711
  etiology of, 709
  oil granuloma vs., 718
  pathology of, 709–710, *710–711*
  vasculitis associated with, 226
PNNG, gastrointestinal carcinoma induction with, 595
Polyadenoma, history of, 548
Polyadenomes polypeaux, history of, 548
Polyarteritis nodosa, gastrointestinal involvement in, 226–227
  gastrointestinal vasculitis in, 226
Polyarthritis, in ulcerative colitis, 654
Polycythemia, gastrointestinal hemorrhage and infarction in, 354
  necrotizing enterocolitis from, 233
Polyfoam pads, biopsy specimen damage by, 41, *41*
Polymyositis, pseudo-obstruction in, 206
Polyp(s), adenomatous, gastric, flat, 551–552, *552–554*
    histogenesis of, 550
    histologic classification of, 549, 549(t), 550–551, *551*
      comparison of, 549–550, 550(t)
    history of, 548–549
    hyperplastic, 559
    incidence of, 550
    malignant change in, 554–555, 561(t)
    papillary (villous), 552, *554–556*
    pathology of, 550–552, *551–556*, 554–555
    subtypes of, 550–552, *551–556*, 554–555
    schematic presentation of, 551, *551*
  benign, gastric, frequency of, 547, 548(t)
    intestinal, 786–812
  benign epithelial, as precancerous conditions, 824–826, *825–826*
  benign neoplastic, gastric, histologic classification of, 549, 549(t)
  colonic, cytology of, 62
    hyperplastic, collagenous colitis vs., 700
  epithelial, gastric, 547–566
    as carcinoma precursors, 587
    classification of, 587
    definition of, 547
    histologic classification of, 549(t)–550(t), 549–550
    in chronic gastritis, 498
  esophageal, 474
  fibrovascular, esophageal, 474
  filiform, in ulcerative colitis, 648
  foveolar, 564–565
  gastric, biopsy of, interpretation of, 548
    classification of, 547
    clinical aspects of, 547
    epithelial cell proliferation in, 101–102
    focal mucosal hypertrophy from, 537–538
    histologic diagnosis of, 548
    historical review of, 548–549
    incidence of, 547
    malignant, histologic classification of, 549, 549(t)
    regenerative, history of, 549
  gastrointestinal, in carcinoma, genetic basis of, 89, 89(t)
  giant fibrovascular, esophageal, 342, *344*
  hamartomatous, gastric, histologic classification of, 549, 549(t)
    in hereditary gastrointestinal polyposis syndromes, 561
    in Peutz-Jeghers syndrome, 561–563, *562*
    intestinal, in Peutz-Jeghers syndrome, 810
  inverted, 806
  heterotopic, gastric, 565–566
    histologic classifications of, 549, 549(t)
  hyperplasiogenous, gastric, 549
  hyperplastic (regenerative), colorectal, 786
    gastric, as precancerous lesion, 582, *582*
      carcinomatous lesion in, 560, *562*
      dysplastic (adenomatous), 559
      dysplastic change in, 559, *560*
      forms of, 557, *557*
      globoid cells in, 559, *560*

Polyp(s) (*Continued*)
  hyperplastic (regenerative), gastric, histogenesis of, 557
    histologic classifications of, 549, 549(t)
      comparison of, 549–550, 550(t)
    histologic features of, 558–559, *558–559*
    history of, 548–549
    malignant potential of, 560–561, 561(t), *562*
    pathology of, 557–559, *558–560*
    size of, 557–558, *558*
  intestinal, 786–790, *788–790*
    adenomatous change in, 787
    clinical aspects of, 787
    epidemiology of, 787
    etiology of, 787
    glycoconjugate changes in, 789–790
    gross appearance of, 787–788, *788*
    incidence of, 786–787
    pathogenesis of, 787
    pathology of, 787–788, *788–790*
    serrated appearance of, 788, *789*
    sialomucin distribution in, 788–789
    special studies of, 788–790
    star-shaped appearance of glands in, 788, *790*
  malignant potential of, 825–826
  in Cowden's disease, 811
  in Cronkhite-Canada syndrome, 810, *811*
  inflammatory, gastric, 565
    histologic classification of, 549, 549(t)
  intestinal, 792–793, *793–794*
  inflammatory cloacogenic, 703, 885, *886*
  inflammatory fibroid, gastric, 339, *340–341*, 341
    ileal vs., 339(t)
    histogenesis of, 342
    ileal, 341–342, *341–343*
      gastric vs., 339(t)
    intestinal, clinical aspects of, 792
      general aspects of, 792
      pathology of, 792
  intestinal, classification of, 786, 787(t)
    definition of, 786
  intraluminal, gastric, 547
  intramural, gastric, 547
  juvenile, cause of, 563
    clinical presentation of, 563, 563(t)
    colonic, 795–796
    gastric, 563, *563*
      histology of, 563–564, *564*
    intestinal, adenomatous change in, 794–795
      clinical aspects of, 793
      epidemiology of, 793
      etiology of, 793
      incidence of, 793
      pathogenesis of, 793
      pathology of, 793–795, *795–796*
  leiomyomatous, rectosigmoid, 329, 333, *333*
  lymphoid, intestinal, 795–796
    rectal, 286, *286–287*
  malignant, colonic, management of, 805–806
    intestinal, definition of, 804
      lymphatic invasion in, *806*
      tumor emboli in, *807*
  metaplastic, 550
  neoplastic, intestinal, 796–807. See also *Adenoma*.
  nonneoplastic, malignant potential of, 825–826
  of fundic gland, 564
  Peutz-Jeghers. See *Peutz-Jeghers syndrome*.
  rectal, in solitary ulcer syndrome, 704, *705*
    differential diagnosis of, 706
  retention, 565
  umbilical, 130–131, *131*
Polypoid carcinoma, esophageal, 471
Polyposis, colonic, fundic gland polyps in, 564
  familial, adenomatous, genetic basis of, 89–90
    tumorigenesis of, 91

Polyposis (*Continued*)
  familial, DNA synthesis abnormalities in, 105
    juvenile, genetic basis of, 90
    manifestations of, 89, 89(t)
    syndromes of, 89–90
    tumor type in, 89, 89(t)
  hamartomatous, genetic basis of, 90
    intestinal carcinoma in, 826, *826*
  hyperplastic, gastric, 558
  lymphoid colonic, 811–812, *812*
  multiple lymphomatous, nodular lymphoid hyperplasia vs., 290, 297
Polyposis coli, familial (adenomatosis), 807–808, *809*
Polyposis syndrome, 807–812, *809, 811–812*
  genetic basis of, 822
  juvenile, 563–564, *563–565*
    carcinoma in, 564, *565*, 826
    causes of, 563
    differeniation of polyps in, 809
    histology of, 563–564, *564*
    subtypes of, 563, 563(t)
Portal vein, thrombosis of, varices from, 219
Potassium chloride, enteric-coated, gastrointestinal ulceration from, 152
  gastrointestinal ischemia from, 236
Pouchitis, after ileostomy, 654
Pregnancy, gastrointestinal effects of, 356
Prevertebral ganglia, gastrointestinal control by, 189
Proctitis, allergic, 182–185, *183–184*, 185(t)
  adult cases of, 185
  childhood cases of, clinical and laboratory features of, 183
    diagnosis of, 184
    differential diagnosis of, 184
    pathologic features of, 183–184, *183–184*
  definition of, 182–183
  rectal biopsy in, 185
  terminology for, 172
  enemas and, 152, 157
  herpes simplex virus and, in male homosexuals, 630
  in diversion-related colitis, 701, *701–702*
  localized, 703
  ulcerative, 644–646
    increased IgE-bearing cells in, 184–185
Proctitis cystica profunda, localized, 703
Proctocolitis, ulcerative, definition of, 644
Progesterone, colonic injury from, 155
  gastrointestinal lesions from, 147(t), 148
Prolapse, rectal, 703, 885, *886*
Prolapse syndrome, mucosal, 885
Proliferative compartment, esophageal, 99
  of epithelial cells, 99
Prostaglandin(s), effects on colonic epithelial cell proliferation of, 105
  gastrointestinal effects of, 352
  mucosal levels of, gastric NSAID toxicity and, 143–144
  synthesis of, reduction of, aspirin and, 148
Prostaglandin E_1, in gastric epithelial renewal, 101, 101(t)
  in reduction of bowel ischemia, 233
Prostaglandin E_2, in gastric epithelial renewal, 101, 101(t)
  in small-intestinal epithelial cell proliferation, 103, 103(t)
Protease, in mechanisms of cell injury, 142
Protein, dietary, as risk factor for colonic carcinoma, 822
Protein-calorie deficiency, jejunal effects of, 743
Protein deficiency, small-intestinal mucosal alterations from, 743, 743–744
Protein-losing enteropathy. See *Enteropathy, protein-losing*.
Protein loss, in hypertrophic hypersecretory gastropathy, 543
Protozoa, phase contrast microscopy of, 50
Protozoan infections, intestinal, malabsorption from, 749–751, *750–751*
  pathology of, *638–639*, 638–640
Psammoma bodies, in D-cell duodenal tumors, 251
Pseudodiverticula, colonic, 773–774, *774*

Pseudoleukemia, gastrointestinal. See *Lymphoid hyperplasia, nodular.*
Pseudolymphoma, gastric, 282. See also *Lymphoid hyperplasia, gastric.*
Pseudomelanin deposition, 365
Pseudomelanosis coli, 706
Pseudomembranous colitis, antibiotic-associated, 625, 625–626
    Clostridium difficile infection and, as gastrointestinal ecologic perturbation, 624–626, *625*
    type I and II lesions in, 625, *625*
Pseudo-obstruction, intestinal, 196–211
    acute forms of, 196–197
    adynamic ileus in, 196–197
    chronic forms of, 196, 196(t)
    clinical features of, 197, *197*
    definition of, 196
    drug-induced, 155, 157(t)
    idiopathic, systemic disease vs., 203
    morphology of, 196
    Ogilvie's syndrome in, 197
    primary, 197–198, *197–205*, 200–204
        categories of, 196, 196(t)
        secondary vs., 204–205
        visceral myopathy in, 197–198, *197–202*, 200–201. See also *Myopathy, visceral.*
        visceral neuropathy in, 201–204, *203–205.* See also *Neuropathy, visceral.*
    secondary, 204–211, 205(t), *206–210*
        amyloidosis in, 208, *208*
        categories of, 204–205, 205(t)
        ceroidosis in, 206–207, *207*
        Chagas' disease in, 209–210
        definition of, 204
        diabetes mellitus in, 210
        endocrine disorders in, 210–211
        Hirschsprung's disease in, 208, *209*
        hypothyroidism in, 210
        miscellaneous lesions in, 211
        muscle diseases in, 204–208, *206–208*
        myotonic dystrophy in, 206
        neural diseases in, 208–210, *209–210*
        neuronal intestinal dysplasia in, 208–209, *210*
        Parkinson's disease in, 210
        pharmacologic agents in, 211
        progressive muscular dystrophy in, 206
        scleroderma in, 204–205, *206*
        small-intestinal diverticulosis in, *207*, 207–208
    stasis syndrome in, 741
Pseudopolyp(s), in ischemic colitis, *233*, 234
    in ulcerative colitis, 677
        gross features of, 646, *647–648*, 648
    inflammatory, 565
        colonic, 794
        etiology of, 792
        in ulcerative colitis, 648, *650*, 792, *793*
        incidence of, 792
        pathogenesis of, 792
        pathology of, 792–793, *793–794*
    inflammatory fibroid, 565
Pseudoxanthoma elasticum, gastrointestinal bleeding in, 222–223
Pus, in acute appendicitis, 865, *865*
Pyloric atresia, 116
Pyloric stenosis, hypertrophic congenital, clinical features of, 116
    genetic basis of, 87–88
    gross features of, 116–117
    heterotopic pancreatic tissue and, 117
    microscopic features of, 117
    pathogenesis of, 117
Pylorus, myenteric plexus of, degenerative changes in, 117
Pyoderma gangrenosum, in ulcerative colitis, 654

Rad, 158
Radiation, as intestinal carcinogen, 821
    background, 157
    damage from, gastric, 505
    doses of, esophageal, 405
    effects of, gastric, 505
        synergistic, in drug disorders, 144
    gastrointestinal sensitivity to, 158
    localized, acute features of, 159, 159(t), *160–161*
        chronic features of, 159(t), 159–160
    measurements of, 158
    sources of, 157
    tolerance doses for, 158
    types of, 156–158, 157(t)
        electromagnetic wave, 157, 157(t)
        particulate matter, 157, 157(t)
Radiation effect, definition of, 159
Radiation injury, clinical features of, 161–162
    colonic, *164*, 164–165
    definition of, 159
    diagnosis of, 162
    differential diagnosis of, 162
    duodenal, 694
    esophageal, 162, *405*, 405–406
    gastric, 162–163
    gastrointestinal, ischemic necrosis from, fibrosis with, 235
    histologic features of, 159(t), 159–160, *160–161*
    mechanisms of, 158
    motility disorders in, 211
    pathologic features of, 158–161, 159(t), *160–161*
        cellular alterations in, 158–159
        localized radiation in, 159(t), 159–160, *160–161*
        opportunistic infections in, 160
        radiation type and dose in, 159
        tumor development in, 160–161, *161*
        whole-body irradiation in, 159
    rectal, 164–165
        histologic changes in, 164
    small-intestinal, *163*, 163–164
    specific organ involvement in, 162–165, *163–164*
Radioallergosorbent test (RAST), in allergic gastroenteritis, 176
    in food allergies, 172
Radiology, in gastrointestinal bleeding diagnosis, 215
Radionuclide studies, in gastrointestinal bleeding diagnosis, 215
Radiotherapy, deleterious effects of, restriction of, 158
    for esophageal carcinoma, 454
        morphologic changes after, 454
        pathologic changes after, 454
        grading of, 455–456, *455–456*
        tissue changes after, 454–455
    gastric injury from, 505
Rappaport's classification, of gastrointestinal malignant lymphoma, 295, *295*
Rappaport's histiocytic lymphoma, in celiac sprue, 290–291
ras gene, mutation of, in colorectal tumors, 91–92
    invasiveness and, 92–93
Raynaud's phenomenon, in small-intestinal diverticulosis, 207
Rectal atresia, 136
Rectal mucosa, *884*
    in diversion-related colitis, 701–702, *701–702*
    in enema-induced colitis, 707, *707*
    in solitary ulcer syndrome, 704, *704*
    prolapse of, 885, *886*
Rectal prolapse, 885, *886*
    in solitary rectal ulcer syndrome, 703
Rectal tonsil. See *Lymphoid hyperplasia, rectal.*
Rectal ulcer syndrome, solitary, 703–704, *704–705*, 706
    clinical features of, 703
    definition of, 703
    etiology of, 703
    pathology of, 703–704, *704–705*, 706
    rectal prolapse and, 885

Rectum, allergic gastroenteritis of, 182
　carcinoids of, 255, 256
　carcinoma of. See *Carcinoma, rectal.*
　cavernous hemangioma of, 224
　cell turnover time in, 104
　Crohn's disease of, ulcerative colitis vs., 677, 677(t)
　cytologic sampling of, 50
　distal, histology of, in aganglionic megacolon, 119–120
　drug injury to, 156
　embryology of, 135–136
　endocrine cells of, classification of, 241(t)
　gastric heterotopic involvement of, 714
　inflammatory pseudopolyps of, 792
　Kaposi's sarcoma of, in AIDS, 280
　leiomyoma of, deep intramural, histology of, 333–335, 334
　lesions of, cytology of, statistical evaluation of, 67, 67(t)
　lymphoid hyperplasia of, 286, 286–287
　metaplasia of, 7(t), 8
　mucosal biopsy of, amyloidosis diagnosis by, 367–368
　　in Crohn's disease vs. ulcerative colitis differentiation, 678
　　in inflammatory bowel disease, 679, 679(t), 680, 681
　muscularis mucosae of, leiomyoma of, histology of, 329, 333, 333
　radiation injury to, 164–165
　sarcoma of, colonic sarcoma vs., 329, 332
　stromal tumors of, site specificity of, 312
　ulcerative colitis of, 645–646, 652
　ulcers of. See *Rectal ulcer syndrome, solitary.*
Regeneration, epithelial, gastrointestinal injury and, 7
Relative biologic effectiveness, of radiation, 158
Rem, 158
Renal disease, gastrointestinal involvement in, 352–353, 353
　immunosupressive therapy for, secondary gastrointestinal infections from, 352–353
Renal transplantation, ischemic colitis from, 236
Reproductive system, disorders of, gastrointestinal effects of, 356
Reserpine, peptic ulcers from, 154
Respiratory system, diseases of, gastrointestinal involvement in, 352
Reticulin, IgA antibodies against, 729
Retinoblastoma, molecular genetic changes in, 91–92
Rheumatoid arthritis, gastrointestinal involvement in, 228, 357
Rheumatoid disease, gastrointestinal disorders with arthritic symptoms vs., 229
　gastrointestinal vasculitis in, 226
Roentgen, 158
Rotation, of midgut, 125
Rubella, esophagitis associated with, 396
Russell bodies, in solitary plasmacytoma, 303

S phase (synthesis phase), of cell proliferation, 98–99
S phase cells, altered distribution of, in colonic preneoplasia, 105
Saffron, for biopsy specimen staining, 42–43, 43(t)
Saint's triad, in colonic diverticular disease, 782
Salmonella infection, in ulcerative colitis, 653
　initial lesions of, at follicular dome epithelium, 33
　mucosal invasion in, with proliferation in lamina propria and lymph nodes, 627–628
　pathology of, 631, 632
　tissue invasion in, 627
Salmonella paratyphi infection, mucosal translocation in, with systemic spread, 628
Salmonella typhi infection, mucosal translocation in, with systemic spread, 628
Salt, in gastric carcinoma risk, 586
Sarcoidosis, appendiceal, 878
　differential diagnosis of, 370
　esophageal involvement in, 427
　pathology of, 369–370
Sarcoma, gastric, 326, 328
　gastrointestinal, gross characteristics of, 314
　intestinal, gross characteristics of, 313, 313–314
　Kaposi's, 225, 279–281, 280
　rectal, colonic sarcoma vs., 329, 332

Schatzki ring, 424, 426
Schistosoma japonicum infection, 640
Schistosoma mansoni infection, 640
Schistosomiasis, colonic, recognition of ova in, 640, 640
　colorectal carcinoma in, 827
　varices from, 219
Schwann cells, in ganglioneuromatosis, 344, 346
Schwannoma, gastrointestinal, 342, 344
Scleroderma, esophageal, 205, 206
　gastrointestinal, morphologic changes in, 205–206, 206
　intestinal, diverticula in, 205–206, 206, 770
　stasis syndrome in, 741
　villous atrophy in, 202
Sclerosing agents, injection of, ulceration and fibrosis from, 153
Sebaceous glands, ectopic, esophageal, 386
Secretin, in gastric epithelial renewal, 101, 101(t)
　in small-intestinal epithelial cell proliferation, 103, 103(t)
Secretory component, synthesis of, 77, 77
Secretory component deficiency, 273
Selenium, tumor reduction by, 821
Sepsis, diverticular, free perforation in, 779
Serosa, structure and function of, 14–15, 15
Serositis, in systemic lupus erythematosus, 227
Serotonin, in small-intestinal epithelial cell proliferation, 103, 103(t)
Sexually transmitted diseases, anal, 888–889
Shigellosis, 627, 631, 632
Shock, intestinal blood flow during, 232
　of gastrointestinal tract, 6
Short bowel syndrome, malabsorption from, normal mucosal histology in, 727
Shunt fascicles, 190
Shy-Drager syndrome, intestinal pseudo-obstruction with, 210
Sialomucin, in hyperplastic polyp, 788
　in intestinal adenomas, 801
　small-intestinal, 588
Sigmoidoscopy, cytologic sampling with, 50
Signet-ring cell carcinoma, gastric, tumor cell clusters in, 59, 60
　in Barrett's epithelium, 465, 467
　intestinal, 835, 836
Signet-ring cells, in appendiceal adenocarcinoid, 875–876, 876
Silicon rubber, vascular lesion study with, 216
Sinus, umbilical, 130
Sinus tracts, in Crohn's disease, 666–667, 667, 677(t)
　inflammatory, 669–670, 670
β-Sitosterol, effect on colonic epithelial cell proliferation of, 105
Sjögren's syndrome, esophageal involvement in, 425
　gastrointestinal effects of, 358
Skeletal muscle, esophageal, 190
Skin diseases, gastrointestinal effects of, 356
Small bowel. See *Small intestine.*
Small cell carcinoma, colonic, 844–845, 845
　esophageal, 471–472, 472
　gastric, 609, 609
　intestinal, 844–845, 845–846
Small-intestinal mucosa, alcohol-induced damage to, 147
　allergic gastroenteritis of, 180–181, 181–182
　alterations of, protein deficiency and, 743, 743–744
　chemotherapeutic drug injury to, 150
　in acrodermatitis enteropathica, 744
　lesions of, diseases associated with, 755–761, 756–761
　malabsorption involvement of, biopsy and, 726
　vascular organization of, 24
　villous loss in, radiation injury and malabsorption from, 163, 163–164
Small intestine, absorptive cells of, histology of, 26(t), 26–28, 27–28. See also *Absorptive cells, small-intestinal.*
　allergic gastroenteritis of, 180–182, 181–182
　　diagnosis of, 181–182
　　differential diagnosis of, 182
　　mucosal changes in, 180–181, 181–182
　argentaffin (EC cell) carcinoids of, 253, 254
　bacterial overgrowth in, in familial visceral myopathy, 200, 202
　　in immunocompromised patient, 268, 270, 271

Small intestine (Continued)
  biopsy of, in malabsorptive disorders, special considerations in, 725–727
  caveolated cells of, 33
  contamination of, 624, 624
  Crohn's disease of, 665
    differential diagnosis of, 672
    gross features of, 667
    lymphatic dilatation in, 668, 669
    recurrent lesions in, 675–676
  cup cells of, 33
  diverticula of, 769
  duplications of, 135
  embryology of, 118–119
  endocrine cells of, classification of, 241(t)
  epithelial cells of, functions of, 26(t)
    mucin profiles of, 31(t)
    proliferation of, effect of humoral factors on, 103(t)
      in disease states, 103–104
      in normal states, 102–103
    types of, 26(t), 26–33, 27–32, 31(t), 102–103
    ultrastructural characteristics of, 26(t)
  epithelium of, Brunner's glands of, 25–26
    crypts of, 24–25, 25
    degeneration of, in allergic gastroenteritis, 181, 182
    follicular dome, 25, 32, 32
    general structure of, 24–26, 25
    regeneration of, 103
    villi of, 24–25, 25
  goblet mucous cells of, 30–31, 30–32, 31(t)
  gross anatomy of, 24
  hemangioma of, 224
  immunoproliferative disease of. See Immunoproliferative small-intestinal disease (IPSID).
  infarction of. See Infarction, gastrointestinal.
  inflammatory disorders of, 696–697
  iron absorption by, iron deficiency anemia and, 354
  ischemic lesions of, estrogen usage and, 148
    progesterone usage and, 148
  leiomyoma of, histology of, 326, 329, 329–331
  leiomyosarcoma of, histology of, 326, 331
  lymphoid hyperplasia of, 285–286
  malignant lymphoma of, 293, 294
  membranous (M) cells of, 25, 32, 32–33
  metaplasia of, 7(t), 8
  neuromuscular structure of, 191–192, 194
  nodular lymphoid hyperplasia of, without hypogammaglobulinemia, 289–290
  obstruction of, inflammatory fibroid polyps in, in Malawi, 341
  Paneth cells of, 32
    role in antigen processing of, 75
  Peutz-Jeghers polyp of, 791, 792
  plexiform neurofibroma of, in von Recklinghausen's disease, 344, 345
  radiation injury to, acute, 163
    chronic, 163, 163–164
  rapid transit of foodstuffs through, malabsorption from, 727
  resection of, epithelial cell proliferation in, 103
  stromal tumors of, site specificity of, 312
  structure of, similarity to colon of, 816–817
  susceptibility to carcinoma of, 824
  ulcers of, in refractory sprue and celiac disease, 735–736, 737
    systemic disease and, 697
  undifferentiated crypt cells of, 26(t), 29–30, 30
Smoking, role in esophageal cancer of, 443
Smooth muscle cell tumors. See also Mesenchymal tumors; Stromal tumors.
  endometriosis vs., 713
  gastric, frequency of, 585, 585(t)
Smooth muscle cells, small-intestinal, function of, 192
Sodium nitrate, in gastric carcinoma risk, 586
Soft tissue diseases, gastrointestinal effects of, 357
Solitary rectal ulcer syndrome, 703–704, 704–705, 706. See also Rectal ulcer syndrome, solitary.
Somatostatin (D) cell tumors, 249–251, 251
  classification of, 244(t)
Somatostatinoma, hyperfunctional syndrome with, 243, 243(t)
  relationship between duodenal paragangliomas and, 252, 252–253
Somatostatinoma syndrome, with duodenal D-cell tumors, 249, 251
Soy protein allergy, definition of, 175
  in infants, 183
Soybean products, gastric carcinoma risk and, 586
Spasm, colonic, relationship to diverticulosis of, 771–772
Sphincter, esophageal, 190
  pyloric, 191
Spindle cell carcinoma, cellular, gastric, 321, 322–323
  esophageal, 451, 451
  gastrointestinal, differentiation of, 311
  rectal, cellularity of, 333–335, 334
Spindle cells, in colonic leiomyoma, 332
  in esophageal granular cell tumor, 346, 348
  in small-intestinal leiomyomas, 326, 329
Spirochete(s), esophageal location of, 387(t)
  in appendix, 868–869
  in colon, 635–636
  in syphilitic esophagitis, 400–401
  intestinal, in AIDS, 279, 280
    incidence of, 636
    pathology of, 635–636, 635–636
Splanchnic vessels, chronic narrowing of, effect of, 236
Spondylarthropathy, gastrointestinal manifestations of, 357–358
Spondylitis, ankylosing, in ulcerative colitis, 654
Sprue, celiac. See also Celiac disease.
  malignant lymphoma with, histology of, 290–291
    pathology of, 290–291
    risk of, 290
    treament of, 291
  collagenous, 737–738
  definition of, 727
  hypogammaglobulinemic, pathology of, 271–272
  idiopathic. See Celiac disease.
  nontropical. See Celiac disease.
  refractory, 735–737, 735–737
    definition of, 735, 736
    ulcerations accompanying, 735–736, 737
  tropical, chronic malabsorption in, 739
    clinicopathologic correlation of, 741
    definition of, 739
    differential diagnosis of, 741
    epithelial changes in, malabsorption from, 739, 741
    etiology of, 739
    folate deficiency in, 354
    forms of, 739
    gastritis in, 741
    geographic distribution of, 739
    lymphocytic infiltration in, 739
    pathogenesis of, 739
    pathology of, 739, 740, 741
    small-intestinal crypts and villi in, 739, 740
Squamous cell carcinoma, anal canal, 896–899, 898–899
  anal margin, 897, 898
  esophageal, 439–456
    achalasia with, 443
    advanced, 448–450, 448–451
      fungating, 448, 449
      grade classification of, 450, 450–451
      grade I, 450, 450
      grade III, 450, 451
      intraluminal (polypoid), 449, 449–450
      medullary, 448, 448
      scirrhous (stenosing), 449, 449
      ulcerative, 449, 449
    associated conditions with, 443–444
    benign stricture with, 443–444
    celiac disease with, 444
    chronic esophagitis with, 443
    clinical presentation of, diagnosis and, 453

Squamous cell carcinoma (*Continued*)
  esophageal, clinicopathologic correlation of, 453–456, *454–456*
    complications of, 453–454, *454*
    contiguous involvement of neighboring organs in, 452
    cytology of, 55, *55*
    death from, 453–454, *454*
    distribution of, age, 440
      geogaphic, 440–441, *440–441*
      sex, 440
    diverticula with, 444
    early, erosive, 446, *446*
      gross types of, 446(t), 446–447, *446–447*
      histologic types of, 446(t), 447–448, *447–448*
      intraepithelial (in situ), 447, *447*
      intramucosal, 447–448, *448*
      occult, 446, *446*
      papillary, 446–447, *447*
      plaque, 446, *447*
      submucosal, 448
    epidemiology of, 440–442, *440–442*
      mass surveys in China in, *441*, 441–442
      migrant studies in, 442
    etiology of, alcohol in, 443
      dietary factors in, 442–443
      genetic factors in, 443
      nitrosamines in, 443
      smoking in, 443
      trace elements in, 443
    genetic basis of, 88
    hiatal hernia with, 444
    incidence of, in fowl of China, 442, *442*, 442(t)
    location of, 445–446
    metastases in, hematogenous, 452
    pathology of, 445–453
    Plummer-Vinson syndrome with, 444
    precancerous lesions in, 444–445, *444–445*
    prognosis of, 439
      cellular ploidy and, 453
      growth pattern and, 453
      histologic grade and, 453
      location and, 453
      pathologic factors affecting, 452–453
      size and, 453
      stage and, 452–453
      stromal reaction and, 453
    radiation therapy for, 454
      morphologic changes after, factors affecting, 454
      pathologic changes after, grading of, 455–456, *455–456*
      tissue changes after, 454–455
    spread of, intramural, 452
      lymphatic, 452
    staging of, clinicopathologic system of, 451–452
      TNM system of, 451, 452(t)
    surgery for, 454
    treatment of, 454–456, *455–456*
    variants of, 450–451
  gastric, 580, 607–608
  in situ, anal, 894, *895*
  intestinal, 843–844, *843–844*
  metastatic, jejunal, 845, *846*
  of cardia, cytology of, 59
Squamous cells, esophageal, dysplastic, 54, *55*
  nuclear area of, 63(t)
Stagnant loop syndrome. See *Stasis syndrome*.
Staphylococcus spp., enterocolitis from, 236
Starch, granulomatous reaction to, 716
Starvation, decreased epithelial proliferation from, 103
Stasis syndrome, bacterial overgrowth in, 742, *742*
  conditions associated with, 741, 741(t)
  pathogenesis of, 742, *742*
  pathology of, 742, *742–743*
  synonyms for, 741
Steatorrhea, idiopathic. See *Celiac disease*.

Stem cells, of gastric mucosa, carcinoma origination in, 102
  division of, 100
Stenosis, anal, 136
  congenital pyloric, gastric inflammation in, 506
  duodenal, 124
    incidence of, 122
    pathogenesis of, 123
  ileal, 124
  in Crohn's disease, 677
  intestinal, clinical manifestations of, 124
    pathogenesis of, *122*, 122–123
    types of, *122*, 122–123
  pyloric. See *Pyloric stenosis*.
Steroids, gastrointestinal lesions from, 147(t), 148
  in colon carcinoma etiology, 823
Sterols, fecal, colonic carcinoma risk and, 822
Stevens-Johnson syndrome, 357
Stoma, gastrointestinal, varices from, 219
Stomach, actinomycosis of, 502
  allergic gastroenteritis of, 178–180, *179–180*
  anisakiasis of, 504
  atony of, 506
  atrophy of, 487
  benign polypoid lesions of, frequency of, 547, 548(t)
  bezoar retention in, 506
  body (corpus) of, 19
  candidiasis of, 503, *503*
  carcinoma of. See *Gastric carcinoma*.
  carcinosarcoma of, 608, *609*
  cardia of, 19
  chemical injury to, 153–154
    pathogenesis of, mechanisms of, 142
  choriocarcinoma of, 608
  chronic peptic ulcer of, active, histology of, 524, *525–527*
    carcinoma vs., 527, *527–528*
    gross features of, 523–524, *523–524*
    healed, 524, *525*
  Crohn's disease of, 507–508, 673, *673–674*
  cytologic sampling of, 49
  cytomegalovirus infection of, 500, *501*
  diverticula of, 506, 769
  drug injury to, 153–154
  duplications of, 135
  embryology of, 116
  endocrine cells of, classification of, 241(t)
  epithelial polyps of, 547–566. See also *Polyp(s)*.
  erosions of, cell damage in, 56–57, *58*
  functions of, 19–20
  fundus of, 19
  glomus tumors of, histology of, 338, *338–339*
  granulomatous diseases of, 507–508, *508*
  gross anatomy of, 19
  Helicobacter pylori infection of, 500
  herpesvirus infection of, 500
  histoplasmosis of, 503
  in Ménétrier's disease, 541, *543*
  infections of, 500(t), 500–504
    acute gastritis vs., 485
    bacterial, 500–503
    fungal, 503, *503*
    viral, 500
  lesions of, cytology of, 55–60, *56–59*, 58(t)–59(t)
  lymphoid hyperplasia of, 282, *282–285*, 284–285, 285(t). See also *Lymphoid hyperplasia, gastric*.
  malformations of, 223
  Mallory-Weiss syndrome of, 504, *504–505*
  metaplasia of, 7(t), 7–8
  mucormycosis of, 503
  mucosa of. See *Gastric mucosa*.
  Mycobacterium avium-intracellulare infection of, 502
  neuromuscular structure of, 191
  peptic ulcer of, 522
  pH of, acid, as defense mechanism, 623
  phycomycosis of, 503

Stomach (*Continued*)
  pyloric antrum of, 19
  radiation injury to, 162–163
  rugae of, 19
  sarcoma of, 326, *328*
  secretions of, normal, in etiology of chronic peptic ulcer disease, 521
  small- to intermediate-cell endocrine carcinoma of, 257, *257*
  spontaneous rupture of, 117–118
  stress ulcers of, 519, *520*
  stromal tumors of, 321–323, *322–328*
    site specificity of, 312
  syphilis of, 502–503
  teratoma of, 608
  toxic injury to, pathogenesis of, 143–144
  tuberculosis of, 501–502
  tumors of. See *Gastric carcinoma; Gastric tumors.*
  ulceration of, 229
Storage disease, conditions stimulating, 360–362, *361–362*
  gastrointestinal, nature and localization of deposits in, 363, 363(t)
  glycolipid, 362–364, 363(t)
  melanosis coli vs., 706
Strangulation, gastrointestinal, 6
Streptococcus spp., esophagitis from, 398, *399*
  immune protection against, secretory IgA in, 77
Stress, gastrointestinal symptoms associated with, 352
Stress ulcer(s), gastric-duodenal, 517–519
  clinical features of, 518
  definition of, 517
  differential diagnosis of, 519
  etiology of, 517–518
  pathogenesis of, 235, *236*, 517–518
  pathology of, gross features in, 518, *518–519*
    histologic features in, 518–519, *519–520*
Stricture, fibrous, duodenal, 694
  in necrotizing enterocolitis, 234, *235*
  small-intestinal, Crohn's disease and, 196, *196*
Stroma, vascularized, in ileal inflammatory fibroid polyp, 342, *343*
Stromal tumors, at myenteric plexus–muscularis propria interface, histology of, 335–336, *335–336*
  esophageal, 320–321, *321*
  gastric, 321–323, *322–328*
  gastrointestinal, cell origin of, 311–312
    clinical features of, 312
    differentiation of, 311–312
    dissection of, 312–313
    frozen section of, role of, 320
    gross characteristics of, 313–314, *313–315*
    malignant, diagnosis of, 316–320, *319*
    microscopic features of, 314–315, *316–318*
    operating room consultation for, 320
    sites of, 312, 320–336. See also specific site and *Leiomyoma; Leiomyosarcoma.*
    undifferentiated cells in, 311–312
  intestinal, 326, 329, *329–334*, *333–335*
  small-intestinal, gross characteristics of, 313, *314–315*
Strongyloides stercoralis, geographic distribution of, 752
Strongyloidiasis, autoinfection (hyperinfection) in, 752, *753*
  capillariasis vs., 753
  diagnosis of, 752, *752–753*
  rhabditiform larva in, *752*
Submucosa, arteriovenous malformation in, 220, *222–223*
  endoscopic biopsy of, 39
  structure and function of, 14–15, *15*
Submucosal plexus (Meissner's plexus), colonic, histology of, 189, *189*
  ganglion cells of, absence of, in Hirschsprung's disease, 208
  hyperplasia of, in neuronal intestinal dysplasia, 209
  neurons of, eosinophilic intranuclear inclusions in, in familial visceral neuropathy, 203
Substance P, as marker of EC cell carcinoids, 253
Sulfatidosis, lipid deposition in, 364
Sulfomucins, colonic, 588
  in intestinal adenomas, 801

Superoxide radicals, in pathogenesis of ischemic bowel disease, 232–233
Surface-foveolar mucous cells, histology of, 20(t)–21(t), 20–21, *21*
Surgery, cardiac, necrotizing enterocolitis after, 234
Suture, colonic wall reaction to, 716, *716*
Sympathectomy, chemical, effect on epithelial cell proliferation of, 104
Syphilis, anal, 888
  esophagitis from, 400–401
  gastric, 502–503
Systemic disease, gastrointestinal and renal involvement in, 353
  small-intestinal ulcers in, 697

T cells, circulating, in immunodeficiency disorders diagnosis, 267
  dysfunction of, development of, 274
    immunodeficiency disorders from, 266
    in Crohn's disease, 677
    susceptibility to infections from, 267
  effects on human immunodeficiency virus (HIV) of, 754
  in GALT, antigen-specific suppressor function of, 76
  role in secretory immune response of, 75–76
  in Peyer's patches, 71
Taeniae coli, histology of, 192, *194*
Talc, granulomatous reaction to, 716
Tangier disease, diagnostic signs of, 362
Telangiectasia, gastrointestinal, CRST syndrome and, 222
  hereditary hemorrhagic, 221–222, *223*
  radiation and, 159, *160*
Temperature, systemic alterations in, gastrointestinal effect of, 165
Teratoma, gastric, 608
Testosterone, effect on colon carcinoma of, 823
Thalidomide, duodenal stenosis or atresia from, 123
Theliolymphocyte(s), 265, *265–266*
Thermal injury, esophageal, 406
Thoracoabdominal ectopia cordis, 128
Thrombosis, bowel infarcts from, 230
  in chemical and drug disorders, 145
Thumbprint sign, in ischemic colitis, *233*
Thyroid disease, gastrointestinal involvement in, 355
Tissue injury, inflammatory reaction to, 8–9
  ischemia and, 142
  pathogenesis of, free radicals in, 142
Toxin(s), microbial, as virulence factors in exogenous infection, 627
Trabecular (L) cell tumors, hindgut, 255, *256*
  classification of, 244(t)
  hyperfunctional syndrome with, 255
Trabecular (L) cells, in rectal carcinoids, 255, *256*
Tracheoesophageal fistula, with esophageal atresia, *114*, 114, 114(t)
  without esophageal atresia, 114(t), 115
Tracheoesophageal septum, deviation of, esophageal atresia and tracheoesophageal fistula from, 114
Trauma, esophageal, 404–405
  gastrointestinal, 165
Treponema pallidum infection (syphilis), anal, 888
  esophagitis from, 400–401
  gastric, 502–503
Triparanol, lesions from, resemblance to celiac disease of, 734
Trisomy 13, Meckel's diverticulum in, 130
Trisomy 18, Meckel's diverticulum in, 130
  thoracoabdominal ectopia cordis in, 128
Trisomy 21, annular pancreas with, 124
  duodenal stenosis or atresia with, 122
  Hirschsprung's disease with, 87
Trisomy syndrome(s), gastrointestinal involvement in, 85, 85(t)
Tuberculosis, anorectal, *889*, 889–890
  appendiceal, 867–868
  esophagitis from, 399–400
  gastrointestinal, 501–502
  ileocecal, *634*
  intestinal, 633–634, *634*
    Crohn's disease vs., 672
  verrucous, anal, *889*
Tumor-associated antigen, in study of intestinal adenomas, 803
Tumorigenesis, colorectal, mutational events in, 91–92

Tumors, adenocarcinoma-carcinoid, endocrine components of, 259
  adnexal, perianal, 890, 892
  anal, transitional epithelium in, 883, *884*
  argentaffin. See *Argentaffin (EC cell) tumors.*
  assessment of, terminology in, 8
  colonic, cytogenetic changes in, 92
  cytology of. See *Cytology.*
  duodenal, cytology of, 60
  endocrine cell. See *Endocrine cell tumors.*
  endocrine-exocrine, 258, *258*–259
  enterochromaffin-like (ECL) cell. See *Enterochromaffin-like (ECL) cell tumors.*
  epithelial, esophageal, type and origin of, 460(t)
  epithelioid cell, gastric, gross characteristics of, 314, *315*
  esophageal, 88, 473–474
  fibrous tissue, 339, 339(t), *340–344, 341–342*
  gastric. See *Gastric tumors.*
  gastrin cell. See *Gastrin (G) cell tumors.*
  gastrointestinal, categories of, 4(t), 6–7
    development of, in radiation injury, 160–161, *161*
    genetic basis of, 89(t), 89–93
    hereditary syndromes of, 89(t)
  glomus, 338, *338–339*
  granular cell. See *Granular cell tumors.*
  inappropriate, classification of, 244(t)
  intestinal, incidence of, 817, 817(t)
    type and frequency of, 817–818, 818(t)
  malignant, of anal region, 892–901, 894(t), *895–900*
  mesenchymal. See *Mesenchymal tumors.*
  metastatic, anal, 901
    appendiceal, 877–878
    intestinal, 846, *846*
  necrotic, cytology of, 59–60
  nervous tissue, 342, *343–348*, 344, 346
  stromal. See *Stromal tumors.*
  vascular, 224–225, 338–339, *338–339*
    malignant, gastrointestinal, 225
Turcot's syndrome, adenomas in, 809
  genetic basis of, 90
Turnbull's classification, of intestinal carcinoma, 836, 837(t)
Turner's syndrome, gastrointestinal hemorrhagic telangiectasia in, 222
Typhoid, immunization against, history of, 69–70

Ulcer(s), anal, 886
  aphthous, in Crohn's disease, 666, *666*
    disease progression and, 668
  cecal, pathology of, 708–709
  colonic, 708–709
    nonspecific, 708–709
    secondary, 709
  duodenal, blood group O associated with, 84
    cytology of, 60
    epithelial cell proliferation in, 104
    familial, subtypes of, 86
    genetic basis of, 85–86
    HLA complex associated with, 84, 86
    stress, 518, *518–519*
  esophageal, pill-induced, 153
  gastric, 229
    benign vs. malignant, 597, 598(t)
    chronic, as precancerous lesions, 590, *590*
      simple hyperplasia with, *592*
    epithelial cell damage in, 57, *58*
    epithelial cell proliferation in, 101
    in alleric gastroenteritis, 176
    in early carcinoma, 581
  gastrointestinal, in chemotherapeutic drug injury, 150
    uremia and, 352
  in chemical and drug disorders, 145
  in ulcerative colitis, 646, *647*
  ischemic, in rheumatoid disease, 229
  jejunal, 696

Ulcer(s) (*Continued*)
  mucosal, in aganglionic megacolon, 120, *120*
    in etiology of acute appendicitis, 864
  nonspecific, small-intestinal, 697
  peptic. See *Peptic ulcer(s); Peptic ulcer disease.*
  pill-induced, 153
  radiation and, 159, *160*
  rectal. See also *Rectal ulcer syndrome, solitary.*
    localized, 708
  small-intestinal, in refractory sprue and celiac disease, 735–736, *737*
    systemic disease and, 697
  stercoraceous, 708
  stomal, 530–531, *531*
  stress. See *Stress ulcer(s).*
Ulcerative colitis, 643–663, 677, 677(t)
  active, dysplasia in, overdiagnosis of, mucosal features and, 658, *659*
    mucosal changes in, 648, *649*
    pseudopolyp in, 648, *650*
    ulcers in, 648, *649*
  anal lesions in, 887
  appendiceal, 646, 866–867
  Campylobacter enterocolitis vs., 632
  carcinoma in, colonic, 826–827
    dysplasia with, pathology of, 656–657, *657*
    early detection of, 663
    histology of, 656, *656*
    incidence of, 106, 655, 655(t)
    pathology of, 655–656, *656*
    risk factors for, 655, 655(t)
  categorization of, 650
  chronic, dysplasia in, histologic classification of, 657–658, *658*, 658(t)
    histologic features of, 649, 650(t)
    mucosal changes in, 649–650, *651–652*
  clinical applications in, 663
  clinical features of, 644–645
  colitis cystica in, 654
  colonic involvement in, 677, 677(t)
  complications of, 653, 653–655
  Crohn's disease vs., 653
    biopsy differentiation of, 46
    clinical course in, 678
    discriminating features in, 677, 677(t)
    indeterminate colitis in, 678
    mucosal features in, 670–671
    rectocolonic mucosal biopsy in, 679, *680*
    shared features in, 643, 677–678
    surgical specimen examination in, 678
  cytology of, 61
  definition of, 643–644
  diagnosis of, criteria for, 644, 644(t)
  differential diagnosis of, 652–653
  distribution of, 645, 645–646
  diverticular disease in, 781
  DNA synthesis abnormalities in, 105
  dysplasia in, 656–659, *657–663*, 658(t), *662–663*
    high-grade, 659, *661–662*, 662
    "indefinite," 658, *660–661*
    low-grade, 658–659, *661*
    "negative," 658, *658–659*
    surveillance of, 663
  endoscopic biopsy of, 663
  epidemiology of, 644
  epithelial cell proliferation in, 106, 106(t)
  etiology of, 644
  general aspects of, 643–644, 644(t)
  gross features of, 646, *646–648*, 648
  histologic features of, 648–650, *649–652*, 650(t), *652*
  ileal involvement in, 646
  inactive, 648
  increased IgE-bearing cells in, 184–185
  inflammation in, 677, 677(t)
    extraintestinal, 654–655

Ulcerative colitis (*Continued*)
  labeling index in, 106(t)
  mucosal injury in, 650, 652
  pathogenesis of, 644
  pathologic diagnosis of, 652
  pathology of, 645–646, *645–652*, 648–650, 650(t), 652
  prophylactic colectomy for, 663
  pseudopolyps in, 646, *647–648*, 648, 677
    inflammatory, *792, 793*
  rectal, 645, 677, 677(t)
  sclerosing cholangitis in, 655
  secondary infections in, 653–654
  submucosal injury in, 652
  toxic megacolon from, 653, *653*
  treatment of, 645
  ulcers in, 646, *647*, 652
Ulcer-cancer, definition of, 590
Uremia, chronic, ischemic colitis associated with, 236
  gastrointestinal effects of, 352
Ureterosigmoidostomy, complications of, colonic neoplasms in, 353, *353*
Urinary system, diseases of, gastrointestinal involvement in, 352–353, *353*
Urogenital sinus, embryology of, 135–136
Urorectal septum, embryology of, 136–137
Uveitis, in ulcerative colitis, 654

Vacuolar change, 200, *201*
Vacuolization, intestinal, defects in, atresia from, 123
  failure of, atresia and stenosis from, 122
    duplications from, 134
Varicella, esophagitis associated with, 396
Varices, esophageal, causes of, 218
  location of, 217–218, *217–218*
  gastrointestinal, bleeding from, 215
    portal hypertension of extrahepatic origin associated with, 219
    portal hypertension of hepatic origin associated with, *217–218*, 217–219
  stomal, 219
Variola, esophagitis associated with, 396
Vascular abnormalities, gastrointestinal, 219–224, *220–224*
  classification of, 219, 219(t)
Vascular disorders, duodenal, 694–695
  gastritis associated with, 506–507
  gastrointestinal, 214–239
    nomenclature and classification of, 5(t), 5–6
    pathology of, injection techniques in, 11
    renal involvement with, 353
    specimen examination in, blood vessel injection studies in, 216
      lymphatic demonstration in, 216–217
Vascular ectasia, antral, 224
Vascular insufficiency, in mediation of cellular injury, 142
Vascular lakes, in gastroesophageal reflux, 408
Vascular lesions, chemical- and drug-induced, 144
Vascular malformations, gastrointestinal, acquired and congenital, *217–218*, 217–224, 219(t), *220–224*
Vasculitic lesions, gastrointestinal, 226–229
  differentiation of, from other diseases with vasculitis, 229
Vasculitis, classification of, 225
  differential diagnosis of, 226
  etiology of, 225
  gastrointestinal, diagnosis of, ^{111}In-granulocyte scanning in, 226
    mucosal biopsy in, 226, *227*
    renal involvement with, 353
    systemic diseases and, 226(t)
  general considerations in, 224–226
  histologic features of, 226
  necrotizing, in rheumatoid arthritis, 357
  organs involved in, 225–226
  pathology of, 226
  pneumatosis intestinalis associated with, 226
Vasopressin, vasoconstrictive action of, gastrointestinal effects of, 151
VATER complex, imperforate anus and, 136

Vegetables, deficiency of, colonic carcinoma risk and, 822–823
Vein(s), ectatic small, in angiodysplasia, 220
Venous pressure, central, elevated, gastrointestinal effects of, 352
  portal, elevated, 217
Verapamil, in prevention of gastric stress ulcers, 233
Verner-Morrison syndrome, 243(t)
Verrucous carcinoma, esophageal, 450–451
Vibrio cholerae. See *Cholera.*
Villi, small-intestinal, 24–25, *25*
  in tropical sprue, 739, *740*
    loss of, radiation injury and, 163, *163–164*
    shortening of, in allergic gastroenteritis, 181, *181*
  surface and crypt, in celiac disease, 731–732, *731–733*
Villin, in absorptive cells, 29, *29*
Vipoma, hyperfunctional syndrome with, 243, 243(t)
Viral infections, appendiceal, 869
  gastric, 500, *501*
  in immunocompromised patient, 268
  in immunodeficiency disorders, 268, *269*
  intestinal, pathology of, 629–631, *630*
  small-intestinal, enteritis from, 745, 745(t)
Virus(es), as intestinal carcinogen, 821
  esophageal location of, 387(t)
Viscera, displacement of, in congenital posterolateral diaphragmatic hernia, 127, *127*
Vitamin(s), deficiencies of, gastrointestinal effects of, 359–360
  in tropical sprue, mucosal derangements from, 739
  fat-soluble, disorders of, 359–360
  water-soluble, disorders of, 360
Vitamin A, carcinogenesis reduction by, 823
Vitamin B_{12} deficiency, gastrointestinal effects of, 354, 360
  in stasis syndrome, 742
  in tropical sprue, 739
  intestinal megaloblastic changes in, 354
Vitamin C, carcinogenesis reduction with, 821, 823
Vitamin E, carcinogenesis reduction with, 821, 823
  deficiency of, brown bowel syndrome from, 360, 365
  gastrointestinal ceroidosis from, 207
Vitamin K deficiency, gastrointestinal hemorrhage in, 359–360
Volvulus, mechanical obstruction from, 195–196
  meconium ileus with, 132, *132*
  midgut, 125
  sigmoid, 126
  stenosis from, 123
  terminal ileal duplication with, 133, *134*
Vomiting, feculent, in mechanical obstruction, 195
  in allergic gastroenteritis, 175
  in duodenal atresia, 123
  in duodenal obstruction, 125
  in intestinal pseudo-obstruction, 197
  in mechanical obstruction, 195
  pregnancy and, 356
von Recklinghausen's disease, ganglioneuromatous paraganglioma associated with, 252–253
  intramural intestinal neurofibroma in, 344, *345–346*
  neuronal intestinal dysplasia with, 209
  vermiform appendix in, 863

Waldenström's macroglobulinemia, intestinal involvement in, 759–761, *760–761*
  cause of, 760–761, *761*
  gross findings in, 759, *760*
  histology of, 760, *761*
Wart, genital, 890, *891*
Watermelon stomach, 224, 506–507
Wegener's granulomatosis, Churg-Strauss syndrome vs., 228
  gastrointestinal involvement in, 228–229
  gastrointestinal vasculitis in, 226
Weight loss, in allergic gastroenteritis, 175
Wheat bran, effect on colonic epithelial cell proliferation of, 105
Whipple's disease, causative agents of, bacterial, 745
  ultrastructural study of, 746–747, *747*
  isolation of, 748

Whipple's disease (*Continued*)
  clinical presentation of, 745
  diagnosis of, PAS-positive macrophages in, *748*, 748(t), 748–749
    pitfalls in, *748*, 748(t), 748–749
  endoscopic view of, *745*, 745–746
  esophageal involvement in, 400, *400*
  histopathology of, 746, *746*
  malabsorption associated with, 745–748, *745–749*, 748(t)
  Mycobacterium avium-intracellulare infection vs., 277, *279*
  posttreatment findings in, *748*, 748
  ultrastructural findings in, 746–747, *747*
Wiskott-Aldrich syndrome, gastrointestinal manifestations of, 274
Wolman's disease, deposition in, 363(t), 365
World Health Organization, classification of immunodeficiency disorders of, 271
  early gastric carcinoma histologic classification of, 575, 577
  gastric adenocarcinoma typing of, 603
  gastric adenoma classification of, 550–551

Xanthine oxidase, in pathogenesis of ischemic bowel disease, 232–233
Xanthoma, gastric, gross features of, *360*, 361
  in chronic gastritis, 498
X-ray(s), damage from, 159

Yersinia infection, appendiceal, 868
  Crohn's disease vs., 672
  enterocolitis from, pathology of, 633, *633*
  mucosal invasion in, with proliferation in lamina propria and lymph nodes, 627–628

Zinc deficiency, acrodermatitis enteropathica and, 744
Zollinger-Ellison syndrome, clinical features of, 539
  definition of, 539
  diagnosis of, 539–540
  differential diagnosis of, 540
  epithelial cell proliferation in, 102
  etiology of, 539
  gastric argyrophil ECL cell tumors in, 245, *245*
  gastric carcinoma in, incidence of, 591
  gastrin cell tumors in, malignancy rate of, 249
  gastrinomas in, gastrin cell hyperplasia with, *250*
  hyperfunctional syndrome with, 243(t)
  Ménétrier's disease vs., 542
  pathogenesis of, 539
  pathology of, 539, *540*
  peptic ulcer disease from, 531–532, *532–533*
    diagnosis of, 532
    etiology of, 531
    gastric rugae in, 531, *533*
    parietal cell hyperplasia in, 531, *532*
Zymogenic cells, histology of, 20(t), 23, *23*